COMPREHENSIVE ATLAS OF
# Ultrasound-Guided Pain Management Injection Techniques

# COMPREHENSIVE ATLAS OF
# Ultrasound-Guided Pain Management Injection Techniques

## Steven D. Waldman, MD, JD

Clinical Professor of Anesthesiology
Professor of Medical Humanities and Bioethics
University of Missouri–Kansas City School of Medicine
Kansas City, Missouri

Wolters Kluwer Health | Lippincott Williams & Wilkins

Philadelphia · Baltimore · New York · London
Buenos Aires · Hong Kong · Sydney · Tokyo

*Acquisitions Editor*: Brian Brown
*Product Manager*: Nicole T. Dernoski
*Marketing Manager*: Lisa Lawrence
*Production Project Manager*: Alicia Jackson
*Manufacturing Manager*: Beth Welsh
*Design Coordinator*: Teresa Mallon
*Compositor*: SPi Global

© 2014 by LIPPINCOTT WILLIAMS & WILKINS, a WOLTERS KLUWER Business
Two Commerce Square
2001 Market Street
Philadelphia, PA 19103 USA
LWW.com

All rights reserved. This book is protected by copyright. No part of this book may be reproduced in any form or by any means, including photocopying, or utilized by any information storage and retrieval system without written permission from the copyright owner, except for brief quotations embodied in critical articles and reviews. Materials appearing in this book prepared by individuals as part of their official duties as U.S. government employees are not covered by the above-mentioned copyright.

Printed in China

**Library of Congress Cataloging-in-Publication Data**
Waldman, Steven D.
 Comprehensive atlas of ultrasound-guided pain management injection techniques / by Steven D. Waldman. — 1st ed.
   p. ; cm.
 Includes bibliographical references and index.
 ISBN 978-1-4511-8670-3
 I. Title.
 [DNLM: 1. Pain Management.  2. Anesthetics, Local—therapeutic use.  3. Injections—methods.  4. Ultrasonography, Interventional.  WL 704.6]
 RC78.7.U4
 616.07'543—dc23

                                                                                2013014065

Care has been taken to confirm the accuracy of the information presented and to describe generally accepted practices. However, the authors, editors, and publisher are not responsible for errors or omissions or for any consequences from application of the information in this book and make no warranty, expressed or implied, with respect to the currency, completeness, or accuracy of the contents of the publication. Application of this information in a particular situation remains the professional responsibility of the practitioner.

 The authors, editors, and publisher have exerted every effort to ensure that drug selection and dosage set forth in this text are in accordance with current recommendations and practice at the time of publication. However, in view of ongoing research, changes in government regulations, and the constant flow of information relating to drug therapy and drug reactions, the reader is urged to check the package insert for each drug for any change in indications and dosage and for added warnings and precautions. This is particularly important when the recommended agent is a new or infrequently employed drug.

 Some drugs and medical devices presented in this publication have Food and Drug Administration (FDA) clearance for limited use in restricted research settings. It is the responsibility of the health care provider to ascertain the FDA status of each drug or device planned for use in their clinical practice.

To purchase additional copies of this book, call our customer service department at (800) 638-3030 or fax orders to (301) 223-2320. International customers should call (301) 223-2300.

Visit Lippincott Williams & Wilkins on the Internet: at LWW.com. Lippincott Williams & Wilkins customer service representatives are available from 8:30 am to 6 pm, EST.

10 9 8 7 6 5 4 3

*This book is dedicated to
Corey William Waldman, MD,
clinician,
diagnostician,
academician,
musician,*

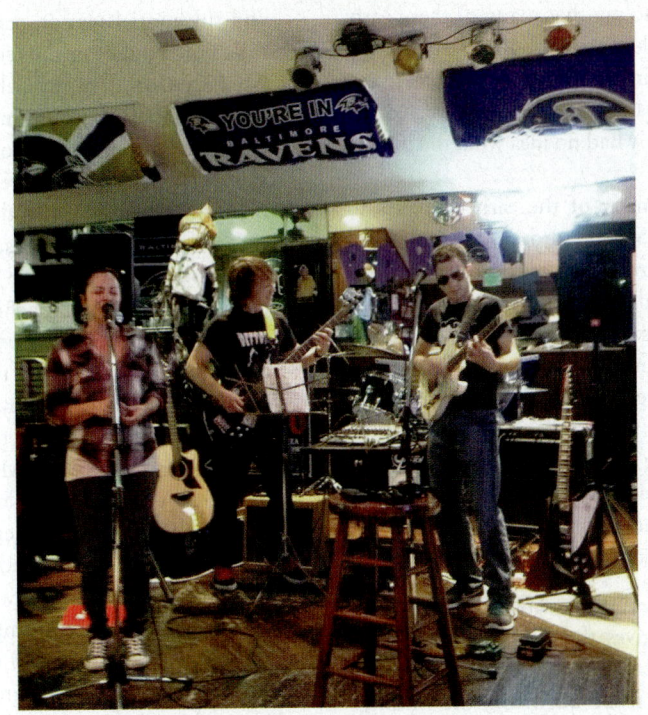

*and the one who makes everything
look so easy!
Dad*

# PREFACE

## ¿HABLA USTED ULTRASOUND?

I have to admit that when articles describing ultrasound-guided pain management procedures started appearing in the pain management literature a few years ago, my first thought was *"don't these guys have anything better to write about?"* This thought was fueled in no small part by my attachment to the things I knew best—landmark-based and fluoroscopic and CT-guided procedures, but to be perfectly honest, my initial resistance and skepticism toward the idea of using ultrasound to guide pain management procedures were probably rooted in the fact that I could not make heads or tails of the ultrasound images presented. I would like to say that many of these early ultrasound images were of less than optimal quality, hence my inability to read them, but the simple truth was that like many other pain management physicians, I had not yet learned the "language of ultrasound." I simply had no idea what the images were "saying."

Thanks to the efforts of many of the early converts to ultrasound such as Philip Peng, Samer Narouze, Andrew Grey, and many others; I began to learn the basic vocabulary of this new language. At first, it was really hard and I missed much of what was being "said." Over time, I began getting more and more of the conversation and found the language of ultrasound to be as rich and nuanced as the languages of landmarks and fluoroscopy ..... different ..... yet very cool!

Although I am still learning the language of ultrasound, I would like to offer some observations about this exciting new addition to the pain management armamentarium and explain why I believe the language of ultrasound is worth learning:

1. **Ultrasound leads to better diagnosis.** Ultrasound is unique in that it not only gives the clinician a real-time snap shot of the painful area, but it also often provides diagnostic information that really augments the findings gleaned from the all important history and physical exam. Nerve entrapments, fluid collections, tendinopathy, infection, foreign bodies, arthritis, and so forth are all easily observed. Ultrasound also allows the clinician to observe the anatomic structure in question dynamically, for example, observing the bicipital tendon sublux during flexion and extension of the biceps, the sciatic nerve becoming entrapped by the piriformis muscle, and so forth. This real-time dynamic information leads to better clinical correlation and diagnosis, which ultimately yields better and safer treatment plans.

2. **Ultrasound leads to better treatment.** Much of the praise surrounding ultrasound-guided pain management procedures centers around "more accurate needle placement." While there is no question in my mind that with many pain management procedures, ultrasound guidance enhances needle placement; to me, the real unsung hero of ultrasound-guided procedures is when the information gleaned from an ultrasound exams tells the clinician NOT to inject a painful condition; for example, when there is significant tendinopathy that includes significant acute inflammation and substantial tendon tears indicating that even a careful injection would put the tendon at the risk of rupture.

3. **No radiation.** It is my belief that many pain management specialists have become inured to the significant risk that daily use of fluoroscopy poses to the pain management specialists. It is a real pleasure to avoid this health risk, not to mention dispensing with the inconvenience and discomfort of lead aprons, lead glasses, and so forth.

4. **Ultrasound is great for teaching.** The ability to easily bring the ultrasound machine to the patient in the office, at the bedside, or in the operating room, makes many procedures into great teaching moments for our staff, residents, and students. Dynamic imaging of the functional anatomy of the rotator cuff or the relationship of the carotid artery to Chassaignac tubercle when performing stellate ganglion block really helps the student learn and remember what he or she needs to know when performing pain management procedures. It also reminds even the most seasoned pain management specialist how easily a needle can go awry.

5. **The equipment keeps improving.** Just compare the digital images in this book to the ultrasound images in earlier pain management literature and you will see what I mean. Not only each new generation of ultrasound machines produces images of infinitely better quality, but the ultrasound machines are lighter, more reliable, and often less expensive.

I hope that this text will help you learn and appreciate the language of ultrasound as it pertains to helping the patient in pain. Oh, I have one more question. ¿HABLA USTED ULTRASOUND?

*Steven D. Waldman, MD, JD*

# ACKNOWLEDGMENTS

## IAMQUE OPUS EXEGI

*Iamque opus exegi* loosely translates to "and now I have finished the work." A great quote (and one that I hope suggests to the reader that I am an erudite and scholarly sort of author … old school, etc.), but one that is in this case surely a misnomer. While it is true that I am the guy whose name is prominently displayed on the cover of this book, this work could not have been possible without the significant efforts and contributions of many dedicated individuals. Without their special expertise, knowledge, and skills, this book simply would not of happened.

In particular, I would like to acknowledge the following individuals:

Dr. Michael Meng, a clinician, diagnostician, and ultrasonographer extraordinaire. Mike produced many of the amazing ultrasound images in this book, and in the process taught all of us the "art of ultrasound," creating images of unsurpassed quality and clarity.

Team Waldman—Izzy Tarantino, Steven Myers, Matt Hendricks, Chelsea Tennison, Shawn Garcia, and many other UMKC School of Medicine students who volunteered and gave of their free time to help organize and produce many of the original photographs in this book. Izzy and Steve both served as project coordinators, and both demonstrated not only superior management skills, but also grace under fire.

The Society for Pain Practice Management Faculty whose expertise and teaching ability is an inspiration. With thanks and friendship to Andres Betts, MD; Ken Candido, MD; Ian Fowler, MD; Capt. Robert Mendez, DO; Thomas Moran, DO; Antoin Nader, MD; Philip Peng, MBBS; Maunak Rana, MD; Michael Verdolin, MD; Erik Voogd, MD.

John Carmody, medical photographer and a longtime friend, whose expertise and efficiency made producing the hundreds of original color photographs used in this text doable. John is always ready to go the extra mile and knows how to keep us moving.

Bernie Kida, a certified medical illustrator, and his team at Kida MediaArt produced many of the original full-color figures for this book. Bernie has the unique ability to translate the technical written word into art that is not only beautiful to look at, but also, at a glance, illustrates sometimes difficult concepts, anatomy, and procedures.

Nicole Dernoski, Senior Product Manager at Lippincott Williams & Wilkins, shepherded this book from conception to completion and not without some weeping and gnashing of teeth. Nicole remained calm in spite of the curve balls and land mines and corrected the myriad errors associated with the production of the first edition of a figure-rich textbook.

And last, but certainly not least, my friend Mark Escarcida of Diagnostic Instruments/Mindray, who convinced me of the need for a comprehensive textbook of ultrasound-guided pain management procedures, and then put his money where his mouth was by not only providing the state-of-the-art Mindray M7 ultrasound machines and transducers used to produce the stunning images in this book, but also providing continued encouragement to all during the writing of this book.

Thanks to all!

*Steven D. Waldman, MD, JD*

# CONTENTS

*Preface vi*
*Acknowledgments vii*

## Section I  Head

1. Ultrasound-Guided Atlanto-Occipital Block — 2
2. Ultrasound-Guided Atlantoaxial Block — 6
3. Ultrasound-Guided Sphenopalatine Ganglion Block — 14
4. Ultrasound-Guided Greater and Lesser Occipital Nerve Block — 19
5. Ultrasound-Guided Auriculotemporal Nerve Block — 27
6. Ultrasound-Guided Greater Auricular Nerve Block — 33
7. Ultrasound-Guided Trigeminal Nerve Block: Coronoid Approach — 39
8. Ultrasound-Guided Maxillary Nerve Block — 46
9. Ultrasound-Guided Mandibular Nerve Block — 52
10. Ultrasound-Guided Supraorbital Nerve Block — 60
11. Ultrasound-Guided Infraorbital Nerve Block — 66
12. Ultrasound-Guided Mental Nerve Block — 74
13. Ultrasound-Guided Temporomandibular Joint Injection — 81
14. Ultrasound-Guided Injection Technique for Eagle Syndrome — 90

## Section II  Neck  99

**15** Ultrasound-Guided Glossopharyngeal Nerve Block  100

**16** Ultrasound-Guided Vagus Nerve Block  107

**17** Ultrasound-Guided Spinal Accessory Nerve Block  112

**18** Ultrasound-Guided Phrenic Nerve Block  118

**19** Ultrasound-Guided Facial Nerve Block  125

**20** Ultrasound-Guided Superficial Cervical Plexus Block  133

**21** Ultrasound-Guided Deep Cervical Plexus Block  137

**22** Ultrasound-Guided Superior Laryngeal Nerve Block  142

**23** Ultrasound-Guided Recurrent Laryngeal Nerve Block  150

**24** Ultrasound-Guided Stellate Ganglion Block  156

**25** Ultrasound-Guided Third Occipital Nerve Block  163

**26** Ultrasound-Guided Cervical Medial Branch Block  171

**27** Ultrasound-Guided Cervical Intra-articular Facet Block  179

**28** Ultrasound-Guided Cervical Selective Nerve Root Block  186

## Section III  Shoulder  191

**29** Ultrasound-Guided Brachial Plexus Block: Interscalene Approach  192

**30** Ultrasound-Guided Brachial Plexus Block: Supraclavicular Approach  198

**31** Ultrasound-Guided Brachial Plexus Block: Infraclavicular Approach  204

| | | |
|---|---|---|
| **32** | Ultrasound-Guided Brachial Plexus Block: Axillary Approach | 209 |
| **33** | Ultrasound-Guided Intra-articular Injection of the Glenohumeral Joint | 215 |
| **34** | Ultrasound-Guided Injection Technique for Acromioclavicular Joint | 221 |
| **35** | Ultrasound-Guided Injection Technique for Subacromial Impingement Syndrome | 227 |
| **36** | Ultrasound-Guided Injection Technique for Supraspinatus Tendonitis | 234 |
| **37** | Ultrasound-Guided Injection Technique for Infraspinatus Tendonitis | 241 |
| **38** | Ultrasound-Guided Injection Technique for Subscapularis Tendonitis | 248 |
| **39** | Ultrasound-Guided Injection Technique for Rotator Cuff Disease | 254 |
| **40** | Ultrasound-Guided Injection Technique for Suprascapular Nerve Block | 261 |
| **41** | Ultrasound-Guided Injection Technique for Radial Nerve Block at the Humerus | 266 |
| **42** | Ultrasound-Guided Injection Technique for Intercostobrachial Nerve Block | 274 |
| **43** | Ultrasound-Guided Injection Technique for Medial Brachial Cutaneous Nerve Block | 281 |
| **44** | Ultrasound-Guided Injection Technique for Bicipital Tendonitis | 288 |
| **45** | Ultrasound-Guided Injection Technique for Axillary Nerve Block in the Quadrilateral Space | 297 |
| **46** | Ultrasound-Guided Injection Technique for Subdeltoid Bursitis Pain | 304 |

**47** Ultrasound-Guided Injection Technique for Subcoracoid Bursitis Pain — 310

**48** Ultrasound-Guided Injection Technique for Pectoralis Major Tear Syndrome — 316

# Section IV  Elbow and Forearm — 324

**49** Ultrasound-Guided Injection Technique for Intra-articular Injection of the Elbow Joint — 325

**50** Ultrasound-Guided Radial Nerve Block at the Elbow — 331

**51** Ultrasound-Guided Median Nerve Block at the Elbow — 336

**52** Ultrasound-Guided Ulnar Nerve Block at the Elbow — 344

**53** Ultrasound-Guided Injection Technique for Cubital Tunnel Syndrome — 351

**54** Ultrasound-Guided Injection Technique for Tennis Elbow Syndrome — 359

**55** Ultrasound-Guided Injection Technique for Golfer's Elbow — 366

**56** Ultrasound-Guided Injection Technique for Radial Tunnel Syndrome — 372

**57** Ultrasound-Guided Injection Technique for Triceps Tendonitis — 380

**58** Ultrasound-Guided Injection Technique for Olecranon Bursitis Pain — 386

**59** Ultrasound-Guided Injection Technique for Pronator Syndrome — 393

**60** Ultrasound-Guided Injection Technique for Anterior Interosseous Syndrome — 401

# Section V  Wrist and Hand    411

**61** Ultrasound-Guided Intra-articular Injection of the Distal Radioulnar Joint    412

**62** Ultrasound-Guided Intra-articular Injection of the Radiocarpal Joint    417

**63** Ultrasound-Guided Radial Nerve Block at the Wrist    424

**64** Ultrasound-Guided Median Nerve Block at the Wrist    430

**65** Ultrasound-Guided Ulnar Nerve Block at the Wrist    438

**66** Ultrasound-Guided Injection Technique for Carpal Tunnel Syndrome    446

**67** Ultrasound-Guided Injection Technique for Ulnar Tunnel Syndrome    454

**68** Ultrasound-Guided Injection Technique for Flexor Carpi Radialis Tendonitis    463

**69** Ultrasound-Guided Injection Technique for Flexor Carpi Ulnaris Tendonitis    471

**70** Ultrasound-Guided Injection Technique for Ganglia Cysts of the Wrist and Hand    478

**71** Ultrasound-Guided Injection Technique for de Quervain's Tenosynovitis    485

**72** Ultrasound-Guided Injection Technique for Intersection Syndrome    493

**73** Ultrasound-Guided Intra-articular Injection of the First Carpometacarpal Joint    501

**74** Ultrasound-Guided Intra-articular Injection of the Carpometacarpal Joints of the Fingers    507

**75** Ultrasound-Guided Injection Technique for Trigger Finger Syndrome    513

| | | |
|---|---|---|
| **76** | Ultrasound-Guided Injection Technique for Dupuytren Contracture | 520 |
| **77** | Ultrasound-Guided Intra-articular Injection of the Metacarpophalangeal Joints | 525 |
| **78** | Ultrasound-Guided Intra-articular Injection of the Interphalangeal Joints | 531 |
| **79** | Ultrasound-Guided Metacarpal and Digital Nerve Block | 537 |

# Section VI  Chest Wall, Trunk, and Abdomen  543

| | | |
|---|---|---|
| **80** | Ultrasound-Guided Injection Technique for Sternoclavicular Joint Pain | 544 |
| **81** | Ultrasound-Guided Injection Technique for Costosternal Joint Pain | 550 |
| **82** | Ultrasound-Guided Injection Technique for Manubriosternal Joint Pain | 555 |
| **83** | Ultrasound-Guided Injection Technique for Xiphisternal Joint Pain | 560 |
| **84** | Ultrasound-Guided Injection Technique for Costotransverse and Costovertebral Joint Pain | 566 |
| **85** | Ultrasound-Guided Thoracic Epidural Block Utilizing the Three-Step Paramedian Sagittal Oblique Approach | 572 |
| **86** | Ultrasound-Guided Thoracic Paravertebral Nerve Block | 583 |
| **87** | Ultrasound-Guided Thoracic Facet Block: Intra-articular Technique | 589 |
| **88** | Ultrasound-Guided Intercostal Nerve Block | 598 |
| **89** | Ultrasound-Guided Injection Technique for Slipping Rib Syndrome | 606 |
| **90** | Ultrasound-Guided Transversus Abdominis Plane Block | 615 |

**91** Ultrasound-Guided Injection Technique for Anterior Cutaneous Nerve Entrapment Syndrome ... 621

**92** Ultrasound-Guided Celiac Plexus Block: Anterior Approach ... 629

**93** Ultrasound-Guided Ilioinguinal Nerve Block ... 639

**94** Ultrasound-Guided Iliohypogastric Nerve Block ... 647

**95** Ultrasound-Guided Genitofemoral Nerve Block ... 655

# Section VII  Low Back ... 663

**96** Ultrasound-Guided Lumbar Facet Block: Medial Branch Technique ... 664

**97** Ultrasound-Guided Lumbar Facet Block: Intra-articular Technique ... 673

**98** Ultrasound-Guided Lumbar Epidural Block Utilizing the Three-Step Paramedian Sagittal Oblique Approach ... 682

**99** Ultrasound-Guided Lumbar Selective Nerve Root Block ... 693

**100** Ultrasound-Guided Lumbar Subarachnoid Block Utilizing the Three-Step Paramedian Sagittal Oblique Approach ... 699

**101** Ultrasound-Guided Caudal Epidural Block ... 710

**102** Ultrasound-Guided Lumbar Plexus Nerve Block ... 719

**103** Ultrasound-Guided Injection Technique for Lumbar Myofascial Pain Syndrome ... 727

**104** Ultrasound-Guided Lumbar Sympathetic Block ... 736

# Section VIII  Hip and Pelvis ... 744

**105** Ultrasound-Guided Intra-articular Injection of the Hip Joint ... 745

**106** Ultrasound-Guided Femoral Nerve Block ... 752

| | | |
|---|---|---|
| **107** | Ultrasound-Guided Lateral Femoral Cutaneous Nerve Block | 758 |
| **108** | Ultrasound-Guided Obturator Nerve Block | 766 |
| **109** | Ultrasound-Guided Injection Technique for Osteitis Pubis | 775 |
| **110** | Ultrasound-Guided Injection Technique for Adductor Tendonitis | 782 |
| **111** | Ultrasound-Guided Injection Technique for Ischial Bursitis Pain | 788 |
| **112** | Ultrasound-Guided Injection Technique for Iliopsoas Bursitis Pain | 795 |
| **113** | Ultrasound-Guided Injection Technique for Iliopectineal Bursitis Pain | 802 |
| **114** | Ultrasound-Guided Injection Technique for Trochanteric Bursitis Pain | 810 |
| **115** | Ultrasound-Guided Injection Technique for Gluteus Medius Bursitis Pain | 817 |
| **116** | Ultrasound-Guided Injection Technique for Piriformis Syndrome | 824 |
| **117** | Ultrasound-Guided Sciatic Nerve Block at the Hip | 835 |
| **118** | Ultrasound-Guided Sacral Nerve Block | 841 |
| **119** | Ultrasound-Guided Hypogastric Plexus Block | 848 |
| **120** | Ultrasound-Guided Ganglion of Walther (Impar) Block | 857 |
| **121** | Ultrasound-Guided Injection Technique for Coccydynia | 865 |
| **122** | Ultrasound-Guided Pudendal Nerve Block | 873 |
| **123** | Ultrasound-Guided Sacroiliac Joint Injection | 881 |
| **124** | Ultrasound-Guided Injection Technique for External Snapping Hip Syndrome | 888 |

# Section IX  Knee and Lower Extremity    896

**125** Ultrasound-Guided Injection Technique for Intra-articular Injection of the Knee Joint    897

**126** Ultrasound-Guided Injection Technique for Intra-articular Injection of the Superior Tibiofibular Joint    903

**127** Ultrasound-Guided Injection Technique for Semimembranosus Insertion Syndrome    909

**128** Ultrasound-Guided Injection Technique for Coronary Ligament Pain    916

**129** Ultrasound-Guided Injection Technique for Medial Collateral Ligament    922

**130** Ultrasound-Guided Injection Technique for Quadriceps Expansion Syndrome    928

**131** Ultrasound-Guided Injection Technique for Jumper's Knee    935

**132** Ultrasound-Guided Injection Technique for Suprapatellar Bursitis Pain    942

**133** Ultrasound-Guided Injection Technique for Prepatellar Bursitis Pain    948

**134** Ultrasound-Guided Injection Technique for Superficial Infrapatellar Bursitis Pain    954

**135** Ultrasound-Guided Injection Technique for Deep Infrapatellar Bursitis Pain    960

**136** Ultrasound-Guided Injection Technique for Pes Anserine Bursitis Pain    966

**137** Ultrasound-Guided Saphenous Nerve Block at the Knee    973

**138** Ultrasound-Guided Sciatic Nerve Block at the Popliteal Fossa    980

**139** Ultrasound-Guided Tibial Nerve Block at the Popliteal Fossa    986

| | | |
|---|---|---|
| **140** | Ultrasound-Guided Common Peroneal Nerve Block at the Popliteal Fossa | 995 |
| **141** | Ultrasound-Guided Injection Technique for Baker Cyst | 1004 |
| **142** | Ultrasound-Guided Injection Technique for Fabella Syndrome | 1011 |

## Section X  Ankle and Foot  1018

| | | |
|---|---|---|
| **143** | Ultrasound-Guided Intra-articular Injection of the Ankle Joint | 1019 |
| **144** | Ultrasound-Guided Intra-articular Injection of the Subtalar Joint | 1025 |
| **145** | Ultrasound-Guided Intra-articular Injection of the Talonavicular Joint | 1030 |
| **146** | Ultrasound-Guided Posterior Tibial Nerve Block at the Ankle | 1035 |
| **147** | Ultrasound-Guided Saphenous Nerve Block at the Ankle | 1042 |
| **148** | Ultrasound-Guided Deep Peroneal Nerve Block at the Ankle | 1048 |
| **149** | Ultrasound-Guided Superficial Peroneal Nerve Block at the Ankle | 1056 |
| **150** | Ultrasound-Guided Sural Nerve Block at the Ankle | 1063 |
| **151** | Ultrasound-Guided Injection Technique for Deltoid Ligament Strain | 1069 |
| **152** | Ultrasound-Guided Injection Technique for Anterior Talofibular Ligament Strain | 1076 |
| **153** | Ultrasound-Guided Injection Technique for Anterior Tarsal Tunnel Syndrome | 1081 |
| **154** | Ultrasound-Guided Injection Technique for Posterior Tarsal Tunnel Syndrome | 1088 |
| **155** | Ultrasound-Guided Injection Technique for Achilles Tendonitis | 1096 |

**156** Ultrasound-Guided Injection Technique for Retrocalcaneal Bursitis Pain     1102

**157** Ultrasound-Guided Injection Technique for Calcaneofibular Ligament     1106

**158** Ultrasound-Guided Injection Technique for Plantar Fasciitis     1110

**159** Ultrasound-Guided Injection Technique for Calcaneal Spurs     1115

**160** Ultrasound-Guided Injection Technique for Posterior Tibialis Tendonitis     1121

**161** Ultrasound-Guided Intra-articular Injection of the Toe Joints     1130

**162** Ultrasound-Guided Metatarsal and Digital Nerve Block of the Foot     1136

**163** Ultrasound-Guided Injection Technique for Hallux Valgus Deformity     1144

**164** Ultrasound-Guided Injection Technique for Bunionette Pain Syndrome     1152

**165** Ultrasound-Guided Injection Technique for Hammertoe Pain Syndrome     1158

**166** Ultrasound-Guided Injection Technique for Morton Neuroma Syndrome     1163

**167** Ultrasound-Guided Injection Technique for Intermetatarsal Bursitis     1170

**168** Ultrasound-Guided Injection Technique for Sesamoiditis Pain     1177

*Index 1185*

# SECTION I

# Head

# CHAPTER 1

# Ultrasound-Guided Atlanto-Occipital Block

## CLINICAL PERSPECTIVES

The atlanto-occipital joint is an often overlooked source of upper posterior neck pain and suboccipital headache. The joint is susceptible to arthritis and is frequently traumatized during acceleration/deceleration injuries. The pain following such injuries is often initially attributed to soft tissue injury such as muscle strain and/or bruising. The pain is ill defined and dull in nature, involving the upper neck and occipital region (Fig. 1.1). Pain emanating from the atlanto-occipital joint is exacerbated with lateral range of motion and flexion and extension of the upper cervical spine. It frequently coexists with pain from the atlantoaxial joint. The patient suffering from pain from the atlanto-occipital joint will frequently complain of neck pain, occipital and suboccipital headaches, preauricular pain, and limited range of motion. The patient may experience an exacerbation of pain at extremes of range of motion as well as sleep disturbance, nausea, and difficulty in concentrating.

## CLINICALLY RELEVANT ANATOMY

The atlanto-occipital joint serves as the articulation between the occiput of the skull and atlas. The atlanto-occipital joint possesses a well-developed joint capsule, cartilage, and synovium. This modified V-shaped joint has a limited range of motion of 35 degrees and functions to aid in the positioning of the sense organs by allowing the head to nod forward and backward. It differs from the true facet joints of the lower cervical spine in that it lacks a true posterior articulation. The atlanto-occipital joint also lacks classic intervertebral foramina. The joint lies anterior to the posterolateral columns of the spinal cord (Fig. 1.2). The vertebral artery ascends within the cervical spine via the transverse foramen and then exits the C1 transverse foramen and turns medially to course diagonally across the posteromedial aspect of the atlanto-occipital joint to join with the contralateral vertebral artery at the level of the medulla to form the basilar artery, which enters the foramen magnum in the midline (Fig. 1.3). The diagonal course of the vertebral artery provides an important landmark when performing ultrasound-guided atlanto-occipital nerve block (Fig. 1.4). The C1 nerve root, which is also known as the suboccipital nerve, exits between the skull and C1 vertebra and lacks the characteristic dorsal sensory root seen with other spinal nerves in most patients. It provides motor innervation to the suboccipital muscles and interconnects with fibers of the C2 and C3 nerves, which may explain the overlapping pain symptomatology when any of these nerves are traumatized or inflamed.

## ULTRASOUND-GUIDED TECHNIQUE

The patient is placed in the prone position with the patient's cervical spine slightly flexed and the skin prepped with antiseptic solution. A high-frequency linear transducer is placed in the transverse position slightly off the midline over the upper cervical vertebra, and the vertebral artery is identified as it passes through the transverse foramina (Figs. 1.4 and 1.5). The artery is then traced cranially by slowly moving the transducer in a cranial direction until the vertebral artery is seen to turn medially in front of the atlanto-occipital joint (Fig. 1.6). In most patients, a needle can be placed into the joint just lateral to the point where the artery makes its turn. In an occasional patient, the vertebral artery blocks the entire extent of the joint as it courses from lateral to medial to join the contralateral vertebral artery, rendering safe needle placement virtually impossible.

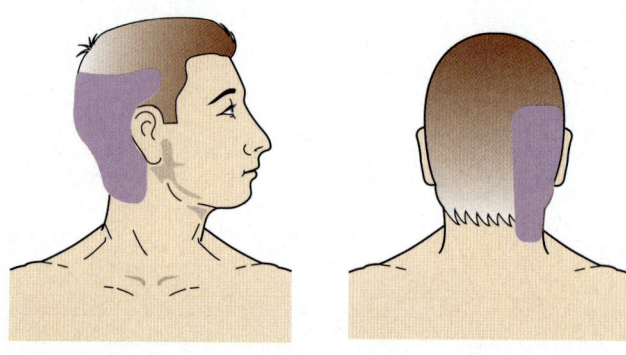

**FIGURE 1.1.** Distribution of pain emanating from the atlanto-occipital joint.

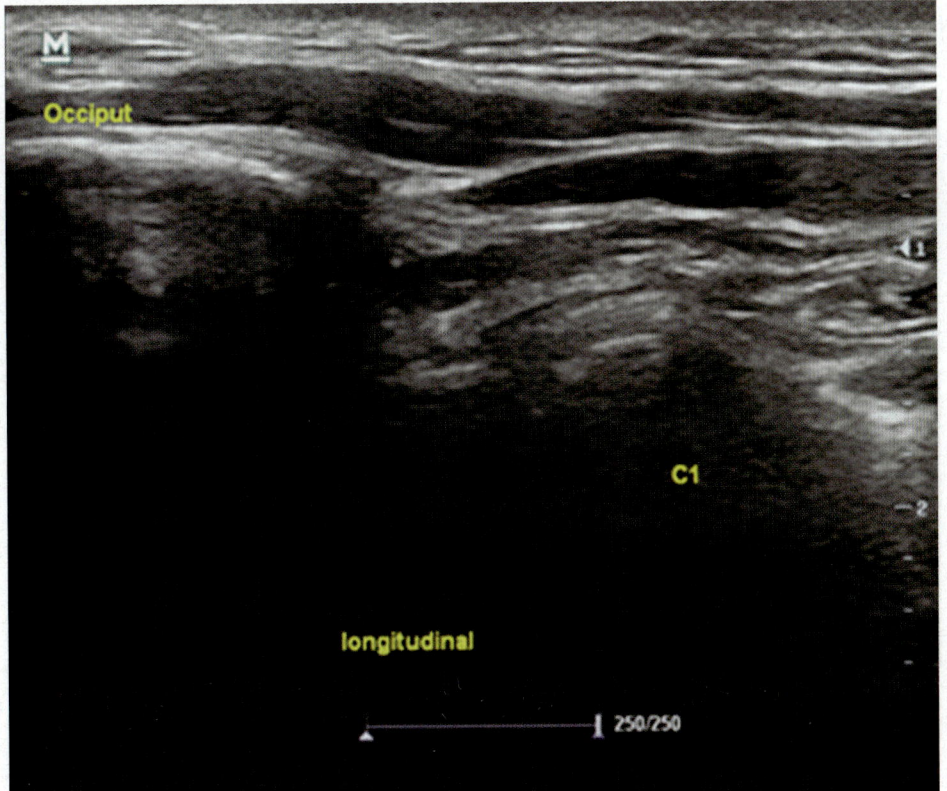

**FIGURE 1.2.** Longitudinal ultrasound image of the atlanto-occipital joint.

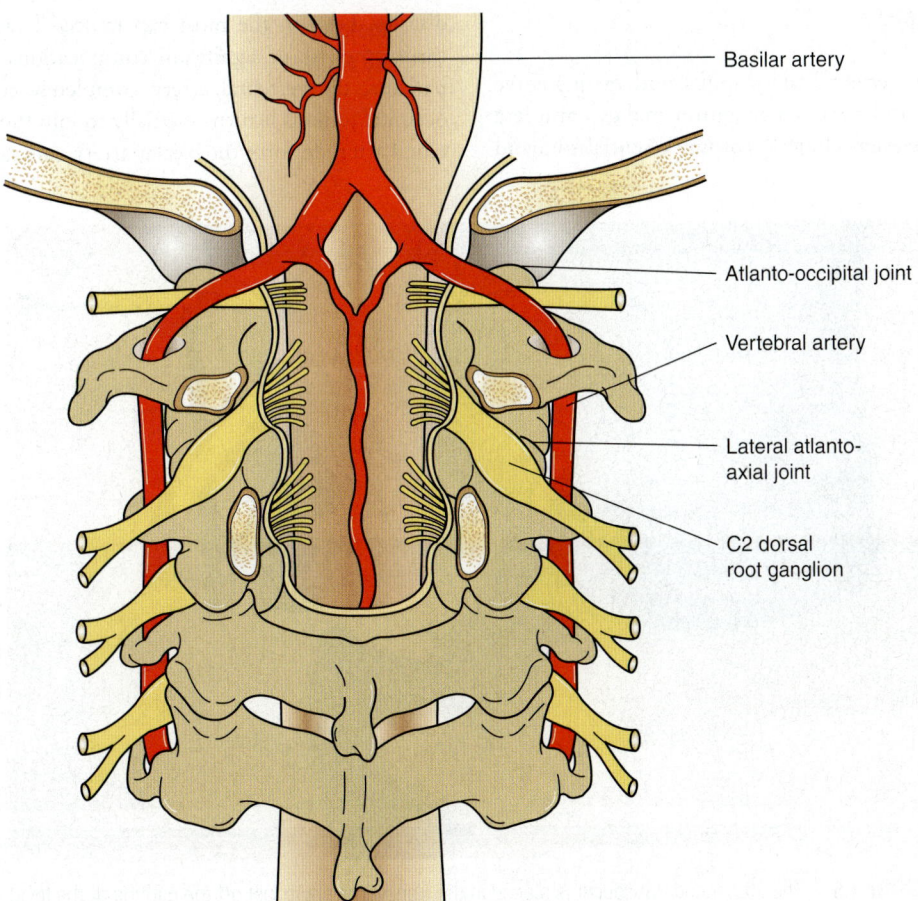

**FIGURE 1.3.** The relationship of the vertebral artery to the atlanto-occipital joint.

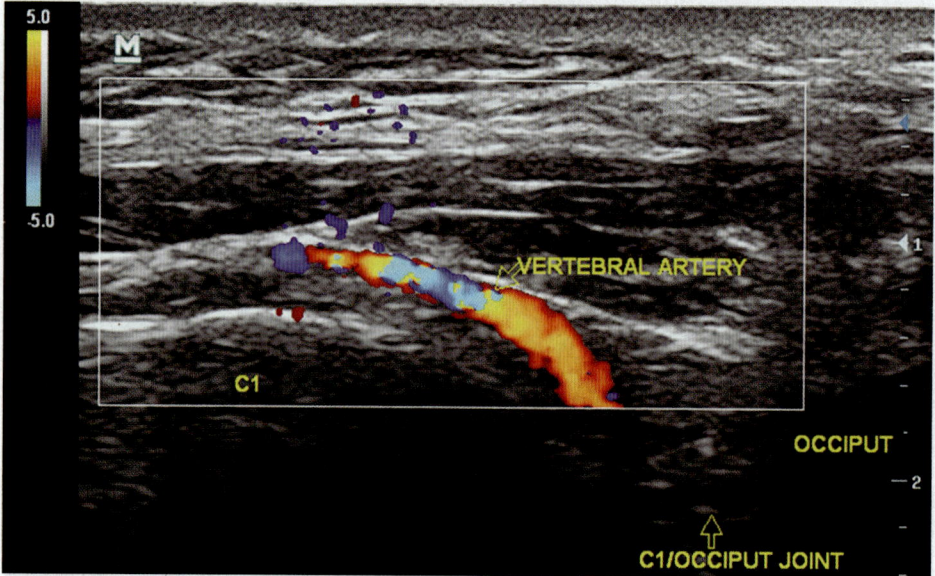

**FIGURE 1.4.** The vertebral artery ascends within the cervical spine via the transverse foramen and then exits the C1 transverse foramen and turns medially to course diagonally across the posteromedial aspect of the atlanto-occipital joint to join with the contralateral vertebral artery at the level of the medulla to form the basilar artery that enters the foramen magnum in the midline. This diagonal turn provides an excellent landmark when performing ultrasound-guided atlanto-occipital nerve block.

## COMPLICATIONS

The proximity of the vertebral artery, spinal cord, exiting nerve roots, brain stem, and foramen magnum makes complete knowledge of the relevant clinical anatomy essential to avoid disaster. Even in the most experienced hands, the procedure carries the risk of significant complications. Because in some patients, the vertebral artery completely covers the atlanto-occipital joint as it turns medially to join the contralateral vertebral artery to form the basilar artery, safe needle placement is

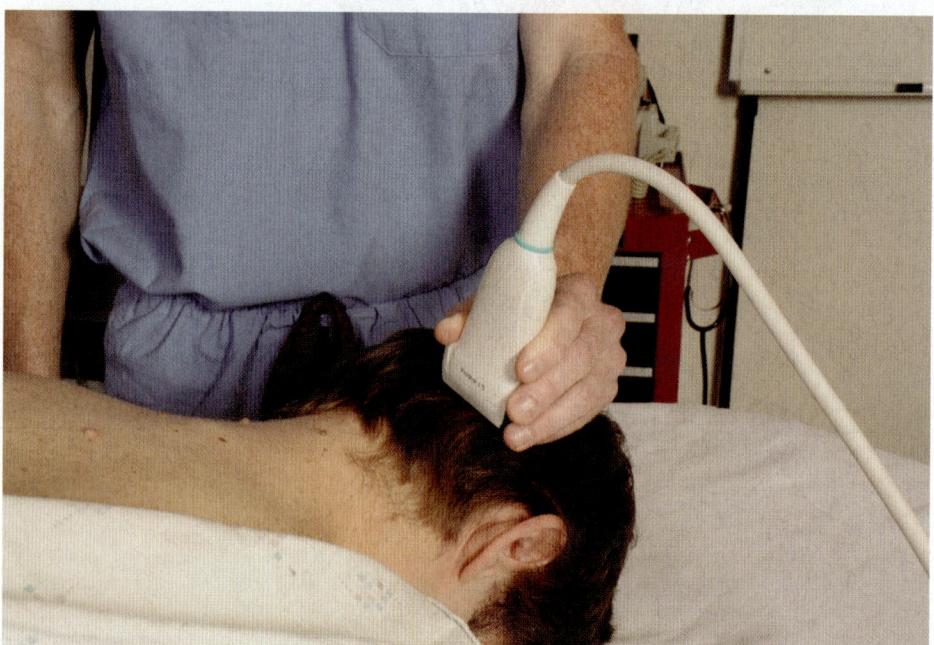

**FIGURE 1.5.** The ultrasound transducer is placed in the transverse plane just off the midline at the level of the upper cervical vertebra, and the vertebral artery is identified.

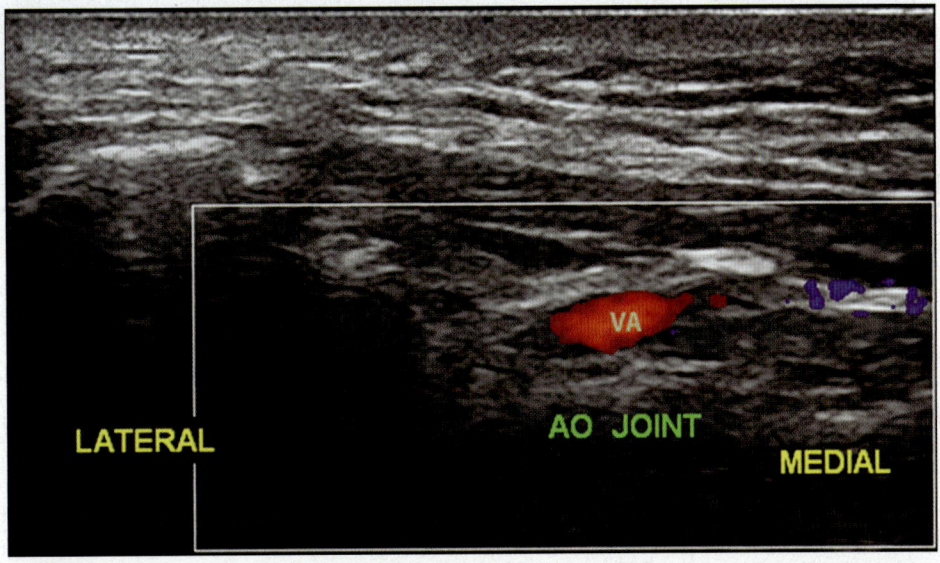

**FIGURE 1.6.** Color Doppler imaging facilitates identification of the vertebral artery as it traverses the transverse processes of the cervical vertebral bodies.

impossible. Even small doses of local anesthetic inadvertently injected into the vertebral or basilar artery can result in immediate local anesthetic–induced seizures and central nervous system toxicity. The particulate nature of steroids can also cause significant side effects if intra-arterial injection occurs. The proximity of the exiting C2 nerve root makes the inadvertent injection of local anesthetic into the dural sleeve with resultant total spinal anesthesia an ever-present possibility.

## CLINICAL PEARLS

Given the significant overlap and cross connections of the fibers of the C1, C2, and C3 nerves, blockade of addition neural structures including the greater and lesser occipital nerves as well as the third occipital nerve may be required to provide the patient with complete pain relief. Blockade of the atlantoaxial joint may also be beneficial, especially if the patient has also sustained trauma to that joint.

The ability of ultrasound imaging to identify the precise position of the vertebral artery relative to the atlanto-occipital joint when performing atlanto-occipital nerve block suggests a significant theoretical advantage over the use of fluoroscopic guidance that more clearly defines the joint but does not delineate the relative position of the artery. Injection of small amounts of iodinated contrast media suitable for use in the central nervous system may help identify intravascular or subdural or subarachnoid placement prior to the injection of local anesthetic if fluoroscopy is utilized concurrently with ultrasound guidance.

## SUGGESTED READINGS

Aprill C, Axinn MJ, Bogduk N. Occipital headaches stemming from the lateral atlanto-axial (C1-2) joint. *Cephalalgia* 2002;22:15–22.
Narouze S. Complications of head and neck procedures. *Tech Reg Anesth Pain Manag* 2007;11:171–177.
Narouze S. Ultrasonography in pain medicine: future directions. *Tech Reg Anesth Pain Manag* 2009;13(3):198–202.
Waldman SD. Atlanto-occipital nerve block. In: *Atlas of interventional pain management*. 3rd ed. Philadelphia, PA: Saunders Elsevier; 2009:3–6.

# CHAPTER 2

# Ultrasound-Guided Atlantoaxial Block

## CLINICAL PERSPECTIVES

The atlantoaxial joint is an often overlooked source of upper posterior neck and suboccipital headache pain. The joint is susceptible to arthritis and is frequently traumatized during acceleration/deceleration injuries. The pain following such injuries is often initially attributed to soft tissue injury such as muscle strain and/or bruising. The pain is ill defined and dull in character involving the upper neck and occipital region (Fig. 2.1). Pain emanating from the atlantoaxial joint is exacerbated with lateral rotation and flexion and extension of the joint and surrounding upper cervical spine. It frequently coexists with pain from the atlanto-occipital joint and the C2/C3 facet joints due to convergence of fibers from these anatomic structures with trigeminal afferent fibers via the trigeminocervical nucleus.

The patient suffering from pain from the atlantoaxial joint will frequently complain of neck pain, occipital and suboccipital headaches, preauricular pain, as well as a limited range of motion with exacerbation of pain at the extremes of range of motion. Sleep disturbance is common as is nausea and difficulty in concentrating. The unique anatomic structure of the atlantoaxial joint also makes it susceptible to instability, which may be exacerbated when the joint is subjected to trauma. A number of diseases are associated with atlantoaxial instability, and they are listed in Table 2.1. The clinician should look carefully for atlantoaxial joint abnormalities and/or instability in patients who have sustained trauma to the joint or who are suffering from the diseases listed in Table 2.1 as failure to identify fractures of the odontoid process and C2 vertebral body and/or disruption of the transverse ligaments with resultant joint instability can have disastrous consequences should the joint sublux (Figs. 2.2 and 2.3).

## CLINICALLY RELEVANT ANATOMY

The atlantoaxial joint serves as the articulation between the C1 and C2 vertebra. The atlantoaxial joint possesses a well-developed capsule, cartilage, and synovium and, like the atlanto-occipital joint, does not possess classic intervertebral foramina seen in the lower cervical vertebrae. The joint allows lateral rotation of the skull of 72 degrees in either direction from the midline and functions to aid in the positioning of the sense organs. It also allows a limited degree of flexion and extension independent of the atlanto-occipital joint and other facet joints of the cervical spine. The vertebral artery ascends via the transverse foramen of the cervical spine, traveling across the lateral one-third of the atlantoaxial joint. The artery ultimately exits the C1 transverse foramen and turns medially to course diagonally across the posteromedial aspect of the atlanto-occipital joint to join with the contralateral vertebral artery at the level of the medulla to form the basilar artery. The basilar artery then ascends to enter the foramen magnum in the midline (Fig. 2.4). The course of the vertebral artery provides an important landmark when performing ultrasound-guided atlantoaxial nerve block (Fig. 2.5). The C2 nerve root exits above the C2 vertebra and provides some motor innervation to the suboccipital muscles. The fibers of the medial branch of the C2 nerve root dorsal primary ramus form the greater occipital nerve. Fibers from the C2 nerve root interconnect with fibers of the C1 and C3 nerves, which may help explain the overlapping pain symptomatology when any of these nerves are traumatized or inflamed.

## ULTRASOUND-GUIDED TECHNIQUE

The patient is placed in prone position with patient's cervical spine slightly flexed and the skin prepped with antiseptic solution. A high-frequency linear transducer is placed in the transverse orientation in the midline at the level of the occiput (Fig. 2.6). The transducer is then slowly moved caudally to identify first the C1 and then the C2 vertebral bodies. The C1 vertebral body has only a vestigial spinous process, and the C2 vertebral body is the first cervical vertebral body with a bifid spinous process making its identification easier (Figs. 2.7 and 2.8). When the C2 vertebra is identified, the transducer is then moved laterally until the exiting C2 nerve root is identified (Figs. 2.9 and 2.10). The transducer is then moved slightly more laterally until the vertebral artery is

CHAPTER 2  ULTRASOUND-GUIDED ATLANTOAXIAL BLOCK  7

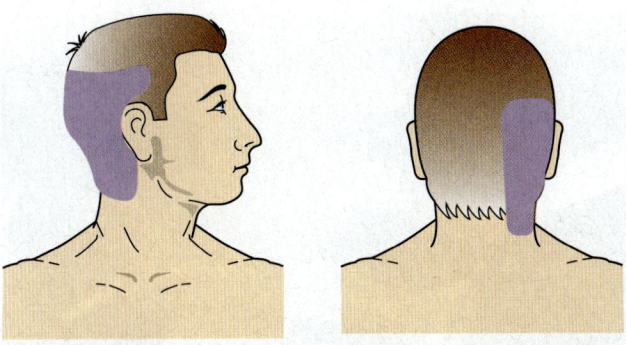

**FIGURE 2.1.** Distribution of pain emanating from the atlantoaxial joint.

**TABLE 2.1  Diseases Associated with Atlantoaxial Joint Instability**

- Rheumatoid arthritis
- Down syndrome
- von Recklinghausen disease
- Osteogenesis imperfect
- Congenital scoliosis
- Morquio syndrome
- Larsen syndrome
- Kniest dysplasia
- Congenital spondyloepiphyseal dysplasia
- Metatropic dysplasia

identified. Color Doppler may be used if the vertebral artery is not readily apparent (Fig. 2.11). The atlantoaxial joint should then be easily identified in between the exiting C2 root and the vertebral artery. A 22-gauge, 3½-inch styletted spinal needle is then advanced into the atlantoaxial joint using an out-of-plane approach under real-time ultrasonography, while constant attention is paid to the location of the vertebral artery laterally and the C2 nerve root medially.

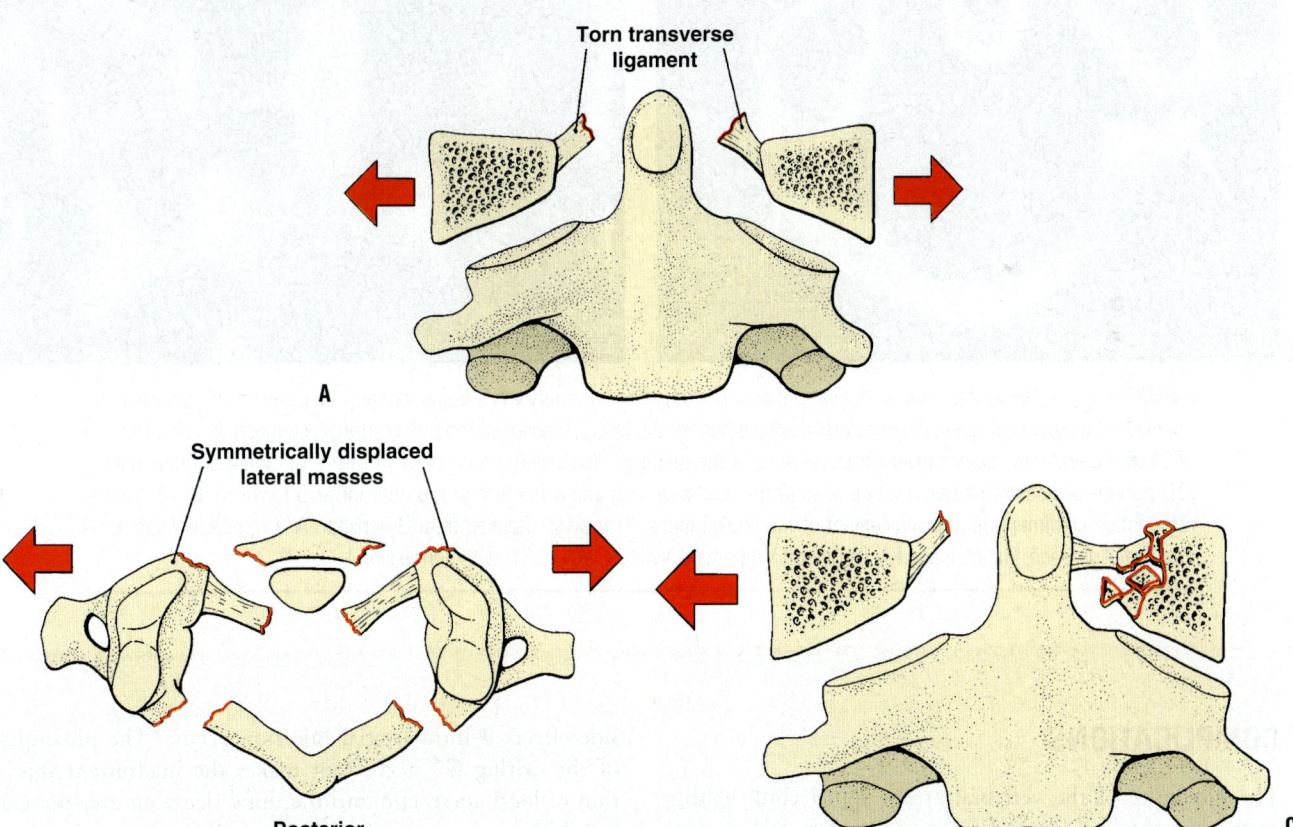

**FIGURE 2.2.** Jefferson fracture. The classic Jefferson fracture, seen here schematically on the anteroposterior (**A**) and axial (**B**) views, exhibits a characteristic symmetric overhang of the lateral masses of C1 over those of C2. Lateral displacement of the articular pillars results in disruption of the transverse ligaments. **C:** On occasion, only unilateral lateral displacement of an articular pillar may be present. (Reused from Greenspan A. *Orthopedic Imaging: A Practical Approach*. Philadelphia, PA: Lippincott Williams & Wilkins; 2011:381, with permission.)

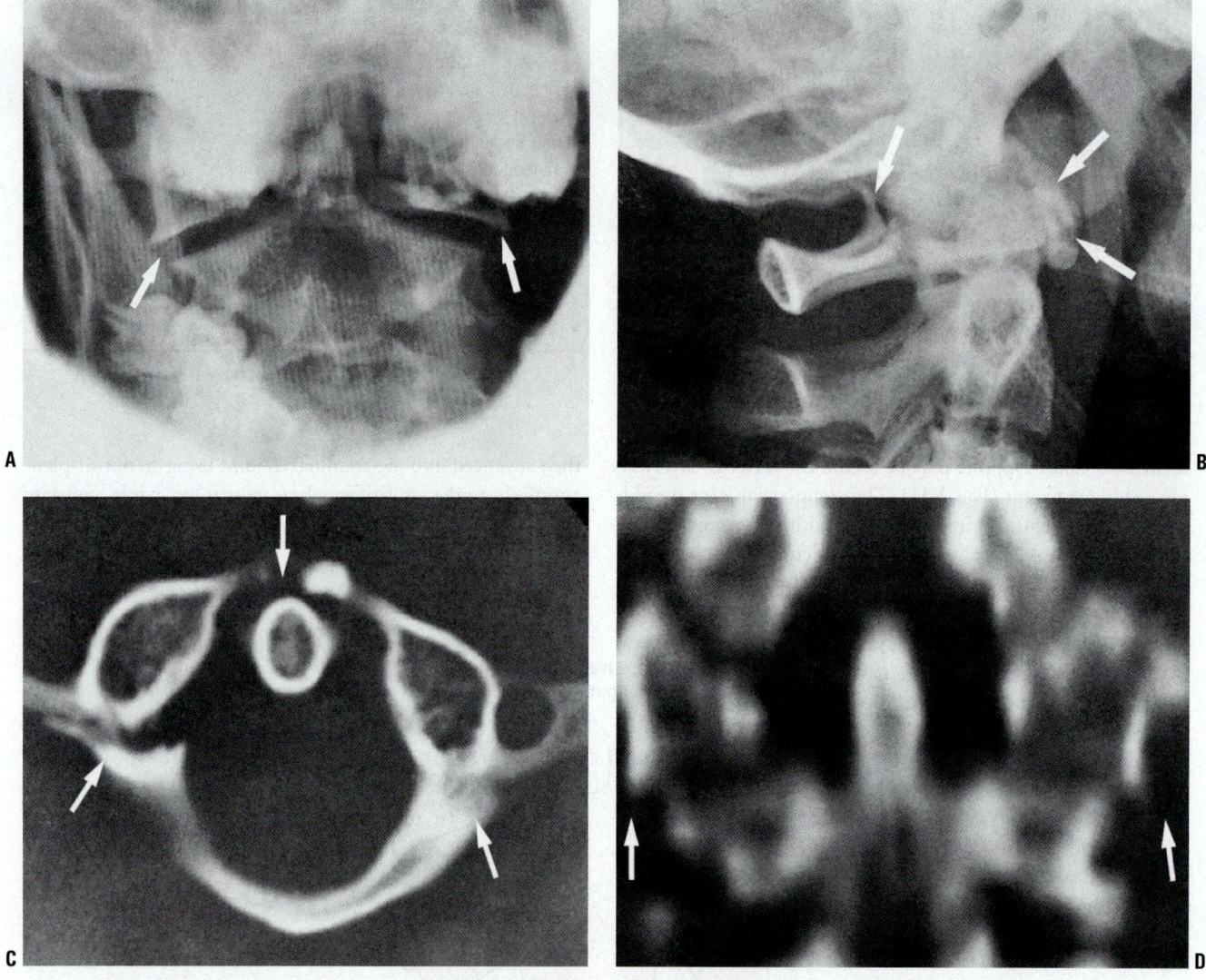

**FIGURE 2.3.** Jefferson fracture. A 19-year-old man sustained a neck injury while being mugged. **A:** Open-mouth anteroposterior view of the cervical spine shows lateral displacement of the lateral masses of the atlas (*arrows*), suggesting a ring fracture of C1. **B:** Lateral view demonstrates fracture lines of the posterior and anterior arch of C1 (*arrows*). **C:** Computed tomography (CT) section demonstrates two fracture lines of the posterior arch and a fracture of the anterior arch (*arrows*). **D:** CT coronal reformation confirms lateral displacement of the lateral masses (*arrows*). (Reused from Greenspan A. *Orthopedic Imaging: A Practical Approach.* Philadelphia, PA: Lippincott Williams & Wilkins; 2011:381, with permission.)

## COMPLICATIONS

The proximity of the vertebral artery, spinal cord, exiting nerve roots, brain stem, and foramen magnum makes complete knowledge of the relevant clinical anatomy essential to avoid disaster. Even in the most experienced hands, the procedure carries the risk of significant complications. Even small doses of local anesthetic inadvertently injected into the vertebral or basilar artery can result in immediate local anesthetic–induced seizures and central nervous system toxicity. The particulate nature of steroids can also cause significant side effects if intra-arterial injection occurs. The proximity of the exiting C2 nerve root makes the inadvertent injection of local anesthetic into the dural sleeve an ever-present possibility.

## CLINICAL PEARLS

Given the significant overlap and cross connections of the fibers of the C1, C2, and C3 nerves, blockade of addition neural structures including the greater and lesser occipital nerves as

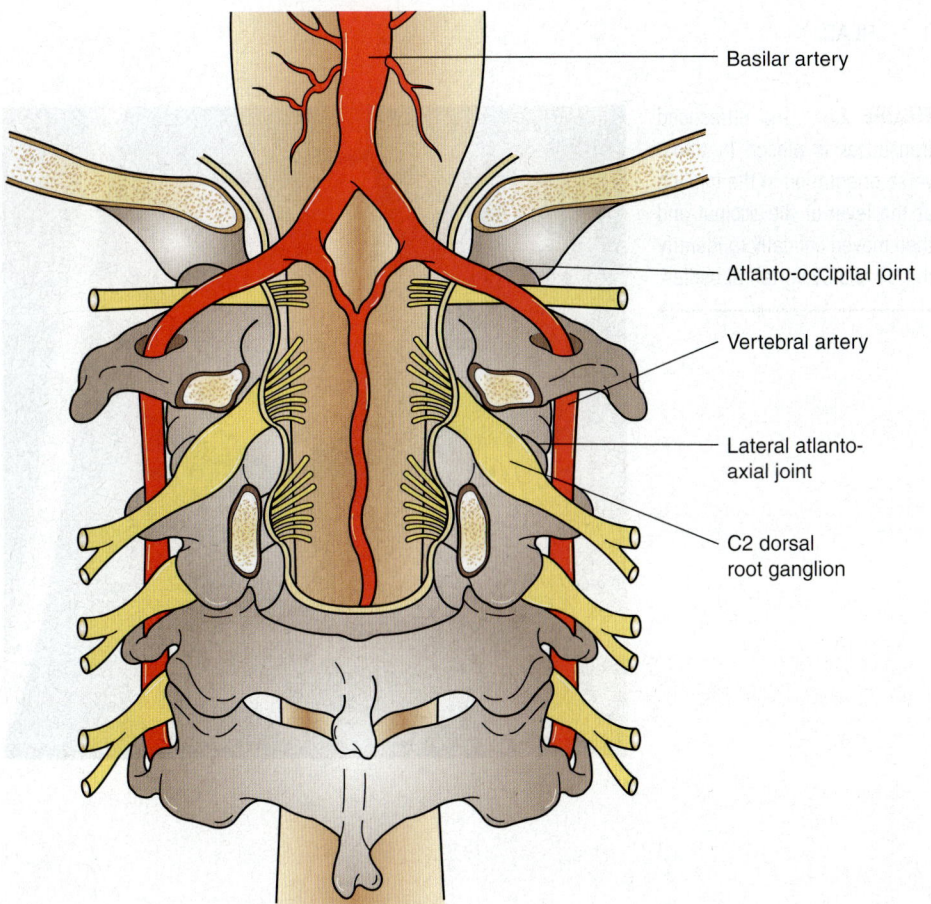

**FIGURE 2.4.** The relationship of the vertebral artery to the atlantoaxial joint.

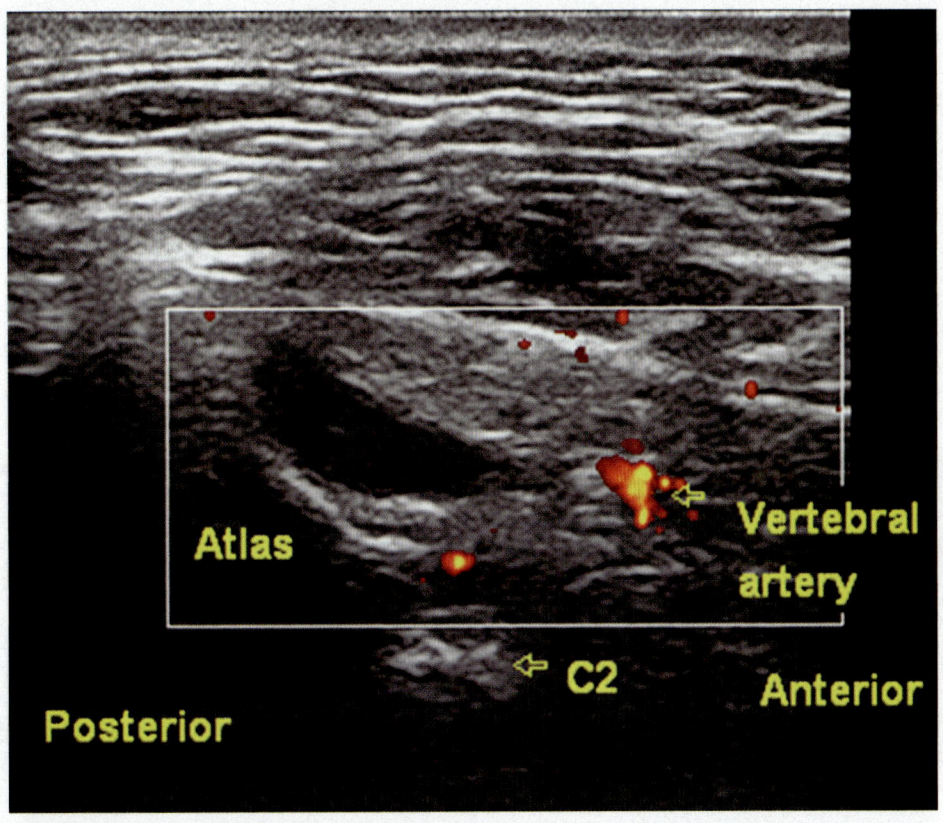

**FIGURE 2.5.** Ultrasound short-axis view showing the relationship of the vertebral artery to the atlanto-axial joint as it ascends through the transverse foramen.

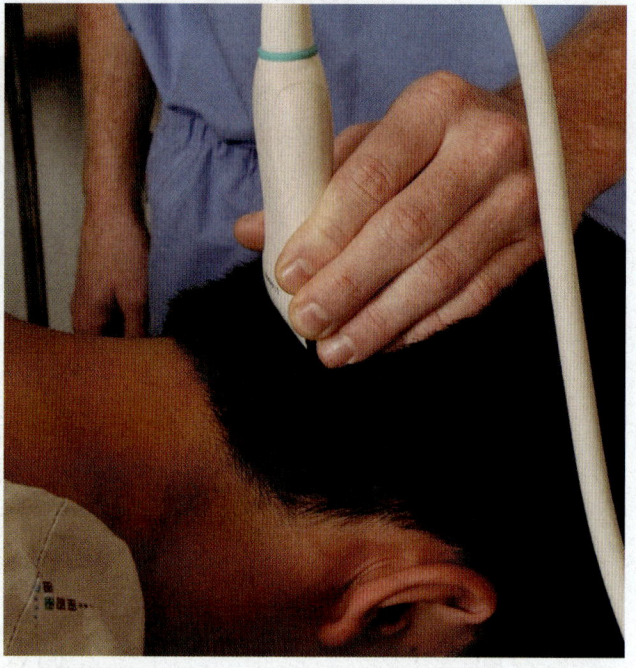

**FIGURE 2.6.** The ultrasound transducer is placed in transverse orientation in the midline at the level of the occiput and then moved caudally to identify the C1 and C2 vertebral bodies.

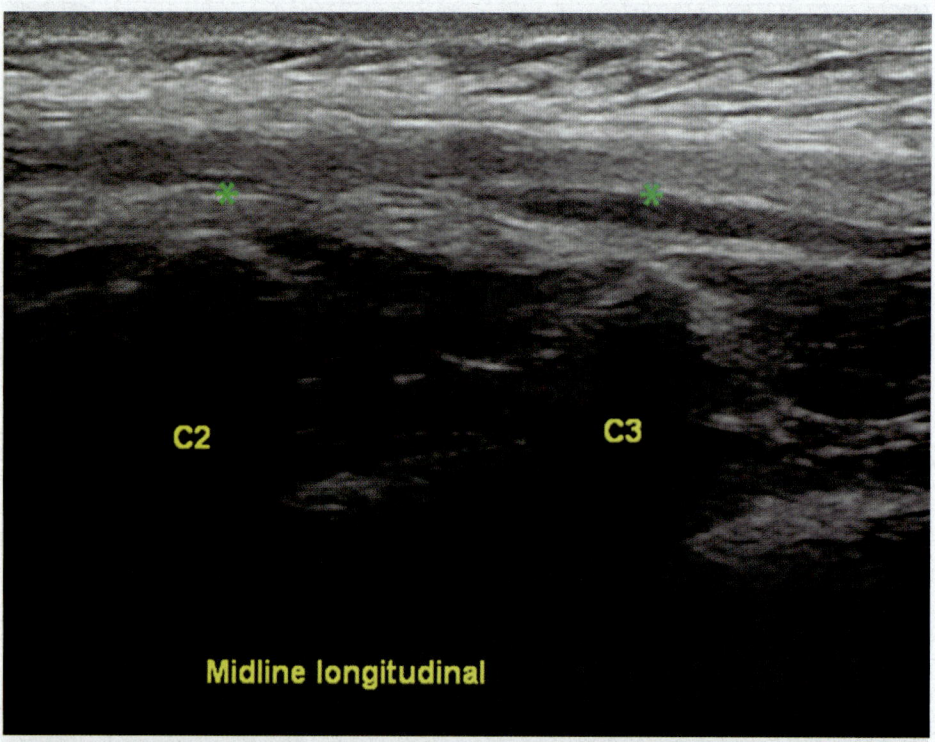

**FIGURE 2.7.** Midline longitudinal view of the spinous processes of the upper cervical vertebra. The C1 vertebra has only a vestigial spinous process as compared with C2 and C3 vertebrae, which have more classic bifid spinous processes (*green asterisk*) (see Fig. 2.8).

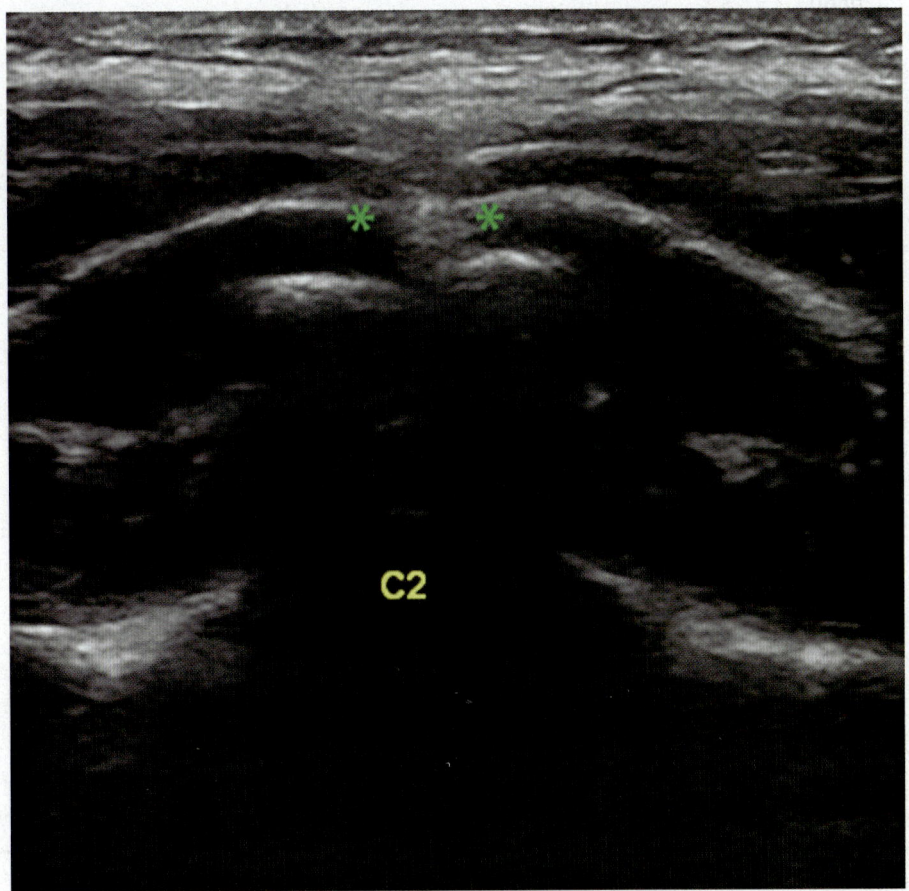

**FIGURE 2.8.** The more classic bifid process (*green asterisk*) of the C2 vertebra is clearly demonstrated on this transverse short-axis scan of the C2 vertebral body.

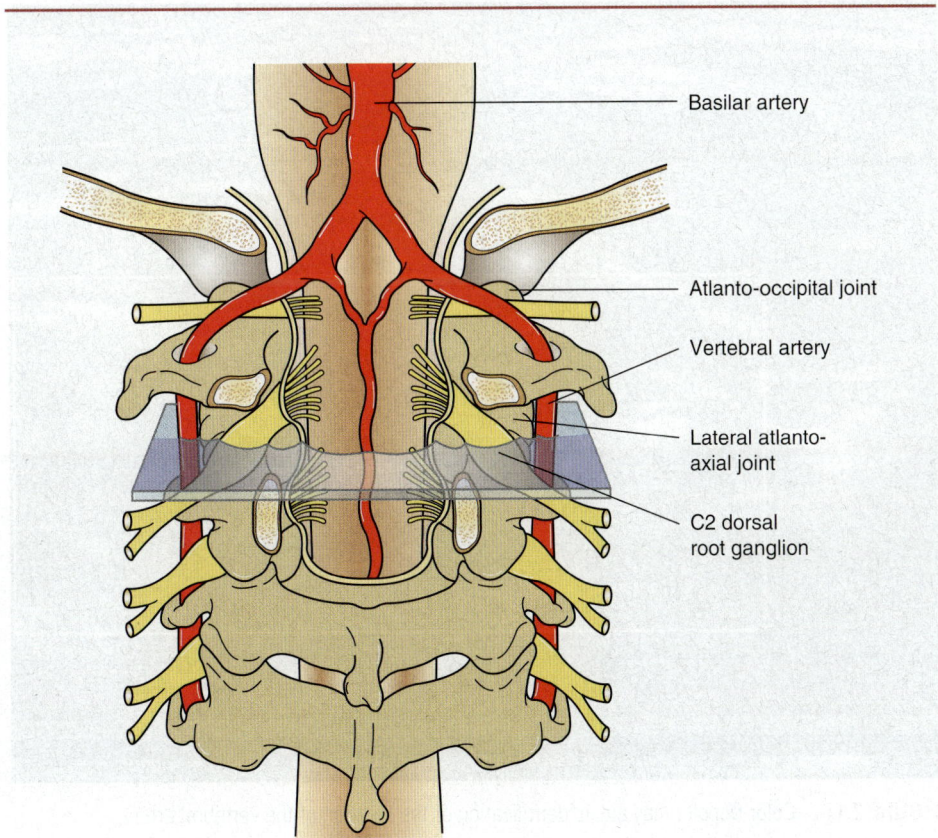

**FIGURE 2.9.** The relationship to the C2 nerve root, vertebral artery, and atlantoaxial joint.

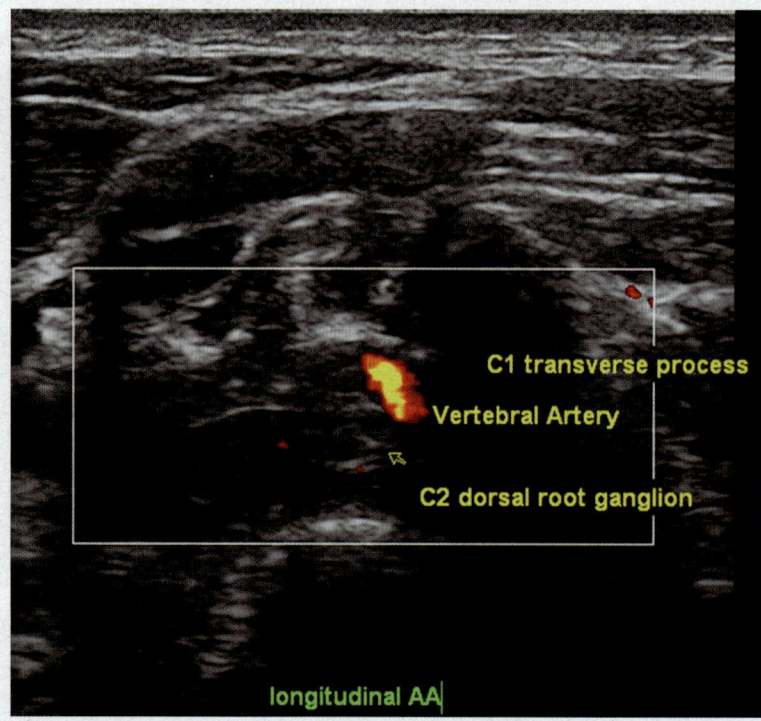

**FIGURE 2.10.** Relationship of the atlantoaxial joint to the exiting C2 nerve root and the vertebral artery.

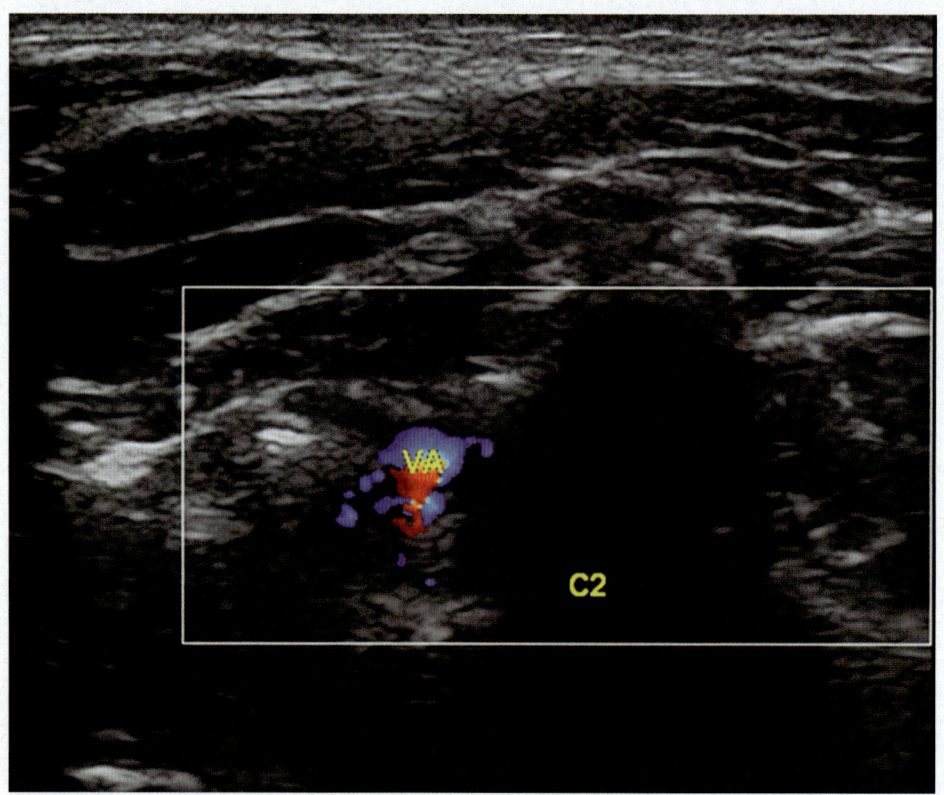

**FIGURE 2.11.** Color Doppler may aid in identification of the location of the vertebral artery.

well as the third occipital nerve may be required to provide the patient with complete pain relief. Blockade of the atlanto-occipital joint may also be beneficial, especially if the patient has sustained trauma to the region.

The ability of ultrasound imaging to identify the precise position of the vertebral artery relative to the atlantoaxial joint suggests a significant theoretical advantage over the use of fluoroscopic guidance, which more clearly defines the joint, but does not delineate the actual position of the artery. Injection of small amounts of iodinated contrast media suitable for use in the central nervous system may help identify intravascular or subdural or subarachnoid placement prior to the injection of local anesthetic if fluoroscopic guidance is utilized concurrently with ultrasound guidance.

## SUGGESTED READINGS

Dreyfuss P, Michaelsen M, Fletcher D. Atlanto-occipital and lateral atlanto-axial joint pain patterns. *Spine (Phila Pa 1976)* 1994;19(10):1125–1131.

Narouze S. Complications of head and neck procedures. *Tech Reg Anesth Pain Manag* 2007;11:171–177.

Narouze S. Ultrasonography in pain medicine: future directions. *Tech Reg Anesth Pain Manag* 2009;13(3):198–202.

Waldman SD. Atlanto-axial nerve block. In: *Atlas of Interventional Pain Management*. 3rd ed. Philadelphia, PA: Saunders Elsevier; 2009:7–11.

Waldman SD, Campbell RSD. Special imaging considerations of the cervical spine. In: *Imaging of Pain*. Philadelphia, PA: Saunders Elsevier; 2010:25–26.

# Ultrasound-Guided Sphenopalatine Ganglion Block

## CLINICAL PERSPECTIVES

Sphenopalatine ganglion block is useful in the treatment of acute migraine headache, acute cluster headache, and a variety of facial neuralgias including Sluder, Vail, and Vidian neuralgia, as well as Gardner syndrome (Table 3.1). The technique has also been utilized in the treatment of status migrainosus and chronic cluster headache. Anecdotal evidence suggests that sphenopalatine ganglion block may also play a role in the palliation of pain secondary to acute herpes zoster involving the trigeminal nerve. The lateral infrazygomatic approach to sphenopalatine ganglion block is indicated in patients who have anatomic abnormalities of the nose that would preclude the use of the transnasal approach to sphenopalatine ganglion block. The lateral infrazygomatic approach is the preferred route for neurodestructive procedures of the sphenopalatine ganglion. Neurodestruction of the sphenopalatine ganglion may be carried out by the injection of neurolytic agents, the use of radiofrequency lesioning, or the use of cryoneurolysis.

## CLINICALLY RELEVANT ANATOMY

The sphenopalatine ganglion, which is also known as the pterygopalatine, nasal, or Meckel ganglion, is located deep within the pterygopalatine fossa lying just posterior to the middle turbinate beneath a thin layer of lateral nasal mucosa (Fig. 3.1). It lies just below the maxillary nerve as it traverses the pterygopalatine fossa, appearing suspended from the maxillary nerve by its two interconnecting branches (Fig. 3.2). It is the largest of the parasympathetic ganglion and provides innervation to the paranasal sinuses, the lacrimal glands, and the glands associated with the mucosa of the nasopharynx and hard palate. It also sends fibers to the carotid plexus, gasserian ganglion, and trigeminal nerves as well as to the facial nerve and the superior cervical ganglion. The sphenopalatine ganglion is triangular in shape and is 5 to 6 mm in size. The sphenopalatine ganglion can be blocked by the topical application of local anesthetic via the transnasal approach, by intraoral injection through the greater palatine foramen, or by the lateral infrazygomatic placement of a needle via the coronoid notch.

## ULTRASOUND-GUIDED TECHNIQUE

Ultrasound-guided sphenopalatine ganglion block via the lateral infrazygomatic approach is a straightforward technique if attention is paid to the clinically relevant anatomy. The success rate of the technique can be increased by the concurrent use of a nerve stimulator to help confirm exact needle placement. To perform ultrasound-guided sphenopalatine ganglion block via the lateral infrazygomatic approach, the patient is placed in supine position with the cervical spine in the neutral position. The mandibular notch provides easy access to the pterygopalatine fossa and the sphenopalatine ganglion (Fig. 3.3). The mandibular notch of the mandible is identified by asking the patient to open and close his or her mouth several times while palpating the area just anterior and slightly inferior to the acoustic auditory meatus. Once the mandibular notch is identified, the patient is asked to hold his or her mouth open in a relaxed, neutral position.

The skin overlying the mandibular notch is prepped with antiseptic solution, and a linear transducer is placed in the transverse plane directly over the mandibular notch (Fig. 3.4). The temporomandibular joint should be readily apparent in the posterior portion of the image with the acoustic shadow of the curved bony mandibular condyle and mandibular neck just below it (Fig. 3.4). Anterior to the neck of the mandible is the maxillary nerve within the pterygopalatine fossa with the

**TABLE 3.1  Indications for Sphenopalatine Ganglion Block**

- Acute migraine headache
- Acute cluster headache
- Chronic cluster headache
- Sluder neuralgia
- Vidian neuralgia
- Vail neuralgia
- Gardner syndrome
- Status migrainosus
- Chronic cluster headache
- Acute herpes zoster involving the trigeminal nerve

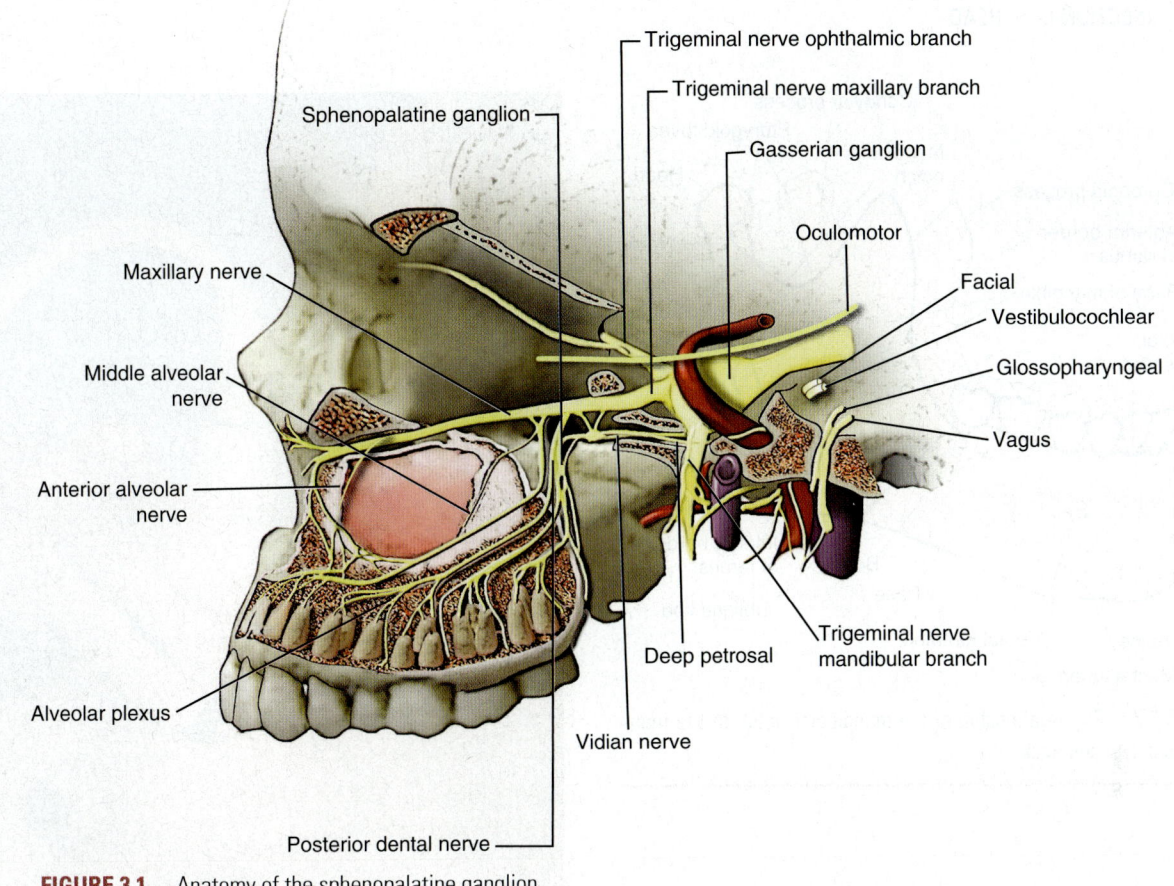

**FIGURE 3.1.** Anatomy of the sphenopalatine ganglion.

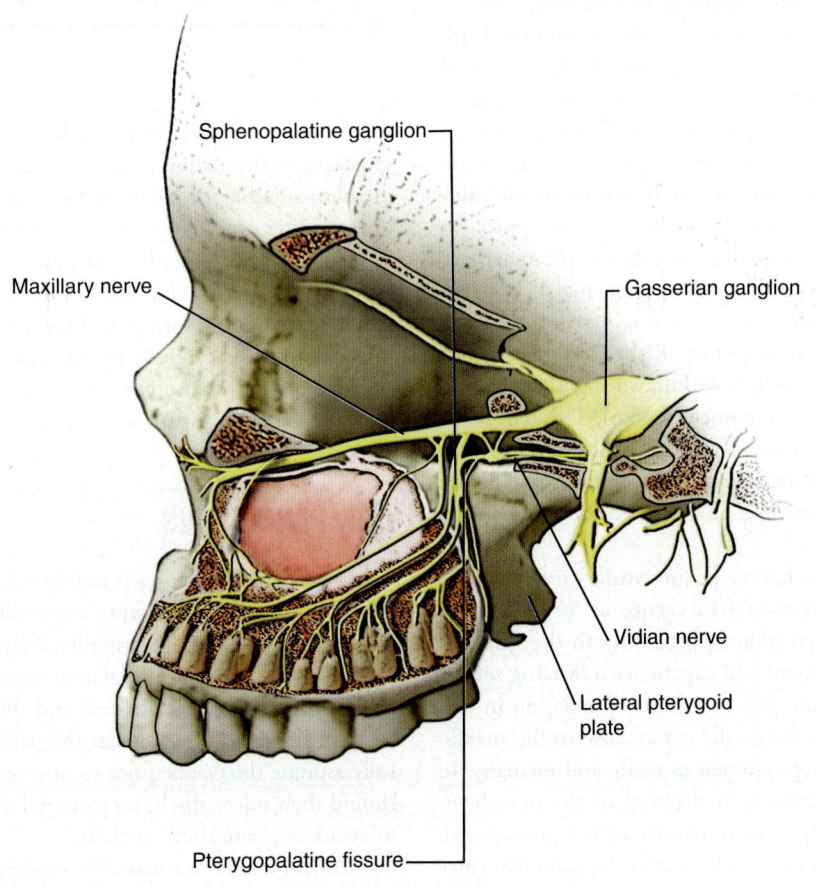

**FIGURE 3.2.** The relationship of the sphenopalatine ganglion and maxillary nerve.

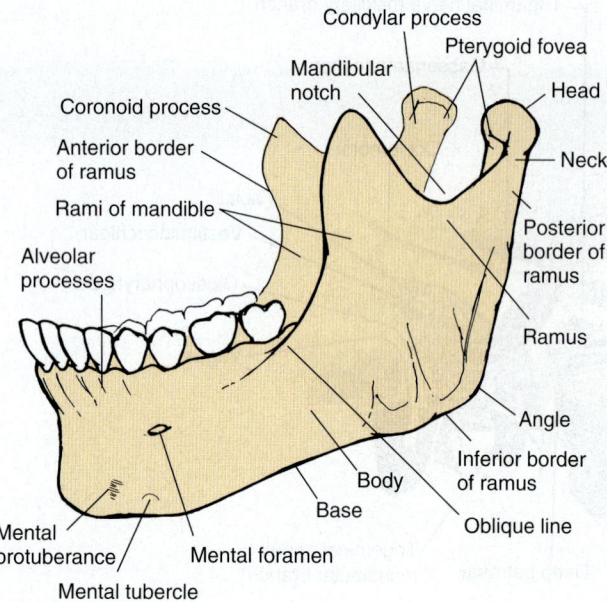

**FIGURE 3.3.** The relationship of the mandibular notch to the mandibular condyle and neck.

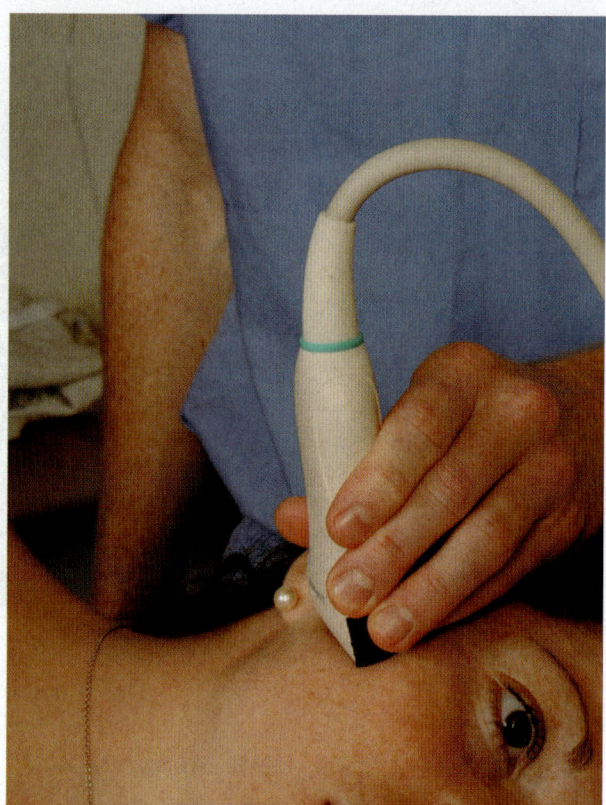

**FIGURE 3.4.** Proper position of the linear transducer for sphenopalatine ganglion block via the lateral infrazygomatic approach.

temporal is and masseter muscles appearing just above it (Fig. 3.5). The body of the masseter muscle can be followed anteriorly to its origin on the zygomatic arch (see Fig. 3.5).

Two milliliters of local anesthetic is drawn up in a 3-mL sterile syringe. Twenty to forty milligrams of depot steroid preparation may be empirically added to the local anesthetic. Under real-time ultrasound guidance, a 22-gauge, 10-cm straight styletted radiofrequency needle with a 2-mm active tip is inserted just below the zygomatic arch directly in the middle of the mandibular notch using an out-of-plane approach. The needle is advanced to an area just below the maxillary nerve. If a paresthesia in the distribution of the maxillary nerve is encountered, the needle is withdrawn and redirected in a more inferior and posterior trajectory. If the lateral pterygoid plate is encountered, the needle is withdrawn slightly and redirected slightly superior and anterior (Fig. 3.6). This will place the needle just above the lower aspect of the lateral pterygoid plate allowing entry into the pterygopalatine fossa just below the maxillary nerve and in close proximity to the sphenopalatine ganglion.

When the needle is felt to be in satisfactory position, stimulation of the needle should be carried at 50 Hz. If the needle is in the correct position in proximity to the sphenopalatine ganglion, the patient will experience a buzzing sensation inside the nose. If the patient reports stimulation in the upper teeth and gingiva, the needle is too close to the maxillary nerve and must be repositioned caudally and medially. If the patient reports stimulation in the roof of the mouth, it means that the needle tip is in proximity to the greater and lesser palatine nerves and the needle must be repositioned caudally and posteromedially. If the procedure is being performed with concurrent fluoroscopic and ultrasound guidance, when a satisfactory stimulation pattern is obtained, 0.5 mL of contrast medium suitable for use in the central nervous system can be injected after careful aspiration to fill the pterygopalatine fossa.

After correct needle placement is confirmed, careful aspiration is carried out and 2 mL of solution is injected in incremental doses. During the injection procedure, the patient must be observed carefully for signs of local anesthetic toxicity. Because of the proximity of the maxillary nerve, the patient may also experience partial blockade of the maxillary nerve.

## COMPLICATIONS

The pterygopalatine fossa is highly vascular, and the potential for trauma to the vasculature, especially the maxillary artery, remains an ever-present possibility. Needle damage to the artery may result in significant facial hematoma formation, which can be very distressing to the patient and clinician alike. The vascularity of the region means that the pain specialist should carefully aspirate the needle prior to injecting any medications and should then inject small, incremental doses of local anesthetic to avoid local anesthetic toxicity.

Patients may occasionally experience profound bradycardia and hypotension when undergoing sphenopalatine

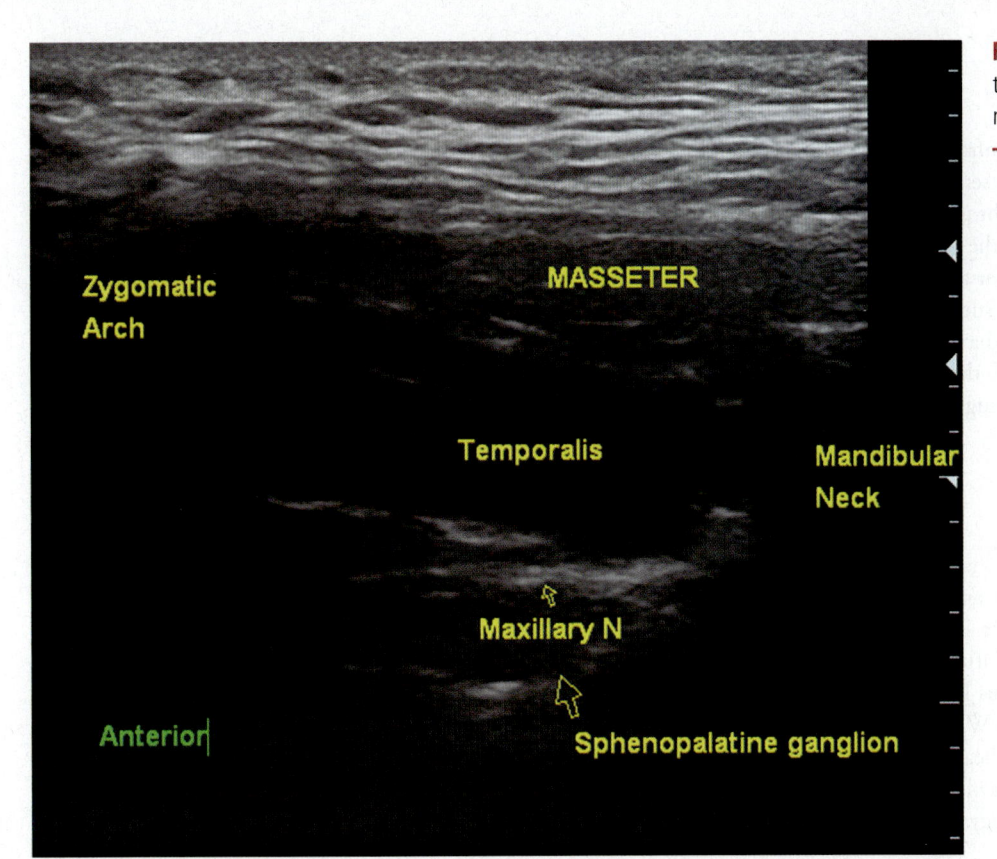

**FIGURE 3.5.** Ultrasound image of the sphenopalatine ganglion and surrounding structures.

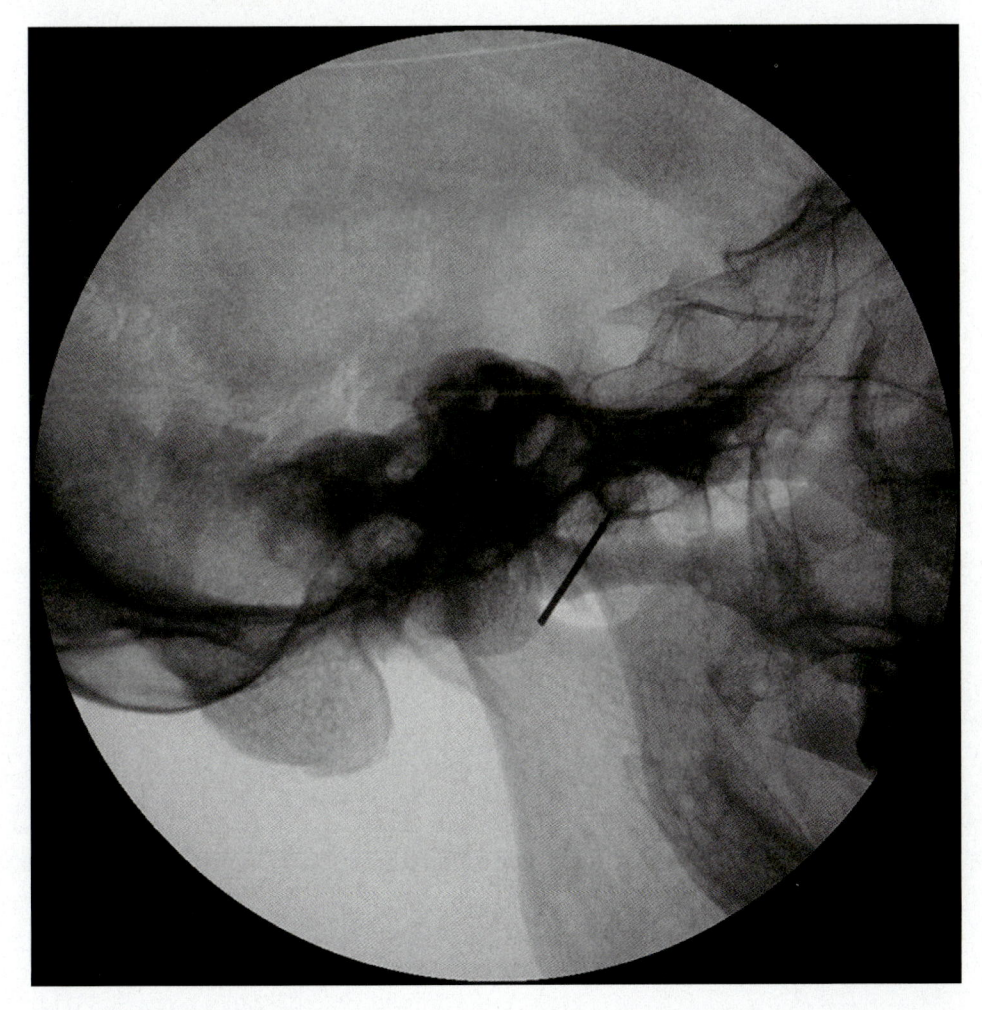

**FIGURE 3.6.** Fluoroscopic image of needle traversing the mandibular notch and resting against the lateral pterygoid plate.

ganglion block via the lateral infrazygomatic approach, and monitoring for these potentially serious side effects is mandatory. These side effects are thought to be due to the widespread parasympathetic influence of the sphenopalatine ganglion when it is stimulated. Atropine or atropine-like drugs such as glycopyrrolate and vasopressors such as ephedrine should be readily available should bradycardia and/or hypotension occur. Following sphenopalatine block, the patient's blood pressure should be monitored when moving the patient from a supine to a sitting or standing position.

## CLINICAL PEARLS

The simplicity of the transnasal approach to sphenopalatine ganglion block lends itself to use in the physician's office or emergency department when treating acute migraine or cluster headache. Two percent viscous lidocaine is a suitable local anesthetic for this application. When using sphenopalatine ganglion block to treat the acute headache sufferer, the concurrent administration of oxygen may hasten the resolution of the patient's headache symptomatology.

If anatomic abnormality, trauma, or tumor makes the use of the transnasal approach to the sphenopalatine ganglion impossible, the injection of local anesthetic and/or steroid via the greater palatine foramen or the lateral infrazygomatic approach represents a reasonable alternative. The lateral zygomatic approach to sphenopalatine block using ultrasound and/or fluoroscopic guidance in combination with nerve stimulation is the preferred approach for neurodestructive procedures of the sphenopalatine ganglion.

## SUGGESTED READINGS

Saunders M, Zuurmond WW. Efficacy of sphenopalatine ganglion blockade in 66 patients suffering from cluster headache: a 12- to 70-month follow-up evaluation. *J Neurosurg* 1997;87:876–880.

Waldman SD. Sphenopalatine ganglion block—80 years later. *Reg Anesth* 1993;18:274–276.

Waldman SD. Sphenopalatine ganglion. In: *Pain Review*. Philadelphia, PA: Saunders Elsevier; 2009:40–41.

Waldman SD. Atlanto-occipital nerve block. In: *Atlas of Interventional Pain Management*. 3rd ed. Philadelphia, PA: Saunders Elsevier; 2009:18–20.

Waldman SD. Cluster headache. In: *Atlas of Common Pain Syndromes*. 3rd ed. Philadelphia, PA: Saunders Elsevier; 2011:11–14.

# CHAPTER 4

# Ultrasound-Guided Greater and Lesser Occipital Nerve Block

## CLINICAL PERSPECTIVES

Ultrasound-guided blockade of the greater and lesser occipital nerves is useful in the diagnosis and treatment of occipital neuralgia and other pain syndromes subserved by the greater and lesser occipital nerves. This technique is also useful in providing surgical anesthesia of the tissues innervated by the greater and lesser occipital nerve for lesion removal and laceration repair and as an adjunct to general anesthesia for surgeries in the occipital region including craniotomies.

## CLINICALLY RELEVANT ANATOMY

The greater occipital nerve is comprised of fibers of the dorsal primary ramus of the second cervical nerve and to a lesser extent from fibers of the third cervical nerve, which is comprised of fibers from the medial branch of the posterior division of the third cervical spinal nerve. As the greater occipital nerve passes in a cephalad direction, it passes between the obliquus capitis inferior and the semispinalis capitis muscles (Fig. 4.1). Along with the occipital artery, the greater occipital nerve ultimately pierces the fascia just below the superior nuchal ridge (Fig. 4.2). The greater occipital nerve provides sensory innervation to the medial portion of the posterior scalp as far anterior as the vertex (Fig. 4.3).

The lesser occipital nerve is comprised of fibers from the ventral primary rami of the second and third cervical nerves. The lesser occipital nerve passes superiorly along the posterior border of the sternocleidomastoid muscle perforating the deep fascia (see Fig. 4.2). The nerve then divides into several cutaneous branches that provide sensory innervation to the lateral portion of the posterior scalp and the cranial surface of the pinna of the ear (see Fig. 4.3). Communicating branches from the lesser occipital nerve to the greater occipital nerve, the greater auricular nerve, and the posterior auricular branch of the facial nerve are common.

## ULTRASOUND-GUIDED TECHNIQUE

Ultrasound-guided occipital nerve block can be carried out using two different techniques. The first technique targets the nerve at the classic block site of the superior nuchal ridge. The second technique targets the nerve as it passes between the obliquus capitis inferior and semispinalis capitis muscles. To perform both techniques, the patient is placed in a sitting position with the cervical spine flexed and the forehead on a padded bedside table (Fig. 4.4). A total of 8 mL of local anesthetic is drawn up in a 12-mL sterile syringe. When treating occipital neuralgia or other painful conditions involving the greater and lesser occipital nerves, a total of 80 mg of depot steroid is added to the local anesthetic with the first block, and 40 mg of depot steroid is added with subsequent blocks.

### Classic Technique

The occipital artery is palpated at the level of the superior nuchal ridge. After preparation of the skin with antiseptic solution, a linear high-frequency ultrasound transducer is placed in the transverse position across the superior nuchal ridge at the point where the pulsation of the occipital artery was identified (Fig. 4.5). Color Doppler can be utilized to help identify the occipital artery if palpation of the pulse is difficult (Fig. 4.6). The greater occipital nerve should be in close proximity to the occipital artery and should appear as a round or ovoid hypoechoic vascular structure that is noncompressible with the ultrasound transducer (Fig. 4.7). When the nerve is identified, a 3½-inch needle is inserted utilizing an in-plane approach and is advanced perpendicularly until the needle approaches the periosteum of the underlying occipital bone. A paresthesia may be elicited and the patient should be warned of such. After gentle aspiration, 4 mL of local anesthetic and/or steroid is injected in a fan-like distribution with care being taken to avoid the foramen magnum, which is located medially. The needle is removed and pressure is placed on the injection site to avoid hematoma formation.

The lesser occipital nerve and a number of superficial branches of the greater occipital nerve are then blocked by directing the needle laterally and slightly inferiorly (Fig. 4.8). After gentle aspiration, an additional 2 to 4 mL of solution is injected.

### Obliquus Capitis Inferior Muscle Approach

After preparation of the skin with antiseptic solution, a linear high-frequency ultrasound transducer is aligned across the long axis of the obliquus capitis inferior muscle (Fig. 4.9). The

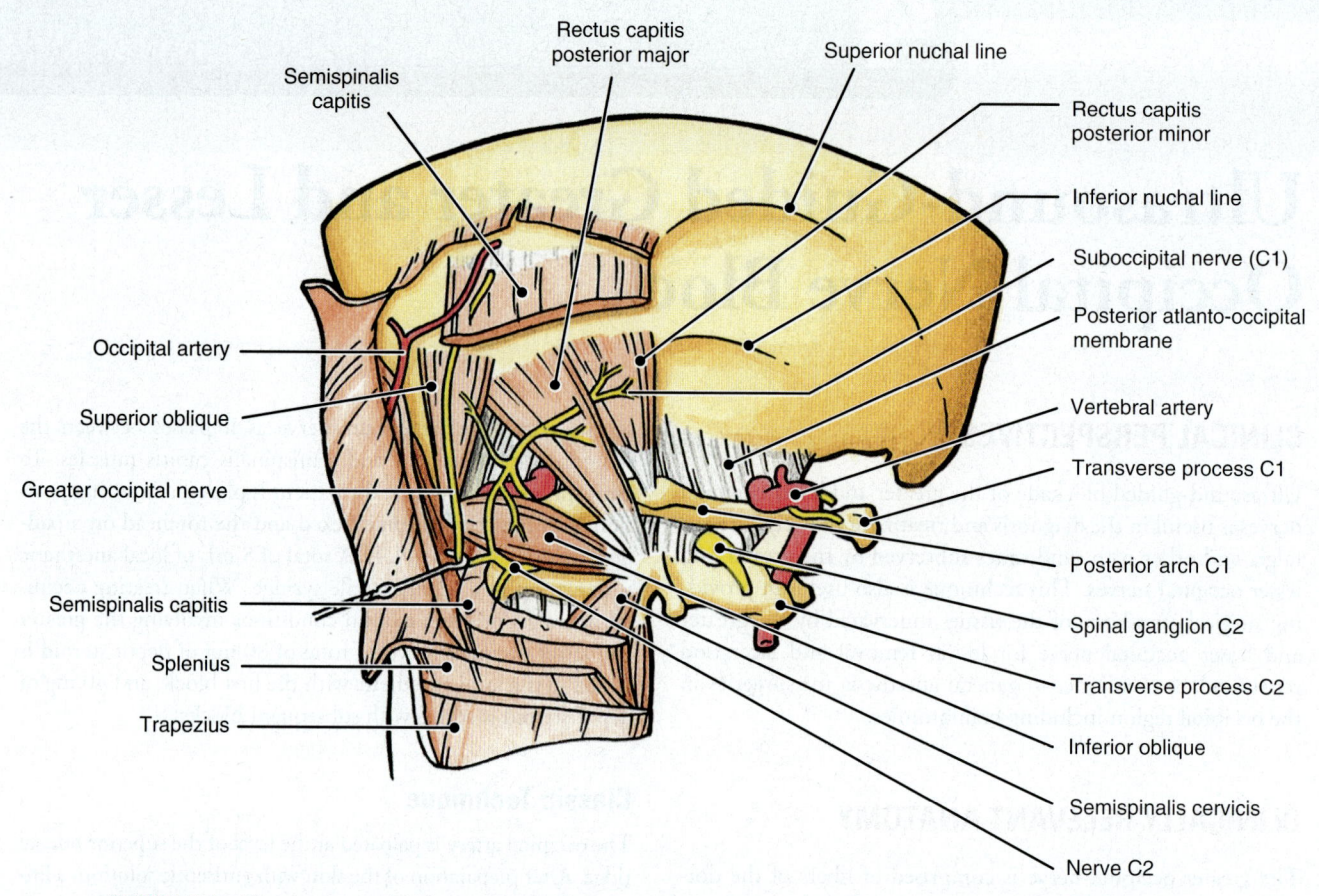

**FIGURE 4.1.** The greater occipital nerve passes between the obliquus capitis inferior and semispinalis capitis muscles. (Reused from Moore KL, Agur AMR. *Essential Clinical Anatomy*. 2nd ed. Baltimore, MD: Lippincott Williams & Wilkins; 2002:300, with permission.)

obliquus capitis inferior muscle is then identified on ultrasound imaging (Fig. 4.10). The semispinalis capitis muscle is then identified just above it (see Fig. 4.10). The greater occipital nerve should be identifiable between the two muscles (see Fig. 4.10). When the nerve is identified, a 3½-inch needle is inserted utilizing an in-plane approach and is advanced until the needle tip is in proximity to the occipital nerve. A paresthesia may be elicited, and the patient should be warned of such. After gentle aspiration, 2 mL of local anesthetic and/or steroid is injected. The needle is removed and pressure is placed on the injection site to avoid hematoma formation.

## COMPLICATIONS

Given the vascularity of the scalp and the proximity of the occipital artery, the clinician should not exceed the recommended safe dosages of local anesthetic when performing ultrasound-guided greater and lesser occipital nerve block. Following injection, pressure should be placed on the injection site to decrease the incidence of postblock ecchymosis and hematoma formation. Application of cold packs for 20-minute periods after the block will also decrease the amount of postprocedure pain and bleeding the patient may experience. Proximity of

CHAPTER 4    ULTRASOUND-GUIDED GREATER AND LESSER OCCIPITAL NERVE BLOCK    21

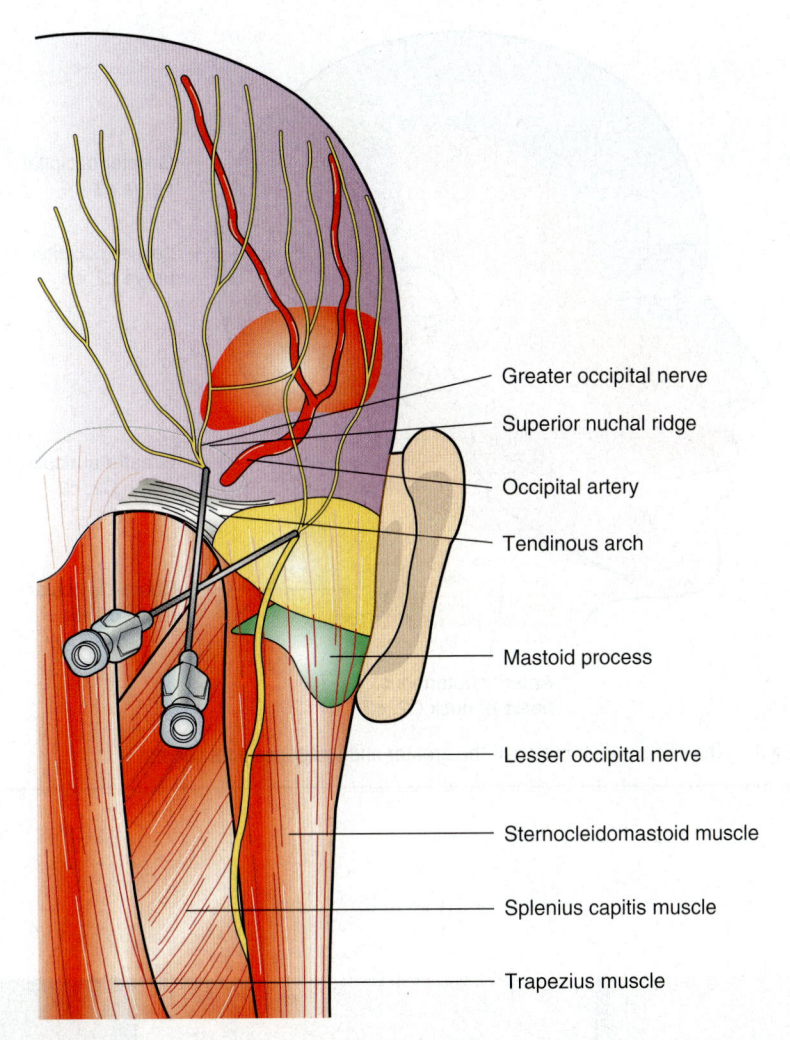

**FIGURE 4.2.** The greater occipital nerve and occipital artery pierce the fascia just below the nuchal ridge.

the C1 and C2 nerves as well as the foramen magnum means that this block should be untaken only by those with complete familiarity of the regional anatomy.

## CLINICAL PEARLS

Occipital neuralgia is one of the most overdiagnosed pain syndromes in clinical medicine. In the absence of trauma to the neck and suboccipital region, the diagnosis becomes one of exclusion with tension-type headache being a much more likely possibility. Tension-type headaches do not respond to occipital nerve blocks but are very amenable to treatment with antidepressant compounds such as amitriptyline in conjunction with cervical steroid epidural nerve blocks.

It is this author's belief that any patient suffering from headaches severe enough to require neural blockade as part of the treatment plan should undergo a magnetic resonance imaging scan of the head to rule out unsuspected intracranial pathology which may mimic the clinical symptoms of occipital neuralgia (Fig. 4.11). Other abnormalities of the cervical spine and cranium such as Arnold-Chiari malformations should also be ruled out with plain radiographs of the cervical spine.

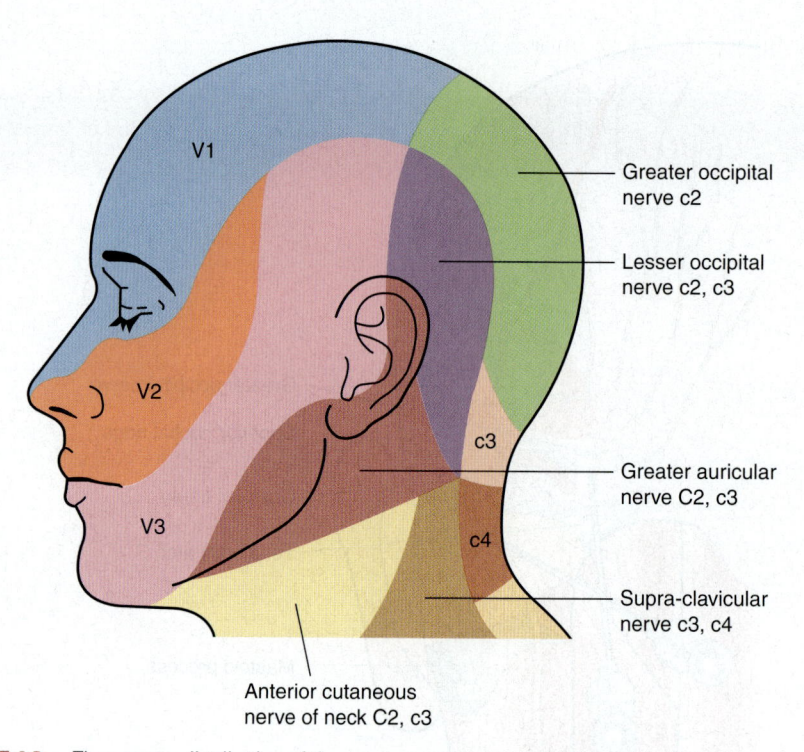

**FIGURE 4.3.** The sensory distribution of the greater and lesser occipital nerves.

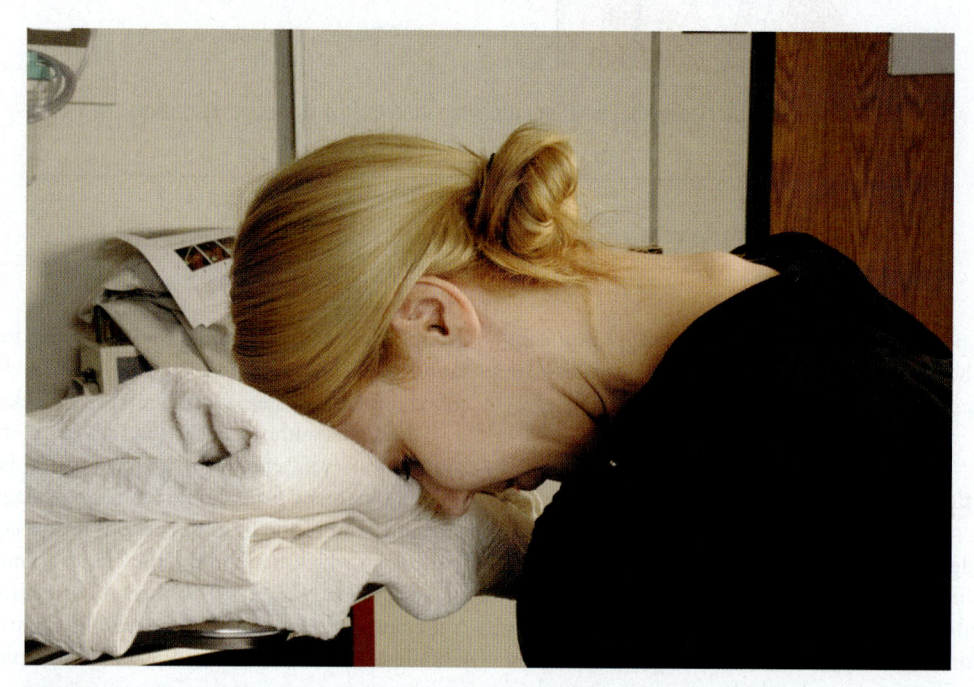

**FIGURE 4.4.** To perform greater and lesser occipital nerve block, the patient is placed in the sitting position with his or her forehead resting on a padded bedside table.

CHAPTER 4   ULTRASOUND-GUIDED GREATER AND LESSER OCCIPITAL NERVE BLOCK   23

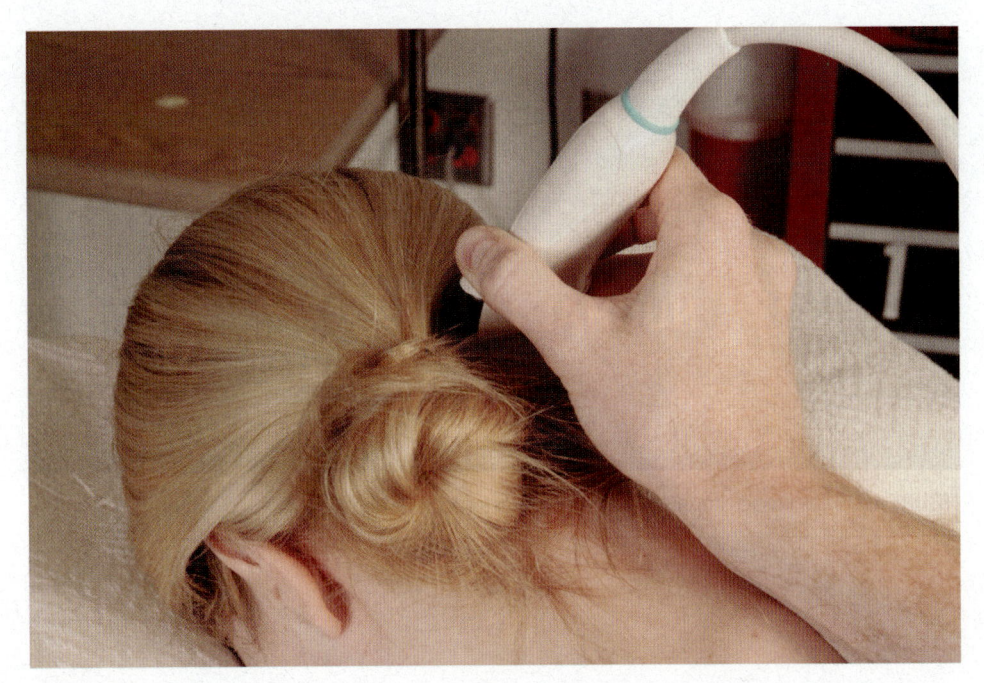

**FIGURE 4.5.** Proper transverse position of the ultrasound transducer to perform the classic approach to the greater occipital nerve block.

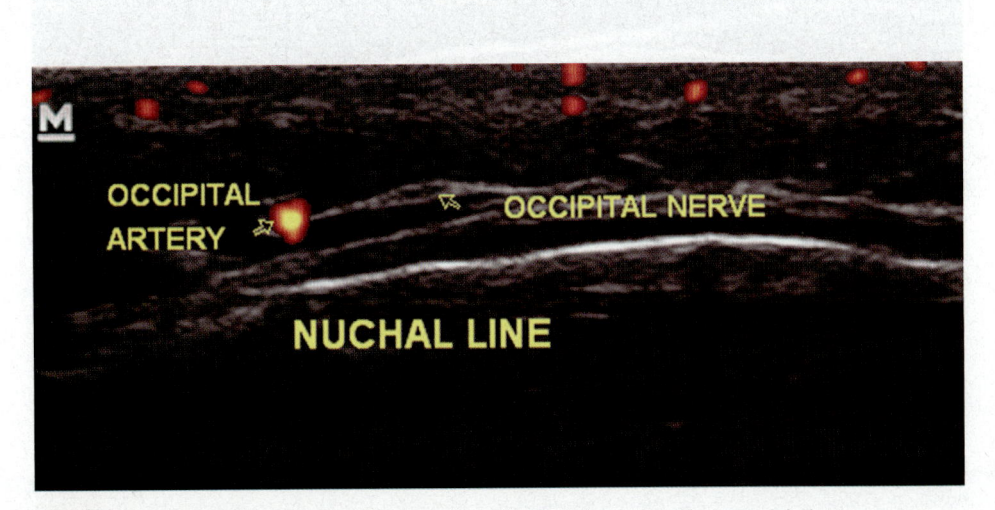

**FIGURE 4.6.** Transverse ultrasound image using color Doppler to identify the occipital artery.

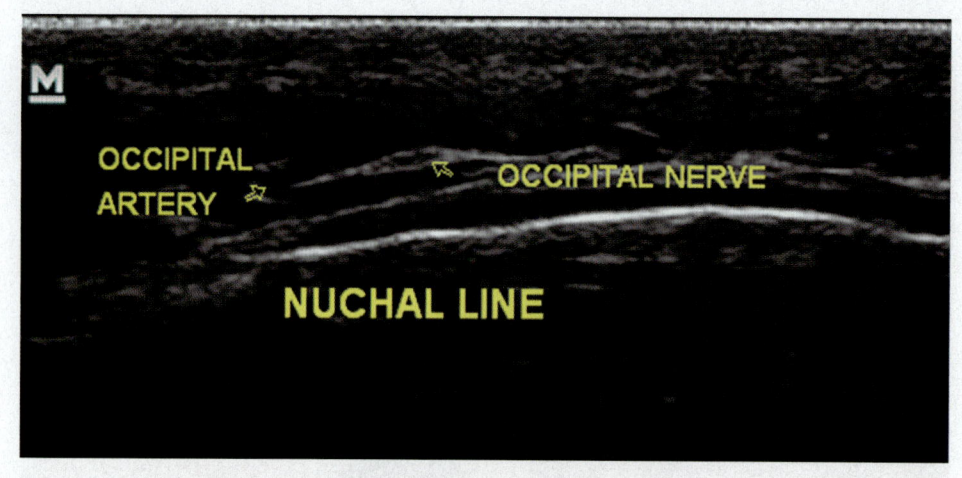

**FIGURE 4.7.** Transverse ultrasound image of the greater occipital nerve.

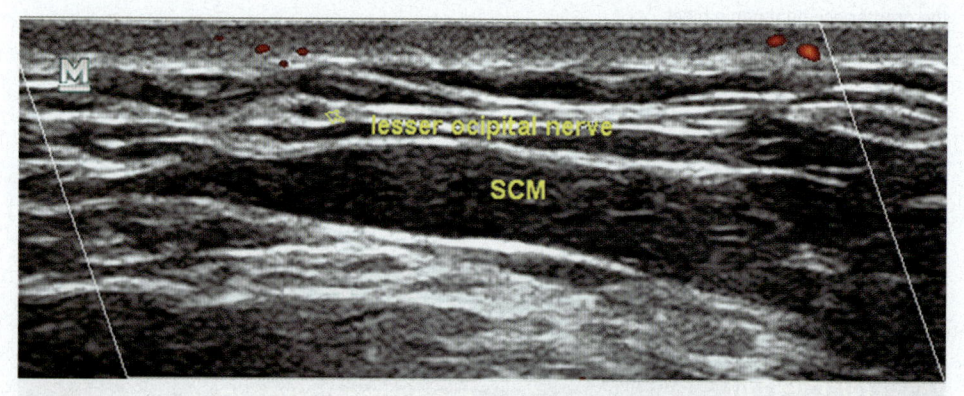

**FIGURE 4.8.** Transverse ultrasound image of the lesser occipital nerve. (SCM, semispinalis capitis muscle)

CHAPTER 4   ULTRASOUND-GUIDED GREATER AND LESSER OCCIPITAL NERVE BLOCK   25

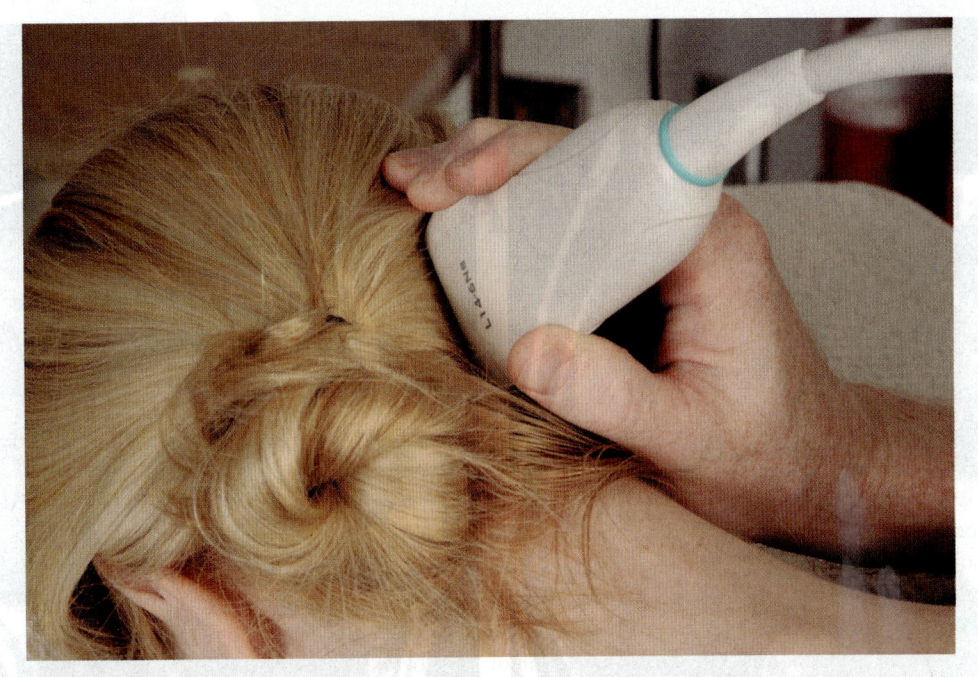

**FIGURE 4.9.** Proper longitudinal position of the ultrasound transducer to perform the obliquus capitis inferior muscle approach for blockade of the greater occipital nerve. The transducer is aligned along the long axis of the obliquus capitis inferior muscle.

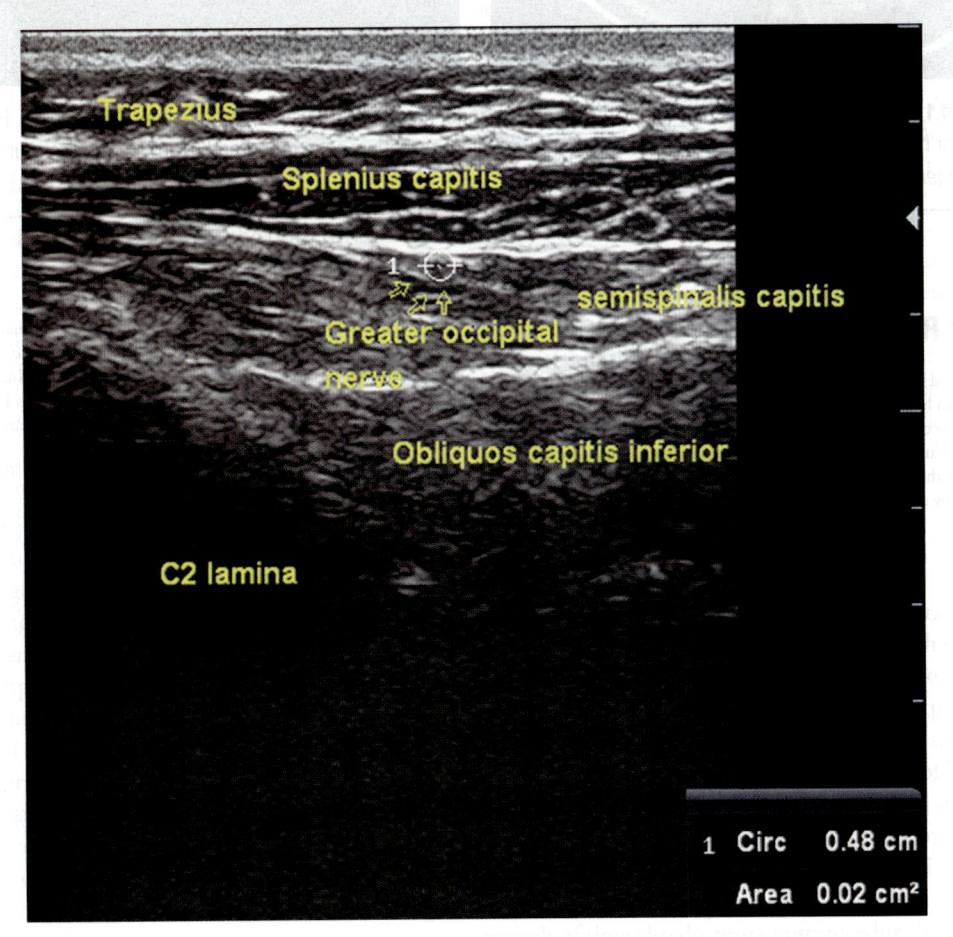

**FIGURE 4.10.** Long-axis ultrasound image of the greater occipital nerve passing between the obliquus capitis inferior and semispinalis capitis muscles.

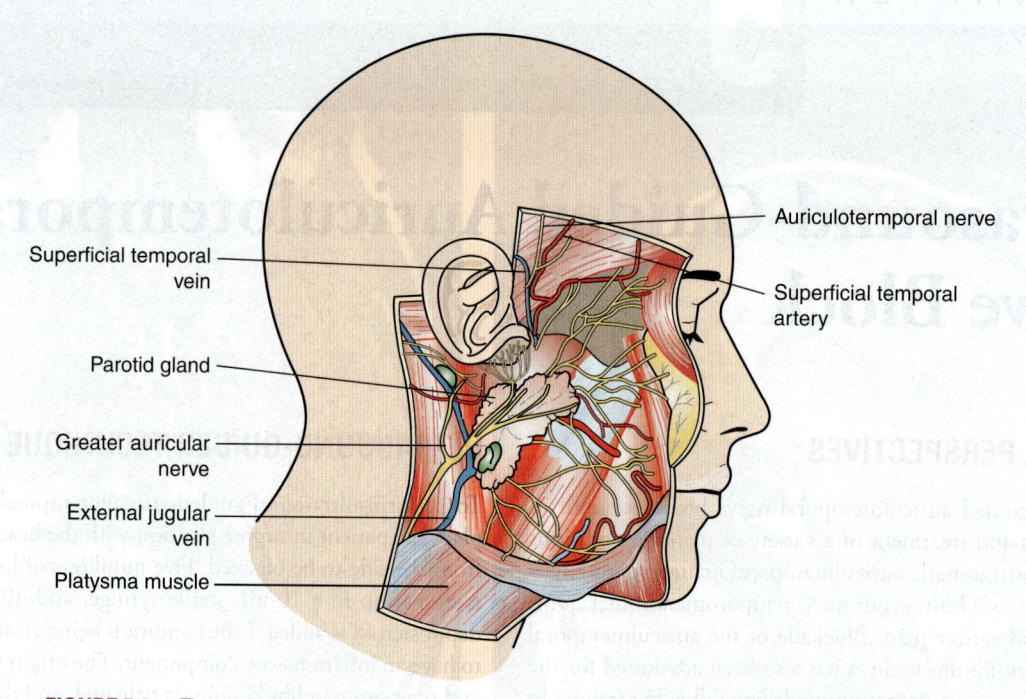

**FIGURE 5.1.** The auriculotemporal nerve ascends in front of the ear along with the superficial temporal artery.

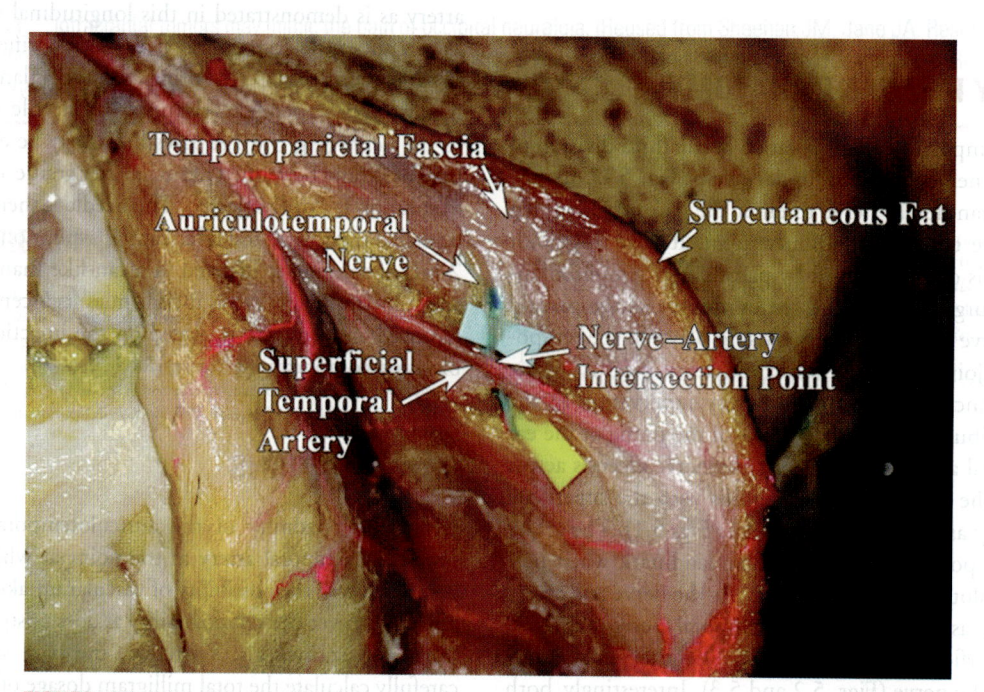

**FIGURE 5.2.** The relationship of the auriculotemporal nerve and the superficial temporal artery. Dissection in the left temple region. The flap has been dissected deep to the temporoparietal fascia. The superficial temporal fat pad lies down. The auriculotemporal nerve can be seen crossing on top of the superficial temporal artery. This illustrates a "single cross" type of nerve–artery relationship. (Reused from Janis JE, Hatef DA, Ducic I, et al. Anatomy of the auriculotemporal nerve: variations in its relationship to the superficial temporal artery and implications for the treatment of migraine headaches. *Plast Reconstr Surg* 2010;125(5):1422–1428, with permission.)

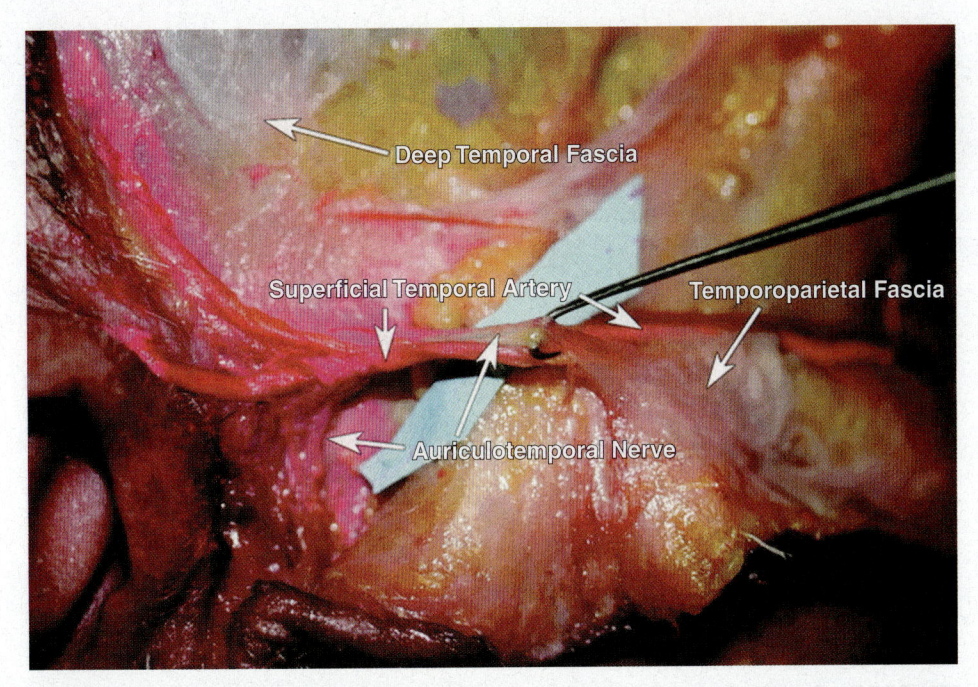

**FIGURE 5.3.** The relationship of the auriculotemporal nerve and the superficial temporal artery. Dissection in the right temple. The superficial temporal artery and auriculotemporal nerve are wrapping around each other. This illustrates an "intertwining" type of nerve–artery relationship. (Reused from Janis JE, Hatef DA, Ducic I, et al. Anatomy of the auriculotemporal nerve: variations in its relationship to the superficial temporal artery and implications for the treatment of migraine headaches. *Plast Reconstr Surg* 2010;125(5):1422–1428, with permission.)

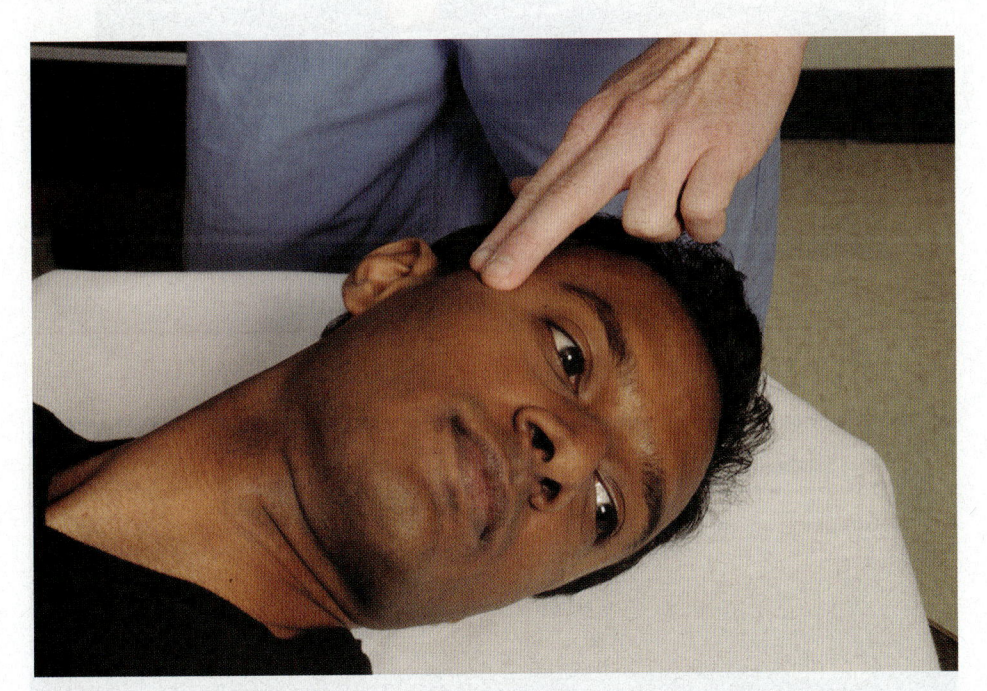

**FIGURE 5.4.** The pulse of the temporal artery is identified just superior to origin of the zygoma.

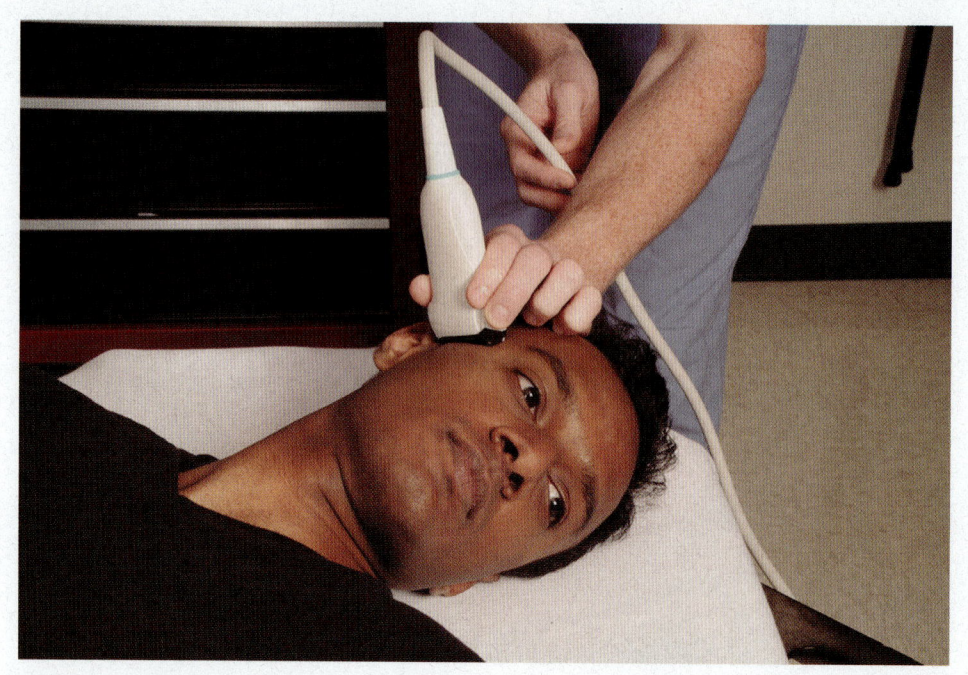

**FIGURE 5.5.** Proper transverse placement of the linear ultrasound transducer over the previously identified pulse of the temporal artery.

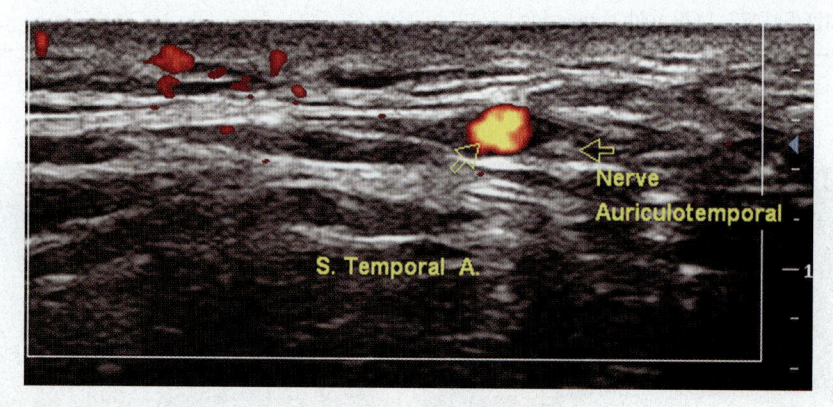

**FIGURE 5.6.** Color Doppler image of the superficial temporal artery.

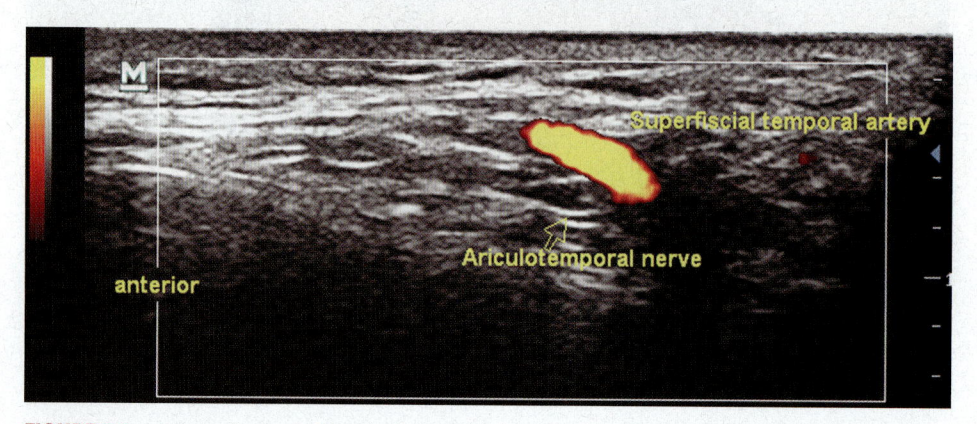

**FIGURE 5.7.** Longitudinal color Doppler image of the temporal artery and the auriculotemporal nerve.

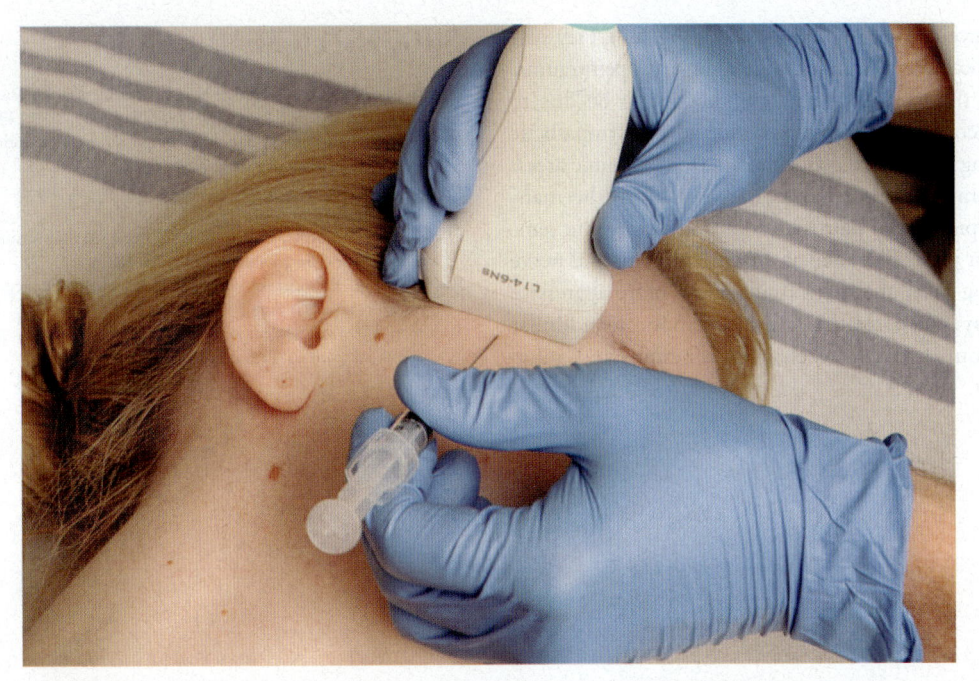

**FIGURE 5.8.** Out-of-plane approach for ultrasound-guided injection of the auriculotemporal nerve.

## CLINICAL PEARLS

Auriculotemporal nerve block is useful in the palliation of pain secondary to acute herpes zoster involving the geniculate ganglion, such as Ramsay-Hunt syndrome, when combined with facial nerve block. Aluminum acetate solution used as tepid soaks several times a day is especially effective in helping dry weeping lesions of the external auditory meatus and enhancing patient comfort.

Auriculotemporal nerve block is also useful in the management of Frey syndrome. Frey syndrome (which is also known as Baillarger syndrome, Dupuy syndrome, salivosudoriparous syndrome, auriculotemporal syndrome, and gustatory sweating syndrome) is an unusual syndrome involving the sympathetic and parasympathetic nervous system that is characterized by postgustatory unilateral hyperhidrosis and flushing of the malar region and pinna of the ear. The symptoms are most pronounced when the patient eats or drinks spicy, sour, or tart foods, which strongly

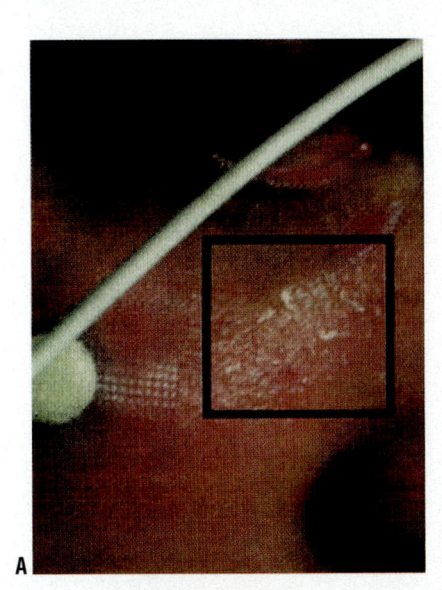

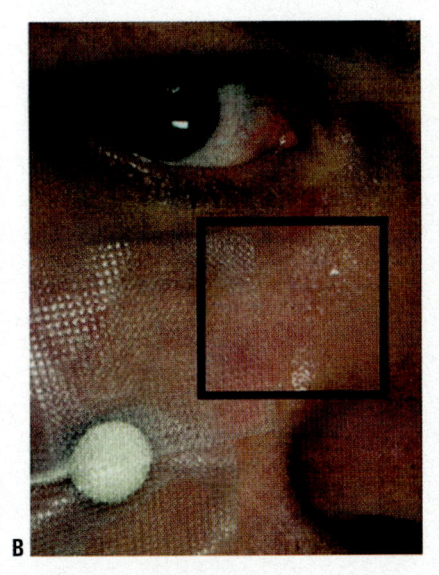

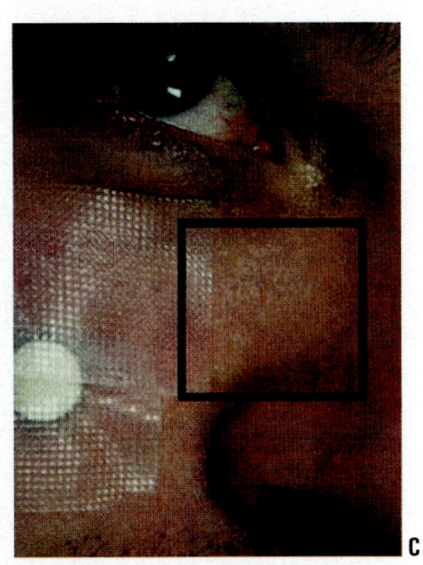

**FIGURE 5.9.** Photographs of the patient's right face **(A)** after drinking orange juice, **(B)** after 2 mg of edrophonium IV, and **(C)** during IV infusion of trimethaphan. Note gustatory and edrophonium-induced sweating, in contrast with dry skin during trimethaphan infusion. (Reused from Goldstein DS, Pechnik S, Moak J, et al. Painful sweating. *Neurology* 2004;63(8):1471–1475, with permission.)

stimulate the parotid gland to produce saliva (Fig. 5.9). Frey syndrome usually occurs 2 to 6 months after surgery, open trauma, or infection of the parotid gland. It is thought to be due to improper regeneration of the sympathetic and parasympathetic nerves subserving the parotid gland and affected anatomic areas.

Auriculotemporal nerve block is also useful in the management of atypical facial pain syndromes involving the temporomandibular joint. Blockade of the auriculotemporal nerve with long-acting local anesthetics may allow more aggressive physical therapy when treating painful temporomandibular joint dysfunction, especially when joint adhesions and ankylosis are present.

## SUGGESTED READINGS

Cantarella G, Berlusconi A, Mele V, et al. Treatment of Frey's syndrome with botulinum toxin type B. *Otolaryngol Head Neck Surg* 2010;143(2):214–218.

Hoff SR, Mohyuddin N, Yao M. Complications of parotid surgery. *Oper Tech Otolaryngol Head Neck Surg* 2009;20(2):123–130.

Morena-Arias GA, Grimalt R, Llusa M, et al. Frey's syndrome. *J Pediatr* 2001;138(2):294.

O'Neill JP, Condron C, Curran A, et al. Lucja Frey—historical relevance and syndrome review. *Surgeon* 2008;6(3):178–181.

Rustemeyer J, Eufinger H, Bremerich A. The incidence of Frey's syndrome. *J Craniomaxillofac Surg* 2008;36(1):34–37.

Waldman SD. Auriculotemporal block. In: *Atlas of Pain Management Injection Techniques*. 3rd ed. Philadelphia, PA: 2012:40–41.

# CHAPTER 6

# Ultrasound-Guided Greater Auricular Nerve Block

## CLINICAL PERSPECTIVES

Ultrasound-guided greater auricular nerve block is most commonly utilized in conjunction with lesser occipital nerve and auriculotemporal nerve block to provide complete surgical anesthesia and/or postoperative pain relief for the surgery of the external ear. As a stand-alone technique, ultrasound-guided greater auricular nerve block is useful in the diagnosis and treatment of painful conditions in areas subserved solely by the greater auricular nerve including greater auricular neuralgia, red ear syndrome, and pain secondary to acute herpes zoster and postherpetic neuralgia (Fig. 6.1). This technique can also be utilized to provide surgical anesthesia in the distribution of the greater auricular nerve for lesion removal and laceration repair.

## CLINICALLY RELEVANT ANATOMY

The largest sensory branch of the cervical plexus, the greater auricular nerve, arises from fibers of the primary ventral ramus of the second and third cervical nerves (Fig. 6.2). At a point just inferior and lateral to the lesser occipital nerve, the greater auricular nerve pierces the cervical fascia and passes superiorly and forward and then curves around the sternocleidomastoid muscle. The greater auricular nerve then pierces the superficial cervical fascia to move more superiorly and superficially to provide cutaneous sensory innervation to both surfaces of the auricle, the external auditory canal, angle of the jaw, and the skin overlying a portion of the parotid gland (Figs. 6.3 and 6.4).

## ULTRASOUND-GUIDED TECHNIQUE

The patient is placed in the supine position with the head turned away from the side to be blocked. Five milliliters of local anesthetic is drawn up in a 10-mL sterile syringe, and 40 to 80 mg of depot steroid is added to the local anesthetic if there is thought to be an inflammatory component to the patient's pain symptomatology.

The posterior border of the sternocleidomastoid muscle at the level of the cricoid notch is then identified, and the skin overlying the area is prepped with antiseptic solution. A high-frequency linear ultrasound transducer is then placed over the posterior border of the sternocleidomastoid muscle at the level of the cricoid in a transverse oblique position at essentially a right angle to the posterior border of the sternocleidomastoid muscle (Fig. 6.5). At this point, the greater auricular nerve will be visible twice in the same image and once in its position deep to the sternocleidomastoid muscle and then again in its superficial position as it curves back around the more superficial surface of the muscle (Fig. 6.6). Ultrasound imaging will also help the practitioner identify the relationship of the carotid artery and jugular vein to the greater auricular nerve to help avoid inadvertent intravascular injection (Fig. 6.7). It is at this point that the greater auricular nerve is blocked utilizing an in-plane approach by advancing a 22-gauge, 1½-inch needle in proximity to the superficial portion of the nerve (Fig. 6.8). A paresthesia may be elicited, and the patient should be warned of such. After gentle aspiration, 2 mL of solution is injected under real-time ultrasound imaging. The needle is removed and pressure is placed on the injection site to avoid hematoma or ecchymosis.

## COMPLICATIONS

Given the proximity of the external jugular view and carotid artery, the clinician should carefully calculate the total milligram dosage of local anesthetic that may be safely given, especially if bilateral nerve blocks are being performed. Postblock ecchymosis and hematoma formation are a distinct possibility if these major vascular structures are injured during the procedure. Damage to the brachial plexus can also occur if the needle is placed too deeply.

## CLINICAL PEARLS

The use of ultrasound guidance greatly increases the accuracy and safety of greater auricular nerve block and allows the use

**FIGURE 6.4.** The sensory distribution of the greater auricular nerve.

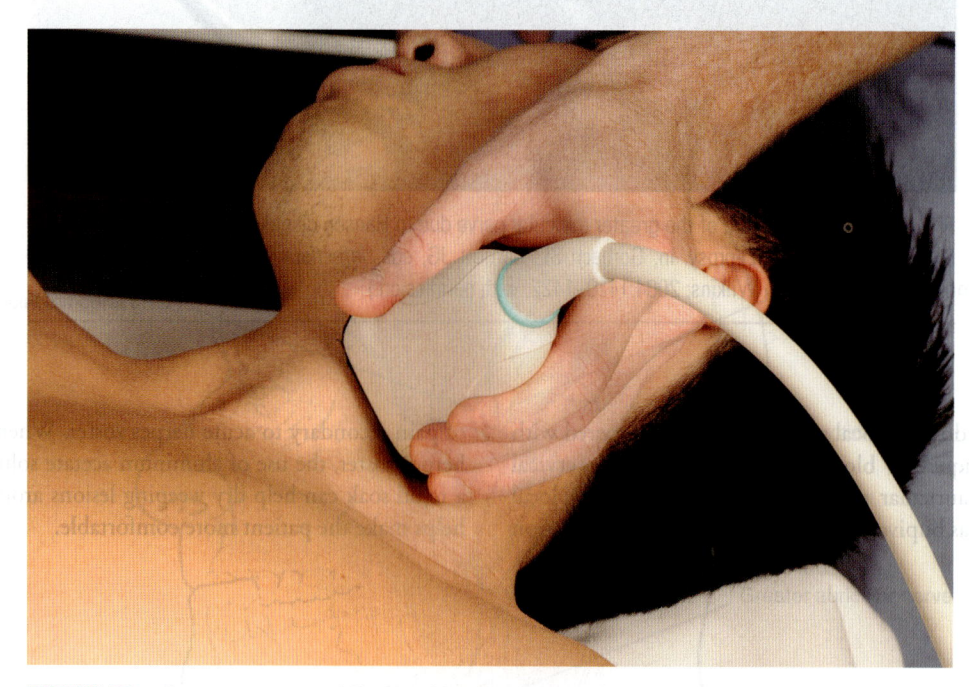

**FIGURE 6.5.** Correct transverse oblique position of the linear ultrasound transducer at a right angle to the sternocleidomastoid muscle at the level of the cricoid to perform greater auricular nerve block.

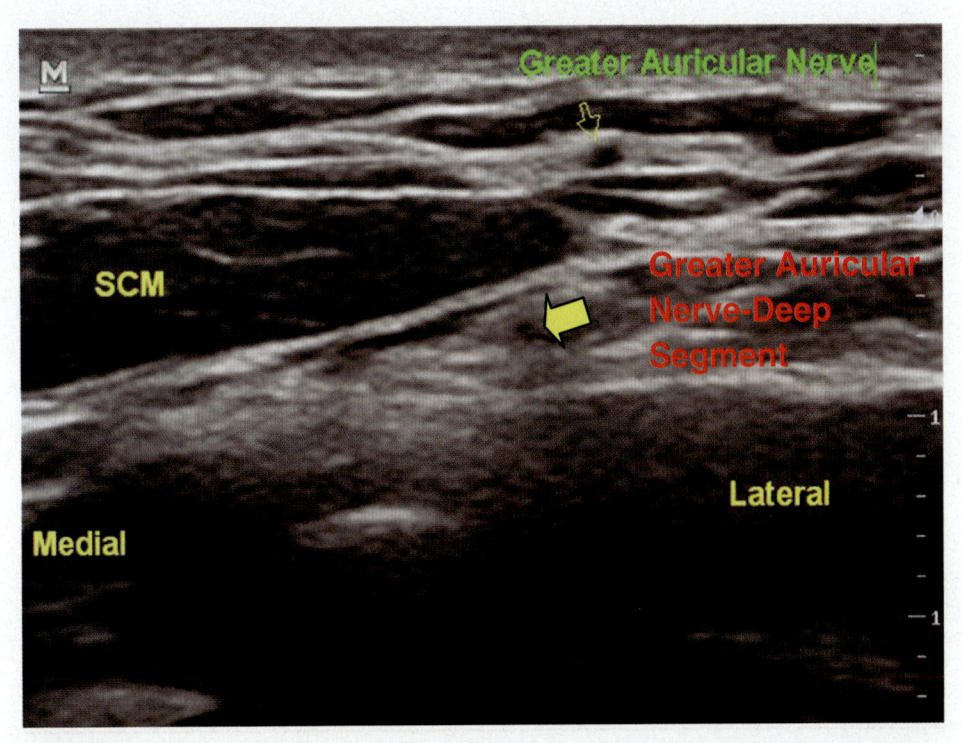

**FIGURE 6.6.** Transverse short-axis ultrasound image demonstrating both the deep and superficial segments of the greater auricular nerve and the nerves relationship to the sternocleidomastoid muscle (SCM).

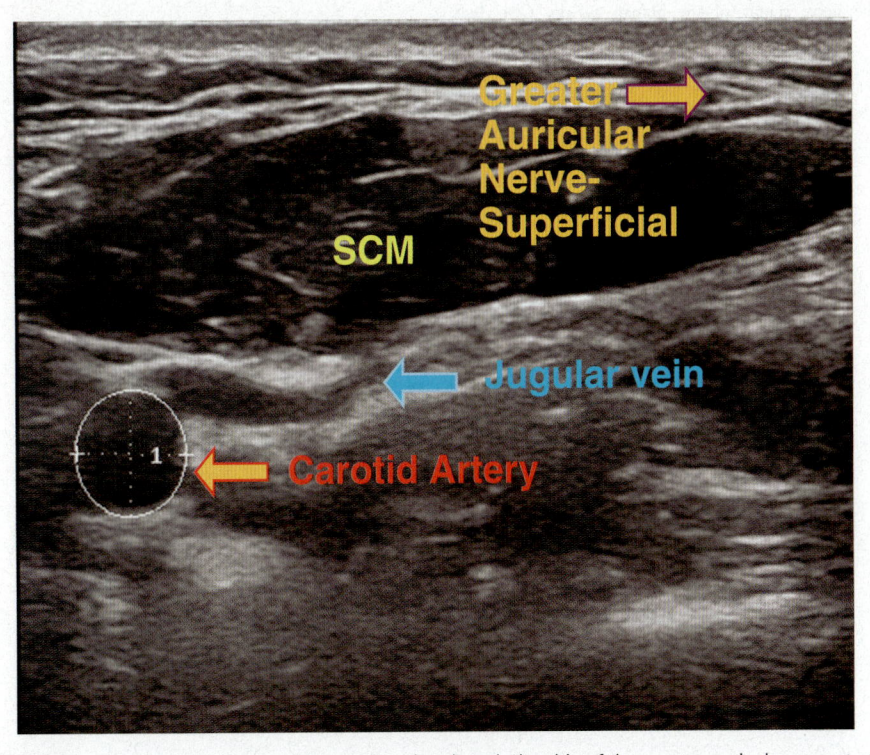

**FIGURE 6.7.** Transverse ultrasound image showing the relationship of the greater auricular nerve to the carotid artery and jugular vein. (SCM, sternocleidomastoid muscle.)

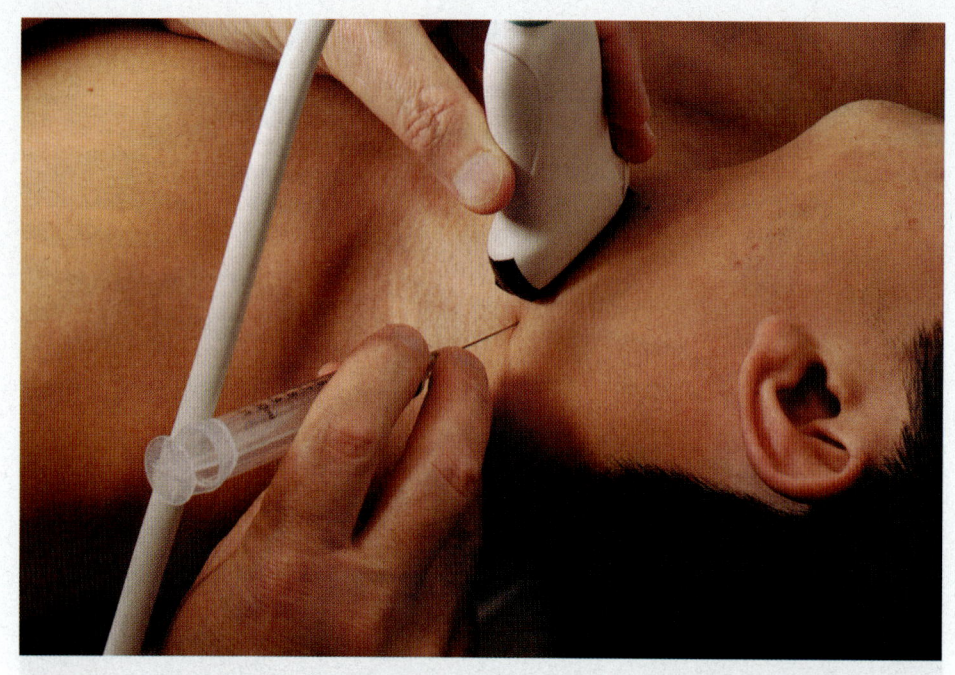

**FIGURE 6.8.** In-plane needle trajectory to perform ultrasound-guided greater auricular nerve block.

## SUGGESTED READINGS

Almand J, Boydell CL, Parry SW, et al. The greater auricular nerve revisited: pertinent anatomy for SMAS-Platysma rhytidectomy. *Ann Plast Surg* 1990;27:44–48.

Peuker ET, Filler TJ. The nerve supply of the human auricle. *Clin Anat* 2002;15:35–37.

Thallaj A, Marhofer P, Moriggl B, et al. Great auricular nerve blockade using high resolution ultrasound: a volunteer study. *Anaesthesia* 2010;65:836–840.

Waldman SD. Greater auricular nerve block. In: *Atlas of Interventional Pain Management*. 3rd ed. Philadelphia, PA: Saunders Elsevier; 2009:86–89.

# CHAPTER 7

# Ultrasound-Guided Trigeminal Nerve Block: Coronoid Approach

## CLINICAL PERSPECTIVES

Ultrasound-guided trigeminal nerve block via the coronoid approach allows blockade of the maxillary and mandibular nerve as they pass through the pterygopalatine space. The simplicity and safety of this technique lend itself to the diagnosis and treatment of a variety of painful conditions subserved by the maxillary and mandibular divisions of the trigeminal nerve (Table 7.1). This technique is useful in the setting of acute pain secondary to trauma, pain of malignant origin, postsurgical pain, dental pain, breakthrough pain of trigeminal neuralgia, atypical facial pain, trismus, and the pain of acute herpes zoster. It can be used in the setting of chronic pain to help manage atypical facial pain including temporomandibular joint dysfunction and postherpetic neuralgia.

## CLINICALLY RELEVANT ANATOMY

The trigeminal nerve is the fifth cranial nerve, and it derives its name from its three branches, the ophthalmic (V1), the maxillary (V2), and the mandibular (V3) (Fig. 7.1). The ophthalmic and maxillary nerves are comprised solely of sensory fibers, while the mandibular nerve has both sensory and motor fibers. The trigeminal nerve exits the pons as a single nerve root on each side of the pons. These bilateral nerve roots travel forward and laterally from the pons to form the gasserian ganglion (also known as the trigeminal ganglion), which is located in Meckel cave in the middle cranial fossa (Fig. 7.2). The canoe-shaped gasserian ganglion is bathed in cerebrospinal fluid and is surrounded by dura mater.

Three sensory divisions exit the anterior convex portion of the gasserian ganglion, the ophthalmic (V1), the maxillary (V2), and the mandibular (V3) divisions, with a small motor root coalescing with the V3 division sensory fibers as the mandibular nerve leaves the middle cranial fossa via the foramen ovale (see Fig. 7.2). The sensory fibers of the trigeminal nerve provide afferent light touch and proprioceptive and nociceptive functions, while the motor fibers of the mandibular nerve provide efferent innervation of the muscles of mastication, the mylohyoid muscle, the anterior belly of the digastric muscle, and the tensor tympani and tensor veli palatini muscles. While the mandibular nerve is responsible for the light touch, proprioception, and pain and temperature sensation within its area of innervation, it does not transmit taste sensation, which is transmitted by the chorda tympani.

The ophthalmic division (V1) of the trigeminal nerve exits the cranial fossa via the superior orbital fissure and transmits sensory information from the scalp, forehead, upper eyelid, the conjunctiva and cornea of the eye, most of the nose except the nasal ala, the nasal mucosa, the frontal sinuses, and the dura and some intracranial vessels. The maxillary division of the trigeminal nerve (V2) exits the cranial fossa via the foramen rotundum and transmits afferent sensory information from the lower eyelid and cheek; the nasal ala; the upper lip, upper dentition, and gingiva; the nasal mucosa; the palate and roof of the pharynx; the maxillary, ethmoid, and sphenoid sinuses; and portions of the meninges. The mandibular division of the trigeminal nerve (V3) exits the cranial fossa via the foramen ovale and transmits sensory information from the lower lip, the lower dentition and gingiva, the chin and jaw (except the angle of the jaw, which is supplied by C2–C3), parts of the external ear, and parts of the meninges. The nerve also transmits sensory information from the dorsal aspect of the anterior two-thirds of the tongue and associated mucosa of the oral cavity.

**TABLE 7.1  Indication for Trigeminal Nerve Block via the Coronoid Approach**

**Acute Pain**
- Trauma
- Pain of malignant origin
- Postsurgical pain
- Dental pain
- Trigeminal neuralgia
- Atypical facial pain
- Trismus
- Acute herpes zoster

**Chronic Pain**
- Atypical facial pain
- Temporomandibular joint dysfunction
- Postherpetic neuralgia

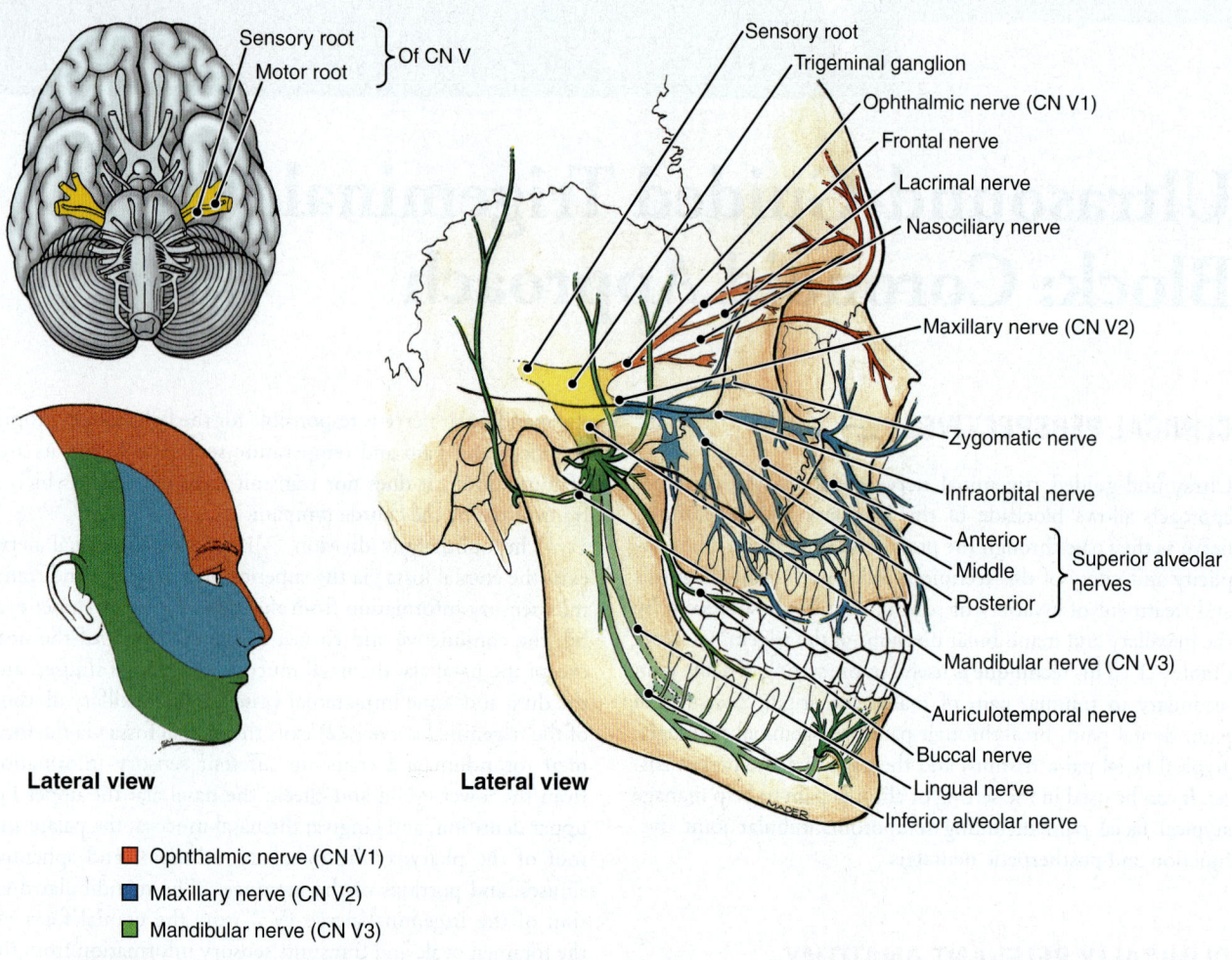

**FIGURE 7.1.** The anatomy of the trigeminal nerve. (Reused from Moore KL, Dalley AF. *Clinically Oriented Anatomy*. 5th ed. Baltimore, MD: Lippincott Williams & Wilkins; 2006:1140, with permission.)

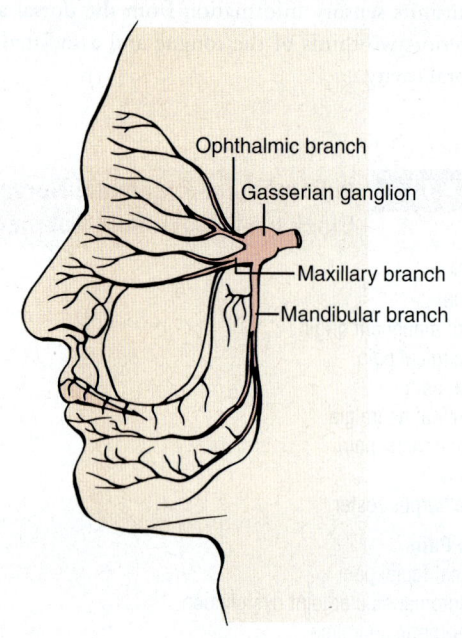

**FIGURE 7.2.** The gasserian ganglion. (Reused from Nettina SM. *The Lippincott Manual of Nursing Practice*. 7th ed. Philadelphia, PA: Lippincott Williams & Wilkins; 2001, with permission.)

## ULTRASOUND-GUIDED TECHNIQUE

Ultrasound-guided trigeminal nerve block via the coronoid approach is a straightforward technique if attention is paid to the clinical relevant anatomy. To perform ultrasound-guided trigeminal nerve block via the coronoid approach, the patient is placed in supine position with the cervical spine in the neutral position. The coronoid (mandibular) notch provides easy access to the pterygopalatine fossa and the maxillary and mandibular nerves (Fig. 7.3). The coronoid notch of the mandible is identified by asking the patient to open and close his or her mouth several times while palpating the area just anterior and slightly inferior to the acoustic auditory meatus (Fig. 7.4). Once the coronoid notch is identified, the patient is asked to hold his or her mouth open in a relaxed, neutral position.

The skin overlying the mandibular notch is prepped with antiseptic solution, and a linear transducer is placed directly in the transverse position over the coronoid notch (Fig. 7.5). The temporomandibular joint should be readily apparent in the posterior portion of the image with the acoustic shadow of the curved bony mandibular condyle and mandibular neck just below it (Fig. 7.6).

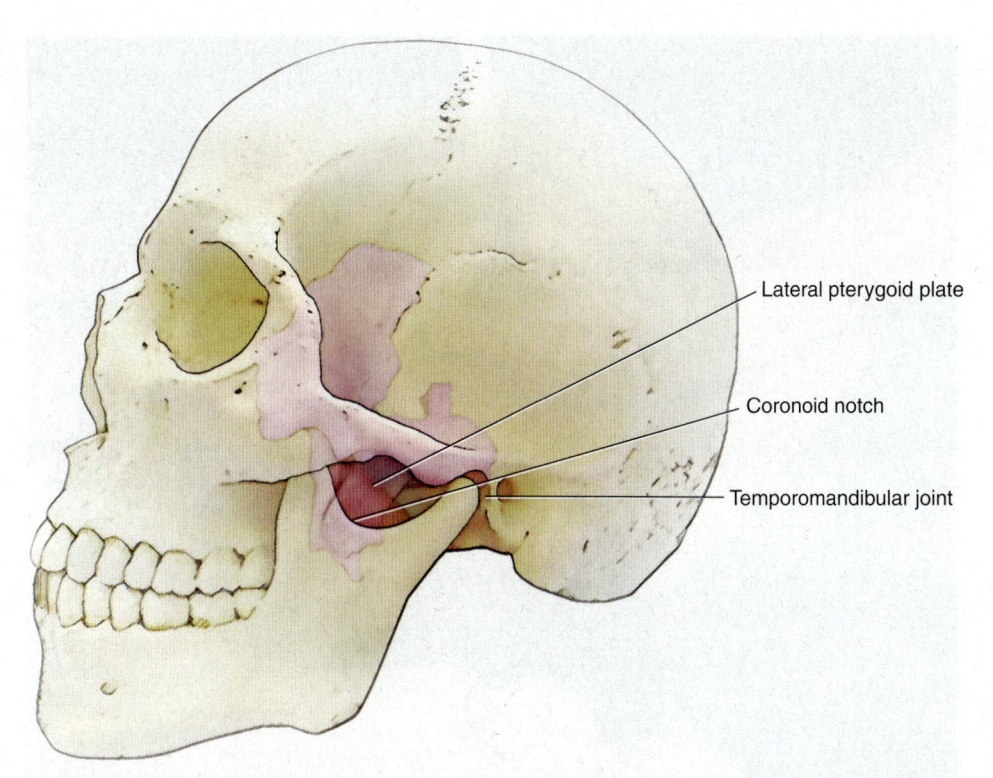

**FIGURE 7.3.** The relationship of the coronoid notch and the lateral pterygoid plate. (Adapted from LifeART image. Philadelphia, PA: Lippincott Williams & Wilkins.)

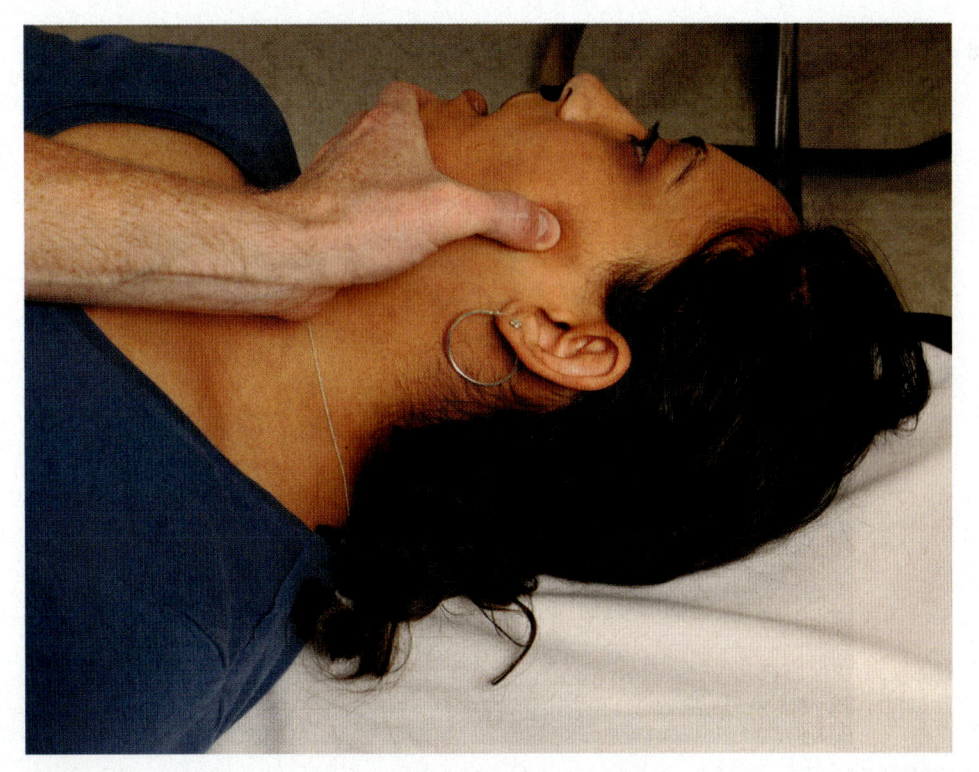

**FIGURE 7.4.** Palpation of the coronoid notch.

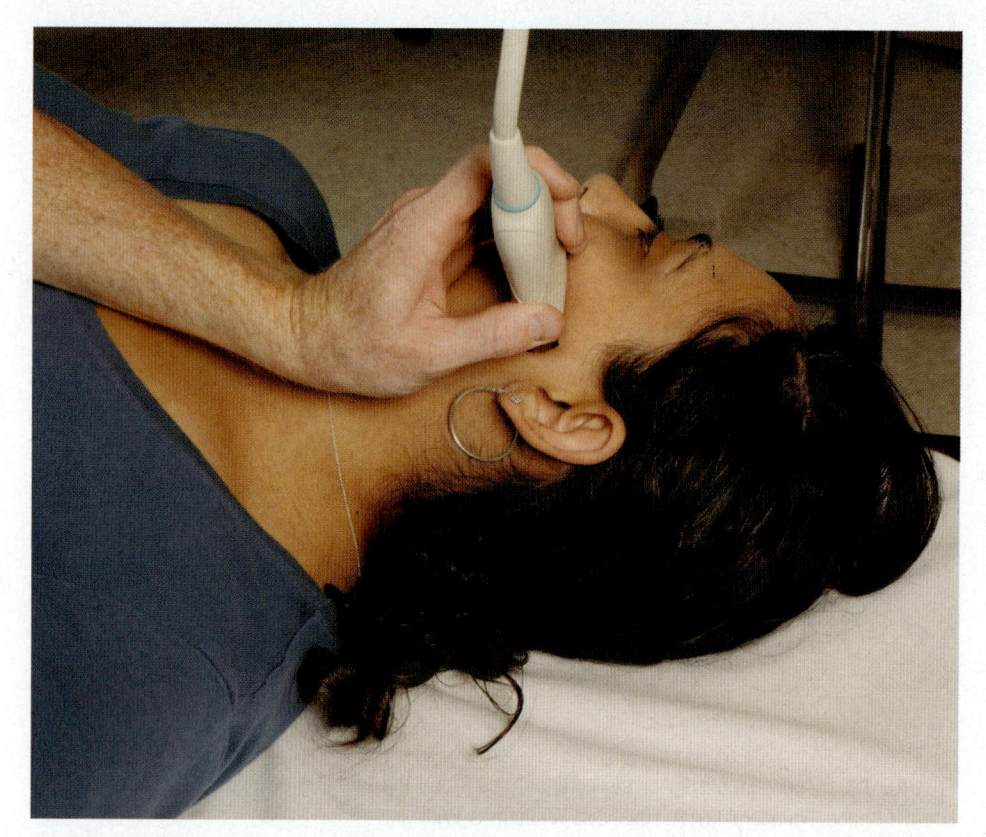

**FIGURE 7.5.** Proper transverse position of the linear transducer for trigeminal nerve block via the coronoid approach.

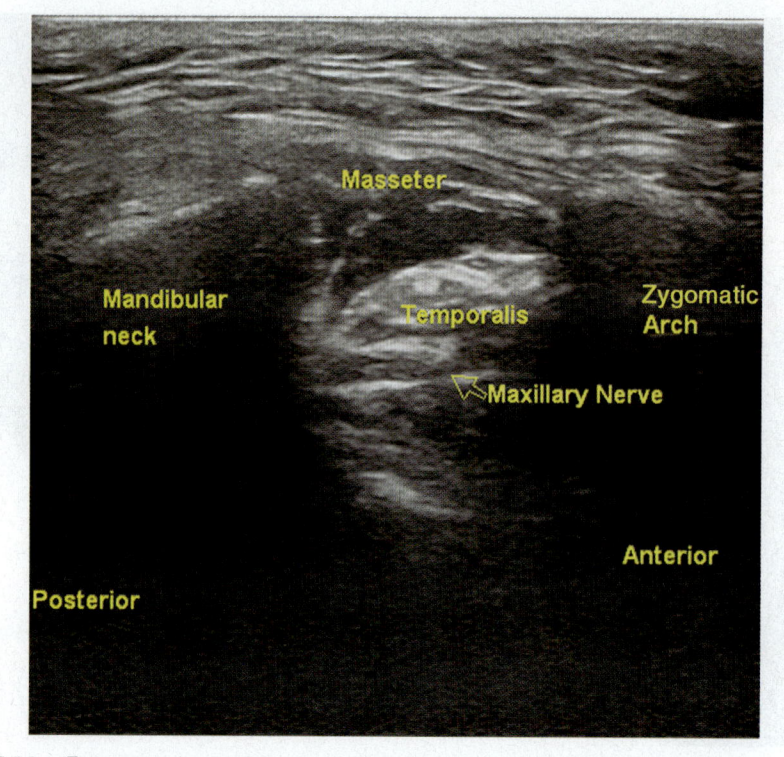

**FIGURE 7.6.** Transverse ultrasound image of the pterygopalatine fossa via the coronoid notch.

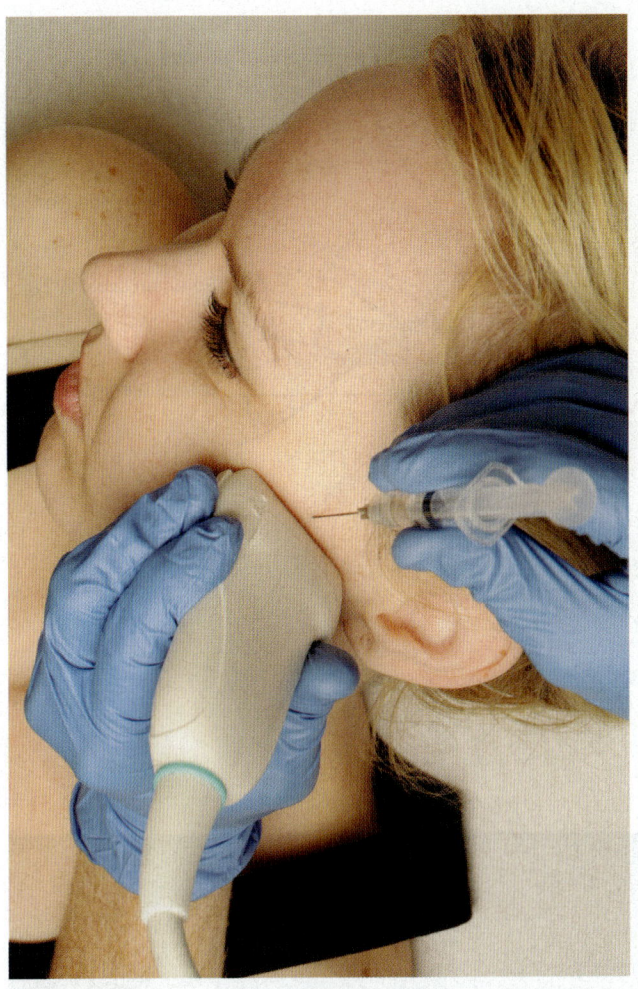

**FIGURE 7.7.** Out-of-plane approach for ultrasound-guided trigeminal nerve block via the coronoid notch.

Seven milliliters of local anesthetic is drawn up in a 10-mL sterile syringe. Forty to eighty milligrams of depot steroid preparation may be added to the local anesthetic if it is thought that there is an inflammatory component to the patient's pain symptomatology. Under real-time ultrasound guidance, a 22-gauge, 1½-inch needle is inserted just below the zygomatic arch directly in the middle of the coronoid notch using an out-of-plane approach (Fig. 7.7). The needle is advanced until it impinges on the lateral pterygoid plate. When the lateral pterygoid plate is encountered, the needle is withdrawn slightly out of the periosteum (Figs. 7.8 and 7.9).

After careful aspiration is carried out, 7 mL of solution is slowly injected in incremental doses. During the injection procedure, the patient must be observed carefully for signs of local anesthetic toxicity.

## COMPLICATIONS

The pterygopalatine fossa is highly vascular, and the potential for trauma to the vasculature, especially the maxillary artery, remains an ever-present possibility. Needle damage to the artery may result in significant facial hematoma formation, which can be very distressing to the patient and clinician alike. The vascularity of the region means that the pain specialist should carefully aspirate the needle prior to injecting any medications and should then inject small, incremental doses of local anesthetic to avoid local anesthetic toxicity.

## CLINICAL PEARLS

Trigeminal nerve block via the coronoid approach with local anesthetic and steroid represents an excellent option for those patients suffering from the uncontrolled pain or breakthrough pain of trigeminal neuralgia and cancer pain while waiting for pharmacotherapy to take effect. The vascular nature of this anatomic region mandates care when injecting local anesthetics into the area. Careful gentle aspiration and attention to the total milligram dose of local anesthetic is crucial to avoid complications.

Small punctate facial scars secondary to needle trauma to the skin overlying the coronoid notch may occur, and the patient should be warned of this possibility. Infection, although rare, remains an ever-present possibility, especially in the immunocompromised patient. Early detection of infection is crucial to avoid potential life-threatening sequelae including spread of the infection to the central nervous system. Unexplained pain in areas subserved by the trigeminal nerve and its branches requires careful evaluation as tumors anywhere along the path of the nerve may cause pain (Fig. 7.10).

**FIGURE 7.8.** The proper needle placement for trigeminal nerve block via the coronoid approach.

Foramen rotundum (V3)

Gasserian ganglion

Foramen ovale (V2)

Lateral pterygoid plate

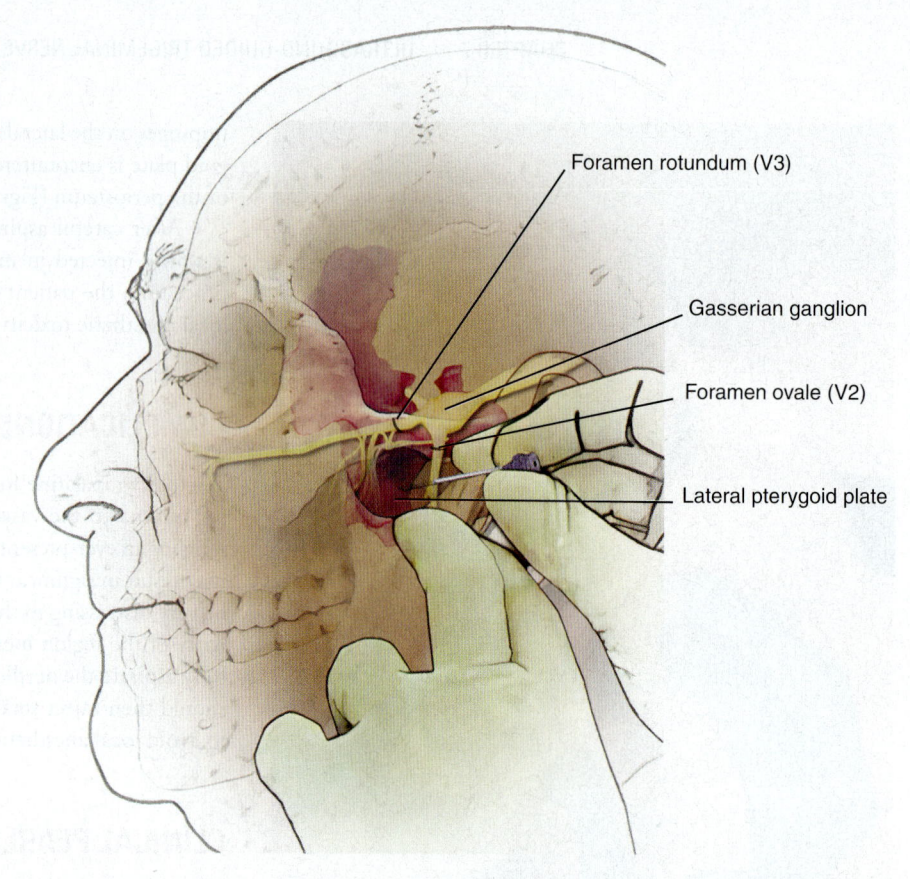

**FIGURE 7.9.** Fluoroscopic image of needle traversing the mandibular notch and resting against the lateral pterygoid plate.

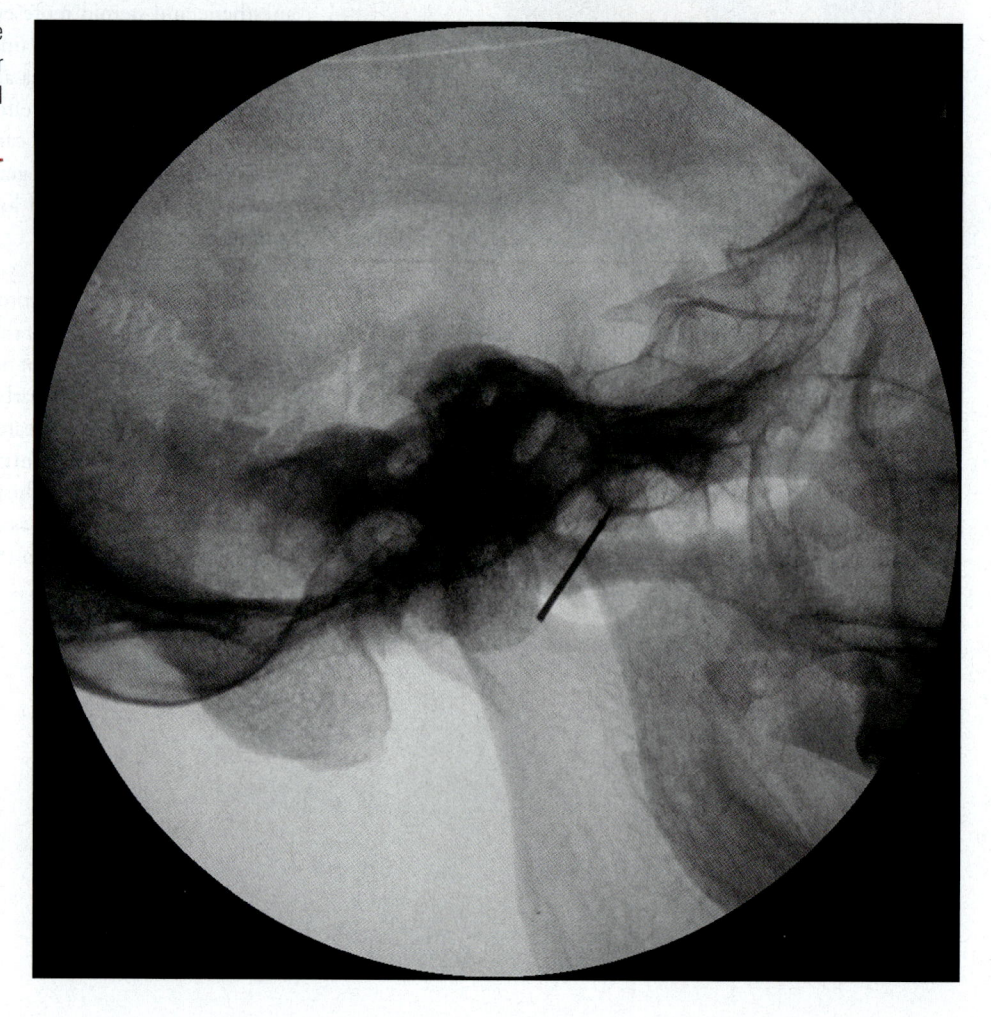

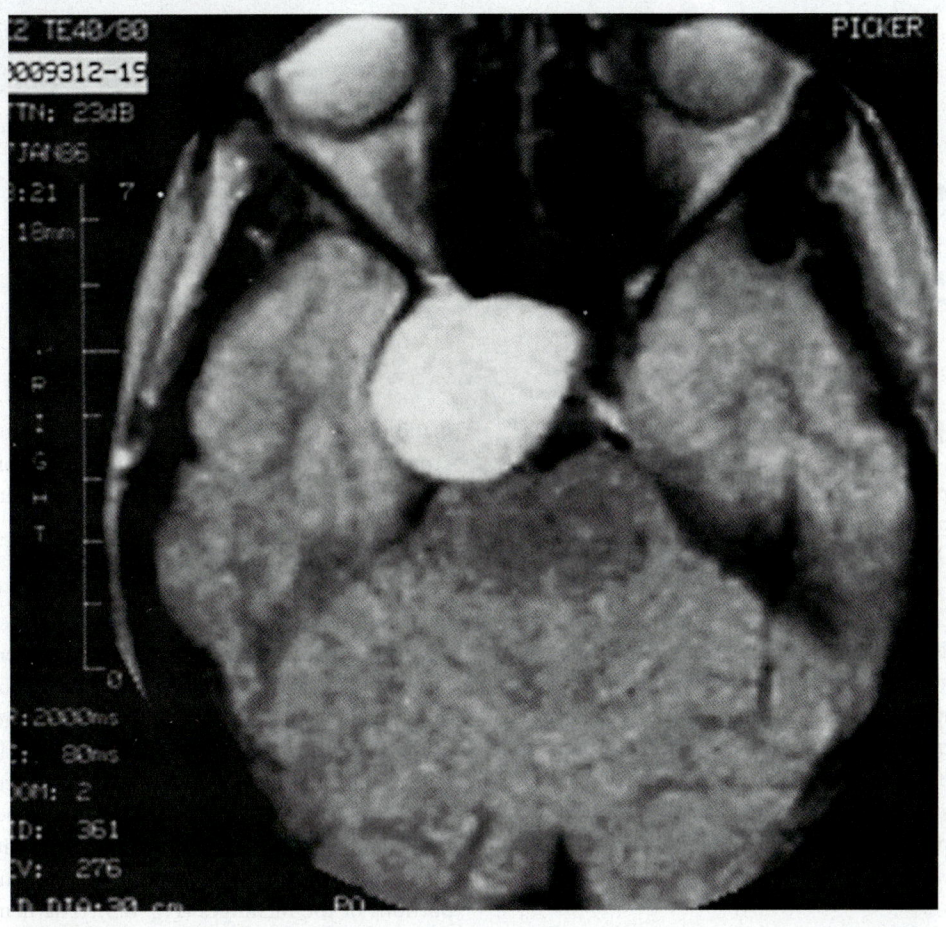

**FIGURE 7.10.** Trigeminal schwannoma of the right gasserian ganglion. T1-weighted coronal image shows the mass to be of relatively low signal intensity and to involve the mandibular division (*arrow*). (Reused from Eisenberg RL. *An Atlas of Differential Diagnosis*. 4th ed. Philadelphia, PA: Lippincott Williams & Wilkins; 2003, with permission.)

## SUGGESTED READINGS

Waldman SD. Selective maxillary nerve block: coronoid approach. In: *Atlas of Interventional Pain Management*. 3rd ed. Philadelphia, PA: Saunders Elsevier; 2009:51–58.

Waldman SD. The trigeminal nerve. In: *Pain Review*. Philadelphia, PA: Saunders Elsevier; 2009:15–17.

Waldman SD. Atypical facial pain. In: *Atlas of Common Pain Syndromes*. 3rd ed. Philadelphia, PA: Saunders Elsevier; 2011:36–38.

Waldman SD. Trigeminal neuralgia. In: *Atlas of Common Pain Syndromes*. 3rd ed. Philadelphia, PA: Saunders Elsevier; 2011:29–32.

# CHAPTER 8

# Ultrasound-Guided Maxillary Nerve Block

## CLINICAL PERSPECTIVES

Ultrasound-guided selective maxillary nerve block via the coronoid approach allows selective blockade of the maxillary nerve as it passes through the pterygopalatine space. The simplicity and safety of this technique lend itself to the diagnosis and treatment of a variety of painful conditions subserved by the maxillary division of the trigeminal nerve. This technique is useful in the setting of acute pain secondary to trauma, pain of malignant origin, postsurgical pain, dental pain, breakthrough pain of trigeminal neuralgia, atypical facial pain, and the pain of acute herpes zoster (Fig. 8.1). It can be used in the setting of chronic pain to help manage atypical facial pain including temporomandibular joint dysfunction and postherpetic neuralgia.

## CLINICALLY RELEVANT ANATOMY

The trigeminal nerve is the fifth cranial nerve, and it derives its name from its three branches, the ophthalmic (V1), the maxillary (V2), and the mandibular (V3). The ophthalmic and maxillary nerves are comprised solely of sensory fibers, while the mandibular nerve has both sensory and motor fibers. The trigeminal nerve exits the pons as a single nerve root on each side of the pons. These bilateral nerve roots travel forward and laterally from the pons to form the gasserian ganglion (also known as the trigeminal ganglion), which is located in Meckel cave in the middle cranial fossa. The canoe-shaped gasserian ganglion is bathed in cerebrospinal fluid and is surrounded by dura mater.

Three sensory divisions exit the anterior convex portion of the gasserian ganglion, the ophthalmic (V1), the maxillary (V2), and the mandibular divisions, with as small motor root coalescing with the V3 division sensory fibers as the mandibular nerve leaves the middle cranial fossa via the foramen ovale (Fig. 8.2). The sensory fibers of the trigeminal nerve provide afferent light touch and proprioceptive and nociceptive functions, while the motor fibers of the mandibular nerve provide efferent innervation of the muscles of mastication, the mylohyoid muscle, the anterior belly of the digastric muscle, and the tensor tympani and tensor veli palatini muscles. While the mandibular nerve is responsible for the light touch, proprioception, and pain and temperature sensation within its area of innervation, it does not transmit taste sensation, which is transmitted by the chorda tympani.

The ophthalmic division (V1) of the trigeminal nerve exits the cranial fossa via the superior orbital fissure and transmits sensory information from the scalp, forehead, upper eyelid, the conjunctiva and cornea of the eye, most of the nose except the nasal ala, the nasal mucosa, the frontal sinuses, and the dura and some intracranial vessels. The maxillary division of the trigeminal nerve (V2) exits the cranial fossa via the foramen rotundum and transmits sensory information from the lower eyelid and cheek; the nasal ala; the upper lip, upper dentition, and gingiva; the nasal mucosa; the palate and roof of the pharynx; the maxillary, ethmoid, and sphenoid sinuses; and portions of the meninges (Fig. 8.3). The mandibular division of the trigeminal nerve (V3) exits the cranial fossa via the foramen ovale and transmits sensory information from the lower lip, the lower dentition and gingiva, the chin and jaw (except the angle of the jaw, which is supplied by C2–C3), parts of the external ear, and parts of the meninges. The nerve also transmits sensory information from the dorsal aspect of the anterior two-thirds of the tongue and associated mucosa of the oral cavity.

## ULTRASOUND-GUIDED TECHNIQUE

Ultrasound-guided selective maxillary nerve block via the coronoid approach is a straightforward technique if attention is paid to the clinical relevant anatomy. To perform ultrasound-guided selective maxillary nerve block via the coronoid approach, the patient is placed in supine position with the cervical spine in the neutral position. The coronoid (mandibular) notch provides easy access to the pterygopalatine fossa and the maxillary and mandibular nerves (Fig. 8.4). The coronoid notch of the mandible is identified by asking the patient to open and close his or her mouth several times while palpating the area just anterior and slightly inferior to the acoustic auditory meatus (Fig. 8.5). Once the coronoid notch is identified, the patient is asked to hold his or her mouth open in a relaxed, neutral position.

CHAPTER 8 ULTRASOUND-GUIDED MAXILLARY NERVE BLOCK 47

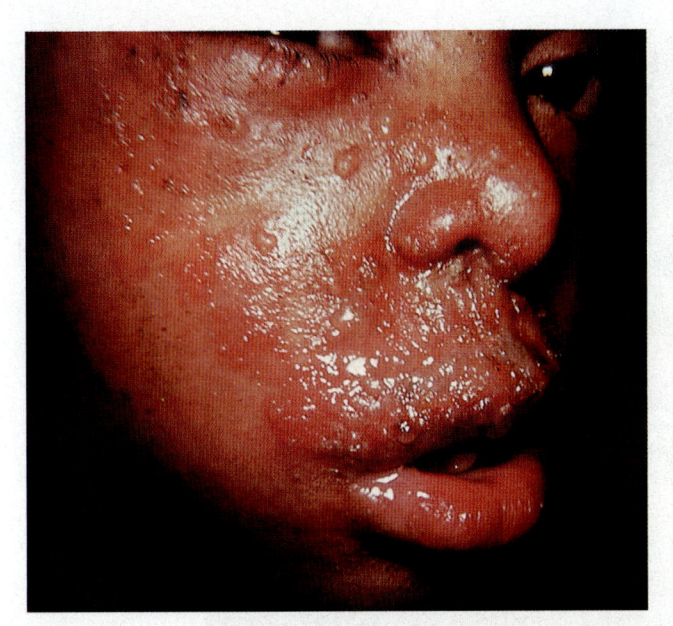

**FIGURE 8.1.** Acute herpes zoster involving the maxillary nerve. (Reused from Fleisher GR, Ludwig W, Baskin MN. *Atlas of Emergency Medicine*. Philadelphia, PA: Lippincott Williams & Wilkins; 2004, with permission.)

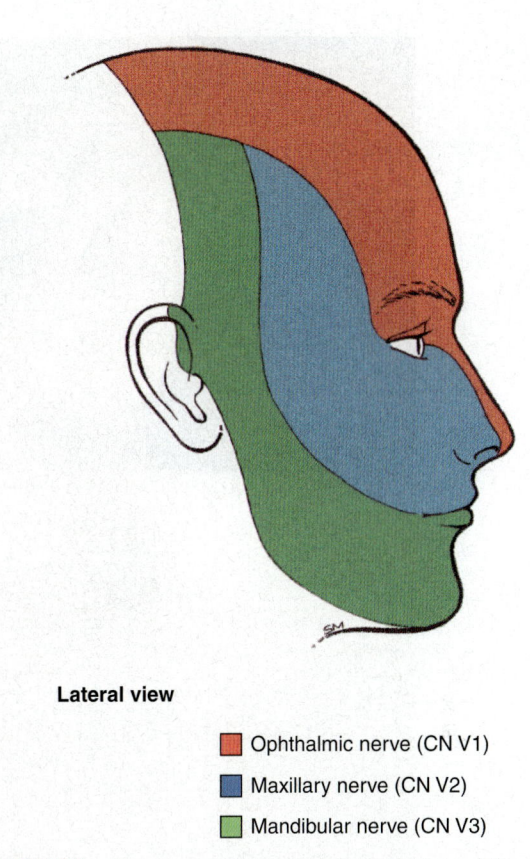

Lateral view

- Ophthalmic nerve (CN V1)
- Maxillary nerve (CN V2)
- Mandibular nerve (CN V3)

**FIGURE 8.3.** The sensory distribution of the divisions of the trigeminal nerve. (Reused from Moore KL, Dalley AF. *Clinically Oriented Anatomy*. 5th ed. Baltimore, MD: Lippincott Williams & Wilkins; 2006:1140, with permission.)

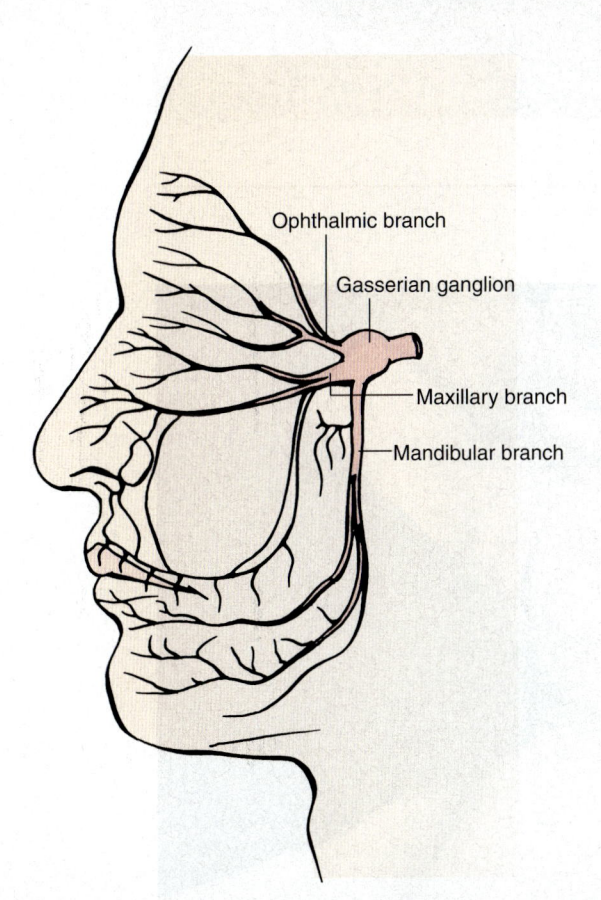

**FIGURE 8.2.** The gasserian ganglion and divisions of the trigeminal nerve. (Reused from Nettina SM. *The Lippincott Manual of Nursing Practice*. 7th ed. Philadelphia, PA: Lippincott Williams & Wilkins; 2001, with permission.)

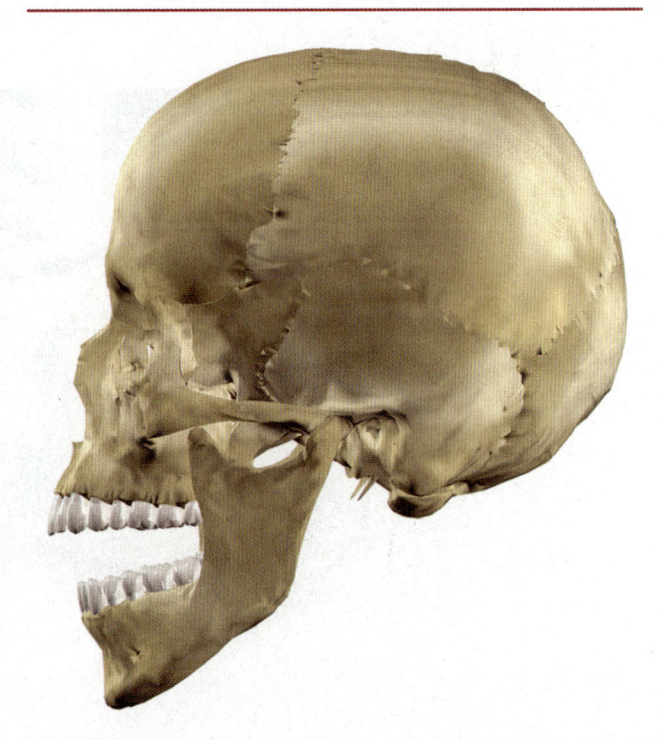

**FIGURE 8.4.** The relationship of the coronoid notch and the lateral pterygoid plate. (Adapted from LifeART image. Philadelphia: Lippincott Williams & Wilkins.)

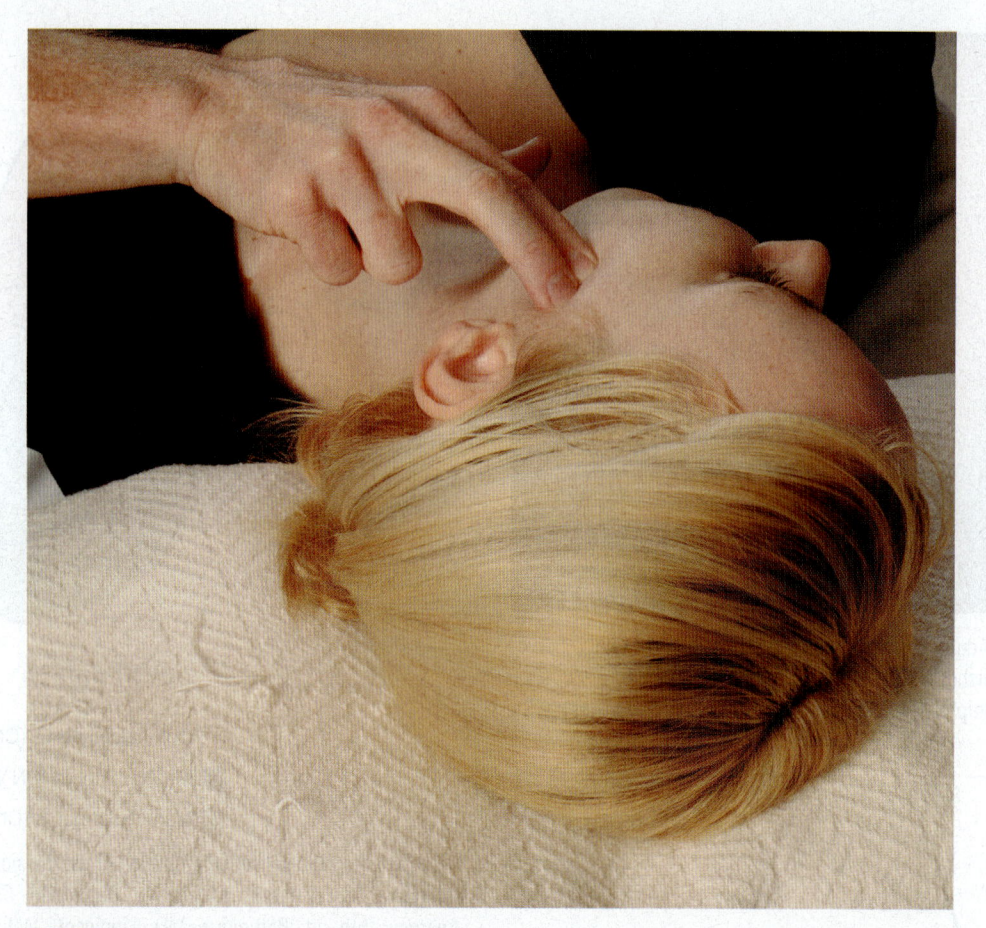

**FIGURE 8.5.** Palpation of the coronoid notch.

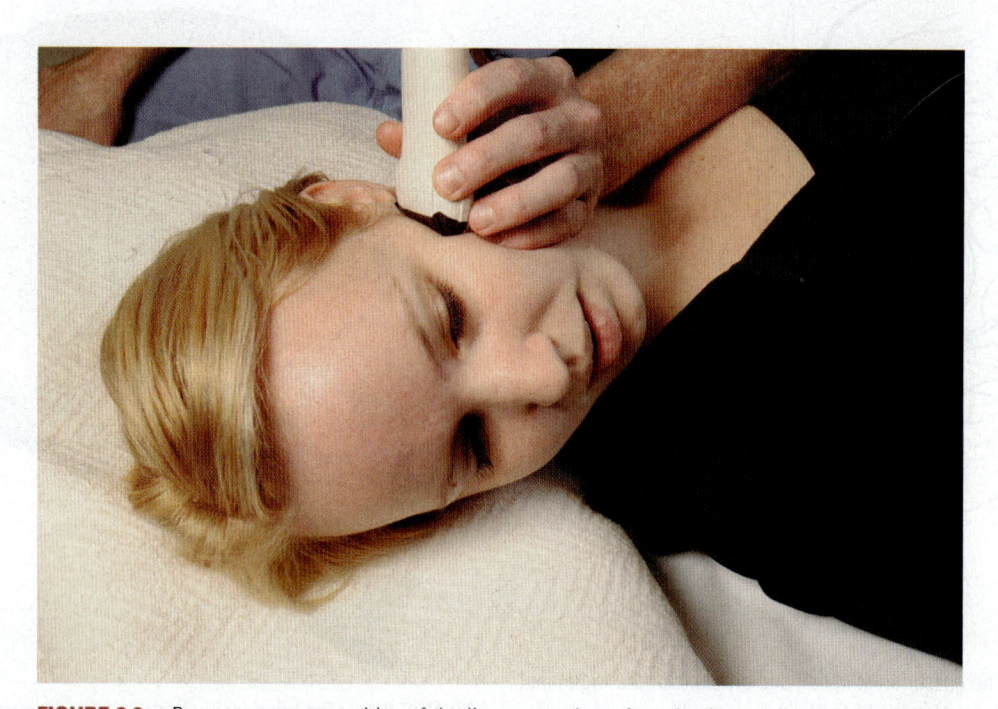

**FIGURE 8.6.** Proper transverse position of the linear transducer for selective maxillary nerve block via the coronoid approach.

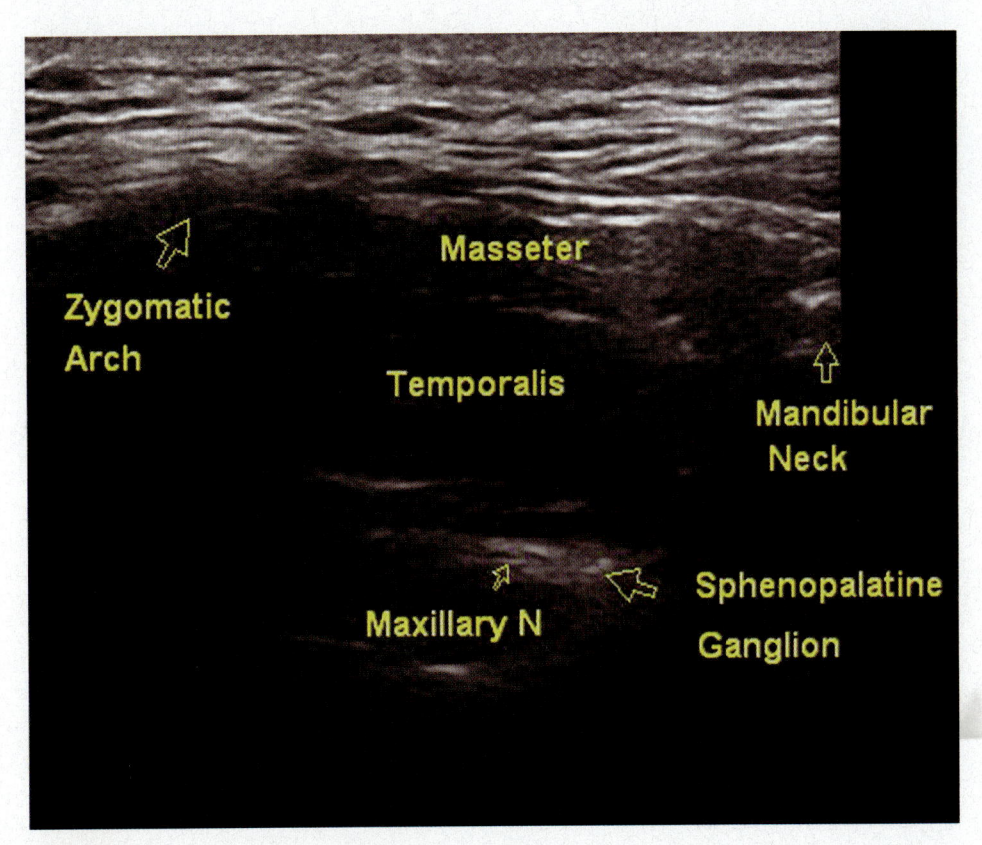

**FIGURE 8.7.** Ultrasound image of the pterygopalatine fossa via the coronoid notch.

The skin overlying the mandibular notch is prepped with antiseptic solution, and a linear transducer is placed in the transverse position directly over the coronoid notch (Fig. 8.6). The temporomandibular joint should be readily apparent in the posterior portion of the image with the acoustic shadow of the curved bony mandibular condyle and mandibular neck just below it (Fig. 8.7).

Seven milliliters of local anesthetic is drawn up in a 10-mL sterile syringe. Forty to eighty milligrams of depot-steroid preparation may be added to the local anesthetic if it is thought that there is an inflammatory component to the patient's pain symptomatology. Under real-time ultrasound guidance, a 22-gauge, 3½-inch styletted spinal needle is inserted just below the zygomatic arch directly in the middle of the coronoid notch using an out-of-plane approach. The needle is advanced until it impinges on the lateral pterygoid plate (Fig. 8.8). When the lateral pterygoid plate is encountered, the needle is withdrawn slightly and redirected toward the pupil of the eye until it slips past the anterosuperior margin of the lateral pterygoid plate into the pterygopalatine fissure and into proximity of the maxillary nerve (Fig. 8.9). A paresthesia may be elicited and the patient should be warned of such.

After careful aspiration is carried out, 4 to 5 mL of solution is injected in incremental doses. During the injection procedure, the patient must be observed carefully for signs of local anesthetic toxicity. Because of the proximity of the sphenopalatine ganglion, the patient may also experience partial blockade of this structure.

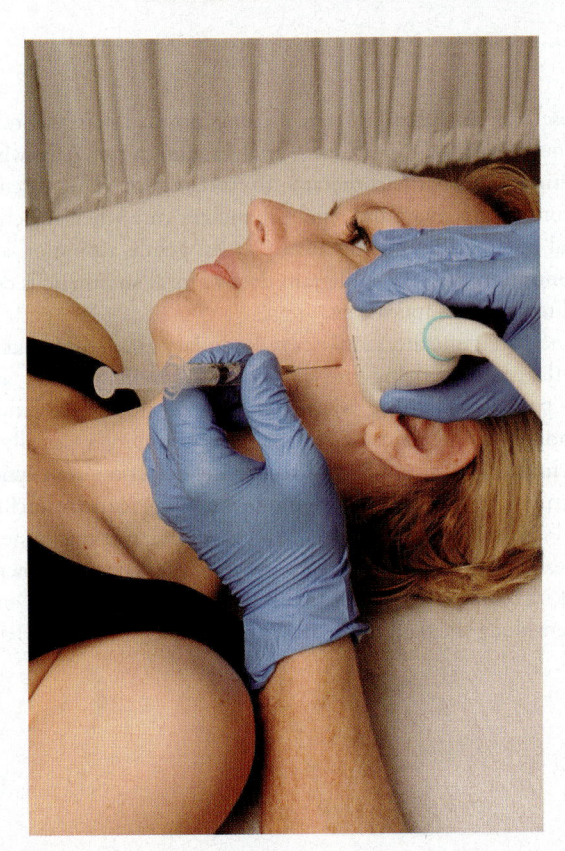

**FIGURE 8.8.** Out-of-plane approach for ultrasound-guided selective maxillary nerve block via the coronoid notch.

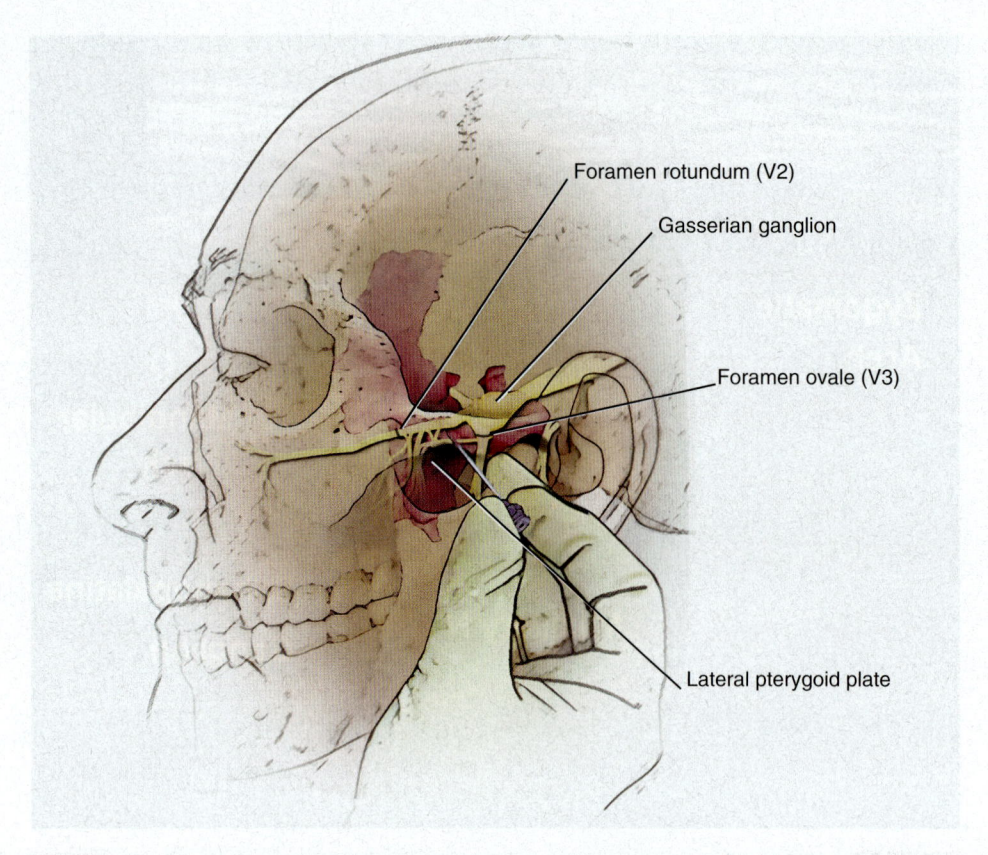

**FIGURE 8.9.** The proper needle placement for selective maxillary nerve block via the coronoid approach.

## COMPLICATIONS

The pterygopalatine fossa is highly vascular, and the potential for trauma to the vasculature, especially the maxillary artery, remains an ever-present possibility. Needle damage to the artery may result in significant facial hematoma formation, which can be very distressing to the patient and clinician alike. The vascularity of the region means that the pain specialist should carefully aspirate the needle prior to injecting any medications and should then inject small, incremental doses of local anesthetic to avoid local anesthetic toxicity.

## CLINICAL PEARLS

Selective maxillary nerve block via the coronoid approach with local anesthetic and steroid represents an excellent option for those patients suffering from the uncontrolled pain or breakthrough pain of trigeminal neuralgia and cancer pain while waiting for pharmacotherapy to take effect. The vascular nature of this anatomic region mandates care when injecting local anesthetics into the area. Careful gentle aspiration and attention to the total milligram dose of local anesthetic is crucial to avoid complications.

Small punctate facial scars secondary to needle trauma to the skin overlying the coronoid notch may occur, and the patient should be warned of this possibility. Infection, although rare, remains an ever-present possibility, especially in the immunocompromised patient. Early detection of infection is crucial to avoid potential life-threatening sequelae including spread of the infection to the central nervous system. Unexplained pain in areas subserved by the trigeminal nerve and its branches requires careful evaluation as pathology anywhere along the path of the nerve may cause pain (Fig. 8.10).

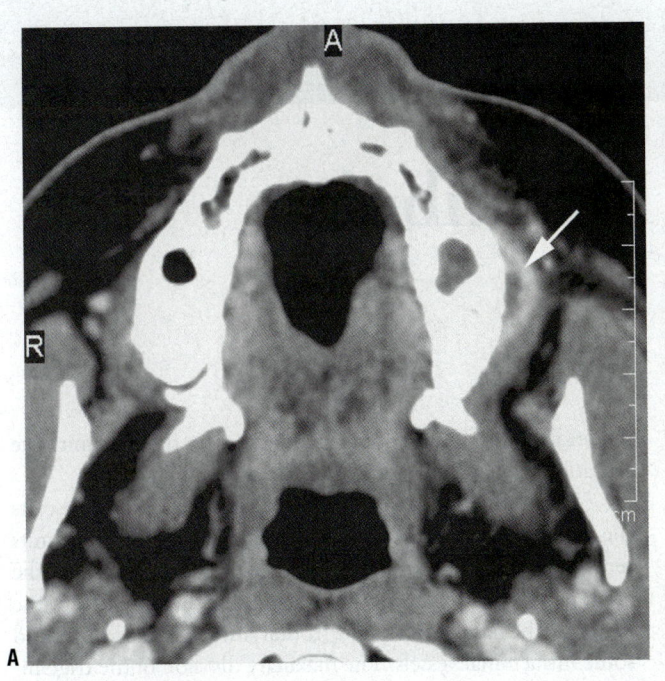

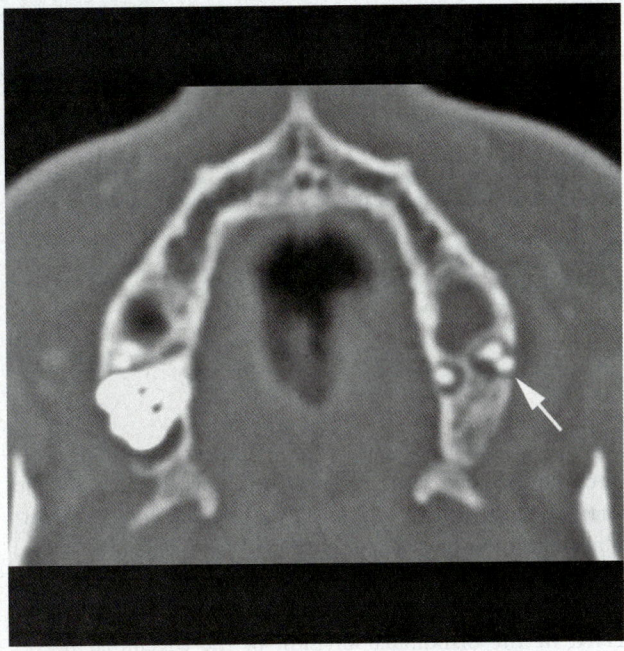

**FIGURE 8.10.** A patient presenting with atypical facial pain limited mainly to what was believed to be a V2 distribution. The findings were slowly progressive over months. **A:** Contrast-enhanced computed tomography showing a subperiosteal abscess adjacent to the maxilla (*arrow*). **B:** Bone windows showing periodontal disease extending through the buccal cortex, explaining the pain as due to a periapical dental abscess with secondary subperiosteal spread. (Reused from Mancuso AA, Verbist BM. Trigeminal neuralgia and other trigeminal neuropathies. In: Mancuso AA, Hanafee WN, eds. *Head and Neck Radiology*. Philadelphia, PA: Lippincott Williams & Wilkins; 2010:505, with permission.)

## SUGGESTED READINGS

Waldman SD. Selective maxillary nerve block: coronoid approach. In: *Atlas of Interventional Pain Management*. 3rd ed. Philadelphia, PA: Saunders Elsevier; 2009:51–58.

Waldman SD. The Trigeminal nerve. In: *Pain Review*. Philadelphia, PA: Saunders Elsevier; 2009:15–17.

Waldman SD. Atypical facial pain. In: *Atlas of Common Pain Syndromes*. 3rd ed. Philadelphia, PA: Saunders Elsevier; 2011:36–38.

Waldman SD. Trigeminal neuralgia. In: *Atlas of Common Pain Syndromes*. 3rd ed. Philadelphia, PA: Saunders Elsevier; 2011:29–32.

# CHAPTER 9

# Ultrasound-Guided Mandibular Nerve Block

## CLINICAL PERSPECTIVES

Ultrasound-guided selective mandibular nerve block via the coronoid approach allows selective blockade of the mandibular nerve as it passes through the pterygopalatine space. The simplicity and safety of this technique lends itself to the diagnosis and treatment of a variety of painful conditions subserved by the mandibular division of the trigeminal nerve. This technique is useful in the setting of acute pain secondary to trauma, pain of malignant origin, postsurgical pain, dental pain, breakthrough pain of trigeminal neuralgia, atypical facial pain, trismus, and the pain of acute herpes zoster. It can be used in the setting of chronic pain to help manage atypical facial pain including chronic dental pain and postherpetic neuralgia (Fig. 9.1).

## CLINICALLY RELEVANT ANATOMY

The trigeminal nerve is the fifth cranial nerve, and it derives its name from its three branches, the ophthalmic (V1), the maxillary (V2), and the mandibular (V3). The ophthalmic and maxillary nerves are comprised solely of sensory fibers, while the mandibular nerve has both sensory and motor fibers. The trigeminal nerve exits the pons as a single nerve root on each side of the pons. These bilateral nerve roots travel forward and laterally from the pons to form the gasserian ganglion (also known as the trigeminal ganglion), which is located in Meckel cave in the middle cranial fossa. The canoe-shaped gasserian ganglion is bathed in cerebrospinal fluid and is surrounded by dura mater.

Three sensory divisions exit the anterior convex portion of the gasserian ganglion, the ophthalmic (V1), the maxillary (V2), and the mandibular divisions, with as small motor root coalescing with the V3 division sensory fibers as the mandibular nerve leaves the middle cranial fossa via the foramen ovale (Fig. 9.2). The sensory fibers of the trigeminal nerve provide afferent light touch and proprioceptive and nociceptive functions, while the motor fibers of the mandibular nerve provide efferent innervation of the muscles of mastication, the mylohyoid muscle, the anterior belly of the digastric muscle, and the tensor tympani and tensor veli palatini muscles. While the mandibular nerve is responsible for the light touch, proprioception, and pain and temperature sensation within its area of innervation, it does not transmit taste sensation, which is transmitted by the chorda tympani.

The ophthalmic division (V1) of the trigeminal nerve exits the cranial fossa via the superior orbital fissure and transmits sensory information from the scalp, forehead, upper eyelid, the conjunctiva and cornea of the eye, most of the nose except the nasal ala, the nasal mucosa, the frontal sinuses, and the dura and some intracranial vessels. The maxillary division of the trigeminal nerve (V2) exits the cranial fossa via the foramen rotundum and transmits sensory information from the lower eyelid and cheek; the nasal ala; the upper lip, upper dentition, and gingiva; the nasal mucosa; the palate and roof of the pharynx; the maxillary, ethmoid, and sphenoid sinuses; and portions of the meninges. The mandibular division of the trigeminal nerve (V3) exits the cranial fossa via the foramen ovale and transmits sensory information from the lower lip, the lower dentition and gingiva, the chin and jaw (except the angle of the jaw, which is supplied by C2–C3), parts of the external ear, and parts of the meninges (Fig. 9.3). The nerve also transmits sensory information from the dorsal aspect of the anterior two-thirds of the tongue and associated mucosa of the oral cavity.

## ULTRASOUND-GUIDED TECHNIQUE

Ultrasound-guided selective mandibular nerve block via the coronoid approach is a straightforward technique if attention is paid to the clinical relevant anatomy. To perform ultrasound-guided selective mandibular nerve block via the coronoid approach, the patient is placed in the supine position with the cervical spine in the neutral position. The coronoid (mandibular) notch provides easy access to the pterygopalatine fossa and the maxillary and mandibular nerves (Fig. 9.4). The coronoid notch of the mandible is identified by asking the patient to open and close his or her mouth several times while palpating the area just anterior and slightly inferior to the acoustic auditory meatus (Fig. 9.5). Once the coronoid notch is identified, the patient is asked to hold his or her mouth open in a relaxed, neutral position.

The skin overlying the mandibular notch is prepped with antiseptic solution, and a linear transducer is placed in a transverse position directly over the coronoid notch (Fig. 9.6). The temporomandibular joint should be readily apparent in the posterior portion of the image with the acoustic shadow of the

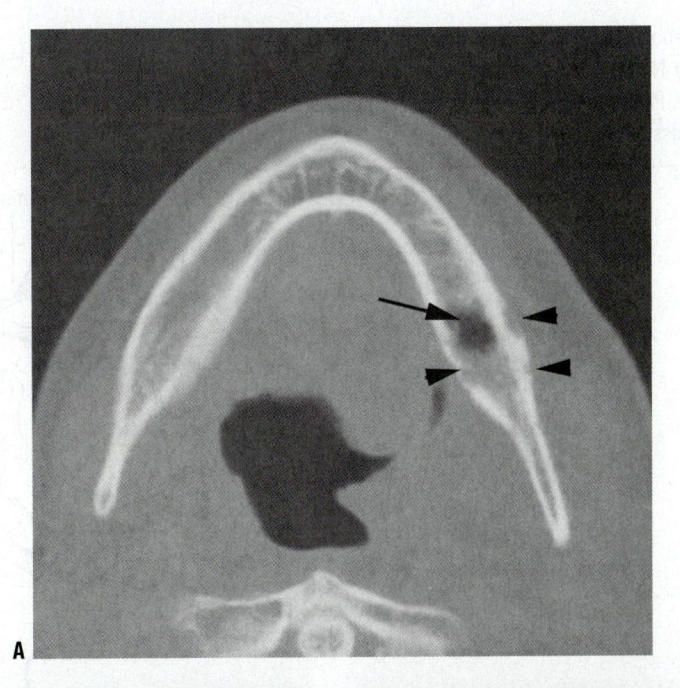

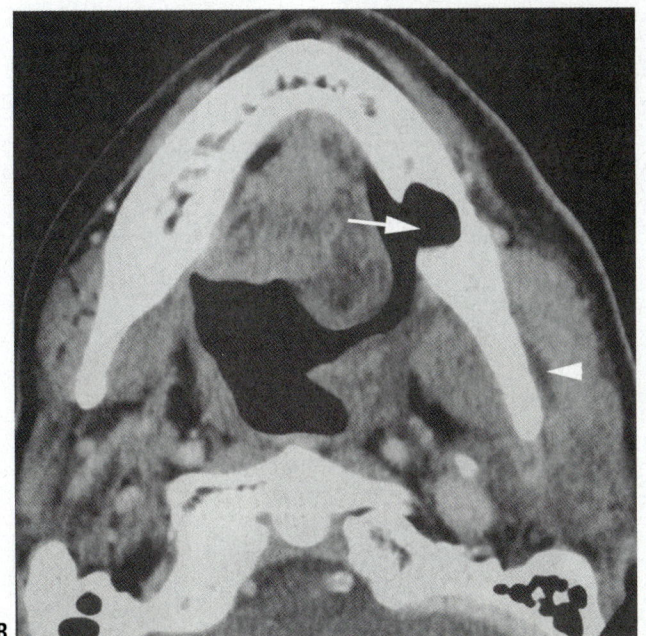

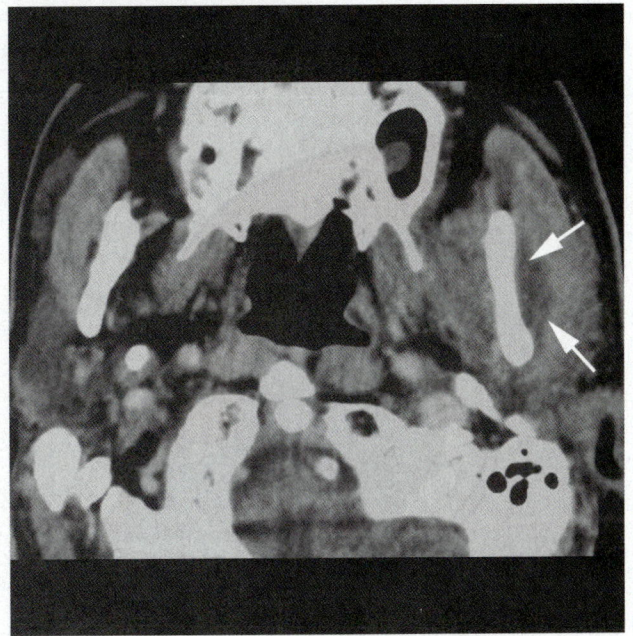

**FIGURE 9.1.** Sometimes, a dental-related abscess may not be immediately contiguous with the causative tooth. This computed tomography study was done in a patient with chronic left jaw pain. **A:** The prior extraction site (*arrow*) is irregular, and there is chronic erosion and periosteal thickening on its buccal surface and loss of endosteal bone on the buccal surface (*arrowheads*). **B:** There is no evidence of significant soft tissue swelling within what appears to almost be a dry socket (*arrow*). A subperiosteal abscess has actually manifested more near the angle to the mandible (*arrowhead*). **C:** That subperiosteal abscess continues to spread between the masseter and ascending ramus of the mandible (*arrows*). (Reused from Mancuso AA, Pettigrew JC, Nair MK. Acute and subacute mandibular and dental infections and noninfectious inflammatory conditions. In: Mancuso AA, Hanafee WN, eds. *Head and Neck Radiology*. Philadelphia, PA: Lippincott Williams & Wilkins; 2010:525, with permission.)

curved bony mandibular condyle and mandibular neck just below it (Fig. 9.7).

Five milliliters of local anesthetic is drawn up in a 10-mL sterile syringe. Forty to eighty milligrams of depot steroid preparation may be added to the local anesthetic if it is thought that there is an inflammatory component to the patient's pain symptomatology. Under real-time ultrasound guidance, a 22-gauge, 3½-inch stylletted spinal needle is inserted

**FIGURE 9.2.** The gasserian ganglion and divisions of the trigeminal nerve. (Reused from Nettina SM. *The Lippincott Manual of Nursing Practice*. 7th ed. Philadelphia, PA: Lippincott Williams & Wilkins; 2001, with permission.)

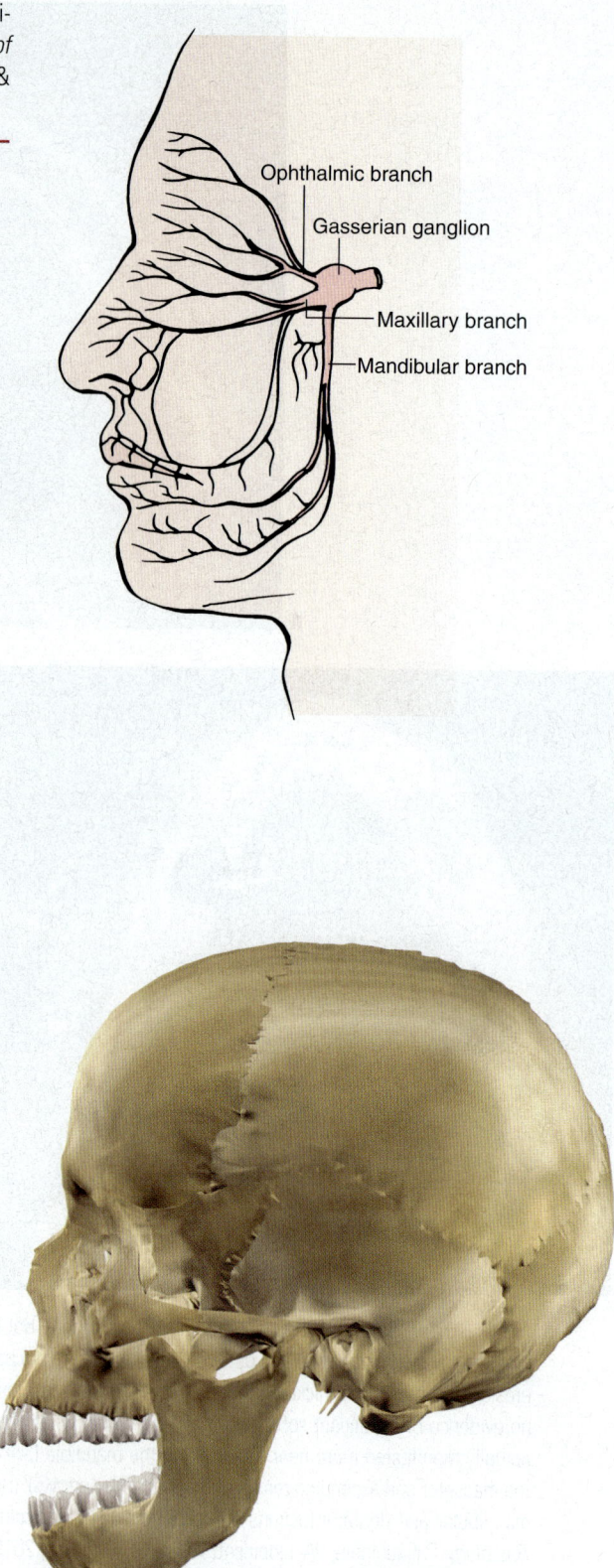

**Lateral view**

- Ophthalmic nerve (CN V1)
- Maxillary nerve (CN V2)
- Mandibular nerve (CN V3)

**FIGURE 9.3.** The sensory distribution of the divisions of the trigeminal nerve. (Reused from Moore KL, Dalley AF. *Clinically Oriented Anatomy*. 5th ed. Baltimore, MD: Lippincott Williams & Wilkins; 2006:1140, with permission.)

**FIGURE 9.4.** The relationship of the coronoid notch and the lateral pterygoid plate. (Adapted from LifeART image. Philadelphia, PA: Lippincott Williams & Wilkins.)

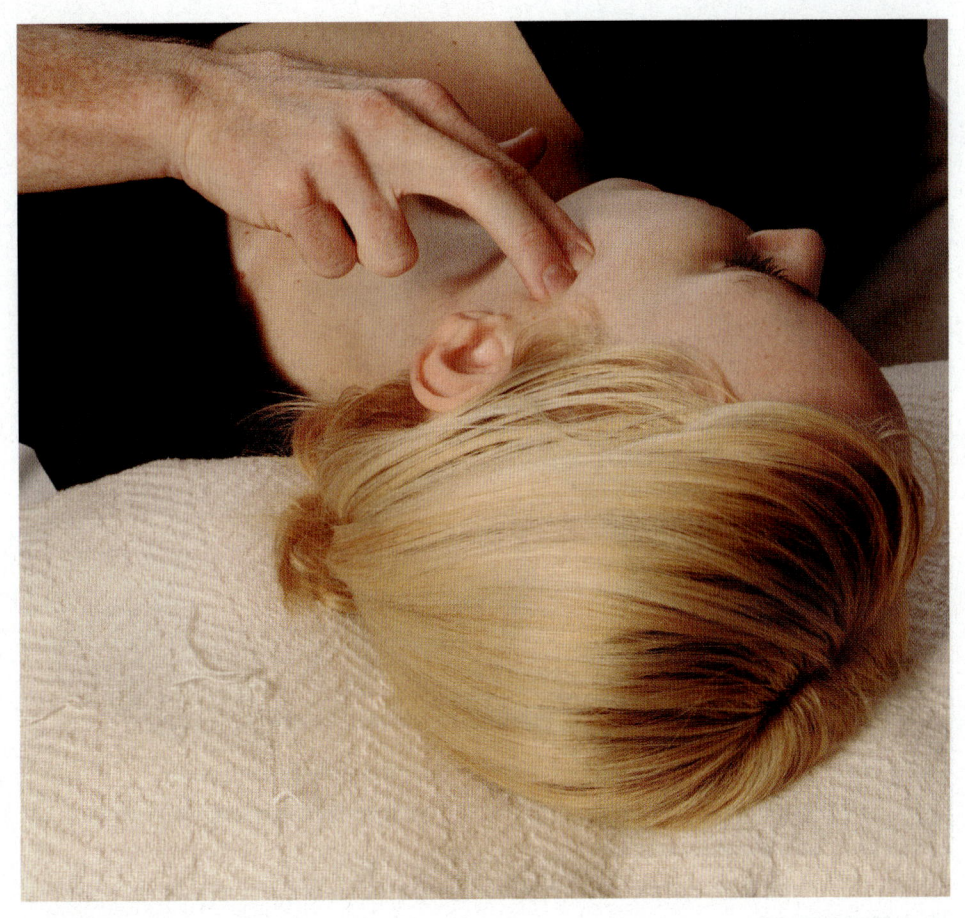

**FIGURE 9.5.** Palpation of the coronoid notch.

just below the zygomatic arch directly in the middle of the coronoid notch using an out-of-plane approach. The needle is advanced until it impinges on the lateral pterygoid plate (Fig. 9.8). When the lateral pterygoid plate is encountered, the needle is withdrawn slightly and redirected toward the mastoid process until it slips past the posterior–inferior margin of the lateral pterygoid plate into the pterygopalatine fissure and into proximity of the mandibular nerve (Figs. 9.9 and 9.10). A paresthesia may be elicited and the patient should be warned of such.

After careful aspiration is carried out, 4 to 5 mL of solution is injected in incremental doses. During the injection procedure, the patient must be observed carefully for signs of local anesthetic toxicity.

## COMPLICATIONS

The pterygopalatine fossa is highly vascular, and the potential for trauma to the vasculature, especially the maxillary artery, remains an ever-present possibility. Needle damage to the artery may result in significant facial hematoma formation, which can be very distressing to the patient and clinician alike. The vascularity of the region means that the pain specialist should carefully aspirate the needle prior to injecting any medications and should then inject small, incremental doses of local anesthetic to avoid local anesthetic toxicity.

## CLINICAL PEARLS

Selective mandibular nerve block via the coronoid approach with local anesthetic and steroid represents an excellent option for those patients suffering from the uncontrolled pain or breakthrough pain of trigeminal neuralgia and cancer pain while waiting for pharmacotherapy to take effect. The vascular nature of this anatomic region mandates care when injecting local anesthetics into the area. Careful gentle aspiration and attention to the total milligram dose of local anesthetic is crucial to avoid complications.

Small punctate facial scars secondary to needle trauma to the skin overlying the coronoid notch may occur, and the patient should be warned of this possibility. Infection, although rare, remains an ever-present possibility, especially in the immunocompromised patient. Early detection of infection is crucial to avoid potential life-threatening sequelae including spread of the infection to the central nervous system. Unexplained pain in areas subserved by the trigeminal nerve and its branches requires careful evaluation as pathology anywhere along the path of the nerve may cause pain (Fig. 9.11).

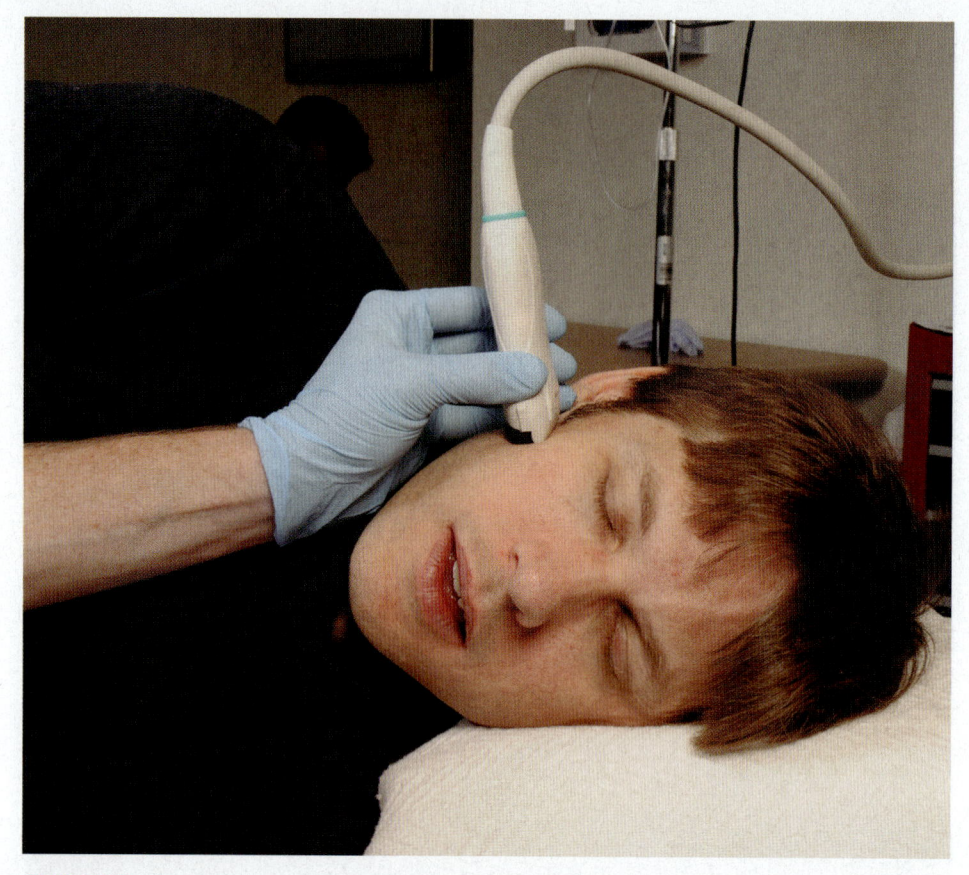

**FIGURE 9.6.** Proper transverse position of the linear transducer for selective mandibular nerve block via the coronoid approach.

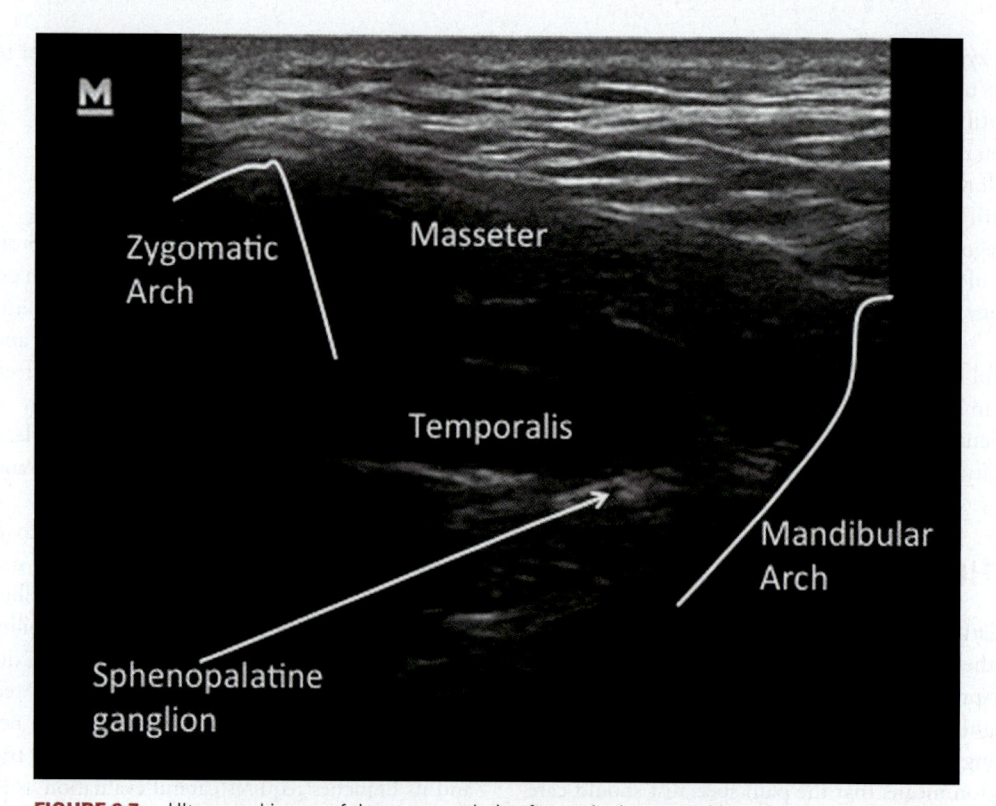

**FIGURE 9.7.** Ultrasound image of the pterygopalatine fossa via the coronoid notch.

CHAPTER 9   ULTRASOUND-GUIDED MANDIBULAR NERVE BLOCK

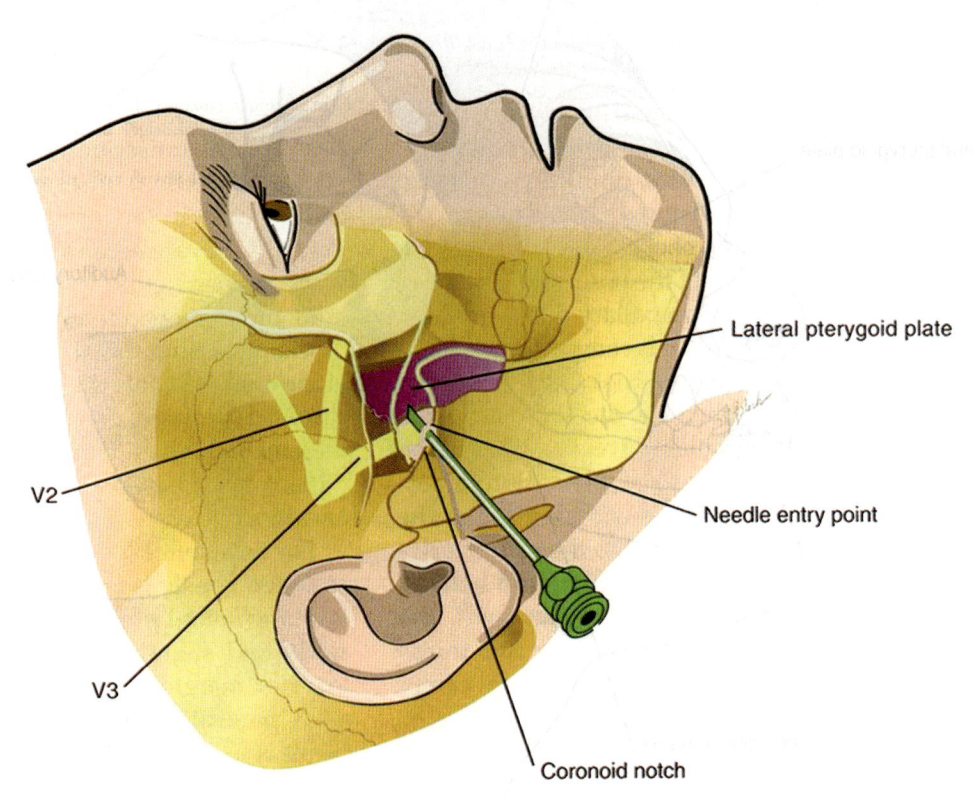

**FIGURE 9.8.** Needle tip resting against the inferior portion of the lateral pterygoid plate.

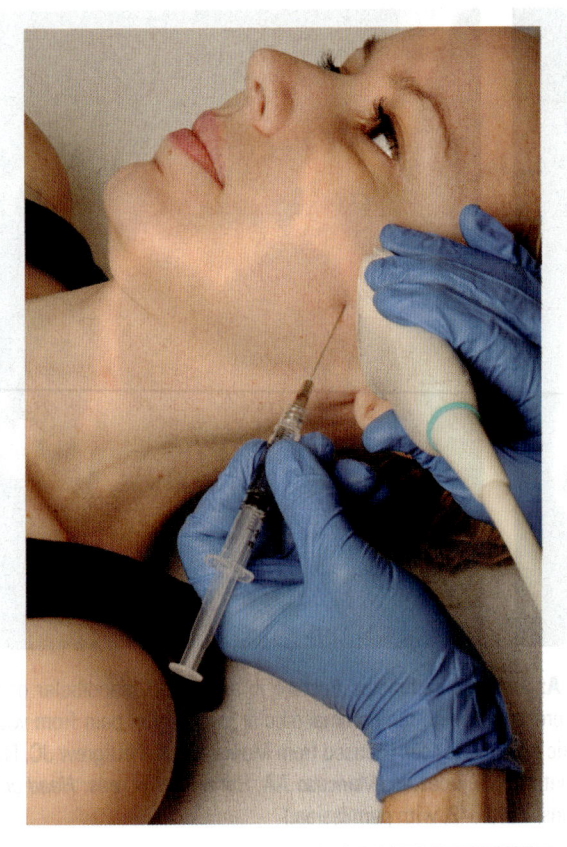

**FIGURE 9.9.** Out-of-plane approach for ultrasound-guided selective mandibular nerve block via the coronoid notch.

# CHAPTER 10

# Ultrasound-Guided Supraorbital Nerve Block

## CLINICAL CONSIDERATIONS

Ultrasound-guided supraorbital nerve block is useful in the diagnosis and treatment of a variety of painful conditions in areas subserved by the supraorbital nerve, including supraorbital neuralgia, supraorbital nerve entrapment, swimmer's headache, and pain secondary to herpes zoster (Fig. 10.1). This technique is also useful in providing surgical anesthesia in the distribution of the supraorbital nerve for lesion removal, cosmetic procedures, and laceration repair.

## CLINICALLY RELEVANT ANATOMY

The supraorbital nerve is a pure sensory nerve. It arises from fibers of the frontal nerve, which is the largest branch of the ophthalmic nerve. The frontal nerve enters the orbit via the superior orbital fissure and passes anteriorly beneath the periosteum of the roof of the orbit. The frontal nerve gives off a larger lateral branch, the supraorbital nerve, and a smaller medial branch, the supratrochlear nerve. Both nerves exit the orbit anteriorly along with the supraorbital artery via the supraorbital foramen (Fig. 10.2). The supraorbital nerve provides sensory innervation to the forehead, upper eyelid, and anterior scalp all the way to the vertex of the skull (Fig. 10.3).

## ULTRASOUND-GUIDED TECHNIQUE

The patient is placed in a supine position. A total of 2 mL of local anesthetic is drawn up in a 5-mL sterile syringe. When treating conditions involving the supraorbital nerve thought to have an inflammatory component such as supraorbital neuralgia, acute herpes zoster, neuritis, and postherpetic neuralgia, 40 to 80 mg of depot steroid may be added to the local anesthetic.

The basis for the use of ultrasound when performing supraorbital nerve block is its ability to easily identify the discontinuity of the hyperechoic image associated with the supraorbital foramen when imaging the supraorbital ridge. To perform ultrasound-guided supraorbital nerve block, the supraorbital foramen on the affected side is identified by palpation (Fig. 10.4). The foramen can usually be found 2.5 to 2.8 cm laterally from the midline. The skin overlying the supraorbital foramen is then prepped with antiseptic solution. Care must be taken to avoid allowing the antiseptic solution to flow into the eye. A high-frequency small linear or hockey stick transducer is then placed in a transverse plane over the previously identified supraorbital notch and slowly moved from a cephalad to caudad direction until a discontinuity in the supraorbital ridge is identified (Figs. 10.5 and 10.6). In most patients, color Doppler can be utilized to identify the supraorbital artery, which exits the supraorbital foramen along with the supraorbital nerve (Fig. 10.7).

Once the nerve and artery are identified, a 22-gauge, 1½-inch needle is inserted in the middle of the inferior border of the ultrasound transducer under real-time ultrasound imaging utilizing an out-of-plane approach and advanced toward the nerve with care being taken to avoid entering the foramen. The needle is advanced until it approaches the periosteum of the underlying bone. A paresthesia may be elicited, and the patient should be warned of such. The needle should not enter the supraorbital foramen, and should this occur, the needle should be withdrawn and redirected slightly more medially.

Prior to injecting the solution, a gauze sponge should be used to apply gentle pressure on the upper eyelid and supraorbital tissues to prevent the injectate from dissecting inferiorly into these tissues (Fig. 10.8). This pressure should be maintained after the procedure to avoid periorbital hematoma and ecchymosis. After gentle aspiration, 2 mL of solution is injected around the nerve.

## COMPLICATIONS

The area surrounding the supraorbital nerve is highly vascular, and the clinician should carefully calculate the total milligram dosage of local anesthetic that may be safely given, especially if bilateral nerve blocks are being performed. Because of the proximity of the supraorbital artery combined with the vascularity of the regions, postblock ecchymosis and hematoma formation can occur even in the best of hands. These bleeding complications can be decreased if manual pressure is applied to the area of the block immediately after injection. Application of cold packs for 20-minute periods after the block also decreases the amount of postprocedure pain and bleeding the patient may experience.

## CLINICAL PEARLS

Supraorbital nerve block is especially useful in the palliation of pain secondary to acute herpes zoster involving the ophthalmic division or the trigeminal nerve and its branches. In this setting, blockade of the supratrochlear nerve is also advisable. The use of tepid aluminum acetate solution applied as a soak can speed the drying of the weeping herpetic lesions and enhance patient comfort. Care should be taken to avoid spillage of the aluminum acetate solution into the eye. It is important to note that patients with acute herpes zoster involving the first division of the trigeminal nerve may first experience vesicular eruptions on the tip of the nose (positive Hutchinson sign), which may presage a particularly severe bout of herpes zoster with ocular complications such as acute glaucoma and keratitis (Fig. 10.9).

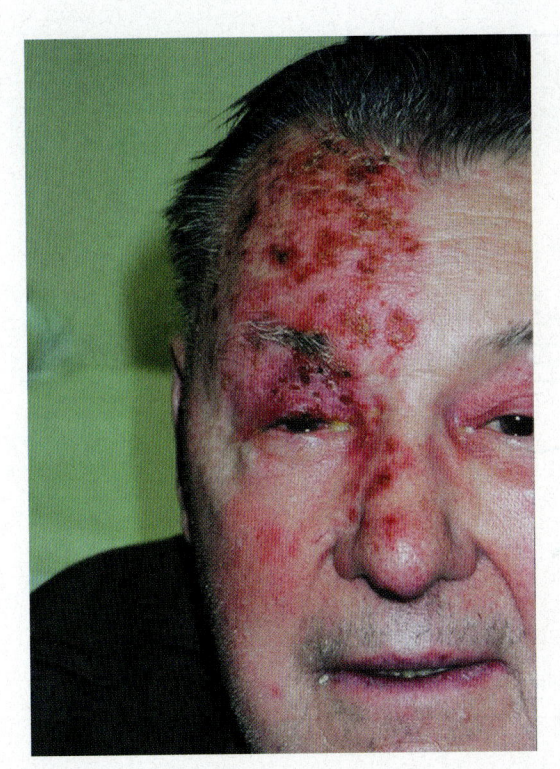

**FIGURE 10.1.** Acute herpes zoster involving the first division of the trigeminal nerve. Note the lesions on the tip of the nose (positive Hutchinson sign).

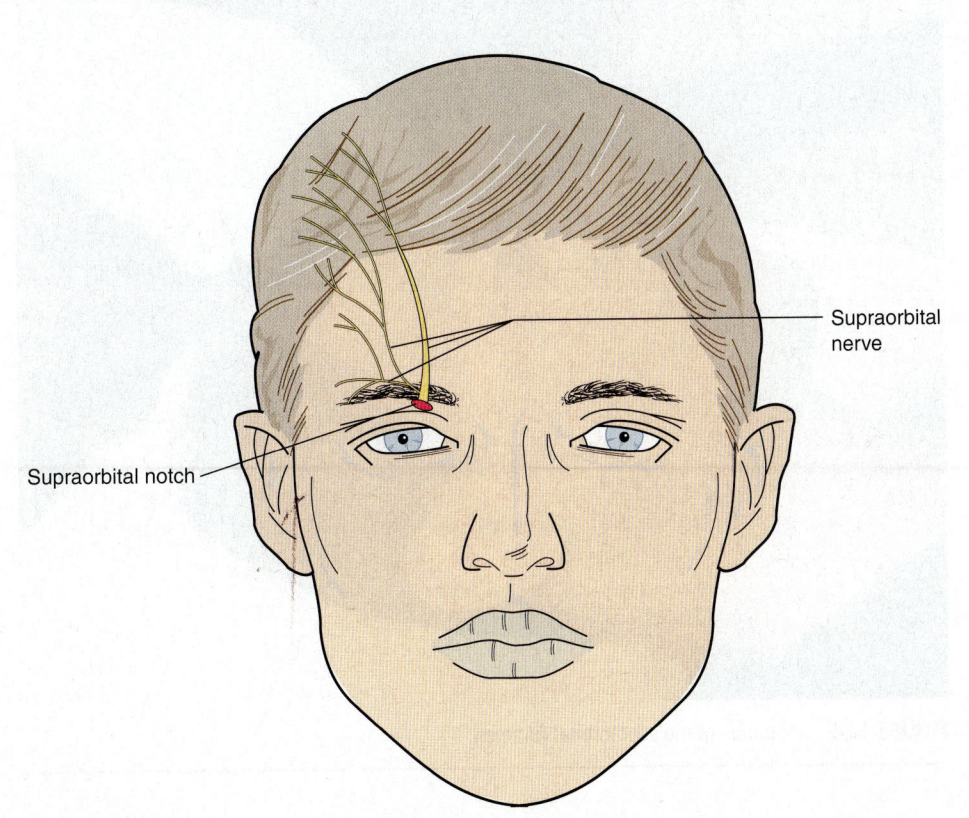

**FIGURE 10.2.** The supraorbital nerve and a smaller medial branch, the supratrochlear nerve, exit the orbit anteriorly along with the supraorbital artery via the supraorbital foramen.

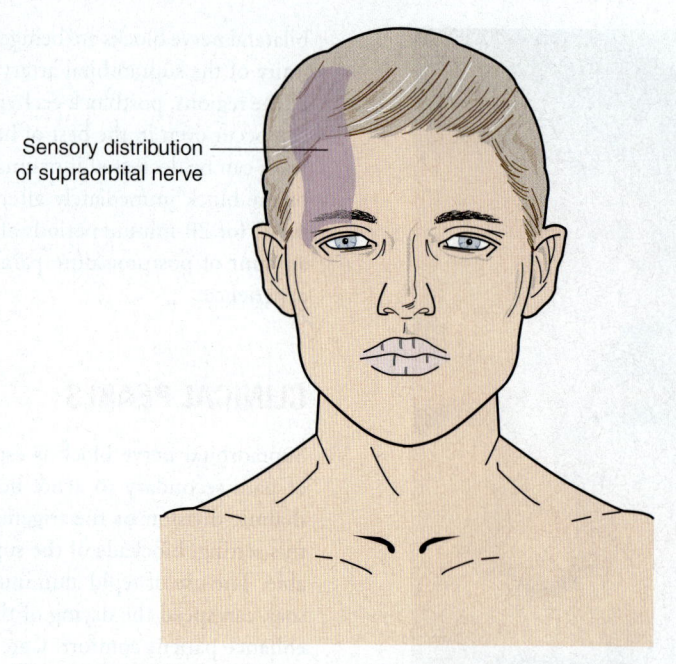

**FIGURE 10.3.** The sensory distribution of the supraorbital nerve.

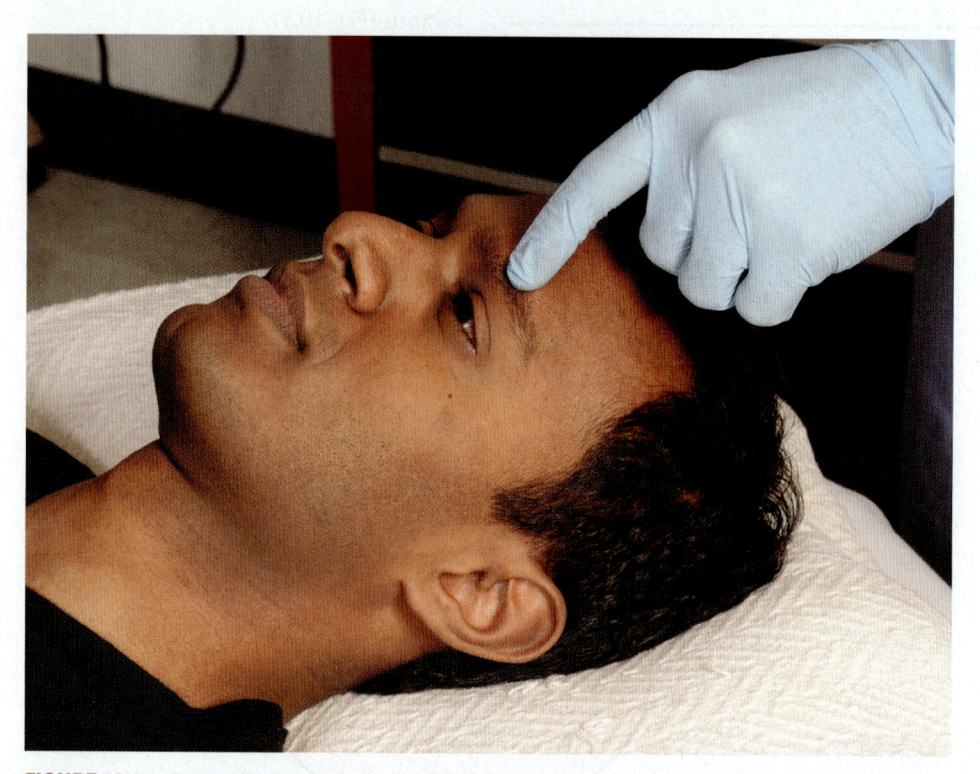

**FIGURE 10.4.** Palpation of the supraorbital foramen.

CHAPTER 10   ULTRASOUND-GUIDED SUPRAORBITAL NERVE BLOCK

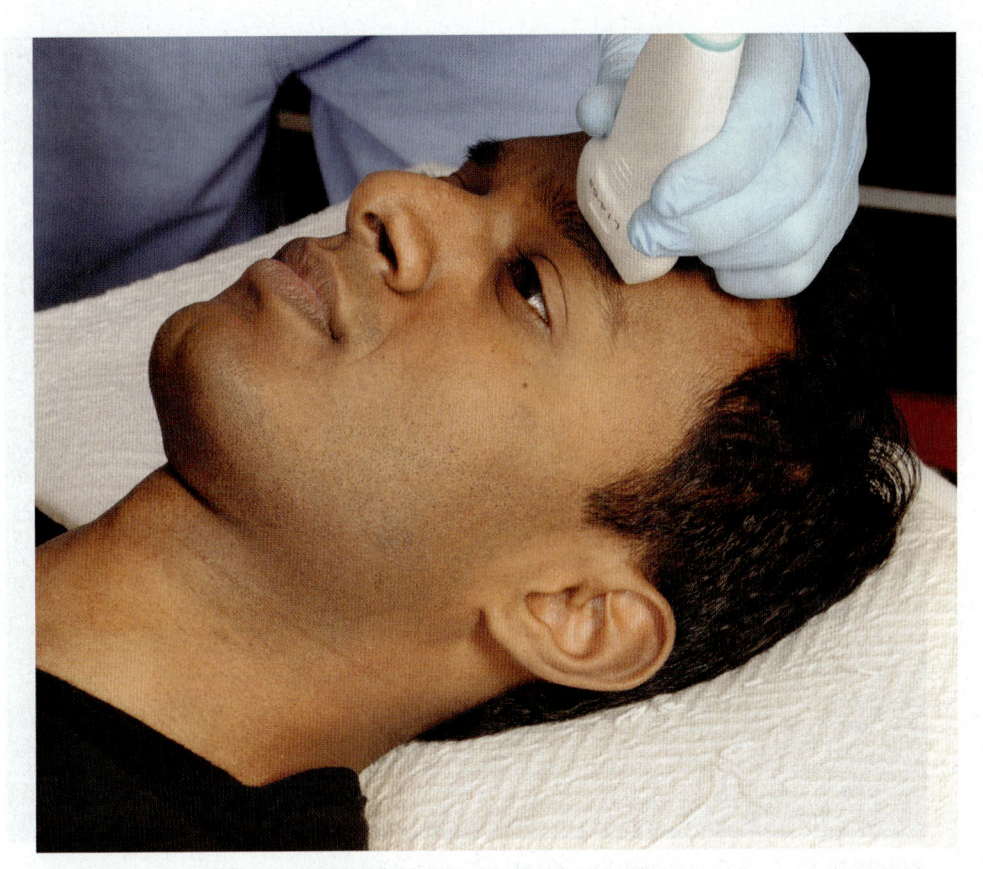

**FIGURE 10.5.** The high-frequency small linear transducer is placed in the over the supraorbital foramen.

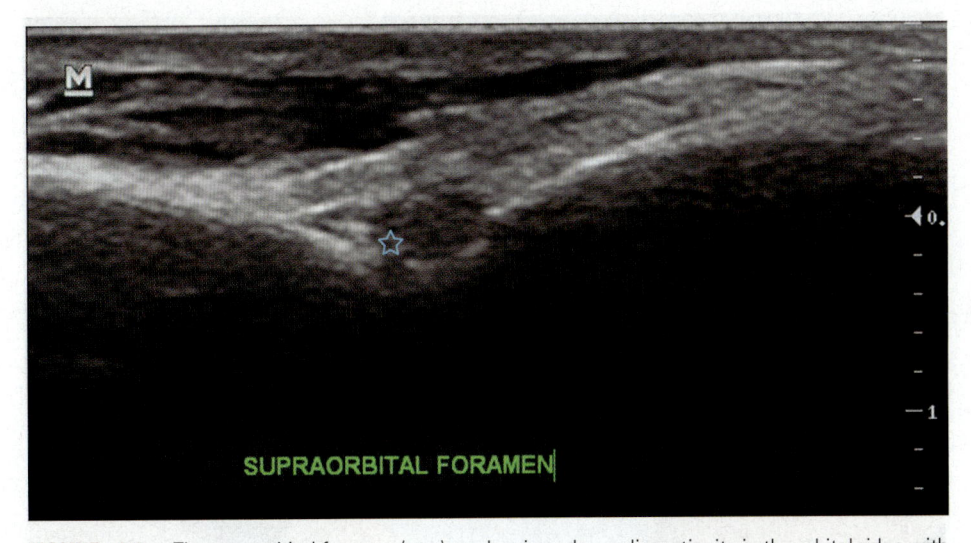

**FIGURE 10.6.** The supraorbital foramen (*star*) can be viewed as a discontinuity in the orbital ridge with the nerve and artery exiting through it.

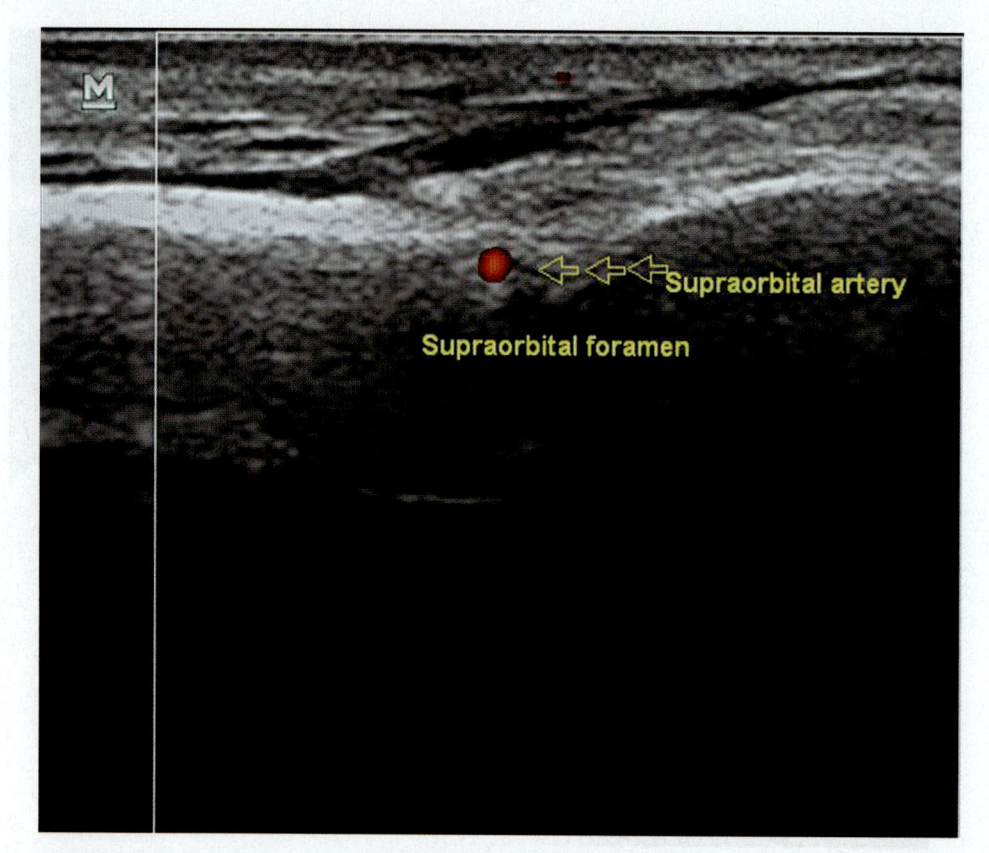

**FIGURE 10.7.** Color Doppler may help identify the supraorbital artery.

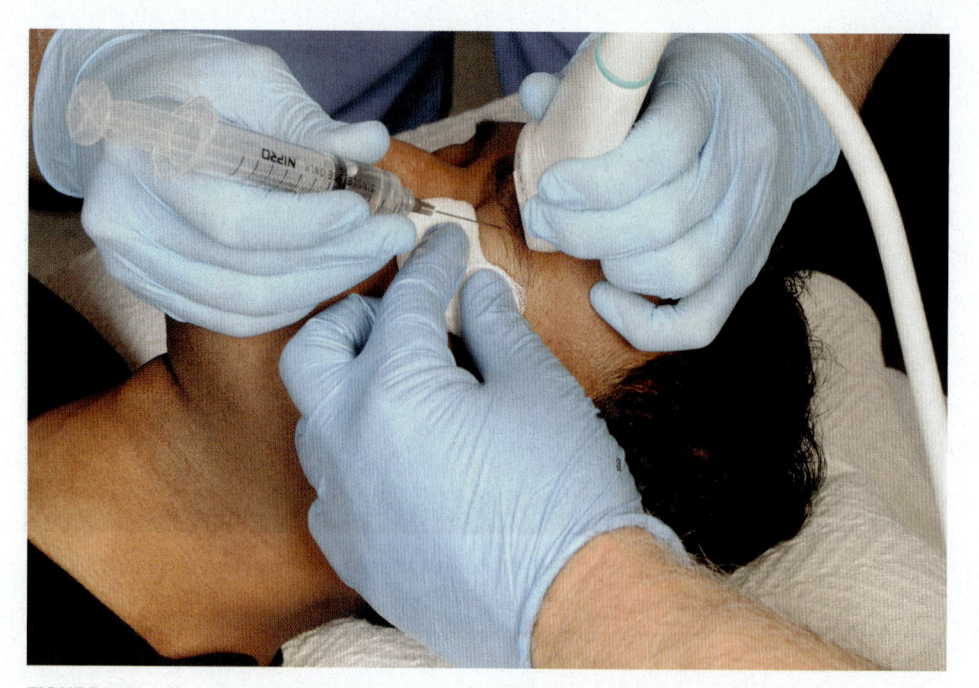

**FIGURE 10.8.** A gauze sponge should be used to apply gentle pressure on the upper eyelid and supraorbital tissues to prevent the injectate from dissecting inferiorly into these tissues.

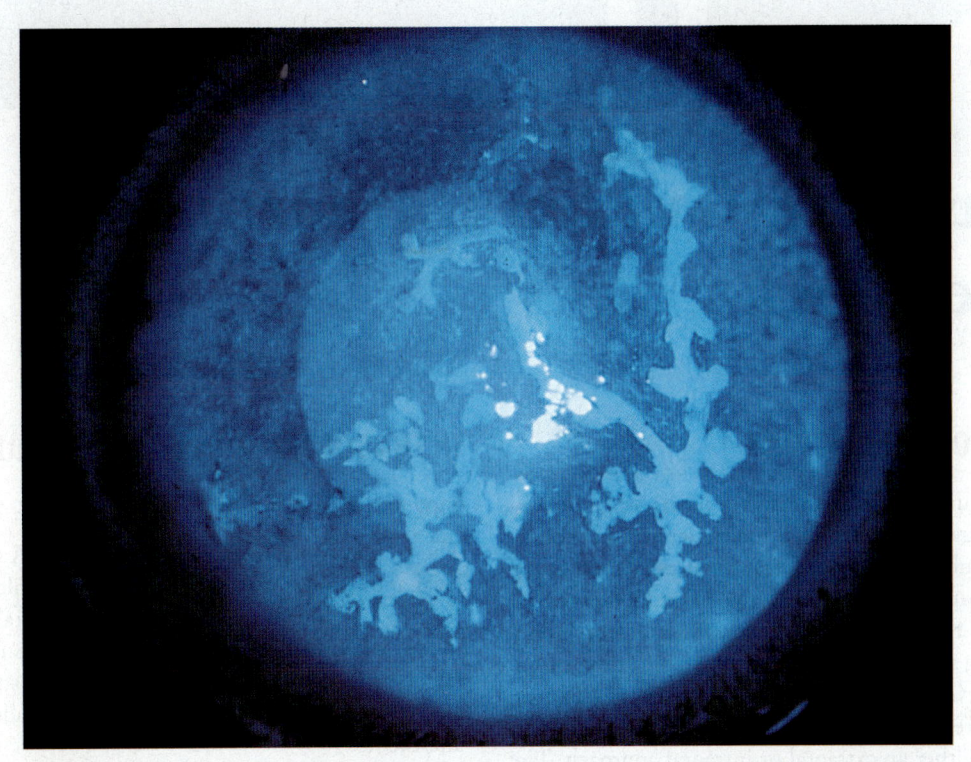

**FIGURE 10.9.** Keratitis. Note pseudodendritic uptake of fluorescein. (Reused from Cohen EJ, Rapuano CJ, Laibson PR. External diseases. In: Tasman W, Jaeger EA, eds. *The Wills Eye Hospital Atlas of Clinical Ophthalmology*. 2nd ed. Philadelphia, PA: Lippincott Williams & Wilkins; 2001:8, with permission.)

## SUGGESTED READINGS

Waldman SD. Supraorbital nerve block: coronoid approach. In: *Atlas of Interventional Pain Management*. 3rd ed. Philadelphia, PA: Saunders Elsevier; 2009:59–65.

Waldman SD. The trigeminal nerve. In: *Pain Review*. Philadelphia, PA: Saunders Elsevier; 2009:15–17.

Waldman SD. Acute herpes zoster of the first division of the trigeminal nerve. In: *Atlas of Common Pain Syndromes*. 3rd ed. Philadelphia, PA: Saunders Elsevier; 2011:1–4.

Waldman SD. Swimmer's headache. In: *Atlas of Common Pain Syndromes*. 3rd ed. Philadelphia, PA: Saunders Elsevier; 2011:13–14.

# CHAPTER 11

# Ultrasound-Guided Infraorbital Nerve Block

## CLINICAL CONSIDERATIONS

Ultrasound-guided infraorbital nerve block is useful in the diagnosis and treatment of a variety of painful conditions in areas subserved by the infraorbital nerve, including infraorbital neuralgia, infraorbital nerve entrapment, and pain secondary to herpes zoster. This technique is also useful in providing surgical anesthesia in the distribution of the infraorbital nerve for lesion removal, cosmetic procedures, and laceration repair (Fig. 11.1). The infraorbital nerve can be blocked via either an extraoral or intraoral approach. The intraoral approach to infraorbital nerve block is especially useful in providing surgical anesthesia in the distribution of the infraorbital nerve for lesion removal and laceration repair when a cosmetic result is desired, because this approach avoids distortion of the facial anatomy from local anesthetic infiltration at the surgical site. The intraoral approach is also useful in the pediatric population as the oral mucosa can be anesthetized with topical application of local anesthetic prior to needle placement.

## CLINICALLY RELEVANT ANATOMY

The infraorbital nerve is a pure sensory nerve arising from fibers from the maxillary nerve. Entering the orbit via the inferior orbital fissure, the infraorbital nerve passes along the floor of the orbit in the infraorbital groove. Along with the infraorbital artery, the infraorbital nerve exits the orbit via the infraorbital foramen (Fig. 11.2). The nerve then divides into a superior alveolar branch, which provides sensory innervation to the upper incisor, canine, and associated gingiva and a cutaneous branch that fans out to provide sensory innervation to the lower eyelid, lateral naris, and upper lip (Fig. 11.3). In rare instances, the infraorbital nerve may bifurcate within the orbit and exit via separate infraorbital foramen (Fig. 11.4). A patient with five separate infraorbital foramina and nerves has been reported.

## ULTRASOUND-GUIDED TECHNIQUES

### Extraoral Approach

The patient is placed in a supine position. A total of 2 mL of local anesthetic is drawn up in a 5-mL sterile syringe. When treating conditions involving the infraorbital nerve thought to have an inflammatory component such as infraorbital neuralgia, acute herpes zoster, neuritis, and postherpetic neuralgia, 40 to 80 mg of depot steroid may be added to the local anesthetic.

The basis for the use of ultrasound when performing infraorbital nerve block is its ability to easily identify the discontinuity of the hyperechoic image associated with the infraorbital foramen when imaging the infraorbital ridge. To perform ultrasound-guided infraorbital nerve block, the infraorbital foramen on the affected side is identified by palpation (Fig. 11.5). The foramen can usually be found ~2.5 to 2.8 cm laterally from the midline. The skin overlying the infraorbital foramen is then prepped with antiseptic solution. Care must be taken to avoid allowing the antiseptic solution to flow into the eye. A high-frequency small linear or hockey stick transducer is then placed in the transverse plane over the previously identified infraorbital notch and slowly moved from a medial to lateral direction until a discontinuity in the infraorbital ridge is identified (Figs. 11.6 and 11.7). Alternatively, a longitudinal view can be utilized. In most patients, color Doppler can be utilized to identify the infraorbital artery, which exits the infraorbital foramen along with the infraorbital nerve (see Fig. 11.8).

Once the nerve and artery are identified, a 22-gauge, 1½-inch needle is inserted under real-time ultrasound imaging utilizing an in-plane approach and advanced toward the nerve with care being taken to avoid entering the foramen. The needle is advanced until it approaches the periosteum of the underlying bone. A paresthesia may be elicited, and the patient should be warned of such. The needle should not enter the infraorbital foramen, and should this occur, the needle should be withdrawn and redirected slightly more medially.

CHAPTER 11 ULTRASOUND-GUIDED INFRAORBITAL NERVE BLOCK 67

Prior to injecting the solution, a gauze sponge should be used to apply gentle pressure on the lower eyelid and infraorbital tissues to prevent the injectate from dissecting inferiorly into these tissues (Fig. 11.9). This pressure should be maintained after the procedure to avoid periorbital hematoma and ecchymosis. After gentle aspiration, 2 mL of solution is injected around the nerve.

## Intraoral Approach

The infraorbital foramen is identified using palpation and ultrasound as described with the extraoral approach above. After the infraorbital foramen is identified, the upper lip is then retracted and a cotton ball soaked in 10% cocaine solution, or 2% viscous lidocaine is placed in the superior alveolar sulcus, directly inferior to the infraorbital foramen (Fig. 11.10). After adequate topical anesthesia of the mucosa is obtained, the cotton ball is removed and a 22-gauge, 1½-inch needle is advanced through the anesthetized mucosa toward the infraorbital foramen under real-time ultrasound guidance (Fig. 11.11). A paresthesia may be elicited and the patient should be warned of such. Because of the loose alveolar tissue of the eyelid, a gauze sponge should be used to apply gentle pressure on the lower eyelid and infraorbital tissues before injection of solution to prevent the injectate from dissecting upward into these tissues. This pressure should be maintained after the procedure to avoid periorbital hematoma and ecchymosis. After gentle aspiration, 3 mL of solution is injected in a fan-like distribution.

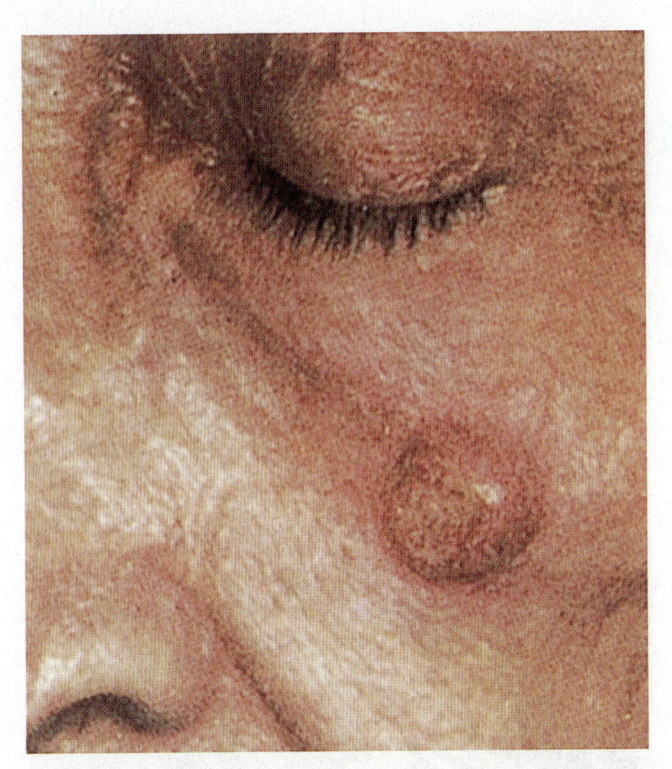

**FIGURE 11.1.** Squamous cell carcinoma in the sensory distribution of the infraorbital nerve. (Reprinted from Bickley LS. *Bate's Guide to Physical Examination and History Taking*. 8th ed. Philadelphia, PA: Lippincott Williams & Wilkins; 2003, with permission.)

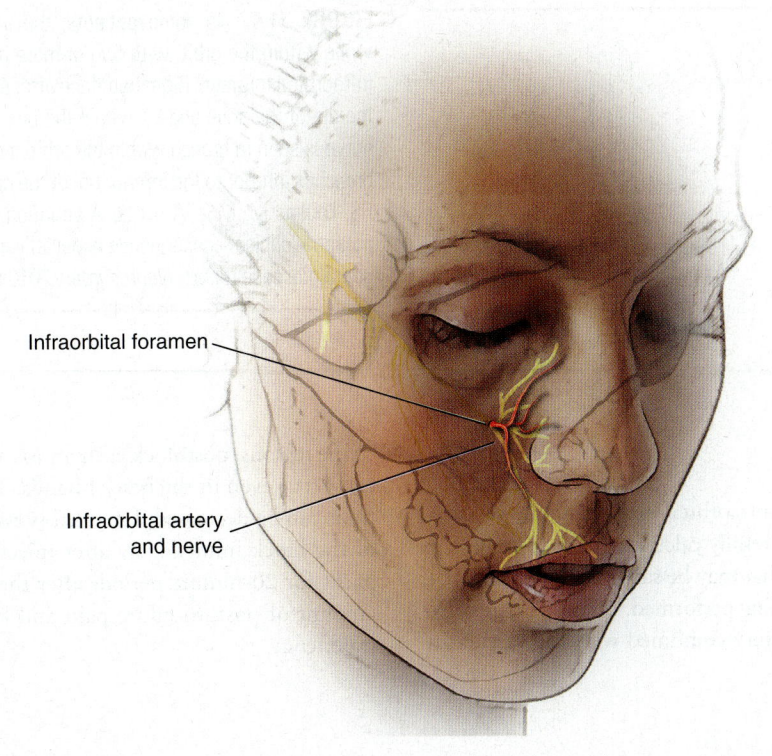

**FIGURE 11.2.** Infraorbital artery exiting the infraorbital foramen along with nerve.

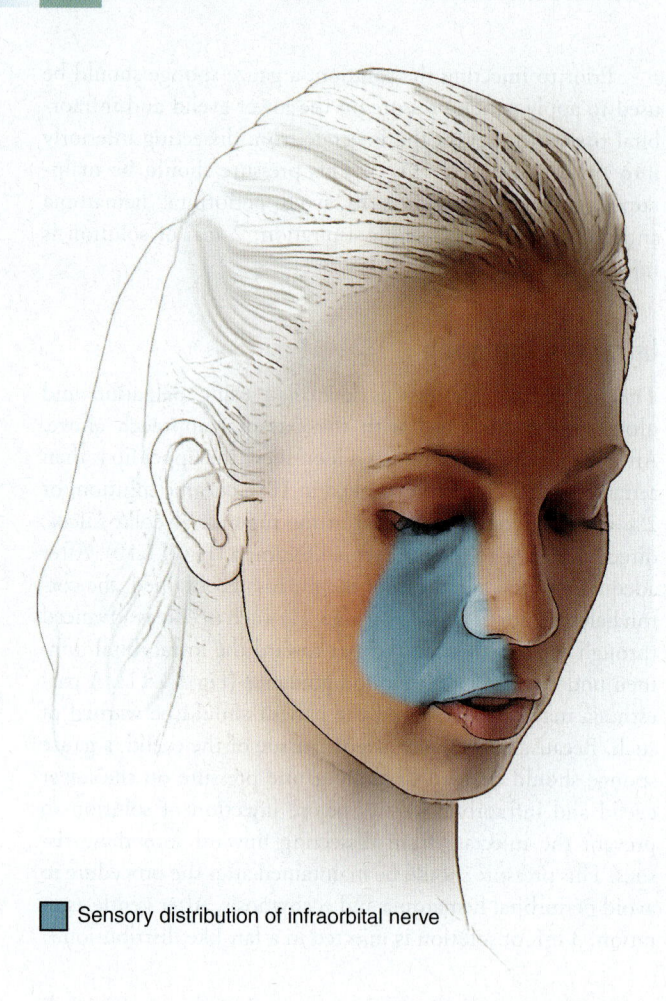

**FIGURE 11.3.** The sensory distribution of the infraorbital nerve.

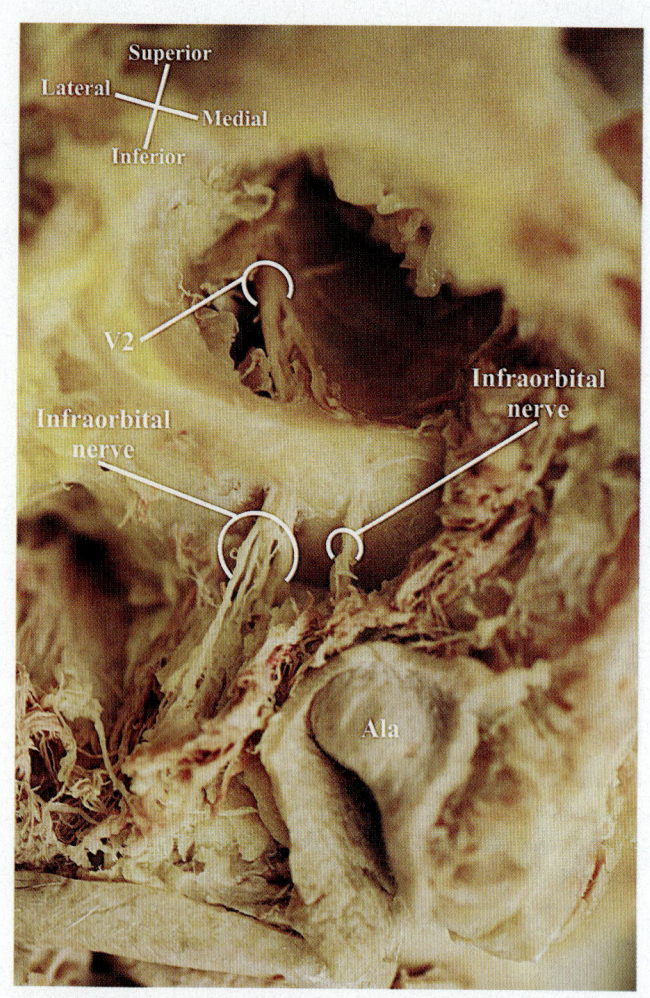

**FIGURE 11.4.** In some patients, the infraorbital nerve may divide while within the orbit, with two or more branches exiting via separate infraorbital foramen. Right hemiface after enucleation of the globe. Note the ala of the nose and V2 within the posterior aspect of the orbit. The nerve is seen to branch within the orbit and then leave as two separate branches inferior to the inferior rim of the right orbit. (Reused from Tubbs RS, Loukas M, May W, et al. A variation of the infraorbital nerve: its potential clinical consequence especially in the treatment of trigeminal neuralgia: case report. *Neurosurgery* 2010;67(3):E315, with permission.)

## COMPLICATIONS

The area surrounding the infraorbital nerve is highly vascular, and the clinician should carefully calculate the total milligram dosage of local anesthetic that may be safely given, especially if bilateral nerve blocks are being performed. Because of the proximity of the infraorbital artery combined with the vascularity of the regions, postblock ecchymosis and hematoma formation can occur even in the best of hands. These bleeding complications can be decreased if manual pressure is applied to the area of the block immediately after injection. Application of cold packs for 20-minute periods after the block also decreases the amount of postprocedure pain and bleeding the patient may experience.

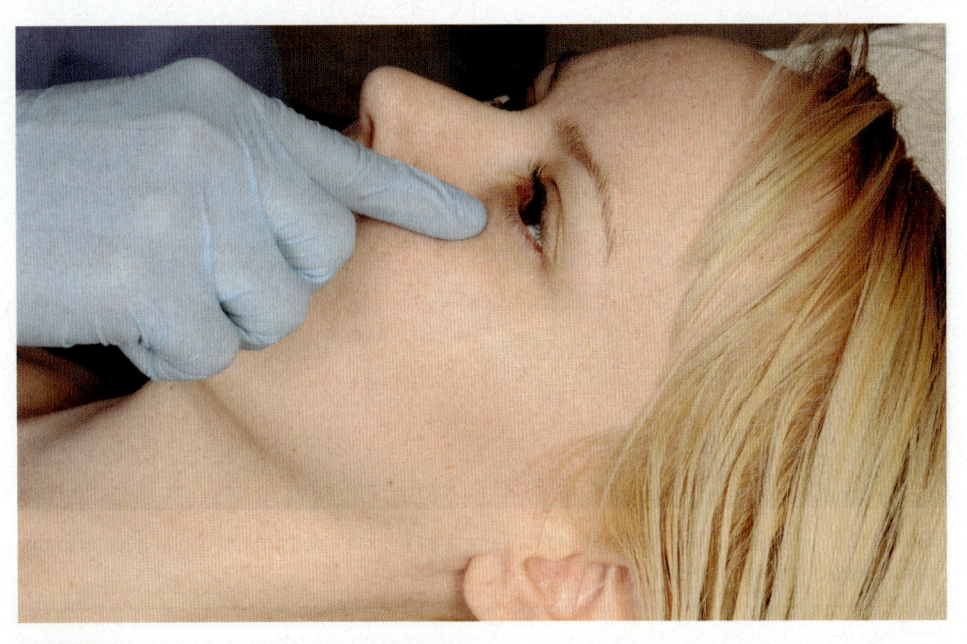

**FIGURE 11.5.** Palpation of the infraorbital foramen.

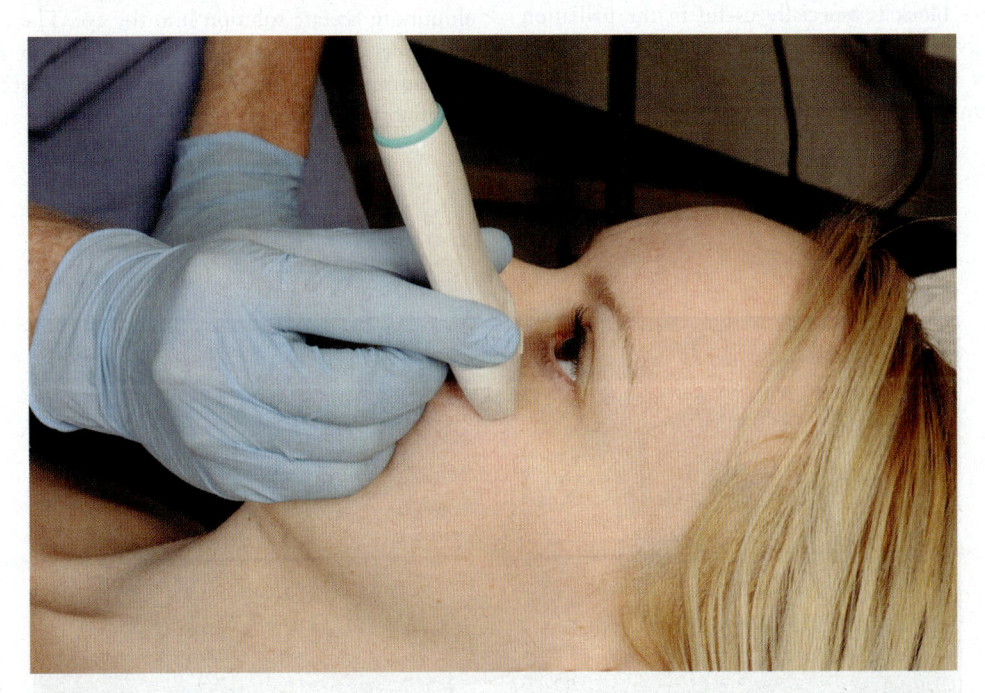

**FIGURE 11.6.** The high-frequency small transducer is placed in the transverse plane over the infraorbital foramen.

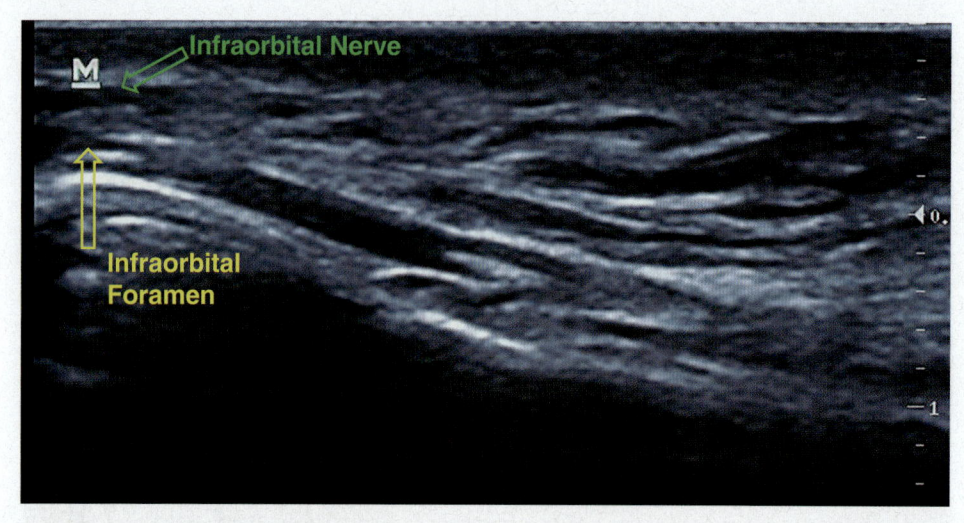

**FIGURE 11.7.** The infraorbital foramen can be viewed as a discontinuity in the orbital ridge with the nerve and artery exiting through it.

## CLINICAL PEARLS

Infraorbital nerve block is especially useful in the palliation of pain secondary to acute herpes zoster involving the maxillary division of the trigeminal nerve and its branches. The use of tepid aluminum acetate solution applied as a soak can speed the drying of the weeping herpetic lesions and enhance patient comfort. Care should be taken to avoid spillage of the aluminum acetate solution into the eye. The clinician should remember that trauma, tumors, or infection anywhere along the course of the infraorbital nerve can produce the symptoms of infraorbital neuralgia (Fig. 11.12).

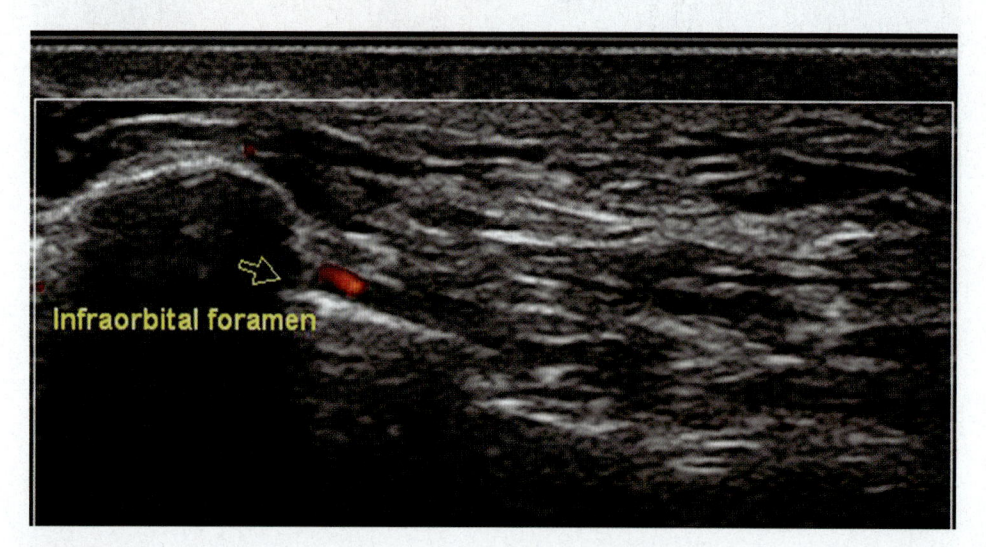

**FIGURE 11.8.** Color Doppler may help identify the infraorbital artery.

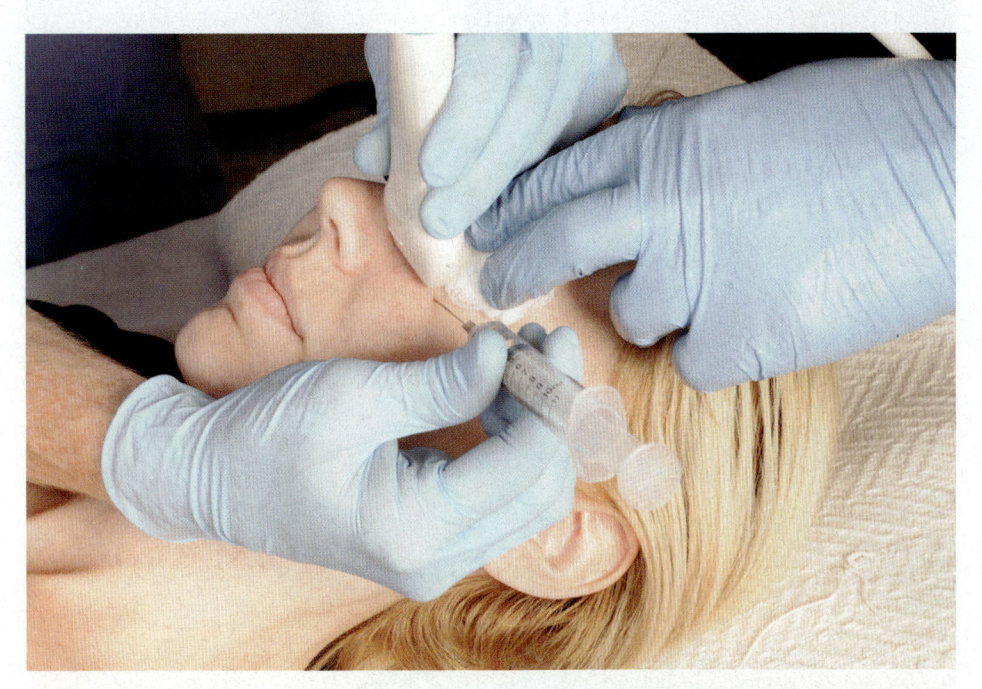

**FIGURE 11.9.** A gauze sponge should be used to apply gentle pressure on the lower eyelid and infraorbital tissues to prevent the injectate from dissecting inferiorly into these tissues. An in-plane approach may be utilized with the ultrasound transducer in transverse plane.

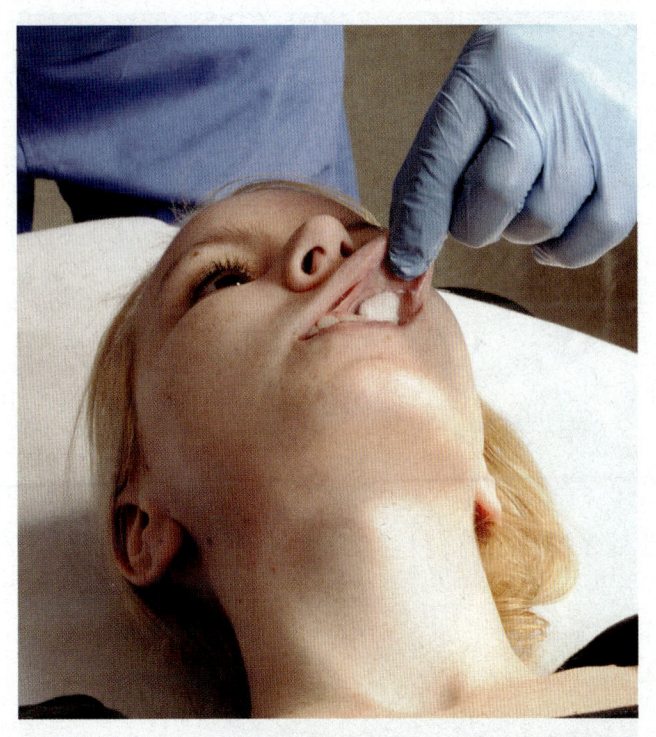

**FIGURE 11.10.** A cotton ball soaked in local anesthetic suitable for topical application is placed in the superior alveolar sulcus.

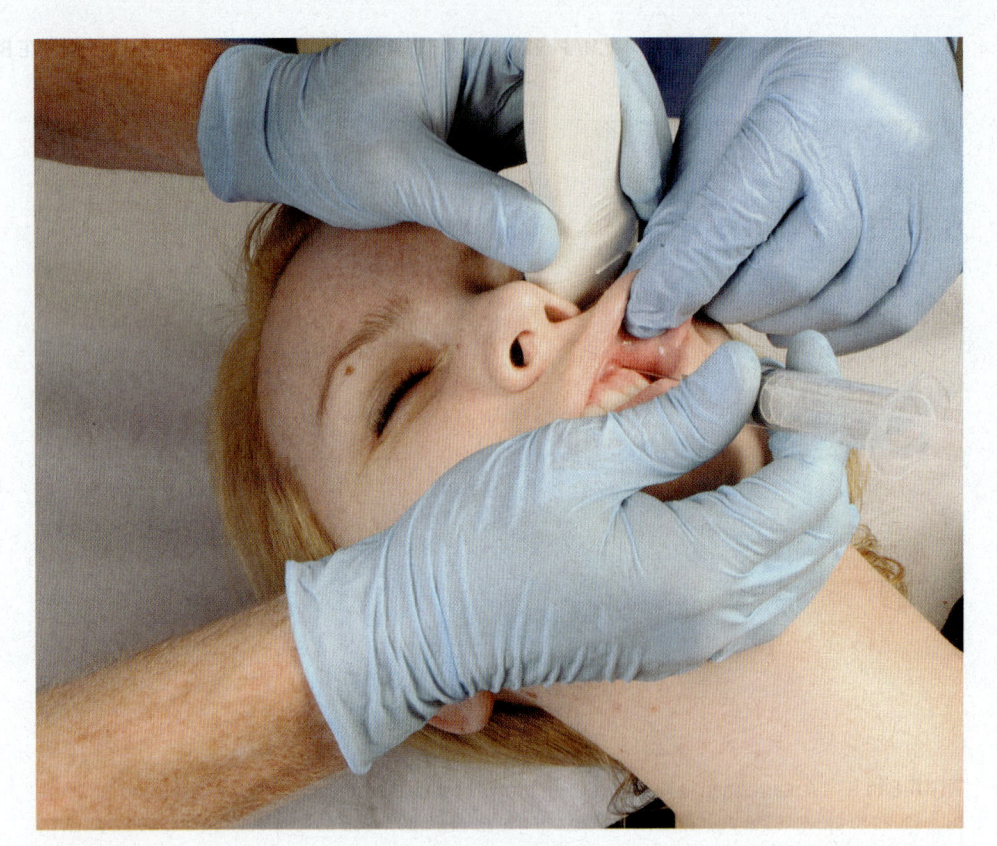

**FIGURE 11.11.** The needle is placed through the previously anesthetized area and advanced under real-time ultrasound guidance toward the infraorbital nerve.

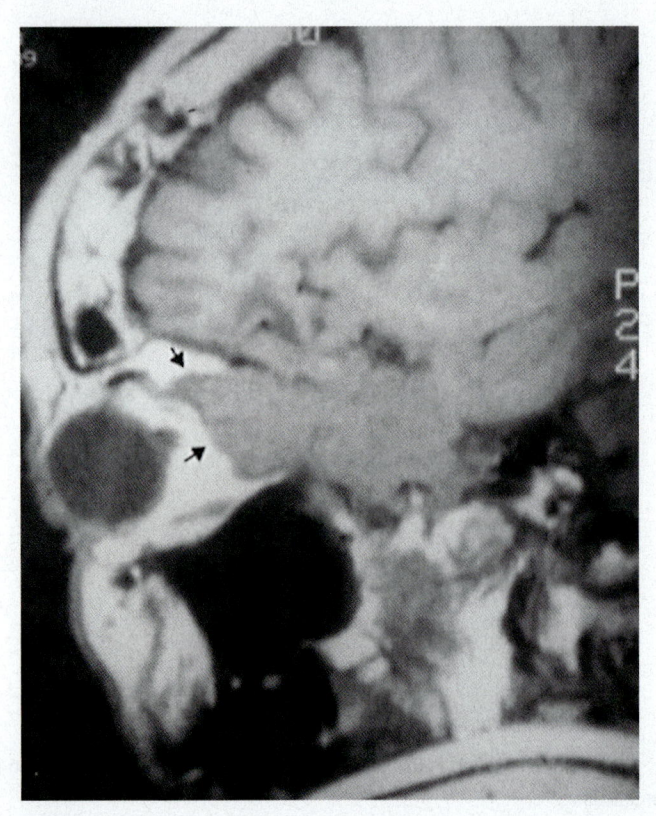

**FIGURE 11.12.** Magnetic resonance image shows a large mass virtually isointense to brain that arose from the planum sphenoidale and extended into the posterior aspect of the orbit (*arrows*). (Reused from Eisenberg RL. *Clinical Imaging: An Atlas of Differential Diagnosis.* Philadelphia, PA: Lippincott Williams & Wilkins; 2010:1370, with permission.)

## SUGGESTED READINGS

Saeedi OJ, Wang H, Blomquist PH. Penetrating globe injury during infraorbital nerve block. *Arch Otolaryngol Head Neck Surg* 2011;137(4):396–397.

Waldman SD. Infraorbital nerve block: coronoid approach. In: *Atlas of Interventional Pain Management*. 3rd ed. Philadelphia, PA: Saunders Elsevier; 2009:59–65.

Waldman SD. The trigeminal nerve. In: *Pain Review*. Philadelphia, PA: Saunders Elsevier; 2009:15–17.

Waldman SD. Swimmer's headache. In: *Atlas of Common Pain Syndromes*. 3rd ed. Philadelphia, PA: Saunders Elsevier; 2011:13–14.

Waldman SD. Trigeminal neuralgia. In: *Atlas of Common Pain Syndromes*. 3rd ed. Philadelphia, PA: Saunders Elsevier; 2011:29–32.

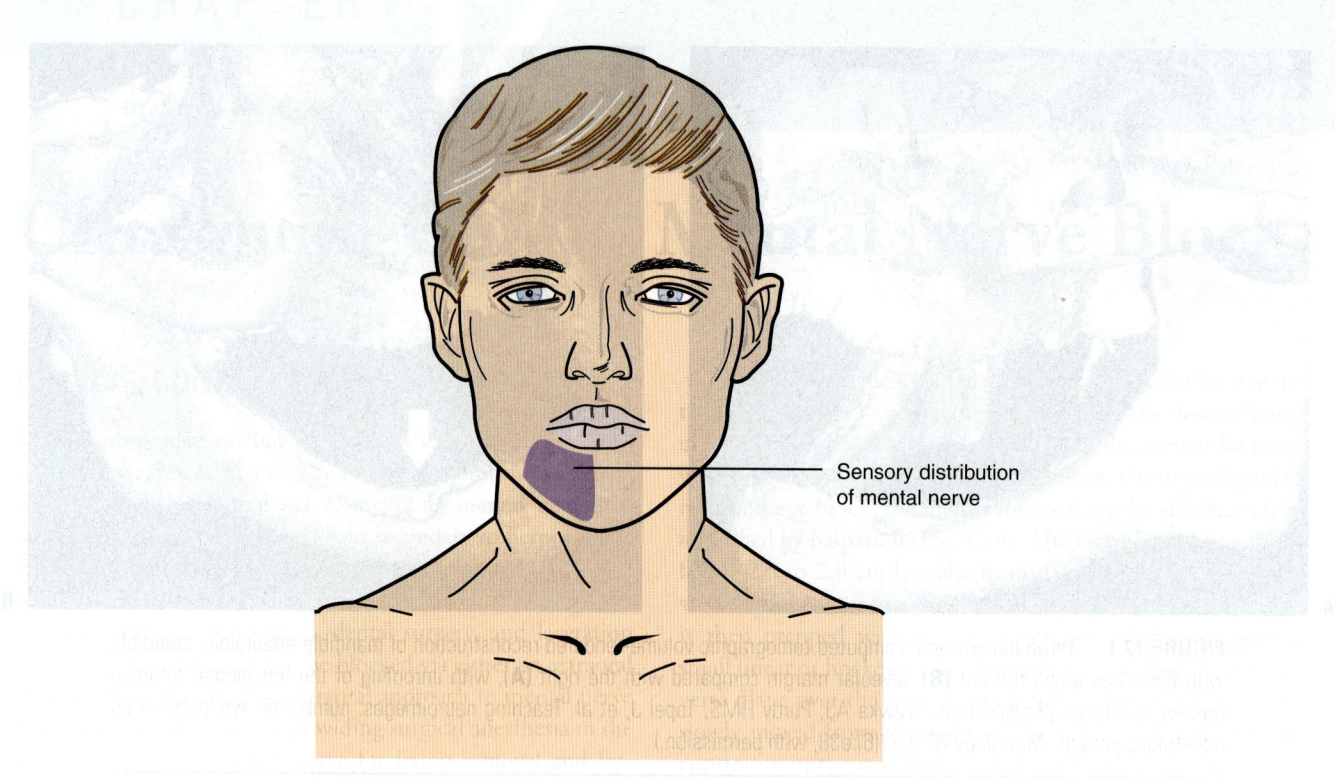

**FIGURE 12.3.** The sensory distribution of the mental nerve.

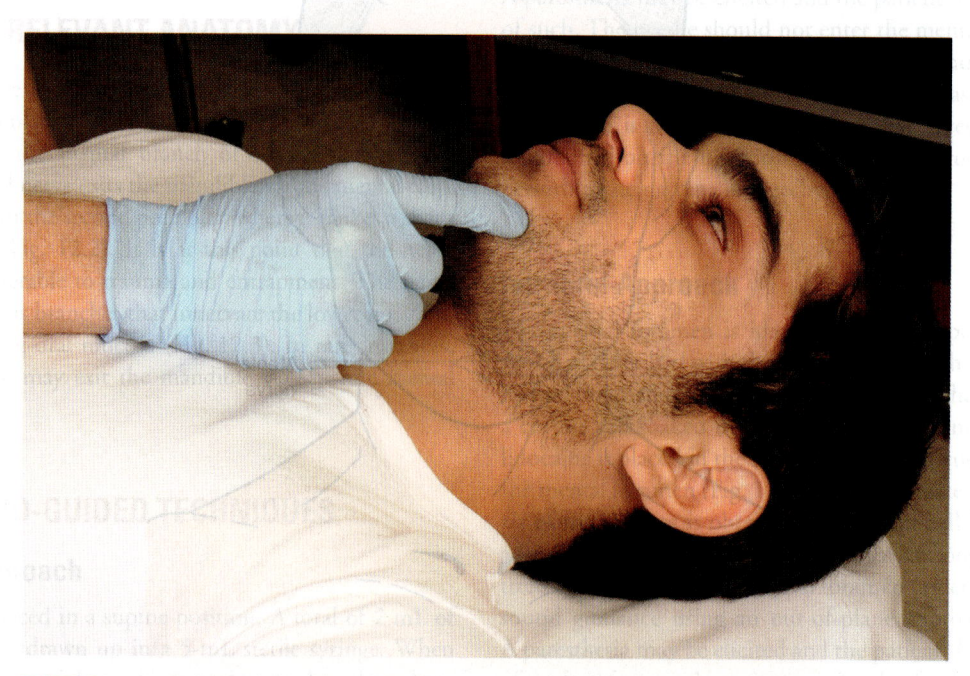

**FIGURE 12.4.** Palpation of the mental foramen.

CHAPTER 12    ULTRASOUND-GUIDED MENTAL NERVE BLOCK    77

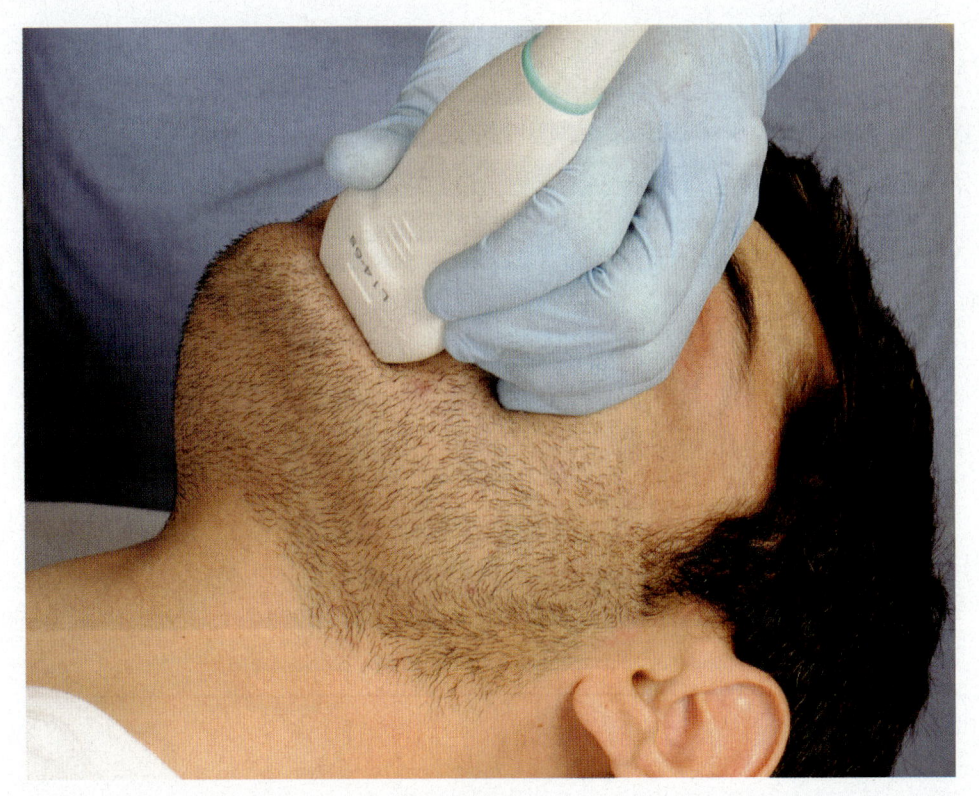

**FIGURE 12.5.** The high-frequency small linear transducer is placed in the transverse plane over the mental foramen.

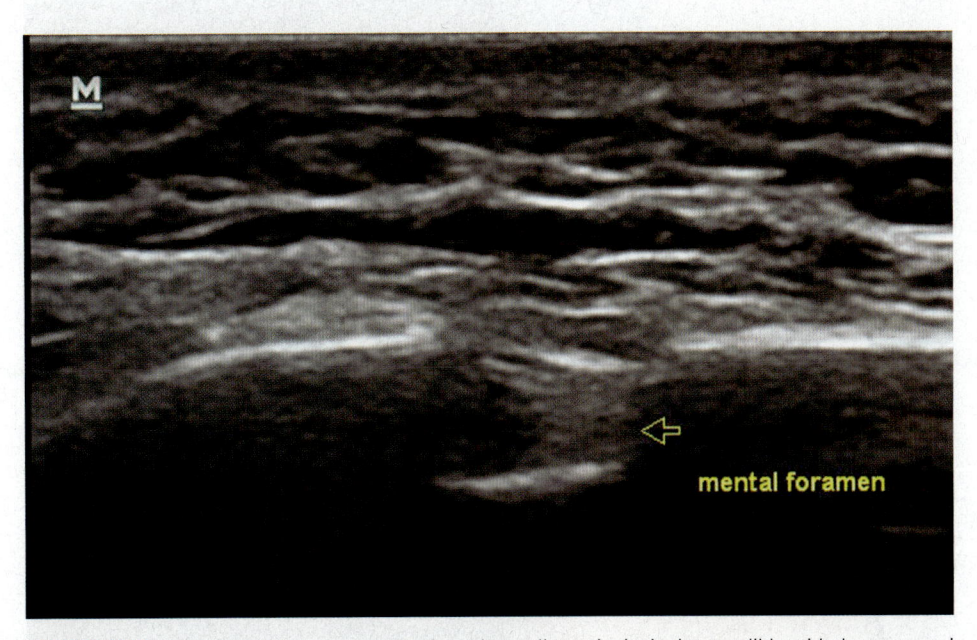

**FIGURE 12.6.** The mental foramen can be viewed as a discontinuity in the mandible with the nerve and artery exiting through it.

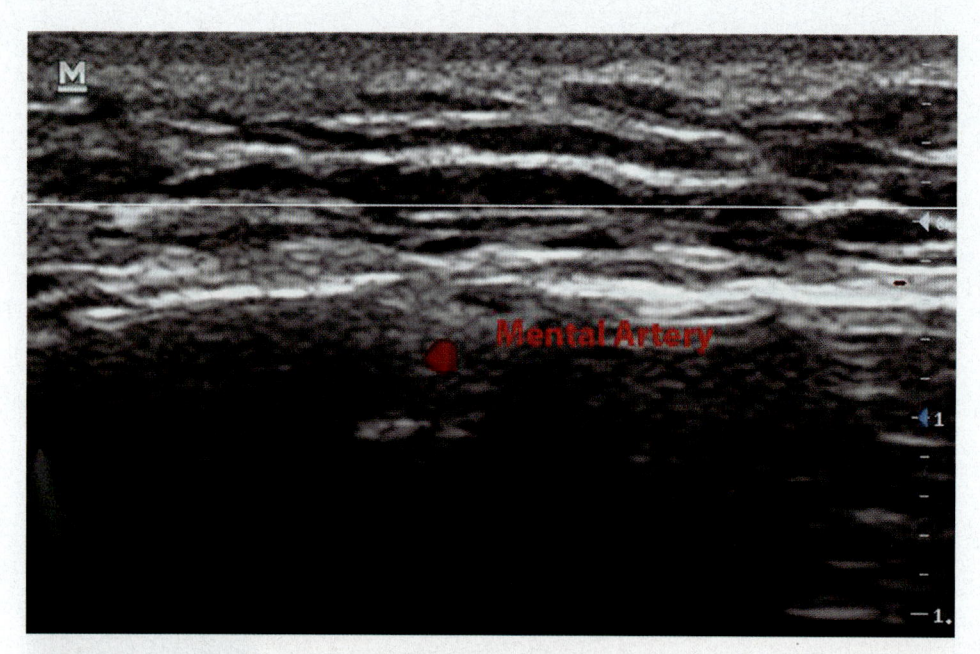

**FIGURE 12.7.** Color Doppler may help identify the mental artery.

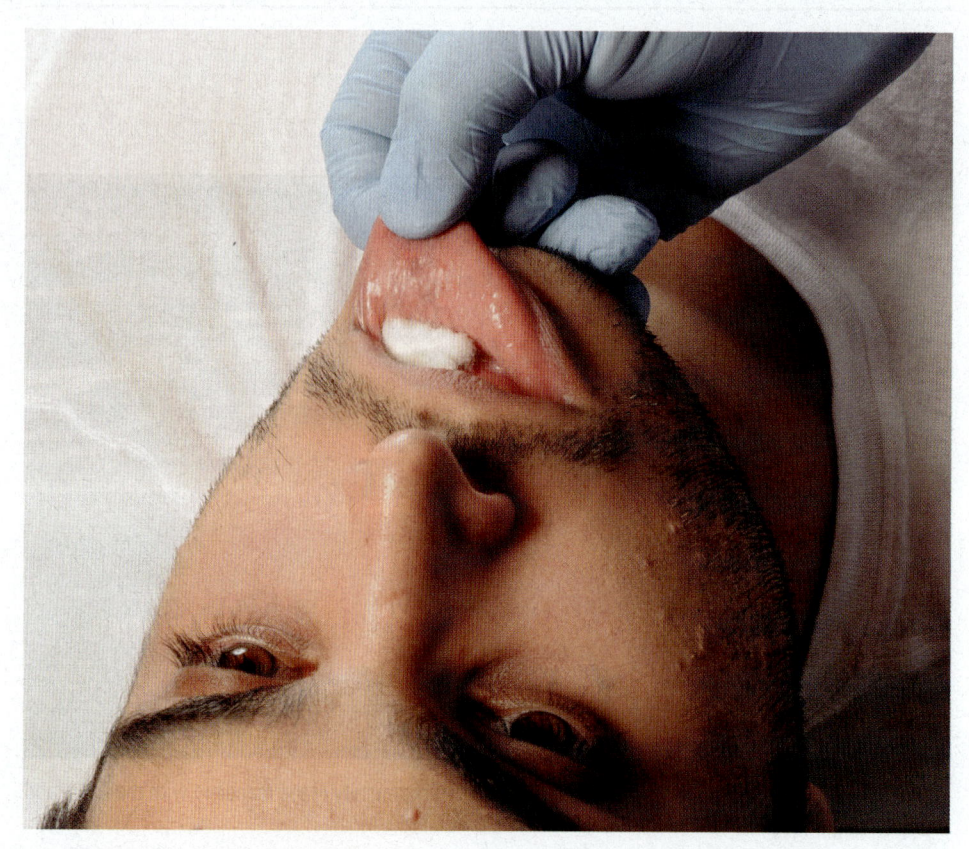

**FIGURE 12.8.** A cotton ball soaked in local anesthetic suitable for topical application is placed in the superior alveolar sulcus.

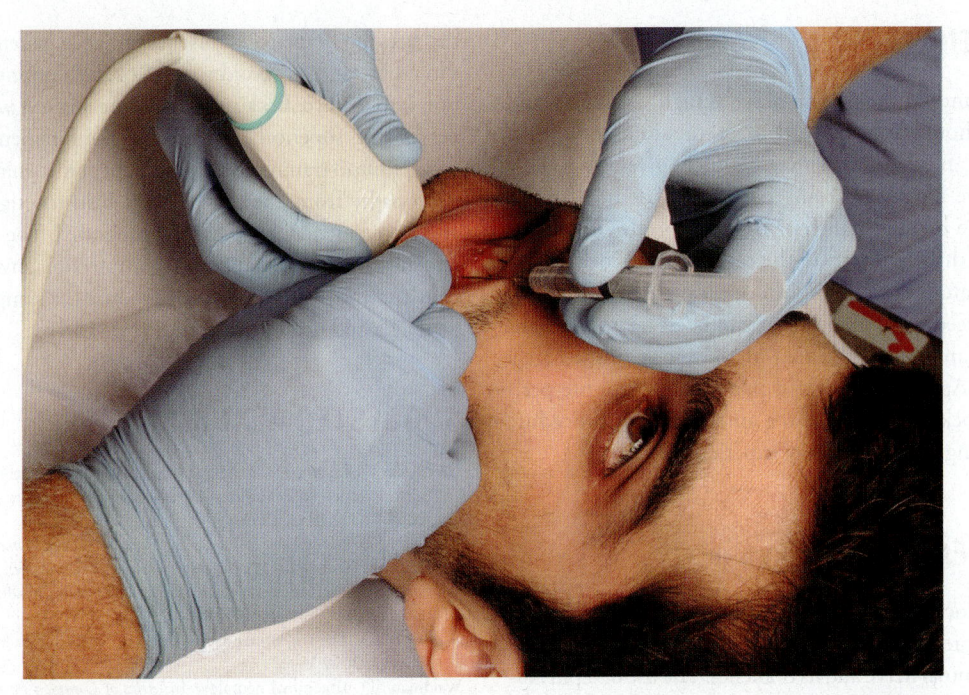

**FIGURE 12.9.** The needle is placed through the previously anesthetized area and advanced under real-time ultrasound guidance in an out-of-plane trajectory toward the mental nerve.

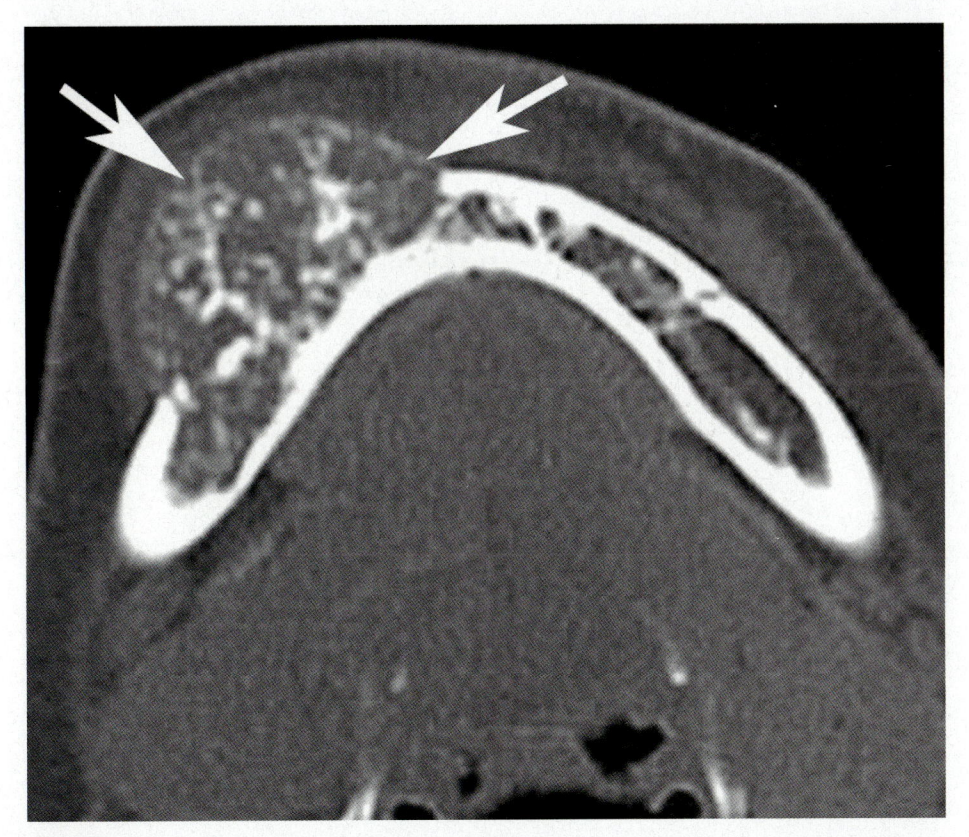

**FIGURE 12.10.** Aggressive ameloblastoma. Expansile enhancing lesion within the right mandibular body (*arrows*) that causes significant buccal cortical destruction. (Courtesy of Akifumi Fujita, M.D., Jichi Medical University, Shimotsuke, Japan.) (Reused from Eisenberg RL. *Clinical Imaging*. 5th ed. Philadelphia, PA: Lippincott Williams & Wilkins, 2010: 1384, with permission.)

## COMPLICATIONS

The area surrounding the mental nerve is highly vascular, and the clinician should carefully calculate the total milligram dosage of local anesthetic that may be safely given, especially if bilateral nerve blocks are being performed. Because of the proximity of the mental branch of the inferior alveolar artery combined with the vascularity of the regions, postblock ecchymosis and hematoma formation can occur even in the best of hands. These bleeding complications can be decreased if manual pressure is applied to the area of the block immediately after injection. Application of cold packs for 20-minute periods after the block also decreases the amount of postprocedure pain and bleeding the patient may experience.

## CLINICAL PEARLS

Mental nerve block is especially useful in the palliation of pain secondary to acute herpes zoster involving the mandibular division of the trigeminal nerve and its branches. The use of tepid aluminum acetate solution applied as a soak can speed the drying of the weeping herpetic lesions and enhance patient comfort. Care should be taken to avoid spillage of the aluminum acetate solution into the eye. Because of the acute angle at which the mental nerves turn superiorly after exiting the foramen, it is extremely susceptible to trauma and entrapment at this point. Compression neuropathy from anesthesia masks held too tightly against the area of the mental nerve has been reported. The clinician should remember that trauma, tumors, or infection anywhere along the course of the mental nerve can produce the symptoms of mental neuralgia and must be ruled out (Fig. 12.10).

## SUGGESTED READINGS

Greenstein G, Tarnow D. The mental foramen and nerve: clinical and anatomical factors related to dental implant placement: a literature review. *J Periodontol* 2006;77(12):1933–1943.

Waldman SD. Mental nerve block. In: *Atlas of Interventional Pain Management*. 3rd ed. Philadelphia, PA: Saunders Elsevier; 2009:66–69.

Waldman SD. Mental nerve block. In: *Pain Review*. Philadelphia, PA: Saunders Elsevier; 2009:404–405.

Waldman SD. The trigeminal nerve. In: *Pain Review*. Philadelphia, PA: Saunders Elsevier; 2009:15–17.

Waldman SD. Trigeminal neuralgia. In: *Atlas of Common Pain Syndromes*. 3rd ed. Philadelphia, PA: Saunders Elsevier; 2011:29–32.

# CHAPTER 13

# Ultrasound-Guided Temporomandibular Joint Injection

## CLINICAL PERSPECTIVES

Ultrasound-guided temporomandibular joint (TMJ) injection is useful in the diagnosis and management of a variety of painful disorders of the TMJ including arthritis, myofascial pain, and TMJ disk dysfunction (Fig. 13.1; Table 13.1). This technique can be utilized to inject autologous blood into the joint when treating joint hypermobility and recurrent joint dislocation as well as to inject viscosupplementation agents such as hyaluronic acid derivatives. Recently, the use of botulinum toxin injections to treat TMJ disk dysfunction has been advocated when more conservative treatment options have failed to provide palliation of the patient's pain and joint dysfunction. Internal derangement of the intra-articular disk may manifest itself clinically as popping, clicking, catching, or locking of the joint (see Fig. 13.1). Dental malocclusion or bruxism may exacerbate these problems. Patients suffering from TMJ pain may also complain of otalgia and headache, which is often worse in the morning in contradistinction to tension-type headache that often worsens as the day progresses.

## CLINICALLY RELEVANT ANATOMY

The TMJ is a ginglymoarthrodial joint, meaning that it is a two-compartment joint (Fig. 13.2). Like the sternoclavicular joint, the TMJ has two synovial-lined compartments divided by a fibroelastic cartilaginous articular disk (Fig. 13.3). When the mouth initially opens, the movement occurs primarily in the lower compartment of the joint as the condylar head rotates. As the mouth opens more widely, the upper compartment begins to function by allowing a secondary forward and downward gliding motion known as translation. The intra-articular disk changes position during mouth opening, and internal derangement of this disk may result in pain and TMJ dysfunction (Fig. 13.4). It should be noted that extracapsular causes of TMJ pain are much more common than internal disk derangement. The sensory innervation of the TMJ is provided by branches of the mandibular nerve. The muscles involved in TMJ dysfunction include the temporalis, masseter, and external pterygoid and internal pterygoid muscles, which are innervated by motor fibers of the mandibular nerve and may also include the trapezius and sternocleidomastoid (Fig. 13.5). Trigger points may be identified when palpating these muscles. The articular joint space between the mandibular condyle and the glenoid fossa of the zygoma is easily accessible for injection utilizing the ultrasound-guided technique described below.

## ULTRASOUND-GUIDED TECHNIQUE

Ultrasound-guided TMJ injection is a straightforward technique if attention is paid to the clinical relevant anatomy. To perform ultrasound-guided TMJ injection, the patient is placed in the supine position with the cervical spine in the neutral position. The TMJ is identified by drawing an imaginary line between the tragus of the ear and the ala of the nose (Camper line) (Fig. 13.6). The joint is then identified by gentle palpation along this line while the patient open and closes his or her mouth (Fig. 13.7). Once the TMJ is identified, the patient is asked to close his or her mouth, but not to clench their teeth. The skin overlying the TMJ is prepped with antiseptic solution, and a high-frequency linear transducer is placed directly over the joint in a transverse position (Fig. 13.8). The TMJ should be readily apparent with the acoustic shadow of the curved bony mandibular condyle and mandibular neck just below it (Fig. 13.9). In order to most clearly see the joint space, the ultrasound transducer may need to be tilted slightly in a cephalad or caudad direction to align the ultrasound beam in a true perpendicular plane relative to the joint.

A total of 0.5 mL of local anesthetic is drawn up in a 3-mL sterile syringe. When treating TMJ dysfunction, internal derangement of the TMJ, arthritis pain of the TMJ, or other painful conditions involving the TMJ that are thought to have an inflammatory component, 10 to 20 mg of depot corticosteroid is added to the local anesthetic. Under real-time ultrasound guidance, a 22-gauge, 1½-inch needle is inserted into the previously identified joint using an out-of-plane approach (Fig. 13.10). It should be noted that the joint space is relatively superficial with a depth of half to three-fourth of an inch. The clinician may appreciate a pop when the joint is entered. After careful aspiration, 1 mL of solution is slowly injected.

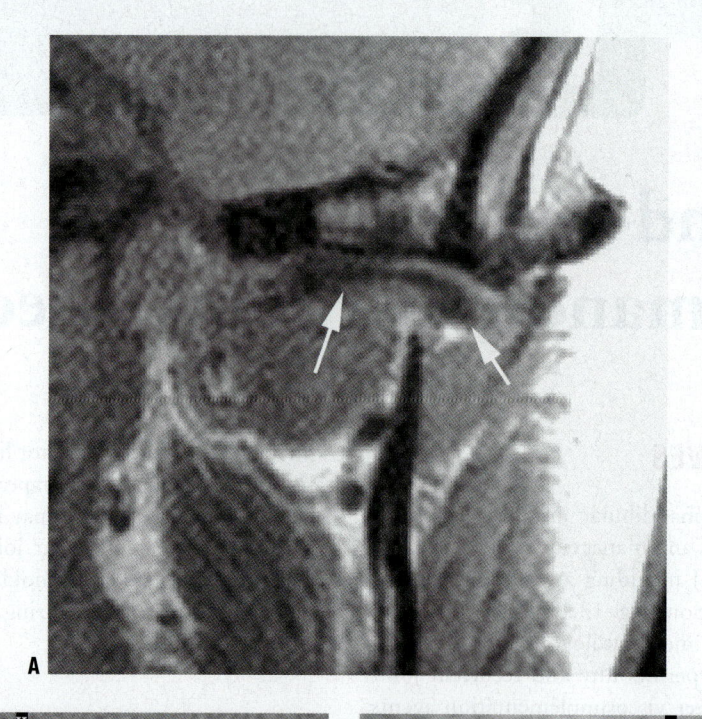

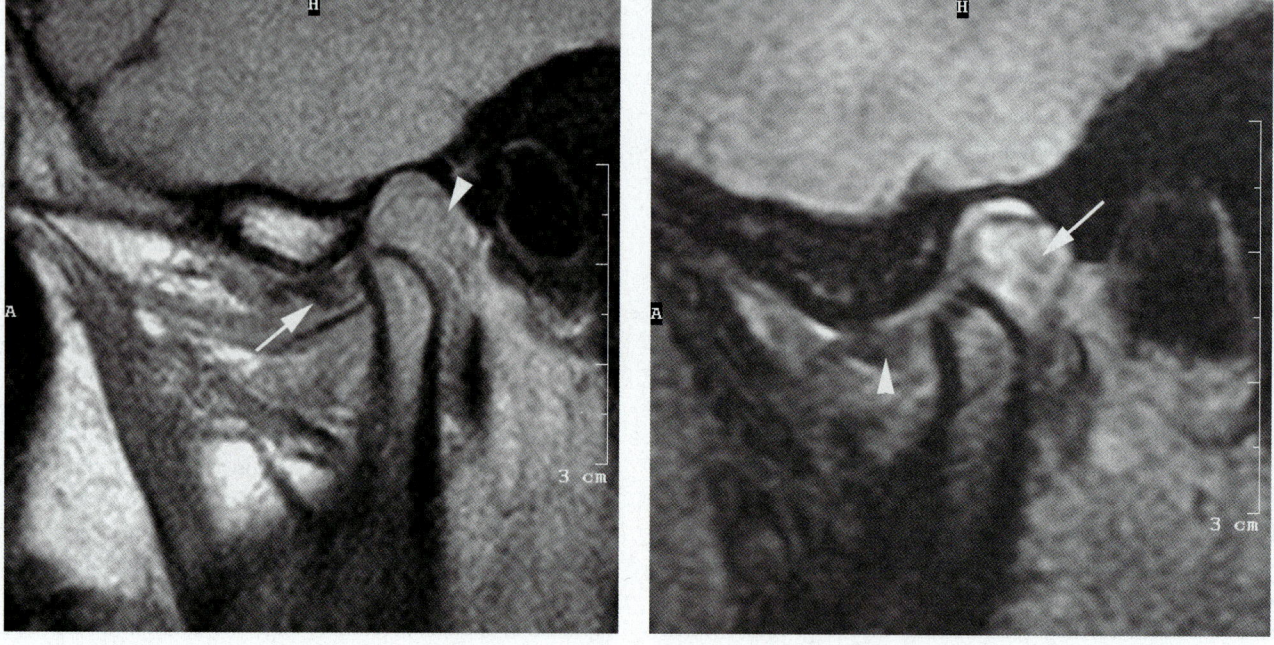

**FIGURE 13.1.** A patient presenting with TMJ pain. **A:** T1-weighted (T1W) coronal image showing the anteriorly dislocated articular disk (*arrows*). **B:** Sagittal T1W image showing limited opening with lack of recapture of the articular disk (*arrow*) and what appears to be a relatively normal appearance of the bilaminar zone (*arrowhead*). **C:** T2-weighted image in the open position again showing the displaced articular disk (*arrowhead*), but the bilaminar zone (*arrow*) is obviously edematous. (Reused from Mancuso AA, Pettigrew JC, Nair MK, et al. Temporomandibular joint: introduction, general principles, and internal derangements. In: Mancuso AA, Hanafee WN, eds. *Head and Neck Radiology*. Vol. 1. Philadelphia, PA: Lippincott Williams & Wilkins; 2011:574, with permission.)

| TABLE 13.1 | Common Causes of TMJ Pain and Dysfunction |
|---|---|

- Arthritis
- Myofascial pain
- Capsulitis
- Trauma
- Myositis
- Neuralgia
- Disk derangement
- Synovitis
- Tumor
- Malocclusion

Injection of the joint may be repeated in 5- to 7-day intervals if the symptoms persist.

## COMPLICATIONS

This anatomic region is highly vascular, and the potential for significant facial hematoma formation and ecchymosis exists, and the patient should be warned of such. The vascularity of the region means that the pain specialist should carefully aspirate the needle prior to injecting any medications and should then inject small, incremental doses of local anesthetic to avoid local anesthetic toxicity. Should the needle inadvertently be advanced through the TMJ, the facial nerve (cranial nerve VII) may be blocked resulting in facial paralysis, which can be distressing for the clinician and patient alike if the cause is not quickly ascertained.

## CLINICAL PEARLS

Ultrasound-guided TMJ injection with local anesthetic and steroid represents an excellent option in the treatment of patients suffering from TMJ pain and dysfunction. It can be used in the acute setting to provide pain relieve while waiting for pharmacotherapy to take effect. The vascular nature of this anatomic region mandates care when injecting local anesthetics into the area. Careful gentle aspiration and attention to the total milligram dose of local anesthetic is crucial to avoid complications.

Small punctate facial scars secondary to needle trauma to the skin overlying the joint may occur, and the patient

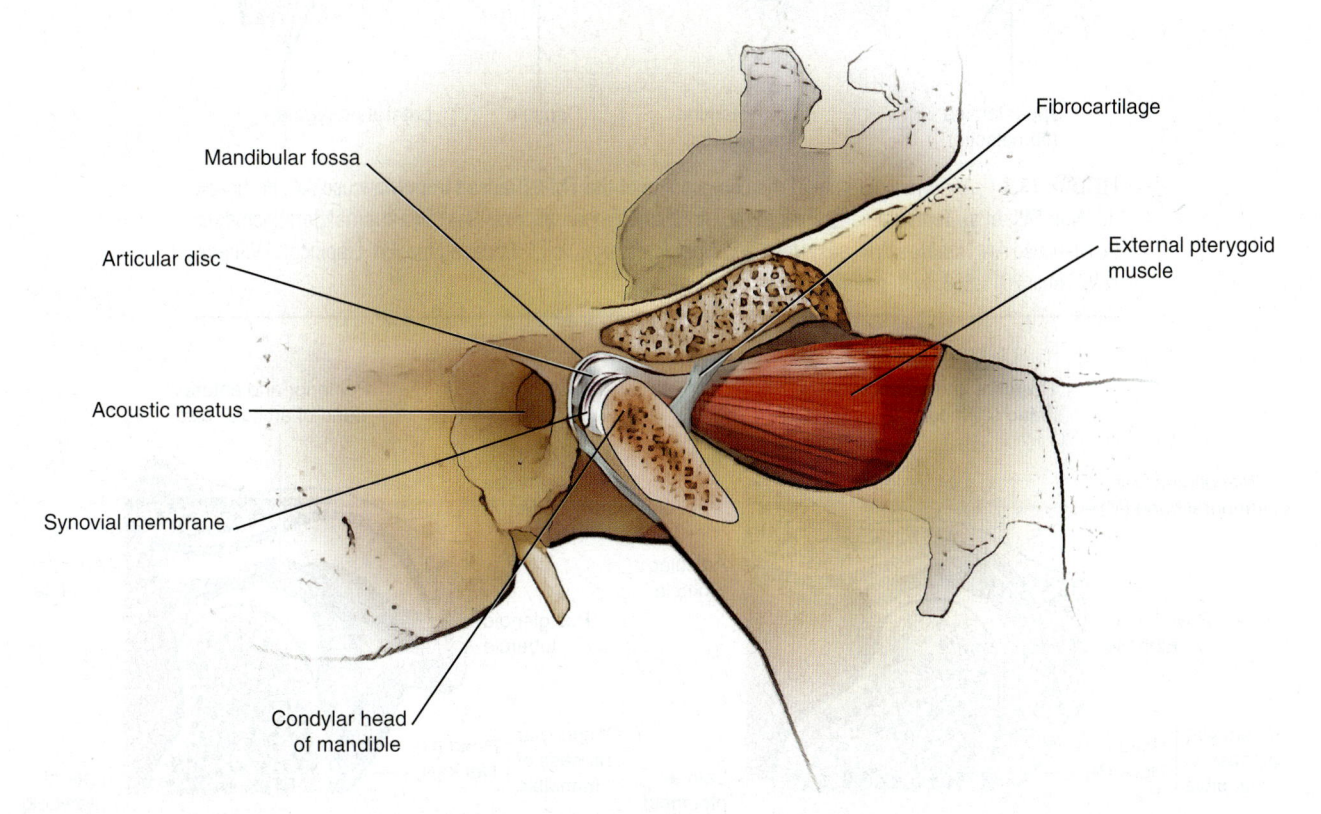

**FIGURE 13.2.** Anatomy of the TMJ. (Modified from *Stedman's Medical Dictionary.* 27th ed. Baltimore, MD: Lippincott Williams & Wilkins; 2000, with permission.)

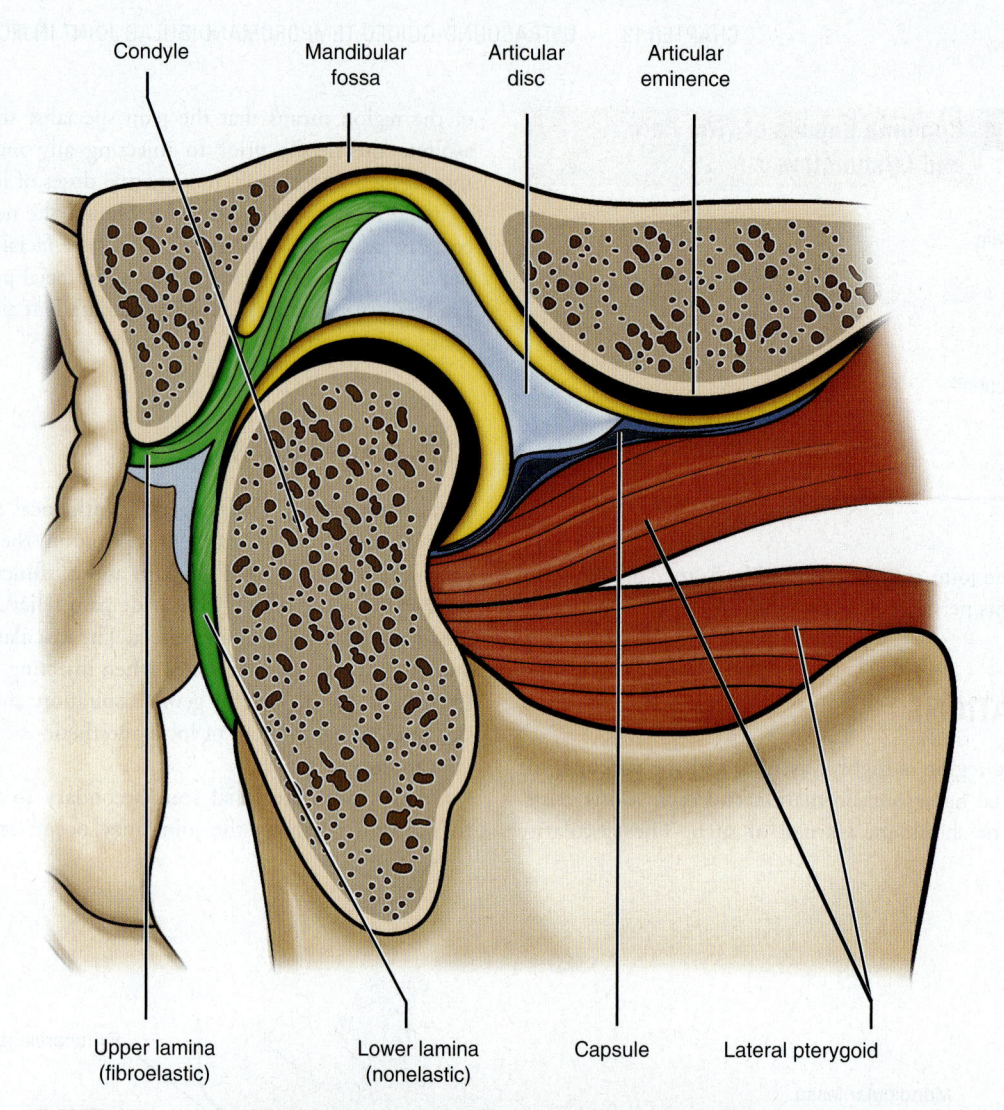

**FIGURE 13.3.** Anatomic diagram of the components of the TMJ. (Reused from Mancuso AA, Pettigrew JC, Nair MK, et al. Temporomandibular joint: introduction, general principles, and internal derangements. In: Mancuso AA, Hanafee WN, eds. *Head and Neck Radiology*. Vol. 1. Philadelphia, PA: Lippincott Williams & Wilkins; 2011:568, with permission.)

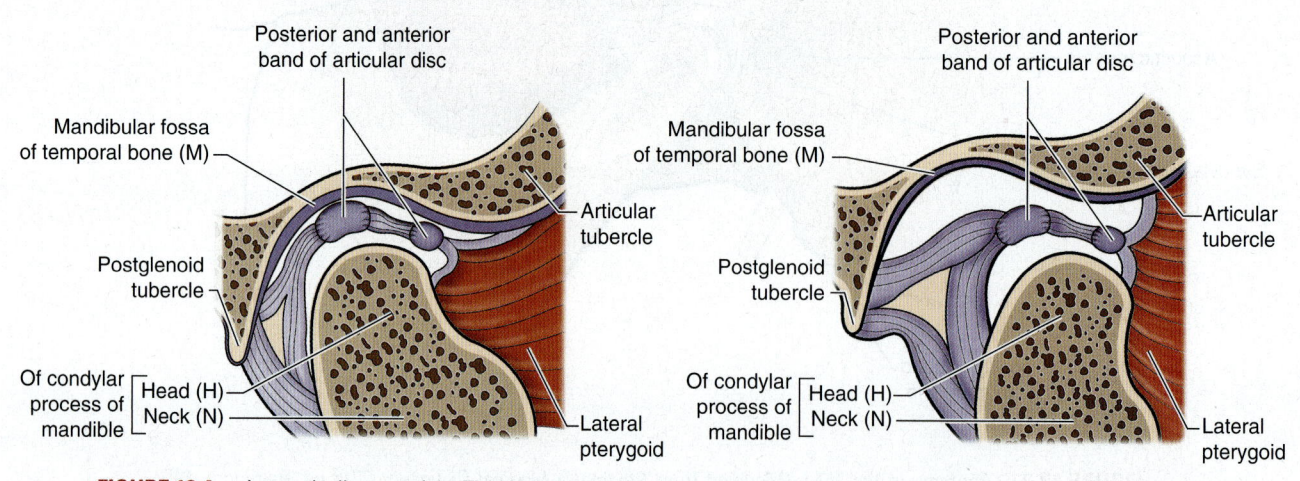

**FIGURE 13.4.** Anatomic diagram of the TMJ in the open and closed position. The particular relationships of interest are that of the condylar head and articular disk and their relationship to the bilaminar zone and joint spaces. (Reused from Mancuso AA, Pettigrew JC, Nair MK, et al. Temporomandibular joint: introduction, general principles, and internal derangements. In: Mancuso AA, Hanafee WN, eds. *Head and Neck Radiology*. Vol. 1. Philadelphia, PA: Lippincott Williams & Wilkins; 2011:569, with permission.)

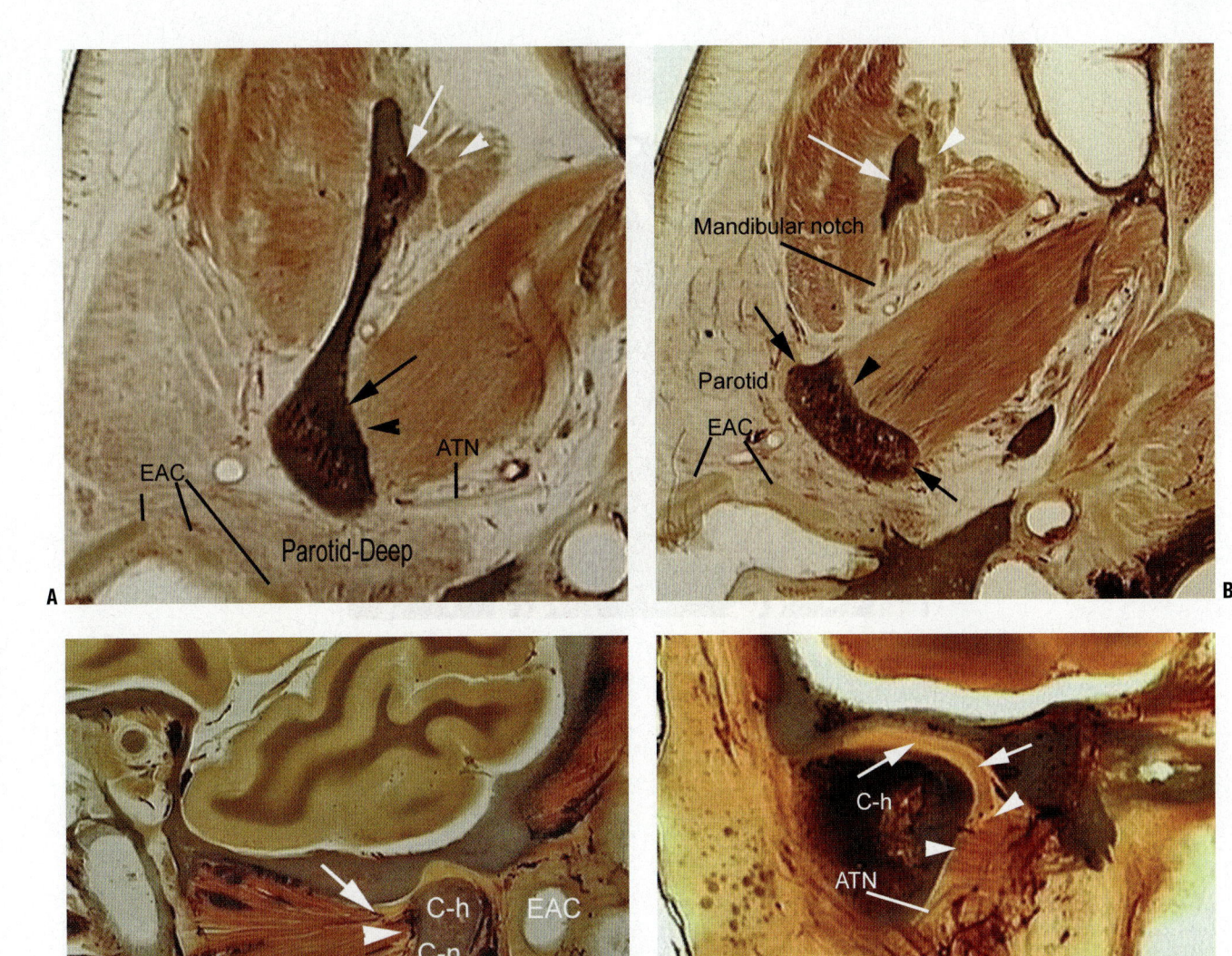

**FIGURE 13.5.** A series of whole-organ sections to illustrate important relationships of and around the TMJ. **A:** Axial section at the junction of the condylar head and neck showing the fovea region (*arrow*) and the attachment of the lateral pterygoid muscle along the condyle (*arrowhead*). It is at this level that the auriculotemporal nerve (ATN) ramifies from the mandibular nerve toward its distal points of innervations. Important anatomic landmarks at this level include the cartilage portion of the external auditory canal (EAC) and deep portion of the parotid gland (parotid deep). **B:** A section at the level of the condylar head more cephalad than in (A). Medial and lateral poles of the condylar head are shown by the *black arrows*. The medial pterygoid muscle attaches at the junction of the condylar head and neck (*black arrowhead*). The coronoid process of the mandible (*white arrow*) is a point of attachment of the temporalis muscle tendon (*white arrowhead*). The parotid gland is situated just laterally, its capsule tightly adherent to the cartilage portion of the external auditory canal (EAC). **C:** Oblique whole-organ section showing the condylar head (C-h) situated within the mandibular fossa. The lateral pterygoid muscle attaches to the TMJ capsule (*arrow*). The other bellies of the lateral pterygoid muscle (*arrowheads*) attach to the condylar neck (C-n). As in (A) and (B), note the very close relationship of the external auditory canal to the TMJ. **D:** Coronal section through the TMJ. The articular disk lies slightly more medial than lateral (*white arrows*). At the margin of the disk is the attachment of the superior belly of the lateral pterygoid muscle to the joint capsule (*arrowheads*). The auriculotemporal nerve (ATN) is generally located near the transition from the condylar head (C-h) to its neck.

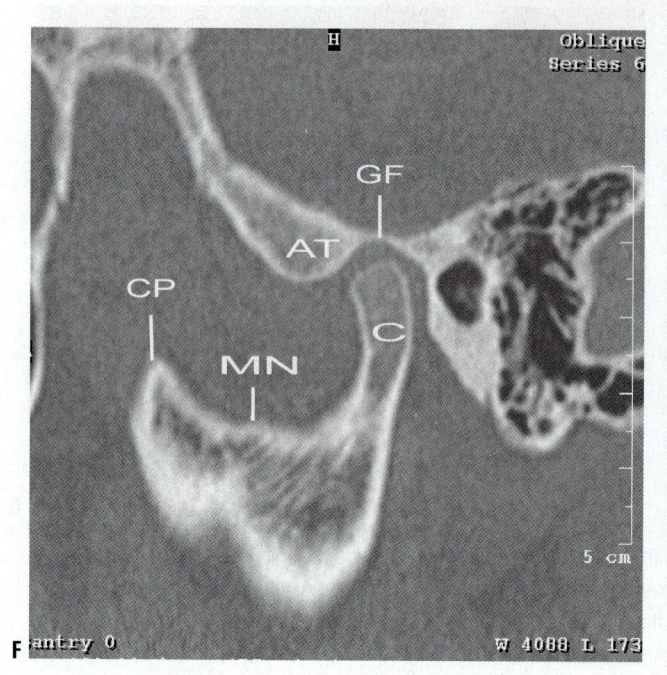

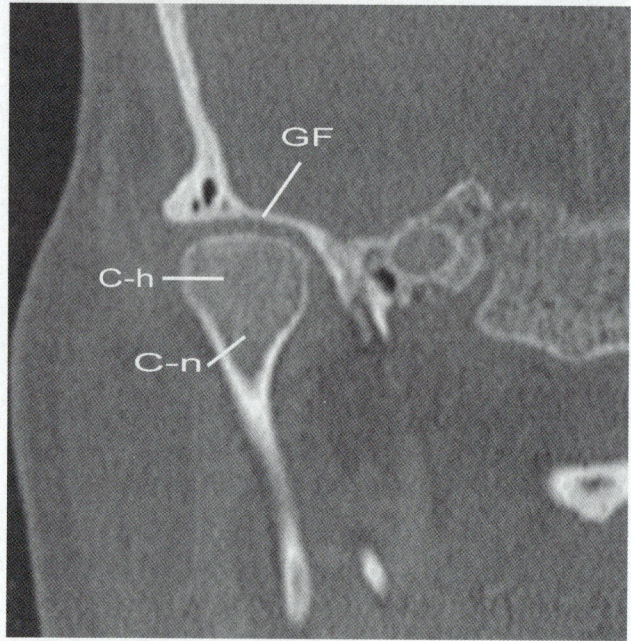

**FIGURE 13.5.** (*Continued*) **E:** Magnified section of the TMJ as originally seen in (C). The anterior and posterior bands (*white arrowheads*) are connected by the thin portion (*arrow*) of the disk. The bilaminar zone is composed of fibrovascular tissue. Note the attachments of the pterygoid muscles as pointed out in (C). **F,G:** Two computed tomography sections illustrating bony anatomy of the TMJ. In (F), the sagittal reformations show the condyle (C) within the glenoid or mandibular fossa (GF). The articular tubercle (AT) is at the anterior limit of the TMJ. The mandibular notch (MN) is between the coronoid process (CP) and the condylar head. In (G), the coronal reformations show the relationship of the glenoid fossa (GF) to the condylar head (C-h) and condylar neck (C-n). (Reused from Mancuso AA, Pettigrew JC, Nair MK, et al. Temporomandibular joint: introduction, general principles, and internal derangements. In: Mancuso AA, Hanafee WN, eds. *Head and Neck Radiology*. Vol. 1. Philadelphia, PA: Lippincott Williams & Wilkins; 2011:569–571, with permission.)

CHAPTER 13   ULTRASOUND-GUIDED TEMPOROMANDIBULAR JOINT INJECTION

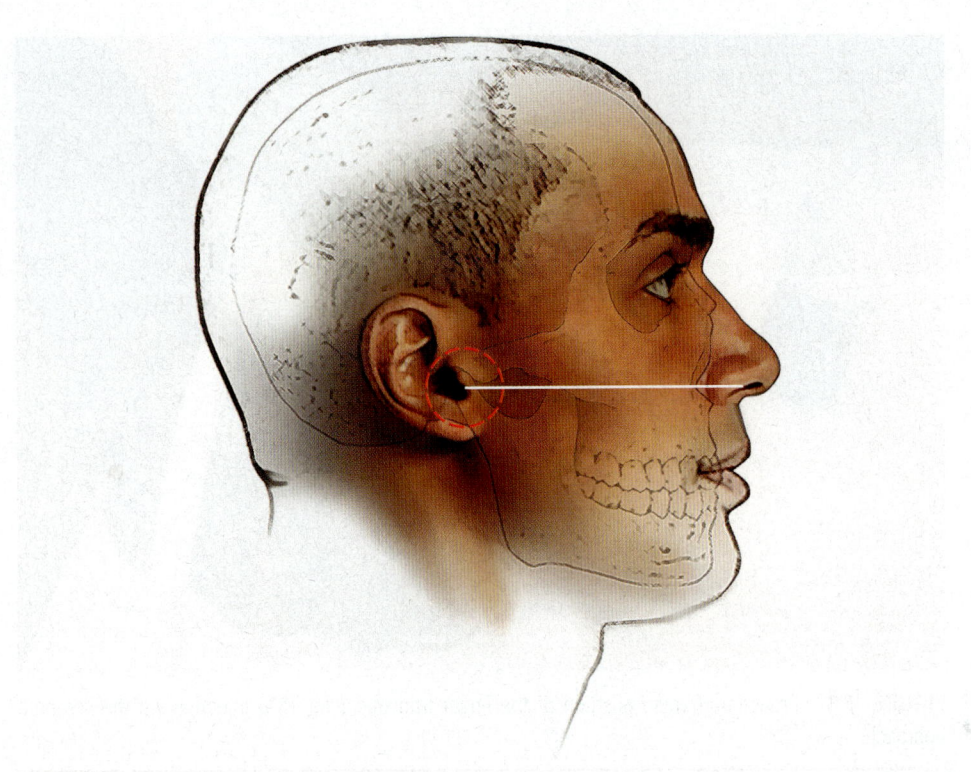

**FIGURE 13.6.** To locate the TMJ, an imaginary line is drawn from the ala of the nose to the tragus of the ear. This line is known as Camper line.

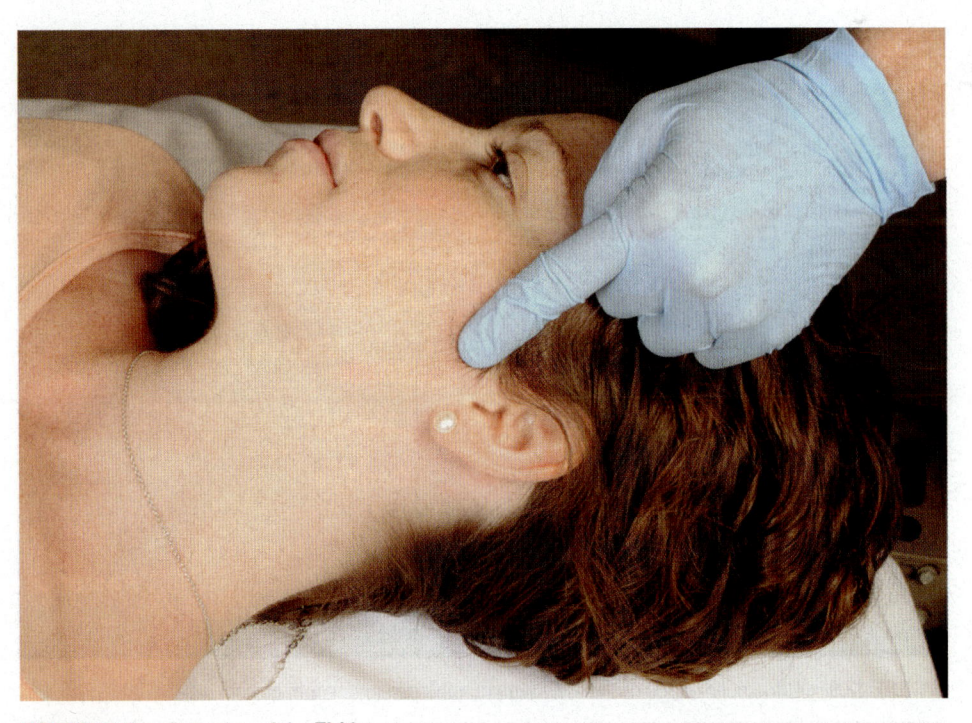

**FIGURE 13.7.** Palpation of the TMJ.

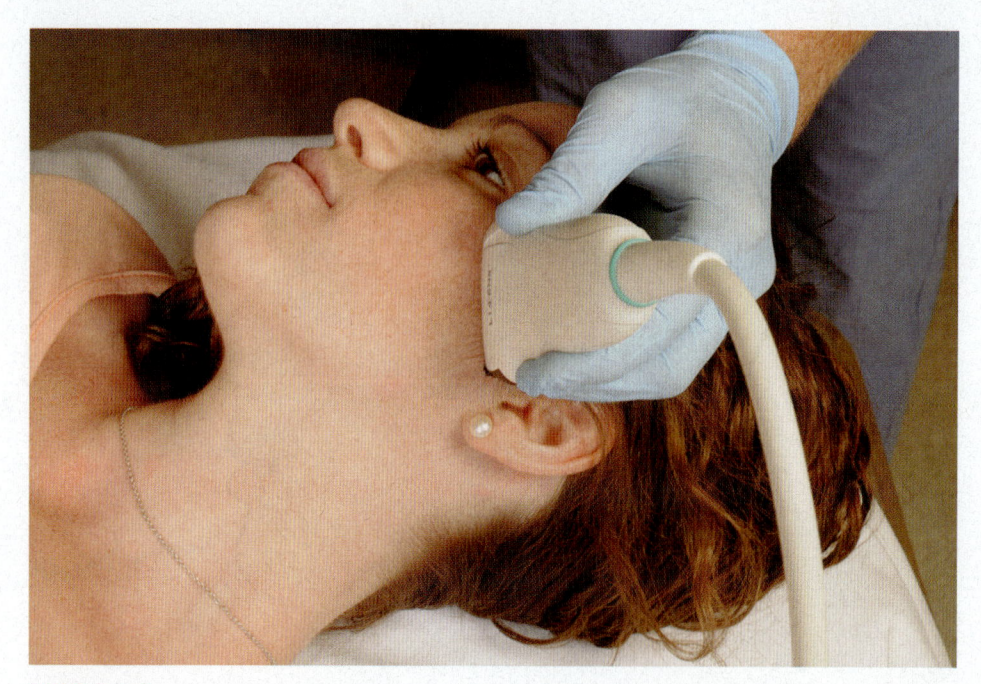

**FIGURE 13.8.** Proper transverse position of the linear transducer for TMJ injection via the coronoid approach.

should be warned of this possibility. Infection, although rare, remains an ever-present possibility, especially in the immunocompromised patient. Early detection of infection is crucial to avoid potential life-threatening sequelae including spread of the infection to the central nervous system. Unexplained pain in this anatomic region requires careful evaluation as pathology anywhere along the path of the nerve may cause pain (Fig. 13.11).

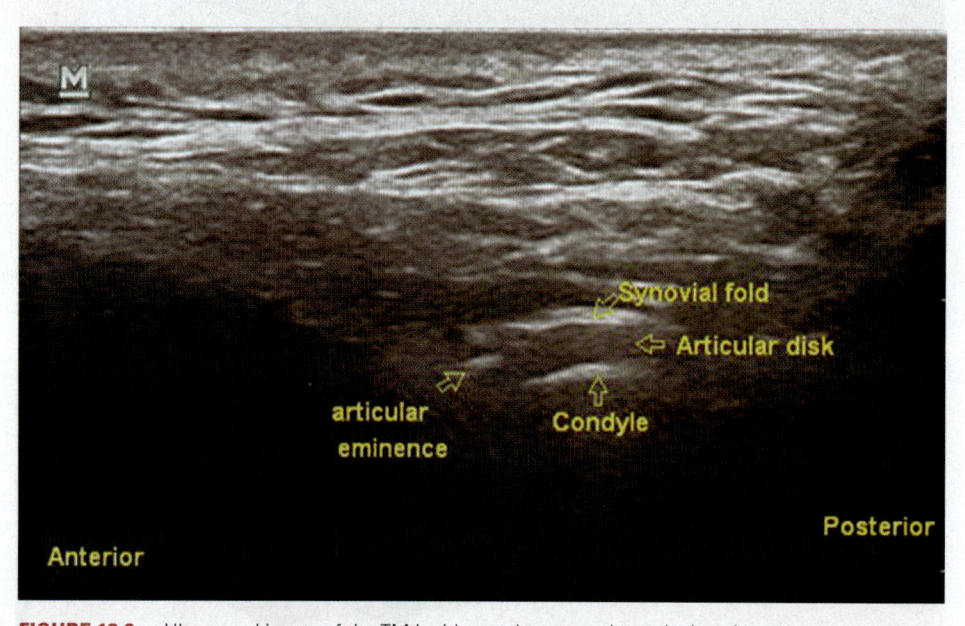

**FIGURE 13.9.** Ultrasound image of the TMJ with mouth open and mouth closed.

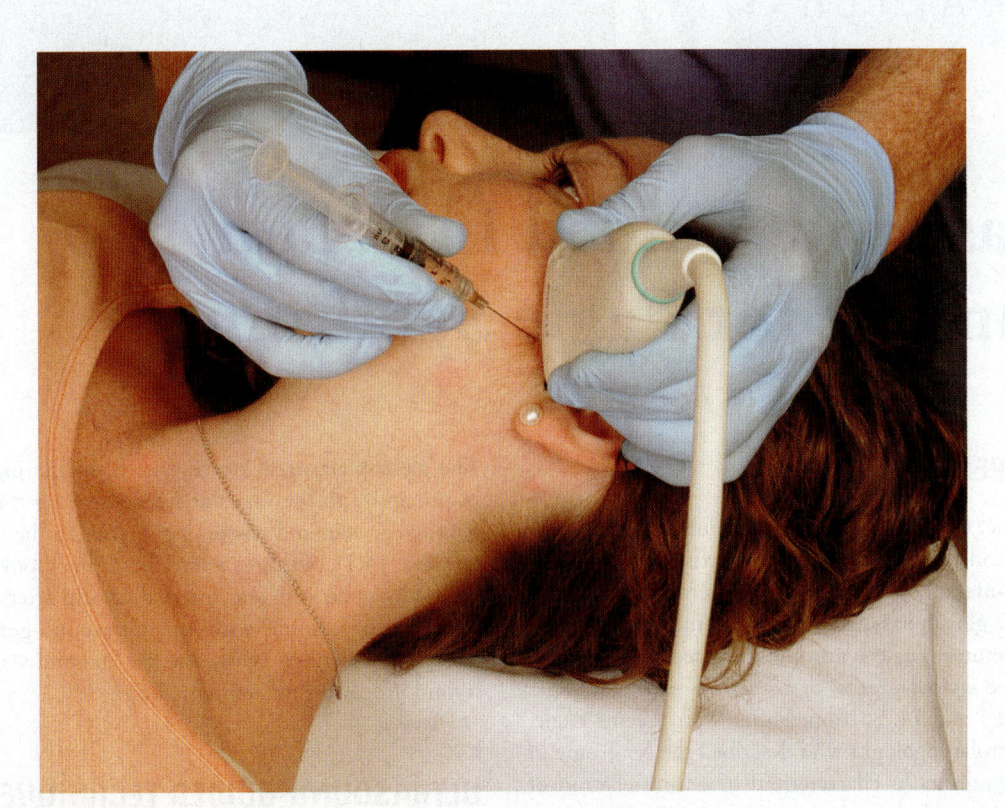

**FIGURE 13.10.** Out-of-plane approach for ultrasound-guided TMJ injection.

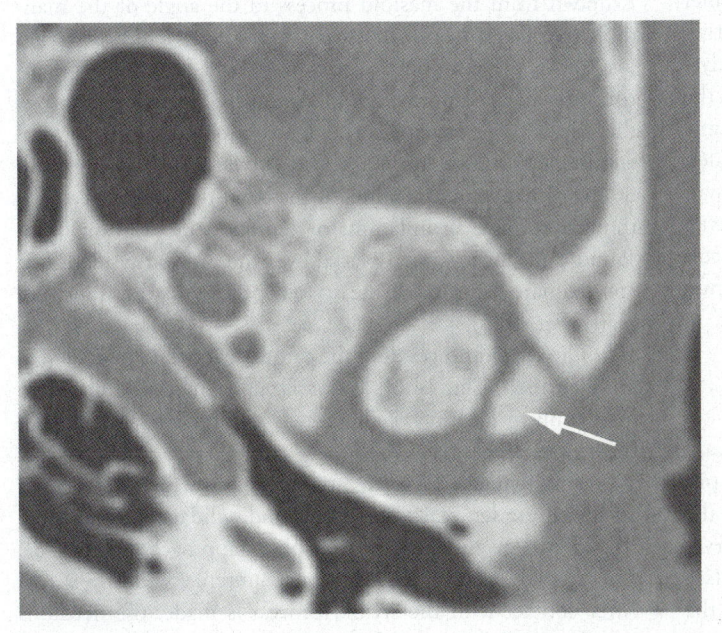

**FIGURE 13.11.** This patient presented with otalgia but not specifically with signs of TMJ dysfunction. Eventually, the ear pain was shown to be due to this loose body (*arrow*), an area of osteitis dissecans. Following this study, the patient remembered a prior episode of TMJ trauma. The fragment was removed and the ear pain resolved. (Reused from Mancuso AA, Pettigrew JC, Nair MK, et al. Temporomandibular joint: inflammatory, degenerative, and traumatic conditions. In: Mancuso AA, Hanafee WN, eds. *Head and Neck Radiology*. Vol. 1. Philadelphia, PA: Lippincott Williams & Wilkins; 2011:588, with permission.)

## SUGGESTED READINGS

Waldman SD. The temporomandibular joint. In: *Pain Review*. Philadelphia, PA: Saunders Elsevier; 2009:42–43.

Waldman SD. Atypical facial pain. In: *Atlas of Common Pain Syndromes*. 3rd ed. Philadelphia, PA: Saunders Elsevier; 2011:36–38.

Waldman SD. Temporomandibular joint dysfunction. In: *Atlas of Common Pain Syndromes*. 3rd ed. Philadelphia, PA: Saunders Elsevier; 2011:33–35.

Waldman SD. Temporomandibular joint injection. In: *Atlas of Pain Management Injection Techniques*. 3rd ed. Philadelphia, PA: Saunders Elsevier; 2013:1–3.

# Ultrasound-Guided Injection Technique for Eagle Syndrome

## CLINICAL PERSPECTIVES

Eagle syndrome, which is also known as stylohyoid syndrome, is caused by compression of various structures of the neck including the internal carotid artery, the internal jugular vein, branches of the glossopharyngeal nerve, and their surrounding anatomic structures. Eagle syndrome is caused by an abnormally elongated styloid process or a calcified stylohyoid ligament (Figs. 14.1 and 14.2). Named after Watt Weems Eagle, an American otolaryngologist who described the syndrome in 1937, Eagle syndrome is characterized by a constellation of symptoms which include a sharp stabbing pain that occurs with turning of the neck or mandible. The pain starts below the angle of the mandible and radiates into the tonsillar fossa, temporomandibular joint, and the base of the tongue. A trigger point may be present in the tonsillar fossa in a manner analogous to glossopharyngeal neuralgia. Patients suffering from Eagle syndrome may also complain of otalgia, dysphagia, and tinnitus. Eagle syndrome is a syndrome of the third to fifth decade although the syndrome can occur at any age. Eagle syndrome is slightly more common in females. The ultrasound-guided injection technique for Eagle syndrome serves as both a diagnostic and therapeutic maneuver. Ultimately, surgical resection of the elongated styloid process and/or calcified stylohyoid ligament may be required to cure the syndrome.

## CLINICALLY RELEVANT ANATOMY

The word styloid is derived from the Greek word for pillar, *stylos*. The temporal styloid process extends from the temporal bone in a caudad and ventral direction and serves as the cephalad attachment of the stylohyoid ligament (see Figs. 14.1 and 14.2). The ligament attaches caudally to the hyoid bone. Patients suffering from Eagle syndrome have either an abnormally elongated styloid process or a calcified stylohyoid ligament which in certain positions of the head and neck has the potential to compress the internal carotid artery, the internal jugular vein, branches of the glossopharyngeal nerve, and surrounding structures (Figs. 14.3 and 14.4).

The glossopharyngeal nerve exits from the jugular foramen in proximity to the vagus and accessory nerve and the internal jugular vein and passes just inferior to the styloid process (see Fig. 14.1). All three nerves lie in the groove between the internal jugular vein and internal carotid artery. When treating Eagle syndrome with the ultrasound-guided injection technique described below, the key anatomic landmark is the styloid process of the temporal bone.

## ULTRASOUND-GUIDED TECHNIQUE

To perform ultrasound-guided injection technique for Eagle syndrome, place the patient in supine position with the head turned away from the side to be blocked. An imaginary line is drawn from the mastoid process to the angle of the mandible (see Fig. 14.1). In most patients, the styloid process lies just above the midpoint of this line. After preliminary identification of the approximate location of the styloid process, the skin is prepped with antiseptic solution and 5 mL of local anesthetic is drawn up in a 10-mL sterile syringe, with 40 to 80 mg of depot steroid added if the condition being treated is thought to have an inflammatory component. A linear ultrasound transducer is then placed over the previously identified approximate location of the styloid process in the transverse plane (Fig. 14.5).

The styloid process and the carotid artery and jugular vein are identified (Fig. 14.6). Color Doppler may be utilized to help confirm location of the vessels and their relationship to the styloid process (Fig. 14.7).

A 22-gauge, 3½-inch styletted spinal needle is then advanced under real-time ultrasound guidance toward the styloid process using an out-of-plane approach (Fig. 14.8). The styloid process should be encountered within ~3 cm. After contact with the styloid process is made, the needle is withdrawn slightly out of the periosteum or substance of the calcified ligament. After careful aspiration reveals no blood or cerebrospinal fluid, 5 mL of solution should be slowly injected. The needle is removed and pressure is placed on the injection site to avoid bleeding complications. Subsequent daily nerve blocks are carried out in a similar manner.

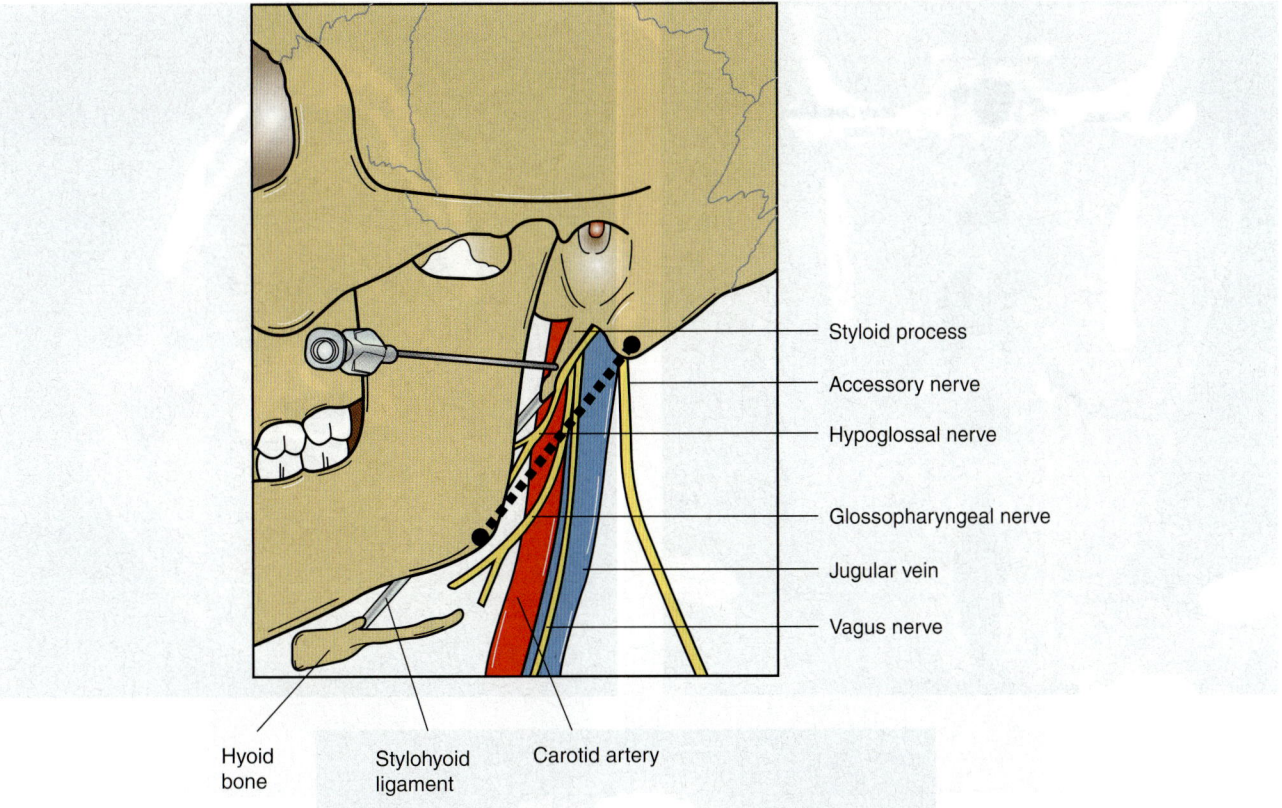

**FIGURE 14.1.** The anatomy of the styloid process and stylohyoid ligament and their surrounding anatomic structures.

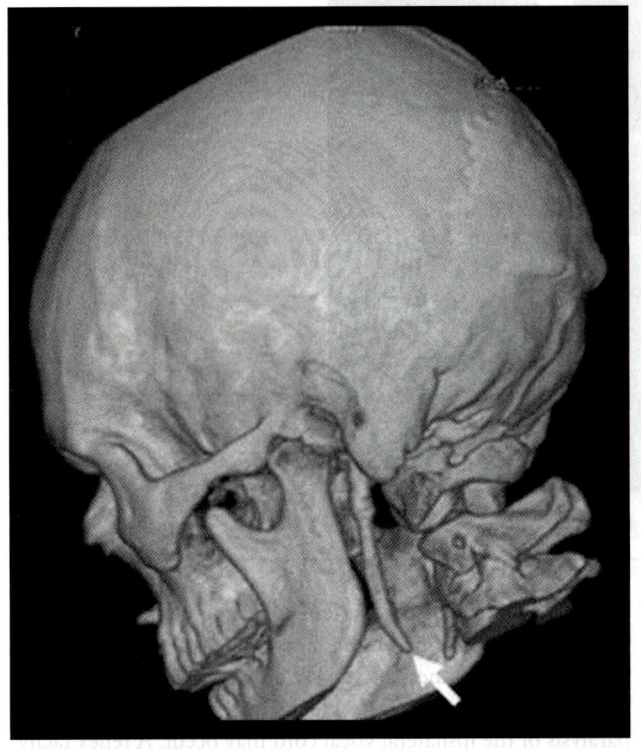

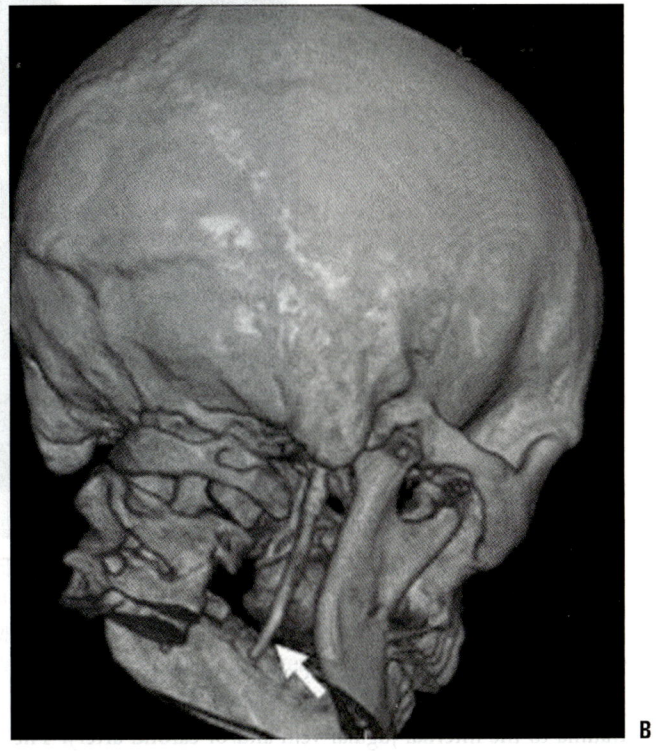

**FIGURE 14.2.** **A–E:** Bilateral hypertrophied styloid processes as shown with three-dimensional computed tomography (CT) scan. (Reused from Dashti SR, Nakaji P, Hu Y, et al. Styloidogenic jugular venous compression syndrome: diagnosis and treatment: case report. *Neurosurgery* 2012;70(3):E795–E799, with permission.)

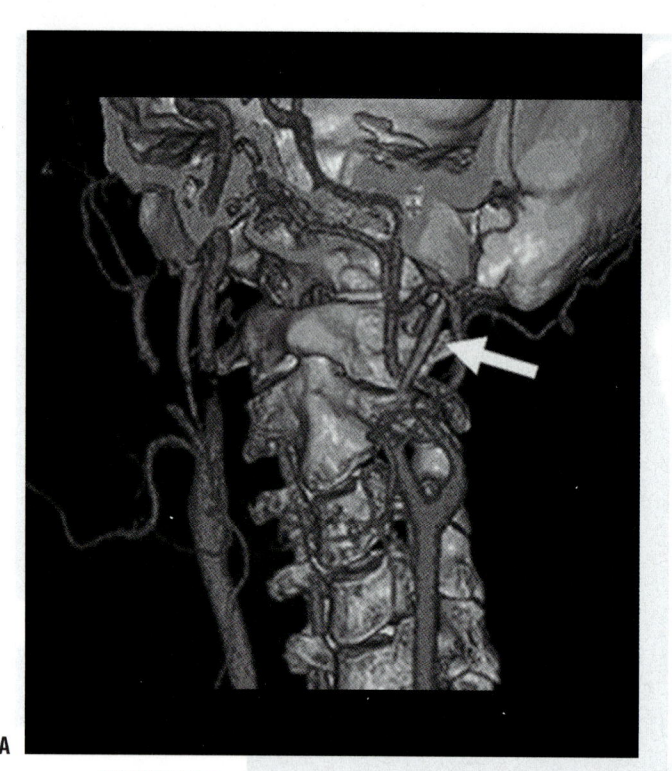

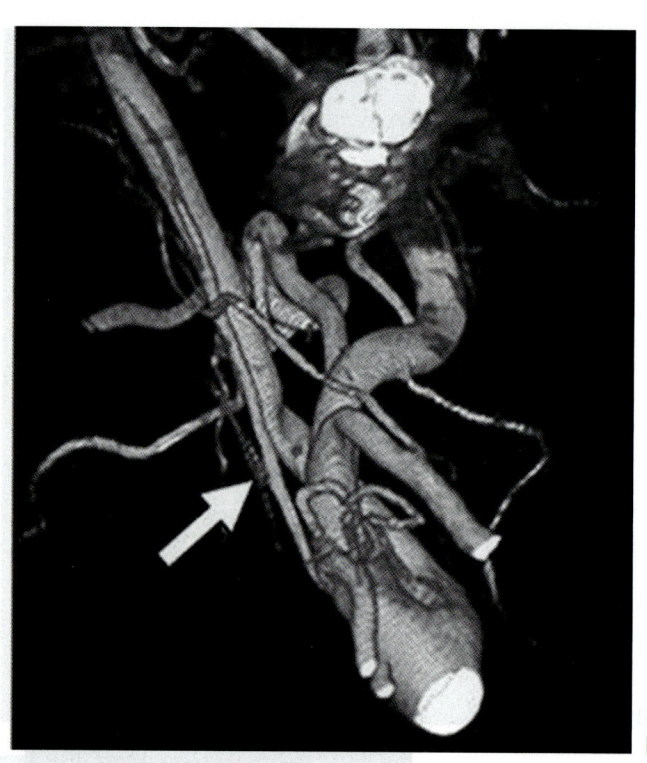

**FIGURE 14.4** **A:** Three-dimensional computed tomography. Bilateral elongated styloid processes (right, 38 mm; left, 35 mm). The styloid process (*arrow*) and internal carotid artery (ICA) crossed at the lower level of C1. **B:** With the patient's neck flexed, three-dimensional angiography showed a compressive dent in the cervical portion of the left ICA (*arrow*) caused by the styloid process. (Reused from Nakagawa D, Ota T, Iijima A, et al. Diagnosis of eagle syndrome with 3-dimensional angiography and near-infrared spectroscopy: case report. *Neurosurgery* 2011;68(3):E847–E849, with permission.)

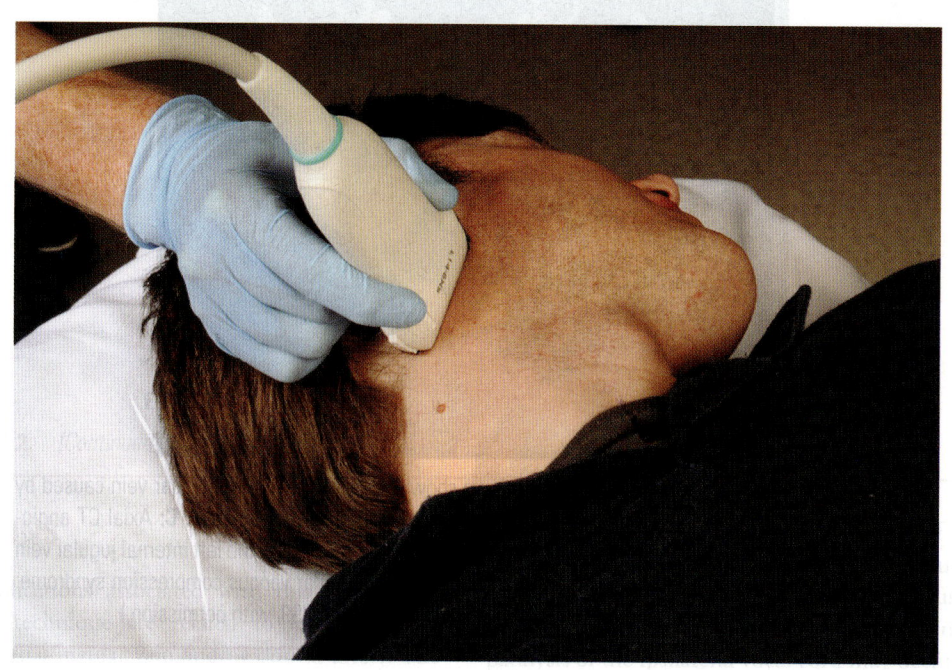

**FIGURE 14.5.** Proper placement of the linear ultrasound transducer over the previously identified styloid process.

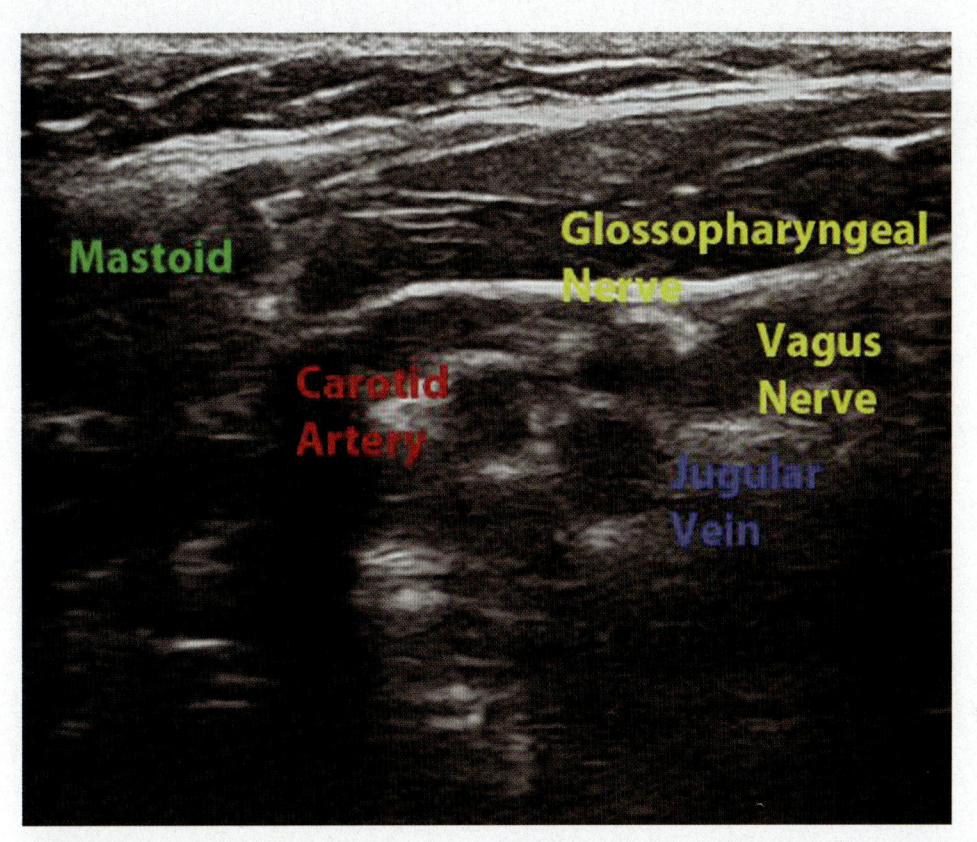

**FIGURE 14.6.** Transverse ultrasound image demonstrating the relationship of the carotid artery, jugular vein, glossopharyngeal nerve, and vagus nerve to the mastoid bone.

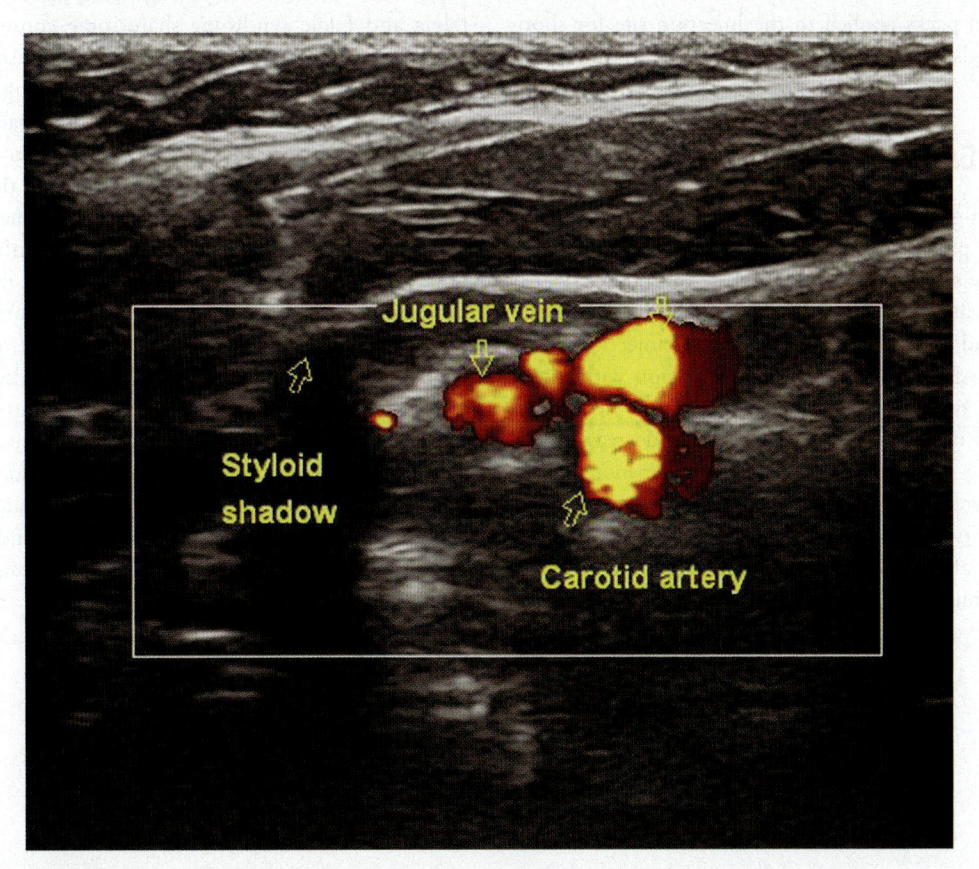

**FIGURE 14.7.** Color Doppler image of the carotid artery and jugular vein.

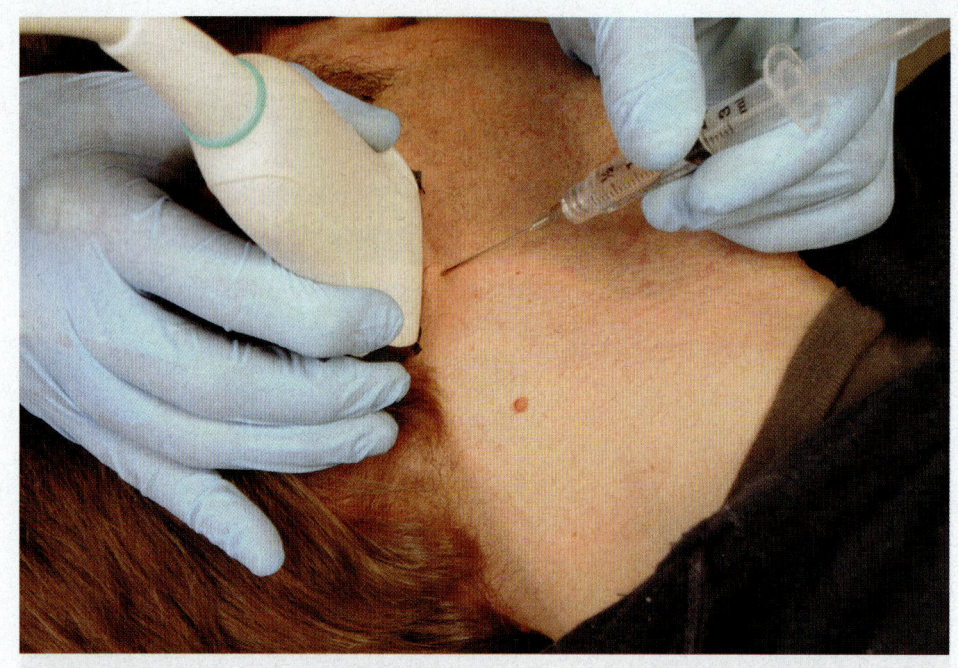

**FIGURE 14.8.** Out-of-plane approach for ultrasound-guided injection of the styloid process.

weakness of the tongue and trapezius muscle. Bleeding complications associated with this technique can be decreased if pressure is applied to the injection site following the injection. The use of cold packs applied to the injection site for short periods of time also decreases postprocedure bleeding and pain.

## CLINICAL PEARLS

This ultrasound-guided injection technique can produce dramatic relief for patients suffering from Eagle syndrome. The proximity of the styloid process to both the carotid artery and jugular vein means that the possibility for needle trauma to these vessels and/or inadvertent intravascular injection is an ever-present possibility. The careful identification with ultrasound imaging of all structures in proximity to the styloid process prior to needle placement is crucial to decreasing the incidence of the potentially fatal complications. Incremental dosing while carefully monitoring the patient for signs of local anesthetic toxicity can further decrease the risk to the patient. Even in the best of hands, postblock hematoma and ecchymosis can occur. Although these complications are usually transitory in nature, their dramatic appearance can be quite upsetting to the patient; therefore, the patient should be warned of such prior to the procedure. Although both glossopharyngeal neuralgia and Eagle syndrome share some common symptoms, glossopharyngeal neuralgia can be distinguished from Eagle syndrome in that the pain of glossopharyngeal neuralgia is characterized by paroxysms of shock-like pain in a manner more analogous to trigeminal neuralgia rather than the sharp, shooting pain on head and neck movement that is associated with Eagle syndrome. Because both glossopharyngeal neuralgia and Eagle syndrome may be associated with serious cardiac bradyarrhythmias and syncope, the clinician must distinguish between the two syndromes as the ultimate curative treatments for each of these syndromes are very different.

Given the low incidence of Eagle syndrome relative to other causes of pain in this anatomic region including pain secondary to malignancy, Eagle syndrome must be considered a diagnosis of exclusion. The clinician should always evaluate the patient who suffers from pain in this anatomic region for occult tumors of the larynx, hypopharynx, and anterior triangle of the neck as may present with clinical symptoms that may mimic Eagle syndrome (Fig. 14.9).

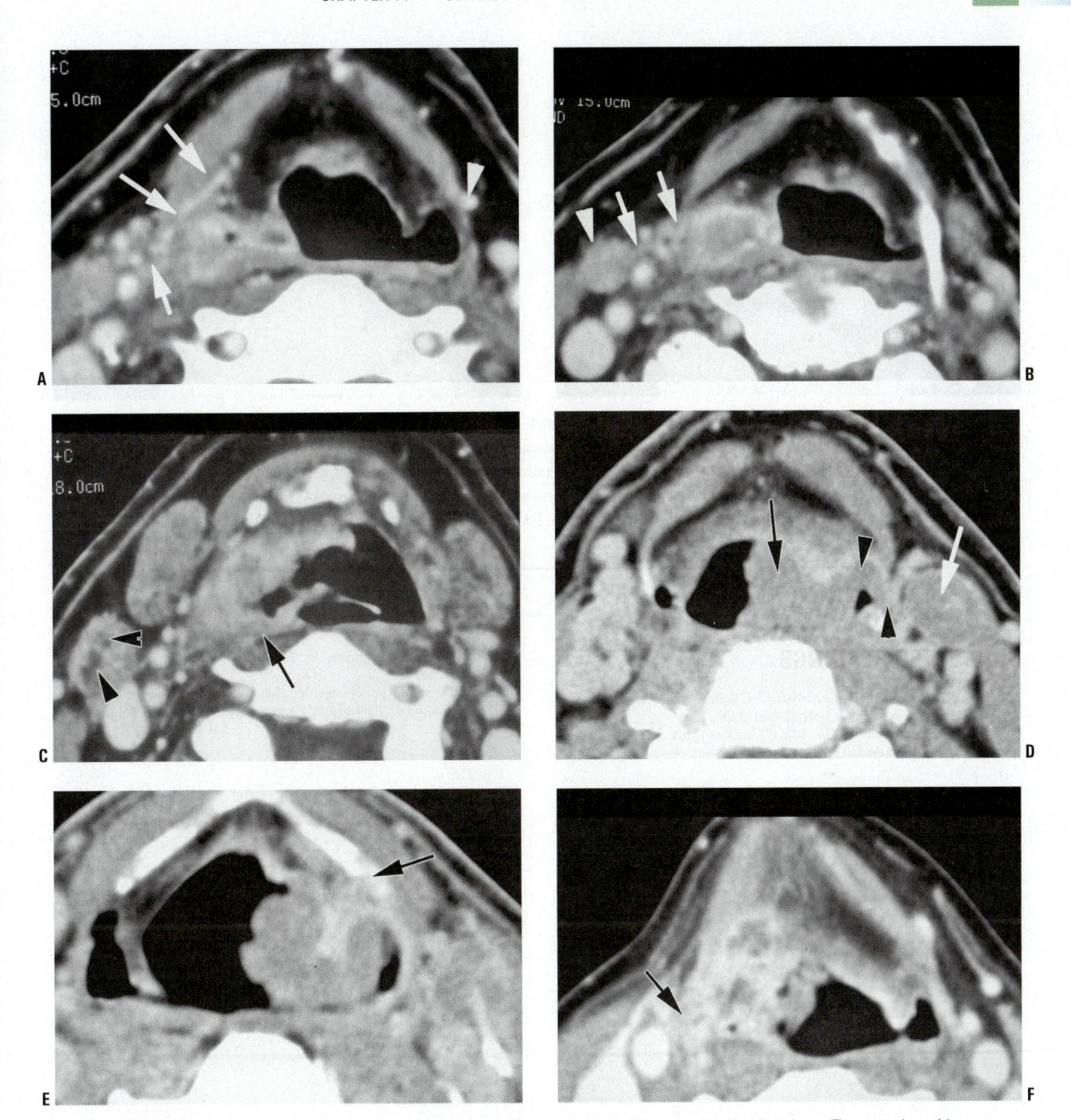

**FIGURE 14.9.** Three patients demonstrating extralaryngeal spread. CT studies were done in all patients. The spread outside the pharynx was not detectable in any of the patients on the basis of the clinical examination. **A–C:** Patient 1. A low-volume but locally aggressive-appearing pyriform sinus carcinoma invading the right superior laryngeal neurovascular bundle (*arrows* in A) and spreading outside the larynx. In (**B**), that spread pattern along the superior neurovascular bundle can be seen again (*arrows*) with an associated metastatic lymph node. In (**C**), submucosal spread to the junction of the hypopharyngeal and oropharyngeal posterior walls is present (*arrow*), and there is a positive level 2 lymph node containing multiple peripheral metastatic deposits (*arrowheads*). **D,E:** Patient 2. There is an almost entirely exophytic pyriform sinus and aryepiglottic fold cancer (*arrow*). However, the tumor can be seen spreading along the superior laryngeal neurovascular bundle outside the larynx (*arrowhead*). There is an associated level 3 metastatic lymph node that is completely replaced by tumor (*white arrow*). In (**E**), the tumor, which on its surface appears relatively lobulated and exophytic, shows evidence of probable early thyroid lamina invasion (*arrow*).

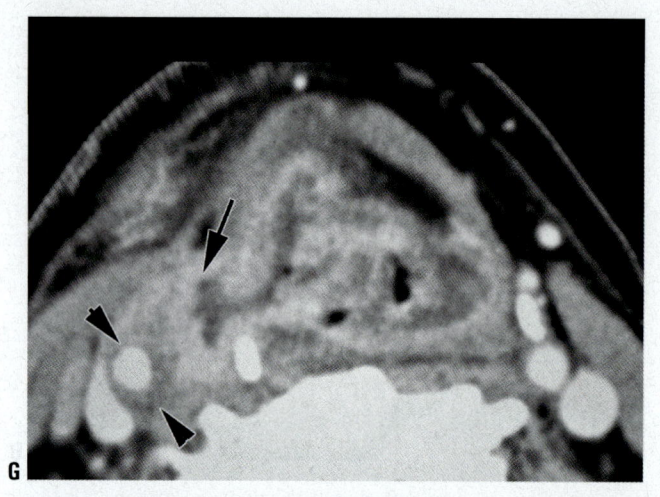

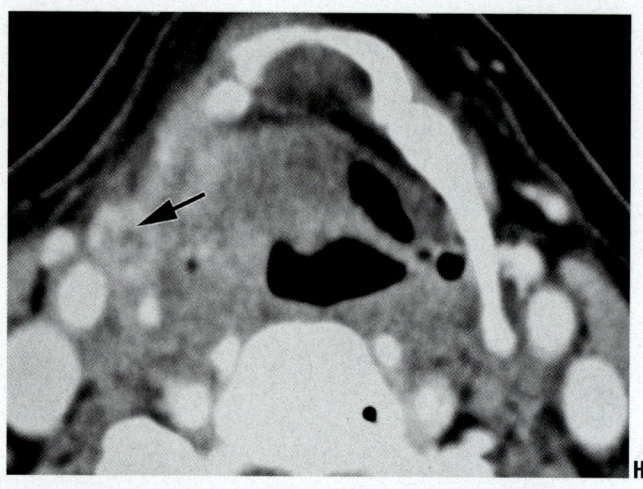

**FIGURE 14.9.** *(Continued)* **F–H:** Patient 3. A very aggressive cancer can be seen growing through the thyrohyoid membrane along the superior laryngeal neurovascular bundle (*arrows* in **F** and **G**). The carotid artery is encased by this tumor growth, as seen in (**G**). Spread along the superior laryngeal neurovascular bundle is sometimes associated with or due to lymph nodes (*arrow*) along this bundle, as demonstrated in (**H**). (Reused from Hermans R, Mancuso AA, Collins WO. Hypopharynx: benign noninflammatory masses and tumors. In: Mancuso AA, Hannafee WN, eds. *Head and Neck Radiology.* Philadelphia, PA: Lippincott Williams & Wilkins; 2011:2157, with permission.)

## SUGGESTED READINGS

Murtagha RD, Caraccioloa JT, Fernandeza G. CT findings associated with eagle syndrome. *Am J Neuroradiol* 2001;22:1401–1402.

Waldman SD. Eagle's syndrome. In: *Atlas of Uncommon Pain Syndromes.* 2nd ed. Philadelphia, PA: Saunders Elsevier; 2008:27–29.

Waldman SD. Eagle's syndrome. In: *Pain Review.* Philadelphia, PA: Saunders Elsevier; 2009:231.

Waldman SD. Styloid process injection. In: *Atlas of Pain Management Injection Techniques.* 3rd ed. Philadelphia, PA: Saunders Elsevier;2013:29–32.

# SECTION II

# Neck

# CHAPTER 15

# Ultrasound-Guided Glossopharyngeal Nerve Block

## CLINICAL PERSPECTIVES

Ultrasound-guided glossopharyngeal nerve block is useful in the management of the pain secondary to glossopharyngeal neuralgia as well as in the palliation of pain of malignant origin emanating from tumors of the posterior tongue, hypopharynx, and tonsils. This technique is also useful as an adjunct when performing awake intubation as well as to attenuate the gag reflex in posttonsillectomy patients and in those patients who are having difficulty tolerating an endotracheal tube during mechanical ventilation and during the weaning process from mechanical intubation when a decrease in sedation is desirable. Ultrasound-guided glossopharyngeal nerve block can also be used in a prognostic manner to determine the degree of neurologic impairment the patient will suffer when destruction of the glossopharyngeal nerve is being considered or when there is a possibility that the nerve may be sacrificed during surgeries in the anatomic region of the glossopharyngeal nerve. This technique may also be useful in those patients suffering symptoms from compromise of the glossopharyngeal nerve by an elongated styloid process and/or calcified stylohyoid ligament secondary to Eagle syndrome (see Chapter 14).

## CLINICALLY RELEVANT ANATOMY

The key landmark when performing glossopharyngeal nerve block is the styloid process of the temporal bone (Fig. 15.1). The temporal styloid process extends from the temporal bone in a caudad and ventral direction and serves as the cephalad attachment of the stylohyoid ligament. The ligament attaches caudally to the hyoid bone. The glossopharyngeal nerve exits from the jugular foramen in proximity to the vagus and accessory nerve and the internal jugular vein and passes just inferior to the styloid process (Fig. 15.2). All three nerves lie in the groove between the internal jugular vein and internal carotid artery. The glossopharyngeal nerve (cranial nerve IX) contains both motor and sensory fibers (Fig. 15.3). The motor fibers innervate the stylopharyngeus muscle. The sensory portion of the nerve innervates the posterior third of the tongue, palatine tonsil, and the mucous membranes of the mouth and pharynx. Special visceral afferent sensory fibers transmit information from the taste buds of the posterior third of the tongue. Information from the carotid sinus and body that helps control blood pressure, pulse, and respiration is carried via the carotid sinus nerve, which is a branch of the glossopharyngeal nerve. Parasympathetic fibers pass via the glossopharyngeal nerve to the otic ganglion. Postganglionic fibers from the ganglion carry secretory information to the parotid gland.

## ULTRASOUND-GUIDED TECHNIQUE

To perform ultrasound-guided injection technique for glossopharyngeal nerve block, place the patient in supine position with the head turned away from the side to be blocked. An imaginary line is drawn from the mastoid process to the angle of the mandible (see Fig. 15.1). In most patients, the styloid process lies just above the midpoint of this line. After preliminary identification of the approximate location of the styloid process, the skin is prepped with antiseptic solution and 3 mL of local anesthetic is drawn up in a 10-mL sterile syringe, with 40 to 80 mg of depot steroid added if the condition being treated is thought to have an inflammatory component. A linear ultrasound transducer is then placed over the previously identified approximate location of the styloid process in the transverse plane (Fig. 15.4).

The styloid process, the carotid artery, and the jugular vein are identified (Fig. 15.5). Color Doppler may be utilized to help confirm location of the vessels and their relationship to the styloid process (Fig. 15.6). A 22-gauge, 3½-inch styletted spinal needle is then advanced under real-time ultrasound guidance toward the styloid process using an out-of-plane approach (Fig. 15.7). The styloid process should be encountered within ~3 cm. After contact with the styloid process is made, the needle is withdrawn slightly out of the periosteum, or substance of the calcified ligament and under real-time ultrasound guidance is walked off the posterior aspect of the styloid process/ligament and advanced slightly so the needle tip rests in proximity to the glossopharyngeal nerve. After careful aspiration reveals no blood or cerebrospinal fluid, 3 mL of solution should be slowly injected. The needle is removed

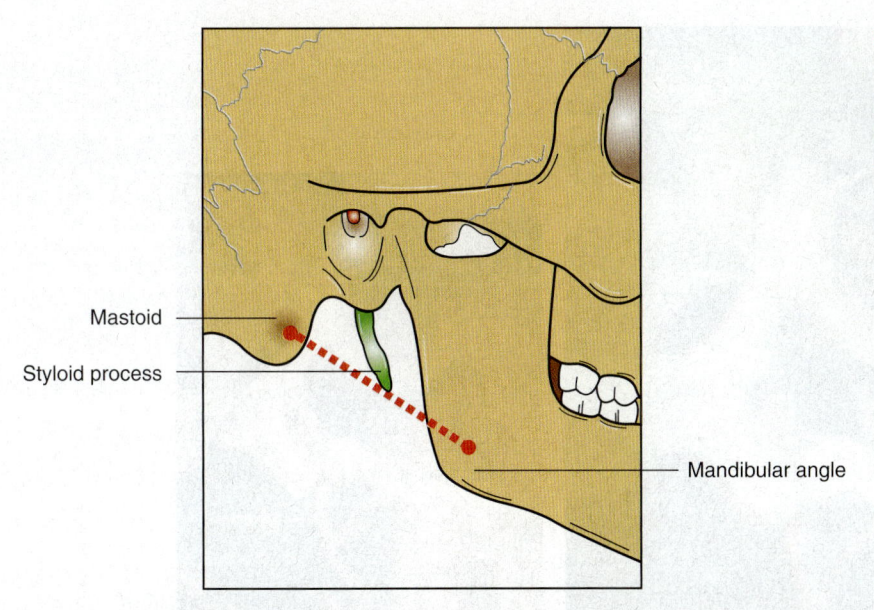

**FIGURE 15.1.** To identify the location of the styloid process, an imaginary line is drawn between the mastoid process and the angle of the mandible.

and pressure is placed on the injection site to avoid bleeding complications. Subsequent daily nerve blocks are carried out in a similar manner.

## COMPLICATIONS

The major complications associated with this ultrasound-guided injection technique are related to needle-induced trauma to the internal jugular vein and/or carotid artery. The incidence of injury to these vessels and the inadvertent intravascular injection of local anesthetic with subsequent toxicity are less common complication of this technique when ultrasound guidance is utilized. Inadvertent blockade of the motor portion of the glossopharyngeal nerve can result in dysphagia secondary to weakness of the stylopharyngeus muscle. If the vagus nerve is inadvertently blocked, dysphonia secondary to paralysis of the ipsilateral vocal cord may occur. A reflex tachycardia secondary to vagal nerve block is also observed in some patients. Inadvertent block of the hypoglossal and spinal accessory nerves during glossopharyngeal nerve block will result in weakness of the tongue and trapezius and sternocleidomastoid muscles. Bleeding complications associated with this technique can be decreased if pressure is applied to the injection site following the injection. The use of cold packs applied to the injection site for short periods of time also decreases postprocedure bleeding and pain.

## CLINICAL PEARLS

This ultrasound-guided injection technique can produce dramatic relief for patients suffering from the pain of glossopharyngeal neuralgia and from cancer pain from tumors of

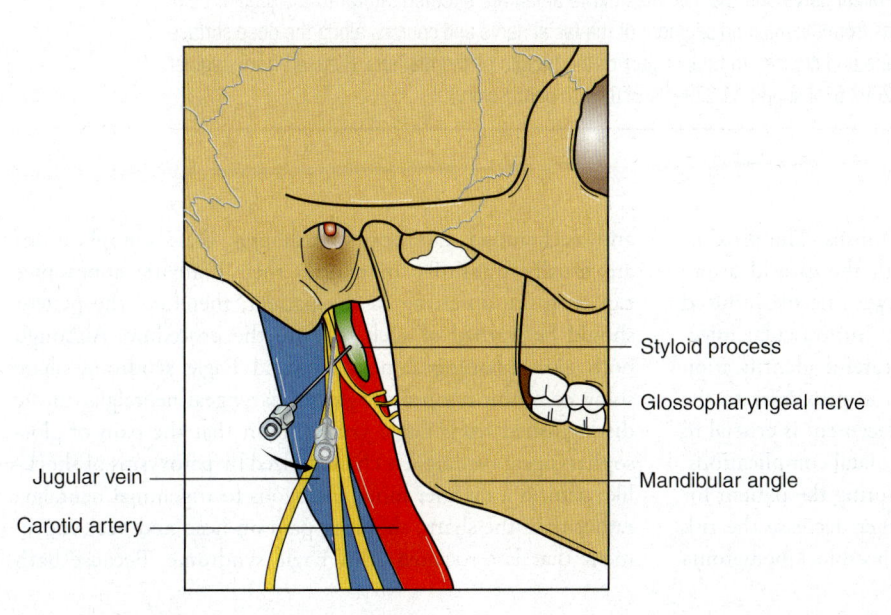

**FIGURE 15.2.** The anatomy of the glossopharyngeal nerve and its relationship to the carotid artery and jugular vein.

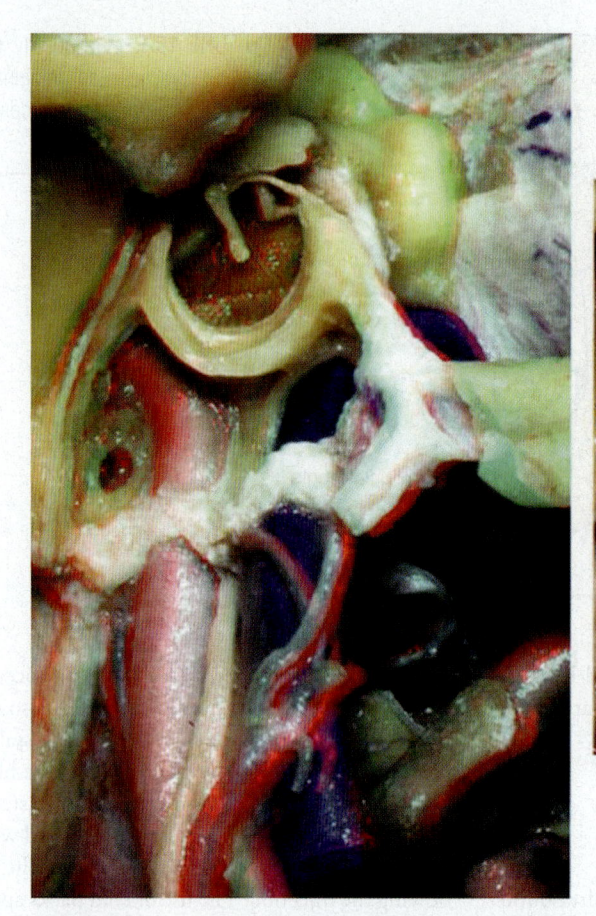

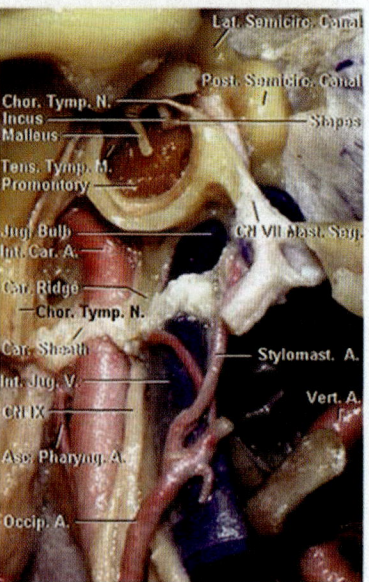

**FIGURE 15.3.** Lateral view of the left tympanic cavity and mastoid area. The tympanic part of the temporal bone, which forms the lower and anterior margin of the external meatus, has been removed, but the tympanic sulcus and osseous ring to which the tympanic membrane attaches have been preserved. The carotid ridge separates the carotid canal and jugular foramen. Meningeal branches of the ascending pharyngeal and occipital arteries enter the jugular foramen. The glossopharyngeal, vagus, and accessory nerves pass through the jugular foramen on the medial side of the jugular bulb. The malleus, incus, and stapes are exposed in the tympanic cavity. The stylomastoid branch of the occipital artery joins the facial nerve at the stylomastoid foramen. The surface of the temporal and occipital bones surrounding the jugular foramen and carotid canal has an irregular surface that serves as the site of attachment of the upper end of the carotid sheath. The mastoid segment of the facial nerve and the stylomastoid foramen are situated lateral to the jugular bulb. The chorda tympani arises from the mastoid segment of the facial nerve and courses along the deep surface of the tympanic membrane and crosses the upper part of the handle of the malleus. (Reused from Jugular Foramen. *Neurosurgery* 2007;61(4 suppl):S4-229–S4-250, with permission.)

the posterior tongue, hypopharynx, and tonsils. The proximity of the glossopharyngeal nerve to both the carotid artery and jugular vein means that the possibility for needle-induced trauma to these vessels and/or inadvertent intravascular injection is an ever-present possibility. The careful identification with ultrasound imaging of all structures in proximity to the glossopharyngeal nerve prior to needle placement is crucial to decreasing the incidence of the potentially fatal complications. Incremental dosing while carefully monitoring the patient for signs of local anesthetic toxicity can further decrease the risk to the patient. Even in the best of hands, postblock hematoma and ecchymosis can occur. Although these complications are usually transitory in nature, their dramatic appearance can be quite upsetting to the patient; therefore, the patient should be warned of such prior to the procedure. Although both glossopharyngeal neuralgia and Eagle syndrome share some common symptoms, glossopharyngeal neuralgia can be distinguished from Eagle syndrome in that the pain of glossopharyngeal neuralgia is characterized by paroxysms of shock-like pain in a manner more analogous to trigeminal neuralgia rather than the sharp, shooting pain on head and neck movement that is associated with Eagle syndrome. Because both

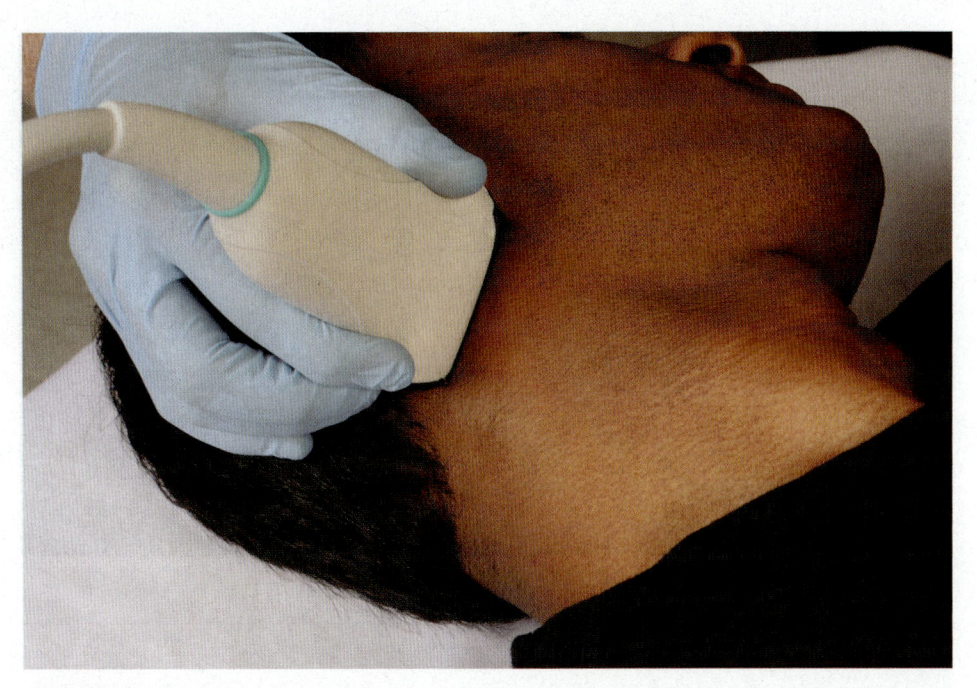

**FIGURE 15.4.** Proper transverse placement of the linear ultrasound transducer over the previously identified styloid process.

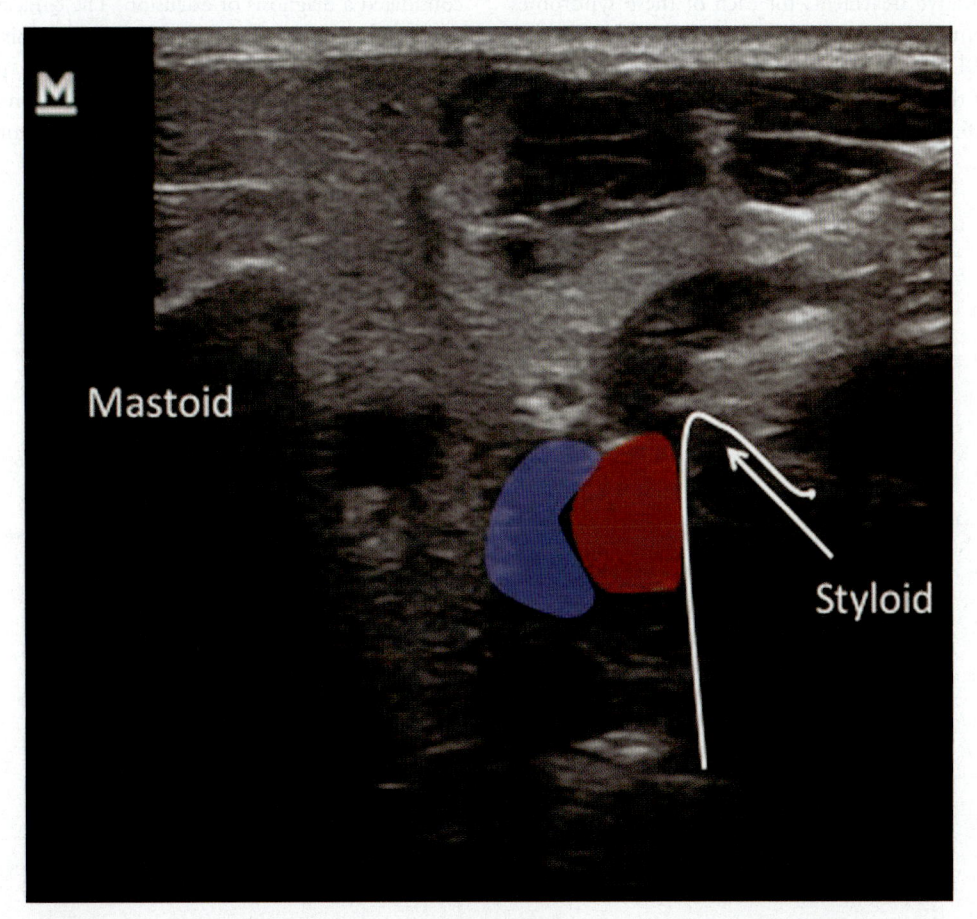

**FIGURE 15.5.** Transverse ultrasound view of the styloid process, carotid artery, and jugular vein.

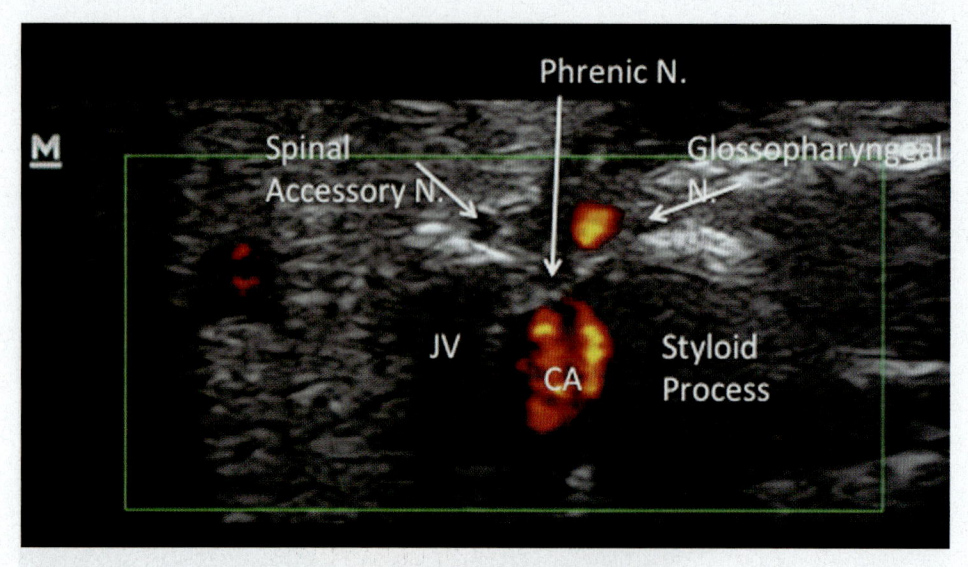

**FIGURE 15.6.** Color Doppler image of the carotid artery and jugular vein.

glossopharyngeal neuralgia and Eagle syndrome may be associated with serious cardiac bradyarrhythmias and syncope, the clinician must distinguish between the two syndromes as the ultimate curative treatments for each of these syndromes are very different. All patients thought to be suffering from glossopharyngeal neuralgia should be evaluated for multiple sclerosis due to the high incidence of both diseases occurring together (Fig. 15.8).

Given the low incidence of glossopharyngeal neuralgia relative to other causes of pain in this anatomic region including pain secondary to malignancy, glossopharyngeal neuralgia must be considered a diagnosis of exclusion. The clinician should always evaluate the patient who suffers from pain in this anatomic region for occult tumors of the larynx, hypopharynx, posterior tongue, and anterior triangle of the neck as they may present with clinical symptoms that can mimic glossopharyngeal neuralgia (Fig. 15.9).

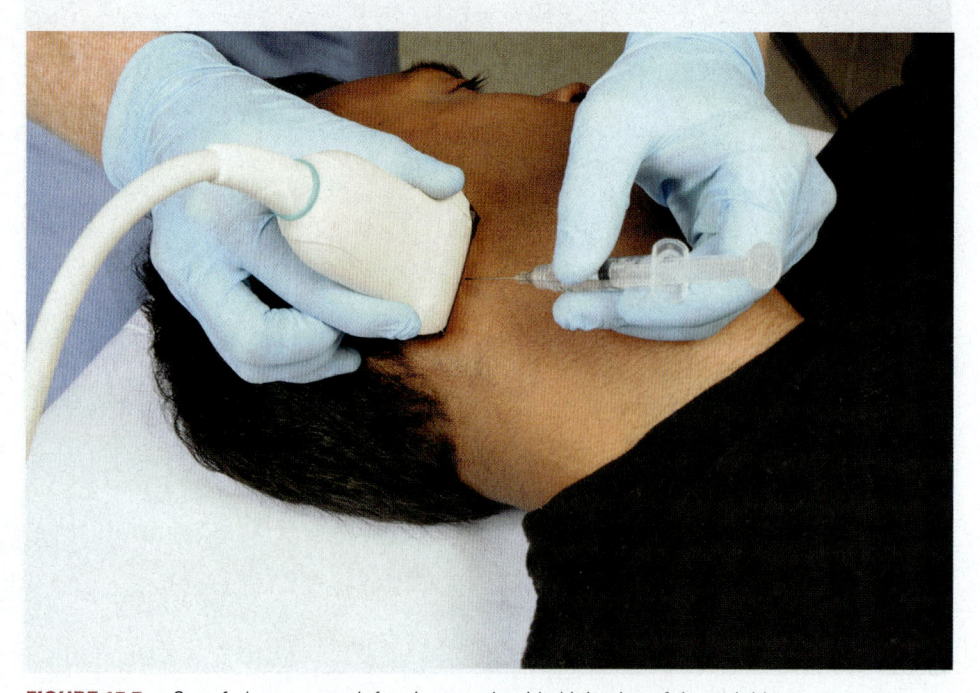

**FIGURE 15.7.** Out-of-plane approach for ultrasound-guided injection of the styloid process nerve.

# CHAPTER 15  ULTRASOUND-GUIDED GLOSSOPHARYNGEAL NERVE BLOCK

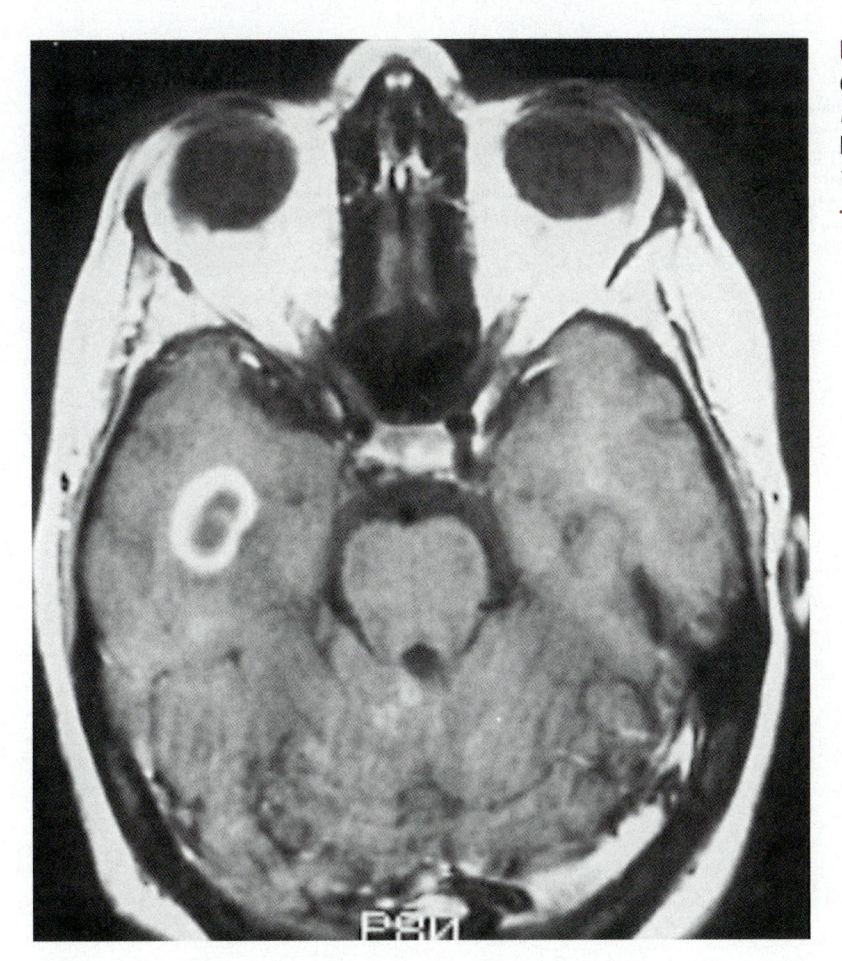

**FIGURE 15.8.** Multiple sclerosis. Single large ring-enhancing lesion. (Reused from Eisenberg RL. *Clinical Imaging: An Atlas of Differential Diagnosis.* 5th ed. Philadelphia, PA: Lippincott Williams & Wilkins; 2010: 1254, with permission.)

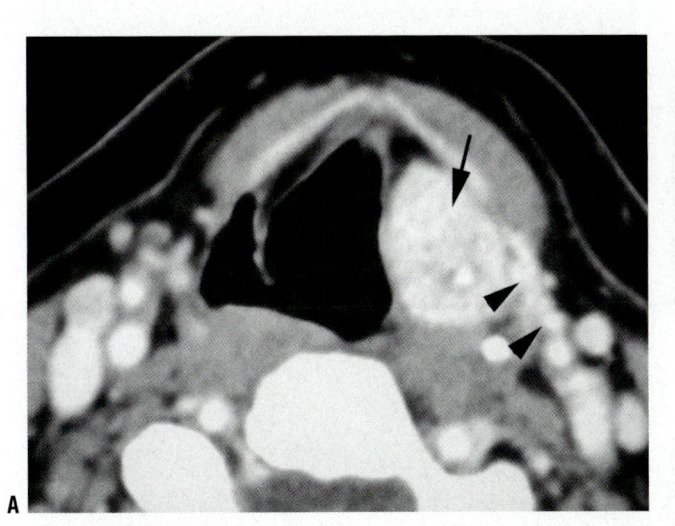

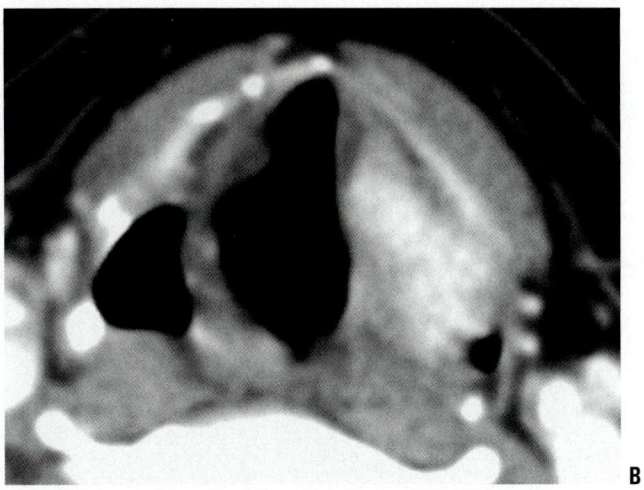

**FIGURE 15.9.** A patient presenting with a submucosal supraglottic mass and vocal cord dysfunction. **A,B:** Contrast-enhanced computed tomography shows an excessively enhancing mass centered in the aryepiglottic fold (*arrow*). There is also a very prominent superior laryngeal neurovascular bundle (*arrowheads*) that identifies this as an arterialized lesion, subsequently shown to be a paraganglioma. (Reused from Hermans R, Mancuso AA, Collins WO. Larynx: infectious and noninfectious inflammatory diseases. In: Mancuso AA, Hanafee WN, eds. *Head and Neck Radiology.* Philadelphia, PA: Lippincott Williams & Wilkins; 2011:1967, with permission.)

## SUGGESTED READINGS

Carrieri PB, Montella S, Petracca M. Glossopharyngeal neuralgia as onset of multiple sclerosis. *Clin J Pain* 2009;25(8):737–739.

Park H-P, Hwang J-W, Park S-H, et al. The effects of glossopharyngeal nerve block on postoperative pain relief after tonsillectomy: the importance of the extent of obtunded gag reflex as a clinical indicator. *Anesth Analg* 2007;105(1):267–271.

Waldman SD. Glossopharyngeal neuralgia. In: *Atlas of Uncommon Pain Syndromes*. 2nd ed. Philadelphia, PA: Saunders Elsevier; 2008:30–32.

Waldman SD. The glossopharyngeal nerve. In: *Pain Review*. Philadelphia, PA: Saunders Elsevier; 2009:25–28.

Waldman SD. Glossopharyngeal nerve block. In: *Pain Review*. Philadelphia, PA: Saunders Elsevier; 2009:407–408.

Waldman SD. The trigeminal nerve. In: *Pain Review*. Philadelphia, PA: Saunders Elsevier; 2009:15–17.

Waldman SD. Glossopharyngeal nerve block. In: *Atlas of Interventional Pain Management*. 3rd ed. Philadelphia, PA: Saunders Elsevier; 2009:93–96.

# CHAPTER 16

# Ultrasound-Guided Vagus Nerve Block

## CLINICAL PERSPECTIVES

Ultrasound-guided vagus nerve block is useful in the management of the acute pain emergencies as an adjunct to pharmacologic, surgical, and antiblastic measures. In combination with glossopharyngeal nerve block, ultrasound-guided vagus nerve block is useful in the palliation of pain of malignant origin emanating from tumors of the posterior tongue, hypopharynx, and tonsils. This technique may also be utilized as a diagnostic maneuver when performing differential neural blockade on an anatomic basis when evaluating difficult-to-diagnose head and neck pain syndromes and when considering a diagnosis of vagal neuralgia. If destruction of the vagus nerve is being considered, this technique is useful as a prognostic indicator of the degree of motor and sensory impairment that the patient may experience.

## CLINICALLY RELEVANT ANATOMY

The key landmark when performing vagus nerve block is the styloid process of the temporal bone (Fig. 16.1). The temporal styloid process extends from the temporal bone in a caudad and ventral direction and serves as the cephalad attachment of the stylohyoid ligament. The ligament attaches caudally to the hyoid bone. The vagus nerve exits from the jugular foramen in proximity to the vagus and accessory nerve and the internal jugular vein and passes just inferior to the styloid process (Fig. 16.2). All three nerves lie in the groove between the internal jugular vein and internal carotid artery with vagus nerve lying caudad to the glossopharyngeal nerve with its downward course superficial to the jugular vein.

## ULTRASOUND-GUIDED TECHNIQUE

To perform ultrasound-guided injection technique for vagus nerve block, place the patient in supine position with the head turned away from the side to be blocked. An imaginary line is drawn from the mastoid process to the angle of the mandible (see Fig. 16.1). In most patients, the styloid process lies just above the midpoint of this line. After preliminary identification of the approximate location of the styloid process, the skin is prepped with antiseptic solution and 3 mL of local anesthetic is drawn up in a 10-mL sterile syringe, with 40 to 80 mg of depot steroid added if the condition being treated is thought to have an inflammatory component. A linear ultrasound transducer is then placed over the previously identified approximate location of the styloid process in the transverse plane (Fig. 16.3).

The styloid process and the carotid artery and jugular vein are identified (Fig. 16.4). Color Doppler may be utilized to help confirm location of the vessels and their relationship to the styloid process (Fig. 16.5).

A 22-gauge, 1½-inch spinal needle is then advanced under real-time ultrasound guidance toward the styloid process using an out-of-plane approach (Fig. 16.6). The styloid process should be encountered within 3 cm. After contact with the styloid process is made, the needle is withdrawn slightly out of the periosteum, or substance of the calcified ligament and under real-time ultrasound guidance is walked off the posterior aspect of the styloid process/ligament in a posterior and slightly inferior trajectory and advanced slightly so the needle tip rests in proximity to the vagus nerve. After careful aspiration reveals no blood or cerebrospinal fluid, 3 mL of solution should be slowly injected. The needle is removed and pressure is placed on the injection site to avoid bleeding complications. Subsequent daily nerve blocks are carried out in a similar manner.

## COMPLICATIONS

The major complications associated with this ultrasound-guided injection technique are related to needle-induced trauma to the internal jugular vein and/or carotid artery. The incidence of injury to these vessels and the inadvertent intravascular injection of local anesthetic with subsequent toxicity are less common complication of this technique when ultrasound guidance is utilized. Blockade of the motor portion of the vagus nerve can result in dysphonia and difficulty coughing due to blockade of the superior and recurrent laryngeal nerves. A reflex tachycardia secondary to vagal nerve block is also observed in some patients. Inadvertent block of the glossopharyngeal, hypoglossal, and spinal accessory nerves during vagus nerve block will result in weakness of the tongue and trapezius and sternocleidomastoid muscle and numbness

**FIGURE 16.1.** To identify the location of the styloid process when performing vagus nerve block, an imaginary line is drawn between the mastoid process and the angle of the mandible.

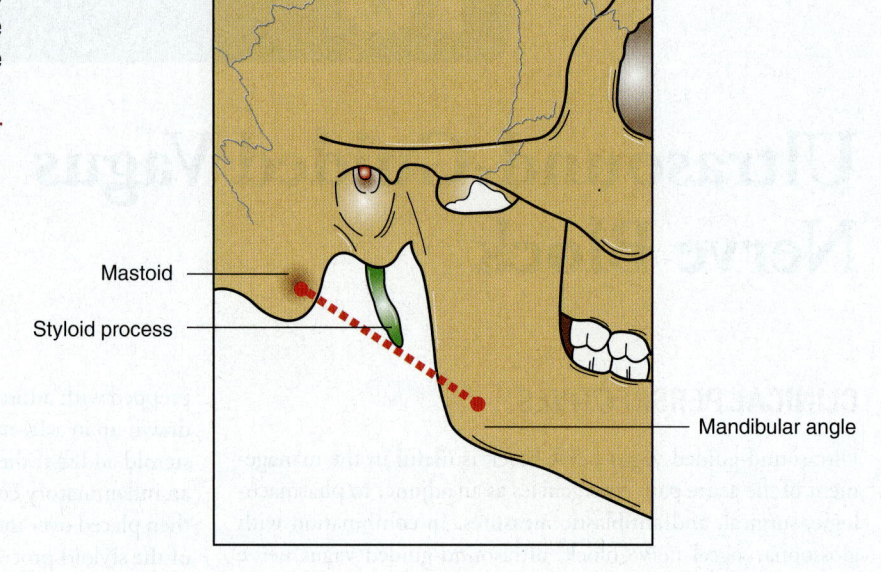

in the distribution of the glossopharyngeal nerve. Bleeding complications associated with this technique can be decreased if pressure is applied to the injection site following the injection. The use of cold packs applied to the injection site for short periods of time also decreases postprocedure bleeding and pain.

## CLINICAL PEARLS

This ultrasound-guided injection technique can produce dramatic relief for patients suffering from the pain of vagal neuralgia and from cancer pain from tumors of the posterior tongue, hypopharynx, and tonsils. Vagal neuralgia is clinically analogous to trigeminal and glossopharyngeal neuralgia. It is characterized by paroxysms of shock-like pain into the thyroid and laryngeal areas. Pain may occasionally radiate into the jaw and upper thoracic region. Attacks of vagal neuralgia may be precipitated by coughing, yawning, and swallowing. Excessive salivation may also be present. This is a rare pain syndrome and should be considered a diagnosis of exclusion. The proximity of the vagus nerve to both the carotid artery and jugular vein means that the possibility for needle-induced trauma to these vessels and/or inadvertent

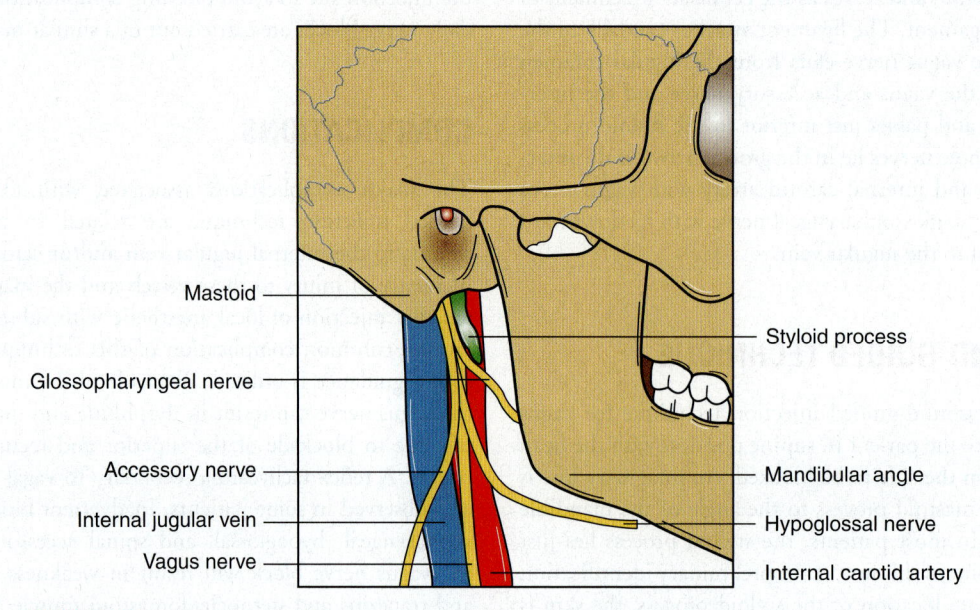

**FIGURE 16.2.** The anatomy of the vagus nerve and its relationship to the carotid artery and jugular vein.

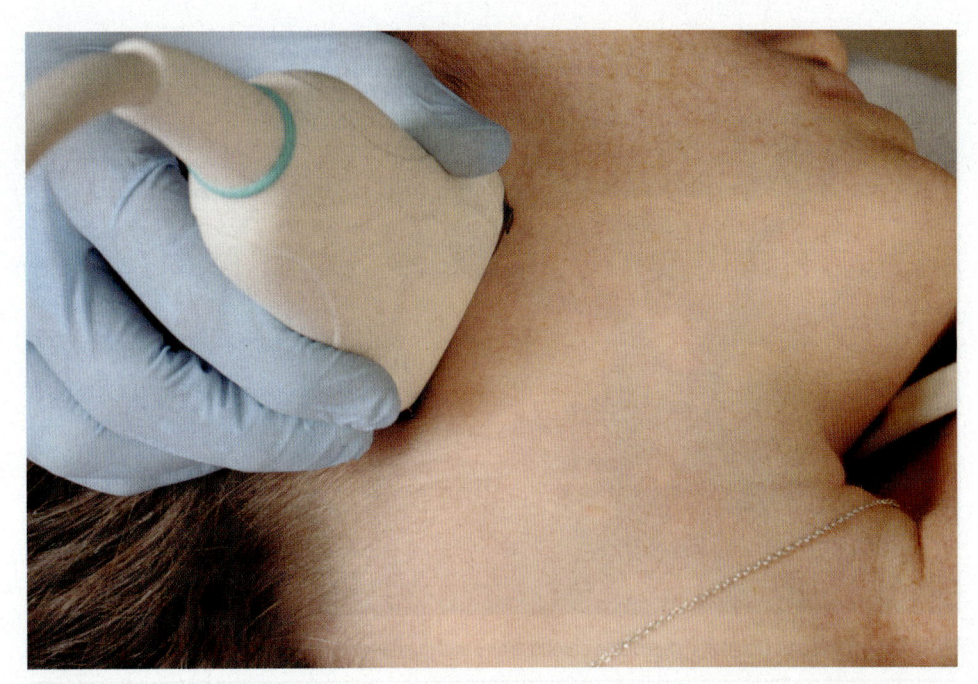

**FIGURE 16.3.** Proper placement of the linear ultrasound transducer over the previously identified styloid process.

intravascular injection is an ever-present possibility. The careful identification with ultrasound imaging of all structures in proximity to the vagus nerve prior to needle placement is crucial to decreasing the incidence of the potentially fatal complications. Incremental dosing while carefully monitoring the patient for signs of local anesthetic toxicity can further decrease the risk to the patient. Even in the best of hands, postblock hematoma and ecchymosis can occur. Although

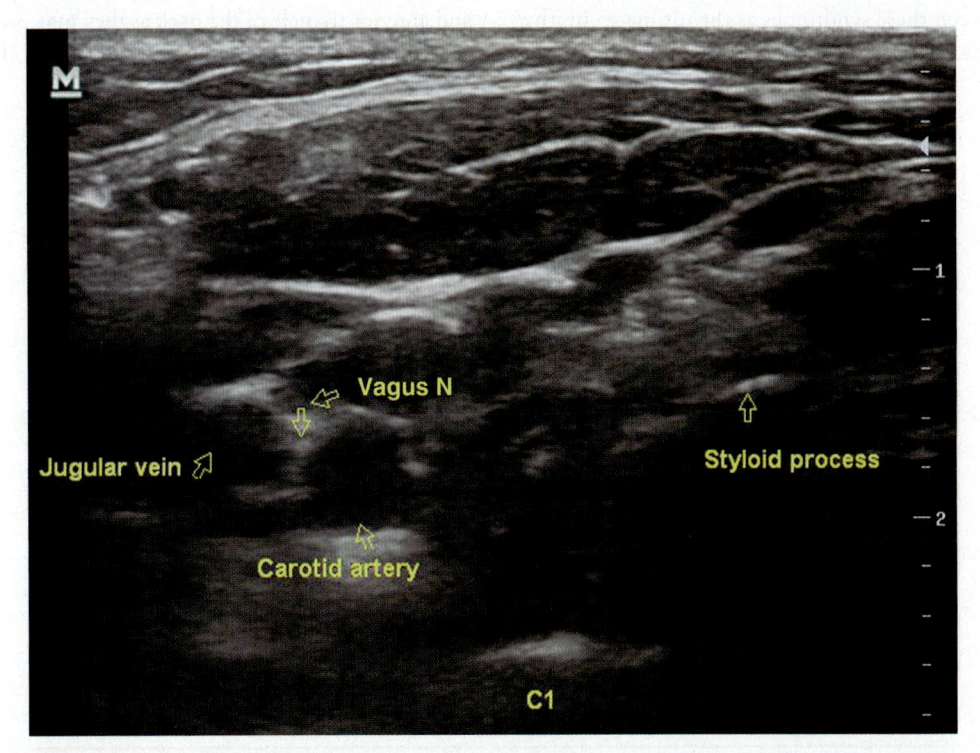

**FIGURE 16.4.** Ultrasound image demonstrating relationship of vagus nerve to the jugular vein and carotid artery.

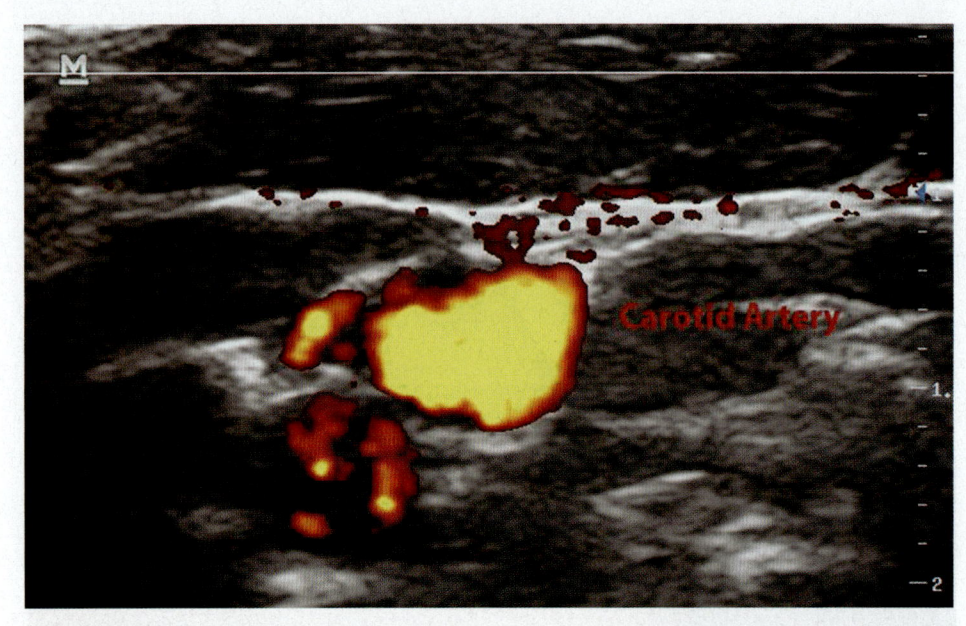

**FIGURE 16.5.** Color Doppler image of the carotid artery and jugular vein.

these complications are usually transitory in nature, their dramatic appearance can be quite upsetting to the patient; therefore, the patient should be warned of such prior to the procedure. Because vagus neuralgia, glossopharyngeal neuralgia, and Eagle syndrome may be associated with serious cardiac bradyarrhythmias and syncope, the clinician must distinguish between these syndromes as the ultimate curative treatments for each are very different.

Given the exceedingly low incidence of vagus neuralgia relative to other causes of pain in this anatomic region including pain secondary to malignancy, vagus neuralgia must be considered a diagnosis of exclusion. The clinician should always evaluate the patient who suffers from pain in this anatomic region for occult tumors of the larynx, hypopharynx, posterior tongue, and anterior triangle of the neck as they may present with clinical symptoms that can mimic vagus neuralgia (Fig. 16.7).

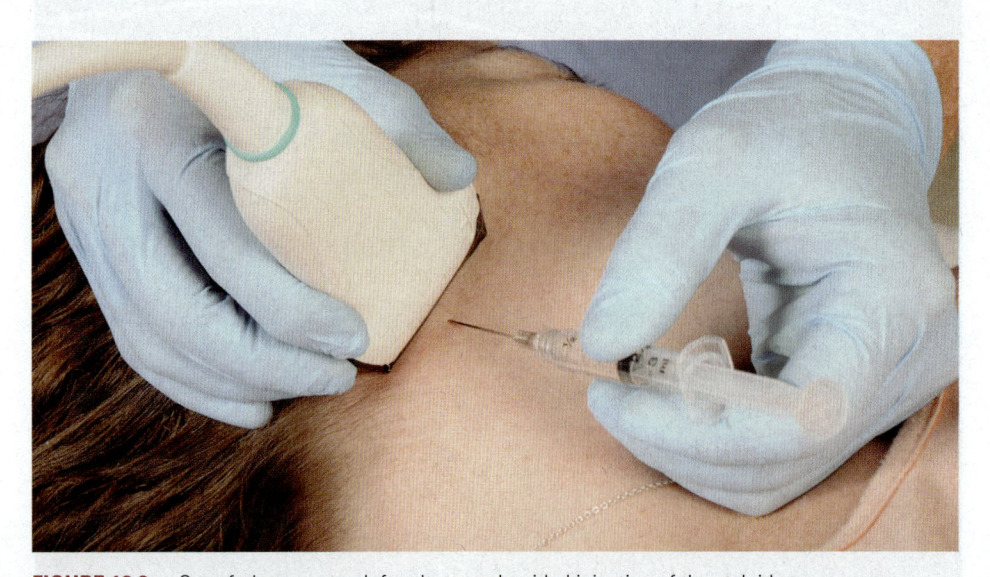

**FIGURE 16.6.** Out-of-plane approach for ultrasound-guided injection of the styloid process nerve.

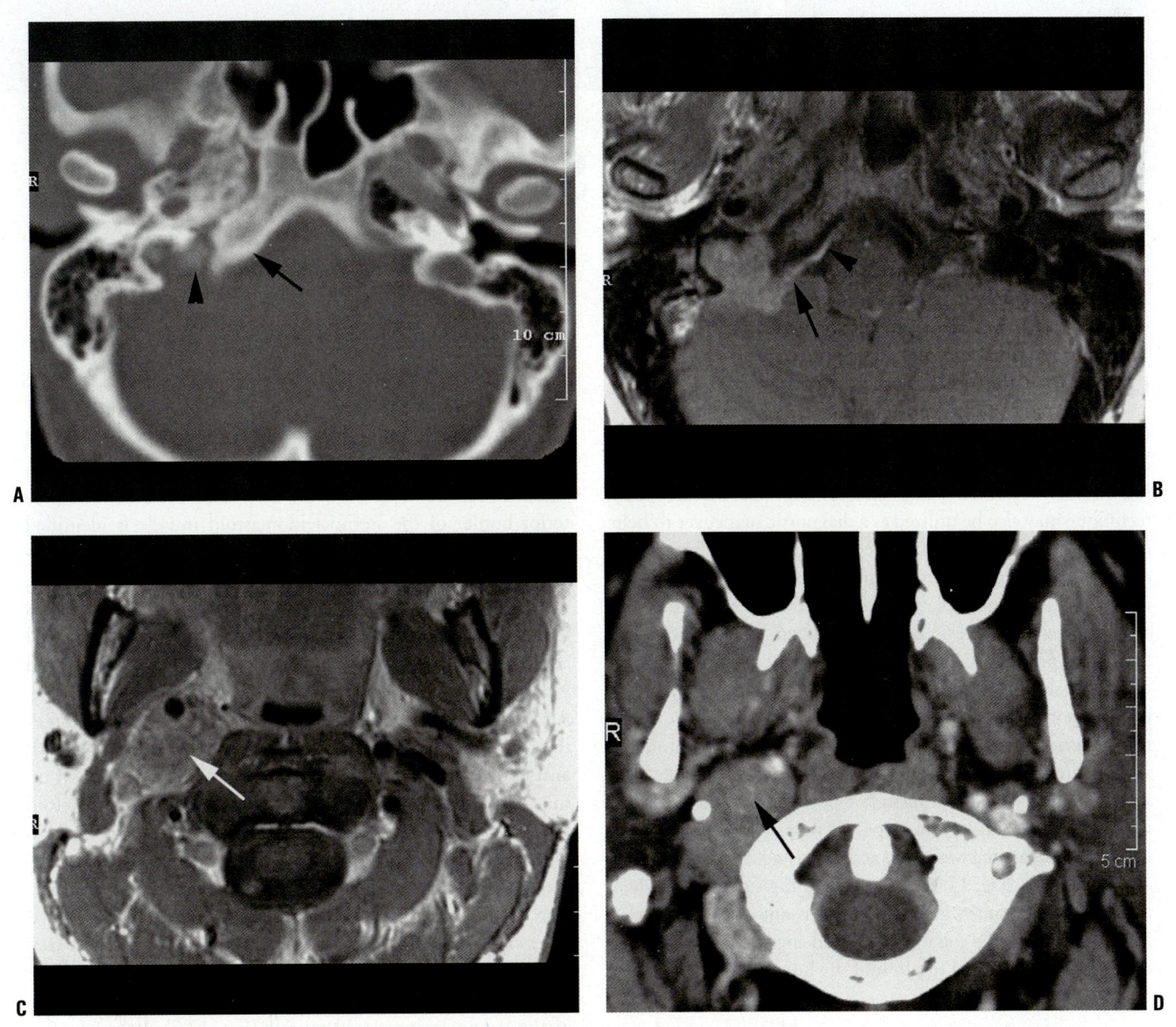

**FIGURE 16.7.** Lower cranial neuropathies by disease location—lesions producing jugular fossa and other skull base syndromes. **A–D:** Jugular fossa. This patient developed a complex neuropathy (cranial nerves IX to XI) on the right due to a meningioma with extension to the retrostyloid parapharyngeal space (*arrows* in C and D) through the jugular foramen (*arrowhead* in A) and producing reactive bone sclerosis as a clue to its etiology along the lower clivus (*arrow*). Note also the dural involvement (*arrow*) and probable reactive dural changes (*arrowhead*) on the contrast-enhanced T1-weighted (T1W) image in (B). (Reused from Verbist BM, Mancuso AA, Antonelli PJ. Vagal neuropathy, vocal cord weakness, and referred otalgia. In: Mancuso AA, Hanafee WN, eds. *Head and Neck Radiology*. Philadelphia, PA: Lippincott Williams & Wilkins; 2011:1063, with permission.)

## SUGGESTED READINGS

Waldman SD. Glossopharyngeal neuralgia. In: *Atlas of Uncommon Pain Syndromes*. 2nd ed. Philadelphia, PA: Saunders Elsevier; 2008:30–32.

Waldman SD. The vagus nerve. In: *Pain Review*. Philadelphia, PA: Saunders Elsevier; 2009:29–33.

Waldman SD. Vagus nerve block. In: *Atlas of Interventional Pain Management*. 3rd ed. Philadelphia, PA: Saunders Elsevier; 2009:104–107.

Waldman SD. Vagus nerve block. In: *Pain Review*. Philadelphia, PA: Saunders Elsevier; 2009:409–410.

# CHAPTER 17

# Ultrasound-Guided Spinal Accessory Nerve Block

## CLINICAL PERSPECTIVES

Ultrasound-guided spinal accessory nerve block is useful in the diagnosis and management of the acute pain and spasm involving the sternocleidomastoid and/or trapezius muscle. This technique may also be utilized as a diagnostic maneuver to help identify the exact location and course of the spinal accessory nerve when surgical procedures in the posterior triangle of the neck are being contemplated. If destruction or sacrifice of the spinal accessory nerve is being considered, this technique is useful as a prognostic indicator of the degree of motor impairment that the patient may experience. Compromise of the spinal accessory nerve will result in pain, stiffness, and ptosis of the ipsilateral shoulder with associated loss of full abduction and winging of the scapula. Patients with isolated spinal accessory nerve palsy will demonstrate a positive scapular flip sign, which is the finding of the scapular "flipping" or winging off the posterior thoracic wall with active resisted external rotation of the humerus (Fig. 17.1). The scapular flip sign occurs when the pull of the contracting infraspinatus and deltoid muscles is unopposed by the paralyzed or weakened trapezius muscle during resisted external rotation of the humerus.

## CLINICALLY RELEVANT ANATOMY

The fibers that comprise the spinal accessory nerve (cranial nerve XI) arise from lower motor neurons of the spinal accessory nucleus, which are located in the lateral horn of the spinal cord. The fibers coalesce to form the spinal accessory nerve, which ascends through the foramen magnum and travels along the inner skull to exit the cranium via the jugular foramen along with the glossopharyngeal and vagus nerves. The spinal accessory nerve has two branches: a small cranial root and a larger spinal root. The fibers of the larger spinal root pass inferiorly and posteriorly to exit beneath the posterior border of the sternocleidomastoid muscle at the junction of the upper and middle third of the muscle to lie on top of the levator scapulae and middle scalene muscles ventral as it passes in an inferiocaudal course toward the anterior border of the trapezius muscle (Fig. 17.2). The spinal accessory nerve provides motor innervation to the sternocleidomastoid and trapezius muscles while providing minimal sensory innervation.

## ULTRASOUND-GUIDED TECHNIQUE

To perform ultrasound-guided injection technique for spinal accessory nerve block, place the patient in supine position with the head turned away from the side to be blocked. The posterior border of the sternocleidomastoid muscle is identified by having the patient raise his or her head against the resistance of the clinician's hand (Fig. 17.3). The junction of the upper and middle third of the posterior margin of the muscle is identified, which is the approximate point at which the spinal accessory nerve emerges from behind the sternocleidomastoid muscle and is most easily identified on ultrasound imaging. After preliminary identification of the approximate location of the nerve utilizing surface landmarks, the skin is prepped with antiseptic solution and 2 mL of local anesthetic is drawn up in a 10-mL sterile syringe, with 40 to 80 mg of depot steroid added if the condition being treated is thought to have an inflammatory component. A linear ultrasound transducer is then placed over the previously identified approximate location of the nerve in the transverse plane (Fig. 17.4). The spinal accessory nerve should appear as a 2- to 3-mm hypoechoic oval structure with a hyperechoic perineurium lying on top of the levator scapula muscle as it exits beneath the posterior margin of the sternocleidomastoid muscle (Fig. 17.5). Its course can be traced in a posterior and caudad direction toward the anterior margin of the trapezius muscle. When the nerve is identified, a 22-gauge, 2-inch stimulating needle is advanced under real-time ultrasound guidance using an in-plane approach (Fig. 17.6). When the needle tip is in proximity to the nerve, stimulation is carried out with isolated contraction of trapezius muscle indicating satisfactory needle placement. After careful aspiration reveals no blood or cerebrospinal fluid, 2 mL of solution should be slowly injected. The needle is removed and pressure is placed on the injection site to avoid bleeding complications. Subsequent daily nerve blocks are carried out in a similar manner.

## COMPLICATIONS

The major complications associated with this ultrasound-guided injection technique are related to needle-induced trauma to the external jugular vein and the deep vessels of the

CHAPTER 17    ULTRASOUND-GUIDED SPINAL ACCESSORY NERVE BLOCK    113

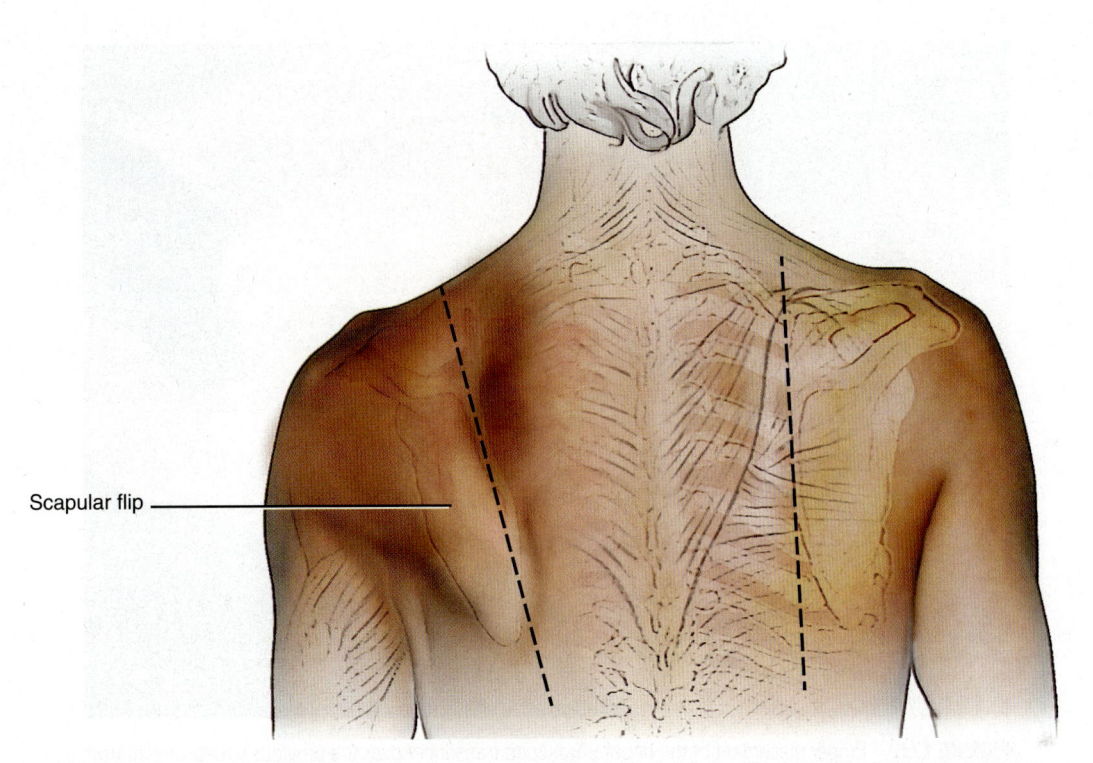

**FIGURE 17.1.**    Spinal accessory nerve palsy may result as a positive scapular flip sign on the left during bilateral resisted shoulder external rotation.

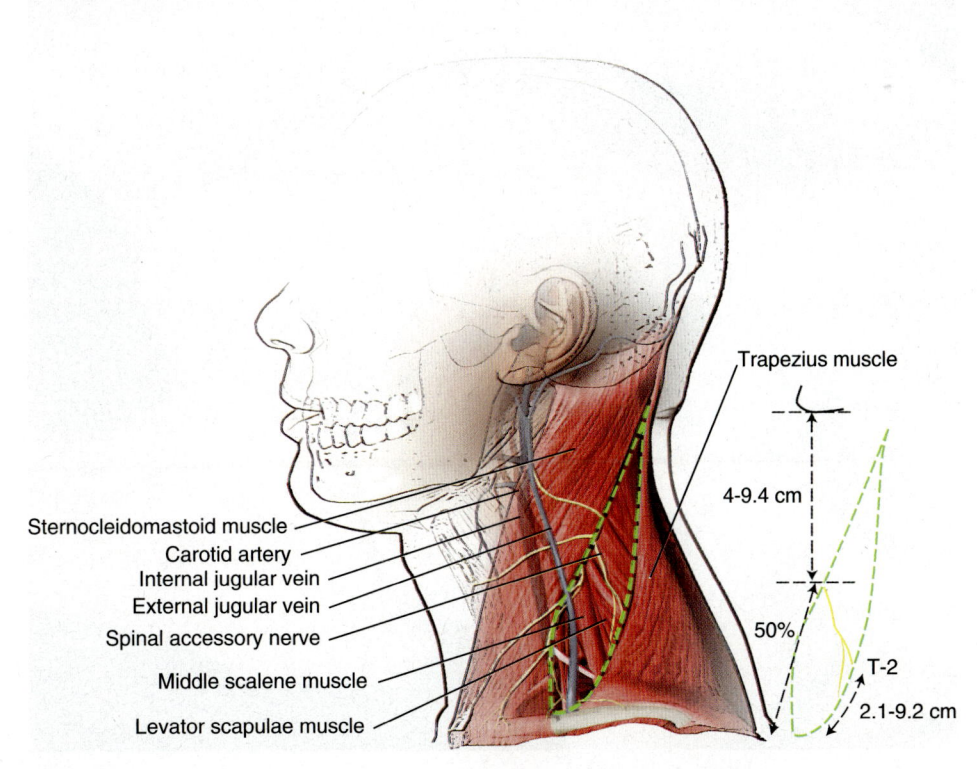

**FIGURE 17.2.**    The anatomy of the spinal accessory nerve and its relationship to the sternocleidomastoid and trapezius muscles and the carotid artery and jugular vein.

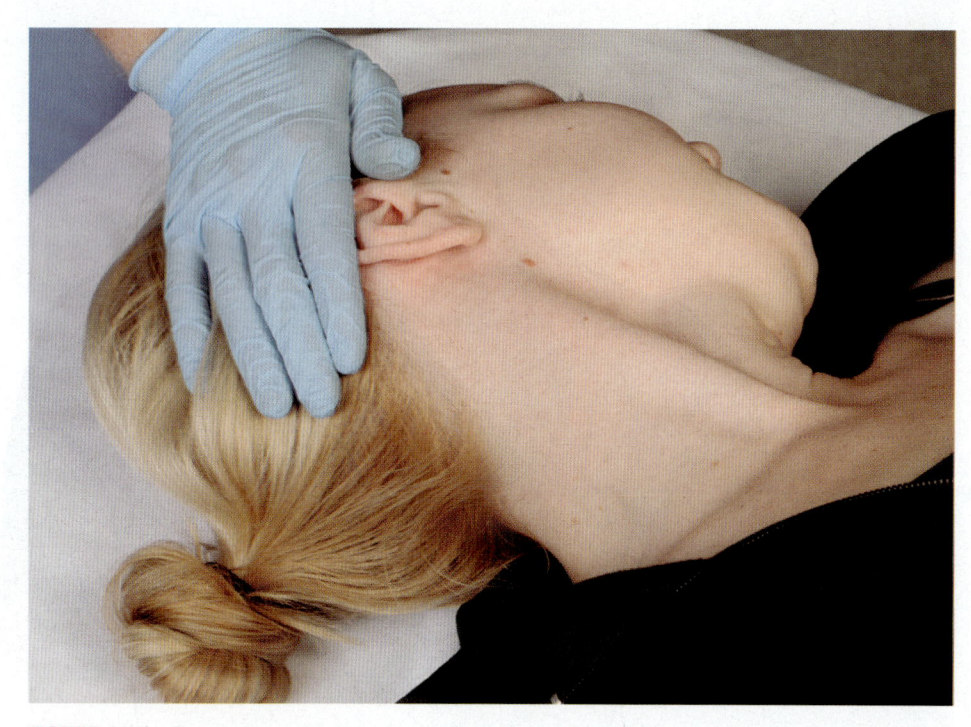

**FIGURE 17.3.** Proper placement of the linear ultrasound transducer over the previously identified margin of the sternocleidomastoid muscle.

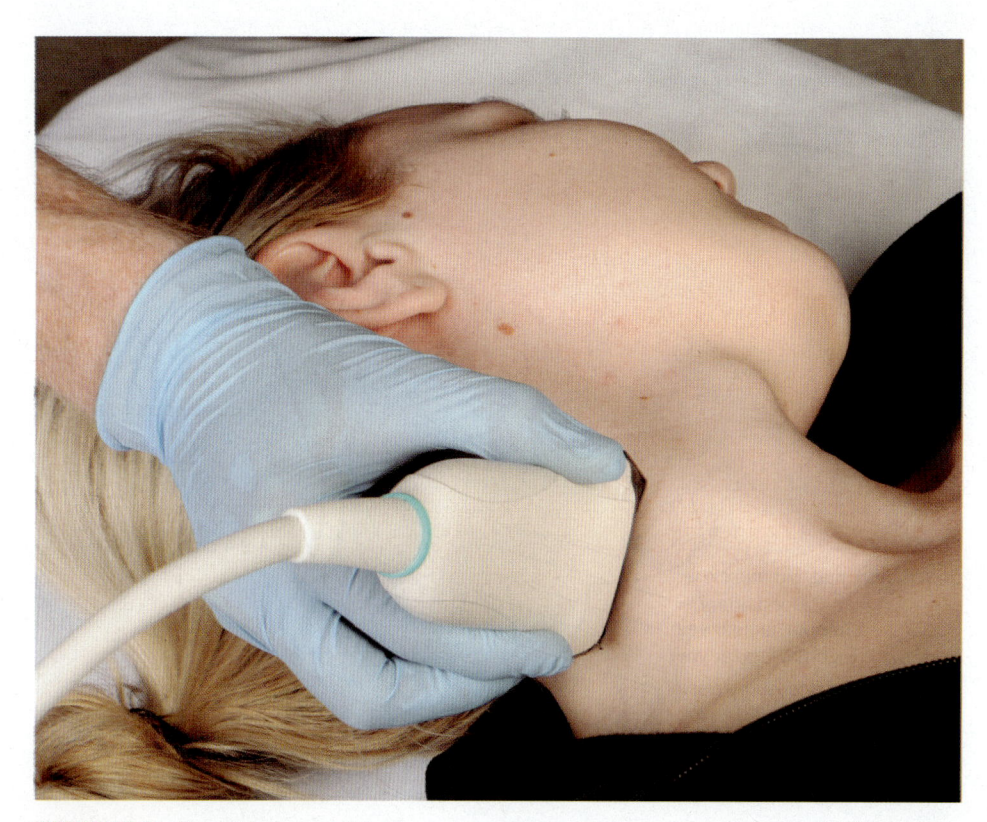

**FIGURE 17.4.** Proper placement of the linear ultrasound transducer over the previously identified margin of the sternocleidomastoid muscle.

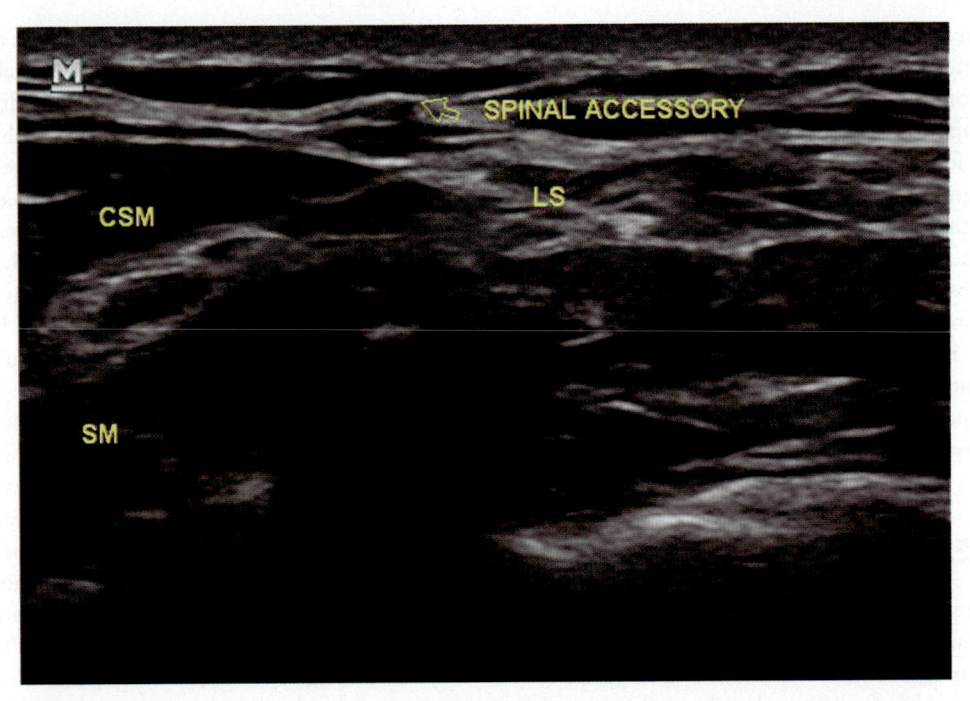

**FIGURE 17.5.** Transverse ultrasound view of the spinal accessory nerve as it lies above the levator scapulae muscle.

neck. The incidence of injury to these vessels and the inadvertent intravascular injection of local anesthetic with subsequent toxicity occur less commonly when ultrasound guidance is utilized when performing this technique. Bleeding complications associated with this technique can be decreased if pressure is applied to the injection site following the injection. The use of cold packs applied to the injection site for short periods of time also decreases postprocedure bleeding and pain.

In addition to the potential for complications involving the vasculature, the proximity of the spinal accessory nerve to

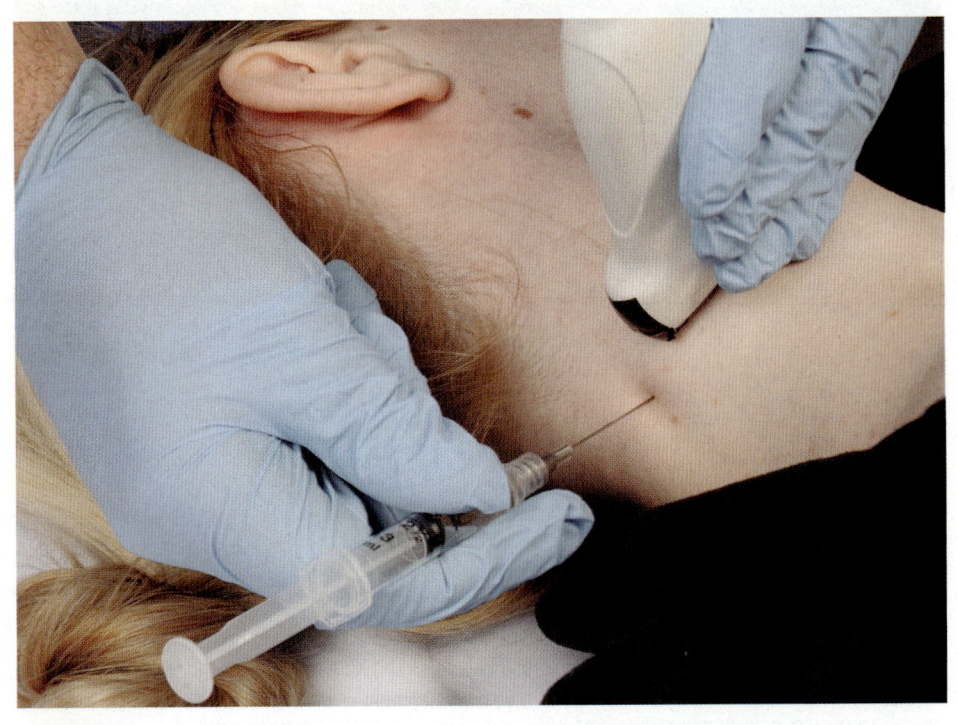

**FIGURE 17.6.** In-plane approach for ultrasound-guided injection of the styloid process nerve.

the central neuraxial structures and the phrenic nerve can result in serious side effects and complications. If the needle is placed too deep, the potential for inadvertent epidural, subdural, or subarachnoid injection is a possibility. If the volume of local anesthetic used for this block is accidentally placed in any of these spaces, significant motor and sensory block will result. Unrecognized, these complications could be fatal. Blockade of the phrenic nerve may occur during spinal accessory nerve block. In the absence of significant pulmonary disease, unilateral phrenic nerve block should rarely create respiratory embarrassment. However, inadvertent blockade of the recurrent laryngeal nerve with its attendant vocal cord paralysis combined with paralysis of the diaphragm may make the clearing of pulmonary and upper airway secretions difficult.

## CLINICAL PEARLS

This ultrasound-guided injection technique can produce dramatic relief for patients suffering from the pain and spasm of the trapezius and sternocleidomastoid muscles. The use of this technique to accurately identify the exact location and course of the spinal accessory nerve prior to surgery in the posterior triangle of the neck can avoid iatrogenic damage to the nerve. The proximity of the spinal accessory nerve to both carotid artery and jugular vein as well as the central neuraxial structures, emerging nerve roots, and the phrenic nerve means that the possibility for needle trauma to these vessels and nerves as well as the potential for inadvertent intravascular or epidural, subdural, or subarachnoid injection remains an ever-present possibility. The careful identification with ultrasound imaging of all structures in proximity to the spinal accessory nerve prior to needle placement is crucial to decreasing the incidence of the potentially fatal complications. Incremental dosing while carefully monitoring the patient for signs of local anesthetic toxicity can further decrease the risk to the patient. Even in the best of hands, postblock hematoma and ecchymosis can occur. Although these complications are usually transitory in nature, their dramatic appearance can be quite upsetting to the patient; therefore, the patient should be warned of such prior to the procedure.

Given the exceedingly low incidence of primary spinal accessory nerve pathology relative to other causes of pain and spasm in this anatomic region, primary lesions of the spinal accessory nerve must be considered a diagnosis of exclusion. The clinician should always evaluate the patient who suffers from pain and spasm in this anatomic region for occult tumors anywhere along the course of the spinal accessory nerve as they may present with clinical symptoms that can mimic the clinical presentation of primary lesions of the spinal accessory nerve (Fig. 17.7). Stretch injuries and compression of the spinal accessory nerve by aberrant arteries, muscle bands, etc. can be difficult to identify, and the use of electromyography and nerve

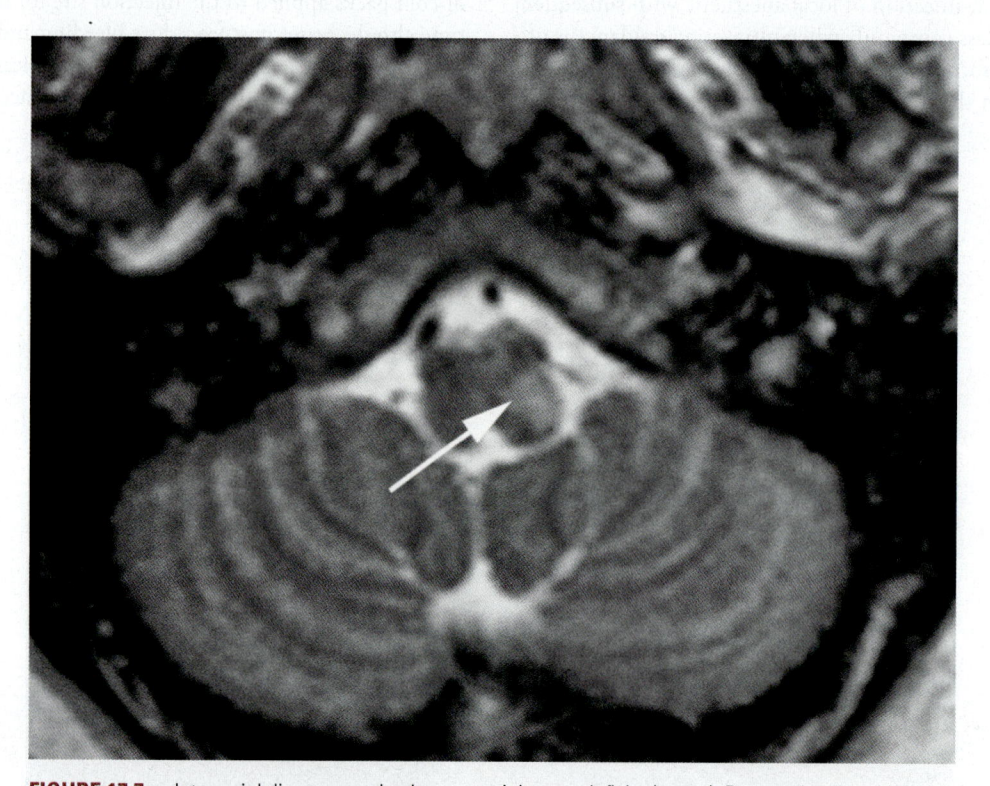

**FIGURE 17.7.** Intra-axial disease causing lower cranial nerve deficits (*arrow*). Progressive demyelinating disease involving the left brain stem causing cranial nerve XI and XII neuropathies clinically. (Reused from Verbist BM, Mancuso AA, Antonelli PJ. Spinal accessory neuropathy. In: Mancuso AA, Hanafee WN, eds. *Head and Neck Radiology.* Philadelphia, PA: Lippincott Williams & Wilkins; 2011:1070, with permission.)

conduction testing may be beneficial in clarifying the diagnosis. Other diseases that must be ruled out include spasmodic torticollis, demyelinating disease, and cervical dystonias.

The use of botulinum toxin administered directly into symptomatic muscles under electromyographic guidance may allow better control of the amount of muscle weakness produced when treating spasticity of the cervical musculature when compared with neurodestructive procedures of the spinal accessory nerve.

## SUGGESTED READINGS

Waldman SD. Glossopharyngeal neuralgia. In: *Atlas of Uncommon Pain Syndromes*. 2nd ed. Philadelphia, PA: Saunders Elsevier; 2008:30–32.

Waldman SD. The spinal accessory nerve. In: *Pain Review*. Philadelphia, PA: Saunders Elsevier; 2009:29–33.

Waldman SD. Spinal accessory nerve block. In: *Atlas of Interventional Pain Management*. 3rd ed. Philadelphia, PA: Saunders Elsevier; 2009:104–107.

Waldman SD. Spinal accessory nerve block. In: *Pain Review*. Philadelphia, PA: Saunders Elsevier; 2009:409–410.

# CHAPTER 18

# Ultrasound-Guided Phrenic Nerve Block

## CLINICAL PERSPECTIVES

Ultrasound-guided phrenic nerve block is useful in the management of intractable hiccups. This technique may also be utilized as both a diagnostic and therapeutic maneuver to help identify if the phrenic nerve is subserving subdiaphragmatic pain from tumor, abscess, or other pathology. The use of ultrasound imaging can identify the exact location and course of the phrenic nerve when surgical procedures in the posterior triangle of the neck are being contemplated. If destruction or sacrifice of the phrenic nerve is being considered, this technique is useful as a prognostic indicator of the degree of respiratory impairment from paralysis of the hemidiaphragm that the patient may experience. Neurodestruction of the phrenic nerve may be carried out by chemoneurolysis, cryoneurolysis, radiofrequency lesioning, surgical crushing, or resection of the nerve.

## CLINICALLY RELEVANT ANATOMY

The fibers that comprise the phrenic nerve arise primarily from the fourth cervical nerve root, with the nerve also receiving contributions from the third and fifth cervical roots as well (Fig. 18.1). The left and right phrenic nerves contains motor, sensory, and sympathetic fibers, which provide the motor and sensory innervation to their respective hemidiaphragm as well as the diaphragmatic central tendon. The phrenic nerve provides sympathetic and sensory fibers to the pericardium and mediastinal pleura.

The phrenic nerve descends in proximity to the internal jugular vein with the phrenic nerve passing inferiorly beneath the sternocleidomastoid muscle. At the level of the cricoid cartilage (the level where classic interscalene brachial plexus block is performed), the phrenic nerve is in very close proximity to the brachial plexus (see Figs. 18.1 and 18.2). As the phrenic nerve courses downward, it moves in an inferior medial trajectory away from the exiting nerves of the brachial plexus making selective blockade of the phrenic nerve a possibility. At the junction of the middle and lower posterior border of the sternocleidomastoid muscle, the phrenic nerve emerges from behind the sternocleidomastoid muscle and lies on top of the anterior scalene muscle where it is easily identified on ultrasound imaging (Figs. 18.3 and 18.4).

The phrenic nerves exits the root of the neck between the subclavian artery and vein to enter the mediastinum. The right phrenic nerve follows the course of the vena cava to provide motor innervation to the right hemidiaphragm. The left phrenic nerve descends across the pericardium of the left ventricle to provide motor innervation to the left hemidiaphragm in a course parallel to that of the vagus nerve.

## ULTRASOUND-GUIDED TECHNIQUE

To perform ultrasound-guided injection technique for phrenic nerve block, place the patient in supine position with the head turned away from the side to be blocked. The posterior border of the sternocleidomastoid muscle is identified by having the patient raise his or her head against the resistance of the clinician's hand (Fig. 18.5). The junction of the middle and lower middle third of the posterior margin of the muscle is identified, which is the approximate point at which the phrenic nerve emerges from beneath the sternocleidomastoid muscle, lying on top of the anterior scalene muscle where it is easily identified on ultrasound imaging (see Fig. 18.3). After preliminary identification of the approximate location of the nerve utilizing surface landmarks, the skin is prepped with antiseptic solution and 3 mL of local anesthetic is drawn up in a 10-mL sterile syringe, with 40 to 80 mg of depot steroid added if the condition being treated is thought to have an inflammatory component. A linear ultrasound transducer is then placed over the previously identified location of the nerve in the transverse plane (Fig. 18.6). The phrenic nerve should appear as a 2- to 3-mm hypoechoic oval monofascicular structure with a hyperechoic perineurium lying on top of the anterior scalene muscle as it exits beneath the posterior margin of the sternocleidomastoid muscle (see Fig. 18.3). If the phrenic nerve at this level is still in too close of proximity to the brachial plexus, its course can be traced in a posterior and caudad direction as it travels away from the brachial plexus. The internal jugular vein should be easily identifiable using color Doppler and may help the clinician identify the phrenic nerve, which lies in close proximity (Fig. 18.7). When the phrenic nerve is identified, a 22-gauge, 3½-inch styletted needle is advanced under real-time ultrasound guidance using an in-plane approach until the needle tip is in proximity to the nerve (Fig. 18.8). After careful

CHAPTER 18   ULTRASOUND-GUIDED PHRENIC NERVE BLOCK   119

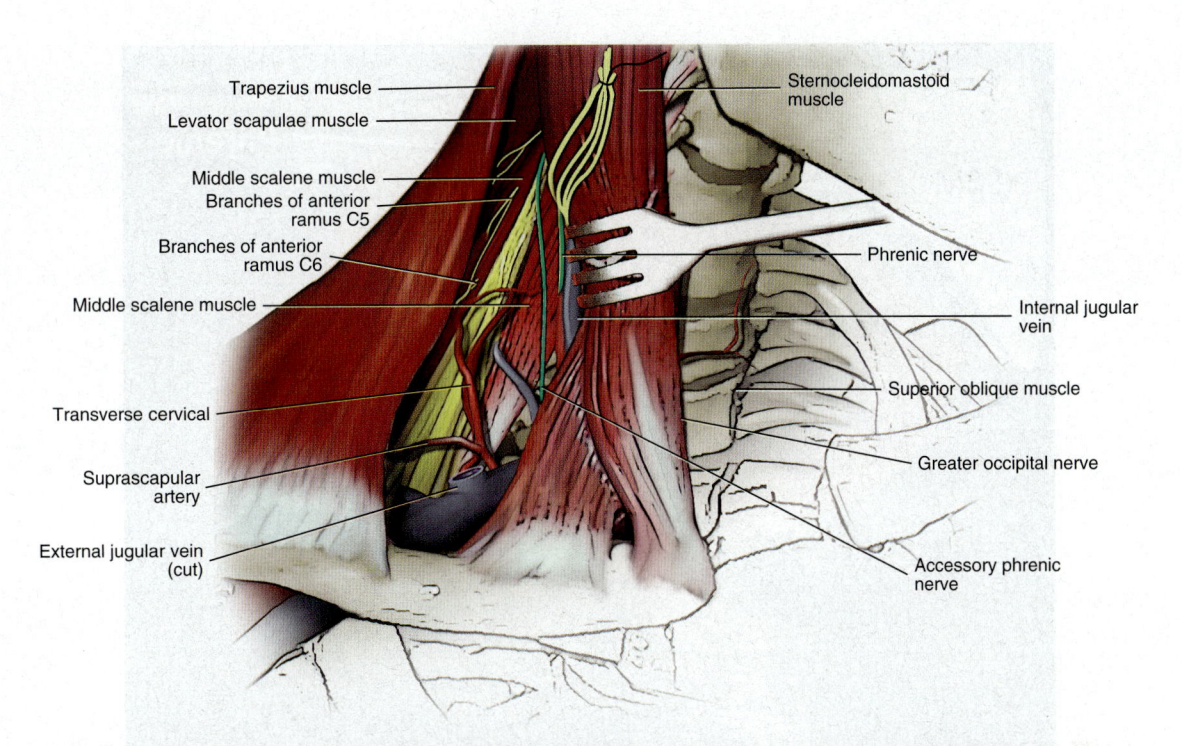

**FIGURE 18.1.** The anatomy of the phrenic nerve and surrounding structures. Note the relationship of the phrenic nerve to the brachial plexus and internal jugular vein.

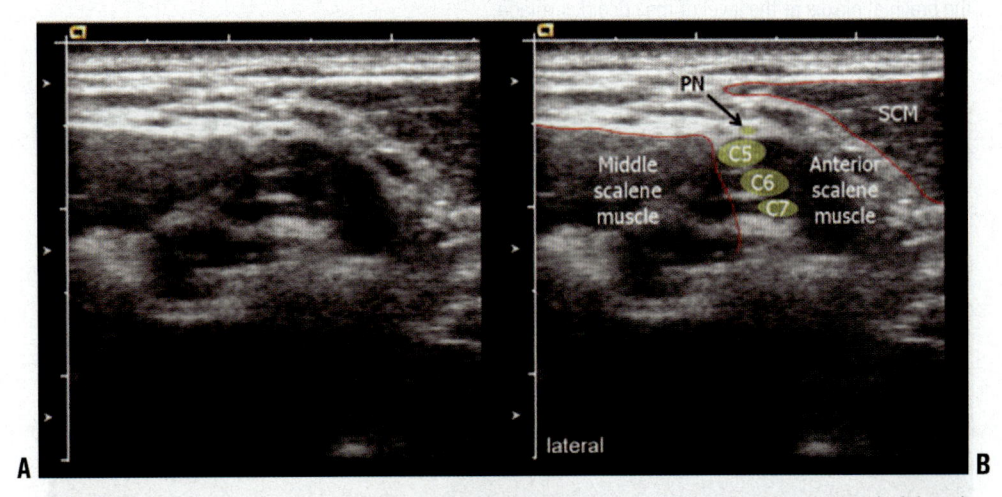

**FIGURE 18.2.** Sonogram showing (**A**) the phrenic nerve and cervical ventral rami at the level of the cricoid cartilage with (**B**) corresponding labeled image. In (B), the phrenic nerve (PN) is identified adjacent to the brachial plexus. Large tick marks are spaced 10 mm. (SCM, sternocleidomastoid muscle.) The borders of the sternocleidomastoid and middle scalene muscles are shown in *red*.

**FIGURE 18.3.** Transverse ultrasound image demonstrating the close proximity of the phrenic nerve to the brachial plexus at the level of the cricoid cartilage.

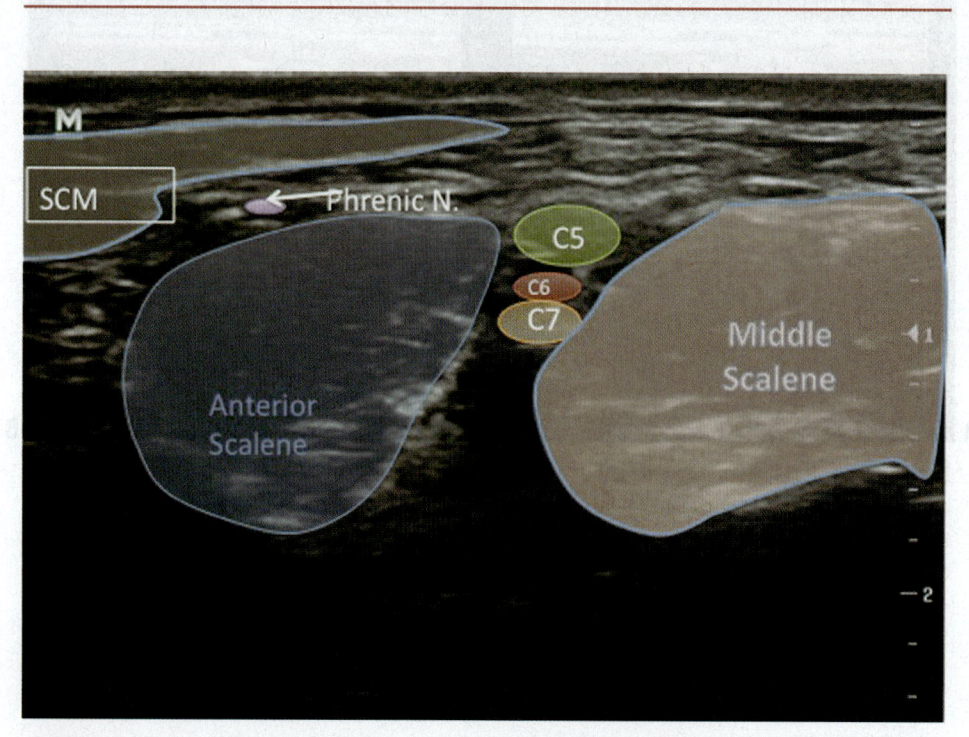

**FIGURE 18.4.** Transverse ultrasound image demonstrating how the phrenic nerve moves away from the brachial plexus as it courses inferiorly.

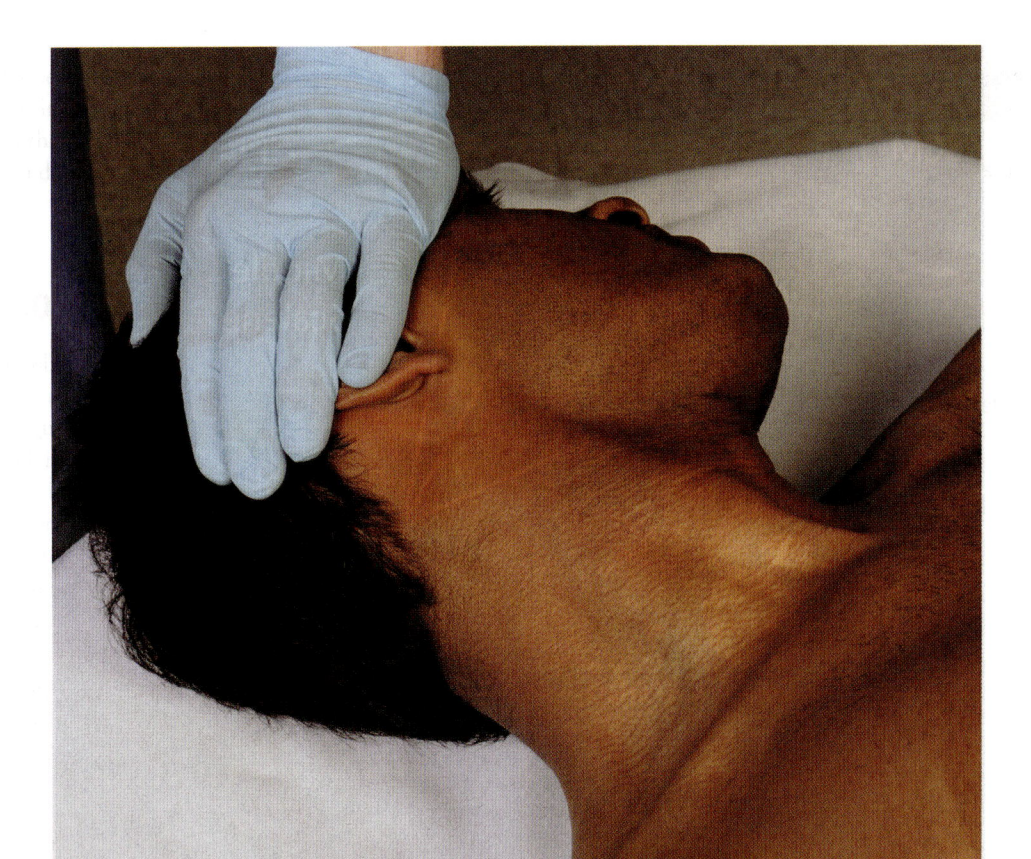

**FIGURE 18.5.** Having the patient raise his or her head against resistance will aid in identification of the sternocleidomastoid muscle.

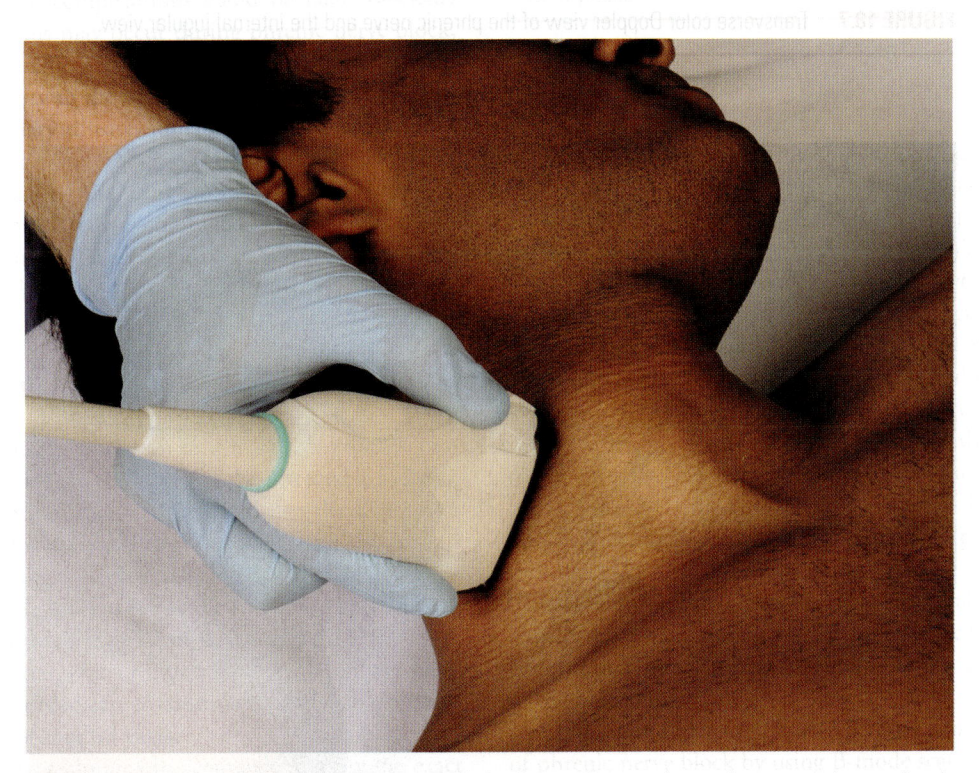

**FIGURE 18.6.** Proper transverse placement of the linear ultrasound transducer over the previously identified margin of the sternocleidomastoid muscle.

## SUGGESTED READINGS

Kessler J, Schafhalter-Zoppoth I, Gray AT. An ultrasound study of the phrenic nerve in the posterior cervical triangle: implications for the interscalene brachial plexus block. *Reg Anesth Pain Med* 2008;33(6):545–550.

Lam SHF, Roche C, Sarko J. Evaluation and management of coughs and hiccups. *Emerg Med Rep* 2012;33(17):193–203.

Michalek P, Kautznerova D. Combined use of ultrasonography and neurostimulation for therapeutic phrenic nerve block. *Reg Anesth Pain Med* 2002;27(3):306–308.

Waldman SD. The phrenic nerve. In: *Pain Review*. Philadelphia, PA: Saunders Elsevier; 2009:72–74.

Waldman SD. Phrenic nerve block. In: *Atlas of Interventional Pain Management*. 3rd ed. Philadelphia, PA: Saunders Elsevier; 2009:111–113.

# Ultrasound-Guided Facial Nerve Block

## CLINICAL PERSPECTIVES

Ultrasound-guided facial nerve block is useful in the diagnosis and management of a variety of painful conditions, which are subserved by the facial nerve. These conditions include geniculate neuralgia, atypical facial neuralgias, herpes zoster, and postherpetic neuralgia involving the geniculate ganglion (Ramsay Hunt syndrome) and the pain associated with Bell palsy (Fig. 19.1). Ultrasound-guided facial nerve block is also useful in the management of hemifacial spasm and may serve as an adjunctive treatment for essential blepharospasm, Meige syndrome, and other uncommon cranial dystonias (Fig. 19.2).

This technique may also be utilized as a diagnostic maneuver when performing differential neural blockade on an anatomic basis when evaluating difficult-to-diagnose head and neck pain syndromes and when considering a diagnosis of geniculate neuralgia. If sacrifice of the facial nerve is being considered in patients scheduled to undergo surgery on the base of the skull, this technique is useful as a prognostic indicator of the degree of motor and sensory impairment that the patient may experience.

## CLINICALLY RELEVANT ANATOMY

The facial nerve is the seventh cranial nerve, providing sensory, motor, and preganglion parasympathetic fibers to the head. The motor portion of the nerve arises from the facial nerve nucleus of the pons. The sensory portion of the nerve arises from the nervus intermedius at the inferior margin of the pons. It is at the point where the sensory portion of the nerve leaves the pons that it is susceptible to compression by aberrant blood vessels, which can cause a trigeminal neuralgia–like syndrome known as geniculate neuralgia and a facial dystonia known as hemifacial spasm (Fig. 19.3). After leaving the pons, the motor and sensory fibers of the facial nerve join to travel across the subarachnoid space and enter the internal auditory meatus to pass through the petrous temporal bone. It is at this point that swelling and inflammation of the facial nerve can cause Bell palsy (Fig. 19.4). The nerve then exits the base of the skull via the stylomastoid foramen (Fig. 19.5). It passes downward and then turns forward to pass through the parotid gland, where it divides into fibers that provide innervation to the muscles of facial expression.

## ULTRASOUND-GUIDED TECHNIQUE

To perform ultrasound-guided facial nerve block, the patient is placed in supine position with the head turned away from the side to be blocked. The mastoid process and the external acoustic auditory meatus are then identified by palpation (Fig. 19.6). After preliminary identification of these anatomic landmarks, the skin is prepped with antiseptic solution and 3 mL of local anesthetic is drawn up in a 10-mL sterile syringe, with 40 to 80 mg of depot steroid added if the condition being treated is thought to have an inflammatory component. A linear ultrasound transducer is then placed over the previously identified approximate location in the transverse plane (Fig. 19.7). The anteroinferior border of the mastoid bone at a point just below the external auditory meatus is then identified with ultrasound imaging (Fig. 19.8). The hyperechoic margin of the bone and its acoustic shadow should be easily identifiable. The facial nerve can then be identified as it exits the stylohyoid foramen (Fig. 19.9). Color Doppler can be utilized to identify major blood vessels in proximity to the facial nerve (Fig. 19.10).

A 22-gauge, 3½-inch styletted spinal needle is then advanced under real-time ultrasound guidance to a point just in front of the anteroinferior border of the mastoid bone and advanced ½ inch beyond the edge of the mastoid bone using an out-of-plane approach (Fig. 19.11). After careful aspiration reveals no blood or cerebrospinal fluid, 3 mL of solution should be slowly injected. The needle is removed and pressure is placed on the injection site to avoid bleeding complications. Subsequent daily nerve blocks are carried out in a similar manner.

## COMPLICATIONS

The major complications associated with this ultrasound-guided injection technique are related to needle-induced trauma to the internal jugular vein and/or carotid artery. The incidence of injury to these vessels and the inadvertent intravascular injection of local anesthetic with subsequent toxicity are less common complication of this technique when ultrasound guidance is utilized. Blockade of the motor portion of the facial nerve can result to paralysis of the muscles of facial

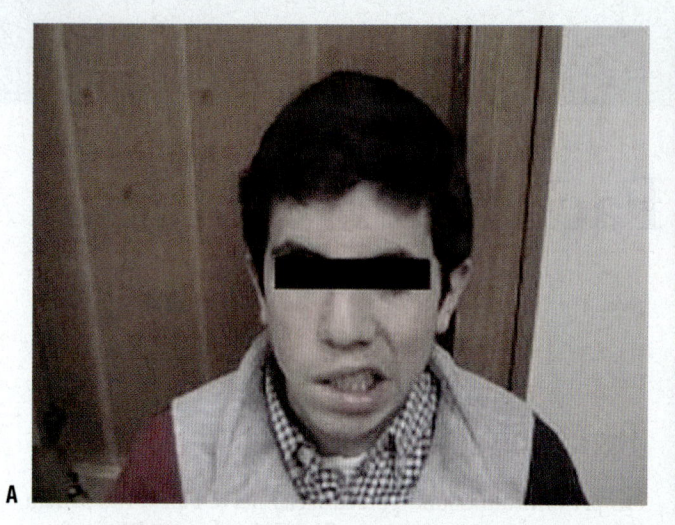

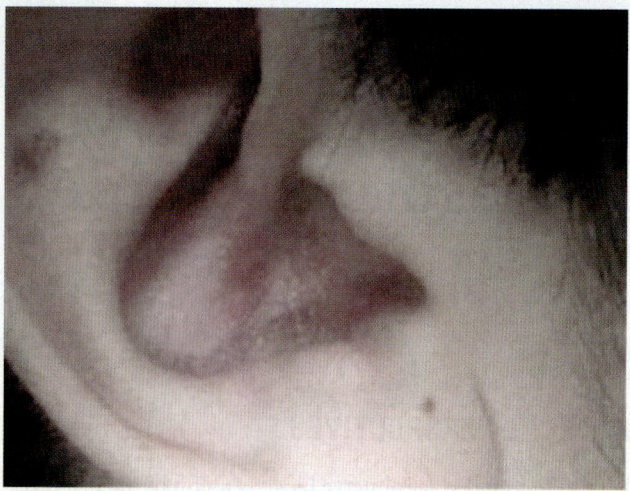

**FIGURE 19.1.** Ramsay Hunt syndrome **(B)**. Note the characteristic herpetic lesions of the external ear and **(A)** the facial drop secondary to facial nerve involvement. (Photo courtesy of Carolyn Beesley, O.D.)

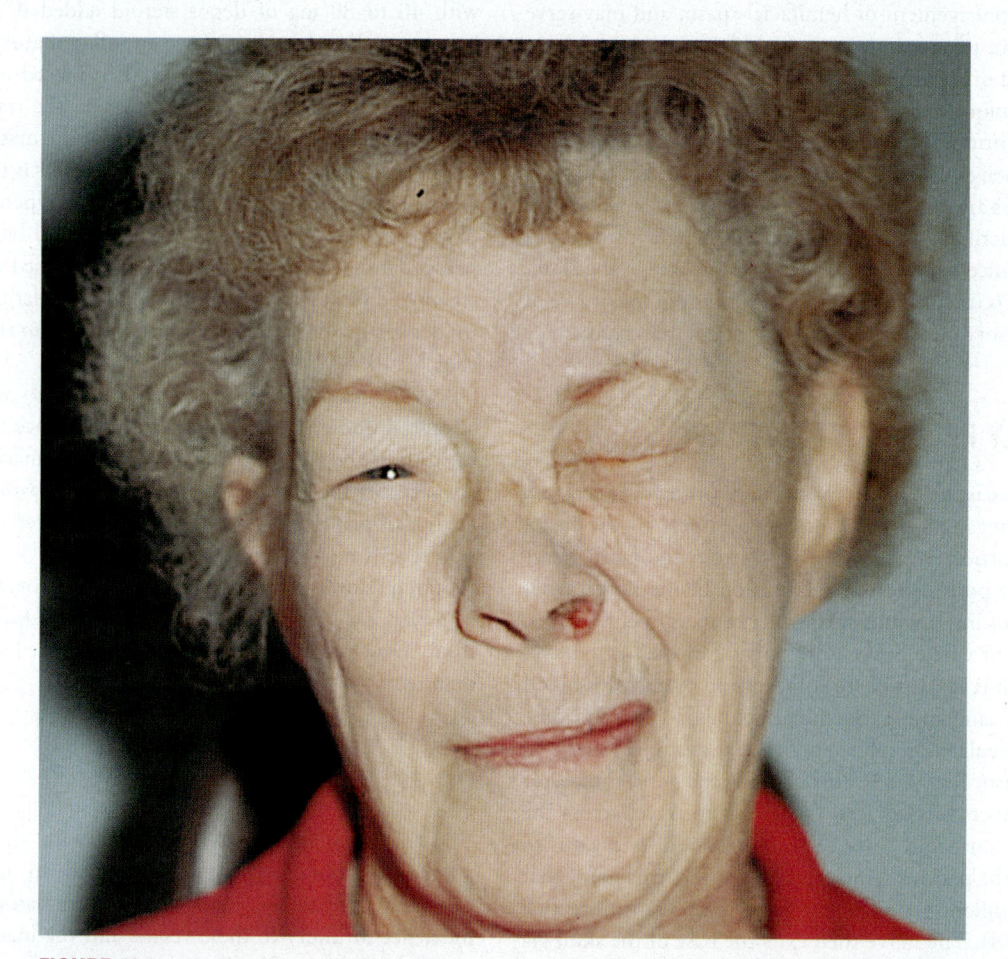

**FIGURE 19.2.** Hemifacial spasm. (Reused from Tasman W, Jaeger E. *The Wills Eye Hospital Atlas of Clinical Ophthalmology.* 2nd ed. Philadelphia, PA: Lippincott Williams & Wilkins; 2001, with permission.)

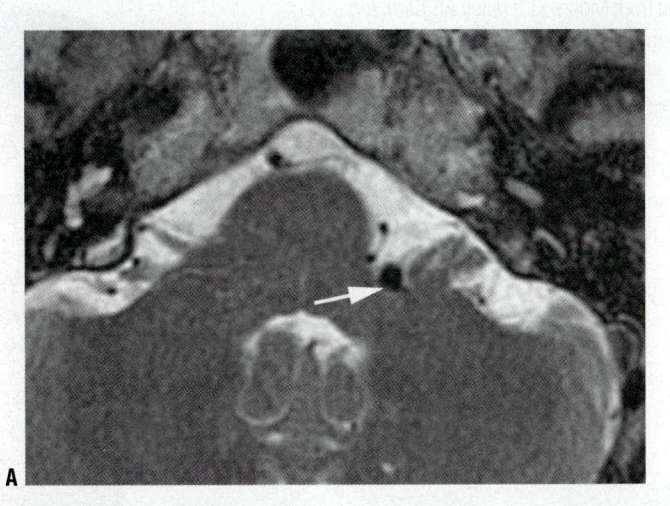

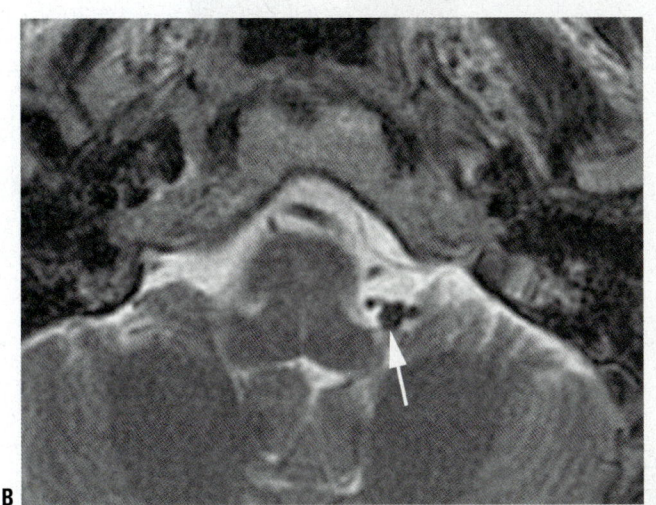

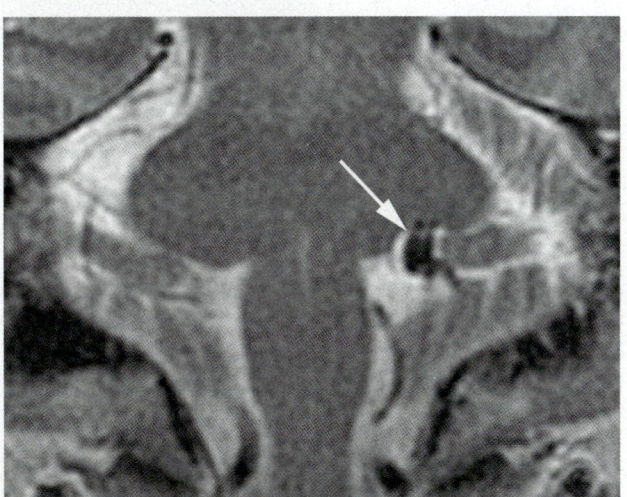

**FIGURE 19.3.** Hemifacial spasm as the presenting symptom of neurovascular compression (conflict) caused by a posterior inferior cerebellar artery (PICA) aneurysm. T2-weighted images show the aneurysm (*arrows*) compressing the nerve at its root entry zone **(A)** and its PICA origin **(B,C)**. (Reused from Verbist BM, Mancuso AA, Antonelli PJ. Facial nerve: vascular conditions. In: Mancuso AA, Hanafee WN, eds. *Head and Neck Radiology.* Philadelphia, PA: Lippincott Williams & Wilkins; 2011:984, with permission.)

expression. Inadvertent block of the glossopharyngeal, hypoglossal, and spinal accessory nerves during facial nerve block will result in weakness of the tongue and trapezius and sternocleidomastoid muscles and numbness in the distribution of the glossopharyngeal nerve. Bleeding complications associated with this technique can be decreased if pressure is applied to the injection site following the injection. The use of cold packs applied to the injection site for short periods of time also decreases postprocedure bleeding and pain.

## CLINICAL PEARLS

This ultrasound-guided injection technique can produce dramatic relief for patients suffering from the pain of geniculate neuralgia and from the symptoms of hemifacial spasm and facial dystonias. Geniculate neuralgia is clinically analogous to trigeminal and glossopharyngeal neuralgia. It is characterized by paroxysms of shock-like pain deep in the ear. Patients suffering from geniculate neuralgia often describe the pain as like having an ice pick stuck deep into their ear. This is a rare pain syndrome and should be considered a diagnosis of exclusion. The proximity of the facial nerve to both the carotid artery and jugular vein means that the possibility for needle trauma to these vessels and/or inadvertent intravascular injection is an ever-present possibility. The careful identification with ultrasound imaging of all structures in proximity to the facial nerve prior to needle placement is crucial to decreasing the incidence of the potentially fatal complications. Incremental dosing while carefully monitoring the patient for signs of local anesthetic

**FIGURE 19.4.** Bell palsy. (Reused from Moore KL, Dalley AF. *Clinically Oriented Anatomy.* 4th ed. Baltimore, MD: Lippincott Williams & Wilkins; 1999, with permission.)

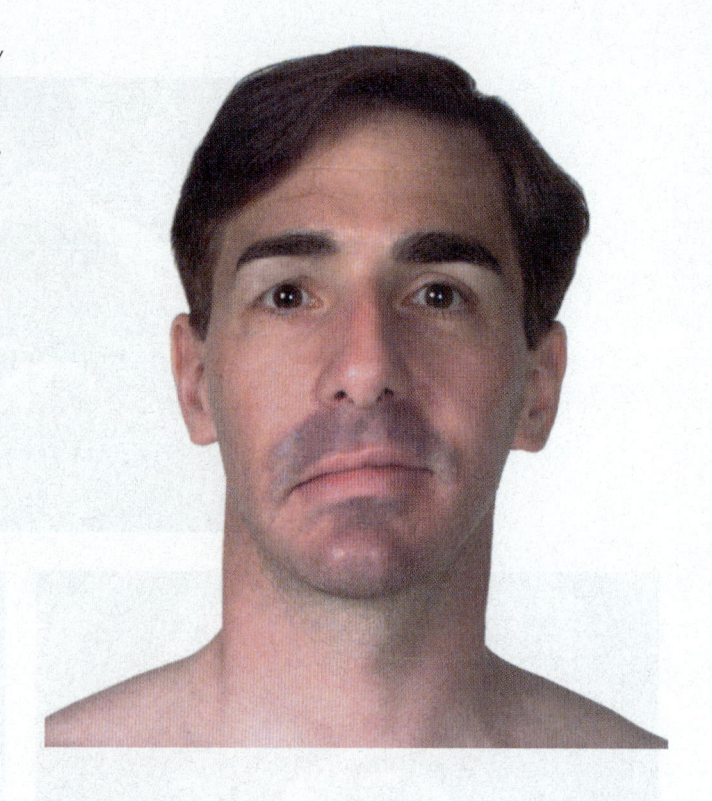

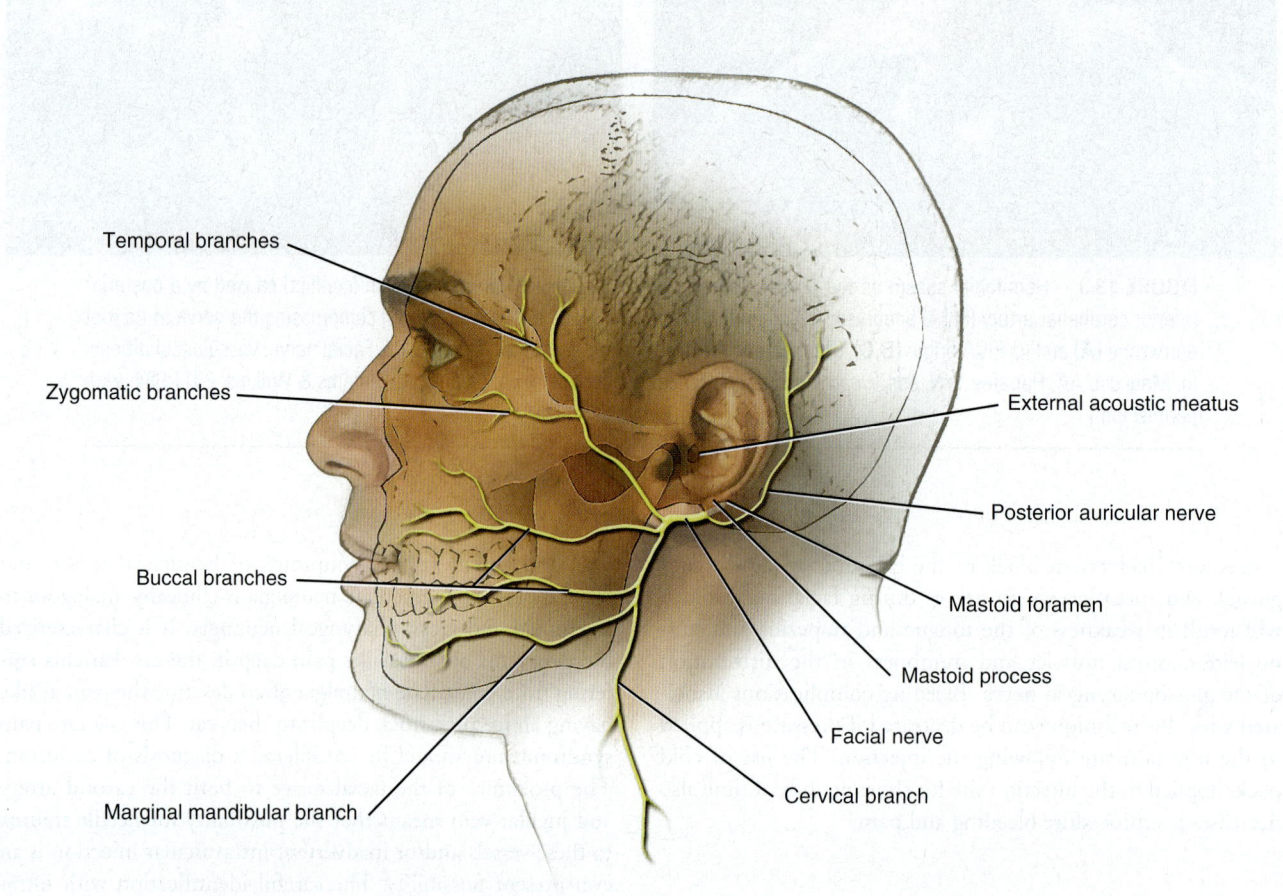

**FIGURE 19.5.** The anatomy of the facial nerve and its relationship to the mastoid process and external auditory meatus.

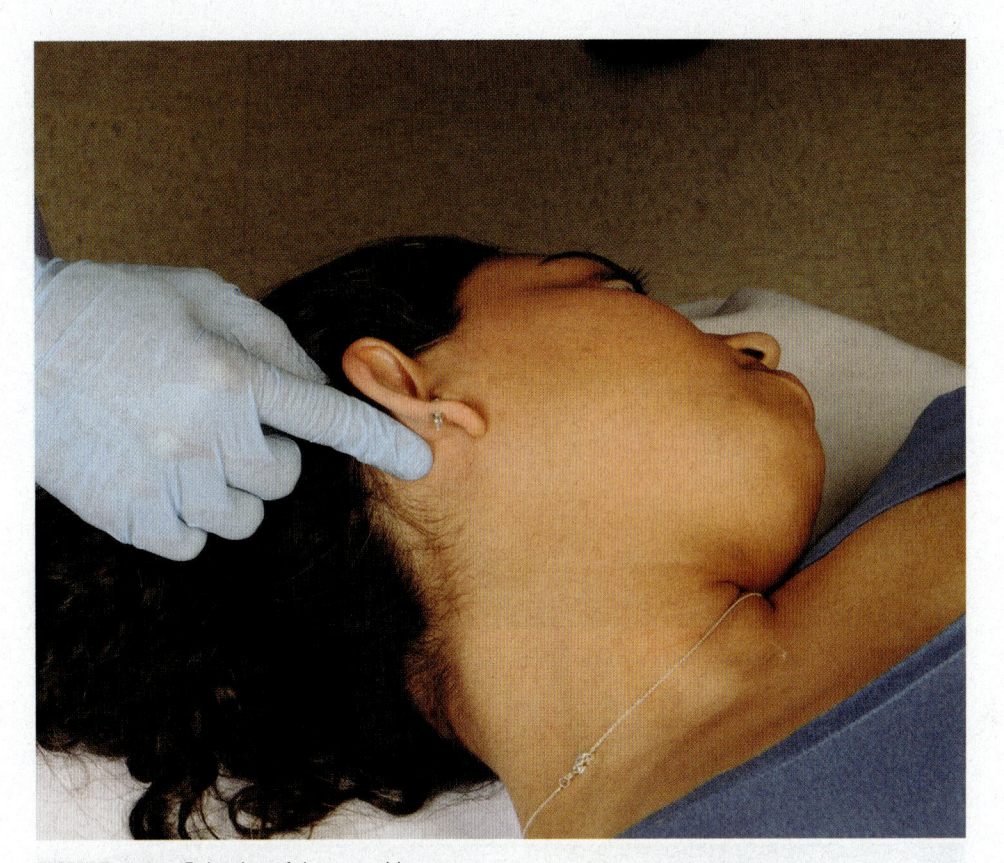

**FIGURE 19.6.** Palpation of the mastoid process.

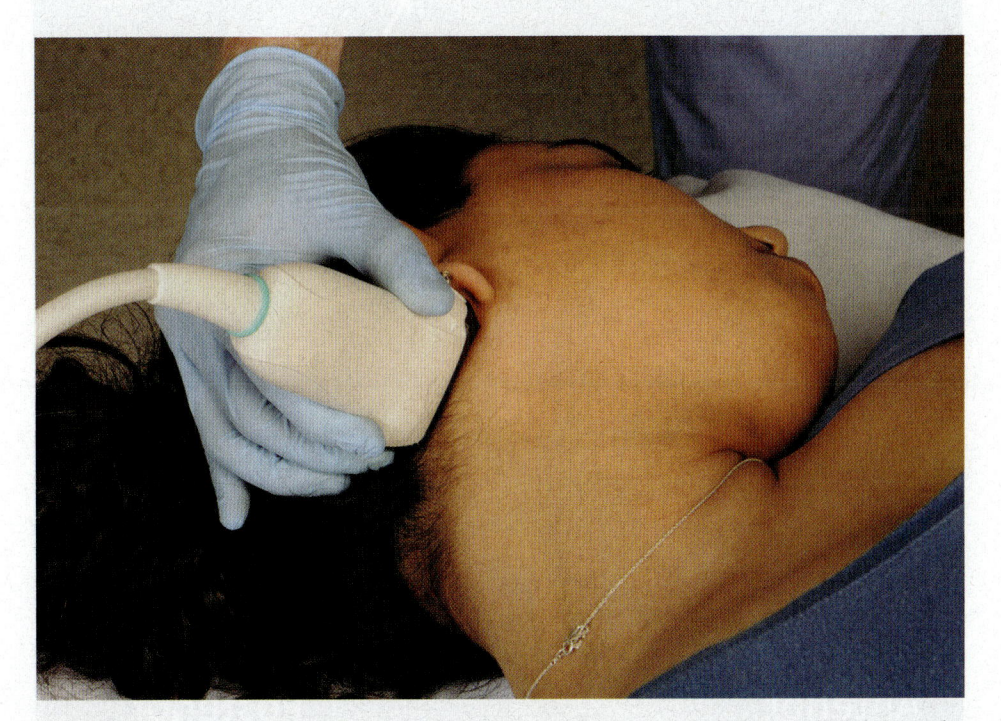

**FIGURE 19.7.** Proper transverse placement of the linear ultrasound transducer over the inferoanterior border of the mastoid process.

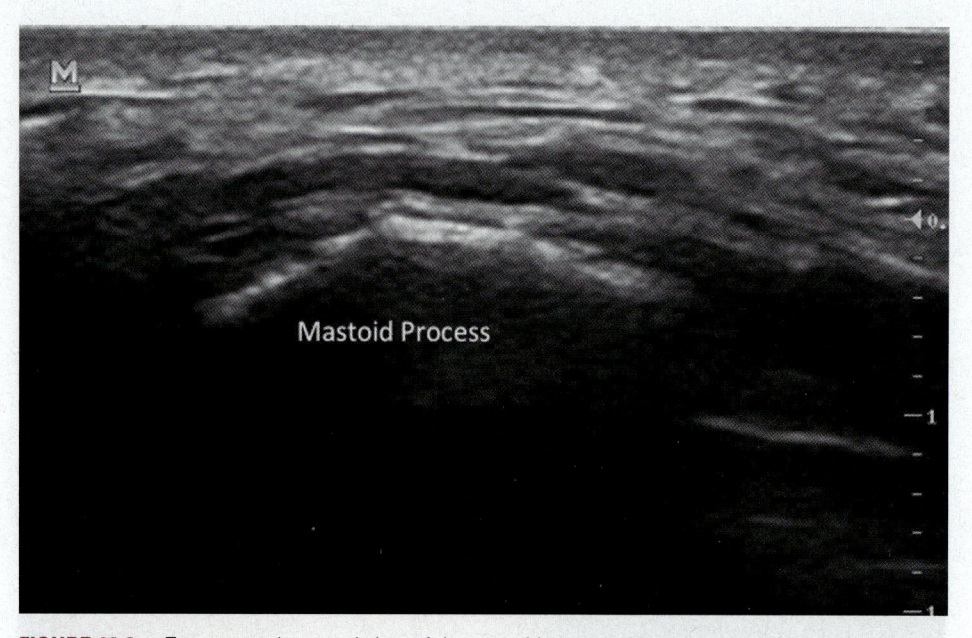

**FIGURE 19.8.** Transverse ultrasound view of the mastoid process. Note the curved hyperechoic border of the mastoid process.

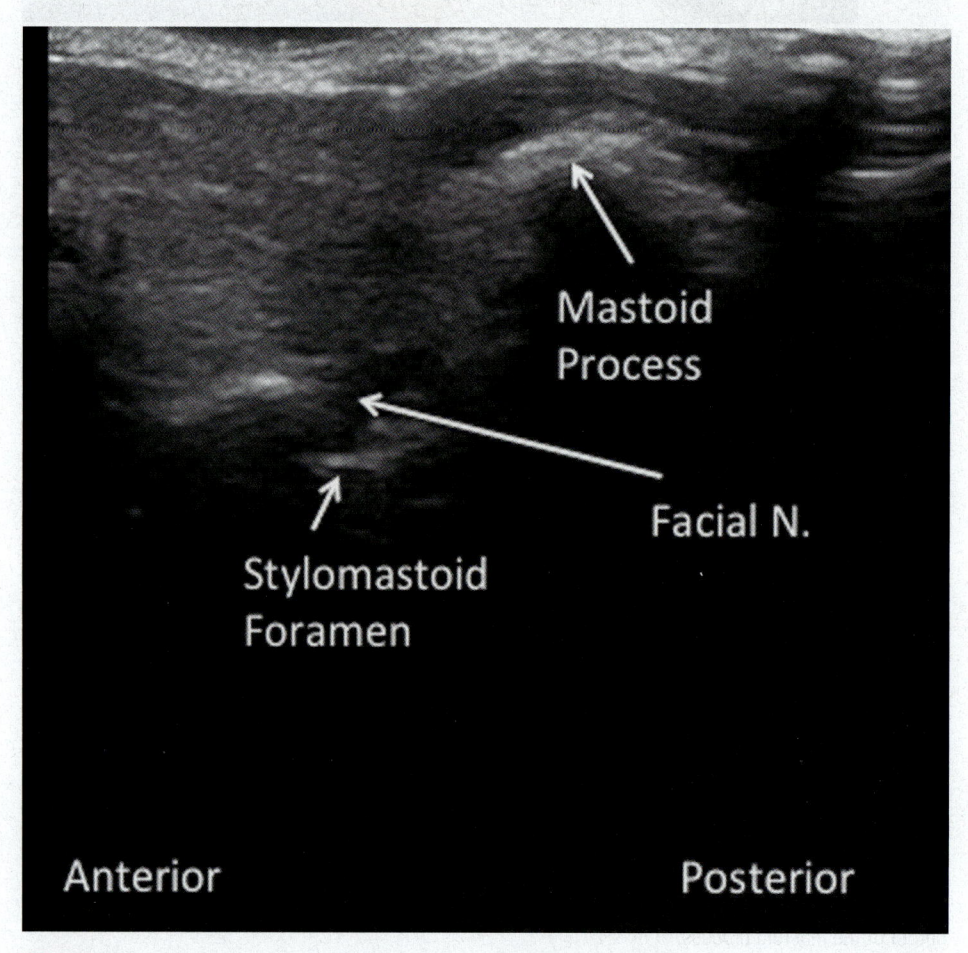

**FIGURE 19.9.** Transverse ultrasound view of the facial nerve.

CHAPTER 19    ULTRASOUND-GUIDED FACIAL NERVE BLOCK    131

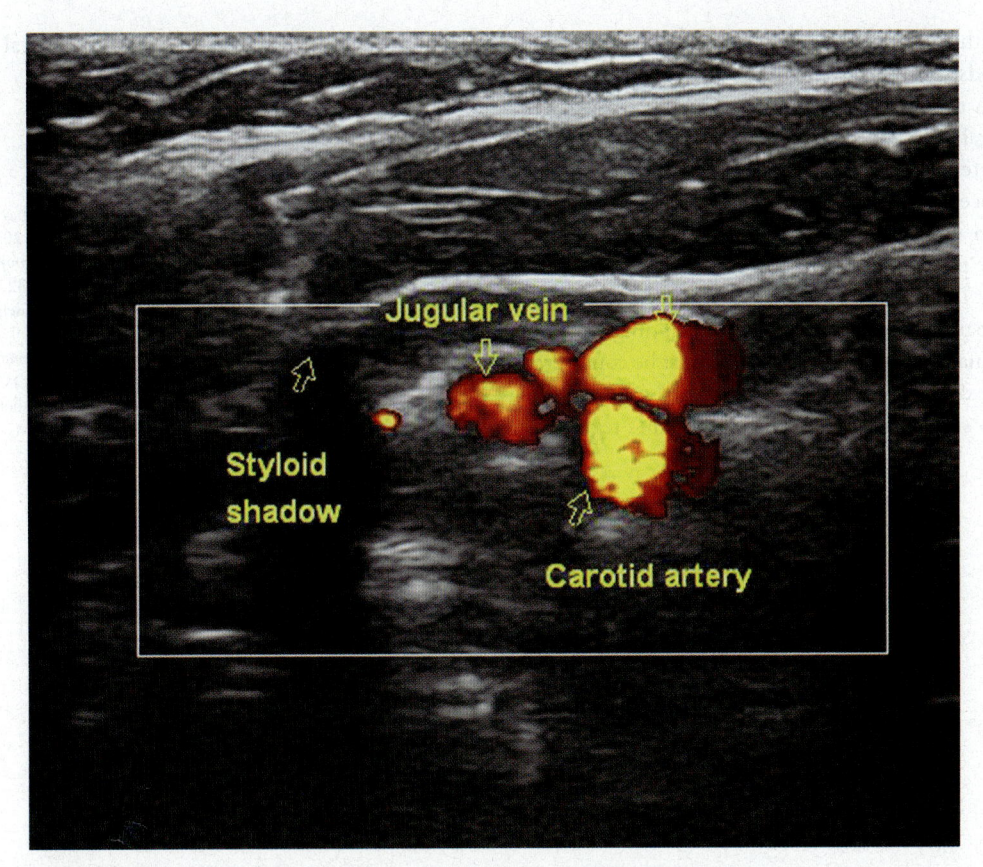

**FIGURE 19.10.** Color Doppler image of the carotid artery and jugular vein.

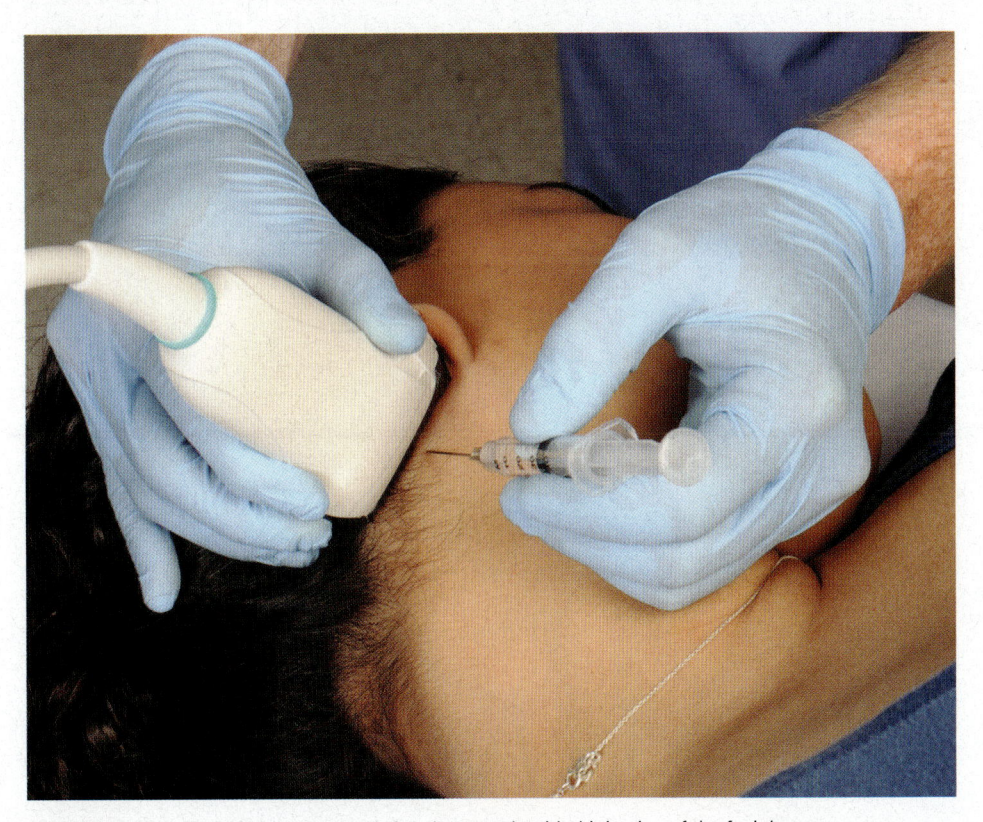

**FIGURE 19.11.** Out-of-plane approach for ultrasound-guided injection of the facial nerve.

toxicity can further decrease the risk to the patient. Even in the best of hands, postblock hematoma and ecchymosis can occur. Although these complications are usually transitory in nature, their dramatic appearance can be quite upsetting to the patient; therefore, the patient should be warned of such prior to the procedure. Since paralysis of the muscles of facial expression is an expected result of ultrasound-guided facial nerve block, the patient should be warned of such. Given the exceedingly low incidence of geniculate neuralgia relative to other causes of pain in this anatomic region including pain secondary to malignancy, geniculate neuralgia must be considered a diagnosis of exclusion. The clinician should always evaluate the patient who suffers from pain in this anatomic region for occult tumors as they may present with clinical symptoms that can mimic facial neuralgia (Fig. 19.7).

## SUGGESTED READINGS

Saers SJF, Han KS, de Ru JA. Microvascular decompression may be an effective treatment for nervus intermedius neuralgia. *J Laryngol Otol* 2011;125:520–522.

Waldman SD. Glossopharyngeal neuralgia. In: *Atlas of Uncommon Pain Syndromes*. 2nd ed. Philadelphia, PA: Saunders Elsevier; 2008:30–32.

Waldman SD. The facial nerve. In: *Pain Review*. Philadelphia, PA: Saunders Elsevier; 2009:19–21.

Waldman SD. Facial nerve block. In: *Atlas of Interventional Pain Management*. 3rd ed. Philadelphia, PA: Saunders Elsevier; 2009:114–117.

Waldman SD. Facial nerve block. In: *Pain Review*. Philadelphia, PA: Saunders Elsevier; 2009:414–415.

# CHAPTER 20

# Ultrasound-Guided Superficial Cervical Plexus Block

## CLINICAL PERSPECTIVES

Ultrasound-guided superficial cervical plexus block is useful in the diagnosis and treatment of painful conditions subserved by the nerves of the superficial cervical plexus, including post-trauma pain of the ear, neck, and clavicular region as well as pain of malignant origin. This technique is also used to provide surgical anesthesia in the distribution of the superficial cervical plexus for lesion removal, laceration repair, treatment of clavicular fractures, acromioclavicular joint dislocations, and carotid endarterectomy (Fig. 20.1). Neurodestructive procedures of the superficial cervical plexus may be indicated for pain of malignant origin that fails to respond to conservative measures.

## CLINICALLY RELEVANT ANATOMY

The superficial cervical plexus arises from fibers of the primary ventral rami of the first, second, third, and fourth cervical nerves. Each nerve divides into an ascending and a descending branch providing fibers to the nerves above and below, respectively. This collection of nerve branches makes up the cervical plexus, which provides both sensory and motor innervation. The most important motor branch is the phrenic nerve, with the plexus also providing motor fibers to the spinal accessory nerve and to the paravertebral and deep muscles of the neck. Each nerve, with the exception of the first cervical nerve, provides significant cutaneous sensory innervation. The four terminal branches of the cervical plexus are the (1) greater auricular, (2) lesser occipital, (3) transverse cervical, and (4) suprascapular nerves. These nerves converge at the midpoint of the sternocleidomastoid muscle at its posterior margin at the level of the superior pole of the thyroid cartilage to provide sensory innervation to the skin of the lower mandible, neck, and supraclavicular fossa (Fig. 20.2). Terminal sensory fibers of the superficial cervical plexus contribute to nerves including the greater auricular and lesser occipital nerves.

## ULTRASOUND-GUIDED TECHNIQUE

The patient is placed in the supine position with the head turned away from the side to be blocked. Nine milliliters of local anesthetic is drawn up in a 10-mL sterile syringe, and 40 to 80 mg of depot steroid is added to the local anesthetic if there is thought to be an inflammatory component to the patient's pain symptomatology. The posterior border of the sternocleidomastoid muscle at the level of the cricoid cartilage is then identified, and the skin overlying the area is prepped with antiseptic solution. A high-frequency linear ultrasound transducer is then placed over this point in a transverse oblique position at essentially a right angle to the posterior border of the sternocleidomastoid muscle (Fig. 20.3). At this point, the greater auricular nerve, which is one of the terminal branches of the superficial cervical plexus, will be visible twice in the same image, once in its position deep to the sternocleidomastoid muscle and then again in its superficial position as it curves back around the more superficial surface of the muscle (Fig. 20.4). It is at this point that the superficial cervical plexus is blocked utilizing an in-plane approach by placing a 22-gauge, 2-inch needle at the posterior border of the sternocleidomastoid muscle and advanced under the tapered belly of the muscle toward the carotid artery keeping the needle tip above the deeper fascia of the levator scapulae muscle (Fig. 20.5). A paresthesia may be elicited, and the patient should be warned of such. When the needle is in proximity to the greater auricular nerve, the stylet is removed, and after gentle aspiration, 9 mL of solution is injected in incremental doses under real-time ultrasound imaging. The needle is removed and pressure is placed on the injection site to avoid hematoma or ecchymosis.

## COMPLICATIONS

Given the proximity of the external jugular view and carotid artery, the clinician should carefully calculate the total milligram dosage of local anesthetic that may be safely given, especially if bilateral nerve blocks are being performed. Postblock ecchymosis and hematoma formation are a distinct possibility if these major vascular structures are injured during the procedure. Damage to the brachial plexus can also occur if the needle is placed too deep.

## CLINICAL PEARLS

The use of ultrasound guidance greatly increases the accuracy and safety of superficial cervical plexus block and allows

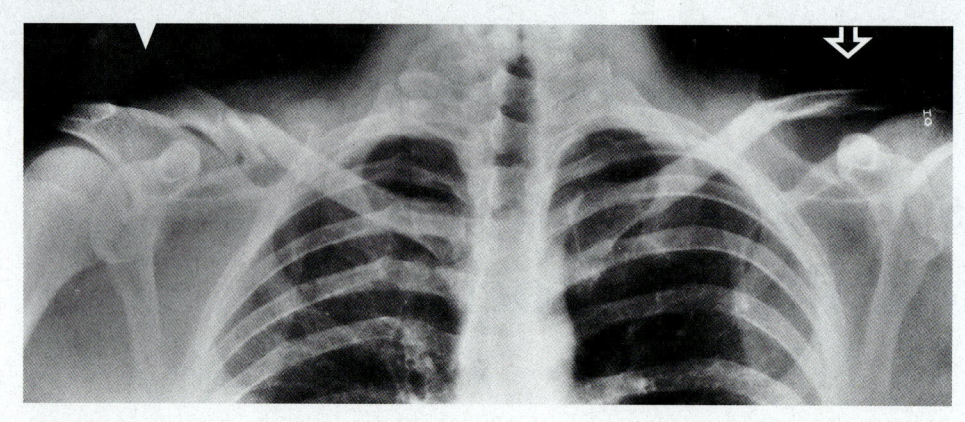

**FIGURE 20.1.** Superficial cervical plexus block is useful in the palliation of pain secondary to clavicular fractures. Fracture of both clavicles. A 22-year-old man sustained multiple traumas in a motorcycle accident. Anteroposterior view of both shoulders demonstrates a comminuted fracture of the middle third of the right clavicle (*arrow*) and a simple fracture of the middle third of the left clavicle (*open arrow*). (Reused from Greenspan A. Upper limb I: shoulder girdle. In: *Orthopaedic Imaging: A Practical Approach*. Philadelphia, PA: Lippincott Williams & Wilkins; 2011:111, with permission.)

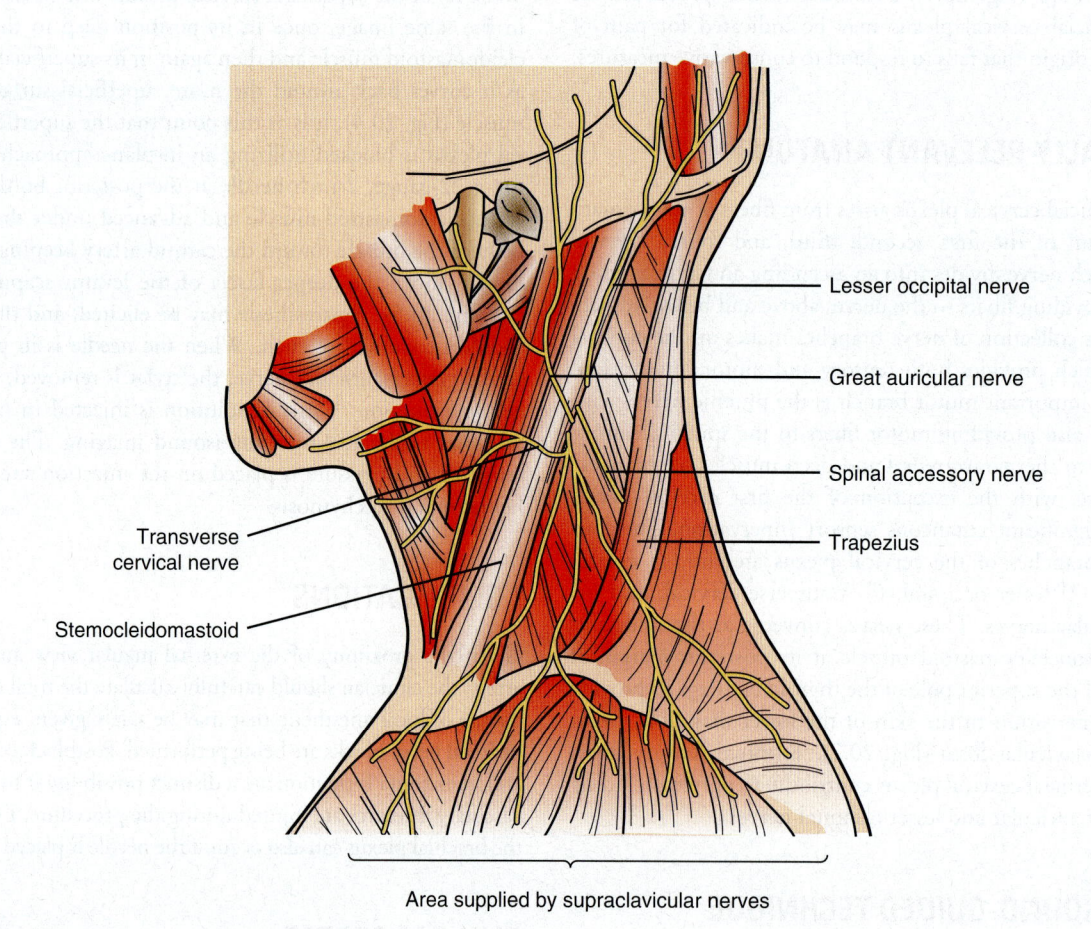

**FIGURE 20.2.** The anatomy of the superficial cervical plexus.

CHAPTER 20    ULTRASOUND-GUIDED SUPERFICIAL CERVICAL PLEXUS BLOCK    **135**

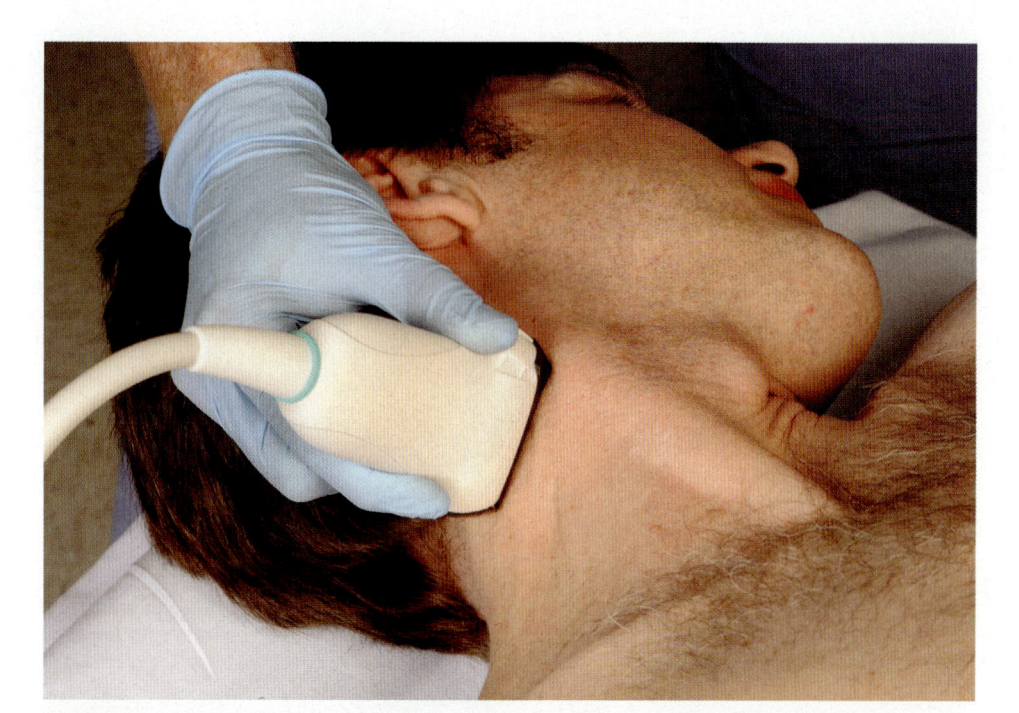

**FIGURE 20.3.** Correct position of the linear ultrasound transducer to perform superficial cervical plexus block.

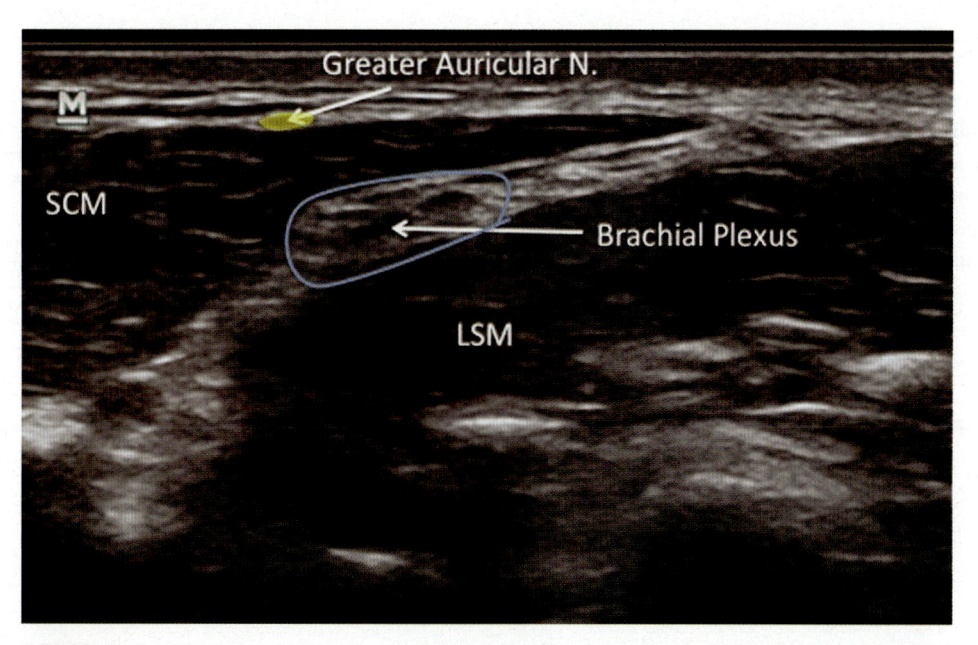

**FIGURE 20.4.** Transverse short-axis ultrasound image demonstrating both the deep and superficial segments of the superficial cervical plexus and the nerves relationship to the sternocleidomastoid muscle.

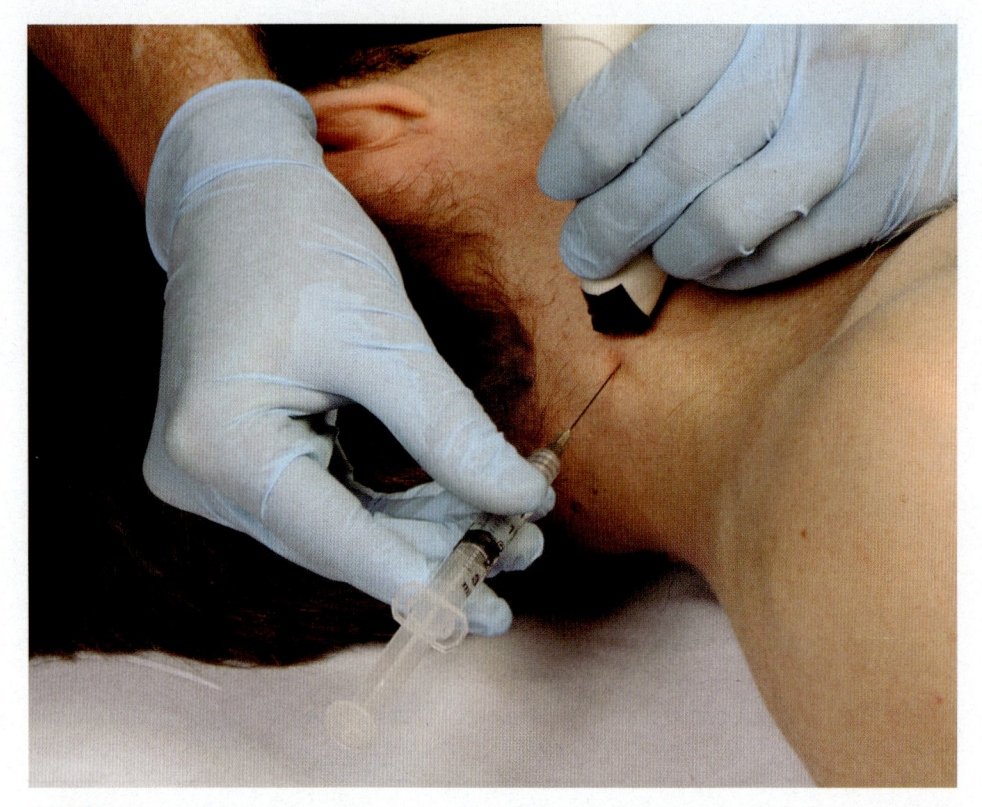

**FIGURE 20.5.** In-plane needle trajectory to perform ultrasound-guided superficial cervical plexus block.

the use of much smaller doses of local anesthetic when compared with landmark techniques. This technique provides excellent palliation of pain secondary to acute herpes zoster. When treating acute herpes zoster, the use of aluminum acetate solution applied as a tepid soak can help dry weeping lesions around the ear and helps make the patient more comfortable.

## SUGGESTED READINGS

Herring AA, Stone MB, Frenkel O, et al. The ultrasound-guided superficial cervical plexus block for anesthesia and analgesia in emergency care settings. *Am J Emerg Med* 2012;30(7):1263–1267.

Waldman SD. Superficial cervical plexus block. In: *Atlas of Interventional Pain Management*. 3rd ed. Philadelphia, PA: Saunders Elsevier; 2009:118–120.

Waldman SD. Superficial cervical plexus block. In: *Pain Review*. Philadelphia, PA: Saunders Elsevier; 2009:115–116.

Waldman SD. The superficial cervical plexus block. In: *Pain Review*. Philadelphia, PA: Saunders Elsevier; 2009:44.

# Ultrasound-Guided Deep Cervical Plexus Block

## CLINICAL PERSPECTIVES

Ultrasound-guided deep cervical plexus block is useful in the diagnosis and treatment of painful conditions subserved by the nerves of the deep cervical plexus, including posttrauma pain of the neck and supraclavicular fossa. This technique is also used to provide surgical anesthesia in the distribution of the deep cervical plexus for lesion removal, laceration repair, thyroid biopsy and thyroidectomy, deep lymph node biopsies and excisions, plastic surgery procedures of the neck, and carotid endarterectomy. Ultrasound-guided deep cervical plexus block may also be useful in the diagnosis and palliation of some cervical dystonias. Neurodestructive procedures of the deep cervical plexus may be indicated for pain of malignant origin that fails to respond to conservative measures.

## CLINICALLY RELEVANT ANATOMY

The deep cervical plexus arises from fibers of the primary ventral rami of the first, second, third, and fourth cervical nerves (Fig. 21.1). Each nerve divides into an ascending and a descending branch providing fibers to the nerves above and below, respectively. This collection of nerve branches makes up the cervical plexus, which provides both sensory and motor innervation. The most important motor branch of the cervical plexus is the phrenic nerve. The plexus also provides motor fibers to the spinal accessory nerve and to the paravertebral muscles and deep muscles of the neck. Each nerve, with the exception of the first cervical nerve, provides significant cutaneous sensory innervation. Terminal sensory fibers of the deep cervical plexus contribute fibers to the greater auricular and lesser occipital nerves. The fibers of the deep cervical plexus are in close proximity to the carotid artery and internal jugular vein, which provide excellent landmarks when performing ultrasound-guided deep cervical plexus block (Fig. 21.2).

## ULTRASOUND-GUIDED TECHNIQUE

The patient is placed in the supine position with the head turned away from the side to be blocked. Eleven milliliters of local anesthetic is drawn up in a 12-mL sterile syringe, and 40 to 80 mg of depot steroid is added to the local anesthetic if there is thought to be an inflammatory component to the patient's pain symptomatology. The posterior border of the sternocleidomastoid muscle at the level of the superior thyroid cartilage (corresponding to approximately the C4 level) is then identified, and the skin overlying the area is prepped with antiseptic solution. A high-frequency linear ultrasound transducer is then placed over this point in a transverse oblique position at essentially a right angle to the posterior border of the sternocleidomastoid muscle (Fig. 21.3). At this point, the ultrasound transducer is slowly moved medially until the carotid artery and internal jugular vein are identified and their positions confirmed with power Doppler (Fig. 21.4). It is at this point that the deep cervical plexus is blocked utilizing an in-plane approach by placing a 22-gauge, 3½-inch styletted spinal needle at the posterior border of the sternocleidomastoid muscle and advanced under the tapered belly of the muscle toward the carotid artery keeping the needle tip above the more lateral internal jugular vein (see Figs. 21.2 and 21.5). When the needle tip is in proximity to the lateral border of the carotid artery, the stylet is removed, and after gentle aspiration, 9 to 10 mL of solution is injected in incremental doses under real-time ultrasound imaging. The needle is removed and pressure is placed on the injection site to avoid hematoma or ecchymosis.

## COMPLICATIONS

Given the proximity of the external jugular view and carotid artery, the clinician should carefully calculate the total milligram dosage of local anesthetic that may be safely given. Postblock ecchymosis and hematoma formation are a distinct possibility if these major vascular structures are injured during the procedure. Damage to the brachial plexus can also occur if the needle is placed too deep.

## CLINICAL PEARLS

The use of ultrasound guidance greatly increases the accuracy and safety of deep cervical plexus block and allows the use of

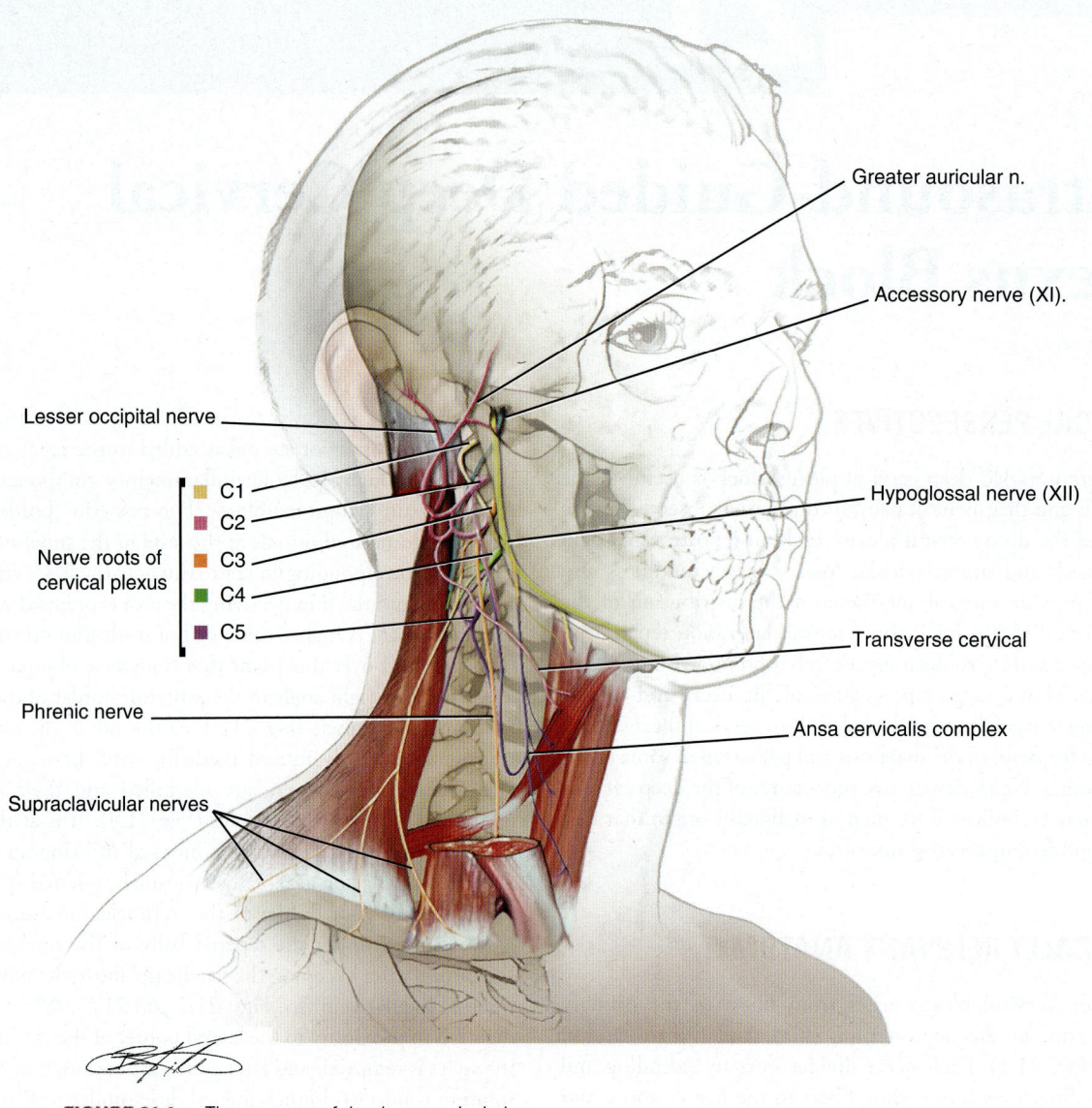

**FIGURE 21.1.** The anatomy of the deep cervical plexus.

smaller doses of local anesthetic when compared with landmark techniques. This ultrasound-guided technique allows the clinician to avoid placing the needle tip in proximity to the exiting nerve roots and neuroaxial structures as is done when performing a traditional landmark-guided approach to the deep cervical plexus. Given the close proximity of the cervical sympathetic chain, inadvertent block of this anatomic structure with resultant Horner syndrome can occur.

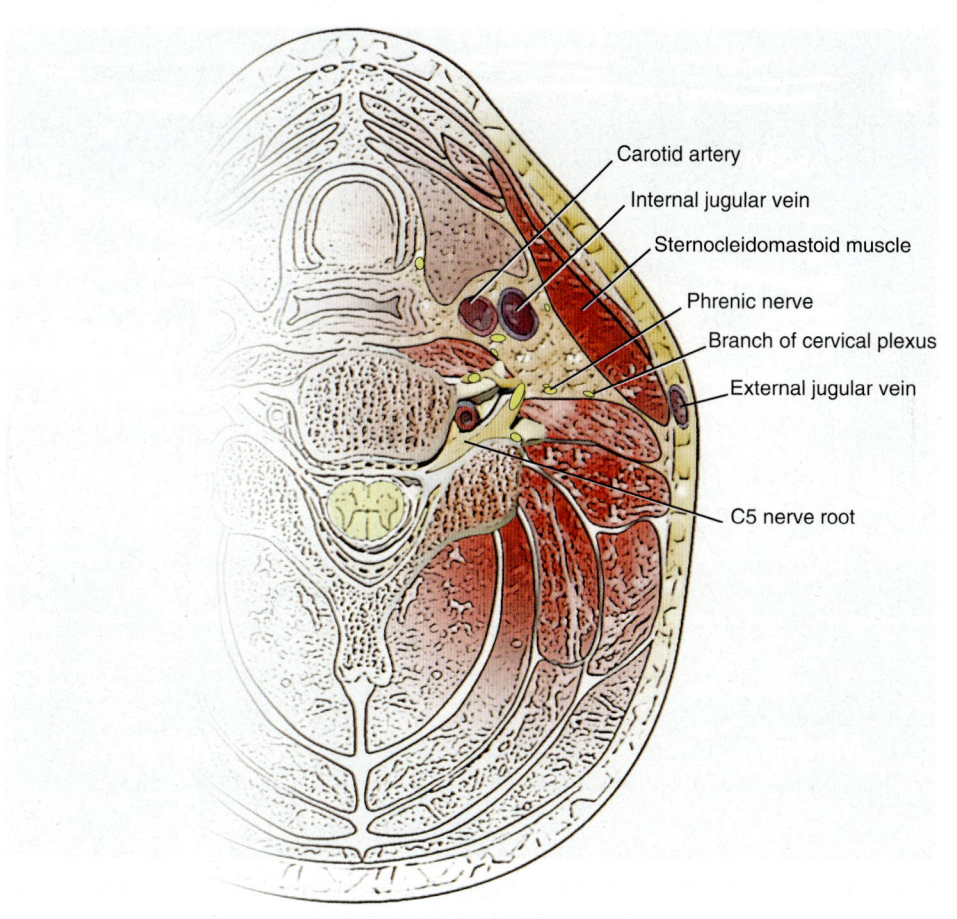

**FIGURE 21.2.** The cross-sectional anatomy of the deep cervical plexus illustrating the relationship of the carotid artery and jugular vein at the level of the superior thyroid cartilage.

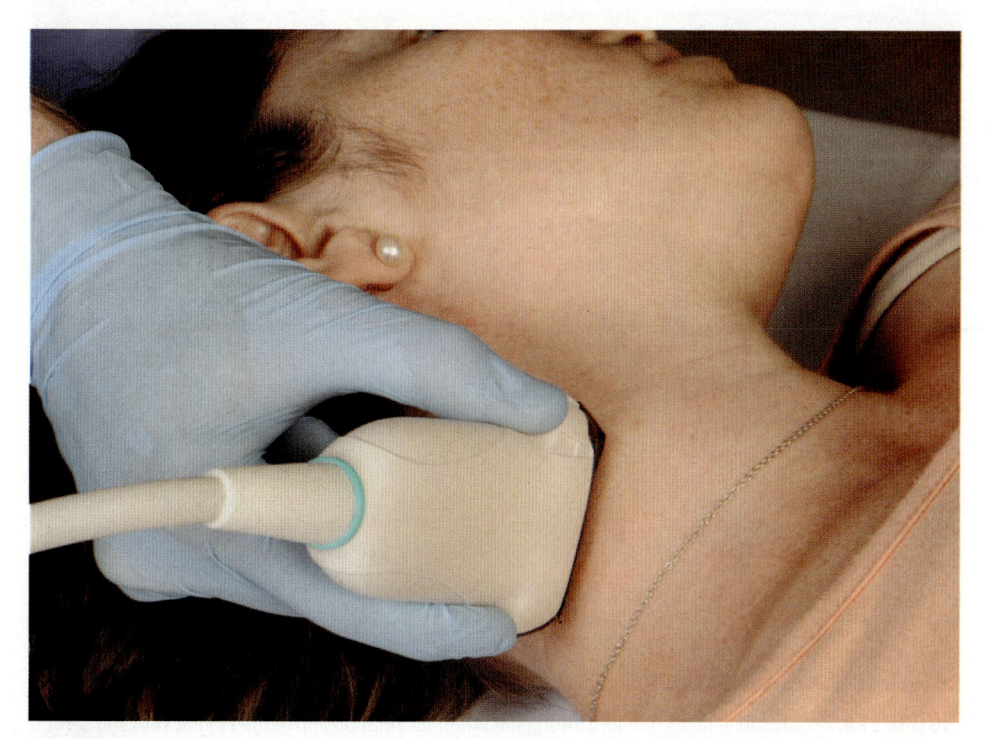

**FIGURE 21.3.** Correct position of the linear ultrasound transducer to perform deep cervical plexus block.

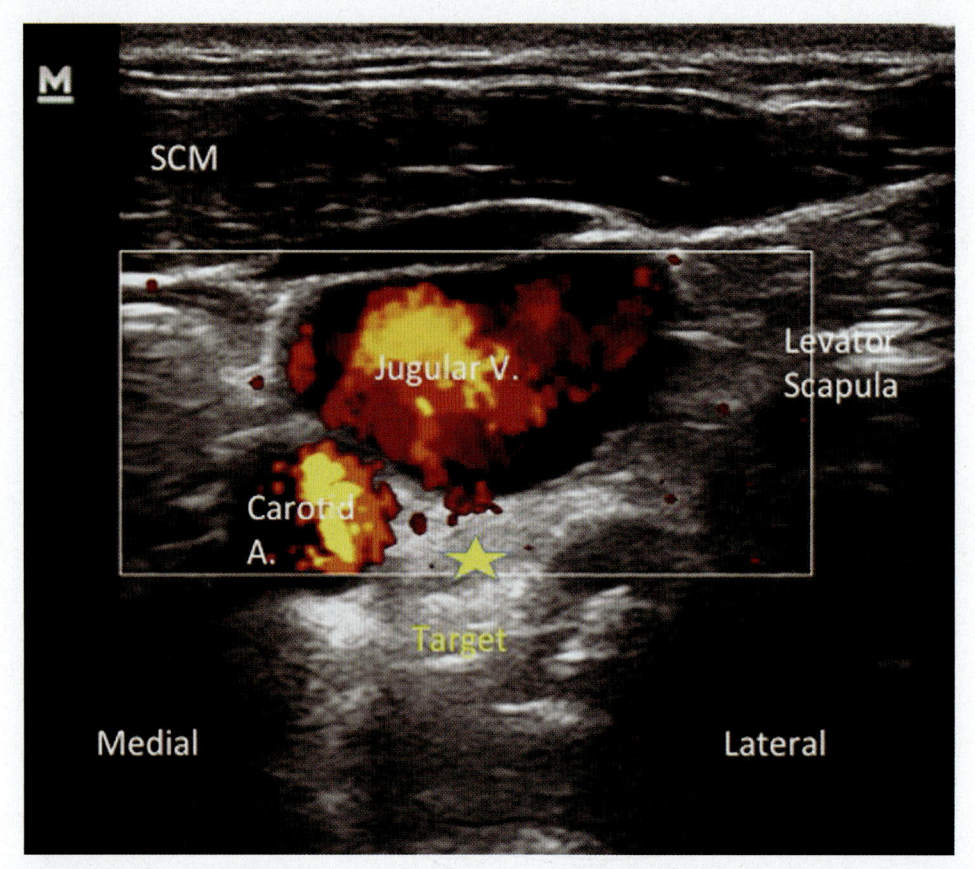

**FIGURE 21.4.** Power Doppler image demonstrating the anatomic relationship of the jugular vein and carotid artery to the target injection site for deep brachial plexus block.

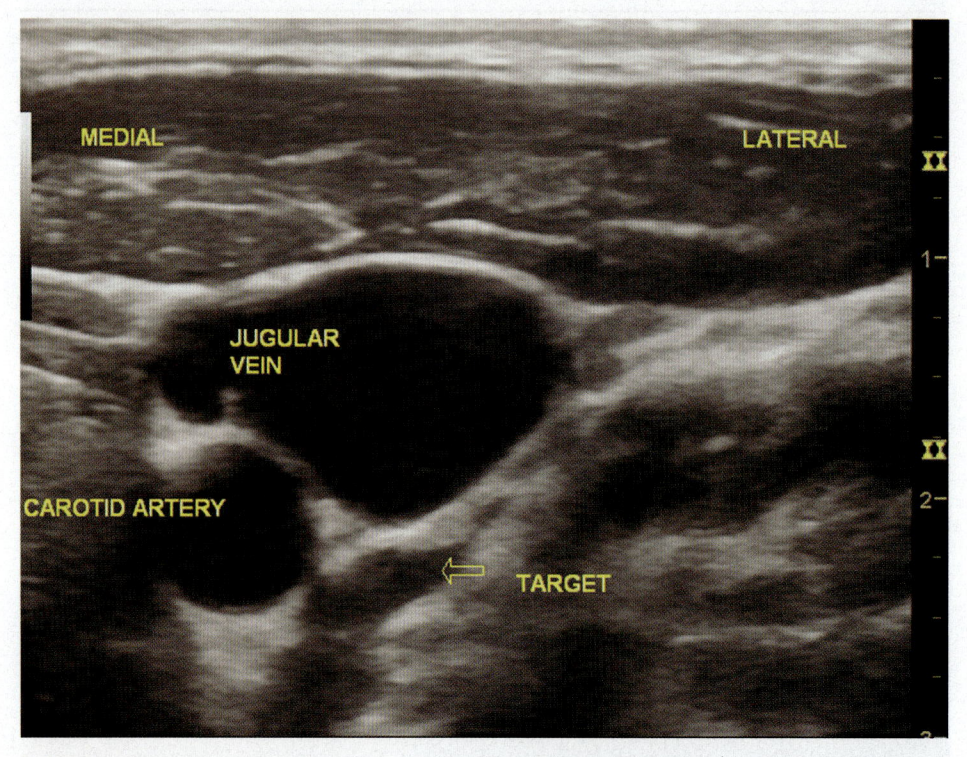

**FIGURE 21.5.** Ultrasound image demonstrating the anatomic relationship of the jugular vein and carotid artery to the target injection site for deep brachial plexus block.

## SUGGESTED READINGS

Herring AA, Stone MB, Frenkel O, et al. The ultrasound-guided superficial cervical plexus block for anesthesia and analgesia in emergency care settings. *Am J Emerg Med* 2012;30(7):1263–1267.

Usui Y, Kobayaski T, Kakinuma H, et al. An anatomical basis for blocking of the deep cervical plexus and cervical sympathetic tract using an ultrasound-guided technique. *Anesth Analg* 2010;110(3):964–968.

Waldman SD. Deep cervical plexus block. In: *Atlas of Interventional Pain Management*. 3rd ed. Philadelphia, PA: Saunders Elsevier; 2009:121–123.

Waldman SD. Deep cervical plexus block. In: *Pain Review*. Philadelphia, PA: Saunders Elsevier; 2009:417–418.

Waldman SD. The deep cervical plexus block. In: *Pain Review*. Philadelphia, PA: Saunders Elsevier; 2009:45.

# CHAPTER 22

# Ultrasound-Guided Superior Laryngeal Nerve Block

## CLINICAL PERSPECTIVES

Ultrasound-guided superior laryngeal nerve bock is useful in the diagnosis and treatment of painful conditions subserved by the superior laryngeal nerve, including posttrauma pain in the region of hyoid bone and thyroid gland, superior laryngeal neuralgia, hyoid syndrome, as well as painful conditions of the larynx and pharynx above the glottis and pain of malignant origin (Fig. 22.1). This technique is also used as an adjunct to awake endotracheal intubation and laryngobronchoscopy.

## CLINICALLY RELEVANT ANATOMY

The superior laryngeal nerve arises from the vagus nerve with a small contribution from the superior cervical ganglion. The nerve passes inferiorly and anteriorly behind the carotid arteries along the side of the pharynx to pass the lateral extent of the hyoid bone where it is accessible for nerve block (Fig. 22.2). Along with the superior laryngeal artery, which is a branch of the superior thyroid artery, the internal branch of the superior laryngeal nerve enters the larynx and pharynx through a foramen in the posteroinferior portion of the thyrohyoid membrane (see Fig. 22.2). It is at this penetration that malignancies tend to spread from the supraglottic region into the larynx (Fig. 22.3). The internal branch of the superior laryngeal nerve provides sensory innervation to the base of the tongue, both surfaces of epiglottis, the aryepiglottic folds, and the vestibule of the larynx to the level of the vocal folds. There are also secretomotor fibers that travel within the internal branch of the superior laryngeal nerve. An external branch provides motor innervation to the internal constrictor and cricothyroid muscles. The superior laryngeal nerve and its branches are susceptible to damage during thyroid surgery and compression from tumors.

## ULTRASOUND-GUIDED TECHNIQUE

The patient is placed in the supine position with the head in neutral position, and the patient is asked to minimize swallowing, which moves the position of the hyoid bone. Four milliliters of local anesthetic is drawn up in a 10-mL sterile syringe, and 40 to 80 mg of depot steroid is added to the local anesthetic if there is thought to be an inflammatory component to the patient's pain symptomatology. The lateral margin of the hyoid bone, which lies above the thyroid cartilage, is identified by palpation, and the skin overlying the area is prepped with antiseptic solution (Figs. 22.4 and 22.5). A high-frequency linear ultrasound transducer is then placed over the hyoid bone in the transverse position (Fig. 22.6). In patients with thinner necks, an acoustic standoff of ultrasound gel may be needed to optimize image quality. A characteristic triangular acoustic shadow helps to identify the body of the hyoid bone with the echogenic periosteum of the lesser cornua just cephalad (Fig. 22.7). In some patients, it may be helpful to have an assistant manually displace the hyoid bone toward the side to be blocked (Fig. 22.8). Just caudad to the body of the hyoid bone is the approximate location of the superior laryngeal nerve (Fig. 22.9). It is at this point that the superior laryngeal nerve is blocked utilizing an in-plane approach by placing a 22-gauge, 1½-inch needle lateral to the hyoid bone and advancing it to a point just caudad to the triangular acoustic shadow of the body of the hyoid bone (Fig. 22.10). If the periosteum of the bone is encountered, the needle is withdrawn and directed in a slightly more caudad direction. In some patients, the superior laryngeal artery, which lies just below the superior laryngeal nerve, may be identified with color Doppler (Fig. 22.11). When the needle is in proximity to the superior laryngeal nerve, after gentle aspiration, 4 mL of solution is injected in incremental doses under real-time ultrasound imaging. The needle is removed and pressure is placed on the injection site to avoid hematoma or ecchymosis.

## COMPLICATIONS

Given the proximity of the superior laryngeal, superior thyroid, and external carotid artery, the clinician should carefully calculate the total milligram dosage of local anesthetic that may be safely given, especially if bilateral nerve blocks are being performed. Postblock ecchymosis and hematoma formation are a distinct possibility if these vascular structures are injured during the procedure.

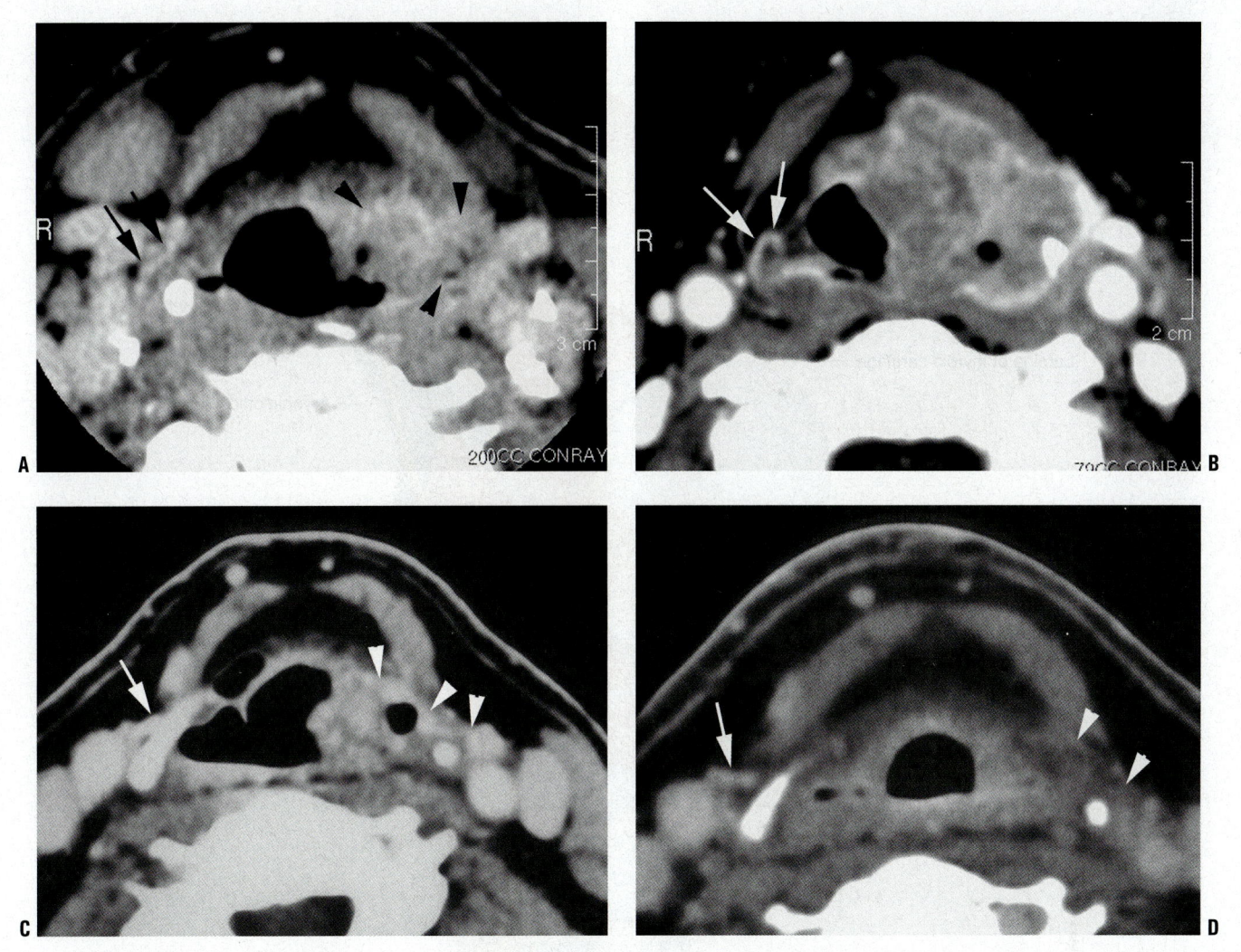

**FIGURE 22.1.** Contrast-enhanced computed tomography study of three patients with marginal supraglottic lesions showing a tendency for the lesions to spread out of the larynx through an area of inherent weakness along the region of penetration of the superior laryngeal neurovascular bundle. **A:** Patient 1. A highly infiltrating-appearing lesion (*arrowheads*) involves the infrahyoid strap muscles and grows to surround veins in the deep neck compared to the normal superior laryngeal vascular bundle on the opposite side (*arrows*). **B:** Patient 2. With a tumor that has more pushing type of margins but showing the same tendency to grow out of the larynx along with superior laryngeal neurovascular bundle. Note the normal superior laryngeal vessels as they penetrate the thyrohyoid membrane on the right (*arrows*). **C,D:** Patient 3. Showing spread of tumor along the superior laryngeal neurovascular bundle toward the carotid artery in the left neck (*arrowheads*) compared to the normal vessels on the right side (*arrow*). This was a relatively low-volume lesion treated with radiotherapy (RT). In (D), following RT, there is restoration of the normal anatomy around the superior laryngeal vessels (*arrowheads*) except for some vague soft tissue swelling. (NOTE: The normal vessel on the right (*arrow*). These are minor post-RT changes seen within the larynx. The patient was controlled with RT alone.) (Reused from Hermans R, Mancuso AA, Mendenhall WM, et al. Larynx: malignant tumors. In: Mancuso AA, Hanafee WN, eds. *Head and Neck Radiology.* Philadelphia, PA: Lippincott Williams & Wilkins; 2011:1994, with permission.)

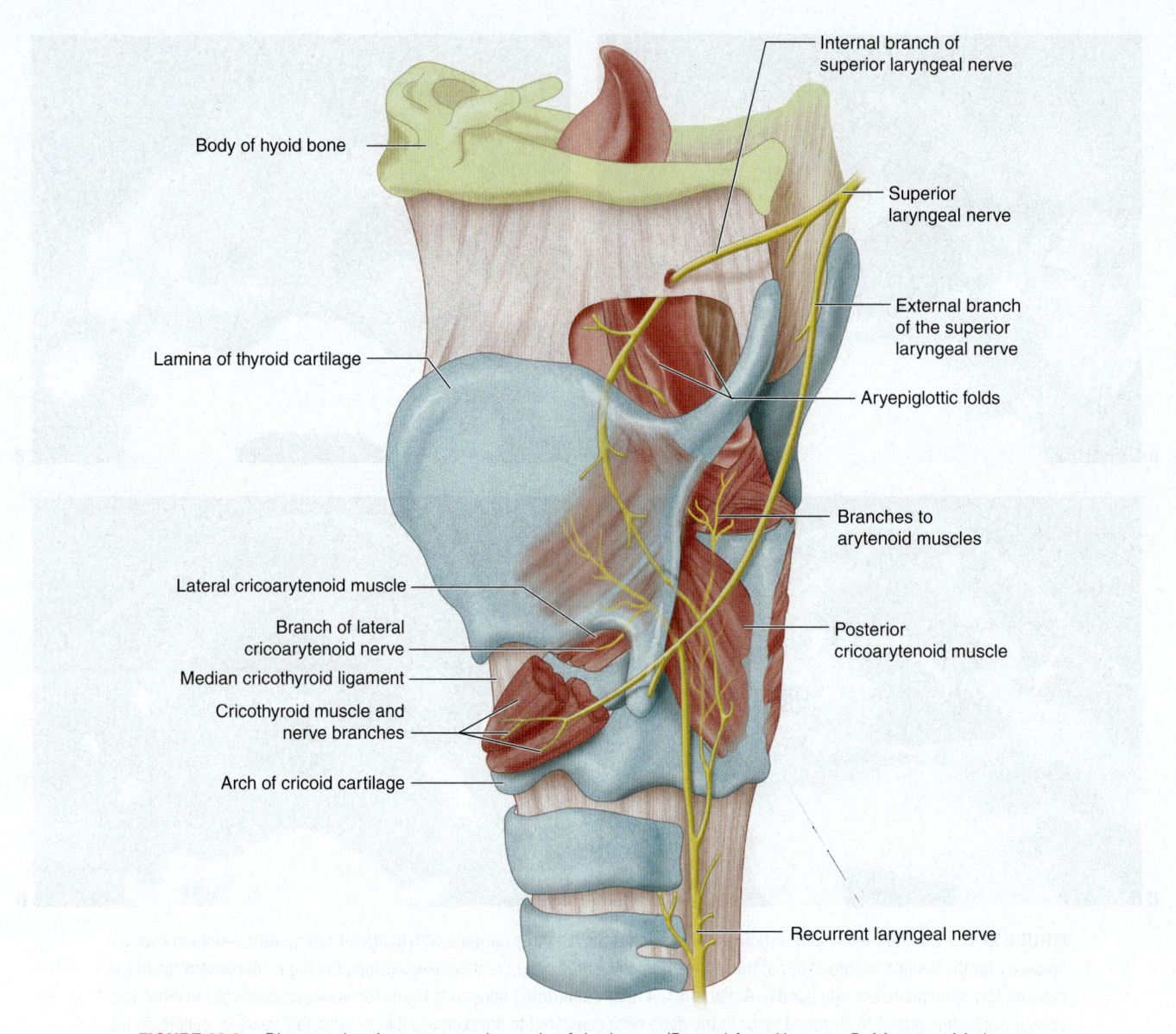

**FIGURE 22.2.** Diagram showing nerves and vessels of the larynx. (Reused from Hermans R, Mancuso AA. Larynx: introduction, normal anatomy, and function. In: Mancuso AA, Hanafee WN, eds. *Head and Neck Radiology.* Philadelphia, PA: Lippincott Williams & Wilkins; 2011:1923, with permission.)

# CLINICAL PEARLS

The use of ultrasound guidance increases the accuracy and potentially the safety of superior laryngeal nerve bock. It is a useful adjunct when performing awake intubation or laryngobronchoscopy. It is useful in the treatment of the pain of superior laryngeal neuralgia when medication management with membrane stabilizers such as carbamazepine and gabapentin has failed. It should be remembered that the risk of aspiration following superior laryngeal nerve block is increased and the patient should be warned of such.

CHAPTER 22 ULTRASOUND-GUIDED SUPERIOR LARYNGEAL NERVE BLOCK 145

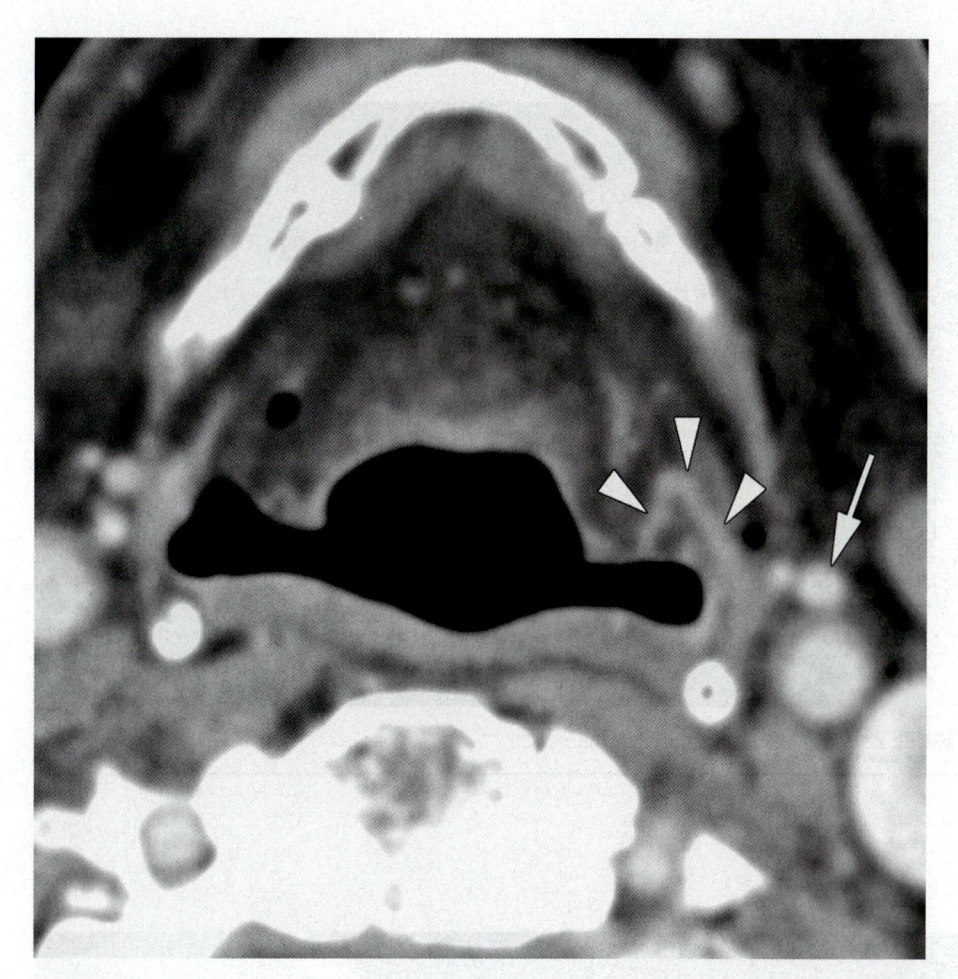

**FIGURE 22.3.** Contrast-enhanced computed tomography study showing the superior laryngeal neurovascular bundle external to the larynx (*arrow*) and then its branches extending into the supraglottis and continuing into the aryepiglottic fold (*arrowheads*). (Reused from Hermans R, Mancuso AA. Larynx: introduction, normal anatomy, and function. In: Mancuso AA, Hanafee WN, eds. *Head and Neck Radiology*. Philadelphia, PA: Lippincott Williams & Wilkins; 2011:1923, with permission.)

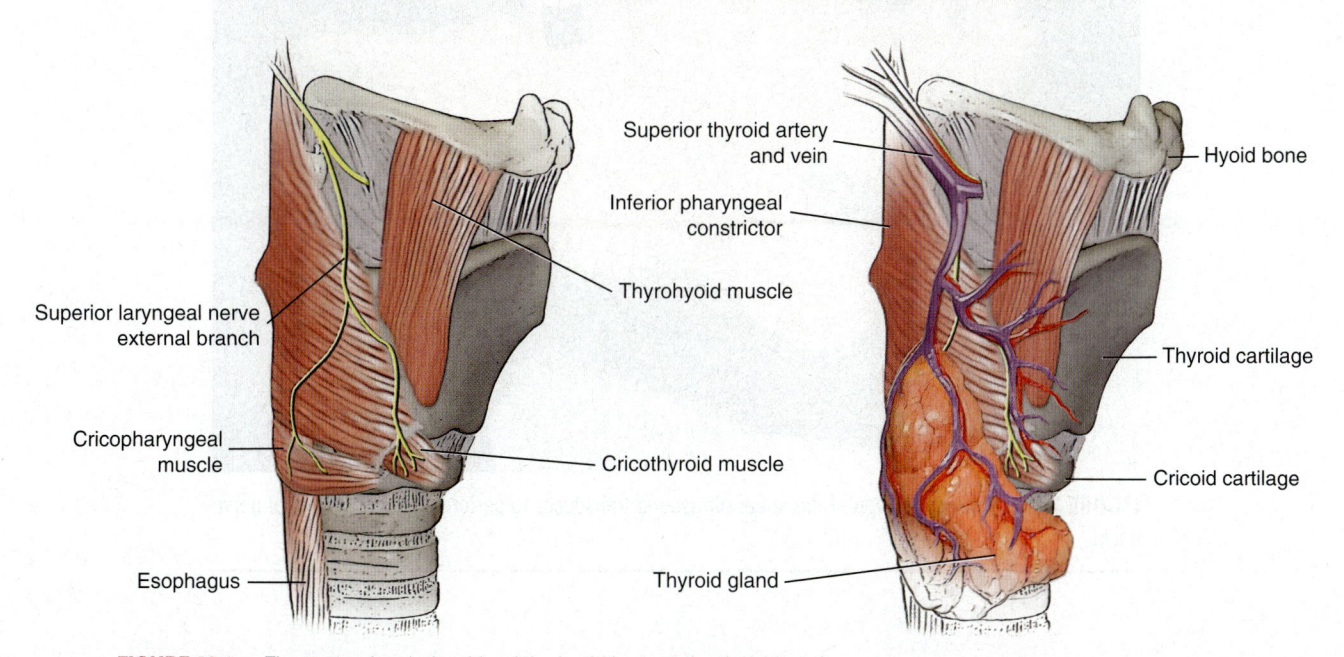

**FIGURE 22.4.** The anatomic relationship of the hyoid bone to the thyroid cartilage.

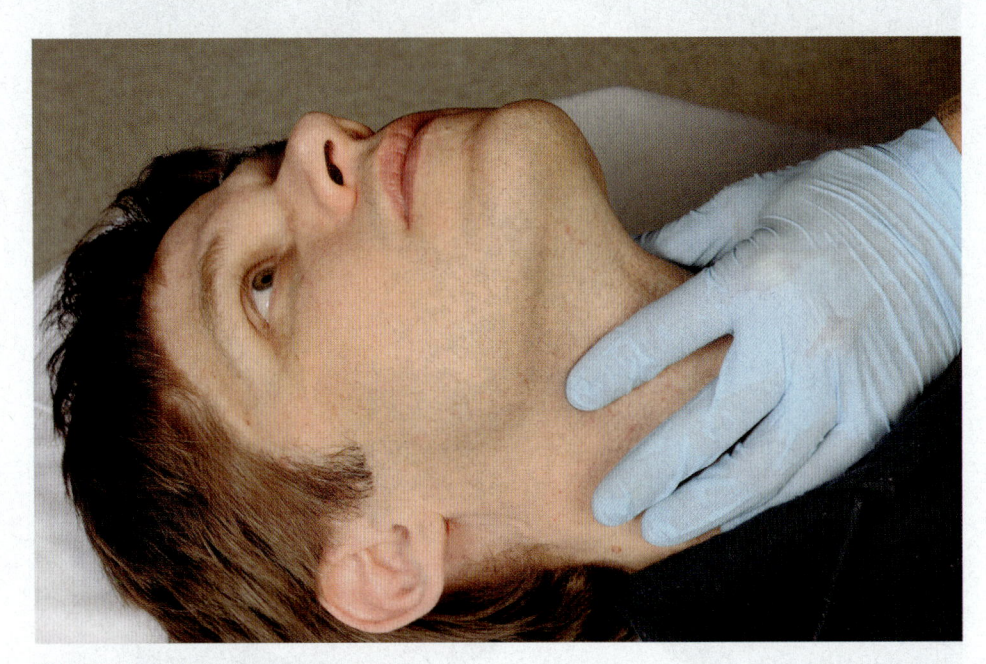

**FIGURE 22.5.** Palpation of the hyoid bone.

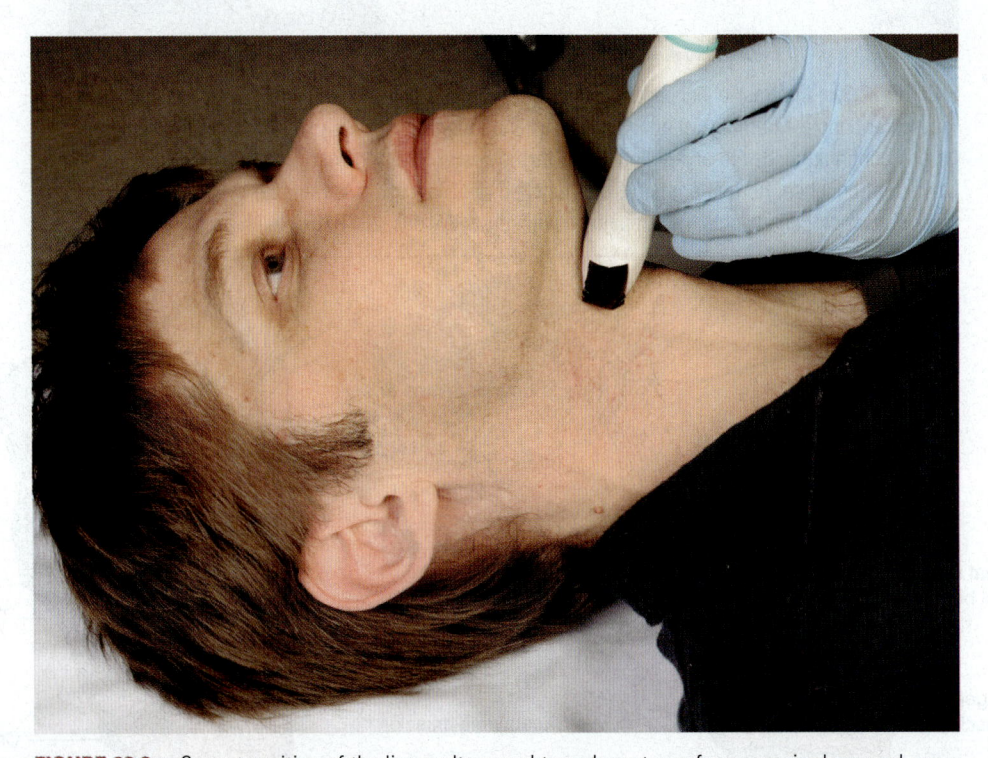

**FIGURE 22.6.** Correct position of the linear ultrasound transducer to perform superior laryngeal nerve bock.

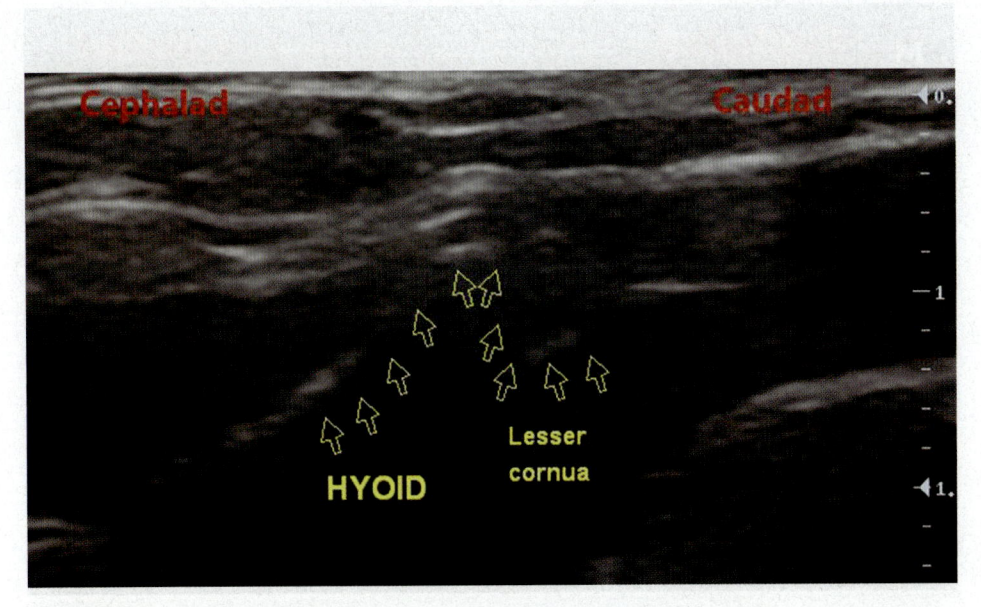

**FIGURE 22.7.** The characteristic triangular acoustic shadow of the hyoid bone.

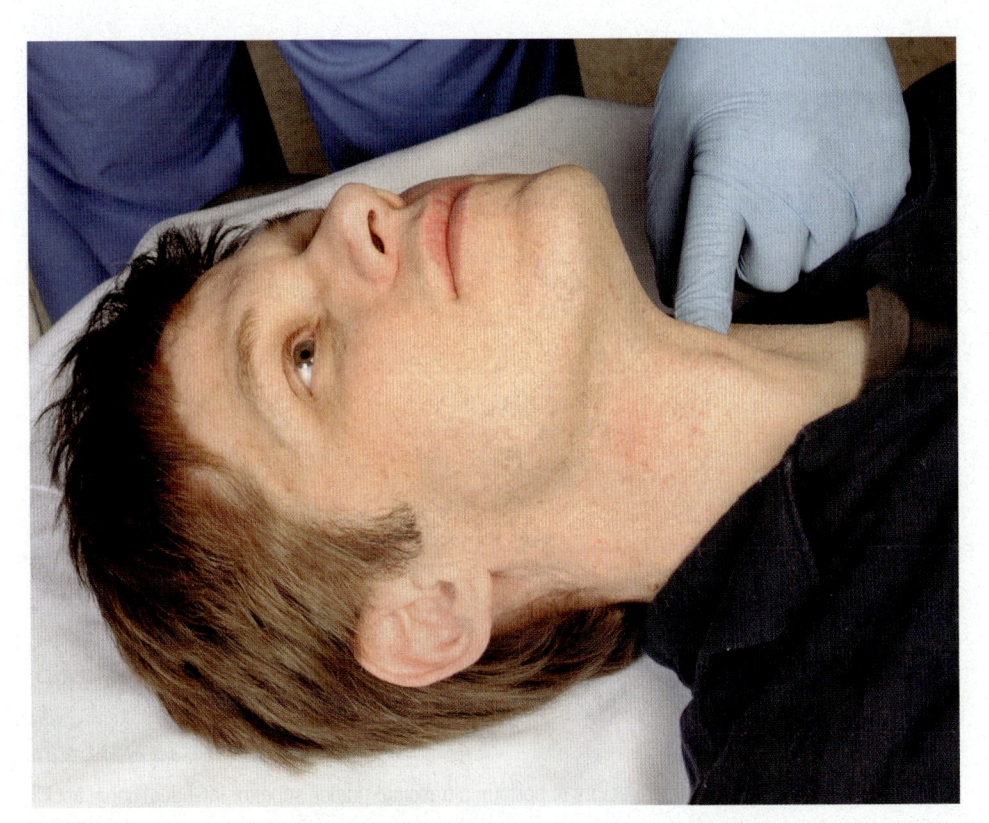

**FIGURE 22.8.** Manual displacement of the hyoid bone may make it easier to image.

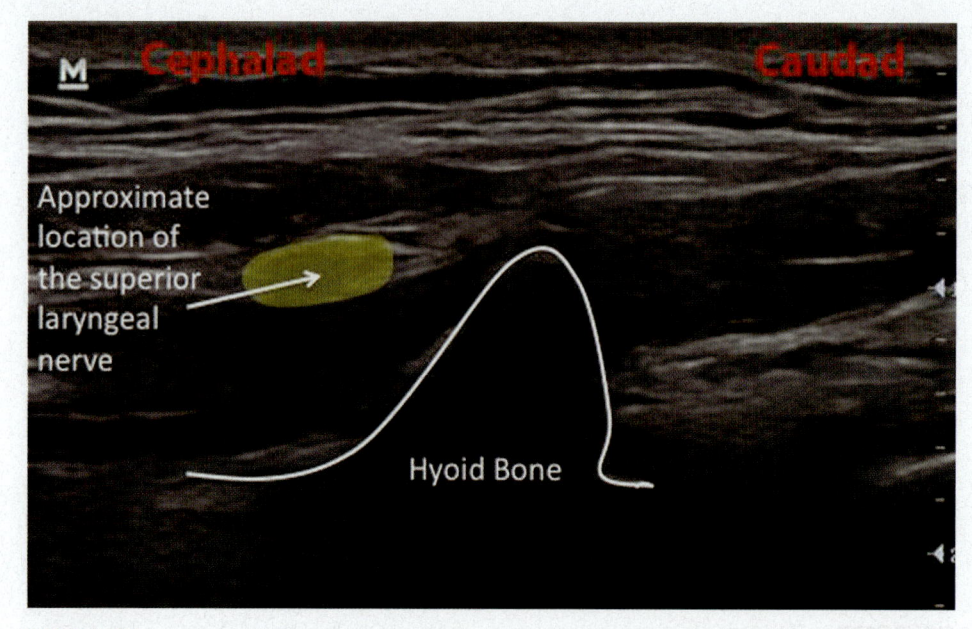

**FIGURE 22.9.** Location of the superior laryngeal nerve just caudad to the body of the hyoid bone.

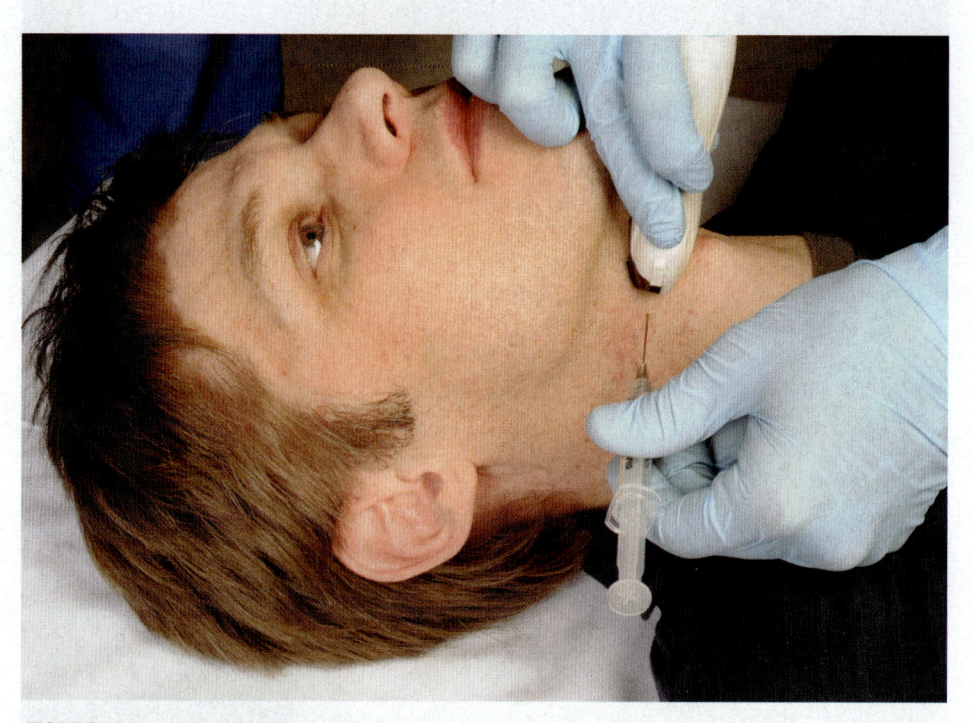

**FIGURE 22.10.** In-plane needle trajectory to perform ultrasound-guided superior laryngeal nerve bock.

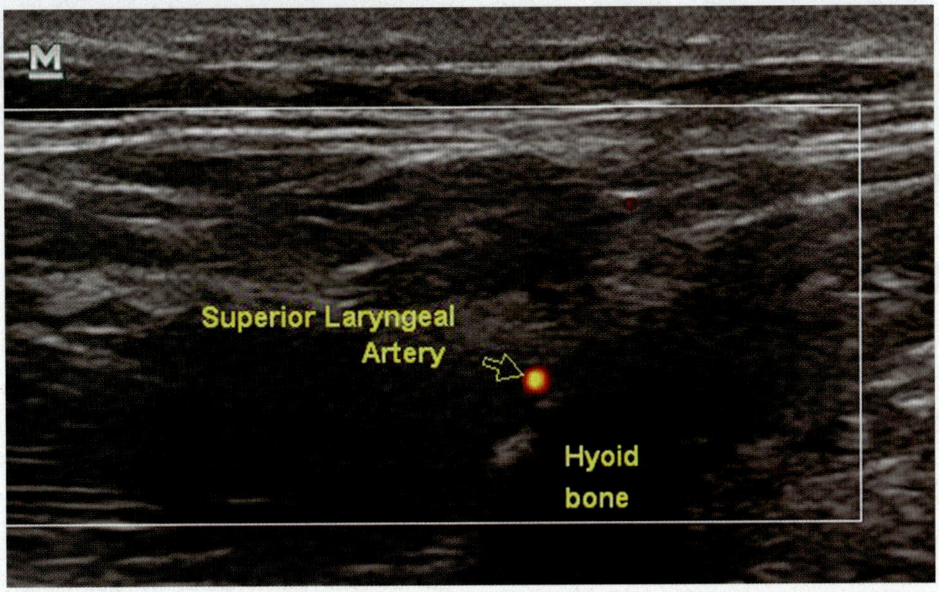

**FIGURE 22.11.** Color Doppler may aid in identification of the superior laryngeal artery that is adjacent to the superior laryngeal nerve.

## SUGGESTED READINGS

Manikandan S, Neema PK, Rathod RC. Ultrasound guided bilateral superior laryngeal nerve block to aid awake endotracheal intubation in a patient with cervical spine disease for emergency surgery. *Anaesth Intensive Care* 2010;38(5):946–948.

Monfared A, Gorti G, Kim D. Microsurgical anatomy of the laryngeal nerves as related to thyroid surgery. *Laryngoscope* 2002;112(2):386–392.

Sato KT, Suzuki M, Izuha A, et al. Two cases of idiopathic superior laryngeal neuralgia treated by superior laryngeal nerve block with a high concentration of lidocaine. *J Clin Anesth* 2007;19(3):237–238.

Stockwell M, Lozanoff S, Lang SA, et al. Superior laryngeal nerve block: an anatomical study. *Clin Anat* 1995;8(2):89–95.

Waldman SD. Superior laryngeal nerve bock. In: *Atlas of Interventional Pain Management*. 3rd ed. Philadelphia, PA: Saunders Elsevier; 2009:124–126.

# CHAPTER 23

# Ultrasound-Guided Recurrent Laryngeal Nerve Block

## CLINICAL PERSPECTIVES

Ultrasound-guided recurrent laryngeal nerve block is useful in the diagnosis and treatment of painful conditions subserved by the recurrent laryngeal nerve, including posttrauma pain in the region, as well as painful conditions of the larynx and pharynx below the glottis and pain of malignant origin (Fig. 23.1).

## CLINICALLY RELEVANT ANATOMY

The recurrent laryngeal nerves arise from the vagus nerve. The right and left recurrent laryngeal nerves follow different paths to reach the larynx and trachea. The right recurrent laryngeal nerve loops underneath the innominate artery and then ascends in the lateral groove between the trachea and esophagus to enter the inferior portion of the larynx. The left recurrent laryngeal nerve loops below the arch of the aorta and then ascends in the lateral groove between the trachea and esophagus to enter the inferior portion of the larynx (Fig. 23.2). It is at this point when traveling superiorly in this lateral groove between the trachea and esophagus at the level of the first tracheal ring that the nerve is most accessible for neural blockade (Figs. 23.3 and 23.4). The recurrent laryngeal nerves provide the innervation to all the intrinsic muscles of the larynx except the cricothyroid muscle as well as providing the sensory innervation for the mucosa below the vocal cords. The nerve is susceptible to damage during thyroid surgery and compression from tumors.

## ULTRASOUND-GUIDED TECHNIQUE

The patient is placed in the supine position with the head in neutral position. Three milliliters of local anesthetic is drawn up in a 10-mL sterile syringe, and 40 to 80 mg of depot steroid is added to the local anesthetic if there is thought to be an inflammatory component to the patient's pain symptomatology. The medial border of the sternocleidomastoid muscle at the level of the cricothyroid notch is identified by palpation as is the first tracheal ring just below it. A high-frequency linear ultrasound transducer is then placed over medial border of the sternocleidomastoid muscle in the transverse position at the level of the first tracheal ring (Fig. 23.5). In patients with thinner necks, an acoustic standoff of ultrasound gel may be needed to optimize image quality. The trachea and esophagus are then visualized and the relative position of the carotid artery is noted (Fig. 23.6). Color Doppler is then utilized to further delineate the carotid artery as well as to identify any significant vessels including branches of the thyroid artery that could be injured during needle placement. The recurrent laryngeal nerve is located in the lateral groove between the trachea and esophagus and may be identified on ultrasound as a monofascicular hypoechoic bundle with a hyperechoic perineurium in some patients (Fig. 23.7). Longitudinal ultrasound views may help confirm the identification of the nerve (Fig. 23.8).

The point where the recurrent laryngeal nerve lies in the lateral groove is the target for needle placement (see Fig. 23.2). The recurrent laryngeal nerve is blocked utilizing an in-plane approach by placing a 22-gauge, 1½-inch needle at the medial margin of the transversely placed ultrasound transducer and advancing it to a point where the recurrent laryngeal nerve lies in the lateral groove between the trachea and esophagus while avoiding the carotid artery and other vessels previously identified by color Doppler (Fig. 23.9). When the needle is in proximity to the recurrent laryngeal nerve, after gentle aspiration, 3 mL of solution is injected in incremental doses under real-time ultrasound imaging. The needle is removed and pressure is placed on the injection site to avoid hematoma or ecchymosis.

## COMPLICATIONS

Given the proximity of the superior thyroid and carotid arteries, the clinician should carefully calculate the total milligram dosage of local anesthetic that may be safely given, especially if bilateral nerve blocks are being performed. Postblock ecchymosis and hematoma formation are a distinct possibility if these vascular structures are injured during the procedure. Because the recurrent laryngeal nerves provide the innervation to all the

CHAPTER 23  ULTRASOUND-GUIDED RECURRENT LARYNGEAL NERVE BLOCK    151

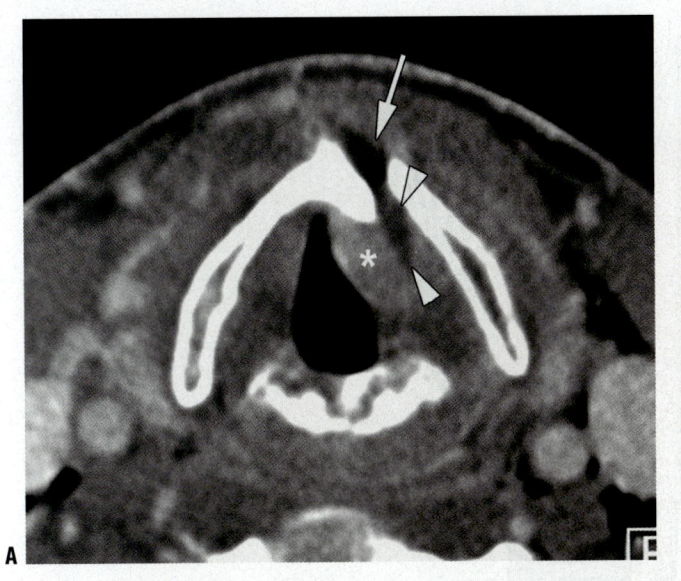

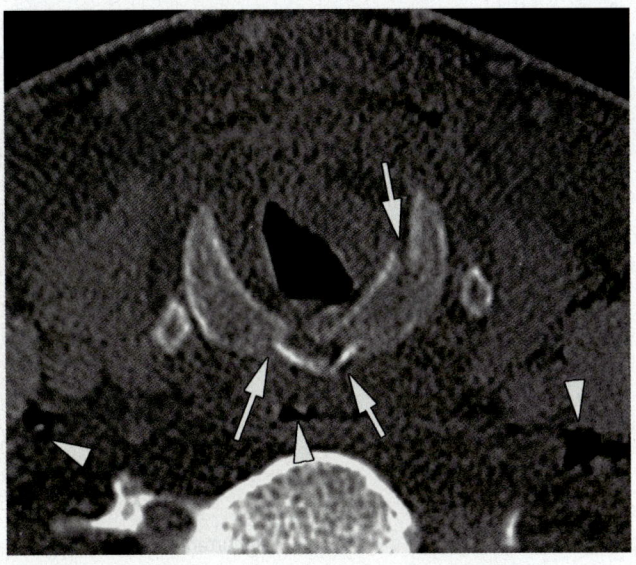

**FIGURE 23.1.** Axial computed tomography images in a patient suffering dyspnea and dysphonia after a motor vehicle accident. **A:** At the glottis level, there is a displaced fracture of the thyroid cartilage (*arrow*) and a soft tissue tear (*arrowheads*) with partial avulsion of left true vocal cord (*asterisk*). **B:** At the subglottic level, there are several fractures of the cricoid arch (*arrows*). The associated soft tissue thickening causes narrowing of the subglottic lumen. Several air bubbles are present in the soft tissues of the neck (*arrowheads*). (Reused from Hermans R, Mancuso AA, Collins WO. Larynx: acute and chronic effects of blunt and penetrating trauma. In: Mancuso AA, Hanafee WN, eds. *Head and Neck Radiology*. Philadelphia, PA: Lippincott Williams & Wilkins; 2011:2028, with permission.)

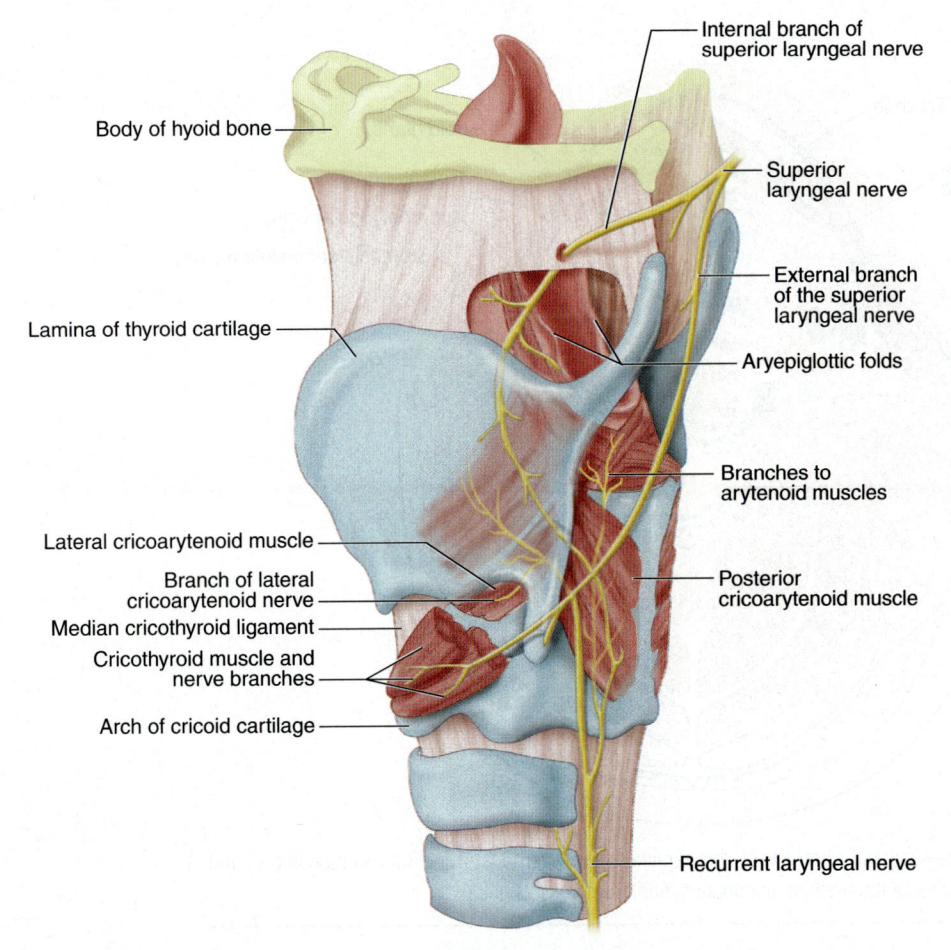

**FIGURE 23.2.** Diagram showing nerves and vessels of the larynx. (Reused from Hermans R, Mancuso AA. Larynx: introduction, normal anatomy, and function. In: Mancuso AA, Hanafee WN, eds. *Head and Neck Radiology*. Philadelphia, PA: Lippincott Williams & Wilkins; 2011:1923, with permission.)

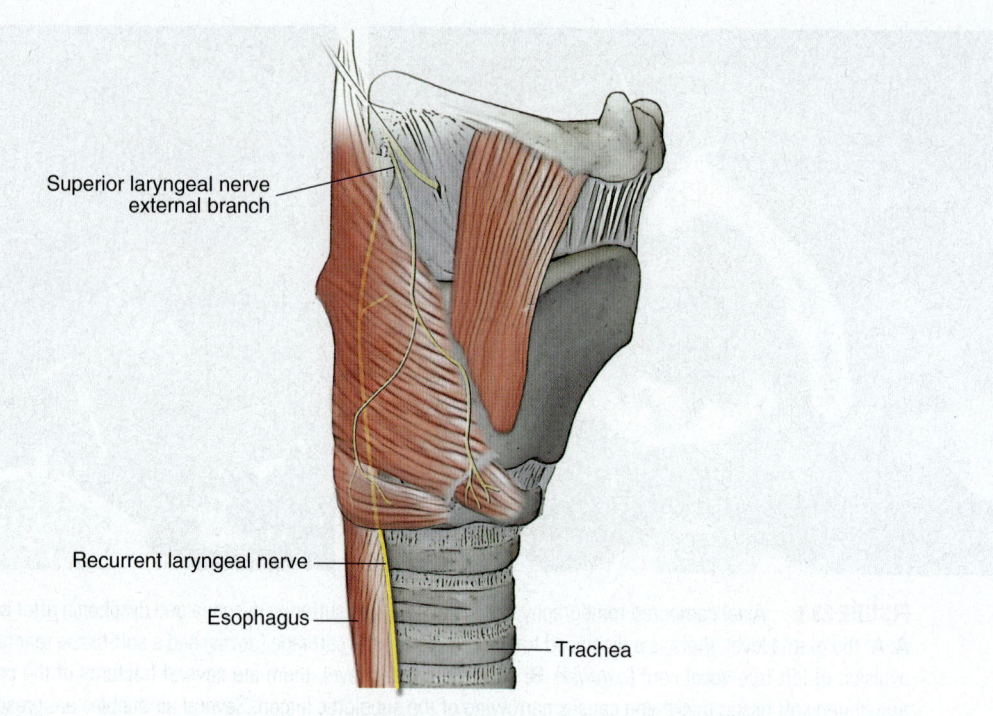

**FIGURE 23.3.** The recurrent laryngeal nerve runs in the lateral groove between the trachea and esophagus.

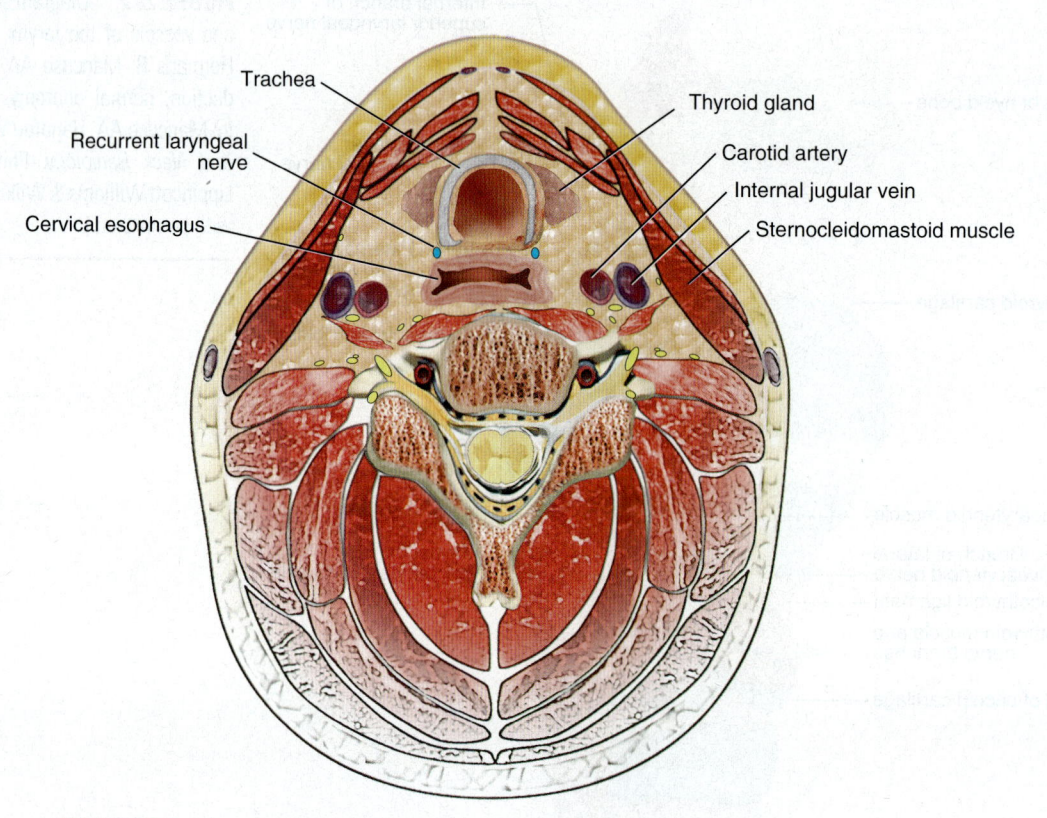

**FIGURE 23.4.** Cross-sectional anatomy of the cervical region demonstrating the relationship of the recurrent laryngeal nerve to the trachea, esophagus, and great vessels.

CHAPTER 23    ULTRASOUND-GUIDED RECURRENT LARYNGEAL NERVE BLOCK    153

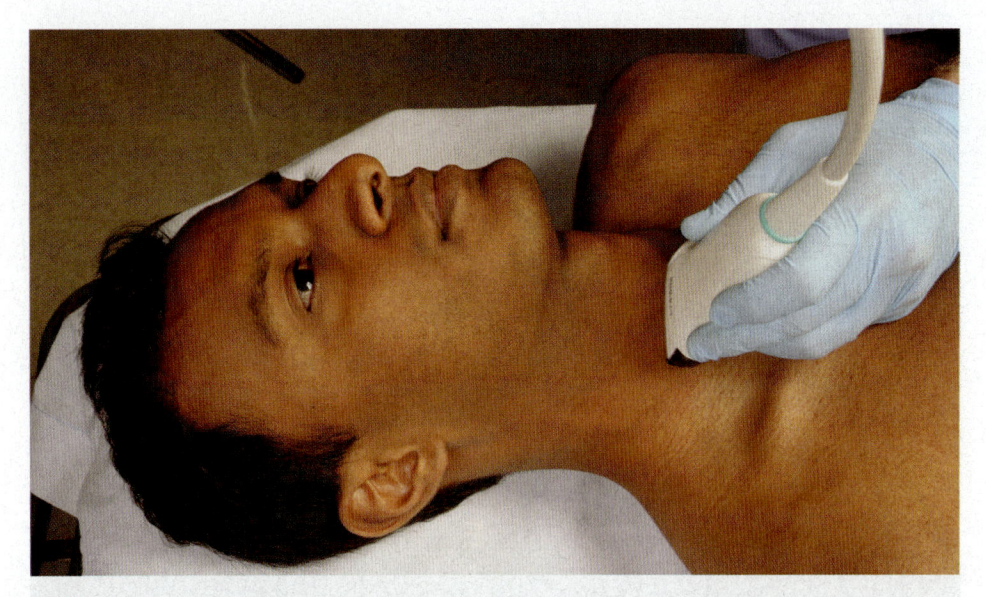

**FIGURE 23.5.** Correct position of the linear ultrasound transducer to perform recurrent laryngeal nerve block.

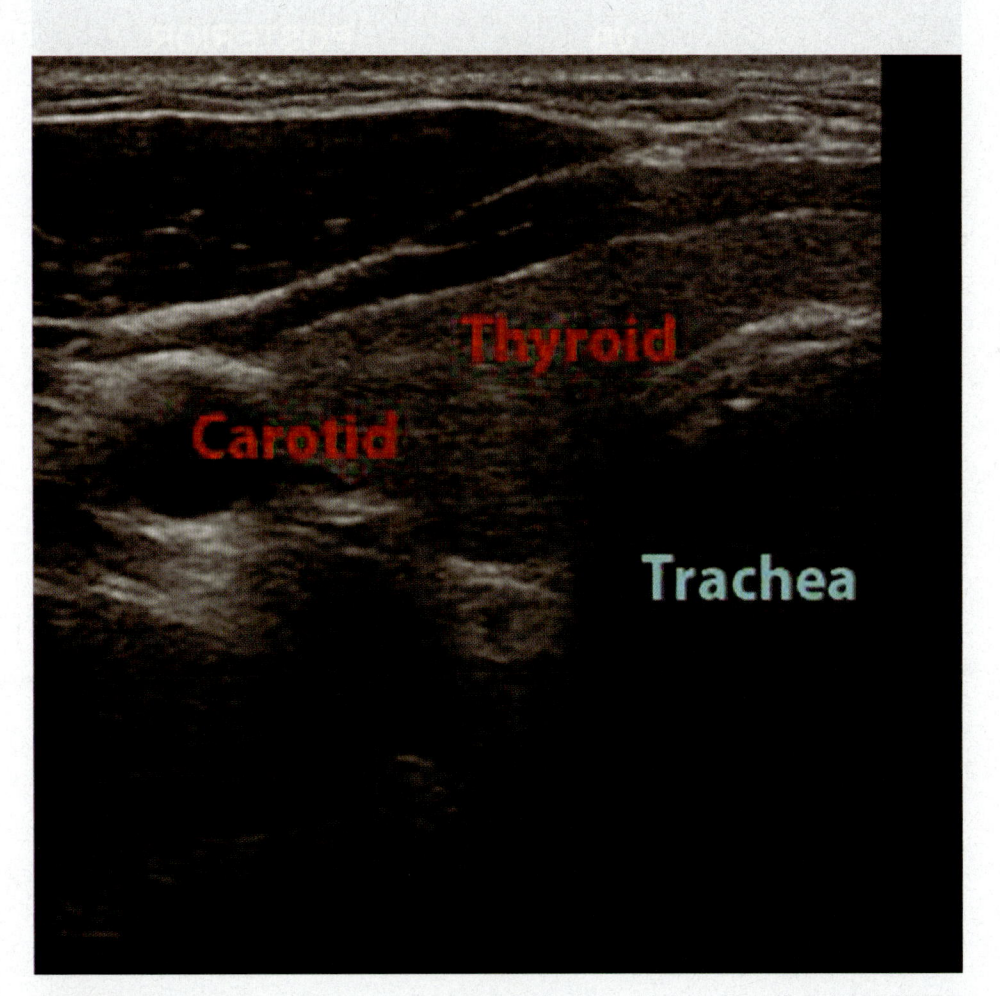

**FIGURE 23.6.** Transverse ultrasound view demonstrating the relationship of recurrent laryngeal nerve to trachea and carotid artery.

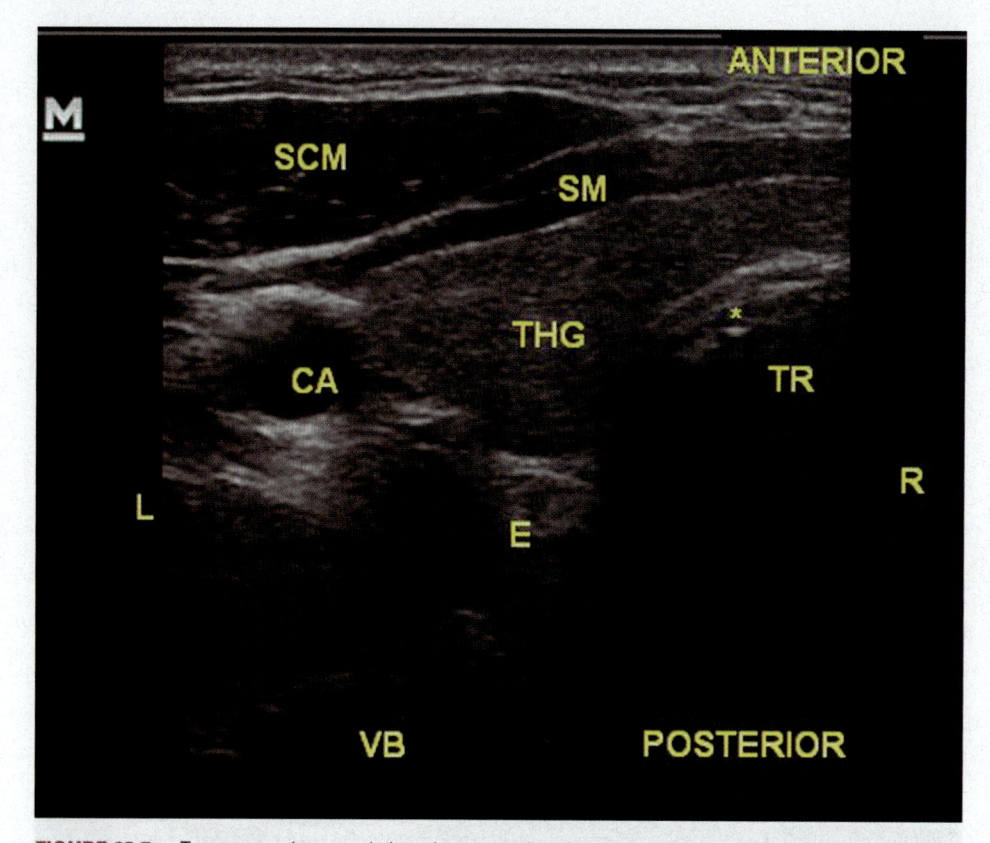

**FIGURE 23.7.** Transverse ultrasound view demonstrating the relationship between the recurrent laryngeal nerve and the tracheal, esophagus, thyroid gland, and carotid artery. (*, recurrent laryngeal nerve; TR, trachea; TG, thyroid gland; E, esophagus; CA, carotid artery; SCM, sternocleidomastoid muscle; VB, vertical body; R, right; L, left; SM, scalenus medius.)

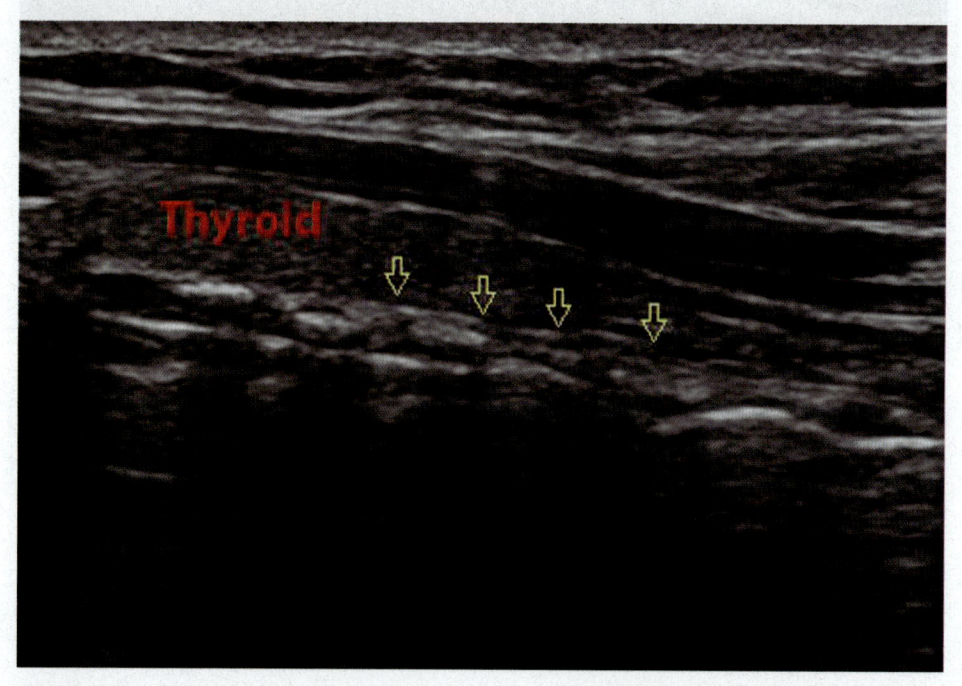

**FIGURE 23.8.** Longitudinal ultrasound view demonstrating the relationship of the thyroid gland, recurrent laryngeal nerve, and trachea. *Open arrows* indicate recurrent laryngeal nerve.

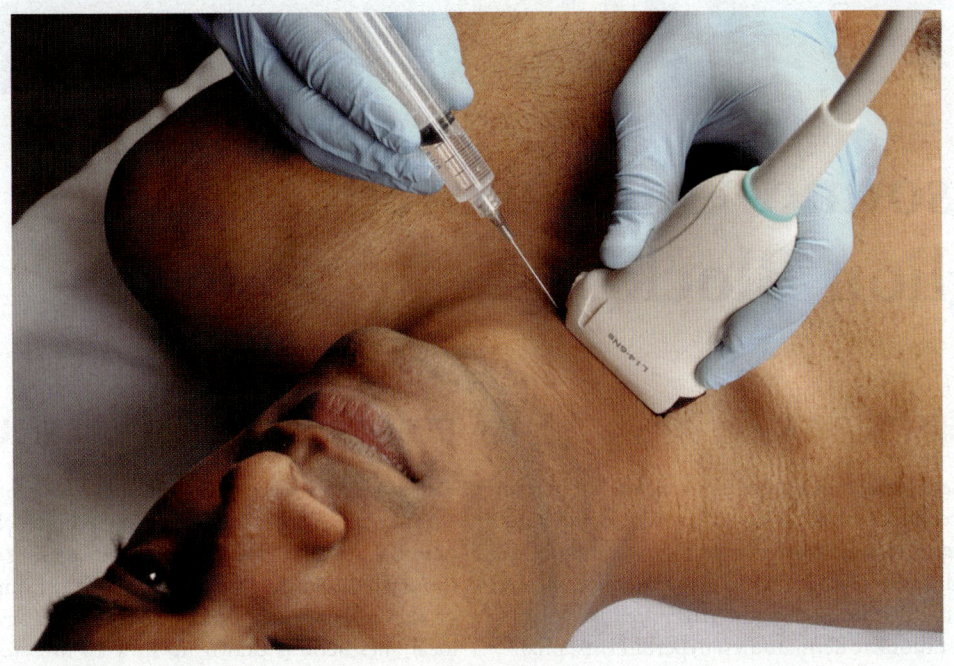

**FIGURE 23.9.** Proper in-plane needle placement for ultrasound-guided block of the recurrent laryngeal nerve.

intrinsic muscles of the larynx except the cricothyroid muscle, bilateral recurrent laryngeal nerve block is reserved for those patients who have undergone laryngectomy and/or tracheostomy because the resulting bilateral vocal cord paralysis could result in airway obstruction.

## CLINICAL PEARLS

The use of ultrasound guidance increases the accuracy and potentially the safety of recurrent laryngeal nerve block. It should be remembered that the risk of aspiration following recurrent laryngeal nerve block is increased and the patient should be warned of such. Bilateral block should be reserved for those patients who have undergone previous laryngectomy to avoid airway obstruction from bilateral vocal cord paralysis. When treating cancer pain of the larynx and upper trachea, recurrent laryngeal nerve block often has to be combined with superior laryngeal nerve block to obtain adequate pain control.

## SUGGESTED READINGS

Kundra P, Kumar K, Allampalli V, et al. Use of ultrasound to assess superior and recurrent laryngeal nerve function immediately after thyroid surgery. *Anaesthesia* 2012;67(3):301–302.

Monfared A, Gorti G, Kim D. Microsurgical anatomy of the laryngeal nerves as related to thyroid surgery. *Laryngoscope* 2002;112(2):386–392.

Singh M, Chin KJ, Chan VWS, et al. Use of sonography for airway assessment: an observational study. *J Ultrasound Med* 2010;29:79–85.

Waldman SD. Recurrent laryngeal nerve block. In: *Atlas of Interventional Pain Management*. 3rd ed. Philadelphia, PA: Saunders Elsevier; 2009:124–129.

# CHAPTER 24

# Ultrasound-Guided Stellate Ganglion Block

## CLINICAL PERSPECTIVES

Ultrasound-guided stellate ganglion block is useful in the diagnosis and treatment of a variety of painful conditions including reflex sympathetic dystrophy of the face and upper extremity, causalgia involving the upper extremity, acute herpes zoster in the distribution of the trigeminal nerve and cervical and upper thoracic dermatomes, hyperhidrosis, phantom limb pain, postmyocardial sympathetically mediated pain, sympathetically mediated pain of malignant origin, and sudden idiopathic sensorineural hearing loss. Ultrasound-guided stellate ganglion block is useful in the diagnosis and treatment of a number of diseases that have in common their ability to cause acute vascular insufficiency. These diseases include acute frostbite, acute angina, ergotism, obliterative vascular disease, Raynaud disease, scleroderma, vasospastic disorders, posttraumatic vascular insufficiency, and embolic phenomenon (Fig. 24.1; Table 24.1). Ultrasound-guided stellate ganglion block can also be used in a prognostic manner to determine the effect of blockade of the stellate ganglion prior to surgical sympathectomy in the cervical and upper thoracic region.

## CLINICALLY RELEVANT ANATOMY

The stellate ganglion, which is also known as the cervicothoracic or inferior cervical ganglion, is formed by the fusion of the inferior cervical and first thoracic sympathetic ganglia. The stellate ganglion is located on the anterior surface of the longus colli muscle (Fig. 24.2). This muscle lies just anterior to the transverse processes of the seventh cervical and first thoracic vertebrae (Fig. 24.3). The stellate ganglion lies anteromedial to the vertebral artery and is medial to the common carotid artery and jugular vein. The stellate ganglion is lateral to the trachea and esophagus. Although the stellate ganglion is located at the level of the seventh cervical and first thoracic vertebrae, when using the landmark technique, it is most commonly blocked at the C6 level to avoid the possibility of pneumothorax as the dome of the lung lies at the C7–T1 interspace in many patients (Fig. 24.4).

## ULTRASOUND-GUIDED TECHNIQUE

The patient is placed in the supine position with the head turned slightly away from the side to be blocked. Turning the head has the dual advantages of (1) increasing distance between the trachea and the carotid artery and (2) improving the view of the anatomy on ultrasound imaging. Seven milliliters of local anesthetic is drawn up in a 10-mL sterile syringe, and 40 to 80 mg of depot steroid is added to the local anesthetic if there is thought to be an inflammatory component to the patient's pain symptomatology.

The medial border of the sternocleidomastoid muscle at the level of the cricothyroid notch is identified by palpation. A high-frequency linear ultrasound transducer is then placed

**TABLE 24.1  Indications for Ultrasound-Guided Stellate Ganglion Block**

**Painful Conditions**
- Reflex sympathetic dystrophy of the face and upper extremity
- Causalgia involving the upper extremity
- Acute herpes zoster in the distribution of the trigeminal nerve and cervical and upper thoracic dermatomes
- Hyperhidrosis
- Phantom limb pain
- Postmyocardial sympathetically mediated pain
- Sympathetically mediated pain of malignant origin

**Miscellaneous Conditions**
- Sudden idiopathic sensorineural hearing loss

**Acute Vascular Insufficiency**
- Acute frostbite
- Acute angina
- Ergotism
- Obliterative vascular disease
- Raynaud disease
- Scleroderma
- Vasospastic disorders
- Posttraumatic vascular insufficiency
- Embolic phenomenon
- Prognostic stellate ganglion block prior to surgical sympathectomy

CHAPTER 24  ULTRASOUND-GUIDED STELLATE GANGLION BLOCK   157

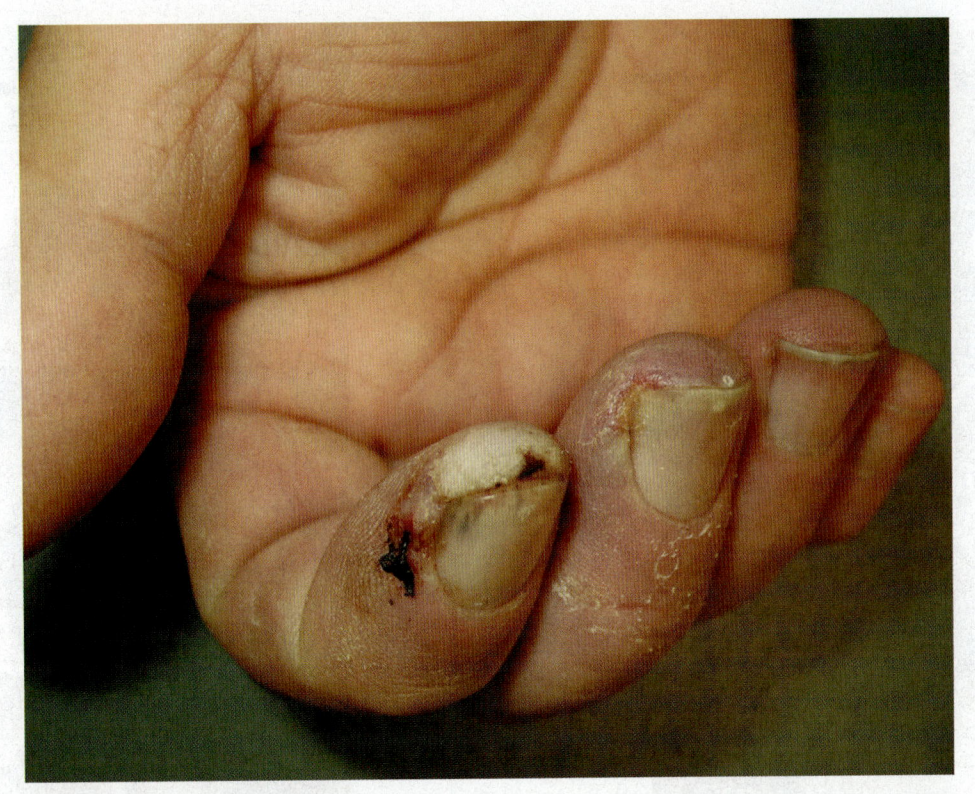

**FIGURE 24.1.** Acrocyanosis in scleroderma patient. (Image provided by Stedman's.)

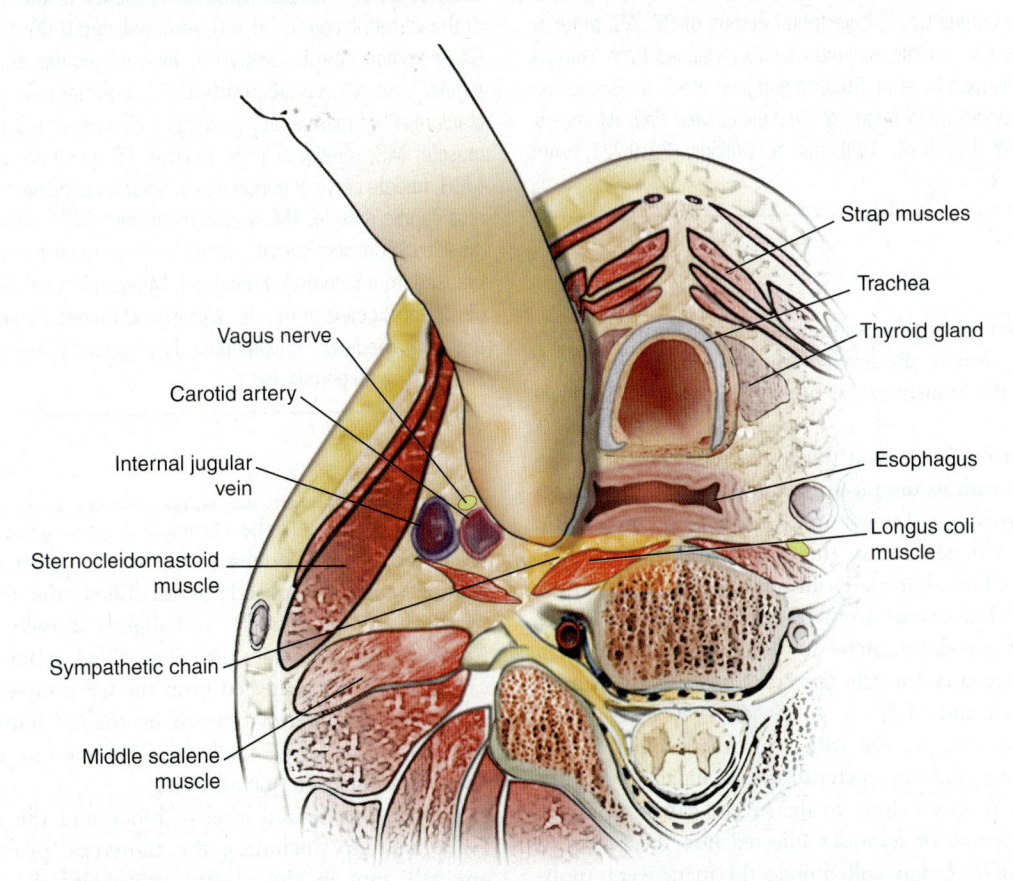

**FIGURE 24.2.** Cross-sectional anatomy of the C6 level. Note the relative locations of the sympathetic chain, the longus colli muscle beneath it, and the location of the carotid artery, jugular vein, and vertebral artery.

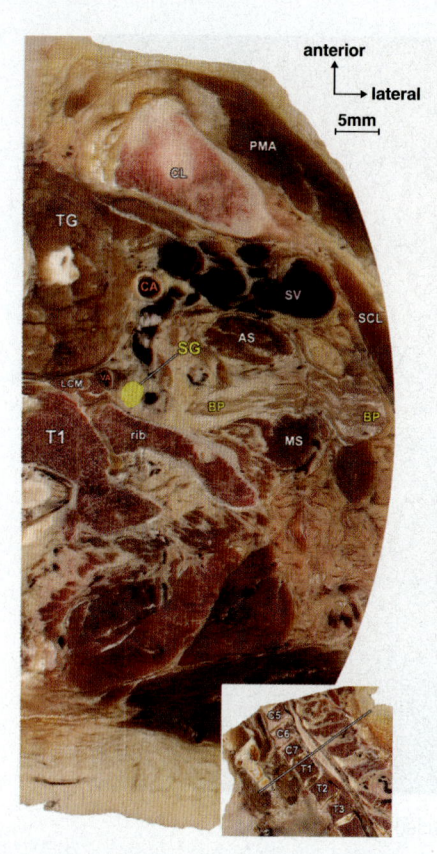

**FIGURE 24.3.** Reconstructed cross-section of the neck at the level of the vertebral corpus C7. (C7, vertebral corpus of C7; AS, anterior scalene muscle; MS, middle scalene muscle.) (Reused from Shibata Y, Komatsu T, Moayeri N, et al. Stellate ganglion block. In: Bigeleisen PE, ed. *Ultrasound-Guided Regional Anesthesia and Pain Medicine*. Philadelphia, PA: Lippincott Williams & Wilkins; 2010:221, with permission.)

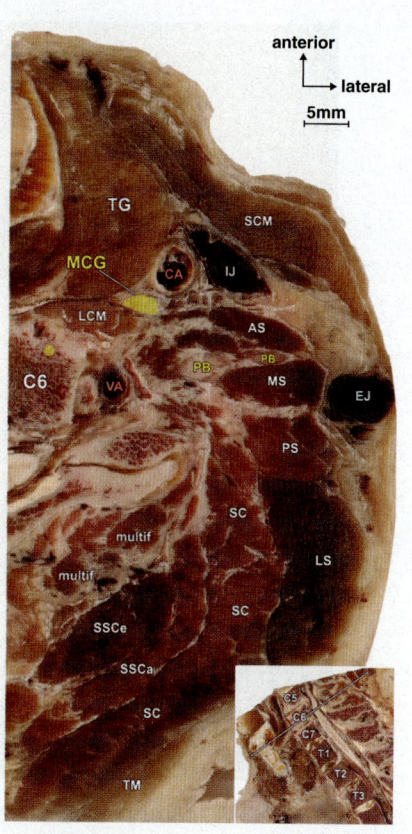

**FIGURE 24.4.** Reconstructed cross-section of the neck at the level of the vertebral corpus C6. (C6, vertebral corpus C6; TG, thyroid gland; CA, common carotid artery; IJ, internal jugular vein; EJ, external jugular vein; VA, vertebral artery; PB, brachial plexus; SCM, sternocleidomastoid muscle; LCM, longus colli muscle; AS, anterior scalene muscle; MS, middle scalene muscle; PS, posterior scalene muscle; MCG, middle cervical ganglion; LS, levator scapulae muscle; SC, splenius capitis muscle; TM, trapezius muscle; SSCa, semispinalis capitis muscle; SSCe, semispinalis cervicis muscle; multif, multifidus muscle.) (Reused from Shibata Y, Komatsu T, Moayeri N, et al. Stellate ganglion block. In: Bigeleisen PE, ed. *Ultrasound-Guided Regional Anesthesia and Pain Medicine*. Philadelphia, PA: Lippincott Williams & Wilkins; 2010:221, with permission.)

over medial border of the sternocleidomastoid muscle in the transverse position at the level of the cricoid notch, which should place the transducer at approximately the C6 level (Fig. 24.5).

The ultrasound images at this level should reveal the C6 vertebral body with its unique-appearing camel-humped anterior tubercle (which is known as Chassaignac or the carotid tubercle), the C6 nerve root, the carotid artery, the longus colli muscle, and the short posterior tubercle (Fig. 24.6). If the carotid artery blocks access to the cervical sympathetic chain, the ultrasound transducer can be slowly moved laterally to help delineate a more lateral needle trajectory to avoid the carotid artery (Figs. 24.7 and 24.8).

Many clinicians proceed with sympathetic block at this level, while some clinicians prefer to move caudally to the C7 vertebral body to move closer to the stellate ganglion. Given the extent of spread of solutions injected into the prefascial space in front of the longus colli muscle, this maneuver is probably one more of personal preference than of one that yields increased efficacy. If the clinician desires to inject at the C7 level, once the C6 vertebral body with its characteristic camel-humped anterior tubercle is identified, the transducer can be slowly moved caudally and slightly dorsally until the C7 transverse process comes into view. The C7 transverse process can be easily distinguished from the C6 transverse process by the lack of an anterior tubercle on the C7 transverse process (Fig. 24.9). At the C7 level, the C7 nerve root is located just anterior to the posterior tubercle.

Once the desired level of block and the clinically relevant anatomy including the transverse process, the longus colli muscle, the carotid artery, and the exiting nerve root have been identified, a careful scan at the chosen level

CHAPTER 24    ULTRASOUND-GUIDED STELLATE GANGLION BLOCK    159

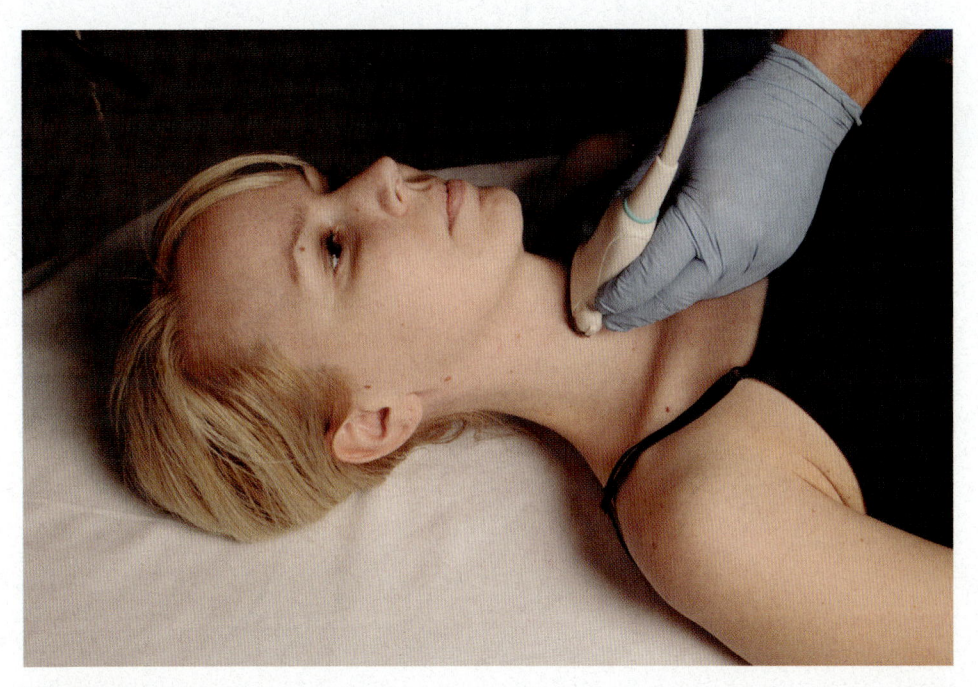

**FIGURE 24.5.**   Correct position of the linear ultrasound transducer to perform stellate ganglion block at the C6 level.

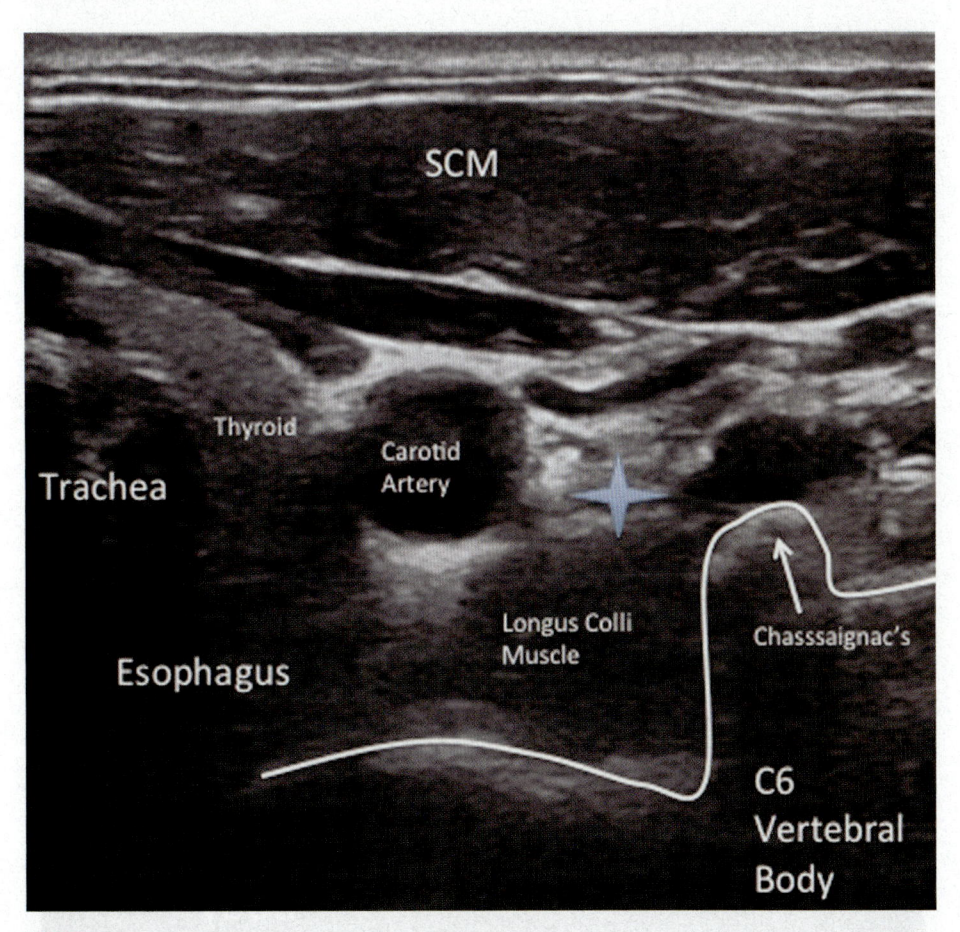

**FIGURE 24.6.**   Transverse ultrasound view of the C6 vertebral body and adjacent anterior anatomic structures. Note the characteristic camel's hump appearance of the anterior tubercle (Chassaignac tubercle) indicating that this is in fact the C6 vertebral body.

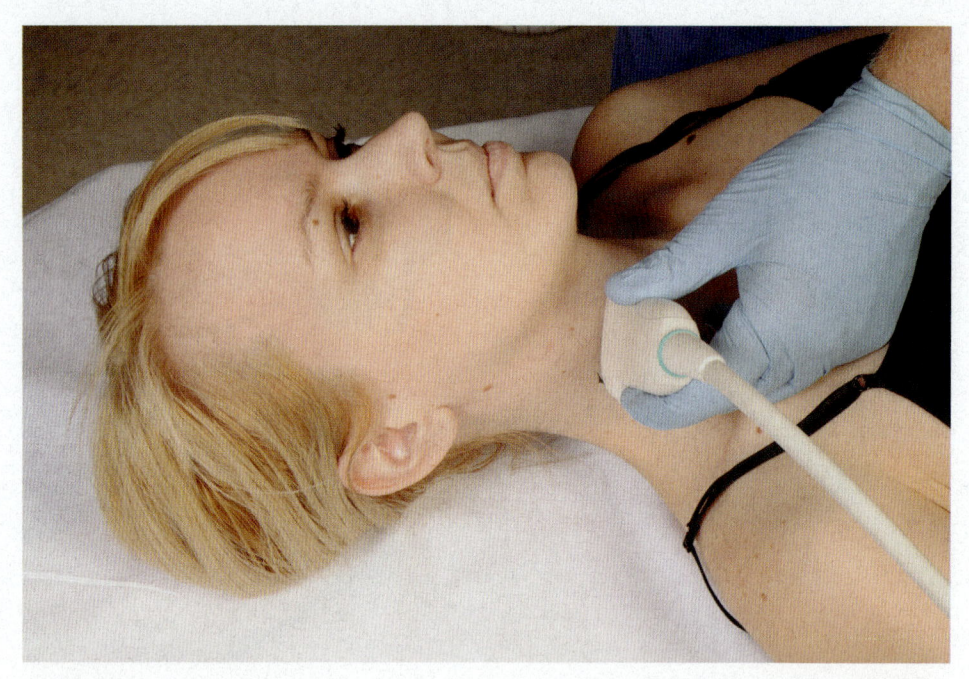

**FIGURE 24.7.** More lateral placement of the ultrasound transducer may help delineate a needle trajectory that avoids the carotid artery.

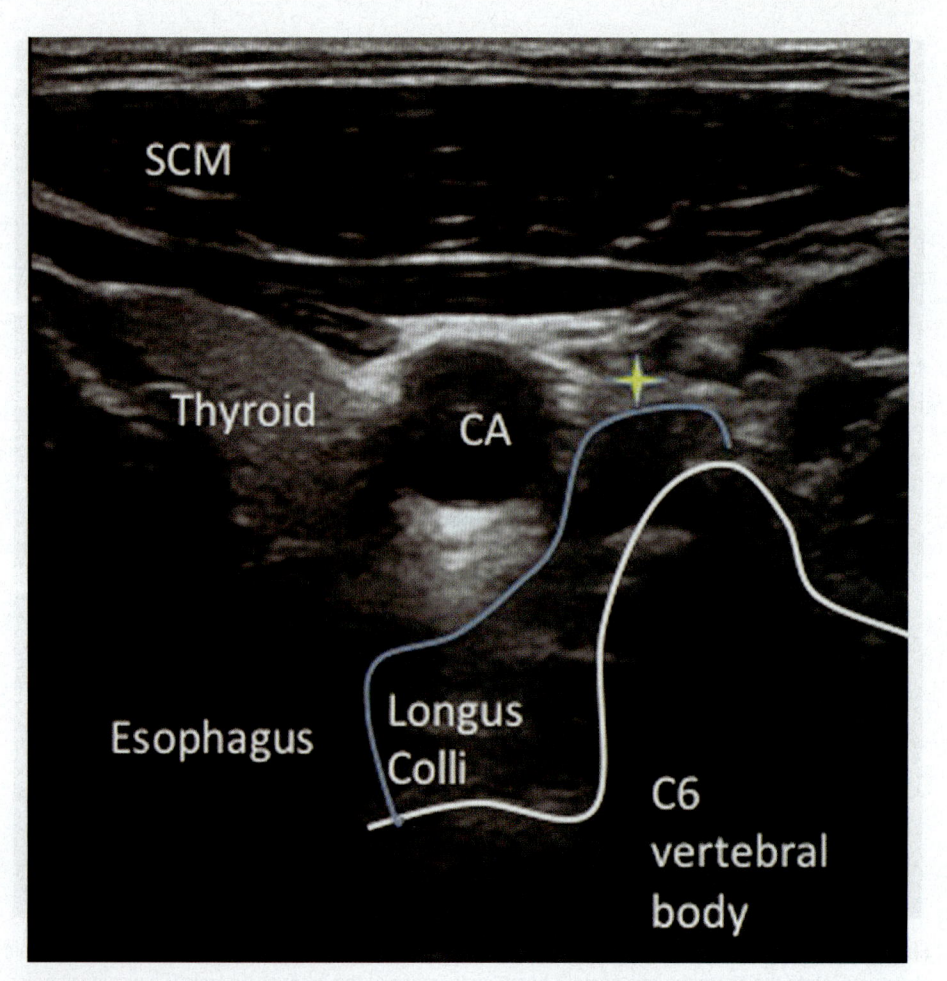

**FIGURE 24.8.** Transverse anterolateral ultrasound view of the C6 vertebral body. Compare the relationship of the carotid artery to the longus colli muscle in this image as compared with Figure 24.6.

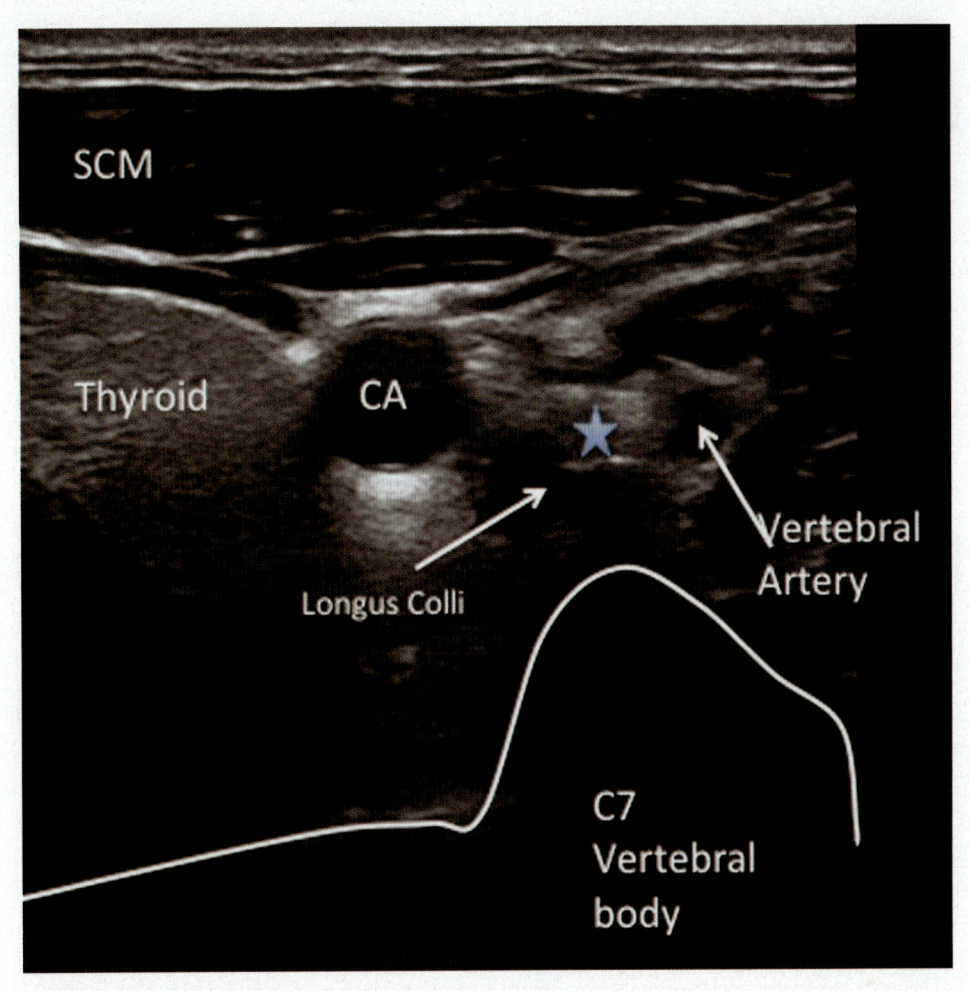

**FIGURE 24.9.** Transverse ultrasound image of the C7 vertebral body.

using color Doppler is carried out to identify if the inferior thyroid artery is not in proximity to the intended path of the needle (Fig. 24.10). The target for the needle tip is the anterior prefascial surface of the longus colli muscle where the sympathetic nerves and ganglion are located. The skin is prepped with antiseptic solution and utilizing an out-of-plane approach, a 22-gauge, 3½-inch styletted spinal needle is inserted and advanced under continuous ultrasound guidance toward the anterior prefascial surface of the longus colli muscle while avoiding the carotid artery and other vessels previously identified by color Doppler. Gentle pressure against the skin with the ultrasound transducer will decrease the distance between the skin and the anterior prefascial space of the longus colli muscle. When the needle is in proximity to the prefascial surface of the longus colli muscle, after gentle aspiration, a small amount of solution is injected under real-time ultrasound imaging to observe the ballooning of the anterior prefascial space of the longus colli muscle. If the solution is seen within the muscle substance or between the muscle and the transverse process, the needle is withdrawn slightly, and this maneuver is repeated until satisfactory needle placement is confirmed. Once this is accomplished, 7 mL of solution is injected in incremental doses under real-time ultrasound imaging. The needle is removed and pressure is placed on the injection site to avoid hematoma or ecchymosis.

## COMPLICATIONS

Given the proximity of the inferior thyroid and carotid artery, the clinician should carefully calculate the total milligram dosage of local anesthetic that may be safely given. Postblock ecchymosis and hematoma formation are a distinct possibility if these vascular structures are injured during the procedure. The application of cold packs for 20-minute periods after the block will also decrease the amount of postprocedure pain and bleeding the patient may experience. The clinician should

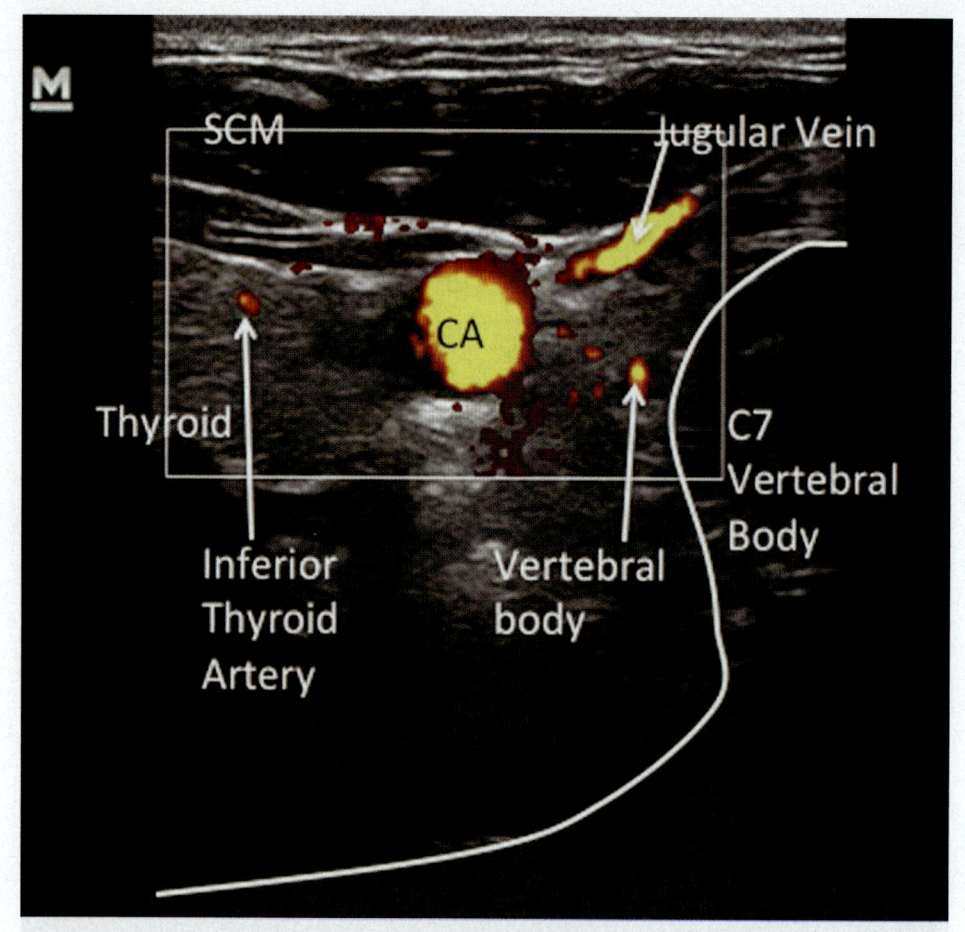

**FIGURE 24.10.** Transverse color Doppler image of the carotid and inferior thyroid artery.

remember that the vertebral artery lies posterior to the target area for stellate ganglion block, but if the needle is placed between the transverse processes of two adjacent vertebra, the artery may be injured.

Because of the proximity to the neural axis, inadvertent injection of the local anesthetic solution into the epidural, subdural, or subarachnoid space remains an ever-present possibility. At this level, even small amounts of local anesthetic placed into the subarachnoid space may result in total spinal anesthesia. If needle placement is too inferior, pneumothorax is possible because the dome of the lung lies at the level of the C7–T1 interspace.

Additional side effects associated with stellate ganglion block include inadvertent block of the recurrent laryngeal nerve with associated hoarseness and dysphagia and the sensation that there is a lump in the throat when swallowing. Horner syndrome occurs when the superior cervical sympathetic ganglion is also blocked during stellate ganglion block. The patient should be forewarned of the possibility of these complications prior to stellate ganglion block.

## CLINICAL PEARLS

The use of ultrasound guidance increases the accuracy and potentially the safety of stellate ganglion block. However, improperly performed, stellate ganglion block can be one of the most dangerous regional anesthetic techniques used in pain management. To safely perform this procedure, the clinician must be thoroughly familiar with the region anatomy and carefully identify all key ultrasound landmarks before needle placement.

## SUGGESTED READINGS

Kundra P, Kumar K, Allampalli V, et al. Use of ultrasound to assess superior and stellate ganglion function immediately after thyroid surgery. *Anaesthesia* 2012;67(3):301–302.

Monfared A, Gorti G, Kim D. Microsurgical anatomy of the laryngeal nerves as related to thyroid surgery. *Laryngoscope* 2002;112(2):386–392.

Singh M, Chin KJ, Chan VWS, et al. Use of sonography for airway assessment: an observational study. *J Ultrasound Med* 2010;29:79–85.

Waldman SD. Stellate ganglion block. In: *Atlas of Interventional Pain Management*. 3rd ed. Philadelphia, PA: Saunders Elsevier; 2009:124–129.

# CHAPTER 25

# Ultrasound-Guided Third Occipital Nerve Block

## CLINICAL PERSPECTIVES

Ultrasound-guided blockade of the third occipital nerve is useful in the diagnosis and treatment of cervicogenic headache, cervicalgia, and other pain syndromes subserved by the third occipital nerves. This technique is also useful as a prognostic indicator of the potential efficacy of destruction of the third occipital nerve with neurolytic agents such as phenol or radiofrequency lesioning. Traditionally, third occipital nerve block is performed under fluoroscopic guidance, but recent investigations by Narouze and others have demonstrated the utility of ultrasound guidance when performing this technique.

## CLINICALLY RELEVANT ANATOMY

The third occipital nerve arises from medial branch fibers of the posterior division of the third cervical nerve at the level of the trapezius muscle (Fig. 25.1). The third occipital nerve courses dorsomedially around the superior articular process of the C3 vertebra (Fig. 25.2). Fibers from the third occipital nerve provide the primary innervation of the C2–C3 facet joints with some contribution from the C3 medial branch and small communicating fibers from the second cervical nerve. Fibers of third occipital nerve then course superiorly at a point medial to the greater occipital nerve to provide sensory innervation to the ipsilateral suboccipital region (Fig. 25.3). In most patients, there are communicating branches from the third occipital nerve with the greater occipital nerve.

## ULTRASOUND-GUIDED TECHNIQUE

Ultrasound-guided third occipital nerve block can be carried out by placing the patient in the lateral position. A total of 2 mL of local anesthetic is drawn up in a 10-mL sterile syringe. If the painful condition being treated is thought to have an inflammatory component, 40 to 80 mg of depot steroid is added to the local anesthetic.

The mastoid process on the side to be blocked is then identified by palpation (Fig. 25.4). After preparation of the skin with antiseptic solution, a linear high-frequency ultrasound transducer is placed in a longitudinal plane with the cephalad end of the transducer resting at the base of the mastoid process, and the inferior border of the mastoid process is identified on ultrasound (Figs. 25.5 and 25.6). The transducer is then slowly moved in a posterior direction ¾ inch until the arch of C1 (atlas) and the articular pillar of C2 (axis) can be identified (Figs. 25.7 and 25.8). The transducer is then slowly moved in a caudad direction until the C2–C3 facet joints are visualized (Fig. 25.9). The ultrasound transducer is then slowly rotated toward the acoustic auditory meatus until the third occipital nerve is identified crossing just above the "hill" of the C2–C3 facet joint. The third occipital nerve will appear like a hyperechoic dot within a hypoechoic halo. The larger medial branch of the C3 can also be visualized in the "valley" between the articulations of the C2–C3 facet and the C3–C4 facet joints (Fig. 25.10).

When the third occipital nerve is identified, a 3½-inch needle is inserted anterior to the ultrasound transducer utilizing an out-of-plane approach and is advanced from an anterior to posterior trajectory until the needle approaches the third occipital nerve. After gentle aspiration, 2 mL of solution is injected with care being taken to avoid the vertebral artery, which is located anteriorly in relation to the facet joints. The needle is removed and pressure is placed on the injection site to avoid hematoma formation.

## COMPLICATIONS

This area is highly vascular and this coupled with the fact that the third occipital nerves are in close proximity to the vertebral arteries means that the pain specialist should carefully calculate and observe the patients undergoing third occipital nerve block for inadvertent intravascular injection, which could cause significant central nervous system side effects including ataxia, dizziness, and, on rare occasions, seizures (Fig. 25.11). Proximity of the third occipital nerve to exiting spinal nerve roots makes trauma to the nerve roots as well as inadvertent subarachnoid, subdural, and/or epidural injection a distinct possibility. Care must be taken to avoid inadvertent needle placement into the foramen magnum, as the subarachnoid administration of local anesthetic in this region will result in an immediate total spinal anesthetic.

**SECTION II  NECK**

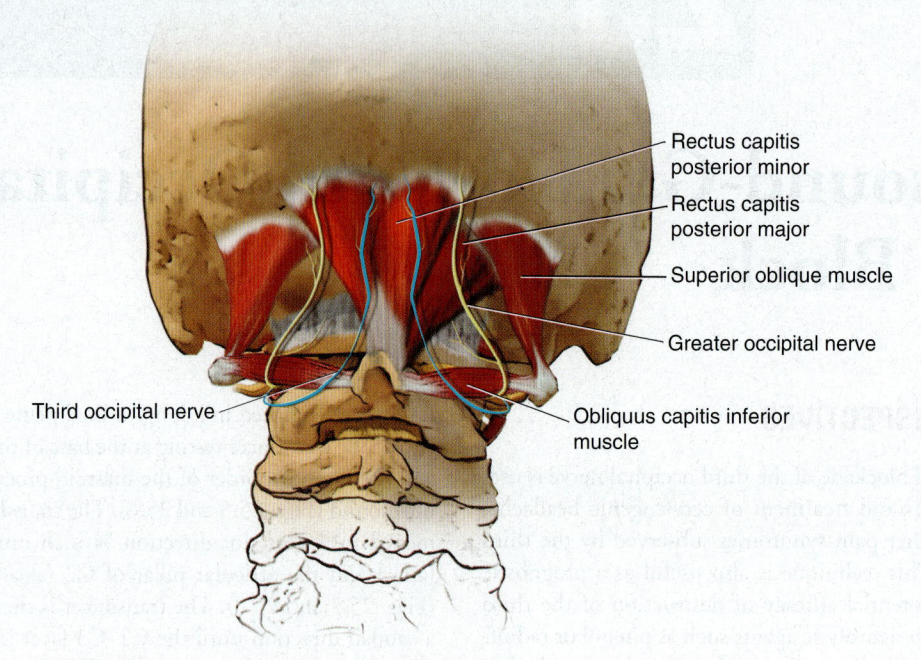

**FIGURE 25.1.** The anatomy of the third occipital nerve.

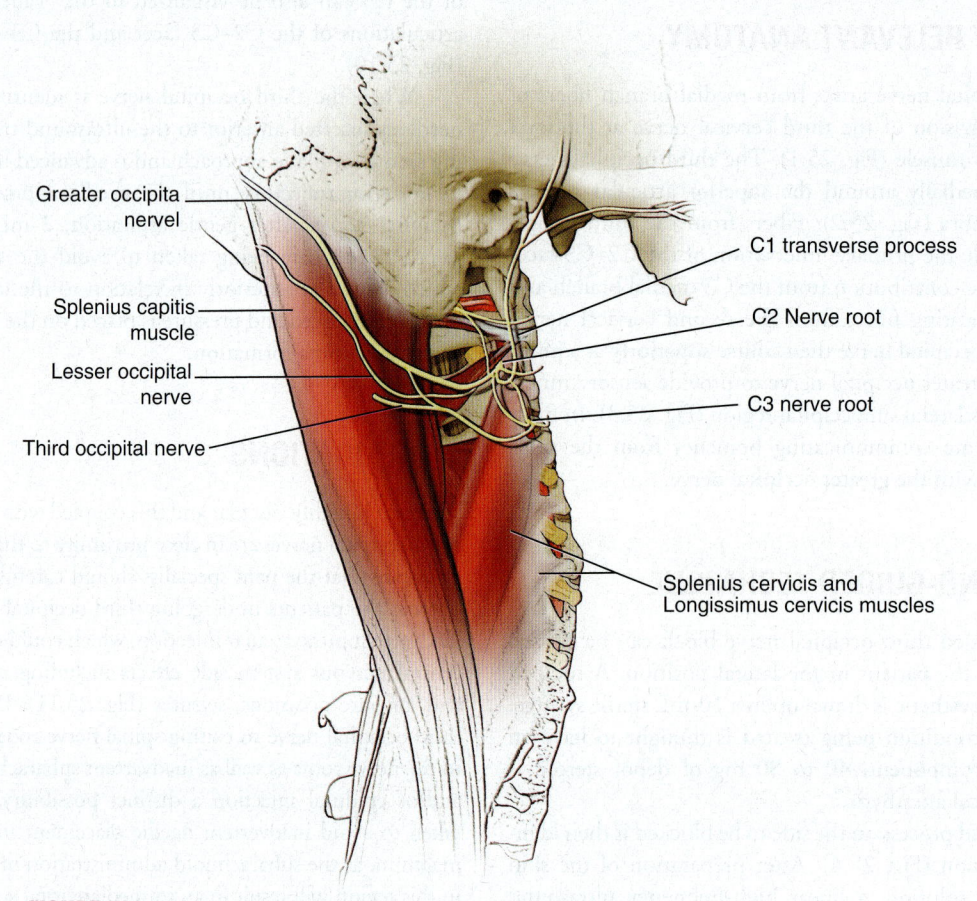

**FIGURE 25.2.** Lateral view of the anatomy of the third occipital nerve.

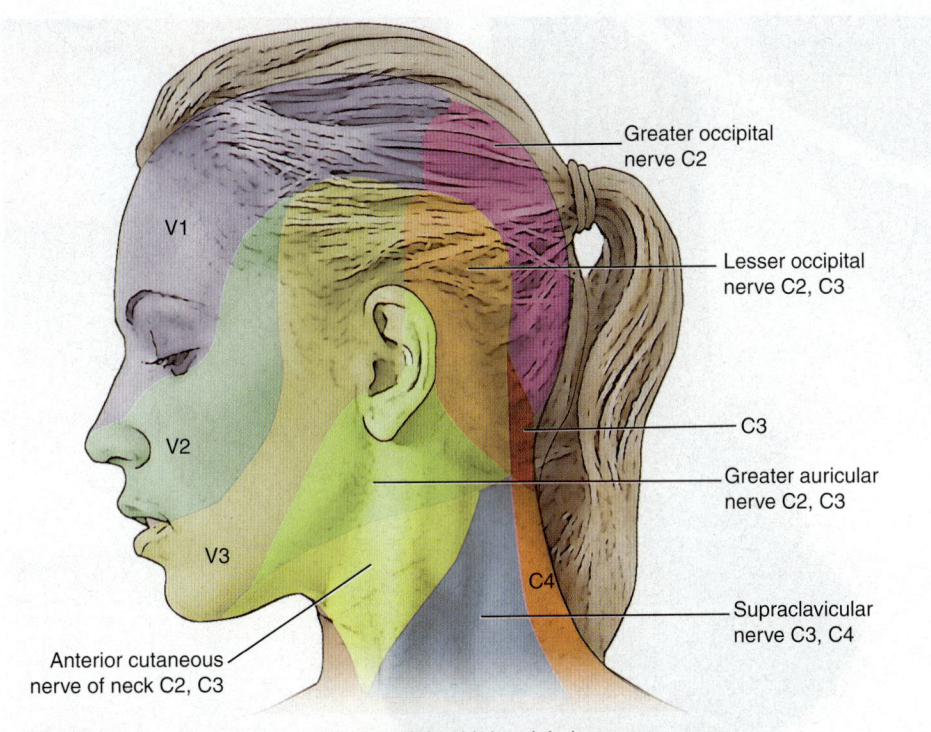

**FIGURE 25.3.** The sensory distribution of the third occipital nerves.

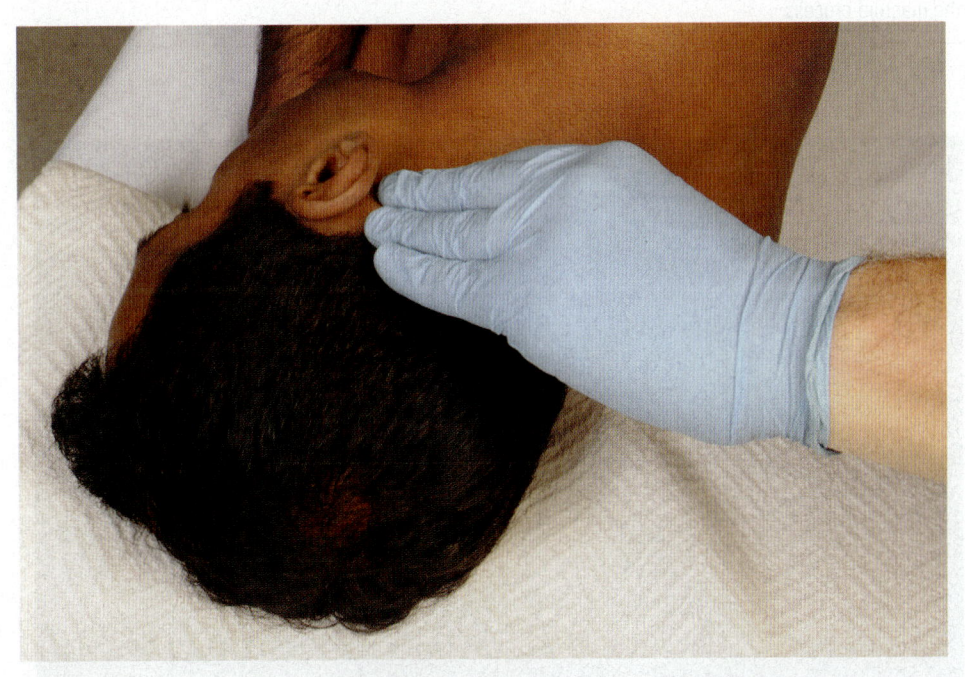

**FIGURE 25.4.** Palpation of the mastoid process with the patient in lateral position.

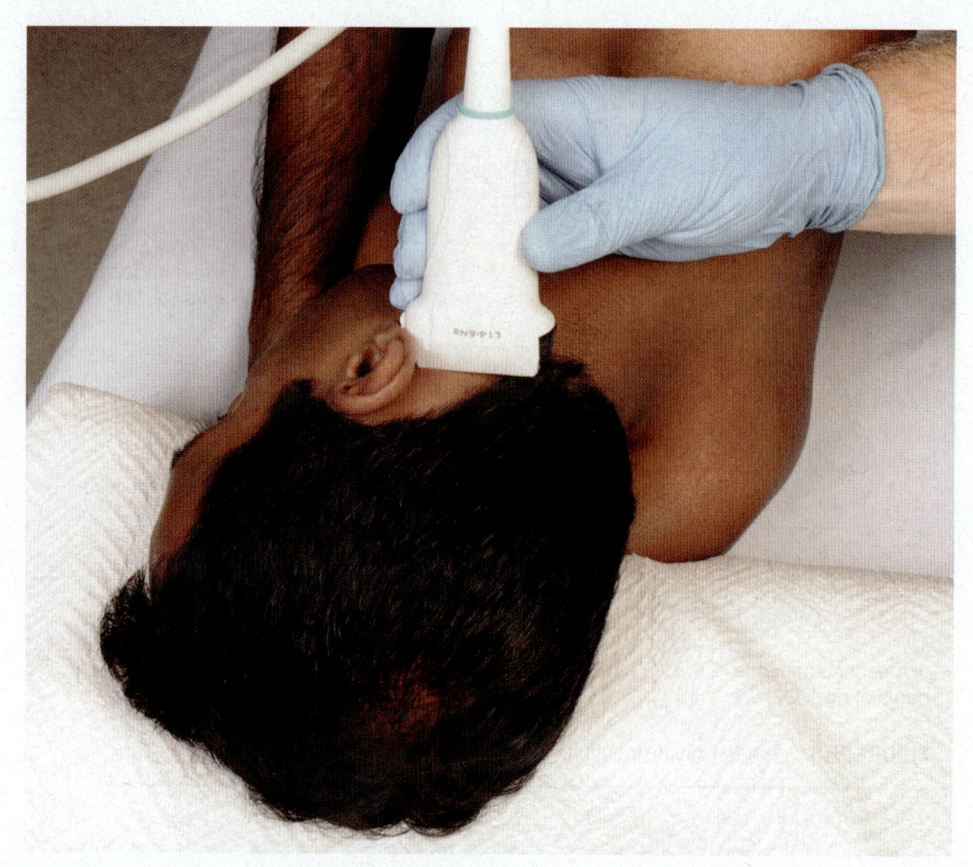

**FIGURE 25.5.** Placement of the ultrasound transducer in the longitudinal plane at the inferior margin of the mastoid process.

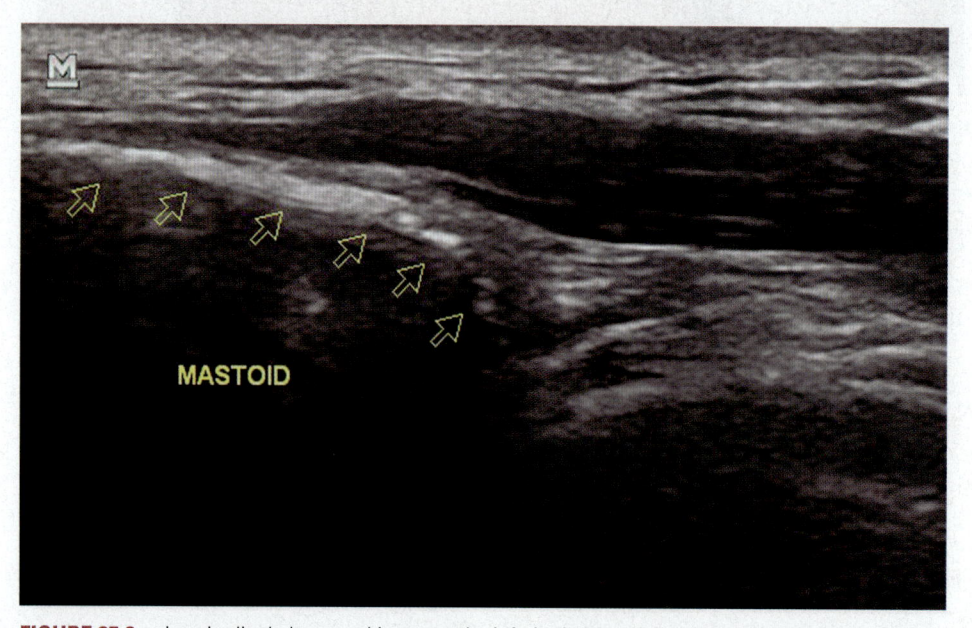

**FIGURE 25.6.** Longitudinal ultrasound image at the inferior border of the mastoid process.

CHAPTER 25 ULTRASOUND-GUIDED THIRD OCCIPITAL NERVE BLOCK 167

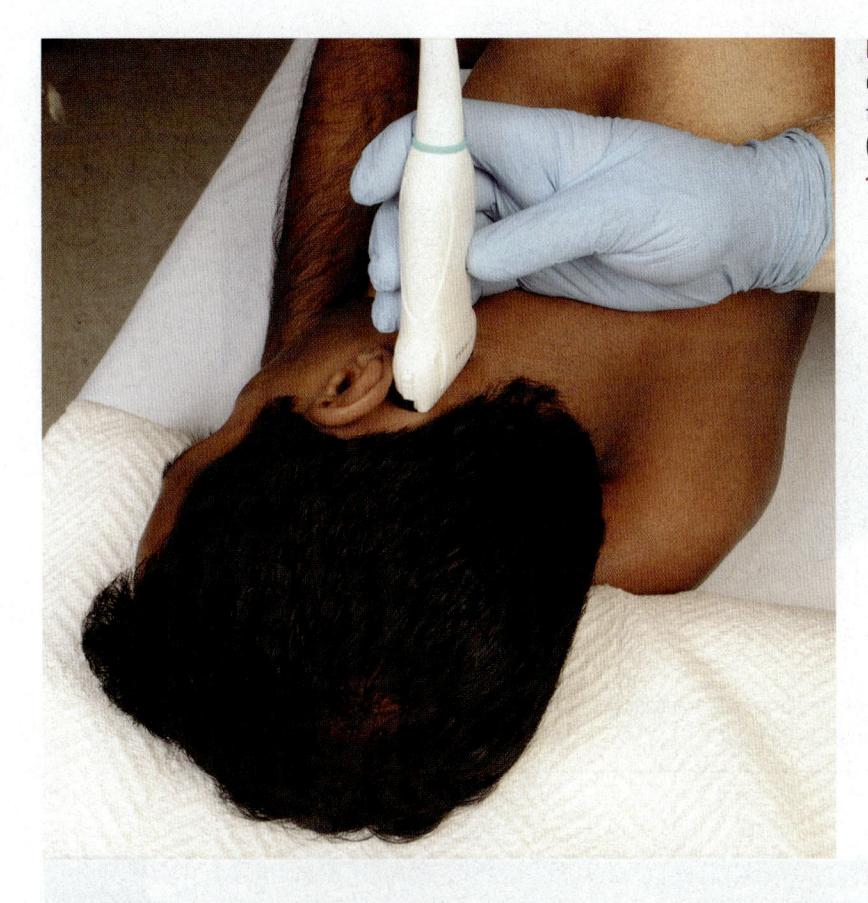

**FIGURE 25.7.** Placement of the ultrasound transducer in the longitudinal plane in position to identify the arch of atlas (C1) and the articular pillar of axis (C2).

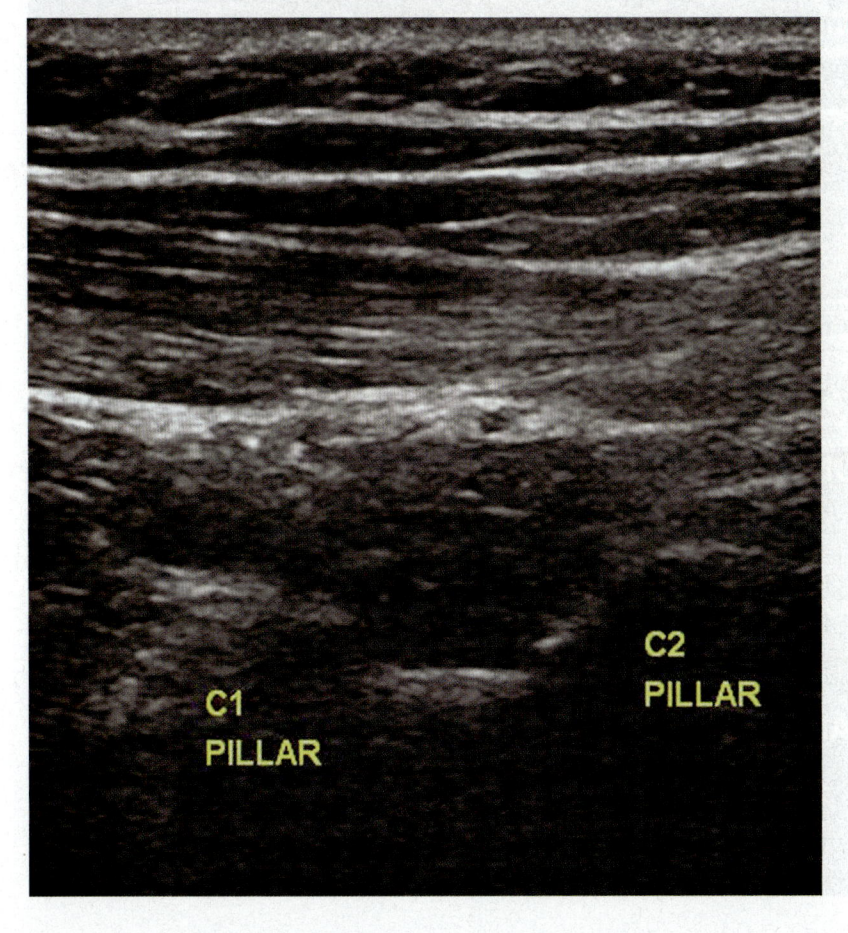

**FIGURE 25.8.** Longitudinal ultrasound image of the arch of atlas (C1) and the articular pillar of axis (C2).

**SECTION II** NECK

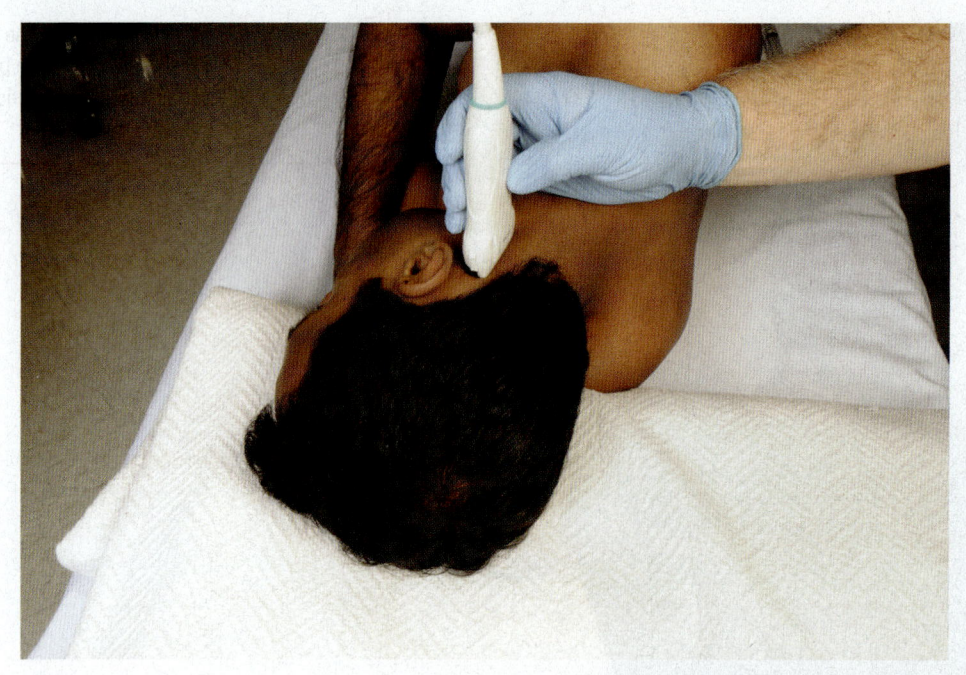

**FIGURE 25.9.** Proper position of the ultrasound transducer to perform the third occipital nerve block. The transducer is aligned across the C2–C3 facet.

**FIGURE 25.10.** Longitudinal ultrasound image of the C2–C3 facet joint with the third occipital nerve traveling across the joint and the medial branch of C3 in the valley between the articulations of C2–C3 and C3–C4.

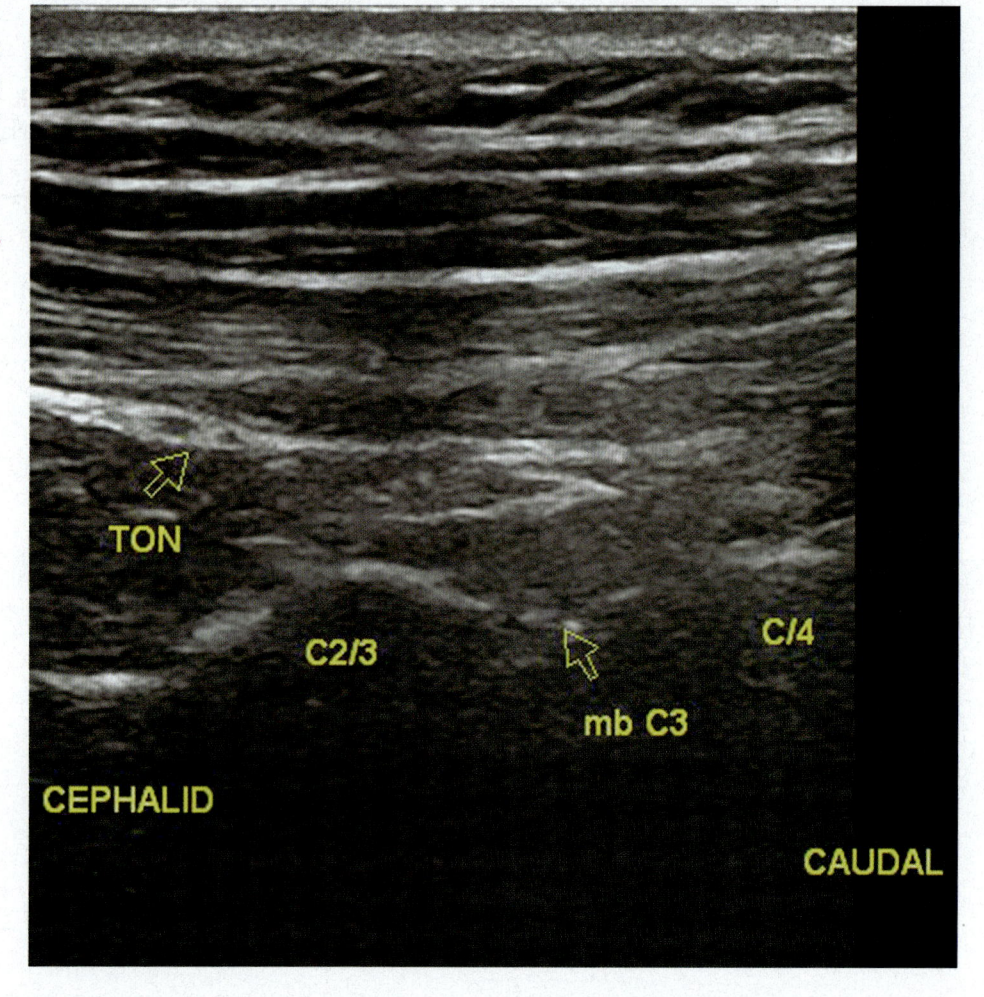

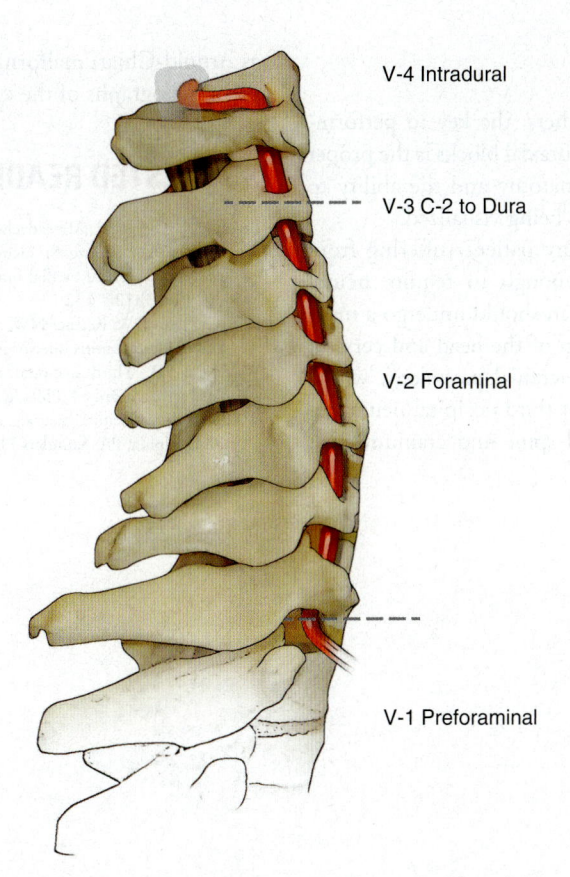

**FIGURE 25.11.** The relationship of the vertebral artery to the cervical facet joints.

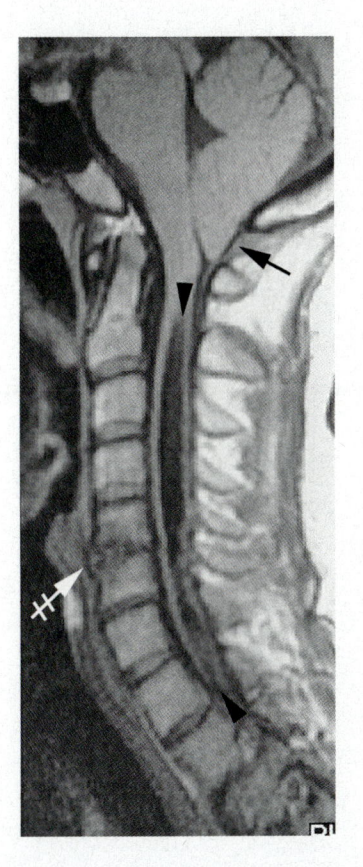

**FIGURE 25.12.** Arnold-Chiari malformation with syrinx. T1-Weighted MRI, sagittal cervical spine. Observe the ectopic cerebellar tonsils projecting caudally to the C1 level (*arrow*) and the uniformly low-signal intensity syrinx that enlarges the entire cervical spinal cord (*arrowhead*). Note that the borders of the syrinx are well defined. Also note the unrelated changes of degenerative spondylosis at C5–C6 (*crossed arrow*). NOTE: MRI is the most sensitive imaging modality to determine the presence of Arnold-Chiari malformations with or without syrinx. It provides a noninvasive means of obtaining this diagnosis. (Reused from Yochum TR, Rowe LJ. *Yochum and Rowe's Essentials of Skeletal Radiology.* 3rd ed. Philadelphia, PA: Lippincott Williams & Wilkins; 2004, with permission.)

## CLINICAL PEARLS

As pointed out by Narouze and others, the key to performing successful ultrasound cervical neuraxial blocks is the proper identification of the sonographic anatomy and the ability to properly identify the spinal segment being visualized.

It is this author's belief that any patient suffering from headaches and neck pain severe enough to require neural blockade as part of the treatment plan should undergo a magnetic resonance imaging (MRI) scan of the head and cervical spine to rule out unsuspected intracranial pathology, which may mimic the clinical symptoms of third occipital neuralgia. Other abnormalities of the cervical spine and cranium such as Arnold-Chiari malformations should also be ruled out with plain radiographs of the cervical spine (Fig. 25.12).

## SUGGESTED READINGS

Bogduk N. The neck and headaches. *Neuro Clin* 2004;22(1):151–171.

Siegenthaler A, Narouze S, Eichenberger U. Ultrasound-guided third occipital nerve and cervical medial branch nerve blocks. *Tech Reg Anesth Pain Manag* 2009;13(3):128–132.

Suk JC, Haun DW, Kettner NW. Sonography of the normal greater occipital nerve and obliquus capitis inferior muscle. *J Clin Ultrasound* 2010;38(6):299–304.

Waldman SD. Third occipital nerve block. In: *Atlas of Interventional Pain Management.* 3rd ed. Philadelphia, PA: Saunders Elsevier; 2009:146–150.

Waldman SD. Occipital neuralgia. In: *Atlas of Common Pain Syndromes.* 3rd ed. Philadelphia, PA: Saunders Elsevier; 2011:19–21.

# CHAPTER 26

# Ultrasound-Guided Cervical Medial Branch Block

## CLINICAL PERSPECTIVES

Ultrasound-guided blockade of the cervical medial branch is useful in the diagnosis and treatment of cervicogenic headache, cervicalgia, arthritis of the cervical facet joints, and other pain syndromes subserved by the cervical medial branches. These disease processes present clinically as neck pain, suboccipital headache, and occasionally shoulder and supraclavicular pain. This technique is also useful as a prognostic indicator of the potential efficacy of destruction of the cervical medial branch with neurolytic agents such as phenol or with radiofrequency lesioning.

## CLINICAL RELEVANT ANATOMY

Except for the atlanto-occipital and atlantoaxial joints, the cervical facet joints (which are also known as the zygapophyseal joints) are formed by the articulations of the superior and inferior articular facets of adjacent vertebrae. The cervical facet joints are true joints, which are lined with synovium, contain cartilage, menisci, and are enclosed in a true joint capsule. This joint capsule is richly innervated and supports the notion of the facet joint as a pain generator. The cervical facet joint is susceptible to arthritic changes and trauma caused by acceleration–deceleration injuries. Such damage to the joint results in pain secondary to synovial joint inflammation and adhesions.

Each facet joint receives innervation from two spinal levels, receiving fibers from the dorsal ramus at the same level as the vertebra as well as fibers from the dorsal ramus of the vertebra above (Fig. 26.1). This fact is important clinically for two reasons: (1) It provides an explanation for the ill-defined nature of facet-mediated pain and (2) it also explains why the medial branch from the vertebra above the painful joint as well as the medial branch at the level of the painful joint must both be blocked to provide complete pain relief. At each level, the dorsal ramus provides a medial branch that wraps around the convexity of the articular pillar of its respective vertebra (Fig. 26.2). This location is constant for the C3–C4 through the C8–T1 facet joints nerves and allows a simplified approach to ultrasound-guided medial branch block. The atlanto-occipital and atlantoaxial joints are not innervated by medial branches but by branches of the respective C1 and C2 ventral rami (see Chapters 1 and 2). The C2–C3 facet joint is innervated primarily by the third occipital nerve, which arises from medial branch fibers of the posterior division of the third cervical nerve (see Chapter 25).

## ULTRASOUND-GUIDED TECHNIQUE

Ultrasound-guided cervical medial branch block can be carried out by placing the patient in the lateral position. A total of 1 mL of local anesthetic is drawn up in a 10-mL sterile syringe for each medial branch to be blocked. If the painful condition being treated is thought to have an inflammatory component, 40 to 80 mg of depot steroid is added to the local anesthetic.

The mastoid process on the side to be blocked is then identified by palpation (Fig. 26.3). After preparation of the skin with antiseptic solution, a linear high-frequency ultrasound transducer is placed in a longitudinal plane with the cephalad end of the transducer resting at the base of the mastoid process, and the inferior border of the mastoid process is identified on ultrasound (Figs. 26.4 and 26.5). The transducer is then slowly moved in a posterior direction ~¾ inch until the arch of C1 (atlas) and the articular pillar of C2 (axis) can be identified (Figs. 26.6 and 26.7). The transducer is then slowly moved in a caudad direction until the C2–C3 facet joints are visualized (Fig. 26.8). Counting from the C2–C3 facet joints, this process is repeated by slowly moving the ultrasound transducer in a caudad direction while counting the "hills," which represent the articulations of each joint until the specific facet joint to be blocked is identified (Fig. 25.9A and B).

Once the facet joints of the desired level are identified, the ultrasound transducer is then slowly rotated toward the external acoustic meatus until the cervical medial branch is identified in the "valley" between adjacent facet joints. The cervical medial branches will appear like a hyperechoic dot within a hypoechoic halo.

When the cervical medial branch is identified, a 3½-inch needle is inserted anterior to the ultrasound transducer utilizing

SECTION II  NECK

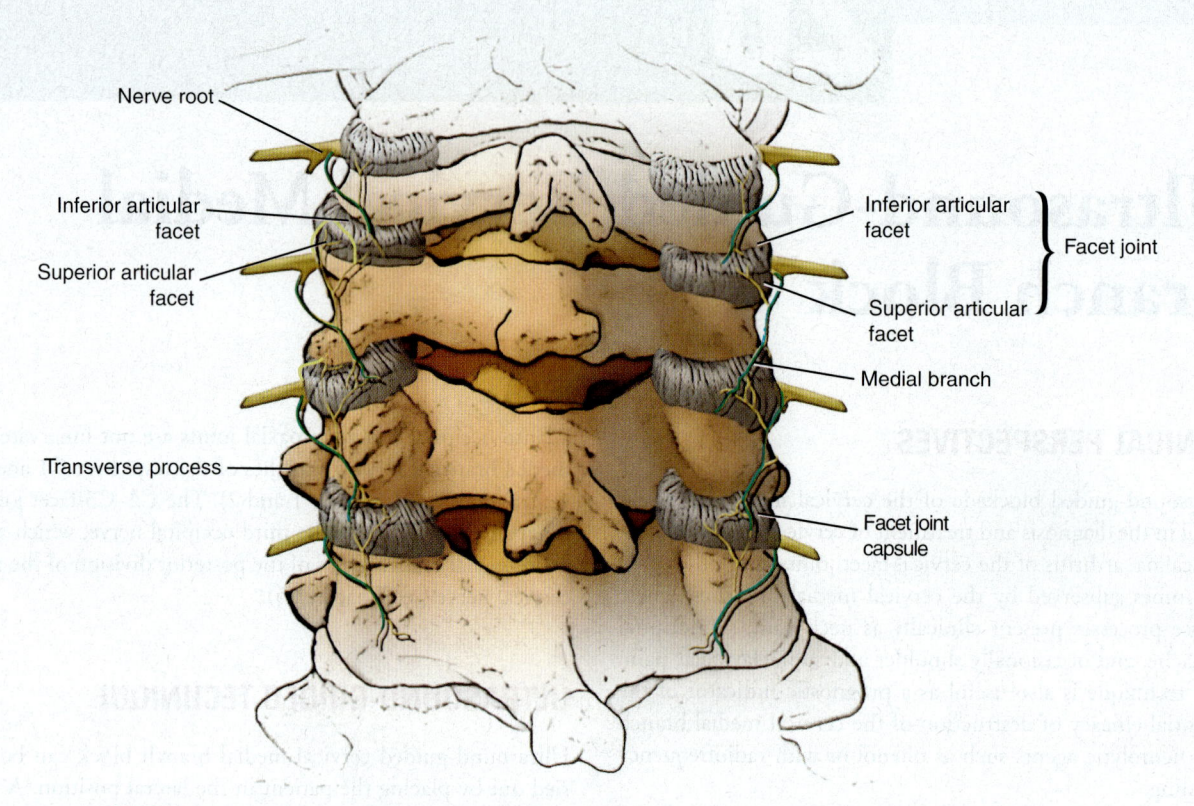

**FIGURE 26.1.** The anatomy of the cervical facet joint. Note that each joint receives innervation from two spinal levels, receiving fibers from the dorsal ramus at the same level as the vertebra as well as fibers from the dorsal ramus of the vertebra above the medial branch.

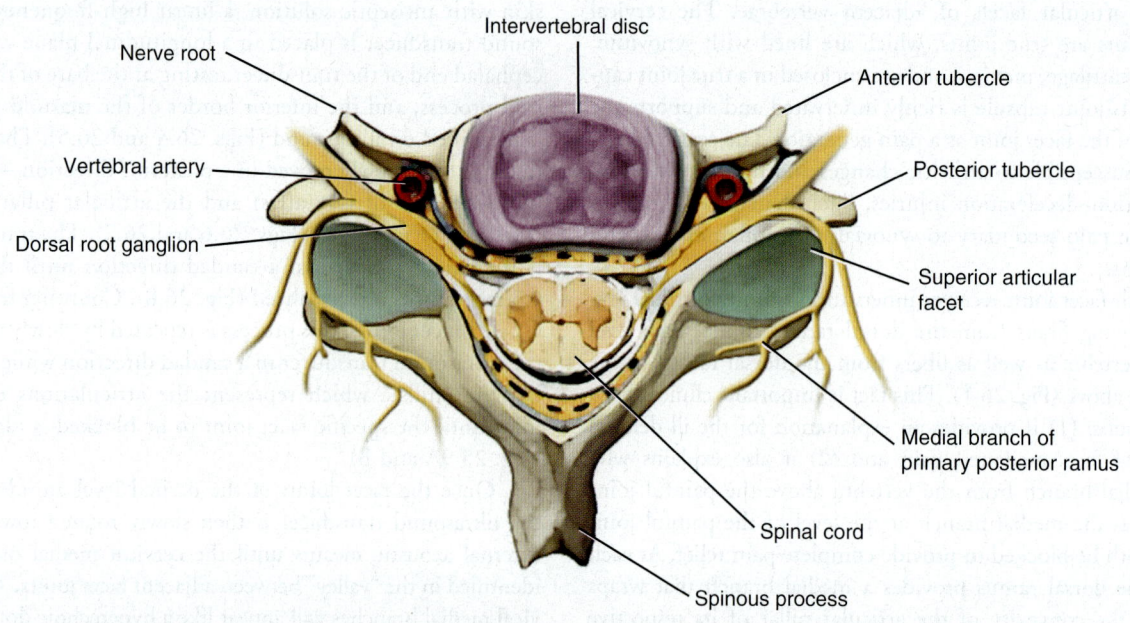

**FIGURE 26.2.** Cross-sectional view of the anatomy of the cervical medial branch and its relationship to the superior articular process.

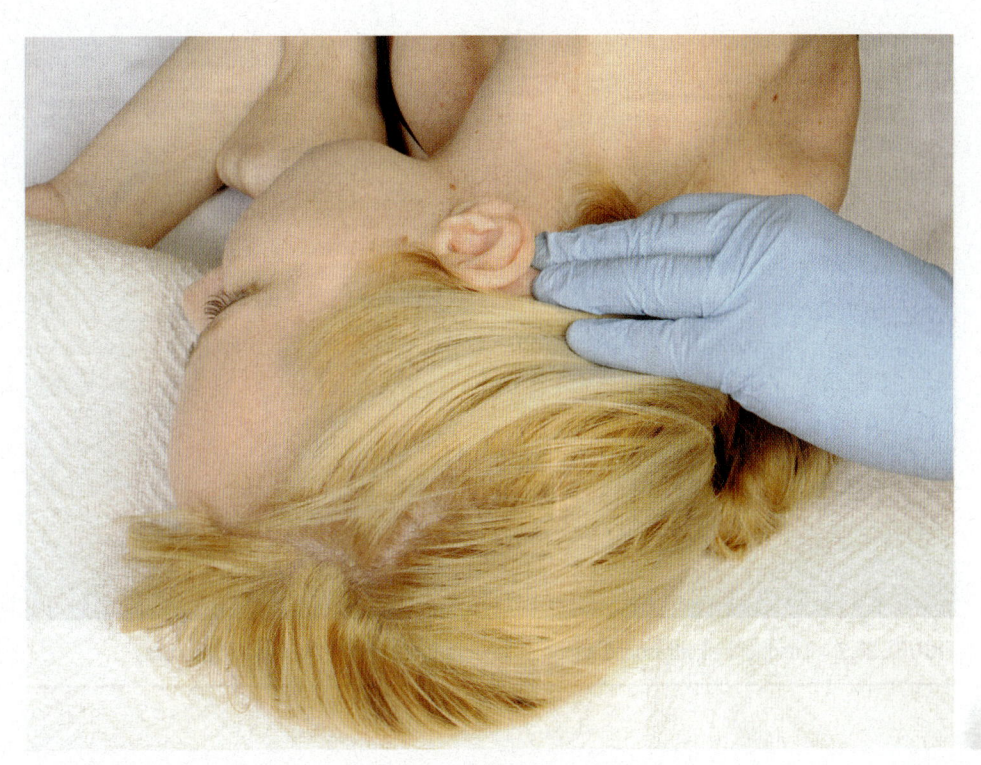

**FIGURE 26.3.** Palpation of the mastoid process with the patient in lateral position.

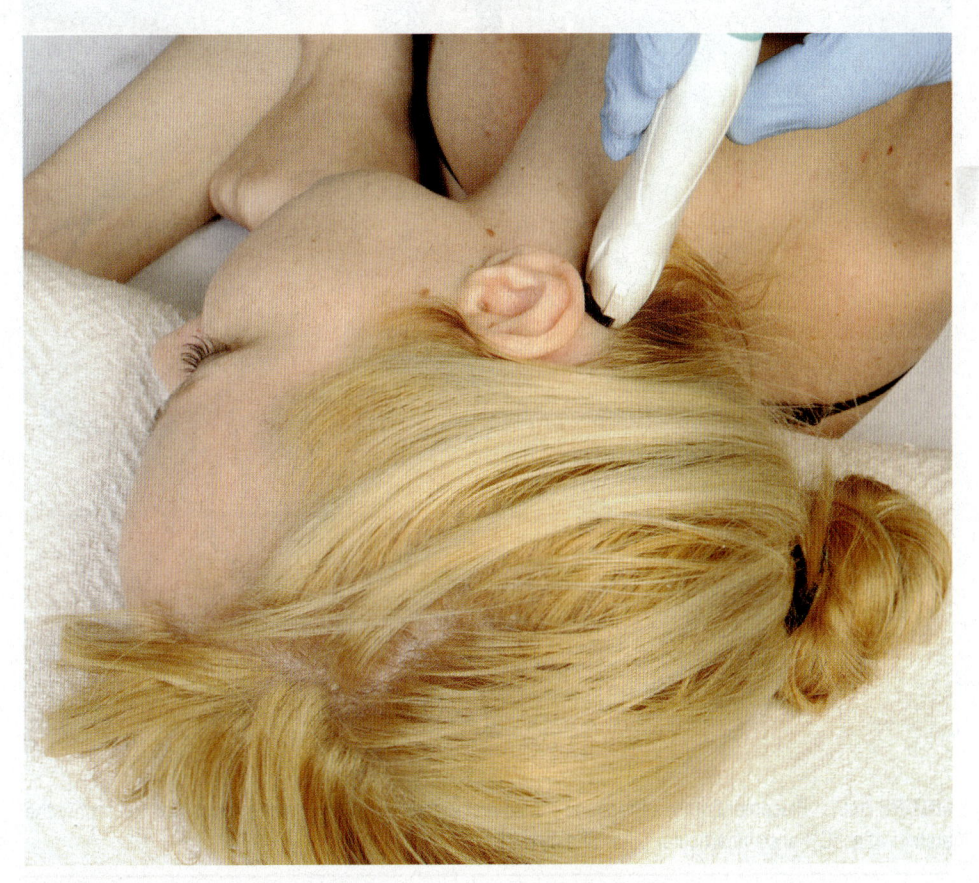

**FIGURE 26.4.** Placement of the ultrasound transducer in the longitudinal plane at the inferior margin of the mastoid process.

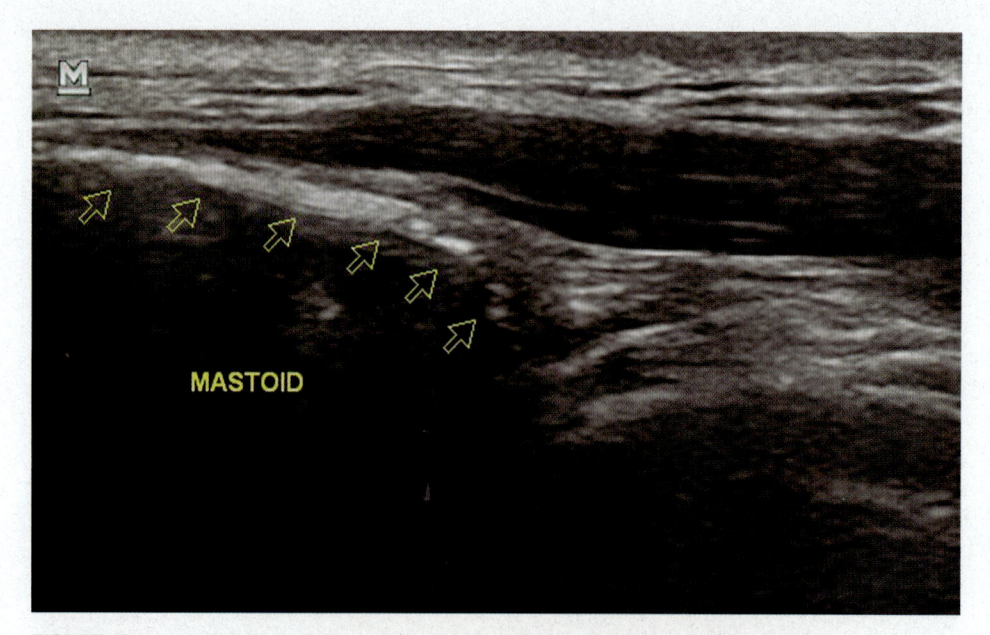

**FIGURE 26.5.** Longitudinal ultrasound image at the inferior border of the mastoid process.

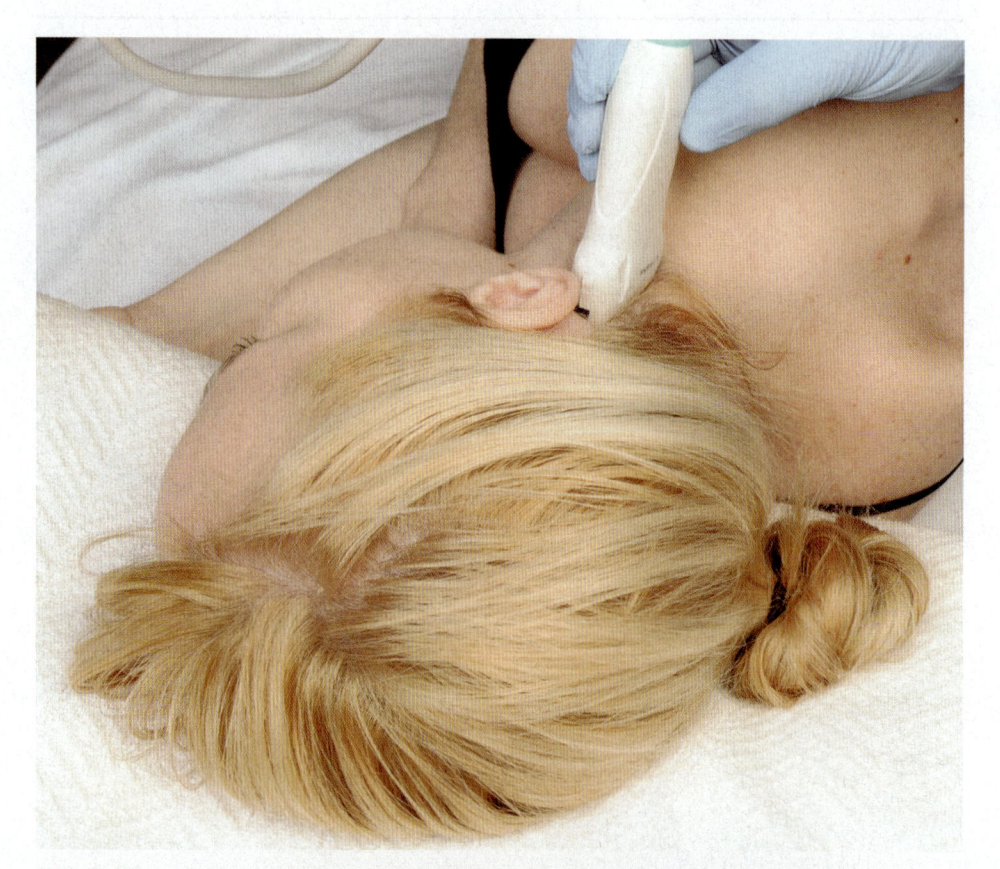

**FIGURE 26.6.** Placement of the ultrasound transducer in the longitudinal plane in position to identify the arch of atlas (C1) and the articular pillar of axis (C2).

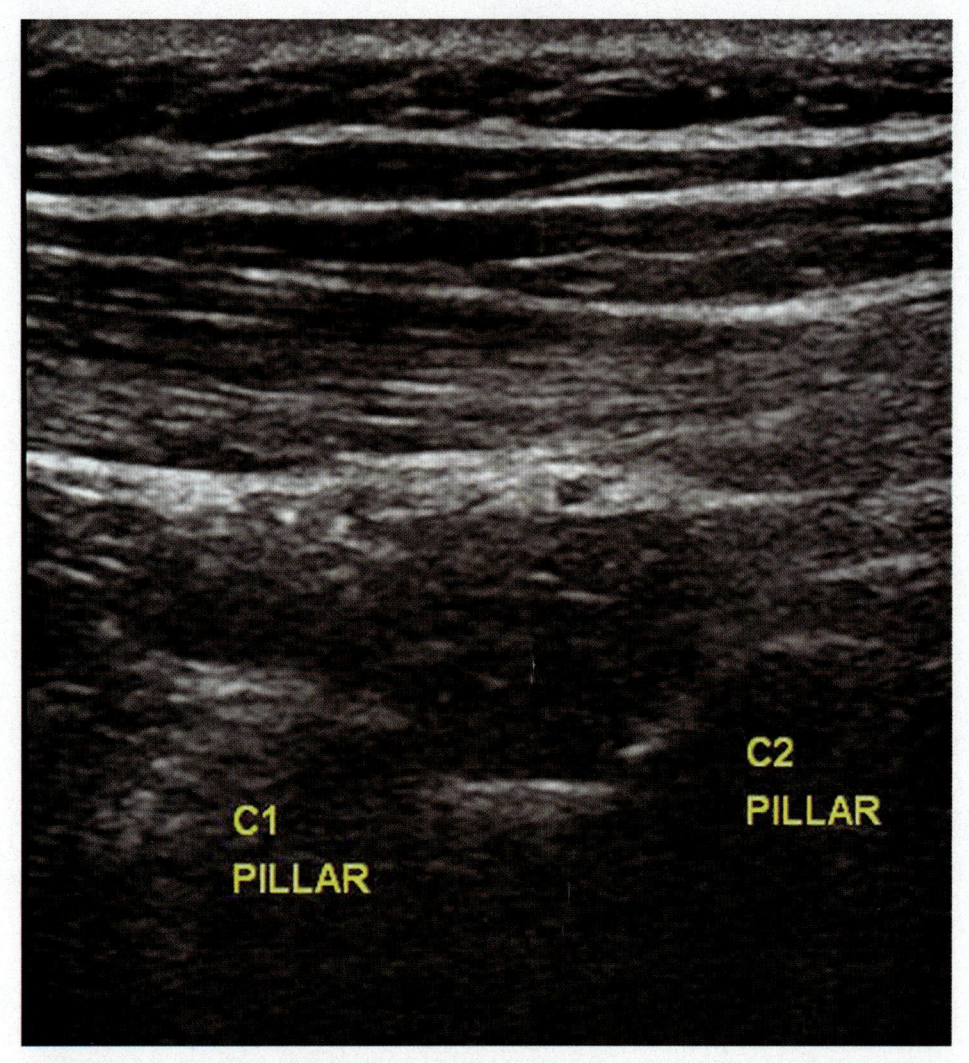

**FIGURE 26.7.** Longitudinal ultrasound image of the arch of atlas (C1) and the articular pillar of axis (C2).

an out-of-plane approach and is advanced from an anterior to posterior trajectory away from the vertebral artery and neuraxial structures until the needle approaches the cervical medial branch. After gentle aspiration, 1 mL of solution is injected with care being taken to avoid the vertebral artery, which is located anteriorly in relation to the facet joints. The needle is removed and pressure is placed on the injection site to avoid hematoma formation.

## COMPLICATIONS

This area is highly vascular and this coupled with the fact that the cervical medial branches are in close proximity to the vertebral artery that lies just anterior to the facet joint means that the pain specialist should carefully calculate the total mg dosage of local anesthetic and observe the patients undergoing cervical medial branch block for inadvertent intravascular injection, which could cause significant central nervous system side effects including ataxia, dizziness, and, on rare occasions, seizures (Fig. 26.10). Proximity of the cervical medial branch to exiting spinal nerve roots makes trauma to the nerve roots, which also lie just anterior to the facet joint, as well as inadvertent subarachnoid, subdural, and/or epidural injection a distinct possibility. Care must be taken to avoid inadvertent needle placement into the foramen magnum, as the subarachnoid administration of local anesthetic in this region will result in an immediate total spinal anesthetic.

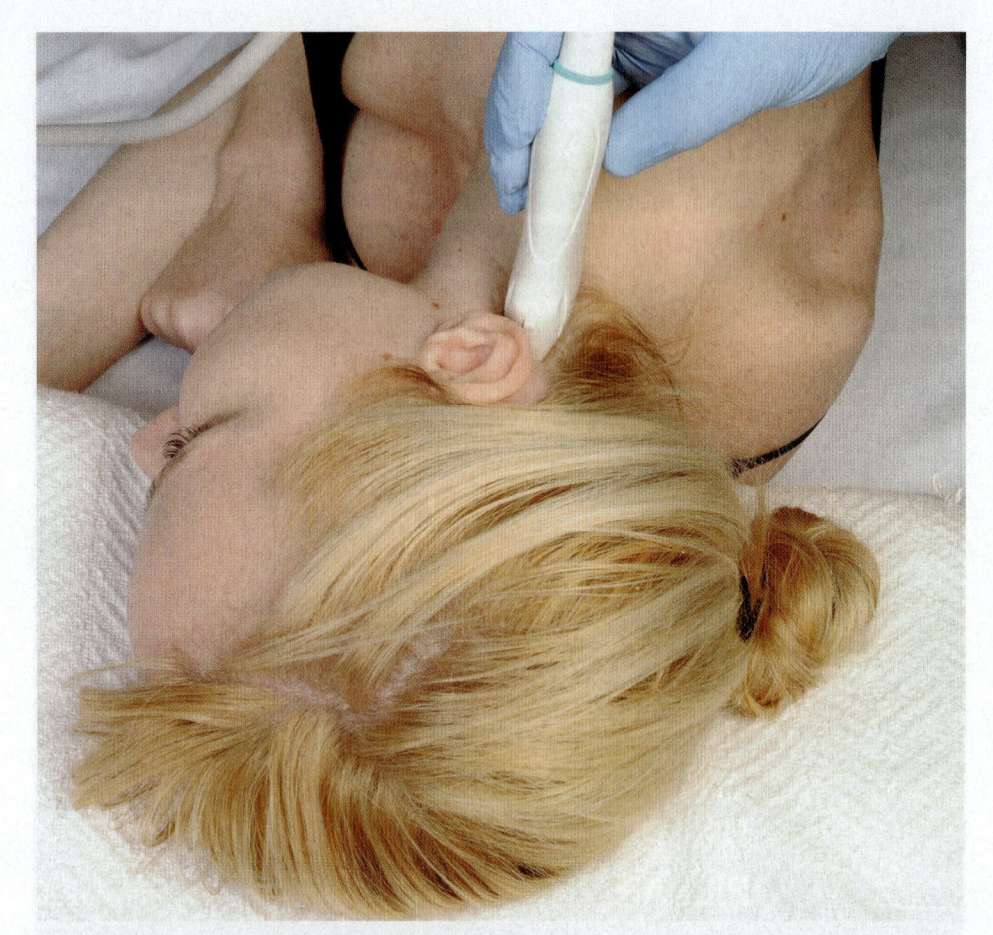

**FIGURE 26.8.** Proper position of the ultrasound transducer to perform the cervical medial branch block. The transducer is aligned across the C2–C3 facet joint.

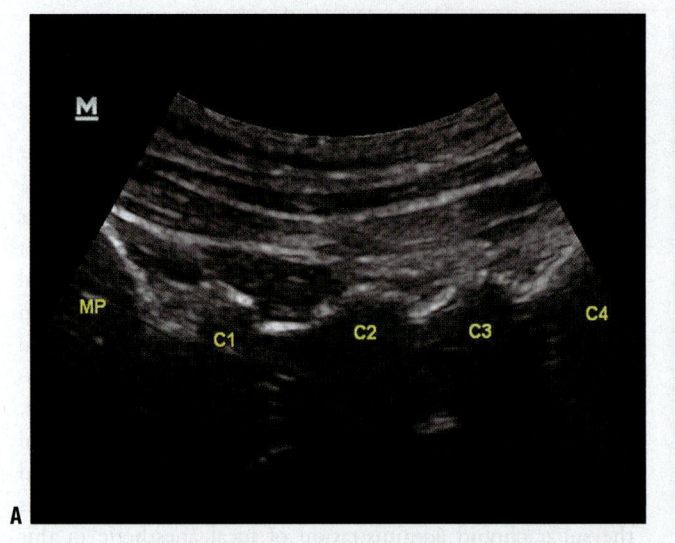

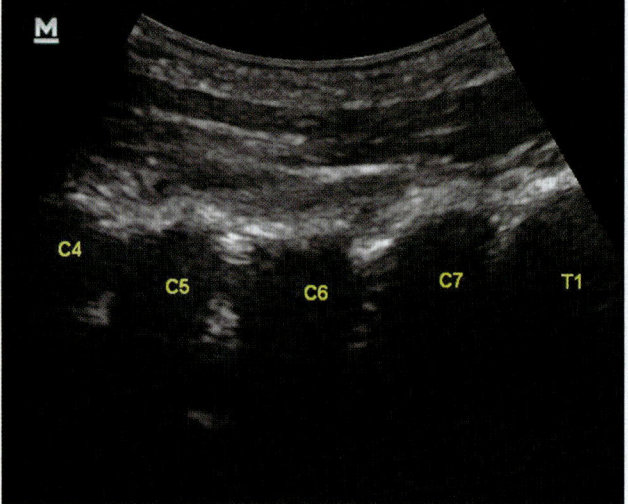

**FIGURE 26.9 A,B:** Longitudinal ultrasound image of the cervical articular processes demonstrating the "hills," which represent the articular processes, and the "valleys" between the adjacent facet joints. A: Demonstrates C1–C4. B: Demonstrates C4–T1. (Reused from Koopman WJ, Moreland LW. *Arthritis and Allied Conditions. A Textbook of Rheumatology.* 15th ed. Philadelphia, PA: Lippincott Williams & Wilkins; 2005, with permission.)

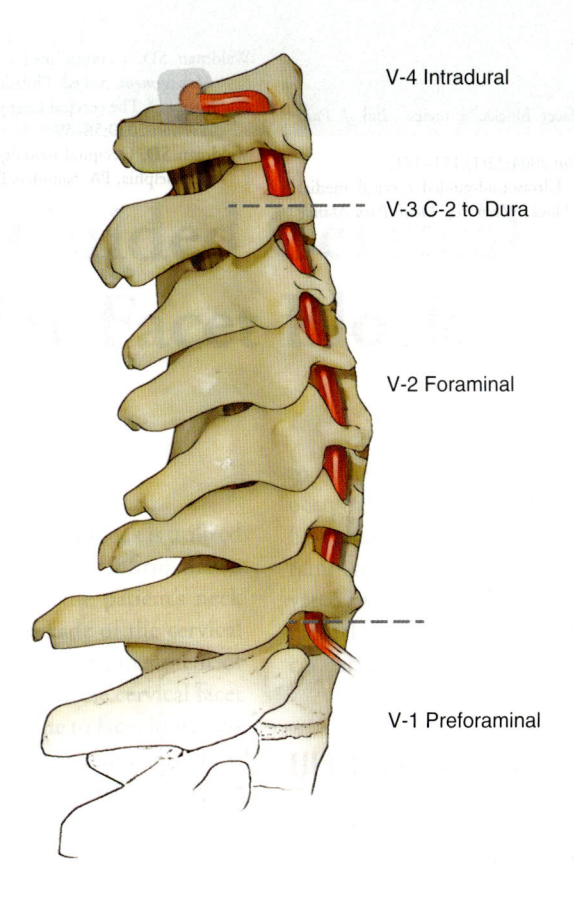

**FIGURE 26.10.** The relationship of the vertebral artery to the cervical facet joints.

## CLINICAL PEARLS

As pointed out by Narouze and others, the key to performing successful ultrasound cervical neuraxial blocks is the proper identification of the sonographic anatomy and the ability to properly identify the spinal segment being visualized. This should not be a problem if the above technique is used. Cervical facet block using the medial branch approach is the preferred technique for treatment of cervical facet syndrome. Although intra-articular placement of the needle into the facet joint is technically feasible, unless specific diagnostic information about that specific joint is required, such maneuvers add nothing to the efficacy of the procedure and in fact may increase the rate of complications.

It is this author's belief that any patient suffering from headaches and neck pain severe enough to require neural blockade as part of the treatment plan should undergo a magnetic resonance imaging scan of the head and cervical spine to rule out unsuspected intracranial pathology, which may mimic the clinical symptoms of third occipital neuralgia. Other abnormalities of the cervical spine and cranium such as Arnold-Chiari malformations, Paget disease, and tumor should also be ruled out with plain radiographs of the cervical spine (Fig. 26.11).

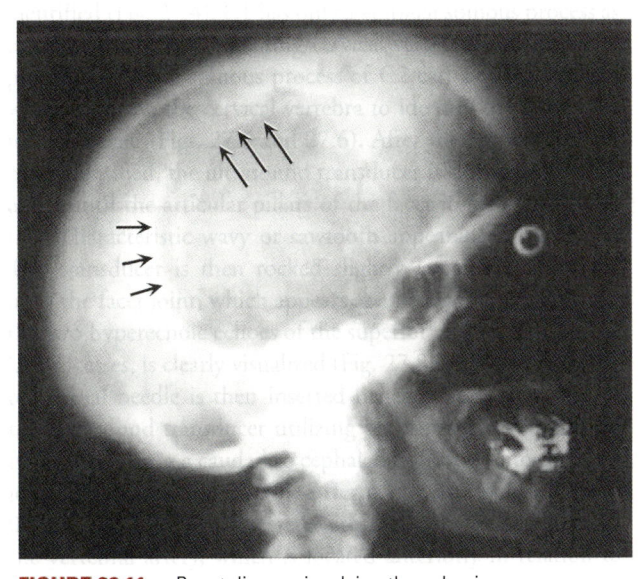

**FIGURE 26.11.** Paget disease involving the calvarium.

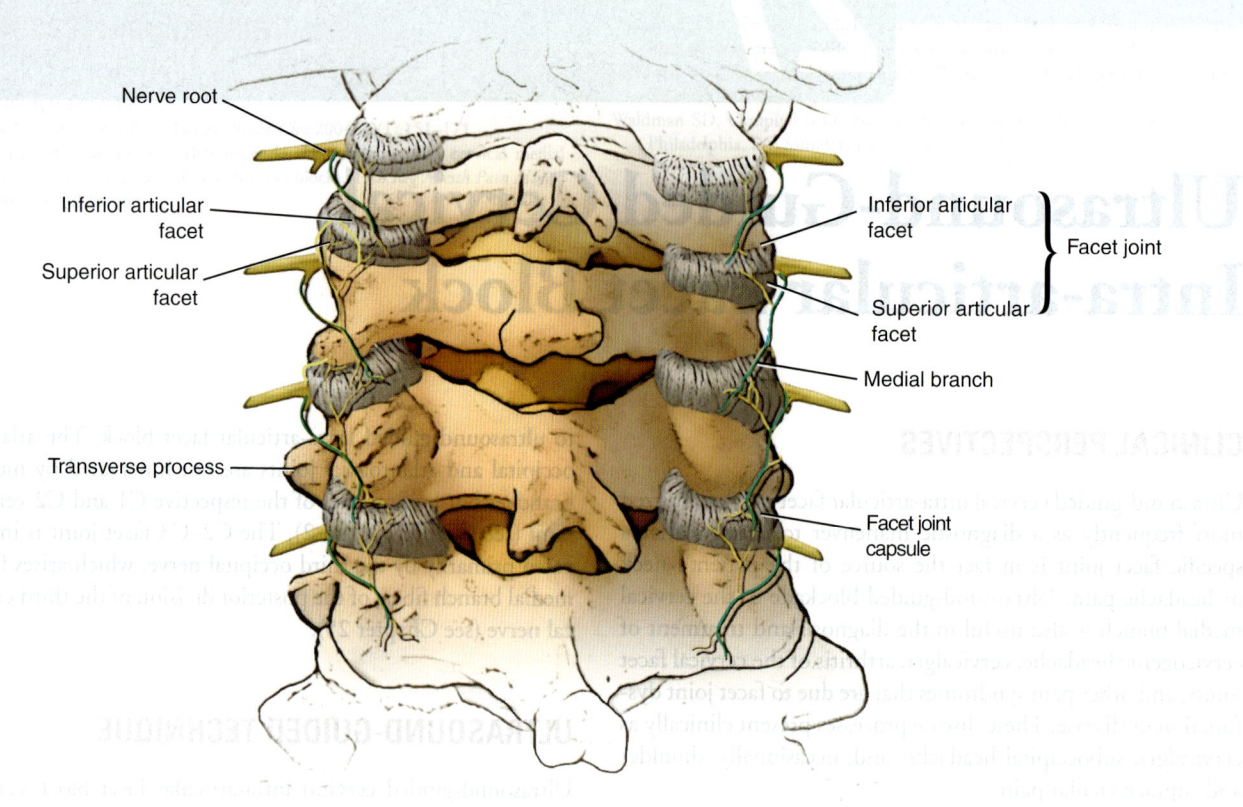

**FIGURE 27.1.** The anatomy of the cervical facet joint. Note that each joint receives innervation from two spinal levels, receiving fibers from the dorsal ramus at the same level as the vertebra as well as fibers from the dorsal ramus of the vertebra above.

the facet joints. The needle is removed and pressure is placed on the injection site to avoid hematoma formation.

## COMPLICATIONS

The cervical facet joints are in close proximity to the spinal cord and exiting nerve roots, and this procedure should be performed only by those well versed in the regional anatomy and skilled at ultrasound-guided interventional pain management procedures (Fig. 27.11). Trauma to the exiting cervical nerve roots, which also lie just anterior to the facet joint, as well as inadvertent subarachnoid, subdural, and/or epidural injection can occur even in the best of hands. The proximity to the vertebral artery combined with the vascular nature of this anatomic region makes the potential for intravascular injection high although the use of color Doppler to identify the vertebral artery and other vascular structures should help the clinician avoid this potentially fatal complication. Even small amounts of injection of local anesthetic into the vertebral arteries will result in seizures. Given the proximity of the brain and brain stem, ataxia due to vascular absorption of local anesthetic is not an uncommon occurrence after cervical facet block. Many patients also complain of a transient increase in headache and cervicalgia after injection of the joint.

## CLINICAL PEARLS

As pointed out by Narouze and others, the key to performing successful ultrasound cervical neuraxial blocks is the proper identification of the sonographic anatomy and the ability to properly identify the spinal segment being visualized. This should not be a problem if the above technique is used. Cervical facet block using the medial branch approach is the preferred technique for treatment of cervical facet syndrome. Although intra-articular placement of the needle into the facet joint is technically feasible, unless specific diagnostic information about that specific joint is required, such maneuvers probably add little to the efficacy of the procedure and in fact may increase the rate of complications.

It is this author's belief that any patient suffering from headaches and neck pain severe enough to require neural blockade as part of the treatment plan should undergo a magnetic resonance imaging scan of the head and cervical spine to rule out unsuspected intracranial pathology, which may mimic the clinical symptoms of third occipital neuralgia. Other abnormalities of the cervical spine and cranium such as Arnold-Chiari malformations, Paget disease, and tumor should also be ruled out with plain radiographs of the cervical spine.

CHAPTER 27   ULTRASOUND-GUIDED CERVICAL INTRA-ARTICULAR FACET BLOCK

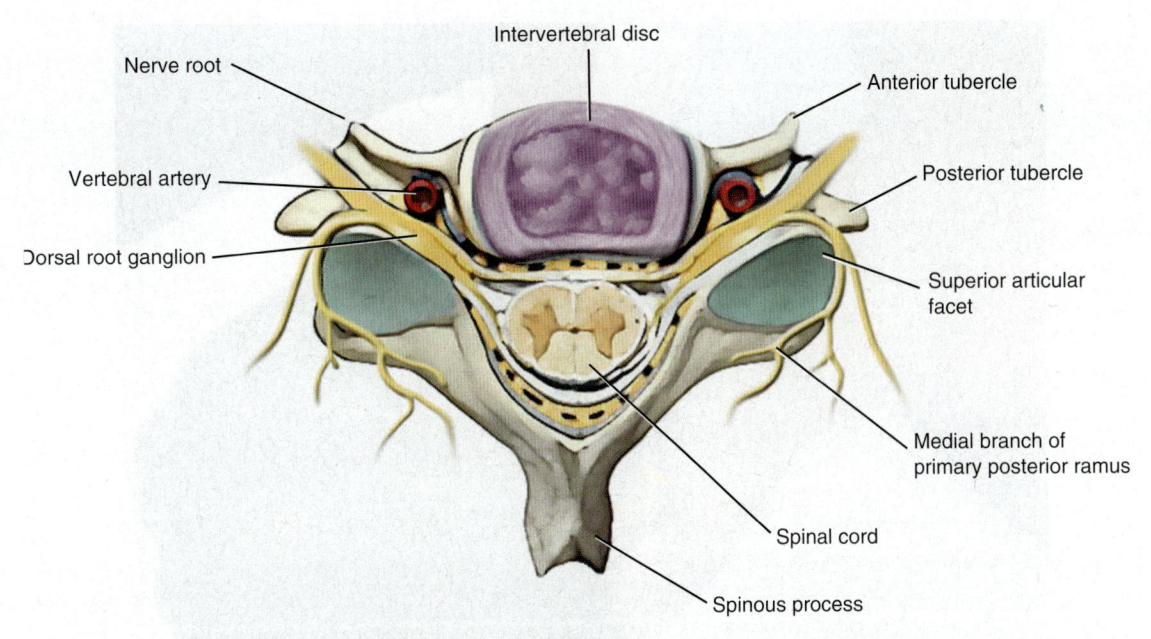

**FIGURE 27.2.** Cross-sectional view of the anatomy of the cervical medial branch and its relationship to the superior articular process.

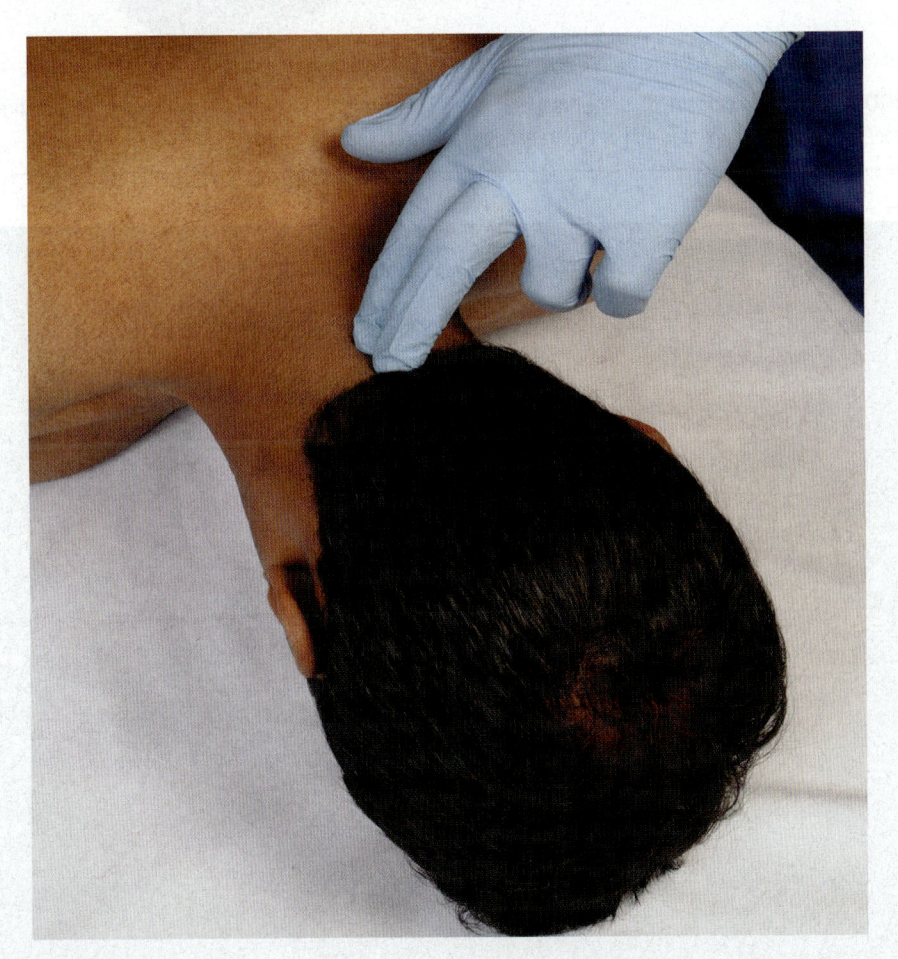

**FIGURE 27.3.** Palpation of the spinous processes of the cervical spine to identify the midline with the patient in the prone position.

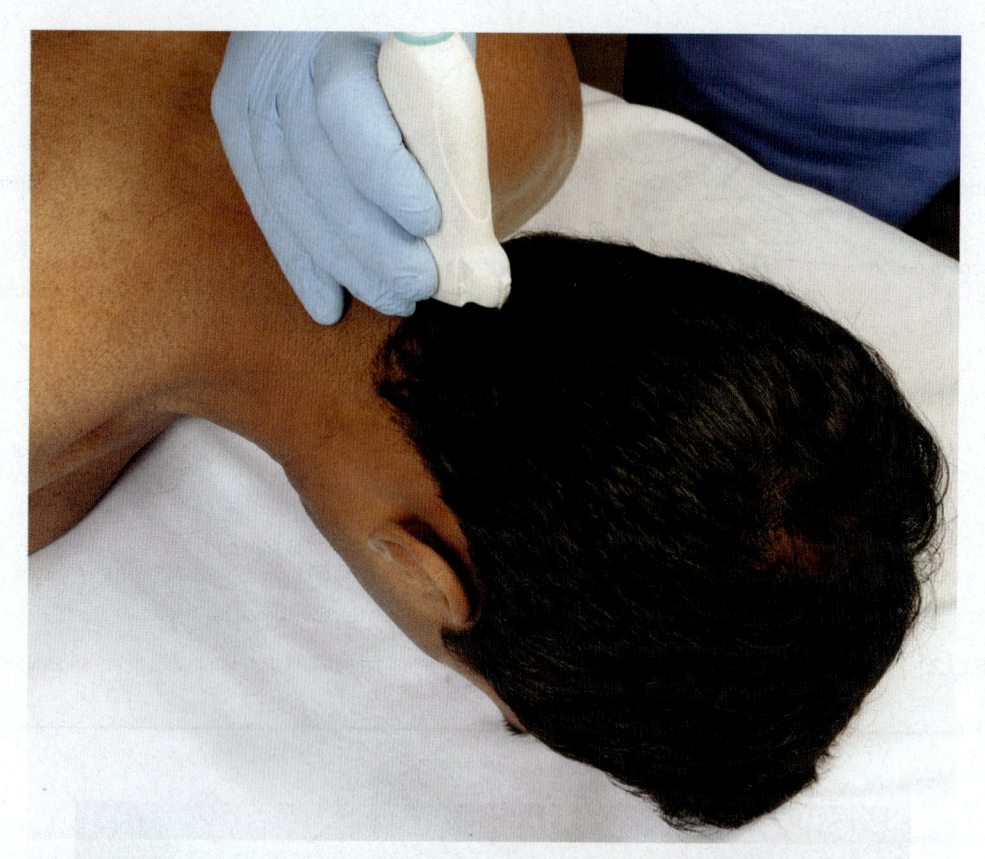

**FIGURE 27.4.** Placement of the ultrasound transducer in the longitudinal plane over the spinous processes with the cephalad end of the transducer at the occiput.

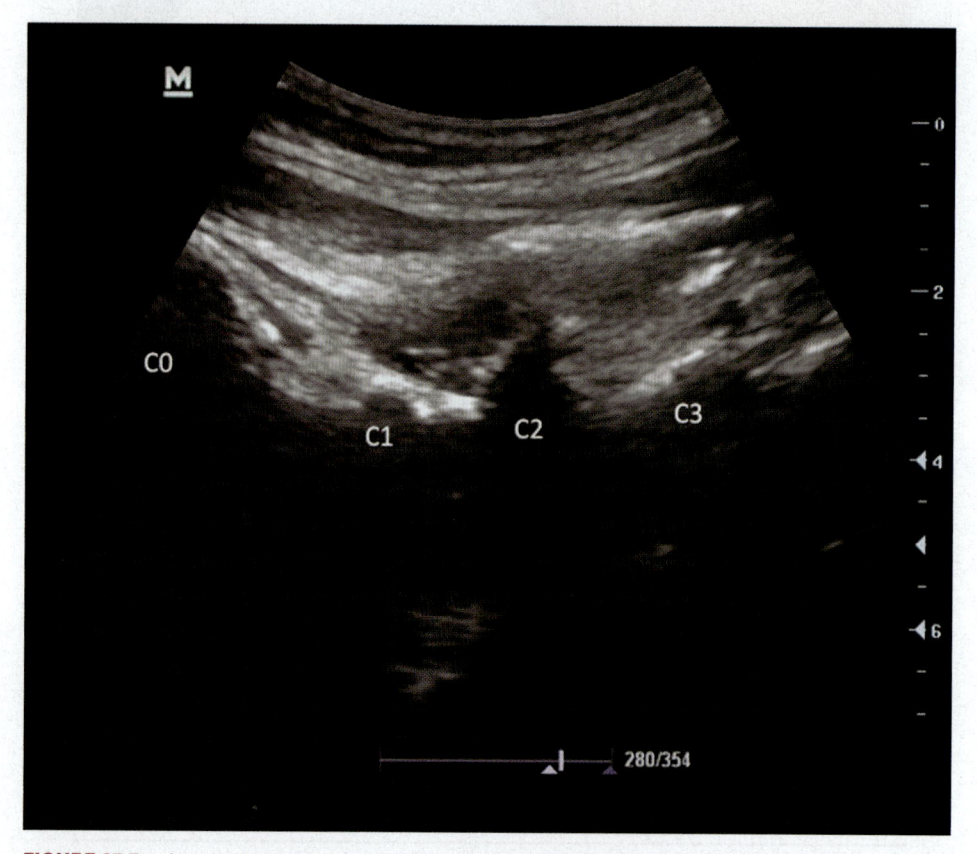

**FIGURE 27.5.** Longitudinal ultrasound image at the inferior border of the mastoid process.

CHAPTER 27    ULTRASOUND-GUIDED CERVICAL INTRA-ARTICULAR FACET BLOCK    183

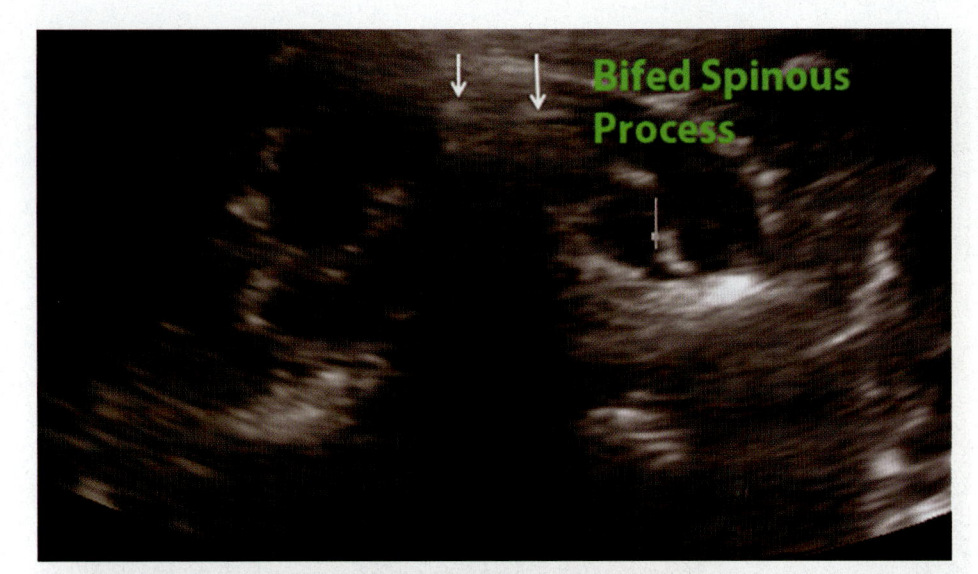

**FIGURE 27.6.** The classic ultrasound appearance of the bifid spinous process of C2.

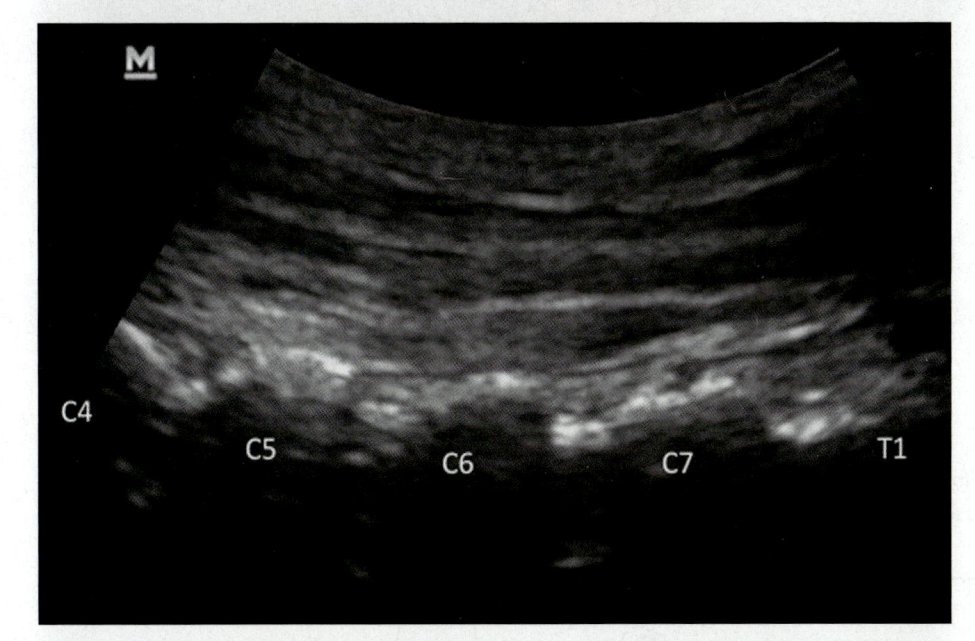

**FIGURE 27.7.** The characteristic wavy or sawtooth appearance of the articular processes of the cervical spine.

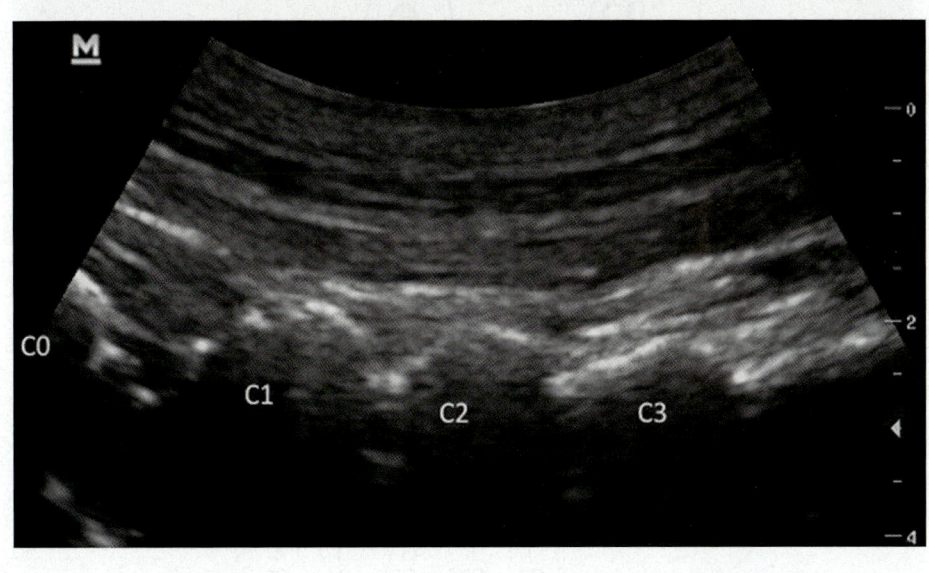

**FIGURE 27.8.** Longitudinal ultrasound image demonstrating the hyperechoic "hills," which are the articular processes, and the "valleys," which are the hyperechoic spaces between two adjacent facet joints. The "valleys" contain the medial branches.

**FIGURE 27.9.** Proper position and trajectory for an in-plane ultrasound-guided needle placement into the cervical facet joint.

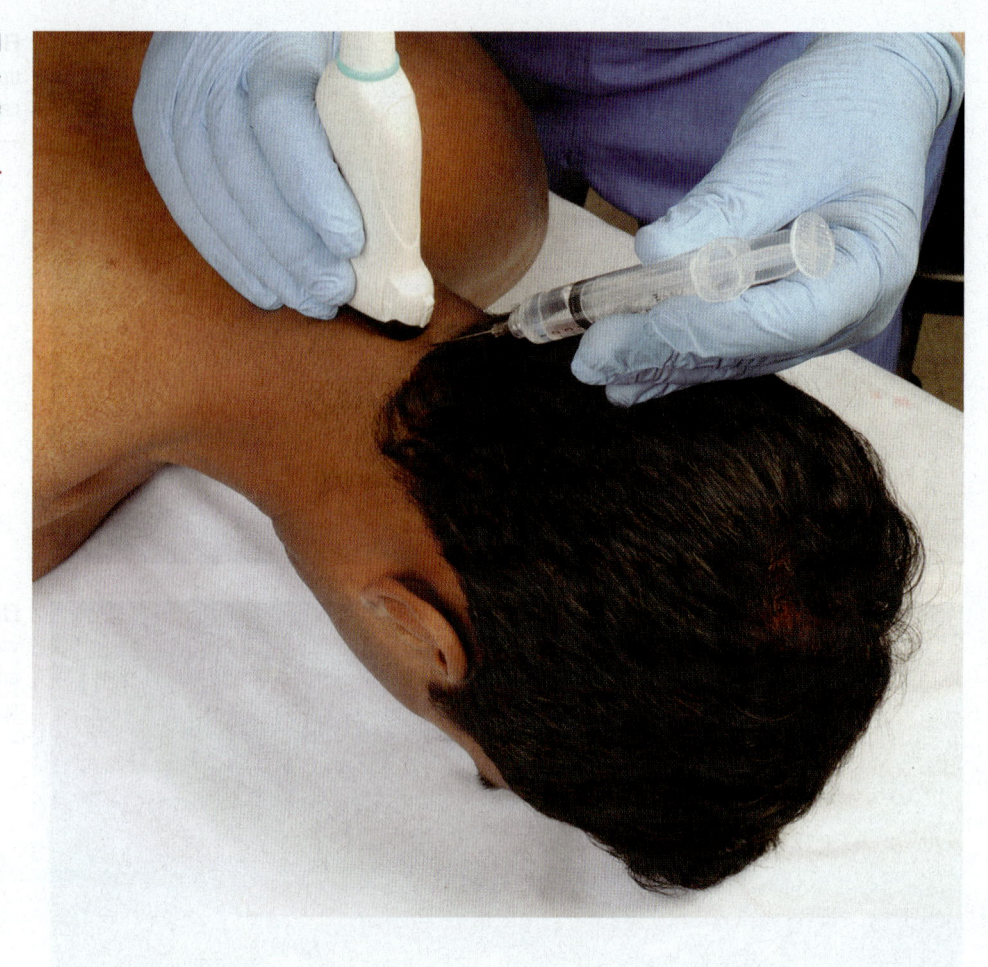

**FIGURE 27.10.** Proper trajectory for an in-plane ultrasound-guided needle placement into the cervical facet joint.

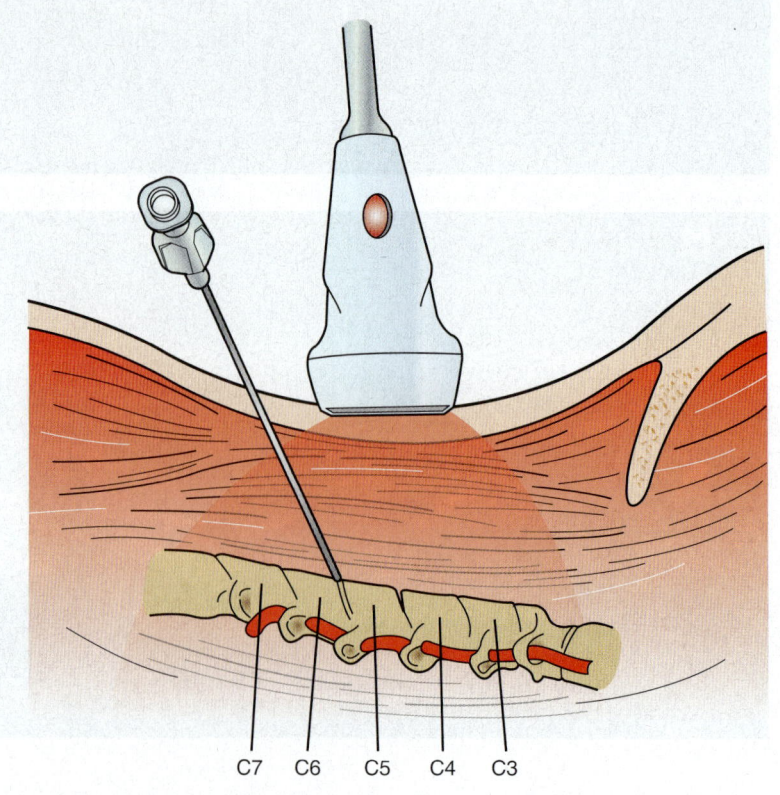

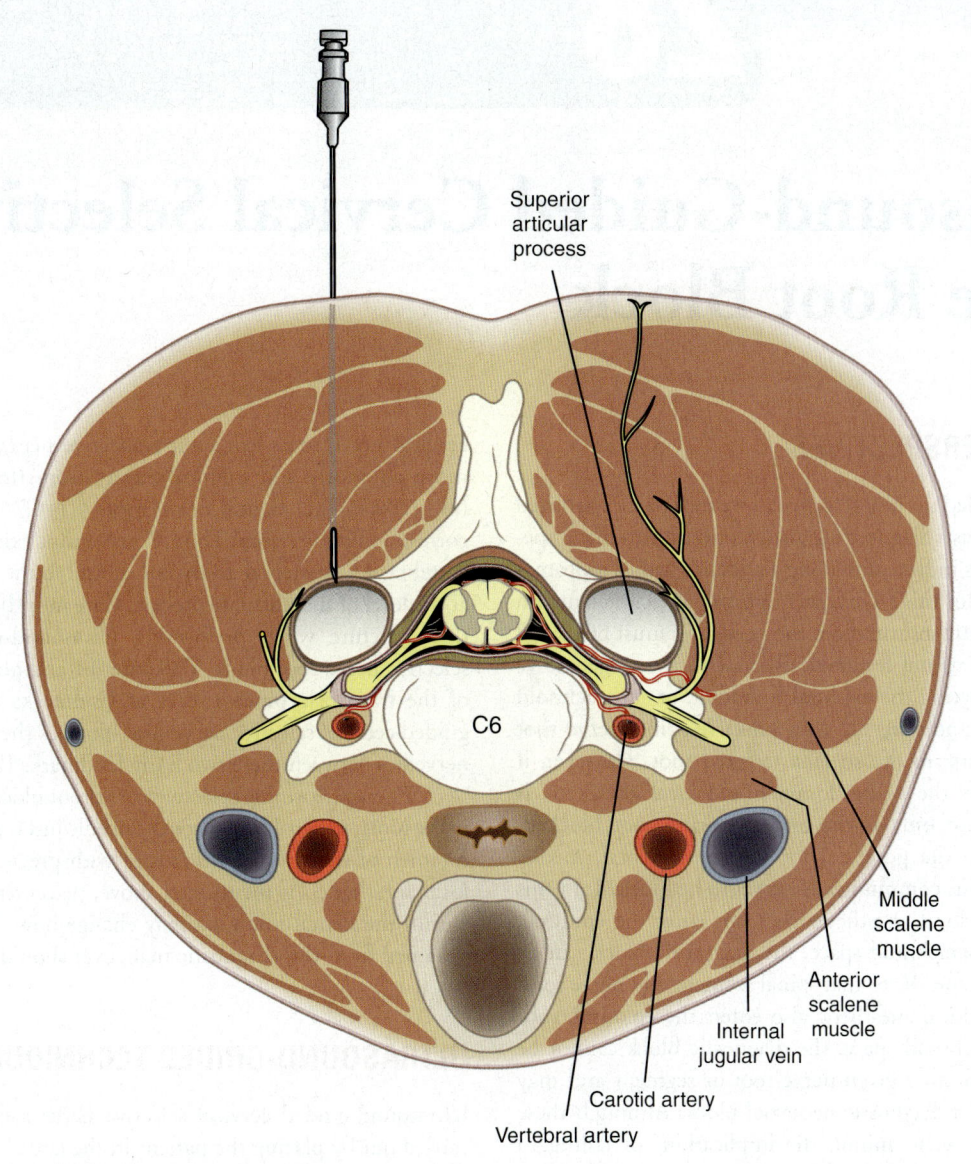

**FIGURE 27.11.** The cervical facet joints are in close proximity to the vertebral artery and neuraxial structures including the exiting nerve roots and spinal cord. (Reused from Rathmell JP. Facet injection: intra-articular injection, medial branch block, and radiofrequency treatment. In: *Atlas of Image-Guided Intervention in Regional Anesthesia and Pain Medicine*. 2nd ed. Philadelphia, PA: Lippincott Williams & Wilkins; 2012:87, with permission.)

## SUGGESTED READINGS

Bertini L, Baciarello M. Ultrasound and facet blocks: a review. *Eur J Pain* 2009;3(2):139–143.

Bogduk N. The neck and headaches. *Neurol Clin* 2004;22(1):151–171.

Narouze S, Vydyanathan A. Ultrasound-guided cervical facet intra-articular injection. *Tech Reg Anesth Pain Manag* 2009;13(3):133–136.

Waldman SD. The cervical facet joints. In: *Pain Review*. Philadelphia, PA: Saunders Elsevier; 2009:58–59.

Waldman SD. Cervical intra-articular facet block. In: *Atlas of Interventional Pain Management*. 3rd ed. Philadelphia, PA: Saunders Elsevier; 2011.

Waldman SD. Occipital neuralgia. In: *Atlas of Common Pain Syndromes*. 3rd ed. Philadelphia, PA: Saunders Elsevier; 2011:19–21.

# Ultrasound-Guided Cervical Selective Nerve Root Block

## CLINICAL PERSPECTIVES

Ultrasound-guided cervical selective nerve root block is utilized most frequently as a diagnostic maneuver to confirm that a specific nerve root is in fact subserving a patient's pain symptomatology. In order for this technique to provide the clinician with accurate diagnostic information, the needle tip must be placed just outside the neural foramen adjacent to the target nerve root *without* entering the epidural, subdural, or subarachnoid space. If these conditions are met, selective spinal nerve root block is diagnostic to the specific targeted root. However, if the needle enters the neural foramen and local anesthetic is injected, then not only is the targeted nerve root blocked, but there is also the potential for the sinovertebral, medial branch, and ramus communicans nerves to be blocked. In this situation, if the local anesthetic does not enter the epidural, subdural, or subarachnoid space, the diagnostic block can be considered to be specific to that spinal segment and nerve root. However, if the local anesthetic also enters the epidural, subdural, or subarachnoid space, the diagnostic block cannot be said to be specific to a given nerve root or segment and may be simply called a diagnostic neuraxial block. Although these distinctions may seem minor, the implications of failing to distinguish these subtle differences relative to technique could lead to surgical interventions that fail to benefit the patient. Ultrasound-guided blockade of the cervical nerve root block is also useful as a therapeutic maneuver when treating radiculitis involving a single nerve root.

## CLINICALLY RELEVANT ANATOMY

The superior boundary of the cervical epidural space is the fusion of the periosteal and spinal layers of dura at the foramen magnum. The epidural space continues inferiorly to the sacrococcygeal membrane. The cervical epidural space is bounded anteriorly by the posterior longitudinal ligament and posteriorly by the vertebral laminae and the ligamentum flavum. The vertebral pedicles and intervertebral foramina form the lateral limits of the epidural space. The cervical epidural space is 3 to 4 mm at the C7–T1 interspace with the cervical spine flexed. The cervical epidural space contains a small amount of fat, veins, arteries, lymphatics, and connective tissue. The eight cervical nerve roots exit their respective neural foramina and move anteriorly and inferiorly away from the cervical spine (Fig. 28.1). The cervical nerve roots C1–C7 exit above their corresponding vertebra. The C8 nerve root exits below the C7 vertebra. The vertebral artery lies ventral to the neural foramen at the level of the uncinate process. Care must be taken to avoid this structure when performing ultrasound-guided cervical selective nerve root block. The anterior and posterior tubercle of the transverse process serve as landmarks for ultrasound-guided cervical selective nerve root block as the exiting cervical nerve lies between these two bony landmarks (Fig. 28.2).

When performing selective nerve root block of the cervical nerve roots, the goal is to place the needle just outside the neural foramen of the affected nerve root with precise application of local anesthetic. As mentioned above, placement of the needle within the neural foramina may change how the information obtained from this diagnostic maneuver should be interpreted.

## ULTRASOUND-GUIDED TECHNIQUE

Ultrasound-guided cervical selective nerve root block can be carried out by placing the patient in the lateral decubitus position. A total of 0.25 to 0.5 mL of local anesthetic is drawn up in a 10-mL sterile syringe for each cervical nerve root to be blocked. If the painful condition being treated is thought to have an inflammatory component, 40 to 80 mg of depot steroid is added to the local anesthetic. The cricothyroid notch is then identified by palpation, which is at the C6 level. After preparation of the skin with antiseptic solution, a linear high-frequency ultrasound transducer is placed in a transverse plane at the level of C6 (Fig. 28.3). A transverse ultrasound view is obtained and the anterior and posterior tubercles of the transverse process are identified. These tubercles have been described as a two-humped camel. The cervical nerve root lies between the two humps (Fig. 28.4). Because the C6 vertebral body can be easily identified by its characteristic camel-humped anterior tubercle (which is known as Chassaignac or the carotid tubercle), the ultrasound transducer is slowly moved in a cephalad or caudad direction until the C6 vertebral body is identified (Fig. 28.5). Once the position of the C6 vertebral body is confirmed, it can serve as a landmark to count from should the clinician desire to block the C5 or C7 nerve root. The C7 transverse process can

CHAPTER 28    ULTRASOUND-GUIDED CERVICAL SELECTIVE NERVE ROOT BLOCK    187

be easily distinguished from the C6 transverse process by the lack of a taller and more pointed anterior tubercle on the C7 transverse process. At the C7 level, the C7 nerve root is located just anterior to the posterior tubercle. At each level, the anterior and posterior tubercle camel humps will appear as a hyperechoic two-humped camel with the hypoechoic nerve located between the two humps. Color Doppler can help identify the vertebral artery (Fig. 28.6). Once the correct level has been confirmed, a 22-gauge, 3½-inch blunt needle is inserted utilizing an in-plane approach and is advanced until the needle tip is in proximity to the nerve root, which is resting between the anterior and posterior tubercle (Fig. 28.7). After gentle aspiration, 0.25 to 0.5 mL of solution is injected with care being taken to avoid the vertebral artery, which is located anteriorly in relation to the facet joints. The needle is removed and pressure is placed on the injection site to avoid hematoma formation.

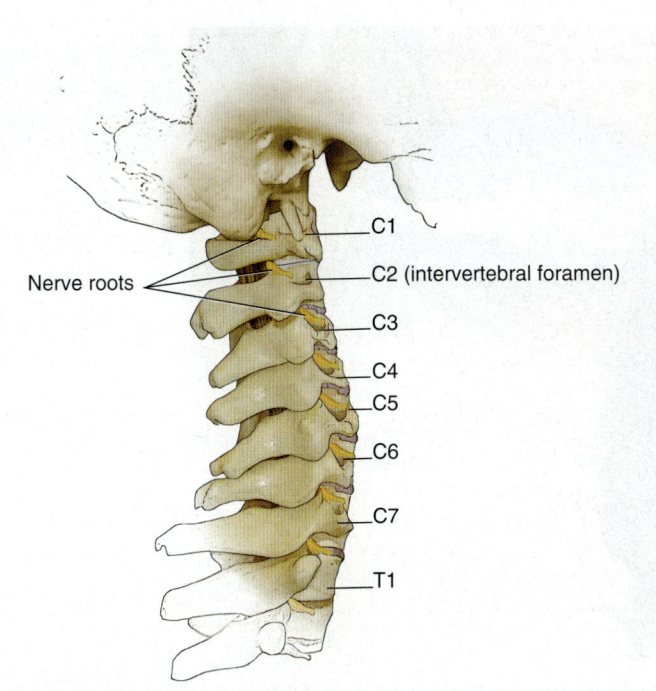

**FIGURE 28.1.** The anatomy of the cervical vertebrae and exiting nerve roots.

## COMPLICATIONS

The cervical nerve roots are in close proximity to the spinal cord and exiting nerve roots, and this procedure should be performed only by those well versed in the regional anatomy and

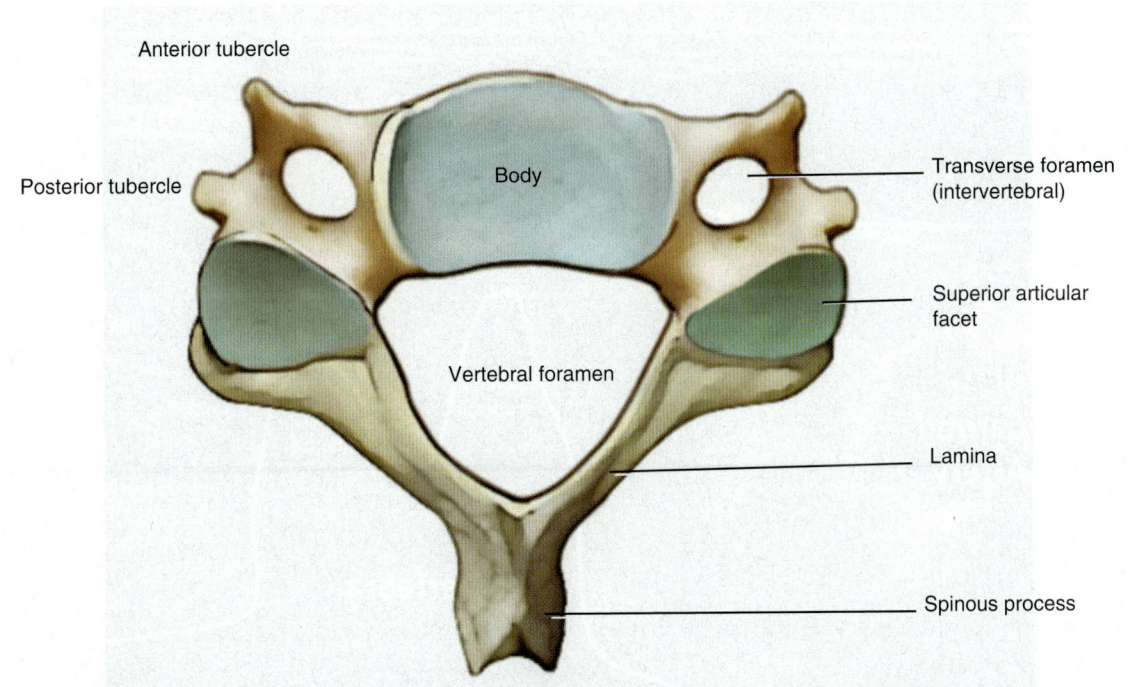

**FIGURE 28.2.** Cross-sectional view of the cervical vertebra. Note the location of the anterior and posterior tubercles and their relationship to nerve root, which lies between them.

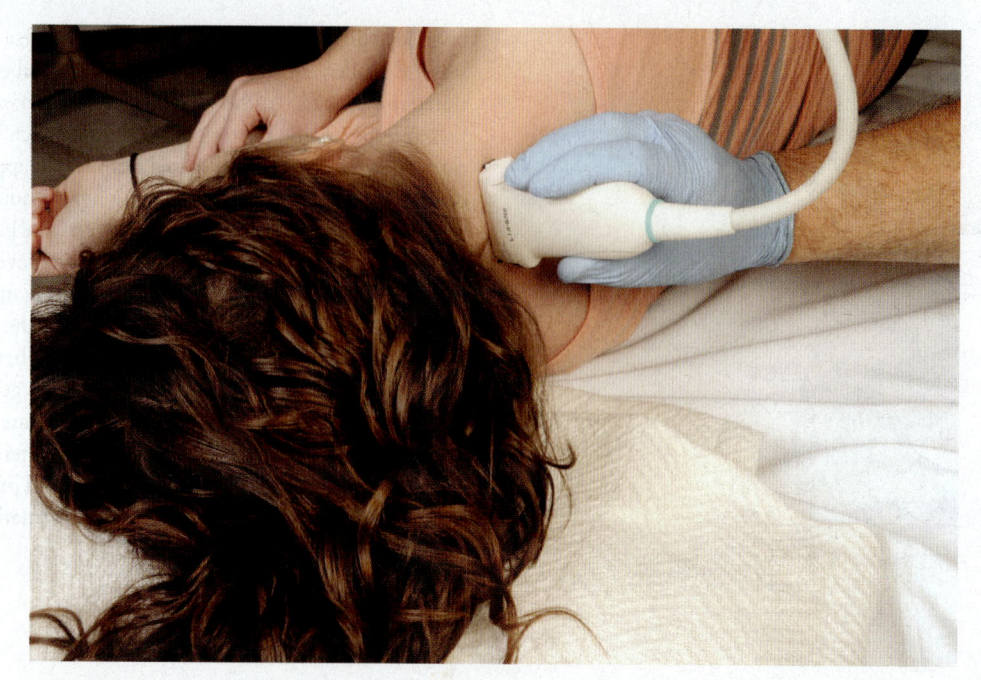

**FIGURE 28.3.** Placement of the ultrasound transducer in the transverse axis at the level of C6.

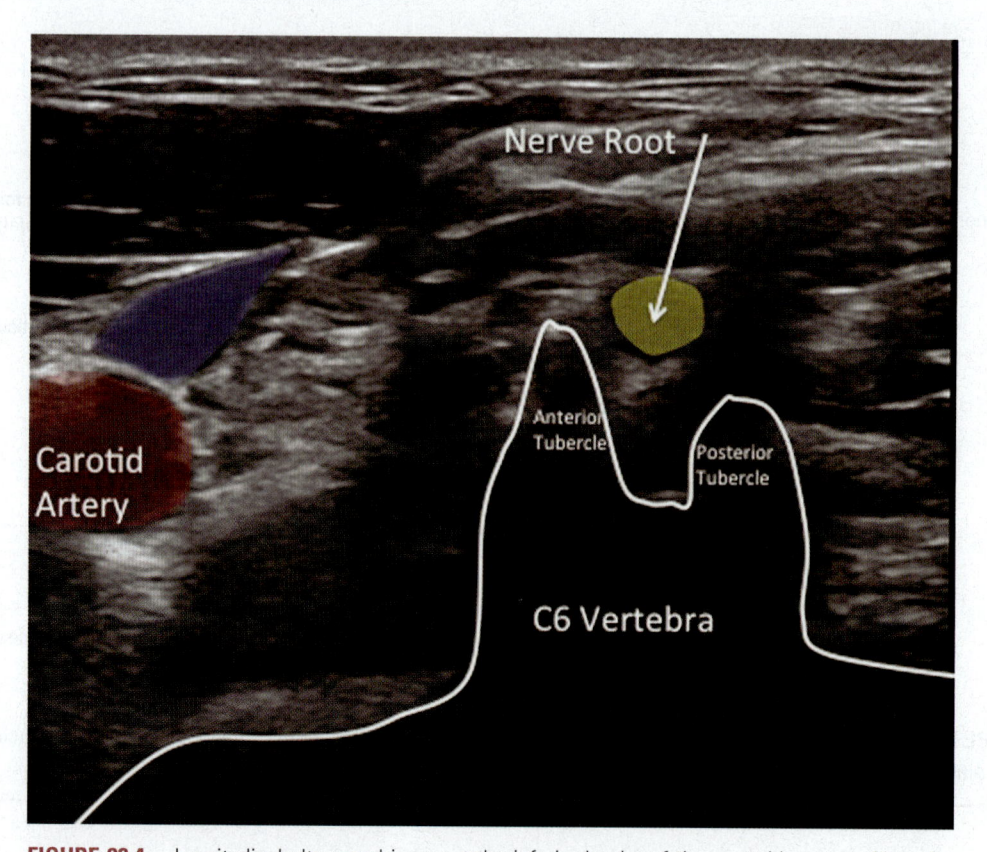

**FIGURE 28.4.** Longitudinal ultrasound image at the inferior border of the mastoid process. Note the "two-humped camel" of the C6 vertebra.

CHAPTER 28   ULTRASOUND-GUIDED CERVICAL SELECTIVE NERVE ROOT BLOCK   **189**

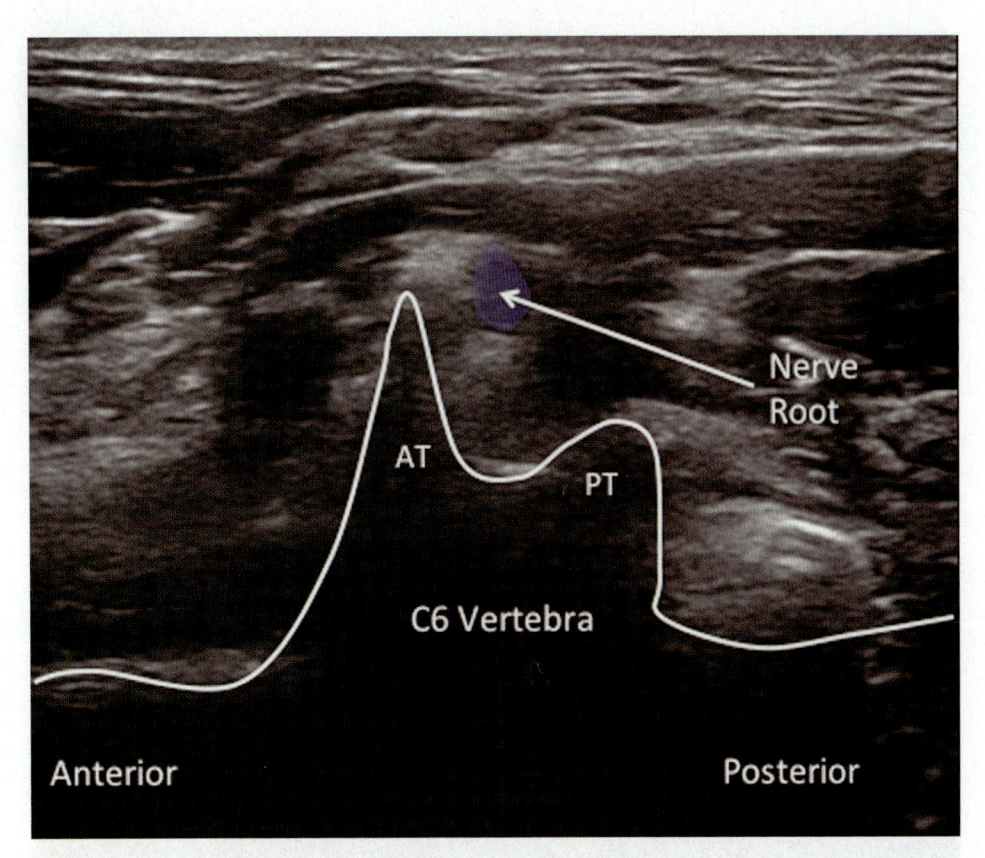

**FIGURE 28.5.** Transverse ultrasound view of the C6 vertebra demonstrating the characteristic taller and pointier anterior tubercle of the transverse process.

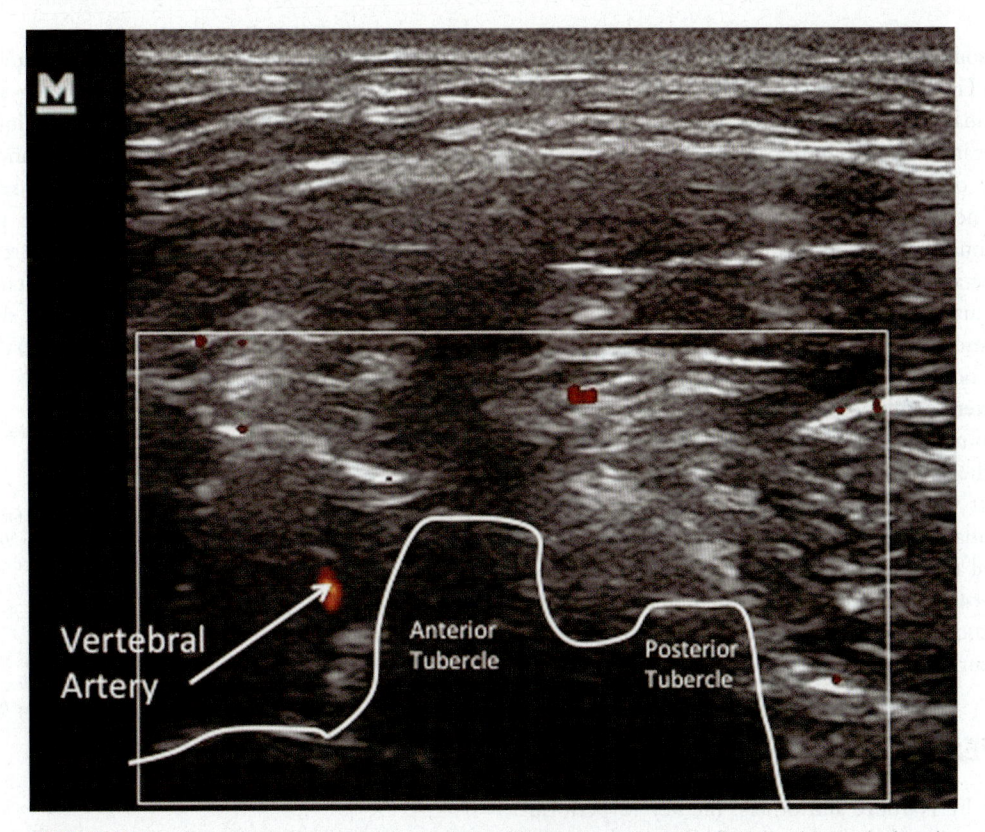

**FIGURE 28.6.** Transverse ultrasound view of the C6 vertebra with color Doppler demonstrating the relationship of the anterior tubercle to the position of the vertebral artery.

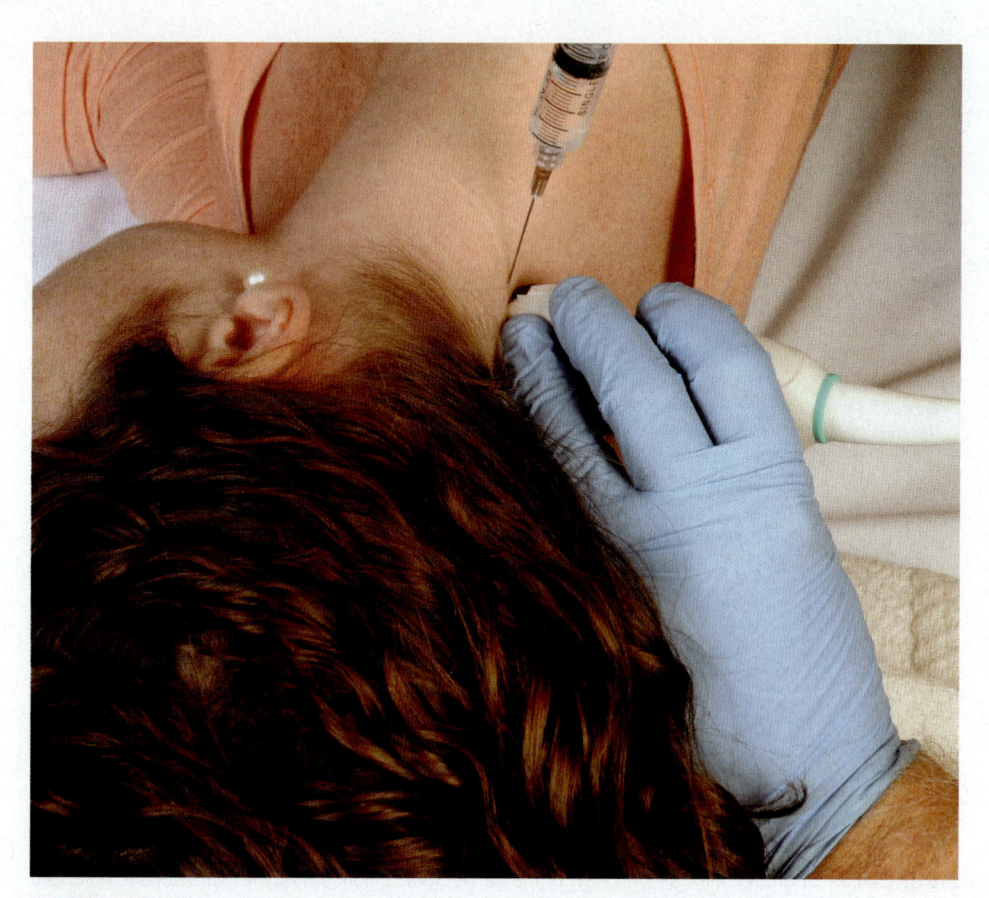

**FIGURE 28.7.** Proper needle position for performing selective cervical nerve root block.

skilled at ultrasound-guided interventional pain management procedures (see Fig. 28.1). Trauma to the exiting cervical nerve roots as well as inadvertent subarachnoid, subdural, and/or epidural injection can occur even in the best of hands. Inadvertent dural puncture occurring during selective nerve root block of the cervical nerve roots should rarely occur if attention is paid to the technical aspects of this procedure. However, failure to recognize an unintentional dural or subdural injection can result in immediate total spinal anesthesia with associated loss of consciousness, hypotension, and apnea. This can be disastrous if not immediately recognized. The proximity to the vertebral artery combined with the vascular nature of this anatomic region makes the potential for intravascular injection high although the use of color Doppler to identify the vertebral artery and other vascular structures should help the clinician avoid this potentially fatal complication. Even small amounts of injection of local anesthetic into the vertebral arteries will result in seizures. Given the proximity of the brain and brain stem, ataxia due to vascular absorption of local anesthetic is not an uncommon occurrence after cervical selective nerve root block.

## CLINICAL PEARLS

As pointed out by Narouze and others, the key to performing successful ultrasound cervical neuraxial blocks is the proper identification of the sonographic anatomy and the ability to properly identify the spinal segment being visualized. This should not be a problem if the above technique is used. Any significant pain or sudden increase in resistance during injection when performing ultrasound-guided selective cervical nerve root block suggests incorrect needle placement, and one should stop injecting immediately and reassess the position of the needle. Because pain is an important indication of improper needle placement, the practitioner should avoid the use of excessive sedation during selective nerve root block of the cervical nerve roots.

## SUGGESTED READINGS

Narouze S, Vydyanathan A. Ultrasound-guided cervical transforaminal injection and selective nerve root block. *Tech Reg Anesth Pain Manag* 2009;13(3):137–141.

Slipman CW, Lipetz JS, Jackson HB, et al. Therapeutic selective nerve root block in the nonsurgical treatment of atraumatic cervical spondylotic radicular pain: a retrospective analysis with independent clinical review. *Arch Phys Med Rehabil* 2000;81(6):741–746.

Waldman SD. Cervical selective nerve root block. In: *Atlas of Interventional Pain Management*. 3rd ed. Philadelphia, PA: Saunders Elsevier; 2009:187–191.

Waldman SD. Cervical selective nerve root block. In: *Pain Review*. Philadelphia, PA: Saunders Elsevier; 2009:434–435.

# SECTION III

# Shoulder

# CHAPTER 29

# Ultrasound-Guided Brachial Plexus Block: Interscalene Approach

## CLINICAL PERSPECTIVES

Ultrasound-guided interscalene brachial plexus block is useful as a diagnostic maneuver to help identify if the brachial plexus is subserving pain from tumor, plexopathy, plexitis, abscess, or other pathology. Interscalene brachial plexus nerve block with local anesthetic may be used to palliate acute pain emergencies, including acute herpes zoster, brachial neuritis, brachial plexopathy including Parsonage-Turner syndrome, shoulder and upper extremity trauma, and cancer pain, while waiting for pharmacologic, surgical, and antiblastic methods to become effective. Interscalene brachial plexus nerve block is also useful as an alternative to stellate ganglion block when treating reflex sympathetic dystrophy of the shoulder and upper extremity. The use of ultrasound imaging can identify the exact location and course of the brachial plexus when surgical procedures of the neck are being contemplated. For surgery of the shoulder and upper extremity, interscalene brachial plexus block is the preferred approach for blockade of the brachial plexus.

## CLINICALLY RELEVANT ANATOMY

The fibers that comprise the brachial plexus arise primarily from the fusion of the anterior rami of the C5, C6, C7, C8, and T1 spinal nerves (Fig. 29.1). In some patients, there may also be a contribution of fibers from C4 to T2 spinal nerves. The nerves that make up the plexus exit the lateral aspect of the cervical spine and pass downward and laterally in conjunction with the subclavian artery. The nerves and artery run between the anterior scalene and middle scalene muscles, passing inferiorly behind the middle of the clavicle and above the top of the first rib to reach the axilla (see Fig. 29.1). The scalene muscles are enclosed in an extension of prevertebral fascia, which helps contain drugs injected into this region and provide the theoretical and anatomic basis for this technique.

## ULTRASOUND-GUIDED TECHNIQUE

To perform ultrasound-guided injection technique for interscalene brachial plexus block, place the patient in the supine position with the head turned away from the side to be blocked. The posterior border of the sternocleidomastoid muscle is identified by having the patient raise his or her head against the resistance of the clinician's hand (Fig. 29.2). In most patients, a groove between the posterior border of the sternocleidomastoid muscle and the anterior scalene muscle can be palpated (Fig. 29.3). Identification of the interscalene groove can be facilitated by having the patient inhale strongly against a closed glottis. Once the interscalene groove is identified, the C6 level is identified by palpation of the cricothyroid notch. If the interscalene groove cannot be identified, the needle is placed just slightly behind the posterior border of the sternocleidomastoid muscle at the C6 level.

After preliminary identification of the approximate location of the brachial plexus utilizing surface landmarks, the skin is prepped with antiseptic solution and 15 mL of local anesthetic is drawn up in a 20-mL sterile syringe, with 40 to 80 mg of depot steroid added if the condition being treated is thought to have an inflammatory component.

A linear ultrasound transducer is then placed over the previously identified location in the transverse plane, and a survey scan is taken (Fig. 29.4).

The superficial triangular-shaped sternocleidomastoid muscle is identified, and then the anterior and middle scalene muscles are identified beneath it (Fig. 29.5). The roots of the brachial plexus lie between the anterior and middle scalene muscles and will appear as hypoechoic round or slightly oval multifascicular structure with a hyperechoic perineurium. The location of the internal jugular vein and the carotid and vertebral arteries can be facilitated by the use of color Doppler (Fig. 29.6). The clinician then moves the ultrasound transducer in a slightly cephalad or caudad direction until the nerves of the brachial plexus can be seen to "align" within the sheath of prevertebral fascia.

When the nerves of the brachial plexus are seen to be aligned within the facial sheath, a 22-gauge, 3½-inch styletted needle is advanced under real-time ultrasound guidance using an in-plane approach until the needle tip is in proximity to the nerve (Fig. 29.7). After careful aspiration for blood or cerebrospinal fluid, 15 mL of solution should be slowly injected. The needle is removed and pressure is placed on the injection site to avoid bleeding complications.

CHAPTER 29   ULTRASOUND-GUIDED BRACHIAL PLEXUS BLOCK: INTERSCALENE APPROACH   193

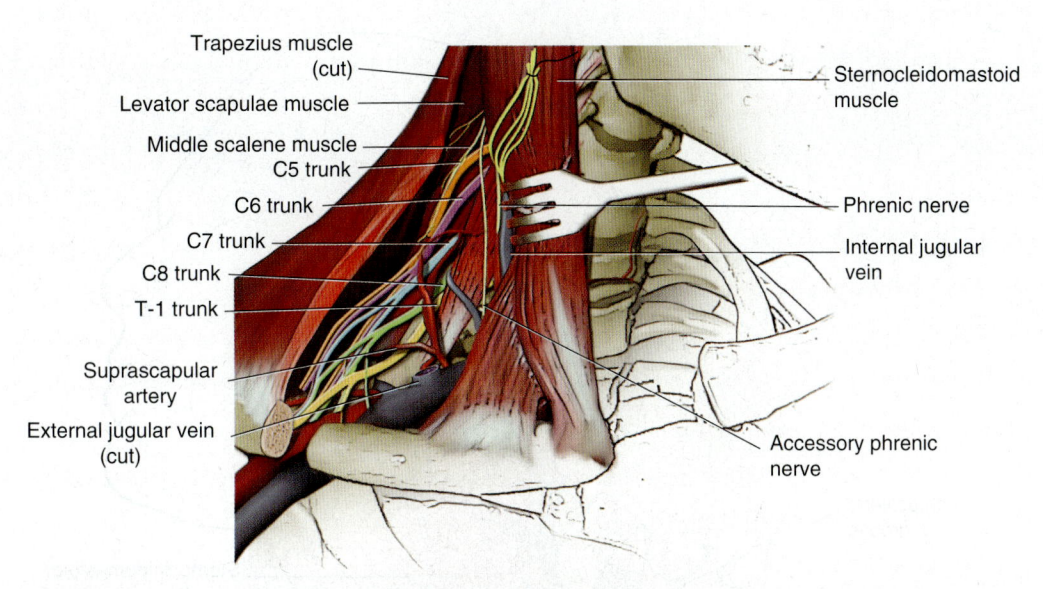

**FIGURE 29.1.**   The anatomy of the brachial plexus and surrounding structures. Note the relationship of the brachial plexus to the phrenic nerve and internal jugular vein.

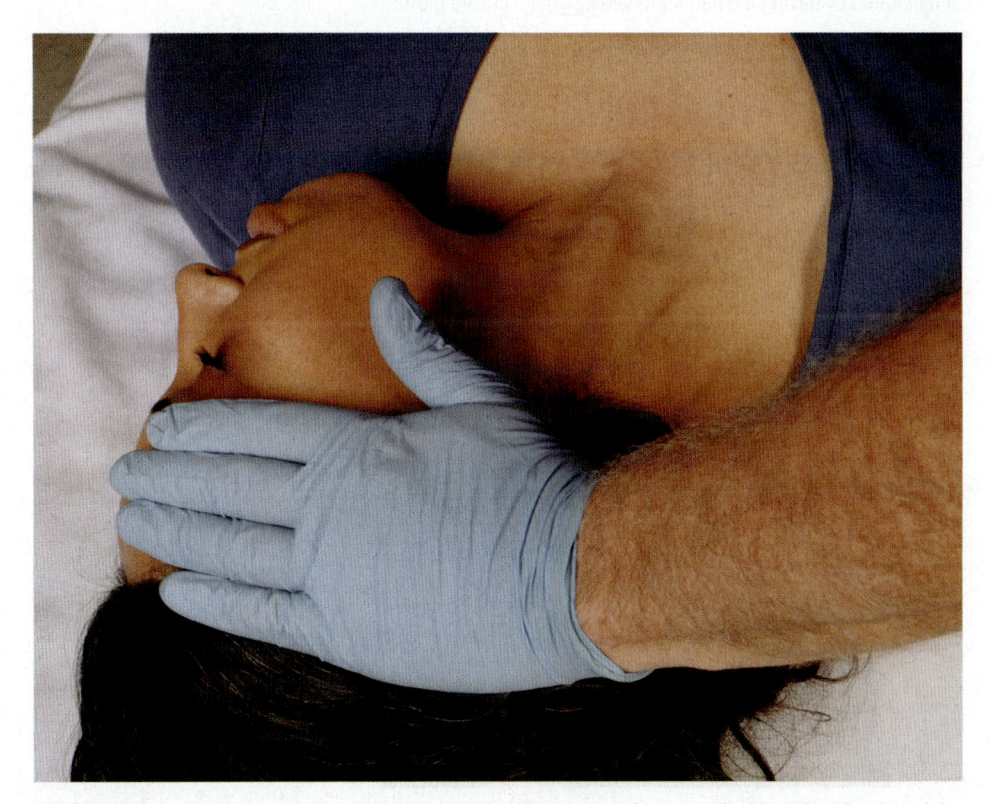

**FIGURE 29.2.**   Having the patient raise his or her head against resistance will aid in identification of the sternocleidomastoid muscle.

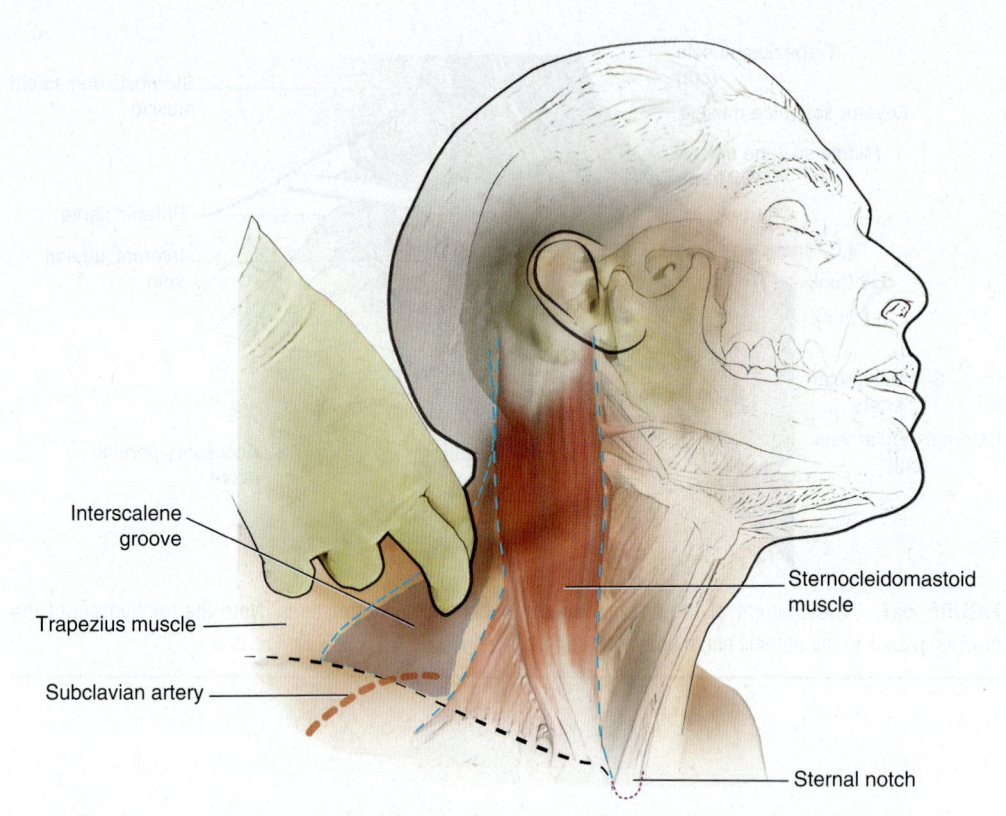

**FIGURE 29.3.** The interscalene groove lies immediately behind the lateral border of the clavicular head of the sternocleidomastoid muscle at the level of the cricoid cartilage (C6). Identification of the groove can be facilitated by having the patient inhale against a closed glottis.

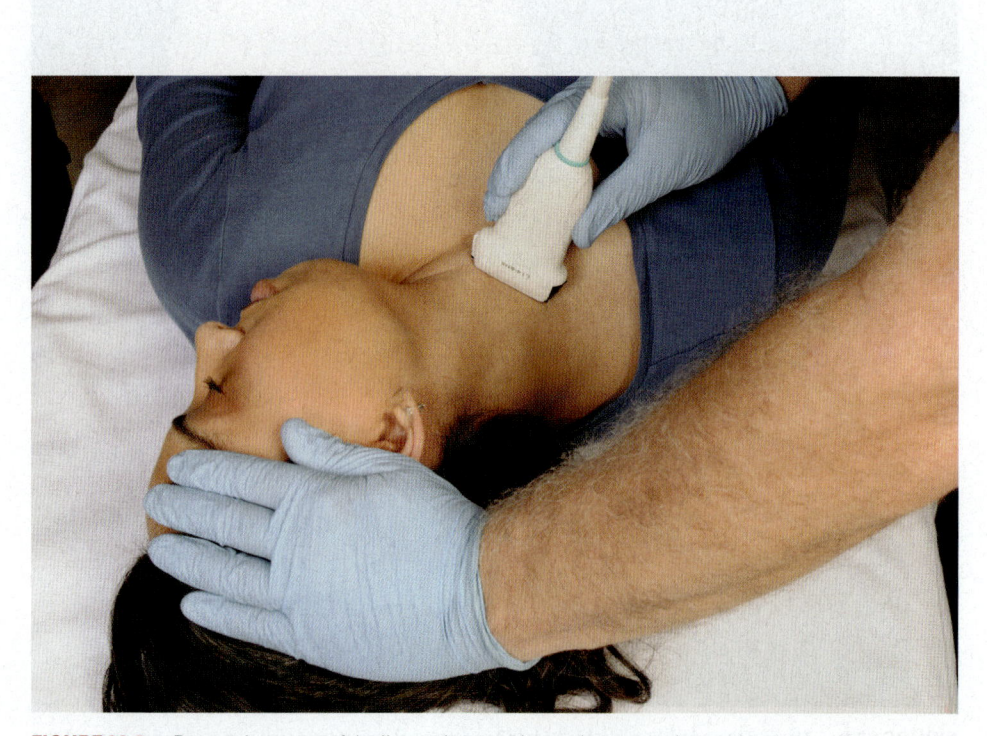

**FIGURE 29.4.** Proper placement of the linear ultrasound transducer over the previously identified posterior margin of the sternocleidomastoid muscle.

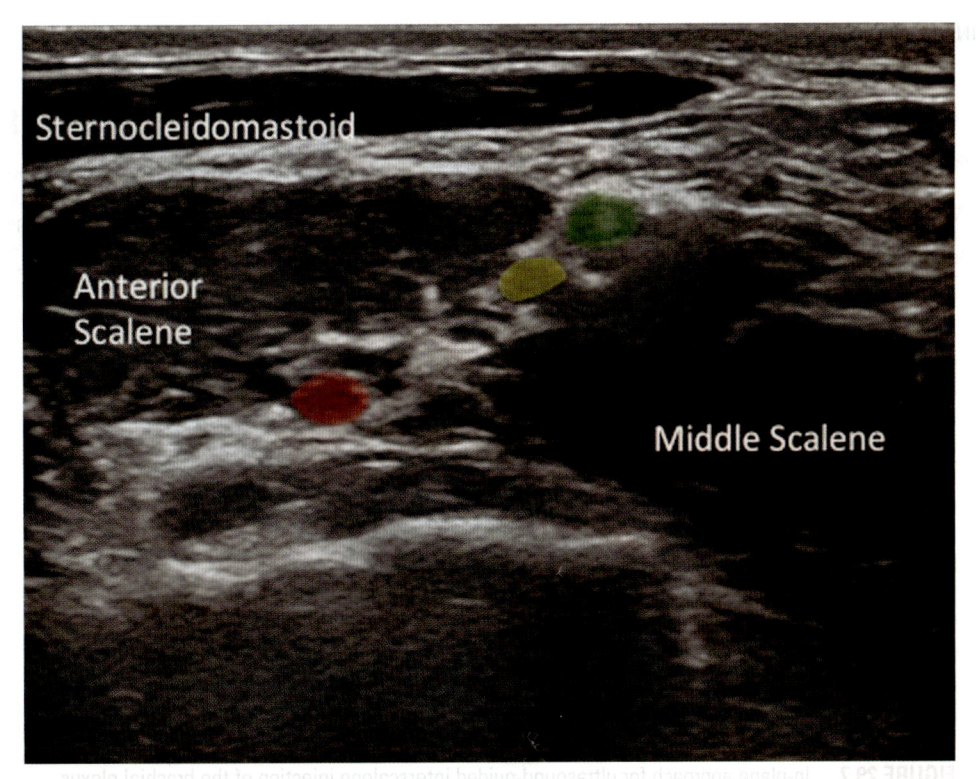

**FIGURE 29.5.** Transverse ultrasound image of the brachial plexus at the level of the cricoid cartilage (*arrows*, brachial plexus; ASM, anterior scalene muscle; MSM, middle scalene muscle).

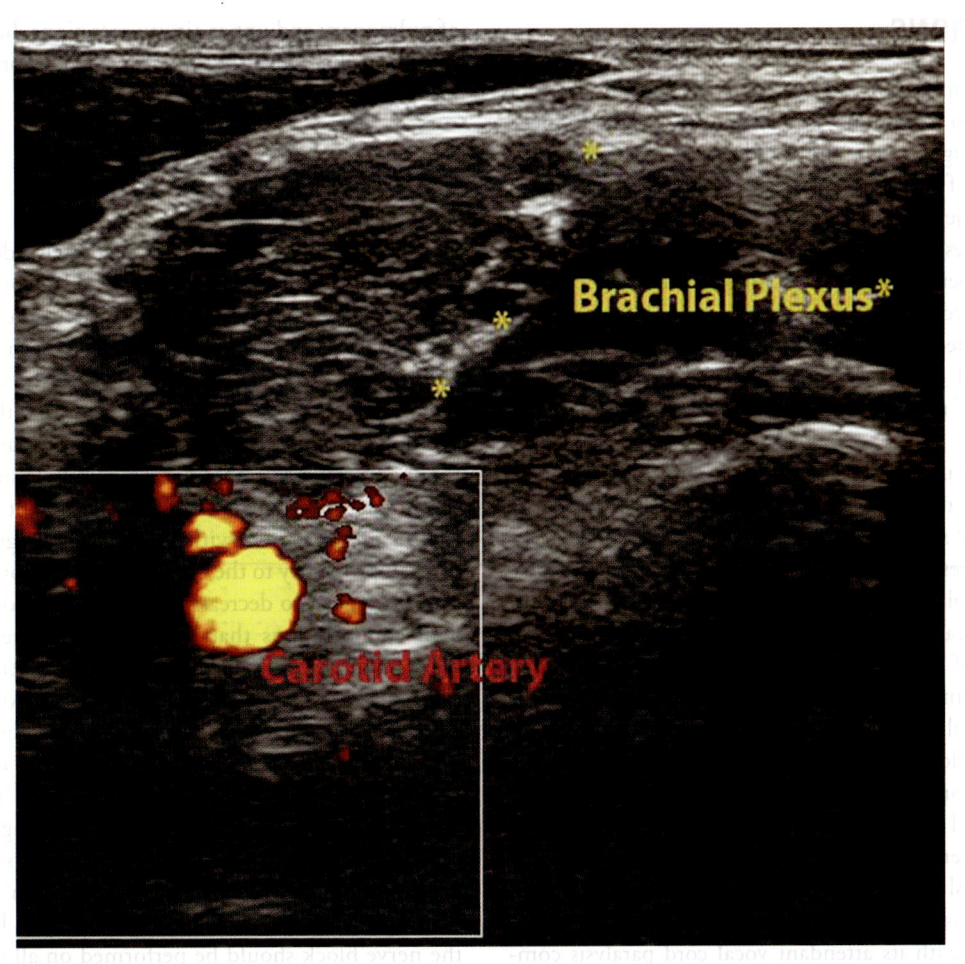

**FIGURE 29.6.** Transverse color Doppler view of the brachial plexus and the internal jugular and carotid artery.

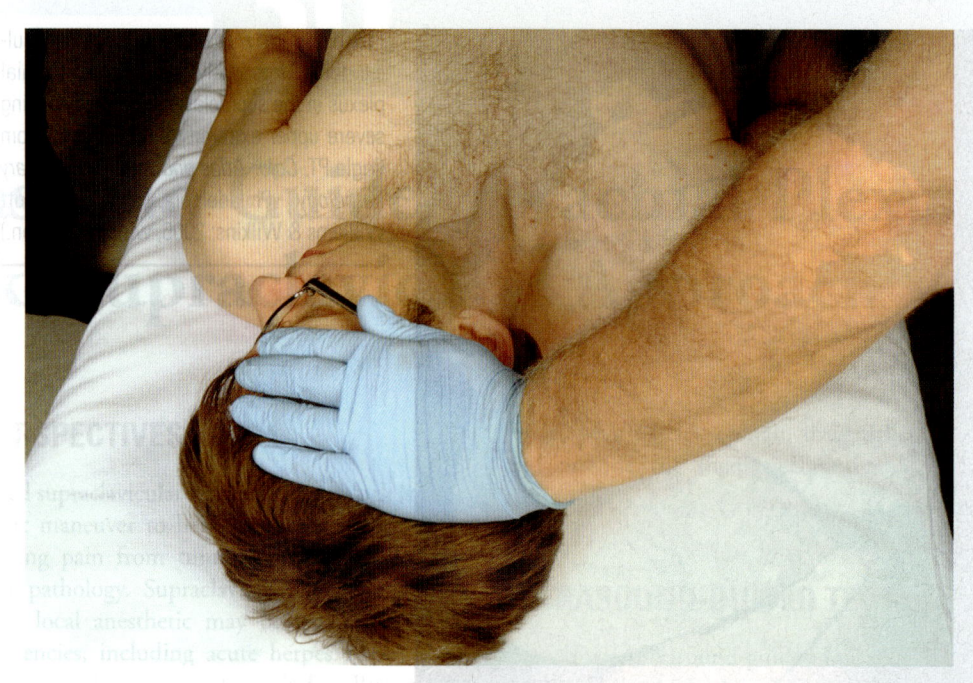

**FIGURE 30.3.** Having the patient raise his or her head against resistance will aid in identification of the sternocleidomastoid muscle.

in-plane approach until the needle tip is resting within the corner pocket between the subclavian artery and the superior border of the first rib placing it in proximity to the brachial plexus (see Figs. 30.8 and 30.9). After careful aspiration for blood or cerebrospinal fluid, 15 mL of solution should be slowly injected in incremental doses. The needle is removed and pressure is placed on the injection site to avoid bleeding complications.

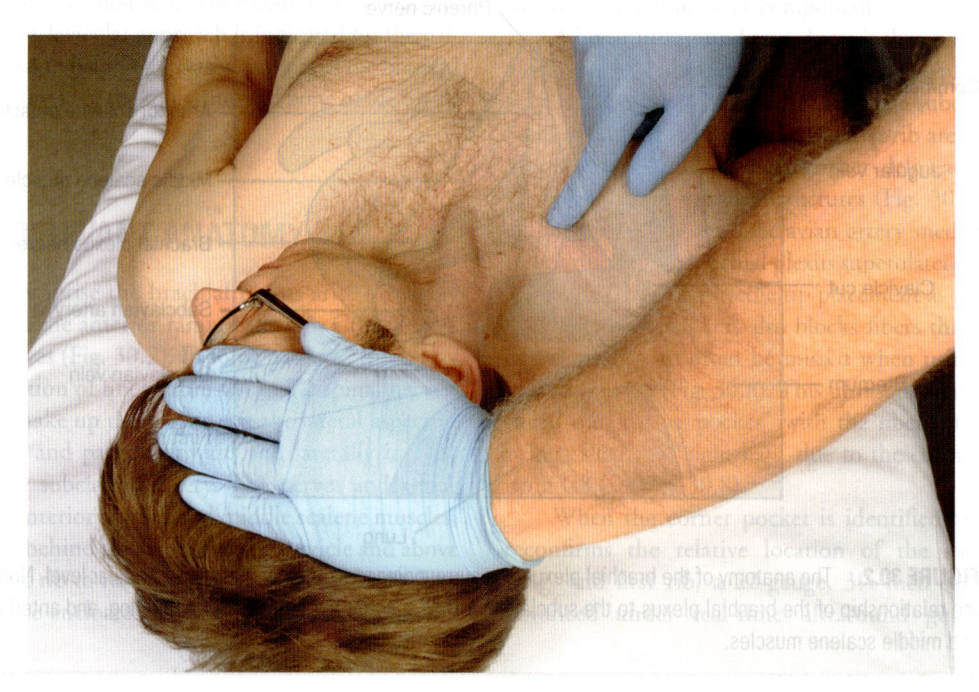

**FIGURE 30.4.** The point at which the lateral border of the sternocleidomastoid attaches to the clavicle.

# CHAPTER 30 ULTRASOUND-GUIDED BRACHIAL PLEXUS BLOCK: SUPRACLAVICULAR APPROACH

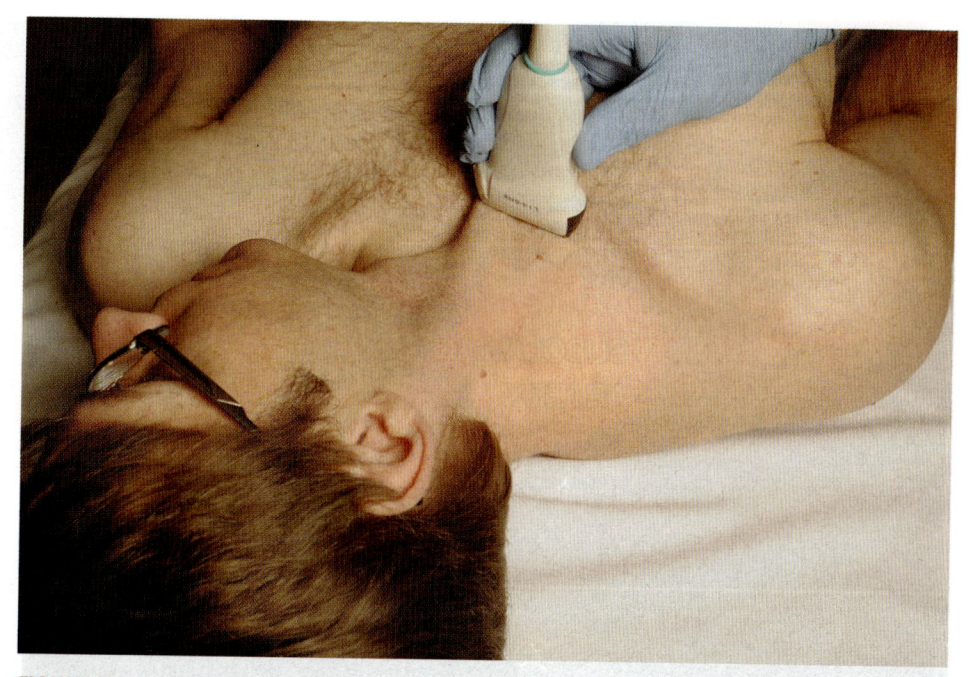

**FIGURE 30.5.** Proper placement of the linear ultrasound transducer over the previously identified margin of the sternocleidomastoid muscle.

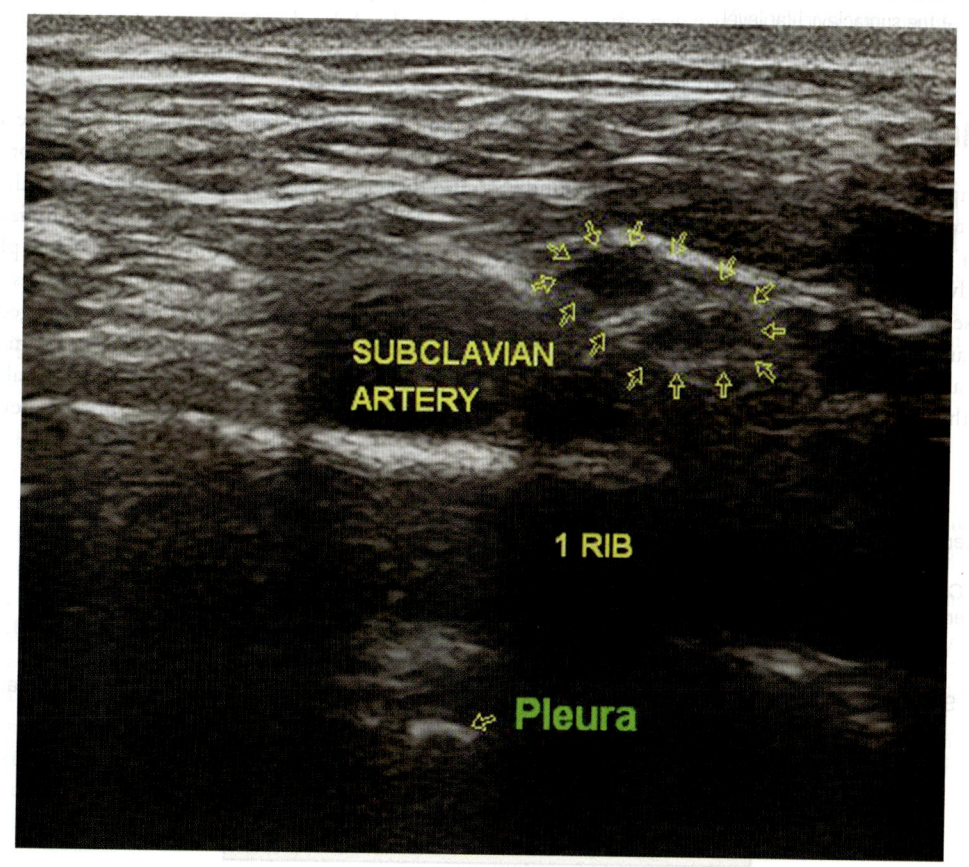

**FIGURE 30.6.** Transverse ultrasound image of the brachial plexus at the level of the cricoid cartilage.

CHAPTER 31

# Ultrasound-Guided Brachial Plexus Block: Infraclavicular Approach

## CLINICAL PERSPECTIVES

Ultrasound-guided infraclavicular brachial plexus block is useful as a diagnostic maneuver to help identify if the brachial plexus is subserving pain from tumor, plexopathy, plexitis, abscess, or other pathology. Infraclavicular brachial plexus nerve block with local anesthetic may be used to palliate acute pain emergencies, including acute herpes zoster, brachial plexus neuritis, brachial plexopathy including Parsonage-Turner syndrome, upper extremity trauma, and cancer pain including Pancoast superior sulcus lung tumor, while waiting for pharmacologic, surgical, and antiblastic methods to become effective (Fig. 31.1). Infraclavicular brachial plexus nerve block is also useful as an alternative to stellate ganglion block when treating reflex sympathetic dystrophy and ischemic conditions of the upper extremity. The use of ultrasound imaging can identify the exact location and course of the brachial plexus when surgical procedures of the neck and clavicle are being contemplated. For surgery of the distal upper extremity, infraclavicular brachial plexus block offers the dual advantages of rapid onset and dense surgical anesthesia. Destruction of the brachial plexus via the infraclavicular approach is indicated for the palliation of cancer pain, including invasive tumors of the brachial plexus as well as tumors of the soft tissue and bone of the upper extremity.

## CLINICALLY RELEVANT ANATOMY

The fibers that comprise the brachial plexus arise primarily from the fusion of the anterior rami of the C5, C6, C7, C8, and T1 spinal nerves. In some patients, there may also be a contribution of fibers from C4 to T2 spinal nerves. The nerves that make up the plexus exit the lateral aspect of the cervical spine and pass downward and laterally in conjunction with the subclavian artery. The nerves and artery run between the anterior scalene and middle scalene muscles, passing inferiorly behind the middle of the clavicle and above the top of the first rib to reach the axilla. After passing over the top of the first rib, the cords of the plexus continue their downward path in proximity to the subclavian artery and then the axillary artery. (Fig. 31.2). In order to inject the brachial plexus at the infraclavicular level, the needle must traverse skin, subcutaneous tissue, and the pectoralis major and minor muscles (Fig. 31.3).

## ULTRASOUND-GUIDED TECHNIQUE

To perform ultrasound-guided injection technique for infraclavicular brachial plexus block, place the patient in the supine position with the ipsilateral arm abducted to bring the artery and plexus closer to the skin facilitating ultrasound visualization. The acromioclavicular joint on the affected side is identified by palpation, and an imaginary line is drawn between the acromioclavicular joint and the ipsilateral nipple as a guide to transducer placement (Fig. 31.4). After preliminary identification of the surface landmarks is completed, the skin is prepped with antiseptic solution and 16 mL of local anesthetic is drawn up in a 20-mL sterile syringe, with 40 to 80 mg of depot steroid added if the condition being treated is thought to have an inflammatory component.

A linear high-frequency ultrasound transducer is then placed over the previously identified imaginary line between the acromioclavicular joint and the ipsilateral nipple, and a survey scan is taken (Fig. 31.5). Placement of the transducer in this position will provide a short-axis view of the axillary artery and cords of the brachial plexus with the artery appearing as a round pulsatile structure surrounded by the medial, lateral, and posterior cords of the brachial plexus (Fig. 31.6). The axillary artery, the cords of the brachial plexus, the intercostal muscle, and the pleura and lung are then identified. Color Doppler can be utilized to further delineate the axillary artery and any other vascular structures (Fig. 31.7). When the axillary artery and surrounding cords of the brachial plexus are identified and the clinician reconfirms the relative location of the intercostal muscle and underlying pleura and lung, a 22-gauge, 3½-inch styletted needle is advanced toward the 12:00 o'clock position of the axillary artery under real-time ultrasound guidance using an in-plane approach until the needle tip rests adjacent to the

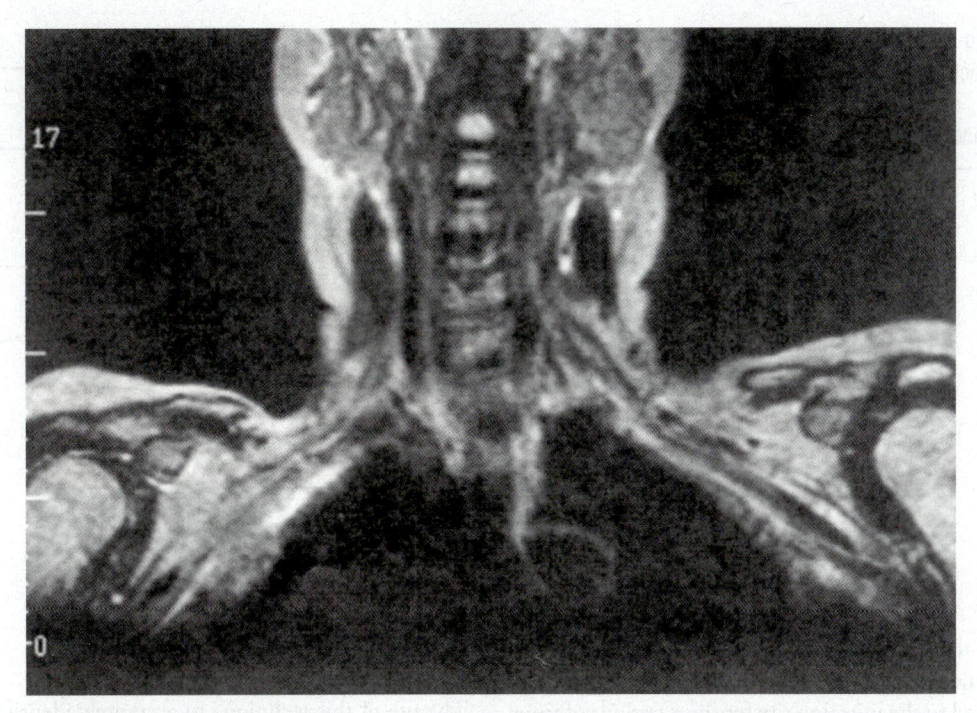

**FIGURE 31.1.** Magnetic resonance imaging demonstrating a mass in the axilla involving the brachial plexus and invading the chest wall.

axillary artery. After careful aspiration for blood or cerebrospinal fluid, 8 mL of solution should be slowly injected in incremental doses. The needle is then repositioned until the needle tip rests at the 6:00 o'clock position, and after careful aspiration for blood or cerebrospinal fluid, an additional 8 mL of solution is slowly injected in incremental doses. A good periarterial flow of local anesthetic should be observed. The needle is removed and pressure is placed on the injection site to avoid bleeding complications.

## COMPLICATIONS

The major complication associated with this ultrasound-guided injection technique is related to needle-induced trauma to the axillary artery. The incidence of injury to these vessels and the inadvertent intravascular injection of local anesthetic with subsequent toxicity occur less commonly when ultrasound guidance is utilized than when performing this technique using anatomic landmarks. Bleeding complications

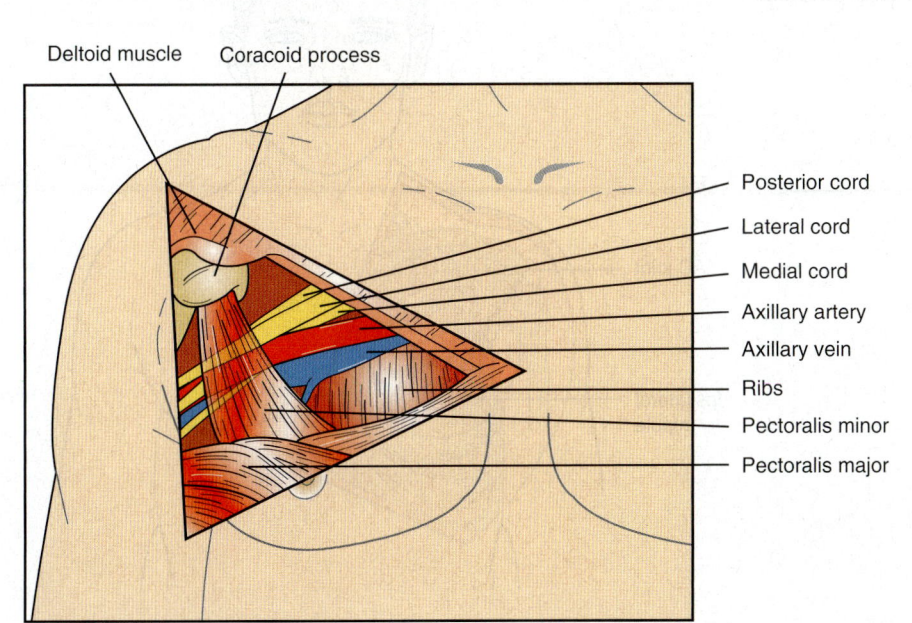

**FIGURE 31.2.** The anatomy of the brachial plexus and surrounding structures at the infraclavicular level. Note the relationship of the brachial plexus to the axillary artery and lung.

**FIGURE 31.3.** To reach the cords of the brachial plexus at the infraclavicular level, the needle must traverse the skin, subcutaneous tissues, and the pectoralis major and minor muscles.

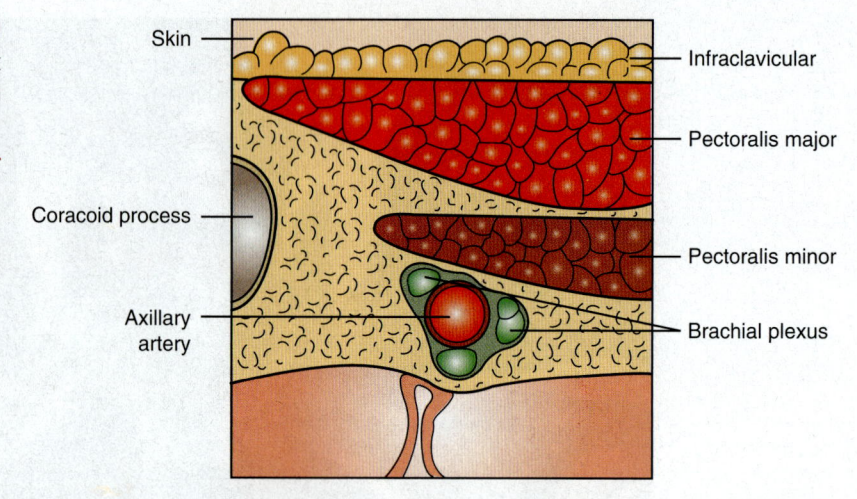

associated with this technique can be decreased if pressure is applied to the injection site following the injection. The use of cold packs applied to the injection site for short periods of time also decreases postprocedure bleeding and pain.

In addition to the potential for complications involving the vasculature, the proximity of the cords of the brachial plexus to the pleura and lung can result in pneumothorax and respiratory embarrassment if these structures are damaged during needle placement. Pneumothorax is a possibility even with the use of ultrasound guidance.

**FIGURE 31.4.** To place the ultrasound transducer for infraclavicular brachial plexus block, an imaginary line is drawn from the acromioclavicular joint to the ipsilateral nipple.

## CLINICAL PEARLS

The use of this technique to accurately identify the exact location and course of the brachial plexus prior to surgery of the neck and clavicle can avoid iatrogenic damage to the brachial plexus. The proximity of the brachial plexus at the infraclavicular level to both the axillary artery and vein as well as the pleura and lung means that the possibility for needle trauma to these vessels as well as the potential for inadvertent pneumothorax intravascular remains an ever-present possibility. While the use of ultrasound

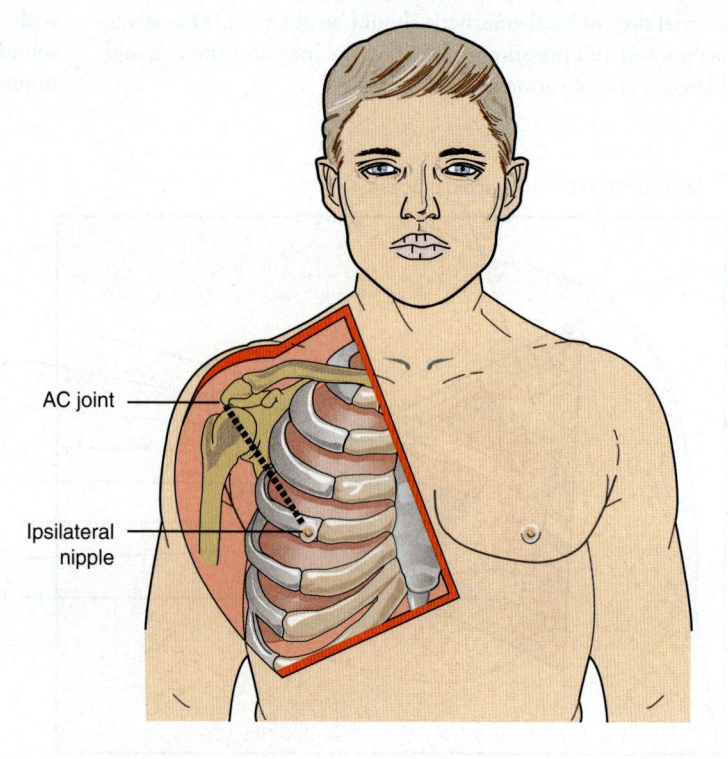

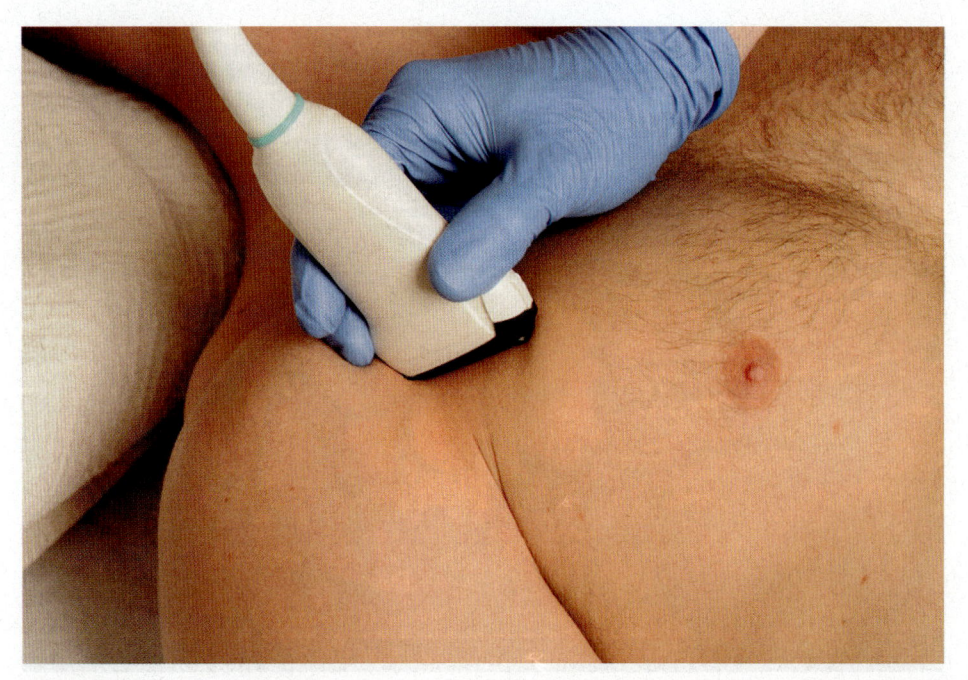

**FIGURE 31.5.** Proper placement of the linear ultrasound transducer over the previously identified margin of the sternocleidomastoid muscle.

guidance decreases the incidence of pneumothorax secondary to needle-induced trauma to the pleura and lung, it does not completely eliminate this risk. The careful identification with ultrasound imaging of all structures in proximity to the brachial plexus prior to needle placement is crucial to decreasing the incidence of the potentially fatal complications. Incremental dosing of local anesthetic while carefully monitoring the patient for signs of local anesthetic toxicity can further decrease the risk to the patient. Even in the best of hands, postblock hematoma and ecchymosis can occur. Although these complications are usually transitory in nature, their dramatic appearance can be quite upsetting to the patient; therefore, the patient should be warned of such prior to the procedure. Careful neurologic examination to identify preexisting neurologic deficits that may later be attributed to the nerve block should be performed on all patients prior to beginning brachial plexus block.

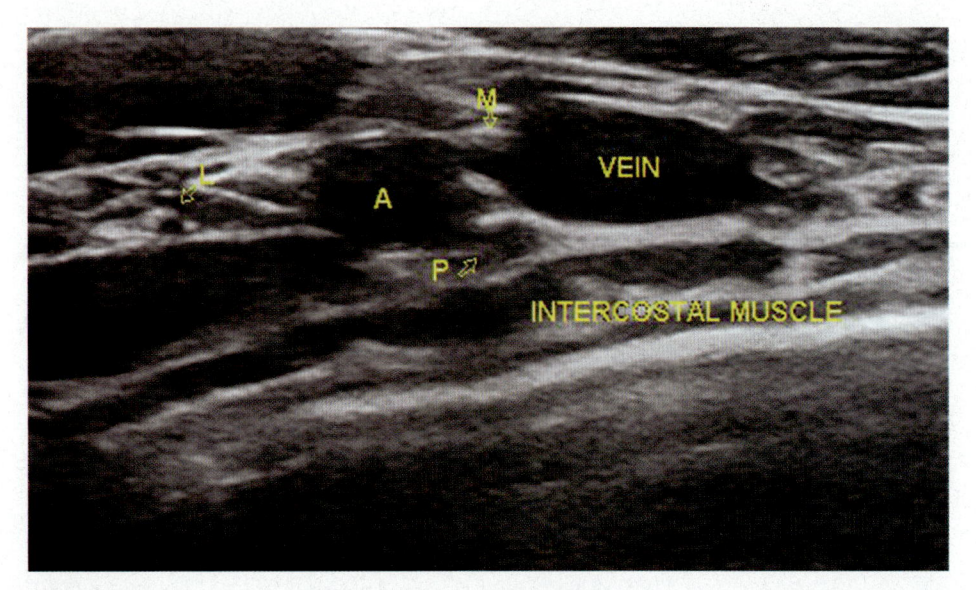

**FIGURE 31.6.** Transverse ultrasound image of the brachial plexus at the infraclavicular level. (A, artery; M, medial cord; P, posterior cord; L, lateral cord.)

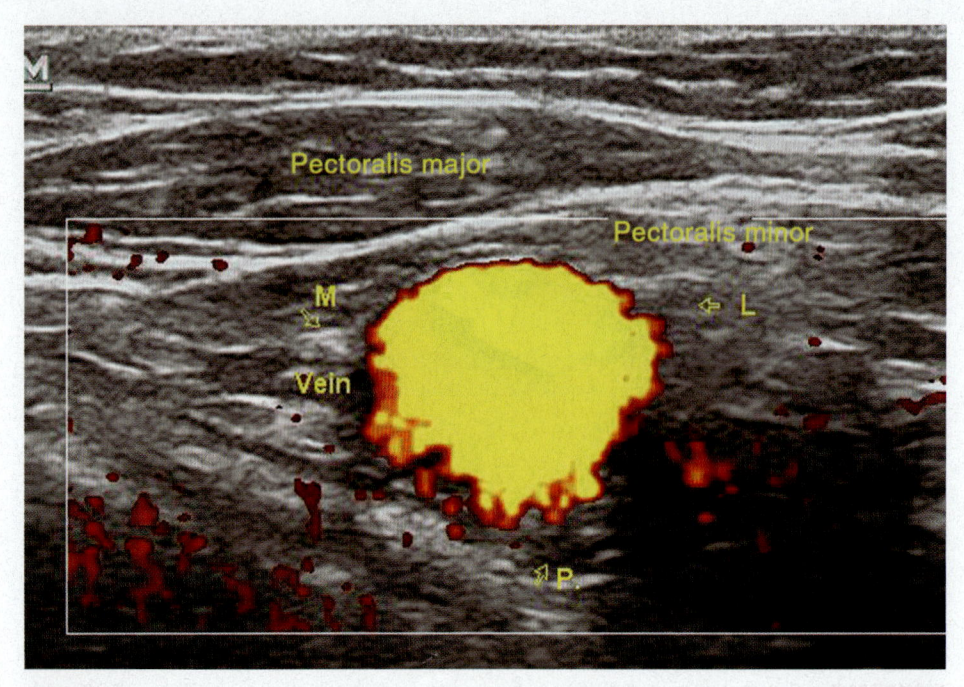

**FIGURE 31.7.** Transverse color Doppler view of the brachial plexus and the axillary artery at the infraclavicular level.

## SUGGESTED READINGS

Bigeleisen P, Wilson M. A comparison of two techniques for ultrasound guided infraclavicular block. *Br J Anaesth* 2006;96:502–507.

Sandhu NS, Bahniwal CS, Capan LM. Feasibility of an infraclavicular block with a reduced volume of lidocaine with sonographic guidance. *J Ultrasound Med* 2006;25:51–56.

Waldman SD. The brachial plexus. In: *Pain Review*. Philadelphia, PA: Saunders Elsevier; 2009:72–74.

Waldman SD. Brachial plexopathy. In: *Pain Review*. Philadelphia, PA: Saunders Elsevier; 2009:260–261.

# Ultrasound-Guided Brachial Plexus Block: Axillary Approach

## CLINICAL PERSPECTIVES

Ultrasound-guided axillary brachial plexus block is useful as a diagnostic maneuver to help identify if the distal brachial plexus is subserving pain from tumor, plexopathy, plexitis, abscess, or other pathology. Axillary brachial plexus nerve block with local anesthetic may be used to palliate acute pain emergencies, including acute herpes zoster, brachial plexus neuritis, brachial plexopathy including Parsonage-Turner syndrome, upper extremity trauma, and cancer pain including Pancoast superior sulcus lung tumor, while waiting for pharmacologic, surgical, and antiblastic methods to become effective. Axillary brachial plexus nerve block is also useful as an alternative to stellate ganglion block when treating reflex sympathetic dystrophy and ischemic conditions of the distal upper extremity (Fig. 32.1). The use of ultrasound imaging can identify the exact location and course of the brachial plexus when surgical procedures of the axilla proximal upper extremity are being contemplated. For surgery of the distal upper extremity, axillary brachial plexus block offers the dual advantages of rapid onset and dense surgical anesthesia. Destruction of the brachial plexus via the axillary approach is indicated for the palliation of cancer pain, including invasive tumors of the brachial plexus as well as tumors of the soft tissue and bone of the upper extremity.

## CLINICALLY RELEVANT ANATOMY

The fibers that comprise the brachial plexus arise primarily from the fusion of the anterior rami of the C5, C6, C7, C8, and T1 spinal nerves. In some patients, there may also be a contribution of fibers from C4 to T2 spinal nerves. The nerves that make up the plexus exit the lateral aspect of the cervical spine and pass downward and laterally in conjunction with the subclavian artery. The nerves and artery run between the anterior scalene and middle scalene muscles, passing inferiorly behind the middle of the clavicle and above the top of the first rib to reach the axilla. After passing over the top of the first rib, the cords of the plexus continue their downward path in proximity to the subclavian artery and then the axillary artery. The sheath that encloses the axillary artery and nerves as it travels downwards through the axilla is less well developed than that, which encloses the brachial plexus at the level at which interscalene and supraclavicular brachial plexus blocks are performed, making a single injection technique less satisfactory in many patients (Fig. 32.2). The median, radial, ulnar, and musculocutaneous nerves surround the artery within this imperfect sheath. David Brown, M.D., has suggested that the position of these nerves relative to the axillary artery can best be visualized by placing them in the quadrants as represented on the face of a clock, with the axillary artery being at the center of the clock (Fig. 32.3). The median nerve is found in the 12:00 o'clock to 3:00 o'clock quadrant, the ulnar nerve is found in the 3:00 o'clock to 6:00 o'clock quadrant, the radial nerve is found in the 6:00 o'clock to 9:00 o'clock quadrant, and the musculocutaneous nerve is found in the 9:00 o'clock to 12:00 o'clock quadrant. To ensure adequate block of these nerves, drugs must be injected in each quadrant to place medication in proximity to each of these nerves (see Fig. 32.3).

## ULTRASOUND-GUIDED TECHNIQUE

To perform ultrasound-guided injection technique for axillary brachial plexus block, place the patient in the supine position with the arm abducted to 90 degrees and externally rotated, which brings the artery and plexus closer to the skin facilitating ultrasound visualization. At a point 2 inches distal to the axillary crease, the pulse of the axillary artery is palpated and the skin overlying the pulsations is marked (Fig. 32.4). After preliminary identification of the surface landmarks is completed, the skin is prepped with antiseptic solution and 20 mL of local anesthetic is drawn up in a 20-mL sterile syringe, with 40 to 80 mg of depot steroid added if the condition being treated is thought to have an inflammatory component.

A linear high-frequency ultrasound transducer is then placed in a transverse orientation over the previously identified arterial pulse, and a survey scan is taken (Fig. 32.5). Placement of the transducer in this position will provide a short-axis view of the axillary artery and nerves of the terminal brachial plexus with the artery appearing as a round pulsatile structure surrounded by the median, ulnar, and radial nerves (Fig. 32.6). The musculocutaneous nerve, which should be at 9:00 o'clock to 10:00 o'clock relative to the axillary artery lying in the flexor compartment between the biceps and the coracobrachialis muscle or in some patients within the body of the coracobrachialis

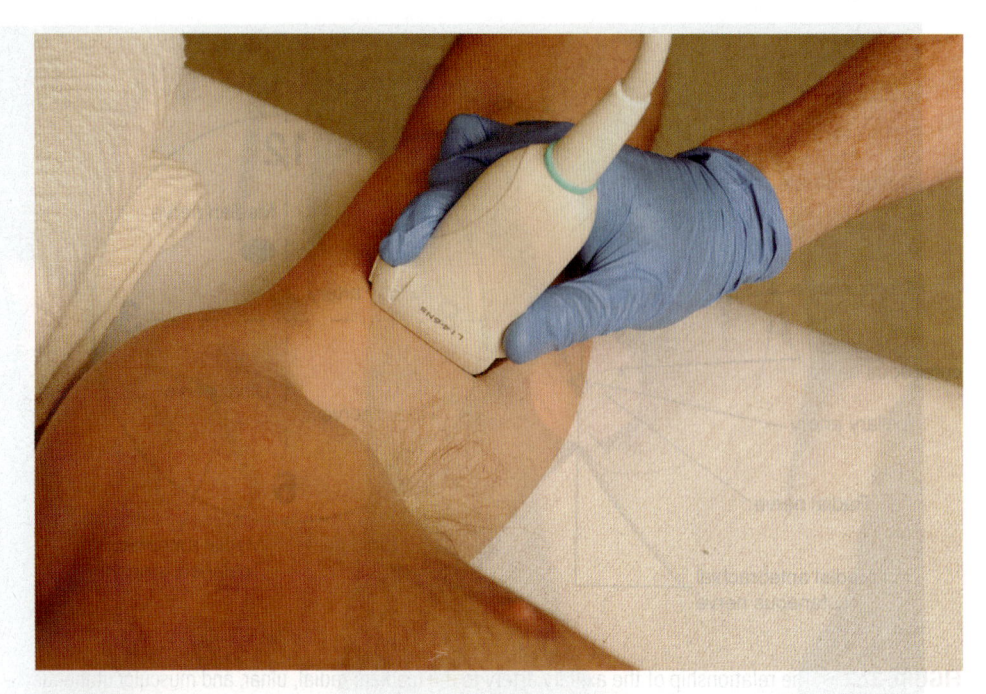

**FIGURE 32.5.** Proper placement of the linear ultrasound transducer over the previously identified pulse of the axillary artery ~2 inches below the axillary crease.

injected in incremental doses. The needle is then repositioned until the needle tip rests at the 3:00 o'clock position relative to the axillary artery and in proximity to the ulnar nerve, and after careful aspiration for blood or cerebrospinal fluid, an additional 5 mL of solution is slowly injected in incremental doses. These steps are repeated with the needle tip being repositioned to the 6:00 o'clock position to block the radial nerve and then to the 9:00 o'clock position to block the musculocutaneous nerve. A good periarterial arterial flow of local anesthetic and/or steroid should be observed, and it may not be necessary to reposition the needle to block all nerves in those patients who have a well-developed neurovascular sheath. The needle is removed and pressure is placed on the injection site to avoid bleeding complications.

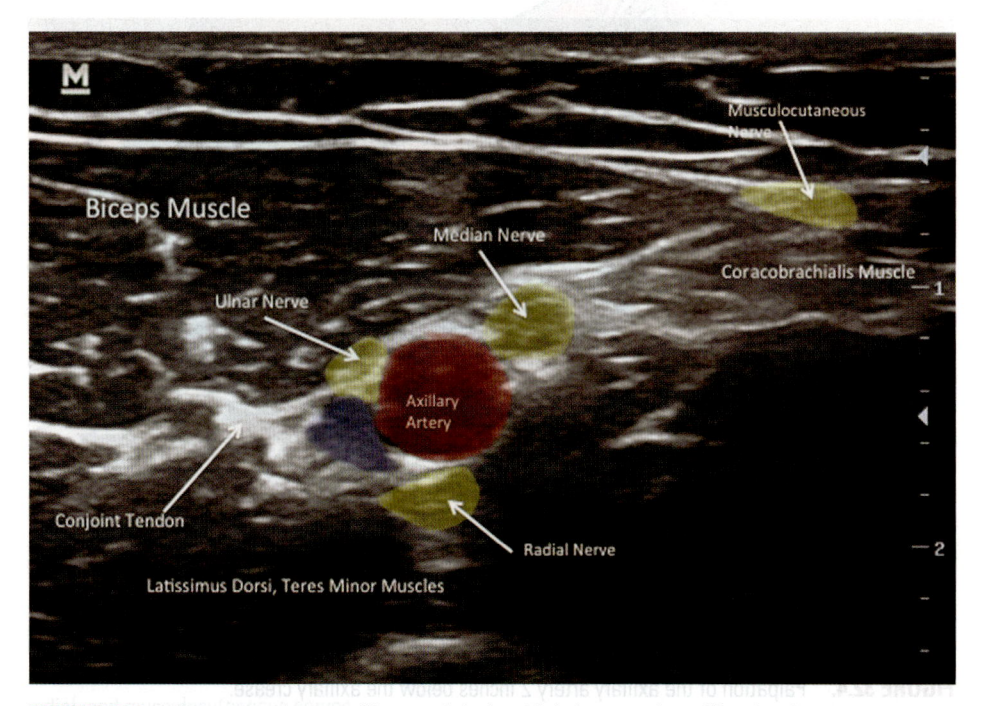

**FIGURE 32.6.** Transverse ultrasound image of the brachial plexus at the axillary level.

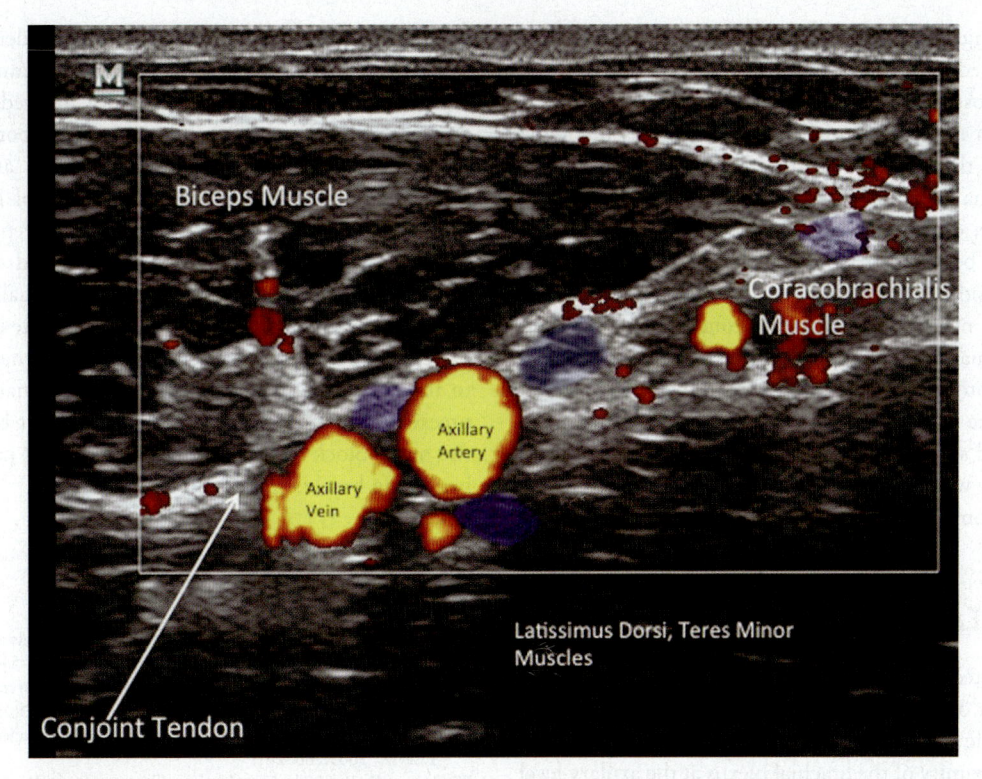

**FIGURE 32.7.** Transverse color Doppler view of the terminal nerves of the brachial plexus and the axillary artery and vein at the axillary level.

## COMPLICATIONS

The major complication associated with this ultrasound-guided injection technique is related to needle-induced trauma to the axillary artery. The incidence of injury to these vessels and the inadvertent intravascular injection of local anesthetic with subsequent toxicity occur less commonly when ultrasound guidance is utilized than when performing this technique using anatomic landmarks. Bleeding complications associated with this technique can be decreased if pressure is

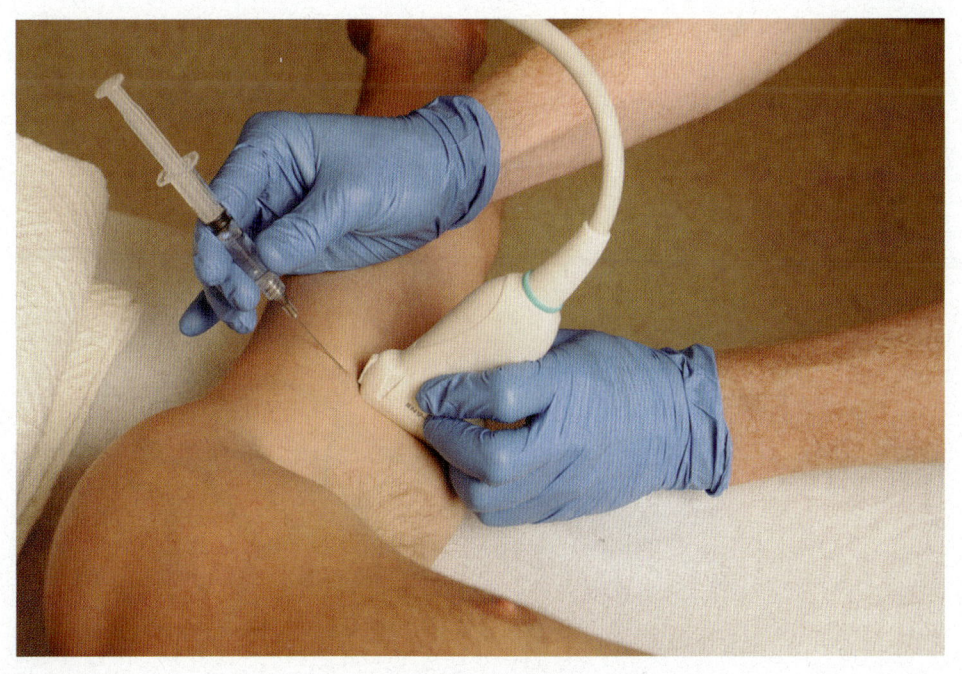

**FIGURE 32.8.** Proper in-plane needle placement for ultrasound-guided axillary brachial plexus block.

applied to the injection site following the injection. The use of cold packs applied to the injection site for short periods of time also decreases postprocedure bleeding and pain.

In addition to the potential for complications involving the vasculature, the nerves of the terminal brachial plexus are subject to trauma if the needle impinges on them. With ultrasound guidance, direct contact with the nerves by the needle tip can usually be avoided although occasionally a paresthesia is elicited, and the patient should be warned of such. The distance of the nerves to be blocked from the neuraxis and phrenic nerve makes the complications associated with injection of drugs onto these structures highly unlikely, which is an advantage of the axillary approach when compared with the interscalene and supraclavicular approaches to brachial plexus block, especially when treating patient who cannot tolerate respiratory compromise.

## CLINICAL PEARLS

The use of this technique to accurately identify the exact location and course of the brachial plexus prior to surgery of the neck and clavicle can avoid iatrogenic damage to the brachial plexus. The proximity of the brachial plexus at the axillary level to both the axillary artery and vein means that the possibility for needle trauma to these remains an ever-present possibility. While the use of ultrasound guidance decreases the incidence of needle-induced trauma to the nerves, it does not completely eliminate this risk. The careful identification with ultrasound imaging of all structures in proximity to the terminal nerves of the brachial plexus prior to needle placement is crucial to decreasing the incidence of these potentially serious complications. Incremental dosing of local anesthetic while carefully monitoring the patient for signs of local anesthetic toxicity can further decrease the risk to the patient. Even in the best of hands, postblock hematoma and ecchymosis can occur. Although these complications are usually transitory in nature, their dramatic appearance can be quite upsetting to the patient; therefore, the patient should be warned of such prior to the procedure. Careful neurologic examination to identify preexisting neurologic deficits that may later be attributed to the nerve block should be performed on all patients prior to beginning brachial plexus block.

## SUGGESTED READINGS

Orebaugh SL, Pennington S. Variant location of the musculocutaneous nerve during axillary nerve block. *J Clin Anesth* 2006;18(7):541–544.
Schafhalter-Zoppoth I, Gray AT. The musculocutaneous nerve: ultrasound appearance for peripheral nerve block. *Reg Anesth Pain Med* 2005;30(4):385–390.
Waldman SD. Brachial plexopathy. In: *Pain Review*. Philadelphia, PA: Saunders Elsevier; 2009:260–261.
Waldman SD. Brachial plexus block: axillary approach. In: *Atlas of Interventional Pain Management*. 3rd ed. Philadelphia, PA: Saunders Elsevier; 2009:203–206.
Waldman SD. Musculocutaneous nerve. In: *Pain Review*. Philadelphia, PA: Saunders Elsevier; 2009:75–76.
Waldman SD. The brachial plexus. In: *Pain Review*. Philadelphia, PA: Saunders Elsevier; 2009:72–74.

# CHAPTER 33

# Ultrasound-Guided Intra-articular Injection of the Glenohumeral Joint

## CLINICAL PERSPECTIVES

The glenohumeral joint is the most mobile joint in the human body. The joint's articular cartilage is susceptible to damage, which if left untreated will result in arthritis with its associated pain and functional disability. Osteoarthritis of the joint is the most common form of arthritis that results in shoulder joint pain and functional disability, with rheumatoid arthritis, posttraumatic arthritis, and rotator cuff tear arthropathy also causing arthritis of the glenohumeral joint (Fig. 33.1). Less common causes of arthritis-induced shoulder joint pain include the collagen vascular diseases, infection, villonodular synovitis, and Lyme disease. Acute infectious arthritis of the glenohumeral joint is best treated with early diagnosis, with culture and sensitivity of the synovial fluid and prompt initiation of antibiotic therapy. The collagen vascular diseases generally manifest as a polyarthropathy rather than a monoarthropathy limited to the glenohumeral joint, although shoulder pain secondary to the collagen vascular diseases responds exceedingly well to ultrasound-guided intra-articular injection of steroid into the glenohumeral joint.

Patients with glenohumeral joint pain secondary to arthritis, rotator cuff tendinopathy, and collagen vascular disease–related joint pain complain of pain that is localized to the shoulder and upper arm. Activity makes the pain worse, with rest and heat providing some relief. The pain is constant and characterized as aching. Sleep disturbance is common with awakening when patients roll over onto the affected shoulder. Some patients complain of a grating, catching, or popping sensation with range of motion of the joint, and crepitus may be appreciated on physical examination.

Functional disability often accompanies the pain associated with many pathologic conditions of the glenohumeral joint. Patients will often notice increasing difficulty in performing their activities of daily living and tasks that require reaching overhead or behind are particularly problematic. If the pathologic process responsible for the patient's pain symptomatology is not adequately treated, the patient's functional disability may worsen and muscle wasting and ultimately a frozen shoulder may occur.

Plain radiographs are indicated in all patients who present with shoulder pain (see Fig. 33.1). Based on the patient's clinical presentation, additional testing may be indicated, including complete blood cell count, sedimentation rate, and antinuclear antibody testing. Magnetic resonance imaging or ultrasound of the shoulder is indicated if a rotator cuff tendinopathy, tear, or other joint pathology is suspected.

## CLINICALLY RELEVANT ANATOMY

The glenohumeral joint is a multiaxial synovial ball and socket joint. The rounded head of the humerus articulates with the pear-shaped glenoid fossa of the scapula (Fig. 33.2). The joint's articular surface is covered with hyaline cartilage, which is susceptible to arthritis and degeneration. The rim of the glenoid fossa is composed of a fibrocartilaginous layer called the glenoid labrum (Fig. 33.3). The labrum is susceptible to damage should the humerus be subluxed or dislocated. The most mobile joint in the human body, the glenohumeral joint, is surrounded by a relatively lax capsule that allows the wide range of motion of the shoulder joint, albeit at the expense of decreased joint stability. The joint capsule is lined with a synovial membrane, which attaches to the articular cartilage. This membrane gives rise to synovial tendon sheaths and bursae that are subject to inflammation. The shoulder joint is innervated by the axillary and suprascapular nerves.

The major ligaments of the shoulder joint are the glenohumeral ligaments in front of the capsule, the transverse humeral ligament between the humeral tuberosities, and the coracohumeral ligament, which stretches from the coracoid process to the greater tuberosity of the humerus (Fig. 33.4). Along with the accessory ligaments of the shoulder, these major ligaments provide strength to the shoulder joint. The strength of the shoulder joint also is dependent on short muscles that surround the joint: the subscapularis, the supraspinatus, the infraspinatus, and the teres minor. These muscles and their attaching tendons are susceptible to trauma and to wear and tear from overuse and misuse.

## ULTRASOUND-GUIDED TECHNIQUE

The benefits, risks, and alternative treatments are explained to the patient, and informed consent is obtained. The patient is then placed in the sitting position with the forearm resting comfortably on the ipsilateral thigh. The skin overlying the

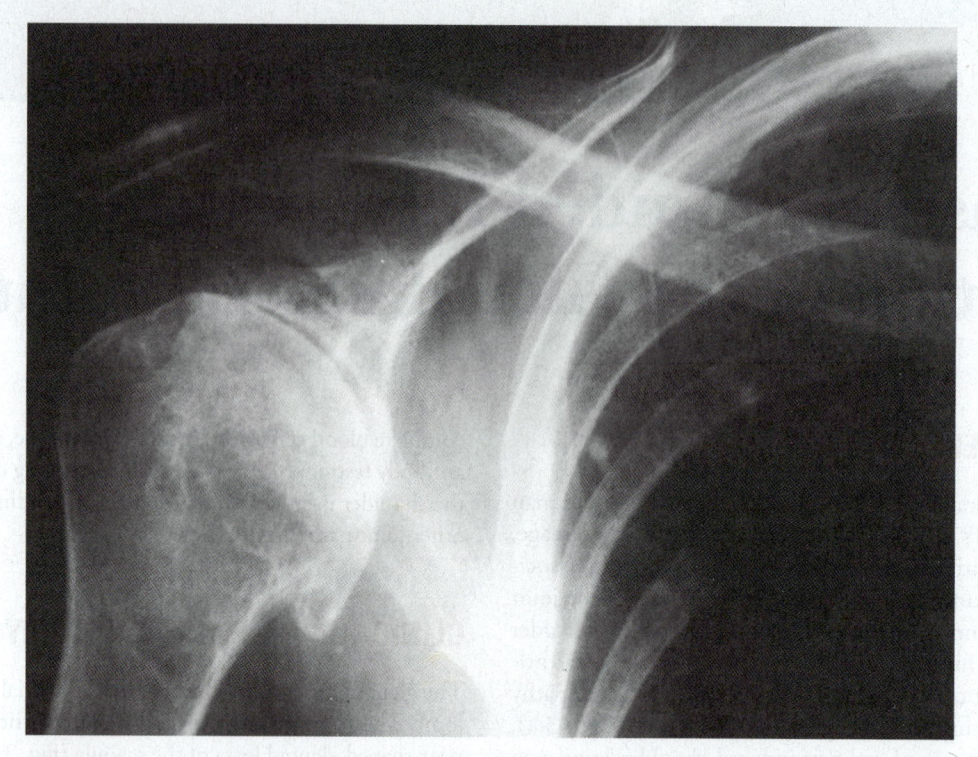

**FIGURE 33.1.** Glenohumeral osteoarthritis in an 87-year-old woman. The joint space is narrowed. Subchondral sclerosis of the humeral head and the glenoid and large inferior osteophytes are present. (Reused from Koopman WJ, Moreland LW. *Arthritis and Allied Conditions. A Textbook of Rheumatology.* 15th ed. Philadelphia, PA: Lippincott Williams & Wilkins; 2005, with permission.)

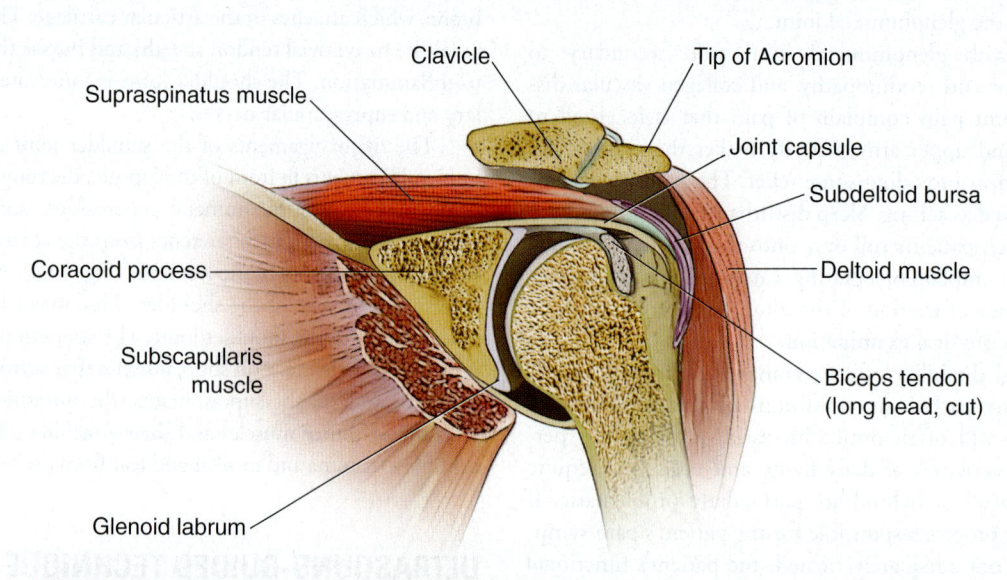

**FIGURE 33.2.** The anatomy of the glenohumeral joint.

CHAPTER 33   ULTRASOUND-GUIDED INTRA-ARTICULAR INJECTION OF THE GLENOHUMERAL JOINT   217

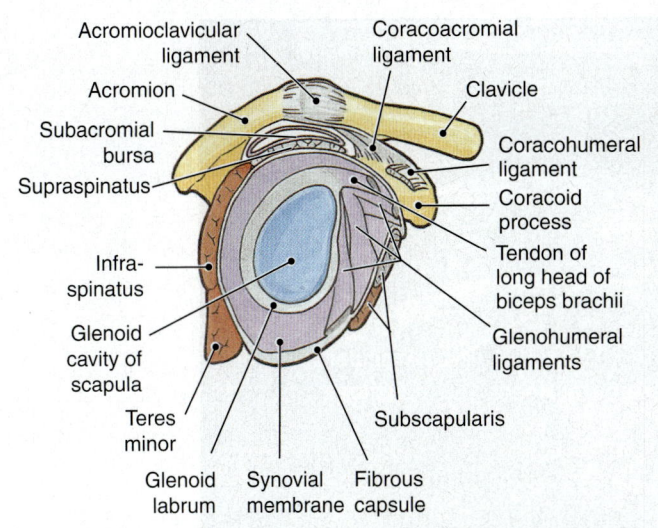

**FIGURE 33.3.** Cross-sectional anatomy of the glenohumeral joint demonstrating the labrum and synovium. (Reused from Moore KL, Agur AMR. *Essential Clinical Anatomy.* 2nd ed. Baltimore, MD: Lippincott Williams & Wilkins; 2002:483, with permission.)

glenohumeral joint is then prepped with antiseptic solution. A sterile syringe containing 2.0 mL of 0.25% preservative-free bupivacaine and 40 mg of methylprednisolone is attached to a 1½-inch, 22-gauge needle using strict aseptic technique. A linear high-frequency ultrasound transducer is placed over the lateral tip of the acromion in the coronal plane and angled slightly toward the scapula (Fig. 33.5). The supraspinatus tendon is then identified as it exits from beneath the acromion and curves over the head of the humerus to attach to the greater tuberosity (Fig. 33.6). The tendon should be carefully examined for calcifications or tendinopathy that may be contributing to the

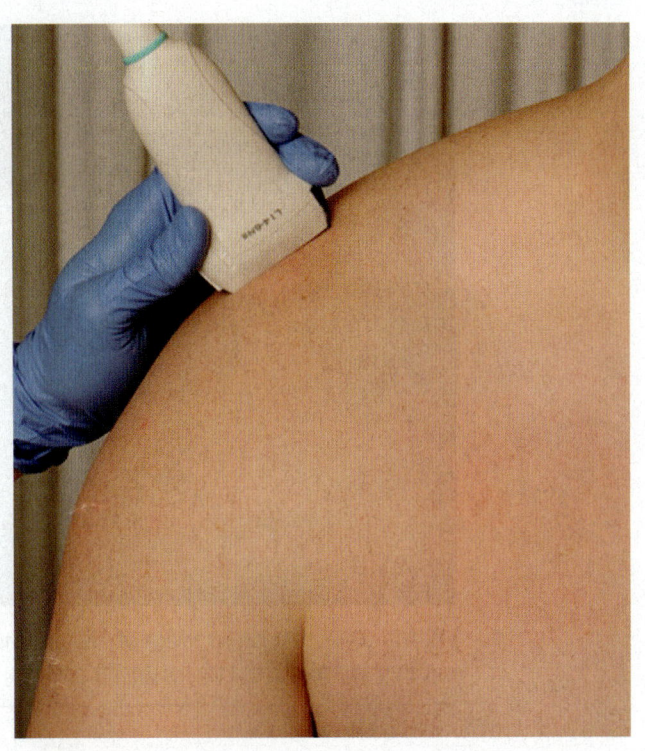

**FIGURE 33.5.** Correct coronal position for ultrasound transducer for ultrasound-guided intra-articular injection of the glenohumeral joint.

patient's shoulder pain. The glenohumeral joint is then identified as a fluid containing structure beneath supraspinatus tendon (see Figs. 33.6 and 33.7). Although the normal or mildly inflamed glenohumeral joint most often appears on ultrasonic imaging as a hypoechoic curvilinear layer of fluid sandwiched between a hyperechoic layer of bursal wall and peribursal fat,

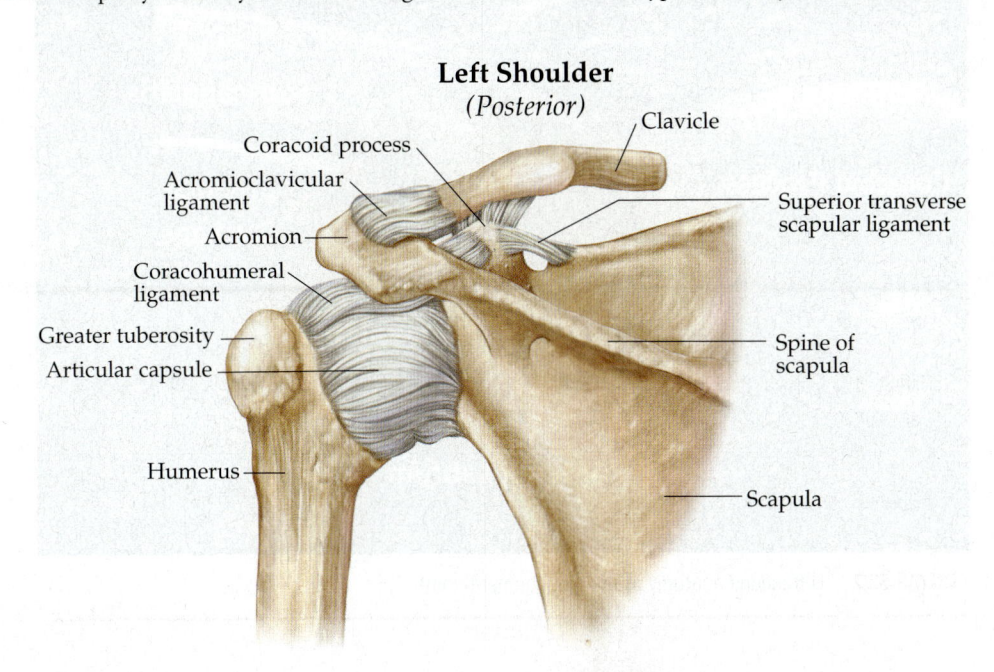

**FIGURE 33.4.** Anterior view of the ligaments of the shoulder. (Provided by Anatomical Chart Company.)

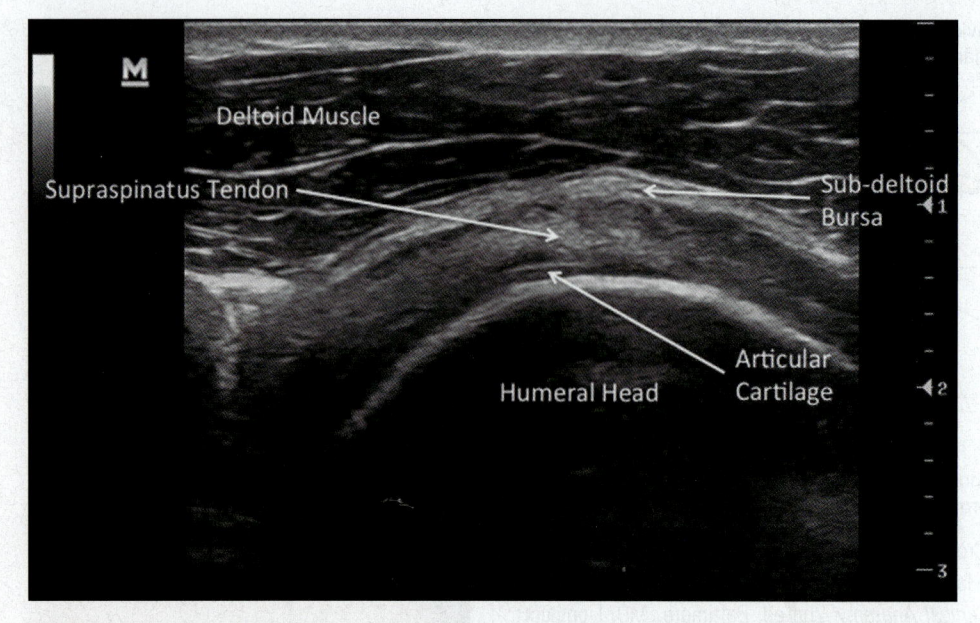

**FIGURE 33.6.** Ultrasound image of the glenohumeral joint demonstrating the relationship of the supraspinatus tendon and the head of the humerus.

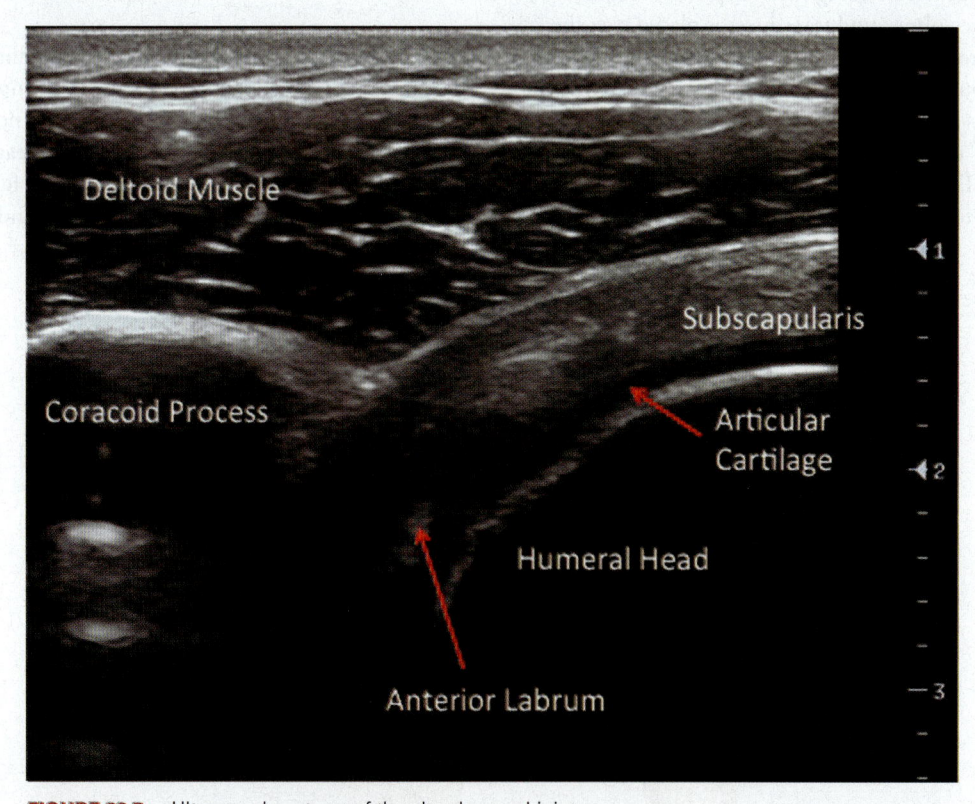

**FIGURE 33.7.** Ultrasound anatomy of the glenohumeral joint.

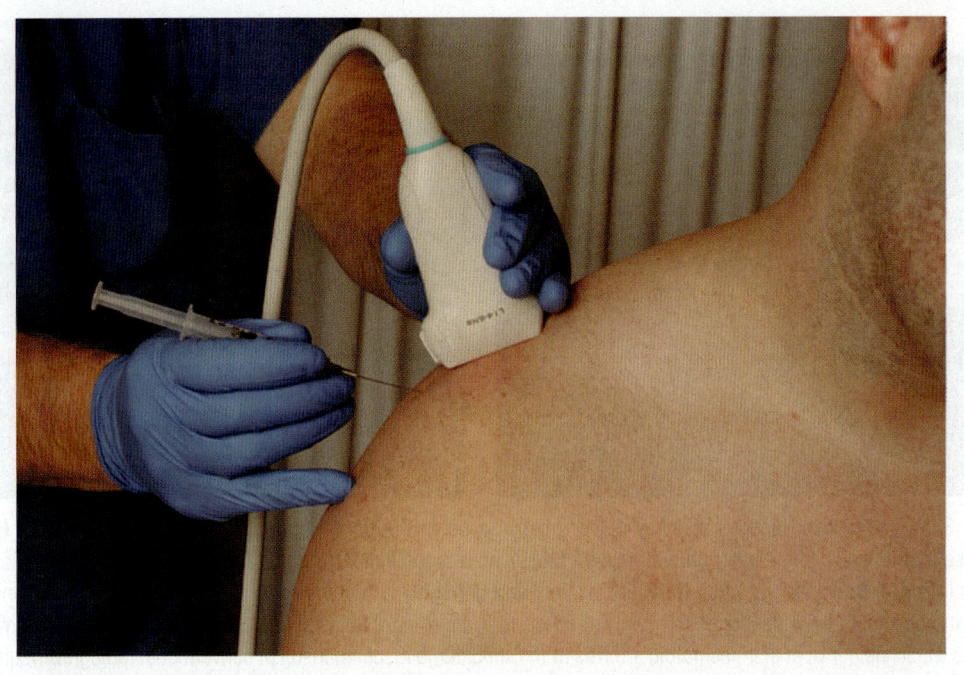

**FIGURE 33.8.** Correct in-plane needle placement for ultrasound-guided glenohumeral joint injection.

inflammation and distention of the bursal sac may make the bursal contents appear anechoic or even hyperechoic. After the joint space is identified, the needle is placed through the skin ~1 cm lateral to the end of the transducer and is then advanced using an in-plane approach with the needle trajectory adjusted under real-time ultrasound guidance to enter the glenohumeral joint just lateral to the acromion (Fig. 33.8). When the tip of needle is thought to be within the joint space, a small amount of local anesthetic and steroid is injected under real-time ultrasound guidance to confirm intra-articular placement by the characteristic spreading swirl of hyperechoic injectate within the joint. After intra-articular needle tip placement is confirmed, the remainder of the contents of the syringe are slowly injected. There should be minimal resistance to injection. If synechiae, loculations, or calcifications are present, the needle may have to be repositioned to ensure that the entire intra-articular space is treated. The needle is then removed, and a sterile pressure dressing and ice pack are placed at the injection site.

## COMPLICATIONS

The major complication of ultrasound-guided injection of the glenohumeral joint is infection. Ecchymosis and hematoma formation may also occur. A transient exacerbation of the patient's pain occurs ~25% of the time following this injection technique, and the patient should be warned of this possibility prior to the procedure.

## CLINICAL PEARLS

Care must be taken not to rotate the ultrasound transducer too far laterally or the clinician may mistake the hyperechoic margin of the lateral epicondyle for the lateral trochlea of the distal humerus. Bursitis, medial and lateral epicondylitis, tendinopathy, entrapment neuropathy osteoarthritis, synovitis, avascular necrosis of the humeral head, impingement syndromes, and other joint pathology may coexist with glenohumeral joint disease and may contribute to the patient's pain symptomatology (Fig. 33.9). Universal precautions should always be observed to protect the operator, and strict adherence to sterile technique must be used to avoid infection. Gentle physical therapy and local heat should be introduced following ultrasound-guided injection of the elbow joint to reduce pain and improve function. Simple analgesics and nonsteroidal anti-inflammatory agents or COX-2 inhibitors may be used concurrently with this injection technique.

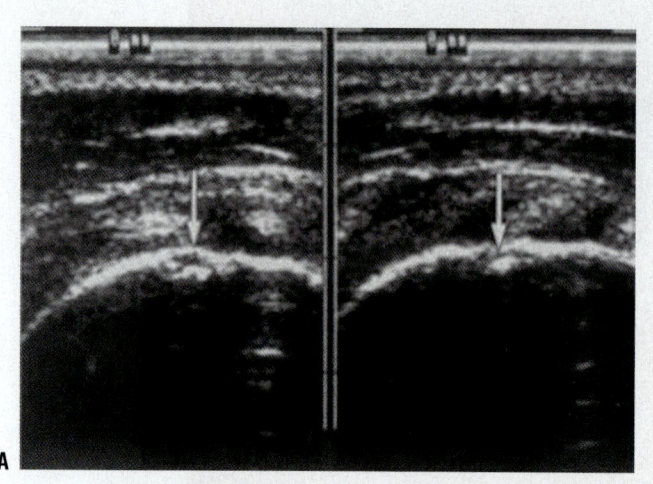

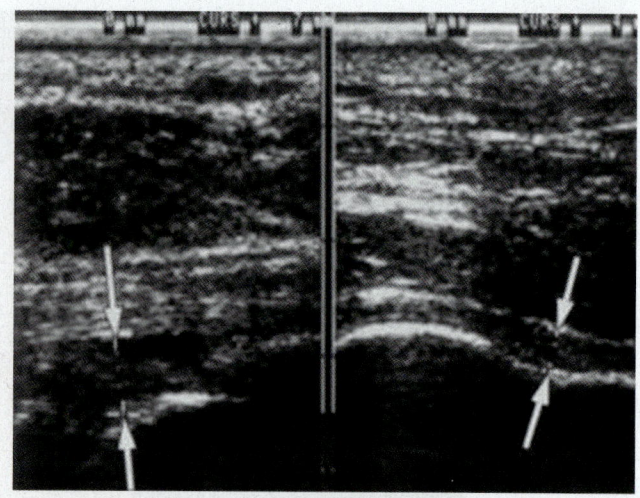

**FIGURE 33.9.** Ultrasound images of the shoulder joint in a patient with rheumatoid arthritis. **A:** Longitudinal **(left)** and transverse **(right)** views of the anterolateral region of the humerus, showing erosion of the anterior portion of the head of the humerus (*arrows*). **B:** Posterior portion **(left)** and axillary recess **(right)** of the shoulder joint, with hypoechogenic indications of synovitis as shown by widening of the synovial space to 7 and 4 mm, respectively (*arrows*). (Reused from Hermann KG, Backhaus M, Schneider U, et al. Rheumatoid arthritis of the shoulder joint: comparison of conventional radiography, ultrasound, and dynamic contrast-enhanced magnetic resonance imaging. *Arthritis Rheum* 2003;48(12):3338–3349, with permission.)

## SUGGESTED READINGS

Lento PH, Strakowski JA. The use of ultrasound in guiding musculoskeletal interventional procedures. *Phys Med Rehab Clin North Am* 2010;21(3):559–583.

Narouze SN. Ultrasound-guided hand, wrist, and elbow injections. In: *Atlas of Ultrasound Guided Procedures in Pain Management*. New York: Springer; 2010:308–321.

Waldman SD. The elbow joint. In: *Pain Review*. Philadelphia, PA: Saunders Elsevier; 2009:90–95.

Waldman SD, Campbell RSD. Anatomy, special imaging considerations of the shoulder. In: *Imaging of Pain*. Philadelphia, PA: Saunders Elsevier; 2011:217–219.

Waldman SD, Campbell RSD. Osteoarthritis of the glenohumeral joint. In: *Imaging of Pain*. Philadelphia, PA: Saunders Elsevier; 2011:221–223.

# CHAPTER 34

# Ultrasound-Guided Injection Technique for Acromioclavicular Joint

## CLINICAL PERSPECTIVES

The acromioclavicular joint is susceptible to injury from acute trauma such as falls directly onto the shoulder as well as repetitive microtrauma from activities that require repeated raising of the arm across the body such as throwing and painting on ladders. Let untreated, the acute inflammation associated with the injury may result in arthritis with its associated pain and functional disability. Patients suffering from acromioclavicular joint dysfunction or inflammation will complain of a marked exacerbation of pain when they perform activities that require raising their arm and reaching across their chest. A grating or grinding sensation with joint movement is often noted, and the patient frequently is unable to sleep on the affected shoulder. Patients with acromioclavicular joint dysfunction and inflammation will exhibit pain on downward traction or passive adduction of the affected shoulder. The chin adduction test is also frequently positive. Palpation of the acromioclavicular joint often reveals swelling or enlargement of the joint secondary to joint effusion (Fig. 34.1). If there is disruption of the ligaments that surround and support the acromioclavicular joint, joint instability may be evident on physical examination. Plain radiographs are indicated in patients suffering from acromioclavicular joint pain. They may reveal narrowing or sclerosis of the joint consistent with osteoarthritis or widening of the joint consistent with ligamentous injury (Fig. 34.2). They may also reveal occult fractures. If joint instability is suspected or detected on physical examination, magnetic resonance imaging and/or ultrasound scanning is a reasonable next step. Ultrasound-guided acromioclavicular joint injection can aid the clinician in both the diagnosis and treatment of acromioclavicular joint pain and dysfunction (Fig. 34.3).

## CLINICALLY RELEVANT ANATOMY

The acromioclavicular joint is the junction of the distal end of the clavicle and the anterior and medial aspects of the acromion of the scapula (Fig. 34.4). In many patients, the space between the distal end of the clavicle and the acromion is filled with an intra-articular disk. The dense coracoclavicular ligament provides the majority of strength of the joint. Additionally, strength is provided by the articular capsule, which completely surrounds the joint. The superior portion of the joint is covered by the superior acromioclavicular ligament, which attaches the distal clavicle to the upper surface of the acromion. The inferior portion of the joint is covered by the inferior acromioclavicular ligament, which attaches the inferior portion of the distal clavicle to the acromion. Both of these ligaments provide further joint stability. On palpation of the joint, a small indentation can be felt where the clavicle abuts the acromion. The acromioclavicular joint may or may not contain an articular disk. The volume of the acromioclavicular joint space is small, and care must be taken not to disrupt the joint by forcefully injecting large volumes of local anesthetic and corticosteroid into the intra-articular space when performing this injection technique.

## ULTRASOUND-GUIDED TECHNIQUE

The benefits, risks, and alternative treatments are explained to the patient, and informed consent is obtained. The patient is then placed in the sitting position with the shoulder relaxed and the forearm resting comfortably on the ipsilateral thigh. The acromioclavicular joint is then identified by palpation (Fig. 34.5). The skin overlying the acromioclavicular joint is then prepped with antiseptic solution. A sterile syringe containing 1.0 mL of 0.25% preservative-free bupivacaine and 40 mg of methylprednisolone is attached to a 1½-inch, 22-gauge needle using strict aseptic technique. A linear high-frequency ultrasound transducer is placed in the coronal plane across the acromioclavicular joint (Fig. 34.6). Slowly move the ultrasound transducer to identify the acromion and the distal end of the clavicle and the acromioclavicular joint in between (Fig. 34.7). To facilitate needle placement, position the ultrasound transducer so the center of the v-shaped hypoechoic joint is in the center of the image between the hyperechoic margins of the acromion and distal end of the clavicle. In some patients, a hyperechoic intra-articular disk can be identified, and if a significant joint effusion is present, bulging of the joint capsule may be apparent (see Figs. 34.1 and 34.7). After the joint space is identified, the needle is placed through the skin and is then advanced using an out-of-plane approach with the needle trajectory adjusted under real-time ultrasound guidance to enter

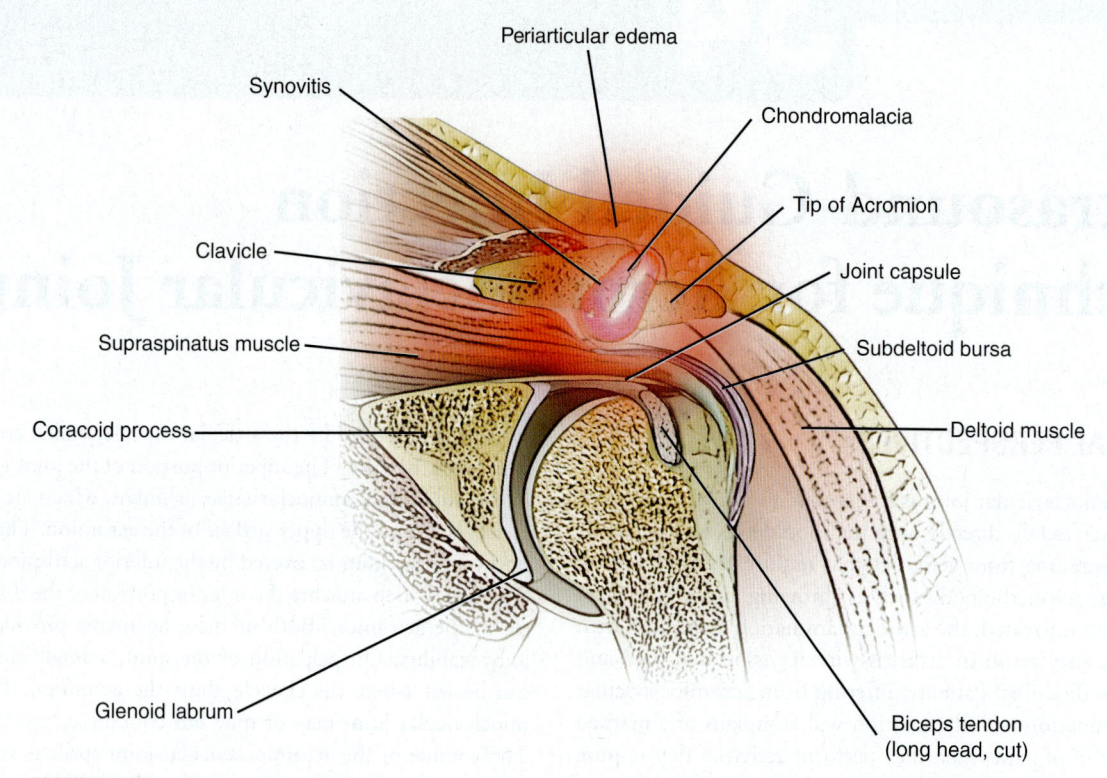

**FIGURE 34.1.** Patients with significant acromioclavicular joint pain often exhibit joint swelling and enlargement secondary to joint effusions.

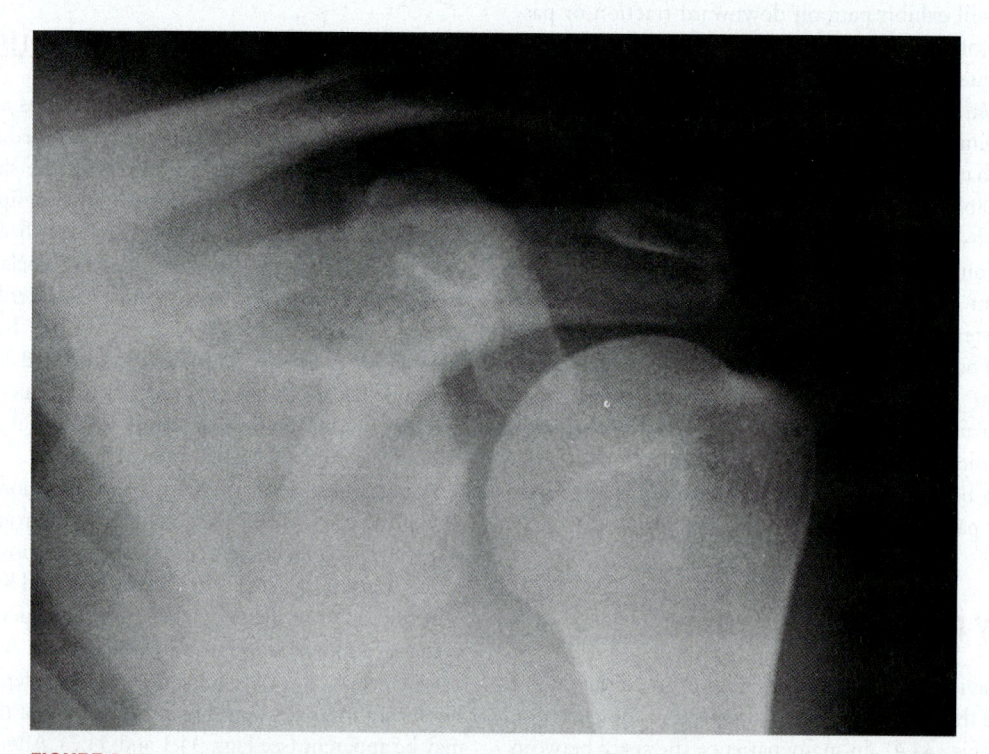

**FIGURE 34.2.** A third-degree acromioclavicular separation with fractured base of the coracoid and a comminuted glenoid fracture. Note the normal coracoclavicular distance, indicating intact ligaments. (Reused from Bucholz RW, Heckman JD. *Rockwood & Green's Fractures in Adults.* 5th ed. Philadelphia, PA: Lippincott Williams & Wilkins; 2001, with permission.)

CHAPTER 34   ULTRASOUND-GUIDED INJECTION TECHNIQUE FOR ACROMIOCLAVICULAR JOINT   223

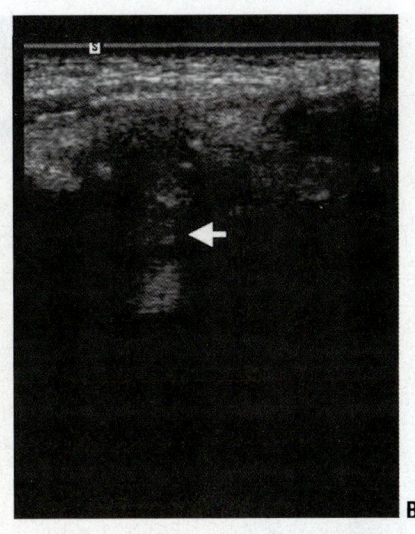

**FIGURE 34.3.** Acromioclavicular joint injection. **A:** In this patient, the needle is seen in cross-section (*arrow*). A faint reverberation artifact may be appreciated deep to the needle. The clavicle (*cl*) and acromion (*ac*) are labeled. **B:** During the injection, while observing in real-time, the appearance of bright echoes within the joint due to the contrast effect of the therapeutic mixture helps to ensure appropriate localization (*arrow*). (Reused from Adler RS, Allen A. Percutaneous ultrasound guided injections in the shoulder. *Tech Shoulder Elbow Surg* 2004;5(2):122–133, with permission.)

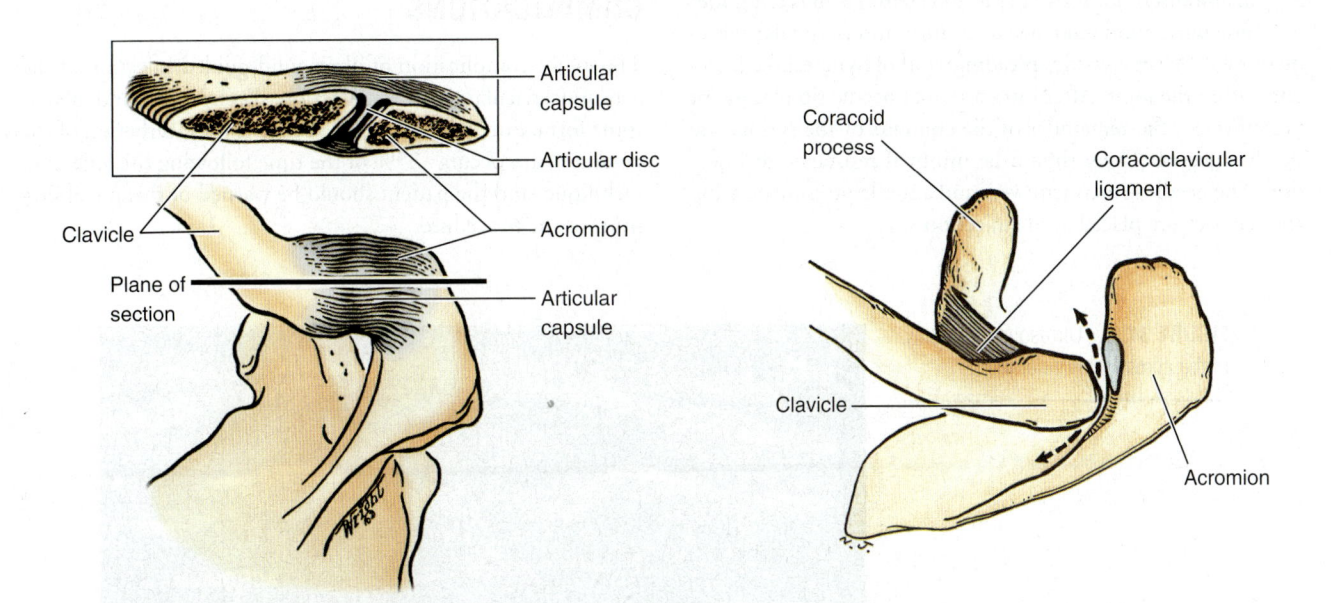

**FIGURE 34.4.** Anatomy of the acromioclavicular joint. Note the supporting ligaments and surrounding joint capsule. (Reused from Moore KL, Agur A. *Essential Clinical Anatomy*. 2nd ed. Philadelphia, PA: Lippincott Williams & Wilkins; 2002, with permission.)

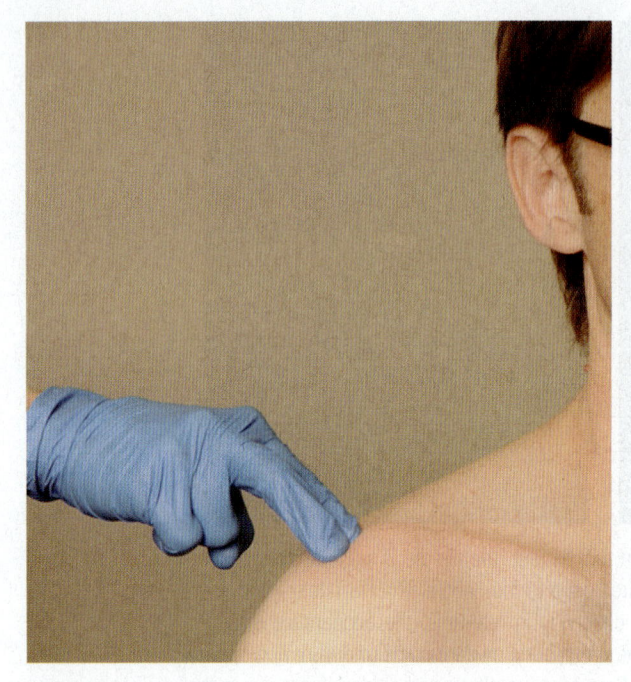

**FIGURE 34.5.** Palpation of the acromioclavicular joint.

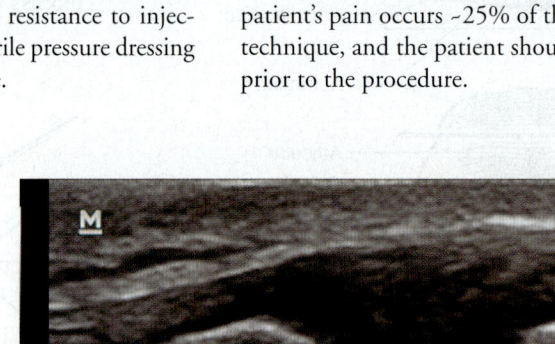

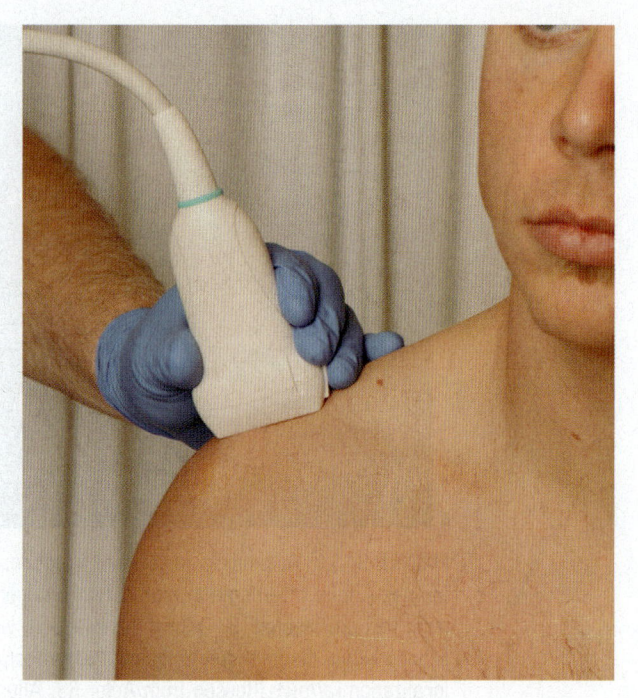

**FIGURE 34.6.** Proper coronal placement of the high-frequency linear ultrasound probe for ultrasound-guided acromioclavicular joint injection.

the center of the acromioclavicular joint (Figs. 34.8 and 34.9). When the tip of needle is thought to be within the joint space, a small amount of local anesthetic and steroid is injected under real-time ultrasound guidance to confirm intra-articular placement by the characteristic spreading swirl of hyperechoic injectate within the joint. After intra-articular needle tip placement is confirmed, the remainder of the contents of the syringe are slowly injected. There should be minimal resistance to injection. The needle is then removed, and a sterile pressure dressing and ice pack are placed at the injection site.

## COMPLICATIONS

The major complication of ultrasound-guided injection of the acromioclavicular joint is infection. Ecchymosis and hematoma formation may also occur. A transient exacerbation of the patient's pain occurs ~25% of the time following this injection technique, and the patient should be warned of this possibility prior to the procedure.

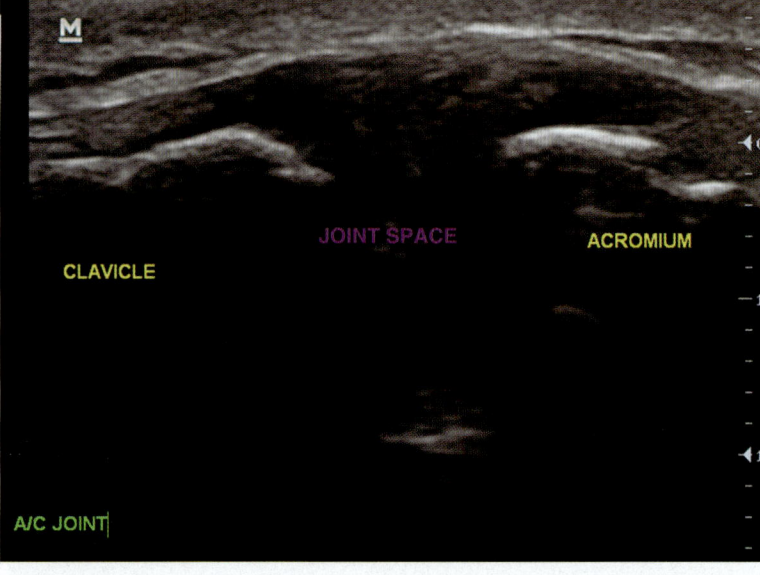

**FIGURE 34.7.** Ultrasound anatomy of the acromioclavicular joint.

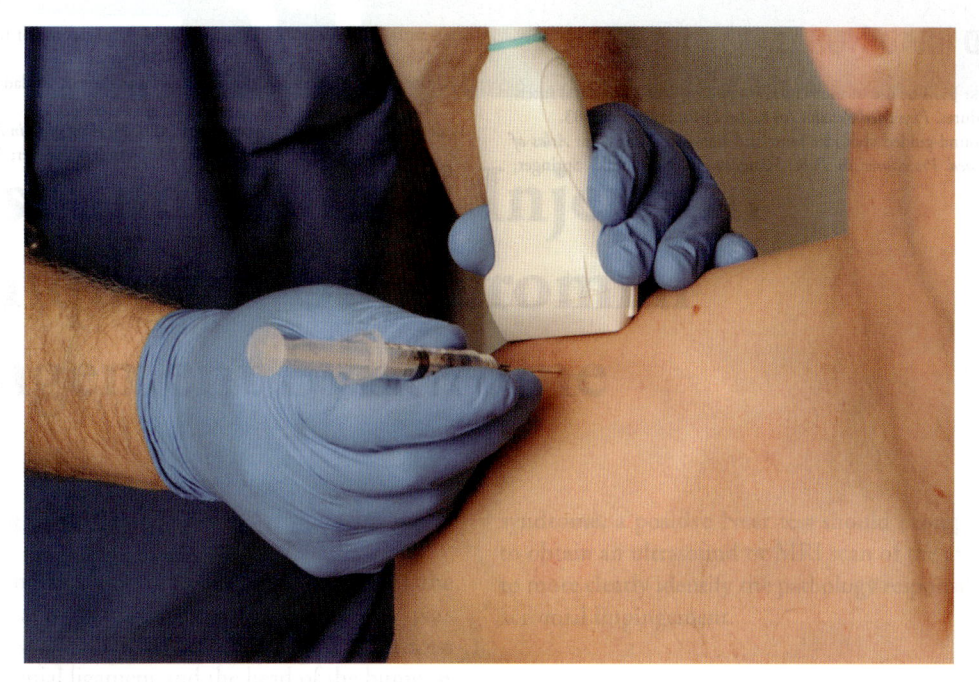

**FIGURE 34.8.** Proper out-of-plane needle placement for ultrasound-guided acromioclavicular joint injection.

## CLINICAL PEARLS

Shoulder pathology including rotator cuff tendinopathy, osteoarthritis, avascular necrosis of the humeral head, and impingement syndromes may coexist with acromioclavicular joint disease and may contribute to the patient's pain symptomatology. Universal precautions should always be observed to protect the operator, and strict adherence to sterile technique must be used to avoid infection. Gentle physical therapy and local heat should be introduced following ultrasound-guided injection of the acromioclavicular joint to reduce pain and improve function. Simple analgesics and nonsteroidal anti-inflammatory agents or COX-2 inhibitors may be used in conjunction with this injection technique.

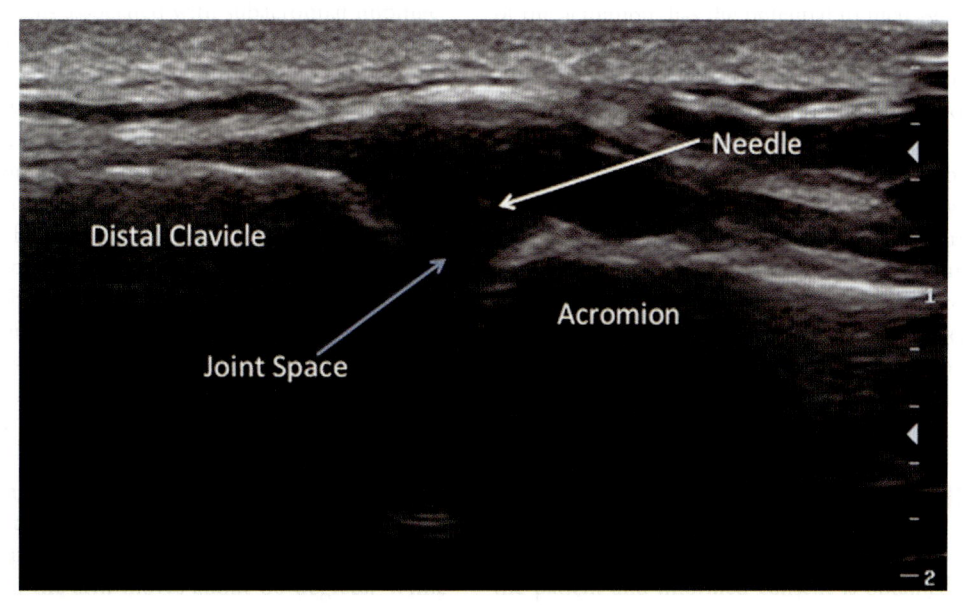

**FIGURE 34.9.** Transverse ultrasound image demonstrating the needle tip within the acromioclavicular joint using an out-of-plane approach.

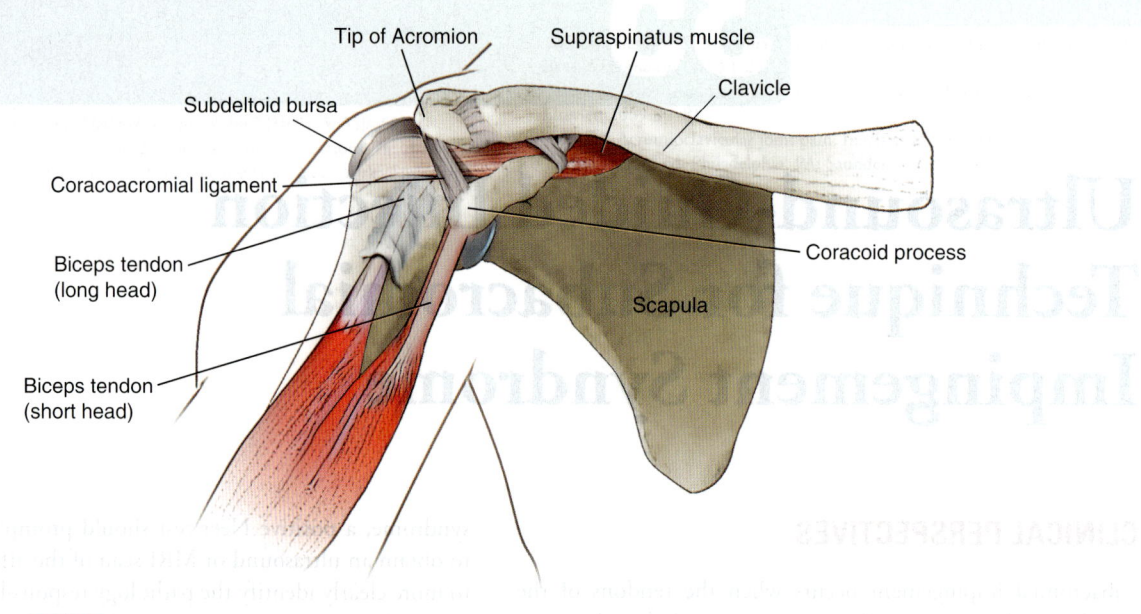

**FIGURE 35.1.** The anatomy of the subacromial space.

and the forearm resting comfortably on the ipsilateral thigh. The acromioclavicular joint is then identified by palpation (Fig. 35.7). The skin overlying the acromion is then prepped with antiseptic solution. A sterile syringe containing 2.0 mL of 0.25% preservative-free bupivacaine and 40 mg of methylprednisolone is attached to a 1½-inch, 22-gauge needle using

strict aseptic technique. A linear high-frequency ultrasound transducer is placed in the coronal plane across the acromioclavicular joint (Fig. 35.8). After the acromioclavicular joint is identified, slowly move the ultrasound transducer laterally to identify the hyperechoic margin of the acromion (Fig. 35.9). After the margin of the acromion is identified, the

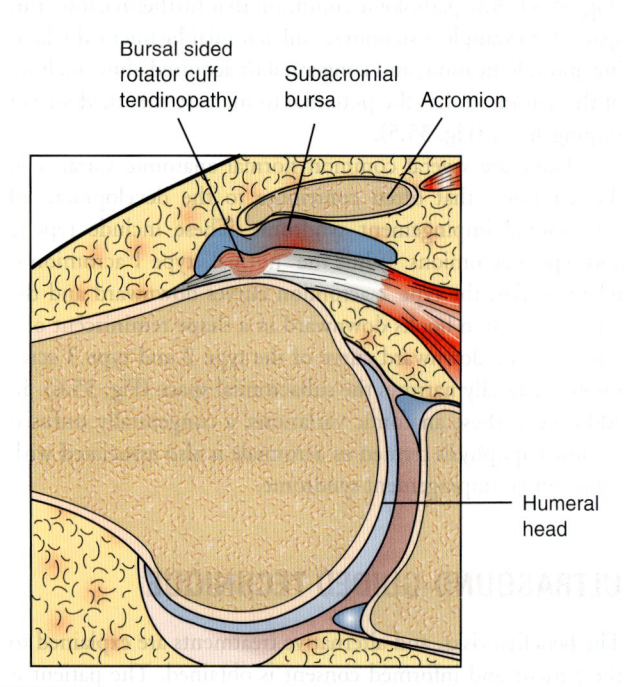

**FIGURE 35.2.** Untreated, subacromial impingement can lead to rotator cuff tendinopathy.

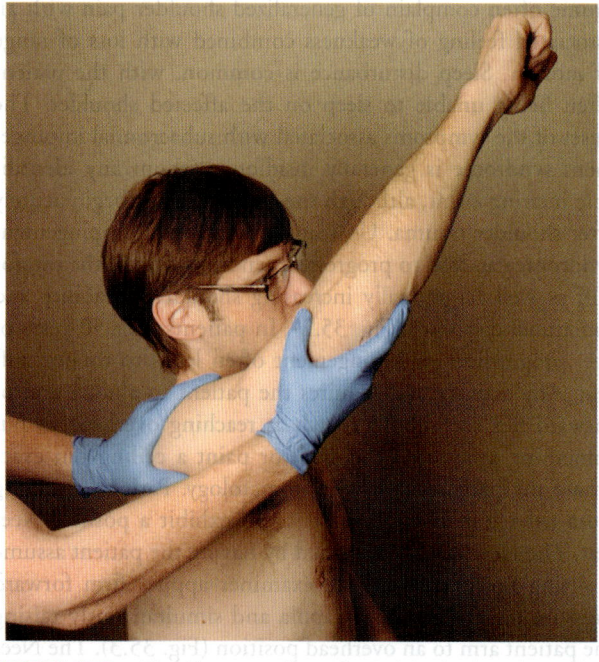

**FIGURE 35.3.** The Neer test is performed by having the patient assume a sitting position while the examiner applies firm forward pressure on the patient's scapula and simultaneously raising the patient arm to an overhead position.

**FIGURE 35.4.** The space between the acromion and the superior aspect of the humeral head is called the impingement interval, and abduction of the arm will further narrow the space. (Reused from Anatomical Chart Company, with permission.)

needle is placed through the skin at the middle of the anterior border of the coronally placed ultrasound transducer and is then advanced using an out-plane approach with the needle trajectory adjusted under real-time ultrasound guidance to enter the subacromial space just beneath the acromion (Fig. 35.10). When the tip of needle is thought to be within the subacromial space, a small amount of local anesthetic and steroid is injected under real-time ultrasound guidance to confirm needle placement. After needle tip placement is confirmed, the remainder of the contents of the syringe are slowly injected. There should be minimal resistance to injection. If synechiae, loculations, or calcifications are present, the needle may have to be repositioned to ensure that the entire subacromial space is treated.

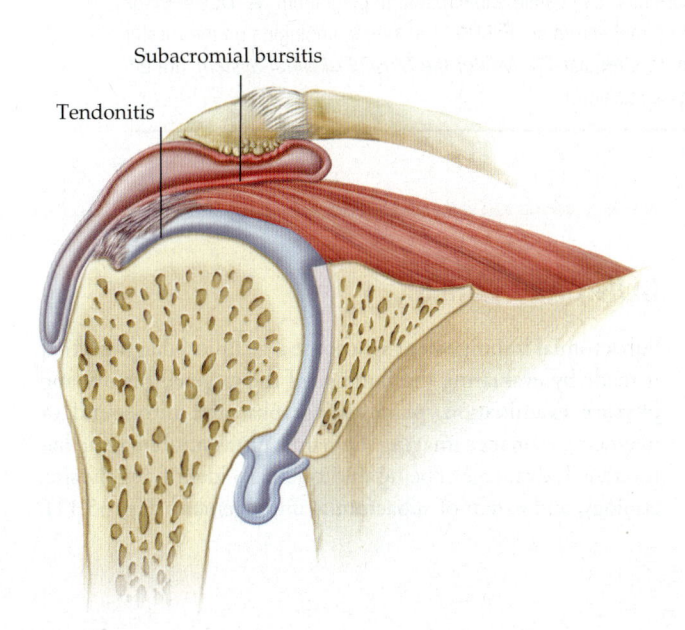

**FIGURE 35.5.** Osteophytes of the acromion can cause rotator cuff tendinopathy due to compromise of the subacromial space. (Reused from Anatomical Chart Company, with permission.)

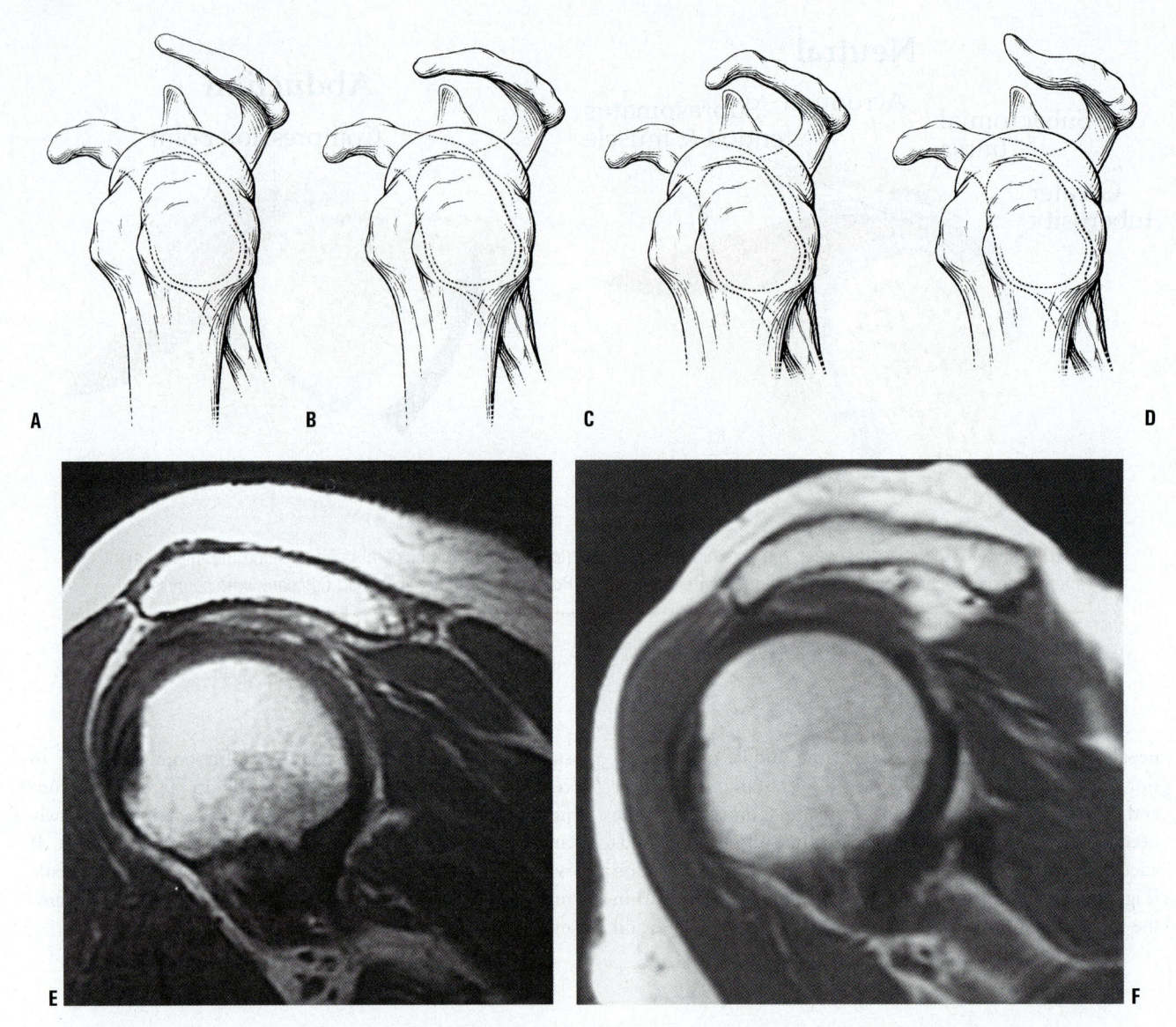

**FIGURE 35.6.** Congenital or acquired abnormalities of the acromion can cause subacromial impingement. **A–D:** Drawings demonstrate common abnormalities of the acromion. **E:** MRI of normal acromion. **F:** MRI of acromion impinging on the rotator cuff. (Reused from Berquist TH, Peterson JJ. Shoulder and arm. In: Berquist TH. *MRI of the Musculoskeletal System*. 6th ed. Philadelphia, PA: Lippincott Williams & Wilkins; 2013:641, with permission.)

## COMPLICATIONS

The major complication of ultrasound-guided injection of the subacromial space is infection. Ecchymosis and hematoma formation may also occur. A transient exacerbation of the patient's pain occurs ~25% of the time following this injection technique, and the patient should be warned of this possibility prior to the procedure.

## CLINICAL PEARLS

Subacromial impingement syndrome is a clinical diagnosis that is made by evaluating the findings of the targeted history and physical examination, plain radiographs, and ultrasound or magnetic resonance imaging. Dynamic ultrasound imaging has the added advantage of being able to actually identifying the site, etiology, and extent of subacromial impingement (Fig. 35.11).

# CHAPTER 35 ULTRASOUND-GUIDED INJECTION TECHNIQUE FOR SUBACROMIAL IMPINGEMENT SYNDROME

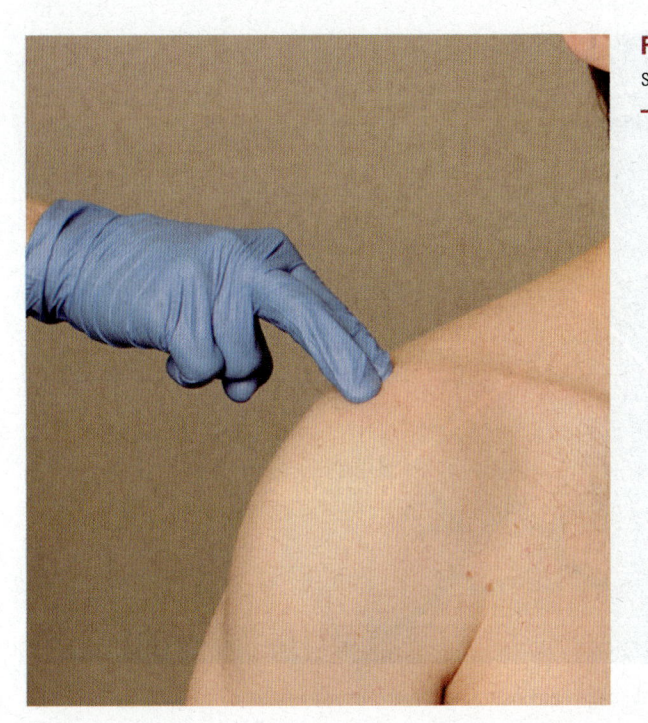

**FIGURE 35.7.** Palpation of the subacromial space.

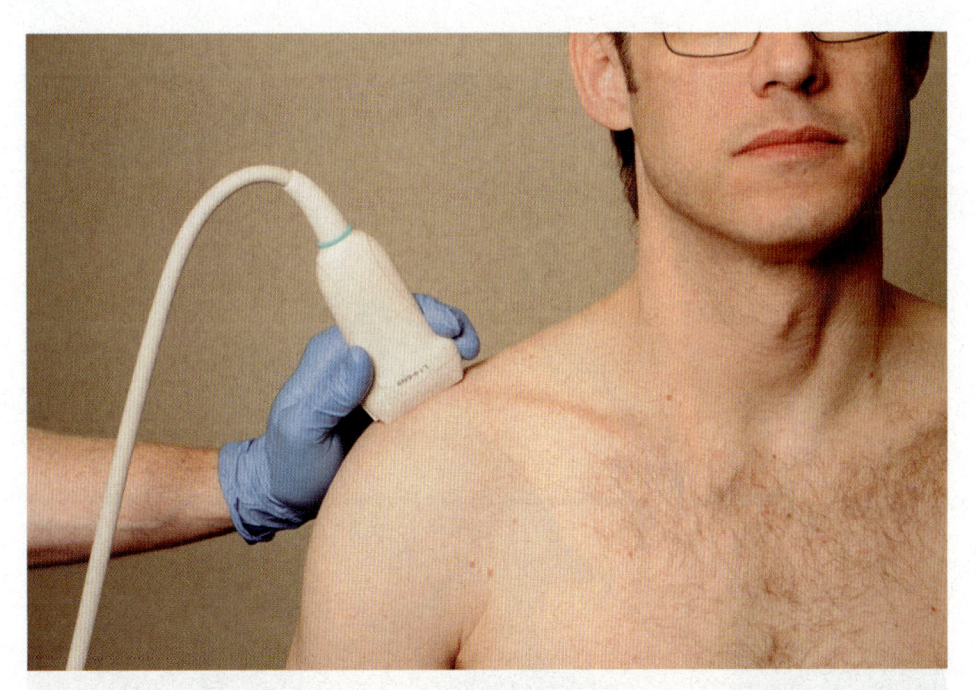

**FIGURE 35.8.** Proper coronal placement of the high-frequency linear ultrasound probe for ultrasound-guided subacromial injection.

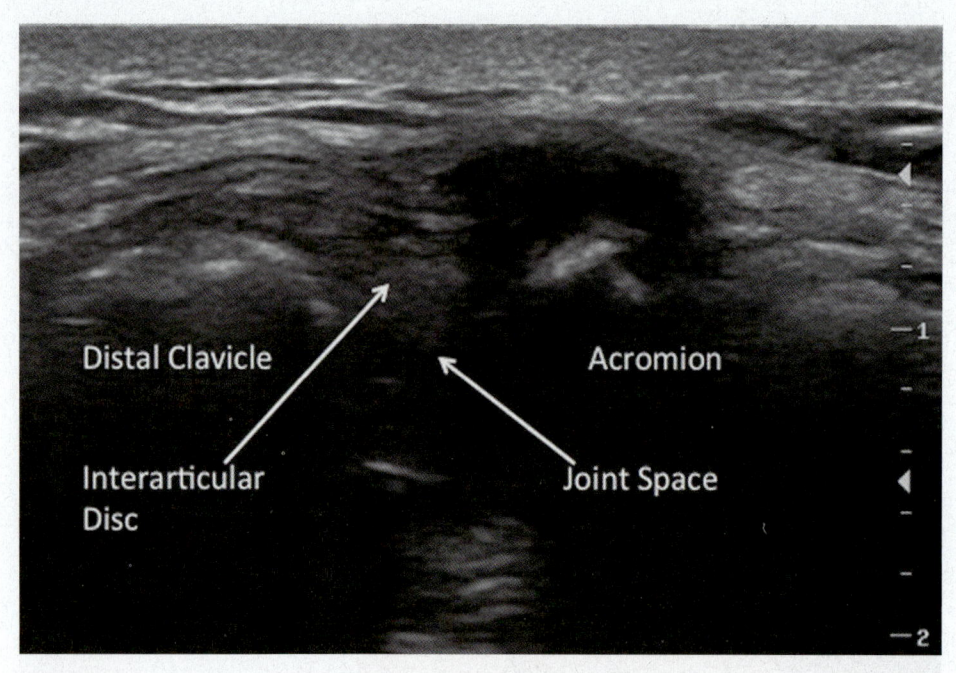

**FIGURE 35.9.** Coronal ultrasound image demonstrating the acromioclavicular joint.

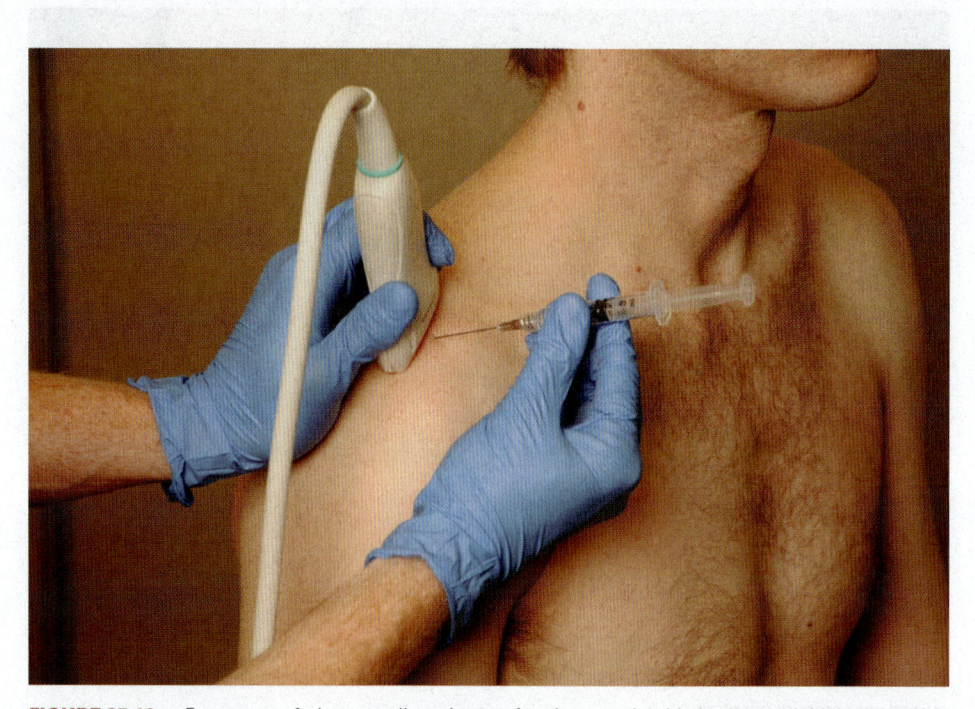

**FIGURE 35.10.** Proper out-of-plane needle trajectory for ultrasound-guided subacromial joint injection.

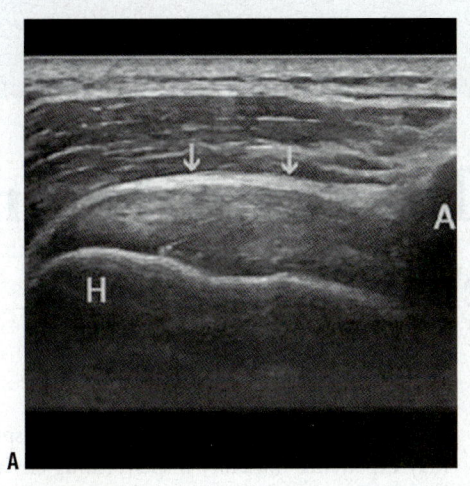

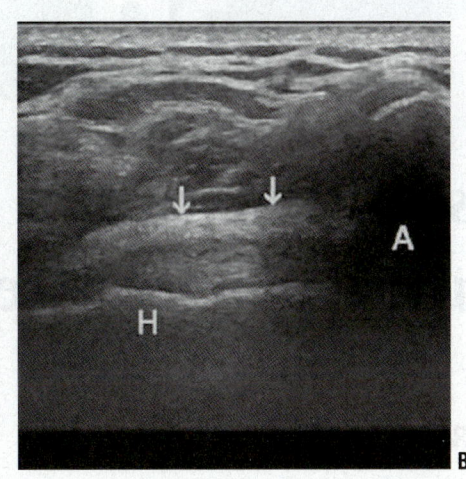

**FIGURE 35.11.** Long axis dynamic ultrasound imaging over supraspinatus **(A)** at rest and **(B)** abduction showing bunching of the supraspinatus tendon and subacromial-subdeltoid bursa (*arrows*) under the acromion (*A*). H, greater tuberosity of humerus. (Reused from Tagg CE, Campbell AS, McNally EG. Shoulder impingement. *Semin Musculoskelet Radiol* 2013;17(1):3–11, with permission.)

Pain syndromes that may mimic or coexist with subacromial impingement syndrome are listed in Table 35.1. A failure to correctly diagnose subacromial impingement syndrome will put the patient at risk of the missed diagnosis of other syndromes that may result in ongoing damage to the shoulder or lead to overlooked pathology in this anatomic region that may harm the patient such as Pancoast tumor or primary or metastatic tumors of the shoulder.

| TABLE 35.1 | Causes of Subacromial Impingement Syndrome |
|---|---|

- Subacromial/subdeltoid bursitis
- Rotator cuff tendinopathy
- Rotator cuff tendonitis
- Thickening of the coracoacromial ligament
- Calcification of the coracoacromial ligament
- Osteophyte formation
- Arthritis affecting any of the shoulder joints
- Synovitis affecting any of the shoulder joints
- Adhesive capsulitis

## SUGGESTED READINGS

Lento PH, Strakowski JA. The use of ultrasound in guiding musculoskeletal interventional procedures. *Phys Med Rehabil Clin N Am* 2010;21(3):559–583.

Narouze SN. Ultrasound-guided shoulder joint and bursa injections. In: *Atlas of Ultrasound Guided Procedures. Pain Management.* New York, NY: Springer; 2010: 298–299.

Precerutti M, Garioni E, Madonia L, et al. US anatomy of the shoulder: pictorial essay. *J Ultrasound* 2010;13(4):179–187.

Waldman SD. The shoulder joint. In: *Pain Review*. Philadelphia, PA: WB Saunders; 2009:80–81.

Waldman SD. Injection technique for os acromiale. *Atlas of Pain Management Injection Techniques*. 3rd ed. Philadelphia, PA: WB Saunders; 2013:92–94.

Waldman SD. Injection technique for subacromial impingement syndrome. In: *Atlas of Pain Management Injection Techniques*. 3rd ed. Philadelphia, PA: WB Saunders; 2013:87–91.

# CHAPTER 36

# Ultrasound-Guided Injection Technique for Supraspinatus Tendonitis

## CLINICAL PERSPECTIVES

The musculotendinous unit of the rotator cuff is subjected to an amazing variation of stresses as it performs its function to allow range of motion of the shoulder while at the same time providing shoulder stability. The relatively poor blood supply limits the ability of these muscles and tendons to heal when traumatized. Over time, muscle tears and tendinopathy develop, further weakening the musculotendinous units and making them susceptible to additional damage. The potential for impingement as the supraspinatus musculotendinous unit passes beneath the coracoacromial arch can further exacerbate the problem and further inflame and damage the structures (Fig. 36.1). Contributing to the susceptibility of the musculotendinous unit of the supraspinatus muscle to microtrauma is the fact that the supraspinatus tendon fibers interpolate themselves in the substance of the supraspinatus muscle in an oblique fashion meaning that eccentric force is applied to the musculotendinous unit when the muscle contracts (Fig. 36.2). Over time, if the inflammation continues, calcium deposition around the tendon with resultant calcific tendonitis may occur, making subsequent treatment more difficult (Fig. 36.3). Tendonitis of the musculotendinous units of the shoulder frequently coexists with bursitis of the associated bursae of the shoulder joint, creating additional pain and functional disability (Fig. 36.4).

The supraspinatus tendon of the rotator cuff is susceptible to the development of tendonitis following even seemingly minor trauma. The onset of supraspinatus tendonitis is usually acute, occurring after overuse or misuse of the shoulder joint. Inciting factors may include carrying heavy loads in front and away from the body or the vigorous use of exercise equipment. The pain of supraspinatus tendonitis is constant and severe. The patient often complains of sleep disturbance and is unable to sleep on the affected shoulder. In an effort to decrease pain, patients suffering from supraspinatus tendonitis often splint the inflamed tendon by elevating the scapula to remove tension from the ligament, giving the patient a "shrugging" appearance. Patients with supraspinatus tendonitis exhibit a positive Dawbarn sign, which is pain to palpation over the greater tuberosity of the humerus when the arm is hanging down and which disappears when the arm is fully abducted.

If untreated, patients suffering from supraspinatus tendonitis may experience difficulty in performing any task that requires initial abduction of the upper extremity, making simple everyday tasks such as brushing ones teeth or eating difficult. Over time, muscle atrophy, calcific tendonitis, and ultimately adhesive capsulitis may result (see Fig. 36.3).

Plain radiographs are indicated in all patients who present with shoulder pain. Based on the patient's clinical presentation, additional testing may be indicated, including complete blood cell count, sedimentation rate, and antinuclear antibody testing. Magnetic resonance imaging or ultrasound imaging of the shoulder is indicated if a rotator cuff tear is suspected (Fig. 36.5). Magnetic resonance imaging or ultrasound imaging of the affected area may also help delineate the presence of calcific tendonitis or other shoulder pathology.

## CLINICALLY RELEVANT ANATOMY

The supraspinatus muscle serves to stabilize the shoulder by helping resist the inferior gravitational forces placed on the shoulder joint due to the downward pull from the weight of the upper limb. Responsible for the first 10 to 15 degrees of abduction of the upper extremity, the supraspinatus muscle abducts the arm at the shoulder by fixing the head of the humerus firmly against the glenoid fossa. The supraspinatus muscle is innervated by the suprascapular nerve, which is comprised of fibers from the superior trunk of the brachial plexus. The muscle finds its origin from the supraspinous fossa of the scapula and inserts into the upper facet of the greater tuberosity of the humerus (Fig. 36.6). The muscle passes across the superior aspect of the shoulder joint beneath the acromion with the inferior portion of the tendon intimately involved with the joint capsule.

## ULTRASOUND-GUIDED TECHNIQUE

The benefits, risks, and alternative treatments are explained to the patient and informed consent is obtained. The patient is then placed in the neutral sitting position with the

# CHAPTER 36  ULTRASOUND-GUIDED INJECTION TECHNIQUE FOR SUPRASPINATUS TENDONITIS

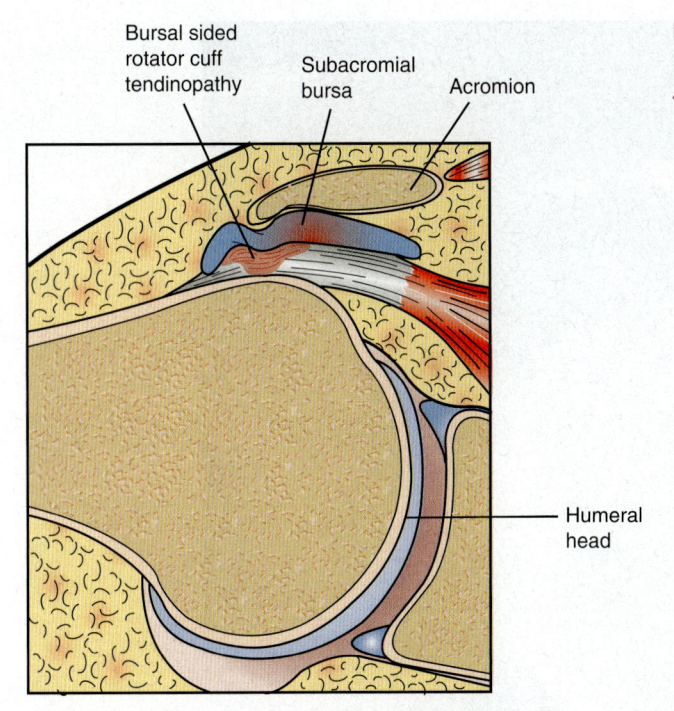

**FIGURE 36.1.** The supraspinatus musculotendinous unit is subject to impingement as it passes beneath the acromion.

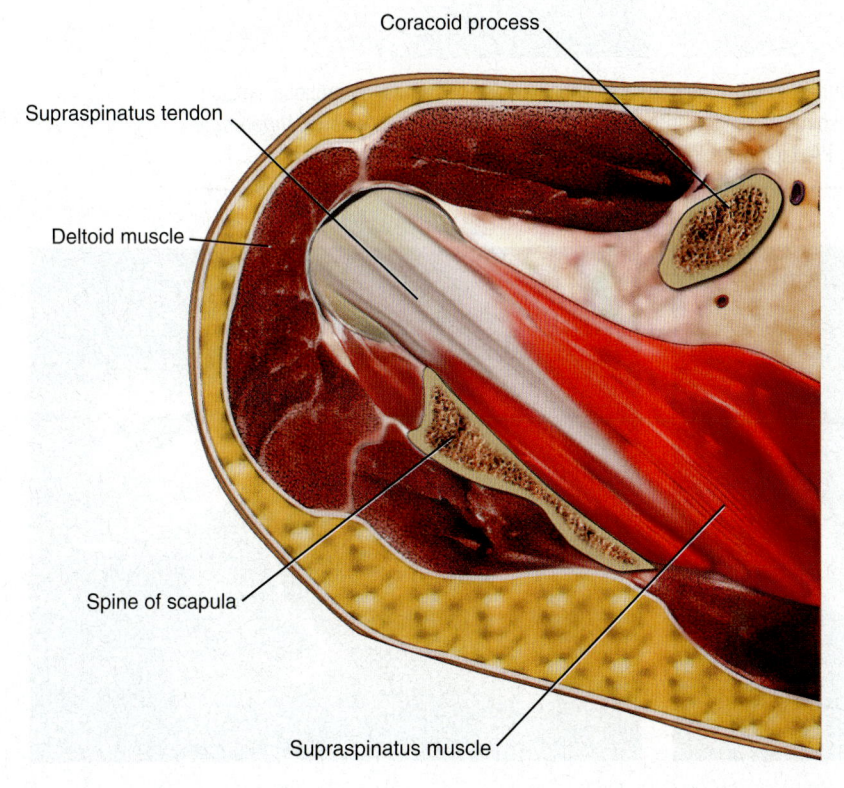

**FIGURE 36.2.** Axial cross section of the musculotendinous unit of the supraspinatus muscle demonstrating the obliquity of the supraspinatus tendon relative to the supraspinatus muscle.

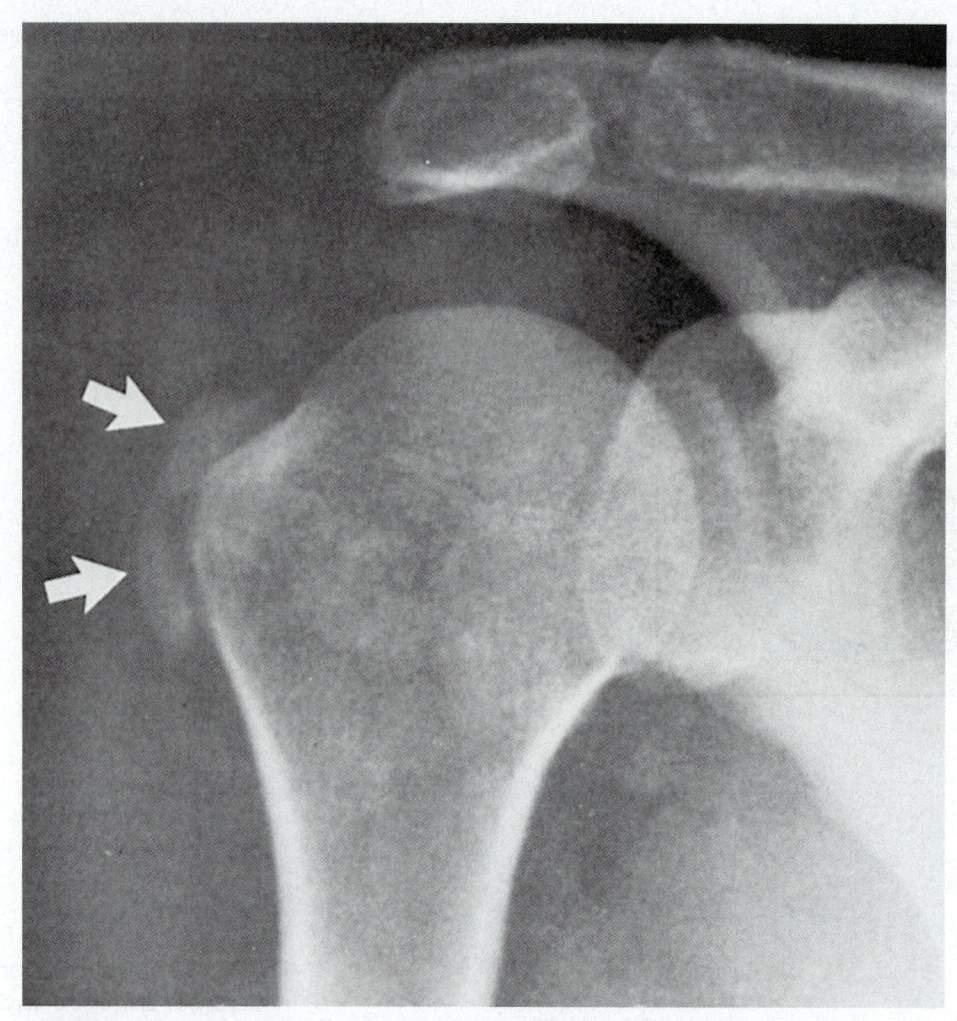

**FIGURE 36.3.** Calcific tendonitis. Frontal view of the shoulder demonstrates amorphous calcium deposits (*arrows*) in the supraspinatus tendon. (Reused from Eisenberg RL. *An Atlas of Differential Diagnosis*. 4th ed. Philadelphia, PA: Lippincott Williams & Wilkins; 2003, with permission.)

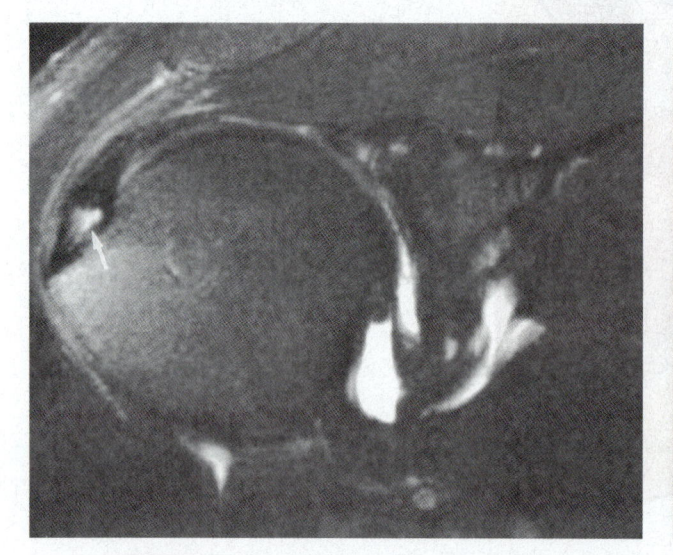

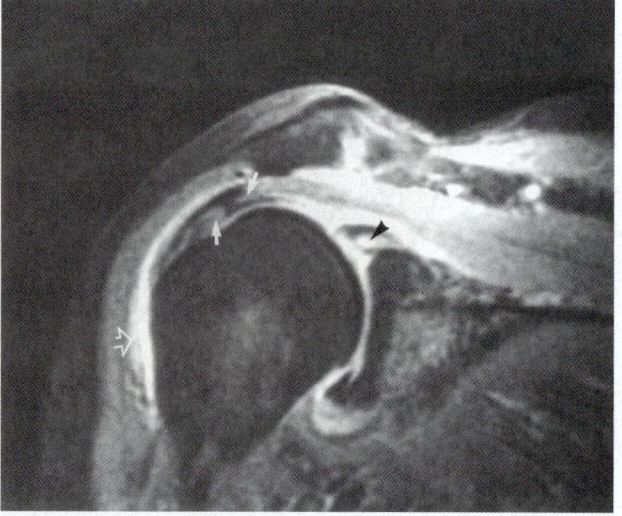

**FIGURE 36.4.** Tendonitis of the musculotendinous units of the shoulder frequently coexists with bursitis of the associated bursae of the shoulder joint, creating additional pain and functional disability. (Reused from Berquist TH, Peterson JJ. Shoulder and arm. In: Berquist TH. *MRI of the Musculoskeletal System*. 6th ed. Philadelphia, PA: Lippincott Williams & Wilkins; 2013:647, with permission.)

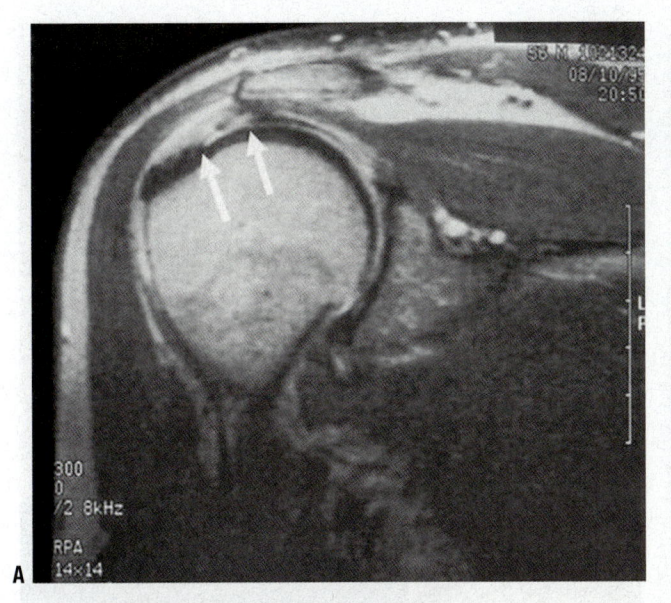

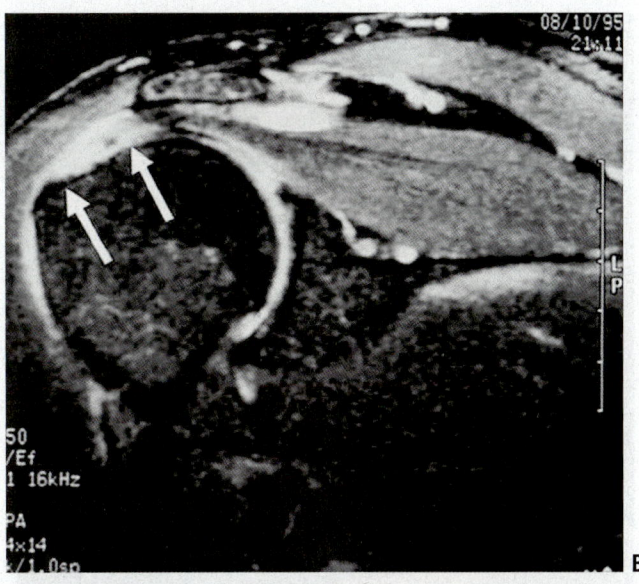

**FIGURE 36.5.** Convention spin echo (CSE) versus fast spin echo (FSE). **A:** Coronal oblique CSE T2-weighted image of the shoulder. A full-thickness defect in the supraspinatus tendon is identified (*arrows*). **B:** Coronal oblique T2-weighted FSE image with fat saturation. The tendon defect is well seen as well, and the addition of fat suppression in fact makes the moderate-sized defect in the supraspinatus tendon more conspicuous (*arrows*). (Reused from Zlatkin MB. *MRI of the Shoulder.* 2nd ed. Philadelphia, PA: Lippincott Williams & Wilkins; 2003, with permission.)

forearm resting comfortably on the ipsilateral thigh (Fig. 36.7). Alternatively, the patient may be placed in the modified Crass position by positioning the hand of the affected extremity over the posterior hip as if reaching into his or her hip pants pocket to retrieve a comb (Fig. 36.8). The modified Crass position aids in visualization of the supraspinatus tendon by internally rotating the head of the humerus so that the tendon is moved from beneath the acromion as its insertion on the greater tuberosity moves anteriorly (Fig. 36.9). The physician stands behind or at the side of the patient.

The skin overlying the lateral aspect of the acromion is then prepped with antiseptic solution. A sterile syringe containing 3.0 mL of 0.25% preservative-free bupivacaine and 40 mg of methylprednisolone is attached to a 1½-inch, 22-gauge needle using strict aseptic technique. With the patient in the neutral position, a high-frequency linear ultrasound transducer

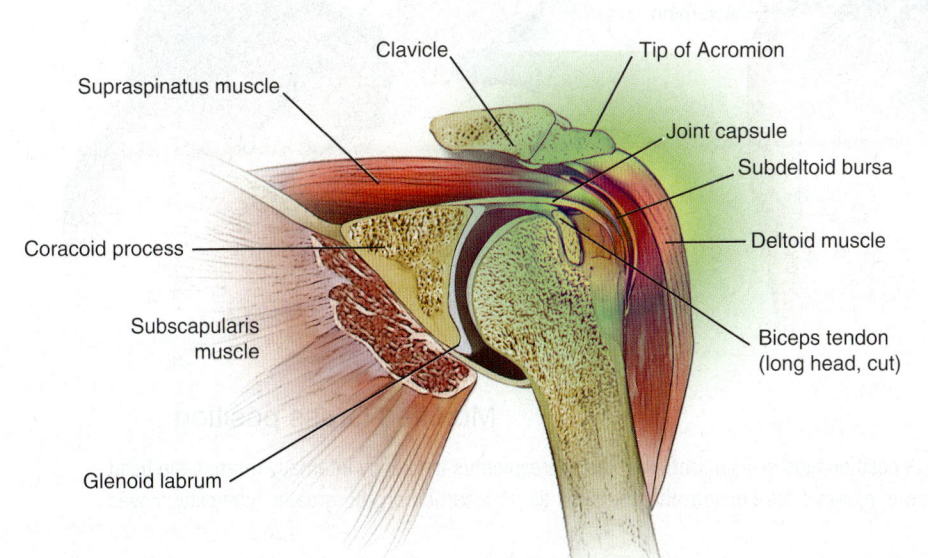

**FIGURE 36.6.** The anatomy of the supraspinatus musculotendinous unit.

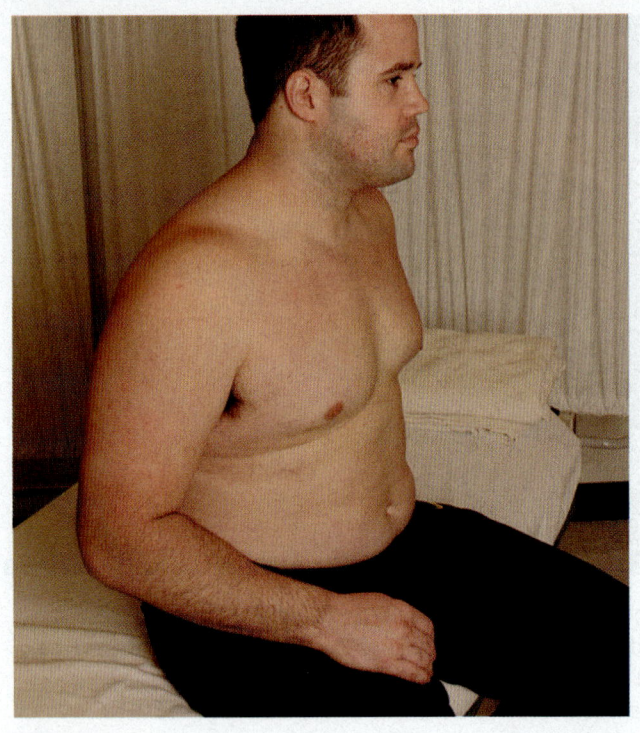

**FIGURE 36.7.** The neutral sitting position for ultrasound-guided injection of the supraspinatus tendon.

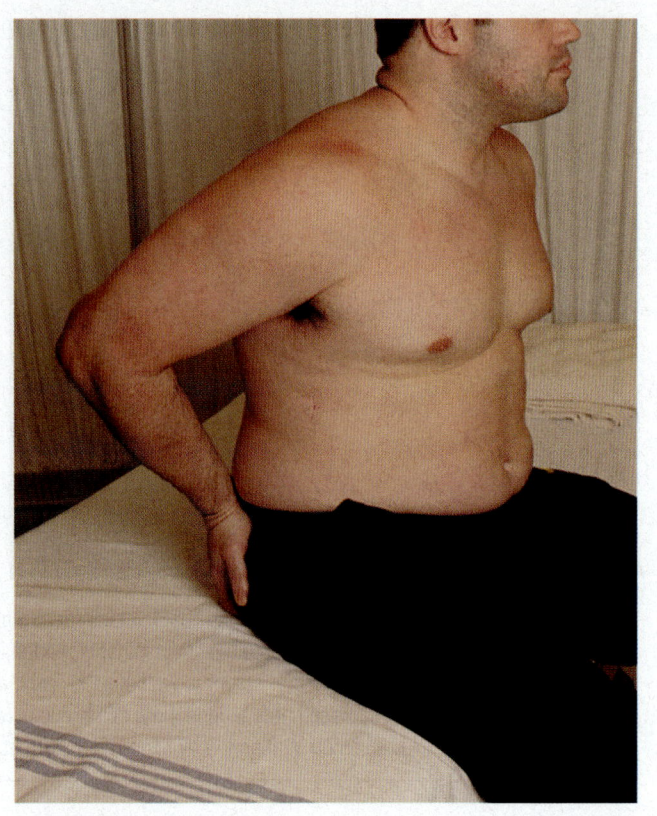

**FIGURE 36.8.** The modified Crass position.

Modified Crass position

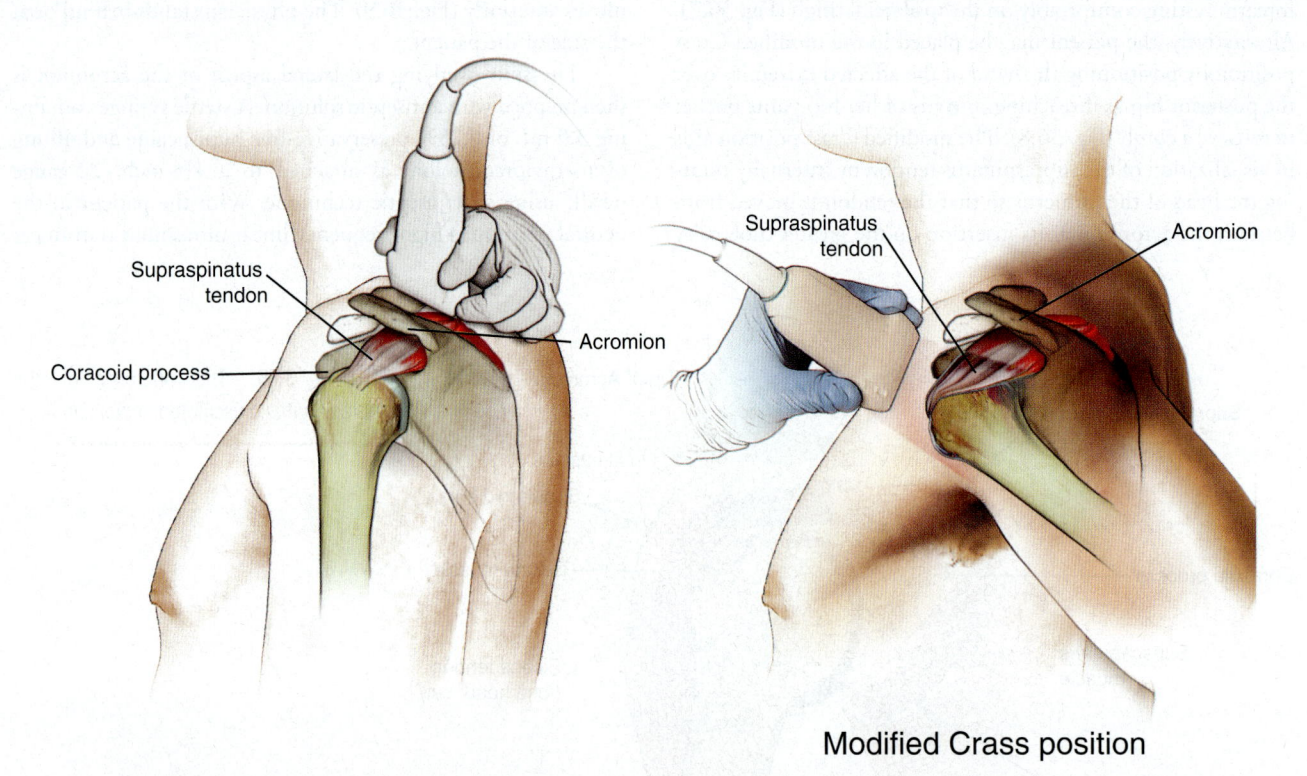

**FIGURE 36.9.** The modified Crass position aids in visualization of the supraspinatus tendon by internally rotating the head of the humerus so that the tendon is moved from beneath the acromion as its insertion on the greater tuberosity moves anteriorly.

CHAPTER 36    ULTRASOUND-GUIDED INJECTION TECHNIQUE FOR SUPRASPINATUS TENDONITIS    239

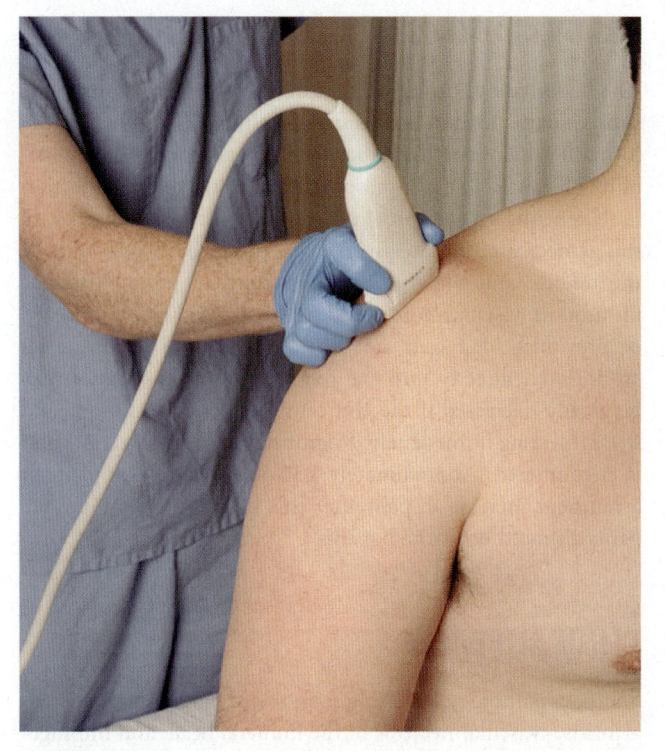

**FIGURE 36.10.** Proper coronal ultrasound transducer position for injection of the supraspinatus tendon with the patient in the neutral sitting position.

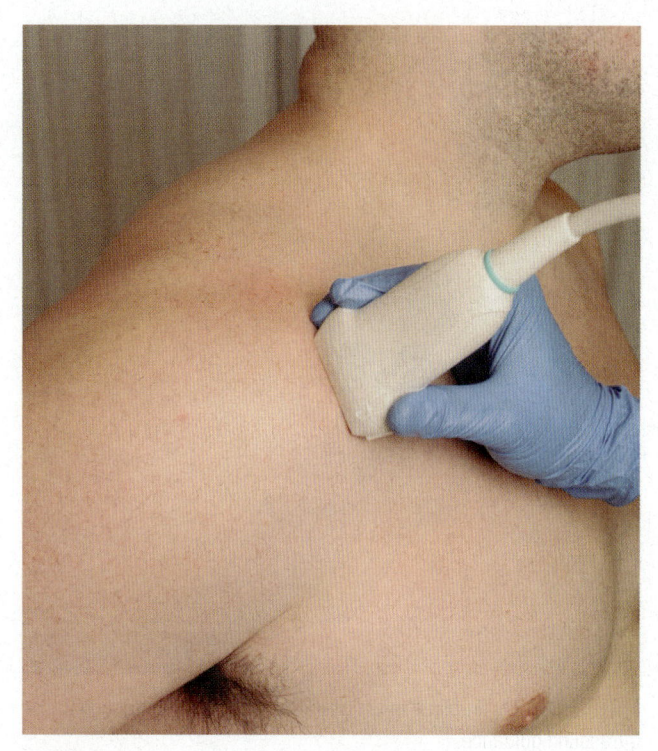

**FIGURE 36.11.** Proper ultrasound transducer position for injection of the supraspinatus tendon with the patient in the modified Crass position.

is placed over the lateral tip of the acromion in the coronal plane and angled slightly toward the scapula (Fig. 36.10). In the modified Crass position, the transducer is placed over the anterior shoulder (Fig. 36.11). The supraspinatus tendon is then identified as it exits from beneath the acromion and curves over the head of the humerus to attach to the greater tuberosity (Fig. 36.12). The tendon has a classic fibular, hyperechoic appearance with a symmetrical convex superior margin making easy to identify. The tendon will exhibit the property of anisotropy. The tendon should be carefully examined for

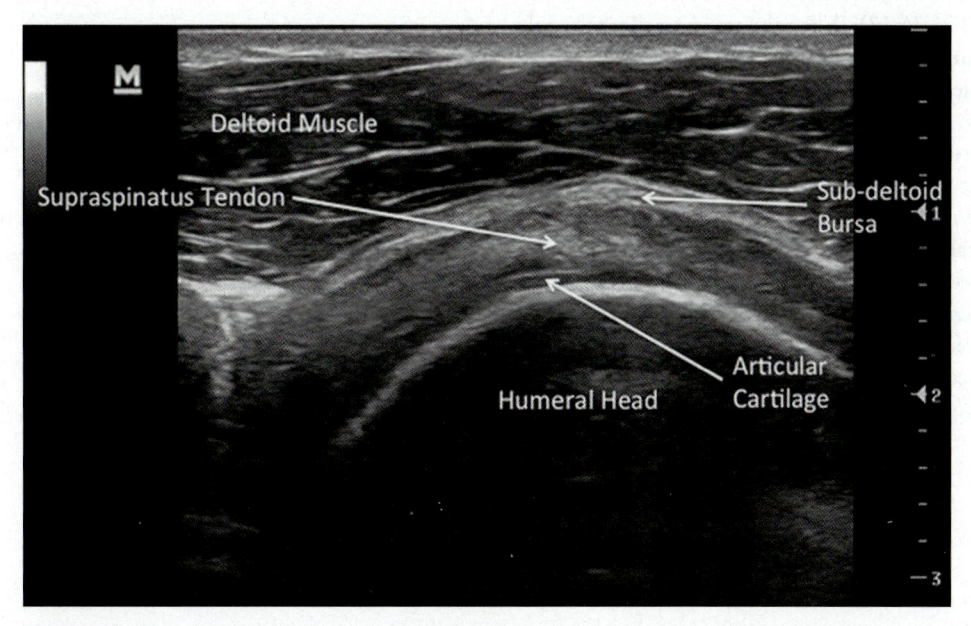

**FIGURE 36.12.** Typical coronal ultrasound appearance of the supraspinatus muscle and tendon.

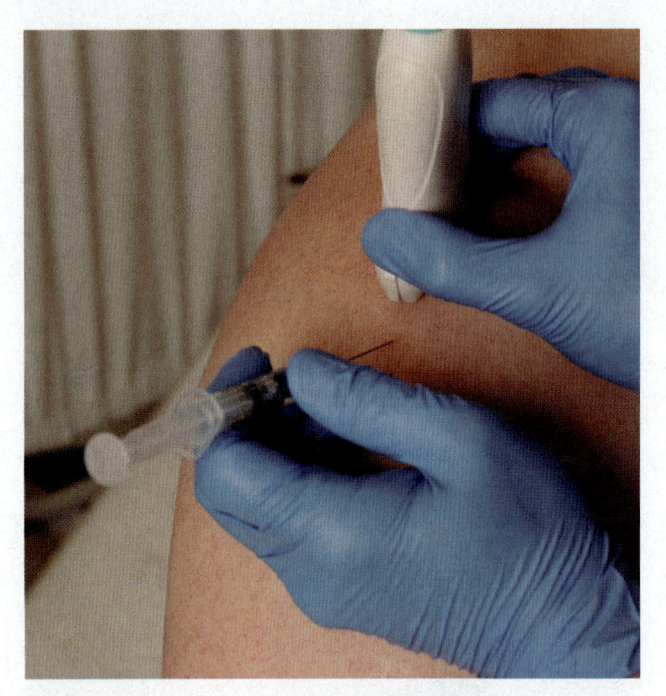

**FIGURE 36.13.** In-plane injection of the supraspinatus tendon under ultrasound guidance.

calcifications or tendinopathy that may be contributing to the patient's shoulder pain. A healthy supraspinatus tendon should have a uniform thickness in both the longitudinal and transverse views.

After the tendon is identified, the needle is placed through the skin ~1 cm lateral to the end of the transducer and is then advanced using an in-plane approach with the needle trajectory adjusted under real-time ultrasound guidance so that the needle tip rests just above the tendon, but not within the tendon substance itself (Fig. 36.13). When the tip of needle is thought to be in satisfactory position, a small amount of local anesthetic and steroid is injected under real-time ultrasound guidance to confirm that the needle tip is not with the substance of the tendon. After proper needle tip placement is confirmed, the remainder of the contents of the syringe are slowly injected. There should be minimal resistance to injection. If synechiae, loculations, or calcifications are present, the needle may have to be repositioned to ensure that the entire tendon is treated. The needle is then removed, and a sterile pressure dressing and ice pack are placed at the injection site. If calcific tendonitis is present, a two-needle ultrasound-guided lavage and aspiration technique may be beneficial.

## COMPLICATIONS

The major complication of ultrasound-guided injection of the supraspinatus tendon is infection. Ecchymosis and hematoma formation following this procedure may also occur. The possibility of trauma to the supraspinatus tendon from the injection itself remains an ever-present possibility, although the risk of this is decreased if care is taken to place the needle outside the tendon and the injection is performed under real-time ultrasound visualization. Tendons that are highly inflamed or previously damaged are subject to rupture if substances are injected directly into the tendon. This complication can be greatly decreased if the clinician uses gentle technique and stops injecting immediately if significant resistance to injection is encountered. Approximately 25% of patients complain of a transient increase in pain after this injection technique; the patient should be warned of this.

## CLINICAL PEARLS

Shoulder pathology including rotator cuff tendinopathy, osteoarthritis, avascular necrosis of the humeral head, and impingement syndromes may coexist with supraspinatus tendonitis and may contribute to the patients pain symptomatology. Universal precautions should always be observed to protect the operator, and strict adherence to sterile technique must be used to avoid infection. Gentle physical therapy and local heat should be introduced following ultrasound-guided injection of the supraspinatus tendon to reduce pain and improve function. Simple analgesics and nonsteroidal anti-inflammatory agents or COX-2 inhibitors may be used concurrently with this injection technique.

## SUGGESTED READINGS

Lento PH, Strakowski JA. The use of ultrasound in guiding musculoskeletal interventional procedures. *Phys Med Rehabil Clin N Am* 2010;21(3):559–583.

Narouze SN. Ultrasound-guided shoulder joint and bursa injections. In: *Atlas of Ultrasound Guided Procedures in Pain Management*. New York, NY: Springer; 2010:295–296.

Precerutti M, Garioni E, Madonia L, et al. US anatomy of the shoulder: pictorial essay. *J Ultrasound* 2010;13(4):179–187.

Waldman SD. The supraspinatus muscle. In: *Pain Review*. Philadelphia, PA: Saunders Elsevier; 2009:86.

Waldman SD. Dawbarn sign. In: *Physical Diagnosis of Pain: An Atlas of Signs and Symptoms*. 2nd ed. Philadelphia, PA: WB Saunders; 2010:88–89.

Waldman SD. Injection technique for supraspinatus tendonitis. In: *Atlas of Pain Management Injection Techniques*. 3rd ed. Philadelphia, PA: Saunders Elsevier; 2013:65–67.

CHAPTER 37

# Ultrasound-Guided Injection Technique for Infraspinatus Tendonitis

## CLINICAL PERSPECTIVES

The musculotendinous unit of the rotator cuff is subjected to an amazing variation of stresses as it performs its function to allow range of motion of the shoulder while at the same time providing shoulder stability. The relatively poor blood supply limits the ability of these muscles and tendons to heal when traumatized. Over time, muscle tears and tendinopathy develop, further weakening the musculotendinous units and making them susceptible to additional damage.

The infraspinatus tendon of the rotator cuff may develop tendonitis after overuse or misuse, especially when performing activities that require repeated upper extremity abduction and lateral rotation. The pain of infraspinatus tendonitis is constant and severe. The patient often complains of sleep disturbance and is unable to sleep on the affected shoulder. Patients with infraspinatus tendonitis exhibit pain with lateral rotation of the humerus and on active abduction of the upper extremity. In an effort to decrease pain, patients suffering from infraspinatus tendonitis often splint the inflamed tendon by rotating the scapular anteriorly to remove tension from the inflamed tendon.

If untreated, patients suffering from infraspinatus tendonitis may experience difficulty in performing any task that requires initial abduction of the upper extremity, making simple everyday tasks such as brushing ones teeth or eating difficult. Over time, muscle atrophy and calcific tendonitis may result.

Plain radiographs are indicated in all patients who present with shoulder pain. Based on the patient's clinical presentation, additional testing may be indicated, including complete blood cell count, sedimentation rate, and antinuclear antibody testing. Magnetic resonance imaging or ultrasound imaging of the shoulder is indicated if a rotator cuff tear is suspected. Magnetic resonance imaging or ultrasound evaluation of the affected area may also help delineate the presence of calcific tendonitis or other shoulder pathology (Fig. 37.1).

## CLINICALLY RELEVANT ANATOMY

The infraspinatus muscle, as part of the rotator cuff, provides shoulder stability (Fig. 37.2). In conjunction with the teres minor muscle, the infraspinatus muscle externally rotates the arm at the shoulder. Like the supraspinatus muscle, the infraspinatus muscle is innervated by the suprascapular nerve, which is comprised of fibers from the superior trunk of the brachial plexus. The infraspinatus muscle finds its origin in the infraspinous fossa of the scapula and inserts into the middle facet of the greater tuberosity of the humerus (Fig. 37.3). It is at this insertion on the greater tuberosity that infraspinatus tendonitis most commonly occurs (see Fig. 37.3).

## ULTRASOUND-GUIDED TECHNIQUE

The benefits, risks, and alternative treatments are explained to the patient and informed consent is obtained. The patient is then placed in the neutral sitting position with the hand resting comfortably palm up on the ipsilateral thigh (Fig. 37.4). The physician stands behind or at the side of the patient.

With the patient in the neutral sitting position, a high-frequency linear ultrasound transducer is placed in an oblique axial plane with top of the transducer angled superiorly toward the head of the humerus (Fig. 37.5). The dense central tendon of the infraspinatus tendon is then identified at its musculotendinous junction just posterior to the glenoid. The tendon is then followed laterally to its insertion on the middle facet on the posterior aspect of the greater tuberosity of the humerus (Fig. 36.6). This is the point where infraspinatus tendonitis most often develops (Fig. 37.7). The tendon should be carefully examined for calcifications or tendinopathy that may be contributing to the patient's shoulder pain.

After the tendinous insertion is identified, the skin overlying the area beneath the ultrasound transducer is prepped with antiseptic solution. A sterile syringe containing 3.0 mL of 0.25% preservative-free bupivacaine and 40 mg of methylprednisolone is attached to a 1½-inch, 22-gauge needle using strict aseptic technique. The needle is placed through the skin 1 cm below the inferior edge of the transducer and is then advanced using an out-of-plane approach with the needle trajectory adjusted under real-time ultrasound guidance so that the needle tip rests just above the tendon, but not within the tendon substance itself (Fig. 37.8). When the tip of needle is thought to be in satisfactory position, after careful aspiration, a small amount of local anesthetic and steroid is injected under

**FIGURE 37.2.** *(Continued)* **E:** Teres minor muscle (TM). (From Lee JP, Joseph KT, Sagel SS, et al. *Computed Body Tomography with MRI Correlation.* 4th ed. Philadelphia, PA: Lippincott Williams & Wilkins; 2006, with permission.)

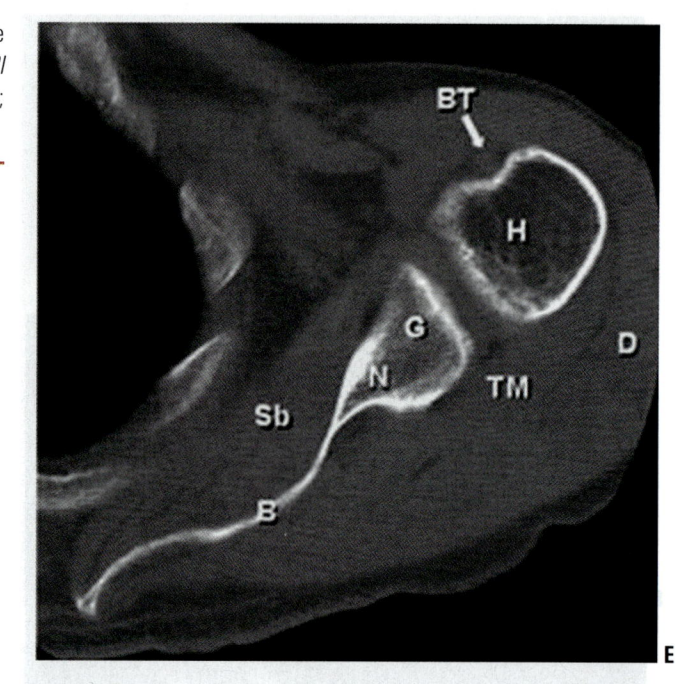

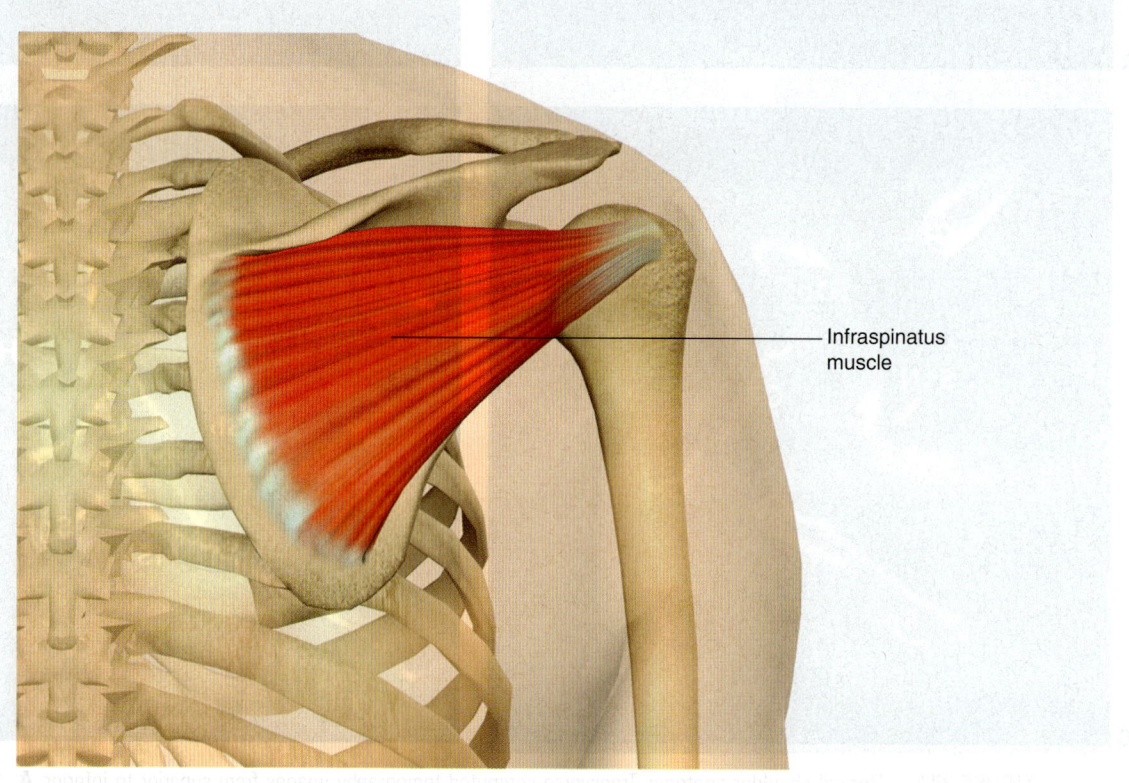

**FIGURE 37.3.** The anatomy of the infraspinatus muscle. (LifeArt Image © 2012, Lippincott Williams & Wilkins, all rights reserved.)

CHAPTER 37  ULTRASOUND-GUIDED INJECTION TECHNIQUE FOR INFRASPINATUS TENDONITIS  245

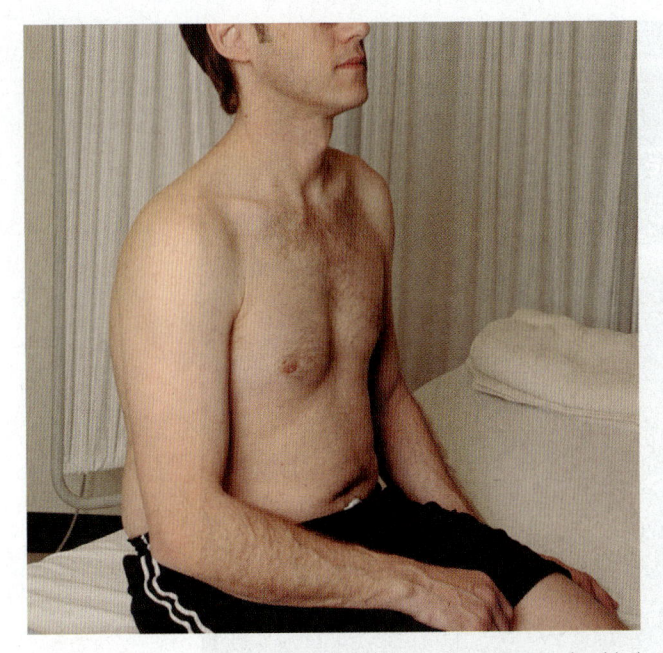

**FIGURE 37.4.** Proper patient positioning for ultrasound-guided injection for infraspinatus tendonitis.

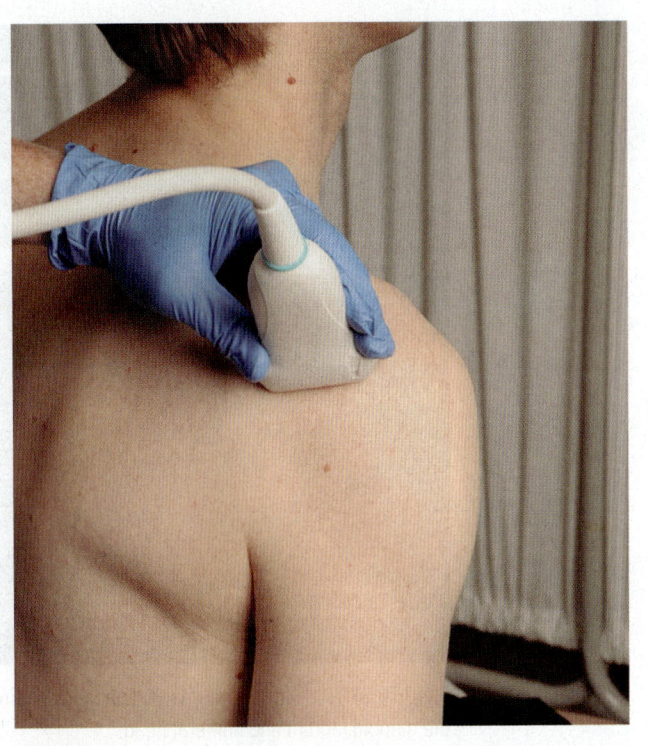

**FIGURE 37.5.** Proper oblique axial ultrasound transducer placement for ultrasound-guided injection for infraspinatus tendonitis.

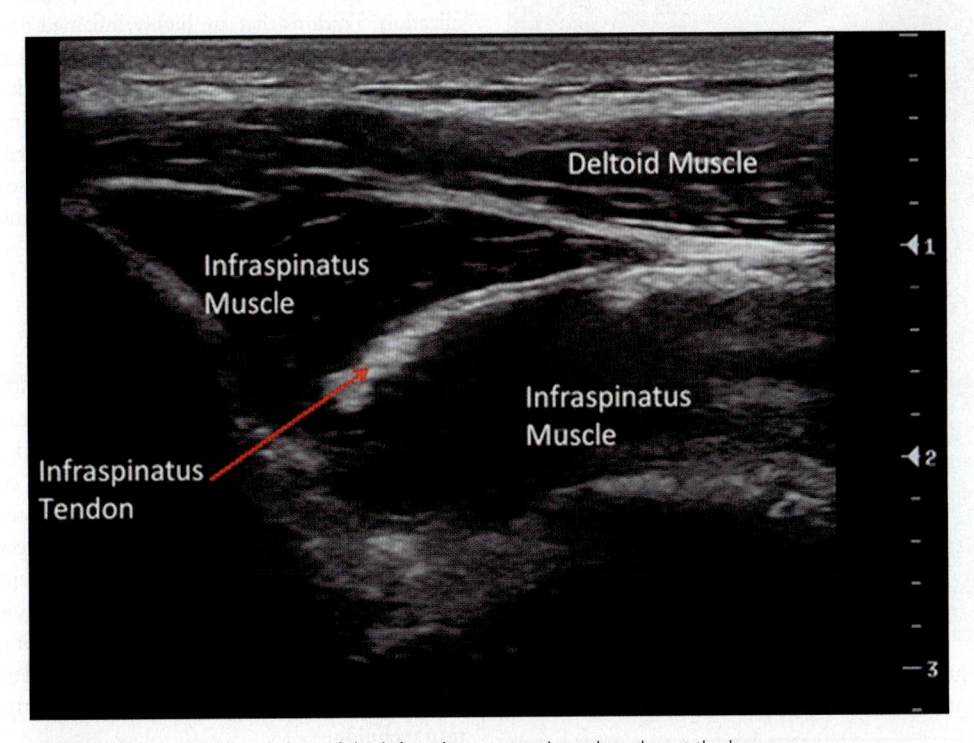

**FIGURE 37.6.** Ultrasound view of the infraspinatus muscle and tendon at the humerus.

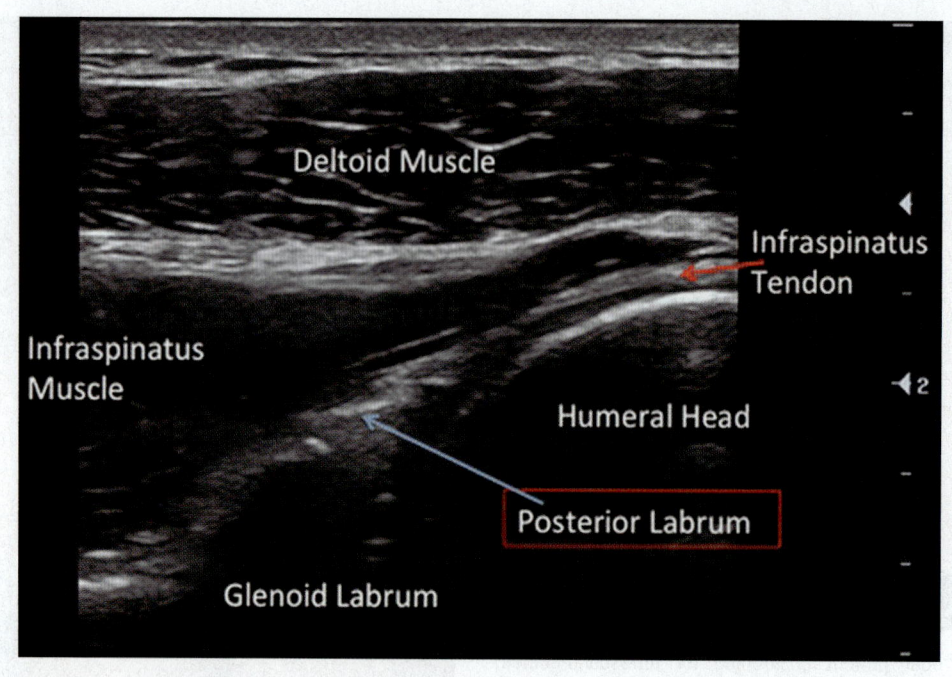

**FIGURE 37.7.** Ultrasound image demonstrating relationship of the infraspinatus muscle and tendon to the glenoid labrum and humeral head.

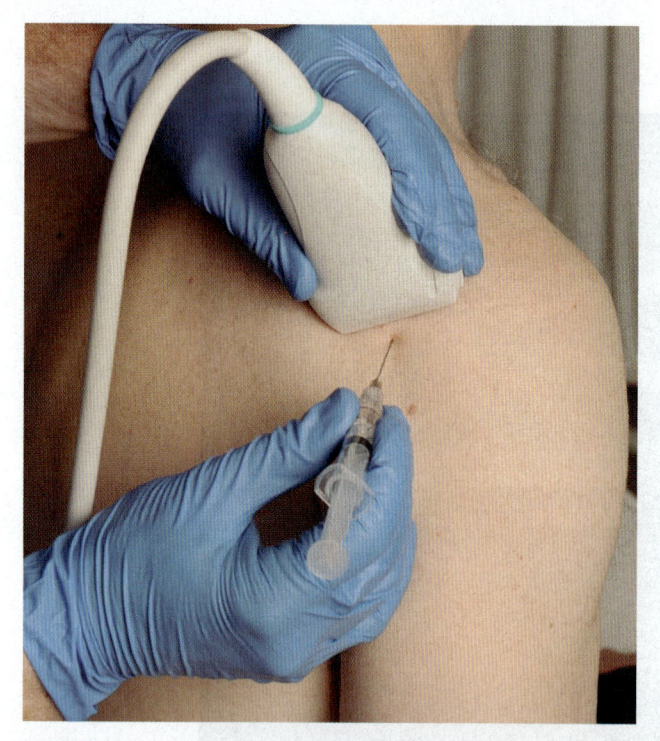

**FIGURE 37.8.** Out-of-plane injection of the supraspinatus tendon under ultrasound guidance.

decreased if care is taken to place the needle outside the tendon and the injection is performed under real-time ultrasound visualization. Tendons that are highly inflamed or previously damaged are subject to rupture if substances are injected directly into the tendon. This complication can be greatly decreased if the clinician uses gentle technique and stops injecting immediately if significant resistance to injection is encountered. Approximately 25% of patients complain of a transient increase in pain after this injection technique; the patient should be warned of this.

## CLINICAL PEARLS

Shoulder pathology including rotator cuff tendinopathy, osteoarthritis, avascular necrosis of the humeral head, and impingement syndromes may coexist with infraspinatus tendonitis and may contribute to the patient's pain symptomatology. Universal precautions should always be observed to protect the operator, and strict adherence to sterile technique must be used to avoid infection. Gentle physical therapy and local heat should be introduced following ultrasound-guided injection of the infraspinatus muscle to reduce pain and improve function. Simple analgesics and nonsteroidal anti-inflammatory agents or COX-2 inhibitors may be used concurrently with this injection technique.

## SUGGESTED READINGS

Lento PH, Strakowski JA. The use of ultrasound in guiding musculoskeletal interventional procedures. *Phys Med Rehabil Clin N Am* 2010;21(3):559–583.

Narouze SN. Ultrasound-guided shoulder joint and bursa injections. In: *Atlas of Ultrasound Guided Procedures in Pain Management*. New York, NY: Springer; 2010:295–296.

Precerutti M, Garioni E, Madonia L, et al. US anatomy of the shoulder: pictorial essay. *J Ultrasound* 2010;13(4):179–187.

Waldman SD. The infraspinatus muscle. In: *Pain Review*. Philadelphia, PA: Saunders Elsevier; 2009:87.

Waldman SD. Mid arc abduction test. In: *Physical Diagnosis of Pain: An Atlas of Signs and Symptoms*. 2nd ed. Philadelphia, PA: WB Saunders; 2010:91–92.

Waldman SD. Injection technique for infraspinatus tendinitis. In: *Atlas of Pain Management Injection Techniques*. 3rd ed. Philadelphia, PA: Saunders Elsevier; 2013:68–70.

# CHAPTER 38

# Ultrasound-Guided Injection Technique for Subscapularis Tendonitis

## CLINICAL PERSPECTIVES

The musculotendinous unit of the rotator cuff is subjected to an amazing variation of stresses as it performs its function to allow range of motion of the shoulder while at the same time providing shoulder stability. The relatively poor blood supply limits the ability of these muscles and tendons to heal when traumatized. Over time, muscle tears and tendinopathy develop, further weakening the musculotendinous units and making them susceptible to additional damage.

The subscapularis tendon of the rotator cuff may develop tendonitis after overuse or misuse, especially when performing activities that require repeated upper extremity adduction and medial rotation of the humerus. The pain of subscapularis tendonitis is constant and severe and is localized to the deltoid region. The patient suffering from subscapularis tendonitis often complains of sleep disturbance and is unable to sleep on the affected shoulder. Patients with subscapularis tendonitis exhibit pain with active resisted medial rotation and on active adduction of the humerus. In an effort to decrease pain, patients suffering from subscapularis tendonitis often splint the inflamed tendon by limiting medial rotation of the humerus to remove tension from the inflamed tendon. The patient with subscapularis tendonitis will exhibit pain on the Gerber lift off test, whereas the patient with complete rupture of the subscapularis tendon or muscle will exhibit weakness (Fig. 38.1). If untreated, patients suffering from subscapularis tendonitis may experience difficulty in performing any task that requires adduction medial rotation of the upper extremity, making simple everyday tasks such as turning off a faucet difficult. Over time, muscle atrophy and calcific tendonitis may result.

Plain radiographs are indicated in all patients who present with shoulder pain. Based on the patient's clinical presentation, additional testing may be indicated, including complete blood cell count, sedimentation rate, and antinuclear antibody testing. Magnetic resonance imaging or ultrasound imaging of the shoulder is indicated if a rotator cuff tear is suspected. Magnetic resonance imaging or ultrasound evaluation of the affected area may also help delineate the presence of calcific tendonitis or other shoulder pathology.

## CLINICALLY RELEVANT ANATOMY

The subscapularis muscle, as part of the rotator cuff, provides shoulder stability in combination with the supraspinatus, infraspinatus, and teres minor muscle (Fig. 38.2). The subscapularis muscle adducts the upper extremity and medially rotates the arm at the shoulder. The subscapularis muscle is innervated by branches of the posterior cord of the brachial plexus and the upper and lower subscapular nerves. The subscapularis muscle finds its origin in the subscapular fossa of the anterior scapula and inserts into the lesser tuberosity of the humerus (Fig. 38.3). It is at this insertion that subscapularis tendonitis and rupture most commonly occurs (Fig. 38.4).

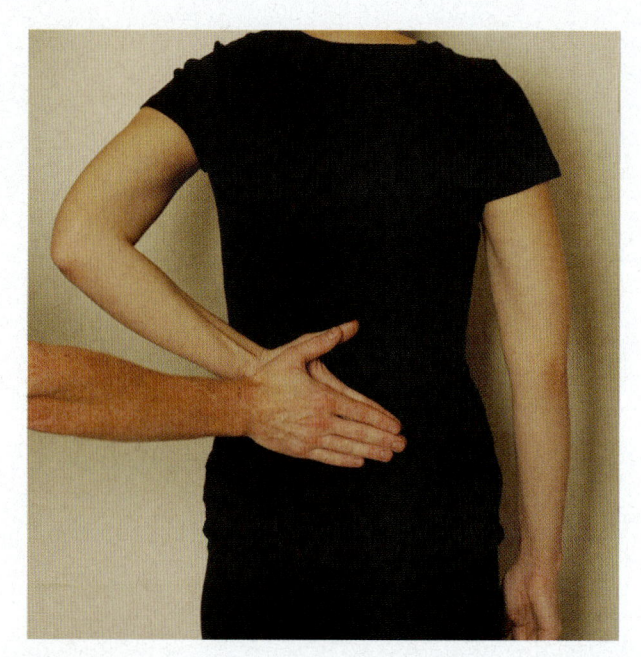

**FIGURE 38.1.** The patient with subscapularis tendonitis will exhibit pain on the Gerber lift off test, whereas the patient with complete rupture of the subscapularis tendon or muscle will exhibit weakness.

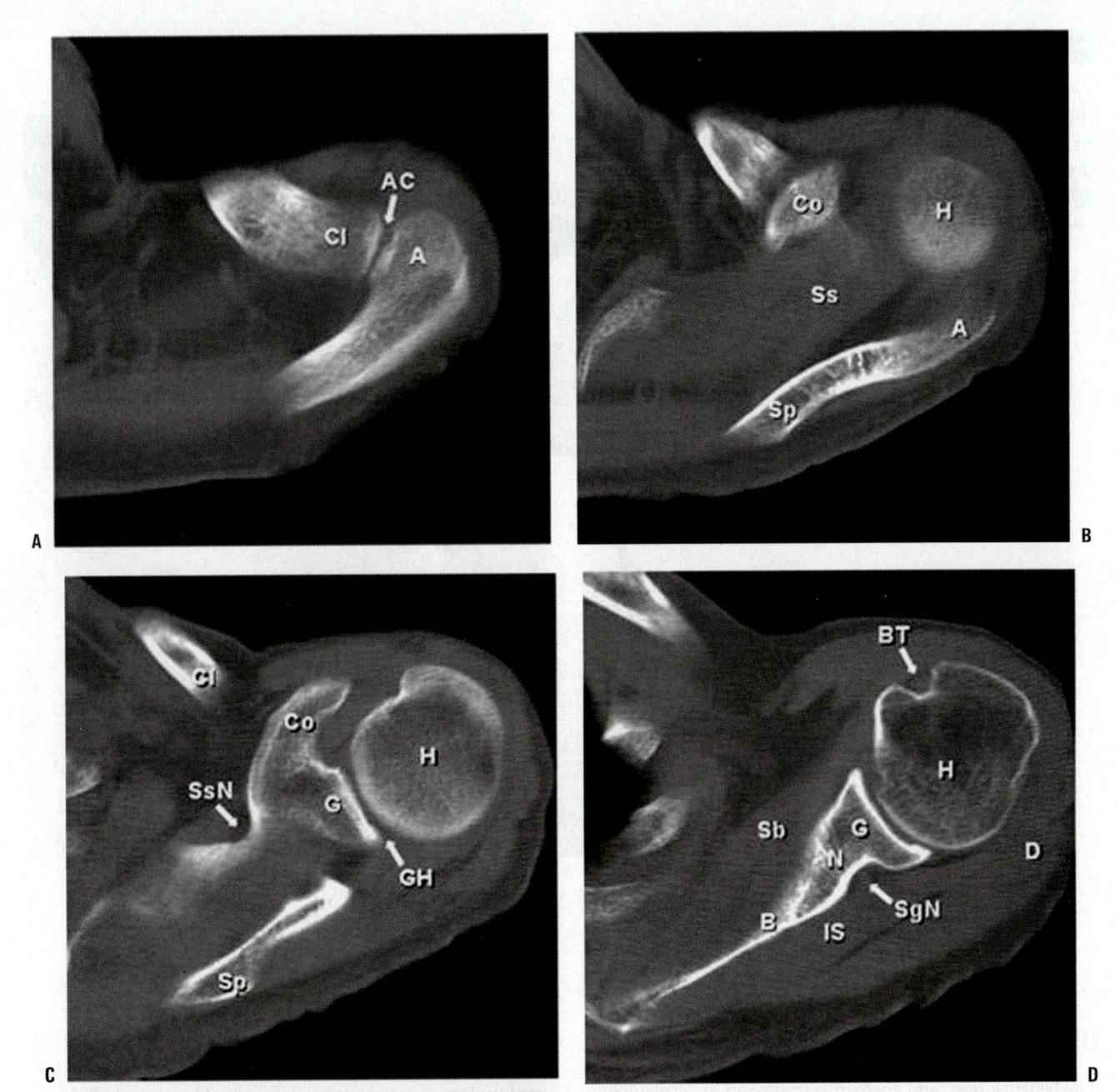

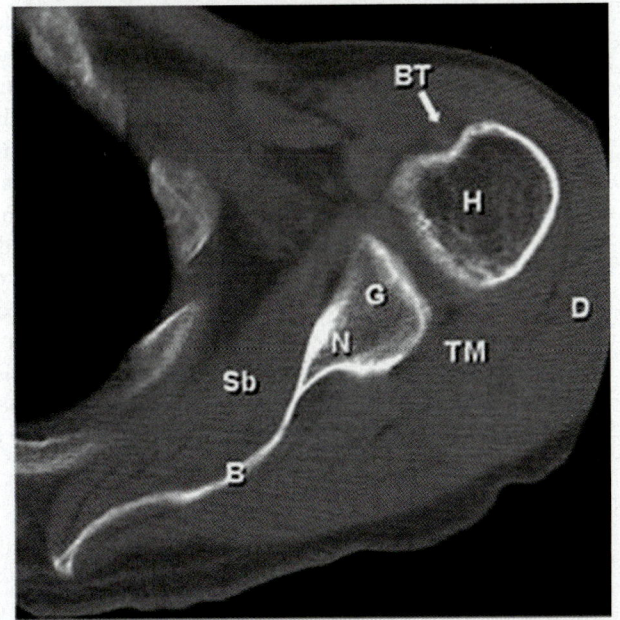

**FIGURE 38.2.** Normal shoulder anatomy. Transverse computed tomography images from superior to inferior. **A:** Acromion (A), clavicle (Cl), AC joint (AC). **B:** Coracoid (Co), humerus (H), supraspinatus muscle (Ss), scapular spine (Sp). **C:** Glenoid (G), glenohumeral joint (GH), suprascapular notch (SsN). **D:** Biceps tendon (BT), deltoid muscle (D), subscapularis muscle (Sb), subscapularis muscle (IS), spinoglenoid notch (SgN), scapular neck (N), scapular body (B). **E:** Teres minor muscle (TM). (Reused from Lee JKT, Sagel SS, Stanley RJ, et al. *Computed Body Tomography with MRI Correlation.* 4th ed. Philadelphia, PA: Lippincott Williams & Wilkins; 2006, with permission.)

**FIGURE 38.3.** The anatomy of the subscapularis muscle. (LifeART image ©2012 Lippincott Williams & Wilkins. All rights reserved.)

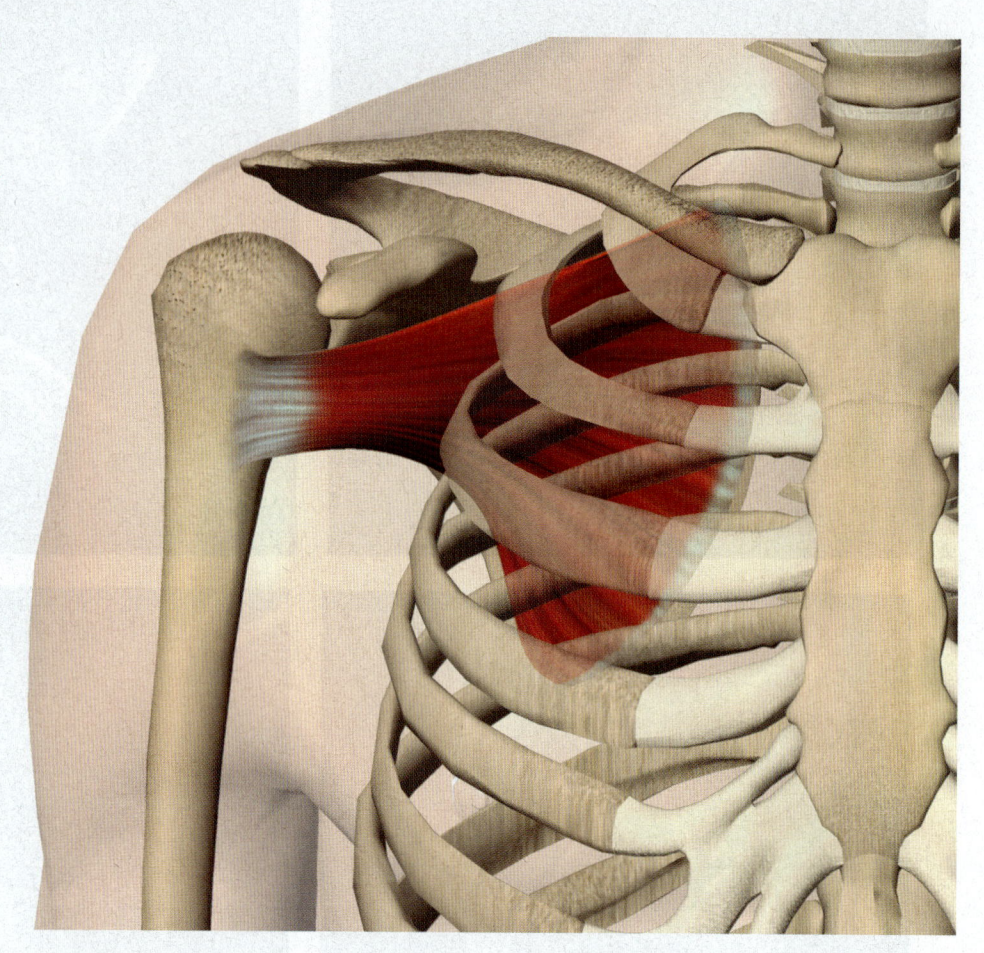

## ULTRASOUND-GUIDED TECHNIQUE

The benefits, risks, and alternative treatments are explained to the patient and informed consent is obtained. The patient is then placed in the sitting position with the shoulder externally rotated (Fig. 38.5). The physician stands behind or at the side of the patient.

With the patient in the above position, a high-frequency linear ultrasound transducer is placed in a transverse plane with the transducer over the lesser tuberosity of the humerus (Fig. 38.6). The distal tendon of the subscapularis muscle is then identified and followed to its insertion on the lesser tuberosity of the humerus. This is the point where subscapularis tendonitis most often develops (Fig. 38.7). The tendon should be carefully examined for calcifications or tendinopathy that may be contributing to the patient's shoulder pain (Fig. 38.8).

After the tendinous insertion is identified, the skin overlying the area beneath the ultrasound transducer is prepped with antiseptic solution. A sterile syringe containing 3.0 mL of 0.25% preservative-free bupivacaine and 40 mg of methylprednisolone is attached to a 1½-inch, 22-gauge needle using strict aseptic technique. The needle is placed through the skin ~1 cm below the superior edge of the transducer and is then advanced using an out-of-plane approach with the needle trajectory adjusted under real-time ultrasound guidance so that the needle tip rests just above the tendon, but not within the tendon substance itself (Fig. 38.9). When the tip of needle is thought to be in satisfactory position, after careful aspiration, a small amount of local anesthetic and steroid is injected under real-time ultrasound guidance to confirm that the needle tip is not with the substance of the tendon. After proper needle tip placement is confirmed, the remainder of the contents of the syringe are slowly injected. There should be minimal resistance to injection. If calcific tendonitis is present, a two needle ultrasound-guided lavage and aspiration technique may be beneficial.

# CHAPTER 38  ULTRASOUND-GUIDED INJECTION TECHNIQUE FOR SUBSCAPULARIS TENDONITIS

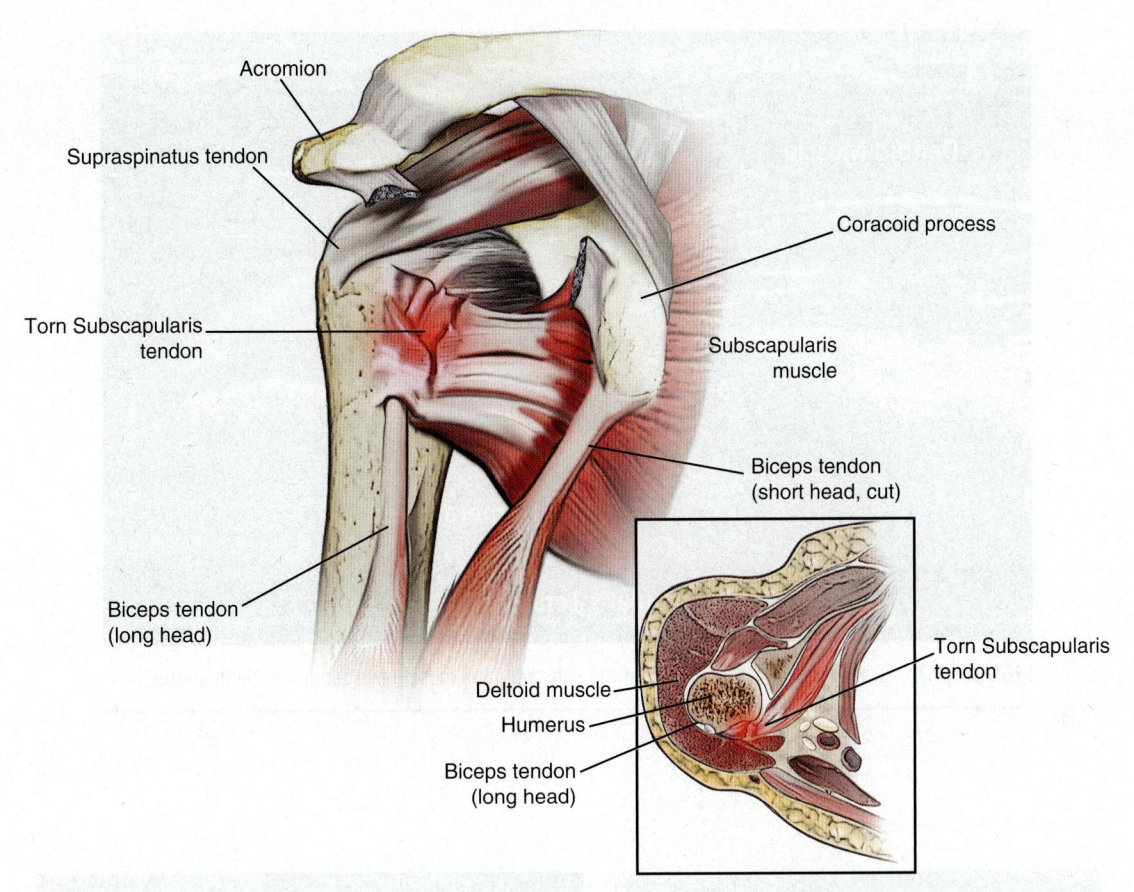

**FIGURE 38.4.** The subscapularis musculotendinous unit inserts into the lesser tuberosity of the humerus, and it is at this point that tendonitis and tears most commonly occur.

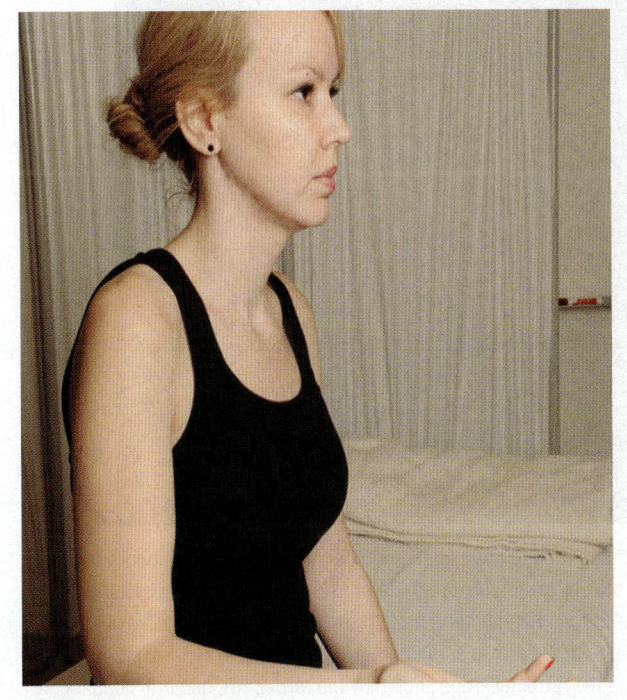

**FIGURE 38.5.** Proper patient positioning for ultrasound-guided injection for subscapularis tendonitis.

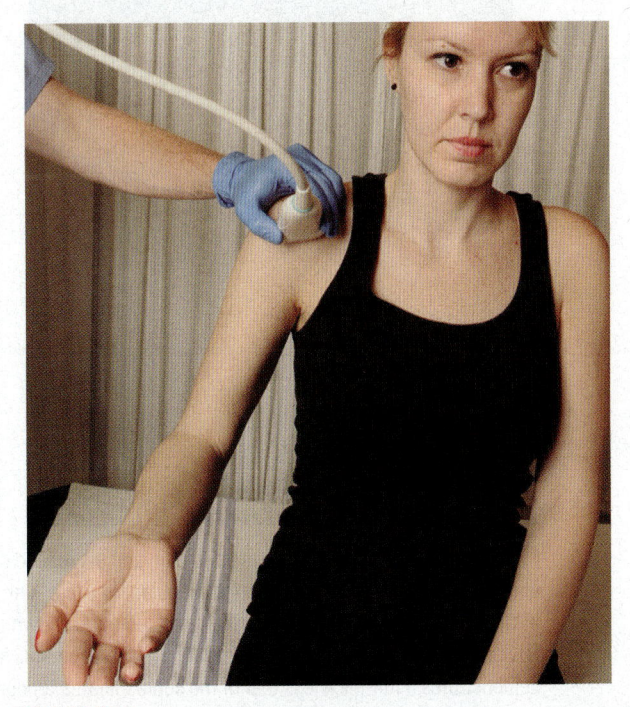

**FIGURE 38.6.** Proper transverse ultrasound transducer placement for ultrasound-guided injection for subscapularis tendonitis.

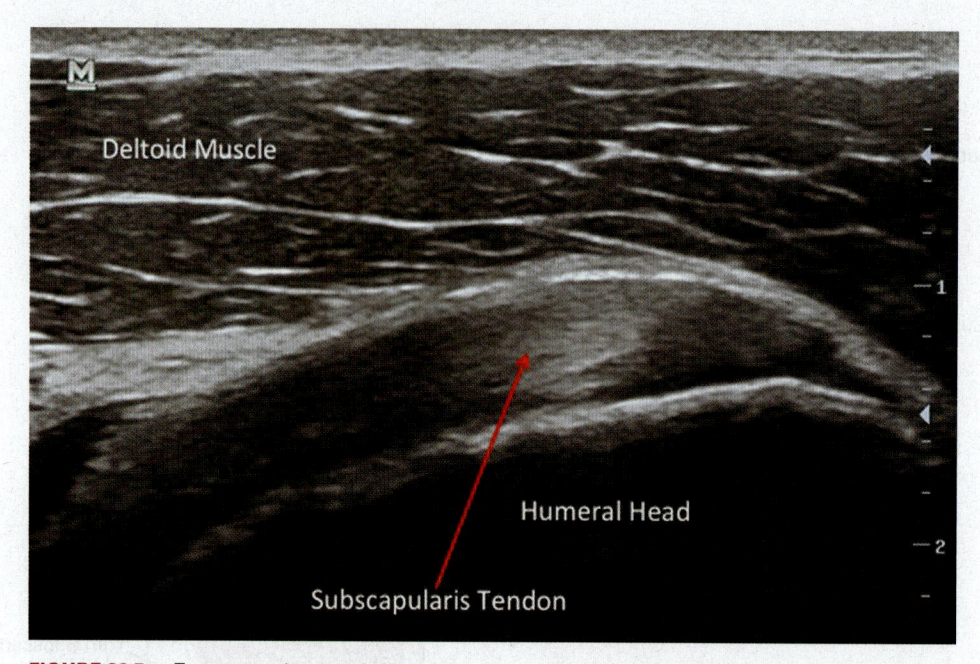

**FIGURE 38.7.** Transverse ultrasound view of the subscapularis muscle and tendon at the humerus.

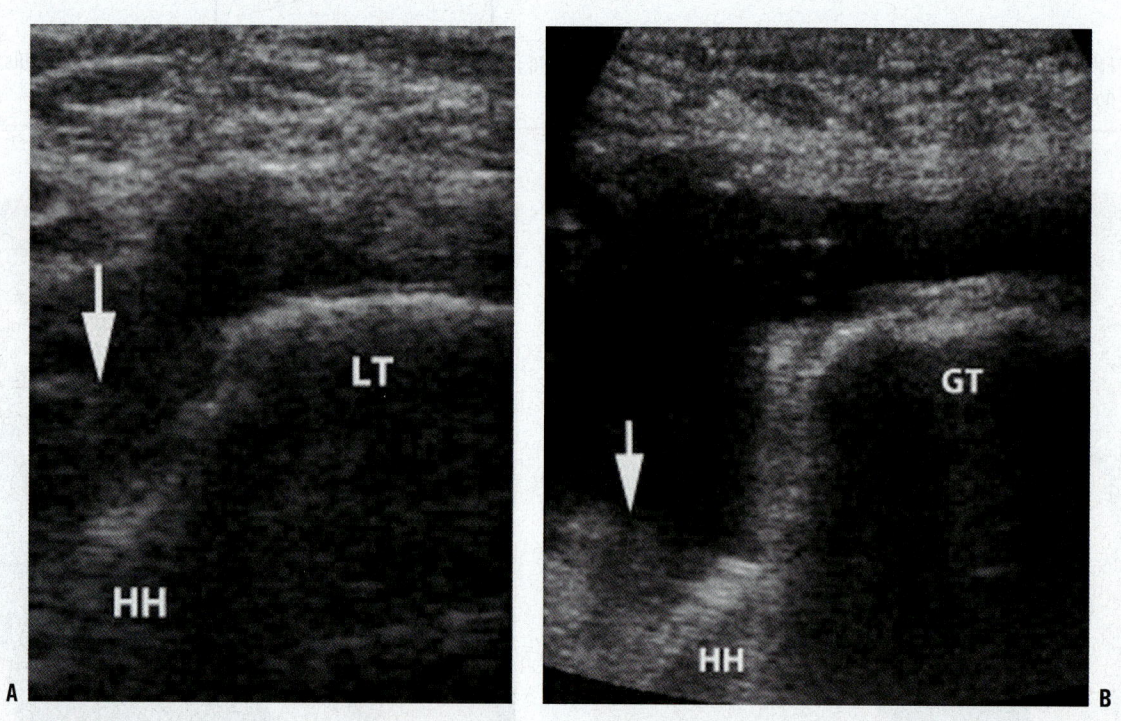

**FIGURE 38.8.** A 50-year-old man with pain and decreased range of motion following left shoulder arthroplasty. **A:** Sonogram aligned with the long axis of the subscapularis muscle with the arm in external rotation demonstrates a full-thickness tear of the subscapularis tendon, with the retracted edge shown by the *arrow*. HH, humeral head prosthesis; LT, lesser tuberosity. **B:** Sonogram aligned with the long axis of the supraspinatus muscle with the arm in adduction, extension, and internal rotation demonstrates a full-thickness tear of the supraspinatus tendon, with the retracted edge shown by the *arrow*. HH, humeral head prosthesis; GT, greater tuberosity. (Reused from Ives EP, Nazarian LN, Parker L, et al. Subscapularis tendon tears: a common sonographic finding in symptomatic postarthroplasty shoulders. *J Clin Ultrasound* 2013;41(3):129–133, with permission.)

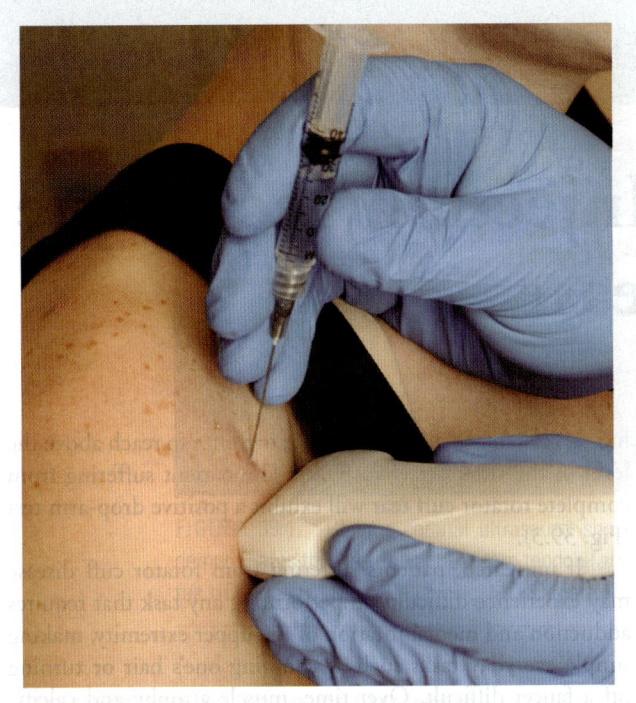

**FIGURE 38.9.** Injection of the subscapularis tendon under ultrasound guidance.

## COMPLICATIONS

The major complication of ultrasound-guided injection of the subscapularis tendon is infection. Ecchymosis and hematoma formation following this procedure may also occur. The possibility of trauma to the subscapularis tendon from the injection itself remains an ever-present possibility, although the risk of this is decreased if care is taken to place the needle outside the tendon and the injection is performed under real-time ultrasound visualization. Tendons that are highly inflamed or previously damaged are subject to rupture if substances are injected directly into the tendon. This complication can be greatly decreased if the clinician uses gentle technique and stops injecting immediately if significant resistance to injection is encountered. Approximately 25% of patients complain of a transient increase in pain after this injection technique; the patient should be warned of this.

## CLINICAL PEARLS

Shoulder pathology including rotator cuff tendinopathy, osteoarthritis, avascular necrosis of the humeral head, and impingement syndromes may coexist with subscapularis tendonitis and may contribute to the patient's pain symptomatology. Universal precautions should always be observed to protect the operator, and strict adherence to sterile technique must be used to avoid infection. Gentle physical therapy and local heat should be introduced following ultrasound-guided injection of the subdeltoid bursa to reduce pain and improve function. Simple analgesics and nonsteroidal anti-inflammatory agents or COX-2 inhibitors may be used concurrently with this injection technique.

## SUGGESTED READINGS

Lento PH, Strakowski JA. The use of ultrasound in guiding musculoskeletal interventional procedures. *Phys Med Rehabil Clin N Am* 2010;21(3):559–583.
Narouze SN. Ultrasound-guided shoulder joint and bursa injections. In: *Atlas of Ultrasound Guided Procedures in Pain Management*. New York, NY: Springer; 2010:295–296.
Precerutti M, Garioni E, Madonia L, et al. US anatomy of the shoulder: pictorial essay. *J Ultrasound* 2010;13(4):179–187.
Waldman SD. The subscapularis muscle. In: *Pain Review*. Philadelphia, PA: Elsevier Saunders; 2009:88.
Waldman SD. Injection technique for subscapularis tendinitis. In: *Atlas of Pain Management Injection Techniques*. 3rd ed. Philadelphia, PA: Elsevier Saunders; 2013:71–72.

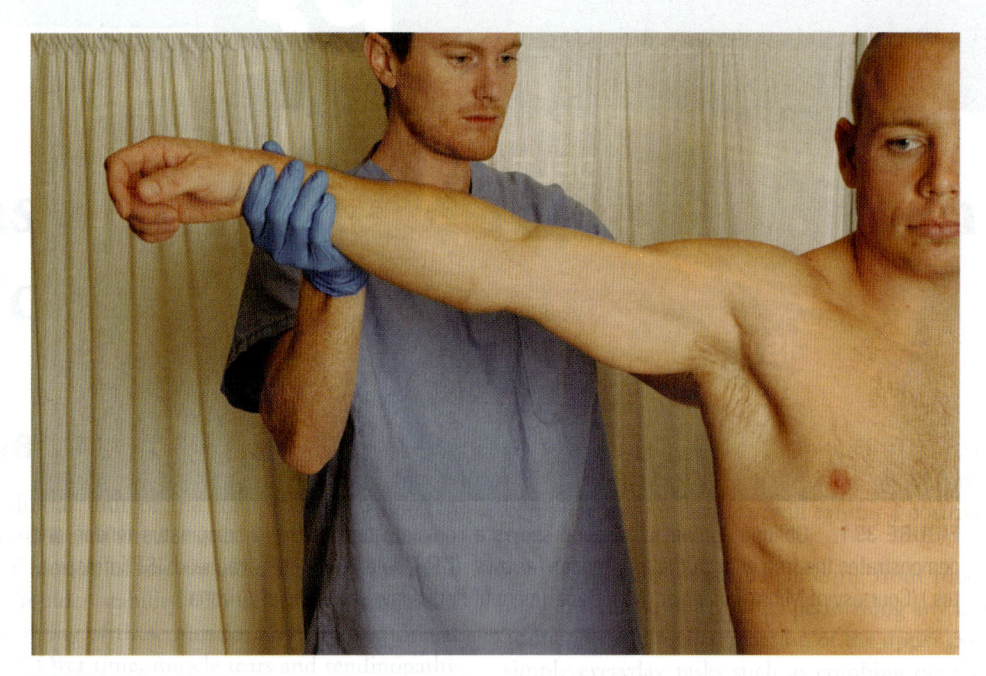

**FIGURE 39.3.** The drop-arm test for rotator cuff tear is positive if the patient is unable to hold the arm abducted at the level of the shoulder after the supported arm is released.

methylprednisolone is attached to a 1½-inch, 22-gauge needle using strict aseptic technique. The needle is placed through the skin ~1 cm below the inferior edge of the transducer and is then advanced using an out-of-plane approach with the needle trajectory adjusted under real-time ultrasound guidance so that the needle tip rests within the rotator interval between the subscapularis and supraspinatus tendons (Figs. 39.11 and 39.12). The biceps tendon should be easily identifiable and can serve as a useful landmark to confirm anatomic position. The clinician should avoid injecting into the substance of the biceps tendons (see Fig. 39.10). When the tip of needle is thought to be in satisfactory position, after careful aspiration, a small amount of local anesthetic and steroid is injected under real-time ultrasound guidance to confirm that the needle tip is not with the substance of the tendon. After proper needle tip placement is confirmed, the remainder of the contents of the syringe are slowly injected. There should be minimal resistance to injection.

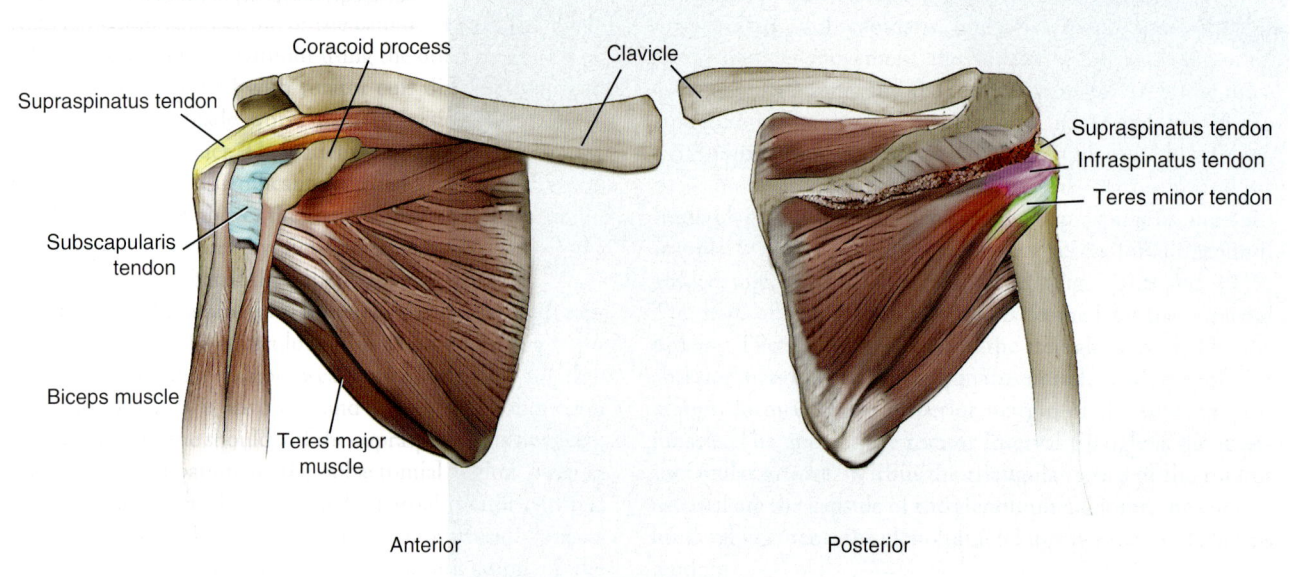

**FIGURE 39.4.** The muscles and tendons of the rotator cuff.

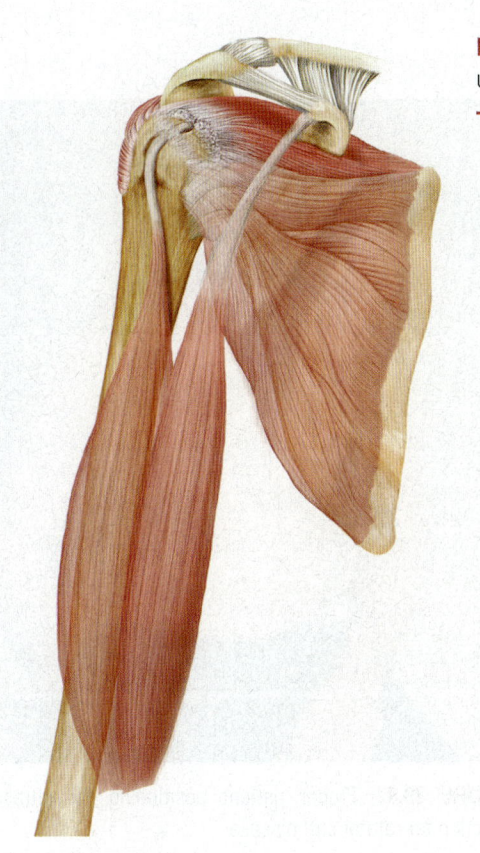

**FIGURE 39.5.** Tear of the supraspinatus musculotendinous unit. (From Anatomical Chart Company.)

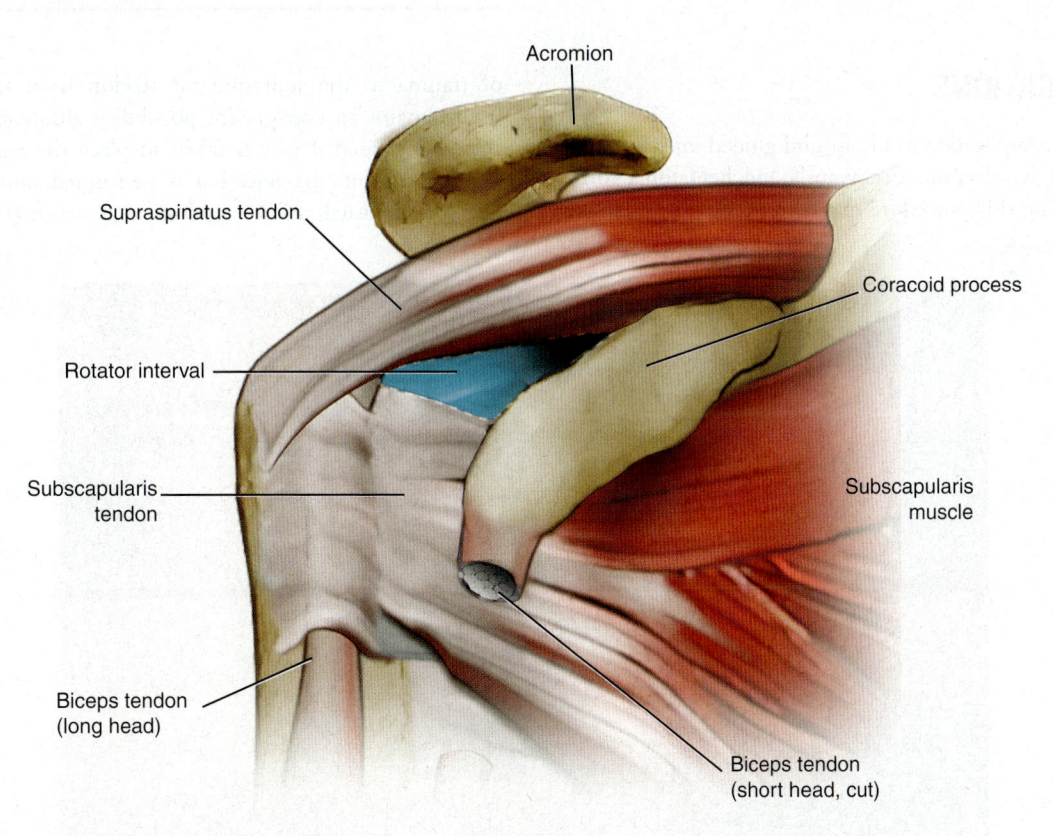

Borders of the Rotator Interval:
**Superior**- Anterior margin of the Supraspinatus tendon
**Inferior** - Superior margin of the Subscapularis tendon
**Apex** - Intertubercular groove
**Base** - Coracoid process

**FIGURE 39.6.** The rotator interval is a triangular-shaped space located between the supraspinatus and subscapularis tendons that provides easy access for ultrasound-guided injections of the rotator cuff.

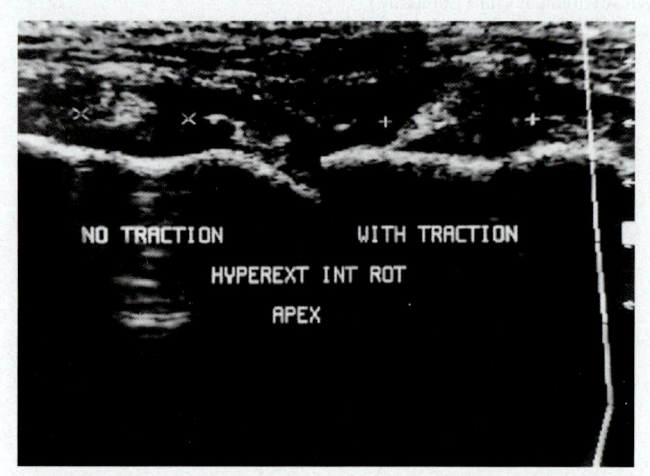

**FIGURE 39.7.** Saggital ultrasound image demonstrating the rotator interval. The X marks the borders of the rotator interval. The change in distance between these areas can be seen. (a) Ultrasound obtained in internal rotation (int rot) and extension without traction. (b) Ultrasound obtained with internal rotation and extension with traction. Hyperext, hyperextension. (Reused from Cole BJ, Rodeo SA, O'Brien SJ, et al. The anatomy and histology of the rotator interval capsule of the shoulder. *Clin Orthop Relat Res* 2001;390:129–137, with permission.)

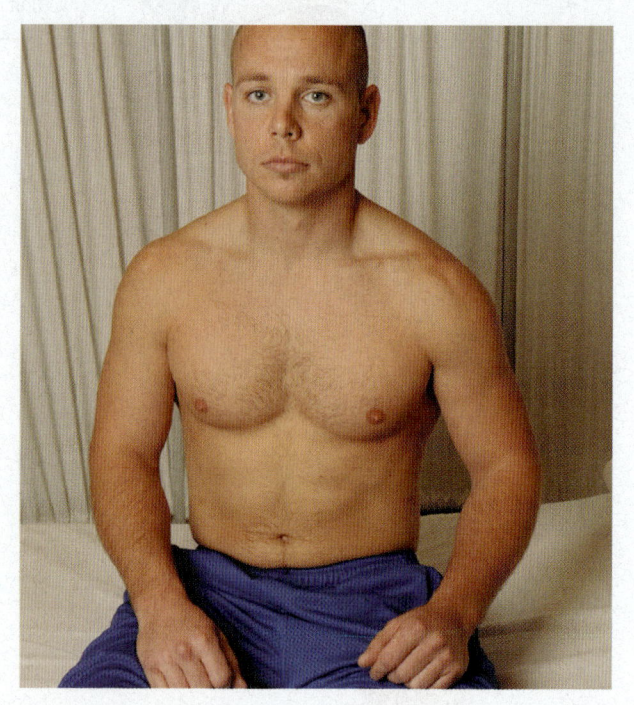

**FIGURE 39.8.** Proper patient positioning for ultrasound-guided injection for rotator cuff disease.

## COMPLICATIONS

The major complication of ultrasound-guided injection of the rotator cuff is infection. Ecchymosis and hematoma formation following this procedure may also occur. The possibility of trauma to the supraspinatus tendon from the injection itself remains an ever-present possibility, although the risk of this is decreased if care is taken to place the needle outside the tendon and the injection is performed under real-time ultrasound visualization. Tendons that are highly inflamed

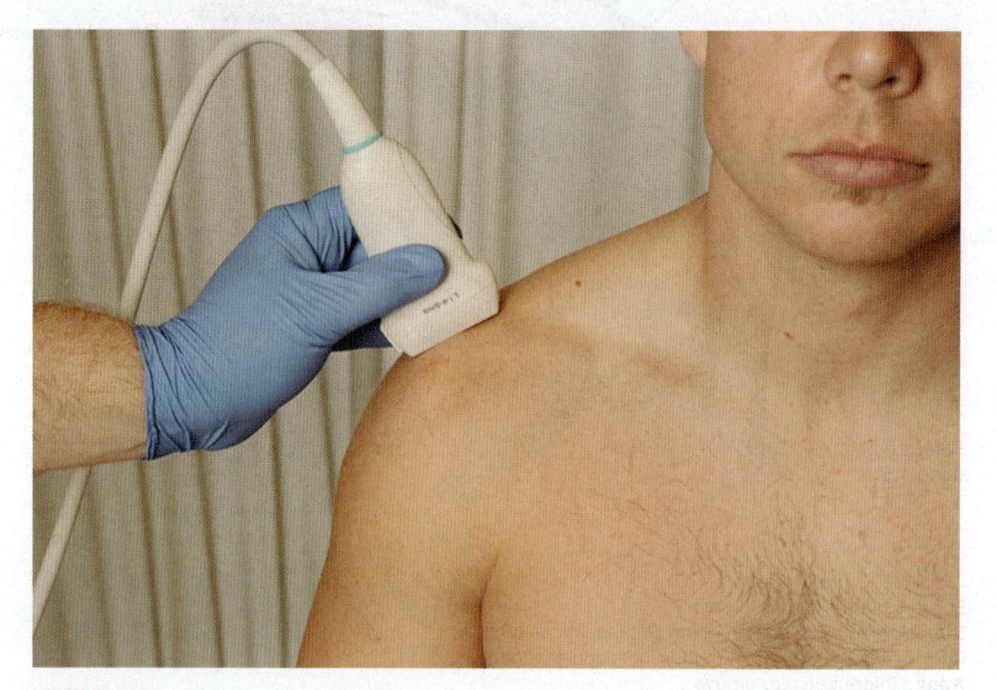

**FIGURE 39.9.** Proper coronal ultrasound transducer placement for ultrasound-guided injection for rotator cuff disease.

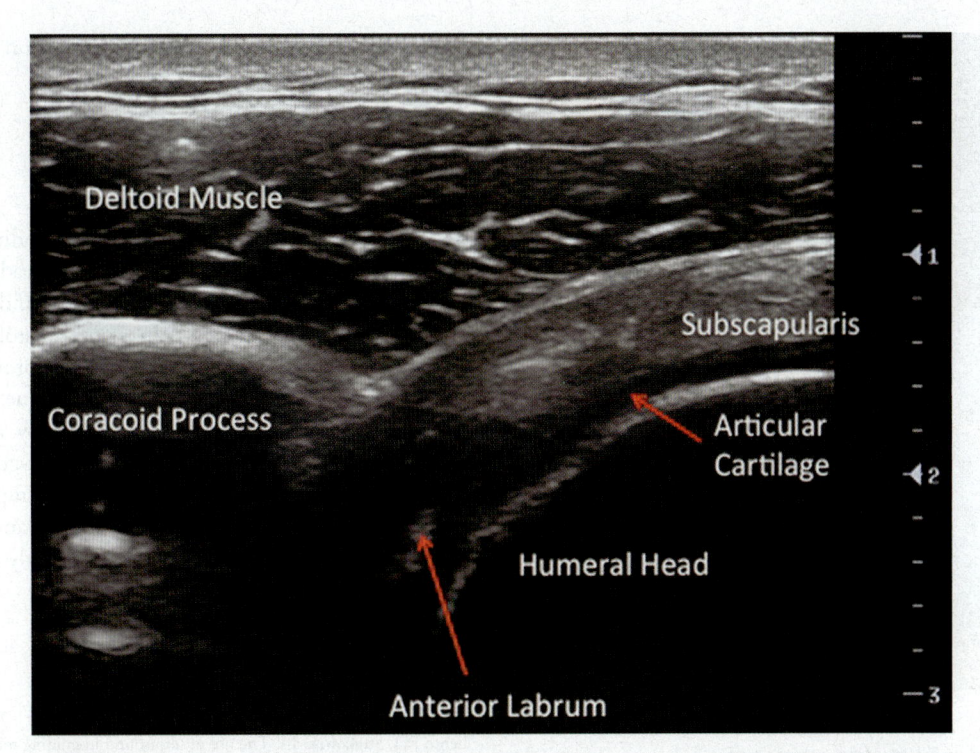

**FIGURE 39.10.** Ultrasound coronal view of the rotator cuff interval identifying the humeral head and the coracoid process.

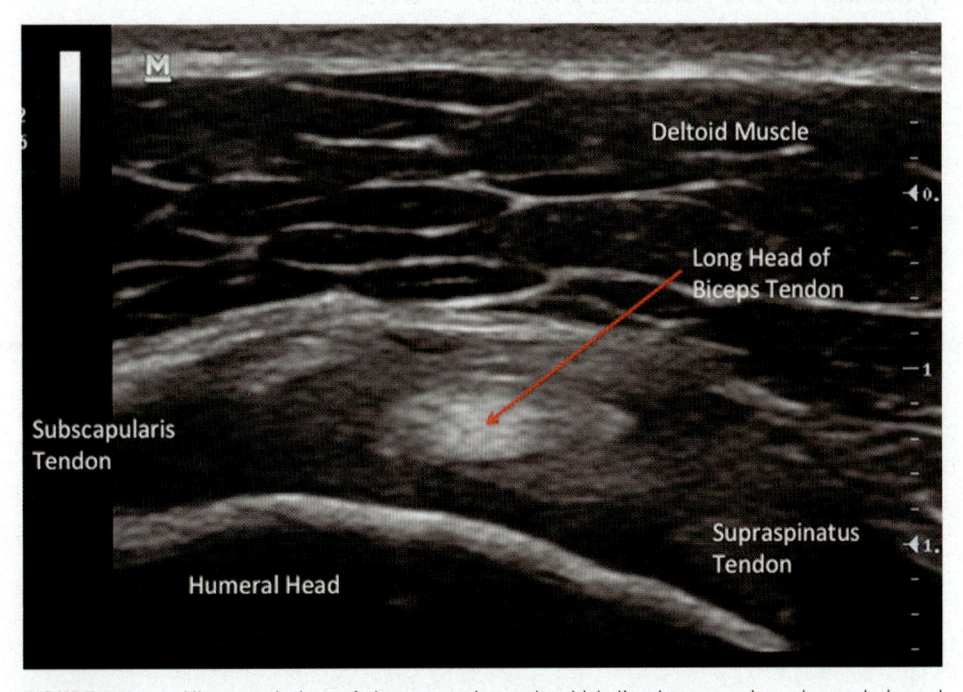

**FIGURE 39.11.** Ultrasound view of the rotator interval, which lies between the subscapularis and supraspinatus tendons. Note the biceps tendon, which passes through the interval.

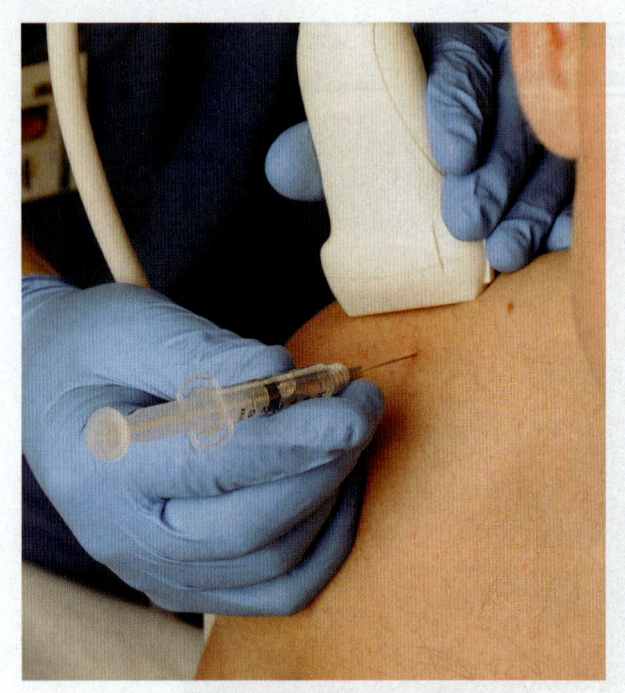

**FIGURE 39.12.** Proper out-of-plane needle placement for ultrasound-guided injection of the rotator cuff.

or previously damaged are subject to rupture if substances are injected directly into the tendon. This complication can be greatly decreased if the clinician uses gentle technique and stops injecting immediately if significant resistance to injection is encountered. Approximately 25% of patients complain of a transient increase in pain after this injection technique; the patient should be warned of this.

## CLINICAL PEARLS

Shoulder pathology including rotator cuff tendinopathy, osteoarthritis, avascular necrosis of the humeral head, and impingement syndromes may coexist with rotator cuff disease and may contribute to the patient's pain symptomatology. Universal precautions should always be observed to protect the operator, and strict adherence to sterile technique must be used to avoid infection. Gentle physical therapy and local heat should be introduced following ultrasound-guided injection of the subdeltoid bursa to reduce pain and improve function. Simple analgesics and nonsteroidal anti-inflammatory agents or COX-2 inhibitors may be used concurrently with this injection technique.

## SUGGESTED READINGS

Lento PH, Strakowski JA. The use of ultrasound in guiding musculoskeletal interventional procedures. *Phys Med Rehabil Clin N Am* 2010;21(3):559–583.

Narouze SN. Ultrasound-guided shoulder joint and bursa injections. In: *Atlas of Ultrasound Guided Procedures in Pain Management.* New York, NY: Springer; 2010:295–296.

Ng AWH, Hung EHY, Griffith JF, et al. Comparison of ultrasound versus fluoroscopic guided rotator cuff interval approach for MR arthrography. *Clin Imaging* 2013;37(3):548–553.

Precerutti M, Garioni E, Madonia L, et al. US anatomy of the shoulder: pictorial essay. *J Ultrasound* 2010;13(4):179–187.

Waldman SD. Injection technique for rotator cuff tears. In: *Atlas of Pain Management Injection Techniques.* 3rd ed. Philadelphia, PA: Elsevier Saunders; 2013:100–102.

# CHAPTER 40

# Ultrasound-Guided Injection Technique for Suprascapular Nerve Block

## CLINICAL PERSPECTIVES

Ultrasound-guided suprascapular nerve block is useful in the management of the scapular and acromioclavicular joint pain as well as shoulder pain subserved by the suprascapular nerve and in the palliation of pain of malignant origin emanating from tumors of the scapula, acromioclavicular joint, and the superior and posterior shoulder. This technique serves as an excellent adjunct to general anesthesia when performing surgery on the abovementioned areas. Suprascapular nerve block with local anesthetic may be used to palliate acute pain emergencies, including postoperative pain, pain secondary to traumatic injuries of the shoulder joint and girdle, and cancer pain, while waiting for pharmacologic, surgical, and antiblastic methods to become effective. Suprascapular nerve block is also useful as an adjunctive therapy when treating the decreased range of motion of the shoulder secondary to reflex sympathetic dystrophy or adhesive capsulitis. Suprascapular nerve block can also be used to allow more aggressive physical therapy after shoulder reconstruction surgery. Ultrasound-guided suprascapular nerve block can also be used in a prognostic manner to determine the degree of neurologic impairment the patient will suffer when destruction of the suprascapular nerve is being considered or when there is a possibility that the nerve may be sacrificed during surgeries in the anatomic region of the suprascapular nerve. This technique may also be useful in those patients suffering from symptoms secondary to compromised suprascapular nerve by ganglion cysts or tumors which the suprascapular notch and entrap the nerve. Ultrasound-guided suprascapular nerve block may also be used to palliate the pain and dysesthesias associated with stretch injuries to the suprascapular nerve such as backpack neuropathy.

Plain radiographs are indicated in all patients who present with shoulder pain. Based on the patient's clinical presentation, additional testing may be indicated, including complete blood cell count, sedimentation rate, and antinuclear antibody testing. Magnetic resonance imaging or ultrasound evaluation of the affected area may also help delineate the presence of ganglion cysts or other masses compressing the suprascapular nerve as it passes through the suprascapular notch (Fig. 40.1).

## CLINICALLY RELEVANT ANATOMY

The key landmark when performing suprascapular nerve block is the suprascapular notch. Arising from fibers from the C5 and C6 nerve roots of the upper trunk of the brachial plexus with some contribution of fibers from the C4 root, the suprascapular nerve travels in an inferior and posterior path from the brachial plexus to pass underneath the coracoclavicular ligament through the suprascapular notch. The suprascapular artery and vein accompany the nerve through the suprascapular notch (Fig. 40.2). The suprascapular nerve provides much of the sensory innervation to the shoulder and acromioclavicular joint and provides innervation to the supraspinatus and infraspinatus muscles of the rotator cuff.

## ULTRASOUND-GUIDED TECHNIQUE

The benefits, risks, and alternative treatments are explained to the patient and informed consent is obtained. The patient is then placed in the sitting position with the forearm resting across the ipsilateral thigh (Fig. 40.3). The physician stands behind or at the side of the patient. With the patient in the neutral sitting position, the spine of the scapula is palpated and a high-frequency linear ultrasound transducer is placed in a coronal position just above and parallel to the scapular spine (Fig. 40.4). Since the spine of the scapula runs at approximately a 40-degree angle to the superior margin of the scapula, the transducer should be rotated with the superior end of the transducer aimed toward the medial aspect of the coracoid process (see Fig. 40.4). When the ultrasound transducer is parallel to the scapular spine, the spine will appear as a bright, linear hyperechoic line that does not move with respiration like the pleura does. After the spine of the scapula is identified, the ultrasound transducer is then slowly moved in a cephalad and lateral trajectory until the "U"-shaped suprascapular notch is identified (Fig. 40.5). The suprascapular nerve should be visible within the notch appearing as a 2- to 3-cm hyperechoic margin beneath the suprascapular ligament (see Fig. 40.5). The suprascapular artery and vein should lie just above the suprascapular nerve, and their exact location relative to the suprascapular nerve can be identified with the use of color Doppler (Fig. 40.6).

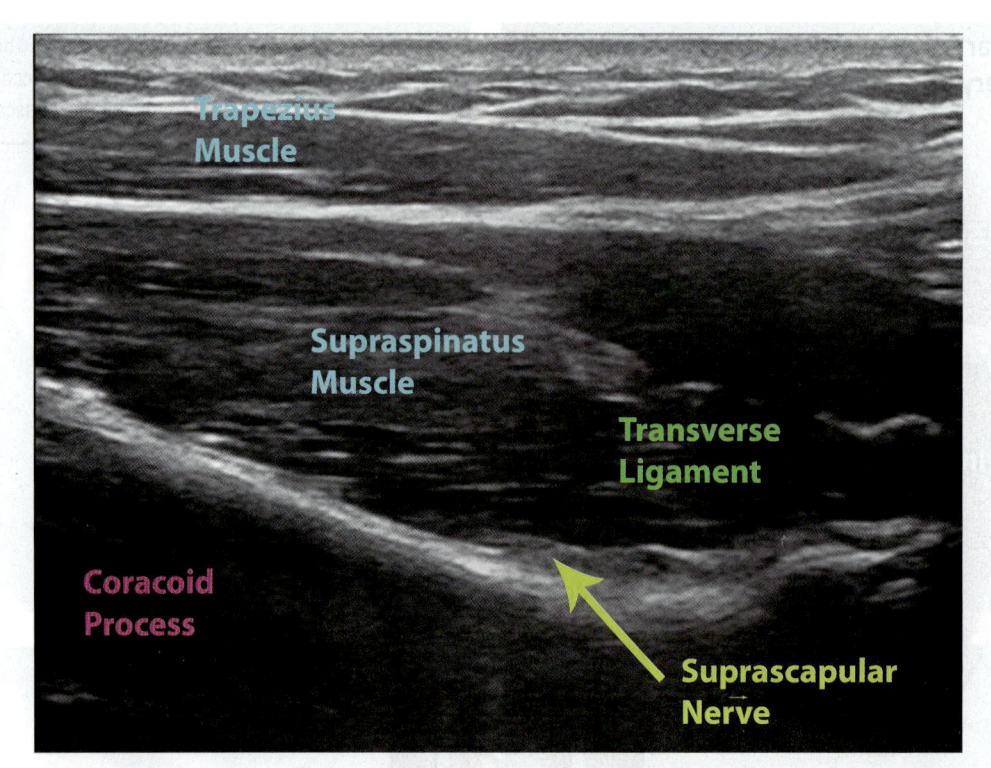

**FIGURE 40.5.** Transverse ultrasound image of the suprascapular notch, nerve, and overlying musculature.

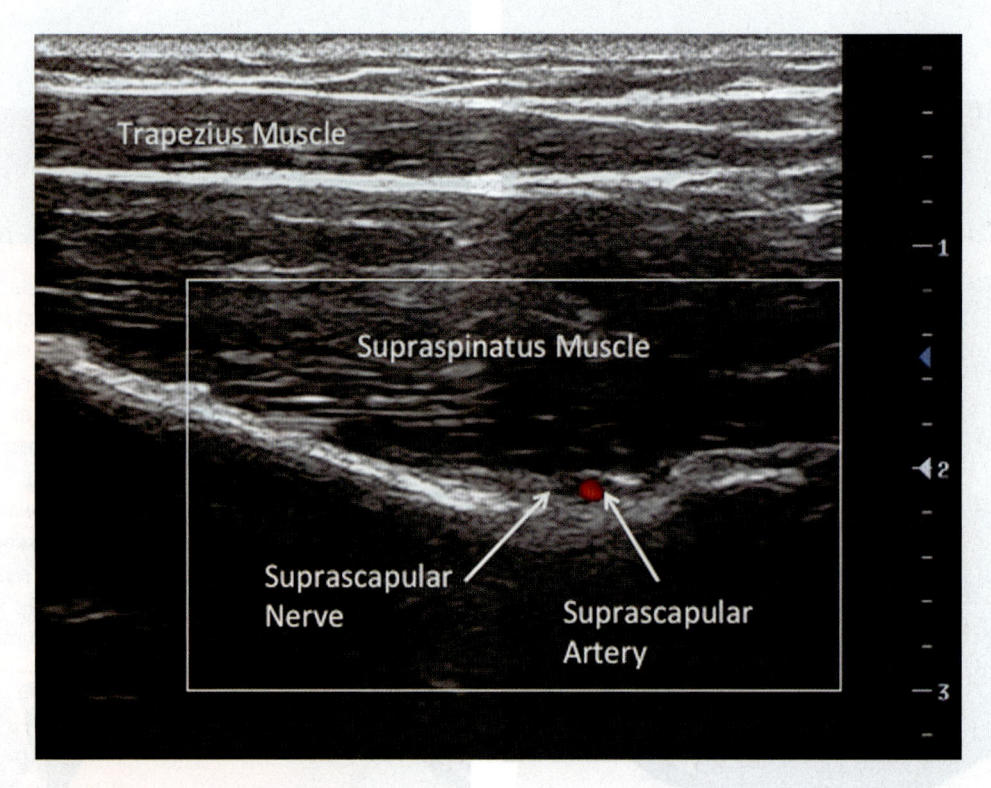

**FIGURE 40.6.** Use of color Doppler can aid in the identification of the suprascapular artery and vein.

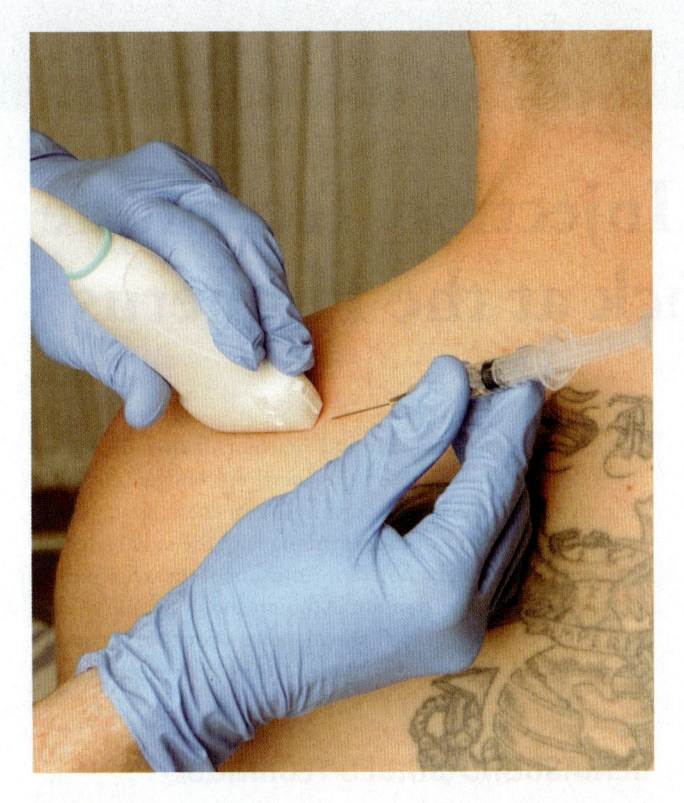

**FIGURE 40.7.** Proper in-plane needle trajectory for ultrasound-guided suprascapular nerve block.

After the suprascapular notch and the suprascapular nerve within it are identified, the skin overlying the area beneath the ultrasound transducer is prepped with antiseptic solution. A sterile syringe containing 5.0 mL of 0.25% preservative-free bupivacaine and 40 mg of methylprednisolone is attached to a 1½-inch, 22-gauge needle using strict aseptic technique. The needle is placed through the skin 1 cm from the medial border of the transducer and is then advanced using an in-plane approach with the needle trajectory adjusted under real-time ultrasound guidance so that the needle tip ultimately rests in proximity to the suprascapular nerve as it lies within the notch (Fig. 40.7). Color Doppler should be used to avoid needle-induced trauma to the suprascapular artery or vein, which lies just above the nerve. When the tip of needle is thought to be in satisfactory position, after careful aspiration, a small amount of local anesthetic and steroid is injected under real-time ultrasound guidance to confirm that the needle tip is in the proper position below the coracoclavicular ligament. After proper needle tip placement is confirmed, the remainder of the contents of the syringe are slowly injected. There should be minimal resistance to injection.

## COMPLICATIONS

The major complications of ultrasound-guided injection of ultrasound-guided suprascapular nerve block are related to improper needle placement. If the needle is placed too medially or too deep, pneumothorax may result. If the suprascapular artery and vein are not properly identified, the potential for needle-induced trauma to these vascular structures and/or intravascular injection is a distinct possibility. Although rare, infection may occur. Ecchymosis and hematoma formation following this procedure may also occur. Approximately 25% of patients complain of a transient increase in pain after this injection technique; the patient should be warned of this.

## CLINICAL PEARLS

Shoulder pathology including rotator cuff tendinopathy, osteoarthritis, avascular necrosis of the humeral head, and bursitis may coexist with pathology involving the suprascapular nerve and may also contribute to the patient's pain symptomatology. Universal precautions should always be observed to protect the operator, and strict adherence to sterile technique must be used to avoid infection. Gentle physical therapy and local heat should be introduced following ultrasound-guided injection of the suprascapular nerve to reduce pain and improve function. Simple analgesics and nonsteroidal anti-inflammatory agents or COX-2 inhibitors may be used concurrently with this injection technique.

## SUGGESTED READINGS

Gorthi V, Moon YL, Kang JH. The effectiveness of ultrasonography-guided suprascapular nerve block for perishoulder pain. *Orthopedics* 2010;33(4):213–216.

Precerutti M, Garioni E, Madonia L, et al. US anatomy of the shoulder: pictorial essay. *J Ultrasound* 2010;13(4):179–187.

Waldman SD. Suprascapular nerve entrapment. In: *Atlas of Uncommon Pain Syndromes*. 2nd ed. Philadelphia, PA: WB Saunders; 2008:77–80.

Waldman SD. Adhesive capsulitis. In: *Atlas of Common Pain Syndromes*. 3rd ed. Philadelphia, PA: Saunders Elsevier; 2012:94–97.

Waldman SD. Injection technique for suprascapular nerve block. In: *Atlas of Pain Management Injection Techniques*. 3rd ed. Philadelphia, PA: Saunders Elsevier; 2013:207–210.

# Ultrasound-Guided Injection Technique for Radial Nerve Block at the Humerus

## CLINICAL PERSPECTIVES

Ultrasound-guided radial nerve block at the humerus is useful in the management of the pain subserved by the radial nerve. This technique serves as an excellent adjunct to brachial plexus block and for general anesthesia when performing surgery at the elbow or below. Ultrasound-guided radial nerve block at the humerus with local anesthetic may be used to palliate acute pain emergencies, including postoperative pain, pain secondary to traumatic injuries of the radius, and cancer pain, while waiting for pharmacologic, surgical, and antiblastic methods to become effective (Figs. 41.1 and 41.2).

Ultrasound-guided radial nerve block can also be used as a diagnostic tool when performing differential neural blockade on an anatomic basis in the evaluation of upper extremity pain as well as in a prognostic manner to determine the degree of neurologic impairment the patient will suffer when destruction of the radial nerve is being considered or when there is a possibility that the nerve may be sacrificed during surgeries in the anatomic region of the radial nerve at the level of the humerus. This technique may also be useful in those patients suffering symptoms from compromise of the radial nerve due to radial tunnel syndrome. Ultrasound-guided radial nerve block at the humerus may also be used to palliate the pain and dysesthesias associated with stretch injuries to the radial nerve.

## CLINICALLY RELEVANT ANATOMY

The key landmark when performing ultrasound-guided radial nerve block at the humerus is the point at which the radial nerve travels sandwiched between the intermuscular septum separating the bellies of the brachialis and brachioradialis muscles (Fig. 41.3). Arising from fibers from the C5–T1 nerve roots of the posterior cord of the brachial plexus, the radial nerve passes through the axilla lying posterior and inferior to the axillary artery. As the radial nerve exits the axilla, it passes between the medial and long heads of the triceps muscle and then curves across the posterior aspect of the humerus, giving off a motor branch to the triceps muscle. Continuing its downward path, the radial nerve gives off a number of sensory branches to the upper arm as it travels in the intermuscular septum separating the bellies of the brachialis and brachioradialis muscles (see Fig. 41.3). At a point above the lateral epicondyle, the radial nerve divides into deep and superficial branches; the superficial branch continues down the arm along with the radial artery to provide sensory innervation to the dorsum of the wrist and the dorsal aspects of a portion of the thumb and index and middle fingers and the deep branch provides the majority of the motor innervation to the extensors of the forearm (Fig. 41.4).

## ULTRASOUND-GUIDED TECHNIQUE

The benefits, risks, and alternative treatments are explained to the patient and informed consent is obtained. The patient is then placed in the supine position with the elbow flexed and the hand resting on the abdomen (Fig 41.5). The physician stands at the side of the patient. With the patient in the above position, at a point 4 inches above the lateral epicondyle, the intermuscular septum separating the bellies of the brachialis and brachioradialis muscles is palpated. A high-frequency linear ultrasound transducer is placed in a transverse position over the previously identified intermuscular septum (Fig. 41.6). An ultrasound survey image is obtained, and the intermuscular septum separating the bellies of the brachialis and brachioradialis muscles and the radial nerve is identified (Fig. 41.7). To confirm that the ultrasound transducer is in fact above the bifurcation of the radial nerve into its terminal deep and superficial branches, the ultrasound transducer is turned to the longitudinal plane, and the path of the radial nerve is traced proximally or distally until the bifurcation of the nerve is identified (Figs. 41.8 and 41.9). Once the bifurcation of the nerve is identified, at a point 11 inches above the bifurcation, the transducer is then returned to the transverse plane, and the radial nerve, which will appear as an oval hyperechoic structure, is reidentified and centered in ultrasound image. Color Doppler is then used to identify any adjacent vasculature including the radial artery (Fig. 41.10). The skin overlying the area beneath the ultrasound transducer is then prepped with antiseptic solution. A sterile syringe containing 3.0 mL of 0.25% preservative-free bupivacaine and 41 mg of methylprednisolone is attached to a 1½-inch, 22-gauge needle using strict aseptic technique. The needle is placed through the skin just above

# CHAPTER 41 ULTRASOUND-GUIDED INJECTION TECHNIQUE FOR RADIAL NERVE BLOCK AT THE HUMERUS

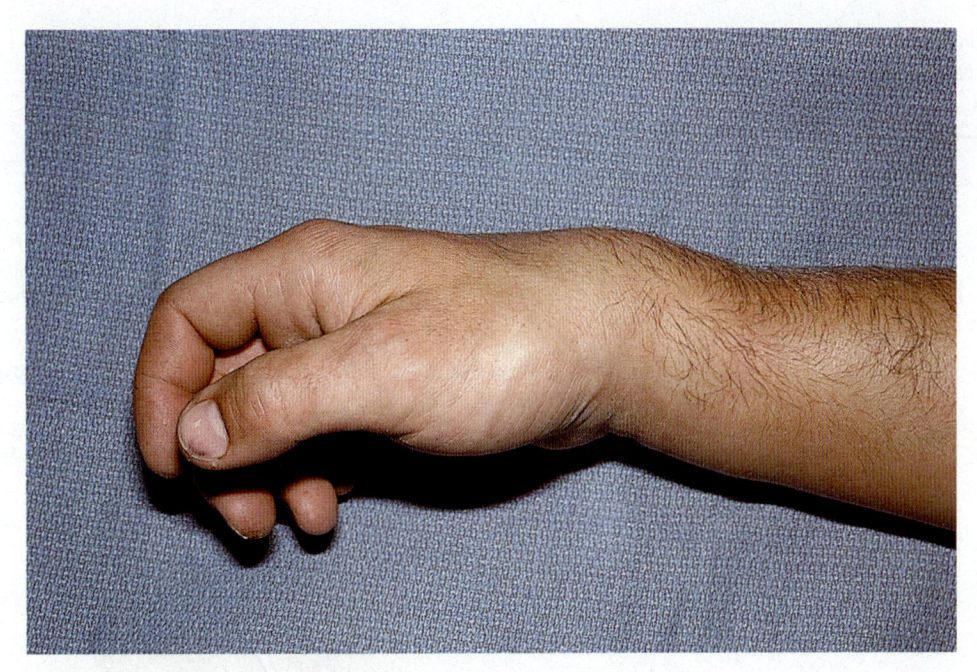

**FIGURE 41.1.** Clinical appearance of acute displaced distal *radius fracture*. (Reused from Koval KJ, Zuckerman JD. *Atlas of Orthopaedic Surgery: A Multimedia Reference*. Philadelphia, PA: Lippincott Williams & Wilkins; 2004, with permission.)

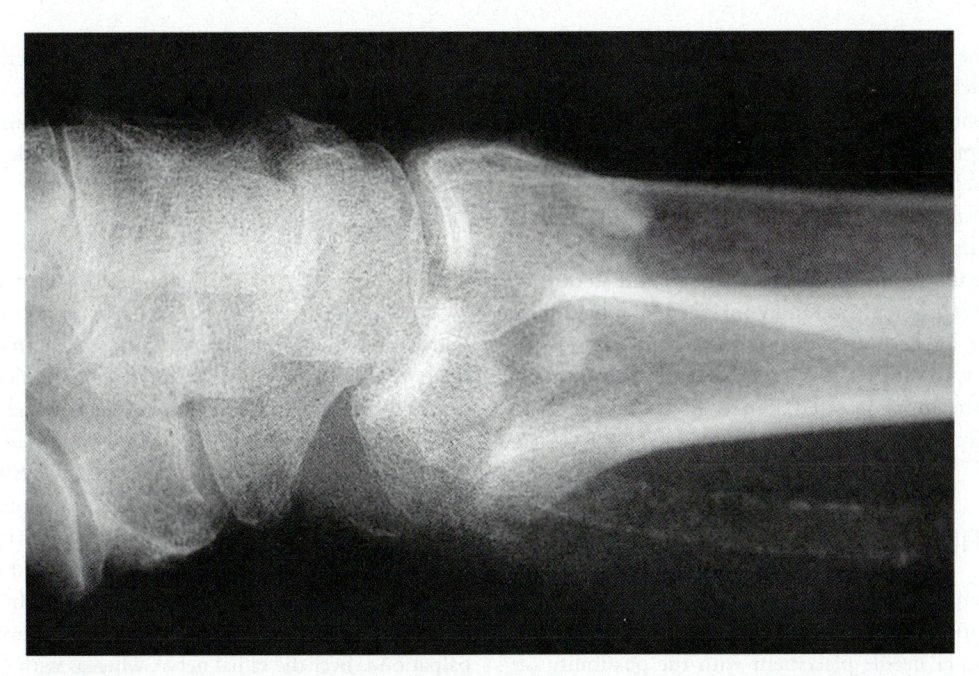

**FIGURE 41.2.** Plain lateral radiograph of underlying unstable distal *radius fracture*. (Reused from Koval KJ, Zuckerman JD. *Atlas of Orthopaedic Surgery: A Multimedia Reference*. Philadelphia, PA: Lippincott Williams & Wilkins; 2004, with permission.)

**FIGURE 41.3.** The radial nerve lies in the intermuscular septum between the brachioradialis and brachialis muscles.

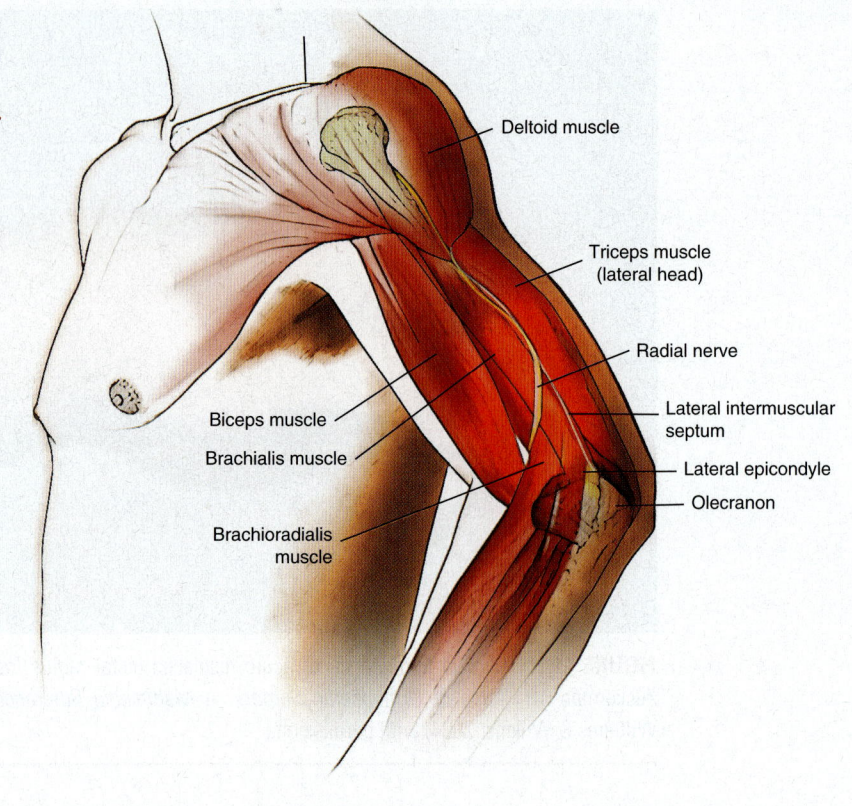

the center of the transducer and is then advanced using an in-plane approach with the needle trajectory adjusted under real-time ultrasound guidance so that the needle tip ultimately rests in proximity to the radial nerve as it lies within intermuscular septum between the bellies of the brachialis and brachioradialis muscles (Fig. 41.11). When the tip of needle is thought to be in satisfactory position, after careful aspiration, a small amount of local anesthetic and steroid is injected under real-time ultrasound guidance to confirm that the needle tip is in the proper position. After proper needle tip placement is confirmed, the remainder of the contents of the syringe are slowly injected. There should be minimal resistance to injection.

## COMPLICATIONS

The major complications of ultrasound-guided injection of ultrasound-guided radial nerve block at the humerus are related to improper needle placement with the possibility of inadvertent intravascular injection and/or persistent paresthesia secondary to needle trauma to the radial nerve. Although rare, infection may occur. Ecchymosis and hematoma formation following this procedure may also occur. These complications can be decreased if manual pressure is applied to the area of the block immediately after injection. Application of cold packs for 20-minute periods after the block will also decrease the amount of postprocedure pain and bleeding the patient may experience.

Approximately 25% of patients complain of a transient increase in pain after this injection technique; the patient should be warned of this.

## CLINICAL PEARLS

Ultrasound-guided radial nerve block at the humerus is a straightforward and relatively safe technique if attention is paid to the clinically relevant anatomy. It is useful as an adjunct to surgical anesthesia and has recently been used with increasing frequency in the emergency department to provide anesthesia for reduction of fractures of the radius. Ultrasound-guided radial nerve block at the humerus is also useful in the management of radial tunnel syndrome, which is often misdiagnosed as tennis elbow. Radial tunnel syndrome can be distinguished from tennis elbow in that with radial tunnel syndrome the maximal tenderness to palpation is over the radial nerve, whereas with tennis elbow, the maximal tenderness to palpation is over the lateral epicondyle (Fig. 41.12). If radial tunnel syndrome is suspected, injection of the radial nerve at the humerus with local anesthetic and steroid will give almost instantaneous relief. Careful neurologic examination to identify preexisting neurologic deficits that may later be attributed to the nerve block should be performed on all patients before beginning radial nerve block at the humerus.

CHAPTER 41 ULTRASOUND-GUIDED INJECTION TECHNIQUE FOR RADIAL NERVE BLOCK AT THE HUMERUS

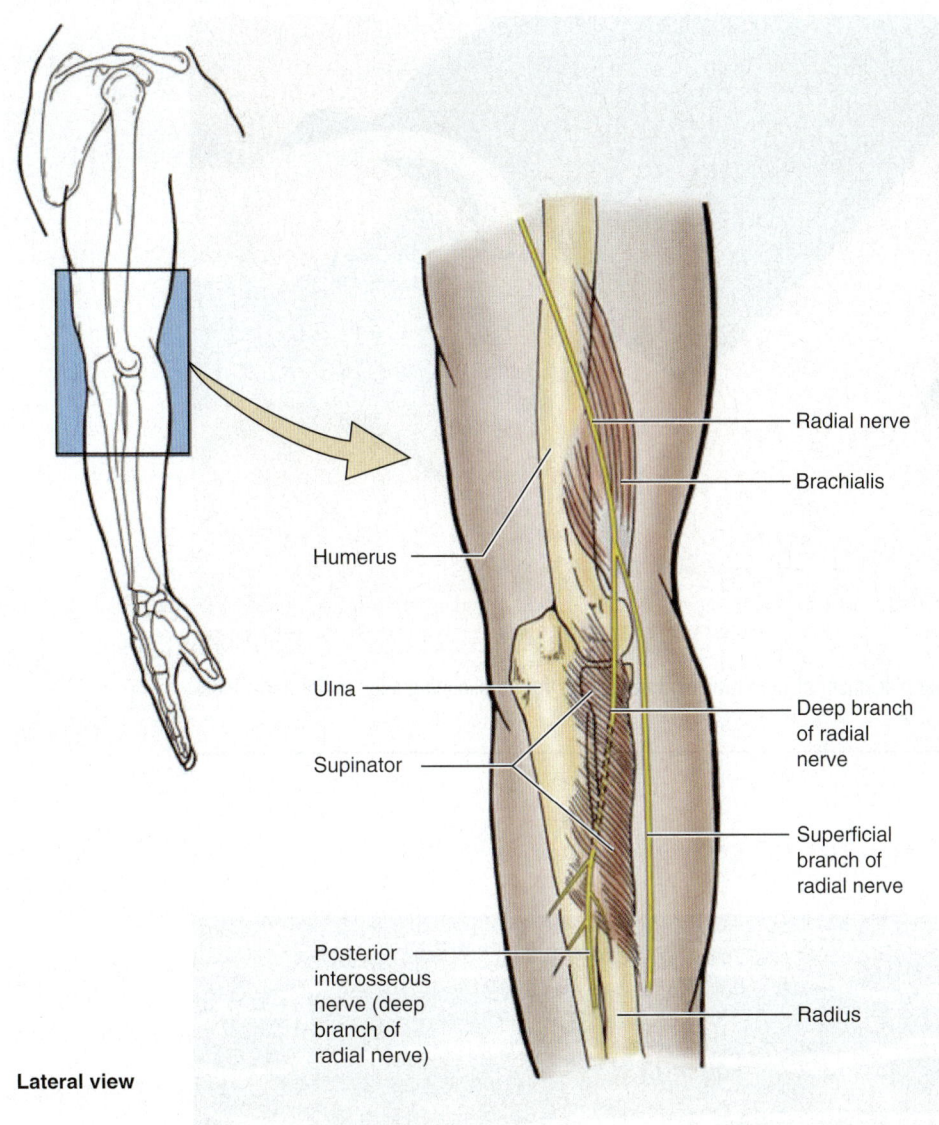

**FIGURE 41.4.** The common radial nerve bifurcates into a deep and superficial branch just above the lateral epicondyle. (Reused from Moore KL, Dalley AF. *Clinical Oriented Anatomy*. 4th ed. Baltimore, MD: Lippincott Williams & Wilkins; 1999, with permission.)

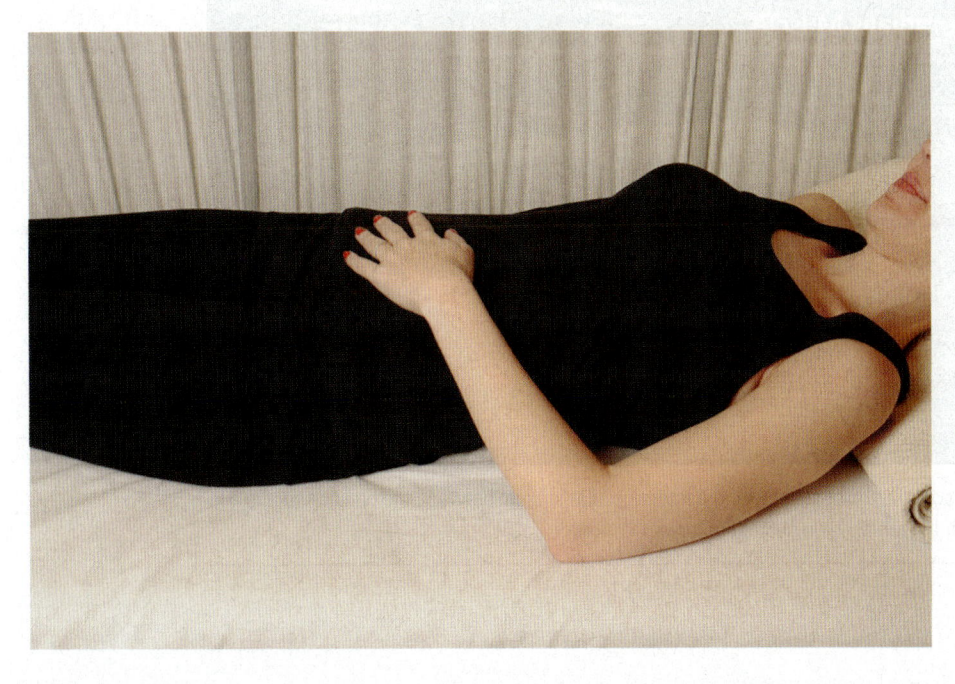

**FIGURE 41.5.** Proper patient positioning for ultrasound-guided radial nerve block at the humerus.

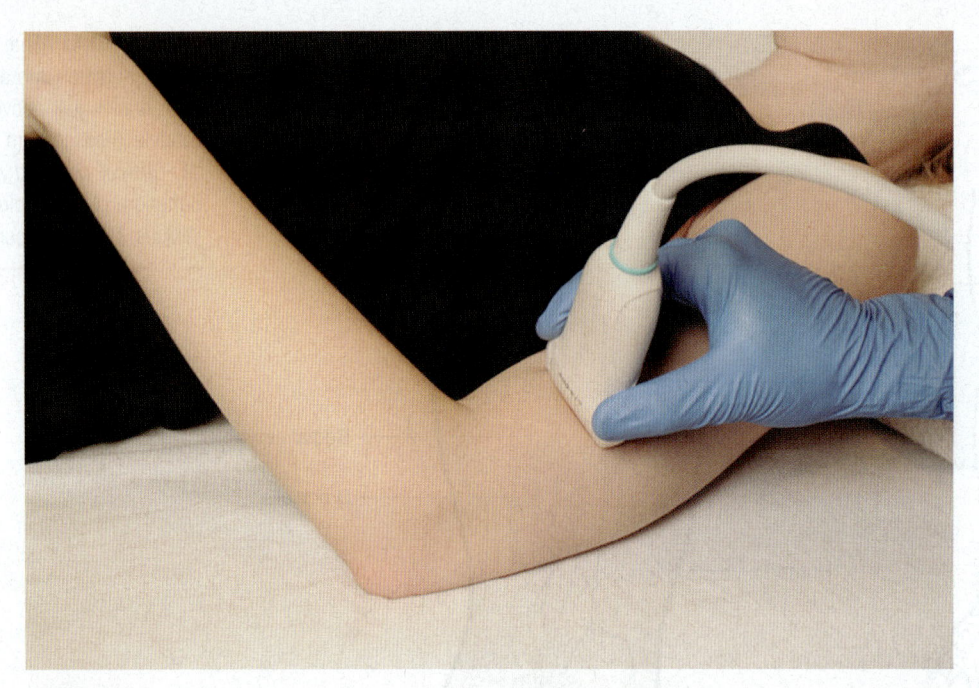

**FIGURE 41.6.** Proper placement of the ultrasound transducer for ultrasound-guided radial nerve block at the elbow.

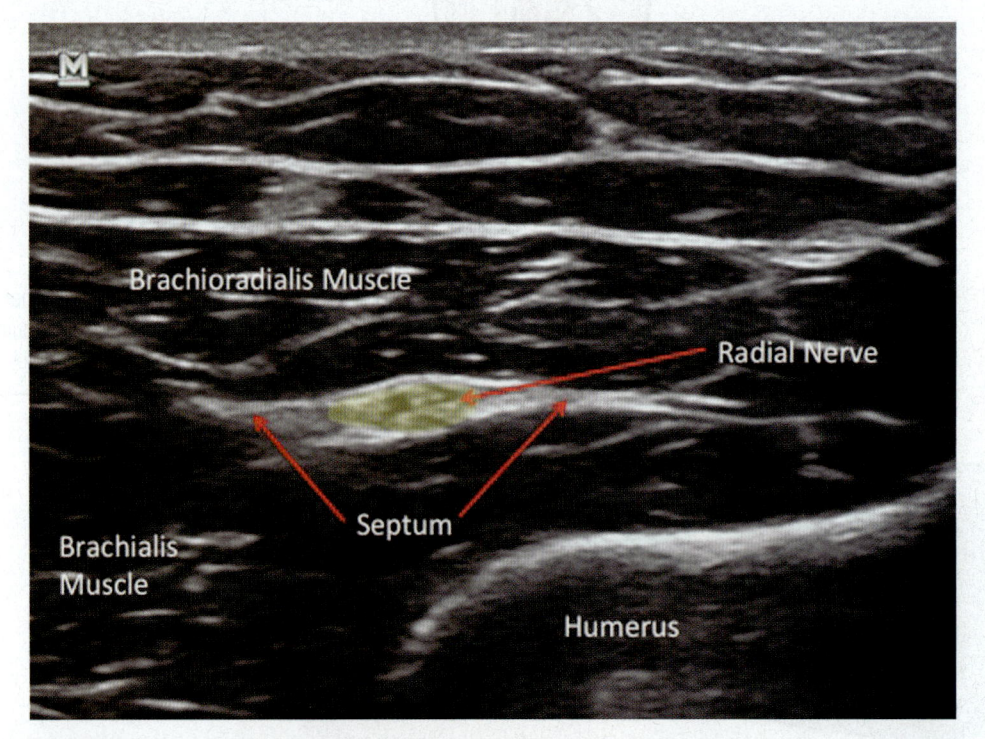

**FIGURE 41.7.** Transverse ultrasound view of the intermuscular septum between the brachioradialis and brachial muscles with the radial nerve nestled between.

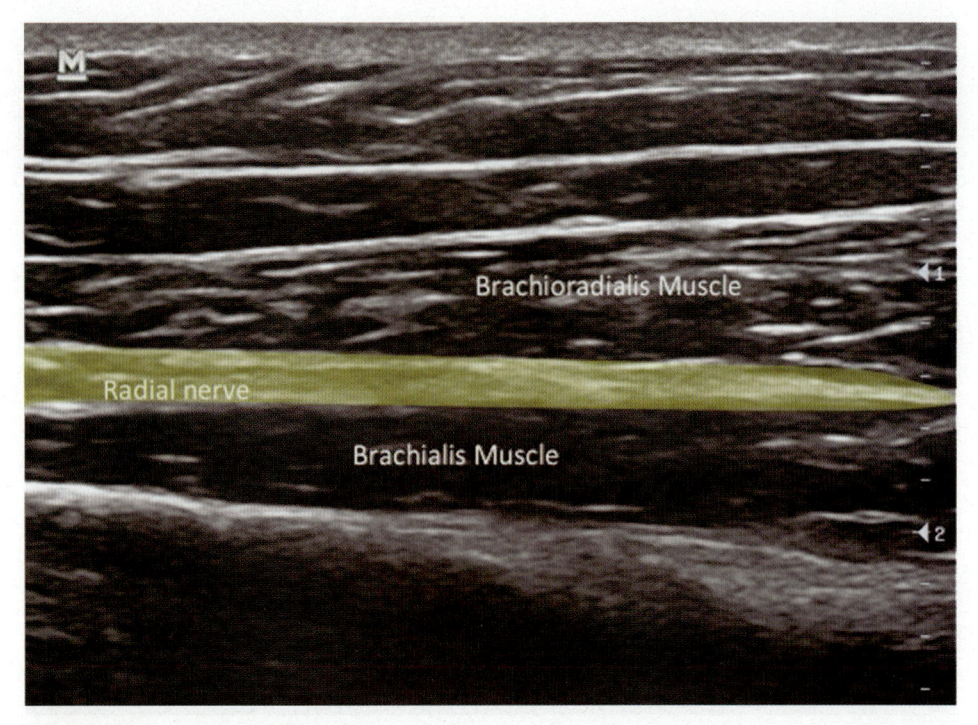

**FIGURE 41.8.** Longitudinal view of the radial nerve within the intermuscular septum between the brachioradialis and brachialis muscles.

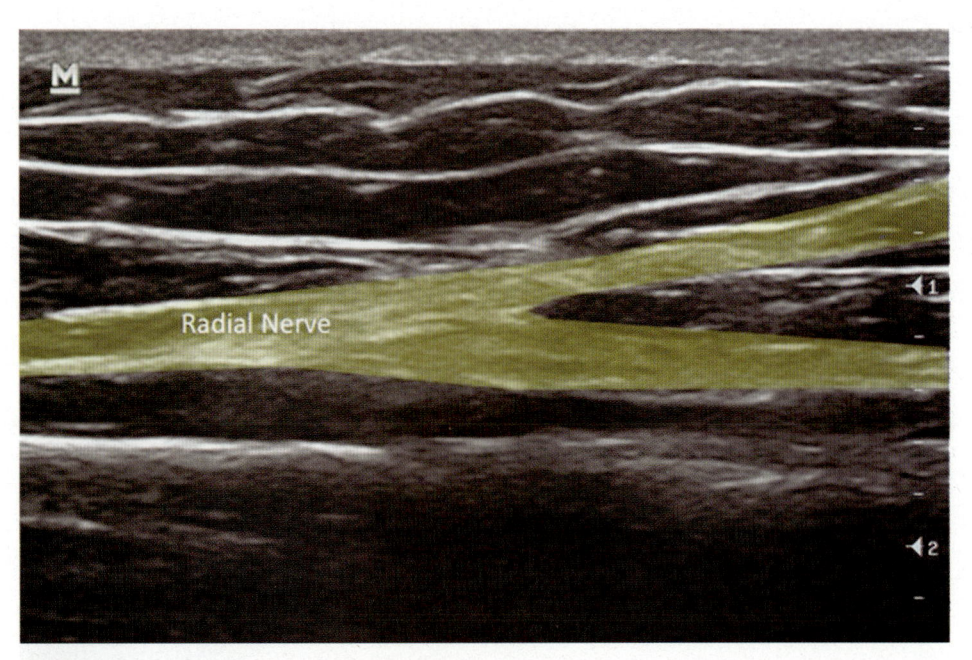

**FIGURE 41.9.** Longitudinal view of the radial nerve within the intermuscular septum between the brachioradialis and brachialis muscles.

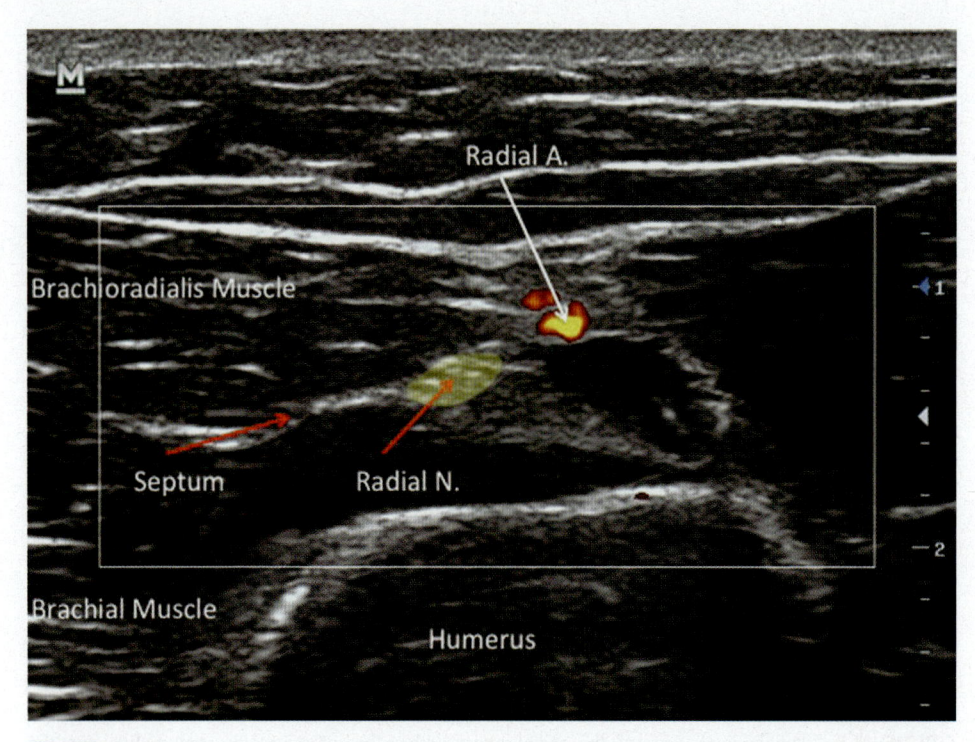

**FIGURE 41.10.** Use of color Doppler can aid in the identification of adjacent vasculature including the radial artery.

**FIGURE 41.11.** Proper in-plane needle placement for ultrasound-guided radial nerve block at the humerus.

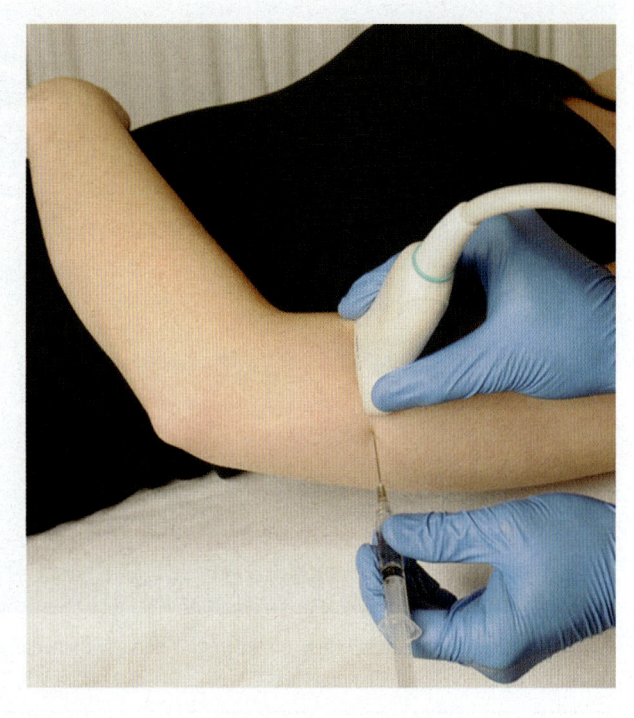

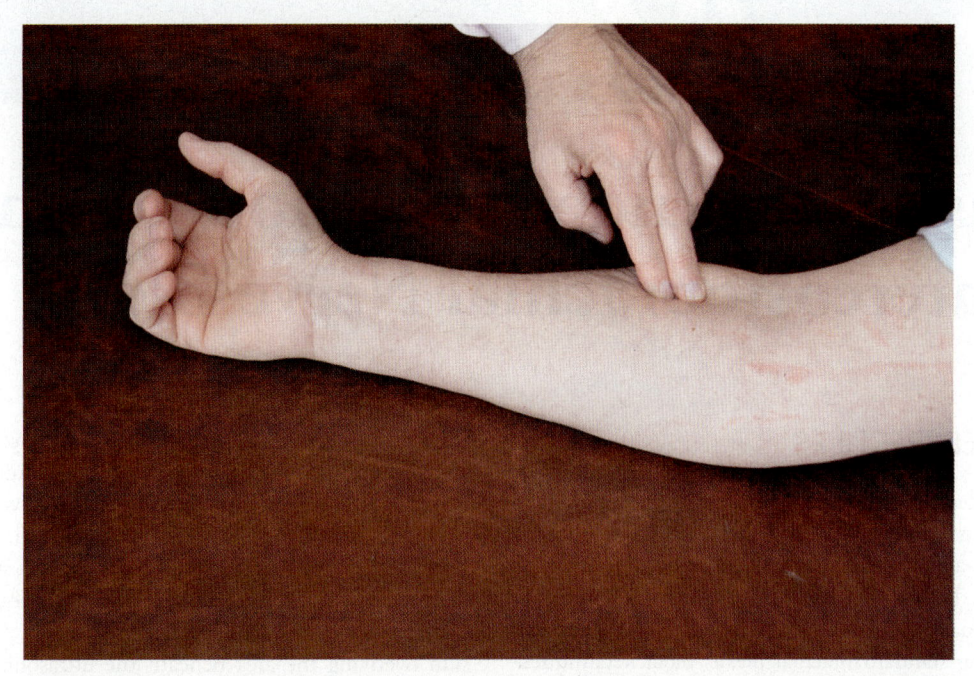

**FIGURE 41.12.** Radial tunnel syndrome is often misdiagnosed as tennis elbow. Patients suffering from radial tunnel syndrome will exhibit maximal tenderness to palpation over the radial nerve, whereas patients with tennis elbow will exhibit maximal tenderness to palpation over the lateral epicondyle.

## SUGGESTED READINGS

Foxall GL, Skinner D, Hardman JG, et al. Ultrasound anatomy of the radial nerve in the distal upper arm. *Reg Anesth Pain Med* 2007;32(3):217–220.

Frenkel O, Herring AA, Fischer J, et al. Supracondylar radial nerve block for treatment of distal radius fractures in the emergency department. *J Emerg Med* 2011;41(4):386–388.

Waldman SD. Radial tunnel syndrome. In: *Atlas of Uncommon Pain Syndromes*. 2nd ed. Philadelphia, PA: WB Saunders; 2008:102–103.

Waldman SD. Injection technique for radial nerve block at the humerus. In: *Atlas of Pain Management Injection Techniques*. 3rd ed. Philadelphia, PA: Elsevier Saunders; 2013:211–214.

# Ultrasound-Guided Injection Technique for Intercostobrachial Nerve Block

## CLINICAL PERSPECTIVES

Ultrasound-guided intercostobrachial cutaneous nerve block is used primarily as an adjunct to brachial plexus block rather than as a stand-alone regional anesthesia and pain management procedure. The intercostobrachial cutaneous nerve is not part of the brachial plexus and is often not adequately blocked when performing standard brachial plexus block techniques. This means that the medial and posterior aspect of the arm just below the axilla remains unanesthetized making prolonged use of a pneumatic tourniquet or the performance of surgical procedures in this region problematic. The intercostobrachial cutaneous nerve is often damaged or transected during radical mastectomy surgery and has been implicated in the evolution of postmastectomy pain syndrome. The nerve may also subserve referred pain from the cardiac region.

## CLINICALLY RELEVANT ANATOMY

The intercostobrachial cutaneous nerve is derived from fibers of the lateral cutaneous branch of the second intercostal nerve. After piercing the intercostalis and serratus anterior muscles, the intercostobrachial cutaneous nerve traverses the axilla where it provides communicating branches to the median cutaneous nerve. The intercostobrachial cutaneous nerve exits the axilla along with the median cutaneous nerve to provide cutaneous sensory innervation to medial and posterior aspect of the upper extremity (Figs. 42.1 and 42.2). The superficial location of this nerve makes it easily accessible for ultrasound-guided nerve block.

## ULTRASOUND-GUIDED TECHNIQUE

The benefits, risks, and alternative treatments are explained to the patient and informed consent is obtained. The patient is then placed in the supine position with the affected upper extremity abducted 90 degrees and the palm facing upward (Fig. 42.3). With the patient in the above position, at a point just below the axilla, the pulsations of the axillary artery are palpated (Fig. 42.4). A high-frequency linear ultrasound transducer is placed in a transverse position over the previously identified arterial pulsations (Fig. 42.5). An ultrasound survey image is obtained, and the axillary artery and vein and the deep fascia are identified (Fig. 42.6). Color Doppler can aid in the identifications of these vessels (Fig. 42.7). Just superficial to the deep fascia lies the intercostobrachial cutaneous nerve, which will appear as an oval hyperechoic structure (Fig. 42.8). The skin overlying the area beneath the ultrasound transducer is then prepped with antiseptic solution. A sterile syringe containing 3.0 mL of 0.25% preservative-free bupivacaine and 40 mg of methylprednisolone is attached to a 1½-inch, 22-gauge needle using strict aseptic technique. The needle is placed through the skin just below the center of the transducer and is then advanced using an out-of-plane approach with the needle trajectory adjusted under real-time ultrasound guidance so that the needle tip ultimately rests in proximity to the intercostobrachial cutaneous nerve (Fig. 42.9). When the tip of needle is thought to be in satisfactory position, after careful aspiration, a small amount of local anesthetic and steroid is injected under real-time ultrasound guidance to confirm that the needle tip is in the proper position. After proper needle tip placement is confirmed, the remainder of the contents of the syringe are slowly injected. There should be minimal resistance to injection.

## COMPLICATIONS

The major complications of ultrasound-guided injection of ultrasound-guided intercostobrachial nerve block are related to improper needle placement with the possibility of inadvertent intravascular injection and/or persistent paresthesia secondary to needle trauma to the nerve. Although rare, infection may occur. Ecchymosis and hematoma formation following this procedure may also occur. These complications can be decreased if manual pressure is applied to the area of the block immediately after injection. Application of cold packs for 20-minute periods after the block will also decrease the amount of postprocedure pain and bleeding the patient may experience.

Approximately 25% of patients complain of a transient increase in pain after this injection technique; the patient should be warned of this.

# CHAPTER 42  ULTRASOUND-GUIDED INJECTION TECHNIQUE FOR INTERCOSTOBRACHIAL NERVE BLOCK

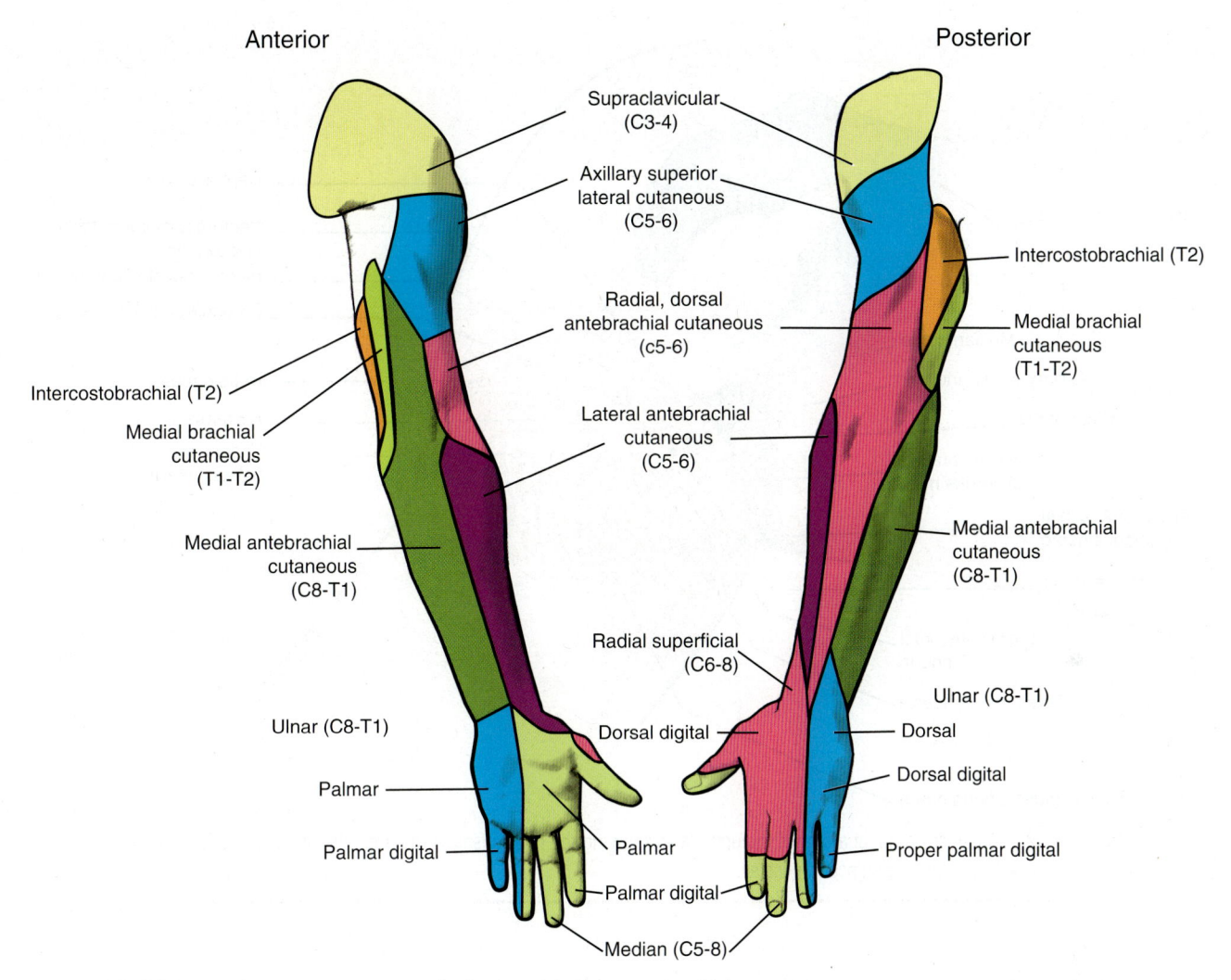

**FIGURE 42.1.** The cutaneous sensory distribution of the intercostobrachial cutaneous nerve.

## CLINICAL PEARLS

Ultrasound-guided intercostobrachial nerve block is a straightforward and relatively safe technique if attention is paid to the clinically relevant anatomy. It is useful as an adjunct to brachial plexus block, often being combined with medial cutaneous nerve block. Careful neurologic examination to identify preexisting neurologic deficits that may later be attributed to the nerve block should be performed on all patients before beginning ultrasound-guided intercostobrachial nerve block especially when surgical exploration of the axilla and chest wall for lymph node dissection during mastectomy is being considered.

**276** SECTION III   SHOULDER

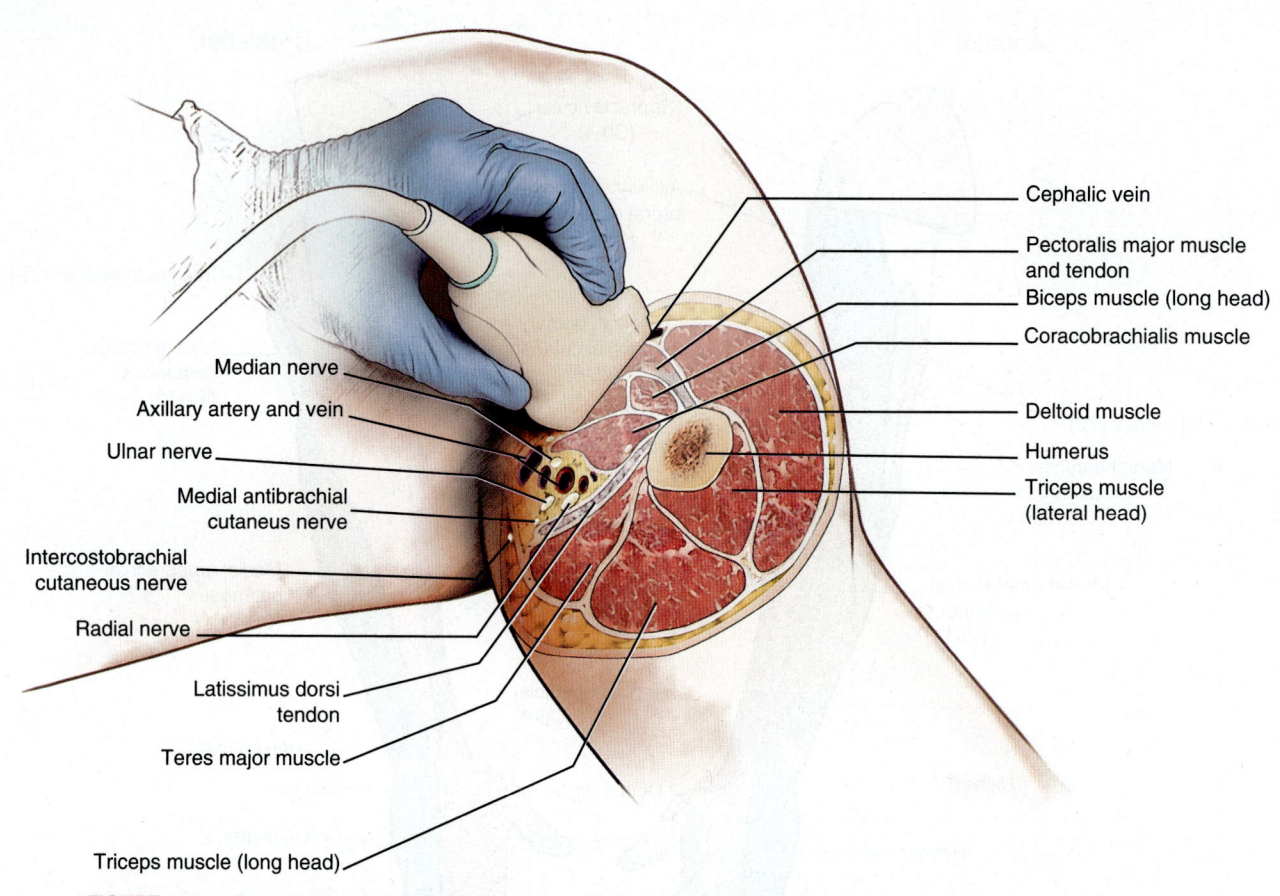

**FIGURE 42.2.** Cross-sectional anatomy of the upper arm showing the relationship of the intercostobrachial cutaneous nerve to the axillary artery, vein, and adjacent muscles.

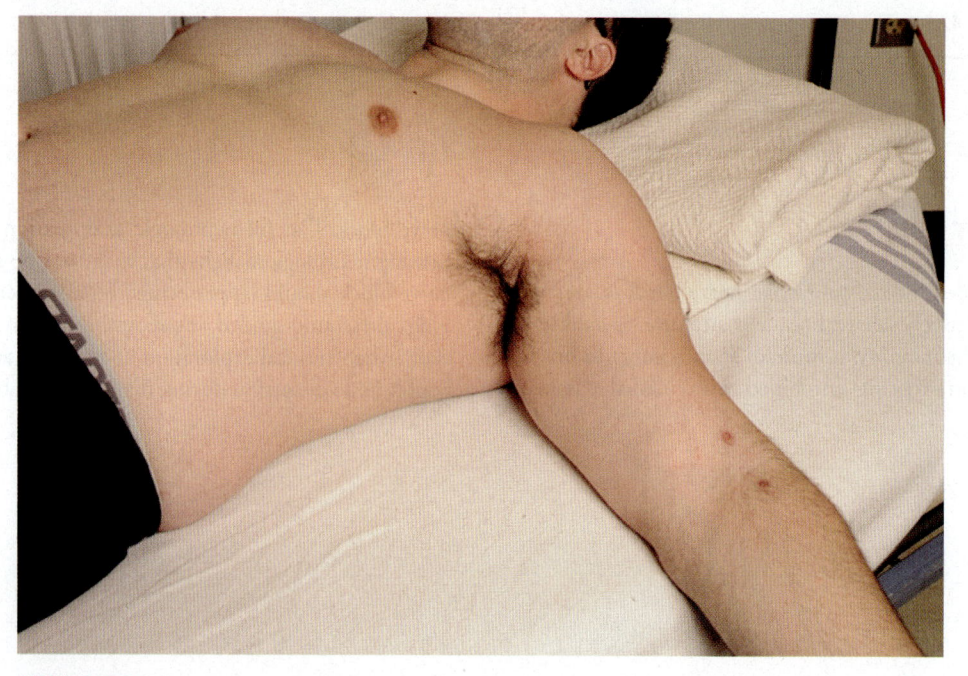

**FIGURE 42.3.** Proper position of the patient for ultrasound-guided intercostobrachial cutaneous nerve block.

CHAPTER 42   ULTRASOUND-GUIDED INJECTION TECHNIQUE FOR INTERCOSTOBRACHIAL NERVE BLOCK   277

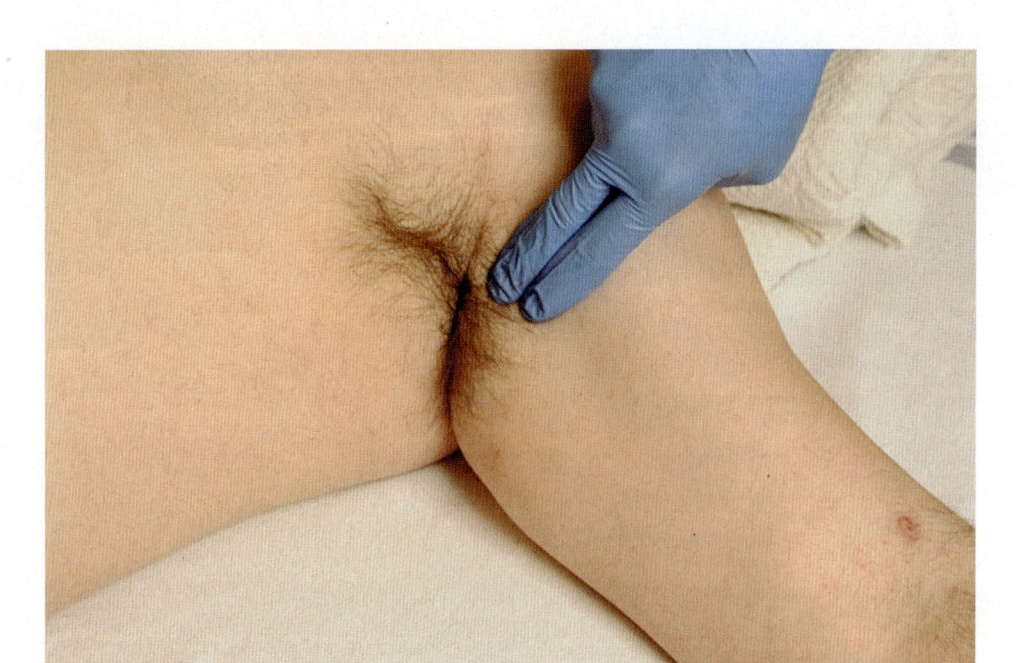

**FIGURE 42.4.**   Palpation of the axillary artery just beneath the axillary fold.

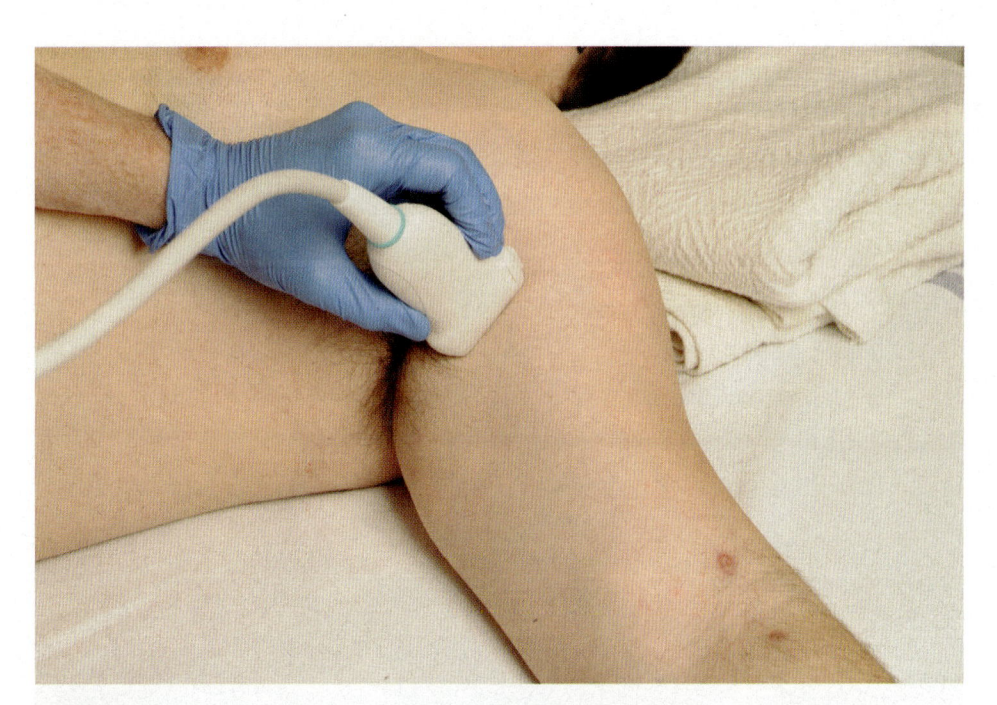

**FIGURE 42.5.**   Proper transverse placement of the ultrasound transducer for ultrasound-guided intercostobrachial cutaneous nerve block.

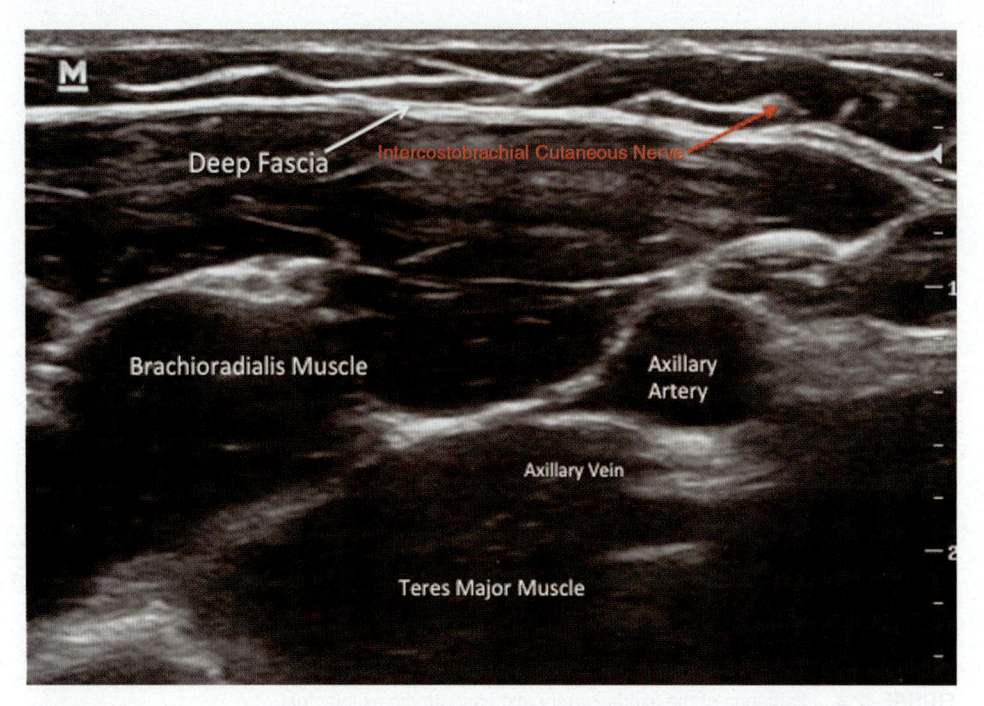

**FIGURE 42.6.** Transverse ultrasound image of the axillary artery and vein and the deep fascia.

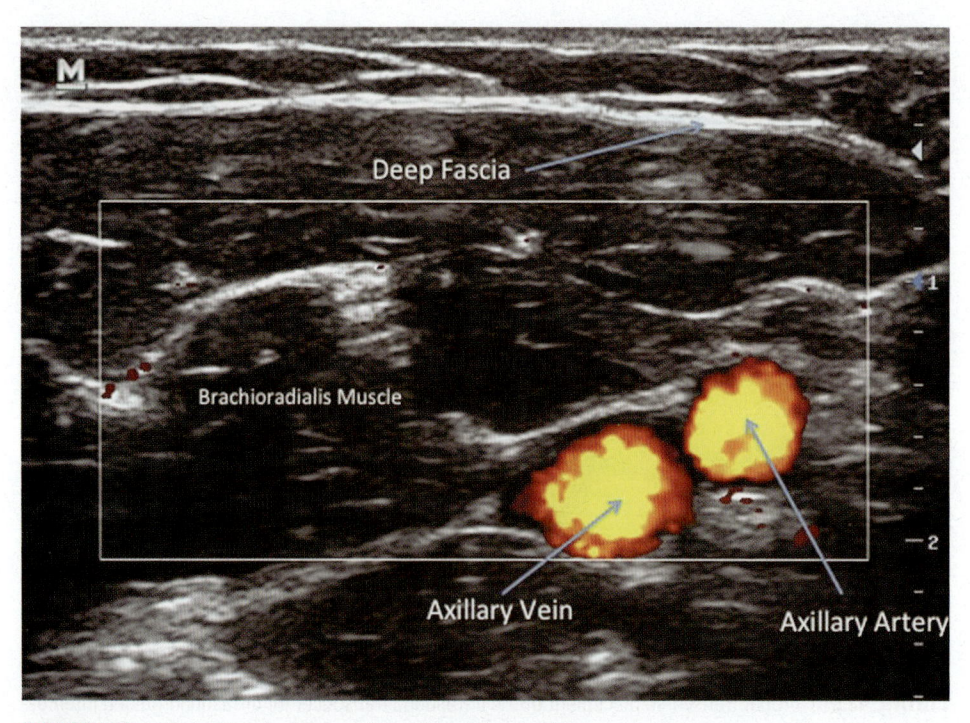

**FIGURE 42.7.** Color Doppler view of the axillary artery and vein.

CHAPTER 42 ULTRASOUND-GUIDED INJECTION TECHNIQUE FOR INTERCOSTOBRACHIAL NERVE BLOCK 279

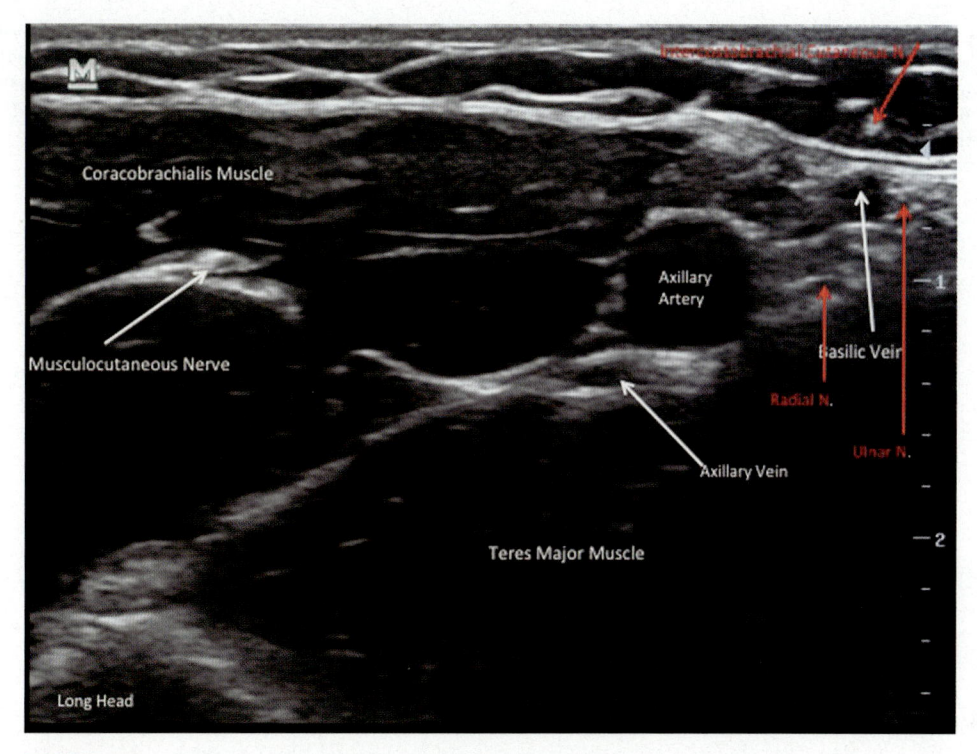

**FIGURE 42.8.** Transverse ultrasound image of the intercostobrachial cutaneous nerve. Note the relationship of the nerve to the deep fascia and the axillary artery and vein.

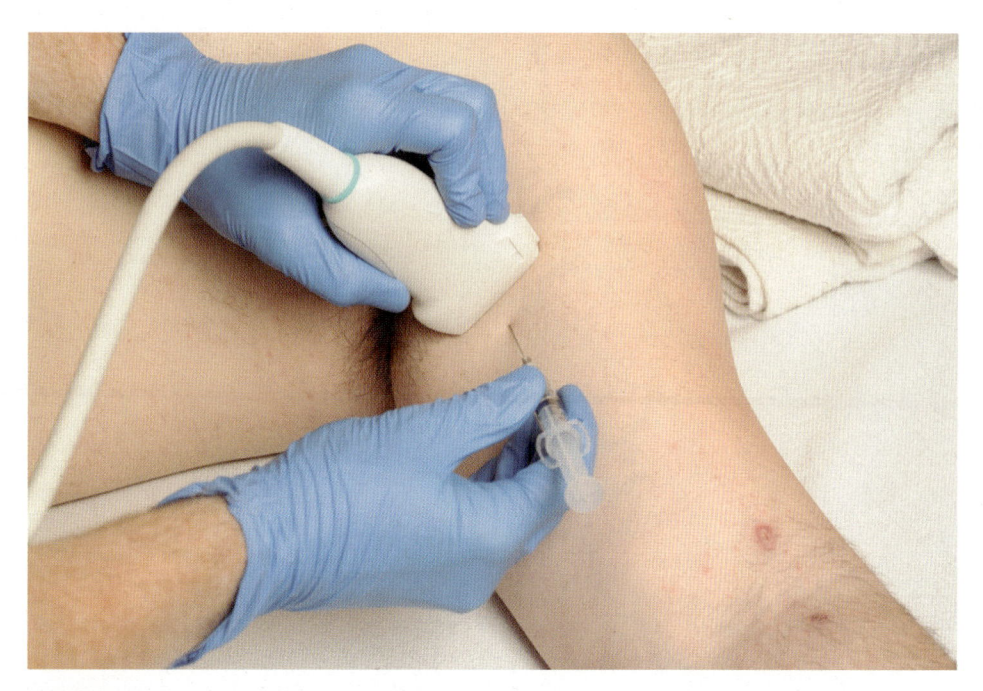

**FIGURE 42.9.** Proper out-of-plane needle placement for ultrasound-guided radial nerve block at the humerus.

## SUGGESTED READINGS

Franco CD, Clark L. Applied anatomy of the upper extremity. *Tech Reg Anesth Pain Manag* 2008;12(3):134–139.

Vries L. Upper limb nerve blocks. *Anaesth Intensive Care Med* 2007;8(4):127–131.

Waldman SD. Post-mastectomy pain. In: *Atlas of Uncommon Pain Syndromes*. 2nd ed. Philadelphia, PA: Saunders Elsevier; 2008:154–156.

Waldman SD. Injection technique for median cutaneous and intercostobrachial nerve block. In: *Atlas of Pain Management Injection Techniques*. 3rd ed. Philadelphia, PA: Saunders Elsevier; 2013:215–217.

CHAPTER 43

# Ultrasound-Guided Injection Technique for Medial Brachial Cutaneous Nerve Block

## CLINICAL PERSPECTIVES

Ultrasound-guided medial brachial cutaneous nerve block is used primarily as an adjunct to brachial plexus block rather than as a stand-alone regional anesthesia and pain management procedure. The medial brachial cutaneous nerve is the smallest branch of the brachial plexus and is often not adequately blocked when performing standard brachial plexus block techniques. This means that the medial and posterior aspect of the arm just below the axilla remains unanesthetized making prolonged use of a pneumatic tourniquet or the performance of surgical procedures in this region problematic.

## CLINICALLY RELEVANT ANATOMY

The medial brachial cutaneous nerve is comprised of fibers from the eighth cervical and first thoracic nerves. It is the smallest branch of the brachial plexus and arises from the medial cord of the brachial plexus. While passing through the axilla on its downward path, it provides communicating branches with the intercostobrachial cutaneous nerve. After leaving the axilla, it passes downward along with the brachial artery to provide cutaneous sensory innervation to medial and posterior aspect of the upper extremity just below the area innervated by the intercostobrachial cutaneous nerve (Figs. 43.1 and 43.2). This nerve can be damaged by surgical procedures, and there are case reports describing damage to the medial brachial cutaneous nerve during placement of long-acting contraceptive implants. The superficial location of this nerve makes it easily accessible for ultrasound-guided nerve block.

## ULTRASOUND-GUIDED TECHNIQUE

The benefits, risks, and alternative treatments are explained to the patient and informed consent is obtained. The patient is then placed in the supine position with the affected upper extremity abducted 90 degrees and the palm facing upward (Fig. 43.3). With the patient in the above position, the medial epicondyle is identified, and at a point ~1 inch above the superomedial margin of the epicondyle, a high-frequency linear ultrasound transducer is placed in the transverse position (Fig. 43.4).

An ultrasound survey image is obtained, and the basilic vein and branches of the medial brachial cutaneous nerve are identified (Fig. 43.5). Color Doppler can aid in the identifications of the basilica vein and any other vasculature in proximity to the medial brachial cutaneous nerve (Fig. 43.6). The ultrasound transducer is then slowly moved proximally to follow the branches of the medial brachial cutaneous nerve until they coalesce into a single ovoid hyperechoic nerve (Fig. 43.7). As the ultrasound transducer is moved more proximally, the medial brachial cutaneous nerve moves from its 6:00 o'clock position in front of the basilic vein to the 9:00 o'clock position next to the vein (Fig. 43.8). It is at this point that ultrasound-guided medial brachial cutaneous nerve block is easiest to perform. Ultimately, as the nerve is followed more proximally, it will move from the 9:00 o'clock to the 12:00 o'clock position making more difficult to block without traversing the basilica vein (Fig. 43.9). Once the medial brachial cutaneous nerve is clearly identified and is felt to be in satisfactory position for ultrasound-guided nerve block, the skin overlying the area beneath the ultrasound transducer is then prepped with antiseptic solution. A sterile syringe containing 3.0 mL of 0.25% preservative-free bupivacaine and 40 mg of methylprednisolone is attached to a 1½-inch, 22-gauge needle using strict aseptic technique. The needle is placed through the skin just below the center of the transducer and is then advanced using an out-of-plane approach with the needle trajectory adjusted under real-time ultrasound guidance so that the needle tip ultimately rests in proximity to the medial brachial cutaneous nerve (Fig. 43.10). When the tip of needle is thought to be in satisfactory position, after careful aspiration, a small amount of local anesthetic and steroid is injected under real-time ultrasound guidance to confirm that the needle tip is in the proper position. After proper needle tip placement is confirmed, the remainder of the contents

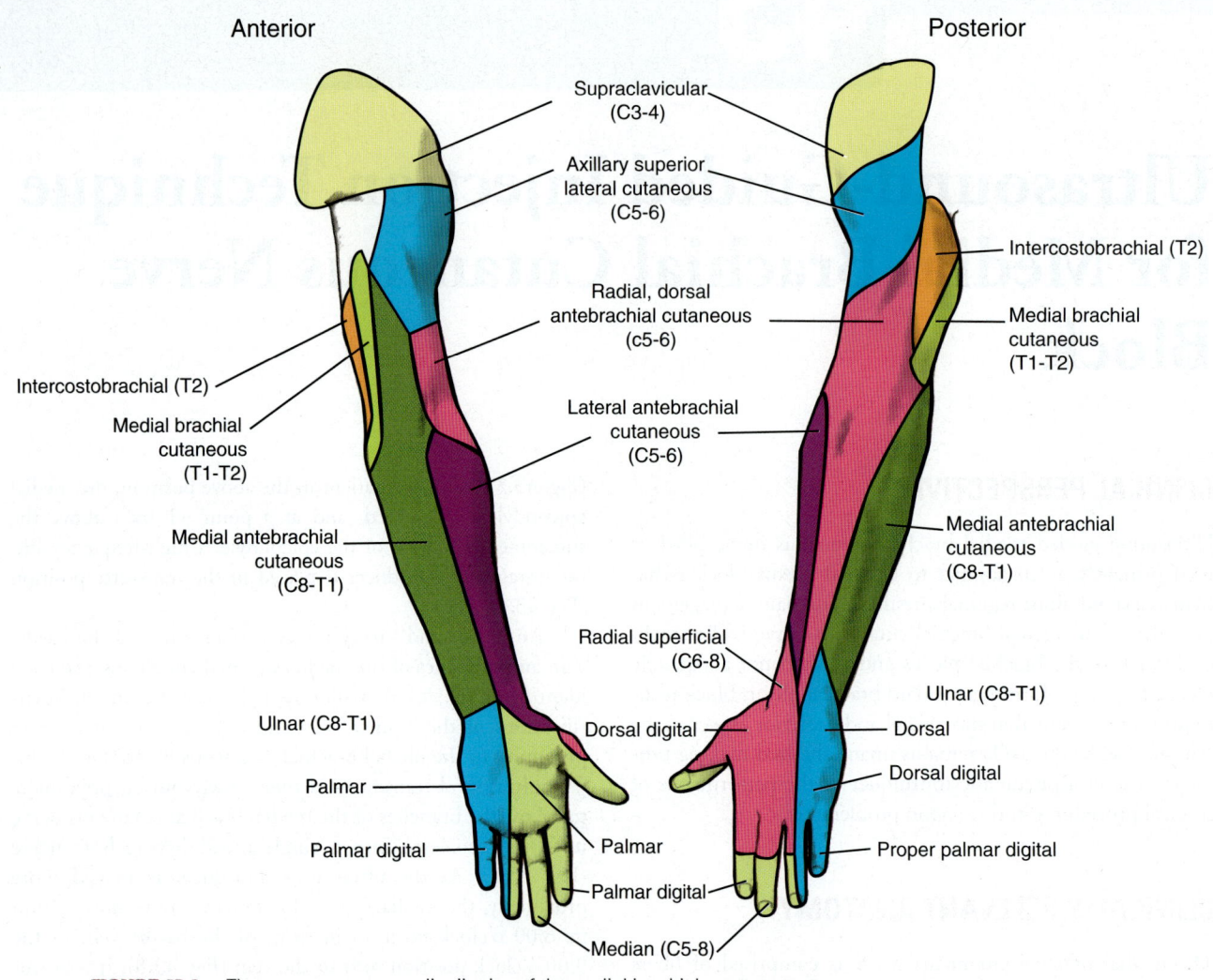

**FIGURE 43.1.** The cutaneous sensory distribution of the medial brachial cutaneous nerve.

of the syringe are slowly injected. There should be minimal resistance to injection.

## COMPLICATIONS

The major complications of ultrasound-guided injection of ultrasound-guided medial brachial cutaneous nerve block are related to improper needle placement with the possibility of inadvertent intravascular injection and/or persistent paresthesia secondary to needle trauma to the nerve. Although rare, infection may occur. Ecchymosis and hematoma formation following this procedure may also occur. These complications can be decreased if manual pressure is applied to the area of the block immediately after injection. Application of cold packs for 20-minute periods after the block will also decrease the amount of postprocedure pain and bleeding the patient may experience.

Approximately 25% of patients complain of a transient increase in pain after this injection technique; the patient should be warned of this.

## CLINICAL PEARLS

Ultrasound-guided medial brachial cutaneous nerve block is a straightforward and relatively safe technique if attention is paid to the clinically relevant anatomy. It is useful as an adjunct to brachial plexus block, often being combined with medial brachial cutaneous nerve block. Careful neurologic examination to identify preexisting neurologic deficits that may later be attributed to the nerve block should be performed on all patients before beginning ultrasound-guided medial brachial cutaneous nerve block especially when surgical exploration of the axilla and chest wall for lymph node dissection during mastectomy is being considered.

CHAPTER 43 ULTRASOUND-GUIDED INJECTION TECHNIQUE FOR MEDIAL BRACHIAL CUTANEOUS NERVE BLOCK 283

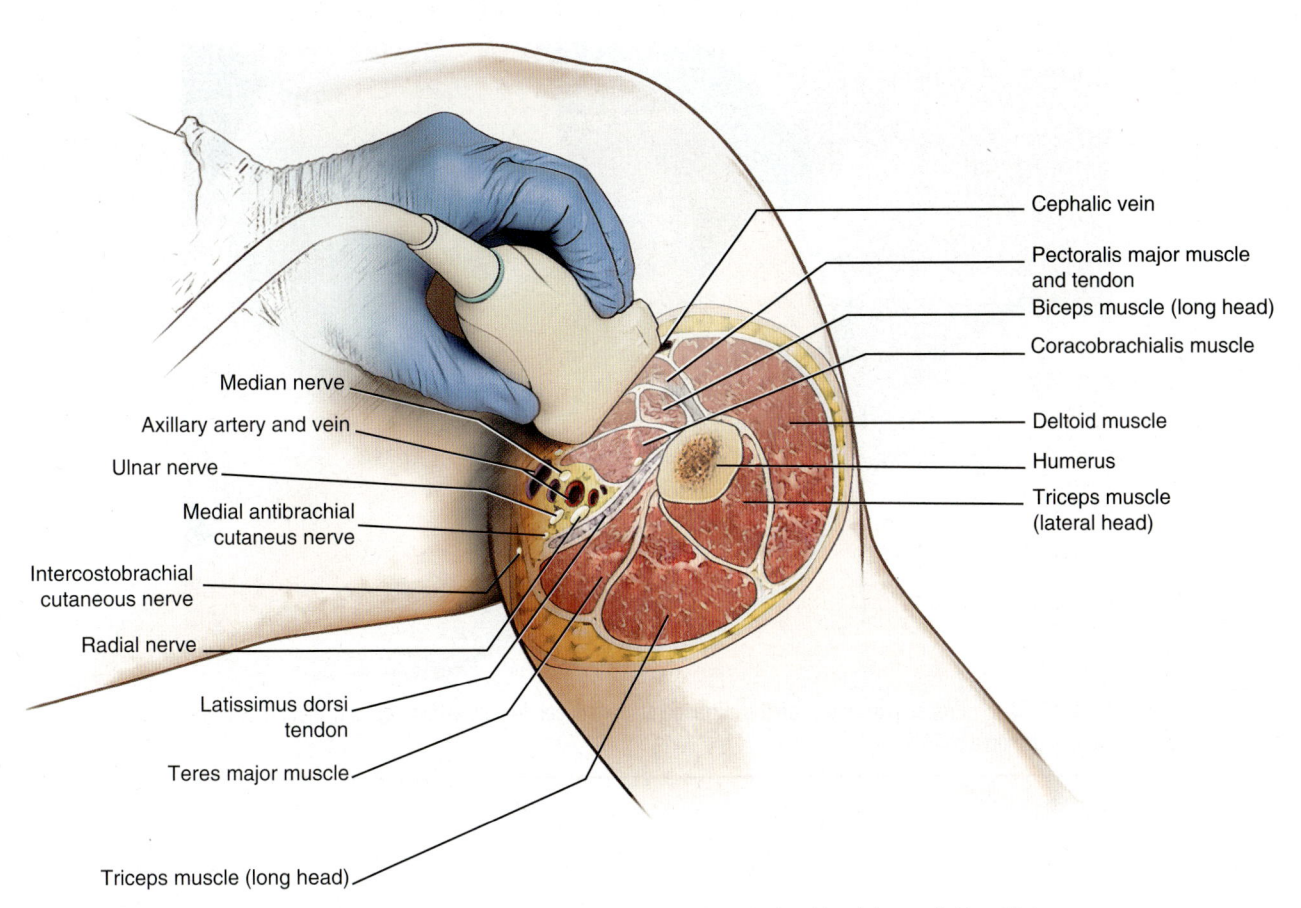

**FIGURE 43.2.** Cross-sectional anatomy of the upper arm showing the relationship of the medial brachial cutaneous nerve to the axillary artery, vein, and adjacent muscles.

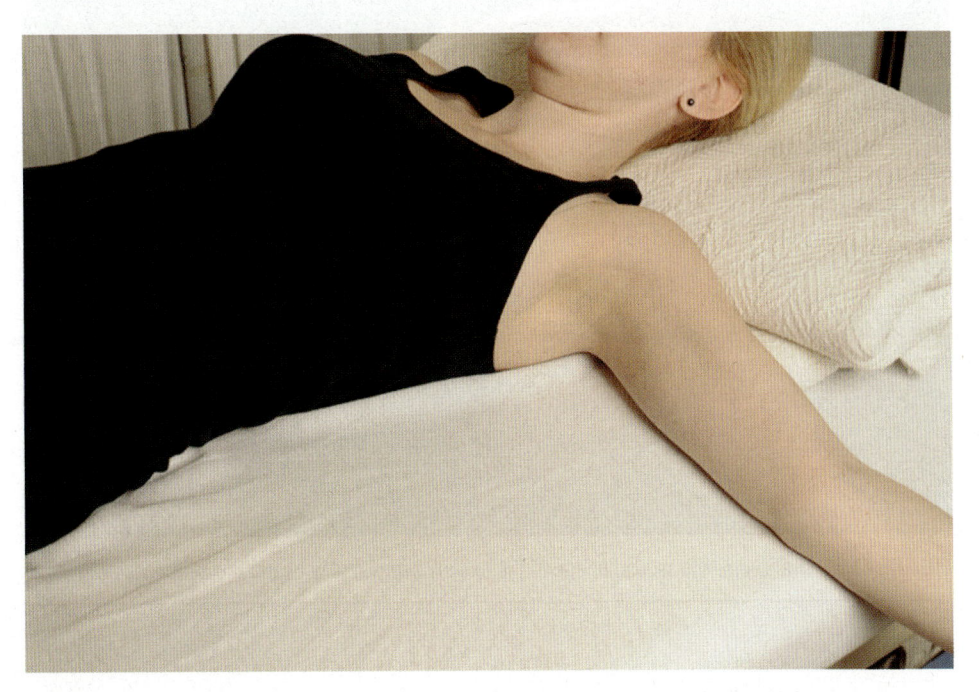

**FIGURE 43.3.** Proper position of the patient for ultrasound-guided medial brachial cutaneous nerve block.

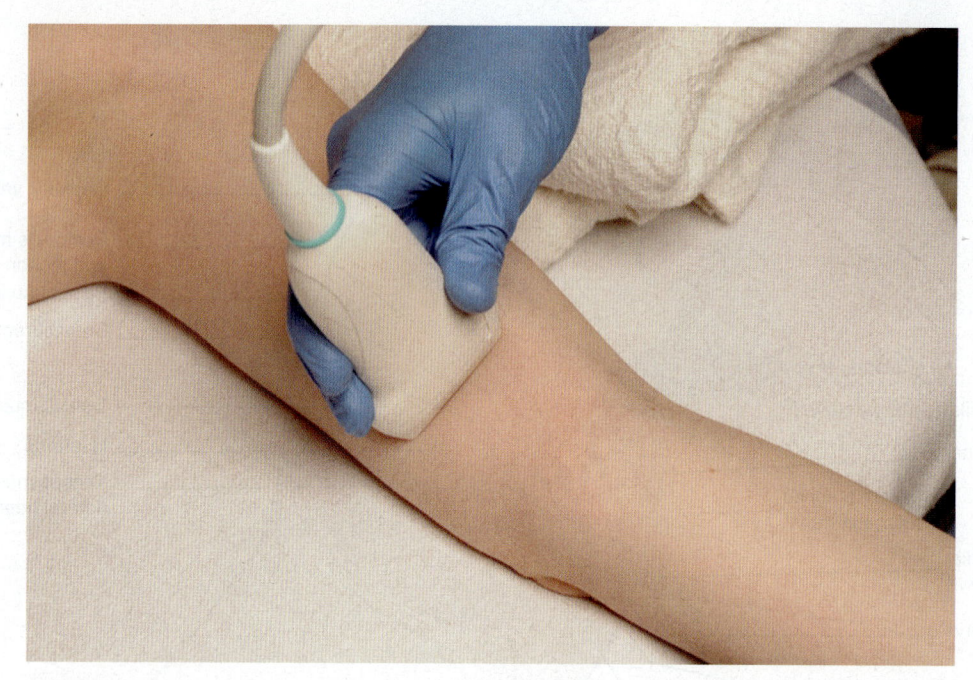

**FIGURE 43.4.** Proper placement of the ultrasound transducer for ultrasound-guided medial brachial cutaneous nerve block.

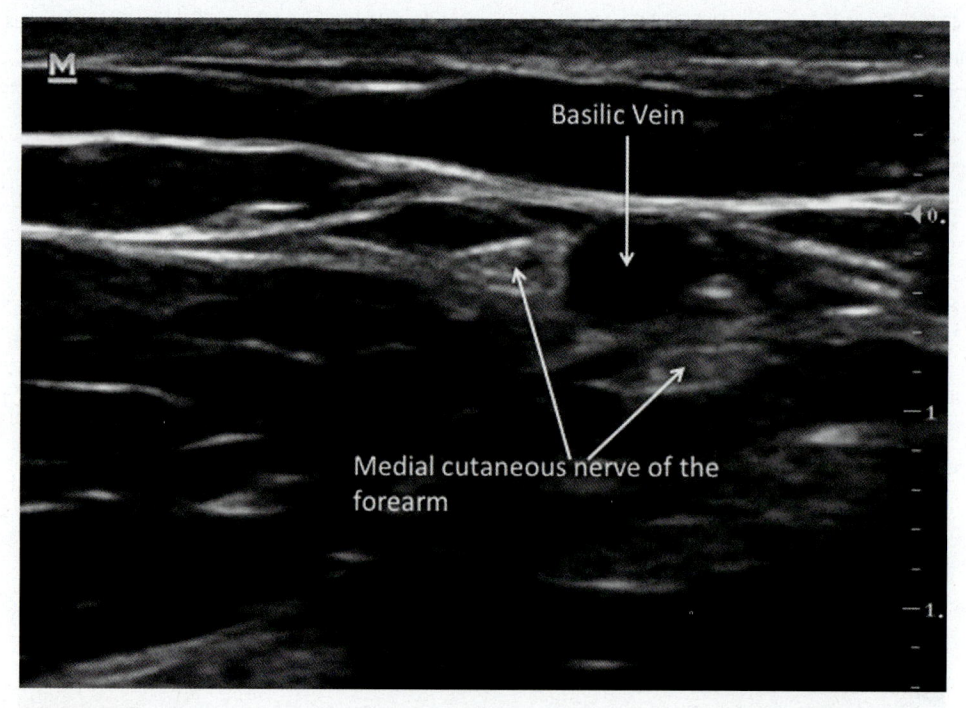

**FIGURE 43.5.** Transverse ultrasound image of the axillary artery and vein and the deep fascia.

CHAPTER 43    ULTRASOUND-GUIDED INJECTION TECHNIQUE FOR MEDIAL BRACHIAL CUTANEOUS NERVE BLOCK    285

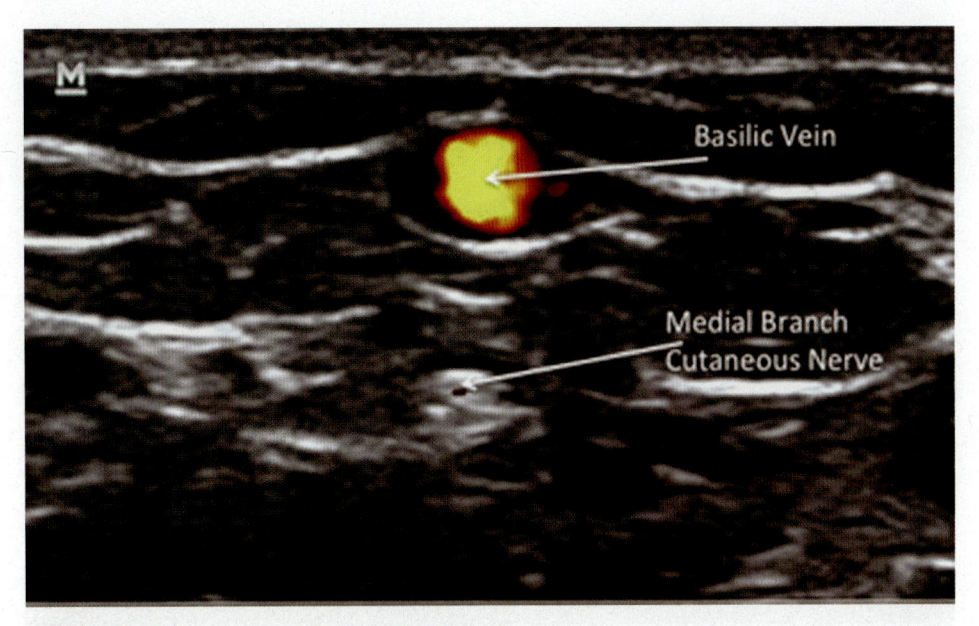

**FIGURE 43.6.** Color Doppler view of the basilic vein.

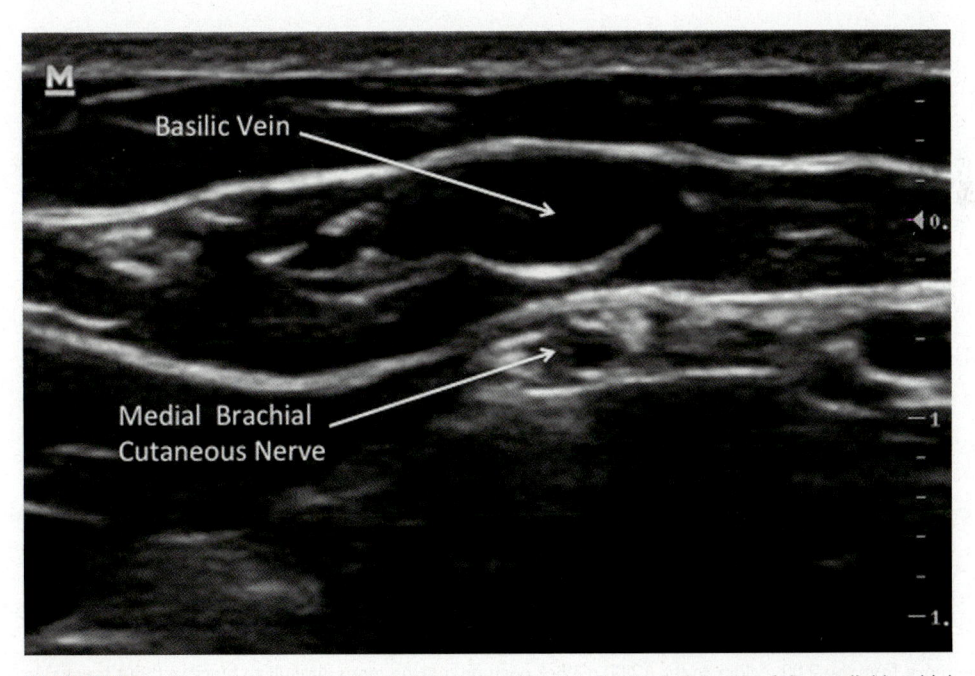

**FIGURE 43.7.** As the ultrasound transducer is moved proximally along the path of the medial brachial cutaneous nerve, the various branches of the nerve will be seen to coalesce into a single ovoid hyperechoic nerve.

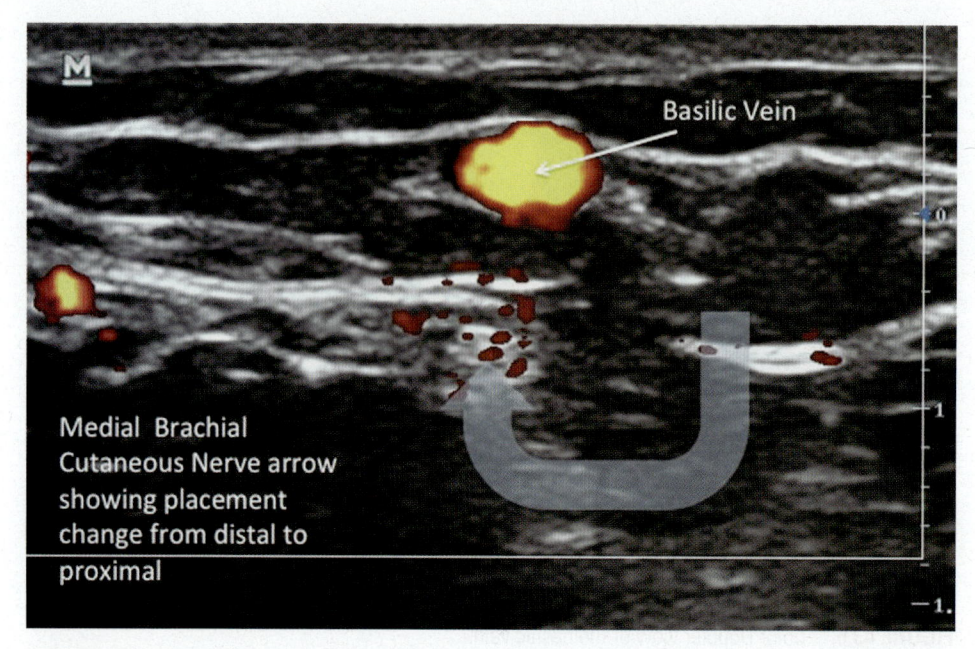

**FIGURE 43.8.** As the ultrasound transducer is moved more proximally, the medial brachial cutaneous nerve moves from its 6:00 o'clock position in front of the basilic vein to the 9:00 o'clock position next to the vein.

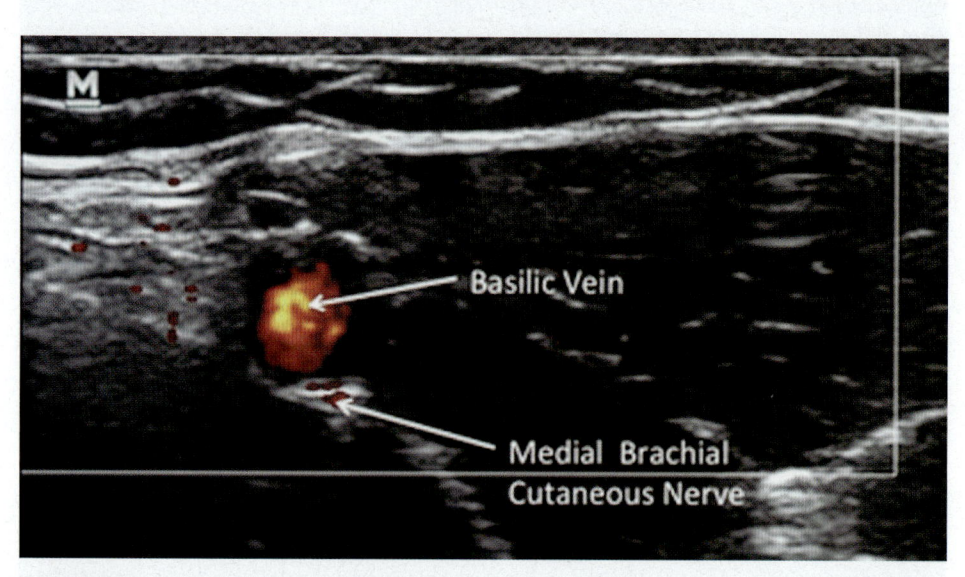

**FIGURE 43.9.** Ultimately, as the medial brachial cutaneous nerve is imaged more proximally, it will move from the 9:00 o'clock to the 12:00 o'clock position making more difficult to block without traversing the basilic vein.

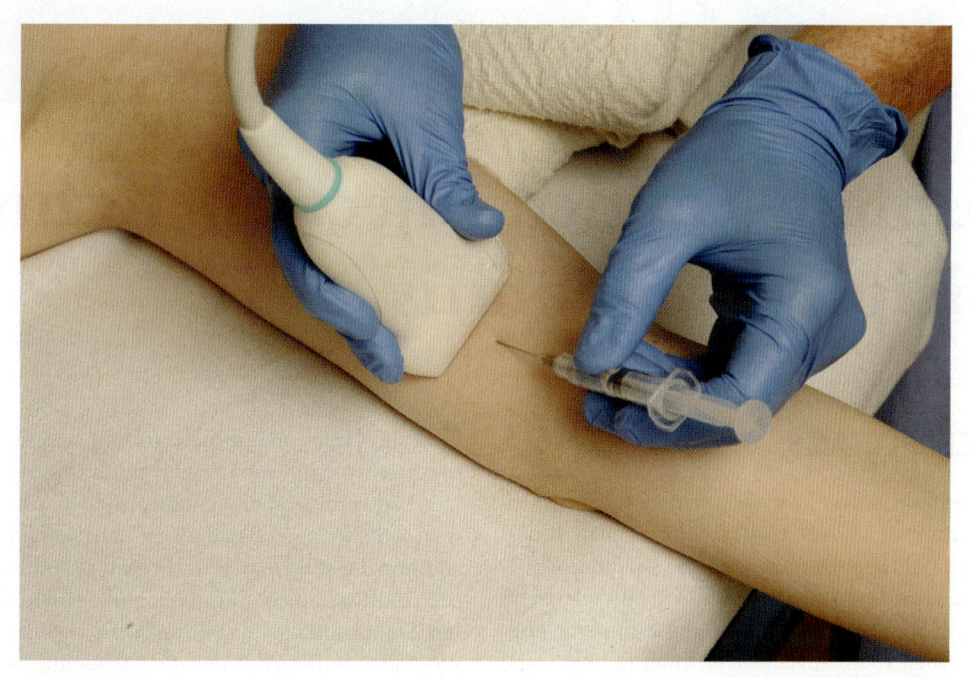

**FIGURE 43.10.** Proper out-of-plane needle placement for ultrasound-guided medial brachial cutaneous nerve block.

## SUGGESTED READINGS

Franco CD, Clark L. Applied anatomy of the upper extremity. *Tech Reg Anesth Pain Manag* 2008;12(3):134–139.

Vries L. Upper limb nerve blocks. *Anaesth Intensive Care Med* 2007;8(4):127–131.

Waldman SD. Post-mastectomy pain. In: *Atlas of Uncommon Pain Syndromes*. 2nd ed. Philadelphia, PA: WB Saunders; 2008:154–156.

Waldman SD. Injection technique for median cutaneous and intercostobrachial nerve block. In: *Atlas of Pain Management Injection Techniques*. 3rd ed. Philadelphia, PA: Saunders Elsevier; 2013:215–217.

# CHAPTER 44

# Ultrasound-Guided Injection Technique for Bicipital Tendonitis

## CLINICAL PERSPECTIVES

The musculotendinous units of the shoulder are subjected to an amazing variation of stresses as they perform their function of allowing a full range of motion of the shoulder while at the same time providing shoulder stability. The relatively poor blood supply limits the ability of these muscles and tendons to heal when traumatized. Over time, muscle tears and tendinopathy develop, further weakening the musculotendinous units and making them susceptible to additional damage. The potential for impingement as the bicipital musculotendinous unit passes beneath the coracoacromial arch can further exacerbate the problem and further inflame and damage the structures (Fig. 44.1). Over time, if the trauma and subsequent inflammation continues, calcium deposition around the tendon with resultant calcific tendonitis may occur, making subsequent treatment more difficult. Tendonitis of the musculotendinous units of the shoulder frequently coexists with bursitis of the associated bursae of the shoulder joint, creating additional pain and functional disability.

The long and short tendons of the biceps are susceptible to the development of tendonitis following even seemingly minor trauma (Fig. 44.2). The onset of bicipital tendonitis is usually acute, occurring after overuse or misuse of the shoulder joint. Inciting factors may include activities such as trying to start a recalcitrant lawn mower, practicing an overhead tennis serve, or overaggressive follow-through when driving golf balls. The pain of bicipital tendonitis is constant, severe, and localized in the anterior shoulder over the bicipital groove. A "catching" sensation also may accompany the pain. Significant sleep disturbance is often reported. The patient may attempt to splint the inflamed tendons by internal rotation of the humerus, which moves the biceps tendon from beneath the coracoacromial arch. Patients suffering from bicipital tendonitis will exhibit a positive Yergason sign, which is elicited by having the patient flex the elbow and supinate the forearm against resistance. Maximal pain will be felt in the bicipital groove (Fig. 44.3). If untreated, patients suffering from bicipital tendonitis may experience difficulty in performing any task that requires initial abduction of the upper extremity, making simple everyday tasks such as brushing ones teeth or eating difficult. Over time, muscle atrophy, calcific tendonitis, and ultimately tendon rupture may result (Fig. 44.4).

Plain radiographs are indicated in all patients who present with shoulder pain. Based on the patient's clinical presentation, additional testing may be indicated, including complete blood cell count, sedimentation rate, and antinuclear antibody testing. Ultrasound imaging or magnetic resonance imaging of the shoulder is indicated if a bicipital tendonitis is suspected as well as to aid in the evaluation of the affected area and may also help delineate the presence of tendinopathy, calcific tendonitis, bursitis, tendon rupture, or other shoulder pathology (Fig. 44.5).

## CLINICALLY RELEVANT ANATOMY

Along with the conjoined tendons of the rotator cuff, the bicipital muscle serves to stabilize the shoulder joint. The biceps muscle, which is named for its two heads, functions to supinate the forearm and flex the elbow joint (Fig. 44.6). The long head finds its origin in the supraglenoid tubercle of the scapula, and the short head finds its origin from the tip of the coracoid process of the scapula. The long head exits the shoulder joint via the bicipital groove, where it is susceptible to trauma and the development of tendonitis. The long head fuses with the short head in the middle portion of the upper arm forming the belly of the biceps muscle. The insertion of the biceps muscle is into the posterior portion of the radial tuberosity. The biceps muscle is innervated by the musculocutaneous nerve, which arises from the lateral cord of the brachial plexus. The fibers of the musculocutaneous nerve are derived from C5, C6, and C7 nerve roots.

The biceps musculotendinous unit is subjected to significant stress during functioning, and misuse or overuse can result in damage. If the damage remains untreated, the musculotendinous unit can rupture (Fig. 44.7). This most commonly occurs with the long head of the biceps, but the short head and the distal tendinous insertion can also rupture. If the long head ruptures, the patient will present with a classic deformity known as the Popeye sign (Fig. 44.8). This deformity can be demonstrated by having the patient perform the Luningston maneuver, which is having the patient place his or her hands behind the head and flex the biceps muscle.

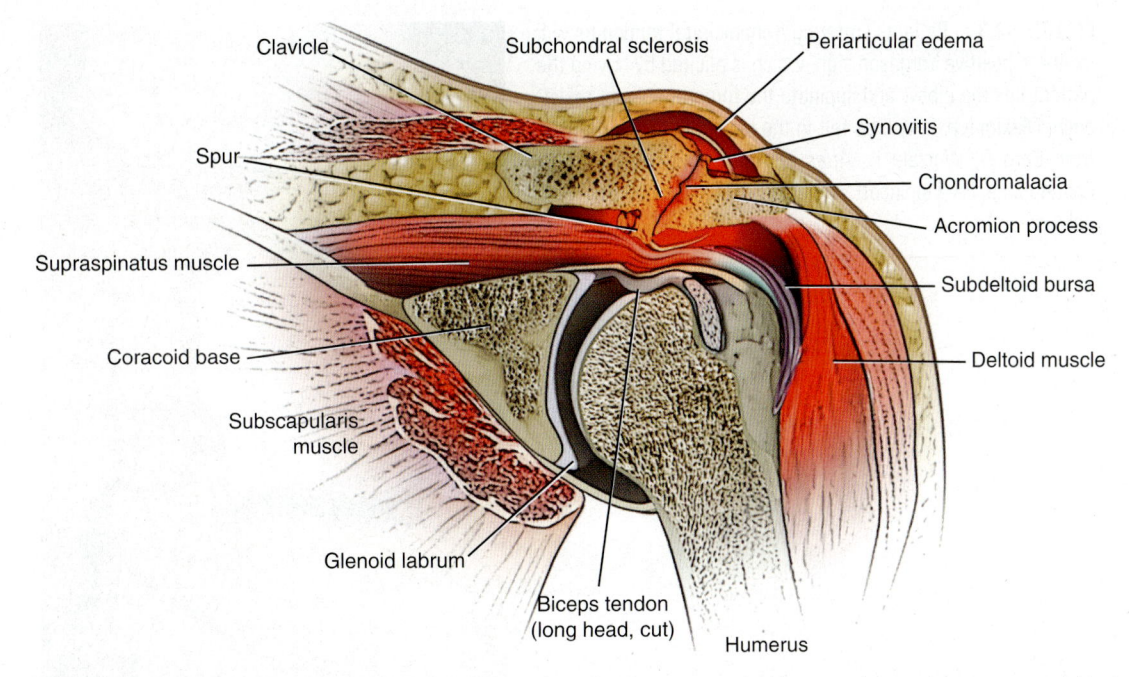

# CHAPTER 44 ULTRASOUND-GUIDED INJECTION TECHNIQUE FOR BICIPITAL TENDONITIS

**FIGURE 44.1.** Bicipital tendonitis is usually, at least in part, due to impingement on the biceps tendons at the coracoacromial arch.

## ULTRASOUND-GUIDED TECHNIQUE

The benefits, risks, and alternative treatments are explained to the patient and informed consent is obtained. The patient is then placed in the sitting position with the forearm resting comfortably on the ipsilateral thigh with the palm up (Fig. 44.9). The bicipital groove is then palpated (Fig. 44.10).

A high-frequency linear ultrasound transducer is placed in the transverse plane centered over the bicipital groove, and an ultrasound survey scan is taken (Fig. 44.11). The bicipital groove is identified with the biceps tendon, which appears as a hyperechoic ovoid structure lying within it (Fig. 44.12). The transverse bicipital ligament, which lies just above the bicipital tendon, is then identified. The tendon will exhibit the property

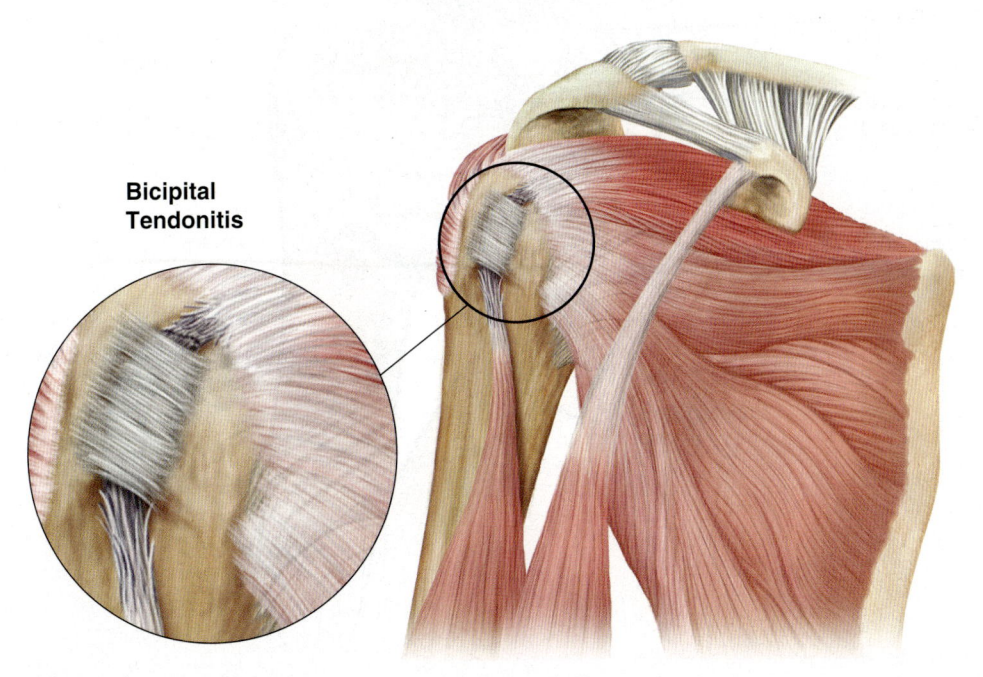

**FIGURE 44.2.** Bicipital tendonitis. (From Anatomical Chart Company.)

**FIGURE 44.3.** Patients suffering from bicipital tendonitis will exhibit a positive Yergason sign, which is elicited by having the patient flex the elbow and supinate the forearm against resistance. Maximal pain will be felt in the bicipital groove. (Reused from Berg D, Worzala K. *Atlas of Adult Physical Diagnosis*. Philadelphia, PA: Lippincott Williams & Wilkins; 2006:240, with permission.)

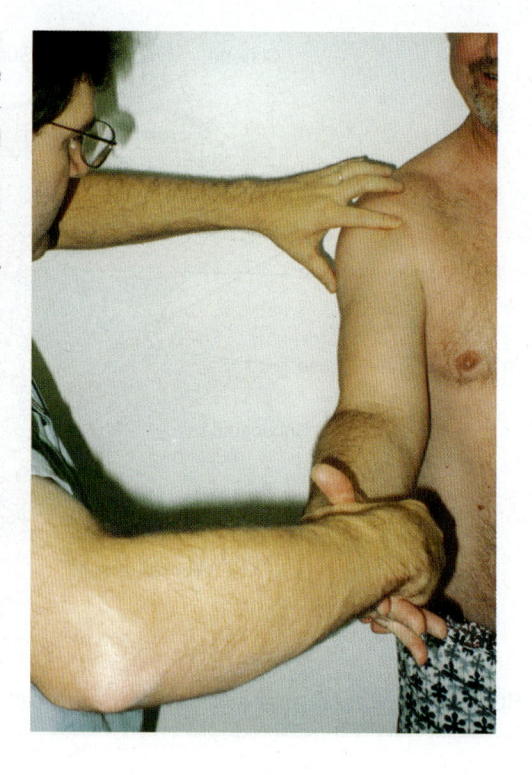

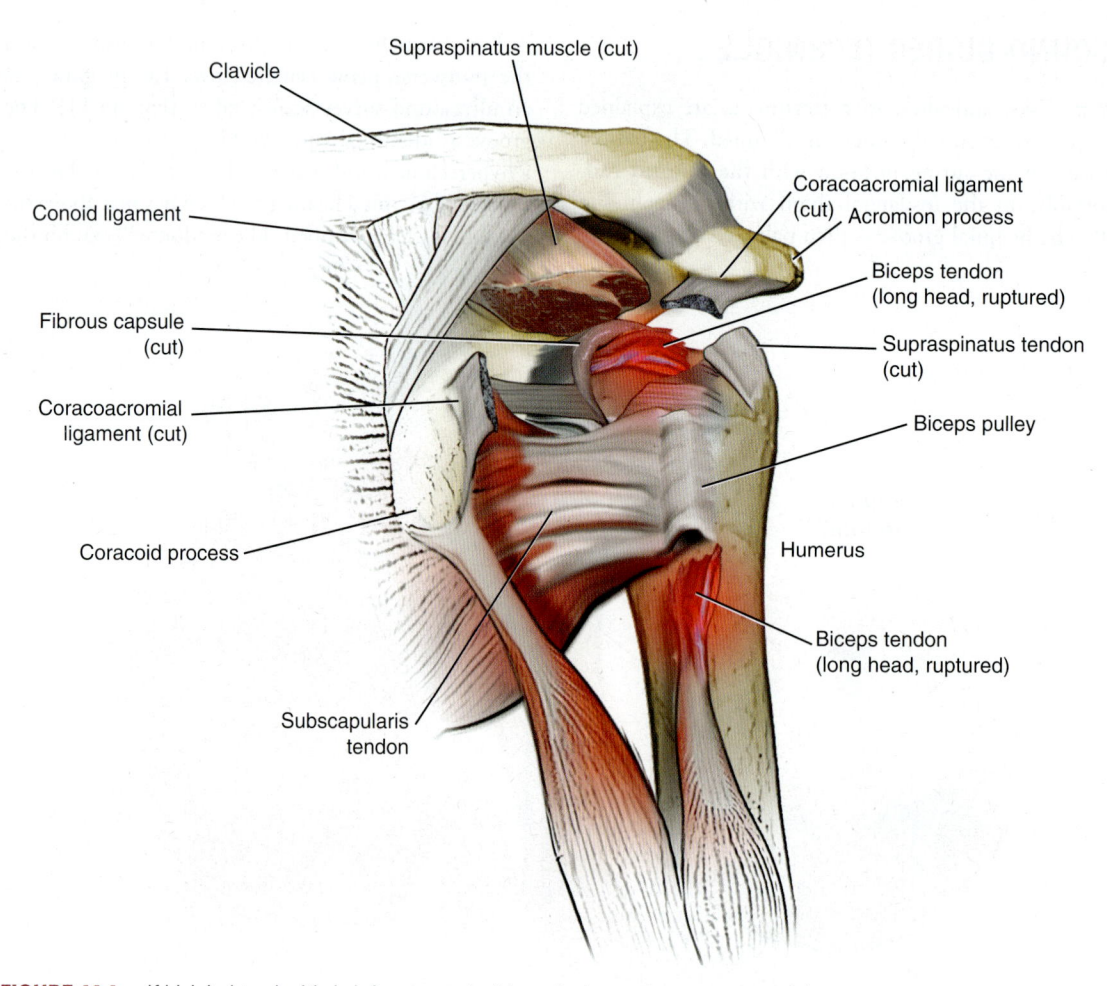

**FIGURE 44.4.** If bicipital tendonitis is left untreated, ultimately the tendon may tear and then rupture.

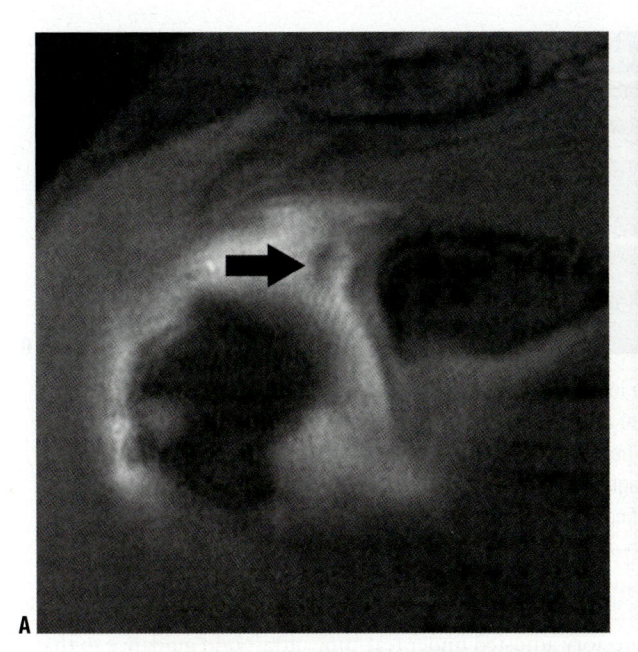

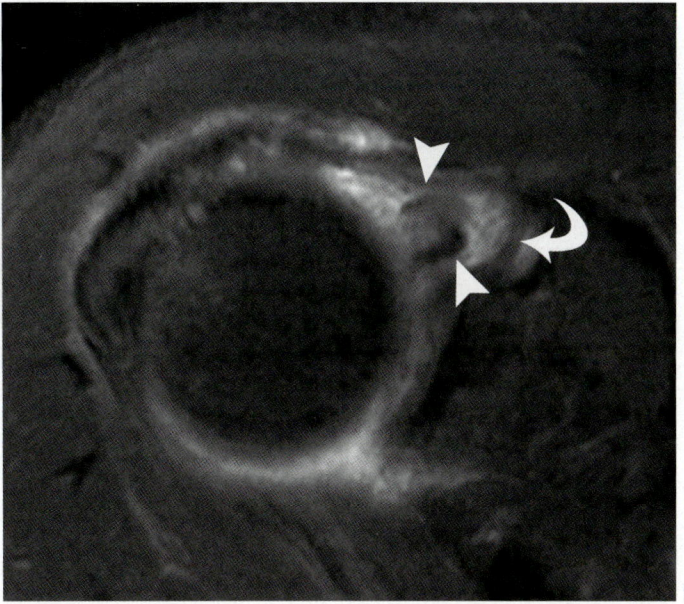

**FIGURE 44.5.** Complete rupture of biceps tendon with free stump. Coronal (**A**) intermediate-weighted fat-suppressed MR image shows the anteriorly displaced torn proximal biceps tendon (*arrow*). Axial (**B**) T2-weighted fat-suppressed MR image profiles the torn proximal biceps tendon (*arrowheads*) that is anteriorly displaced and residing anterior to the superior glenohumeral ligament (*curved arrow*). (Reused from Chung CB, Steinbach L. Long bicipital tendon including superior labral anterior-posterior lesions. In: Chung CB, Steinback L, eds. *MRI of the Upper Extremity: Shoulder, Elbow, Wrist, and Hand.* Philadelphia, PA: Lippincott Williams & Wilkins; 2010:327, with permission.)

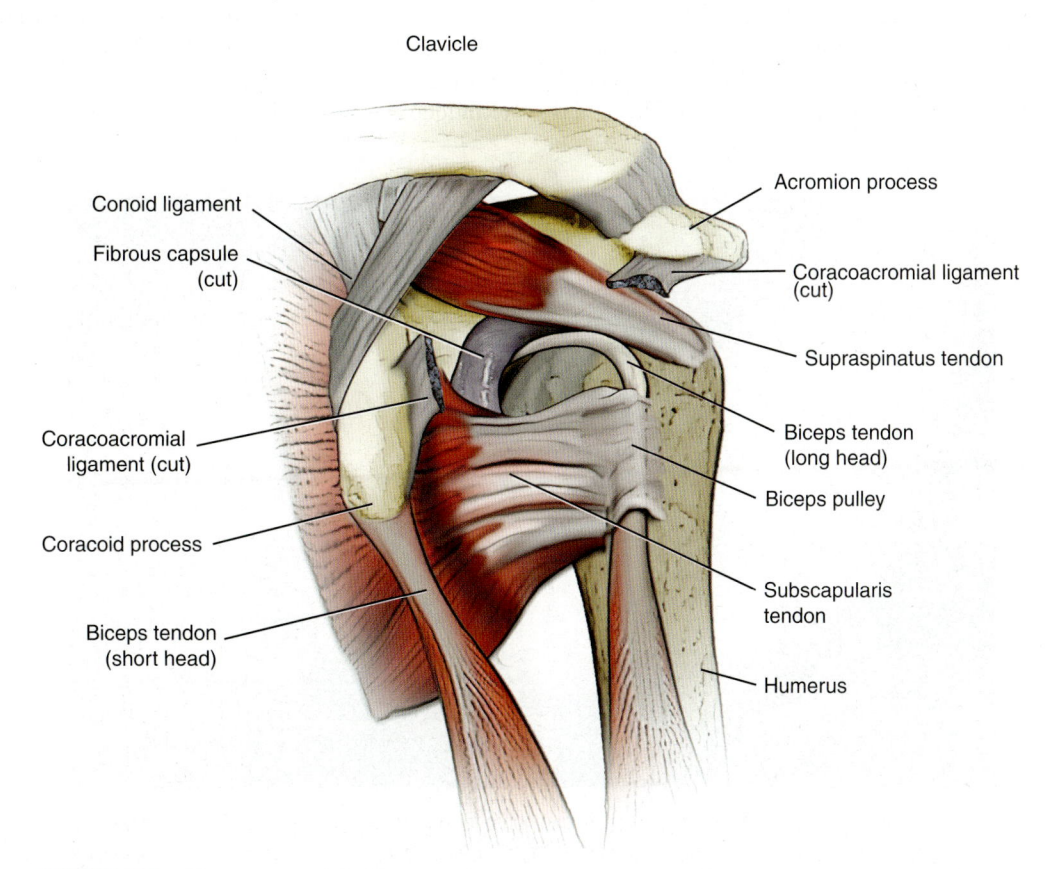

**FIGURE 44.6.** The anatomy of the biceps tendon.

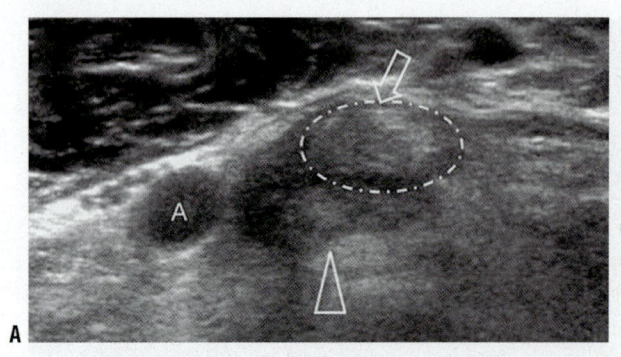

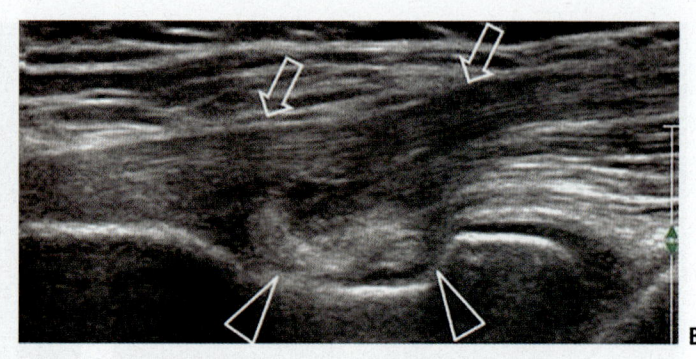

**FIGURE 44.7.** A 65-year-old man with a partial tear involving the long head of the biceps tendon. **A:** The axial ultrasound image demonstrates the rupture of the long head (*arrow*), which also appears surrounded by fluid (*arrowhead*). **B:** In the longitudinal ultrasound image, the distal tendon belonging to the short head is intact (*arrows*), while the tendon of the long head is torn (*arrowheads*). *A* indicates the brachial artery. (Reused from Tagliafico A, Michaud J, Capaccio E, et al. Ultrasound demonstration of distal biceps tendon bifurcation: normal and abnormal findings. *Eur Radiol* 2010;20(1):202–208, with permission.)

of anisotropy when viewed in the longitudinal axis (Figs. 44.13 and 44.14). Any significant amount of peritendinous fluid identified should be considered abnormal and indicative of tendonitis.

After the bicipital tendon within the bicipital groove is identified, the skin overlying the lateral aspect of the acromion is then prepped with antiseptic solution. A sterile syringe containing 3.0 mL of 0.25% preservative-free bupivacaine and 40 mg of methylprednisolone is attached to a 3½-inch, 22-gauge needle using strict aseptic technique. After the bicipital tendon is reidentified, the needle is placed through the skin just below the center of the of the transversely placed transducer and is then advanced using an out-of-plane approach with the needle trajectory adjusted under real-time ultrasound guidance so that the needle tip rests just above the tendon, but not within the tendon substance itself (Fig. 44.15). When the tip of needle is thought to be in satisfactory position, a small amount of local anesthetic and steroid is injected under real-time ultrasound guidance to confirm that the needle tip is not with the substance of the tendon. After proper needle tip placement is confirmed, the remainder of the contents of the syringe are slowly injected. There should be minimal resistance to injection. The needle is then removed, and a sterile pressure dressing and ice pack are placed at the injection site. If calcific tendonitis is present, a two-needle ultrasound-guided lavage and aspiration technique may be beneficial.

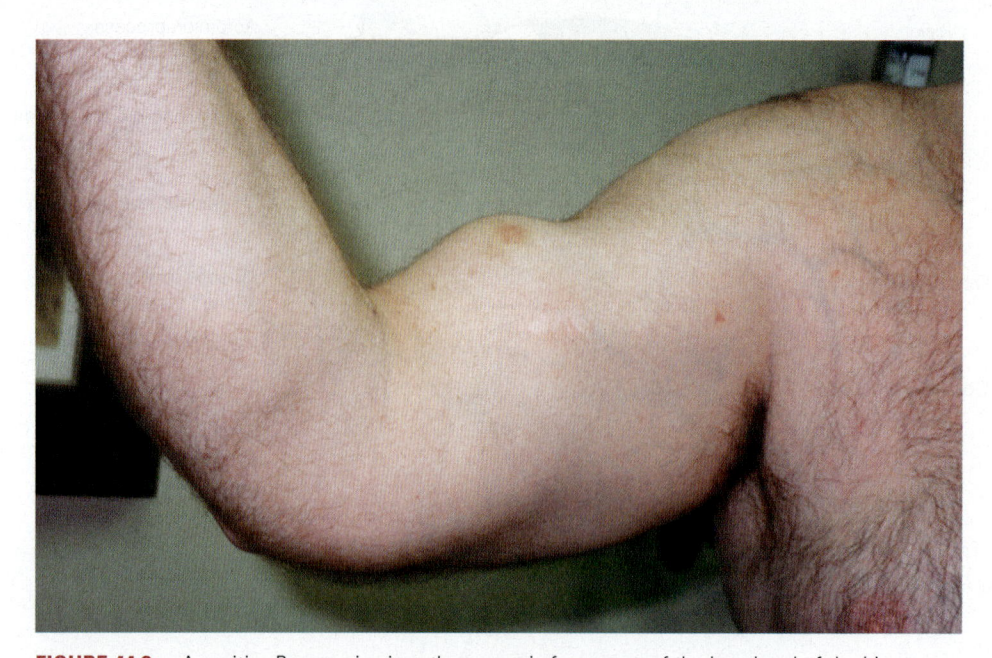

**FIGURE 44.8.** A positive Popeye sign is pathognomonic for rupture of the long head of the biceps tendon. (Reused from Berg D, Worzala K. *Atlas of Adult Physical Diagnosis*. Philadelphia, PA: Lippincott Williams & Wilkins; 2006:241, with permission.)

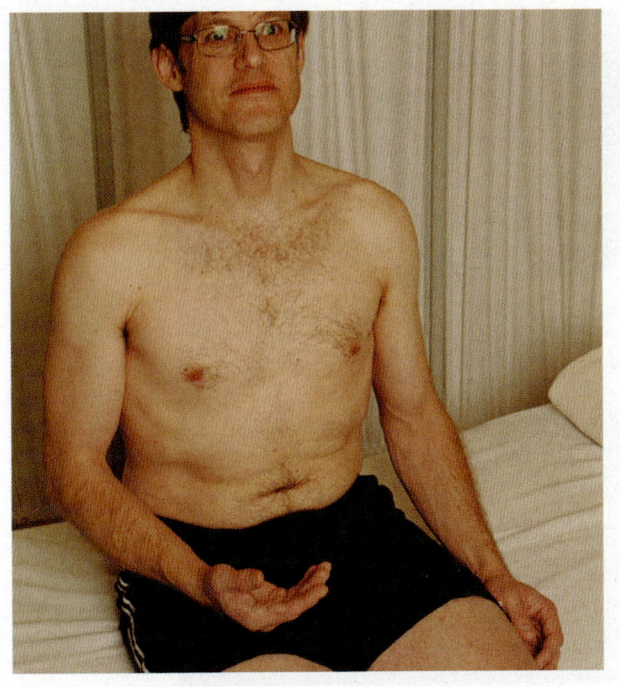

**FIGURE 44.9.** Proper patient positioning for ultrasound-guided injection for bicipital tendonitis.

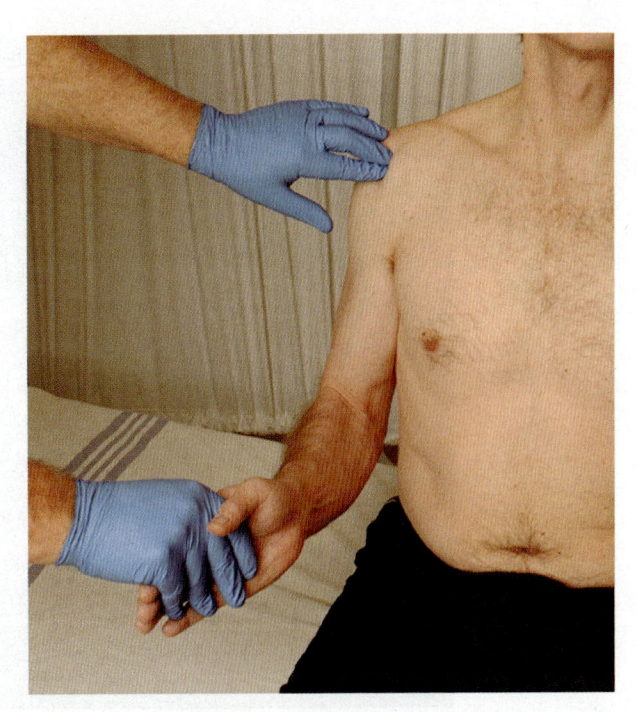

**FIGURE 44.10.** Palpation of the bicipital groove.

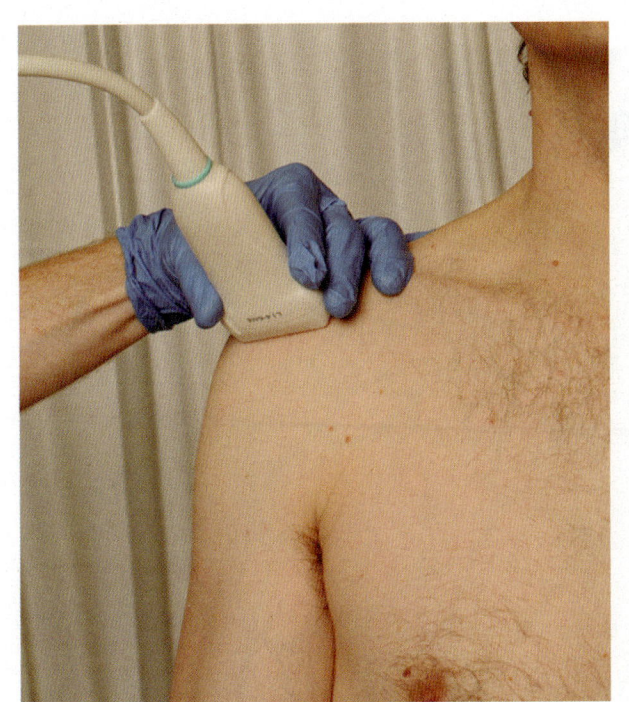

**FIGURE 44.11.** Proper transverse transducer position for ultrasound-guided injection for bicipital tendonitis.

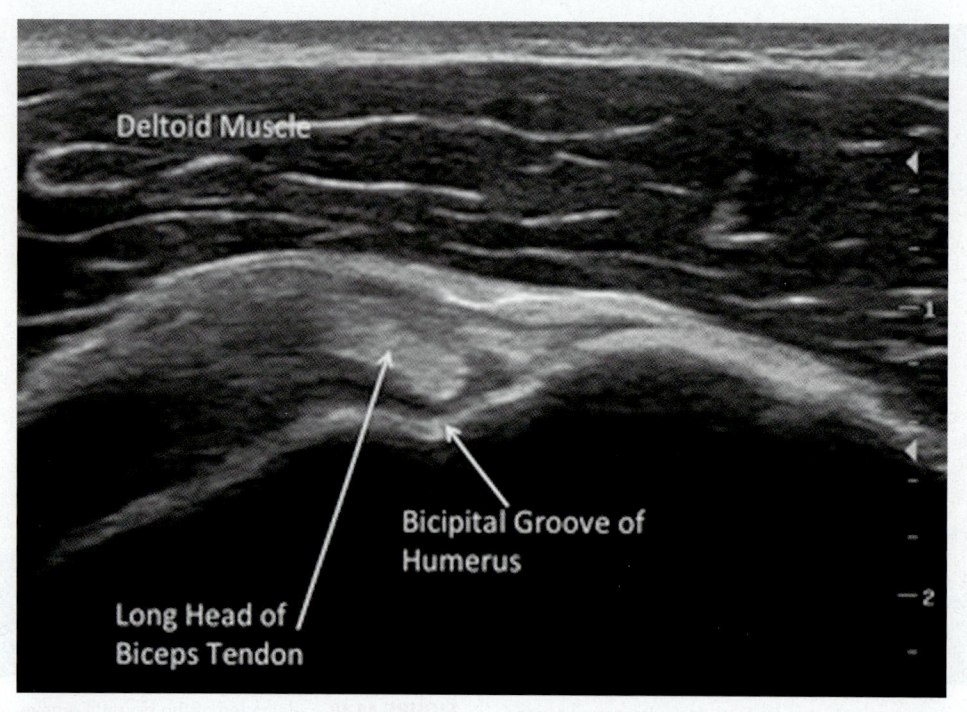

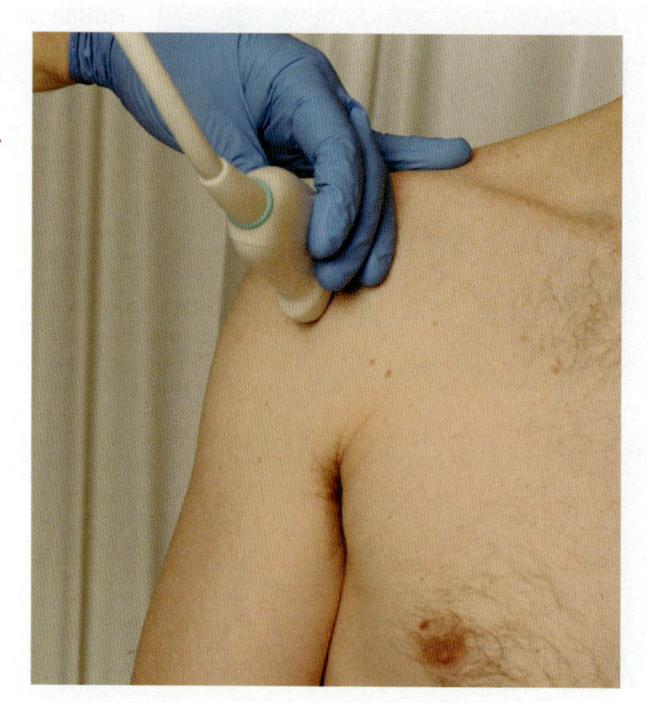

**FIGURE 44.12.** Transverse ultrasound image of the bicipital tendon lying within the bicipital groove. Note the transverse bicipital ligament.

**FIGURE 44.13.** Proper longitudinal transducer position for ultrasound evaluation of bicipital tendonitis.

CHAPTER 44    ULTRASOUND-GUIDED INJECTION TECHNIQUE FOR BICIPITAL TENDONITIS    295

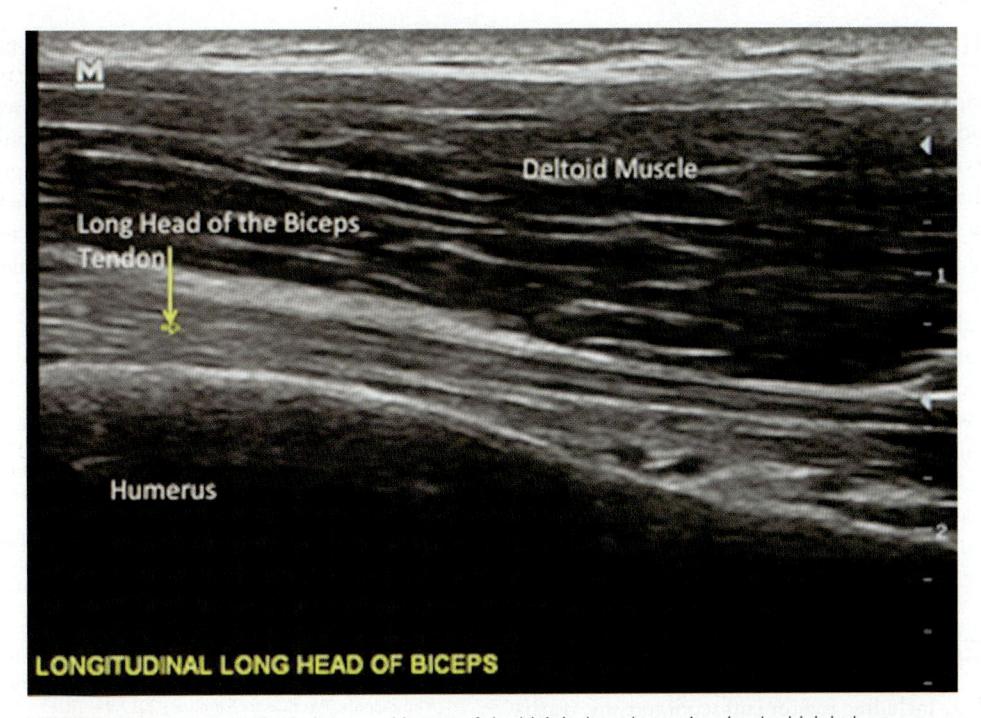

**FIGURE 44.14.**    Longitudinal ultrasound image of the bicipital tendon as it exits the bicipital groove.

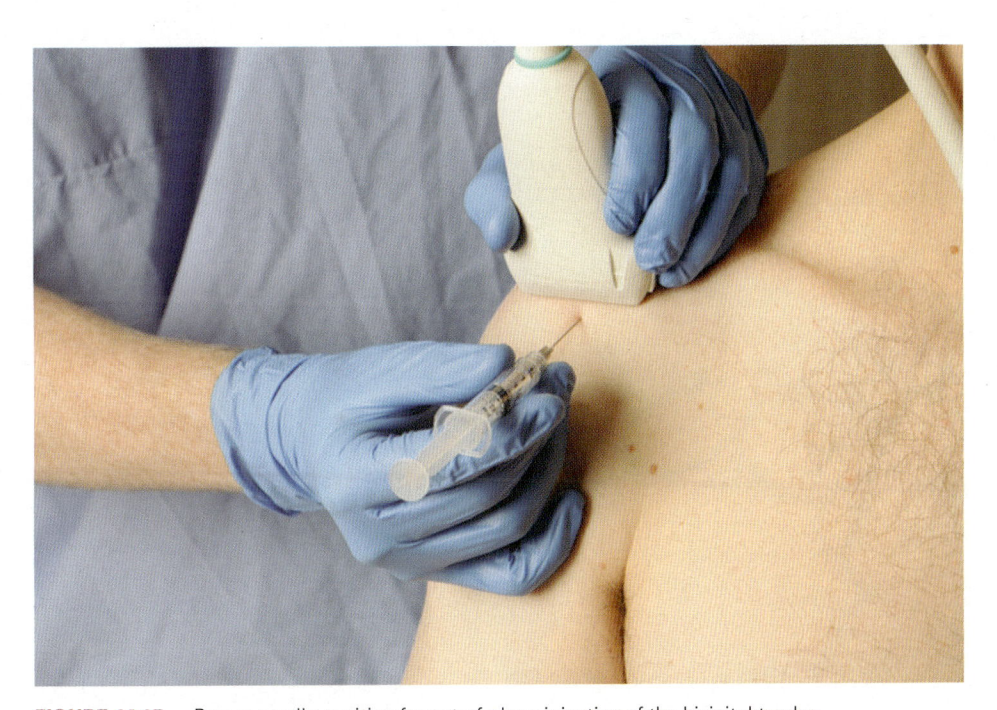

**FIGURE 44.15.**    Proper needle position for out-of-plane injection of the bicipital tendon.

## COMPLICATIONS

The major complication of ultrasound-guided injection of the bicipital tendon is infection. Ecchymosis and hematoma formation following this procedure may also occur. The possibility of trauma to the bicipital tendon from the injection itself remains an ever-present possibility, although the risk of this is decreased if care is taken to place the needle outside the tendon and the injection is performed under real-time ultrasound visualization. Tendons that are highly inflamed or previously damaged are subject to rupture if substances are injected directly into the tendon. This complication can be greatly decreased if the clinician uses gentle technique and stops injecting immediately if significant resistance to injection is encountered. Approximately 25% of patients complain of a transient increase in pain after this injection technique; the patient should be warned of this.

## CLINICAL PEARLS

Shoulder pathology including rotator cuff tendinopathy, osteoarthritis, avascular necrosis of the humeral head, and impingement syndromes may coexist with bicipital tendonitis and may contribute to the patient's pain symptomatology. Universal precautions should always be observed to protect the operator, and strict adherence to sterile technique must be used to avoid infection. Gentle physical therapy and local heat should be introduced following ultrasound-guided injection of bicipital tendonitis to reduce pain and improve function. Simple analgesics and nonsteroidal anti-inflammatory agents or COX-2 inhibitors may be used concurrently with this injection technique.

## SUGGESTED READINGS

Lento PH, Strakowski JA. The use of ultrasound in guiding musculoskeletal interventional procedures. *Phys Med Rehabil Clin N Am* 2010;21(3):559–583.

Narouze SN. Ultrasound-guided shoulder joint and bursa injections. In: *Atlas of Ultrasound Guided Procedures in Pain Management*. New York, NY: Springer; 2010:295–296.

Precerutti M, Garioni E, Madonia L, et al. US anatomy of the shoulder: pictorial essay. *J Ultrasound* 2010;13(4):179–187.

Waldman SD. The biceps tendon. In: *Pain Review*. Philadelphia, PA: Elsevier Saunders; 2009:84–85.

Waldman SD. *Yergason sign*. In: *Physical Diagnosis of Pain: An Atlas of Signs and Symptoms*. 2nd ed. Philadelphia, PA: WB Saunders; 2010:88–70.

Waldman SD. Bicipital tendon tear. In: *Atlas of Common Pain Syndromes*. 3rd ed. Philadelphia, PA: Elsevier Saunders; 2012:98–101.

Waldman SD. Injection technique for bicipital tendinitis. In: *Atlas of Pain Management Injection Techniques*. 3rd ed. Philadelphia, PA: Elsevier Saunders; 2013:84–86.

# CHAPTER 45

# Ultrasound-Guided Injection Technique for Axillary Nerve Block in the Quadrilateral Space

## CLINICAL PERSPECTIVES

Quadrilateral space syndrome is an increasingly recognized cause of shoulder and posterior arm pain that is the result of entrapment or trauma to the axillary nerve as it traverses the quadrilateral space. Cahill and Palmer first described this syndrome in 1983 with the majority of patients being young athletes in their second and third decade of life. The use of magnetic resonance scanning and ultrasound imaging of the quadrilateral space has made the diagnosis of quadrilateral space syndrome more objective, and it is now being diagnosed in all age groups.

Although in some patients, the inciting antecedent trauma responsible for the onset of symptoms of quadrilateral space syndrome is obvious, in many patients the onset of the patient's ill-defined lateral shoulder and posterior upper extremity pain is insidious. The pain is often described as aching in nature with superimposed dysesthesias often present. Adduction and external rotation of the affected upper extremity will make the symptoms worse. If the compromise of the axillary nerve remains untreated, the patient may begin to notice the gradual onset of weakness of the affected upper extremity, particularly when abducting and externally rotating it. In some patients, the weakness is progressive and permanent atrophy of the deltoid and teres minor muscles can be identified on physical examination and medical imaging studies. There often is tenderness to palpation of the quadrilateral space on physical examination.

As with other entrapment neuropathies such as carpal tunnel syndrome, electromyography may help identify compromise of the axillary nerve and help distinguish quadrilateral space syndrome from the brachial plexopathies and cervical radiculopathy, which may both mimic quadrilateral space syndrome. Plain radiographs of the cervical spine and shoulder are indicated in all patients who present with symptoms suggestive of quadrilateral space syndrome to rule out occult bony pathology. Based on the patient's clinical presentation, additional testing including complete blood cell count, uric acid, sedimentation rate, and antinuclear antibody testing may be indicated. Magnetic resonance imaging or ultrasound imaging of the shoulder with special attention to the teres minor muscle is indicated on all patients suspected of suffering from quadrilateral space syndrome as this test is highly specific for this disorder (Fig. 45.1). In the rare patient in whom magnetic resonance scanning is nondiagnostic, subclavian arteriography to demonstrate occlusion of the posterior humeral circumflex artery may be considered as this finding is highly suggestive of a diagnosis of quadrilateral space syndrome.

In addition to treating quadrilateral space syndrome, ultrasound-guided axillary nerve block in the quadrilateral space may be used to palliate acute pain emergencies, including postoperative pain, pain secondary to traumatic injuries of the shoulder, and cancer pain, while waiting for pharmacologic, surgical, and antiblastic methods to become effective. Ultrasound-guided axillary nerve block can also be used as a diagnostic tool when performing differential neural blockade on an anatomic basis in the evaluation of upper extremity pain as well as in a prognostic manner to determine the degree of neurologic impairment the patient will suffer when destruction of the axillary nerve within the quadrilateral space is being considered or when there is a possibility that the nerve may be sacrificed during surgeries in the anatomic region of the quadrilateral space. Ultrasound-guided axillary nerve block in the quadrilateral space may also be used to palliate the pain and dysesthesias associated with stretch injuries to the axillary nerve as it traverses the quadrilateral space.

## CLINICALLY RELEVANT ANATOMY

The quadrilateral space is a four-sided space that is bounded superiorly by the subscapularis and teres minor muscles, medially by the long head of the triceps brachii, laterally by the surgical neck of the humerus, and inferiorly by the teres major muscle (Fig. 45.2). Contained within the quadrilateral space is the axial nerve, which is a branch of the brachial plexus and the posterior circumflex humeral artery. Compromise of either of these structures by tumor, hematoma, aberrant muscle, stretch injury, or heterotopic bone can produce the constellation of symptoms known as quadrilateral space syndrome.

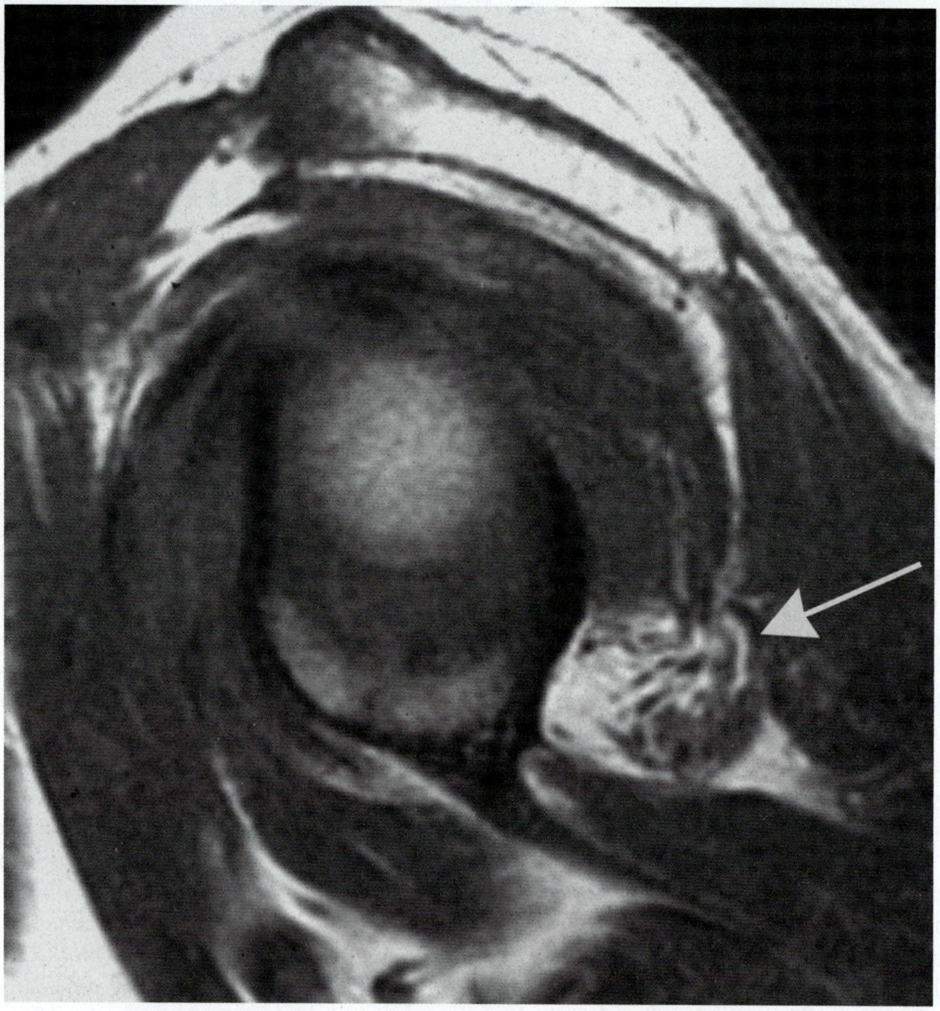

**FIGURE 45.1.** This oblique sagittal T1-weighted magnetic resonance image shows fatty atrophy of the teres minor muscle (*arrow*) consistent with quadrilateral space syndrome. (Reused from Helms CA. Magnetic resonance imaging of the shoulder. In: Brant WE, Helms CA, eds. *Fundamentals of Diagnostic Radiology*. 3rd ed. Philadelphia, PA: Lippincott Williams & Wilkins; 2007:1212, with permission.)

## ULTRASOUND-GUIDED TECHNIQUE

The benefits, risks, and alternative treatments are explained to the patient and informed consent is obtained. The patient is then placed in the sitting position with the forearm resting comfortably on the ipsilateral thigh (Fig 45.3). The physician stands behind or at the side of the patient. With the patient in the above position, at the middle of the posterior arm, a high-frequency linear ultrasound transducer is placed in a longitudinal orientation over the medial side of the posterior humerus (Fig. 45.4). An ultrasound survey image is obtained, and the hyperechoic margin of the shaft of the humerus and the adjacent triceps muscle is identified (Fig. 45.5). The transducer is then slowly moved toward the axilla while tracing the hyperechoic margin of the humerus until the hyperechoic margin curves outward as the transducer approaches the inferior head of the humerus (Fig. 45.6). Below the point of this outward curve lie the axillary nerve and posterior circumflex humeral artery (Fig. 45.7). Color Doppler may be helpful in identifying the posterior circumflex humeral artery (Fig. 45.8). Center the neurovascular bundle in the middle of the ultrasound scan image.

The skin overlying the area beneath the ultrasound transducer is then prepped with antiseptic solution. A sterile syringe containing 3.0 mL of 0.25% preservative-free bupivacaine and 45 mg of methylprednisolone is attached to a 3½-inch, 22-gauge needle using strict aseptic technique. The needle is placed through the skin just above the center of the transducer and is then advanced using an in-plane approach with the needle trajectory adjusted under real-time ultrasound guidance so that the needle tip ultimately rests in proximity to the axillary nerve as it lies within the quadrilateral space (Fig. 45.9). When the tip of needle is thought to be in satisfactory position, after careful aspiration, a small amount of local anesthetic and steroid is injected under real-time ultrasound guidance to confirm that the needle tip is in the proper position. After proper needle

CHAPTER 45 ULTRASOUND-GUIDED INJECTION TECHNIQUE FOR AXILLARY NERVE BLOCK IN THE QUADRILATERAL SPACE 299

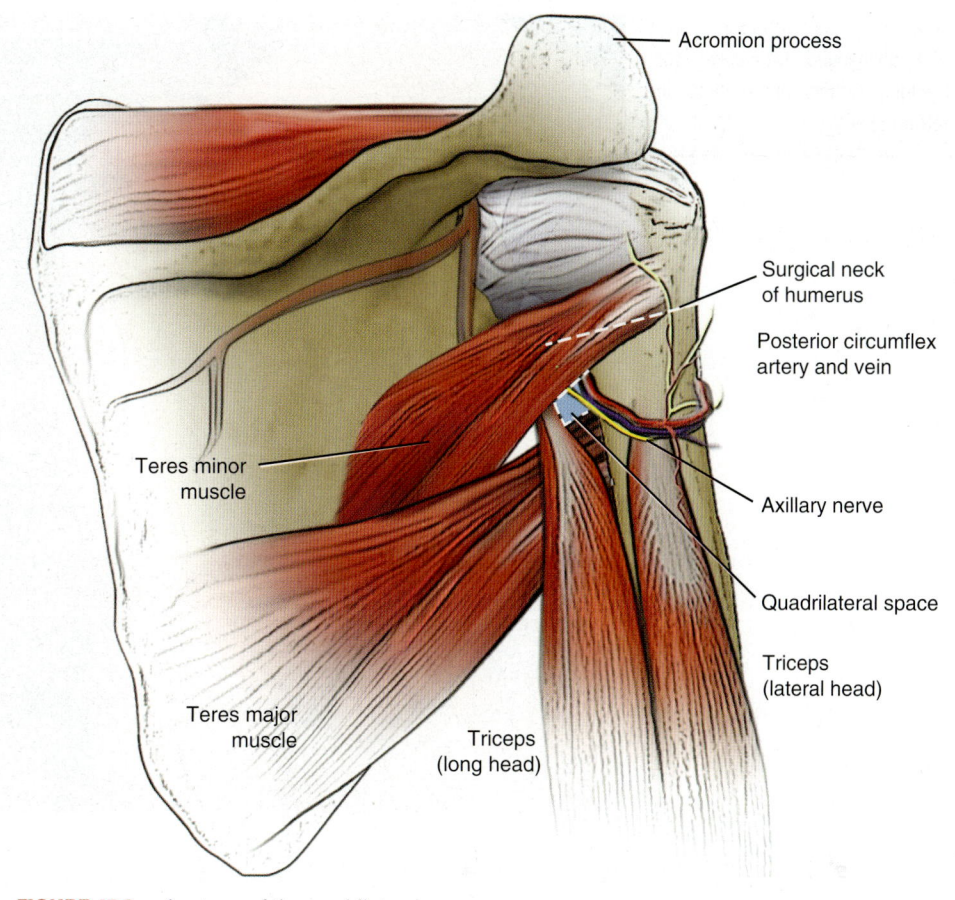

**FIGURE 45.2.** Anatomy of the quadrilateral space.

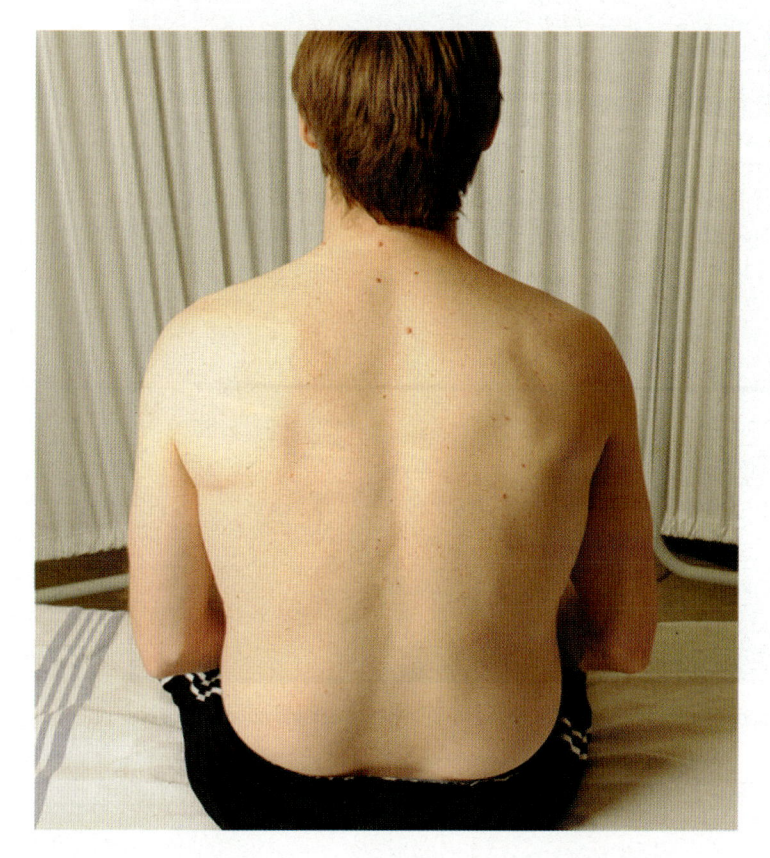

**FIGURE 45.3.** Proper patient positioning for ultrasound-guided axillary nerve block in the quadrilateral space.

**FIGURE 45.4.** Proper longitudinal placement of the ultrasound transducer for ultrasound-guided axillary nerve block in the quadrilateral space.

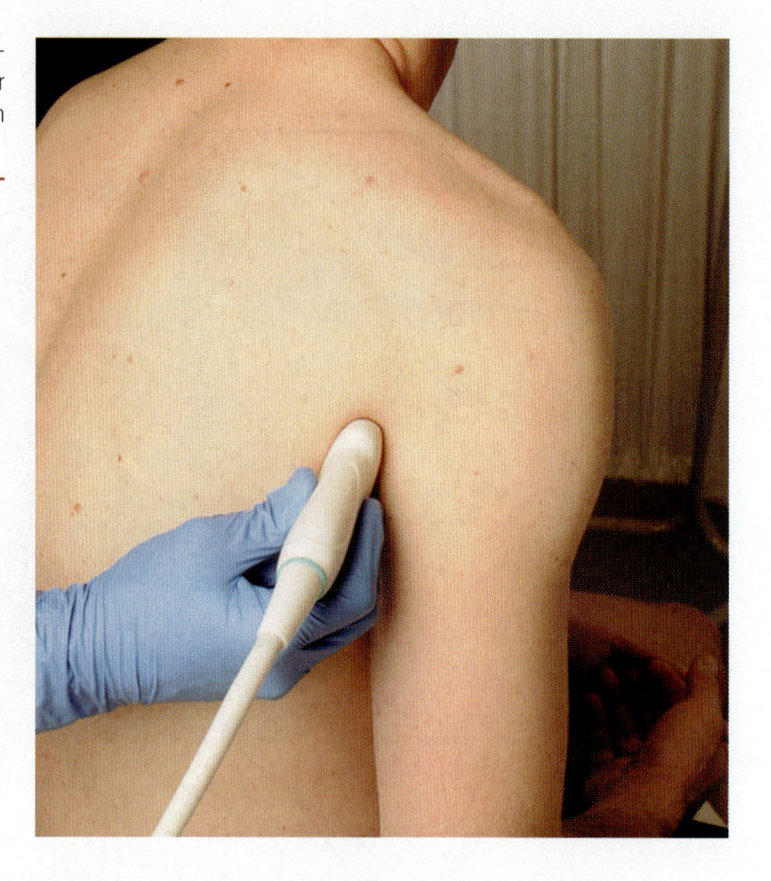

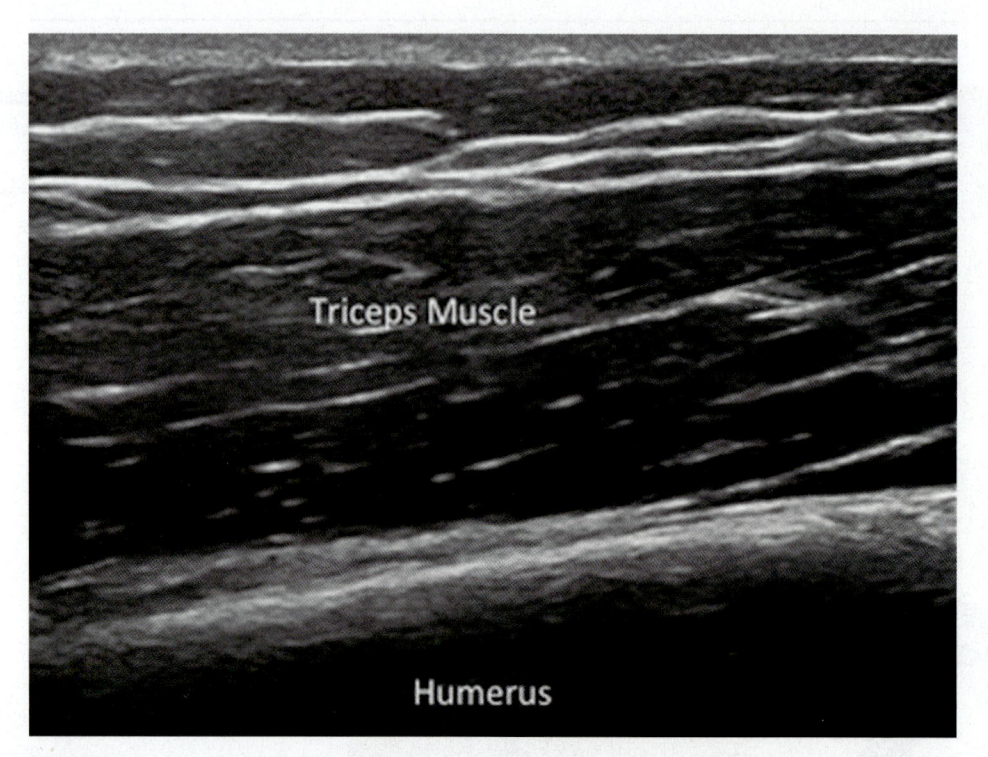

**FIGURE 45.5.** Longitudinal ultrasound view of the margin of the midhumeral shaft and adjacent triceps muscle.

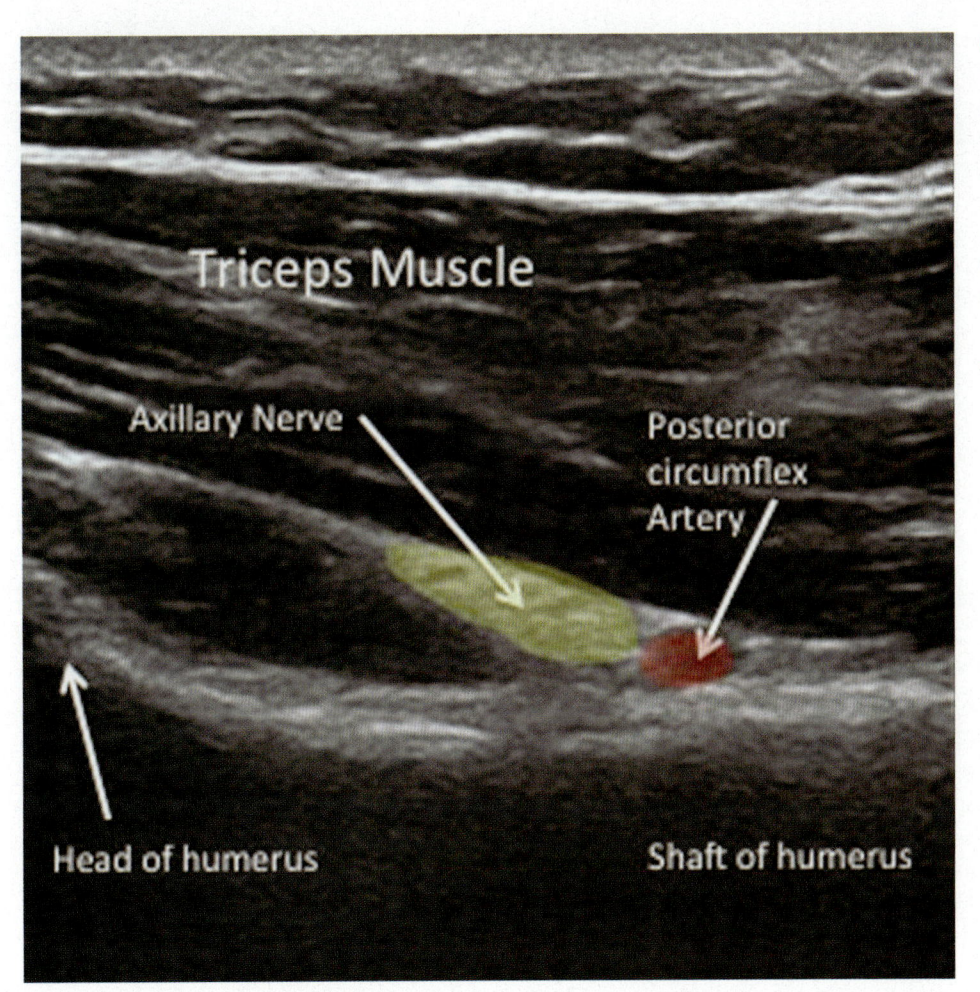

**FIGURE 45.6.** The ultrasound transducer is then slowly moved toward the axilla while tracing the hyperechoic margin of the humerus until the hyperechoic margin curves outward as the transducer approaches the inferior head of the humerus. This below the point of this outward curve lies the axillary nerve and posterior circumflex humeral artery.

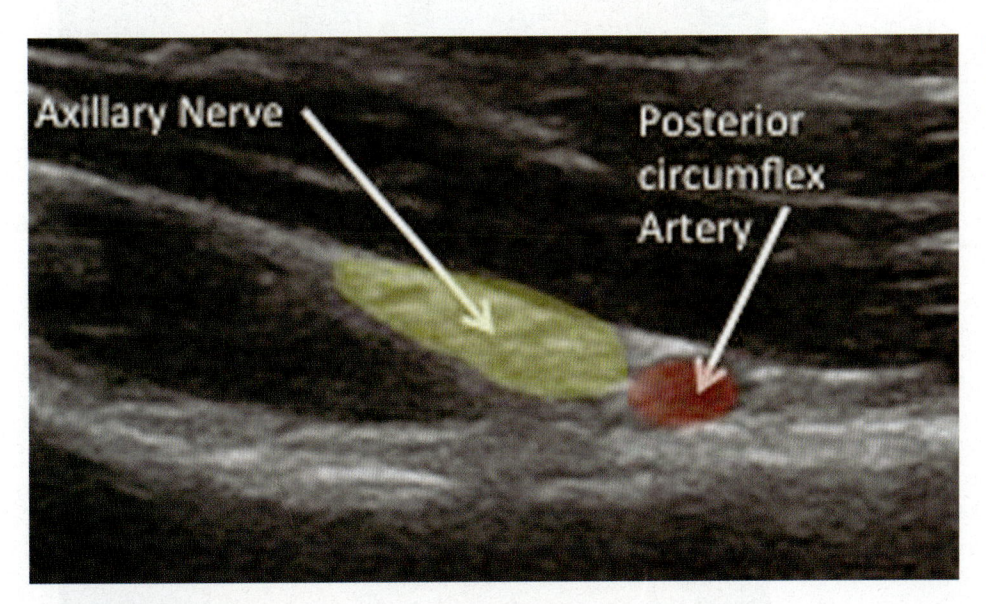

**FIGURE 45.7.** Ultrasound image of the axillary nerve and superior circumflex humeral artery within the quadrilateral space.

**FIGURE 45.8.** Use of color Doppler can aid in the identification of superior circumflex humeral artery.

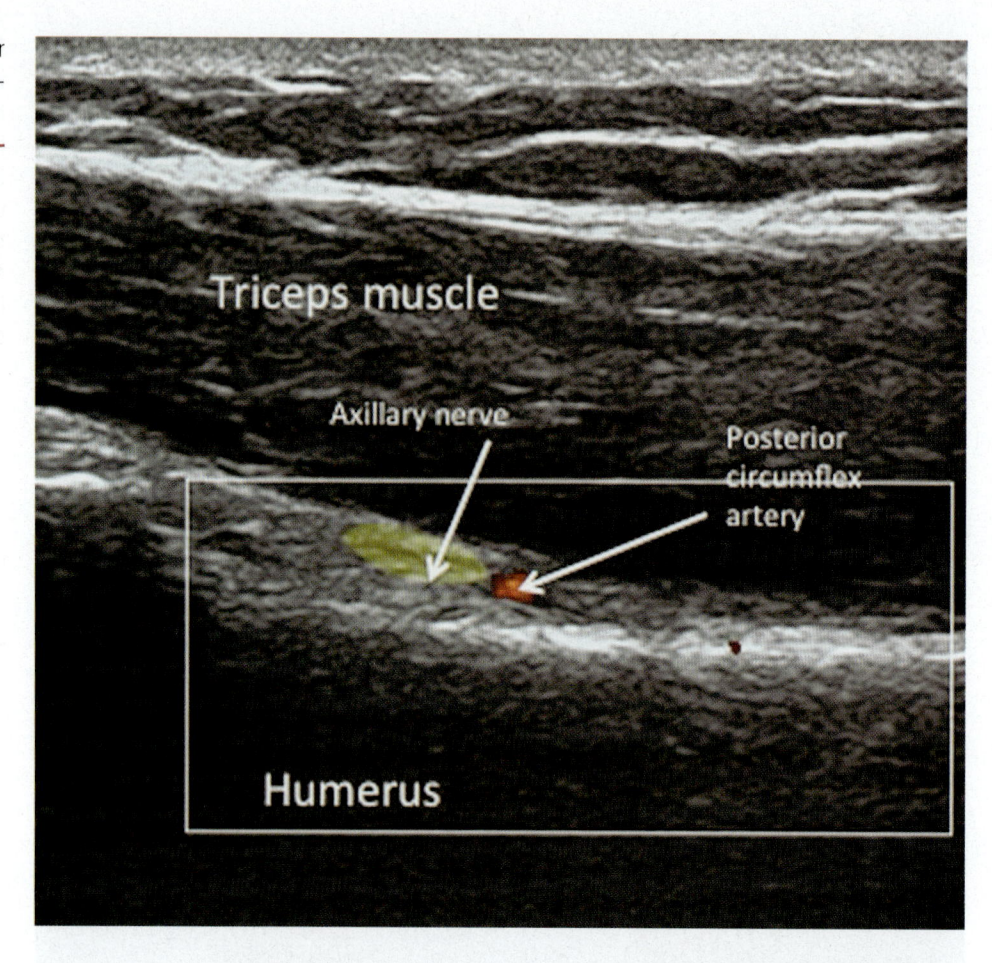

**FIGURE 45.9.** Proper needle placement for ultrasound-guided axillary nerve block in the quadrilateral space.

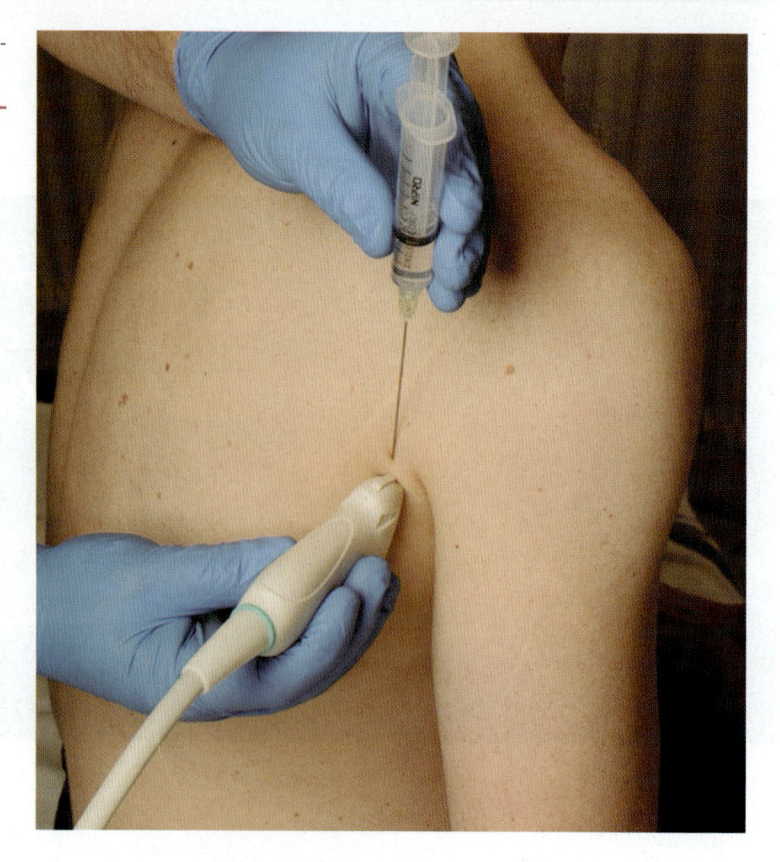

tip placement is confirmed, the remainder of the contents of the syringe are slowly injected. There should be minimal resistance to injection.

## COMPLICATIONS

The major complications of ultrasound-guided injection of ultrasound-guided axillary nerve block in the quadrilateral space are related to improper needle placement with the possibility of inadvertent intravascular injection and/or persistent paresthesia secondary to needle trauma to the axillary nerve. Although rare, infection may occur. Ecchymosis and hematoma formation following this procedure may also occur. These complications can be decreased if manual pressure is applied to the area of the block immediately after injection. Application of cold packs for 20-minute periods after the block will also decrease the amount of postprocedure pain and bleeding the patient may experience.

Approximately 25% of patients complain of a transient increase in pain after this injection technique; the patient should be warned of this.

## CLINICAL PEARLS

Ultrasound-guided axillary nerve block in the quadrilateral space is a straightforward and relatively safe technique if attention is paid to the clinically relevant anatomy. This technique is useful in the management of quadrilateral space syndrome. Careful neurologic examination to identify preexisting neurologic deficits that may later be attributed to the nerve block should be performed on all patients before beginning axillary nerve block in the quadrilateral space.

## SUGGESTED READINGS

Hoskins WT, Pollard HP, McDonald AJ. Quadrilateral space syndrome: a case study and review of the literature. *Br J Sports Med* 2005;39(2):e9.
McClelland D, Paxinos A. The anatomy of the quadrilateral space with reference to quadrilateral space syndrome. *J Shoulder Elbow Surg* 2008;17(1):162–164.
Waldman SD. Quadrilateral space syndrome. In: *Atlas of Uncommon Pain Syndromes*. 2nd ed. Philadelphia, PA: WB Saunders; 2008:80–83.
Waldman SD. Injection technique for quadrilateral space syndrome. In: *Atlas of Pain Management Injection Techniques*. 3rd ed. Philadelphia, PA: Elsevier Saunders; 2013:103–105.

# CHAPTER 46

# Ultrasound-Guided Injection Technique for Subdeltoid Bursitis Pain

## CLINICAL PERSPECTIVES

The subdeltoid bursa is the largest of the ~160 bursae in the human body (Fig. 46.1). Because it is usually contiguous and communicates with the subacromial bursa, the names are often used interchangeably, although each bursa can exist as separate anatomic structures on ultrasound and magnetic resonance images. As its name implies, the subdeltoid bursa lies beneath the deltoid muscle and serves to cushion and facilitate sliding of the supraspinatus muscle as it passes under the acromion process. The bursa is subject to inflammation from a variety of causes with acute shoulder trauma and repetitive microtrauma being the most common (Table 46.1). If the inflammation of the bursa is not treated and the condition becomes chronic, calcification of the bursa with further functional disability may occur. The patient suffering from subdeltoid bursitis most frequently presents with the complaint of severe pain with any movement of the shoulder. Activities requiring abduction of the affected upper extremity are particularly painful, and the patient may complain bitterly of a knife-like catching sensation when using the shoulder upon first awakening. The patient will often be unable to sleep on the affected shoulder. The pain of subdeltoid bursitis is localized to the subdeltoid region and is often referred to the points of insertion of the deltoid muscle along the proximal one-third of the humerus.

Physical examination of the patient suffering from subdeltoid bursitis will reveal point tenderness at the acromion process as well as over the deltoid muscle. If there is significant inflammation, rubor and color may be present and the entire area may feel boggy or edematous to palpation. Passive elevation and rotation of the shoulder may exacerbate the pain of subdeltoid bursitis, and the patient will often exhibit a positive drop-arm test when the affected upper extremity is passively elevated with the elbow flexed and supported by the examiner and then suddenly released. The sudden release of the elevated extremity will cause the patient to cry out in pain. Active resisted abduction and lateral rotation of the affected extremity will also reproduce the patient's pain, and a sudden release in resistance to active abduction will also markedly exacerbate the pain. If calcification has occurred, the examiner may appreciate crepitus with active range of motion of the affected shoulder.

Plain radiographs are indicated in all patients who present with shoulder pain to rule out occult bony pathology. Based on the patient's clinical presentation, additional testing may be indicated, including complete blood cell count, sedimentation rate, and antinuclear antibody testing. Magnetic resonance imaging or ultrasound imaging of the affected area may also help confirm the diagnosis as well as delineate the presence of bursitis, calcific tendonitis, rotator cuff tendinopathy, or other shoulder pathology (Figs. 46.2 and 46.3).

Rarely, the inflamed bursa may become infected and failure to diagnose and treat the acute infection can lead to dire consequences (Fig. 46.4).

## CLINICALLY RELEVANT ANATOMY

The subdeltoid bursa lies primarily under the acromion, extending laterally between the deltoid muscle and supraspinatus muscle (see Fig. 46.1). The acromial arch covers the superior aspect of the shoulder joint and articulates with the clavicle at the acromioclavicular joint. The acromioclavicular joint is formed by the distal end of the clavicle and the anterior and medial aspect of the acromion. The strength of the joint is due to the dense coracoclavicular ligament, which attaches the bottom of the distal end of the clavicle to the coracoid process. The superior portion of the joint is covered by the superior acromioclavicular ligament, which attaches the distal clavicle to the upper surface of the acromion. The inferior portion of the joint is covered by the inferior acromioclavicular ligament, which attaches the inferior portion of the distal clavicle to the acromion.

## ULTRASOUND-GUIDED TECHNIQUE

The benefits, risks, and alternative treatments are explained to the patient and informed consent is obtained. The patient is then placed in the sitting position with the forearm resting comfortably on the ipsilateral thigh (Fig. 46.5). Alternatively, the patient may be placed in the modified Crass position by positioning the hand of the affected extremity over the posterior hip as if reaching into his or her hip pants' pocket to retrieve a comb. The physician stands

CHAPTER 46    ULTRASOUND-GUIDED INJECTION TECHNIQUE FOR SUBDELTOID BURSITIS PAIN

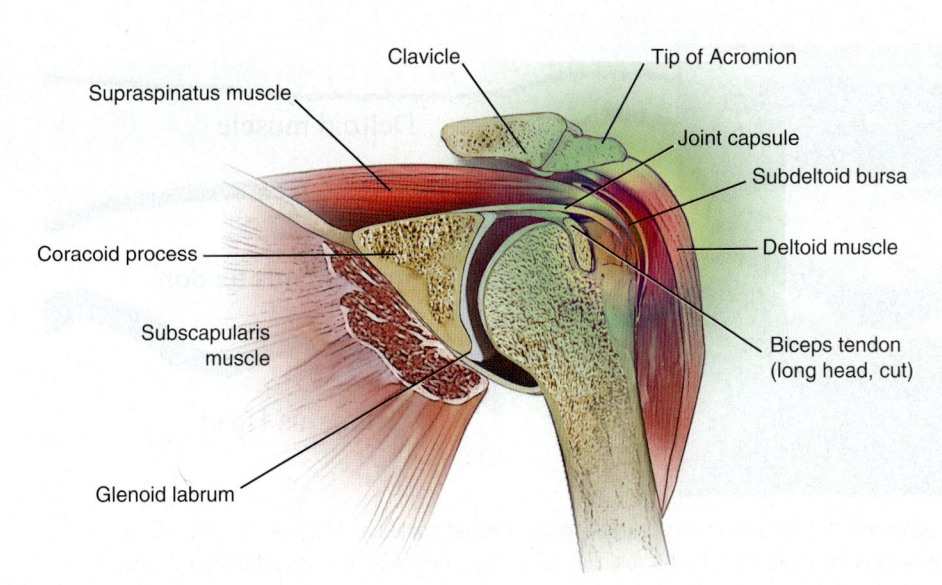

**FIGURE 46.1.** The anatomy of the subdeltoid bursa.

behind or at the side of the patient and palpates the tip of the acromion (Fig. 46.6).

The skin overlying the subdeltoid bursa is then prepped with antiseptic solution. A sterile syringe containing 3.0 mL of 0.25% preservative-free bupivacaine and 40 mg of methylprednisolone is attached to a 1½-inch, 22-gauge needle using strict aseptic technique. The high-frequency ultrasound transducer is placed over the lateral tip of the acromion in the coronal plane and is angled slightly toward the scapula (Fig. 46.7). A survey scan is taken and the supraspinatus tendon is identified as it exits from beneath the acromion and curves over the head of the humerus to attach to the greater tuberosity (Fig. 46.8). The tendon should be carefully examined for calcifications or tendinopathy that may be contributing to the patient's shoulder pain. The subdeltoid bursa is then identified as a fluid-containing structure lying between the deltoid muscle and acromion on top and the supraspinatus tendon below (Fig. 46.9). Although the normal or mildly inflamed subdeltoid bursa most often appears on ultrasonic imaging as a hypoechoic curvilineal layer of fluid sandwiched between a hyperechoic layer of bursal wall and peribursal fat, inflammation and distention of the bursal sac may make the bursal contents appear anechoic or even hyperechoic. After the bursa is identified, the needle is placed

### TABLE 46.1  Causes of Subdeltoid Bursitis

Acute trauma
Repetitive microtrauma
Rotator cuff tendinopathy
Impingement syndromes
Infection
    Bacterial
    Mycoplasma
    Fungal
    Parasitic
Crystal arthropathies
    Uric acid
    Calcium phosphate
    Hydroxyapatite
    Urate
Collagen vascular diseases
    Rheumatoid arthritis
    Polymyalgia rheumatica
Synovial disease
Hemarthrosis

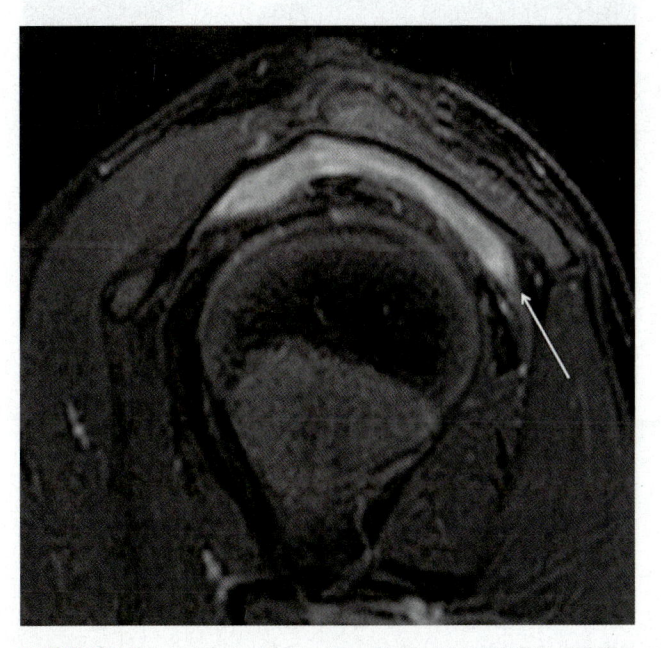

**FIGURE 46.2.** Isolated subacromial–subdeltoid bursitis in a patient with inflammatory arthropathy seen on a sagittal fat-suppressed T2-weighted image (*arrow*). (Reused from Steinbach LS. MRI of the rotator cuff. In: Chung CB, Steinbach LS, eds. *MRI of the Upper Extremity: Shoulder, Elbow, Wrist, and Hand*. Philadelphia, PA: Lippincott Williams & Wilkins; 2010:267, with permission.)

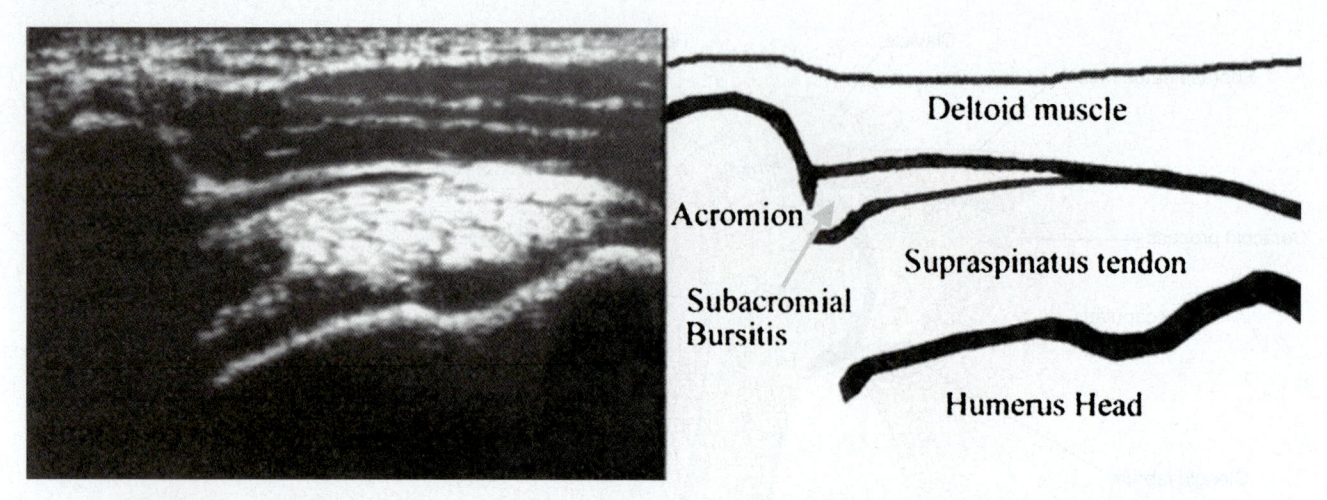

**FIGURE 46.3.** Ultrasound image demonstrating subdeltoid bursitis (subdeltoid). (Reused from Chen MJL, Lew HL, Hsu T-C, et al. Ultrasound-guided shoulder injections in the treatment of subacromial bursitis. *Am J Phys Med Rehabil* 2006;85(1):31–35, with permission.)

through the skin ~1 cm lateral to the end of the transducer and is then advanced using an in-plane approach with the needle trajectory adjusted under real-time ultrasound guidance to enter the subdeltoid bursa just lateral to the acromion (Figs. 46.10 and 46.11). When the tip of needle is thought to be within the bursa cavity, a small amount of local anesthetic and steroid is injected under real-time ultrasound guidance to confirm intrabursal placement by the characteristic spreading swirl of hyperechoic injectate within the bursa. After intrabursal needle tip placement is confirmed, the remainder of the contents of the syringe are slowly injected. There should be minimal resistance to injection. If synechiae, loculations, or calcifications are present, the needle may have to be repositioned to ensure that the entire bursa is treated. The needle is then removed, and a sterile pressure dressing and ice pack are placed at the injection site.

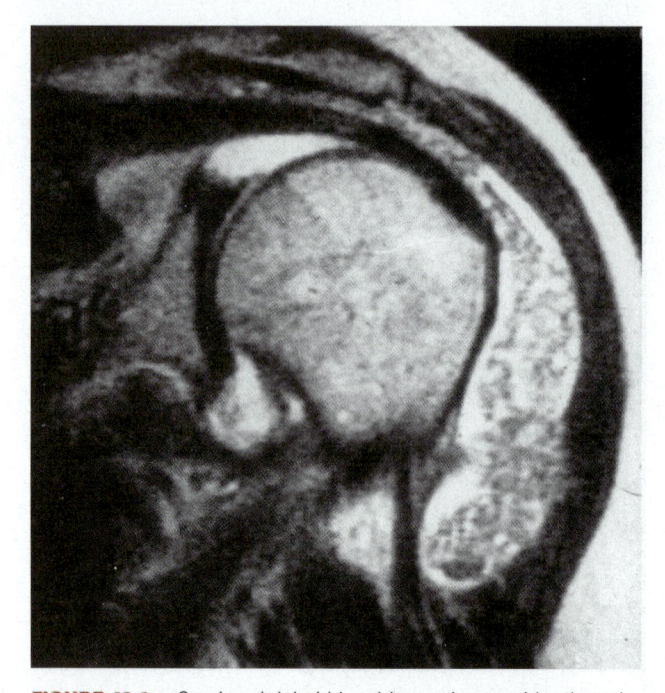

**FIGURE 46.4.** Septic subdeltoid bursitis consistent with tuberculosis infection. Oblique coronal T2-weighted MR image shows extensive subacromial–subdeltoid bursitis with innumerable punctate foci of low signal intensity consistent with rice bodies. (Reused from Zlatkin MB. *MRI of the Shoulder*. 2nd ed. Philadelphia, PA: Lippincott Williams & Wilkins; 2003, with permission.)

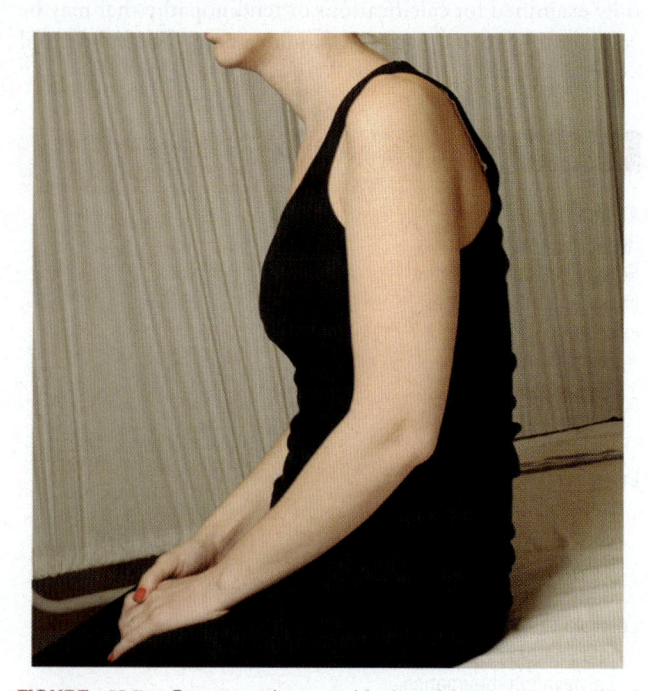

**FIGURE 46.5.** Proper patient positioning for ultrasound-guided injection of the subdeltoid bursa.

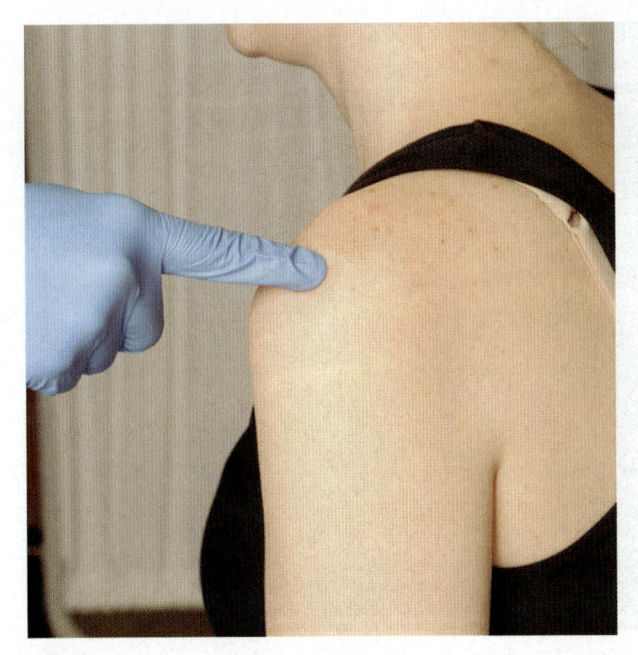

**FIGURE 46.6.** The physician stands in front of the patient and palpates the acromion.

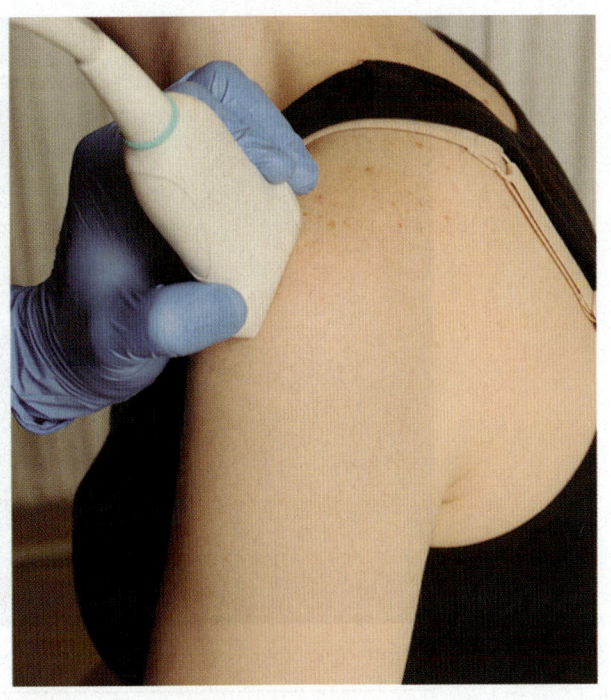

**FIGURE 46.7.** Proper coronal ultrasound transducer position for ultrasound-guided injection of the subdeltoid bursa with the patient in the neutral sitting position.

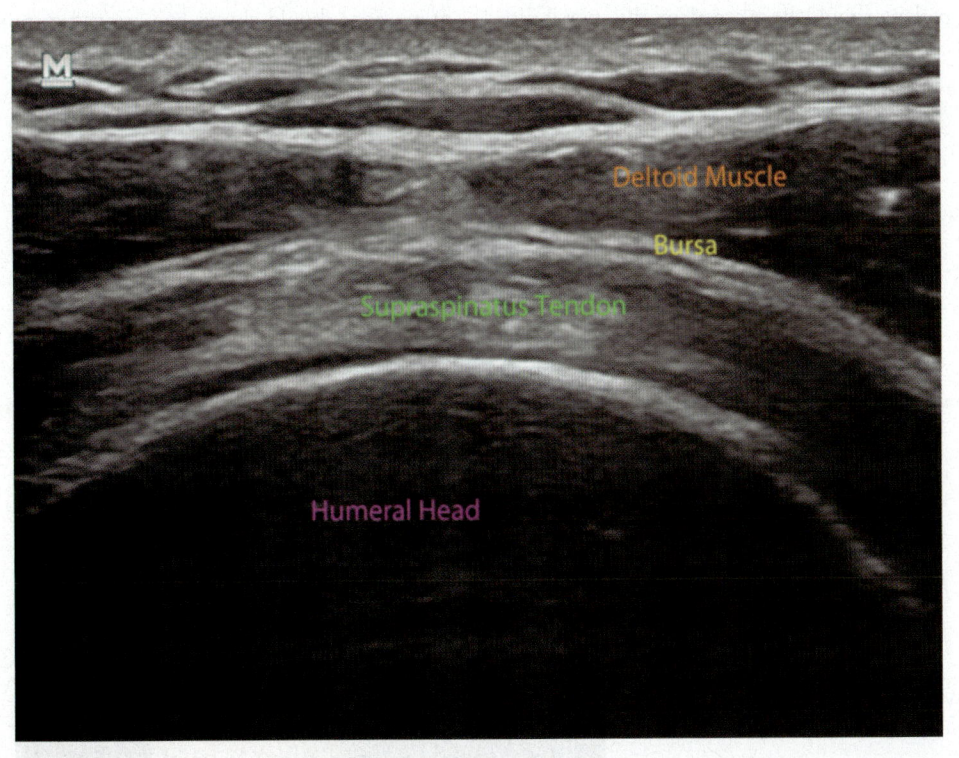

**FIGURE 46.8.** Coronal ultrasound image demonstrating the relationship of the subdeltoid bursa to the deltoid muscle.

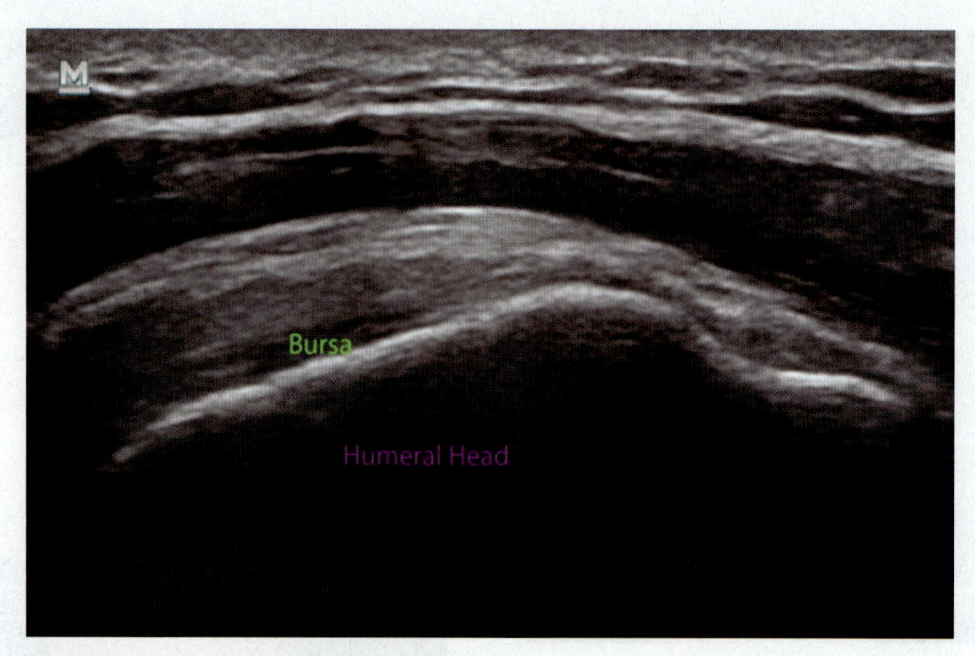

**FIGURE 46.9.** Coronal ultrasound view of the subdeltoid bursa.

## COMPLICATIONS

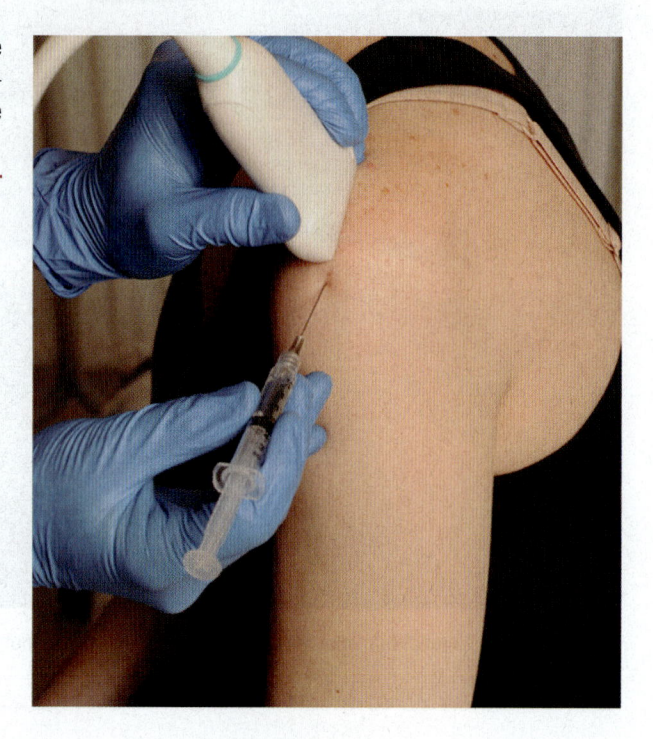

The major complication of ultrasound-guided injection of the subdeltoid bursa is infection. Ecchymosis and hematoma formation may also occur. A transient exacerbation of the patient's pain occurs ~25% of the time following this injection technique, and the patient should be warned of this possibility prior to the procedure.

## CLINICAL PEARLS

Shoulder pathology including rotator cuff tendinopathy, osteoarthritis, avascular necrosis of the humeral head, and impingement syndromes may coexist with subdeltoid bursitis and may contribute to the patients pain symptomatology. Universal precautions should always be observed to protect the operator, and strict adherence to sterile technique must be used to avoid

**FIGURE 46.10.** Proper needle position for injection of the subdeltoid bursa using an in-plane approach.

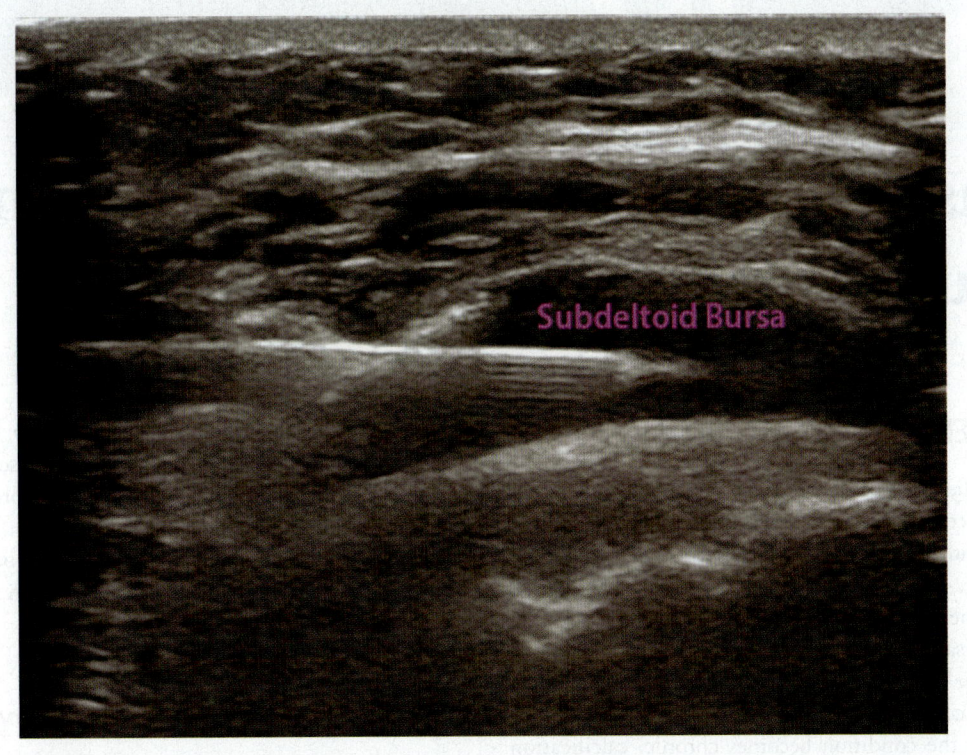

**FIGURE 46.11.** Ultrasound view of needle within the subdeltoid bursa.

infection. Gentle physical therapy and local heat should be introduced following ultrasound-guided injection of the subdeltoid bursa to reduce pain and improve function. Simple analgesics and nonsteroidal anti-inflammatory agents or COX-2 inhibitors may be used concurrently with this injection technique.

## SUGGESTED READINGS

Lento PH, Strakowski JA. The use of ultrasound in guiding musculoskeletal interventional procedures. *Phys Med Rehabil Clin N Am* 2010;21(3):559–583.

Molini L, Mariacher S, Bianchi S. US guided corticosteroid injection into the subacromial-subdeltoid bursa: technique and approach. *J Ultrasound* 2012; 15(1):61–68.

Narouze SN. Ultrasound-guided shoulder joint and bursa injections. In: *Atlas of Ultrasound Guided Procedures in Pain Management*. New York, NY: Springer; 2010:295–296.

Precerutti M, Garioni E, Madonia L, et al. US anatomy of the shoulder: pictorial essay. *J Ultrasound* 2010;13(4):179–187.

Waldman SD. The subdeltoid bursa. In: *Pain Review*. Philadelphia, PA: WB Saunders; 2009:83.

# CHAPTER 47

# Ultrasound-Guided Injection Technique for Subcoracoid Bursitis Pain

## CLINICAL PERSPECTIVES

As its name implies, the subcoracoid bursa lies beneath the joint capsule and the coracoid process between the short head of the biceps muscle and the musculotendinous unit of the subscapularis muscle (Fig. 47.1). The bursa serves to cushion and facilitate sliding of the musculotendinous unit of the subscapularis muscle. The bursa is subject to inflammation from a variety of causes with acute shoulder trauma and repetitive microtrauma being the most common. If the inflammation of the bursa is not treated and the condition becomes chronic, calcification of the bursa with further functional disability may occur. The patient suffering from subcoracoid bursitis most frequently presents with the complaint of severe pain especially with forward movement and abduction of the shoulder. Activities requiring abduction of the affected upper extremity are particularly painful, and the patient may complain bitterly of a knife-like catching sensation when using the shoulder upon first awakening. The patient will often be unable to sleep on the affected shoulder. The pain of subcoracoid bursitis is localized to the area of the coracoid and is often referred to the medial shoulder.

Physical examination of the patient suffering from subcoracoid bursitis will reveal point tenderness at the acromion process as well as in the subcoracoid region. If there is significant inflammation, rubor and color may be present and the entire area may feel boggy or edematous to palpation. Passive elevation and active internal rotation of the shoulder may exacerbate the pain of subcoracoid bursitis, and the patient will often exhibit a positive adduction release test when the affected upper extremity is adducted against the examiner's resistance and the resistance is suddenly and unexpectedly released (Figs. 47.2A and B). If calcification of the bursa and surrounding tendons has occurred, the examiner may appreciate crepitus with active range of motion of the affected shoulder.

Plain radiographs are indicated in all patients who present with shoulder pain to rule out occult bony pathology. Based on the patient's clinical presentation, additional testing may be indicated, including complete blood cell count, sedimentation rate, and antinuclear antibody testing. Magnetic resonance imaging or ultrasound imaging of the affected area may help confirm the diagnosis and also help delineate the presence of subdeltoid bursitis, calcific tendonitis, rotator cuff tendinopathy, or other shoulder pathology (Figs. 47.3 and 47.4). Magnetic resonance imaging or ultrasound imaging of the affected area may also help delineate the presence of calcific tendonitis or other shoulder pathology.

Rarely, the inflamed bursa may become infected, and failure to diagnose and treat the acute infection can lead to dire consequences (Fig. 47.5).

## CLINICALLY RELEVANT ANATOMY

The subcoracoid bursa lies beneath the joint capsule and the coracoid process between the short head of the biceps muscle and the musculotendinous unit of the subscapularis muscle (Fig. 47.6). Compromise of the subcoracoid space by tendonitis, bony deformity following fracture of the coracoid, or osteophytes can irritate the subcoracoid bursa and cause bursitis. It is also susceptible to irritation during extreme arm movement when the short head of the biceps presses against the humeral head. This process can be accelerated if previous trauma to the shoulder joint has compromised its stability and abnormal movement of the head of the humerus in the glenoid fossa occurs.

## ULTRASOUND-GUIDED TECHNIQUE

The benefits, risks, and alternative treatments are explained to the patient and informed consent is obtained. The patient is then placed in the sitting position with the arm resting comfortably at the patients side (Fig. 47.7). A high-frequency ultrasound transducer is placed over the anterior glenohumeral joint in a transverse position and a survey scan is taken (Fig. 47.8). The superior glenohumeral joint is identified, and the ultrasound transducer is slowly moved medially until the coracoid process comes into view (Figs. 47.9 and 47.10). The skin overlying the subcoracoid space is then prepped with antiseptic solution. A sterile syringe containing 3.0 mL of 0.25% preservative-free bupivacaine and 40 mg of methylprednisolone is attached to a 1½-inch, 22-gauge needle using strict aseptic technique. If the subcoracoid bursa is highly inflamed, it may sometimes be identified as a hypoechoic fluid-containing structure with hyperechoic walls lying beneath the coracoid process.

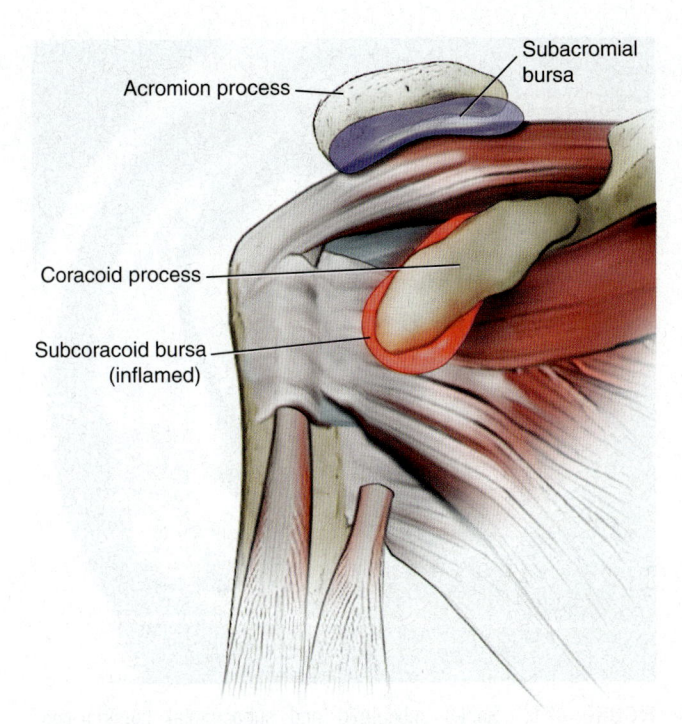

**FIGURE 47.1.** The anatomy of the subcoracoid bursa.

After the subcoracoid space is identified, the needle is placed through the skin ~1 cm below the middle of the transducer and is then advanced using an out-of-plane approach with the needle trajectory adjusted under real-time ultrasound guidance to enter the subcoracoid space (Fig. 47.11). When the tip of needle is thought to be within the subcoracoid space or the subacromial bursa if it is identifiable, a small amount of local anesthetic and steroid is injected under real-time ultrasound guidance to confirm correct needle tip placement. After intrabursal needle tip placement is confirmed, the remainder of the contents of the syringe are slowly injected. There should be minimal resistance to injection. If synechiae, loculations, or calcifications are present, the needle may have to be repositioned to ensure that the entire bursa is treated. The needle is then removed, and a sterile pressure dressing and ice pack are placed at the injection site.

## COMPLICATIONS

The major complication of ultrasound-guided injection of the subcoracoid bursa is infection. Ecchymosis and hematoma formation may also occur. A transient exacerbation of the patient's pain occurs ~25% of the time following this injection technique, and the patient should be warned of this possibility prior to the procedure.

## CLINICAL PEARLS

Shoulder pathology including rotator cuff tendinopathy, osteoarthritis, avascular necrosis of the humeral head, and impingement syndromes may coexist with subcoracoid bursitis and may contribute to the patient's pain symptomatology. Universal precautions should always be observed to protect the operator, and strict adherence to sterile technique must be used to avoid infection. Gentle physical therapy and local heat should be introduced following ultrasound-guided injection of the subcoracoid bursa to reduce pain and improve function. Simple analgesics and nonsteroidal anti-inflammatory agents or COX-2 inhibitors may be used concurrently with this injection technique.

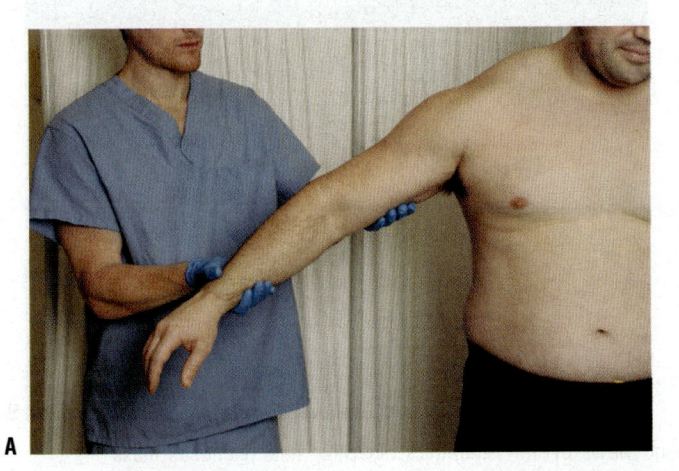

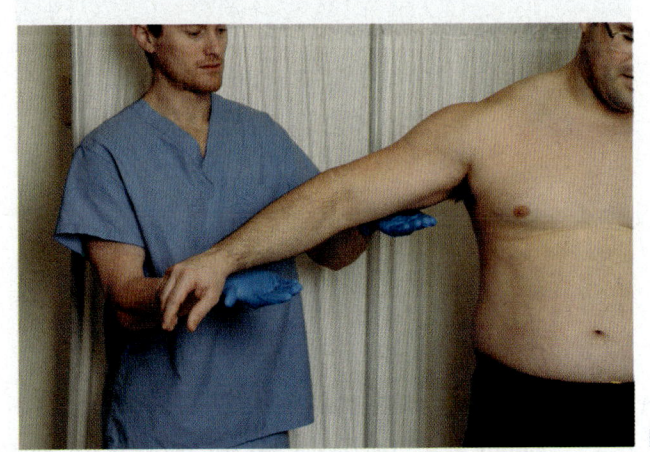

**FIGURE 47.2.** **A:** The adduction release test for subcoracoid bursitis. The affected upper extremity is adducted against the examiner's resistance. **B:** the adduction release test for subcoracoid bursitis. The resistance is suddenly and unexpectedly released causing severe pain.

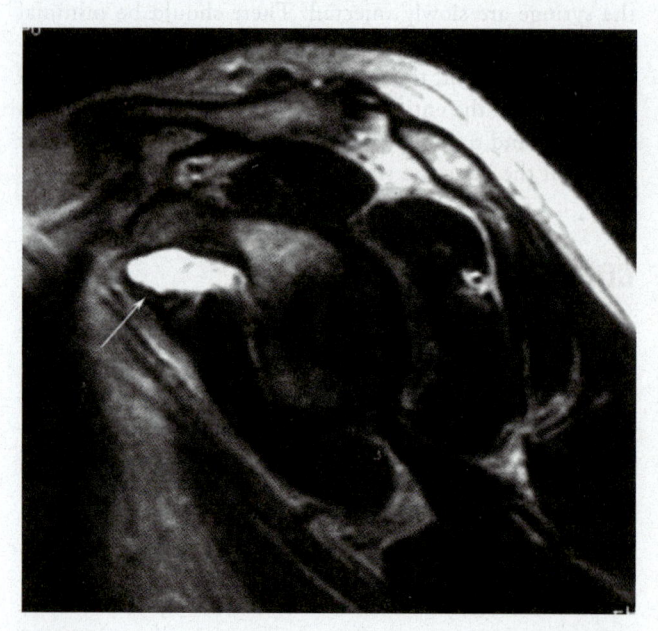

**FIGURE 47.3.** A well-defined fluid collection (*arrow*) extending beneath the coracoid process consistent with subcoracoid bursitis is noted on this oblique sagittal T2-weighted MR image. (Reused from Zlatkin MB. *MRI of the Shoulder*. 2nd ed. Philadelphia, PA: Lippincott Williams & Wilkins; 2003, with permission.)

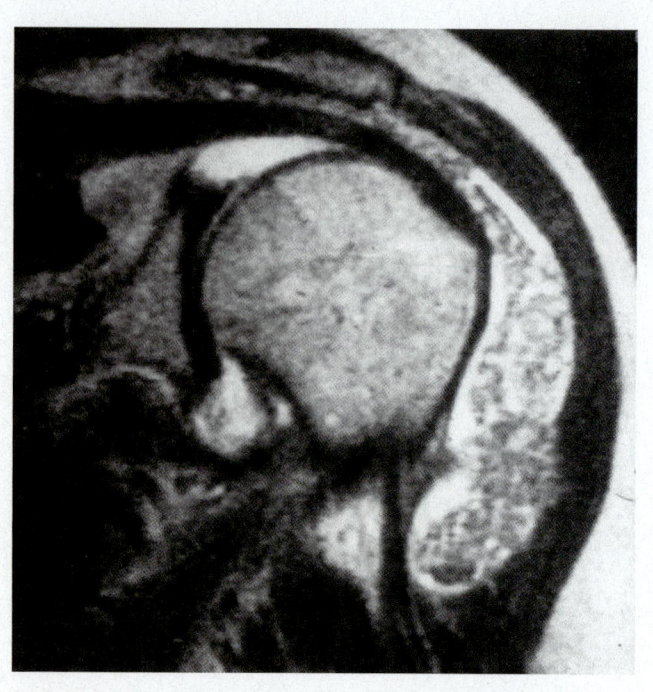

**FIGURE 47.5.** Septic subdeltoid and subacromial bursitis consistent with tuberculosis infection. Oblique coronal T2-weighted MR image shows extensive subacromial subcoracoid bursitis with innumerable punctate foci of low signal intensity consistent with rice bodies. (Reused from Zlatkin MB. *MRI of the Shoulder*. 2nd ed. Philadelphia, PA: Lippincott Williams & Wilkins; 2003, with permission.)

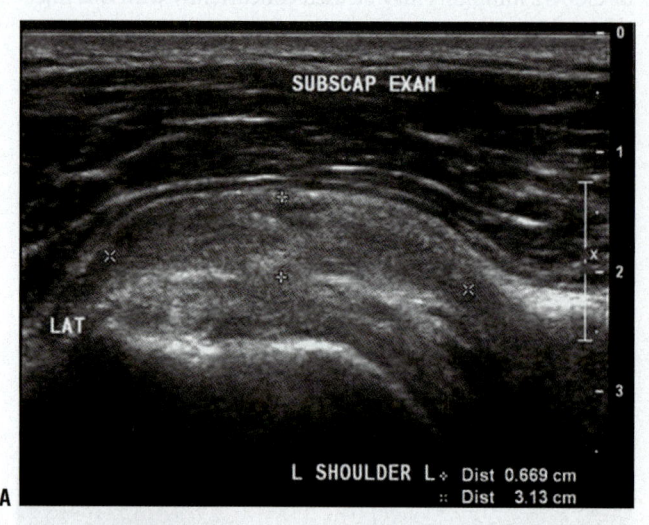

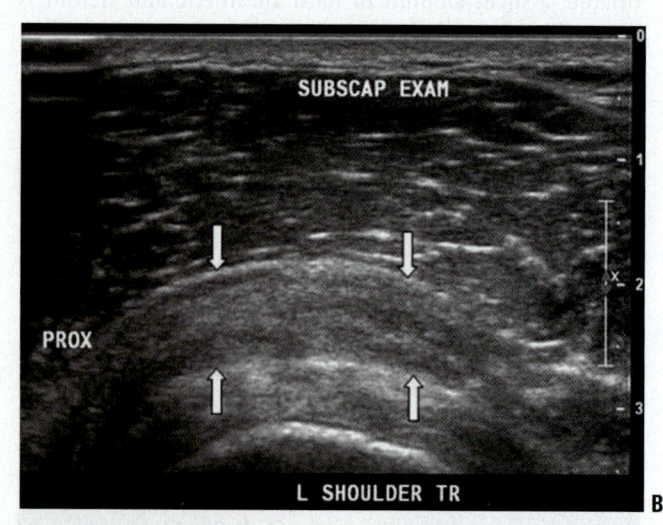

**FIGURE 47.4.** Longitudinal **(A)** and transverse **(B)** ultrasound views of the 7-mm-thick isoechoic heterogeneous mass (between *asterisks* in image **A** and *arrows* in image **B**) superficial to the subscapularis tendon that was proven at surgery to be a large, inflamed subacromial bursa. (Reused from Finnoff JT, Thompson JM, Collins M, et al. Subcoracoid bursitis as an unusual cause of painful anterior shoulder snapping in a weight lifter. *Am J Sports Med* 2010;38(8):1687–1692, with permission.)

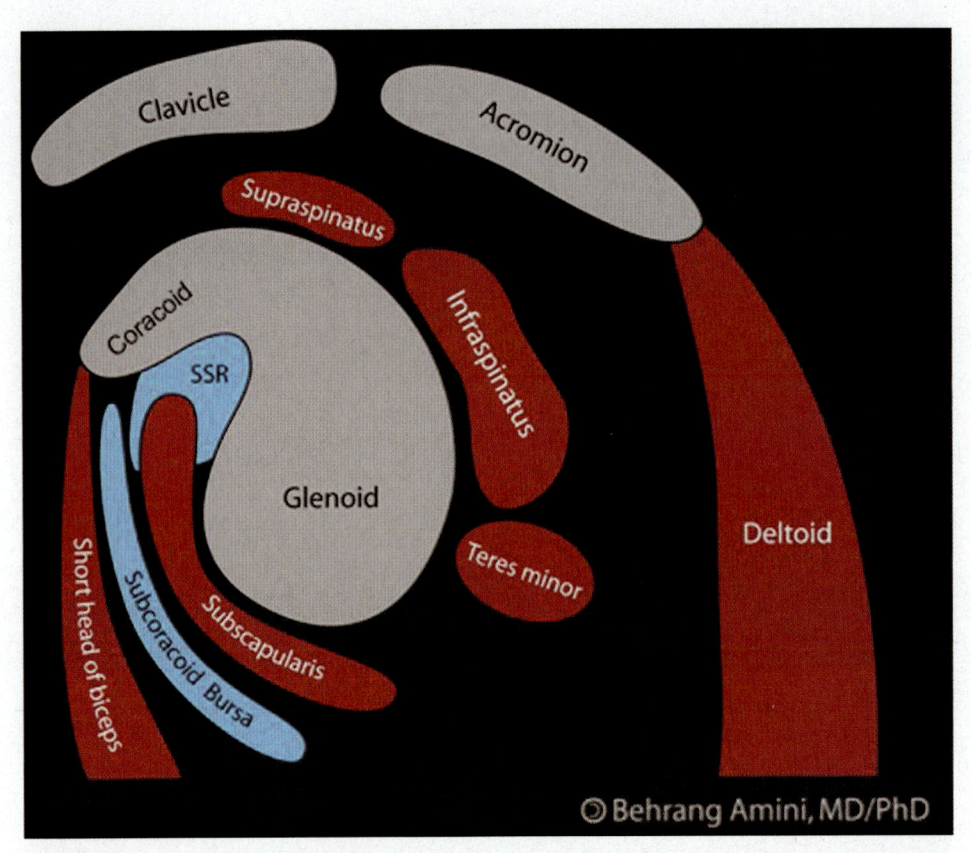

**FIGURE 47.6.** Functional anatomy of the relationship of the subcoracoid bursa to the coronoid process, the glenohumeral joint, and the subscapularis musculotendinous unit and the short head of the biceps. (SSR, superior subscapularis recess.) (Adapted from Grainger AJ, Tirman PFJ, Elliott M, et al. MR anatomy of the subcoracoid bursa and the association of subcoracoid effusion with tears of the anterior rotator cuff and rotator interval. *Am J Roentgenol* 2000;174(5):1377–1380.)

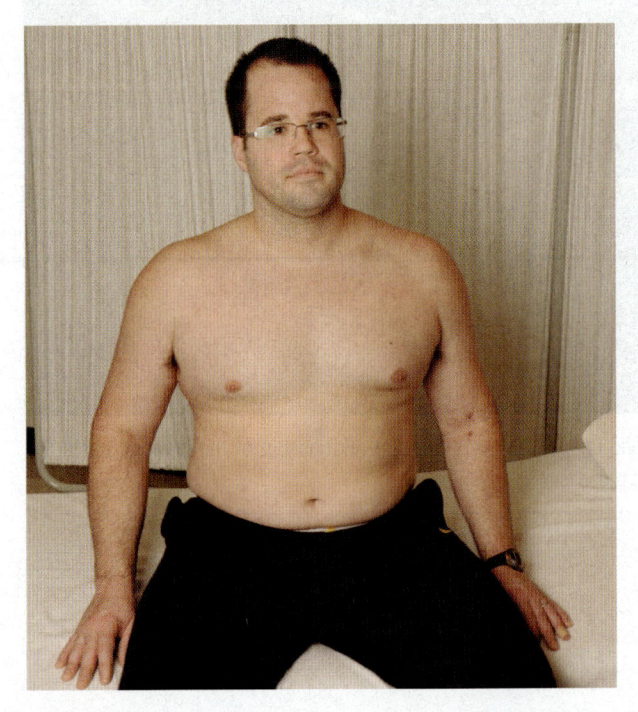

**FIGURE 47.7.** Proper patient positioning for ultrasound-guided injection of the subcoracoid bursa.

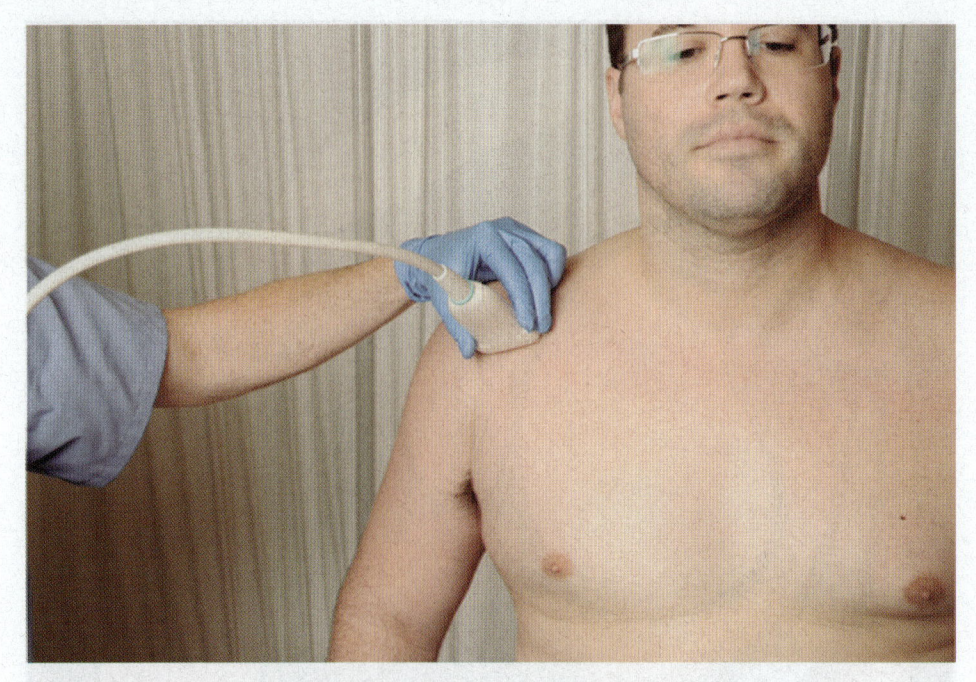

**FIGURE 47.8.** Proper ultrasound transducer position for ultrasound-guided injection of the subcoracoid bursa with the patient in the neutral sitting position.

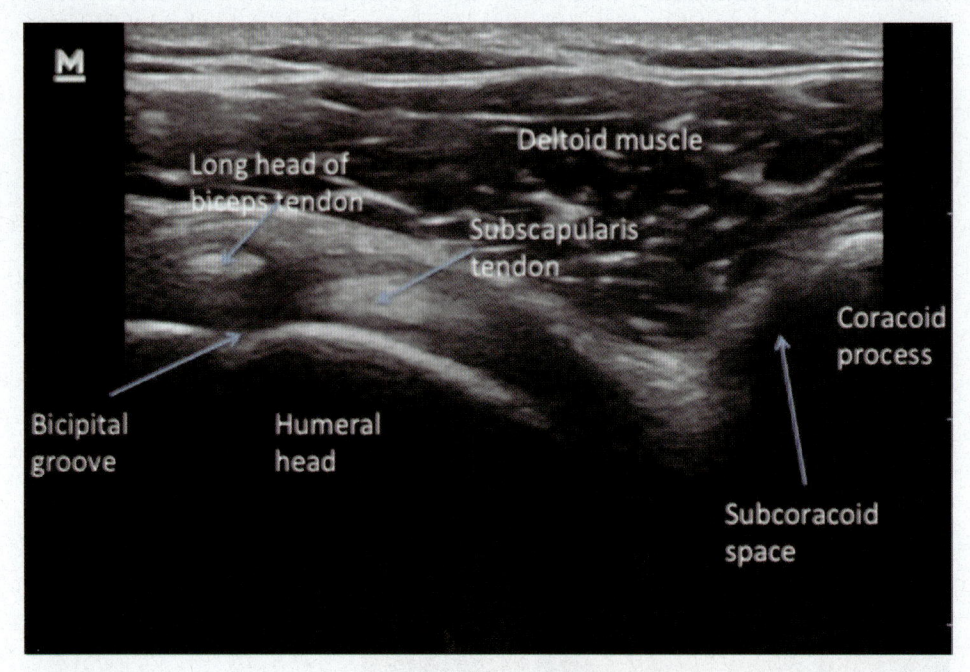

**FIGURE 47.9.** Transverse ultrasound image demonstrating the relationship of the humeral head, the glenohumeral joint, and the coracoid process.

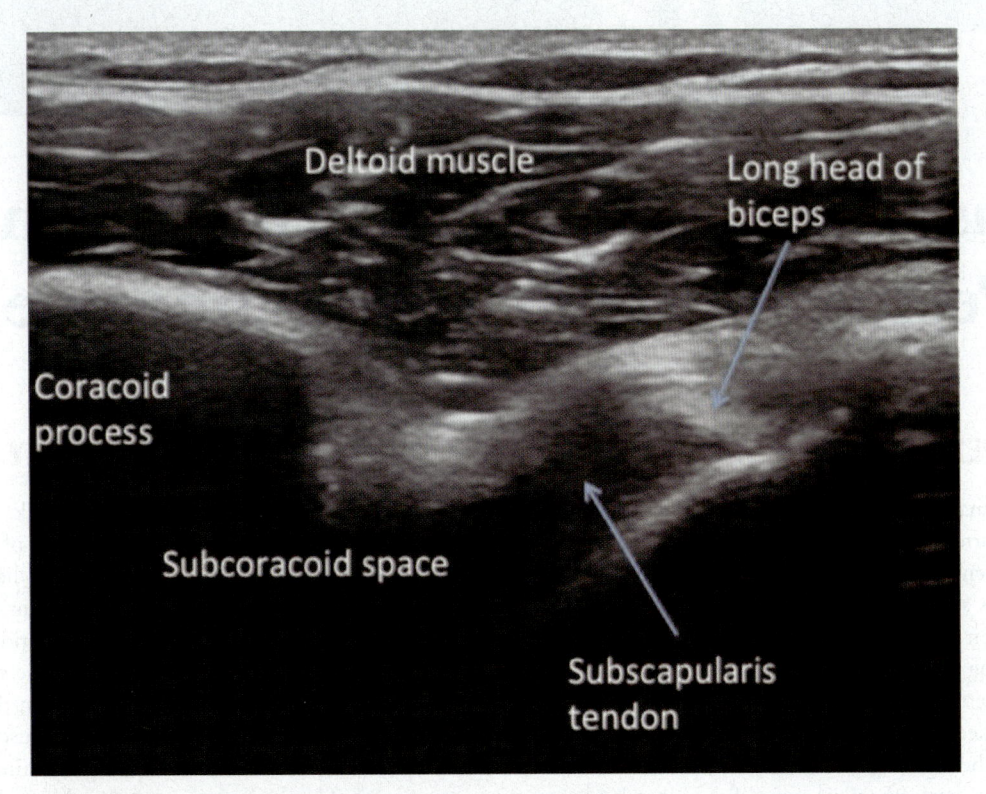

**FIGURE 47.10.** Transverse ultrasound view of the subcoracoid space.

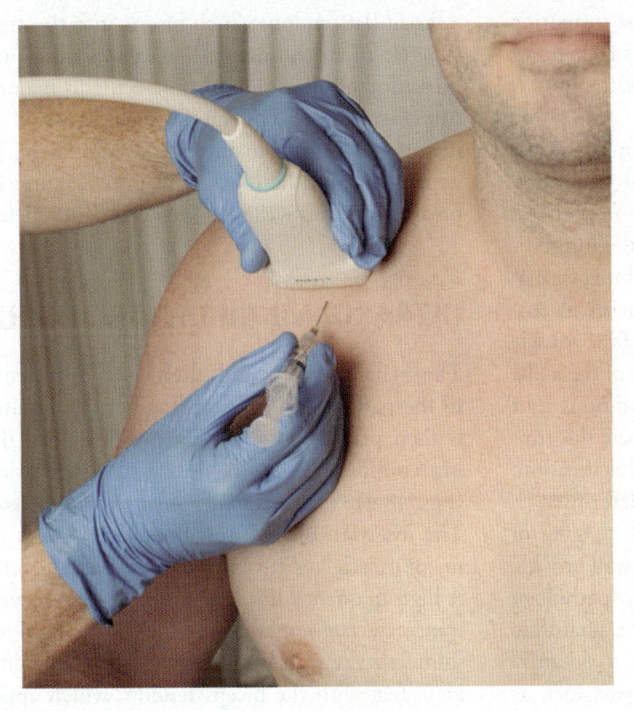

**FIGURE 47.11.** Proper needle position for injection of the subdeltoid bursa using an in-plane approach.

## SUGGESTED READINGS

Lento PH, Strakowski JA. The use of ultrasound in guiding musculoskeletal interventional procedures. *Phys Med Rehabil Clin N Am* 2010;21(3):559–583.

Narouze SN. Ultrasound-guided shoulder joint and bursa injections. In: *Atlas of Ultrasound Guided Procedures in Pain Management*. New York, NY: Springer; 2010:295–296.

Precerutti M, Garioni E, Madonia L, et al. US anatomy of the shoulder: pictorial essay. *J Ultrasound* 2010;13(4):179–187.

Waldman SD. The subcoracoid bursa. In: *Pain Review*. Philadelphia, PA: WB Saunders; 2009:89.

Waldman SD. Injection technique for subcoracoid bursitis. In: *Atlas of Pain Management Injection Techniques*. 3rd ed. Philadelphia, PA: Saunders Elsevier; 2013:109–111.

# CHAPTER 48

# Ultrasound-Guided Injection Technique for Pectoralis Major Tear Syndrome

## CLINICAL PERSPECTIVES

The pectoralis major muscle is a bilaminar muscle of the chest wall that performs five major functions: (1) flexion of the humerus as when lifting a box over one's head, (2) adduction of the humerus as when bringing the arm close to the chest wall, (3) rotation of the humerus medially as when arm wrestling, (4) helping to abduct the humerus at the upper range of the arc of abduction as when reaching for an object on a high shelf, and (5) keeping the arm attached to the trunk of the body. Due to the amazing variation of stresses the muscle is subjected to as it performs these varied functions, the musculotendinous unit is susceptible to injury ranging from microtrauma to individual muscle fibers following overuse or misuse to full-thickness tearing with associated hematoma formation and cosmetic deformity. Most often, full-thickness tears occur at the tendon's point of insertion into the crest of the greater tubercle of the humerus (Fig. 48.1).

Minor tears of the pectoralis muscle present clinically as anterior chest wall pain and require minimal treatment. Complete full-thickness tears occur at the tendon's point of insertion into the crest of the greater tubercle of the humerus present acutely with massive ecchymosis and hematoma formation and weakness of internal rotation of the humerus. A cosmetic deformity is often present with a bunching of the muscle in the anterior chest wall and a webbed appearance of the axilla (Fig. 48.2). Complete rupture of the musculotendinous unit requires prompt surgical repair, and failure to repair the rupture will result in further muscle retraction and calcification, worsening the functional disability and cosmetic deformity.

Magnetic resonance imaging and ultrasound imaging of the shoulder, proximal humerus, and anterior chest wall provide the clinician with the best information regarding any pathology including bursitis, tendonitis, and tumors of these anatomic regions. Both are useful in helping the clinician to identify abnormalities that may require urgent surgical repair such as complete pectoralis major muscle tears and/or tendon rupture. Both magnetic resonance imaging and ultrasound imaging will also help the clinician rule out occult pathology such as primary and metastatic tumors that may harm the patient.

## CLINICALLY RELEVANT ANATOMY

The pectoralis major muscle is a broad, thick, fan-like bilaminar muscle, which makes up the majority of the chest wall muscles (Fig. 48.3). The pectoralis major lies beneath the breast in females. The muscle finds its origins from the anterior surface of the proximal clavicle, the anterior surface of the sternum, the cartilaginous attachments of the second through sixth and occasionally seventh ribs, and from the aponeurotic band of the obliquus externus abdominis muscle. These muscle fibers are laid out in an overlapping bilaminar pattern with some muscle fibers running upward and lateralward and others running horizontally. Other muscle fibers run downward and lateralward. All of this latticework of fibers coalesces into a broad flat tendon, which inserts into the crest of the greater tubercle of the humerus. It is at this distal insertion that the musculotendinous unit of the pectoralis major frequently ruptures (see Fig. 48.1). The motor innervation of the pectoralis major muscle is from the medial and lateral pectoralis nerve, which can both be blocked to provide surgical anesthesia for breast surgery as well postoperative pain relief.

## ULTRASOUND-GUIDED TECHNIQUE

The benefits, risks, and alternative treatments are explained to the patient and informed consent is obtained. The patient is then placed in the sitting position with the forearm resting comfortably on the ipsilateral thigh with the palm up (Fig. 48.4). The bicipital groove is then palpated (Fig. 48.5). The insertion of the musculotendinous unit of the pectoralis major muscle lies just medial to the bicipital tendon (Fig. 48.6). A high-frequency linear ultrasound transducer is placed in the transverse axis centered over the bicipital groove, and an ultrasound survey scan is taken (Fig. 48.7). The bicipital groove is identified with the biceps tendon, which appears as a hyperechoic ovoid structure lying within it (Fig. 48.8). The ultrasound transducer is then turned to a longitudinal axis and is moved inferiorly along the path of the biceps tendon following the margin of the medial aspect of the humeral head as it

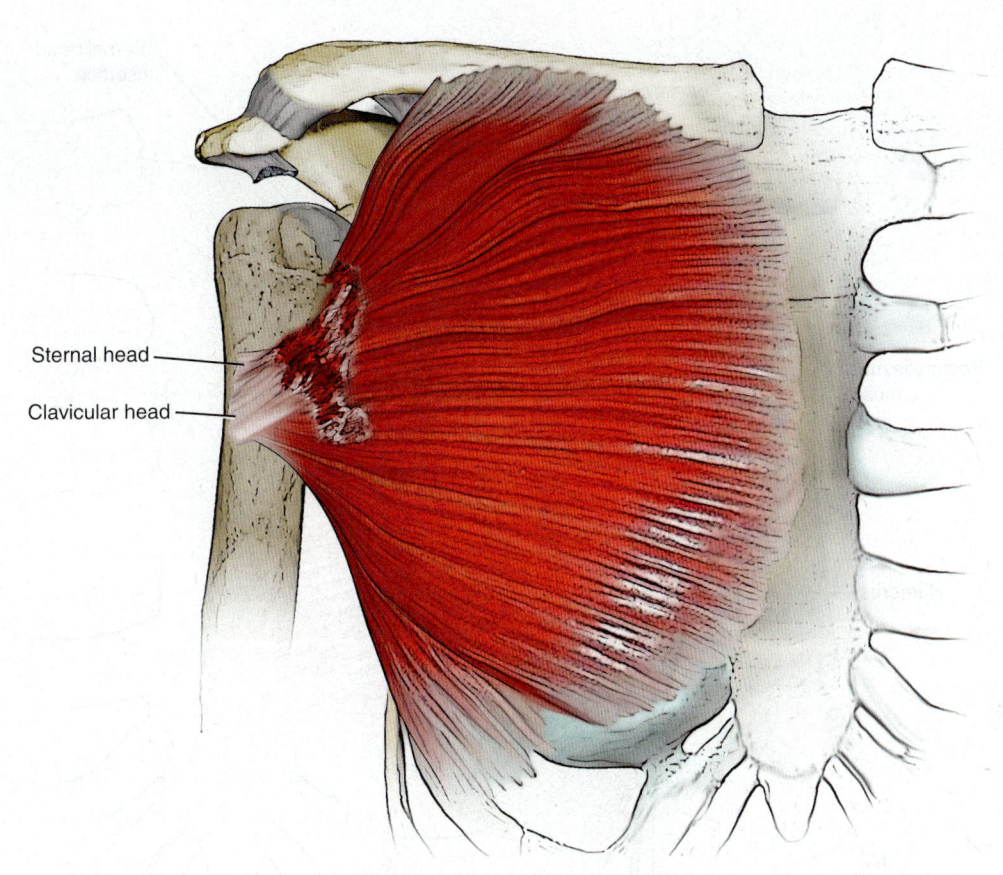

**FIGURE 48.1.** Coronal illustration of the characteristic musculotendinous junction injury involving the clavicular and sternal head tendon contributions.

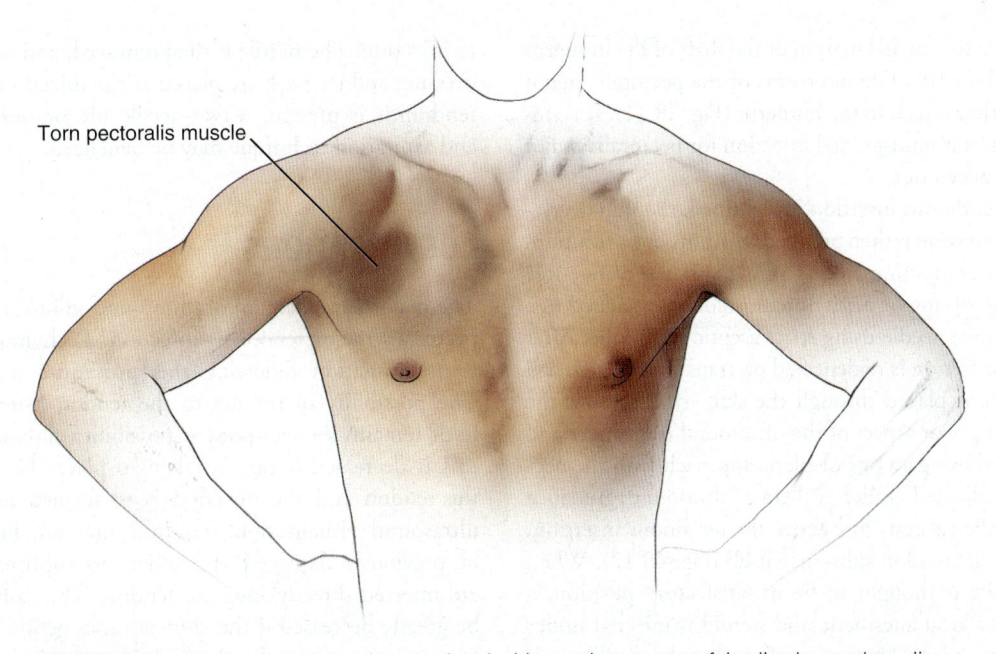

**FIGURE 48.2.** The cosmetic deformity associated with complete rupture of the distal musculotendinous unit of the pectoralis major muscle presents with a bunching of the muscle in the anterior chest wall and a webbed appearance of the axilla.

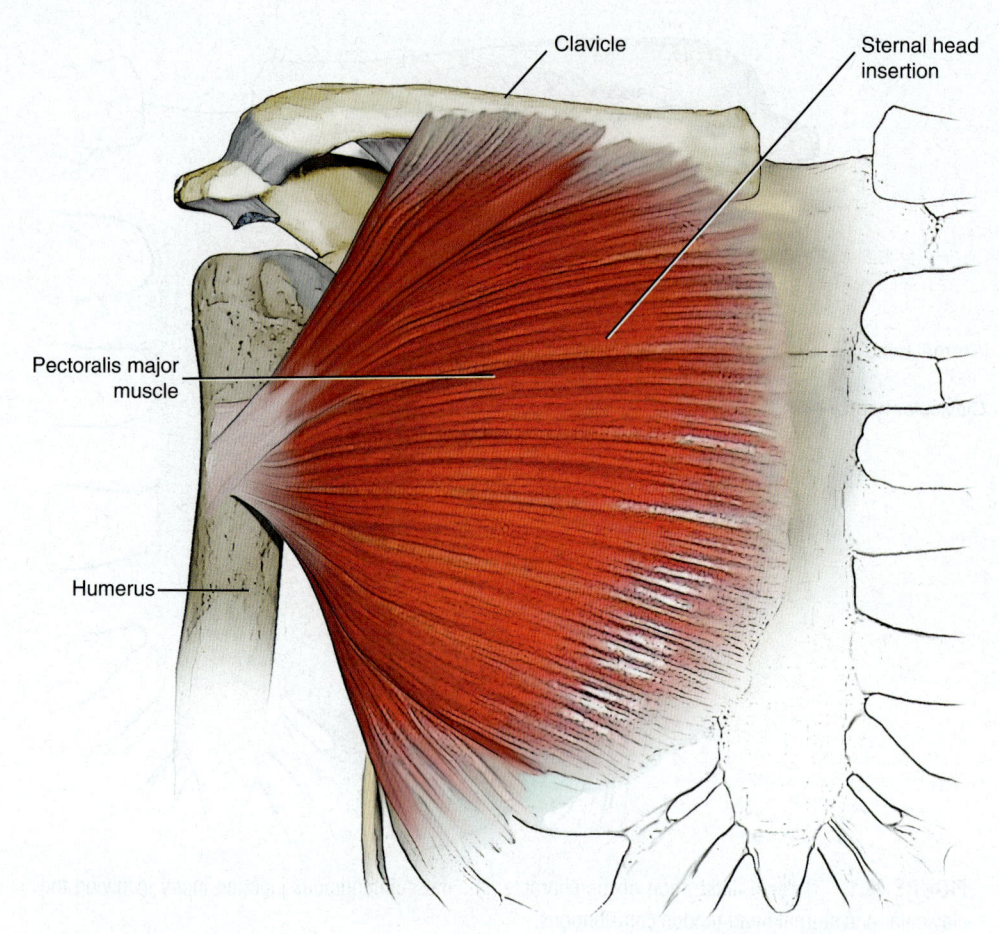

**FIGURE 48.3.** Anatomy of the pectoralis major muscle. (LifeART image ©2012 Lippincott Williams & Wilkins. All rights reserved.)

curves inward to the medial margin of the shaft of the humerus (Figs. 48.9 and 48.10). The insertions of the pectoralis major will be seen as they attach to the humerus (Fig. 48.11). It is this point that the ultrasound-guided injection for pectoralis major muscle tear is carried out.

After the tendinous insertion is identified, the skin overlying the area of insertion is then prepped with antiseptic solution. A sterile syringe containing 5.0 mL of 0.25% preservative-free bupivacaine and 40 mg of methylprednisolone is attached to a 3½-inch, 22-gauge needle using strict aseptic technique. After the tendinous insertion is reidentified on transverse ultrasound scan, the needle is placed through the skin ~1 cm above the middle of the superior aspect of the ultrasound transducer and is then advanced using an out-of-plane approach with the needle trajectory adjusted under real-time ultrasound guidance so that the needle tip rests just above the tendinous insertion, but not within the tendon substance itself (Fig. 48.12). When the tip of needle is thought to be in satisfactory position, a small amount of local anesthetic and steroid is injected under real-time ultrasound guidance to confirm that the needle tip is not with the substance of the tendon. After proper needle tip placement is confirmed, the remainder of the contents of the syringe are slowly injected. There should be minimal resistance to injection. The needle is then removed, and a sterile pressure dressing and ice pack are placed at the injection site. If calcific tendonitis is present, a two-needle ultrasound-guided lavage and aspiration technique may be beneficial.

## COMPLICATIONS

The major complication of ultrasound-guided injection of the pectoralis major tendon is infection. Ecchymosis and hematoma formation following this procedure may also occur. The possibility of trauma to the tendon from the injection itself remains an ever-present possibility, although the risk of this is decreased if care is taken to place the needle outside the tendon and the injection is performed under real-time ultrasound visualization. Tendons that are highly inflamed or previously damaged are subject to rupture if substances are injected directly into the tendon. This complication can be greatly decreased if the clinician uses gentle technique and stops injecting immediately if significant resistance to injection is encountered. Approximately 25% of patients complain of a transient increase in pain after this injection technique; the patient should be warned of this.

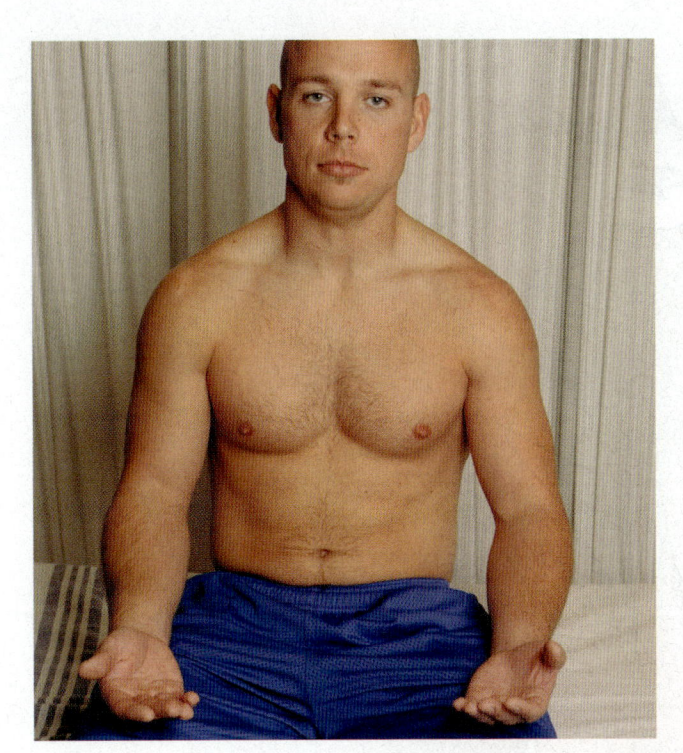

**FIGURE 48.4.** Proper patient positioning for the ultrasound-guided injection for pectoralis major muscle tear.

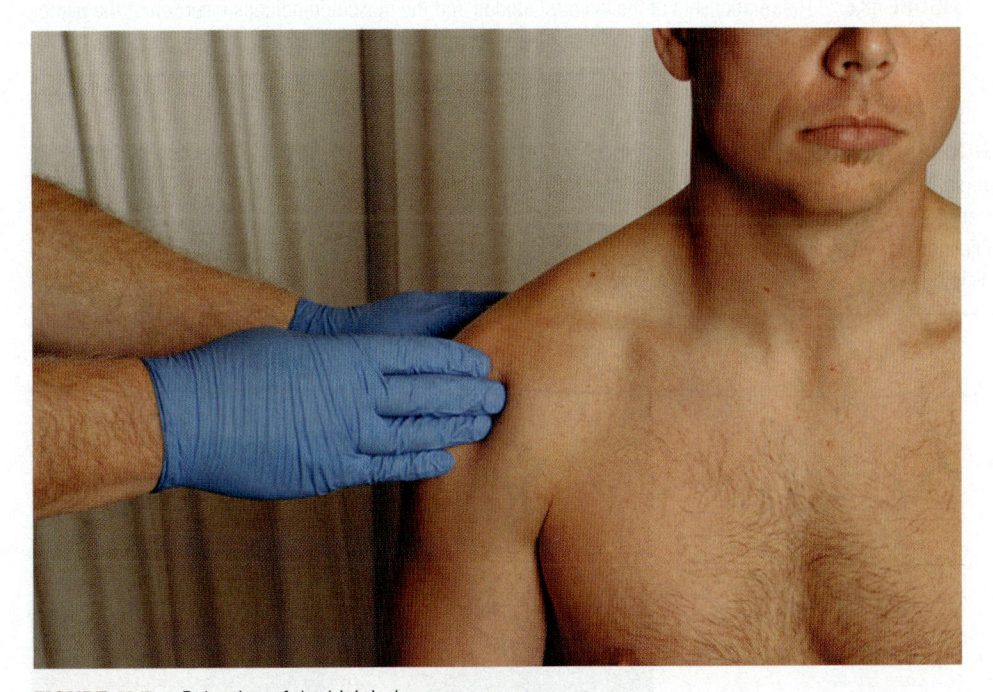

**FIGURE 48.5.** Palpation of the bicipital groove.

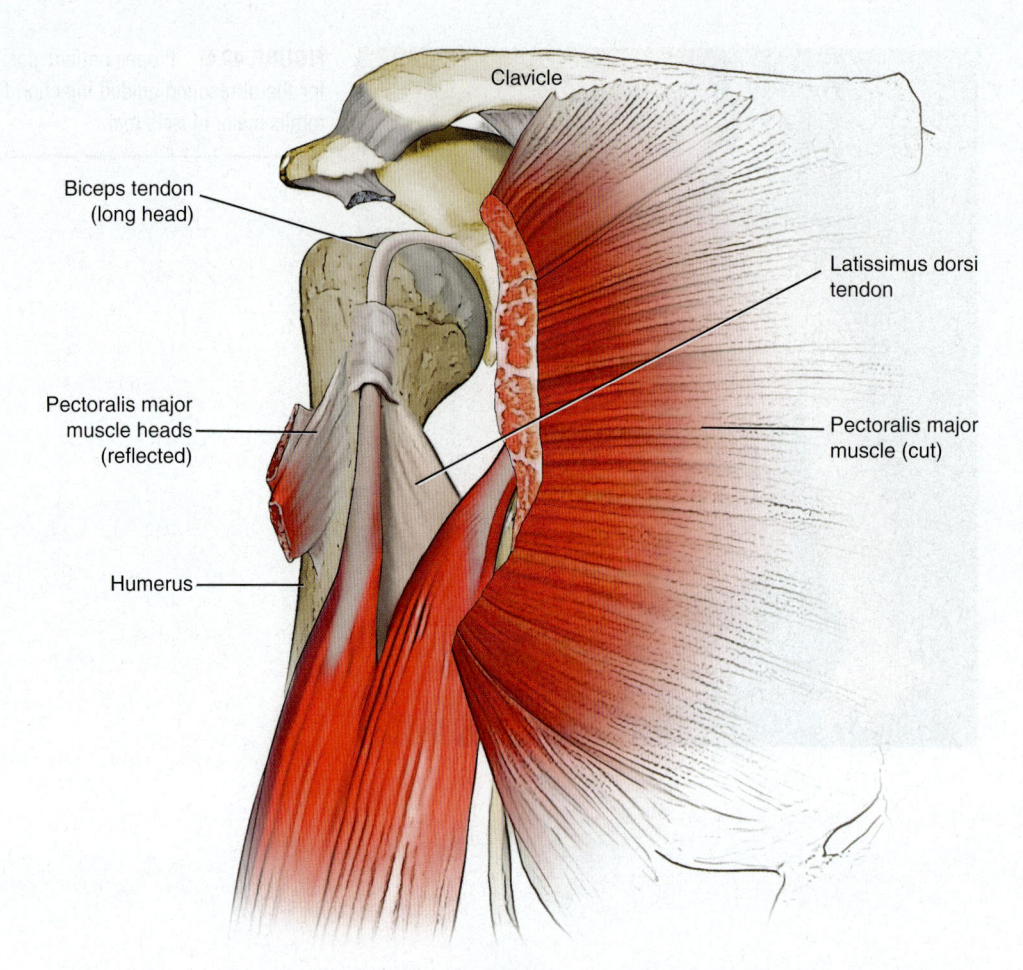

**FIGURE 48.6.** The relationship of the bicipital tendon and the musculotendinous insertion of the pectoralis major muscle. (Adapted from Anatomical Chart Company.)

**FIGURE 48.7.** Proper transverse position of the ultrasound transducer for ultrasound-guided injection for identification of the bicipital groove.

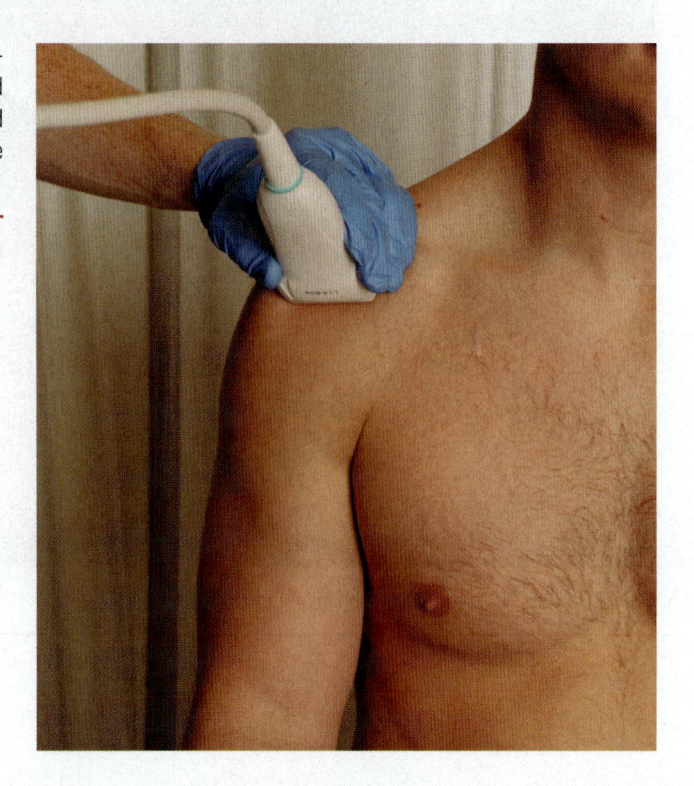

# CHAPTER 48   ULTRASOUND-GUIDED INJECTION TECHNIQUE FOR PECTORALIS MAJOR TEAR SYNDROME

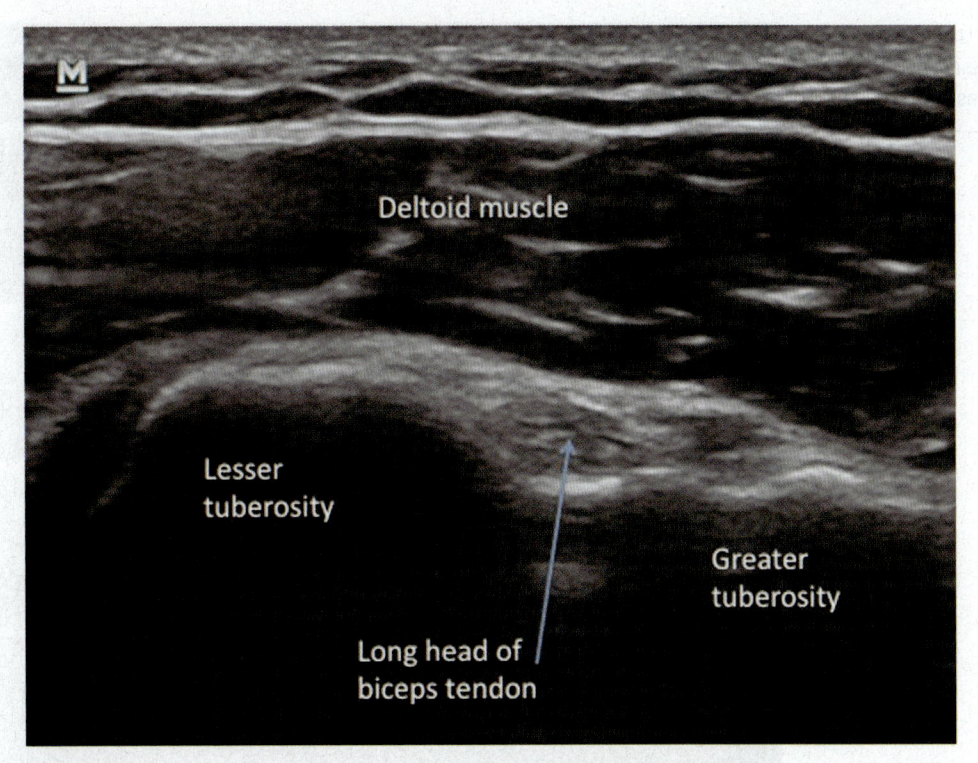

**FIGURE 48.8.** Transverse ultrasound view of the bicipital groove.

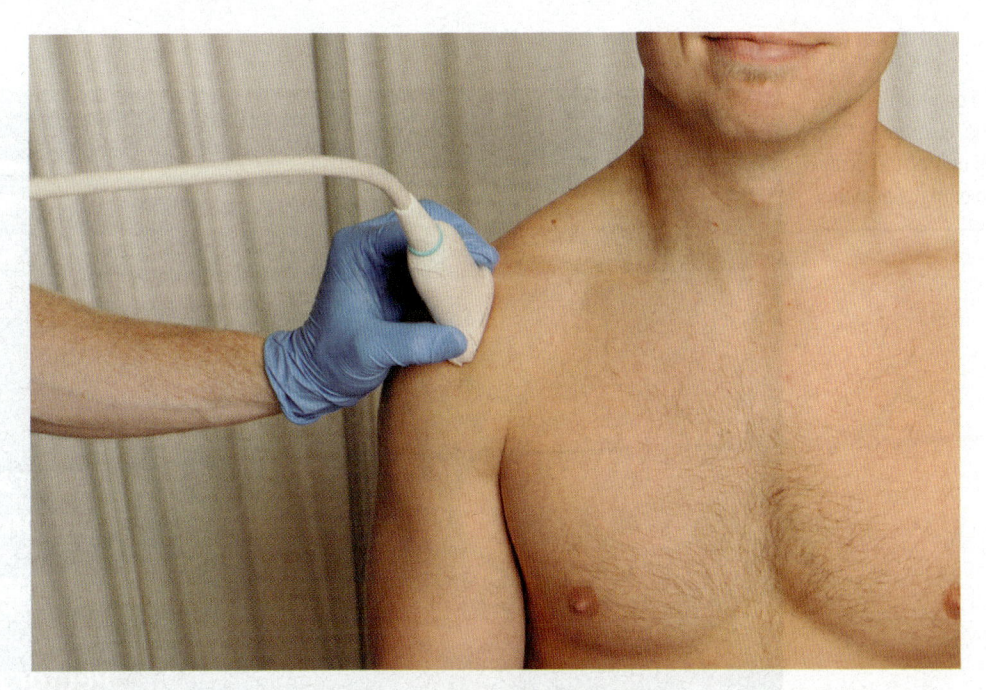

**FIGURE 48.9.** Proper longitudinal position of the ultrasound transducer to follow the bicipital tendon and the medial margin of the humerus.

**FIGURE 48.10.** Longitudinal ultrasound view of the medial aspect of the humeral head as it curves inward.

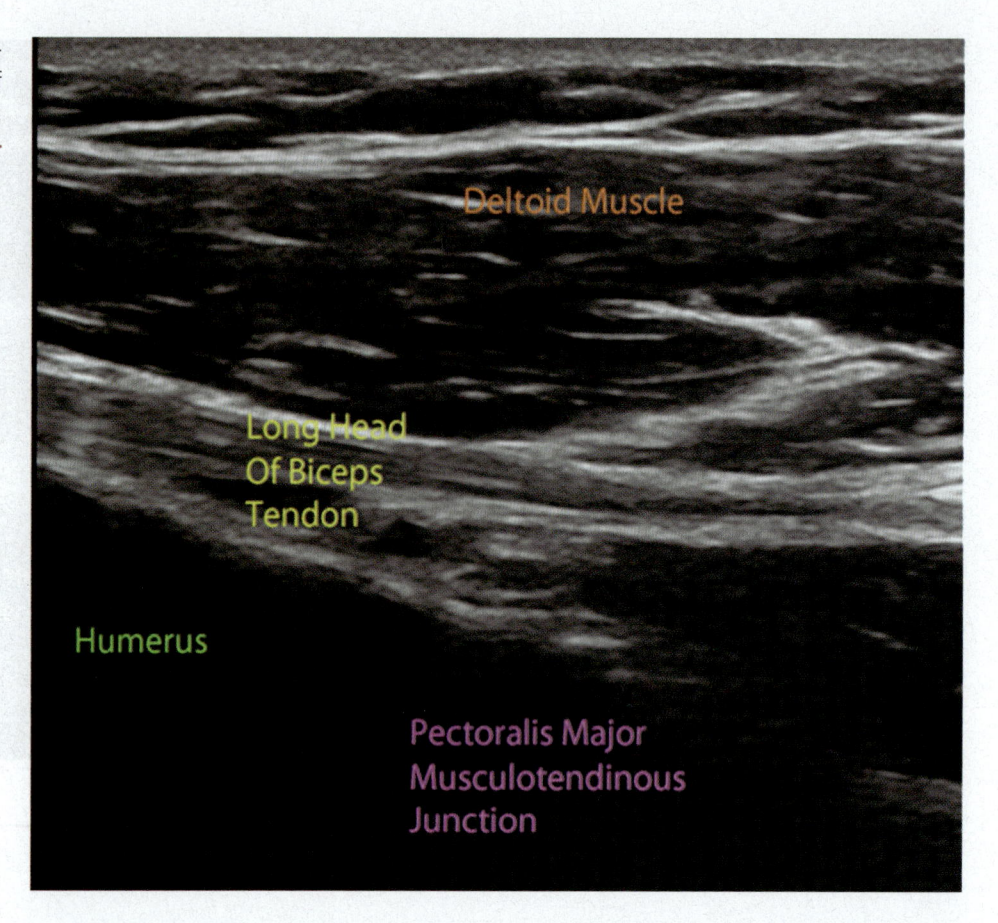

**FIGURE 48.11.** Longitudinal ultrasound view of the insertion of the musculotendinous unit of the pectoralis major muscle onto the humerus.

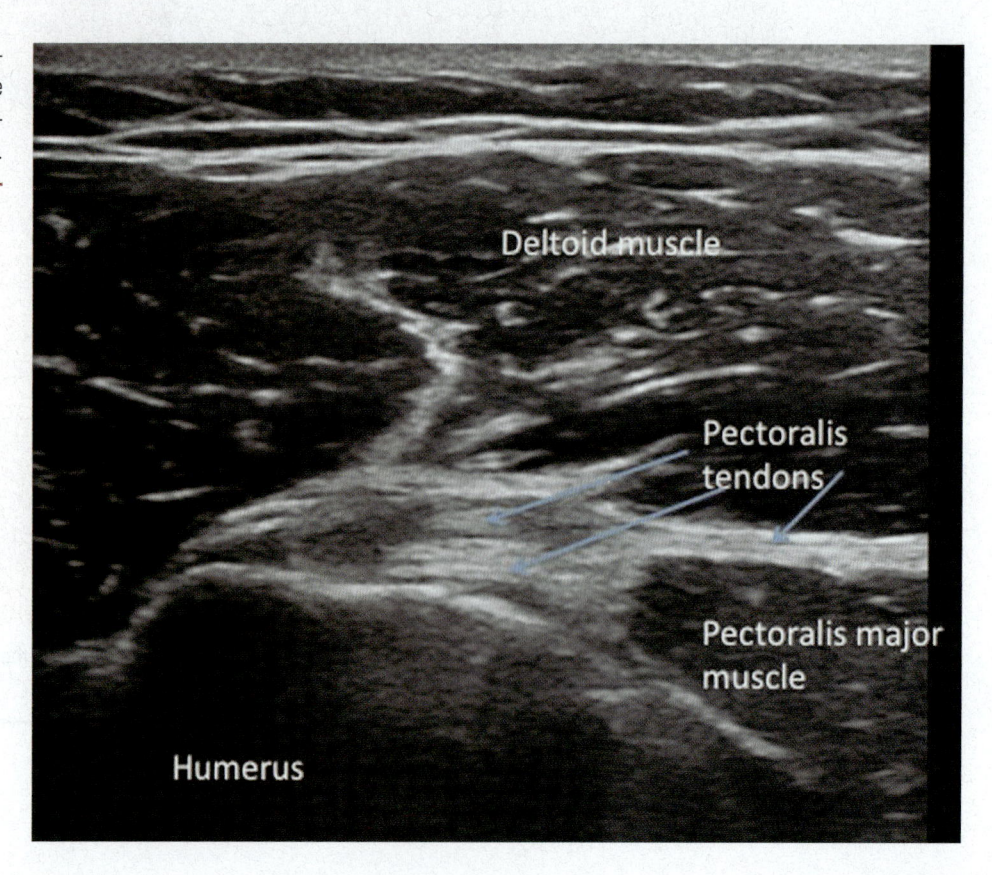

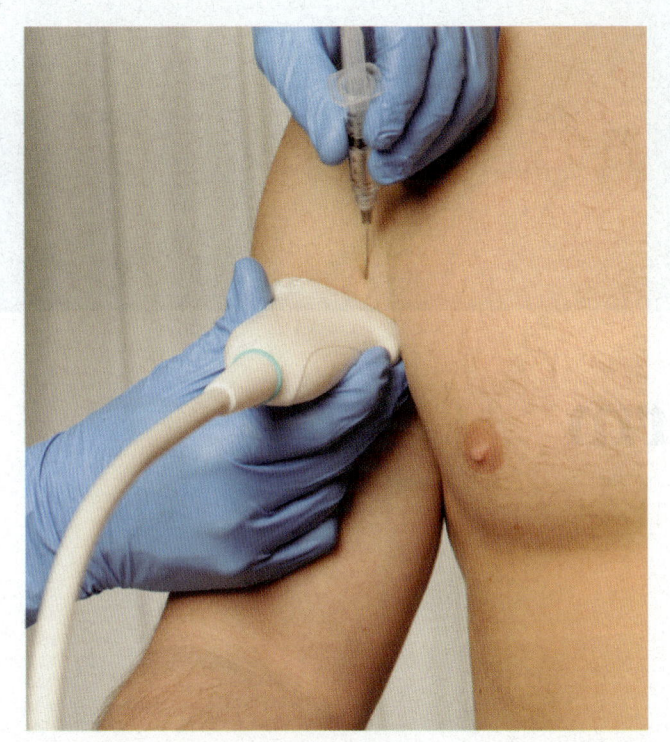

**FIGURE 48.12.** Proper needle and transverse ultrasound transducer position for out-of-plane needle insertion for ultrasound-guided injection for pectoralis major muscle tear.

## CLINICAL PEARLS

Pectoralis major tear syndrome can usually be diagnosed on clinical grounds. While complete rupture of the musculotendinous insertion is uncommon, partial tears occur with reasonable frequency. Complete rupture of the musculotendinous unit of the pectoralis major muscle is accompanied by impressive ecchymosis and hematoma formation that may seem out of proportion to the degree of trauma the muscle has sustained or the pain associated with the injury. Reassurance to the patient is often required. Complete rupture of the musculotendinous unit of the pectoralis major muscle will require surgery to avoid further functional disability and worsening of the cosmetic defect.

Shoulder pathology including rotator cuff tendinopathy, osteoarthritis, avascular necrosis of the humeral head, and impingement syndromes may coexist with pectoralis major tear and may contribute to the patient's pain symptomatology. Universal precautions should always be observed to protect the operator, and strict adherence to sterile technique must be used to avoid infection. Gentle physical therapy and local heat should be introduced following ultrasound-guided injection to reduce pain and improve function. Simple analgesics and nonsteroidal anti-inflammatory agents or COX-2 inhibitors may be used concurrently with this injection technique.

## SUGGESTED READINGS

Precerutti M, Garioni E, Madonia L, et al. US anatomy of the shoulder: pictorial essay. *J Ultrasound* 2010;13(4):179–187.

Vlychou M, Teh J. Ultrasound of muscle. *Curr Probl Diagn Radiol* 2008;37(5):219–230.

Waldman SD. Pectoralis major muscle tear. In: *Atlas of Uncommon Pain Syndromes*. 2nd ed. Philadelphia, PA: Elsevier; 2008:73–74.

Waldman SD. Functional anatomy of the shoulder joint. In: *Pain Review*. Philadelphia, PA: Saunders Elsevier; 2009:80–81.

Waldman SD. Injection technique for pectoralis major tear. In: *Atlas of Pain Management Injection Techniques*. 3rd ed. Philadelphia, PA: Elsevier; 2013:78–80.

# SECTION IV

# Elbow and Forearm

# CHAPTER 49

# Ultrasound-Guided Injection Technique for Intra-articular Injection of the Elbow Joint

## CLINICAL PERSPECTIVES

The elbow joint is a synovial hinge joint whose primary function is to aid in the orientation of the hand in space for crucial functions like eating and drinking. The joint's articular cartilage is susceptible to damage, which left untreated will result in arthritis with its associated pain and functional disability. Osteoarthritis of the joint is the most common form of arthritis that results in elbow joint pain and functional disability, with rheumatoid arthritis, posttraumatic arthritis, and crystal arthropathy also causing arthritis of the elbow joint. Less common causes of arthritis-induced elbow joint pain include the collagen vascular diseases, infection, villonodular synovitis, and Lyme disease. Acute infectious arthritis of the elbow joint is best treated with early diagnosis, with culture and sensitivity of the synovial fluid and prompt initiation of antibiotic therapy. The collagen vascular diseases generally manifest as a polyarthropathy rather than a monoarthropathy limited to the elbow joint, although elbow pain secondary to the collagen vascular diseases responds exceedingly well to ultrasound-guided intra-articular injection of the elbow joint.

Patients with elbow joint pain secondary to arthritis, synovitis, gout, and collagen vascular disease related joint pain complain of pain that is localized to the elbow and forearm. Activity makes the pain worse, with rest and heat providing some relief. The pain is constant and characterized as aching. Sleep disturbance is common with awakening when patients roll over onto the affected elbow. Some patients complain of a grating, catching, or popping sensation with range of motion of the joint, and crepitus may be appreciated on physical examination.

Functional disability often accompanies the pain and many pathologic conditions of the elbow joint. Patients will often notice increasing difficulty in performing their activities of daily living and tasks that require flexing or extending the elbow such as lifting heavy objects and holding a coffee cup. If the pathologic process responsible for the elbow pain is not adequately treated, the patient's functional disability may worsen, and muscle wasting and ultimately a frozen elbow may occur.

Plain radiographs are indicated in all patients who present with elbow pain (Fig. 49.1). Based on the patient's clinical presentation, additional testing may be indicated, including complete blood cell count, sedimentation rate, and antinuclear antibody testing. MRI or ultrasound of the elbow is indicated if tendinopathy, crystal arthropathy, fracture, joint mice, synovitis, bursitis, or ligamentous injury is suspected.

## CLINICALLY RELEVANT ANATOMY

The elbow joint is a synovial hinge-type joint that allows the distal humerus to articulate with the proximal radius and ulna (Fig. 49.2). The joint allows flexion and extension as well as supination and pronation. The joint's articular surface is covered with hyaline cartilage, which is susceptible to arthritis and degeneration. This membrane gives rise to synovial tendon sheaths and bursae that are subject to inflammation. The entire elbow joint is surrounded by ligaments, which coupled with the extremely deep bony articular socket makes the joint stable throughout its range of motion (Figs. 49.3 and 49.4). The joint capsule is lined with a synovial membrane, which attaches to the articular cartilage. This membrane gives rise to synovial tendon sheaths and bursae that are subject to inflammation and swelling, especially in the anterior and posterior aspects of the joint where the joint capsule is less dense. The olecranon bursa lies in the posterior aspect of the joint, while the cubital bursa lies anteriorly. Both are subject to the development of bursitis with misuse or overuse of the elbow joint. The primary innervation of the elbow joint comes from the musculocutaneous and radial nerves with some lesser contribution from the median and ulnar nerves. As the ulnar nerve passes inferiorly down the upper arm, it courses medially at the mid humerus to pass between the olecranon process and medial epicondyle of the humerus. The nerve is extremely susceptible to entrapment and trauma at this point. Anteriorly, the median nerve lies just medial to the brachial artery and occasionally susceptible to damage during puncture of the brachial artery when drawing arterial blood gasses.

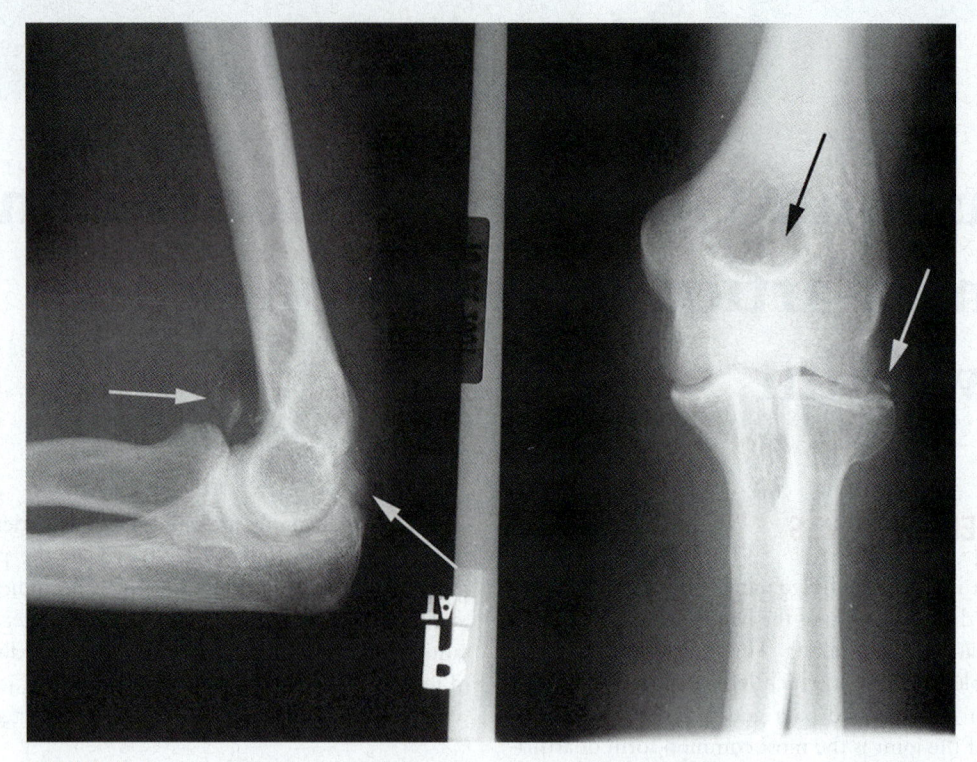

**FIGURE 49.1.** Osteoarthritis of the elbow. Plain radiograph demonstrating olecranon and coronoid osteophytes (*black arrow*) and joint space narrowing (*long white arrow*). Joint mice are also present (*short white arrow*). (Reused from Koopman WJ, Moreland LW. Arthritis and allied conditions: a textbook of rheumatology. 15th ed. Philadelphia, PA: Lippincott Williams & Wilkins; 2005, with permission.)

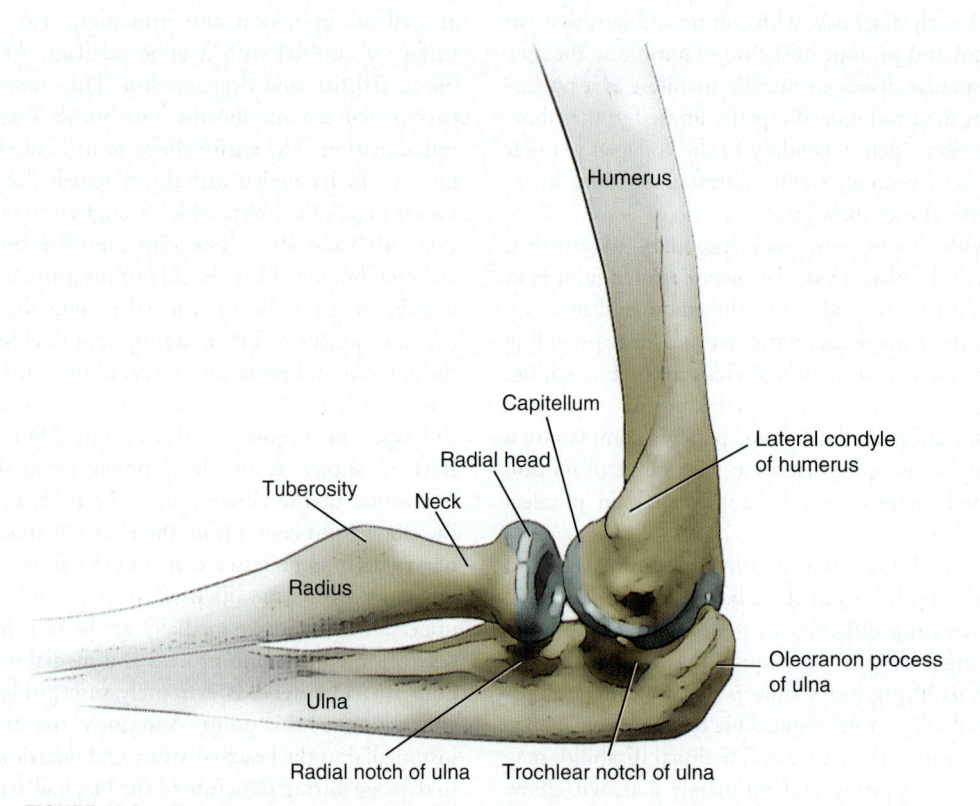

**FIGURE 49.2.** The osseous anatomy of the elbow joint.

CHAPTER 49   ULTRASOUND-GUIDED INJECTION TECHNIQUE FOR INTRA-ARTICULAR INJECTION OF THE ELBOW JOINT

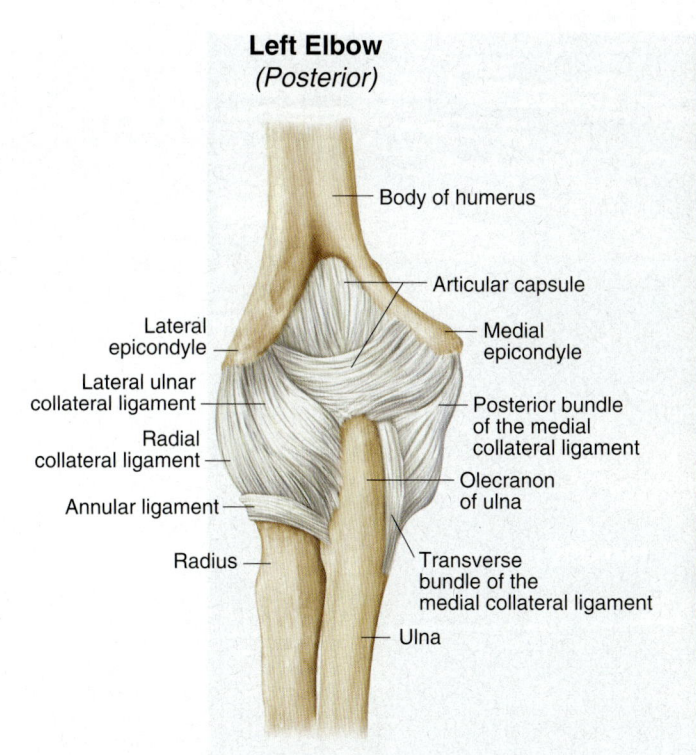

**FIGURE 49.3.** The posterior ligaments of the elbow along with the deep joint socket contribute to the joint's stability. (Anatomical Chart Company.)

## ULTRASOUND-GUIDED TECHNIQUE

The benefits, risks, and alternative treatments are explained to the patient and informed consent is obtained. The patient is

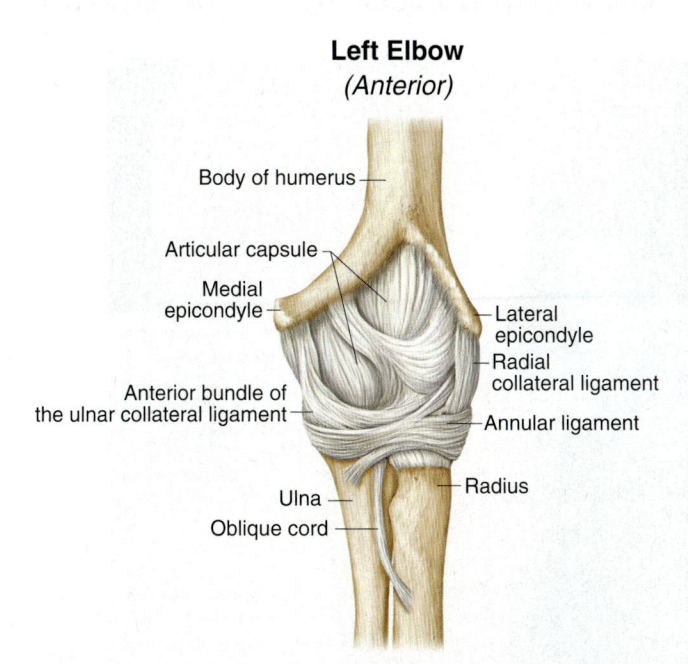

**FIGURE 49.4.** Anterior view of the ligaments of the elbow. (Anatomical Chart Company.)

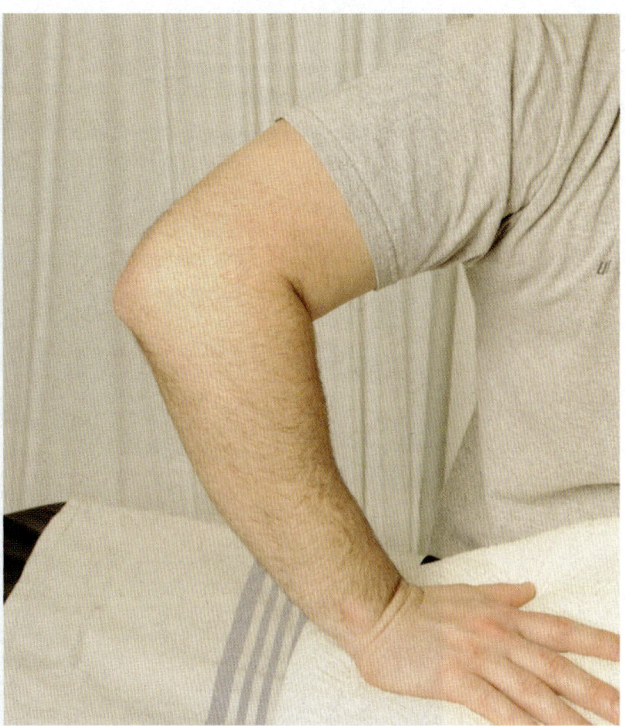

**FIGURE 49.5.** Correct patient position for ultrasound-guided intra-articular injection of the elbow joint.

then placed in the sitting position with the elbow flexed to ~100 degrees with the forearm and hand resting comfortably on a pillow (Fig. 49.5). The skin overlying the posterior elbow joint is then prepped with antiseptic solution. A sterile syringe

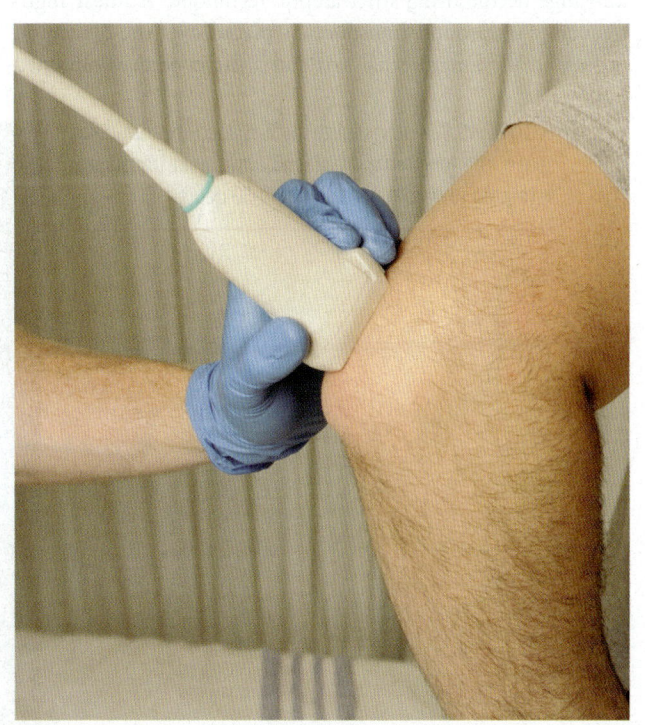

**FIGURE 49.6.** Correct position for ultrasound transducer for ultrasound-guided intra-articular injection of the elbow joint.

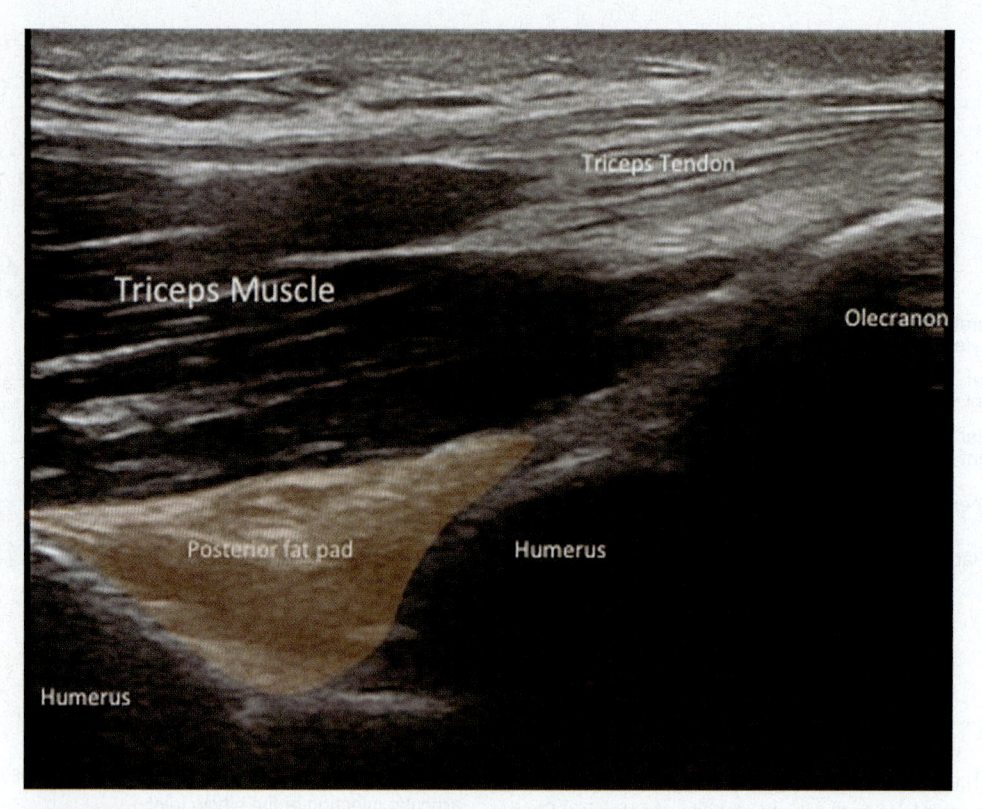

**FIGURE 49.7.** Longitudinal ultrasound view of the elbow demonstrating the olecranon, the humerus, the posterior fat pad, and the triceps muscle and tendon.

containing 2.0 mL of 0.25% preservative-free bupivacaine and 40 mg of methylprednisolone is attached to a 1½-inch, 22-gauge needle using strict aseptic technique. A linear high-frequency ultrasound transducer is placed over the olecranon process in the longitudinal axis and a survey scan is obtained (Fig. 49.6). The olecranon process and triceps tendon are then identified (Fig. 49.7). The superior portion of the ultrasound transducer is slowly rotated toward the little finger until the convex hyperechoic surface of the lateral trochlea of the distal humerus comes into view (Fig. 49.8). The intra-articular

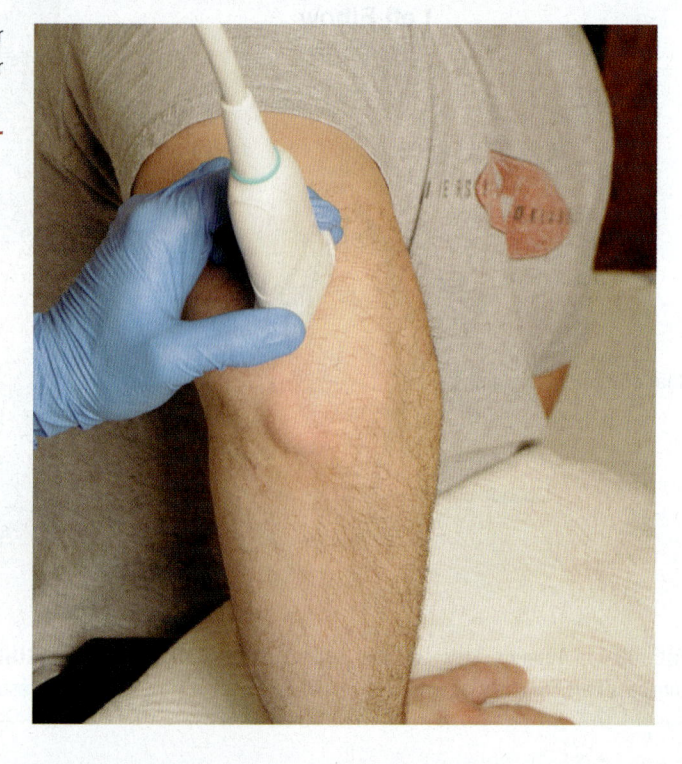

**FIGURE 49.8.** To visualize the V-shaped intra-articular space, the longitudinally placed ultrasound transducer is rotated toward the little finger ~30 degrees.

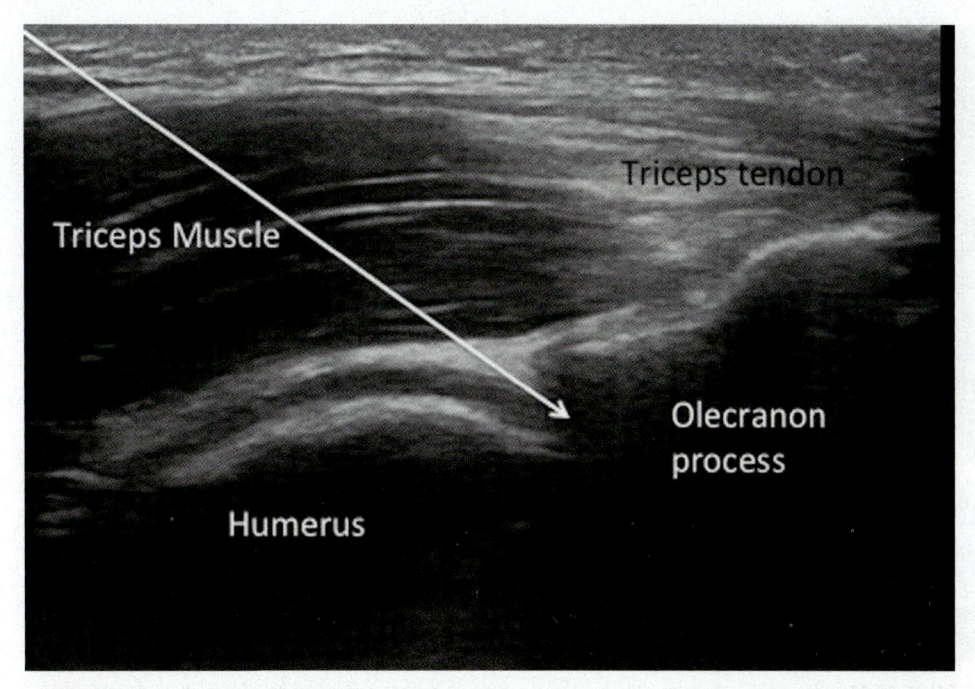

**FIGURE 49.9.** Ultrasound image of the V-shaped intra-articular space of the elbow. Note the relationship of the olecranon, the lateral trochlea of the humerus, and the triceps muscle and tendon.

space will be seen just as a V-shaped notch just in front of the lateral trochlea of the distal humerus and the hyperechoic superior margin of the olecranon process (Fig. 49.9). After the intra-articular notch is identified, the ultrasound transduced is slowly moved inferiorly to place the notch in proximity to the superior aspect of the ultrasound transducer (Fig. 49.10). After the intra-articular notch is reidentified, the needle is placed through the skin ~0.5 cm above the superior end of the

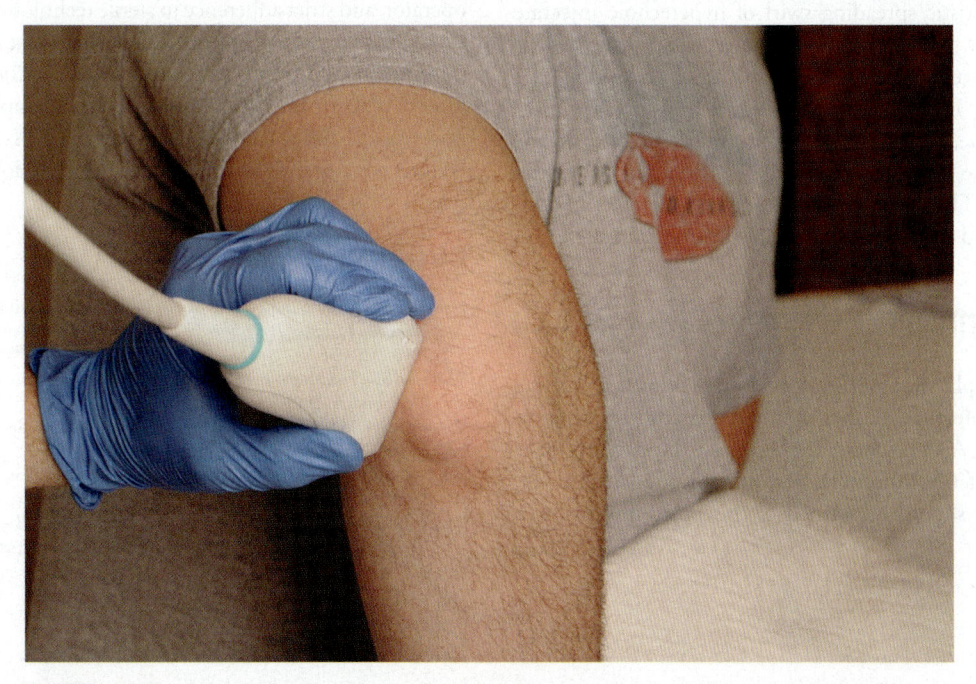

**FIGURE 49.10.** To minimize the distance from the skin to the intra-articular space of the elbow, the ultrasound transducer is moved inferiorly until the V-shaped joint is at the superior margin of the transducer.

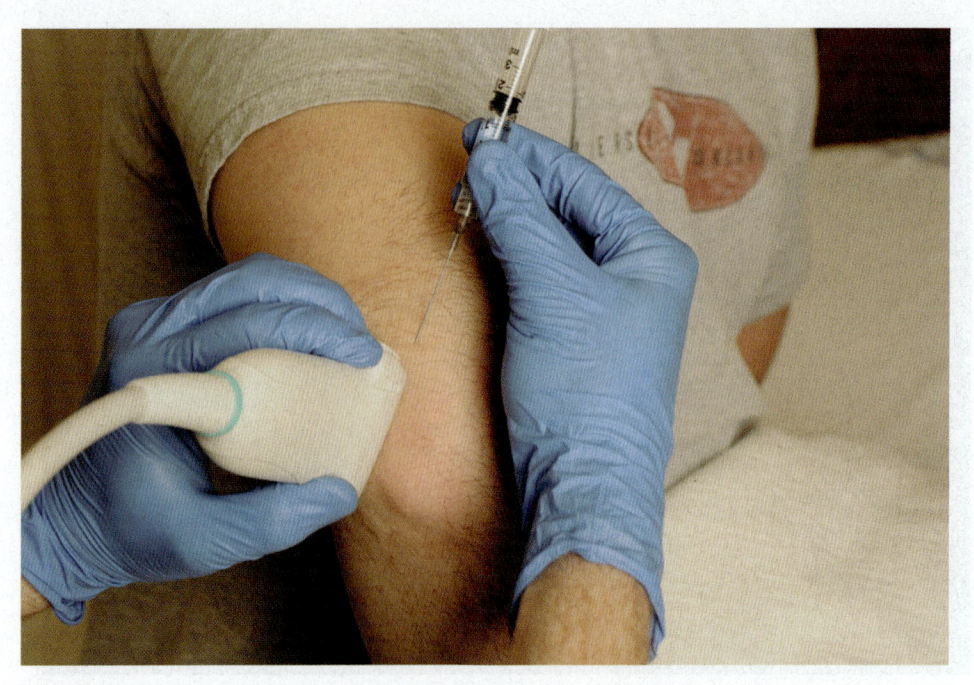

**FIGURE 49.11.** Proper in-plane needle position for ultrasound-guided injection of the elbow joint.

ultrasound transducer and is then advanced using an in-plane approach with the needle trajectory adjusted under real-time ultrasound guidance to enter the elbow joint just in front of the lateral trochlea of the distal humerus (Fig. 49.11). When the tip of needle is thought to be within the joint space, a small amount of local anesthetic and steroid is injected under real-time ultrasound guidance to confirm intra-articular placement by the characteristic spreading swirl of hyperechoic injectate within the joint. After intra-articular needle tip placement is confirmed, the remainder of the contents of the syringe are slowly injected. There should be minimal resistance to injection. If synechiae, loculations, or calcifications are present, the needle may have to be repositioned to ensure that the entire joint is treated. The needle is then removed, and a sterile pressure dressing and ice pack are placed at the injection site.

## COMPLICATIONS

The major complication of ultrasound-guided injection of the elbow joint is infection. Ecchymosis and hematoma formation may also occur. A transient exacerbation of the patient's pain occurs ~25% of the time following this injection technique, and the patient should be warned of this possibility prior to the procedure.

## CLINICAL PEARLS

Elbow pathology including tendinopathy, occult fractures, osteoarthritis, epicondylitis, avascular necrosis of the joint, and impingement syndromes may coexist with elbow joint disease and may contribute to the patient's pain symptomatology. Universal precautions should always be observed to protect the operator, and strict adherence to sterile technique must be used to avoid infection. Gentle physical therapy and local heat should be introduced following ultrasound-guided injection of the elbow joint to reduce pain and improve function. Simple analgesics and nonsteroidal anti-inflammatory agents or COX-2 inhibitors may be used concurrently with this injection technique.

## SUGGESTED READINGS

Narouze SN. Ultrasound-guided elbow joint and bursa injections. In: *Atlas of Ultrasound Guided Procedures in Pain Management*. New York, NY: Springer; 2010:295–296.
Waldman SD. Functional anatomy of the elbow joint. In: *Pain Review*. Philadelphia, PA: Saunders; 2009:90–94.
Waldman SD. Injection technique for intra-articular injection of the elbow. In: *Pain Review*. Philadelphia, PA: Saunders; 2009:457–458.
Waldman SD. Arthritis pain of the elbow. In: *Atlas of Common Pain Syndromes*. 3rd ed. Philadelphia, PA: Elsevier; 2012:120–122.
Waldman SD. Intra-articular injection of the elbow. In: *Atlas of Pain Management Injection Techniques*. 3rd ed. Philadelphia, PA: Elsevier; 2013:119–122.

# CHAPTER 50

# Ultrasound-Guided Radial Nerve Block at the Elbow

## CLINICAL PERSPECTIVES

Ultrasound-guided radial nerve block at the elbow is useful in the management of the pain subserved by the radial nerve. This technique serves as an excellent adjunct to brachial plexus block and for general anesthesia when performing surgery at the elbow or below. Ultrasound-guided radial nerve block at the elbow with local anesthetic may be used to palliate acute pain emergencies, including postoperative pain, pain secondary to traumatic injuries of the radius, and cancer pain, while waiting for pharmacologic, surgical, and antiblastic methods to become effective (Fig. 50.1).

Ultrasound-guided radial nerve block can also be used as a diagnostic tool when performing differential neural blockade on an anatomic basis in the evaluation of upper extremity pain as well as in a prognostic manner to determine the degree of neurologic impairment the patient will suffer when destruction of the radial nerve is being considered or when there is a possibility that the nerve may be sacrificed during surgeries in the anatomic region of the radial nerve at the level of the humerus. This technique may also be useful in those patients suffering symptoms from compromise of the radial nerve due to radial tunnel syndrome. Ultrasound-guided radial nerve block at the elbow may also be used to palliate the pain and dysesthesias associated with stretch injuries to the radial nerve.

## CLINICALLY RELEVANT ANATOMY

The key landmark when performing ultrasound-guided radial nerve block at the elbow is the point at which the radial nerve is just above the point within the substance of the brachioradialis muscle where the radial nerve bifurcates (Fig. 50.2). Arising from fibers from the C5–T1 nerve roots of the posterior cord of the brachial plexus, the radial nerve passes through the axilla lying posterior and inferior to the axillary artery. As the radial nerve exits the axilla, it passes between the medial and long heads of the triceps muscle and then curves across the posterior aspect of the humerus, giving off a motor branch to the triceps muscle. Continuing its downward path, the radial nerve gives off a number of sensory branches to the upper arm as it travels in the intermuscular septum separating the bellies of the brachialis and brachioradialis muscles. The nerve passes into the substance of the brachioradialis muscle, and at a point just above the lateral epicondyle, the radial nerve divides into deep and superficial branches; the superficial branch continues down the arm along with the radial artery to provide sensory innervation to the dorsum of the wrist and the dorsal aspects of a portion of the thumb and index and middle fingers, and the deep branch provides the majority of the motor innervation to the extensors of the forearm (see Fig. 50.2).

## ULTRASOUND-GUIDED TECHNIQUE

The benefits, risks, and alternative treatments are explained to the patient and informed consent is obtained. The patient is then placed in the supine position with the elbow flexed to about 100 degrees and the forearm resting comfortably across the patient's abdomen (Fig. 50.3). The physician stands at the side of the patient. With the patient in the above position, at a point ~2½ inches above the lateral epicondyle, a high-frequency linear ultrasound transducer is placed in a transverse position over the lateral aspect of the humerus, and an ultrasound survey scan is taken (Fig. 50.4). The hyperechoic margin of the humerus is then identified with the radial nerve lying adjacent to the humerus (Fig. 50.5). After the radial nerve has been identified in proximity to the humerus, the ultrasound transducer is slowly moved inferiorly toward the antecubital fossa. The radial nerve will be seen to move away from the humerus and into the substance of the brachioradialis muscle (Fig. 50.6). The skin overlying the area beneath the ultrasound transducer is then prepped with antiseptic solution. A sterile syringe containing 3.0 mL of 0.25% preservative-free bupivacaine and 50 mg of methylprednisolone is attached to a 1½-inch, 22-gauge needle using strict aseptic technique. The needle is placed through the skin just below the inferior border of the transducer and is then advanced using an in-plane approach with the needle trajectory adjusted under real-time ultrasound guidance so that the needle tip ultimately rests in proximity to the radial nerve as it lies within the substance of the brachioradialis

**FIGURE 50.1.** Galeazzi fracture. Note that a comminuted fracture of the radius is present at the junction of the middle and distal thirds, with an associated dislocation of the distal radioulnar joint. There has been an overall shortening of the distal radius, which is a common finding in this fracture–dislocation. (Reused from Rowe LJ, Yochum TR, Maola CJ. Trauma. In: Yochum TR, Rowe LJ, eds. *Yochum and Rowe's Essentials of Skeletal Radiology*. 3rd ed. Philadelphia, PA: Lippincott Williams & Wilkins; 2005:904, with permission.)

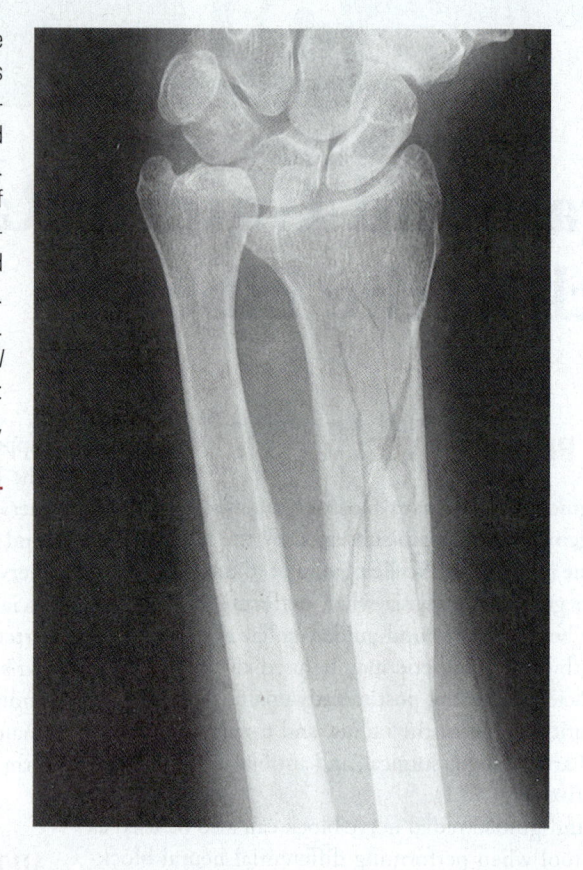

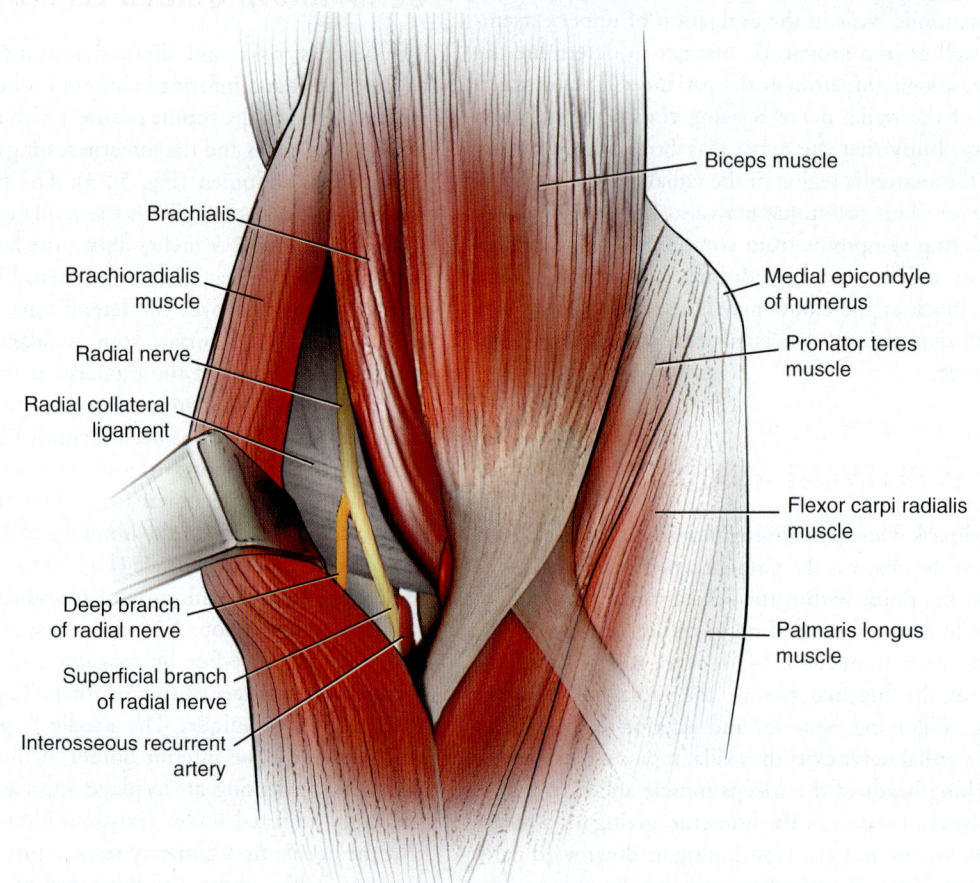

**FIGURE 50.2.** The anatomy of the radial nerve at the elbow. Note the bifurcation of the nerve into a deep and superficial branch.

CHAPTER 50 ULTRASOUND-GUIDED RADIAL NERVE BLOCK AT THE ELBOW **333**

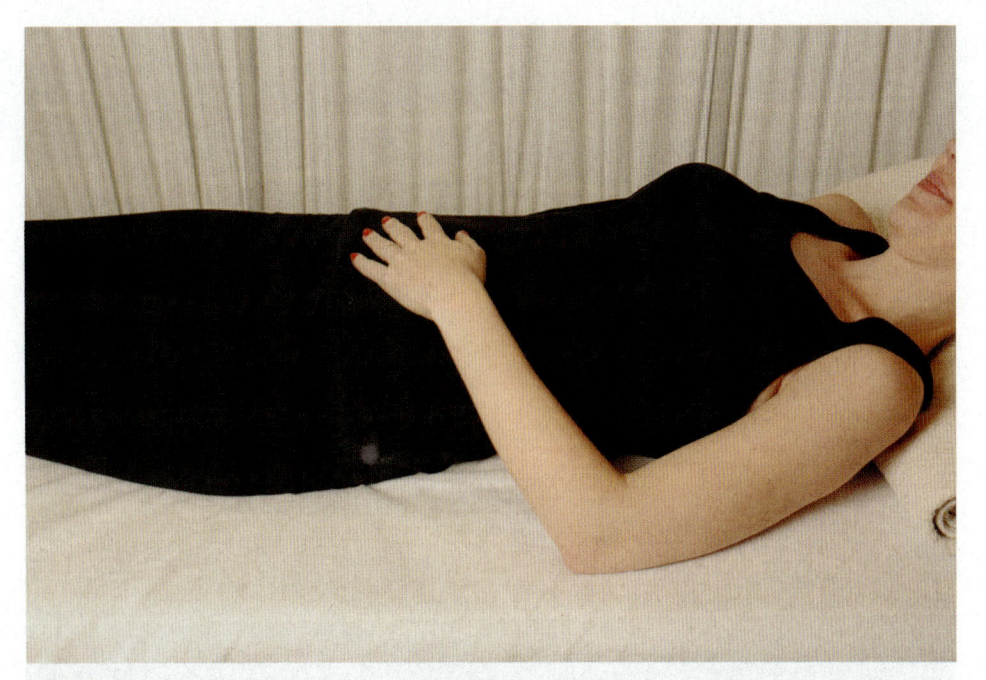

**FIGURE 50.3.** Proper patient positioning for ultrasound-guided radial nerve block at the elbow.

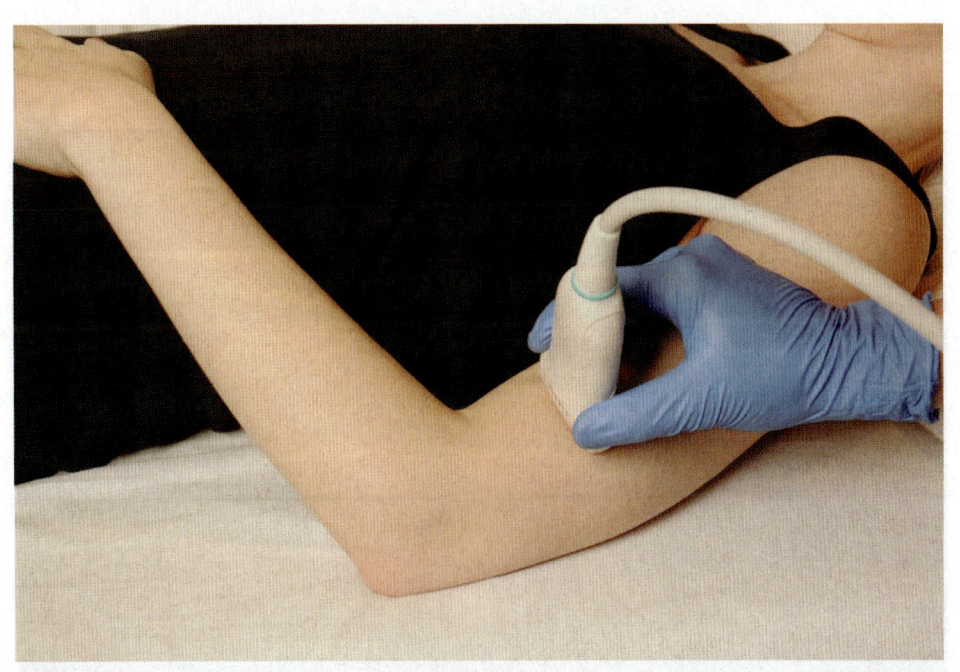

**FIGURE 50.4.** Proper transverse position for the linear high-frequency ultrasound transducer to perform ultrasound-guided radial nerve block at the elbow.

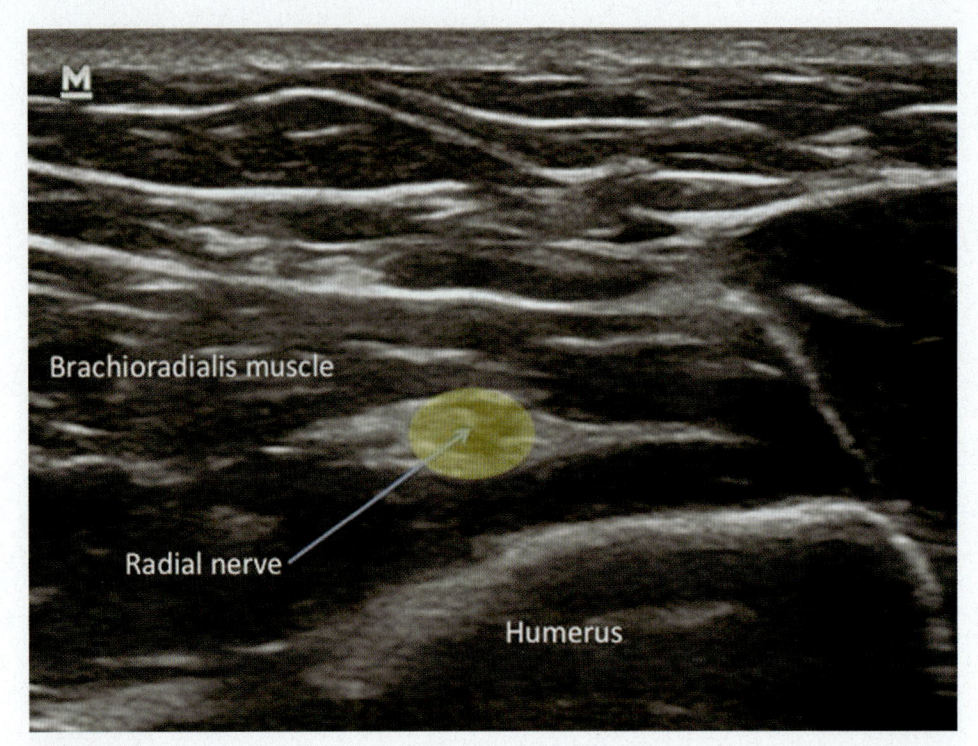

**FIGURE 50.5.** Transverse ultrasound image demonstrating the close proximity of the radial nerve to the humerus.

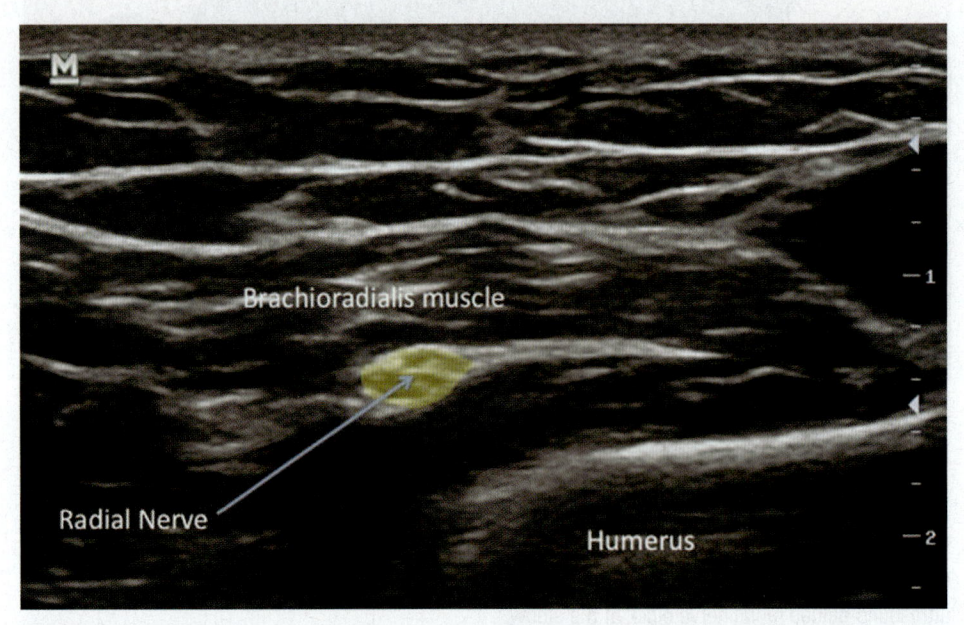

**FIGURE 50.6.** As the ultrasound transducer is moved inferiorly toward the antecubital fossa, the radial nerve is seen to move away from the humerus into the substance of the brachioradialis muscle.

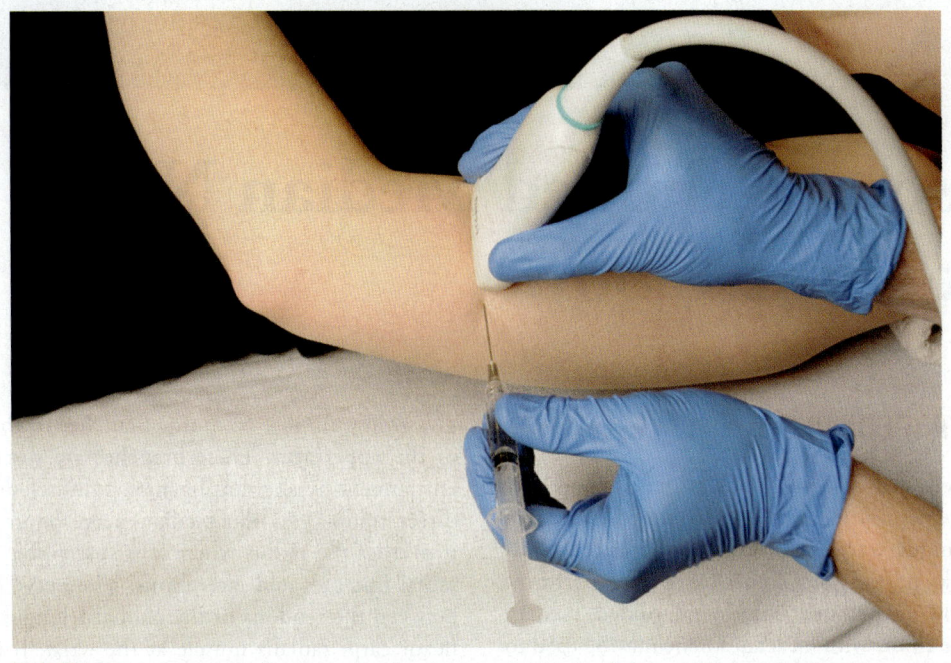

**FIGURE 50.7.** Proper needle placement for ultrasound-guided radial nerve block at the elbow.

muscle (Fig. 50.7). When the tip of needle is thought to be in satisfactory position, after careful aspiration, a small amount of local anesthetic and steroid is injected under real-time ultrasound guidance to confirm that the needle tip is in the proper position. After proper needle tip placement is confirmed, the remainder of the contents of the syringe are slowly injected. There should be minimal resistance to injection.

## COMPLICATIONS

The major complications of ultrasound-guided injection of ultrasound-guided radial nerve block at the elbow are related to improper needle placement with the possibility of inadvertent intravascular injection and/or persistent paresthesia secondary to needle trauma to the radial nerve. Although rare, infection may occur. Ecchymosis and hematoma formation following this procedure may also occur. These complications can be decreased if manual pressure is applied to the area of the block immediately after injection. Application of cold packs for 20-minute periods after the block will also decrease the amount of postprocedure pain and bleeding the patient may experience.

Approximately 25% of patients complain of a transient increase in pain after this injection technique; the patient should be warned of this.

## CLINICAL PEARLS

Ultrasound-guided radial nerve block at the elbow is a straightforward and relatively safe technique if attention is paid to the clinically relevant anatomy. It is useful as an adjunct to surgical anesthesia and has recently been used with increasing frequency in the emergency department to provide anesthesia for reduction of fractures of the radius. Ultrasound-guided radial nerve block at the elbow is also useful in the management of radial tunnel syndrome, which is often misdiagnosed as tennis elbow. Radial tunnel syndrome can be distinguished from tennis elbow in that with radial tunnel syndrome the maximal tenderness to palpation is over the radial nerve, whereas with tennis elbow, the maximal tenderness to palpation is over the lateral epicondyle. If radial tunnel syndrome is suspected, injection of the radial nerve at the elbow with local anesthetic and steroid will give almost instantaneous relief. Careful neurologic examination to identify preexisting neurologic deficits that may later be attributed to the nerve block should be performed on all patients before beginning radial nerve block at the elbow.

## SUGGESTED READINGS

Foxall GL, Hardman JG, Bedforth NM. Three-dimensional, multiplanar, ultrasound-guided, radial nerve block. *Reg Anesth Pain Med.* 2007;32(6): 516–521.
Foxall GL, Skinner D, Hardman JG, et al. Ultrasound anatomy of the radial nerve in the distal upper arm. *Reg Anesth Pain Med.* 2007;32(3):217–220.
Frenkel O, Herring AA, Fischer J, et al. Supracondylar radial nerve block for treatment of distal radius fractures in the emergency department. *J Emerg Med.* 2011;50(4):386–388.
Waldman SD. Radial tunnel syndrome. In: *Atlas of Uncommon Pain Syndromes.* 2nd ed. Philadelphia, PA: WB Saunders; 2008:102–103.
Waldman SD. Radial nerve block at the elbow. In: *Atlas of Interventional Pain Management.* 3rd ed. Philadelphia, PA: WB Saunders; 2009:218–221.

# Ultrasound-Guided Median Nerve Block at the Elbow

## CLINICAL PERSPECTIVES

Ultrasound-guided median nerve block at the elbow is useful in the management of the pain subserved by the median nerve. This technique serves as an excellent adjunct to brachial plexus block and for general anesthesia when performing surgery below the elbow. Ultrasound-guided median nerve block at the elbow with local anesthetic may be used to palliate acute pain emergencies, including postoperative pain, pain secondary to trauma, and cancer pain, while waiting for pharmacologic, surgical, and antiblastic methods to become effective.

Ultrasound-guided median nerve block can also be used as a diagnostic tool when performing differential neural blockade on an anatomic basis in the evaluation of upper extremity pain as well as in a prognostic manner to determine the degree of neurologic impairment the patient will suffer when destruction of the median nerve is being considered or when there is a possibility that the nerve may be sacrificed during surgeries in the anatomic region of the median nerve at the level of the elbow. This technique may also be useful in those patients suffering symptoms from compromise of the median nerve at the elbow due to compression of the median nerve by the ligament of Struthers and the pronator syndrome (Fig. 51.1). Ultrasound-guided median nerve block at the elbow may also be used to palliate the pain and dysesthesias associated with stretch injuries to the median nerve.

## CLINICALLY RELEVANT ANATOMY

The key landmark when performing ultrasound-guided median nerve block at the elbow is pulsation of the brachial artery in the antecubital fossa (Fig. 51.2). Arising from fibers from the ventral roots of C5 and C6 of the lateral cord and C8 and T1 of the medial cord of the brachial plexus, the median nerve lies anterior and superior to the axillary artery in the 12:00 o'clock to 3:00 o'clock quadrant as it passes through the axilla. As the median nerve exits the axilla, it passes inferiorly adjacent to the brachial artery. At the antecubital fossa, the median nerve lies just medial to the brachial artery. Continuing its downward path, the median nerve gives off a number of motor branches to the flexor muscles of the upper arm. These branches are susceptible to nerve entrapment by aberrant ligaments, muscle hypertrophy, and direct trauma. As the median nerve approaches the wrist, it overlies the radius where it is susceptible to trauma from radial fractures and lacerations. The nerve lies deep to and between the tendons of the palmaris longus muscle and the flexor carpi radialis muscle at the wrist. It is susceptible to entrapment as it passes through the carpal tunnel. The terminal branches of the median nerve provide sensory innervation to a portion of the palmar surface of the hand as well as the palmar surface of the thumb, index and middle fingers, and the radial portion of the ring finger (Fig. 51.3). The median nerve also provides sensory innervation to the distal dorsal surface of the index and middle fingers and the radial portion of the ring finger.

## ULTRASOUND-GUIDED TECHNIQUE

The benefits, risks, and alternative treatments are explained to the patient and informed consent is obtained. The patient is then placed in the supine position with the arm resting comfortably at the patient's side with the palm up. The physician stands at the side of the patient. The pulsation of the brachial artery is palpated just medial to the distal biceps tendon at the antecubital fossa (Fig. 51.4). With the patient in the above position, a high-frequency linear ultrasound transducer is placed in a transverse position over the pulsation of the brachial artery, and an ultrasound survey scan is taken (Fig. 51.5). The brachial artery is then identified as is the median nerve lying just medial to the artery (Fig. 51.6). Color Doppler can help identify the artery and other vasculature including the anterior recurrent ulnar artery, which lies just medial to the median nerve at the elbow (Fig. 51.7). After the median nerve has been identified just medial to the brachial artery, the skin overlying the area beneath the ultrasound transducer is then prepped with antiseptic solution. A sterile syringe containing 4.0 mL of 0.25% preservative-free bupivacaine and 40 mg of methylprednisolone is attached to a 1½-inch, 22-gauge needle using strict aseptic technique. The needle is placed through the skin just below

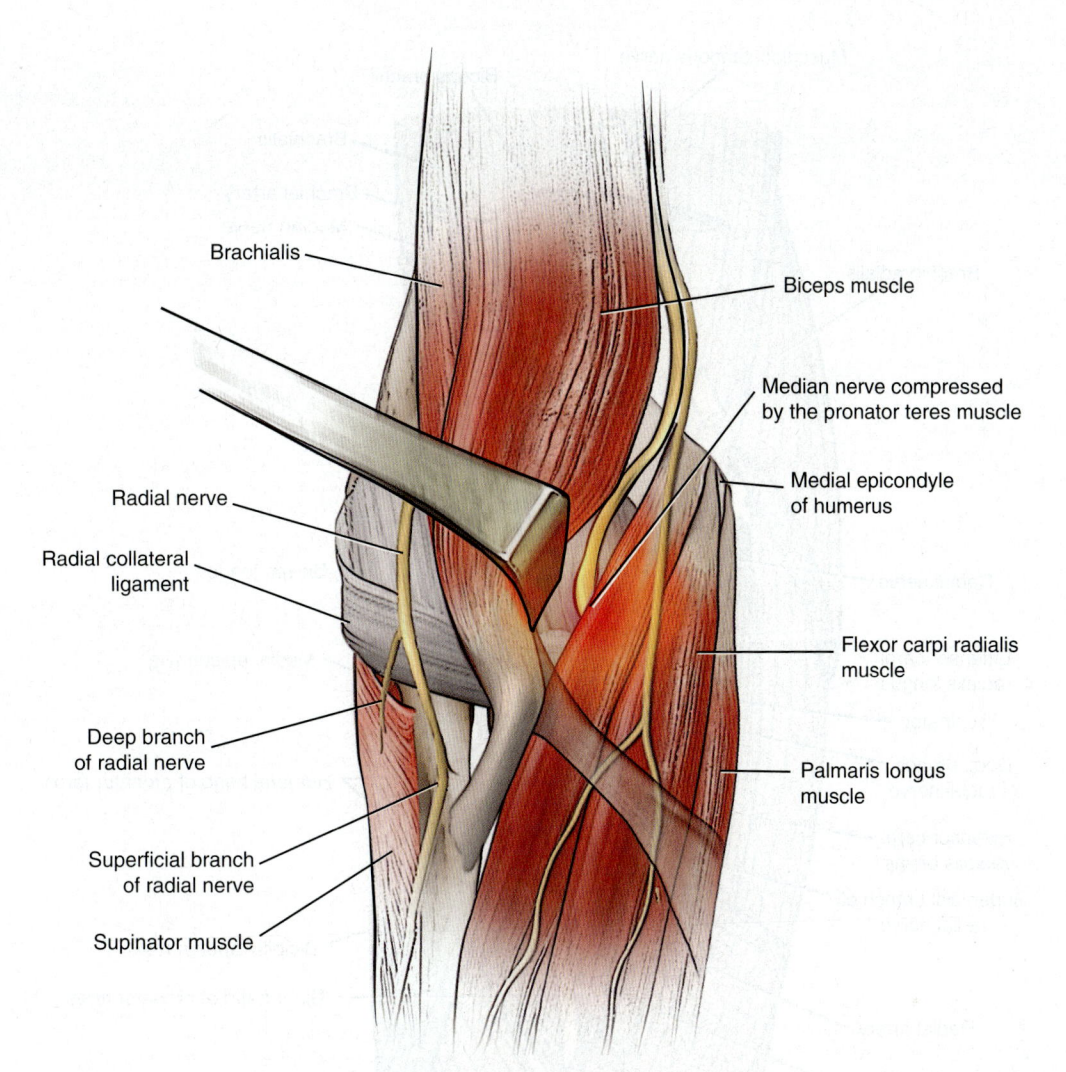

**FIGURE 51.1.** The pronator syndrome is a compressive neuropathy involving the median nerve as it passes beneath the ulnar head of the pronator teres muscle.

the center of the ultrasound transducer and is then advanced using an out-of-plane approach with the needle trajectory adjusted under real-time ultrasound guidance so that the needle tip ultimately rests in proximity to the median nerve (Fig. 51.8). When the tip of needle is thought to be in satisfactory position, after careful aspiration, a small amount of local anesthetic and steroid is injected under real-time ultrasound guidance to confirm that the needle tip is in the proper position. After proper needle tip placement is confirmed, the remainder of the contents of the syringe are slowly injected. There should be minimal resistance to injection.

## COMPLICATIONS

The major complications of ultrasound-guided injection of ultrasound-guided median nerve block at the elbow are related to improper needle placement with the possibility of inadvertent intravascular injection and/or persistent paresthesia secondary to needle trauma to the median nerve. Although rare, infection may occur. Ecchymosis and hematoma formation following this procedure may also occur. These complications can be decreased if manual pressure is applied to the area of the block immediately after injection. Application of cold packs for 20-minute periods after the block will also decrease the amount of postprocedure pain and bleeding the patient may experience. Approximately 25% of patients complain of a transient increase in pain after this injection technique; the patient should be warned of this.

## CLINICAL PEARLS

Ultrasound-guided median nerve block at the elbow is a straightforward and relatively safe technique if attention is paid to the clinically relevant anatomy. It is useful as an adjunct

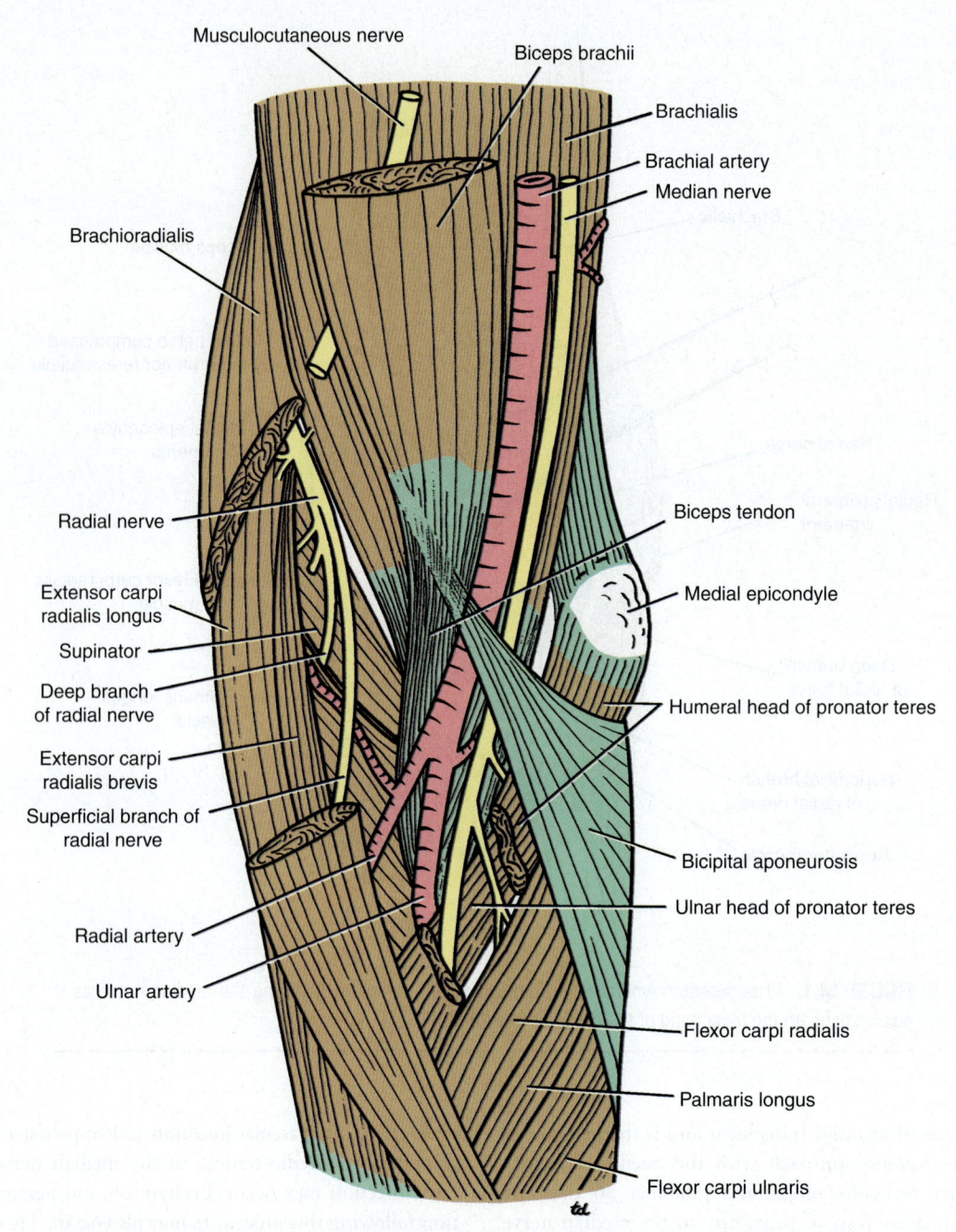

**FIGURE 51.2.** The anatomy of the median nerve at the elbow. Note the relationship of the median nerve to brachial artery. (Reused from Snell. *Clinical Anatomy*. 7th ed. Philadelphia, PA: Lippincott Williams & Wilkins; 2003, with permission.)

CHAPTER 51 ULTRASOUND-GUIDED MEDIAN NERVE BLOCK AT THE ELBOW 339

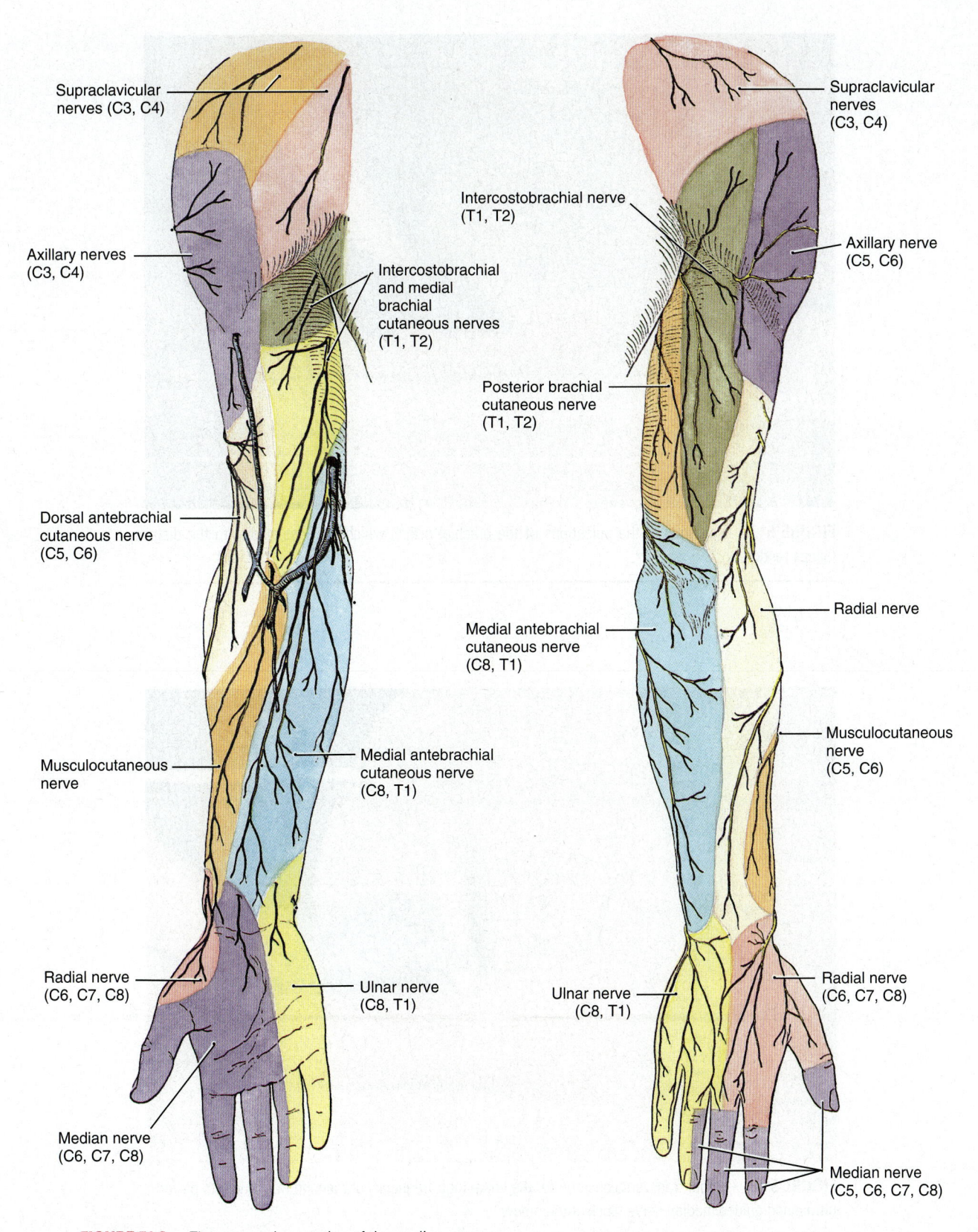

**FIGURE 51.3.** The sensory innervation of the median nerve.

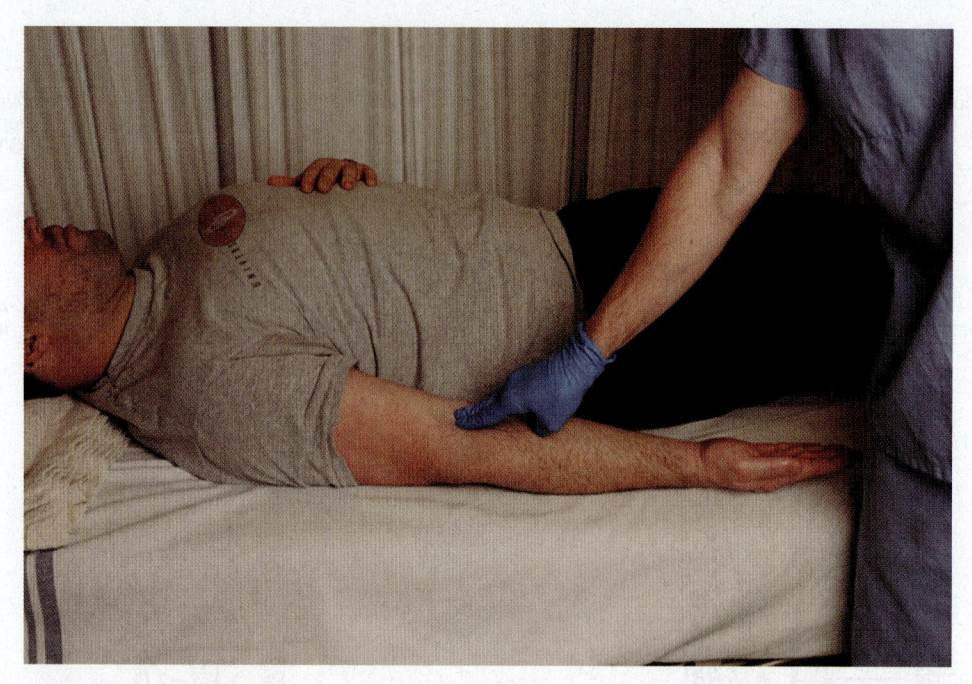

**FIGURE 51.4.** Palpation of the pulsations of the brachial artery, which lies just medial to the distal biceps tendon.

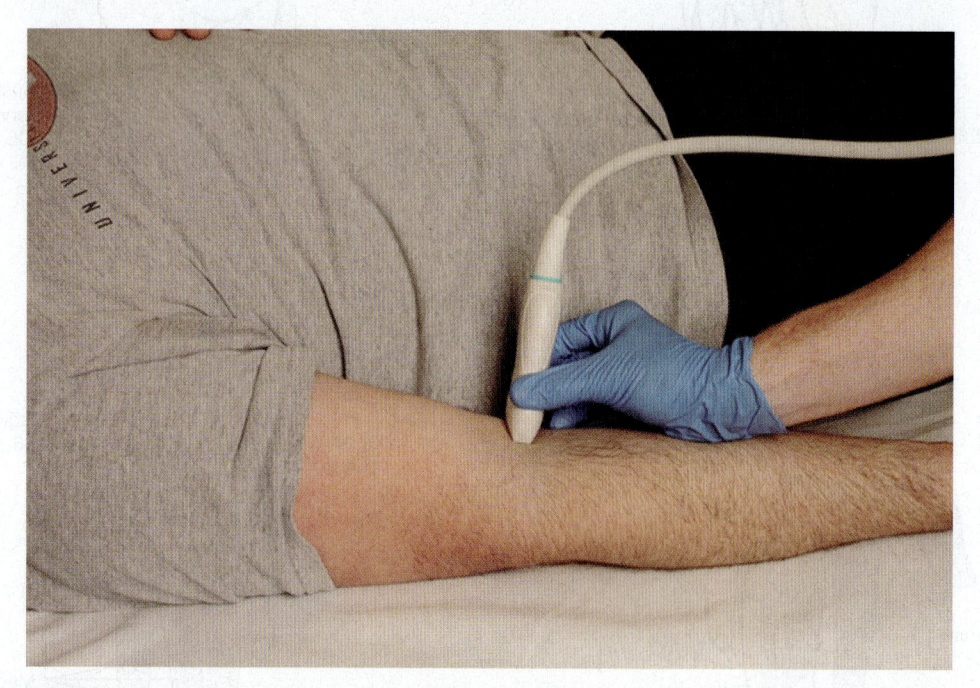

**FIGURE 51.5.** Proper transverse position for the linear high-frequency ultrasound transducer to perform ultrasound-guided median nerve block at the elbow.

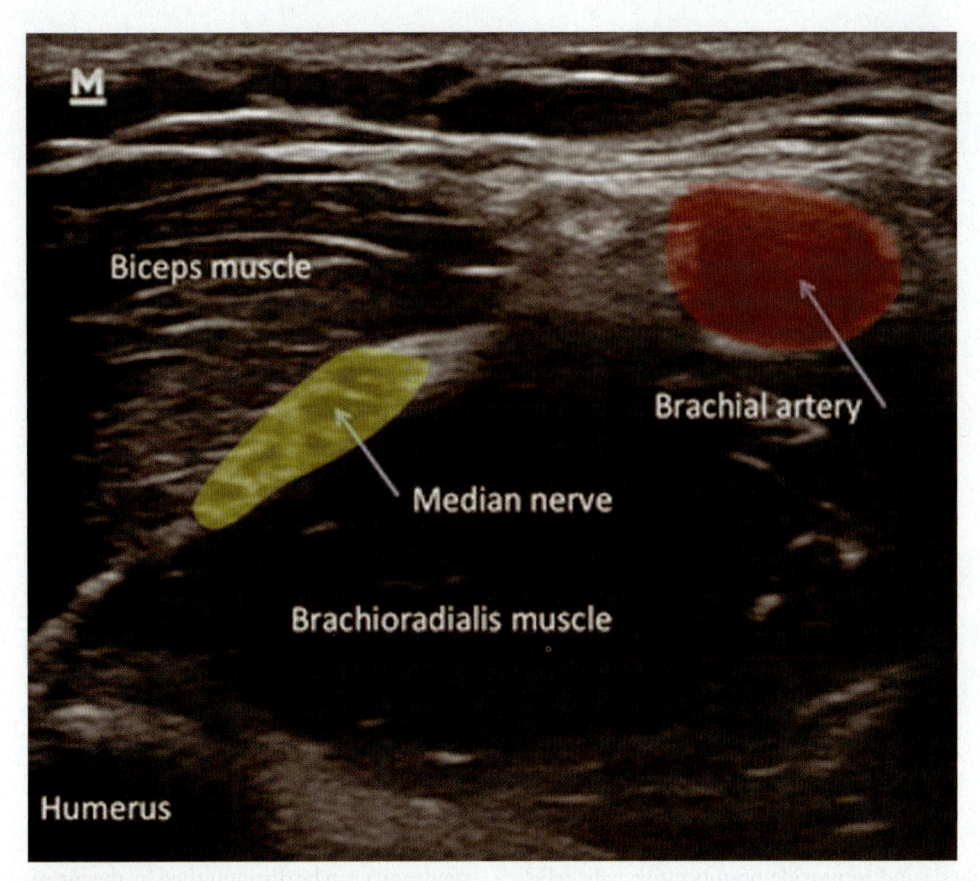

**FIGURE 51.6.** Transverse ultrasound image demonstrating the median nerve lying medially to the brachial artery at the antecubital fossa.

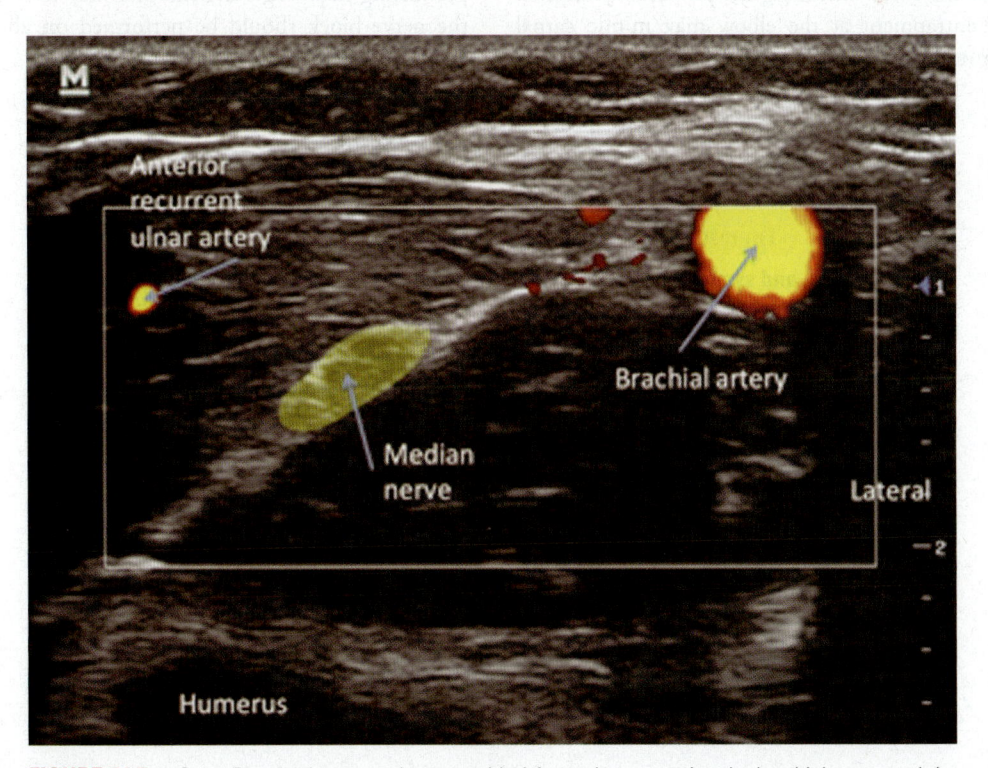

**FIGURE 51.7.** Color Doppler image at the antecubital fossa demonstrating the brachial artery and the median nerve lying just medially.

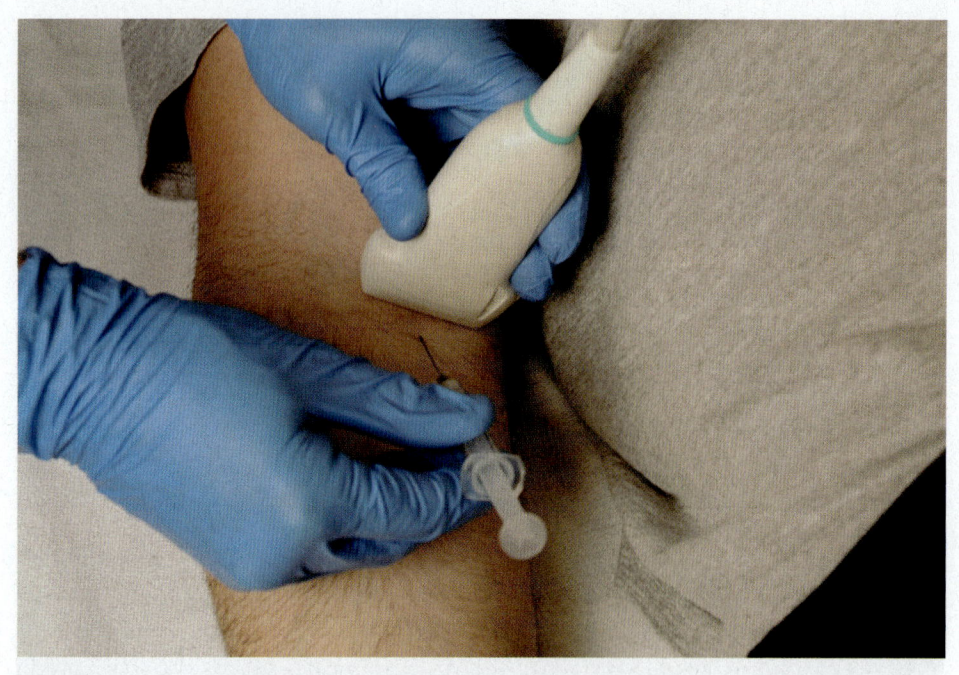

**FIGURE 51.8.** Proper needle placement for ultrasound-guided median nerve block at the elbow.

to surgical anesthesia and to provide postoperative pain relief. Ultrasound-guided median nerve block at the elbow is also useful in the management of compressive neuropathies of the median nerve at the elbow including the pronator syndrome. Median nerve entrapment at the elbow may mimic carpal tunnel syndrome making the diagnosis difficult. These two syndromes can be distinguished by the use of electromyography and nerve conduction testing and a careful physical examination (Table 51.1). Careful neurologic examination to identify preexisting neurologic deficits that may later be attributed to the nerve block should be performed on all patients before beginning median nerve block at the elbow.

**TABLE 51.1 The Differential Diagnosis of Pronator Syndrome and Carpal Tunnel Syndrome**

| Findings, signs, and symptoms | Pronator syndrome | Carpal tunnel syndrome |
| --- | --- | --- |
| Nerve conduction velocity testing | Negative at wrist | Positive at wrist |
| Tinel sign | Positive at forearm | Negative at forearm |
|  | Negative at wrist | Positive at wrist |
| Phalen test | Negative | Positive |
| Symptoms on forearm pronation | Positive | Negative |
| Numbness over palmar thenar eminence | Absent | Present |
| Nocturnal symptomatology | Absent | Present |
| Associated with systemic disease, for example, diabetes, acromegaly | No | Yes |

## SUGGESTED READINGS

Dilger JA, Wells Jr RE. The use of peripheral nerve blocks at the elbow for carpal tunnel release. *J Clin Anesth* 2005;17(8):621–623.

Waldman SD. Pronator syndrome. In: *Atlas of Uncommon Pain Syndromes*. 2nd ed. Philadelphia, PA: WB Saunders; 2008:87–89.

Waldman SD. Median nerve block at the elbow. In: *Atlas of Interventional Pain Management*. 3rd ed. Philadelphia, PA: WB Saunders; 2009:222–228.

Waldman SD. The median nerve. In: *Pain Review*. Philadelphia, PA: Saunders Elsevier; 2009:77–78.

Waldman SD. Median nerve block at the elbow. In: *Pain Review*. Philadelphia, PA: Saunders Elsevier; 2009:442–443.

# CHAPTER 52

# Ultrasound-Guided Ulnar Nerve Block at the Elbow

## CLINICAL PERSPECTIVES

Ultrasound-guided ulnar nerve block at the elbow is useful in the management of the pain subserved by the ulnar nerve. This technique serves as an excellent adjunct to brachial plexus block and for general anesthesia when performing surgery below the elbow. Ultrasound-guided ulnar nerve block at the elbow with local anesthetic may be used to palliate acute pain emergencies, including postoperative pain, pain secondary to trauma, and cancer pain, while waiting for pharmacologic, surgical, and antiblastic methods to become effective.

Ultrasound-guided ulnar nerve block can also be used as a diagnostic tool when performing differential neural blockade on an anatomic basis in the evaluation of upper extremity pain as well as in a prognostic manner to determine the degree of neurologic impairment the patient will suffer when destruction of the ulnar nerve is being considered or when there is a possibility that the nerve may be sacrificed during surgeries in the anatomic region of the ulnar nerve at the level of the elbow. This technique may also be useful in those patients suffering symptoms from compromise of the ulnar nerve at the elbow due to compression of the ulnar nerve by the cubital tunnel retinaculum or anomalous anconeus epitrochlearis muscle (Fig. 52.1). Ultrasound-guided ulnar nerve block at the elbow may also be used to palliate the pain and dysesthesias associated with stretch injuries to the ulnar nerve in this anatomic region.

## CLINICALLY RELEVANT ANATOMY

The key landmark when performing ultrasound-guided ulnar nerve block at the elbow is the ulnar artery in the forearm, which lies in proximity to the ulnar nerve (Fig. 52.2). Arising from fibers from the C8–T1 nerve roots of the medial cord of the brachial plexus, the ulnar nerve lies anterior and inferior to the axillary artery in the 3:00 o'clock to 6:00 o'clock quadrant as it passes through the axilla. As the ulnar nerve exits the axilla, it passes inferiorly adjacent to the brachial artery. At the middle of the upper arm, the ulnar nerve turns medially to pass between the olecranon process and medial epicondyle of the humerus. Continuing its downward path, the ulnar nerve passes between the heads of the flexor carpi ulnaris moving radially along with the ulnar artery. At a point ~1 inch proximal to the crease of the wrist, the ulnar nerve divides into the dorsal and palmar branches. The dorsal branch provides sensation to the ulnar aspect of the dorsum of the hand and the dorsal aspect of the little finger and the ulnar half of the ring finger (Fig. 52.3). The palmar branch provides sensory innervation to the ulnar aspect of the palm of the hand and the palmar aspect of the little finger and the ulnar half of the ring finger.

## ULTRASOUND-GUIDED TECHNIQUE

The benefits, risks, and alternative treatments are explained to the patient and informed consent is obtained. The patient is then placed in the supine position with the arm in the modified bathing beauty position (Fig. 52.4). The ulnar artery is palpated (Fig. 52.5). With the patient in the above position, a high-frequency linear ultrasound transducer is placed in a transverse position over the dorsal surface of the forearm, and an ultrasound survey scan is taken (Fig. 52.6). The ulnar artery is then identified as is the ulnar nerve lying just next to the artery. The ulnar nerve will have a triangular, hyperechoic honeycomb appearance (Fig. 52.7). Color Doppler can help identify the ulnar artery and other vasculature in the area (Fig. 52.8). After the ulnar nerve has been identified adjacent to the ulnar artery, the ultrasound transducer is slowly moved proximally. The ulnar nerve will be seen to move away from the ulnar artery, which moves deeper into the forearm as it approaches the antecubital fossa (Fig. 52.9). After identification of the ulnar nerve is confirmed, the skin overlying the area beneath the ultrasound transducer is then prepped with antiseptic solution. A sterile syringe containing 4.0 mL of 0.25% preservative-free bupivacaine and 40 mg of methylprednisolone is attached to a 1½-inch, 22-gauge needle using strict aseptic technique. The needle is placed through the skin ~0.5 cm lateral to the lateral aspect of the ultrasound transducer and is then advanced using an in-plane approach through the flexor carpi ulnaris muscle with the needle trajectory adjusted under real-time ultrasound guidance so that the needle tip ultimately rests in the hyperechoic fascial cleft between the flexor carpi ulnaris and flexor digitorum profundus muscles. This will place the needle tip proximity to the ulnar nerve

**FIGURE 52.1.** The cubital tunnel syndrome is an entrapment neuropathy involving the ulnar nerve as it passes beneath the cubital tunnel retinaculum.

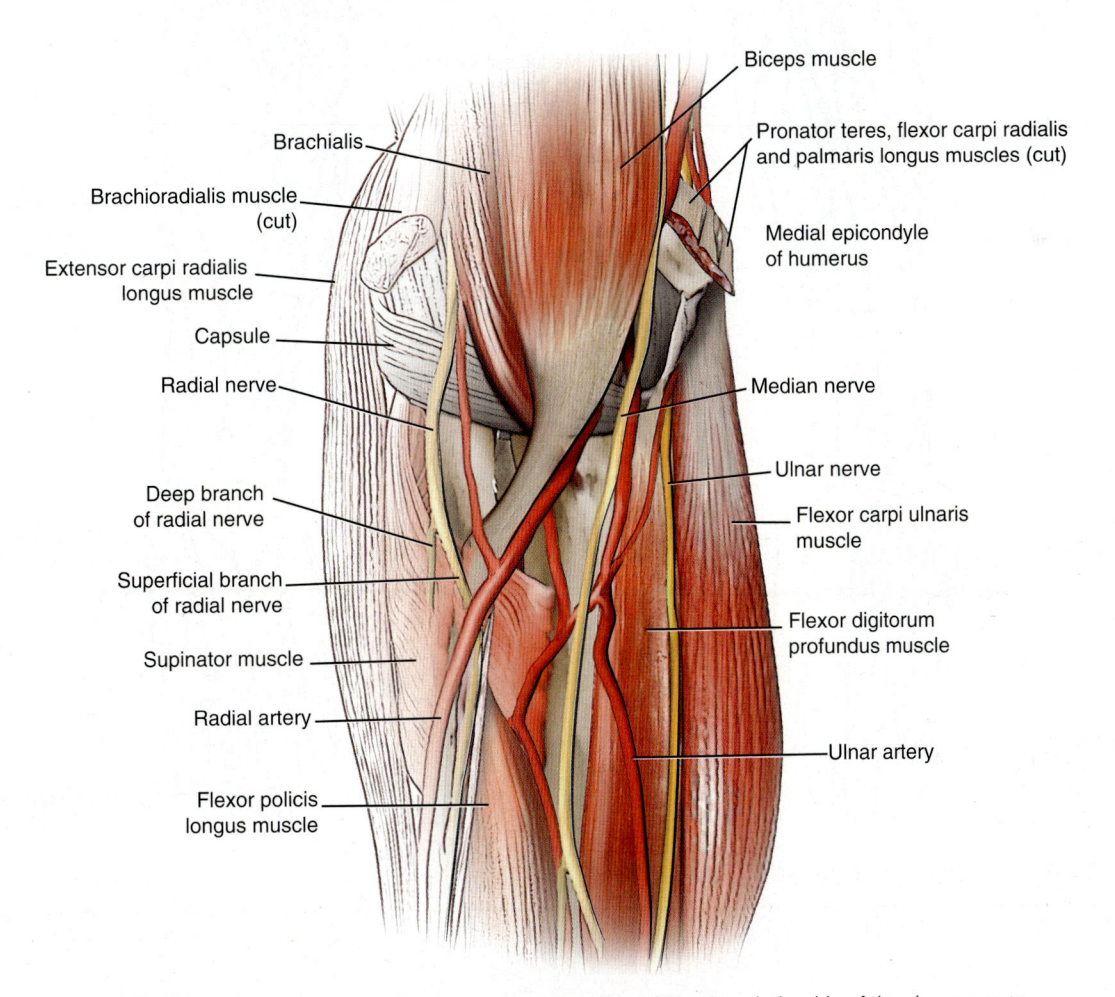

**FIGURE 52.2.** The anatomy of the ulnar nerve at the elbow. Note the relationship of the ulnar nerve to ulnar artery.

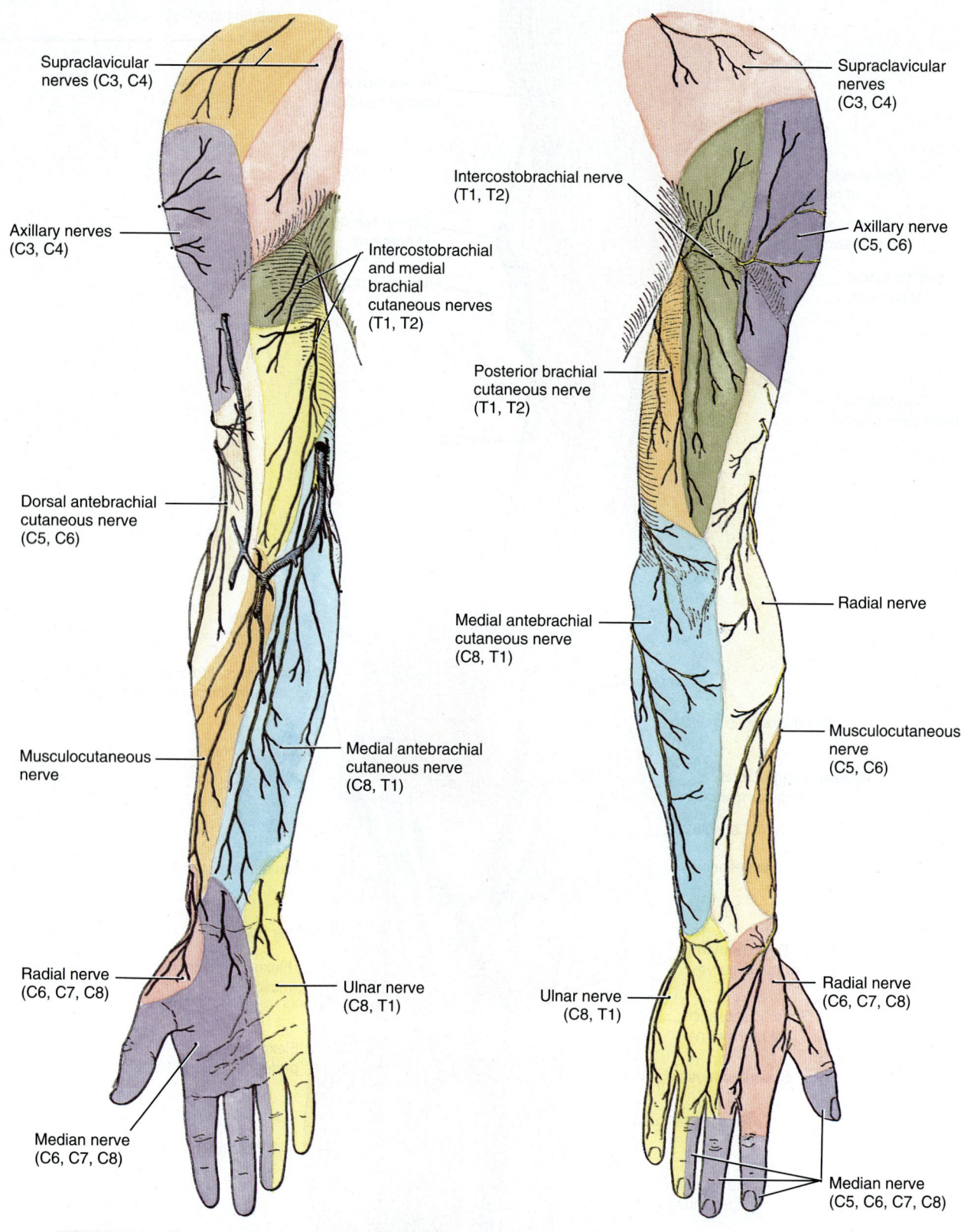

**FIGURE 52.3.** The sensory innervation of the ulnar nerve.

CHAPTER 52    ULTRASOUND-GUIDED ULNAR NERVE BLOCK AT THE ELBOW    347

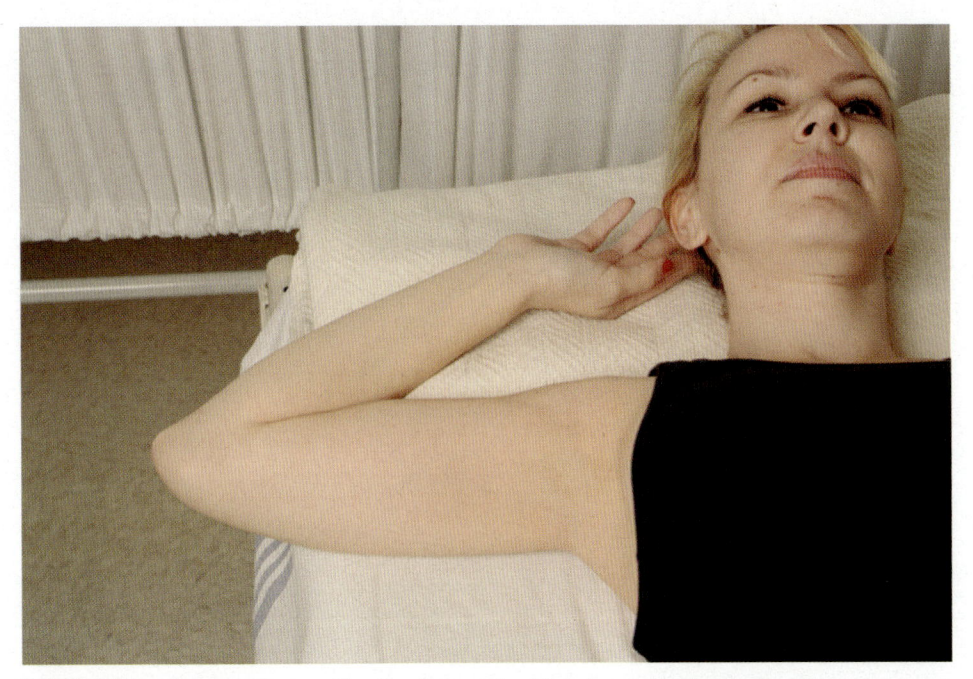

**FIGURE 52.4.** Proper patient position for ultrasound-guided ulnar nerve block at the elbow.

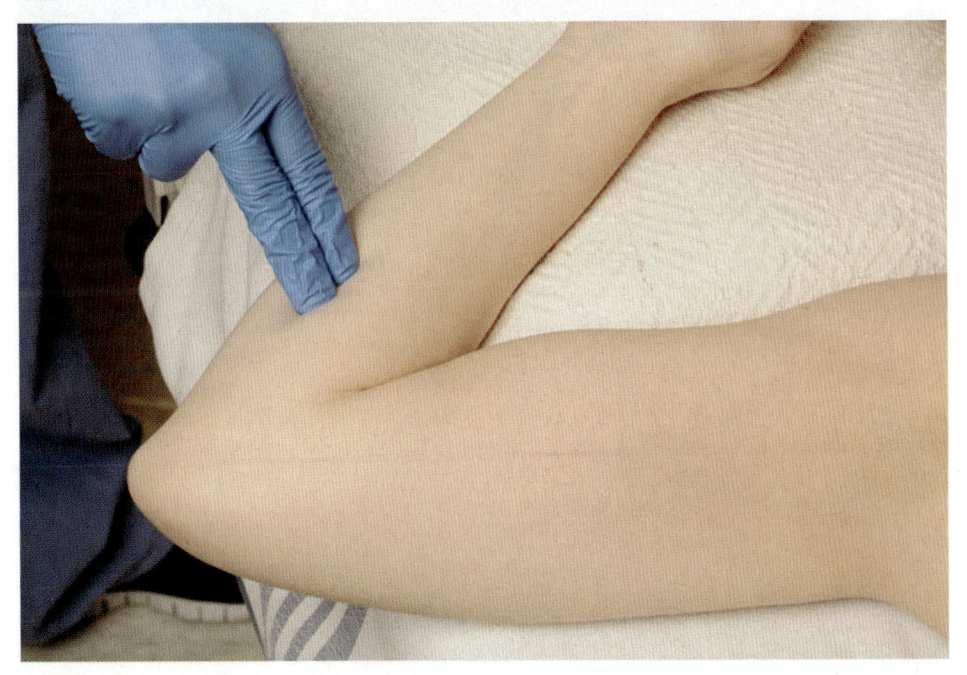

**FIGURE 52.5.** Palpation of the pulsations of the ulnar artery.

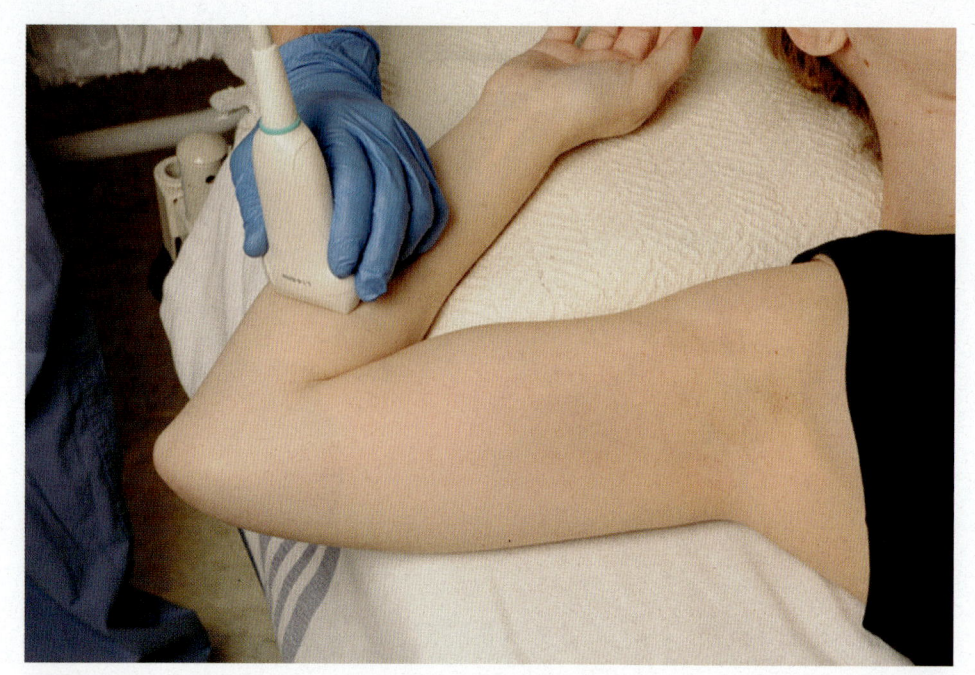

**FIGURE 52.6.** Proper transverse position for the linear high-frequency ultrasound transducer to perform ultrasound-guided ulnar nerve block at the elbow.

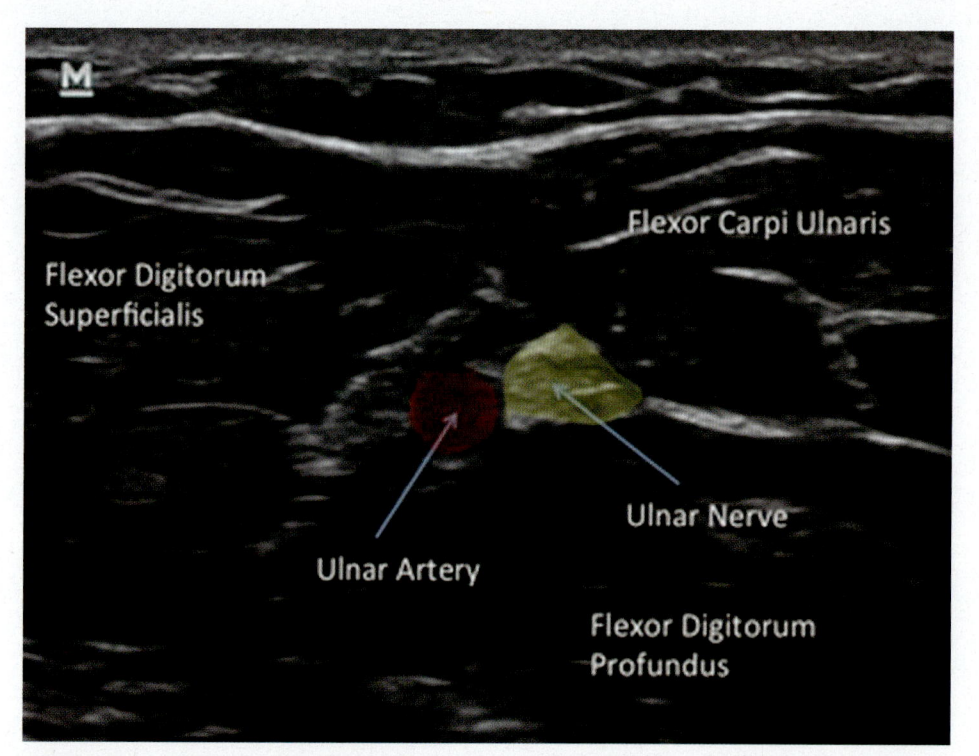

**FIGURE 52.7.** Transverse ultrasound image demonstrating the ulnar nerve lying adjacent to the ulnar artery in the proximal forearm.

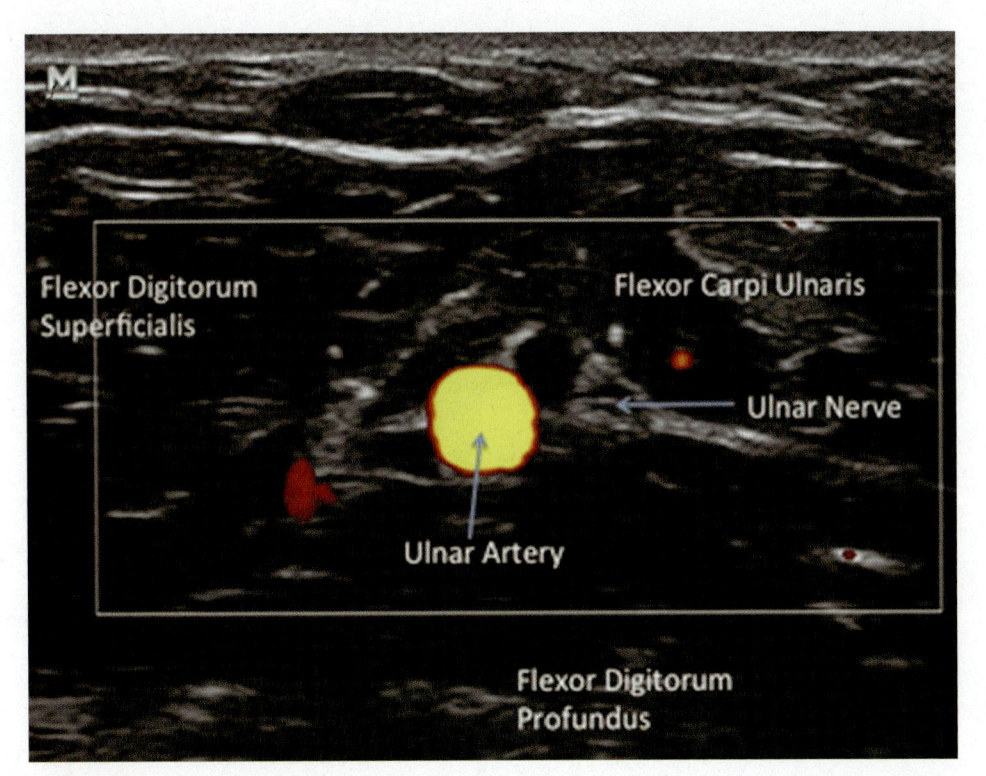

**FIGURE 52.8.** Color Doppler image at the antecubital fossa demonstrating the brachial artery and the ulnar nerve lying just medially.

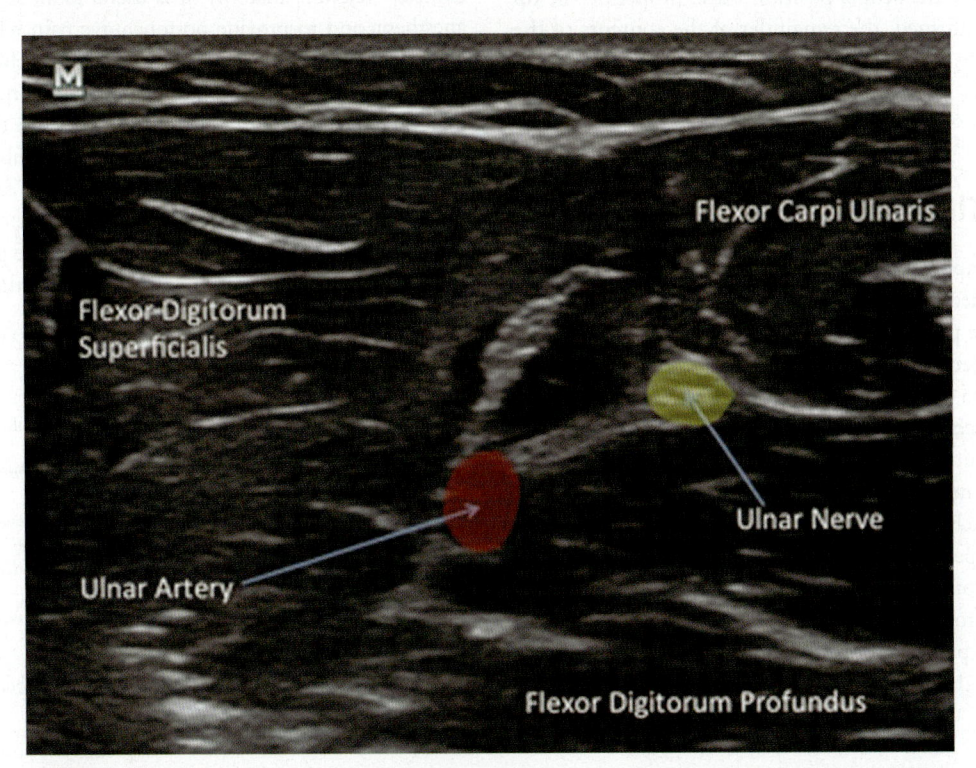

**FIGURE 52.9.** When moving the ultrasound transducer superiorly toward the antecubital fossa in the transverse position, the ulnar nerve will be seen to move away from the ulnar artery, which moves deeper into the forearm as it approaches the antecubital fossa.

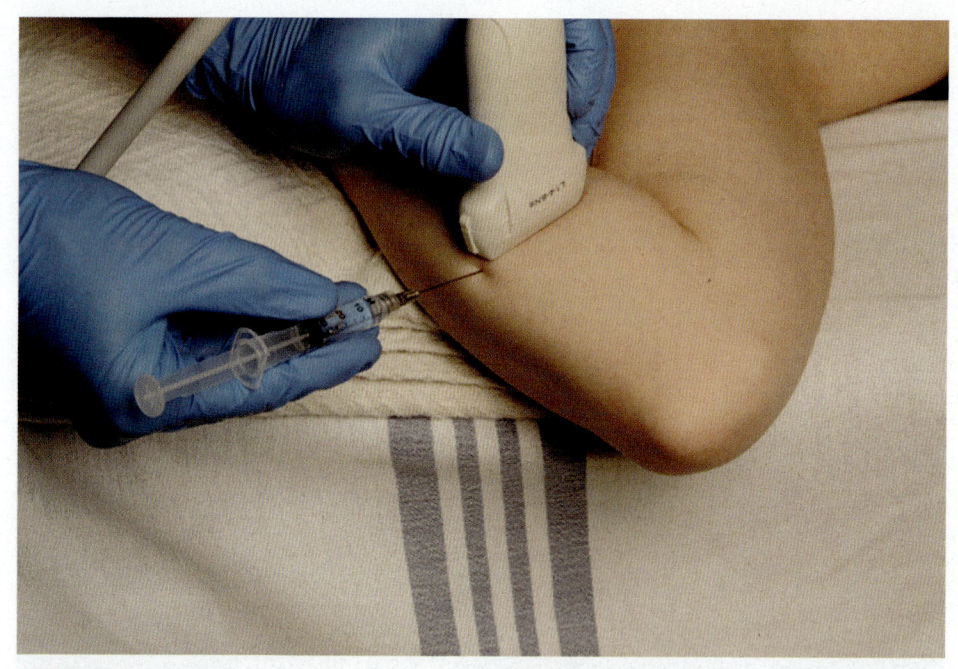

**FIGURE 52.10.** Proper in-plane needle placement for ultrasound-guided ulnar nerve block at the elbow.

just below the antecubital fossa (Fig. 52.10). When the tip of needle is thought to be in satisfactory position, after careful aspiration, a small amount of local anesthetic and steroid is injected under real-time ultrasound guidance to confirm that the needle tip is in the proper position. After proper needle tip placement is confirmed, the remainder of the contents of the syringe are slowly injected. There should be minimal resistance to injection.

## COMPLICATIONS

The major complications of ultrasound-guided injection of ultrasound-guided ulnar nerve block at the elbow are related to improper needle placement with the possibility of inadvertent intravascular injection and/or persistent paresthesia secondary to needle trauma to the ulnar nerve. Although rare, infection may occur. Ecchymosis and hematoma formation following this procedure may also occur. These complications can be decreased if manual pressure is applied to the area of the block immediately after injection. Application of cold packs for 20-minute periods after the block will also decrease the amount of postprocedure pain and bleeding the patient may experience. Approximately 25% of patients complain of a transient increase in pain after this injection technique; the patient should be warned of this.

## CLINICAL PEARLS

Ultrasound-guided ulnar nerve block at the elbow is a straightforward and relatively safe technique if attention is paid to the clinically relevant anatomy. It is useful as an adjunct to surgical anesthesia and to provide postoperative pain relief. Ultrasound-guided ulnar nerve block at the elbow is also useful in the management of compressive neuropathies of the ulnar nerve at the elbow including the cubital tunnel syndrome. Because the ulnar nerve is the largest unprotected nerve in the body, it is subject to trauma at various points along its course. For this reason, careful neurologic examination to identify preexisting neurologic deficits that may later be attributed to the nerve block should be performed on all patients before beginning ulnar nerve block at the elbow.

## SUGGESTED READINGS

Gray AT, Schafhalter-Zoppoth I. Ultrasound guidance for ulnar nerve block in the forearm. *Reg Anesth Pain Med* 2003;28(4):335–339.
Waldman SD. Anconeus epitrochlearis. In: *Atlas of Uncommon Pain Syndromes*. 2nd ed. Philadelphia, PA: WB Saunders; 2008:93–95.
Waldman SD. Cubital tunnel syndrome. In: *Atlas of Uncommon Pain Syndromes*. 2nd ed. Philadelphia, PA: WB Saunders; 2008:104–106.
Waldman SD. The ulnar nerve. In: *Pain Review*. Philadelphia, PA: Saunders Elsevier; 2009:76–77.
Waldman SD. Ulnar nerve block at the elbow. In: *Pain Review*. Philadelphia, PA: Saunders Elsevier; 2009:253.
Waldman SD. Ulnar nerve block at the elbow. In: *Atlas of Interventional Pain Management*. 3rd ed. Philadelphia, PA: WB Saunders; 2009:229–334.

# CHAPTER 53

# Ultrasound-Guided Injection Technique for Cubital Tunnel Syndrome

## CLINICAL PERSPECTIVES

Cubital tunnel syndrome is a common entrapment neuropathy of the ulnar nerve at the elbow that is caused by compression of the ulnar nerve by an aponeurotic band that runs from the medial epicondyle of the humerus to the medial border of the olecranon (Fig. 53.1). Patients suffering from cubital tunnel syndrome will experience pain and dysesthesias radiating from the elbow to the lateral forearm and into the wrist and ring and little finger. The onset of cubital tunnel syndrome can be insidious and is usually the result of misuse or overuse of the elbow joint although direct trauma to the nerve as it passes through the cubital tunnel may also result in a similar clinical scenario. If this entrapment neuropathy is not treated, pain and functional disability may become more severe, and, ultimately, permanent numbness and flexion contractures of the ring and little finger may result.

Physical findings in patients suffering from cubital tunnel syndrome will exhibit weakness of the intrinsic muscles of the forearm and hand that are innervated by the ulnar nerve. A Tinel sign will be present at the point where the ulnar nerve passes through the cubital tunnel and the nerve will be tender to palpation (Fig. 53.2). Weakness of the adductor pollicis muscles can be demonstrated by performing the Froment and Jeanne test (Fig. 53.3). Weakness of the interosseous muscles can be demonstrated by performing the crossed finger, finger flexion, little finger adduction, and Egawa tests (Fig. 53.4). Weakness of the hypothenar muscles can be demonstrated by performing the Wartenberg, Masse, and Pitres-Testut tests. It should be remembered that the ulnar nerve is the largest unprotected nerve in the body and that it is subject to trauma or entrapment at many points along its course and that more than one ulnar nerve lesion may coexist.

Cubital tunnel syndrome often is misdiagnosed as golfer's elbow and can be distinguished from golfer's elbow by determining the site of maximal tenderness to palpation. Patients suffering from cubital tunnel syndrome will experience maximal tenderness to palpation over the ulnar nerve 1 inch below the medial epicondyle, whereas patients suffering from golfer's elbow will experience maximal tenderness to palpation directly over the medial epicondyle. Cubital tunnel syndrome also should be differentiated from cervical radiculopathy involving the C7 or C8 roots and golfer's elbow. Furthermore, it should be remembered that cervical radiculopathy and ulnar nerve entrapment may coexist as the so-called "double crush" syndrome. The double crush syndrome is seen most commonly with median nerve entrapment at the wrist or with carpal tunnel syndrome, but has been reported with the ulnar nerve.

Electromyography and nerve conduction velocity testing are useful in helping in the differentiation of cubital tunnel syndrome from cervical radiculopathy and golfer's elbow. Plain radiographs, ultrasound imaging, and magnetic resonance imaging are indicated in all patients who present with cubital tunnel syndrome in order to rule out occult bony pathology involving the cubital tunnel and to identify occult fractures, masses, or tumors that may be responsible for compromise of the ulnar nerve (Fig. 53.5). Based on the patient's clinical presentation, additional testing may be indicated, including complete blood count, uric acid, sedimentation rate, and antinuclear antibody testing. The ultrasound-guided injection technique described below serves as both a diagnostic and therapeutic maneuver.

## CLINICALLY RELEVANT ANATOMY

The key landmarks when performing ultrasound-guided cubital tunnel syndrome are the medial epicondyle and olecranon process. Arising from fibers from the C8–T1 nerve roots of the medial cord of the brachial plexus, the ulnar nerve lies anterior and inferior to the axillary artery in the 3:00 o'clock to 6:00 o'clock quadrant as it passes through the axilla. As the ulnar nerve exits the axilla, it passes inferiorly adjacent to the brachial artery. At the middle of the upper arm, the ulnar nerve turns medially to pass between the olecranon process and medial epicondyle of the humerus where it passes beneath an aponeurotic band and is subject to entrapment (Fig. 53.6). Continuing its downward path, the ulnar nerve passes between the heads of the flexor carpi ulnaris moving radially along with the ulnar artery. At a point ~1 inch proximal to the crease of the wrist, the ulnar nerve divides into the dorsal and palmar branches. The dorsal branch provides

**FIGURE 53.1.** The cubital tunnel syndrome is an entrapment neuropathy involving the ulnar nerve as it passes beneath the cubital tunnel retinaculum.

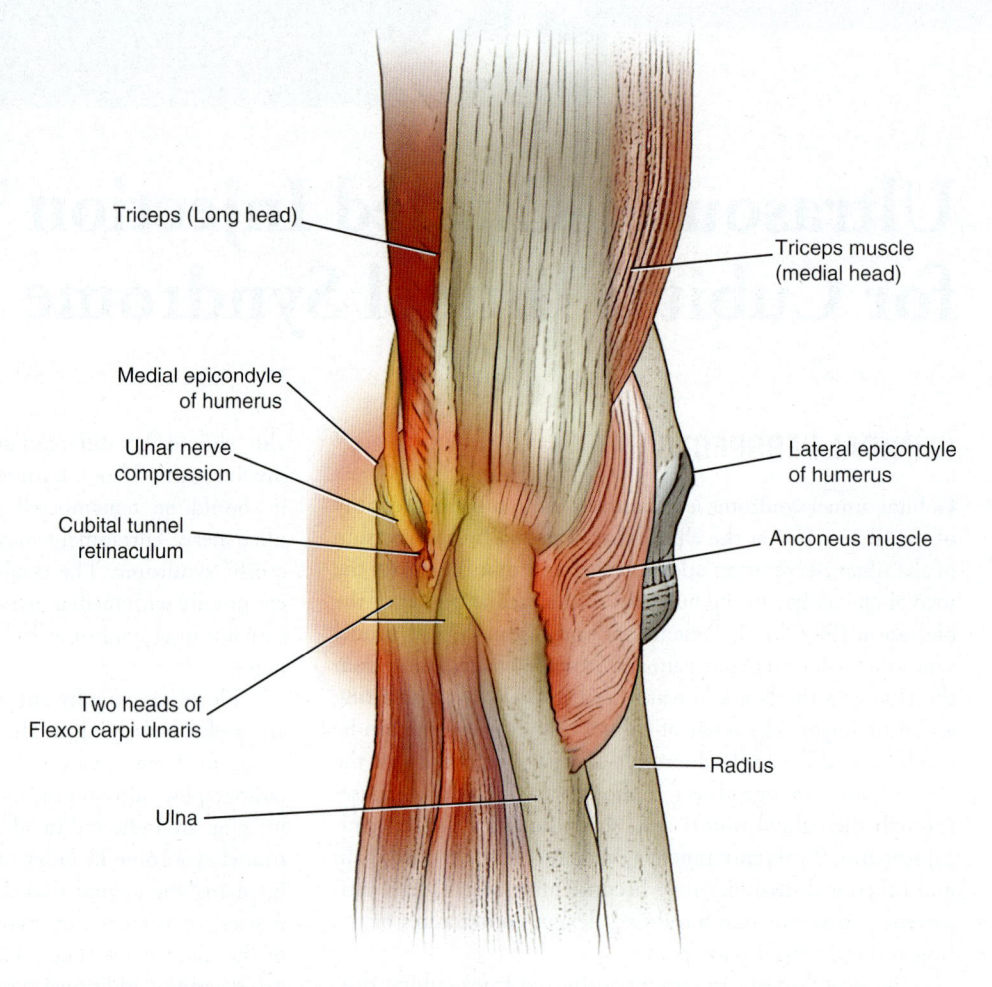

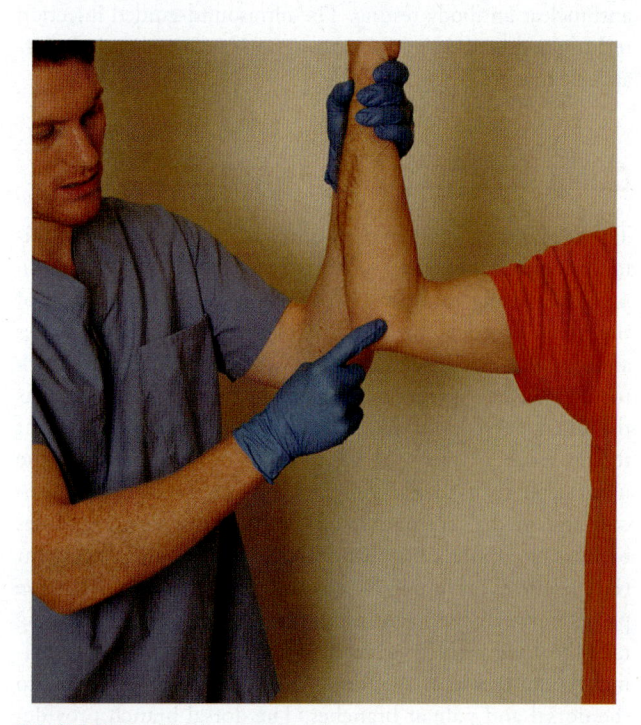

**FIGURE 53.2.** Tinel test at the elbow.

sensation to the ulnar aspect of the dorsum of the hand and the dorsal aspect of the little finger and the ulnar half of the ring finger (Fig. 53.7). The palmar branch provides sensory innervation to the ulnar aspect of the palm of the hand and the palmar aspect of the little finger and the ulnar half of the ring finger.

## ULTRASOUND-GUIDED TECHNIQUE

The benefits, risks, and alternative treatments are explained to the patient and informed consent is obtained. The patient is then placed in the prone position with the elbow flexed ~65 degrees (Fig. 53.8). With the patient in the above position, a high-frequency linear ultrasound transducer is placed in a transverse position over the medial elbow between the medial epicondyle and the olecranon process, and an ultrasound survey scan is taken (Fig. 53.9). The medial epicondyle and olecranon process are identified with the ulnar nerve lying in between these structures just posterior to the medial epicondyle (Fig. 53.10). The ulnar nerve can then be followed distally into the cubital tunnel by slowly moving the ultrasound transducer toward the posterior proximal forearm. The nerve

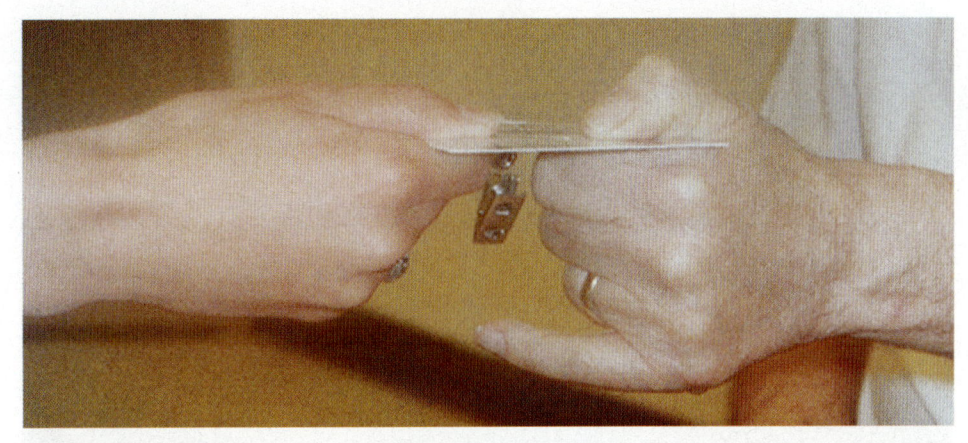

**FIGURE 53.3.** Froment test. Resisted adduction of the thumb (Froment sign). Effectively measures the ulnar nerve and the adductor pollicis muscle. Note patient's hand in a midfist position; note also flexion of interphalangeal joint of thumb to hold paper. (Reused from Berg D, Worzala K. *Atlas of Adult Physical Diagnosis*. Philadelphia, PA: Lippincott Williams & Wilkins; 2006, with permission.)

will be seen to lie between the two heads of the flexor carpi ulnaris muscle and beneath the overlying cubital tunnel retinaculum (Fig. 53.11). The transducer is then rotated longitudinally to evaluate the nerve (Fig. 53.12). After the ulnar nerve has been identified and evaluated, the skin overlying the area beneath the ultrasound transducer is then prepped with antiseptic solution. A sterile syringe containing 2.0 mL of 0.25% preservative-free bupivacaine and 40 mg of methylprednisolone is attached to a 1½-inch, 22-gauge needle using strict aseptic technique. The needle is placed through the skin ~0.5 cm above the lateral aspect of the ultrasound transducer and is then advanced using an in-plane approach with the needle trajectory adjusted under real-time ultrasound guidance so that the needle tip ultimately rests in proximity, but not in contact with the ulnar nerve (Fig. 53.13). When the tip of needle is thought to be in satisfactory position, after careful aspiration, a small amount of local anesthetic and steroid is injected under real-time ultrasound guidance to confirm that the needle tip is in the proper position. After proper needle tip placement is confirmed, the remainder of the contents of the syringe is slowly injected under real-time ultrasound guidance to insure that the injectate is not further compressing and compromising the ulnar nerve within the confines of the cubital tunnel. There should be minimal resistance to injection.

## COMPLICATIONS

The major complications of ultrasound-guided injection of ultrasound-guided cubital tunnel syndrome are related to improper needle placement with the possibility of inadvertent intravascular injection and/or persistent paresthesia secondary to needle trauma to the ulnar nerve. Although rare, infection may occur. Ecchymosis and hematoma formation following this procedure may also occur. These complications can be decreased if manual pressure is applied to the area of the block immediately after injection. Application of cold packs for 20-minute periods after the block will also decrease the amount of postprocedure pain and bleeding the patient may experience. Approximately 25% of patients complain of a transient increase in pain after this injection technique; the patient should be warned of this.

**FIGURE 53.4.** The little finger adduction test evaluated the strength in the interosseous muscles of the hand, which are innervated by the ulnar nerve. It is performed by asking the patient to touch his or her little finger to their index finger.

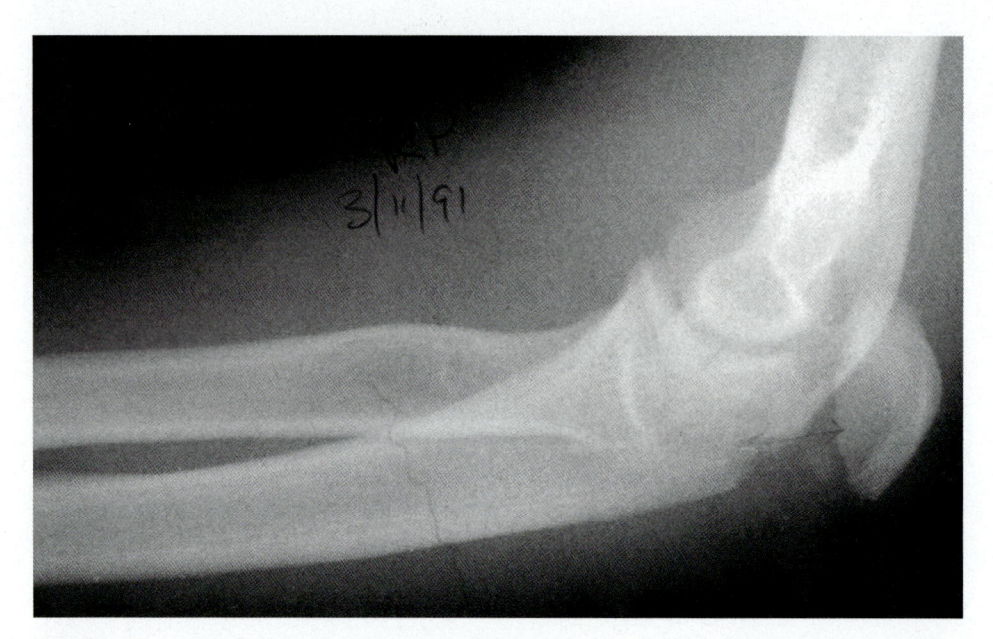

**FIGURE 53.5.** Olecranon fractures can entrap the ulnar nerve as it passes through the cubital tunnel. (From Bucholz RW, Heckman JD. *Rockwood & Green's Fractures in Adults*. 5th ed. Philadelphia, PA: Lippincott Williams & Wilkins; 2001, with permission.)

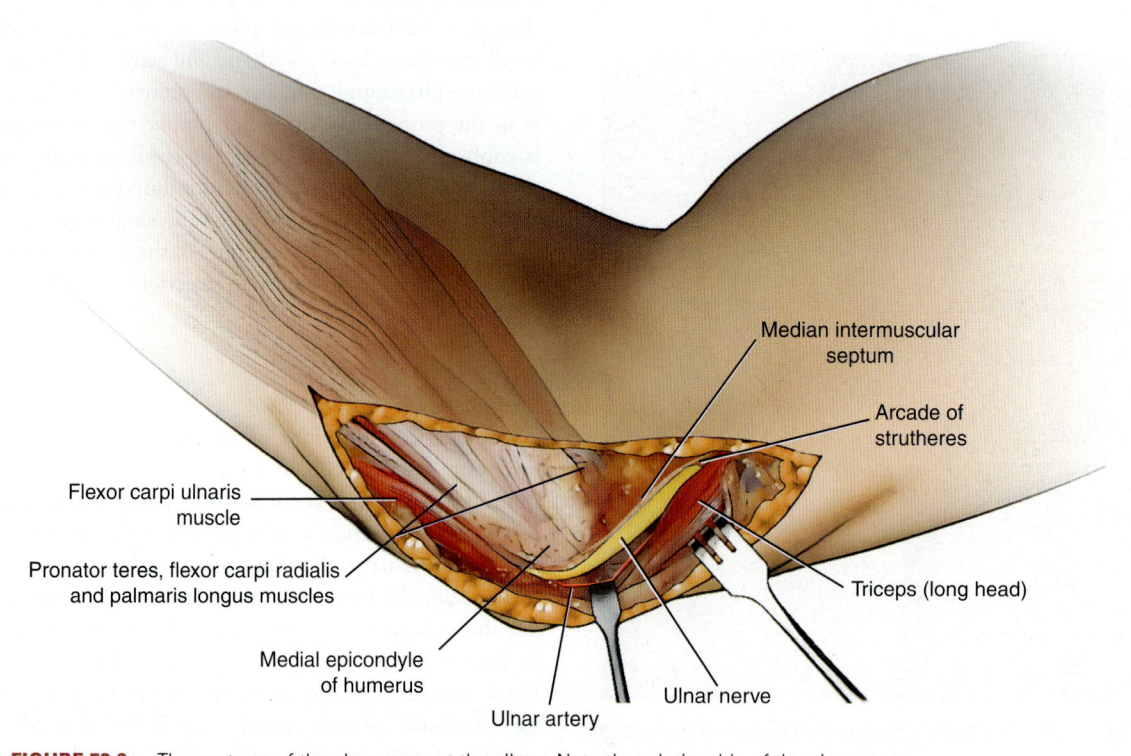

**FIGURE 53.6.** The anatomy of the ulnar nerve at the elbow. Note the relationship of the ulnar nerve.

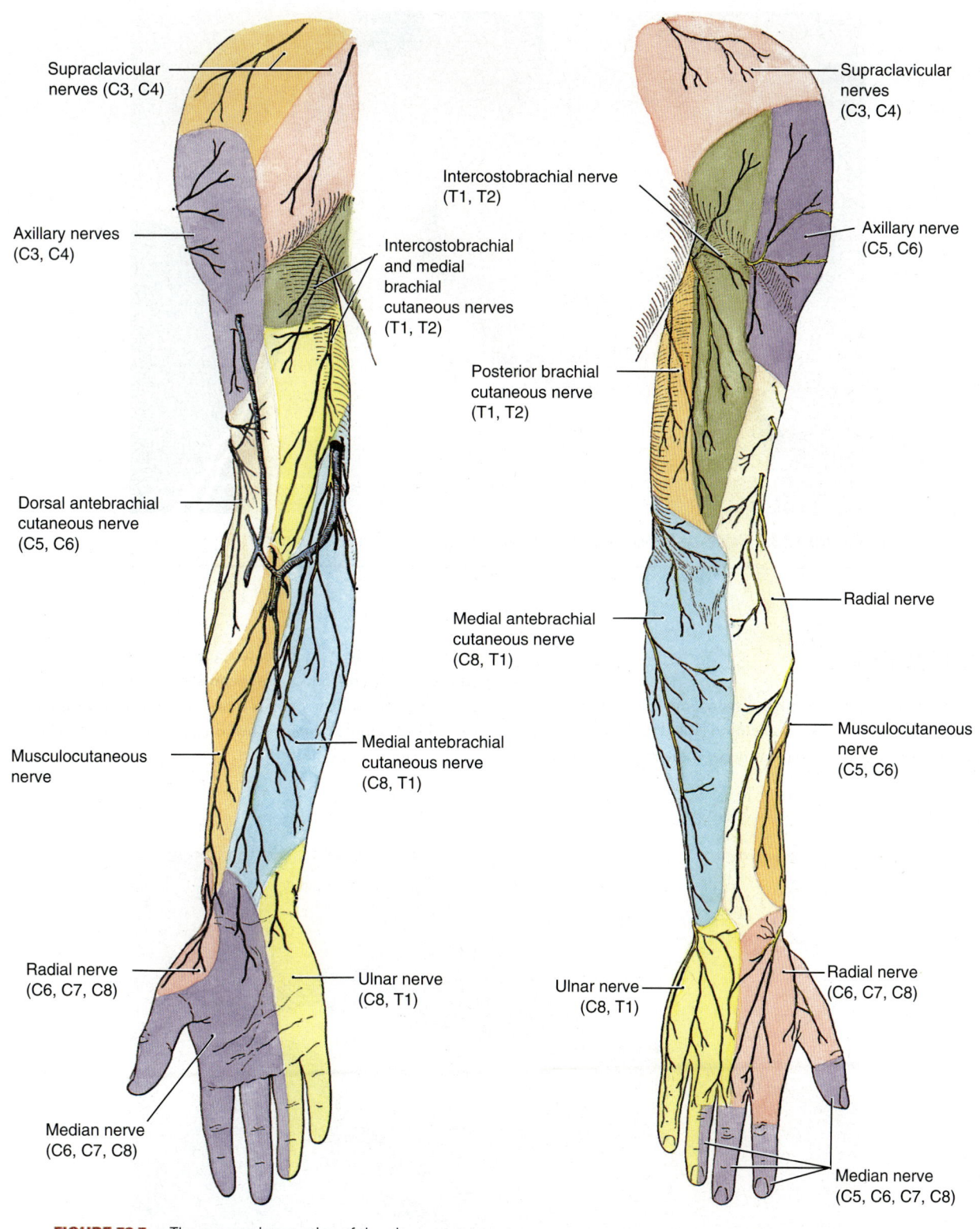

**FIGURE 53.7.** The sensory innervation of the ulnar nerve.

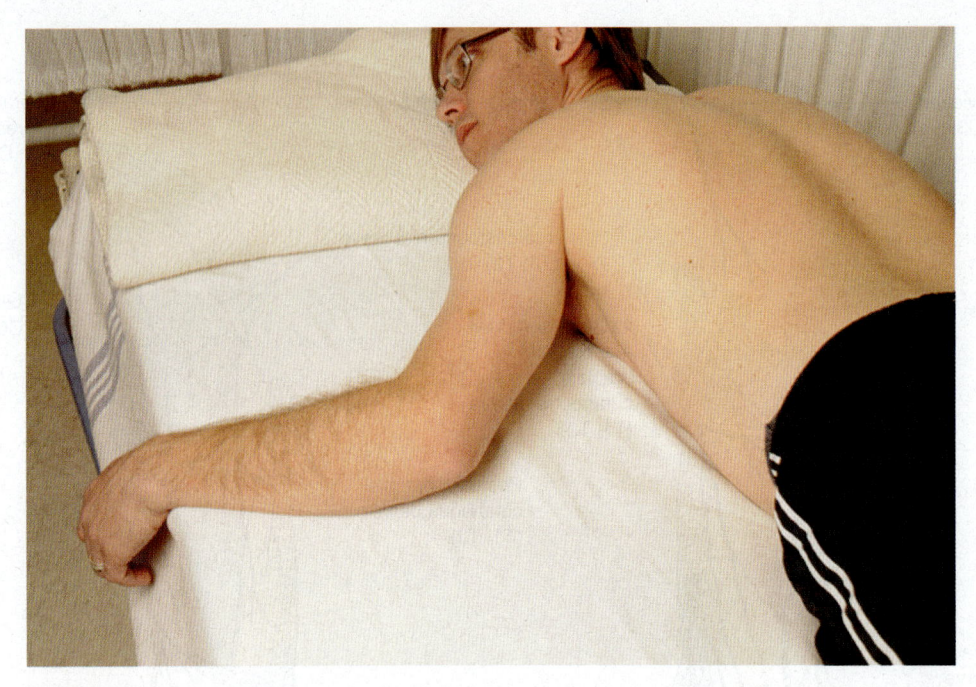

**FIGURE 53.8.** Proper patient position for ultrasound-guided cubital tunnel syndrome.

## CLINICAL PEARLS

Ultrasound-guided cubital tunnel syndrome is a straightforward and relatively safe technique if attention is paid to the clinically relevant anatomy. Because the ulnar nerve is the largest unprotected nerve in the body, it is subject to trauma at various points along its course. For this reason, careful neurologic examination to identify preexisting neurologic deficits that may later be attributed to the nerve block should be performed on all patients before beginning cubital tunnel syndrome.

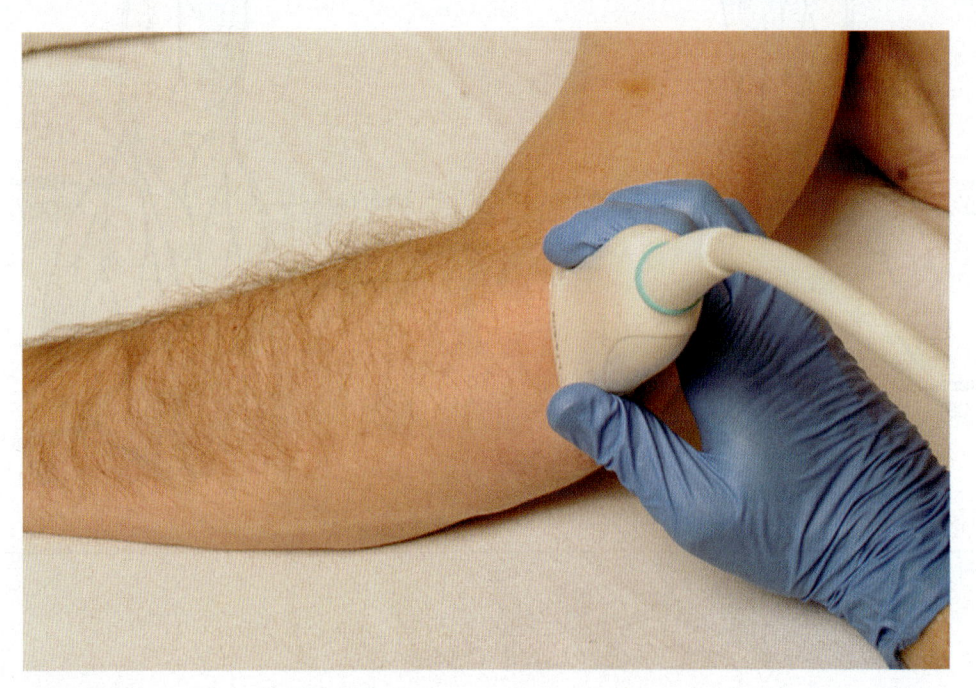

**FIGURE 53.9.** Proper transverse position for the linear high-frequency ultrasound transducer to perform ultrasound-guided cubital tunnel syndrome.

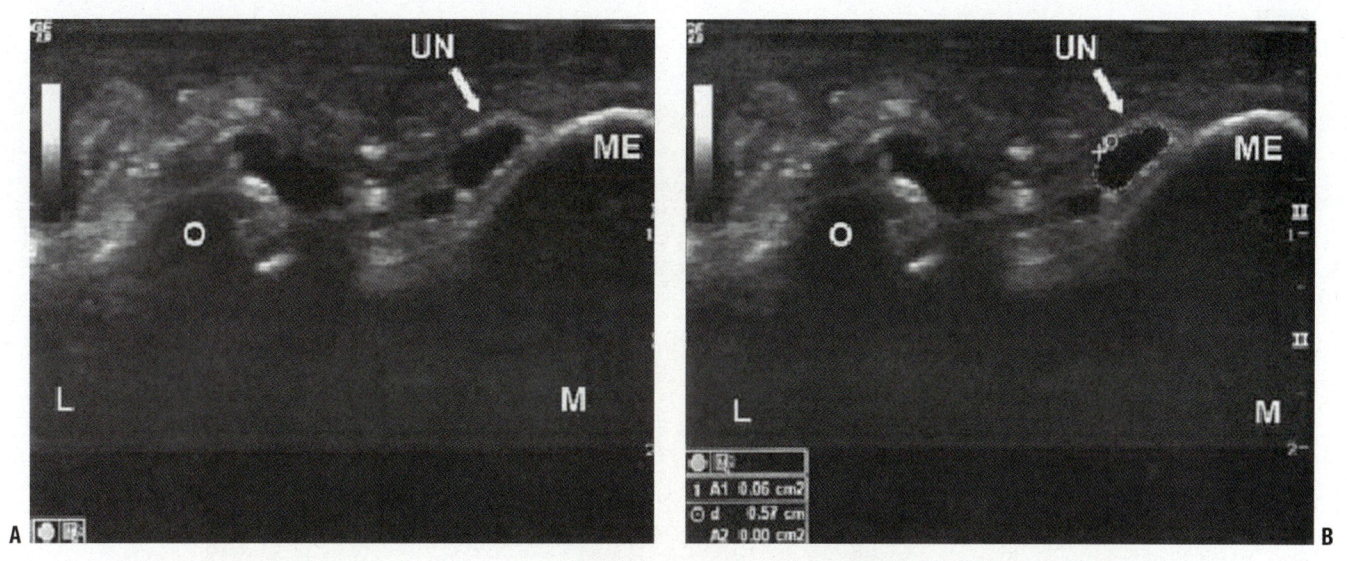

**FIGURE 53.10. A,B:** Transverse ultrasound image demonstrating the ulnar nerve within the cubital tunnel lying next to the medial epicondyle. L, lateral; M, medial; ME, medial epicondyle; O, olecranon; UN, ulnar nerve. (From Ozturk E, Sonmez G, Colak A, et al. Sonographic appearances of the normal ulnar nerve in the cubital tunnel. *J Clin Ultrasound* 2008;36(6):325–329, with permission.)

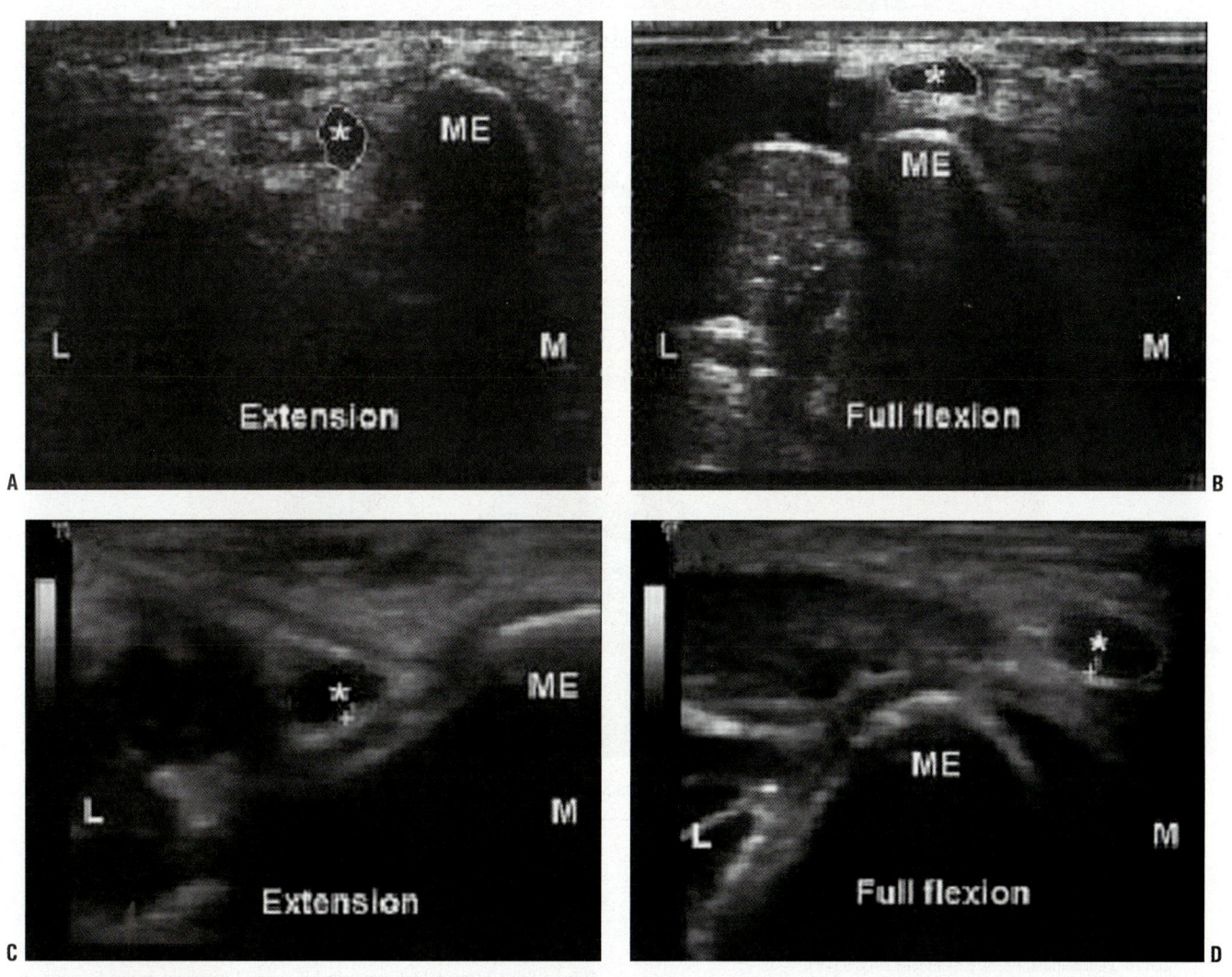

**FIGURE 53.11. A–D:** When moving the ultrasound transducer distally toward the forearm, the ulnar nerve will be seen to lie between the two heads of the flexor carpi ulnaris muscle and beneath the overlying cubital tunnel retinaculum. Note how the ulnar nerve changes position as the extremity moves from flexion to extension. *, ulnar nerve; ME, medial epicondyle; L, lateral; M, medial.

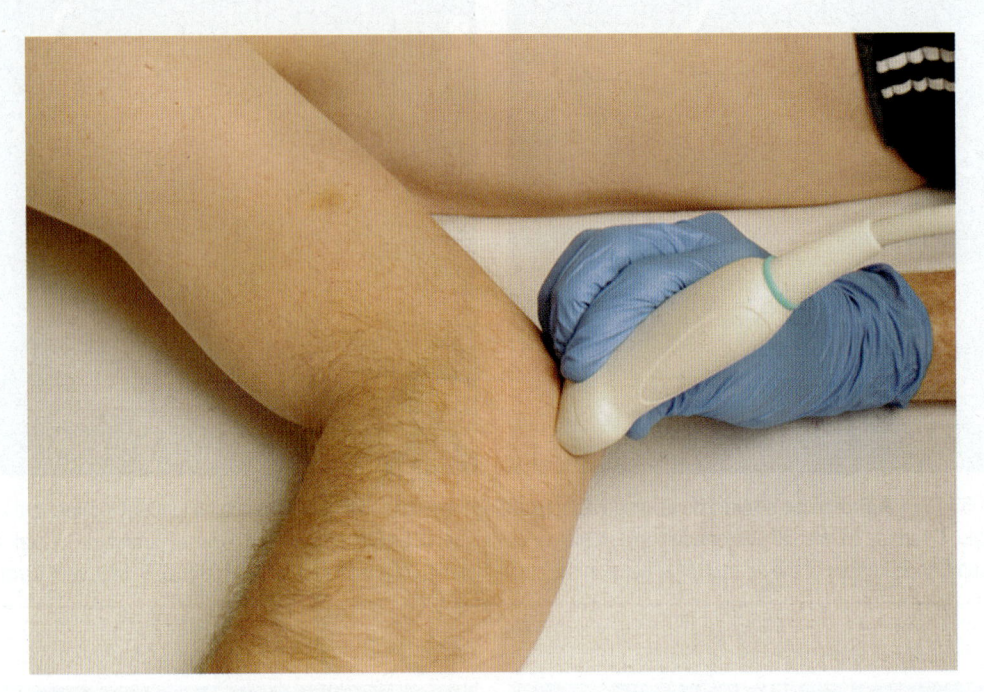

**FIGURE 53.12.** The ultrasound transducer is turned to the longitudinal plane to evaluate the ulnar nerve as it passes through the cubital tunnel.

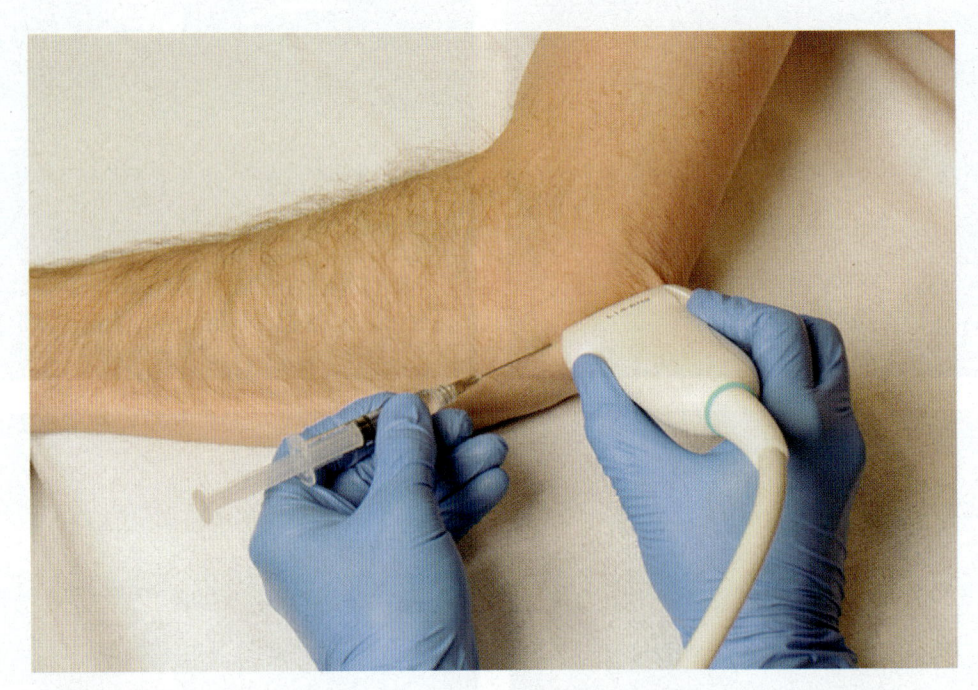

**FIGURE 53.13.** Proper needle placement for ultrasound-guided cubital tunnel syndrome injection.

## SUGGESTED READINGS

Waldman SD. Anconeus epitrochlearis. In: *Atlas of Uncommon Pain Syndromes*. 2nd ed. Philadelphia, PA: WB Saunders; 2008:93–95.

Waldman SD. Cubital tunnel syndrome. In: *Atlas of Uncommon Pain Syndromes*. 2nd ed. Philadelphia, PA: WB Saunders; 2008:104–106.

Waldman SD. Cubital tunnel syndrome. In: *Atlas of Interventional Pain Management*. 3rd ed. Philadelphia, PA: WB Saunders; 2009:229–234.

Waldman SD. The ulnar nerve. In: *Pain Review*. Philadelphia, PA: Saunders Elsevier; 2009:76–77.

Waldman SD. Cubital tunnel syndrome. In: *Pain Review*. Philadelphia, PA: Saunders Elsevier; 2009:253.

Wiesler ER, Chloros GD, Cartwright MS, et al. Ultrasound in the diagnosis of ulnar neuropathy at the cubital tunnel. *J Hand Surg* 2006;31(7):1088–1093.

# CHAPTER 54

# Ultrasound-Guided Injection Technique for Tennis Elbow Syndrome

## CLINICAL PERSPECTIVES

Tennis elbow, which is also known as lateral epicondylitis, is a painful condition of the upper extremity that is caused by repetitive overuse or misuse of the extensor tendons of the forearm. Over time, microscopic tears begin to occur at the origin of the musculotendinous units of the extensor carpi radialis brevis and extensor carpi ulnaris muscles (Fig. 54.1). The repetitive process of tearing and healing of the musculotendinous units of the extensor tendons sets up an inflammatory process that ultimately results in pain and functional disability. If not properly treated, complete rupture of the tendinous insertion of these extensor muscles can occur (Fig. 54.2). It has been postulated that a combination of the poor blood supply of the extensor tendons combined with the significant concentric and eccentric stresses placed on these tendons may be responsible for the evolution of this common pain syndrome.

Activities that require increased grip pressure and high torque twisting of the wrist have been implicated in the evolution of tennis elbow. The biomechanics responsible for the development of tennis elbow in players of racquet sports include the (1) use of an increased grip strength to support a racquet that is too long or too heavy for the player and (2) making backhand shots with a leading shoulder and elbow rather than keeping the shoulder and elbow parallel to the net (Fig. 54.3).

The signs and symptoms frequently observed in patients suffering from tennis elbow include pain that is localized to the lateral epicondyle with maximal point tenderness at the site of the insertion of the musculotendinous units of the extensor carpi radialis brevis and extensor carpi ulnaris muscles. The pain is constant in nature with the patient experiencing an acute exacerbation of pain with any activity that requires gripping with the hand, extending the wrist, or supinating the forearm. The patient suffering from tennis elbow may complain of significant sleep disturbance with awakening when the patient rolls over onto the affected elbow. On physical examination, there is exquisite point tenderness to palpation at or just below the lateral epicondyle. Careful palpation of the area may reveal a band-like thickening of the extensor tendons, and color may be noted. Grip strength is often diminished and patients will exhibit a positive tennis elbow test. The tennis elbow test is performed by stabilizing the patient's forearm and then having the patient clench his or her fist and actively extend the wrist (Fig. 54.4). The examiner then attempts to force the wrist into flexion. Sudden, severe pain is highly suggestive of tennis elbow.

Tennis elbow can be confused with radial tunnel syndrome as well as a C6–C7 radiculopathy. Tennis elbow can be distinguished from radial tunnel syndrome by determining the site of maximal tenderness to palpation. Patients suffering from tennis elbow will experience maximal tenderness to palpation over the lateral epicondyle, whereas patients suffering from radial tunnel syndrome will experience maximal tenderness to palpation distal to the lateral epicondyle over the radial nerve (Fig. 54.5).

Furthermore, it should be remembered that cervical radiculopathy and ulnar nerve entrapment may coexist as the so-called "double crush" syndrome. The double crush syndrome is seen most commonly with median nerve entrapment at the wrist or with carpal tunnel syndrome but has been reported with the radial nerve.

Electromyography and nerve conduction velocity testing are useful in helping in the differentiation of tennis elbow from cervical radiculopathy and radial tunnel syndrome. Plain radiographs, ultrasound imaging, and magnetic resonance imaging are indicated in all patients who are thought to be suffering from tennis elbow in order to confirm the diagnosis as well as to rule out occult bony pathology involving the lateral epicondyle and elbow joint and to identify occult fractures, masses, or tumors that may be responsible for the patient's symptomatology (Fig. 54.6). Based on the patient's clinical presentation, additional testing may be indicated, including complete blood count, uric acid, sedimentation rate, and antinuclear antibody testing. The ultrasound-guided injection technique described below serves as both a diagnostic and therapeutic maneuver as ultrasound imaging can clearly delineate pathology of the extensor musculotendinous units at their insertion on the lateral epicondyle.

**FIGURE 54.1.** Tennis elbow is the result of repetitive stress injury to the extensor musculotendinous units of the extensor carpi radialis brevis and the extensor carpi ulnaris muscles. (From Anatomical Chart Company.)

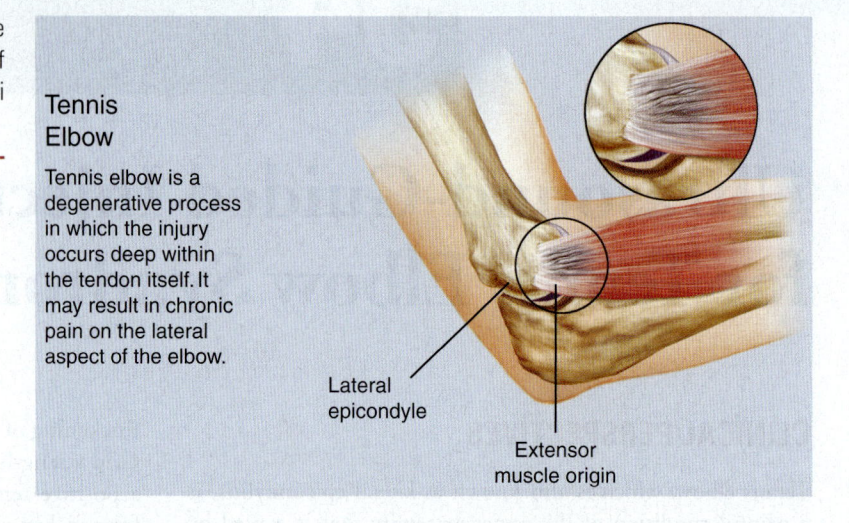

**Tennis Elbow**

Tennis elbow is a degenerative process in which the injury occurs deep within the tendon itself. It may result in chronic pain on the lateral aspect of the elbow.

## CLINICALLY RELEVANT ANATOMY

The key landmarks when performing ultrasound-guided tennis elbow are the extensor tendons of the extensor carpi radialis brevis and extensor carpi ulnaris muscles and their point of origin on anterior facet of the lateral epicondyle of the elbow. The extensor radialis longus musculotendinous unit may also be affected at its origin at the supracondylar crest of the humerus. Confusion in the clinical presentation of cubital and olecranon bursitis may coexist with tennis elbow. The radial nerve passes into the substance of the brachioradialis muscle, and at a point just above the lateral epicondyle, the radial nerve divides into deep and superficial branches; the superficial branch continues down the arm along with the radial artery to provide sensory innervation to the dorsum of the wrist and the dorsal aspects of a portion of the thumb and index and middle fingers, and the deep branch provides the majority of the motor innervation to the extensors of the forearm.

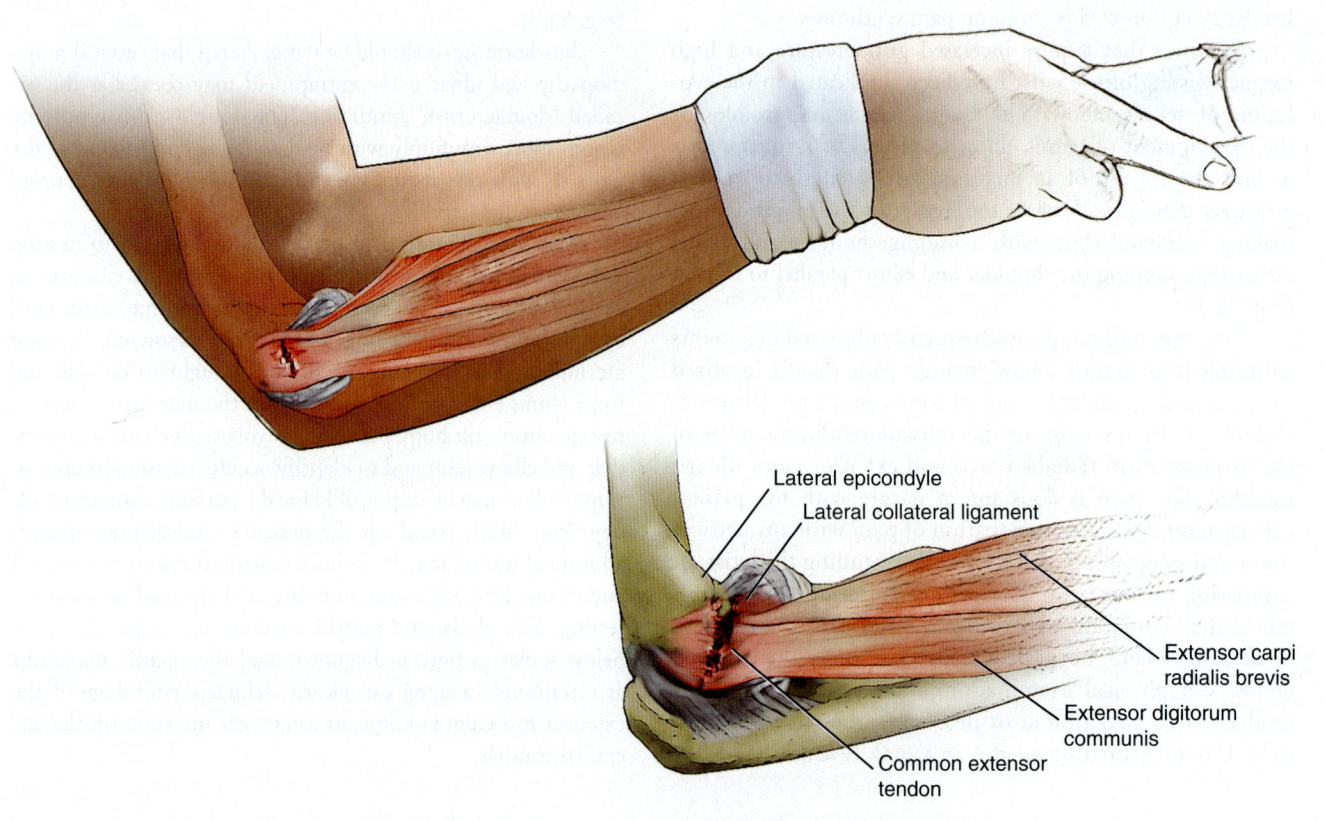

**FIGURE 54.2.** If tennis elbow remains untreated, complete rupture of the extensor tendons can occur.

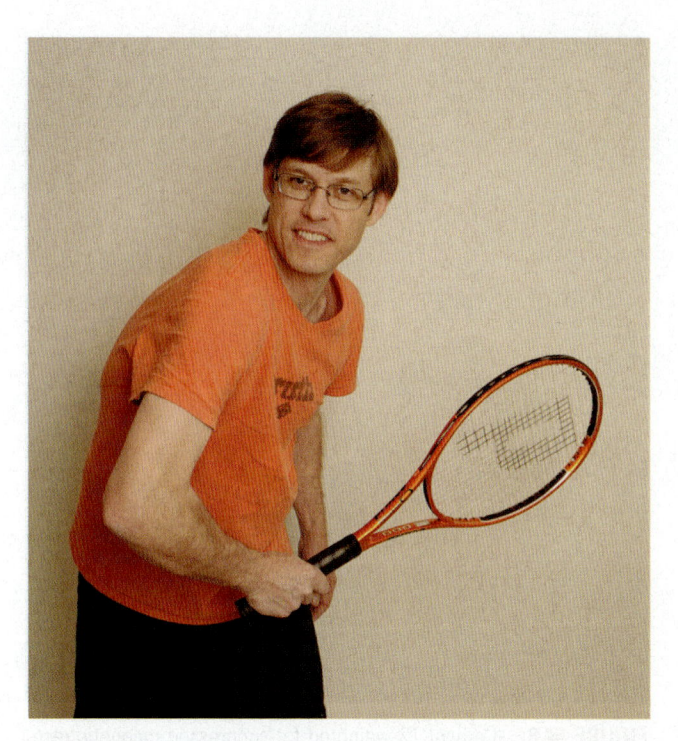

**FIGURE 54.3.** Playing with a racquet that is too heavy and hitting backhand shots with a forward leading shoulder have been implicated in the development of tennis elbow.

## ULTRASOUND-GUIDED TECHNIQUE

The benefits, risks, and alternative treatments are explained to the patient, and informed consent is obtained. The patient is then placed in the supine position with the forearm laying comfortably across the patient's abdomen and the elbow flexed ~75 degrees (Fig. 54.7). With the patient in the above position, the lateral epicondyle is identified and the point of maximal tenderness is then isolated by careful palpation (Fig. 54.8). A high-frequency linear ultrasound transducer is then placed in a longitudinal position over the lateral epicondyle at the point of maximal tenderness (Fig. 54.9). The gentle hyperechoic slope of the lateral epicondyle and the overlying common extensor tendon insertions attaching to the lateral epicondyle are then identified. The radial head will be seen distally as a hyperechoic hill-shaped structure (Fig. 54.10). The area of extensor tendinous insertions on the lateral epicondyle is identified and evaluated for tears, which will appear as hypoechoic areas within the substance of the tendon. The ultrasound transducer is then slowly moved proximally so that the gentle hyperechoic slope of the lateral epicondyle and the overlying common extensor tendon insertions are at the bottom of the ultrasound image to minimize the distance the needle has to travel to reach its target (Fig. 54.11). The skin overlying

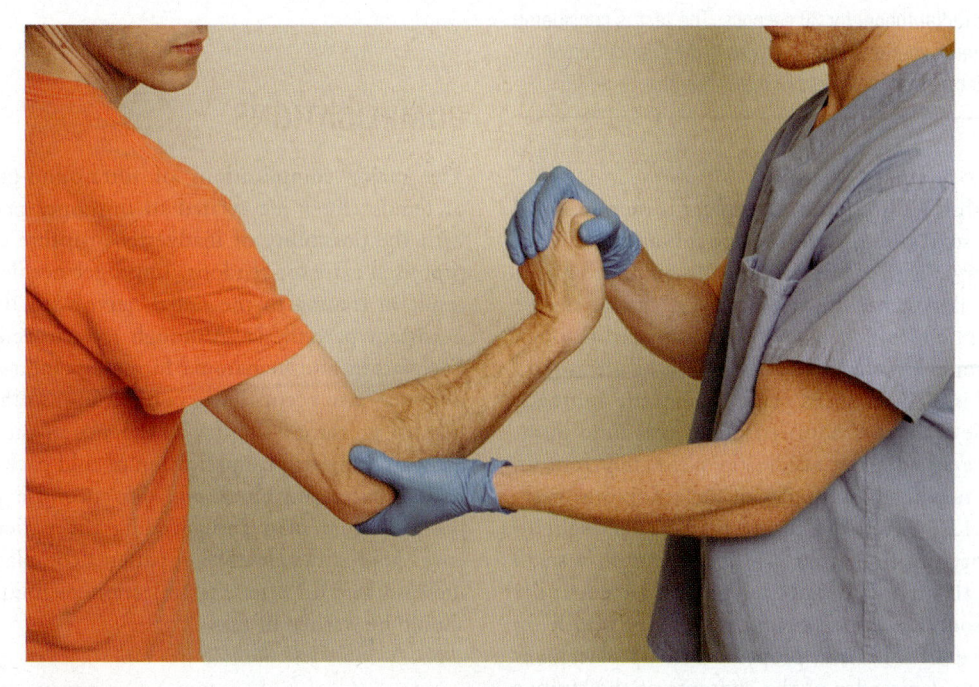

**FIGURE 54.4.** The tennis elbow test is performed by stabilizing the patient's forearm and then having the patient clench his or her fist and actively extend the wrist. The examiner then attempts to force the wrist into flexion. Sudden, severe pain is highly suggestive of tennis elbow.

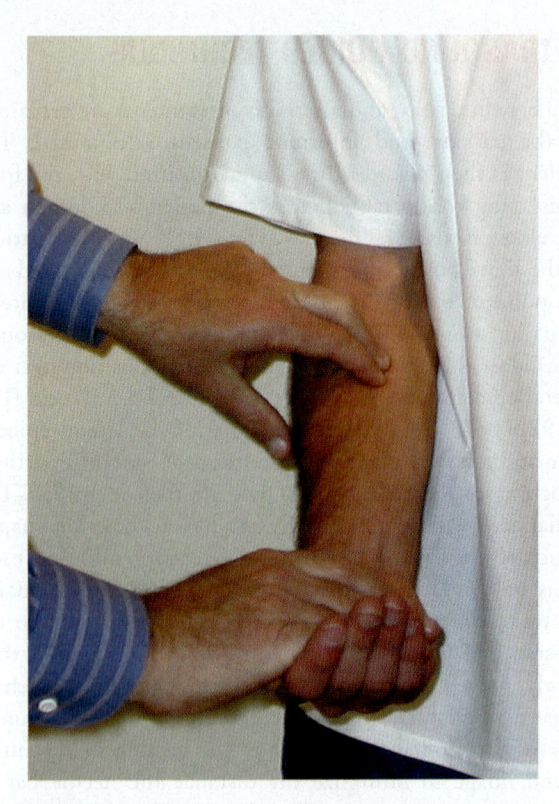

**FIGURE 54.5.** Patients suffering from tennis elbow will experience maximal tenderness to palpation over the lateral epicondyle, whereas patients suffering from radial tunnel syndrome will experience maximal tenderness to palpation distal to the lateral epicondyle over the radial nerve and exhibit a positive radial tunnel compression test. The radial tunnel compression test is performed by tightly compressing the area over the radial tunnel for 30 seconds. The test is considered positive if the patient experience dysesthesias in the distribution of the radial nerve and increasing weakness of grip strength.

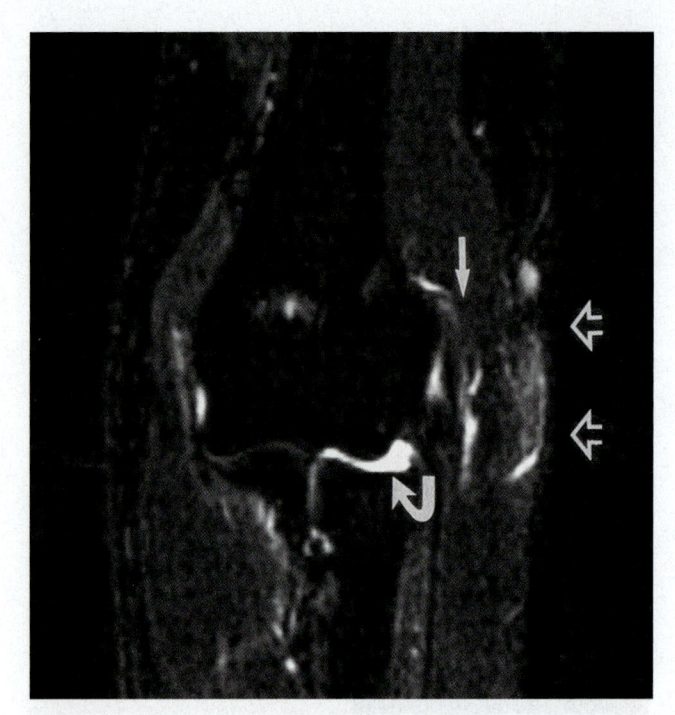

**FIGURE 54.6.** Coronal T2-weighted fat-suppressed magnetic resonance imaging of a patient suffering from tennis elbow. The *arrow* indicated partial tearing of the extensor tendons, with the *open arrows* indicating tissue edema. The *open arrows* indicate an effusion of the elbow joint. (Reused from Greenspan A. *Orthopedic Imaging: A Practical Approach.* Philadelphia, PA: Lippincott Williams & Wilkins; 2011:164, with permission.)

the area beneath the ultrasound transducer is then prepped with antiseptic solution. A sterile syringe containing 4.0 mL of 0.25% preservative-free bupivacaine and 40 mg of methylprednisolone is attached to a 1½-inch, 22-gauge needle using strict aseptic technique. The needle is placed through the skin ~1.0 cm below the inferior aspect of the ultrasound transducer and is then advanced using an in-plane approach with the needle trajectory adjusted under real-time ultrasound guidance so that the needle tip ultimately rests in proximity, but not in the substance of the tendinous insertions (Fig. 54.12). When the tip of needle is thought to be in satisfactory position, after careful aspiration, a small amount of local anesthetic and steroid is injected under real-time ultrasound guidance to confirm that the needle tip is in the proper position. After proper needle tip placement is confirmed, the remainder of the contents of the syringe is slowly injected under real-time ultrasound guidance with the needle being adjusted so that the entire area of the tendon insertion is treated. There should be minimal resistance to injection.

## COMPLICATIONS

The major complications of ultrasound-guided injection of tennis elbow are related to improper needle placement with the possibility of inadvertent rupture of already compromised extensor tendons. Improper needle placement can result in trauma to the radial nerve with the potential for persistent paresthesia. Although rare, infection may occur. Ecchymosis and hematoma formation following this procedure may also occur. These complications can be decreased if manual pressure is applied to the area of the block immediately after injection. Application of cold packs for 20-minute periods after the block will also decrease the amount of postprocedure pain and bleeding the patient may experience. Approximately 25% of patients complain of a transient increase in pain after this injection technique; the patient should be warned of this.

## CLINICAL PEARLS

Ultrasound-guided injection for tennis elbow is a straightforward and relatively safe technique if attention is paid to the

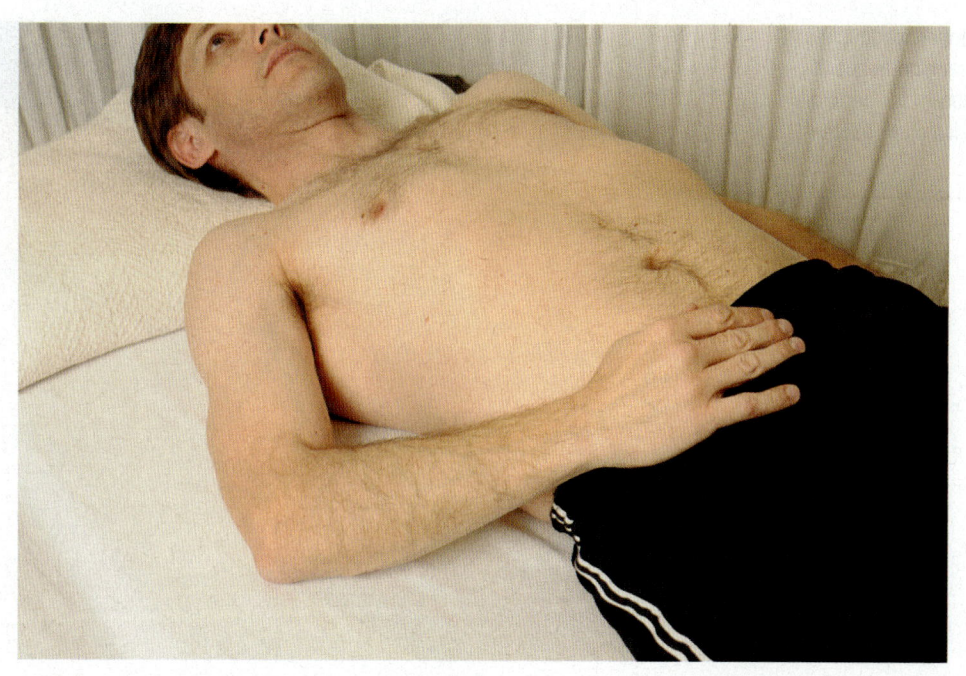

**FIGURE 54.7.** Proper patient position for ultrasound-guided injection for tennis elbow.

clinically relevant anatomy. In addition to injection of local anesthetics and steroids, investigators have also advocated the injection of botulinum toxin and platelet-rich plasma to treat tennis elbow. Because of the proximity of the radial nerve, it is subject to trauma when performing this injection procedure. For this reason, careful neurologic examination to identify preexisting neurologic deficits that may later be attributed to the nerve block should be performed on all patients before performing ultrasound-guided injection for tennis elbow.

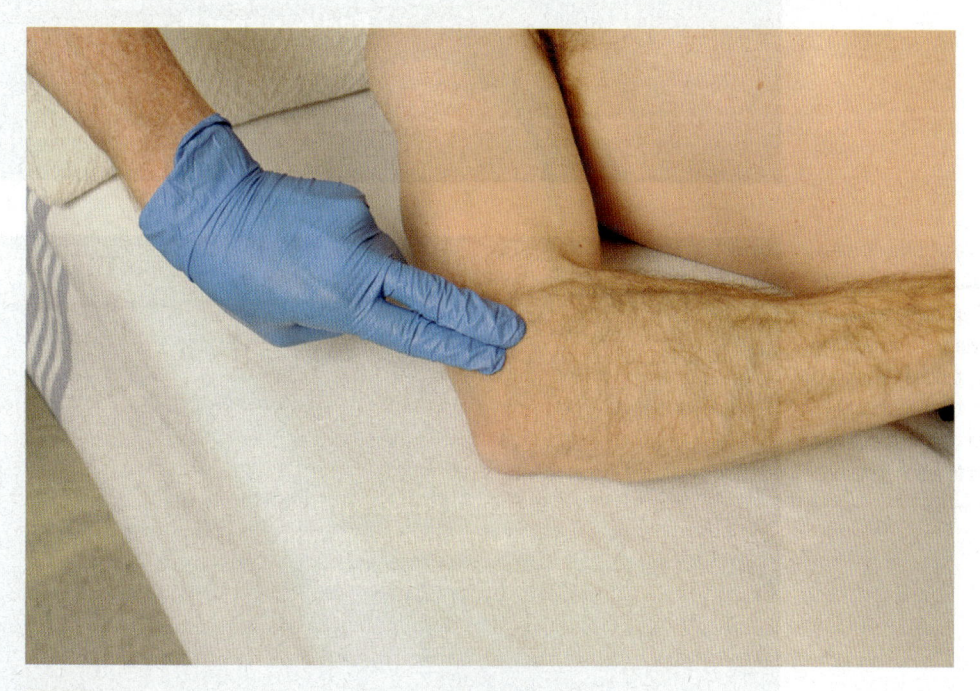

**FIGURE 54.8.** Palpation of the lateral epicondyle of the elbow.

**FIGURE 54.9.** Proper longitudinal position for the linear high-frequency ultrasound transducer to perform ultrasound-guided injection for tennis elbow.

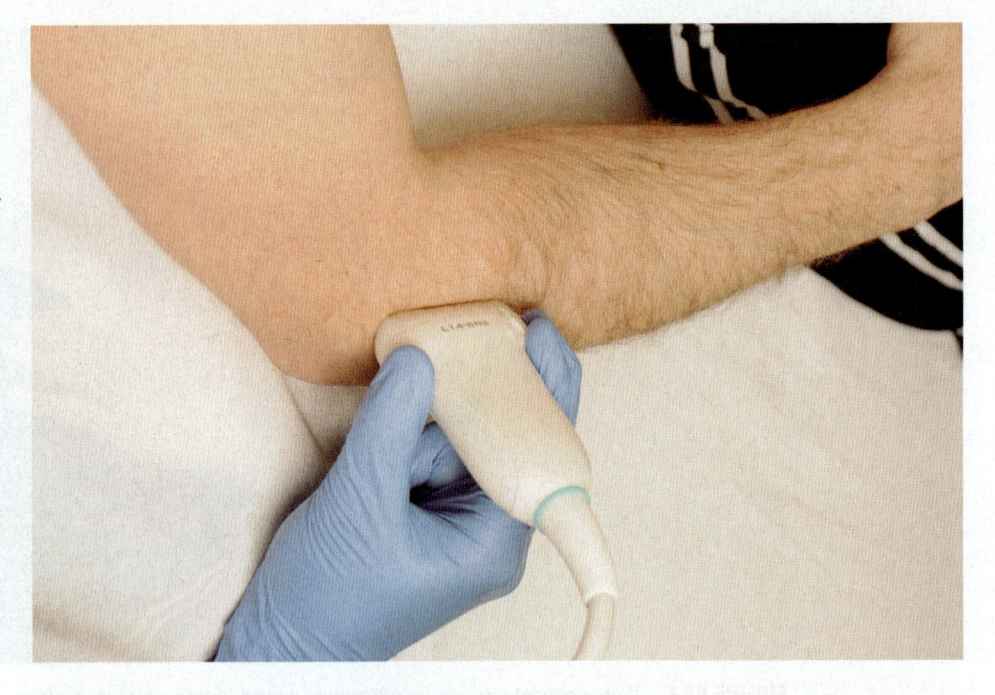

**FIGURE 54.10.** Longitudinal ultrasound image demonstrating the gentle slope of the lateral epicondyle, the river-like–appearing extensor tendons inserting into the lateral epicondyle, and the hill-shaped radial head.

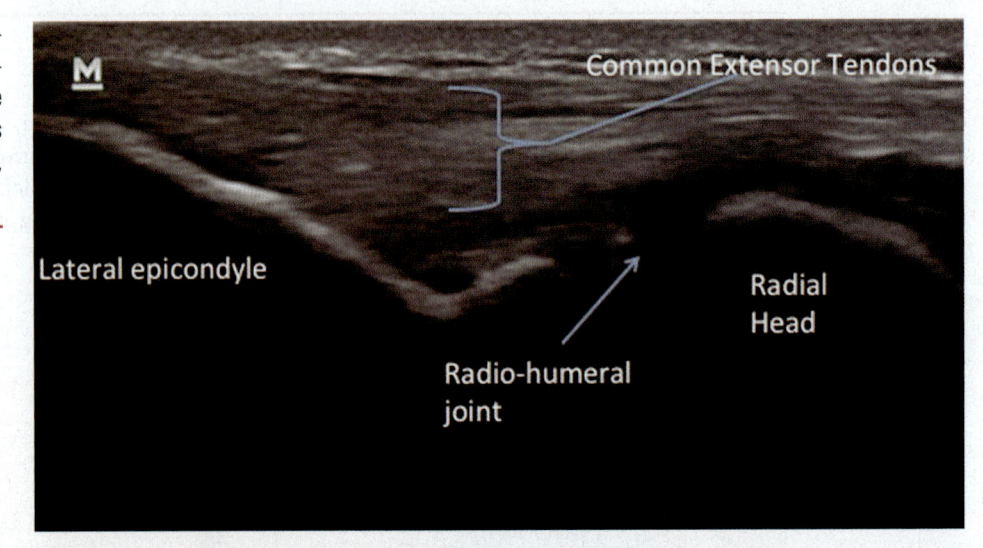

**FIGURE 54.11.** The ultrasound transducer is then slowly moved proximally so that the gentle hyperechoic slope of the lateral epicondyle and the overlying common extensor tendon insertions are at the bottom of the ultrasound image to minimize the distance the needle has to travel to reach its target.

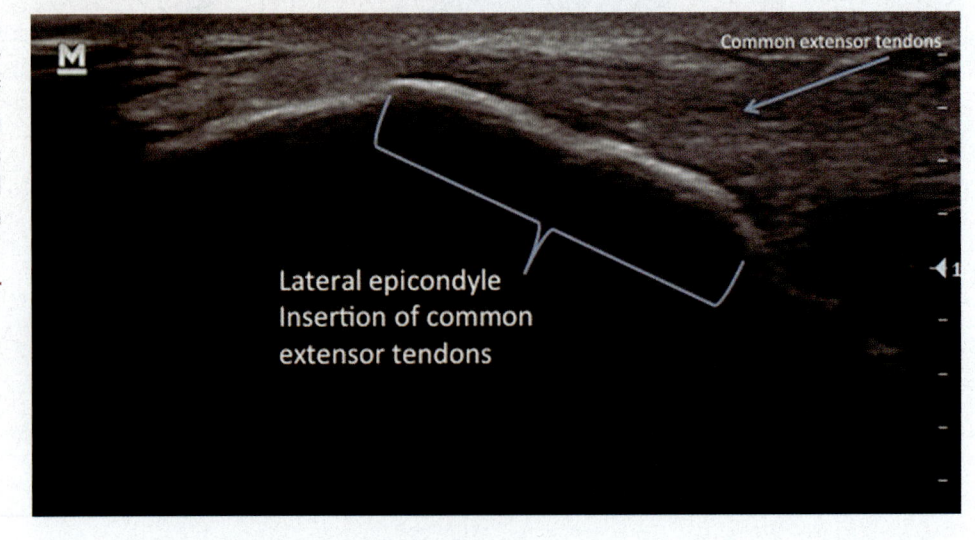

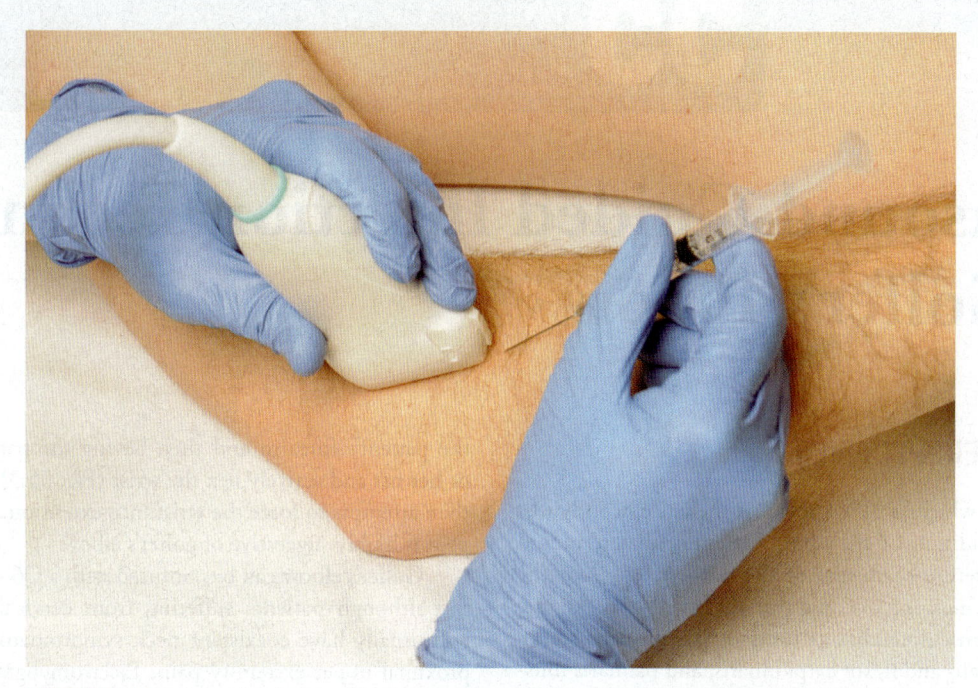

**FIGURE 54.12.** Proper in-plane needle placement for ultrasound-guided tennis elbow injection.

## SUGGESTED READINGS

Waldman SD. Lateral epicondylitis injection. In: *Atlas of Pain Management Injection Techniques*. 3rd ed. Philadelphia, PA: WB Saunders; 2013:139–143.

Waldman SD. Tennis elbow. In: *Atlas of Common Pain Syndromes*. 3rd ed. Philadelphia, PA: WB Saunders; 2012:123–125.

Waldman SD. Radial tunnel syndrome. In: *Atlas of Uncommon Pain Syndromes*. 2nd ed. Philadelphia, PA: WB Saunders; 2008:102–103.

Waldman SD. Tennis elbow. In: *Pain Review*. Philadelphia, PA: Saunders Elsevier; 2009:254.

Waldman SD. The tennis elbow test. In: *Physical Diagnosis of Pain. An Atlas of Signs and Symptoms*. 2nd ed. Philadelphia, PA: WB Saunders; 2010:130–132.

# Ultrasound-Guided Injection Technique for Golfer's Elbow

## CLINICAL PERSPECTIVES

Golfer's elbow, which is also known as medial epicondylitis, is a painful condition of the upper extremity that is caused by repetitive overuse or misuse of the flexor tendons of the forearm. Over time, microscopic tears begin to occur at the origin of the musculotendinous units of the pronator teres, flexor carpi radialis and flexor carpi ulnaris, and palmaris muscles (Fig. 55.1). The repetitive process of tearing and healing of the musculotendinous units of the flexor tendons sets up an inflammatory process that ultimately results in pain and functional disability. If not properly treated, complete rupture of the tendinous insertion of these flexor muscles can occur (Fig. 55.2). It has been postulated that a combination of the poor blood supply of the flexor tendons combined with the significant concentric and eccentric stresses placed on these tendons may be responsible for the evolution of this common pain syndrome.

Activities that require increased grip pressure and high torque twisting of the wrist have been implicated in the evolution of golfer's elbow. The biomechanics responsible for the development of golfer's elbow include activities that have in common repetitive flexion and sudden arrested motion, for example, driving golf balls with too heavy of a golf club and overhead throwing. Carrying heavy suitcases, computer bags, and brief cases have also been implicated.

The signs and symptoms frequently observed in patients suffering from golfer's elbow include pain that is localized to the medial epicondyle with maximal point tenderness at the site of the insertion of the musculotendinous units of the pronator teres, flexor carpi radialis and flexor carpi ulnaris, and palmaris muscles. The pain is constant in nature with the patient experiencing an acute exacerbation of pain with any activity that requires gripping with the hand, extending the wrist, or pronating the forearm. The patient suffering from golfer's elbow may complain of significant sleep disturbance with awakening when the patient rolls over onto the affected elbow. On physical examination, there is exquisite point tenderness to palpation at or just below the medial epicondyle. Careful palpation of the area may reveal a band-like thickening of the flexor tendons, and color may be noted. Grip strength is often diminished and patients will exhibit a positive golfer's elbow test. The golfer's elbow test is performed by stabilizing the patient's forearm and then having the patient clench his or her fist and actively flex the wrist (Fig. 55.3). The examiner then attempts to force the wrist into extension. Sudden, severe pain is highly suggestive of golfer's elbow.

Golfer's elbow can be confused with a C6–C7 radiculopathy although patients suffering from cervical radiculopathy will usually have coexistent neck symptomatology and more proximal upper extremity pain. Electromyography and nerve conduction velocity testing are useful in helping in the differentiation of golfer's elbow from cervical radiculopathy and other nerve entrapment syndromes. Plain radiographs, ultrasound imaging, and magnetic resonance imaging are indicated in all patients who are thought to be suffering from golfer's elbow in order to confirm the diagnosis as well as to rule out occult bony pathology involving the medial epicondyle and elbow joint and to identify occult fractures, masses, or tumors that may be responsible for the patient's symptomatology (Fig. 55.4). Based on the patient's clinical presentation, additional testing may be indicated, including complete blood count, uric acid, sedimentation rate, and antinuclear antibody testing. The ultrasound-guided injection technique described below serves as both a diagnostic and therapeutic maneuver as ultrasound imaging can clearly delineate pathology of the flexor musculotendinous units at their insertion on the medial epicondyle.

## CLINICALLY RELEVANT ANATOMY

The key landmarks when performing ultrasound-guided golfer's elbow are the flexor tendons of the pronator teres, flexor carpi radialis and flexor carpi ulnaris, and palmaris muscles and their point of origin on anterior facet of the medial epicondyle of the elbow (see Fig. 55.1). Cubital and olecranon bursitis may coexist with golfer's elbow further confusing the clinical presentations. The ulnar nerve is in proximity to the medial epicondyle and subject to needle-induced trauma during this injection technique. The nerve exits the axilla, and it passes inferiorly adjacent to the brachial artery. At the middle of the upper arm, the ulnar nerve turns medially to pass between the olecranon process and medial epicondyle of the humerus. Continuing its downward path, the ulnar nerve passes between the heads of the flexor carpi ulnaris moving radially along with the ulnar artery.

# CHAPTER 55   ULTRASOUND-GUIDED INJECTION TECHNIQUE FOR GOLFER'S ELBOW

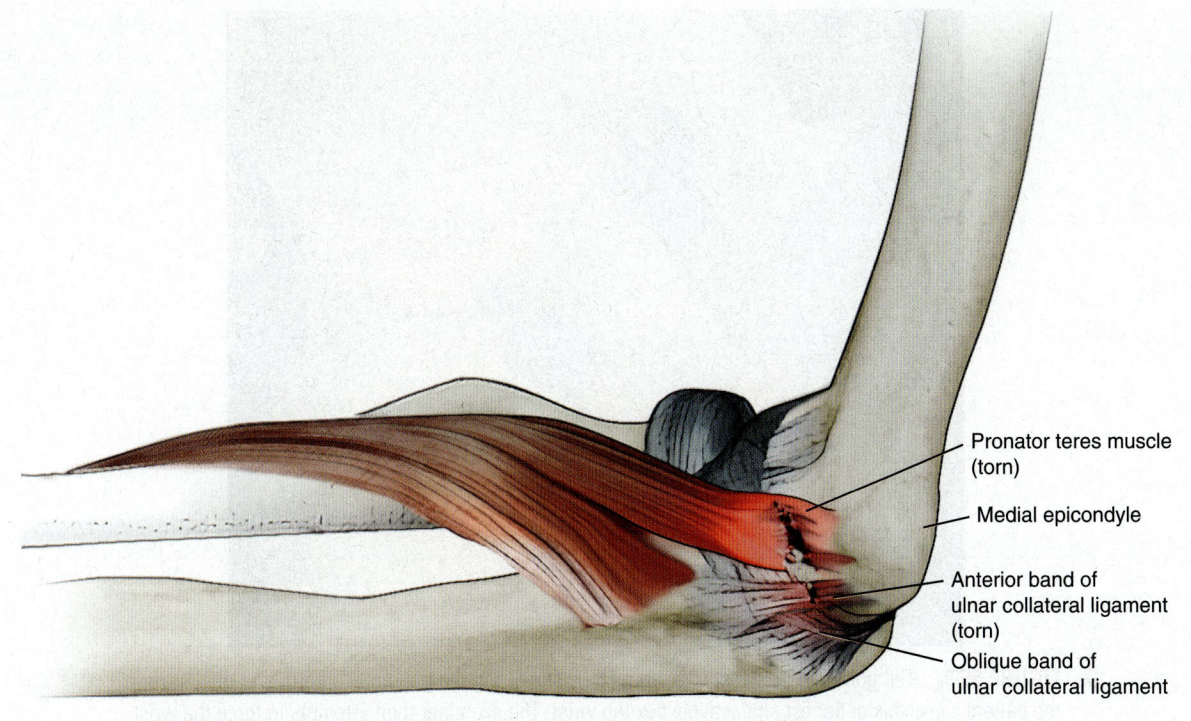

**FIGURE 55.1.** Golfer's elbow is the result of repetitive stress injury to the flexor musculotendinous units of the pronator teres, flexor carpi radialis and flexor carpi ulnaris, and palmaris muscles.

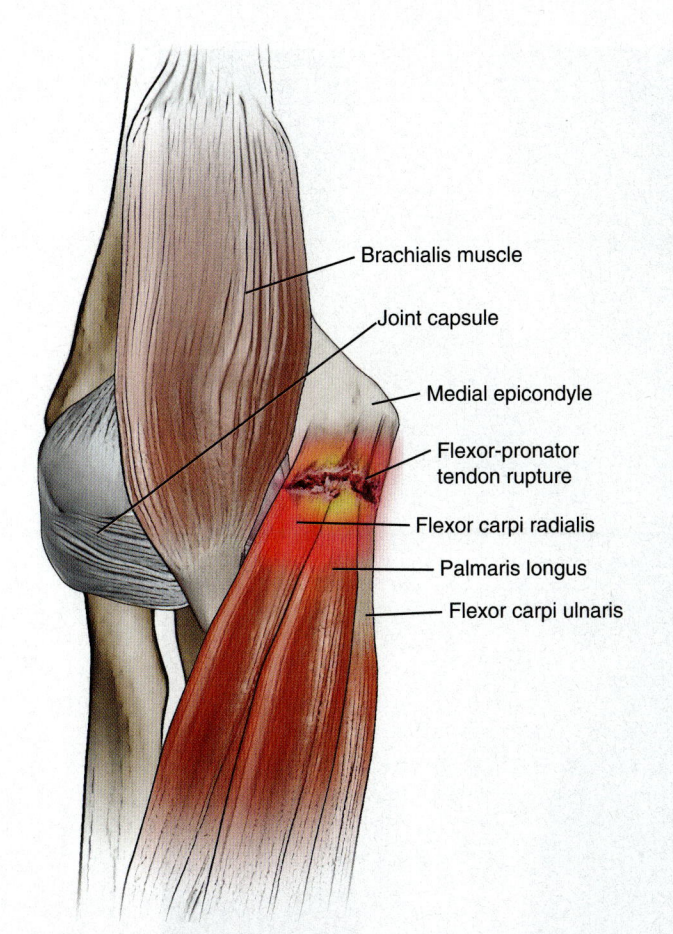

**FIGURE 55.2.** If golfer's elbow remains untreated, complete rupture of the flexor tendons can occur.

## ULTRASOUND-GUIDED TECHNIQUE

The benefits, risks, and alternative treatments are explained to the patient, and informed consent is obtained. The patient is then placed in the supine position with the arm extended at the patient's side and the palm facing up (Fig. 55.5). With the patient in the above position, the medial epicondyle is identified and the point of maximal tenderness is then isolated by careful palpation (Fig. 55.6). A high-frequency linear ultrasound transducer is then placed in a longitudinal position over the medial epicondyle at the point of maximal tenderness (Fig. 55.7). The oval egg-shaped hyperechoic curve of the medial epicondyle and the overlying common flexor tendon insertions attaching to the medial epicondyle are then identified (Fig. 55.8). The trochlea will be seen as a hyperechoic line gently sloping away from the medial epicondyle toward the ulna (see Fig. 55.8). The area of flexor tendinous insertions on the medial epicondyle is identified and evaluated for tears, which will appear as hypoechoic areas within the substance of the tendon. The ultrasound transducer is then slowly moved proximally so that the gentle hyperechoic slope of the medial epicondyle and the overlying common flexor tendon insertions are at the bottom of the ultrasound image to minimize the distance the needle has to travel to reach its target (Fig. 55.9). The skin overlying the area beneath the ultrasound transducer is then prepped with antiseptic solution. A sterile syringe containing 4.0 mL of 0.25% preservative-free bupivacaine and 40 mg of methylprednisolone is attached to a 1½-inch, 22-gauge needle using strict aseptic technique. The needle is placed through the skin ~1.0 cm below the inferior aspect of the ultrasound transducer and is

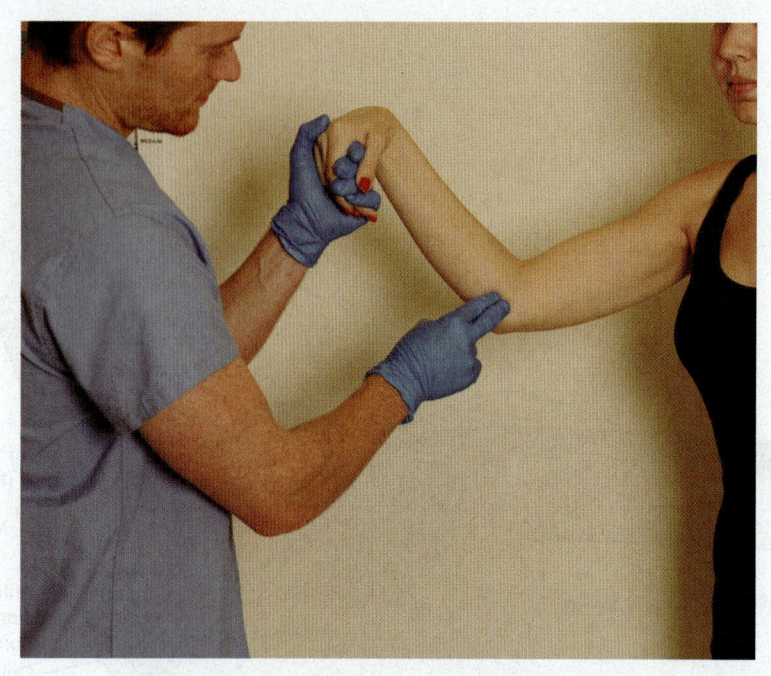

**FIGURE 55.3.** The golfer's elbow test is performed by stabilizing the patient's forearm and then having the patient clench his or her fist and actively flex the wrist. The examiner then attempts to force the wrist into extension. Sudden, severe pain is highly suggestive of golfer's elbow.

**FIGURE 55.4.** Plain radiograph of the elbow demonstrating an avulsion fracture of the medial epicondyle (*arrow*). (From Yochum TR, Rowe LJ. *Yochum and Rowe's Essentials of Skeletal Radiology.* 3rd ed. Philadelphia, PA: Lippincott Williams & Wilkins; 2004, with permission.)

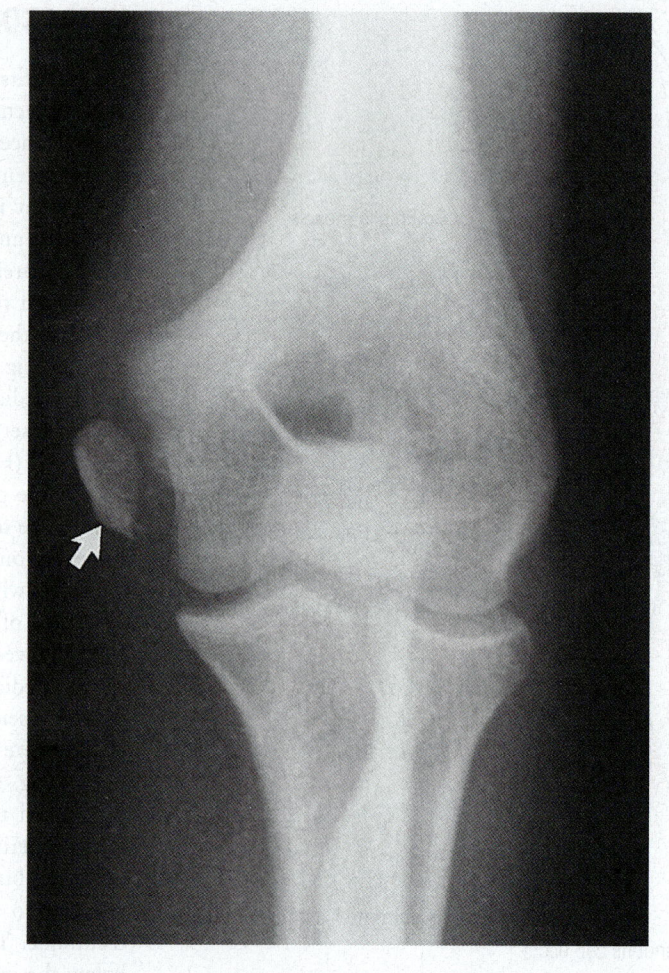

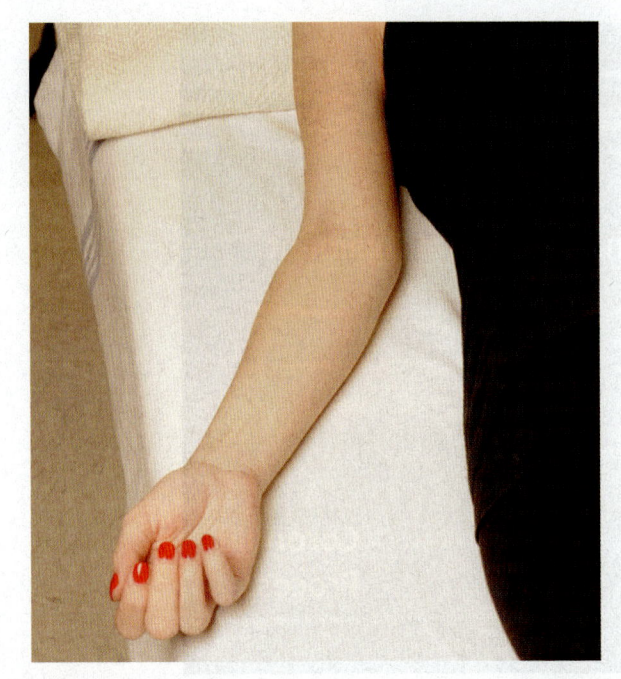

**FIGURE 55.5.** Proper patient position for ultrasound-guided injection for golfer's elbow.

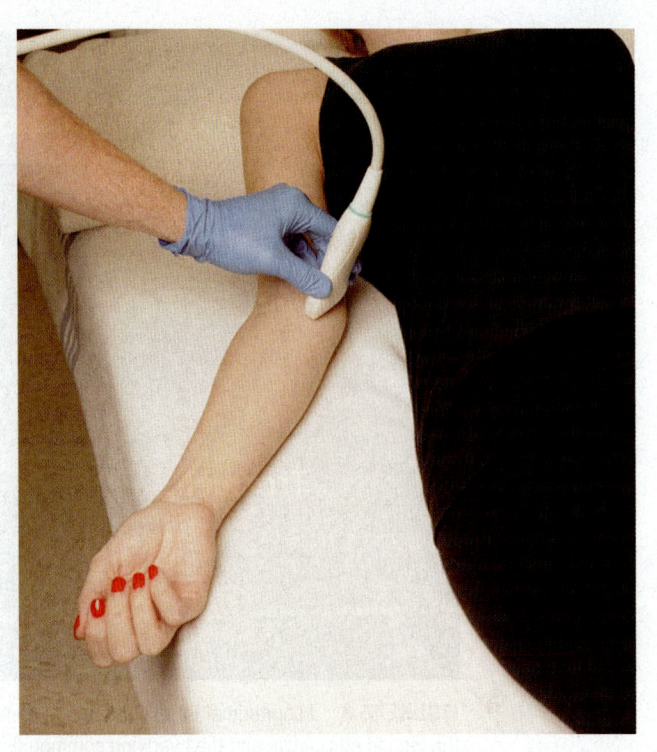

**FIGURE 55.7.** Proper longitudinal position for the linear high-frequency ultrasound transducer to perform ultrasound-guided injection for golfer's elbow.

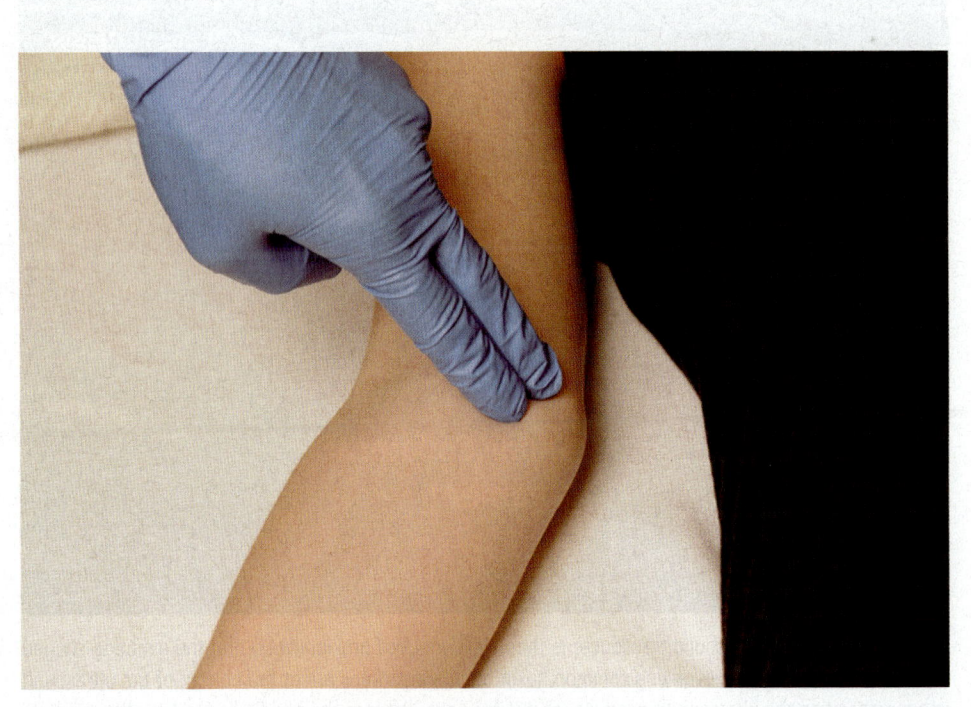

**FIGURE 55.6.** Palpation of the medial epicondyle of the elbow.

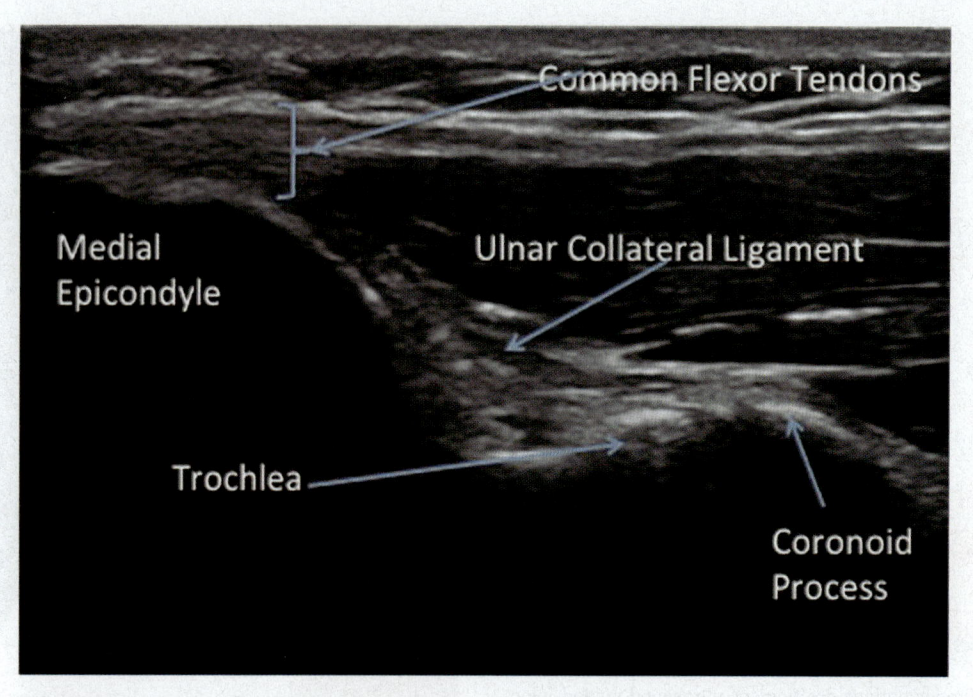

**FIGURE 55.8.** Longitudinal ultrasound image demonstrating the oval egg-shaped hyperechoic curve of the medial epicondyle and the overlying common flexor tendon insertions attaching to the medial epicondyle. The trochlea is seen as a hyperechoic line gently sloping away from the medial epicondyle toward the ulna.

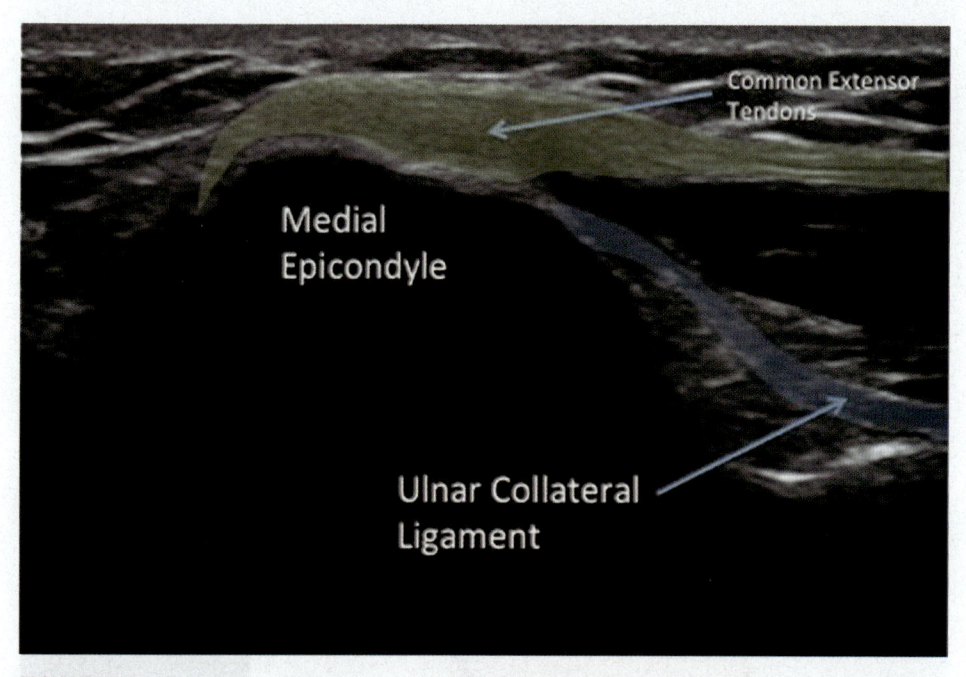

**FIGURE 55.9.** The ultrasound transducer is then slowly moved proximally so that the oval egg-shaped medial epicondyle and the overlying common flexor tendon insertions are at the bottom of the ultrasound image to position the ultrasound transducer to minimize the distance the needle has to travel to reach its target.

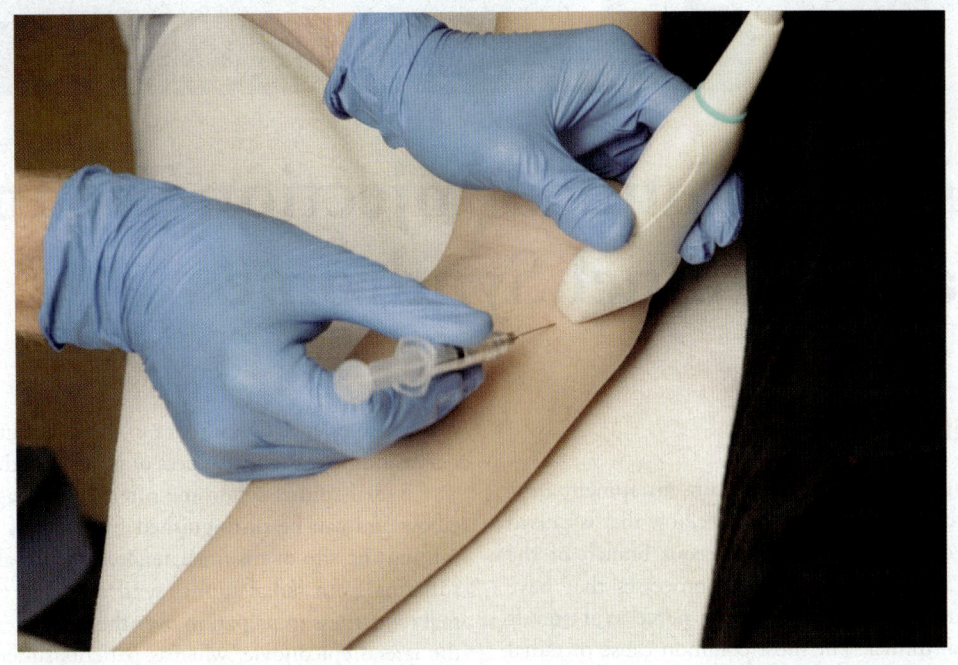

**FIGURE 55.10.** Proper needle placement for ultrasound-guided golfer's elbow injection.

then advanced using an in-plane approach with the needle trajectory adjusted under real-time ultrasound guidance so that the needle tip ultimately rests in proximity, but not in the substance of the tendinous insertions (Fig. 55.10). When the tip of needle is thought to be in satisfactory position, after careful aspiration, a small amount of local anesthetic and steroid is injected under real-time ultrasound guidance to confirm that the needle tip is in the proper position. After proper needle tip placement is confirmed, the remainder of the contents of the syringe are slowly injected under real-time ultrasound guidance with the needle being adjusted so that the entire area of the tendon insertion is treated. There should be minimal resistance to injection.

## COMPLICATIONS

The major complications of ultrasound-guided injection of ultrasound-guided golfer's elbow are related to improper needle placement with the possibility of inadvertent rupture of already compromised flexor tendons. Improper needle placement can result in trauma to the ulnar or radial nerve with the potential for persistent paresthesia. Although rare, infection may occur. Ecchymosis and hematoma formation following this procedure may also occur. These complications can be decreased if manual pressure is applied to the area of the block immediately after injection. Application of cold packs for 20-minute periods after the block will also decrease the amount of postprocedure pain and bleeding the patient may experience. Approximately 25% of patients complain of a transient increase in pain after this injection technique; the patient should be warned of this.

## CLINICAL PEARLS

Ultrasound-guided injection for golfer's elbow is a straightforward and relatively safe technique if attention is paid to the clinically relevant anatomy. In addition to injection of local anesthetics and steroids, investigators have also advocated the injection of botulinum toxin and platelet-rich plasma to treat golfer's elbow. Because of the proximity of the ulnar nerve, it is subject to trauma when performing this injection procedure. For this reason, careful neurologic examination to identify preexisting neurologic deficits that may later be attributed to the nerve block should be performed on all patients before performing ultrasound-guided injection for golfer's elbow.

## SUGGESTED READINGS

Waldman SD. Radial tunnel syndrome. In: *Atlas of Uncommon Pain Syndromes*. 2nd ed. Philadelphia, PA: WB Saunders; 2008:102–103.

Waldman SD. Functional anatomy of the elbow joint. In: *Pain Review*. Philadelphia, PA: Saunders Elsevier; 2009:90–94.

Waldman SD. The Golfer's elbow test. In: *Physical Diagnosis of Pain. An Atlas of Signs and Symptoms*. 2nd ed. Philadelphia, PA: WB Saunders; 2010:132.

Waldman SD. Golfer's Elbow. In: *Atlas of Common Pain Syndromes*. 3rd ed. Philadelphia, PA: WB Saunders; 2012:126–128.

Waldman SD. Medial epicondylitis injection. In: *Atlas of Pain Management Injection Techniques*. 3rd ed. Philadelphia, PA: WB Saunders; 2013:148–152.

# CHAPTER 56

# Ultrasound-Guided Injection Technique for Radial Tunnel Syndrome

## CLINICAL PERSPECTIVES

Radial tunnel syndrome is an uncommon entrapment neuropathy of the radial nerve just below the elbow that is caused by compression of the posterior interosseous branch of the radial nerve by a variety of pathologic processes that have in common their ability to compress the nerve as it travels through the radial tunnel. The most common cause of radial tunnel syndrome is the sharp proximal tendinous margin of the supinator muscle, which is known as the arcade of Frohse (Fig. 56.1). Other pathologic processes that have been implicated in the development of radial tunnel syndrome include anomalous radial recurrent blood vessels that compress the nerve, ganglion cysts, an aberrant aponeurotic band that runs anterior to the radial head, and the sharp tendinous margin of the extensor carpi radialis brevis. These abnormalities may work alone or together to compromise the radial nerve at this anatomic location (Fig. 56.1). Patients suffering from radial tunnel syndrome will experience pain and dysesthesias radiating from the site of compression to the area just below the lateral epicondyle of the humerus. The onset of radial tunnel syndrome can be acute following twisting injuries to the elbow or as a result of direct trauma to the area overlying the radial tunnel. More commonly, the onset of radial tunnel syndrome is insidious and is usually the result of misuse of overuse of the elbow joint and proximal forearm from repetitive pronation and supination. Radial tunnel syndrome has been reported in orchestra conductors, Frisbee players, and swimmers. If this entrapment neuropathy is not treated, pain and functional disability may become more severe, and, ultimately, permanent weakness of the finger extensors and radial deviation of the wrist on extension may result.

Physical findings in patients suffering from radial tunnel syndrome will exhibit weakness of the finger extensors and radial deviation on wrist extension. A Tinel sign will be present at the point where the radial nerve passes through the radial tunnel and the nerve will be tender to palpation. Patients suffering from radial tunnel syndrome exhibit pain on active resisted supination of the forearm and a positive radial tunnel compression test. The radial tunnel compression test is performed by tightly compressing the area over the radial tunnel for 30 seconds (Fig. 56.2). The test is considered positive if the patient experience dysesthesias in the distribution of the radial nerve and increasing weakness of grip strength.

Radial tunnel syndrome often is misdiagnosed as tennis elbow and can be distinguished from tennis elbow by determining the site of maximal tenderness to palpation. Patients suffering from radial tunnel syndrome will experience maximal tenderness to palpation over the radial nerve 1 inch below the lateral epicondyle, whereas patients suffering from tennis elbow will experience maximal tenderness to palpation that is directly over the lateral epicondyle. Radial tunnel syndrome also should be differentiated from C7 cervical radiculopathy. Furthermore, it should be remembered that cervical radiculopathy and radial nerve entrapment may coexist as the so-called "double crush" syndrome. The double crush syndrome is seen most commonly with median nerve entrapment at the wrist or with carpal tunnel syndrome but has been reported with the radial nerve.

Electromyography and nerve conduction velocity testing are useful in helping in the differentiation of radial tunnel syndrome from cervical radiculopathy and golfer's elbow. Plain radiographs, ultrasound imaging, and magnetic resonance imaging are indicated in all patients who present with radial tunnel syndrome in order to rule out occult bony pathology and to identify occult fractures, masses, or tumors that may be responsible for compromise of the radial nerve (Fig. 56.3). Based on the patient's clinical presentation, additional testing may be indicated, including complete blood count, uric acid, sedimentation rate, and antinuclear antibody testing. The ultrasound-guided injection technique described below serves as both a diagnostic and therapeutic maneuver.

## CLINICALLY RELEVANT ANATOMY

The key landmark when performing ultrasound-guided radial nerve block at the elbow is the point at which the radial nerve is just below the point within the substance of the brachioradialis muscle where the radial nerve bifurcates (Fig. 50.4). Arising from fibers from the C5–T1 nerve roots of the posterior cord of the brachial plexus, the radial nerve passes through the axilla lying posterior and inferior to the axillary artery. As the radial nerve exits the axilla, it passes between the medial and long

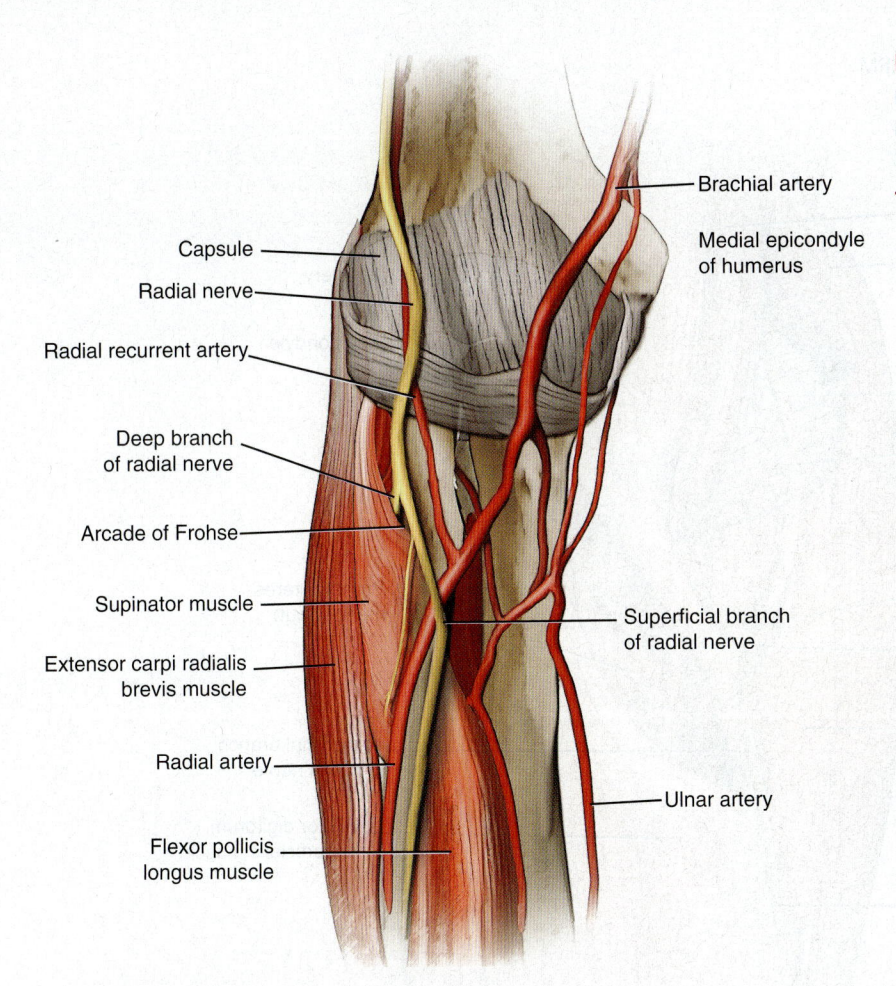

**FIGURE 56.1.** The most common cause of radial tunnel syndrome is an entrapment of the radial nerve as it passes beneath the arcade of Frohse radial tunnel retinaculum.

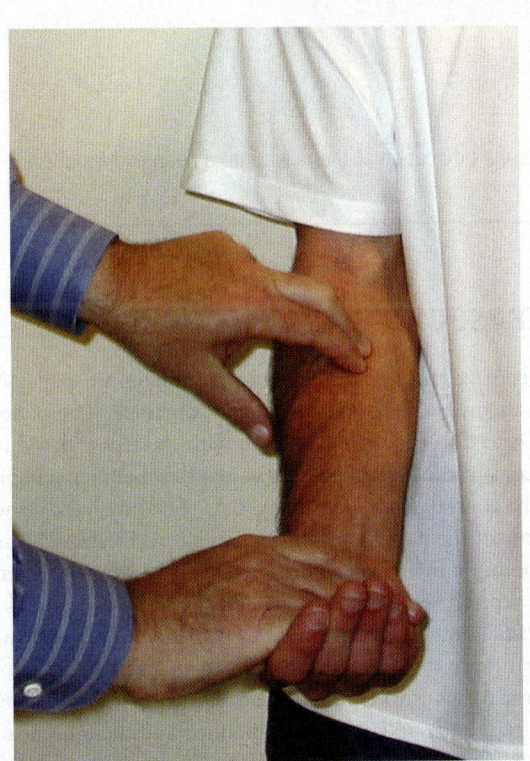

**FIGURE 56.2.** Patients suffering from radial tunnel syndrome will exhibit a positive radial tunnel compression test that is performed by tightly compressing the area over the radial tunnel for 30 seconds. The test is considered positive if the patient experience dysesthesias into the distribution of the radial nerve and increasing weakness of grip strength.

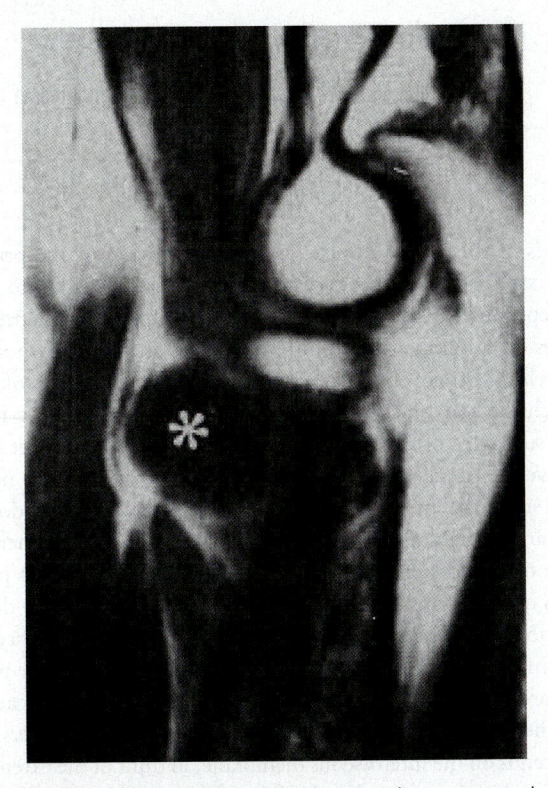

**FIGURE 56.3.** Sagittal T1-weighted magnetic resonance image showing a bursal mass (*asterisk*) at the level of the posterior interosseous nerve causing compression of the nerve.

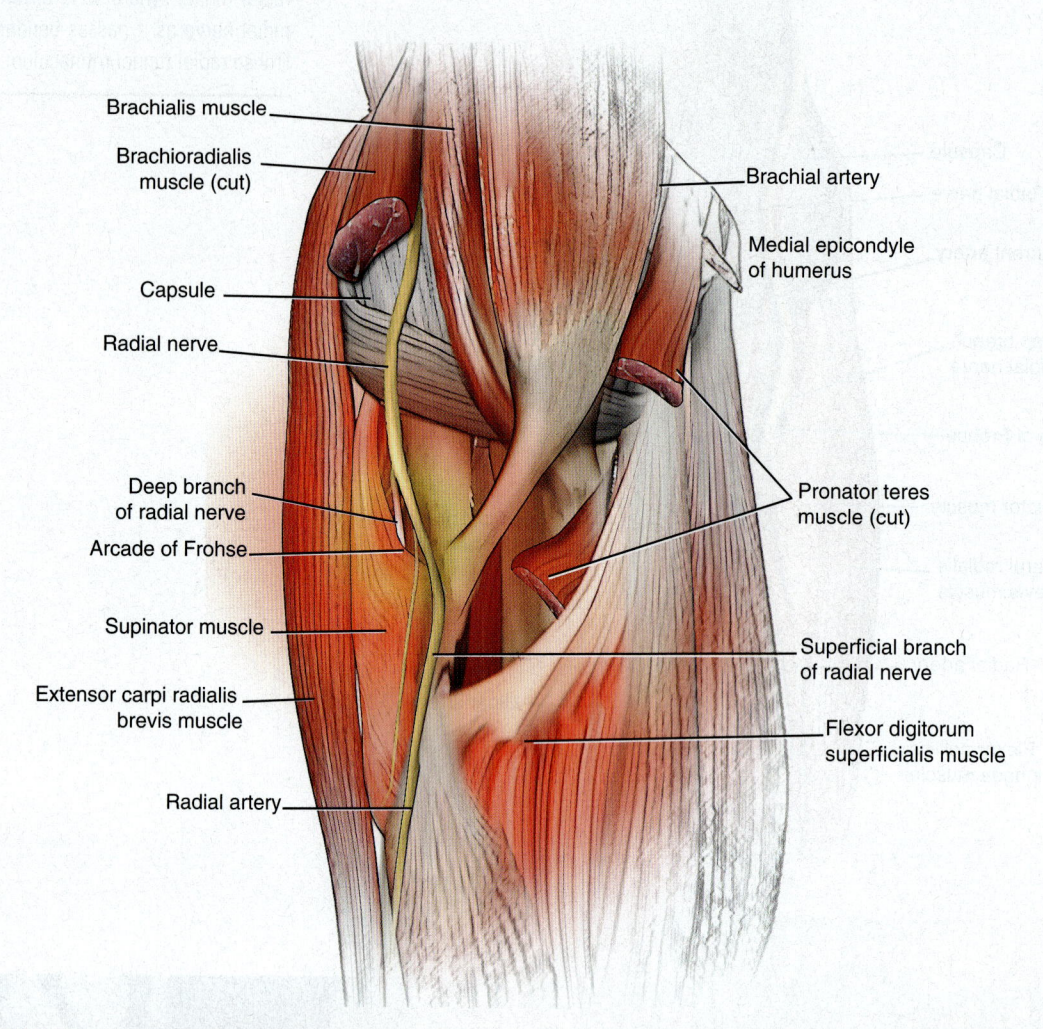

**FIGURE 56.4.** The anatomy of the radial nerve at the elbow. Note the bifurcation of the nerve into a deep and superficial branch.

heads of the triceps muscle and then curves across the posterior aspect of the humerus, giving off a motor branch to the triceps muscle. Continuing its downward path, the radial nerve gives off a number of sensory branches to the upper arm as it travels in the intermuscular septum separating the bellies of the brachialis and brachioradialis muscles. The nerve passes into the substance of the brachioradialis muscle, and at a point just above the lateral epicondyle, the radial nerve divides into deep and superficial branches; the superficial branch continues down the arm along with the radial artery to provide sensory innervation to the dorsum of the wrist and the dorsal aspects of a portion of the thumb and index and middle fingers, and the deep branch crosses the supinator muscle to provide the majority of the motor innervation to the extensors of the forearm. The posterior interosseous nerve is the continuation of the deep branch of the radial nerve, which contains terminal motor fibers. It descends on the interosseous membrane, in front of the extensor pollicis longus, to the dorsal aspect of the carpal bones where it sends off fibers to supply the finger and thumb extensors, extensor carpi ulnaris, and the abductor pollicis longus region.

## ULTRASOUND-GUIDED TECHNIQUE

The benefits, risks, and alternative treatments are explained to the patient, and informed consent is obtained. The patient is then placed in the sitting position with the elbow flexed to 90 degrees and the forearm resting across the abdomen and grasping the contralateral flank (Fig. 56.5). The physician stands at the side of the patient. With the patient in the above position, at a point ~4 inches above the lateral epicondyle, the intermuscular septum separating the bellies of the brachialis and brachioradialis muscles is identified by palpation. A high-frequency linear ultrasound transducer is placed in a transverse position over the previously identified intermuscular septum (Fig. 56.6). An ultrasound survey image is obtained and the intermuscular septum separating the bellies of the brachialis and brachioradialis muscles and the radial nerve is identified (Fig. 56.7). The ultrasound transducer is turned to the longitudinal plane, and the path of the radial nerve is traced distally until the bifurcation of the nerve is identified (Figs. 56.8 and 56.9). Once the bifurcation of the nerve is identified, the ultrasound transducer

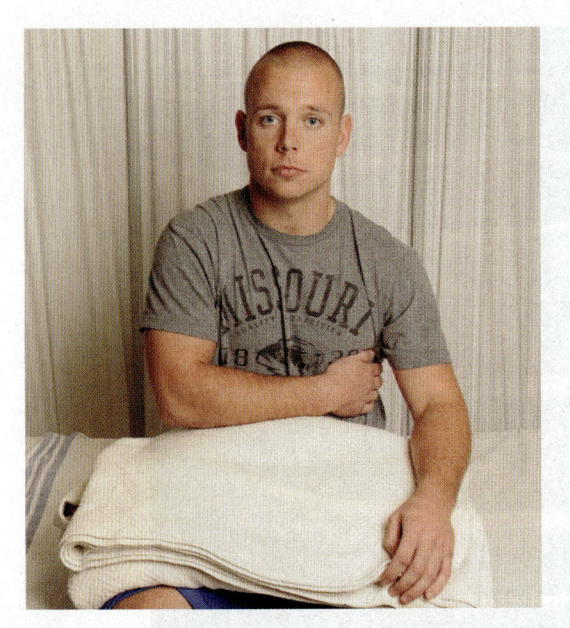

**FIGURE 56.5.** Proper position for ultrasound-guided injection for radial tunnel syndrome.

is turned back to the transverse position, and the superficial and deep nerves will begin to separate appearing on transverse ultrasound scan as two eyes behind spectacles (Fig. 56.10). The deep branch is then followed distally until it penetrated the supinator muscle and becomes the posterior interosseous branch. It is at this point that the nerve is blocked. Color Doppler is then used to identify any adjacent blood vessels that might be injured during the injection procedure (Fig. 56.11).

After the posterior interosseous branch of the radial nerve has been identified and evaluated, the skin overlying the area beneath the ultrasound transducer is then prepped with antiseptic solution. A sterile syringe containing 2.0 mL of 0.25% preservative-free bupivacaine and 40 mg of methylprednisolone is attached to a 1½-inch, 22-gauge needle using strict aseptic technique. The needle is placed through the skin ~1.0 cm above the center of the ultrasound transducer and is then advanced using an out-of-plane approach with the needle trajectory adjusted under real-time ultrasound guidance so that the needle tip ultimately rests in proximity, but not in contact with the radial nerve (Fig. 56.12). When the tip of needle is thought to be in satisfactory position, after careful aspiration, a small amount of local anesthetic and steroid is injected under real-time ultrasound guidance to confirm that the needle tip is in the proper position. After proper needle tip placement is confirmed, the remainder of the contents of the syringe is slowly injected under real-time ultrasound guidance to insure that the injectate is not further compressing and compromising the radial nerve with the confines of the radial tunnel. There should be minimal resistance to injection.

## COMPLICATIONS

The major complications of ultrasound-guided injection of ultrasound-guided radial tunnel syndrome are related to improper needle placement with the possibility of inadvertent intravascular injection and/or persistent paresthesia secondary to needle trauma to the radial nerve. Although rare, infection may occur. Ecchymosis and hematoma formation following this

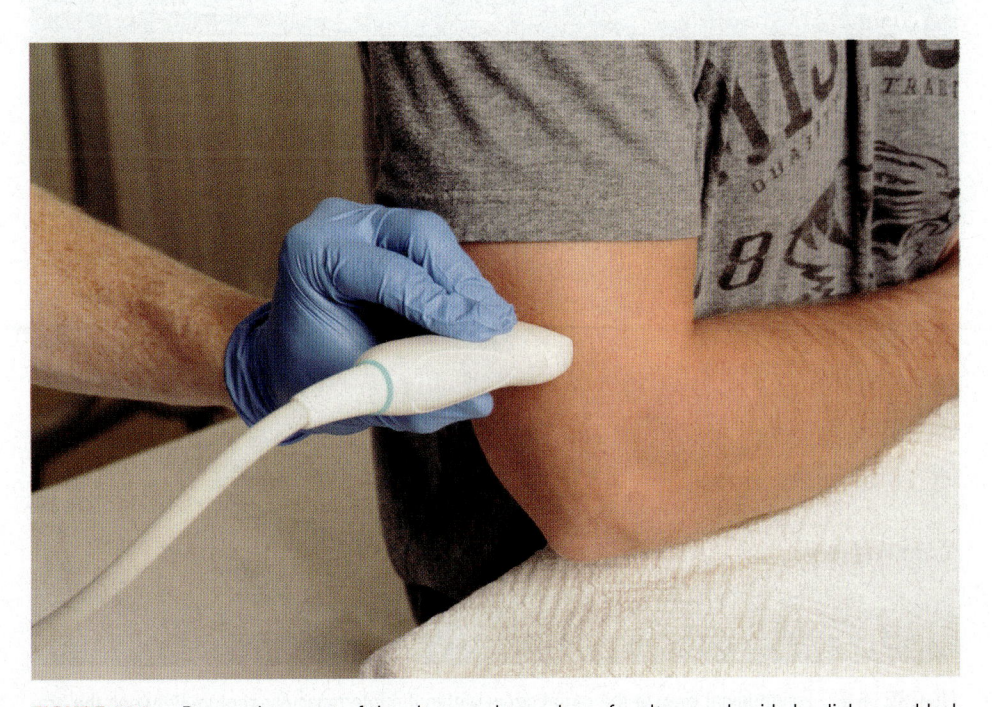

**FIGURE 56.6.** Proper placement of the ultrasound transducer for ultrasound-guided radial nerve block at the elbow.

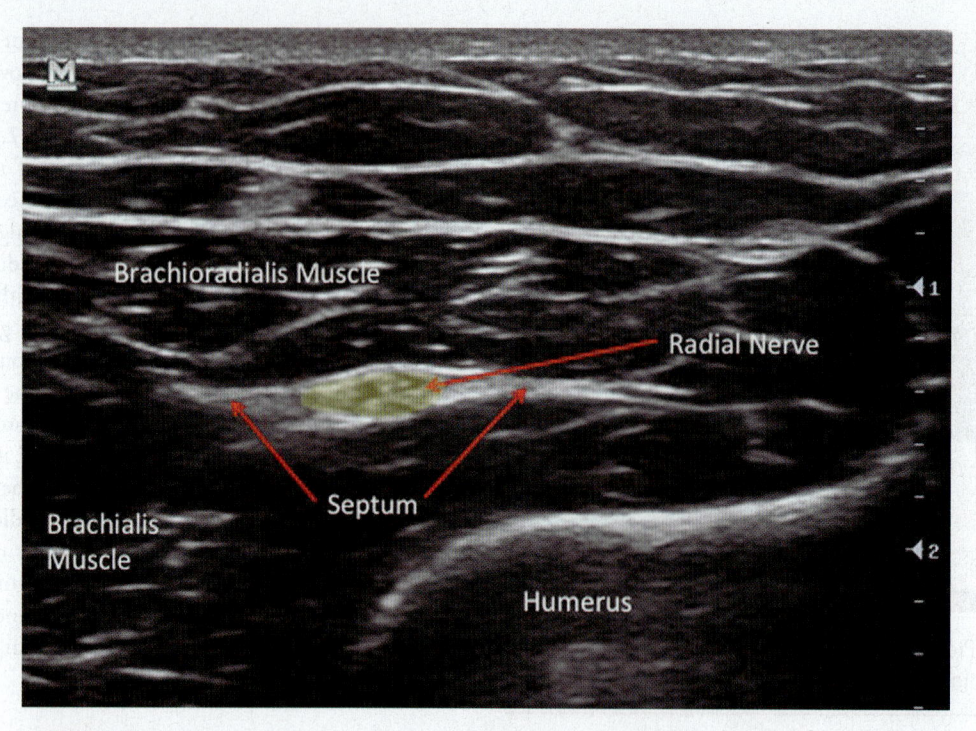

**FIGURE 56.7.** Transverse ultrasound view of the intermuscular septum between the brachioradialis and brachial muscles with the radial nerve nestled between.

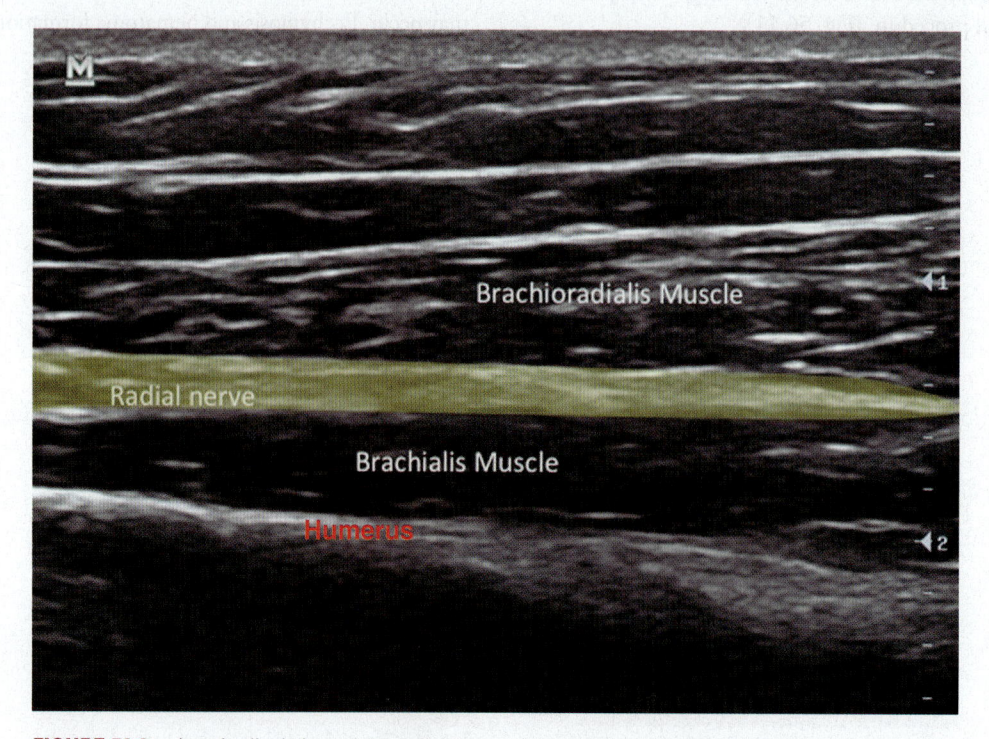

**FIGURE 56.8.** Longitudinal view of the radial nerve within the intermuscular septum between the brachioradialis and brachialis muscles.

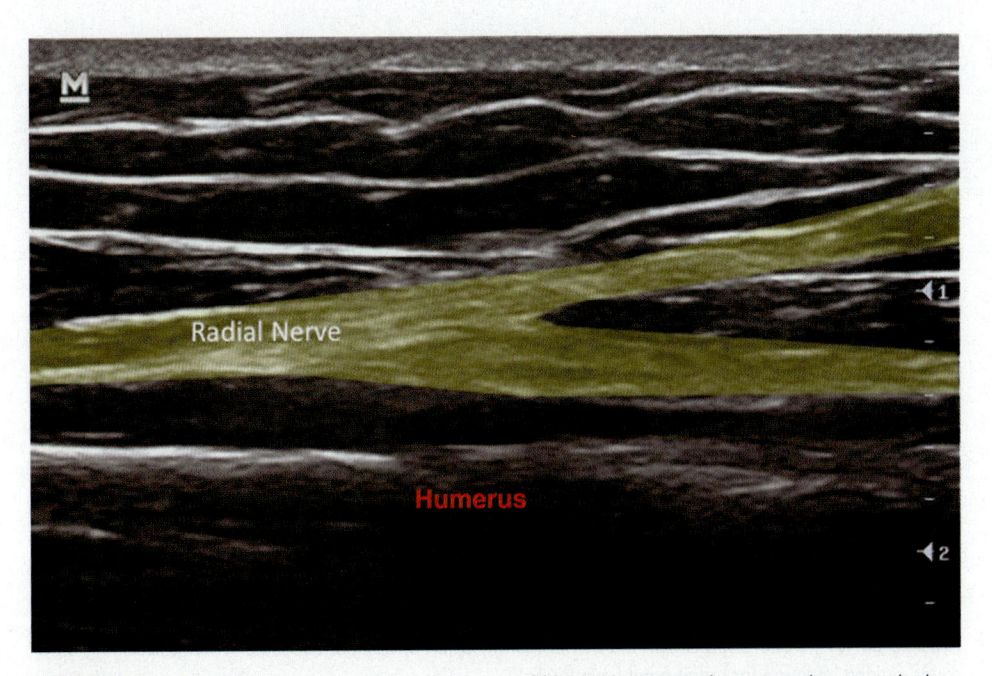

**FIGURE 56.9.** Longitudinal view of the radial nerve within the intermuscular septum between the brachioradialis and brachialis muscles.

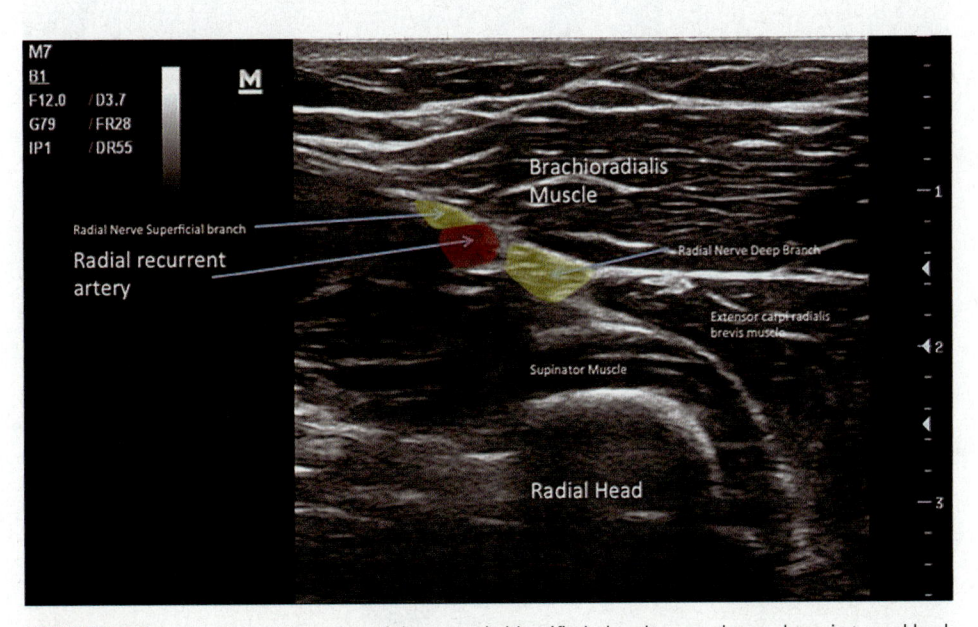

**FIGURE 56.10.** Once the bifurcation of the nerve is identified, the ultrasound transducer is turned back to the transverse position, and the superficial and deep nerves will begin to separate appearing on transverse ultrasound scan as two eyes behind spectacles.

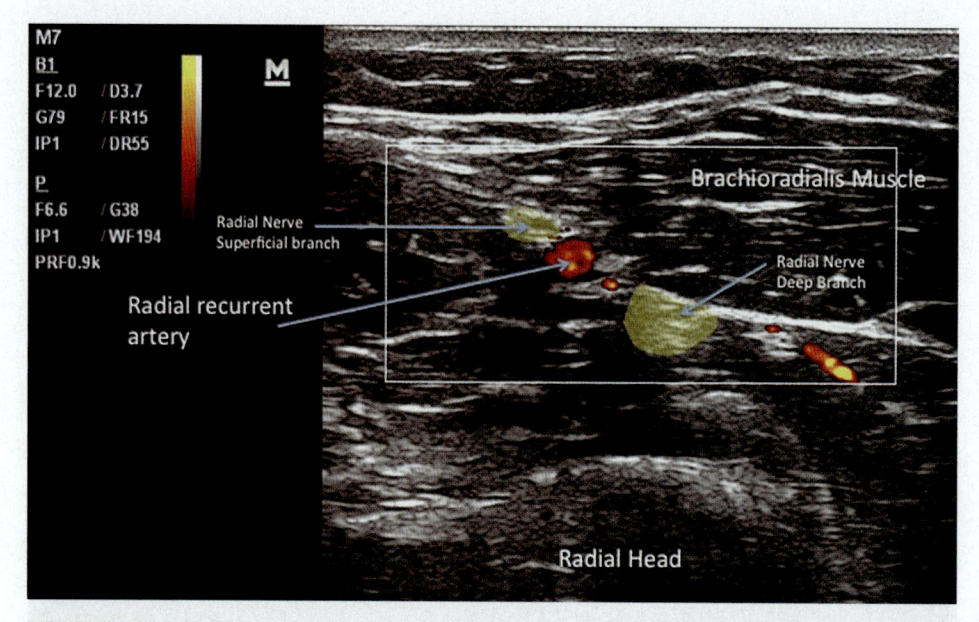

**FIGURE 56.11.** Color Doppler will aid in the identification of adjacent vessels when performing ultrasound-guided injection for radial tunnel syndrome.

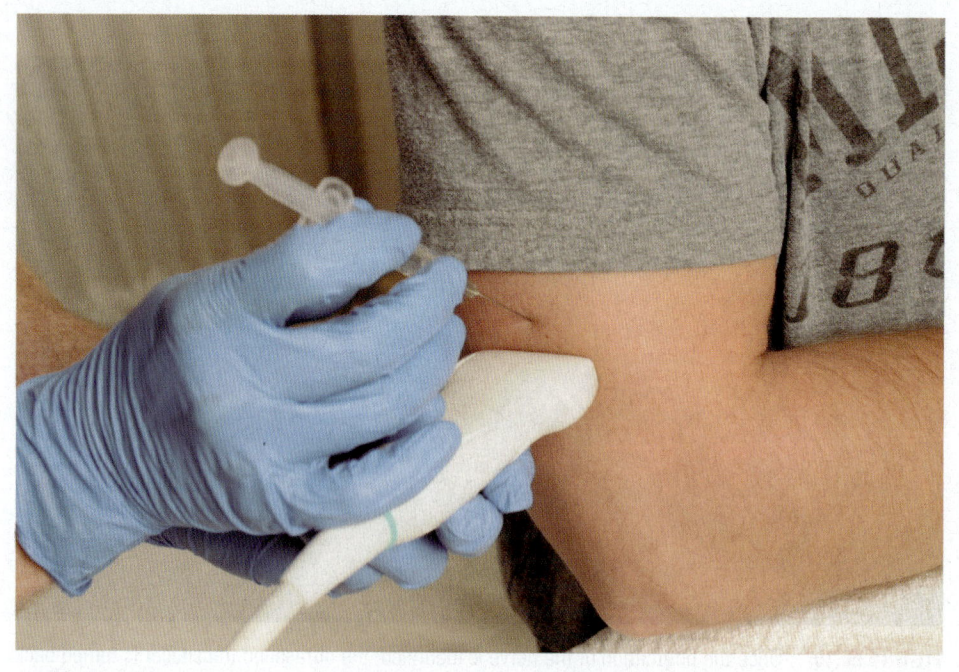

**FIGURE 56.12.** Proper out-of-plane needle position for ultrasound-guided injection for radial tunnel syndrome.

procedure may also occur. These complications can be decreased if manual pressure is applied to the area of the block immediately after injection. Application of cold packs for 20-minute periods after the block will also decrease the amount of postprocedure pain and bleeding the patient may experience. Approximately 25% of patients complain of a transient increase in pain after this injection technique; the patient should be warned of this.

## CLINICAL PEARLS

Ultrasound-guided injection for radial tunnel syndrome is a straightforward and relatively safe technique if attention is paid to the clinically relevant anatomy. Because of the potential for persistent neurologic deficits to occur in patients suffering from radial tunnel syndrome, a careful neurologic examination to identify preexisting neurologic deficits that may later be attributed to the nerve block should be performed on all patients before beginning injection for radial tunnel syndrome.

## SUGGESTED READINGS

Lee JT, Azari K, Jones NF. Long term results of radial tunnel release—the effect of co-existing tennis elbow, multiple compression syndromes and workers' compensation. *J Plast Reconstr Aesthet Surg* 2008;61(9):1095–1099.

Toussaint CP, Zager EL. What's new in common upper extremity entrapment neuropathies. *Neurosurg Clin N Am* 2008;19(4):573–581.

Waldman SD. Radial tunnel syndrome. In: *Atlas of Uncommon Pain Syndromes*. 2nd ed. Philadelphia, PA: WB Saunders; 2008:102–110.

Waldman SD. The radial nerve. In: *Pain Review*. Philadelphia, PA: Saunders Elsevier; 2009:76–77.

CHAPTER 57

# Ultrasound-Guided Injection Technique for Triceps Tendonitis

## CLINICAL PERSPECTIVES

The distal musculotendinous unit of the triceps muscle is subjected to an amazing variation of stresses as it performs its function to allow range of motion of the elbow while at the same time providing elbow stability. The relatively poor blood supply of the distal musculotendinous unit limits the ability of the muscle and tendon to heal when traumatized. Over time, muscle tears and tendinopathy develop, further weakening the musculotendinous unit and making it susceptible to additional damage.

The triceps tendon of the elbow may develop tendonitis after overuse or misuse, especially when performing activities that require repeated flexion and extension of the elbow. Acute triceps tendonitis has been seen in clinical practice with increasing frequency due to the popularity of workouts utilizing exercise machines. Improper stretching of triceps muscle and triceps tendon before exercise has also been implicated in the development of triceps tendonitis as well as acute tendon rupture. Injuries ranging from partial to complete tears of the tendon can occur when the distal tendon sustains direct trauma while it is fully flexed under load or when the elbow is forcibly flexed while the arm is fully extended (Fig. 57.1).

The pain of triceps tendonitis is constant and severe and is localized to the posterior elbow region. The patient suffering from triceps tendonitis often complains of sleep disturbance and is unable to sleep on the affected elbow. Patients with triceps tendonitis exhibit pain with active resisted extension of the elbow. In an effort to decrease pain, patients suffering from triceps tendonitis often splint the inflamed tendon by limiting forearm extension to remove tension from the inflamed tendon. If untreated, patients suffering from triceps tendonitis may experience difficulty in performing any task that requires flexion and extension of the forearm. Over time, if the tendonitis is not treated, muscle atrophy and calcific tendonitis may result, or the muscle may suddenly rupture. Patients who experience complete rupture of the triceps tendon will not be able to fully and forcefully extend the affected arm (Fig. 57.2).

Plain radiographs are indicated in all patients who present with elbow pain (Fig. 57.3). Based on the patient's clinical presentation, additional testing may be indicated, including complete blood cell count, sedimentation rate, and antinuclear antibody testing. Magnetic resonance imaging or ultrasound imaging of the elbow is indicated if triceps tendinopathy or tear is suspected. Magnetic resonance imaging or ultrasound evaluation of the affected area may also help delineate the presence of calcific tendonitis or other elbow pathology.

## CLINICALLY RELEVANT ANATOMY

The triceps brachii muscle is a three-headed muscle that serves as the main extensor of the elbow joint and is the antagonist muscle to the biceps brachii and brachialis muscles (Fig. 57.4). Each of the three heads of the triceps muscle has a different origin. The long head of the triceps finds its origin at the infraglenoid fossa of the scapula and received innervation from the axillary nerve, unlike the rest of the triceps, which is innervated by the radial nerve. The medial head finds its origin at the groove of the radial nerve as well as from the dorsal surface of the humerus, the medial intermuscular septum, and the lateral intermuscular septum. The lateral head finds its origin at the dorsal surface of the humerus at a point lateral and proximal to the grove of the radial nerve as well as the greater tubercle down to the region of the lateral intermuscular septum. The three heads of the triceps muscle coalesce into the dense distal triceps tendon, which inserts onto the olecranon process and the posterior wall of the capsule of the elbow joint (Fig. 57.5). It is at its point of insertion that the distal triceps musculotendinous unit is susceptible to the development of tendonitis, tears, and rupture.

## ULTRASOUND-GUIDED TECHNIQUE

The benefits, risks, and alternative treatments are explained to the patient, and informed consent is obtained. The patient is then placed in the sitting position with the elbow slightly flexed and the hand closed and resting on the exam table (Fig. 57.6). The physician stands or sits at the side of the patient. With the patient in the above position, a high-frequency linear ultrasound transducer is placed in a longitudinal plane with the transducer over the distal triceps tendon and olecranon process, and an ultrasound survey scan is taken (Fig. 57.7). The distal tendon of the triceps muscle is then identified and followed to its insertion on the olecranon process of the ulna (Fig. 57.8). This is the point where triceps tendonitis, tears, and

# CHAPTER 57  ULTRASOUND-GUIDED INJECTION TECHNIQUE FOR TRICEPS TENDONITIS

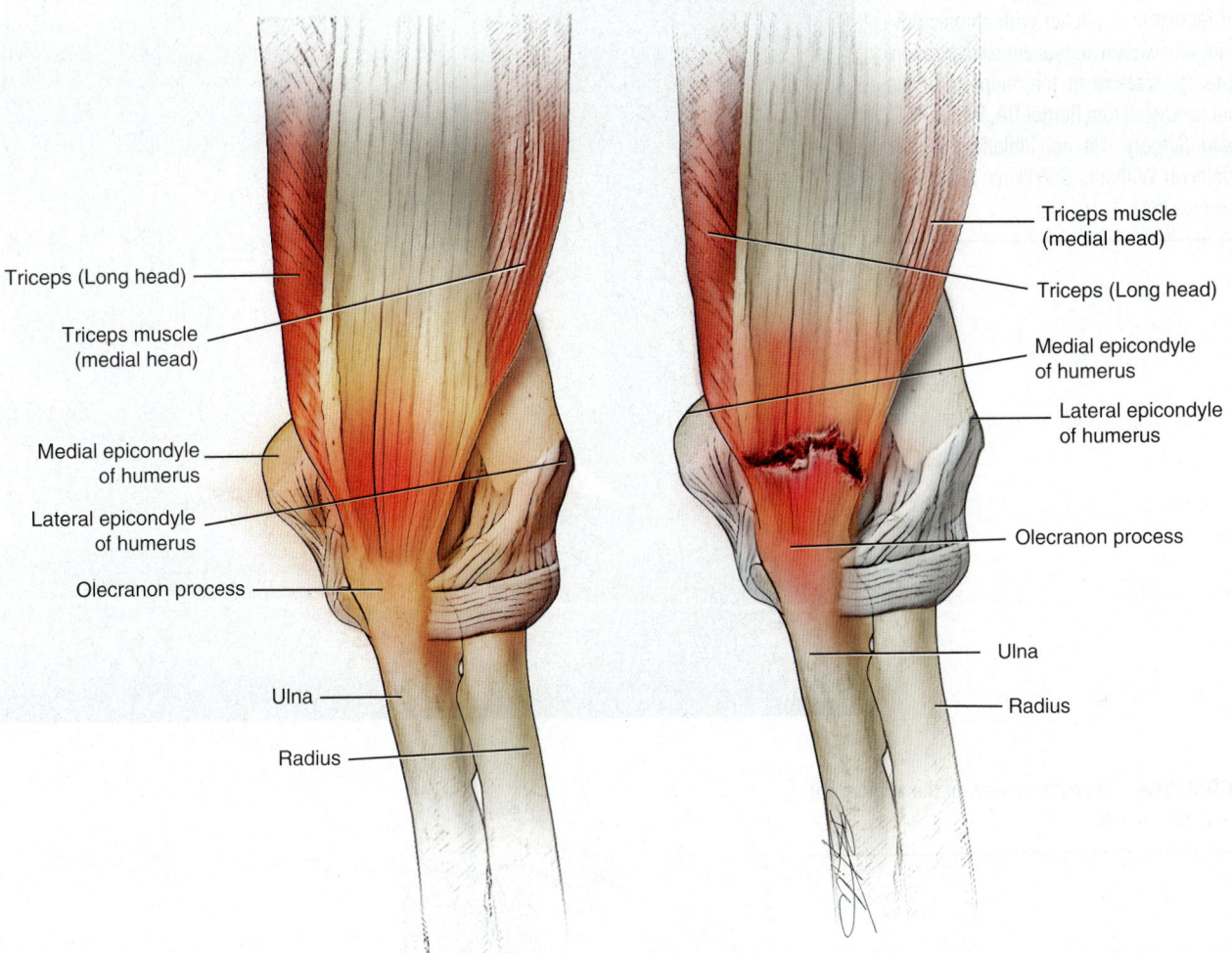

**FIGURE 57.1.** The distal triceps tendinous insertion is subject to the development of tendonitis from overuse or misuse.

**FIGURE 57.2.** If triceps tendonitis remains untreated and the microtrauma responsible for the tendonitis continues, the tendon may suddenly rupture.

rupture most often develop. The tendon should be carefully examined in both the longitudinal and transverse planes for calcifications or tendinopathy that may be contributing to the patient's elbow pain. This is best accomplished by having the patient alternately extend and relax his or her forearm against the examiner's resistance while observing the tendon and its insertion under real-time ultrasound (Fig. 57.9). After the tendon is evaluated and the tendinous insertion is identified, the skin overlying the area beneath the ultrasound transducer is prepped with antiseptic solution. A sterile syringe containing 4.0 mL of 0.25% preservative-free bupivacaine and 40 mg of methylprednisolone is attached to a 1½-inch, 22-gauge needle using strict aseptic technique. The needle is placed through the skin ~1 cm above the superior edge of the transducer and is then advanced using an in-plane approach with the needle trajectory adjusted under real-time ultrasound guidance so that the needle tip rests just above the tendinous insertion on the olecranon process, but not within the tendon substance itself (Fig. 57.10). When the tip of needle is thought to be in satisfactory position, after careful aspiration, a small amount of local anesthetic and steroid is injected under real-time ultrasound guidance to confirm that the needle tip is not with the substance of the tendon. After proper needle tip placement is confirmed, the remainder of the contents of the syringe are slowly injected. There should be minimal resistance to injection. If calcific tendonitis is present, a two-needle ultrasound-guided lavage and aspiration technique may be beneficial.

## COMPLICATIONS

The possibility of trauma to the triceps tendon from this injection technique itself remains an ever-present possibility, although the risk of this is decreased if care is taken to place the needle outside the tendon and the injection is performed under real-time ultrasound visualization. Tendons that are highly inflamed or previously damaged are subject to rupture if substances are injected directly into the tendon. This complication can be greatly decreased if the clinician uses gentle technique and stops injecting immediately if significant resistance

**FIGURE 57.3.** Lateral radiograph that shows a large olecranon spur in a 42-year-old recreational pitcher with chronic posterior elbow pain and recent exacerbation. Note the fracture at the midpoint of the spur (*arrow*). (From Berger RA, Weiss APC. *Hand Surgery*. 1st ed. Philadelphia, PA: Lippincott Williams & Wilkins; 2004, with permission.)

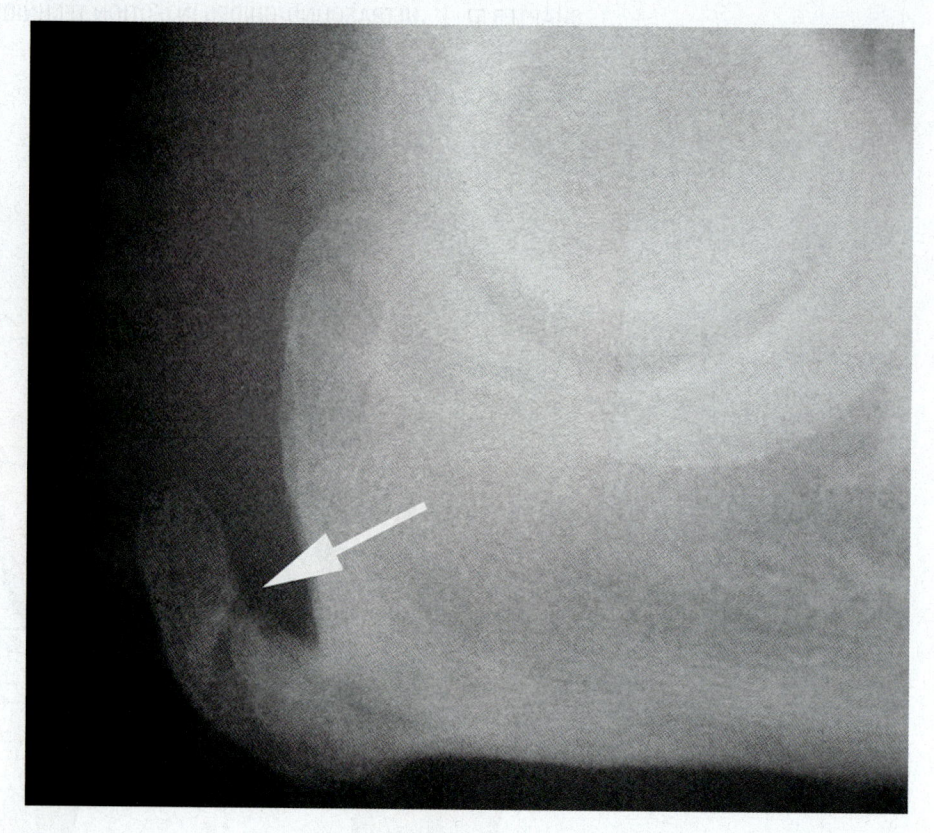

**FIGURE 57.4.** A posterior view of the anatomy of the triceps muscle.

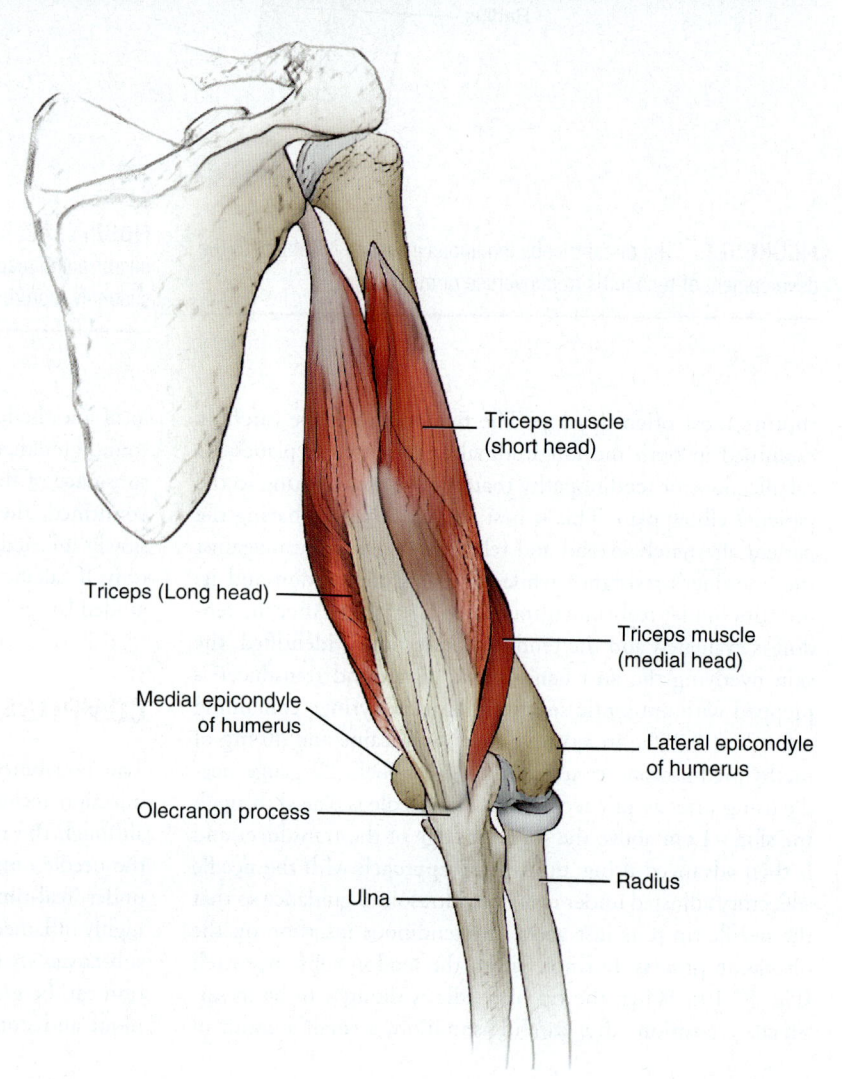

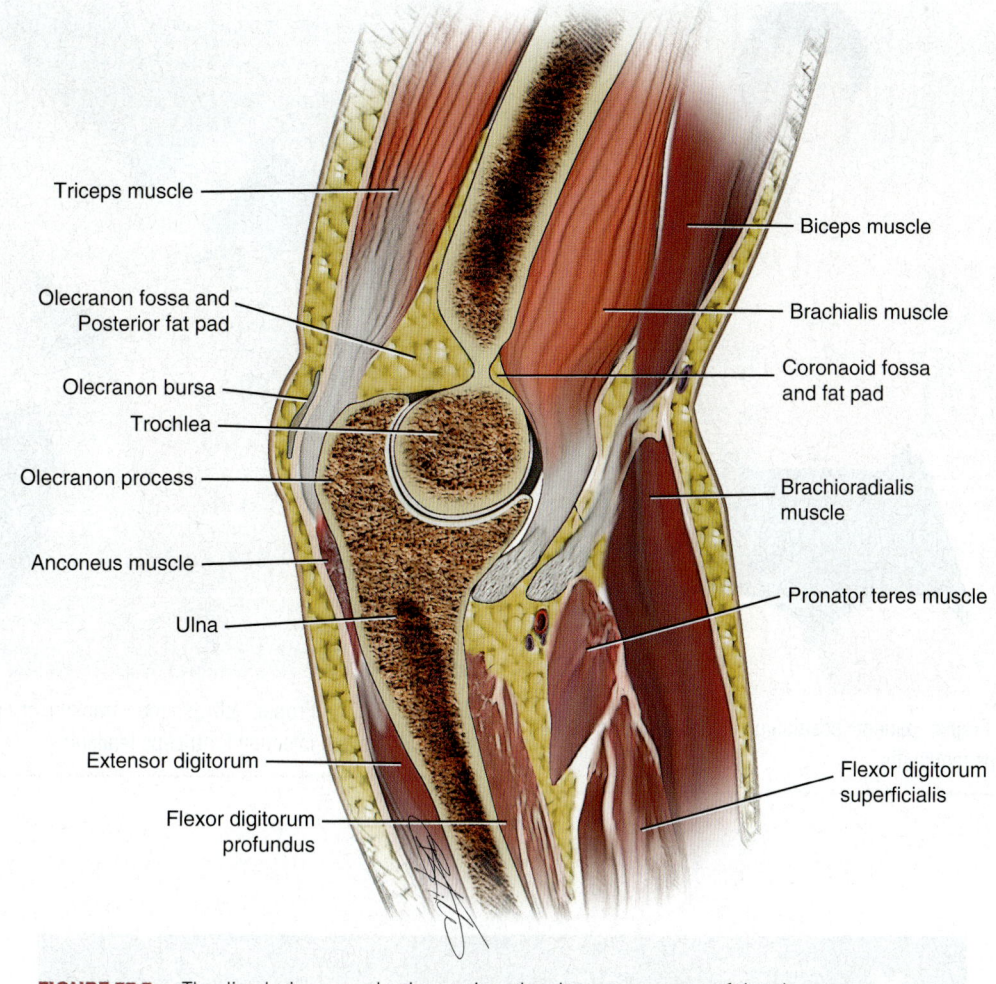

**FIGURE 57.5.** The distal triceps tendon inserts into the olecranon process of the ulna.

to injection is encountered. Approximately 25% of patients complain of a transient increase in pain after this injection technique; the patient should be warned of this. Infection, although uncommon, can occur.

## CLINICAL PEARLS

Elbow pathology including medial and lateral epicondylitis, bursitis, osteoarthritis, avascular necrosis, and entrapment neuropathies may coexist with triceps tendonitis and may contribute to the patient's pain symptomatology. Universal precautions should always be observed to protect the operator, and strict adherence to sterile technique must be used to avoid infection. Gentle physical therapy and local heat should be introduced following ultrasound-guided injection of the distal triceps tendon to reduce pain and improve function. Simple analgesics and nonsteroidal anti-inflammatory agents or COX-2 inhibitors may be used concurrently with this injection technique.

**384** SECTION IV ELBOW AND FOREARM

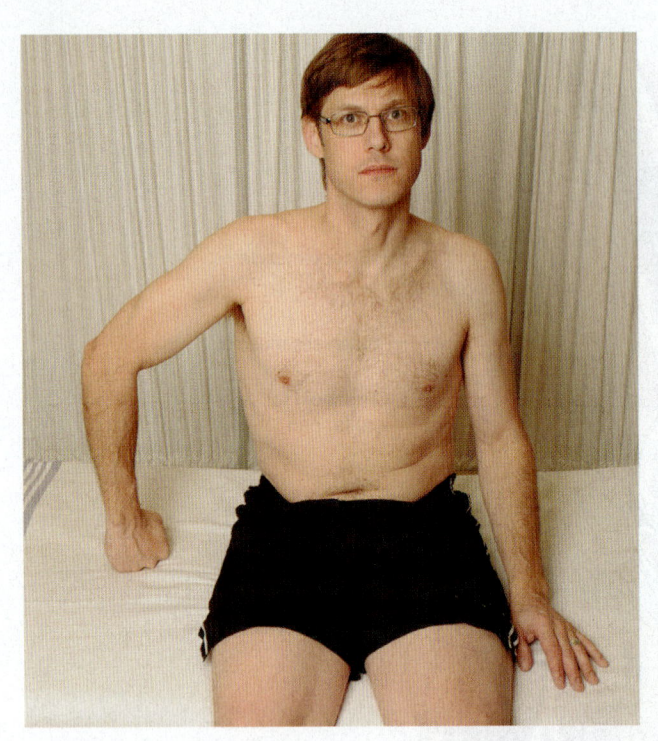

**FIGURE 57.6.** Proper patient positioning for ultrasound-guided injection for triceps tendonitis.

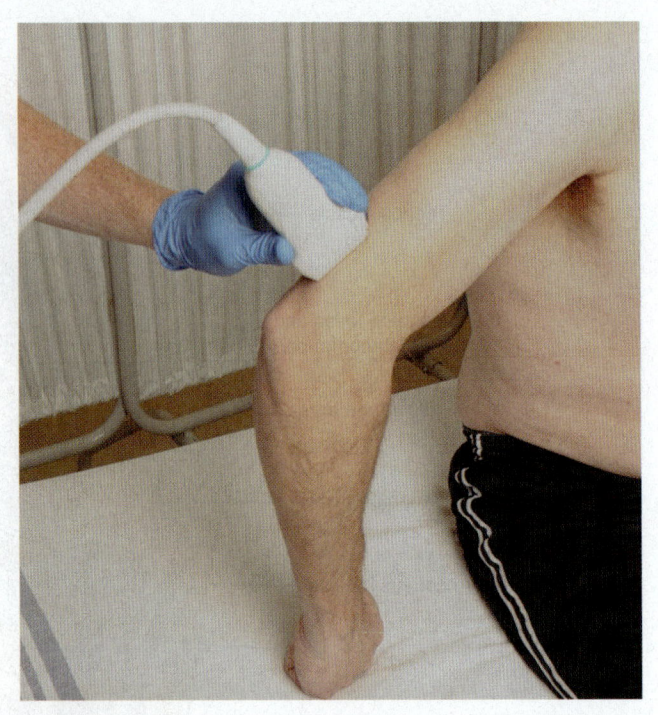

**FIGURE 57.7.** Proper ultrasound transducer placement for ultrasound-guided injection for triceps tendonitis.

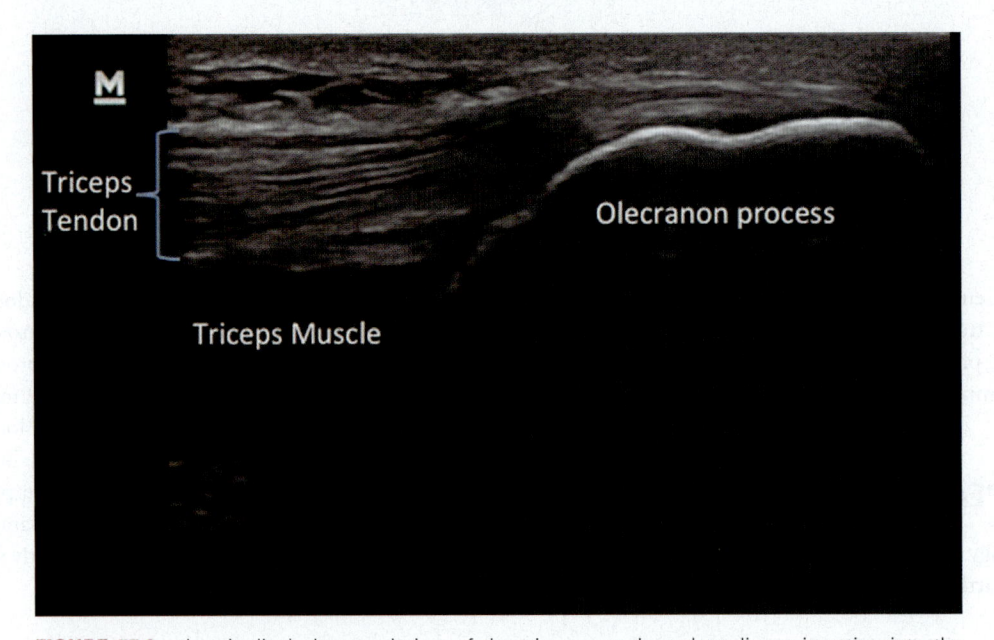

**FIGURE 57.8.** Longitudinal ultrasound view of the triceps muscle and tendinous insertion into the olecranon process.

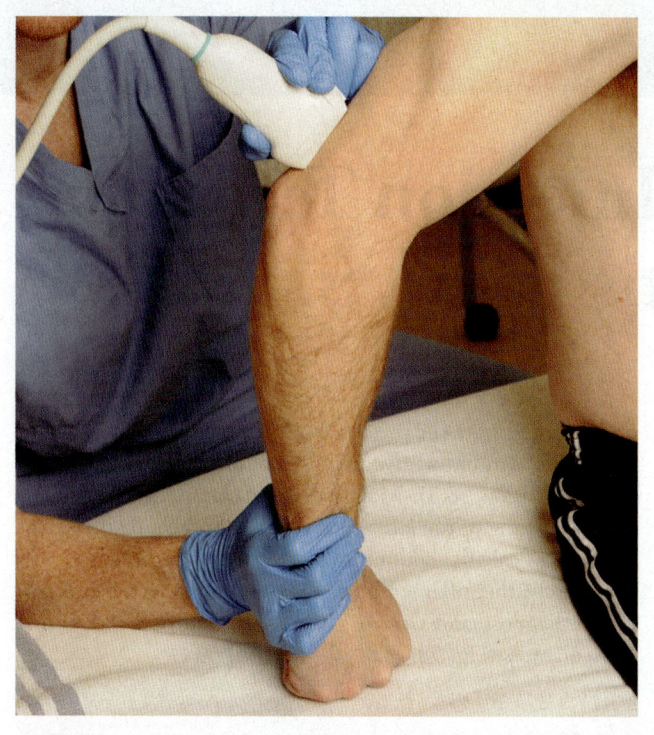

**FIGURE 57.9.** The patient's forearm is stabilized and the patient is then asked to extend his or her arm against resistance to contract the triceps muscle and place tension on the distal musculotendinous unit.

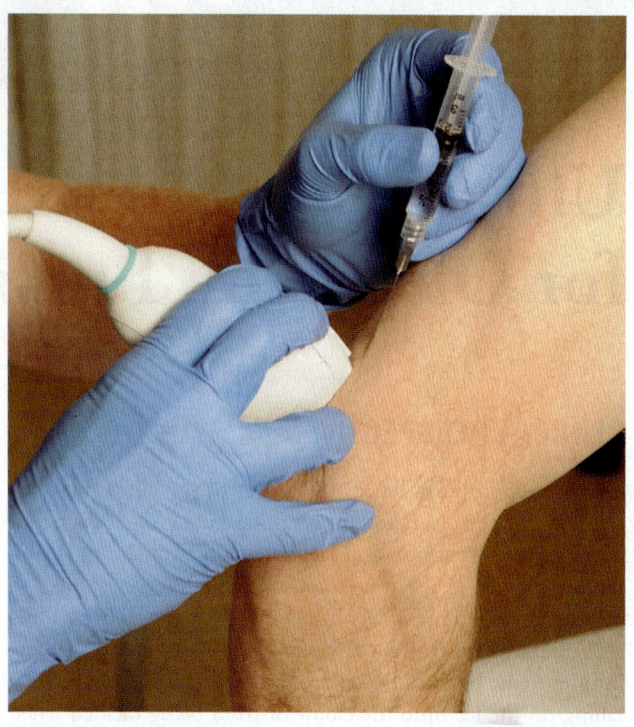

**FIGURE 57.10.** In-plane injection of the distal triceps tendon under ultrasound guidance.

## SUGGESTED READINGS

Gabel GT. Acute and chronic tendinopathies at the elbow. *Curr Opin Rheumatol* 1999;11(2):138–143.

Lento PH, Strakowski JA. The use of ultrasound in guiding musculoskeletal interventional procedures. *Phys Med Rehabil Clin N Am* 2010;21(3):559–583.

Waldman SD. Functional anatomy of the elbow joint. In: *Pain Review*. Philadelphia, PA: WB Saunders; 2009:90–94.

Waldman SD. Injection technique for triceps tendinitis. In: *Atlas of Pain Management Injection Techniques*. 3rd ed. Philadelphia, PA: WB Saunders; 2013:153–156.

# CHAPTER 58

# Ultrasound-Guided Injection Technique for Olecranon Bursitis Pain

## CLINICAL PERSPECTIVES

The olecranon bursa lies in the aspect of the elbow between the skin and the olecranon process of the ulna (Fig. 58.1). The bursa serves to cushion and facilitate sliding of the musculotendinous unit of the triceps muscle. The bursa is subject to inflammation from a variety of causes with acute elbow trauma and repetitive microtrauma being the most common. Acute injuries to the bursa can occur from direct trauma such as when falling on the ice onto the elbow or from being tackled when playing football or checked when playing ice hockey. Direct pressure on the elbow when pushing oneself up with the elbow or working at a drafting table has also been implicated in the development of olecranon bursitis. If the inflammation of the bursa is not treated and the condition becomes chronic, calcification of the bursa with further functional disability may occur. Gout may also precipitate acute olecranon bursitis as may bacterial, tubercular, or fungal infections.

The patient suffering from olecranon bursitis, which is also known as student's and baker's bursitis, most frequently presents with the complaint of severe pain with any movement of the elbow, but extension is often the most painful. Physical examination of the patient suffering from olecranon bursitis will reveal point tenderness over the olecranon process, at the acromion process, as well as in the subacromial region. If there is significant inflammation, rubor and color may be present and the entire area may feel boggy or edematous to palpation (Fig. 58.2). Swelling, which at times can be quite dramatic, is often present (see Fig. 58.2). Passive range of motion, especially extension of the elbow, may exacerbate the pain of olecranon bursitis. If calcification or gouty tophi of the bursa and surrounding tendons are present, the examiner may appreciate crepitus with active range of motion of the affected elbow.

Plain radiographs are indicated in all patients who present with elbow pain to rule out occult boney pathology. Based on the patient's clinical presentation, additional testing may be indicated, including complete blood cell count, sedimentation rate, and antinuclear antibody testing. Magnetic resonance imaging or ultrasound imaging of the affected area may also help delineate the presence of other elbow bursitis, calcific tendonitis, tendinopathy, triceps tendonitis, or other elbow pathology (Fig. 58.3). Magnetic resonance imaging or ultrasound imaging of the affected area may also help delineate the presence of calcific tendonitis or other elbow pathology.

Rarely, the inflamed bursa may become infected and failure to diagnose and treat the acute infection can lead to dire consequences (Fig. 58.4).

## CLINICALLY RELEVANT ANATOMY

The elbow joint is a synovial hinge-type joint that allows the distal humerus to articulate with the proximal radius and ulna (Fig. 58.5). The joint allows flexion and extension as well as supination and pronation. The joint's articular surface is covered with hyaline cartilage, which is susceptible to arthritis and degeneration. This membrane gives rise to synovial tendon sheaths and bursae that are subject to inflammation. The entire elbow joint is surrounded by ligaments, which, coupled with the extremely deep boney articular socket, makes the joint stable throughout its range of motion (Fig. 49.3). The joint capsule is lined with a synovial membrane, which attaches to the articular cartilage. This membrane gives rise to synovial tendon sheaths and bursae that are subject to inflammation and swelling, especially in the anterior and posterior aspects of the joint where the joint capsule is less dense. The olecranon bursa lies in the posterior aspect of the joint, while the cubital bursa lies anteriorly (Fig. 58.6). Both are subject to the development of bursitis with misuse or overuse of the elbow joint. The primary innervation of the elbow joint comes from the musculocutaneous and radial nerves with some lesser contribution from the median and ulnar nerves. As the ulnar nerve passes inferiorly down the upper arm, it courses medially at the mid humerus to pass between the olecranon process and medial epicondyle of the humerus. The nerve is extremely susceptible to entrapment and trauma at this point. Anteriorly, the median nerve lies just medial to the brachial artery and occasionally susceptible to damage during puncture of the brachial artery when drawing arterial blood gasses.

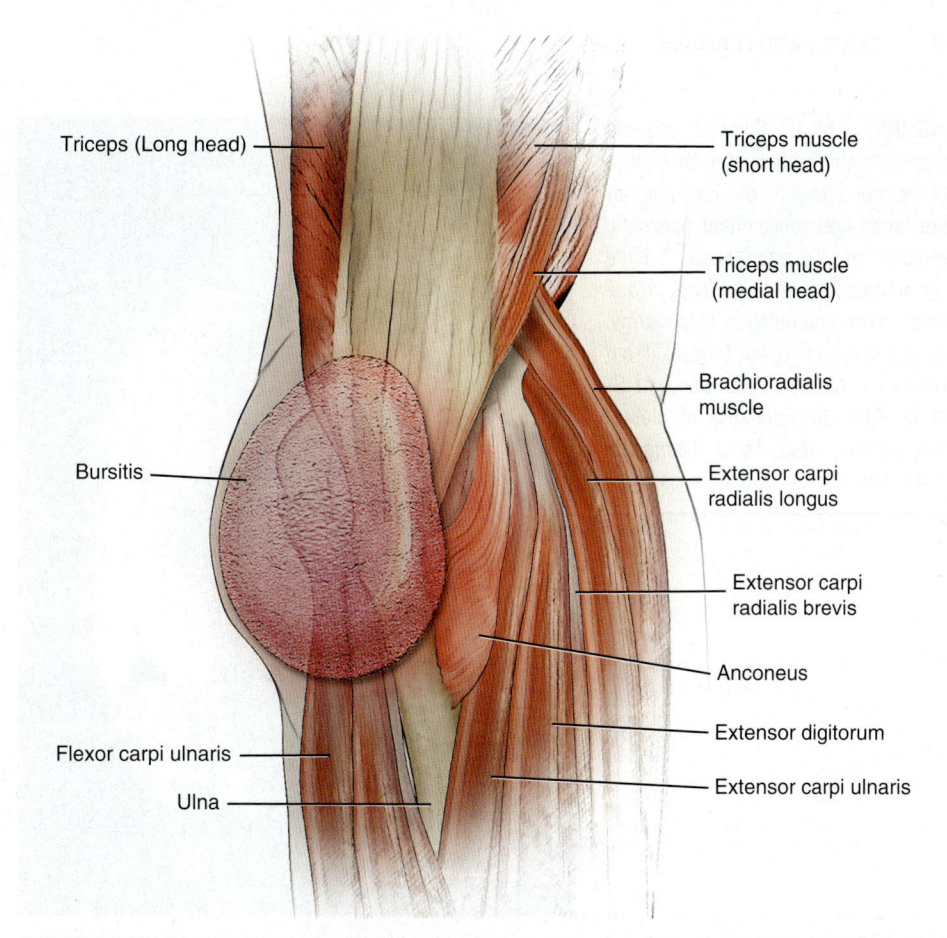

**FIGURE 58.1.** The anatomy of the olecranon bursa.

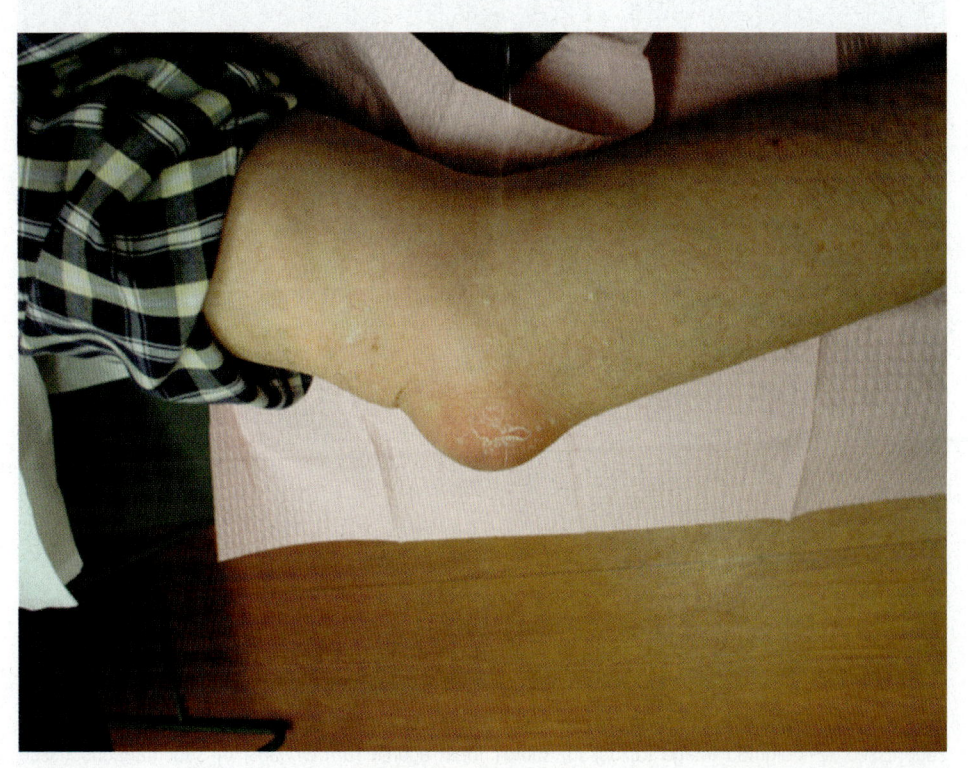

**FIGURE 58.2.** Patients suffering from olecranon bursitis will experience painful swelling, rubor, and color of the posterior elbow. (From Lotke PA, Abboud JA, Ende J. *Lippincott's Primary Care: Orthopaedics*. Philadelphia, PA: Lippincott Williams & Wilkins; 2008, with permission.)

**FIGURE 58.3.** Sixty-one-year-old man with surgically confirmed rupture of triceps tendon at insertion of olecranon and concomitant nonseptic effusion of olecranon bursa. (*White arrowhead*, joint effusion; *black arrowhead*, olecranon bursitis; *black arrow*, effusion beneath triceps tendon). (From Floemer F, Morrison WB, Bongartz G, et al. MRI characteristics of olecranon bursitis. *AMJ Am J Roentgenol* 2004;183(1):29–34, with permission.)

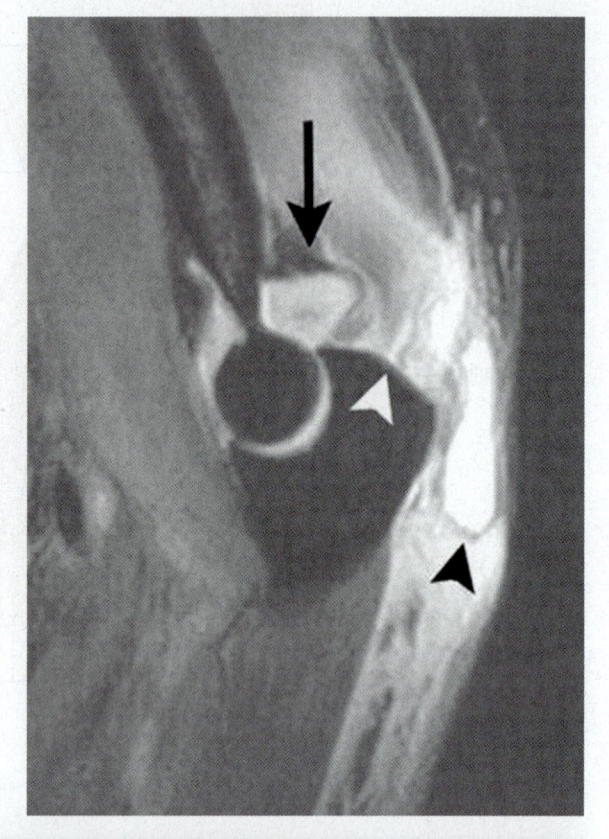

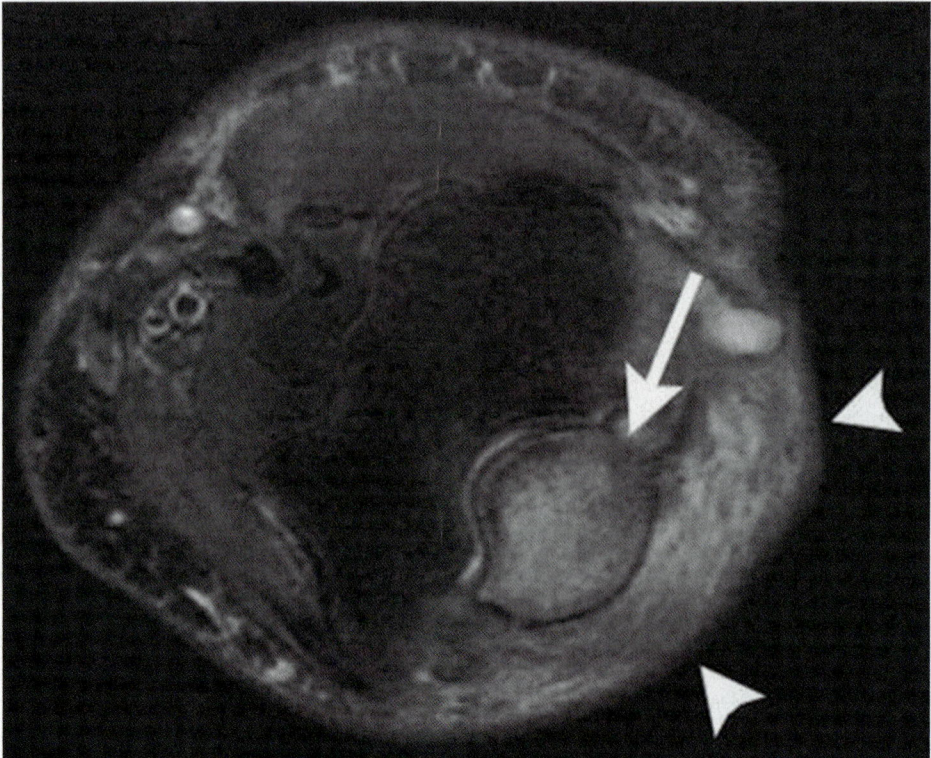

**FIGURE 58.4.** Twenty-six-year-old woman with culture-proven septic olecranon bursitis. Axial fat-suppressed T2-weighted image (5,735/90) shows focal edema (*arrowheads*) of subcutaneous tissue around olecranon bursa. Note also diffuse hyperintense signal (*arrow*) in bone marrow of olecranon indicative of osteomyelitis. (From Floemer F, Morrison WB, Bongartz G, et al. MRI characteristics of olecranon bursitis. *AMJ Am J Roentgenol* 2004;183(1):29–34, with permission.)

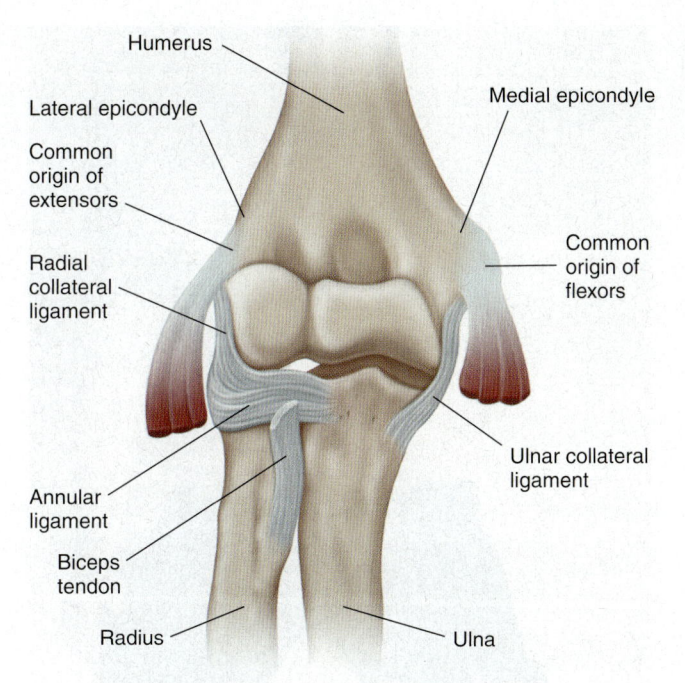

**FIGURE 58.5.** Anatomy of the elbow joint. (Reused from Premkumar K. *The Massage Connection: Anatomy and Physiology.* Baltimore, MD: Lippincott Williams & Wilkins; 2004, with permission.)

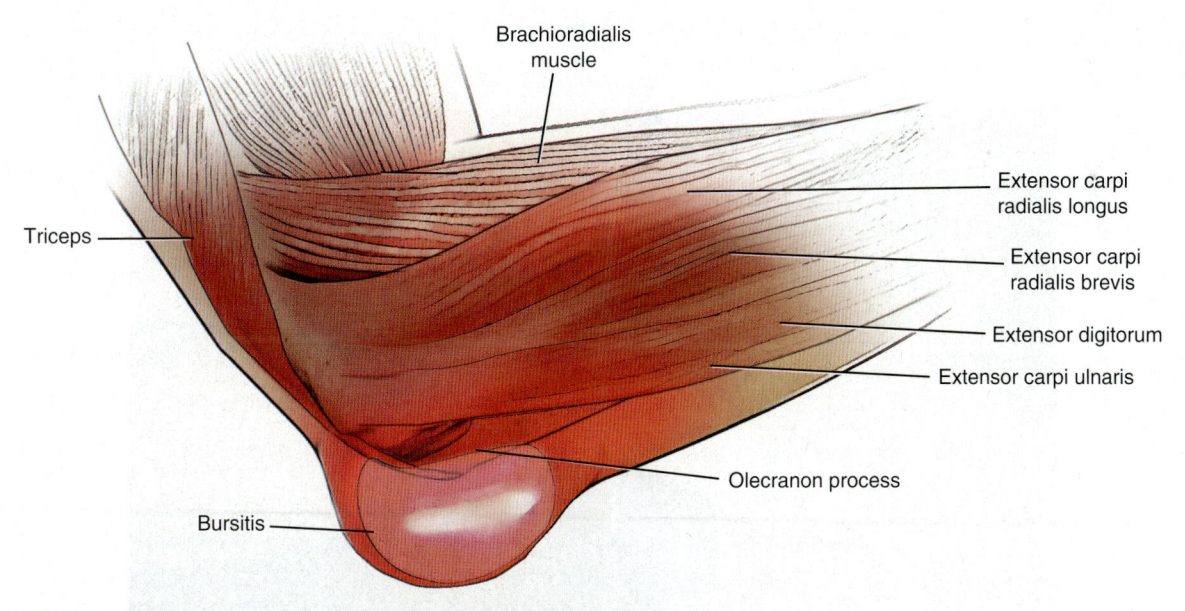

**FIGURE 58.6.** The relationship of the olecranon bursa to the posterior elbow joint.

## ULTRASOUND-GUIDED TECHNIQUE

The benefits, risks, and alternative treatments are explained to the patient, and informed consent is obtained. The patient is then placed in the sitting position with the elbow flexed to 90 degrees and the forearm resting across the abdomen and grasping the contralateral flank (Fig. 58.7). The physician stands or sits at the side of the patient. With the patient in the above position, a high-frequency linear ultrasound transducer is placed in a longitudinal plane with the transducer over the olecranon process, and an ultrasound survey scan is taken (Fig. 57.8). In health, the olecranon bursa may appear as a thin, hypoechoic space between the skin and olecranon. If the bursa is inflamed, it appears as a large, sometimes loculated, fluid-filled sac (Fig. 57.9). After the bursa is identified, the skin overlying the area beneath the ultrasound transducer is prepped with antiseptic solution. A sterile syringe containing 3.0 mL of 0.25% preservative-free bupivacaine and 40 mg of methylprednisolone is attached to a 1½-inch, 22-gauge needle using strict aseptic technique. The needle is placed through the skin ~1 cm above the superior edge of the transducer and is then advanced using an in-plane approach with the needle trajectory adjusted under real-time ultrasound guidance so that the needle tip rests within the bursa sac (Fig. 57.10). When the tip of needle is thought to be in satisfactory position,

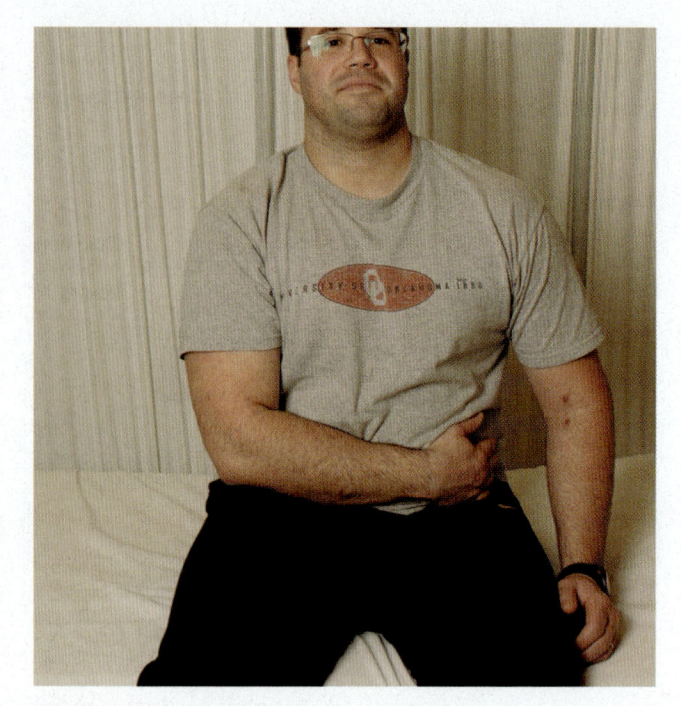

**FIGURE 58.7.** Proper position for ultrasound-guided injection for radial tunnel syndrome.

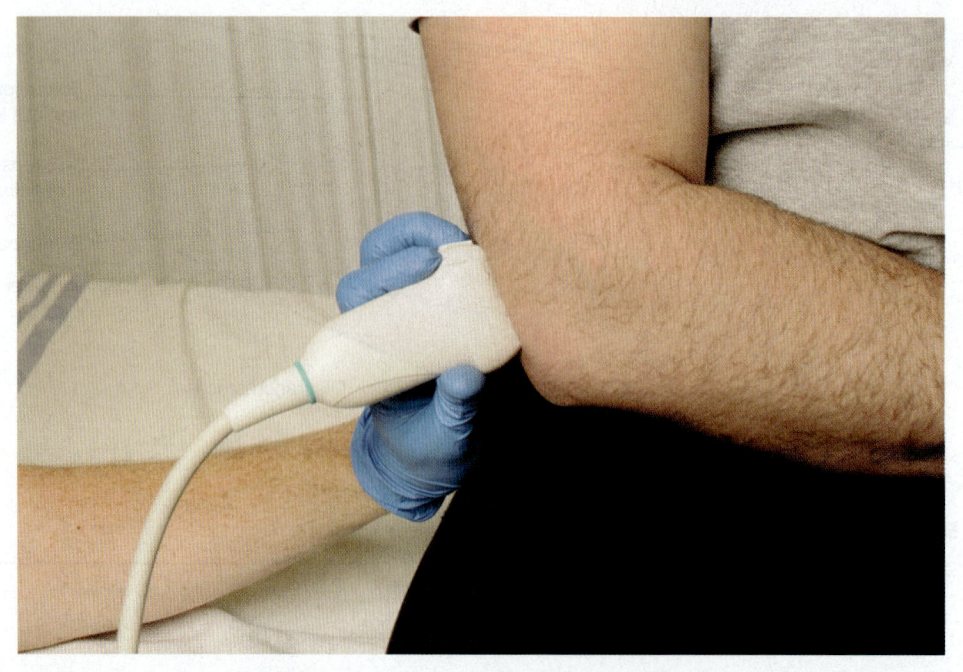

**FIGURE 58.8.** Proper longitudinal placement of the high-frequency ultrasound transducer for ultrasound-guided injection of olecranon bursitis.

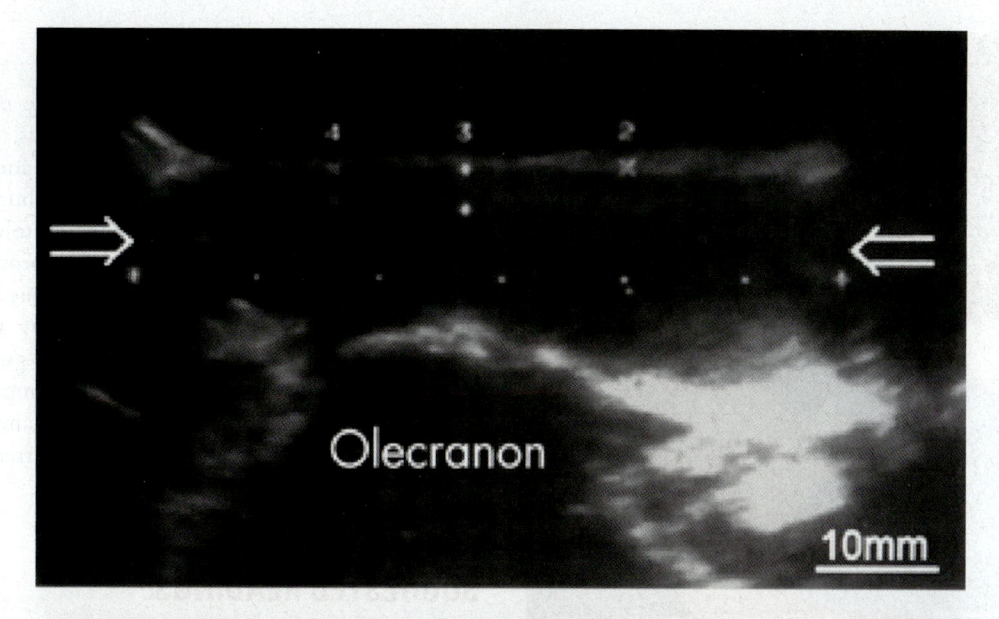

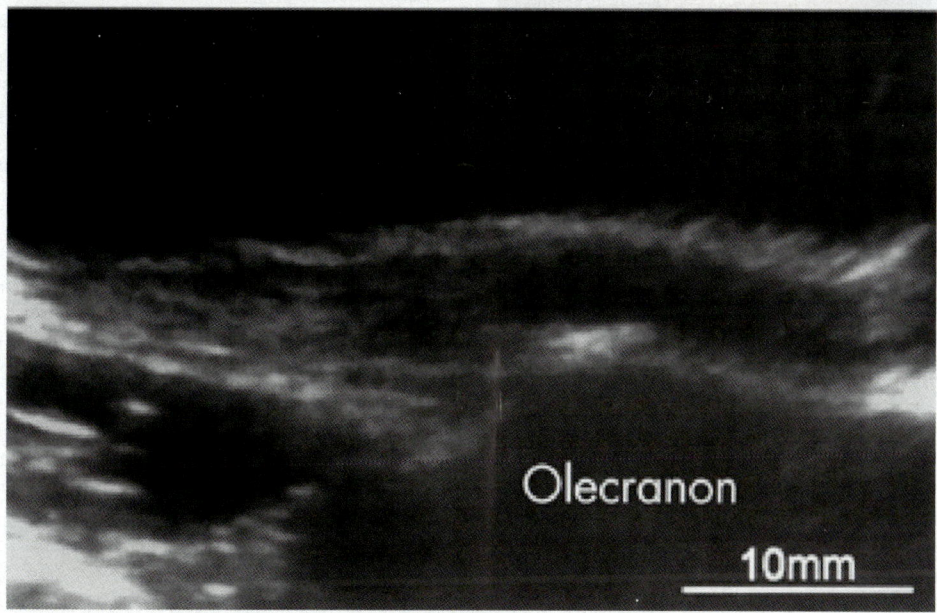

**FIGURE 58.9.** Longitudinal ultrasound view of olecranon bursitis. *Open arrows* delineate the extent of the fluid-filled olecranon bursa. (Reused from Berliner MN, Bretzel RG, Klett R. Successful radiosynoviorthesis of an olecranon bursitis in psoriatic arthritis. *Ann Rheum Dis* 2002;61(2):187–188, with permission.)

after careful aspiration, a small amount of local anesthetic and steroid is injected under real-time ultrasound guidance to confirm that the needle tip is not with the substance of the tendon. After proper needle tip placement is confirmed, the remainder of the contents of the syringe are slowly injected. There should be minimal resistance to injection. If loculations or calcifications are present, the needle may have to be repositioned several times to fully treat and/or aspirate the bursa.

## COMPLICATIONS

The major complication of ultrasound-guided injection of the olecranon bursa is infection. Ecchymosis and hematoma formation may also occur. A transient exacerbation of the patient's pain occurs ~25% of the time following this injection technique, and the patient should be warned of this possibility prior to the procedure.

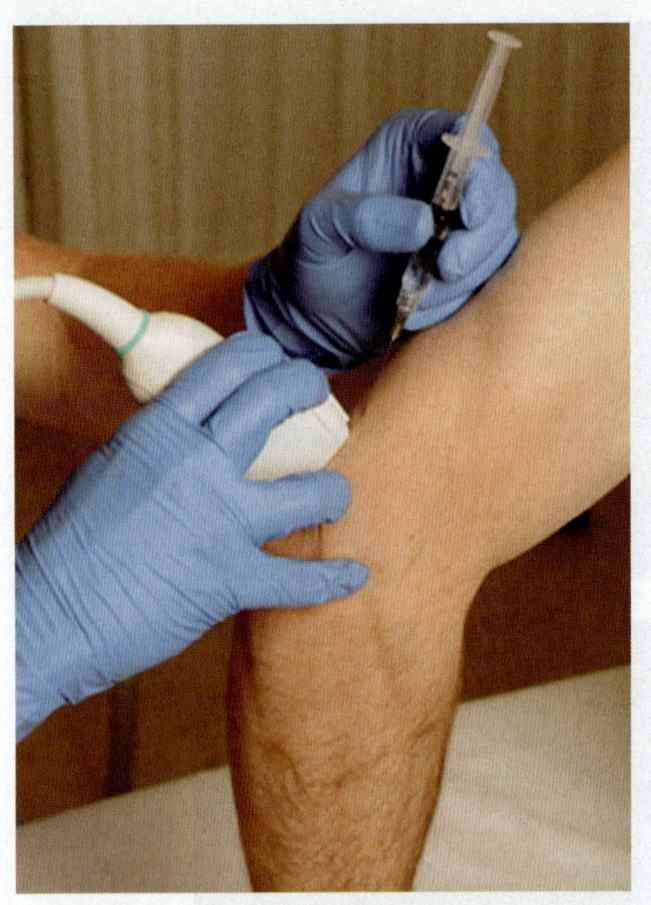

**FIGURE 58.10.** Injection of the distal triceps tendon under ultrasound guidance.

## CLINICAL PEARLS

Elbow pathology including bursitis of the other bursa of the elbow, medial and lateral epicondylitis, tendinopathy, osteoarthritis, avascular necrosis elbow, and entrapment neuropathies may coexist with olecranon bursitis and may contribute to the patient's pain symptomatology. Universal precautions should always be observed to protect the operator, and strict adherence to sterile technique must be used to avoid infection. Gentle physical therapy and local heat should be introduced following ultrasound-guided injection of the olecranon bursa to reduce pain and improve function. Simple analgesics and nonsteroidal anti-inflammatory agents or COX-2 inhibitors may be used concurrently with this injection technique.

## SUGGESTED READINGS

Waldman SD. Olecranon. In: *Pain Review*. Philadelphia, PA: WB Saunders; 2009:272–273.

Waldman SD. The Olecranon Bursa. In: *Pain Review*. Philadelphia, PA: WB Saunders; 2009:95–96.

Waldman SD. Olecranon bursitis. In: *Imaging of Pain*. Philadelphia, PA: WB Saunders; 2011:273–274.

Waldman SD. Injection technique for olecranon bursitis. In: *Atlas of Pain Management Injection Techniques*. 3rd ed. Philadelphia, PA: WB Saunders; 2013:157–159.

# CHAPTER 59

# Ultrasound-Guided Injection Technique for Pronator Syndrome

## CLINICAL PERSPECTIVES

Pronator syndrome is an uncommon entrapment neuropathy of the median nerve just below the elbow that is caused by compression of the median nerve by a variety of anatomic abnormalities including (1) the ligament of Struthers from an anomalous supracondylar process to the medial epicondyle, which may compress the median nerve; (2) the pronator teres muscle; (3) a fibrous arch in the flexor digitorum superficialis (FDS) of the middle finger; (4) posttraumatic hematoma; (5) soft tissue masses, for example, lipomas; (6) prolonged external compression from crush injuries or tourniquet; (7) fractures of the elbow (e.g., Volkman fracture); and rarely (8) the bicipital aponeurosis (the lacertus fibrosus) (Table 59.1; Fig. 59.1). These anatomic abnormalities may work alone or together to compromise the median nerve as it passes through the forearm toward its most common site of entrapment, the carpal tunnel.

Patients suffering from pronator syndrome will experience a dull, aching pain with movement-induced dysesthesias radiating from the site of compression both proximally to the elbow and distally to the anterior forearm. Patients suffering from pronator syndrome frequently complain of a heavy or tired sensation in the muscles of the forearm and clumsiness of the affected extremity. Unlike carpal tunnel syndrome, nighttime symptomatology is uncommon. The onset of pronator syndrome can be acute following twisting injuries to the elbow or as a result of direct trauma to the area overlying the median nerve. More commonly, the onset of pronator syndrome is insidious and is usually the result of misuse overuse of the elbow joint and proximal forearm from repetitive activities like cleaning fish, sculling, or chopping wood. If this entrapment neuropathy is not treated, pain and functional disability may become more severe, and ultimately, permanent weakness of the finger flexors may occur.

Physical findings in patients suffering from pronator syndrome will exhibit weakness of the intrinsic muscles of the forearm and hand innervated by the median nerve. The median nerve will often be tender to palpation at the site of entrapment and a Tinel sign may be present. Hypertrophy of the pronator teres muscle may be noted. Patients suffering from pronator syndrome frequently exhibit positive functional muscle testing that can help localize the site of median nerve entrapment (Fig. 59.2). If flexion of the elbow against resistance between 120 and 135 degrees of elbow flexion causes significant pain, the source of the nerve entrapment is the ligament of Struthers. If the pain is due to compression of the median nerve by the pronator teres muscle, the patient will experience pain on resisted pronation of the forearm with the wrist flexed to relax the flexor digitorum superficialis muscle. If the site compression of the median nerve is the proximal arch flexor digitorum superficialis muscle, resisted flexion of the FDS to the middle finger will exacerbate the pain. If the site of the nerve entrapment is the bicipital aponeurosis (lacertus fibrosus), the patient will experience pain on active flexion of the elbow against resistance with the arm in pronation. Electromyography and nerve conduction velocity testing will aid in determining the exact location of median nerve entrapment in patients who present clinically with signs and symptoms consistent with pronator syndrome. These electrodiagnostic tests will also help distinguish the various causes of pronator syndrome from isolated entrapment of the anterior interosseous nerve. Furthermore, it should be remembered that cervical radiculopathy and median nerve entrapment may coexist as the so-called "double crush" syndrome. The double crush syndrome is seen most commonly with median nerve entrapment at the wrist or with carpal tunnel syndrome but has been reported with the median nerve.

Plain radiographs, ultrasound imaging, and magnetic resonance imaging are indicated in all patients who present with pronator syndrome in order to confirm the clinical diagnosis of pronator syndrome as well as to rule out occult bony pathology and to identify occult fractures, masses, or tumors that may be responsible for compromise of the median nerve (Fig. 59.3). Based on the patient's clinical presentation, additional testing may be indicated, including complete blood count, uric acid, sedimentation rate, and antinuclear antibody testing.

## CLINICALLY RELEVANT ANATOMY

The key landmarks when performing ultrasound-guided median nerve block are the brachial artery in the antecubital fossa at the elbow and the ulnar artery and vein in the proximal forearm. Arising from fibers from the ventral roots of C5 and C6 of the lateral cord and C8 and T1 of the medial cord of the brachial plexus, the median nerve lies anterior and superior to the axillary artery in the 12:00 o'clock to 3:00 o'clock quadrant

### TABLE 59.1 Sites of Compression of the Median Nerve in the Forearm

- The ligament of Struthers from an anomalous supracondylar process to the medial epicondyle
- The pronator teres muscle
- A fibrous arch in the FDS of the middle finger
- The bicipital aponeurosis (the lacertus fibrosus)
- Posttraumatic hematoma
- Soft tissue masses (e.g., lipomas)
- Prolonged external compression from crush injuries or tourniquet
- Fractures of the elbow (e.g., Volkman fracture)

as it passes through the axilla. As the median nerve exits the axilla, it passes inferiorly adjacent to the brachial artery. At the antecubital fossa, the median nerve lies just medial to the brachial artery. Continuing its downward path, the median nerve gives off a number of motor branches to the flexor muscles of the upper arm (Fig. 59.4). These branches are susceptible to nerve entrapment by aberrant ligaments, muscle hypertrophy, and direct trauma. As the median nerve approaches the wrist, it overlies the radius where it is susceptible to trauma from radial fractures and lacerations. The nerve lies deep to and between the tendons of the palmaris longus muscle and the flexor carpi radialis muscle at the wrist. It is susceptible to entrapment as

**FIGURE 59.1.** Sites of compression in the pronator syndrome. **A:** The ligament of Struthers from an anomalous supracondylar process to the medial epicondyle, which may compress the median nerve. **B:** The pronator teres. **C:** The lacertus fibrosus (the least common cause). **D:** A fibrous arch in the FDS of the middle finger. (Adapted from Doyle JR. *Hand and Wrist* Philadelphia, PA: Lippincott Williams & Wilkins; 2006:104, with permission.)

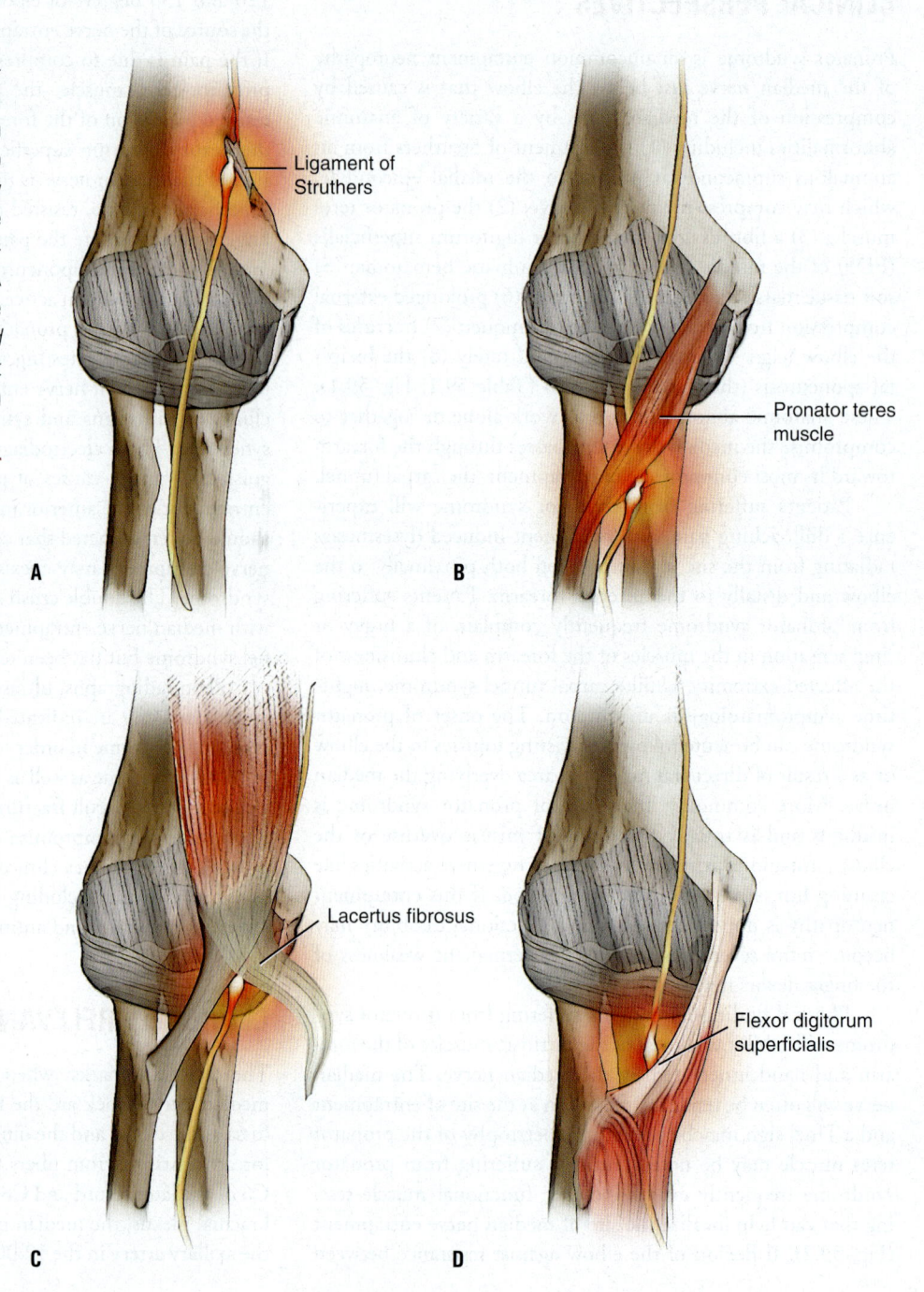

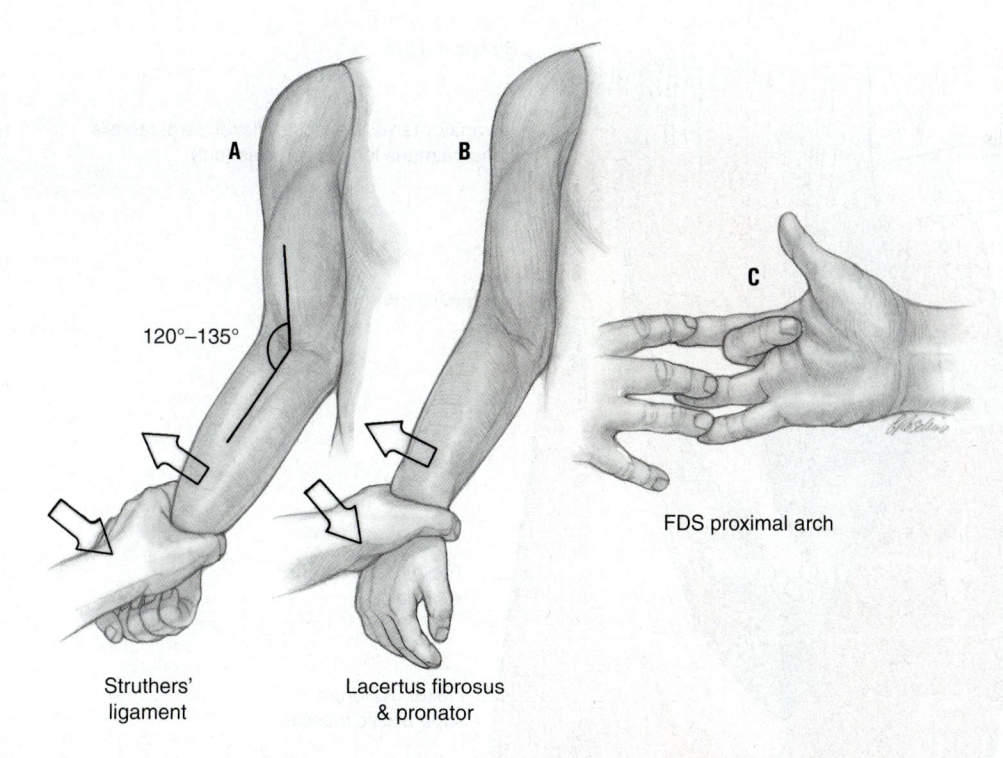

**FIGURE 59.2.** Localizing tests for the pronator syndrome. **A:** Test for presence of ligament of Struthers. **B:** Test for lacertus fibrosus and pronator teres muscle compression. **C:** Test for median nerve compression by a fibrous tissue arch in the FDS of the middle finger. (From Doyle JR. *Hand and Wrist* Philadelphia, PA: Lippincott Williams & Wilkins; 2006:104, with permission.)

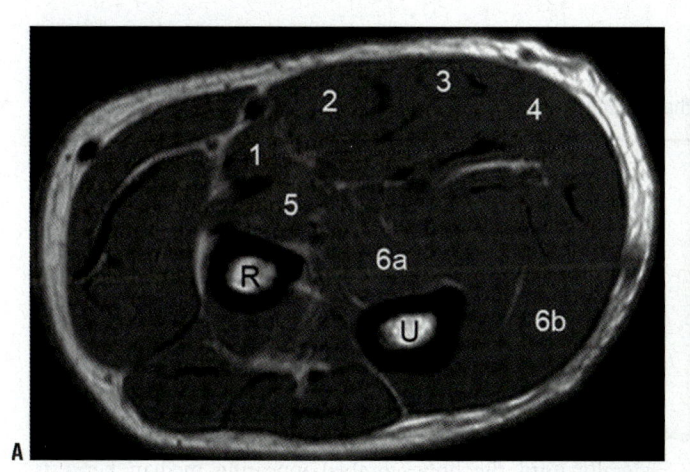

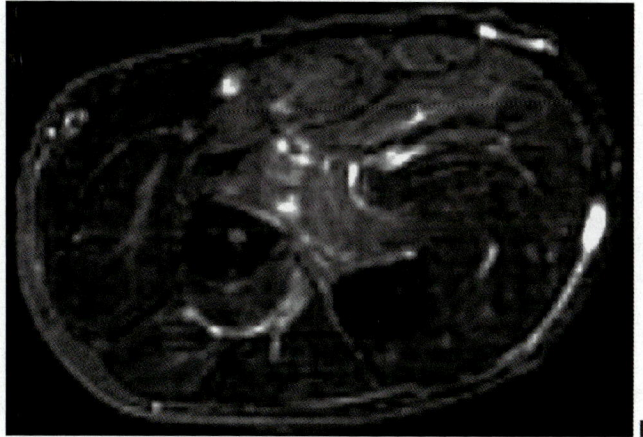

**FIGURE 59.3.** Pronator syndrome in a 58-year-old man after repeated pronation–supination stress from snow shoveling. **A:** Axial T1-weighted SE MR image (repetition time msec/echo time msec, 560/9) at a middle level in the forearm shows normal volume and normal signal intensity of the proximal forearm muscles (*1*, pronator teres; *2*, flexor carpi radialis; *3*, palmaris longus; *4*, flexor digitorum superficialis; *5*, flexor pollicis longus; *6a*, radial part of the flexor digitorum profundus; *6b*, ulnar part of the flexor digitorum profundus) and normal signal intensity of the radius (R) and ulna (U). **B:** Corresponding T2-weighted fat-suppressed fast SE MR image (4340/106; echo train length, eight) demonstrates increased signal intensity indicative of edema in all of the muscles that are innervated by the median nerve. The ulnar part of the flexor digitorum profundus muscle, which is innervated by the ulnar nerve, is unaffected.

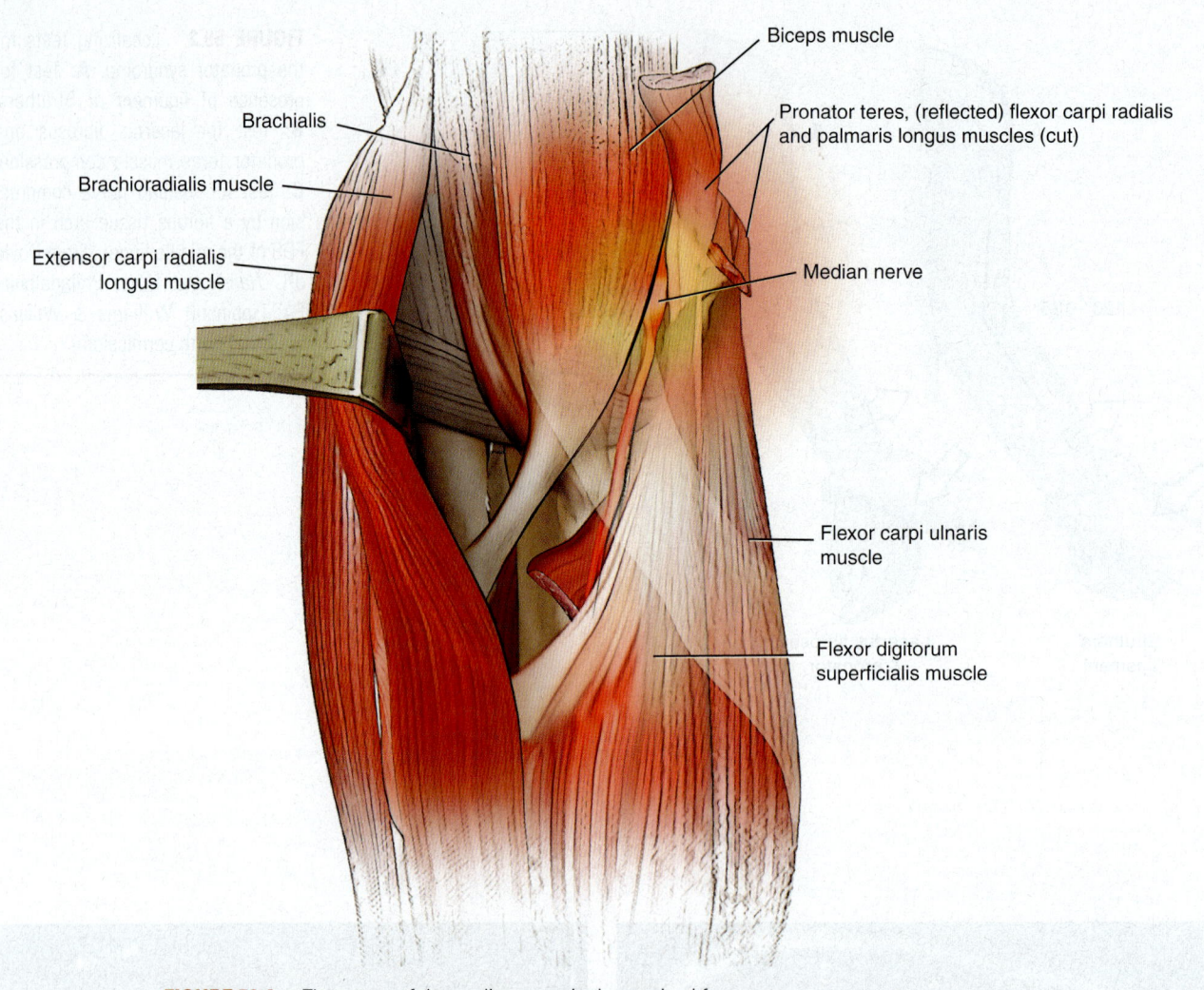

**FIGURE 59.4.** The course of the median nerve in the proximal forearm.

it passes through the carpal tunnel. The terminal branches of the median nerve provide sensory innervation to a portion of the palmar surface of the hand as well as the palmar surface of the thumb, index, and middle fingers and the radial portion of the ring finger (Fig. 59.5). The median nerve also provides sensory innervation to the distal dorsal surface of the index and middle fingers and the radial portion of the ring finger.

## ULTRASOUND-GUIDED TECHNIQUE

The benefits, risks, and alternative treatments are explained to the patient, and informed consent is obtained. The patient is then placed in the supine position with the arm resting comfortably at the patient's side with the palm up (Fig. 59.6). If the median nerve is to be located at the antecubital fossa and then followed distally as it passes into the forearm, the pulsation of the brachial artery is palpated just medial to the distal biceps tendon at the antecubital fossa. A high-frequency linear ultrasound transducer is then placed in a transverse position over the pulsation of the brachial artery, and an ultrasound survey scan is taken (Fig. 59.7). The brachial artery is then identified as is the median nerve lying just medial to the artery. The ultrasound transducer is then slowly moved distally along the course of the nerve as it passes between heads of pronator teres and flexor digitorum superficialis muscles and courses downward (Fig. 59.8). Alternatively, the ulnar nerve and adjacent ulnar artery are identified on transverse ultrasound scan as they pass beneath the FDS, and the ultrasound transducer is then moved laterally until the honeycombed-appearing median nerve is identified (Fig. 59.9). Once the median nerve in the proximal forearm is identified, the skin overlying the area beneath the ultrasound transducer is then prepped with antiseptic solution. A sterile syringe containing 4.0 mL of 0.25% preservative-free bupivacaine and 40 mg of methylprednisolone is attached to a 1½-inch, 22-gauge needle using strict aseptic technique. The needle is placed through the skin ~1.0 cm from the lateral border of the ultrasound transducer and is then advanced using an in-plane approach with the needle trajectory adjusted under real-time ultrasound guidance so that the needle tip ultimately rests in proximity to the median nerve (Fig. 59.10). When the tip of needle is thought to be in satisfactory position,

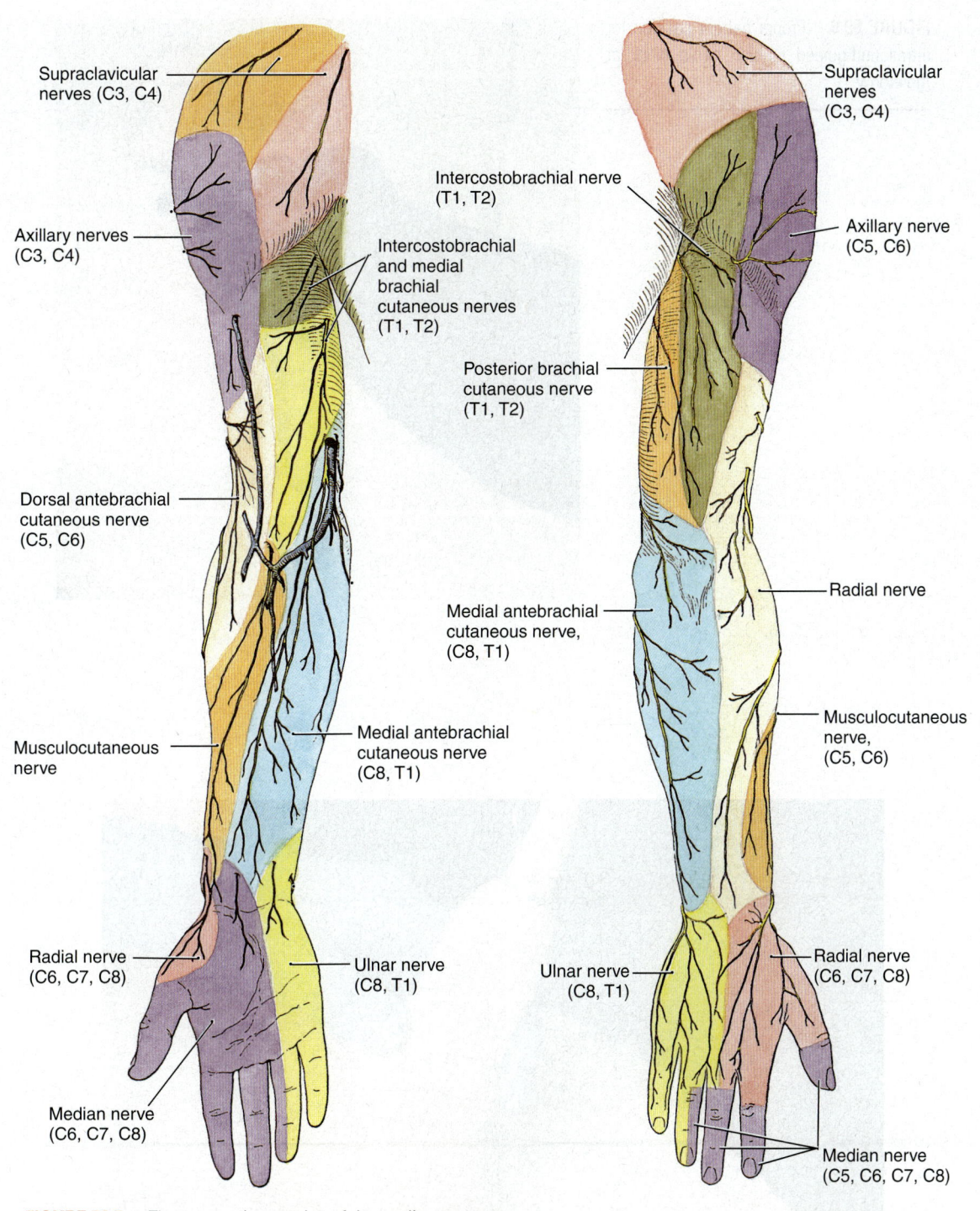

**FIGURE 59.5.** The sensory innervation of the median nerve.

**FIGURE 59.6.** Proper patient position for ultrasound-guided median nerve block at the elbow.

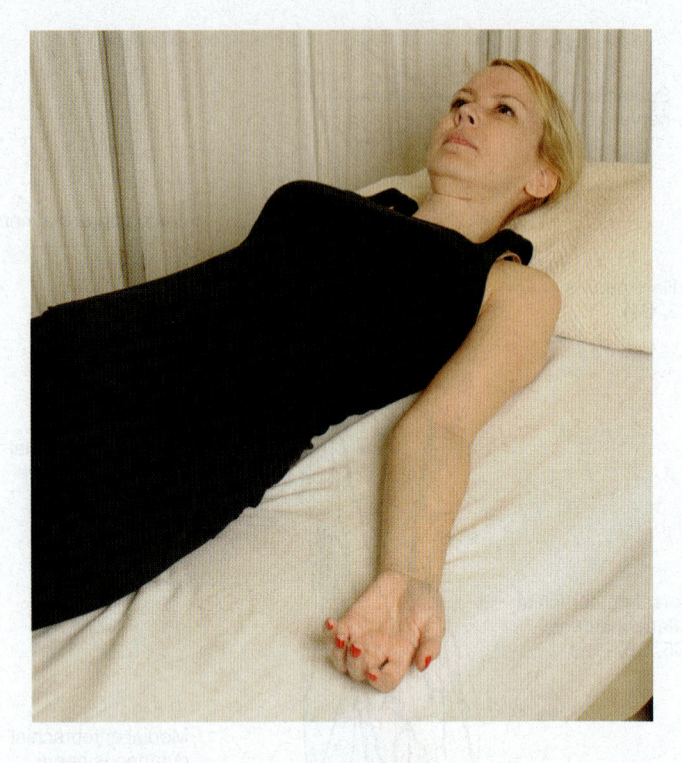

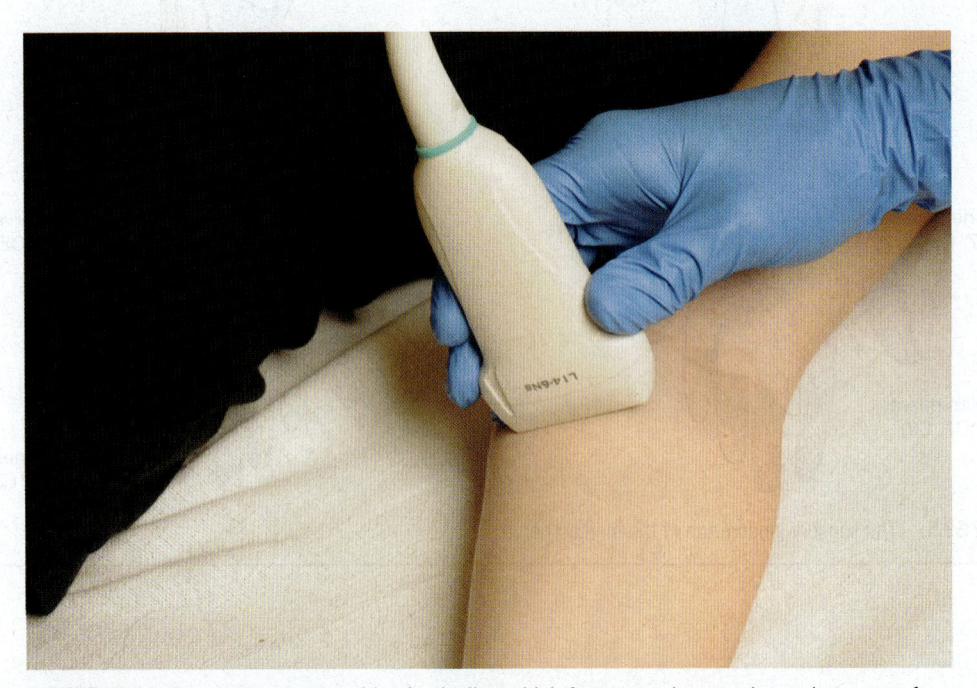

**FIGURE 59.7.** Proper transverse position for the linear high-frequency ultrasound transducer to perform ultrasound-guided median nerve block at the elbow.

CHAPTER 59 ULTRASOUND-GUIDED INJECTION TECHNIQUE FOR PRONATOR SYNDROME

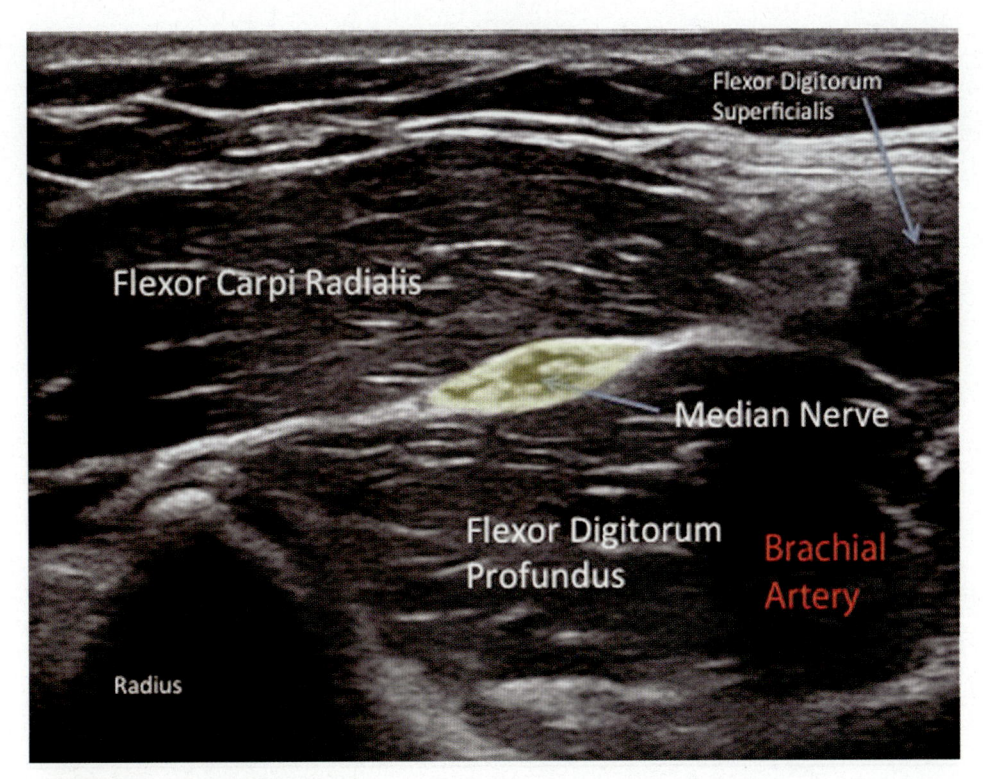

**FIGURE 59.8.** Transverse ultrasound image of the median nerve in the proximal forearm.

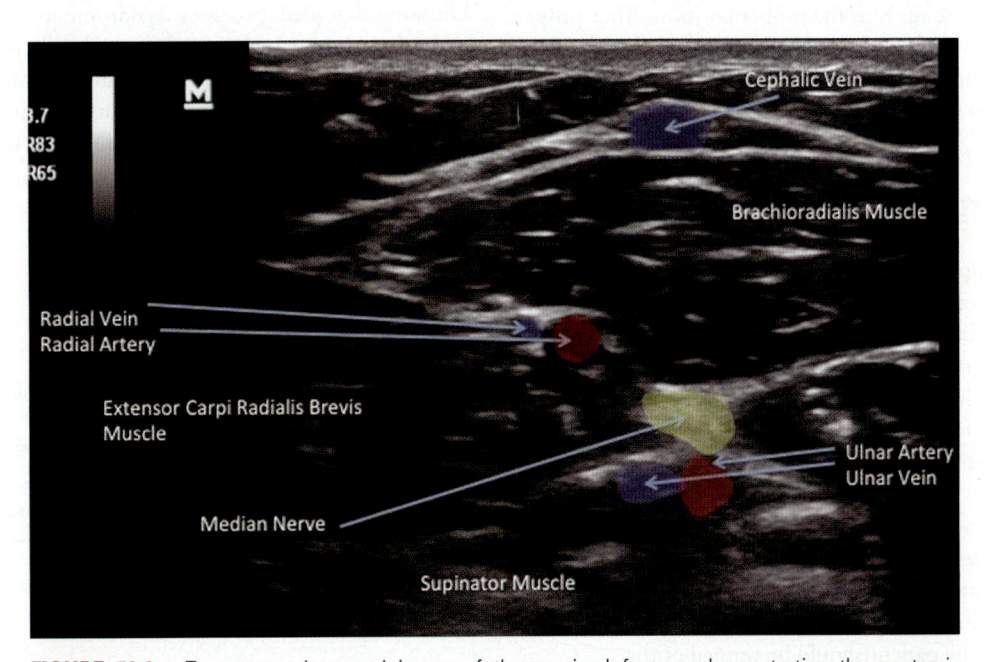

**FIGURE 59.9.** Transverse ultrasound image of the proximal forearm demonstrating the anatomic relationship of the ulnar artery and vein and the median nerve. Note the honeycombed appearance of the median nerve.

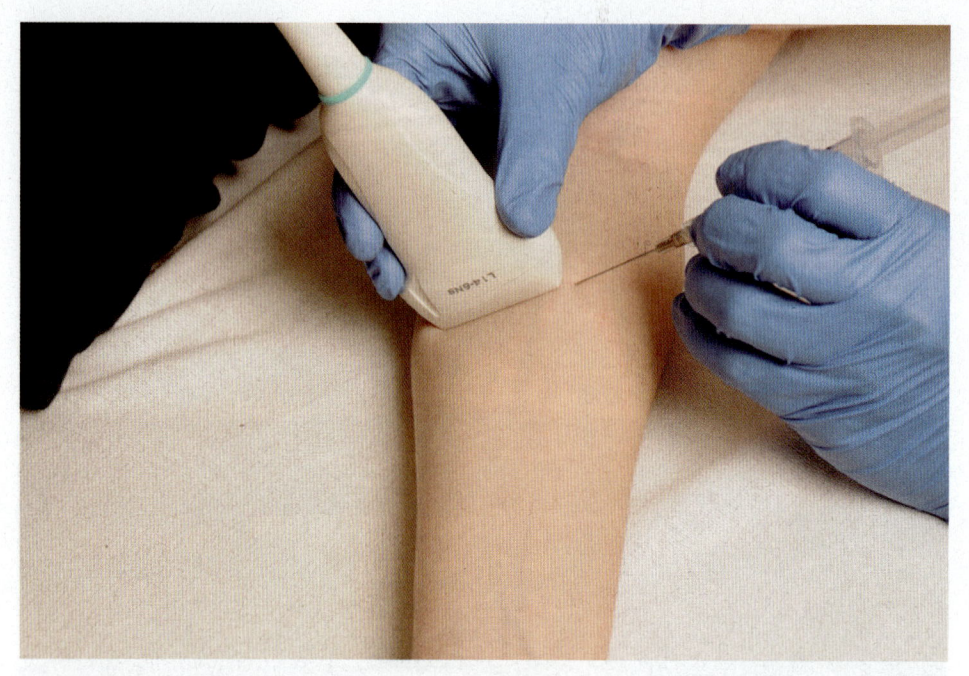

**FIGURE 59.10.** Proper out-of-plane placement of the needle for ultrasound-guided median nerve block at the forearm.

after careful aspiration, a small amount of local anesthetic and steroid is injected under real-time ultrasound guidance to confirm that the needle tip is in the proper position. After proper needle tip placement is confirmed, the remainder of the contents of the syringe are slowly injected. There should be minimal resistance to injection.

## COMPLICATIONS

The major complications of ultrasound-guided injection for pronator syndrome are related to improper needle placement with the possibility of inadvertent intravascular injection and/or persistent paresthesia secondary to needle trauma to the median nerve. Although rare, infection may occur. Ecchymosis and hematoma formation following this procedure may also occur. These complications can be decreased if manual pressure is applied to the area of the block immediately after injection. Application of cold packs for 20-minute periods after the block will also decrease the amount of postprocedure pain and bleeding the patient may experience. Approximately 25% of patients complain of a transient increase in pain after this injection technique; the patient should be warned of this.

## CLINICAL PEARLS

Ultrasound-guided pronator syndrome is a straightforward and relatively safe technique if attention is paid to the clinically relevant anatomy. Because of the potential for persistent neurologic deficits to occur in patients suffering from pronator syndrome, a careful neurologic examination to identify preexisting neurologic deficits that may later be attributed to the nerve block should be performed on all patients before beginning pronator syndrome.

## SUGGESTED READINGS

Lee MJ, LaStayo PC. Pronator syndrome and other nerve compressions that mimic carpal tunnel syndrome. *J Orthop Sports Phys Ther* 2004;34(10):601–609.
Toussaint CP, Zager EL. What's new in common upper extremity entrapment neuropathies. *Neurosurg Clin N Am* 2008;19(4):573–581.
Waldman SD. Anterior interosseous syndrome. In: *Atlas of Uncommon Pain Syndromes*. 2nd ed. Philadelphia, PA: WB Saunders; 2008:107–108.
Waldman SD. Pronator syndrome In: *Atlas of Uncommon Pain Syndromes*. 2nd ed. Philadelphia, PA: WB Saunders; 2008:87–89.
Waldman SD. The median nerve. In: *Pain Review*. Philadelphia, PA: Saunders Elsevier; 2009:76–77.

# CHAPTER 60

# Ultrasound-Guided Injection Technique for Anterior Interosseous Syndrome

## CLINICAL PERSPECTIVES

Anterior interosseous nerve syndrome is an uncommon entrapment neuropathy of the anterior interosseous branch of the median nerve below the elbow that is caused by compression of the anterior interosseous branch of the median nerve by a variety of anatomic abnormalities including (1) the accessory head of flexor pollicis longus (Gantzer muscle); (2) the deep head of the pronator teres muscle; (3) a fibrous arch in the flexor digitorum superficialis of the middle finger; (4) posttraumatic hematoma; (5) soft tissue masses, for example, lipomas; (6) prolonged external compression from crush injuries or tourniquet; (7) fractures of the radius; (8) aberrant origin of the flexor carpi brevis radialis muscle; (9) aberrant origin of the palmaris profundus muscle; (10) an inflammatory neuropathy analogous to Parsonage-Turner syndrome; and (11) thrombosis of the ulnar collateral vessels (Table 60.1; Fig. 60.1). These anatomic abnormalities may work alone, together, or in conjunction with other entrapments of the fibers that ultimately comprise the anterior interosseous nerve as it passes from the neck through the brachial plexus and to the forearm toward its most common site of entrapment, the carpal tunnel.

Patients suffering from anterior interosseous nerve syndrome will experience a dull, aching pain with movement-induced dysesthesias radiating from the site of compression both proximally to the elbow and distally to the anterior forearm. Patients suffering from anterior interosseous nerve syndrome frequently complain of a heavy or tired sensation in the muscles of the forearm and clumsiness of the affected extremity. Unlike carpal tunnel syndrome, nighttime symptomatology is uncommon. The onset of anterior interosseous nerve syndrome can be acute following twisting injuries to the elbow or as a result of direct trauma to the area overlying the anterior interosseous branch of the median nerve. More commonly, the onset of anterior interosseous nerve syndrome is insidious and is usually the result of misuse overuse of the elbow joint and proximal forearm from repetitive activities like chipping ice or shoveling snow. If this entrapment neuropathy is not treated, pain and functional disability may become more severe, and, ultimately, permanent weakness of the deep muscles of the forearm and hand may occur.

Physical findings in patients suffering from anterior interosseous nerve syndrome will exhibit weakness of the intrinsic muscles of the forearm and hand innervated by the anterior interosseous branch of the median nerve. The anterior interosseous branch median nerve will often be tender to palpation at the site of entrapment, and occasionally a Tinel sign 6 to 8 cm below the elbow may be present. Patients suffering from anterior interosseous nerve syndrome frequently exhibit positive functional muscle testing that can help localize the site of median nerve entrapment to the anterior interosseous branch of the median nerve. Patients suffering for anterior interosseous nerve syndrome will exhibit a positive Playboy and Spinner sign. The Playboy bunny sign is positive when the patient is unable to form the A-OK sign with his or her thumb and index finger due to weakness of the flexor pollicis longus and the flexor digitorum profundus muscles causing extension of the distal interphalangeal joint and thumb interphalangeal joint to form the elongated nose of a Playboy bunny (Fig. 60.2). The Spinner sign is positive when the index finger of the affected extremity cannot achieve full flexion to the palmar crease as the middle, ring, and little fingers can when making the thumbs up sign (Fig. 60.3).

Electromyography and nerve conduction velocity testing will aid in determining the exact location of median nerve entrapment in patients who present clinically with signs and symptoms consistent with anterior interosseous nerve syndrome. These electrodiagnostic tests will also help distinguish

**TABLE 60.1 Sites of Compression of the Anterior Interosseous Branch of the Median Nerve in the Forearm**

- The accessory head of flexor pollicis longus (Gantzer muscle)
- The deep head of the pronator teres muscle
- A fibrous arch in the flexor digitorum superficialis of the middle finger
- Fractures of the radius
- Aberrant origin of the flexor carpi brevis radialis muscle
- Aberrant origin of the palmaris profundus muscle
- Inflammatory neuropathy analogous to Parsonage-Turner syndrome
- Thrombosis of the ulnar collateral vessels
- Posttraumatic hematoma
- Soft tissue masses (e.g., lipomas)
- Prolonged external compression from crush injuries or tourniquet

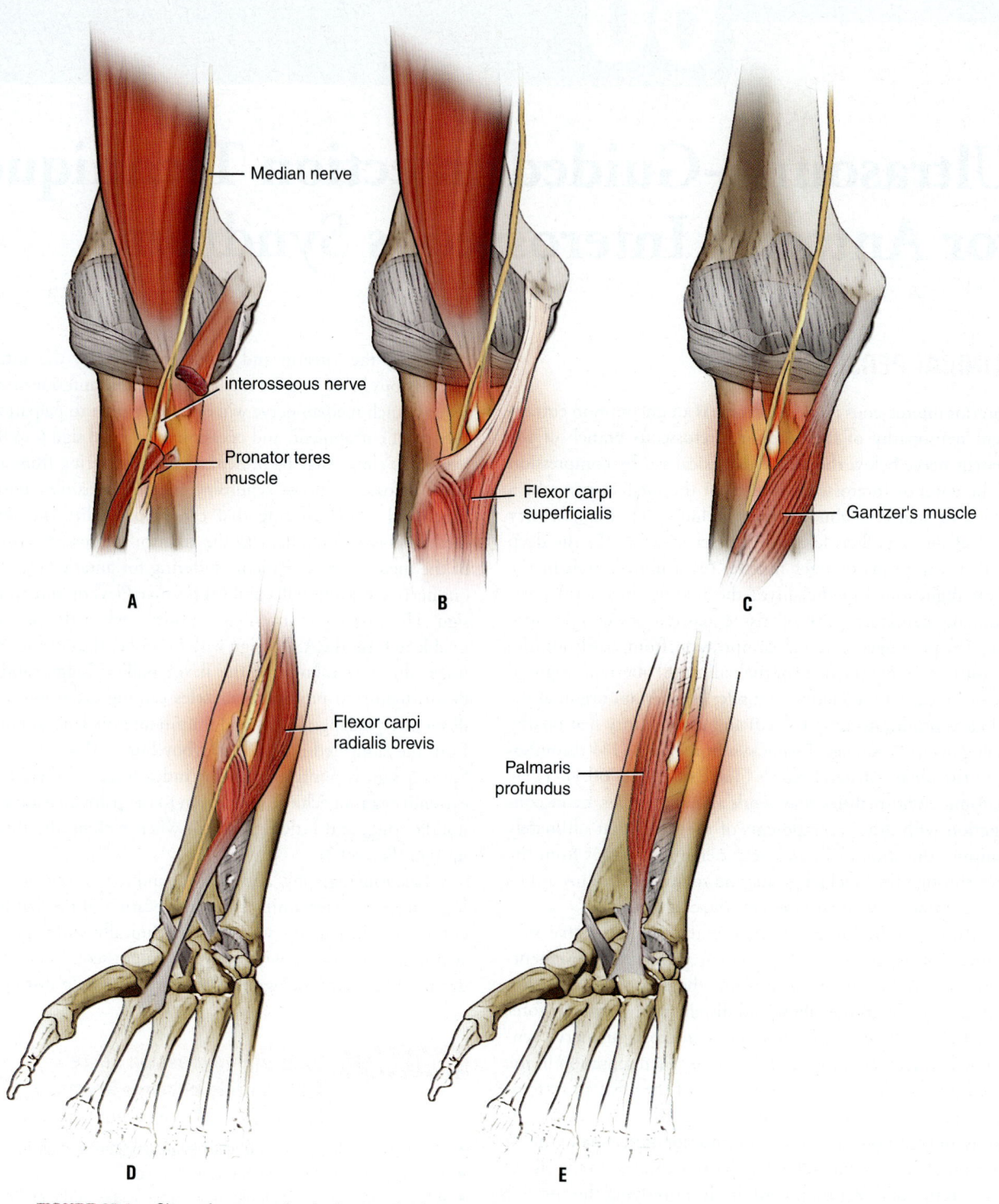

**FIGURE 60.1.** Sites of compression in the anterior interosseous nerve syndrome. Anterior interosseous nerve compression sites. **A:** Deep head of the pronator teres. **B:** Fibrous arch of the middle finger flexor digitorum superficialis. **C:** Gantzer muscle. Presence of abnormal muscles in the form of flexor carpi radialis brevis **(D)** and palmaris profundus **(E)**. (Adapted from Doyle JR. *Hand and Wrist*. Philadelphia, PA: Lippincott Williams & Wilkins; 2006:105.)

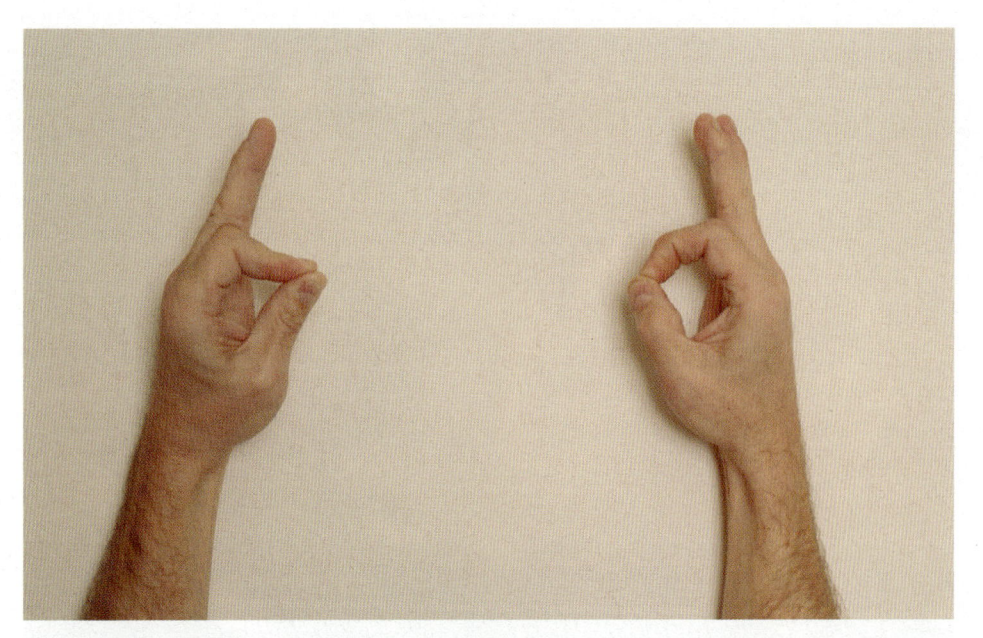

**FIGURE 60.2.** The Playboy bunny sign is positive when the patient is unable to form the A-OK sign with his or her thumb and index finger due to weakness of the flexor pollicis longus and the flexor digitorum profundus muscles causing extension of the distal interphalangeal joint and thumb interphalangeal joint to form the elongated nose of a Playboy bunny.

the various causes of anterior interosseous nerve syndrome from isolated entrapment of other motor branches of the median nerve. Furthermore, it should be remembered that cervical radiculopathy and median nerve entrapment may coexist as the so-called "double crush" syndrome. The double crush syndrome is seen most commonly with median nerve entrapment at the wrist or with carpal tunnel syndrome but has been reported with the median nerve.

Plain radiographs, ultrasound imaging, and magnetic resonance imaging are indicated in all patients who present with

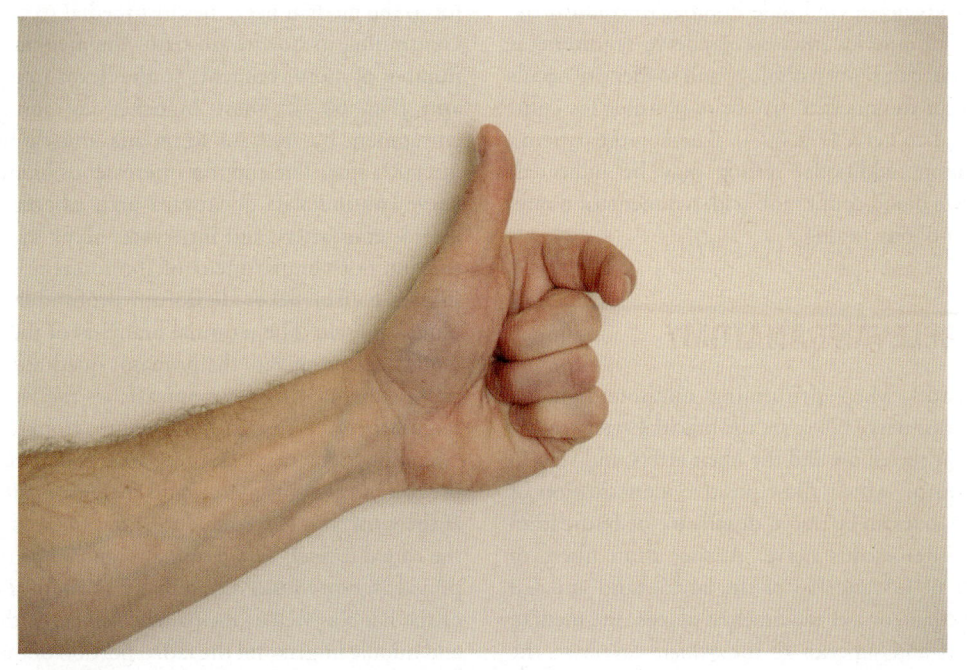

**FIGURE 60.3.** The Spinner sign is positive when the index finger of the affected extremity cannot achieve full flexion to the palmar crease as the middle, ring, and little fingers can when making the thumbs up sign.

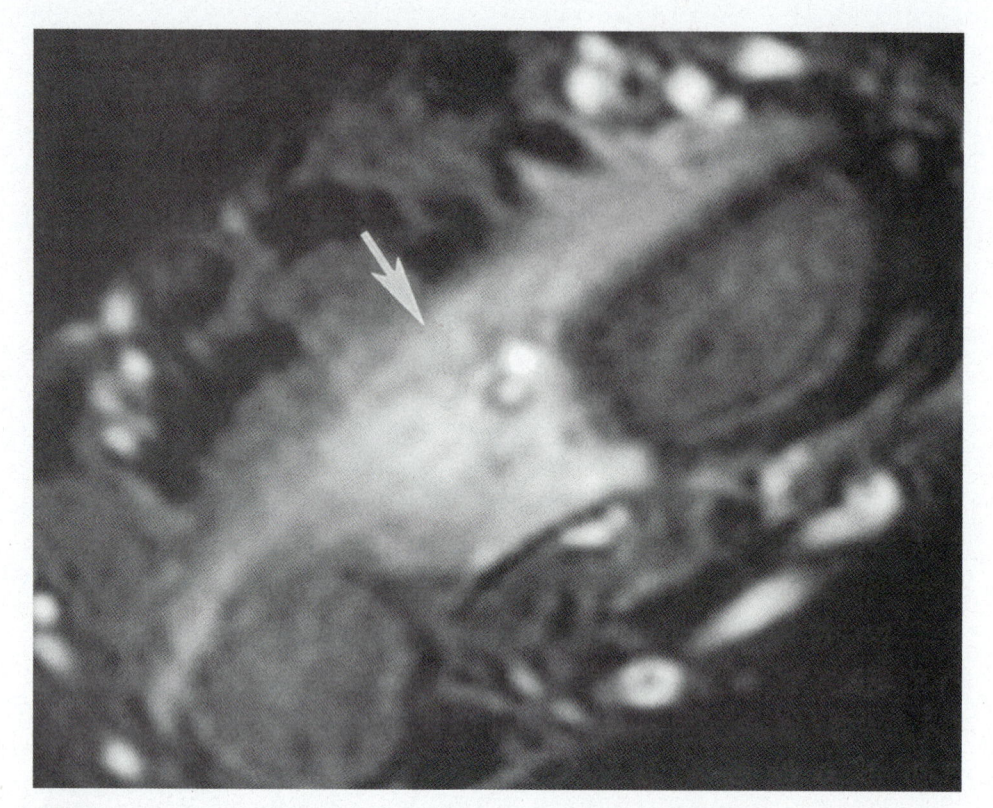

**FIGURE 60.4.** Anterior interosseous nerve compression. Axial T2-weighted sequence shows increased signal intensity in the pronator muscle (*arrow*). (Reused from Berquist TH. *MRI of the Musculoskeletal System*. Philadelphia, PA: Lippincott Williams & Wilkins; 2006, with permission.)

anterior interosseous nerve syndrome in order to confirm the clinical diagnosis of anterior interosseous nerve syndrome as well as to rule out occult bony pathology and to identify occult fractures, masses, or tumors that may be responsible for compromise of the median nerve (Fig. 60.4). Based on the patient's clinical presentation, additional testing may be indicated, including complete blood count, uric acid, sedimentation rate, and antinuclear antibody testing.

## CLINICALLY RELEVANT ANATOMY

The key landmarks when performing ultrasound-guided anterior interosseous nerve block are the brachial artery in the antecubital fossa at the elbow and the ulnar artery and vein in the proximal forearm, which allow positive identification of the median nerve so it can be traced distally to the bifurcation of the anterior interosseous nerve. Arising from fibers of the ventral roots of C5 and C6 of the lateral cord and C8 and T1 of the medial cord of the brachial plexus, the median nerve lies anterior and superior to the axillary artery in the 12:00 o'clock to 3:00 o'clock quadrant as it passes through the axilla. As the median nerve exits the axilla, it passes inferiorly adjacent to the brachial artery. At the antecubital fossa, the median nerve lies just medial to the brachial artery. Continuing its downward path, the median nerve gives off a number of motor branches to the flexor muscles of the upper arm (Fig. 60.5). These branches are susceptible to nerve entrapment by aberrant ligaments, muscle hypertrophy, and direct trauma. The anterior interosseous branch of the median nerve continues its downward path adjacent to the anterior interosseous artery and innervates all of the deep muscles of the anterior compartment of the forearm except the medial (ulnar) half of flexor digitorum profundus and flexor carpi ulnaris muscle. The terminal branches of the anterior interosseous nerve innervate the pronator quadratus muscle.

As the median nerve approaches the wrist, it overlies the radius where it is susceptible to trauma from radial fractures and lacerations. The nerve lies deep to and between the tendons of the palmaris longus muscle and the flexor carpi radialis muscle at the wrist. It is susceptible to entrapment as it passes through the carpal tunnel. The terminal branches of the median nerve provide sensory innervation to a portion of the palmar surface of the hand as well as the palmar surface of the thumb, index, and middle fingers and the radial portion of the ring finger. The median nerve also provides sensory innervation to the distal dorsal surface of the index and middle fingers and the radial portion of the ring finger.

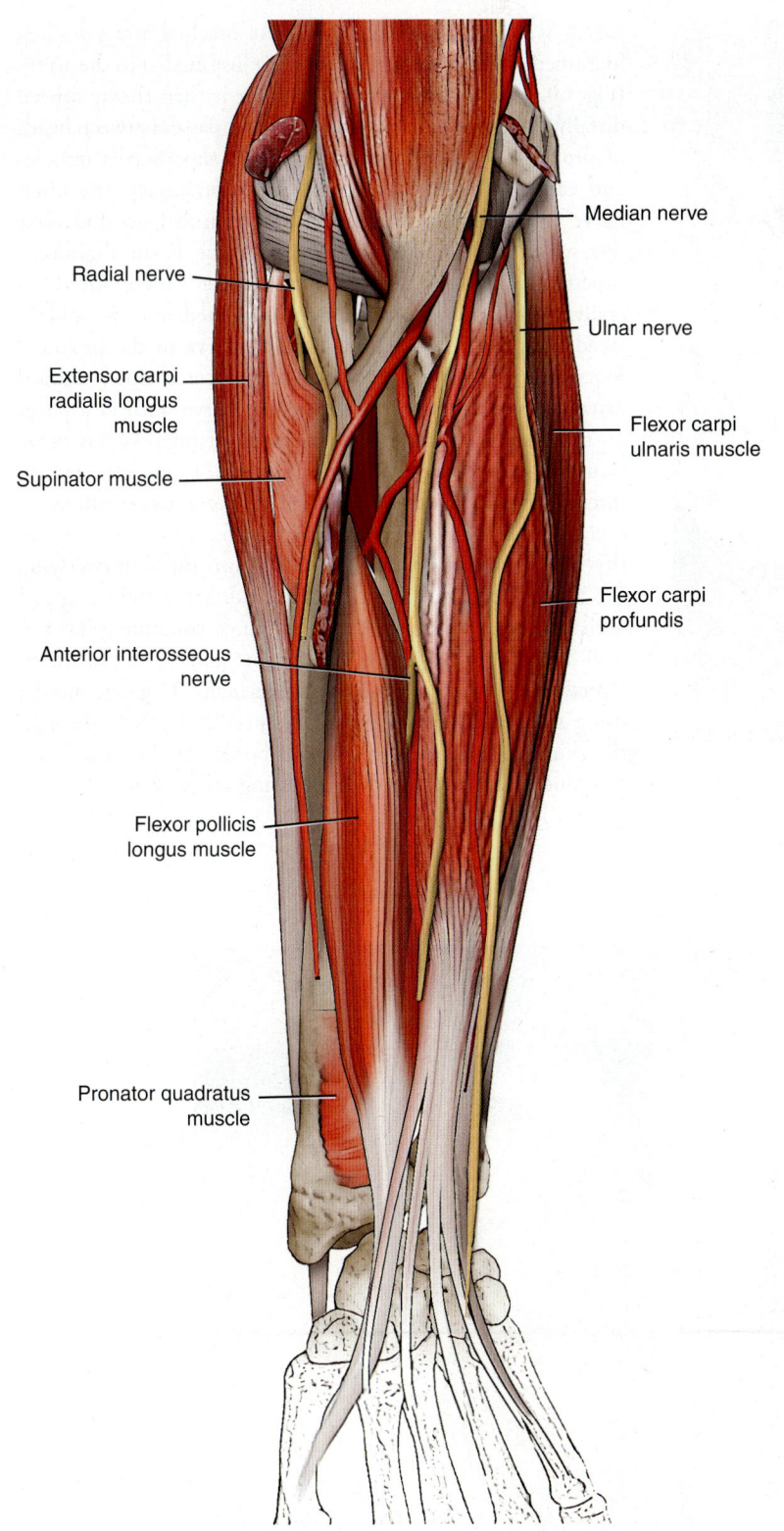

CHAPTER 60   ULTRASOUND-GUIDED INJECTION TECHNIQUE FOR ANTERIOR INTEROSSEOUS SYNDROME    405

**FIGURE 60.5.** The anatomy of the anterior interosseous nerve.

## ULTRASOUND-GUIDED TECHNIQUE

The benefits, risks, and alternative treatments are explained to the patient, and informed consent is obtained. The patient is then placed in the supine position with the arm resting comfortably at the patient's side with the palm up (Fig. 60.6). If the median nerve is to be located at the antecubital fossa and then followed distally as it passes into the forearm, the pulsation of the brachial artery is palpated just medial to the distal biceps tendon at the antecubital fossa. A high-frequency linear ultrasound transducer is then placed in a transverse position over the pulsation of the brachial artery, and an ultrasound survey scan is taken (Fig. 60.7). The brachial artery is then identified as is the median nerve lying just medial to the artery (Fig. 60.8). The ultrasound transducer is then slowly moved distally along the course of the nerve as it passes between heads of pronator teres and flexor digitorum superficialis muscles and courses downward (Fig. 60.9). Alternatively, the ulnar nerve and adjacent ulnar artery are identified on transverse ultrasound scan as they pass beneath the flexor digitorum superficialis, and the ultrasound transducer is then moved laterally until the honeycombed-appearing median nerve is identified (Fig. 60.10). Once the median nerve in the proximal forearm is identified, ultrasound transducer is slowly moved distally along the path of the median nerve until at a point ~6 to 8 cm below the elbow, the anterior interosseous nerve bifurcates from the main nerve (Fig. 60.11). As the anterior interosseous nerve travels adjacent to the anterior interosseous artery, color Doppler may be beneficial in helping identify the nerve (Fig. 60.12). At this point, the skin overlying the area beneath the ultrasound transducer is then prepped with antiseptic solution. A sterile syringe containing 4.0 mL of 0.25% preservative-free bupivacaine and 40 mg of methylprednisolone is attached to a 1½-inch, 22-gauge needle using strict aseptic technique. The needle is placed through the skin ~1.0 cm from the lateral border of the ultrasound transducer and is then advanced using an in-plane approach

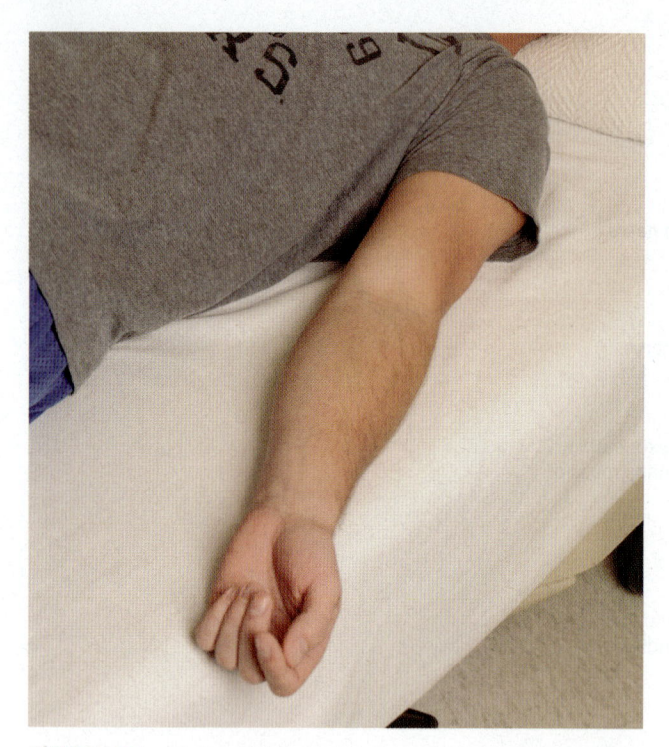

**FIGURE 60.6.** Proper patient position for ultrasound-guided anterior interosseous nerve block at the elbow.

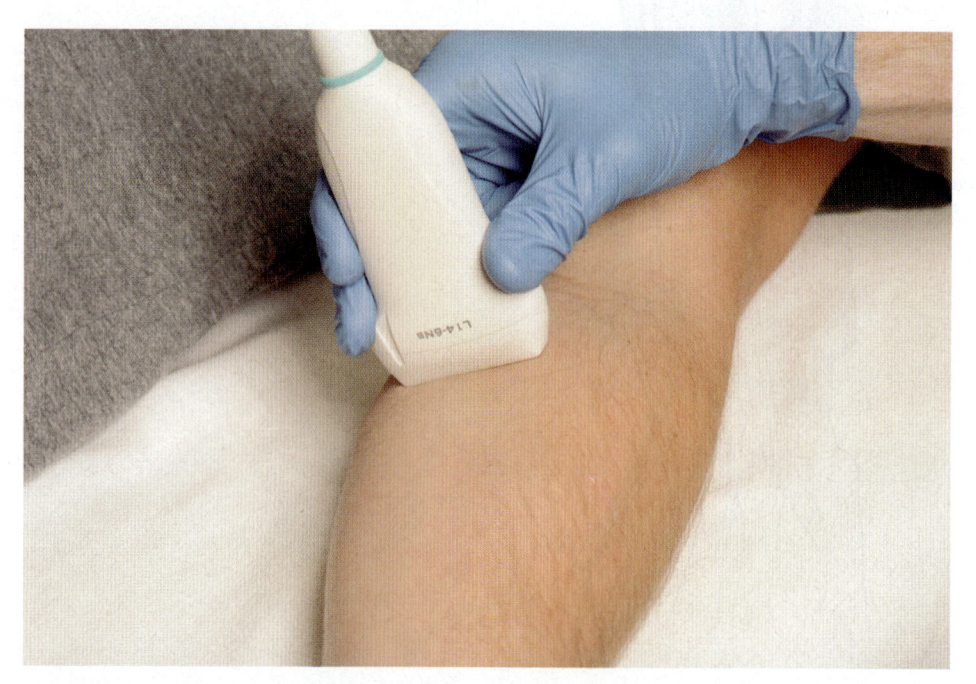

**FIGURE 60.7.** Proper transverse position for the linear high-frequency ultrasound transducer to perform ultrasound-guided median nerve block at the elbow.

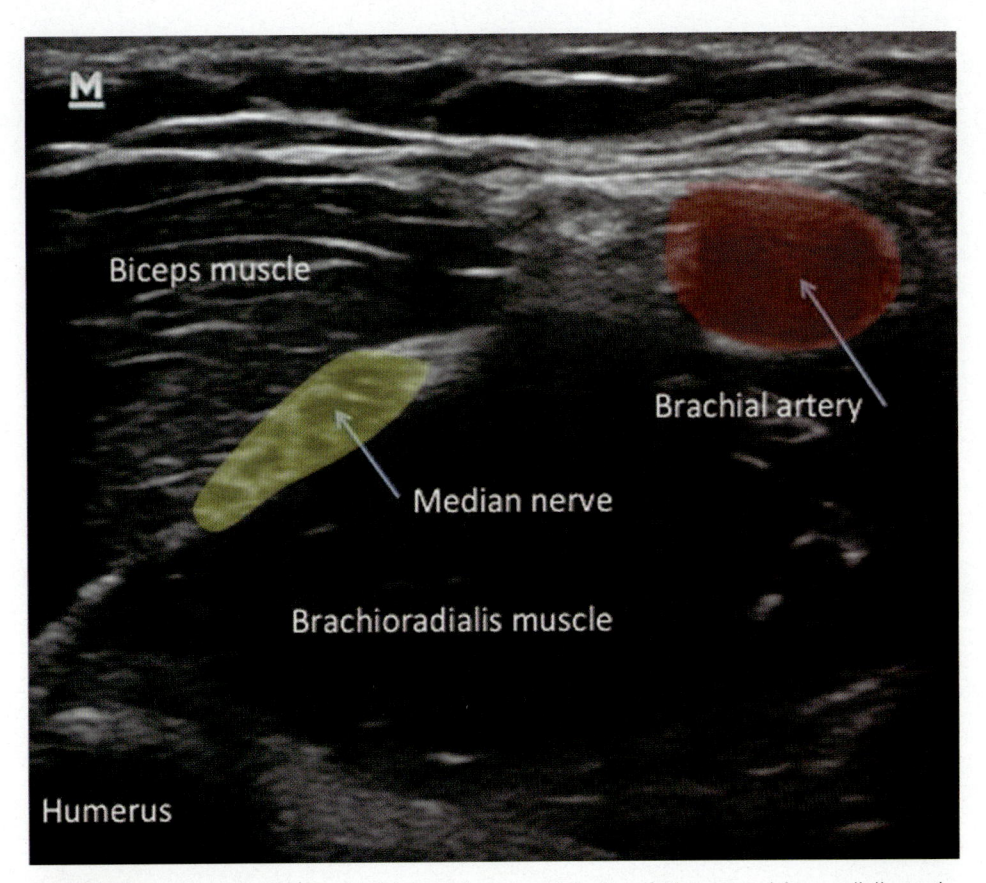

# CHAPTER 60 ULTRASOUND-GUIDED INJECTION TECHNIQUE FOR ANTERIOR INTEROSSEOUS SYNDROME 407

**FIGURE 60.8.** Transverse ultrasound image demonstrating the median nerve lying medially to the brachial artery at the antecubital fossa.

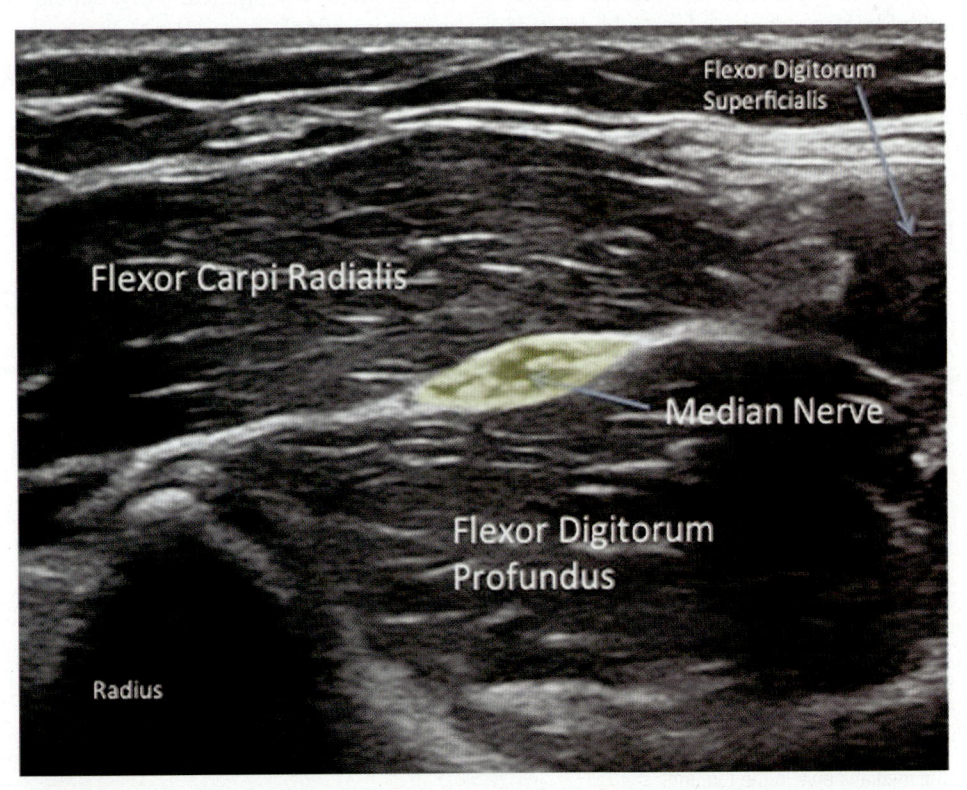

**FIGURE 60.9.** Transverse ultrasound image of the median nerve in the proximal forearm.

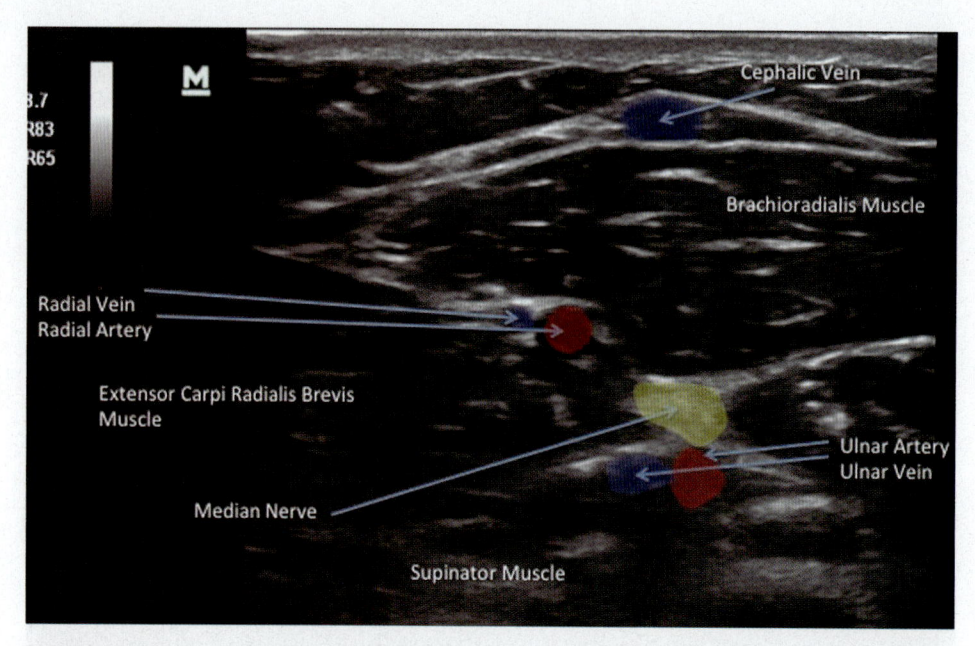

**FIGURE 60.10.** Transverse ultrasound image of the proximal forearm demonstrating the anatomic relationship of the ulnar artery and vein and the median nerve. Note the honeycombed appearance of the median nerve.

with the needle trajectory adjusted under real-time ultrasound guidance so that the needle tip ultimately rests in proximity to the median nerve (Fig. 60.13). When the tip of needle is thought to be in satisfactory position, after careful aspiration, a small amount of local anesthetic and steroid is injected under real-time ultrasound guidance to confirm that the needle tip is in the proper position. After proper needle tip placement is confirmed, the remainder of the contents of the syringe are slowly injected. There should be minimal resistance to injection.

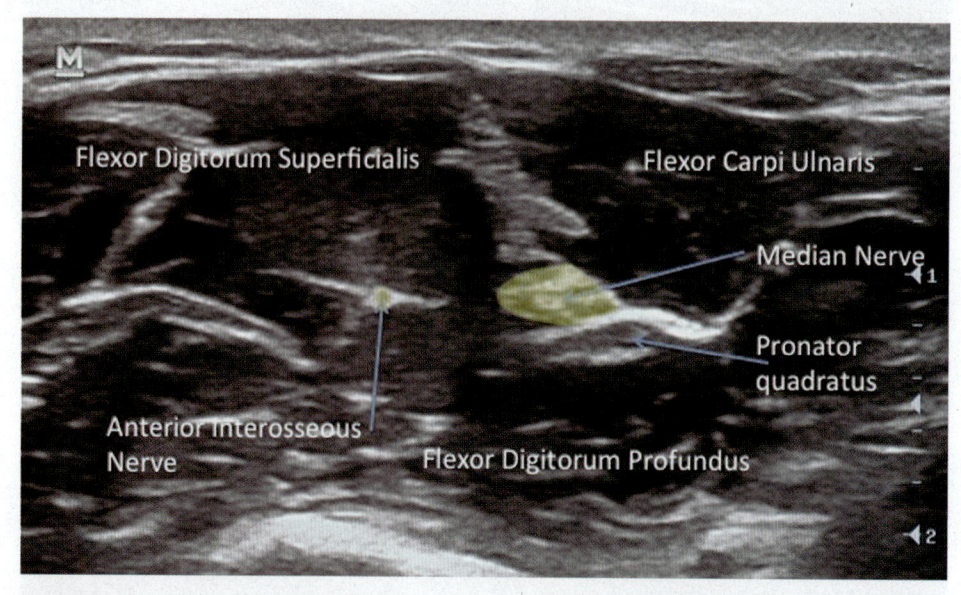

**FIGURE 60.11.** Transverse ultrasound image of the bifurcation of the anterior interosseous nerve from the median nerve in the forearm.

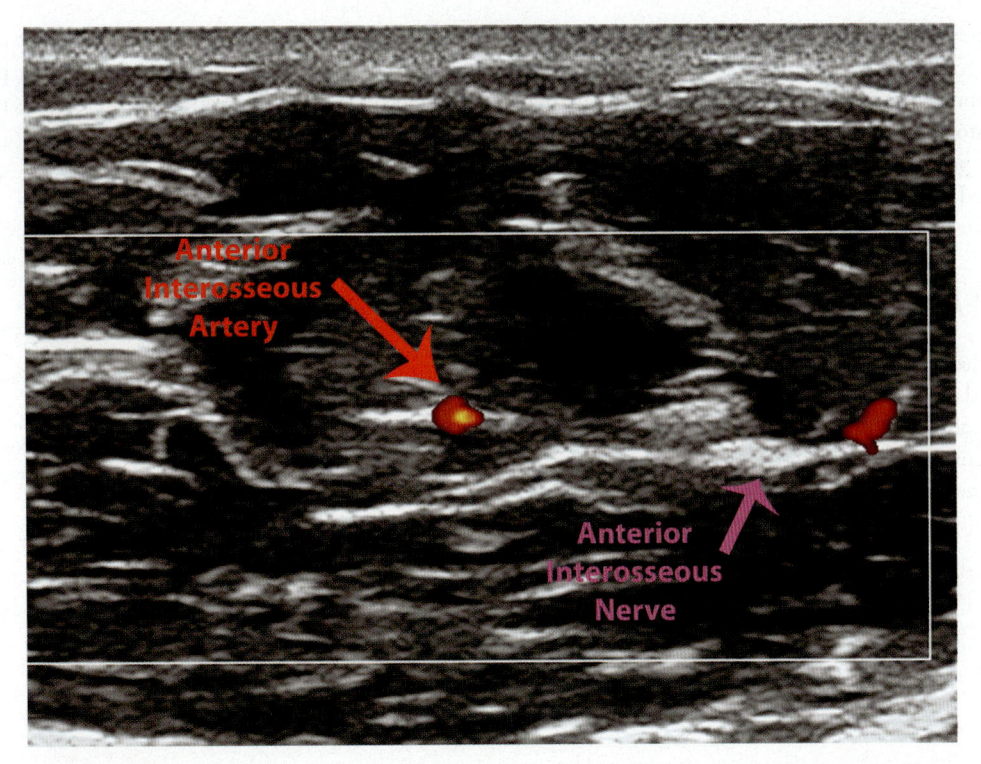

**FIGURE 60.12.** Transverse color Doppler image showing relationship of anterior interosseous artery to the anterior interosseous nerve.

## COMPLICATIONS

The major complications of ultrasound-guided injection for anterior interosseous nerve syndrome are related to improper needle placement with the possibility of inadvertent intravascular injection and/or persistent paresthesia secondary to needle trauma to the median nerve. Although rare, infection may occur. Ecchymosis and hematoma formation following this procedure may also occur. These complications can be decreased if manual pressure is applied to the area of the

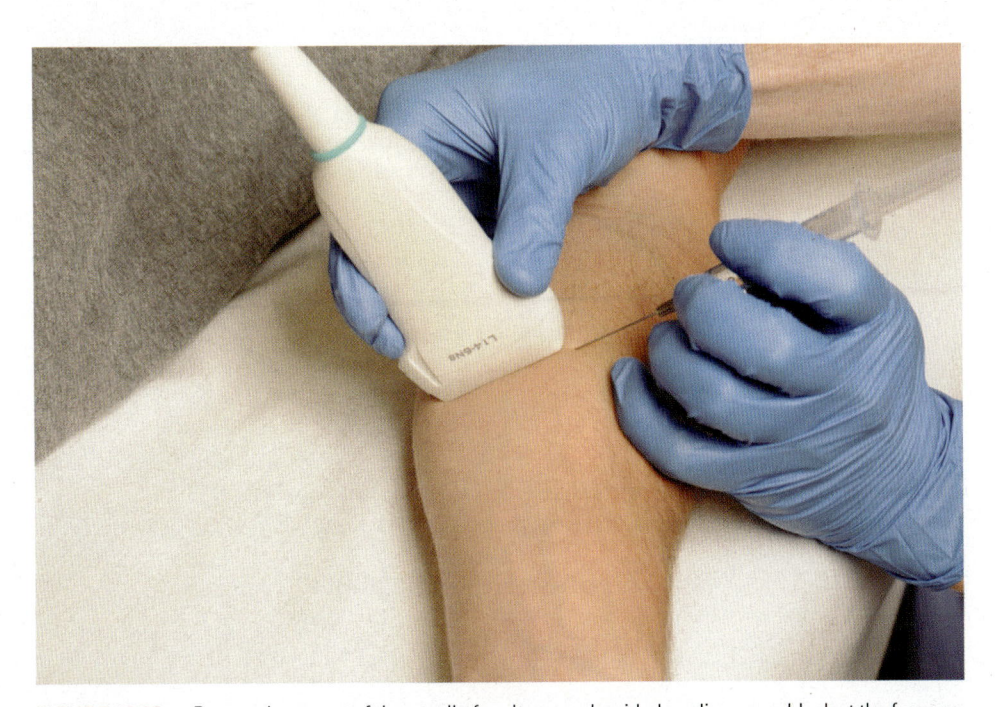

**FIGURE 60.13.** Proper placement of the needle for ultrasound-guided median nerve block at the forearm.

block immediately after injection. Application of cold packs for 20-minute periods after the block will also decrease the amount of postprocedure pain and bleeding the patient may experience. Approximately 25% of patients complain of a transient increase in pain after this injection technique; the patient should be warned of this.

## CLINICAL PEARLS

Ultrasound-guided anterior interosseous nerve syndrome is a straightforward and relatively safe technique if attention is paid to the clinically relevant anatomy. Because of the potential for persistent neurologic deficits to occur in patients suffering from anterior interosseous nerve syndrome, a careful neurologic examination to identify preexisting neurologic deficits that may later be attributed to the nerve block should be performed on all patients before beginning anterior interosseous nerve syndrome.

## SUGGESTED READINGS

Feldman MI, Muhammad K, Beltran J. Preoperative diagnosis of anterior interosseous nerve syndrome resulting in complete recovery. *Eur J Radiol* 2009;69(2):e73–e76.

Toussaint CP, Zager EL. What's new in common upper extremity entrapment neuropathies. *Neurosurg Clin N Am* 2008;19(4):573–581.

Waldman SD. Pronator syndrome. In: *Atlas of Uncommon Pain Syndromes*. 2nd ed. Philadelphia, PA: WB Saunders; 2008:87–89.

Waldman SD. Anterior interosseous syndrome. In: *Atlas of Uncommon Pain Syndromes*. 2nd ed. Philadelphia, PA: WB Saunders; 2008:107–108.

Waldman SD. The median nerve. In: *Pain Review*. Philadelphia, PA: Saunders Elsevier; 2009:76–77.

SECTION V

# Wrist and Hand

# CHAPTER 61

# Ultrasound-Guided Intra-articular Injection of the Distal Radioulnar Joint

## CLINICAL PERSPECTIVES

The distal radioulnar joint is a synovial pivot-type joint whose primary function is to aid in orientation of the hand in space for crucial functions like eating and drinking by allowing pronation and supination of the wrist. The joint's articular cartilage is susceptible to damage, which, if left untreated, will result in arthritis with its associated pain and functional disability. Osteoarthritis of the joint is the most common form of arthritis that results in distal radioulnar joint pain and functional disability, with rheumatoid arthritis, posttraumatic arthritis, and crystal arthropathy also causing arthritis of the distal radioulnar joint. Less common causes of arthritis-induced distal radioulnar joint pain include the collagen vascular diseases, infection, villonodular synovitis, and Lyme disease. Acute infectious arthritis of the distal radioulnar joint is best treated with early diagnosis, with culture and sensitivity of the synovial fluid, and with prompt initiation of antibiotic therapy. The collagen vascular diseases generally manifest as a polyarthropathy rather than a monoarthropathy limited to the distal radioulnar joint, although distal radioulnar pain secondary to the collagen vascular diseases responds exceedingly well to ultrasound-guided intra-articular injection of the distal radioulnar joint.

Patients with distal radioulnar joint pain secondary to arthritis, gout, synovitis, and collagen vascular disease–related joint pain complain of pain that is localized to the distal forearm and wrist. Activity, including pronation and supination, makes the pain worse, with rest and heat providing some relief. The pain is constant and characterized as aching. Sleep disturbance is common with awakening when patients roll over onto the affected upper extremity. Some patients complain of a grating, catching, or popping sensation with range of motion of the joint, and crepitus may be appreciated on physical examination. A distal radioulnar stress test may exacerbate the patient's pain symptomatology and will aid the examiner in identifying instability of the distal radioulnar joint (Fig. 61.1).

Functional disability often accompanies the pain of many pathologic conditions of the distal radioulnar joint. Patients will often notice increasing difficulty in performing their activities of daily living and tasks that require pronating and supinating the forearm such as using a screwdriver and corkscrew or tuning a doorknob. If the pathologic process responsible for the distal radioulnar pain is not adequately treated, the patient's functional disability may worsen and muscle wasting and ultimately a frozen distal radioulnar joint may occur.

Plain radiographs are indicated in all patients who present with distal radioulnar joint pain (see Fig. 61.1). Based on the patient's clinical presentation, additional testing may be indicated, including complete blood cell count, sedimentation rate, and antinuclear antibody testing. Magnetic resonance imaging (MRI) or ultrasound of the distal radioulnar joint is indicated if fracture, effusion, tendinopathy, crystal arthropathy, joint mice, synovitis, bursitis, or ligamentous injury is suspected (Fig. 61.2).

## CLINICALLY RELEVANT ANATOMY

The distal radioulnar joint is a synovial pivot-type joint that allows the pronation and supination of the forearm to optimize the positioning of the hand (Fig. 61.3). The joint's articular surface is covered with hyaline cartilage, which is susceptible to arthritis and degeneration. This membrane gives rise to synovial tendon sheaths and bursae that are subject to inflammation. The distal radioulnar joint is surrounded by a relatively weak joint capsule. The joint capsule is lined with a synovial membrane, which attaches to the articular cartilage. This membrane gives rise to synovial tendon sheaths and occasionally bursae that are subject to inflammation and swelling. The radioulnar joint is innervated primarily by the anterior and posterior interosseous nerves. The joint is bounded anteriorly by the flexor digitorum profundus and posteriorly by the extensor digiti minimi.

## ULTRASOUND-GUIDED TECHNIQUE

The benefits, risks, and alternative treatments are explained to the patient, and informed consent is obtained. The patient is then placed in the sitting position with the elbow flexed and the forearm and hand resting comfortably palm down on a pillow or padded bedside table (Fig. 61.4). The skin overlying the distal radioulnar joint is then prepped with antiseptic solution. A sterile syringe containing 2.0 mL of 0.25% preservative-free bupivacaine and 40 mg of methylprednisolone is attached to a 1½-inch, 22-gauge needle using strict aseptic technique. A linear high-frequency ultrasound transducer is placed over the distal ulna in the transverse axis, and a survey scan is obtained (Fig. 61.5). The hyperechoic dome-shaped distal margin of the

CHAPTER 61  ULTRASOUND-GUIDED INTRA-ARTICULAR INJECTION OF THE DISTAL RADIOULNAR JOINT  413

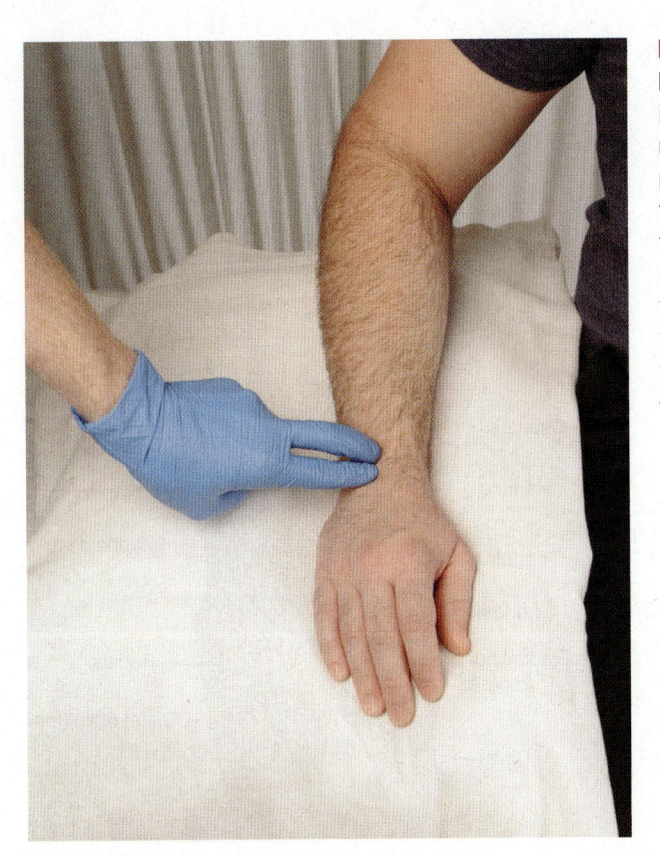

**FIGURE 61.1.** The radioulnar ballottement test is useful in identifying instability of the distal radioulnar joint. It is performed by placing an anterior to posterior force and a posterior to anterior force to the distal radius while stabilizing the distal ulna and then repeating the maneuver with the distal ulna while stabilizing the distal radius.

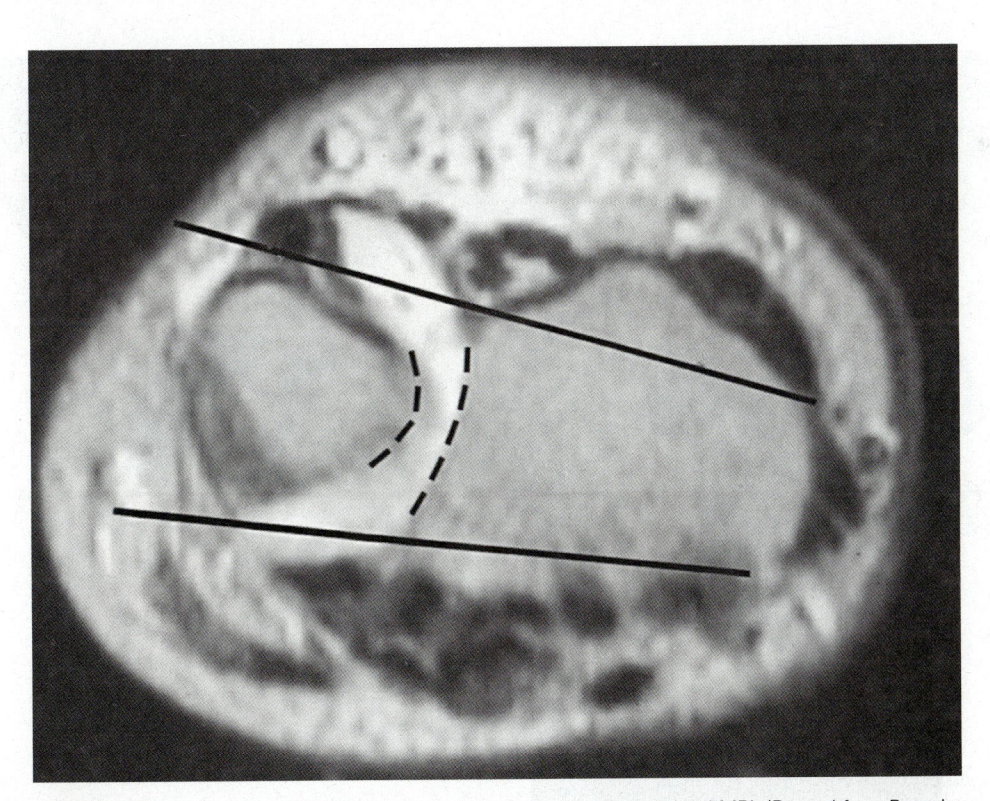

**FIGURE 61.2.** Large effusion of the distal radioulnar joint on T2-weighted MRI. (Reused from Berquist TH. *MRI of the Musculoskeletal System*. Philadelphia, PA: Lippincott Williams & Wilkins; 2006:821, with permission.)

**FIGURE 61.3.** The anatomy of the distal radioulnar joint.

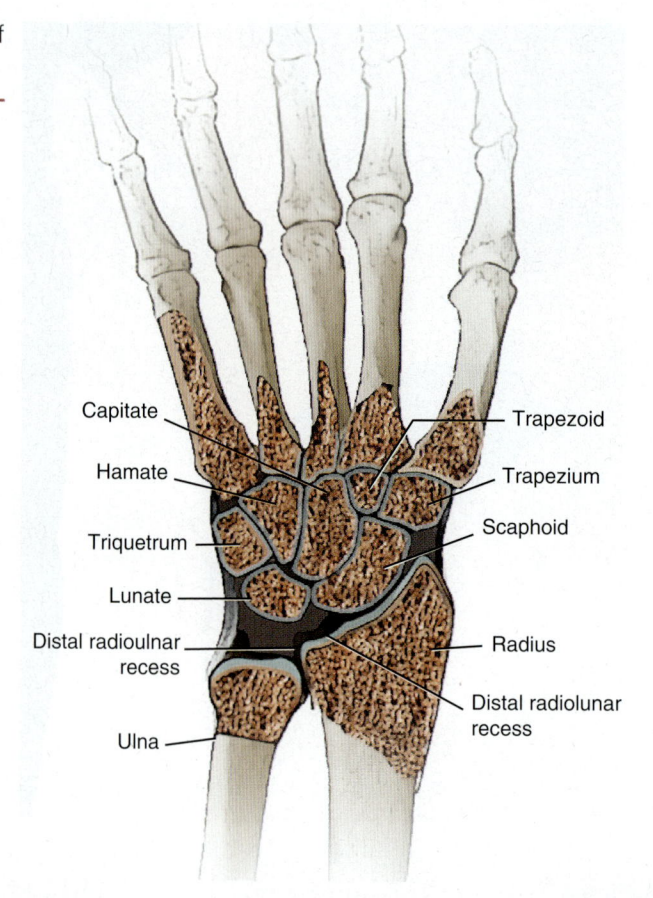

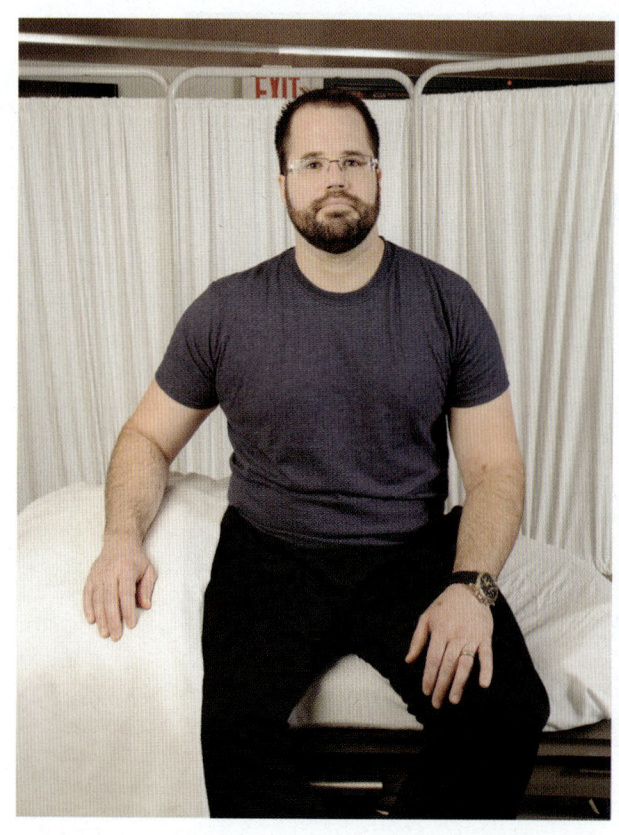

**FIGURE 61.4.** Correct patient position for ultrasound-guided intra-articular injection of the distal radioulnar joint.

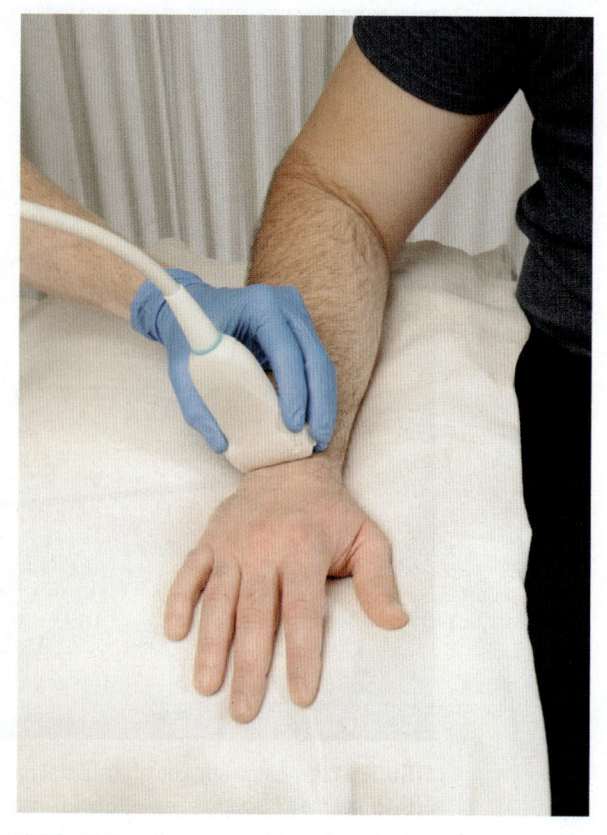

**FIGURE 61.5.** Correct position for ultrasound transducer for ultrasound-guided intra-articular injection of the distal radioulnar joint.

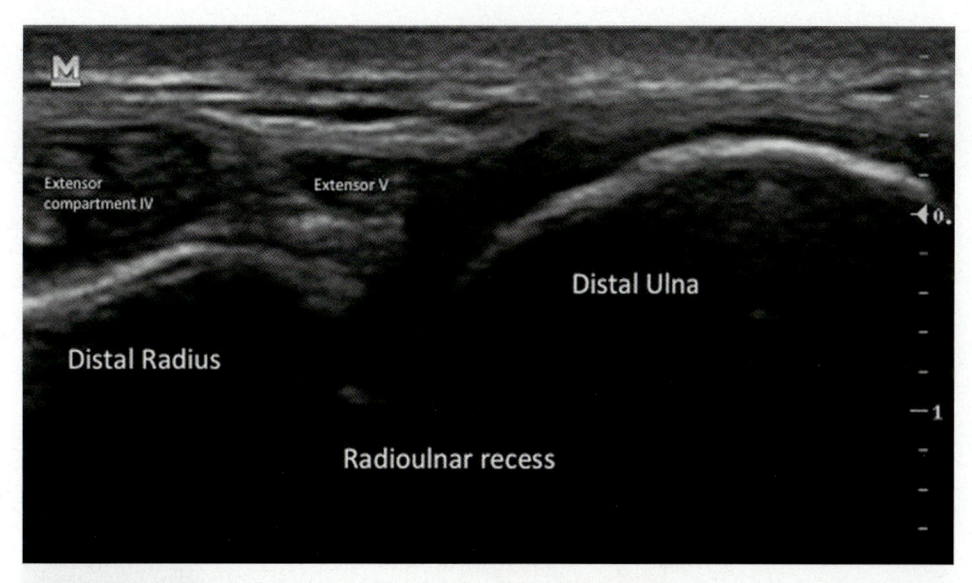

**FIGURE 61.6.** Transverse view of the distal radioulnar demonstrating the distal radius, ulna, and distal radioulnar recess.

ulna is identified as is the hypoechoic intra-articular space just distal to the distal ulna (Fig. 61.6). The ultrasound transducer is slowly moved medially until the crescent-shaped hypoechoic distal radioulnar joint recess is seen lying between the distal radius and ulna (Fig. 61.7). After the distal radioulnar joint recess is identified, it is centered within the ultrasound image, and the needle is placed through the skin ~0.5 cm below the center of the distal aspect of the ultrasound transducer and is then advanced using an out-of-plane approach with the needle trajectory adjusted under real-time ultrasound guidance to enter the distal radioulnar recess (Fig. 61.8). When the tip of needle is thought to be within the recess, a small amount of local anesthetic and steroid is injected under real-time ultrasound guidance to confirm intra-articular placement by the characteristic spreading swirl of hyperechoic injectate within the joint. After intra-articular needle tip placement is confirmed, the remainder of the contents of the syringe are slowly injected. There should be minimal resistance to injection. If synechiae, loculations, or calcifications are present, the needle may have to be repositioned to ensure that the entire joint is treated. The needle is then removed, and a sterile pressure dressing and ice pack are placed at the injection site.

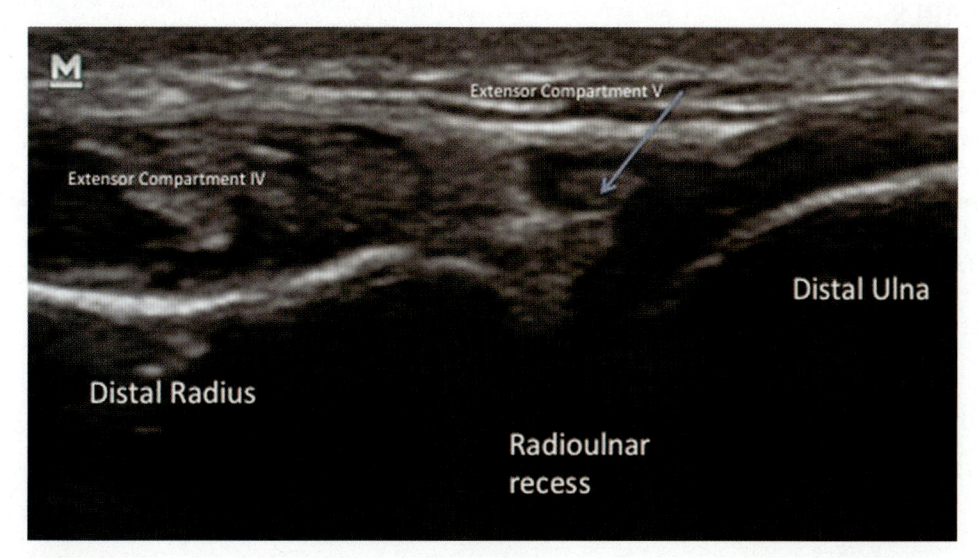

**FIGURE 61.7.** The distal radioulnar recess is identified and the ultrasound transducer is moved so that the recess appears in the center of the image.

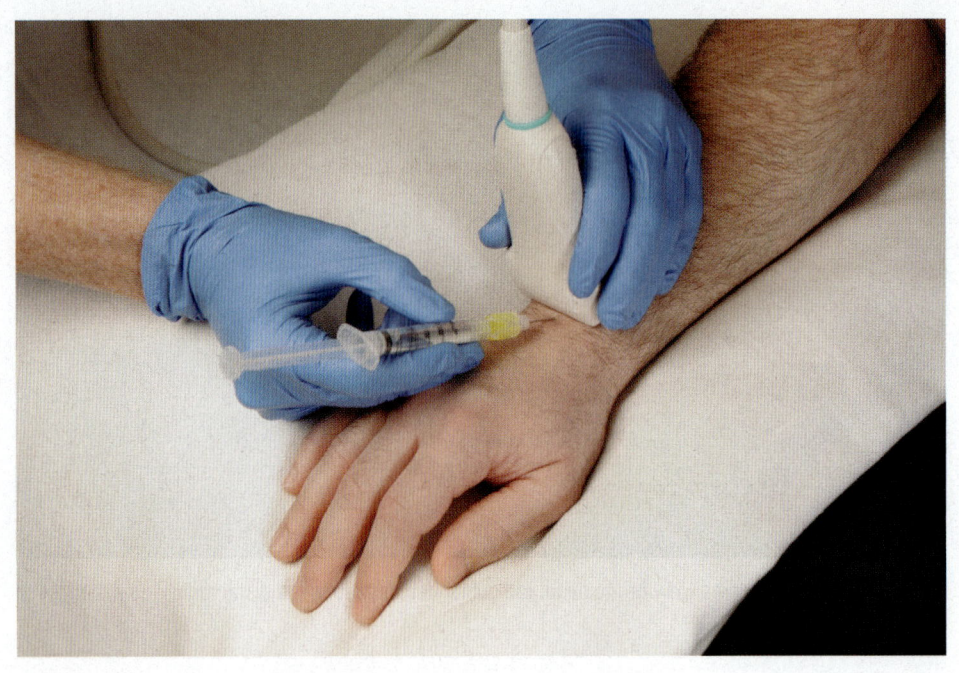

**FIGURE 61.8.** Proper needle position for ultrasound-guided out-of-plane injection of the distal radioulnar joint.

## COMPLICATIONS

The major complication of ultrasound-guided injection of the distal radioulnar joint is infection. Ecchymosis and hematoma formation may also occur. A transient exacerbation of the patient's pain occurs ~25% of the time following this injection technique, and the patient should be warned of this possibility prior to the procedure.

## CLINICAL PEARLS

Wrist pathology including tendinopathy, occult fractures, osteoarthritis, avascular necrosis, bursitis, synovitis, and impingement syndromes may coexist with distal radioulnar joint disease and may contribute to the patient's pain symptomatology. Universal precautions should always be observed to protect the operator, and strict adherence to sterile technique must be used to avoid infection. Gentle physical therapy and local heat should be introduced following ultrasound-guided injection of the distal radioulnar joint to reduce pain and improve function. Simple analgesics and nonsteroidal anti-inflammatory agents or COX-2 inhibitors may be used concurrently with this injection technique.

## SUGGESTED READINGS

Buck FM, Nicol MAC, Ghenol R, et al. Morphology of the distal radioulnar joint: cadaveric study with MRI and MR arthrography with the forearm in neutral position, pronation, and supination. *AJR Am J Roentgenol* 2010;194(2):W202–W207.

Waldman SD. Functional anatomy of the wrist. In: *Pain Review*. Philadelphia, PA: Saunders; 2009:100–103.

Waldman SD. Injection technique for intra-articular injection of the distal radioulnar. In: *Pain Review*. Philadelphia, PA: Saunders Elsevier; 2009:466–467.

Waldman SD. Arthritis pain of the distal radioulnar. In: *Atlas of Common Pain Syndromes*. 3rd ed. Philadelphia, PA: Saunders Elsevier; 2012:190–192.

Waldman SD. Intra-articular injection of the distal radioulnar joint. In: *Atlas of Pain Management Injection Techniques*. 3rd ed. Philadelphia, PA: Saunders Elsevier; 2013:119–122.

# CHAPTER 62

# Ultrasound-Guided Intra-articular Injection of the Radiocarpal Joint

## CLINICAL PERSPECTIVES

The radiocarpal joint is an ellipsoidal joint formed by the radius and the articular disc proximally and the proximal first row of the carpal bones distally (Fig. 62.1). The primary function of the radiocarpal joint is to aid in orientation of the hand in space for crucial functions like eating and drinking by allowing flexion, extension, adduction, and abduction of the wrist. The joint's articular cartilage is susceptible to damage, which, if left untreated, will result in arthritis with its associated pain and functional disability. Osteoarthritis of the joint is the most common form of arthritis that results in radiocarpal joint pain and functional disability, with rheumatoid arthritis, posttraumatic arthritis, and crystal arthropathy also causing arthritis of the radiocarpal joint. Less common causes of arthritis-induced radiocarpal joint pain include the collagen vascular diseases, infection, villonodular synovitis, and Lyme disease. Acute infectious arthritis of the radiocarpal joint is best treated with early diagnosis, with culture and sensitivity of the synovial fluid, and with prompt initiation of antibiotic therapy. The collagen vascular diseases generally manifest as a polyarthropathy rather than a monoarthropathy limited to the radiocarpal joint, although radiocarpal pain secondary to the collagen vascular diseases responds exceedingly well to ultrasound-guided intra-articular injection of the radiocarpal joint.

Patients with radiocarpal joint pain secondary to arthritis, gout, synovitis, and collagen vascular disease–related joint pain complain of pain that is localized to the distal forearm and wrist.

Activity, including flexion, extension, adduction, and abduction, makes the pain worse, with rest and heat providing some relief. The pain is constant and characterized as aching. Sleep disturbance is common with awakening when patients roll over onto the affected upper extremity. Some patients complain of a grating, catching, or popping sensation with range of motion of the joint, and crepitus may be appreciated on physical examination.

Functional disability often accompanies the pain of many pathologic conditions of the radiocarpal joint. Patients will often notice increasing difficulty in performing their activities of daily living and tasks that require flexion, extension, adduction, and abduction of the wrist such as using a computer keyboard, screwdriver, and corkscrew or tuning a doorknob. If the pathologic process responsible for the radiocarpal pain is not adequately treated, the patient's functional disability may worsen and muscle wasting and ultimately a frozen radiocarpal joint may occur.

Plain radiographs are indicated in all patients who present with radiocarpal joint pain (Fig. 62.2). Based on the patient's clinical presentation, additional testing may be indicated,

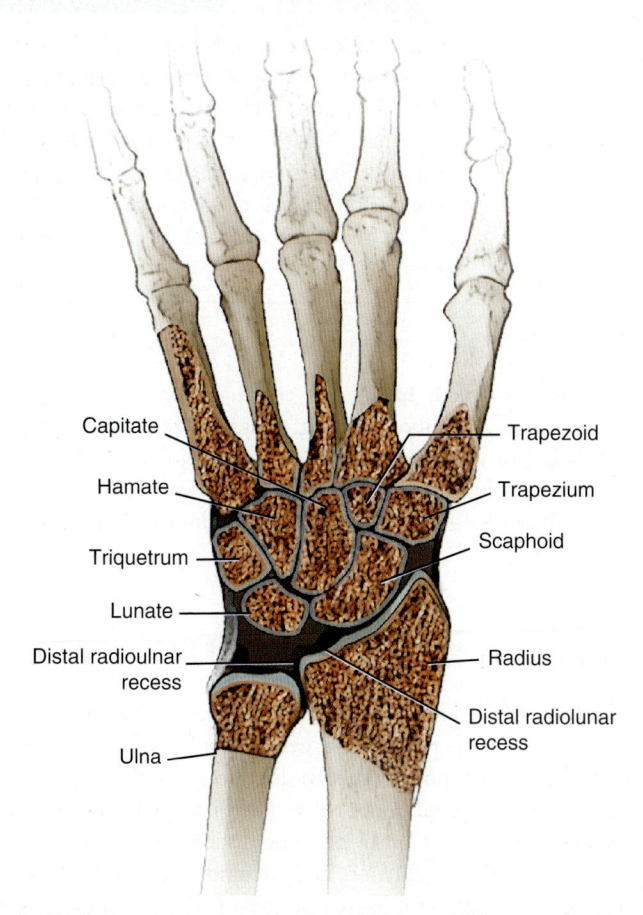

**FIGURE 62.1.** The anatomy of the radiocarpal joint.

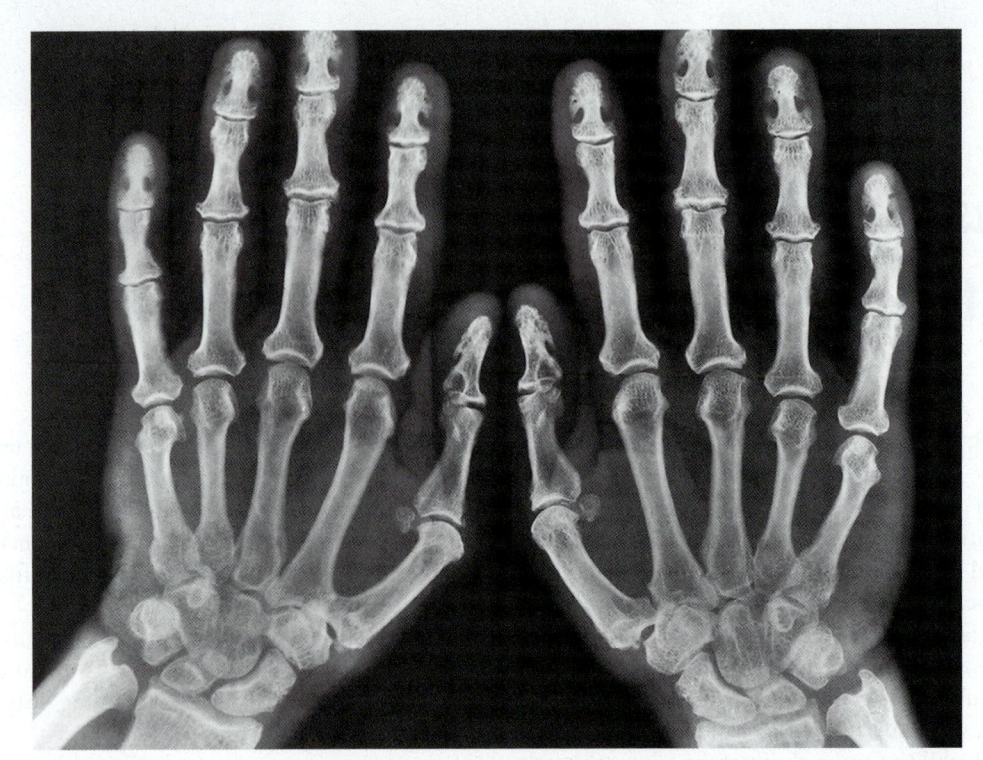

**FIGURE 62.2.** Acromegalic osteoarthritis. Dorsovolar radiograph of both hands of a 42-year-old man with acromegaly shows widening of some and narrowing of other joint spaces, enlargement of the distal tufts and the bases of terminal phalanges, and beak-like osteophytes affecting particularly the heads of the metacarpals. Note the soft tissue prominence and the large sesamoid bones at the first metacarpophalangeal joints. The sesamoid index (derived by multiplying the vertical and horizontal diameters of the sesamoid bone) is 48 in this patient; normally, it should not exceed 20 to 25. (Reused from Greenspan A. *Orthopedic Imaging: A Practical Approach.* 5th ed. Philadelphia, PA: Lippincott Williams & Wilkins; 2011:476, with permission.)

including complete blood cell count, sedimentation rate, and antinuclear antibody testing. Magnetic resonance imaging (MRI) or ultrasound of the radiocarpal joint is indicated if fracture, effusion, tendinopathy, crystal arthropathy, joint mice, synovitis, bursitis, or ligamentous injury is suspected (Fig. 62.3).

## CLINICALLY RELEVANT ANATOMY

The radiocarpal joint of the wrist is a biaxial, ellipsoid-type joint that serves as the concave articulation between the distal end of the radius and the articular disc above and the scaphoid, lunate, and triquetral bones below (see Figs. 62.1). The joint optimizes hand function by allowing flexion and extension as well as abduction, adduction, and circumduction of the wrist. The joint is a synovial-lined true joint with an intra-articular space that allows easy access for intra-articular injection, although septa within the synovial space may limit the flow of injectate. The entire joint is covered by a dense capsule that is attached above to the distal ends of the radius and ulna and below to the proximal row of metacarpal bones. The anterior and posterior joint is strengthened by the anterior and posterior ligaments, with the medial and lateral ligaments strengthening the medial and lateral joint, respectively. The wrist joint also may become inflamed as a result of direct trauma or overuse of the joint.

Primary innervation of the wrist joint is derived from the deep branch of the ulnar nerve, as well as by the anterior interosseous nerve, which is a branch or the median nerve, and the posterior interosseous nerve, which is a continuation of the radial nerve. Anteriorly, the wrist is bounded by the flexor tendons and the median and ulnar nerves. Posteriorly, the wrist is bounded by the extensor tendons. Laterally, the radial artery can be found. The dorsal branch of the ulnar nerve runs medial to the joint; frequently this nerve is damaged when the distal ulna is fractured.

## ULTRASOUND-GUIDED TECHNIQUE

The benefits, risks, and alternative treatments are explained to the patient, and informed consent is obtained. The patient is then placed in the sitting position with the elbow flexed and

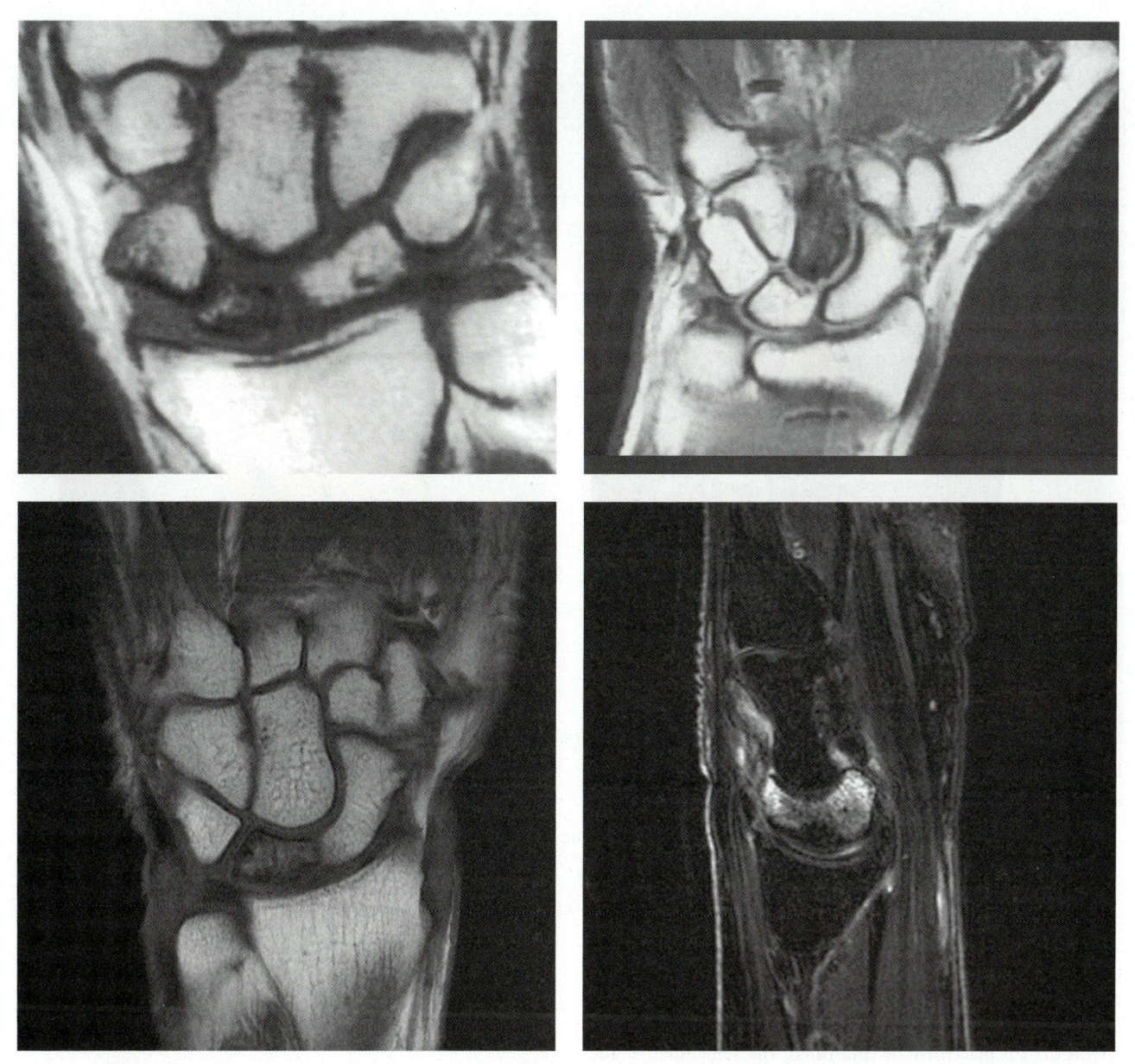

**FIGURE 62.3.** MRI T1- and T2-weighted image demonstrating synovial sarcoma of the wrist. (Reused from Berquist TH. *MRI of the Musculoskeletal System.* 5th ed. Philadelphia, PA: Lippincott Williams & Wilkins; 2006, with permission.)

the forearm and hand resting comfortably palm down on a pillow or padded bedside table (Fig. 62.4). The skin overlying the radiocarpal joint is then prepped with antiseptic solution. A sterile syringe containing 2.0 mL of 0.25% preservative-free bupivacaine and 40 mg of methylprednisolone is attached to a 1½-inch, 22-gauge needle using strict aseptic technique. A linear high-frequency ultrasound transducer is placed over the distal radius in the longitudinal axis, and a survey scan is obtained (Fig. 62.5). The hyperechoic linear plateau of the radius is followed distally until the hypoechoic intra-articular space between the distal radius and the scaphoid bone is identified (Fig. 62.6). After the radiocarpal joint is identified, the ultrasound transducer is slowly moved proximally until the intraarticular joint rests below the distal end on the longitudinally oriented transducer. The needle is placed through the skin ~0.5 cm below the center of the distal aspect of the ultrasound transducer and is then advanced using an in-plane approach with the needle trajectory adjusted under real-time ultrasound guidance to enter the radiocarpal joint between the distal radius and proximal aspect of the scaphoid bone (Fig. 62.7). When the tip of needle is thought to be within the joint, a small amount of local anesthetic and steroid is

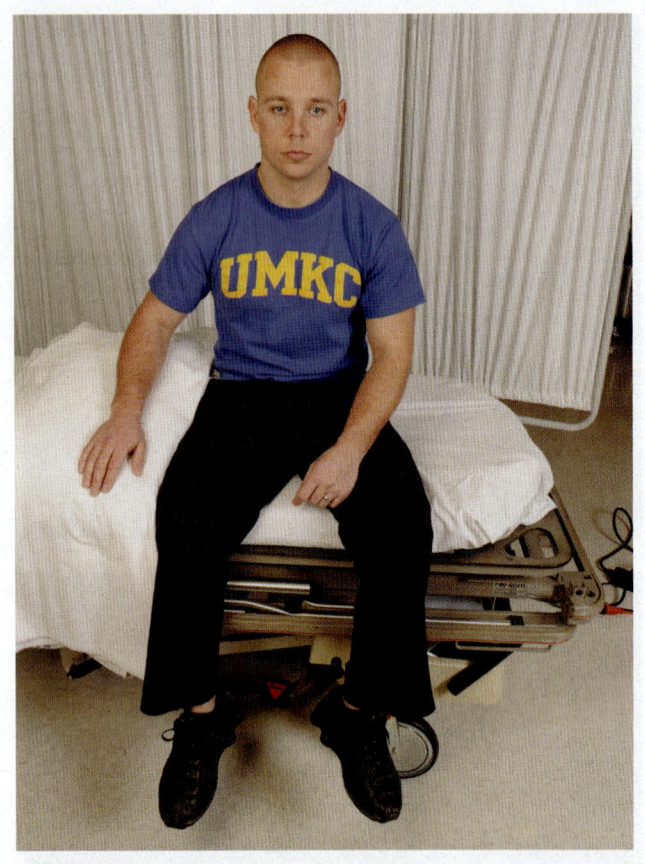

**FIGURE 62.4.** Correct patient position for ultrasound-guided intra-articular injection of the radiocarpal joint.

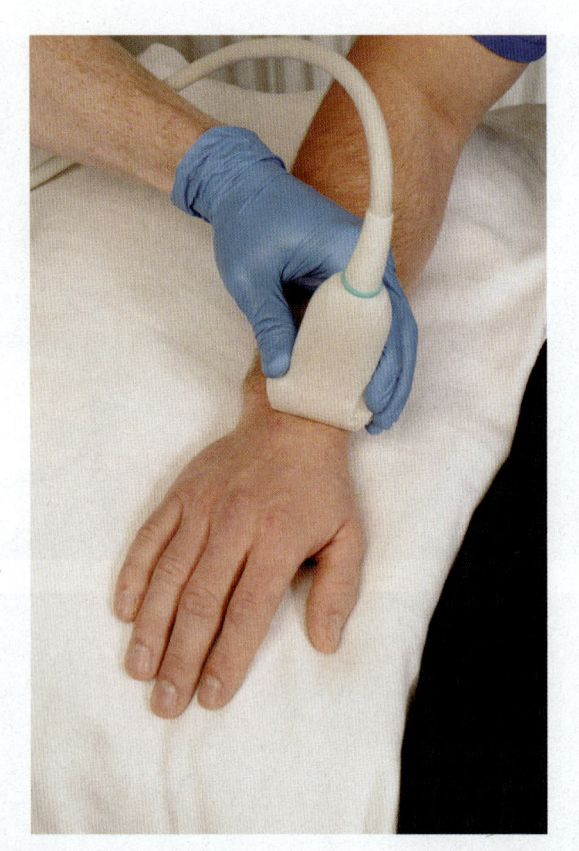

**FIGURE 62.5.** Correct position for ultrasound transducer for ultrasound-guided intra-articular injection of the radiocarpal joint.

injected under real-time ultrasound guidance to confirm intra-articular placement by the characteristic spreading swirl of hyperechoic injectate within the joint. After intra-articular needle tip placement is confirmed, the remainder of the contents of the syringe are slowly injected. There should be minimal resistance to injection. If synechiae, loculations, or calcifications are present, the needle may have to be repositioned to ensure that the entire joint is treated. The needle is then removed, and a sterile pressure dressing and ice pack are placed at the injection site.

## COMPLICATIONS

The major complication of ultrasound-guided injection of the radiocarpal joint is infection. Ecchymosis and hematoma formation may also occur. A transient exacerbation of the patient's pain occurs ~25% of the time following this injection technique, and the patient should be warned of this possibility prior to the procedure.

## CLINICAL PEARLS

Wrist pathology including tendinopathy, occult fractures, osteoarthritis, avascular necrosis (especially of the scaphoid), bursitis, synovitis, and impingement syndromes may coexist with radiocarpal joint disease and may contribute to the patient's pain symptomatology (Figs. 62.8 and 62.9). Universal precautions should always be observed to protect the operator, and strict adherence to sterile technique must be used to avoid infection. Gentle physical therapy and local heat should be introduced following ultrasound-guided injection of the radiocarpal joint to reduce pain and improve function. Simple analgesics and nonsteroidal anti-inflammatory agents or COX-2 inhibitors may be used concurrently with this injection technique.

CHAPTER 62  ULTRASOUND-GUIDED INTRA-ARTICULAR INJECTION OF THE RADIOCARPAL JOINT    421

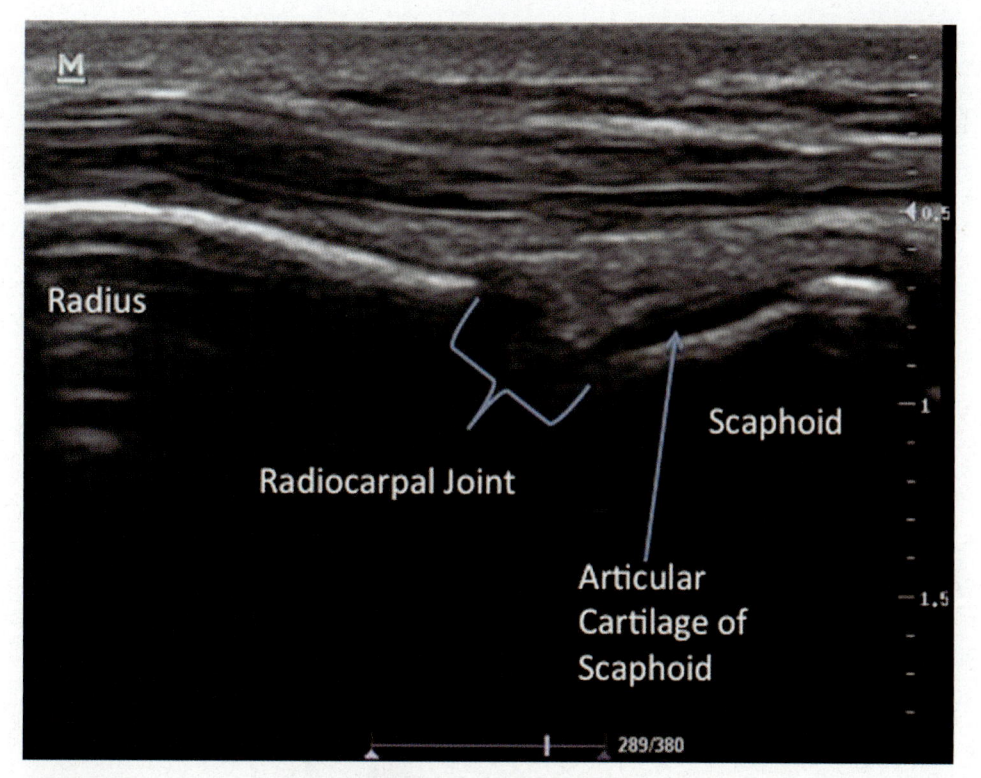

**FIGURE 62.6.** Transverse view of the radiocarpal demonstrating the distal radius, scaphoid, and radiocarpal joint.

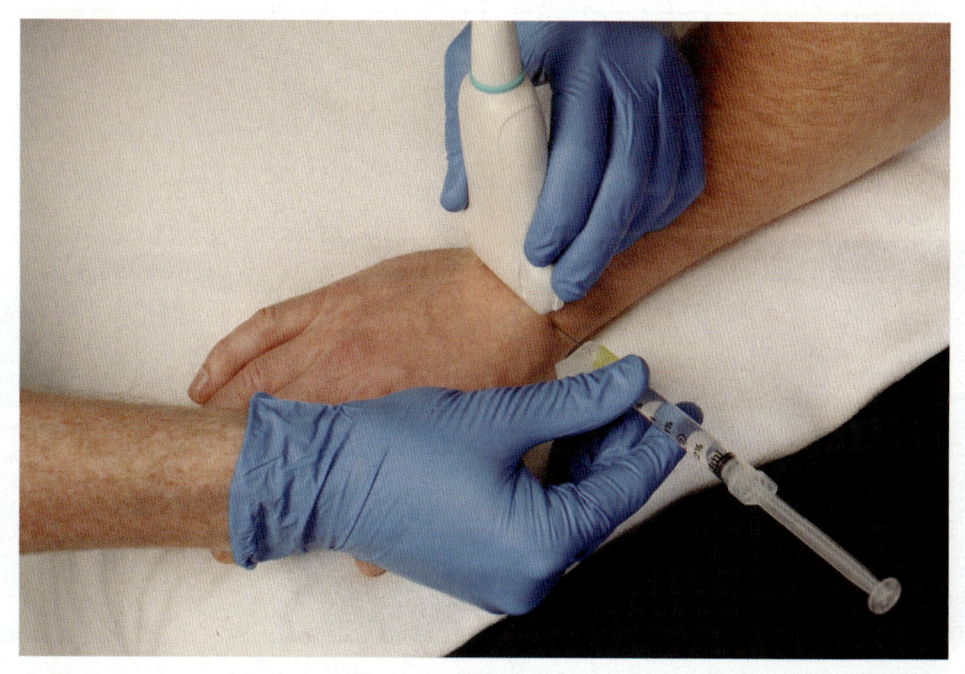

**FIGURE 62.7.** Proper needle position for ultrasound-guided in-plane injection of the radiocarpal joint.

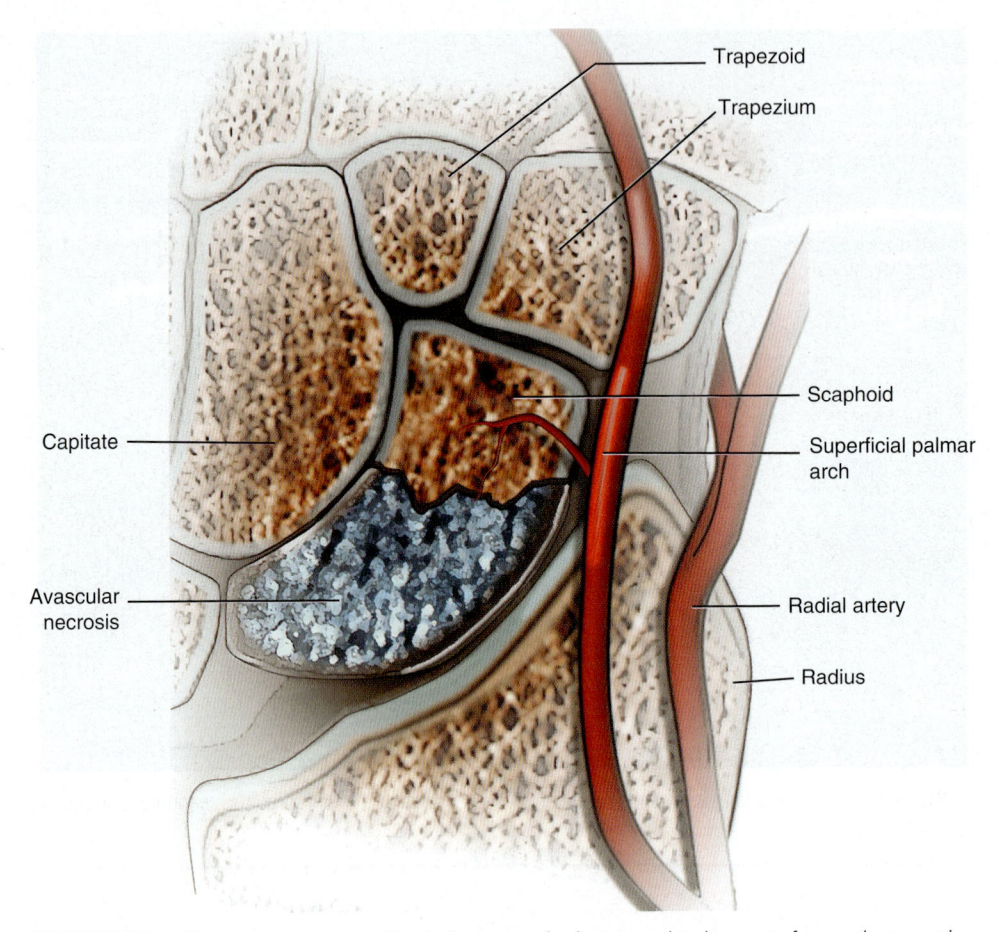

**FIGURE 62.8.** The scaphoid is susceptible to fracture and subsequent development of avascular necrosis.

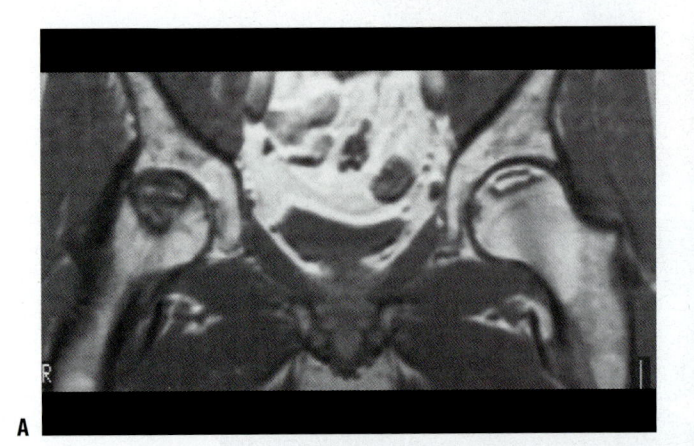

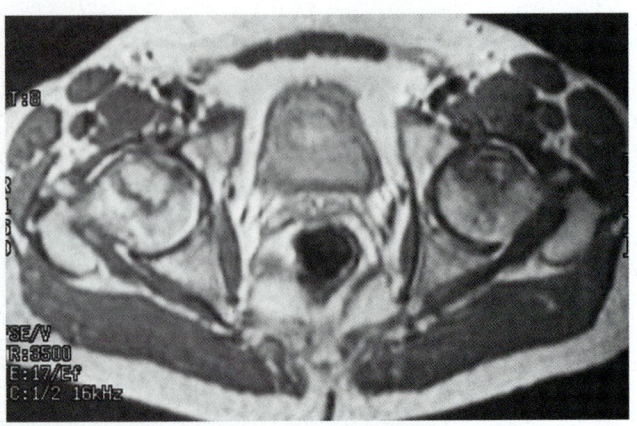

**FIGURE 62.9.** MRI staging of osteonecrosis (class A). **A:** Coronal T1-weighted (SE; TR 600/TE 20 msec) image shows the preservation of a normal bright signal of fat within the lesion, surrounded by a low-signal intensity reactive margin in both femoral heads. **B:** Axial T2-weighted (fast SE; TR 3,500/TE 17 msec/Ef) image shows intermediate signal within an osteonecrotic segment, analogous fat. (Reused from Greenspan A. *Orthopedic Imaging: A Practical Approach.* 5th ed. Philadelphia, PA: Lippincott Williams & Wilkins; 2011:80, with permission.)

## SUGGESTED READINGS

Boesen M, Jensen KE, Torp-Pedersen S, et al. Intra-articular distribution pattern after ultrasound-guided injections in wrist joints of patients with rheumatoid arthritis. *Eur J Radiol* 2009;69(2):331–338.

Waldman SD. Functional anatomy of the wrist. In: *Pain Review*. Philadelphia, PA: Saunders Elsevier; 2009:100–103.

Waldman SD. Injection technique for intra-articular injection of the wrist. In: *Pain Review*. Philadelphia: Saunders Elsevier; 2009:464–465.

Waldman SD. Arthritis pain of the wrist. In: *Atlas of Common Pain Syndromes*. 3rd ed. Philadelphia, PA: Saunders Elsevier; 2012:157–159.

Waldman SD. Intra-articular injection of the wrist joint. In: *Atlas of Pain Management Injection Techniques*. 3rd ed. Philadelphia, PA: Saunders Elsevier; 2013:186–189.

# CHAPTER 63

# Ultrasound-Guided Radial Nerve Block at the Wrist

## CLINICAL PERSPECTIVES

Ultrasound-guided superficial radial nerve block at the wrist is useful in the management of the pain subserved by the radial nerve. This technique serves as an excellent adjunct to brachial plexus block and for general anesthesia when performing surgery at the wrist or below. Ultrasound-guided superficial radial nerve block at the wrist with local anesthetic may be used to palliate acute pain emergencies, including postoperative pain, pain secondary to traumatic injuries of the distal radius, and portions of the wrist and carpal bones innervated by the distal radial nerve, as well as cancer pain, while waiting for pharmacologic, surgical, and antiblastic methods to become effective.

Ultrasound-guided superficial radial nerve block can also be used as a diagnostic tool when performing differential neural blockade on an anatomic basis in the evaluation of distal upper extremity pain as well as in a prognostic manner to determine the degree of neurologic impairment the patient will suffer when destruction of the radial nerve is being considered or when there is a possibility that the nerve may be sacrificed during surgeries in the anatomic region of the radial nerve at the level of the wrist. This technique may also be useful in those patients suffering symptoms from compromise of the radial nerve due to cheiralgia paresthetica. Ultrasound-guided superficial radial nerve block at the wrist may also be used to palliate the pain and dysesthesias associated with stretch injuries to the distal radial nerve.

The superficial sensory branch of the radial nerve at the wrist is susceptible to trauma during surgery for de Quervain tenosynovitis or may be damaged by the wearing of too tight wrist watches or handcuffs or the placement of forearm casts that are too tight, which can compress the nerve against the radius. Entrapment neuropathy of the superficial radial nerve at the wrist is known as cheiralgia paresthetica, Wartenberg syndrome, or prisoner's palsy and presents as pain and dysesthesias with associated numbness of the radial aspect of the dorsum of the hand to the base of the thumb (Fig. 63.1).

Physical findings associated with entrapment or trauma of the superficial radial nerve at the wrist include a positive Tinel sign over the radial nerve at the site of injury (Fig. 63.2). Decreased sensation in the distribution of the sensory branch of the radial nerve often is present although the overlap of the distribution of the lateral antebrachial cutaneous nerve in some patients may result in a confusing clinical presentation. Flexion and pronation of the wrist, as well as ulnar deviation, may elicit in the distribution of the superficial sensory branch of the radial nerve in patients suffering from cheiralgia paresthetica. A positive wristwatch test is highly suggestive of the diagnosis of cheiralgia paresthetica. The wristwatch test is performed by having the patient fully deviate his or her wrist to the ulnar side. The examiner then exerts firm pressure on the skin overlying the ulnar nerve (Fig. 63.3). The patient is then instructed to fully flex the wrist. The test is considered positive if this maneuver elicits dysesthesia, pain, or numbness.

## CLINICALLY RELEVANT ANATOMY

The key landmark when performing ultrasound-guided superficial radial nerve block at the wrist is the location of the radial artery and the bony radial styloid. Arising from fibers from the C5–T1 nerve roots of the posterior cord of the brachial plexus, the radial nerve passes through the axilla lying posterior and inferior to the axillary artery. As the radial nerve exits the axilla, it passes between the medial and long heads of the triceps muscle and then curves across the posterior aspect of the humerus, giving off a motor branch to the triceps muscle. Continuing its downward path, the radial nerve gives off a number of sensory branches to the upper arm as it travels in the intermuscular septum separating the bellies of the brachialis and brachioradialis muscles. The nerve passes into the substance of the brachioradialis muscle, and at a point just above the lateral epicondyle, the radial nerve divides into deep and superficial branches; the superficial branch continues down the arm along with the radial artery to provide sensory innervation to the dorsum of the wrist and the dorsal aspects of a portion of the thumb and index and middle fingers, and the deep branch provides the majority of the motor innervation to the extensors of the forearm (Fig. 63.4).

## ULTRASOUND-GUIDED TECHNIQUE

The benefits, risks, and alternative treatments are explained to the patient, and informed consent is obtained. The patient is then placed in the sitting position with the elbow flexed to about 100 degrees and the forearm resting comfortably palm

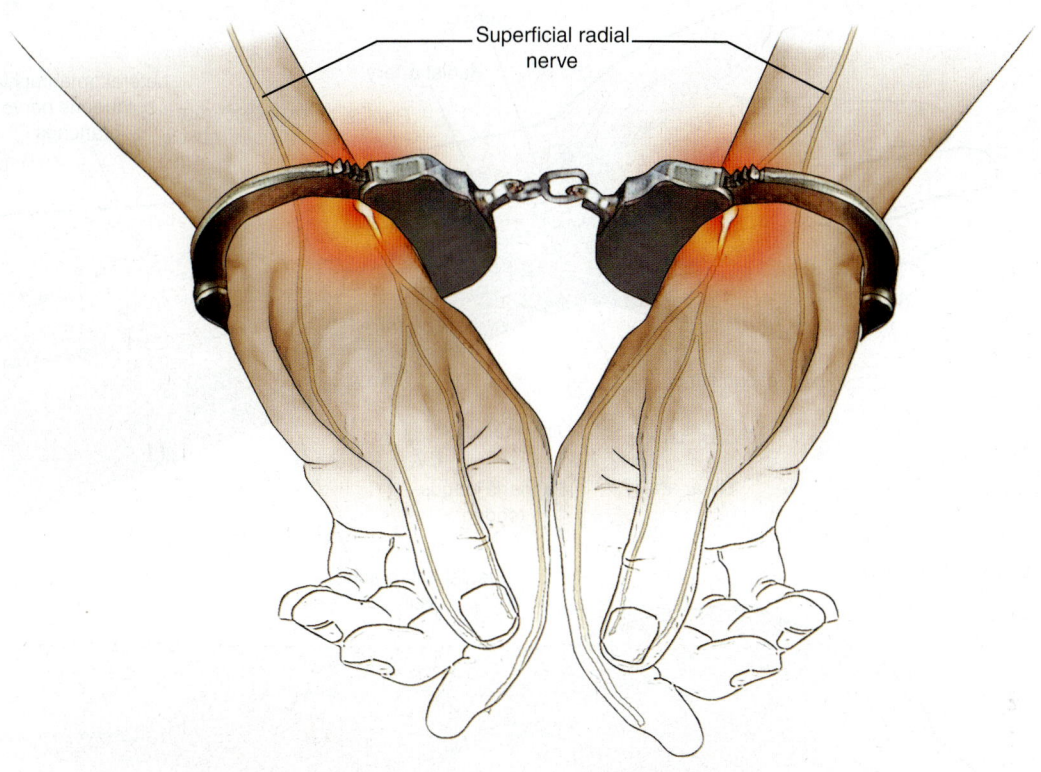

**FIGURE 63.1.** Cheiralgia paresthetica, which is also known as handcuff or prisoner's palsy, is caused by compression of the superficial radial nerve at the wrist.

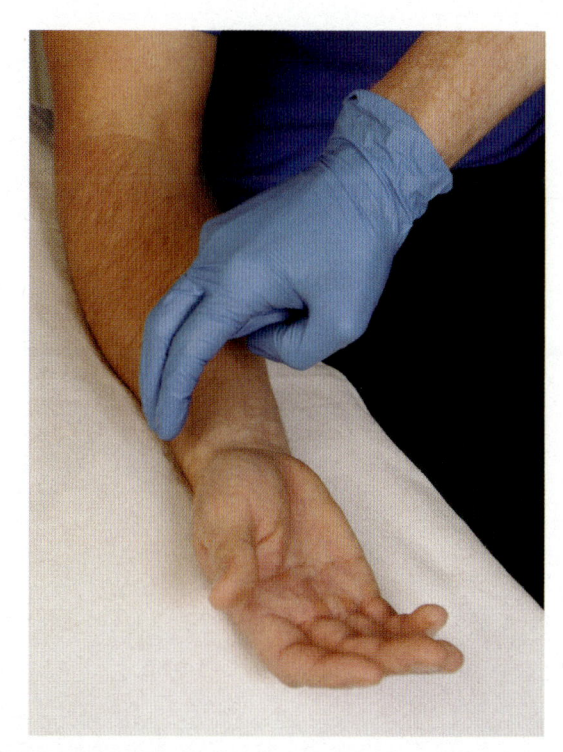

**FIGURE 63.2.** Patients suffering from cheiralgia paresthetica will exhibit a positive Tinel sign over the superficial radial nerve.

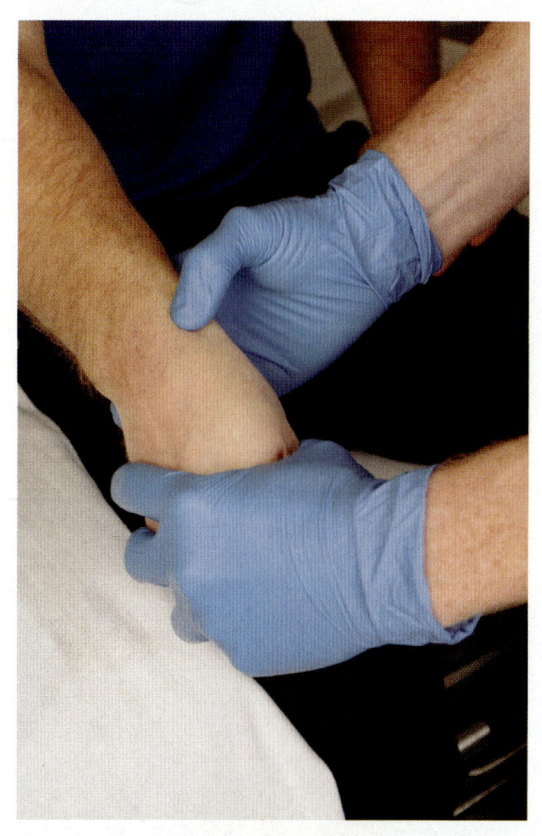

**FIGURE 63.3.** The wristwatch test for cheiralgia paresthetica is performed by having the patient fully deviate his or her wrist to the ulnar side. The examiner then exerts firm pressure on the skin overlying the ulnar nerve.

**A.** Palmar view

Labels: Superficial radial nerve; Radial artery; Radius; Flexor digitorum superficialis muscle; Lateral antebrachial cutaneous nerve branches; Flexor retinaculum; Median nerve; Ulnar nerve; Ulnar artery; Palmaris longus tendon; Medial antebrachial vein

**B.** Dorsoradial view

Labels: Superficial branches of radial nerve; Cephalic vein

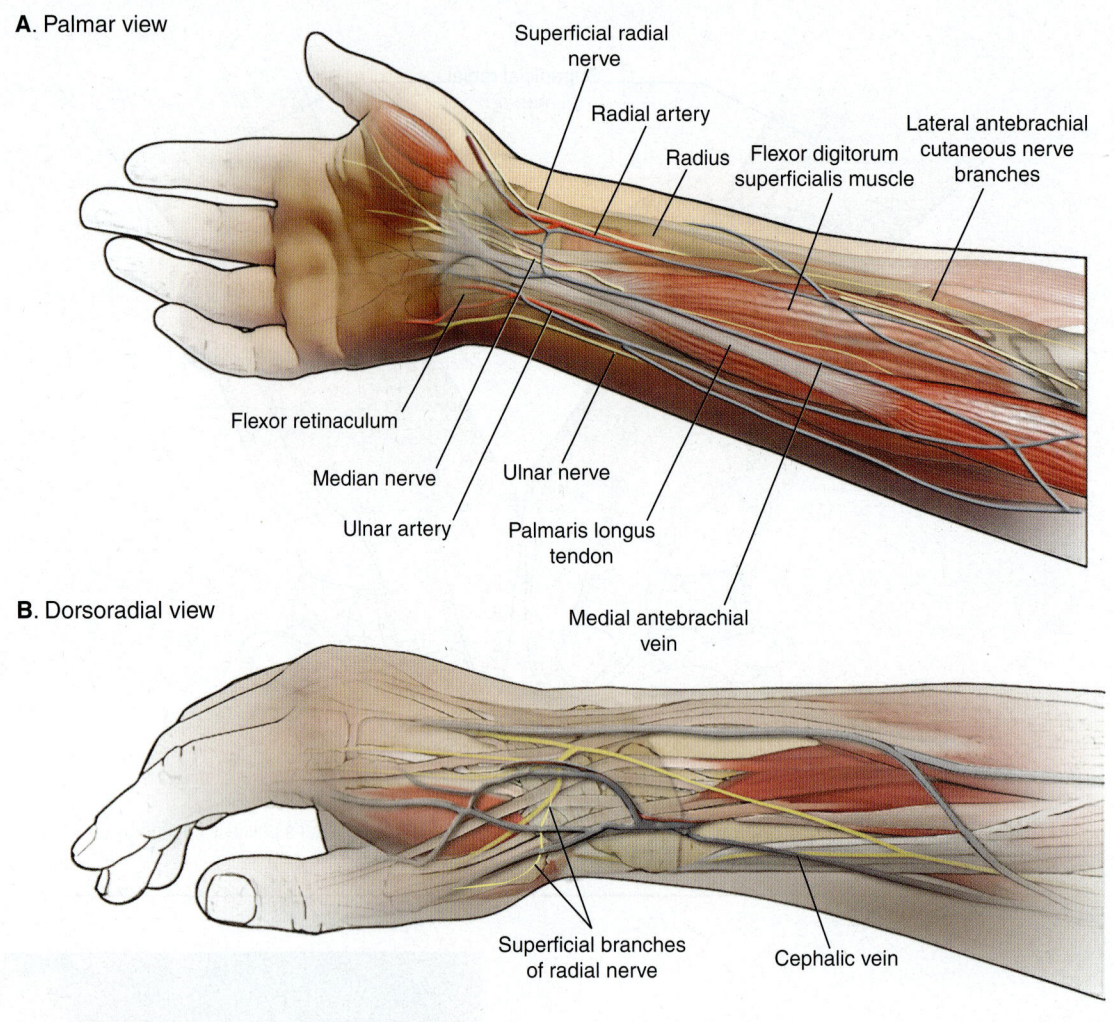

**FIGURE 63.4.** The superficial radial nerve and its relationship to the radial artery.

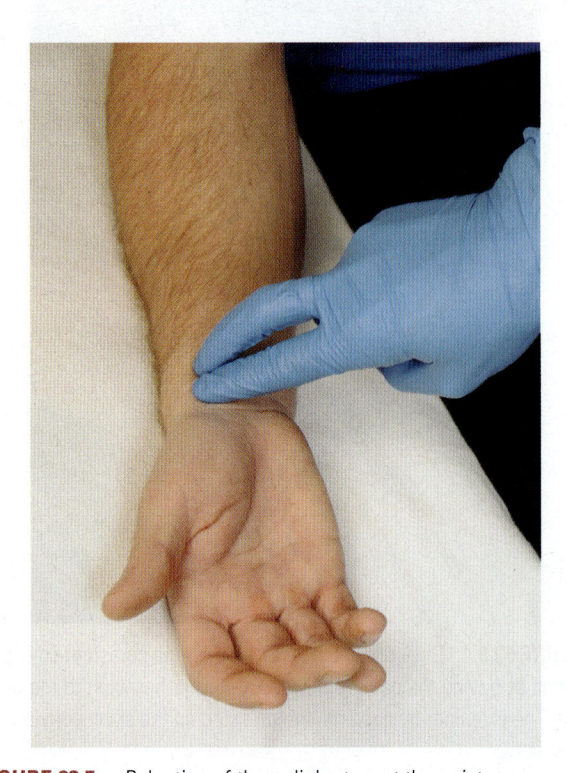

**FIGURE 63.5.** Palpation of the radial artery at the wrist.

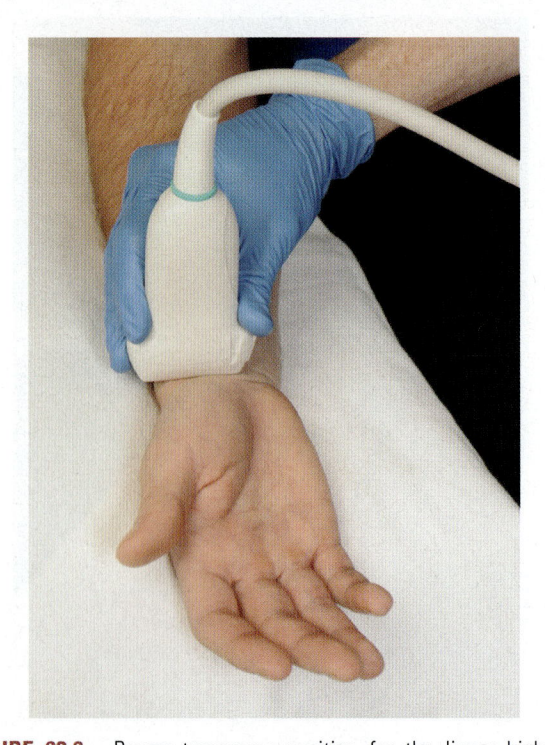

**FIGURE 63.6.** Proper transverse position for the linear high-frequency ultrasound transducer to perform ultrasound-guided superficial radial nerve block at the wrist.

up on a padded bedside table. With the patient in the above position, the radial artery at the wrist is palpated (Fig. 63.5). At a point of maximal pulsation of the radial artery, a high-frequency linear ultrasound transducer is placed in a transverse position over the pulsation at the distal radius, and an ultrasound survey scan is taken (Figs. 63.6 and 63.7). Color Doppler may aid in identification of the radial artery and help separate it with the superficial radial nerve, which lies just radial to the radial artery (Fig. 63.8). The nerve will appear as a bundle of hyperechoic nerve fibers surrounded by a slightly more hyperechoic neural sheath. The skin overlying the area beneath the ultrasound transducer is then prepped with antiseptic solution. A sterile syringe containing 2.0 mL of 0.25% preservative-free bupivacaine and 40 mg of methylprednisolone is attached to a 1½-inch, 22-gauge needle using strict aseptic technique. The needle is placed through the skin just below the inferior border of the transducer and is then advanced using an out-of-plane approach with the needle trajectory adjusted under real-time ultrasound guidance so that the needle tip ultimately rests in proximity to the radial nerve as it lies next to the radial artery (Fig. 63.9). When the tip of needle is thought to be in satisfactory position, after careful aspiration, a small amount of local anesthetic and steroid is injected under real-time ultrasound guidance to confirm that the needle tip is in the proper position. After proper needle tip placement is confirmed, the remainder of the contents of the syringe are slowly injected. There should be minimal resistance to injection.

## COMPLICATIONS

The major complications of ultrasound-guided injection of ultrasound-guided superficial radial nerve block at the wrist are related to improper needle placement with the possibility of inadvertent intravascular injection and/or persistent paresthesia secondary to needle trauma to the radial nerve. Although rare, infection may occur. Ecchymosis and hematoma formation following this procedure may also occur. These complications can be decreased if manual pressure is applied to the area of the block immediately after injection. Application of cold packs for 20-minute periods after the block will also decrease the amount of postprocedure pain and bleeding the patient may experience.

Approximately 25% of patients complain of a transient increase in pain after this injection technique; the patient should be warned of this.

## CLINICAL PEARLS

Ultrasound-guided superficial radial nerve block at the wrist is a straightforward and relatively safe technique if attention is paid to the clinically relevant anatomy. It is useful as an adjunct to surgical anesthesia and has recently been used with increasing frequency in the emergency department to provide anesthesia for reduction of fractures of the radius.

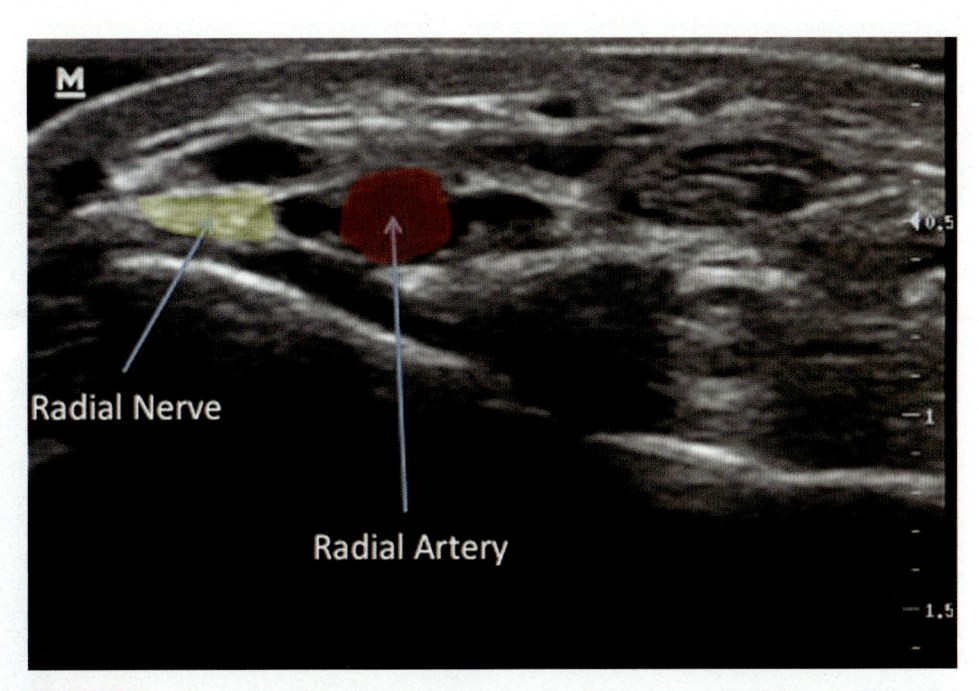

**FIGURE 63.7.** Transverse ultrasound image demonstrating the close proximity of the superficial radial nerve to the radial artery at the wrist.

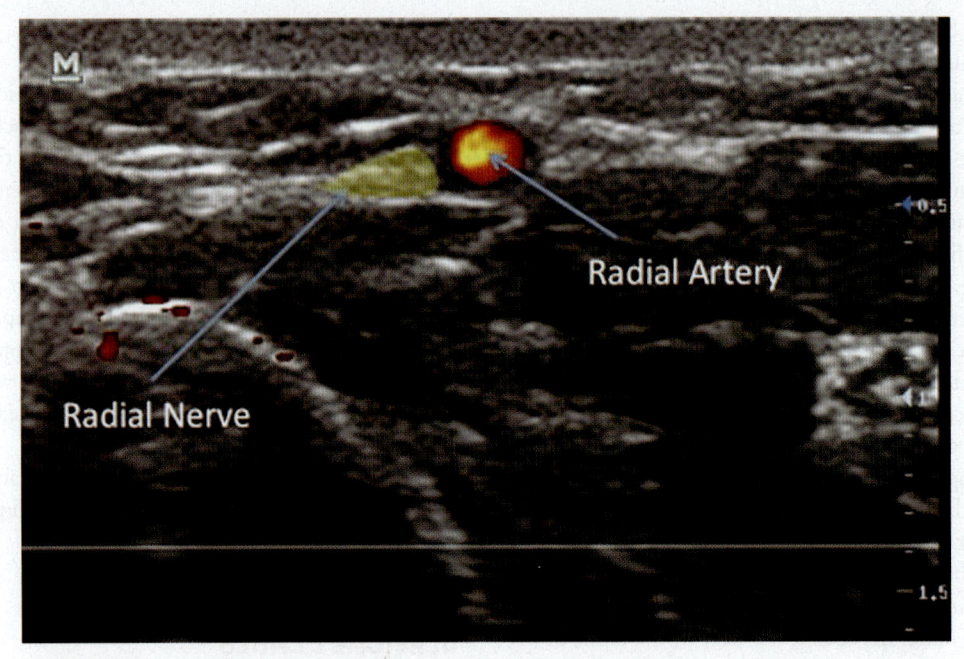

**FIGURE 63.8.** Color Doppler can help distinguish the radial artery from the radial nerve.

Ultrasound-guided superficial radial nerve block at the wrist is also useful in the management of cheiralgia paresthetica, which is also known as handcuff neuropathy. Cheiralgia paresthetica can mimic de Quervain tenosynovitis as both syndromes cause pain when the patient ulnar deviates the wrist. However, de Quervain tenosynovitis pain is more common with activity, while the pain and numbness associated with cheiralgia paresthetica are present at rest. Careful neurologic examination to identify preexisting neurologic deficits that may later be attributed to the nerve block should be performed on all patients before beginning superficial radial nerve block at the wrist.

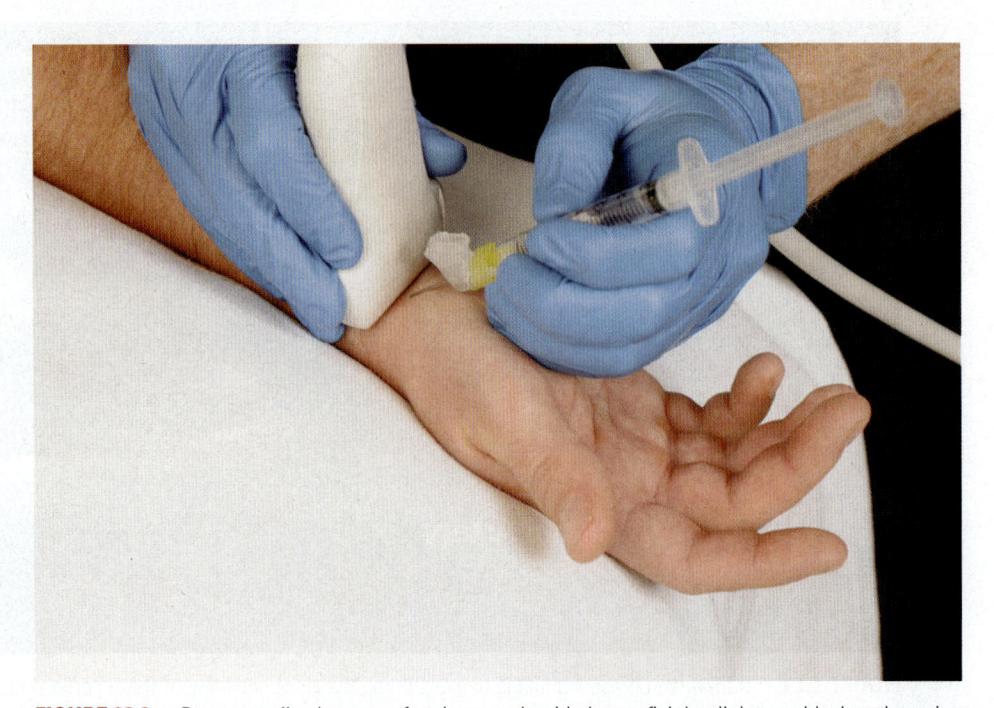

**FIGURE 63.9.** Proper needle placement for ultrasound-guided superficial radial nerve block at the wrist.

## SUGGESTED READINGS

Waldman SD. Cheiralgia paresthetica. In: *Atlas of Uncommon Pain Syndromes*. 2nd ed. Philadelphia, PA: WB Saunders; 2008:114–115.

Waldman SD. Cheiralgia paresthetica. In: *Pain Review*. Philadelphia, PA: Saunders Elsevier; 2009:275–276.

Waldman SD. The radial nerve. In: *Pain Review*. Philadelphia, PA: Saunders Elsevier; 2009:76–77.

Waldman SD. Wristwatch test. In: *Physical Diagnosis of Pain: An Atlas of Signs and Symptoms*. 2nd ed. Philadelphia, PA: WB Saunders; 2010:154–155.

Waldman SD. Superficial radial nerve block at the wrist. In: *Atlas of Pain Management Injection Techniques*. 3rd ed. Philadelphia, PA: WB Saunders; 2012:198–200.

# CHAPTER 64

# Ultrasound-Guided Median Nerve Block at the Wrist

## CLINICAL PERSPECTIVES

Ultrasound-guided median nerve block at the wrist is useful in the management of the pain subserved by the median nerve. This technique serves as an excellent adjunct to brachial plexus block and for general anesthesia when performing surgery at the wrist or below. Ultrasound-guided median nerve block at the wrist with local anesthetic may be used to palliate acute pain emergencies, including postoperative pain, pain secondary to traumatic injuries of the distal radius, and portions of the wrist and carpal bones innervated by the distal median nerve, as well as cancer pain, while waiting for pharmacologic, surgical, and antiblastic methods to become effective.

Ultrasound-guided median nerve block can also be used as a diagnostic tool when performing differential neural blockade on an anatomic basis in the evaluation of distal upper extremity pain as well as in a prognostic manner to determine the degree of neurologic impairment the patient will suffer when destruction of the median nerve is being considered or when there is a possibility that the nerve may be sacrificed during surgeries in the anatomic region of the median nerve at the level of the wrist. This technique may also be useful in those patients suffering symptoms from compromise of the median nerve due to carpal tunnel syndrome. Ultrasound-guided median nerve block at the wrist may also be used to palliate the pain and dysesthesias associated with stretch injuries to the median nerve.

The median nerve at the wrist is susceptible to trauma during surgery for carpal tunnel syndrome or may be damaged by wrist fractures or compressed by mass or tumor (Fig. 64.1). Entrapment neuropathy of the median nerve at the wrist is known as carpal tunnel syndrome and is the most common entrapment neuropathy encountered in clinical practice. Carpal tunnel syndrome presents as pain and dysesthesias with associated numbness and weakness in the hand and wrist that radiate to the thumb, index finger, middle finger, and radial half of the ring finger. These symptoms may also radiate proximal to the level of nerve entrapment into the distal forearm.

Physical findings associated with entrapment or trauma of the median nerve at the wrist include a positive Tinel sign over the median nerve at the site of injury (Fig. 64.2). Decreased sensation in the distribution of the median nerve of the thumb, index finger, middle finger, and radial half of the ring finger is often present as weakness of thumb opposition. A positive Phalen test is highly suggestive of the diagnosis of carpal tunnel syndrome. Phalen test is performed by having the patient place the wrists in complete unforced flexion for at least 30 seconds (Fig. 64.3). The test is considered positive if this maneuver elicits dysesthesia, pain, or numbness in the distribution of the median nerve.

## CLINICALLY RELEVANT ANATOMY

Arising from fibers from the ventral roots of C5 and C6 of the lateral cord and C8 and T1 of the medial cord of the brachial plexus, the median nerve lies anterior and superior to the axillary artery in the 12:00 o'clock to 3:00 o'clock quadrant as it passes through the axilla. As the median nerve exits the axilla, it passes inferiorly adjacent to the brachial artery. At the antecubital fossa, the median nerve lies just medial to the brachial artery. Continuing its downward path, the median nerve gives off a number of motor branches to the flexor muscles of the upper arm. These branches are susceptible to nerve entrapment by aberrant ligaments, muscle hypertrophy, and direct trauma. As the median nerve approaches the wrist, it overlies the radius where it is susceptible to trauma from radial fractures and lacerations. The nerve lies deep to and between the tendons of the palmaris longus muscle and the flexor carpi radialis muscle at the wrist. It is susceptible to entrapment as it passes through the carpal tunnel (Fig. 64.4). The terminal branches of the median nerve provide sensory innervation to a portion of the palmar surface of the hand as well as the palmar surface of the thumb, index, and middle fingers and the radial portion of the ring finger. The median nerve also provides sensory innervation to the distal dorsal surface of the index and middle fingers and the radial portion of the ring finger (Fig. 64.5).

## ULTRASOUND-GUIDED TECHNIQUE

The benefits, risks, and alternative treatments are explained to the patient, and informed consent is obtained. The patient is then placed in the sitting position with the elbow flexed to about 100 degrees and the forearm resting comfortably palm up on a padded bedside table with the fingers slightly flexed,

CHAPTER 64 ULTRASOUND-GUIDED MEDIAN NERVE BLOCK AT THE WRIST 431

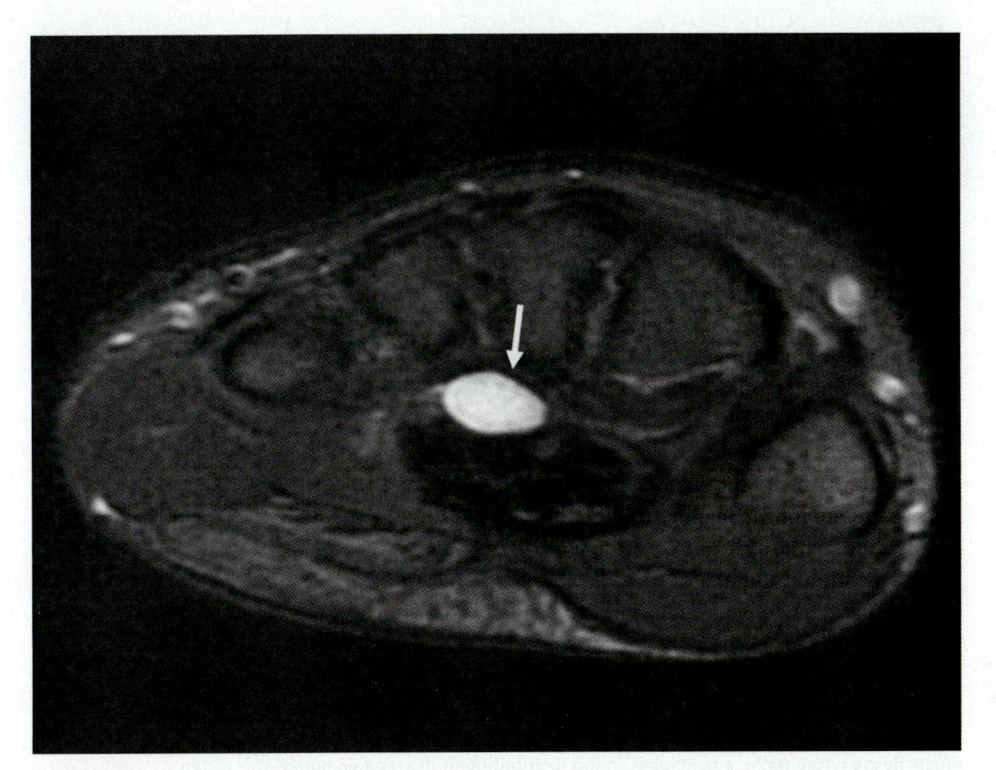

**FIGURE 64.1.** The median nerve is susceptible to compression by a variety of pathologic processes. This axial T2 image demonstrates a high signal mass consistent with a ganglion within the carpal tunnel causing compression of the median nerve. (Reused from Chung CB, Steinbach LS. *MRI of the Upper Extremity*. Philadelphia, PA: Lippincott Williams & Wilkins; 2010:572, with permission.)

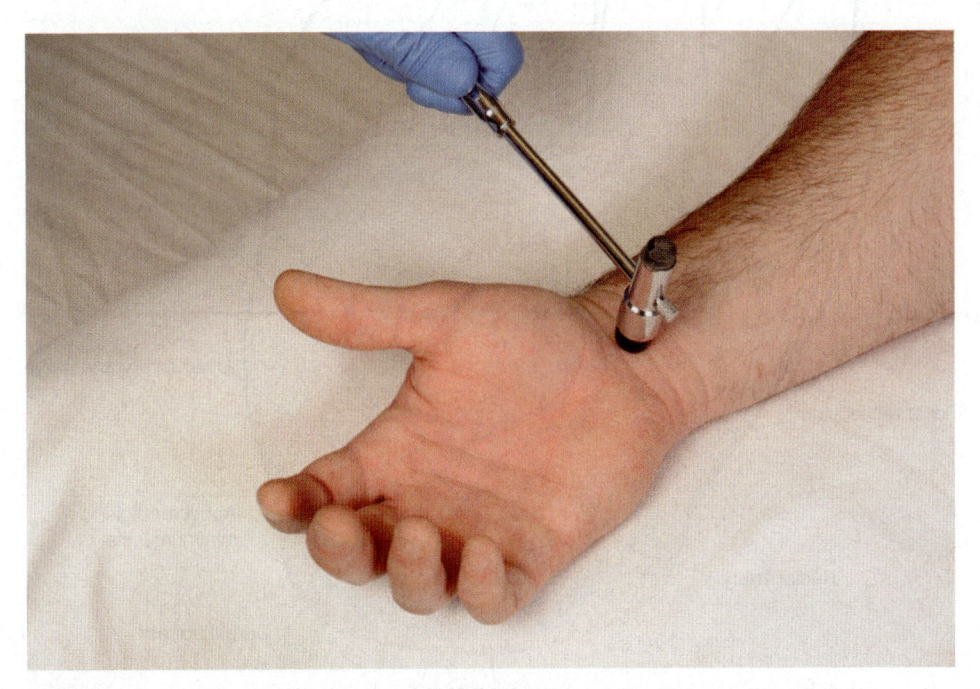

**FIGURE 64.2.** Patients suffering from carpal tunnel syndrome will exhibit a positive Tinel sign over the superficial median nerve.

**SECTION V  WRIST AND HAND**

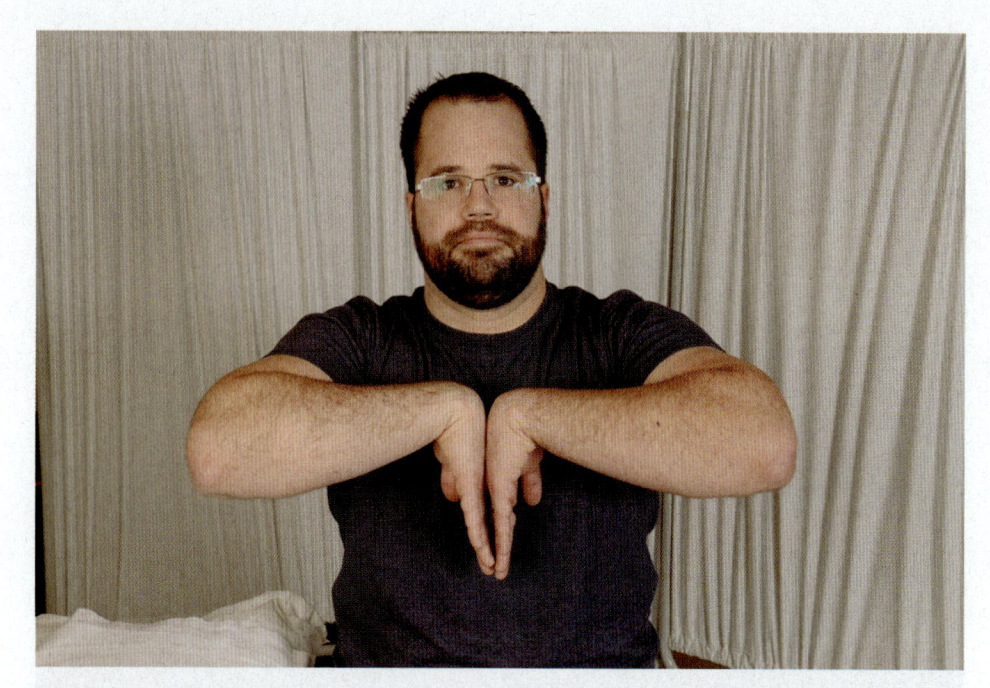

**FIGURE 64.3.** The Phalen test for carpal tunnel syndrome is performed by having the patient place their wrists in complete unforced flexion for at least 30 seconds. The test is considered positive if this maneuver elicits dysesthesia, pain, or numbness in the distribution of the median nerve.

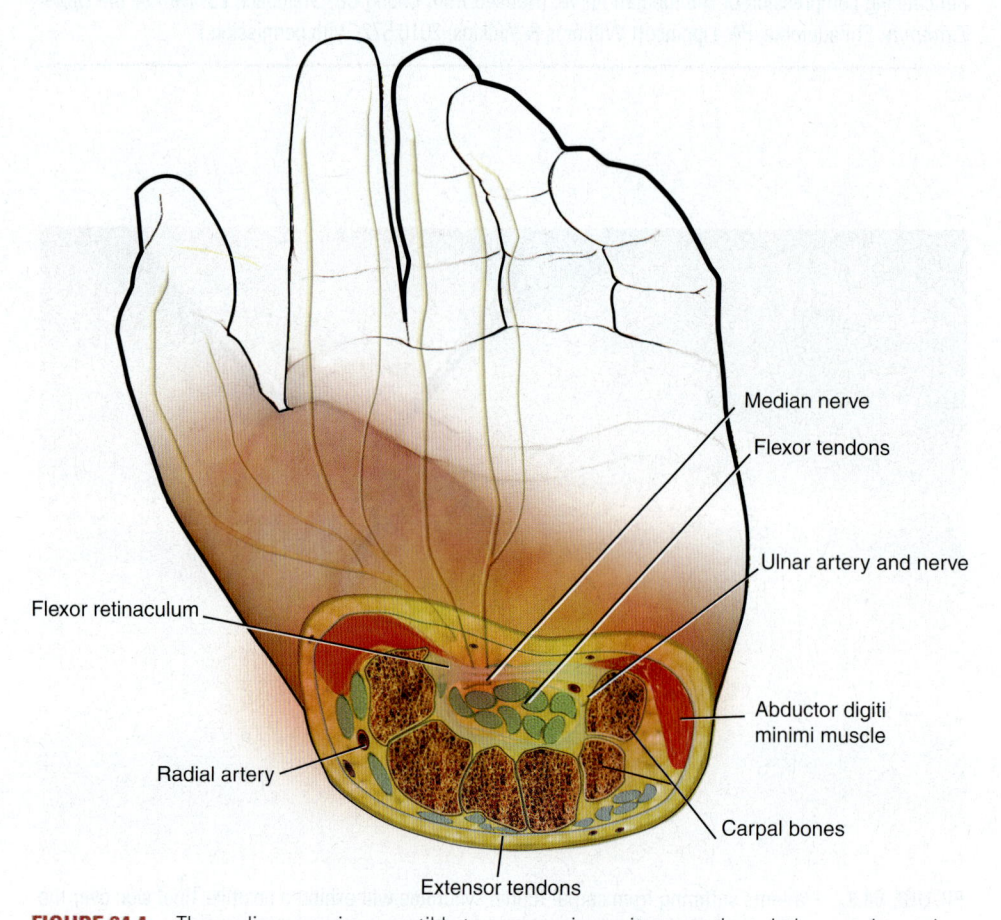

**FIGURE 64.4.** The median nerve is susceptible to compression as it passes through the carpal tunnel.

CHAPTER 64 ULTRASOUND-GUIDED MEDIAN NERVE BLOCK AT THE WRIST 433

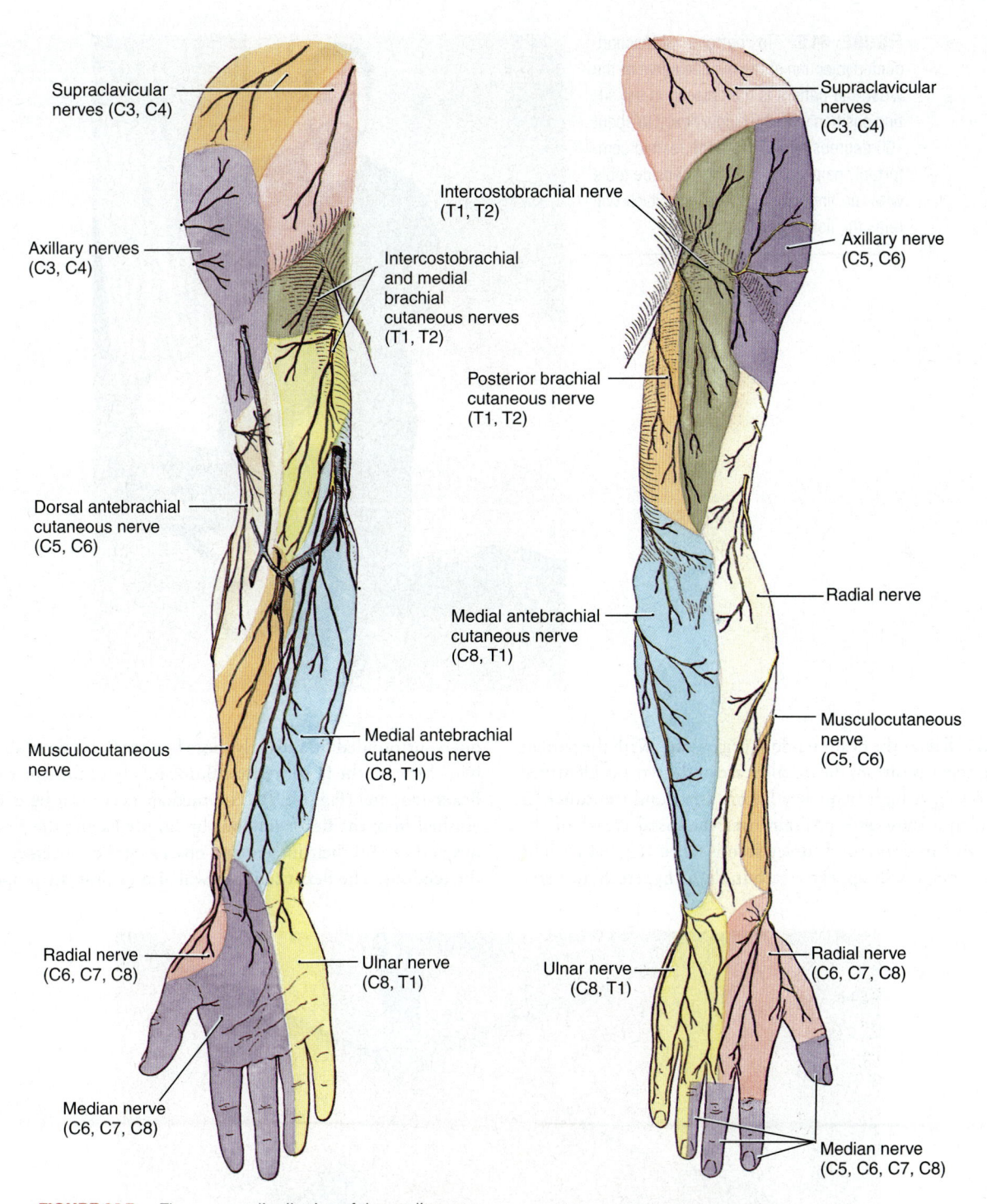

**FIGURE 64.5.** The sensory distribution of the median nerve.

**FIGURE 64.6.** To perform ultrasound-guided injection of the median nerve at the wrist, the patient is then placed in the sitting position with the elbow flexed to about 100 degrees and the forearm resting comfortably palm up on a padded bedside table with the fingers slightly flexed, which will relax the flexor tendons.

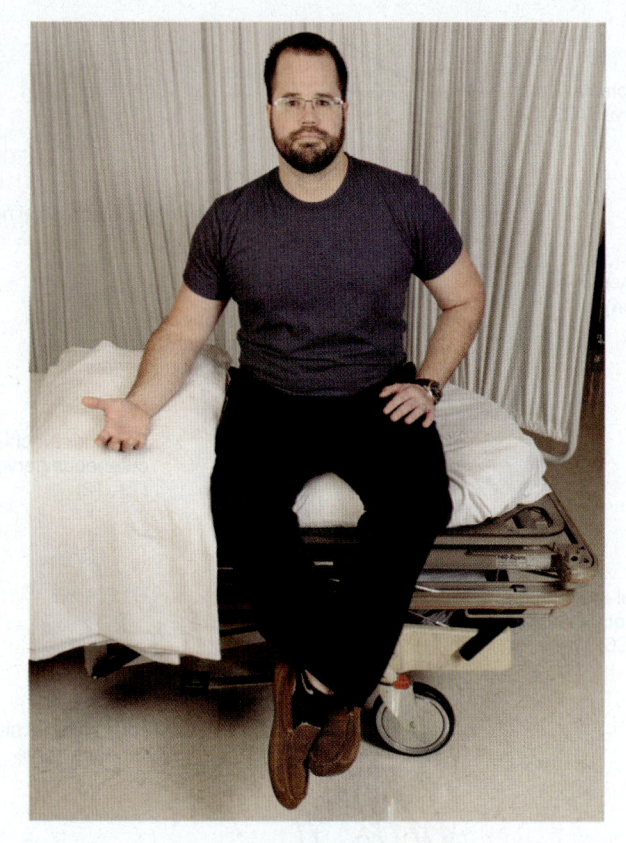

which will relax the flexor tendons (Fig. 64.6). With the patient in the above position, the distal crease of the wrist is identified (Fig. 64.7). A high-frequency linear ultrasound transducer is placed in a transverse position over the distal crease of the wrist, and an ultrasound survey scan is taken (Fig. 64.8). The median nerve will appear as a bundle of hyperechoic nerve fibers surrounded by a slightly more hyperechoic neural sheath lying beneath the flexor retinaculum and above the superficial flexor tendons (Fig. 64.9). The median nerve can be distinguished from the flexor tendons by simply having the patient flex and extend their fingers and observing the movement for the tendons. The flexor tendons will also exhibit the property

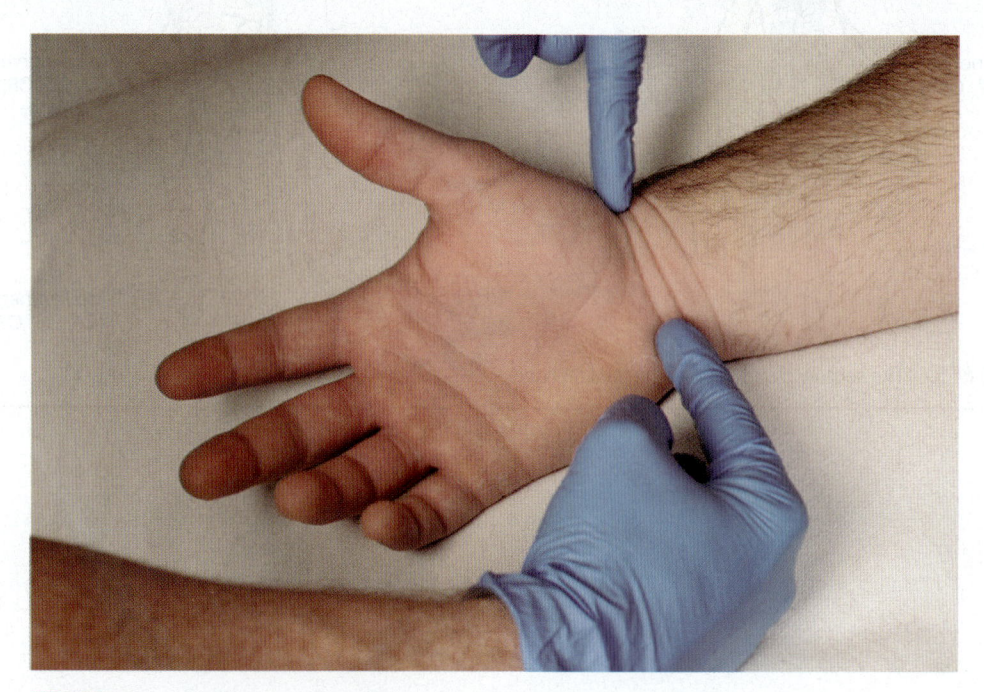

**FIGURE 64.7.** Identification of the distal crease of the wrist.

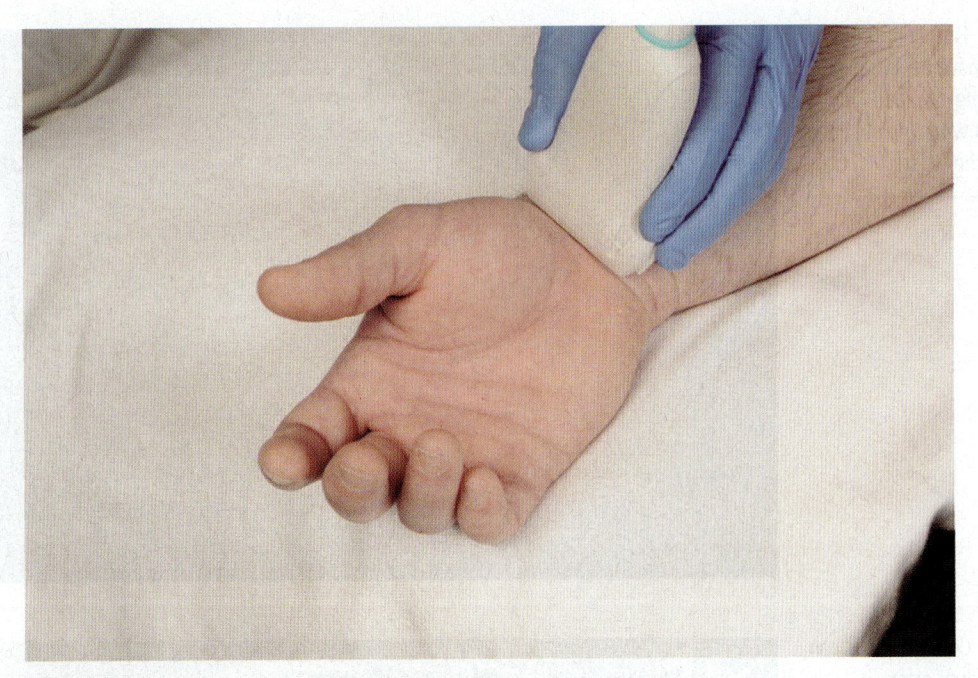

**FIGURE 64.8.** Proper transverse position for the linear high-frequency ultrasound transducer to perform ultrasound-guided median nerve block at the wrist.

of anisotropy with the tipping of the ultrasound transducer back and forth over the tendons. The ulnar artery is then identified on the ulnar side of the wrist (Fig. 64.10). Color Doppler may aid in the identification of the ulnar artery so it can be avoided when performing in-plane needle placement (Fig. 64.11). After the ulnar artery is identified, the ultrasound transducer is slowly moved medially until the median nerve is again easily identifiable in the transverse ultrasound image. The skin overlying the area beneath the ultrasound transducer is then prepped with antiseptic solution. A sterile syringe containing 2.0 mL of 0.25% preservative-free bupivacaine and 40 mg of methylprednisolone is attached to a 1½-inch, 22-gauge needle using strict aseptic technique. The needle is placed through the skin just above the level of where the ulnar artery was previously identified and is advanced using an in-plane approach beneath the ulnar border of the ultrasound transducer with the needle trajectory adjusted under real-time ultrasound guidance so that the needle tip ultimately rests in proximity to the median nerve as it lies within the carpal tunnel beneath the flexor retinaculum (Fig. 64.12).

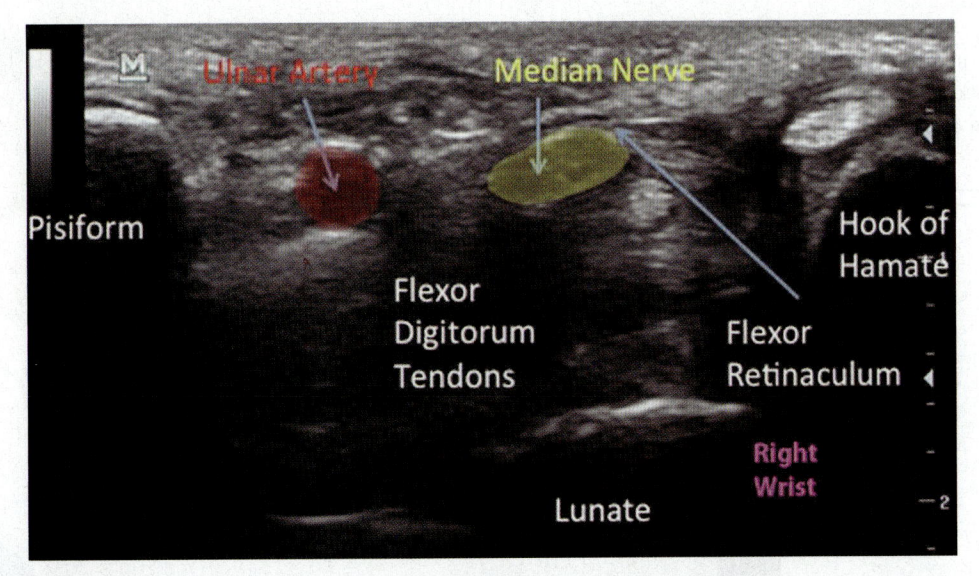

**FIGURE 64.9.** Transverse ultrasound image demonstrating the median nerve lying above the superficial flexor tendons.

**436** SECTION V WRIST AND HAND

**FIGURE 64.10.** The ulnar artery is identified on transverse ultrasound scan so it can be avoided during needle placement when injecting the median nerve at the wrist.

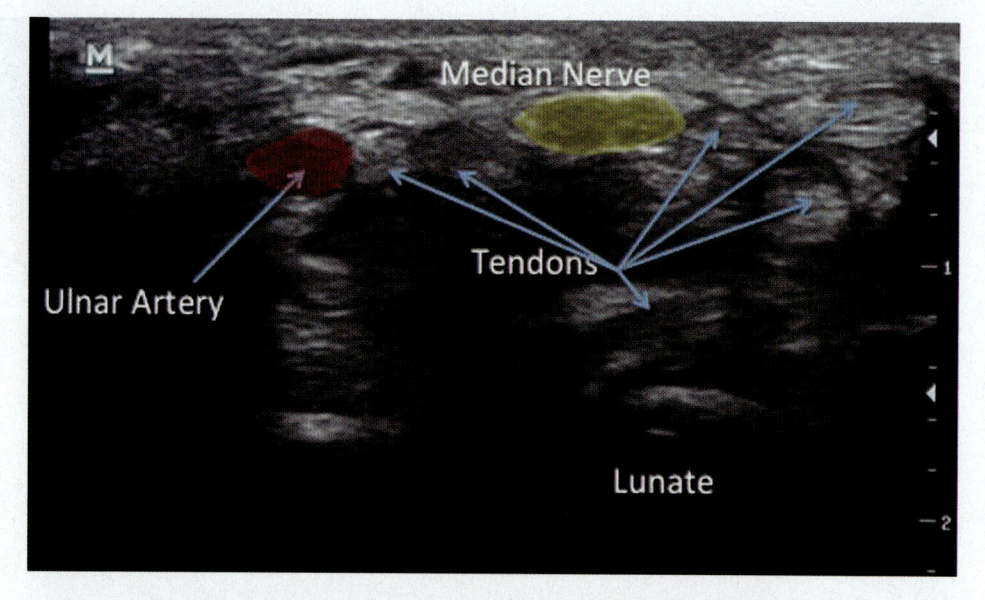

**FIGURE 64.11.** Color Doppler can help identify the ulnar artery.

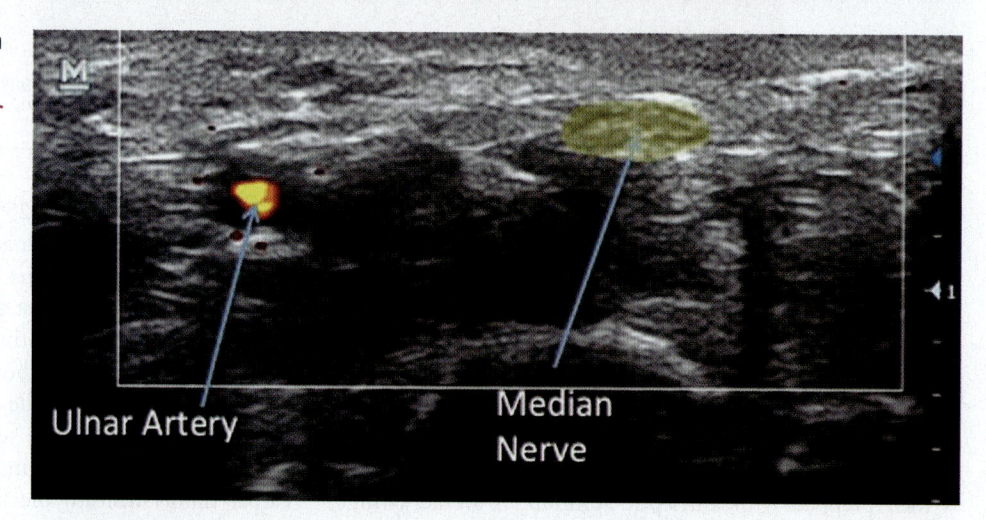

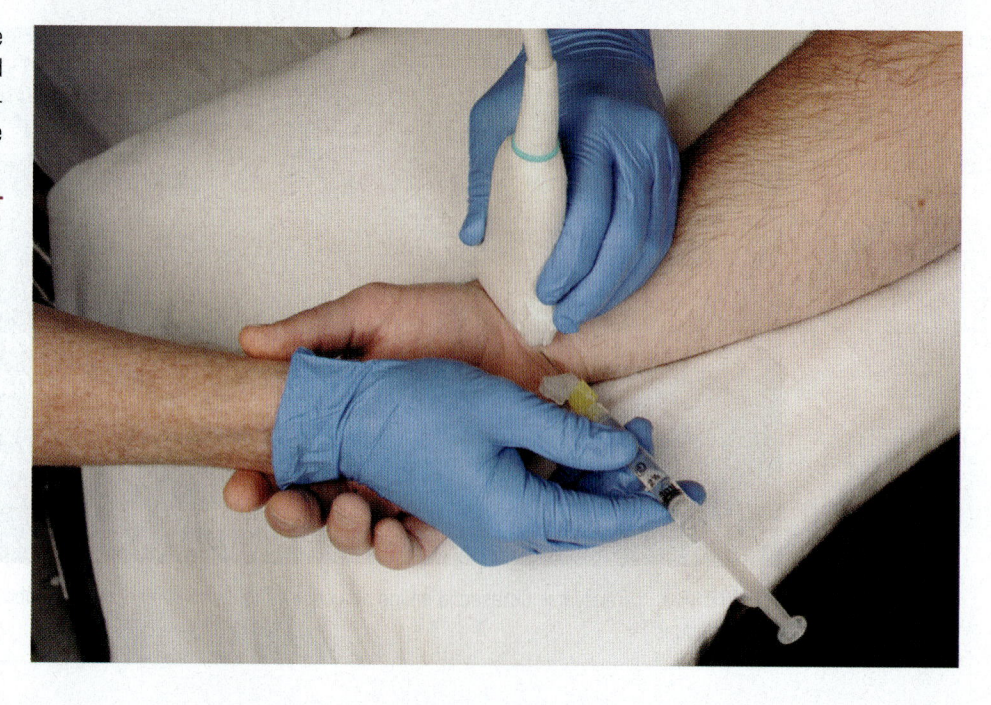

**FIGURE 64.12.** Proper needle placement for ultrasound-guided median nerve block at the wrist utilizing an in-plane approach at the wrist.

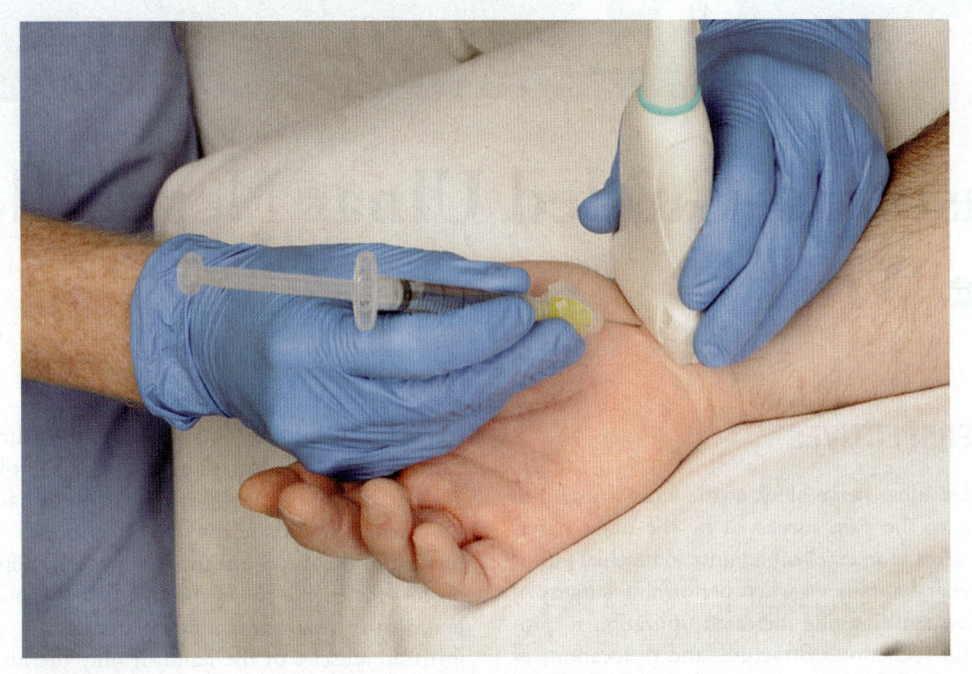

**FIGURE 64.13.** Proper needle placement for ultrasound-guided median nerve block at the wrist utilizing an out-of-plane approach at the wrist.

When the tip of needle is thought to be in satisfactory position, after careful aspiration, a small amount of local anesthetic and steroid is injected under real-time ultrasound guidance to confirm that the needle tip is in the proper position. After proper needle tip placement is confirmed, the remainder of the contents of the syringe are slowly injected. There should be minimal resistance to injection and no paresthesias should be elicited. Alternatively, this injection may be performed utilizing an out-of-plane technique by introducing the needle from the inferior margin of the ultrasound transducer and advancing it under real-time ultrasound guidance (Fig. 64.13).

## COMPLICATIONS

The major complications of ultrasound-guided injection of ultrasound-guided median nerve block at the wrist are related to improper needle placement with the possibility of inadvertent intravascular injection and/or persistent paresthesia secondary to needle trauma to the median nerve. Although rare, infection may occur. Ecchymosis and hematoma formation following this procedure may also occur. These complications can be decreased if manual pressure is applied to the area of the block immediately after injection. Application of cold packs for 20-minute periods after the block will also decrease the amount of postprocedure pain and bleeding the patient may experience.

Approximately 25% of patients complain of a transient increase in pain after this injection technique; the patient should be warned of this.

## CLINICAL PEARLS

Ultrasound-guided median nerve block at the wrist is a straightforward and relatively safe technique if attention is paid to the clinically relevant anatomy. It is useful as an adjunct to surgical anesthesia and has recently been used with increasing frequency in the diagnosis and treatment of carpal tunnel syndrome. Careful neurologic examination to identify preexisting neurologic deficits that may later be attributed to the nerve block should be performed on all patients before beginning median nerve block at the wrist, especially those suffering from carpal tunnel syndrome.

## SUGGESTED READINGS

Waldman SD. Median nerve block at the wrist. In: *Atlas of Interventional Pain Management Injection Techniques*. 3rd ed. Philadelphia, PA: Saunders Elsevier; 2009:239–243.

Waldman SD. The median nerve. In: *Pain Review*. Philadelphia, PA: Saunders Elsevier; 2009:77–78.

Waldman SD. Phalen's test. In: *Physical Diagnosis of Pain: An Atlas of Signs and Symptoms*. 2nd ed. Philadelphia, PA: Saunders Elsevier; 2010:165.

Waldman SD, Campbell RSD. Carpal tunnel syndrome. In: *Imaging of Pain*. Philadelphia, PA: Saunders Elsevier; 2011:319–320.

Waldman SD. Carpal tunnel syndrome. In: *Atlas of Common Pain Syndromes*. 3rd ed. Philadelphia, PA: Saunders Elsevier; 2013:160–163.

# CHAPTER 65

# Ultrasound-Guided Ulnar Nerve Block at the Wrist

## CLINICAL PERSPECTIVES

Ultrasound-guided ulnar nerve block at the wrist is useful in the management of the pain subserved by the ulnar nerve. This technique serves as an excellent adjunct to brachial plexus block and for general anesthesia when performing surgery at the wrist or below and is seeing increased utilization to provide anesthesia for reduction of fractures and dislocations of the fifth metacarpals and phalanges (Fig. 65.1). Ultrasound-guided ulnar nerve block at the wrist with local anesthetic may be used to palliate acute pain emergencies, including postoperative pain, pain secondary to traumatic injuries of the distal radius, and portions of the wrist and carpal bones innervated by the distal ulnar nerve, as well as cancer pain, while waiting for pharmacologic, surgical, and antiblastic methods to become effective.

Ultrasound-guided ulnar nerve block can also be used as a diagnostic tool when performing differential neural blockade on an anatomic basis in the evaluation of distal upper extremity pain as well as in a prognostic manner to determine the degree of neurologic impairment the patient will suffer when destruction of the ulnar nerve is being considered or when there is a possibility that the nerve may be sacrificed during surgeries in the anatomic region of the ulnar nerve at the level of the wrist. This technique may also be useful in those patients suffering symptoms from compromise of the ulnar nerve due to ulnar tunnel syndrome. Ultrasound-guided ulnar nerve block at the wrist may also be used to palliate the pain and dysesthesias associated with stretch injuries to the ulnar nerve.

The ulnar nerve at the wrist is susceptible to trauma during surgery for ulnar tunnel syndrome or may be damaged by wrist fractures or compressed by mass or tumor (Fig. 65.2). Entrapment neuropathy of the ulnar nerve at the wrist as the ulnar nerve passes through Guyon canal is known as ulnar or Guyon tunnel syndrome and is much rarer than ulnar nerve entrapment at the elbow. How ulnar tunnel syndrome presents clinically depends on at what point in its course through Guyon canal the ulnar nerve is compromised. If the ulnar nerve is compromised in the proximal portion of the canal before the bifurcation of the motor and sensory components of the nerve, the patient will experience both motor and sensory symptomatology with pain, dysesthesias, and numbness, which radiate into the ulnar aspect of the palm and dorsum of the hand, the little finger and the ulnar half of the ring finger, and paralysis of the intrinsic muscles of the hand. These symptoms may also radiate proximal to the level of nerve entrapment into the distal forearm. If only the deep palmar branch of the ulnar nerve passes through Guyon canal, a pure motor neuropathy results manifesting as painless paralysis of the intrinsic muscles of the hand. If only the more distal superficial branch of the ulnar nerve is compressed, a pure sensory neuropathy will result.

Physical findings associated with entrapment or trauma of the ulnar nerve at the wrist include a positive Tinel sign over the ulnar nerve at the site of injury. Decreased sensation in the distribution of the ulnar nerve of the palm and dorsum of the hand and the little finger and the ulnar half of the ring finger is common. A positive spread sign test is highly suggestive of the diagnosis of ulnar tunnel syndrome. The spread sign test is performed by having the patient relax the hand on the examination table and then spread his or her fingers as far apart as possible. The sign is considered positive if the patient is unable to spread two or more fingers apart. The little finger is often spared (Figs. 65.3 and 65.4).

## CLINICALLY RELEVANT ANATOMY

The key landmark when performing ultrasound-guided ulnar nerve block at the elbow is ulnar artery at the wrist, which lies in proximity to the ulnar nerve (Fig. 65.5). Arising from fibers from the C8–T1 nerve roots of the medial cord of the brachial plexus, the ulnar nerve lies anterior and inferior to the axillary artery in the 3:00 o'clock to 6:00 o'clock quadrant as it passes through the axilla. As the ulnar nerve exits the axilla, it passes inferiorly adjacent to the brachial artery. At the middle of the upper arm, the ulnar nerve turns medially to pass between the olecranon process and medial epicondyle of the humerus. Continuing its downward path, the ulnar nerve passes between the heads of the flexor carpi ulnaris moving radially along with the ulnar artery. At a point ~1 inch proximal to the crease of the wrist, the ulnar nerve divides into the dorsal and palmar branches. The dorsal branch provides sensation to the ulnar aspect of the dorsum of the hand and the dorsal aspect of the little finger and the ulnar half of the

CHAPTER 65 ULTRASOUND-GUIDED ULNAR NERVE BLOCK AT THE WRIST 439

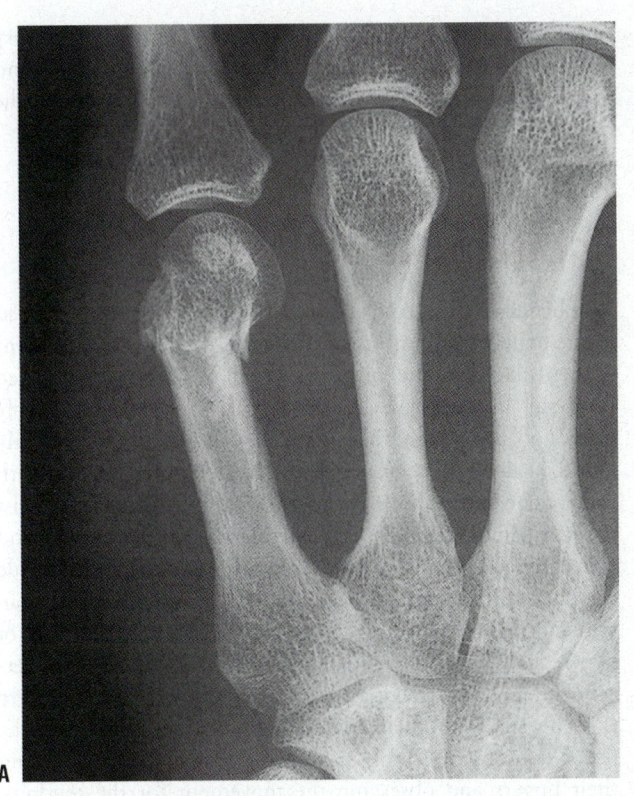

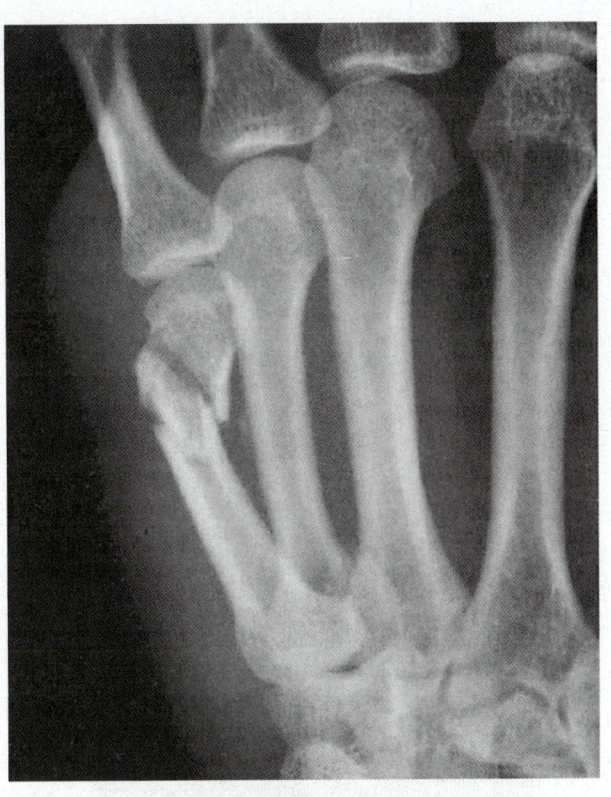

**FIGURE 65.1.** Ultrasound-guided ulnar nerve block at the wrist is useful in providing surgical anesthesia for reduction and fixation of boxer's fractures of the fifth metacarpal and phalanges. (Reused from Greenspan A. *Orthopedic Imaging: A Practical Approach*. 5th ed. Philadelphia, PA: Lippincott Williams & Wilkins; 2011:222, with permission.)

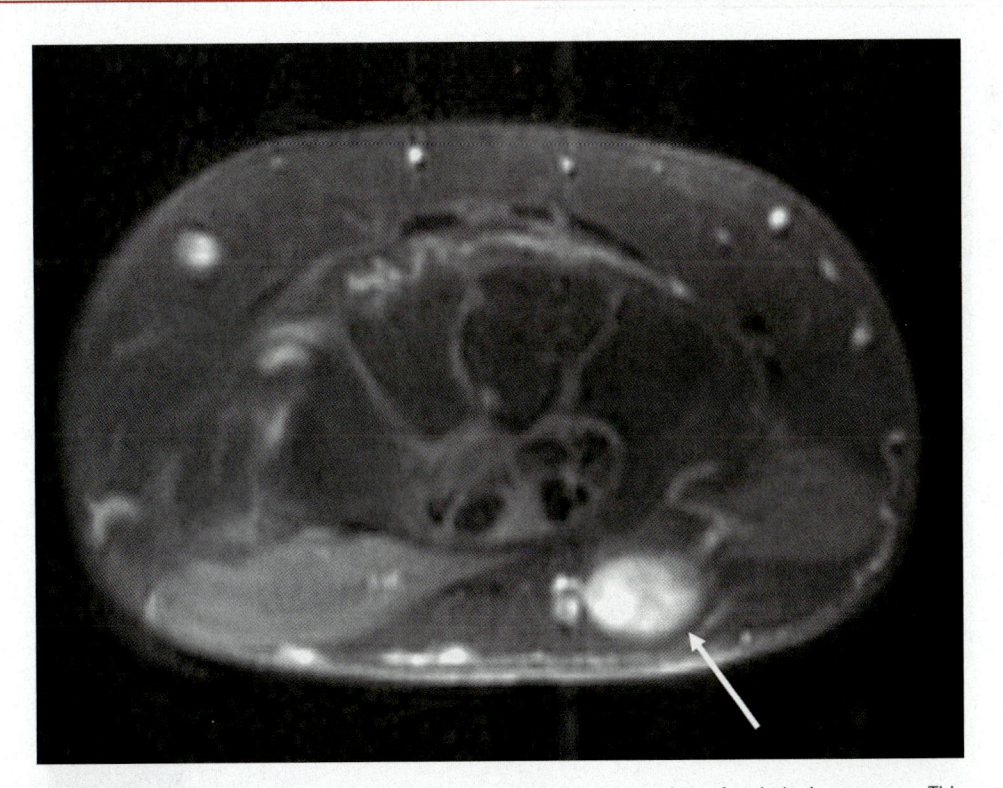

**FIGURE 65.2.** The ulnar nerve is susceptible to compression by a variety of pathologic processes. This axial T2 image demonstrates a high signal mass consistent with a ganglion within the ulnar tunnel causing compression of the ulnar nerve. (Reused from Chung CB, Steinbach LS. *MRI of the Upper Extremity*. Philadelphia, PA: Lippincott Williams & Wilkins; 2010:581, with permission.)

ring finger (Fig. 65.6). The palmar branch provides sensory innervation to the ulnar aspect of the palm of the hand and the palmar aspect of the little finger and the ulnar half of the ring finger.

## ULTRASOUND-GUIDED TECHNIQUE

The benefits, risks, and alternative treatments are explained to the patient, and informed consent is obtained. The patient is then placed in the sitting position with the elbow flexed to about 100 degrees and the forearm resting comfortably palm up on a padded bedside table with the fingers slightly flexed, which will relax the flexor tendons (Fig. 65.7). With the patient in the above position, the distal crease of the wrist is identified (Fig. 65.8). A high-frequency linear ultrasound transducer is placed in a transverse position over the ulnar side of the distal crease of the wrist, and an ultrasound survey scan is taken (Fig. 65.9). The ulnar nerve will appear as a bundle of hyperechoic nerve fibers surrounded by a slightly more hyperechoic neural sheath lying on the ulnar side of the ulnar artery (Fig. 65.10). The ulnar nerve can be distinguished from the flexor tendons by simply having the patient flex and extend their fingers and observing the movement for the tendons. The flexor tendons will also exhibit the property of anisotropy with the tipping of the ultrasound transducer back and forth over the tendons. The ulnar artery is then identified on the ulnar side of the wrist (see Fig. 65.10). Color Doppler may

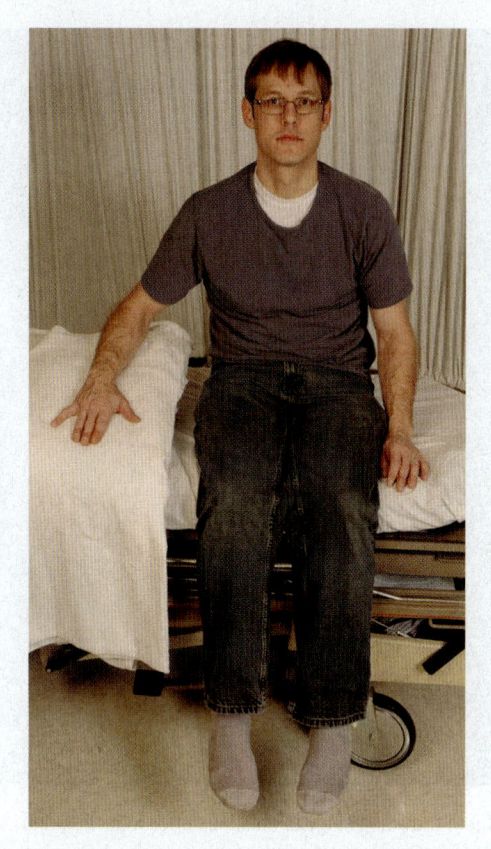

**FIGURE 65.3.** Patients suffering from ulnar tunnel syndrome will exhibit a positive spread sign.

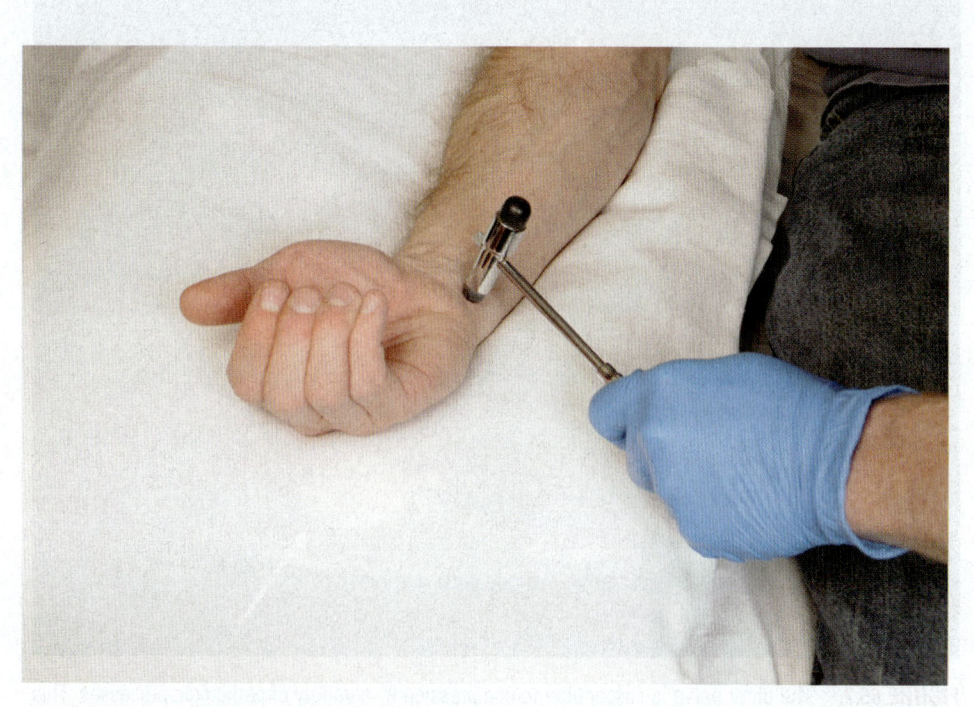

**FIGURE 65.4.** The Tinel sign for carpal tunnel syndrome.

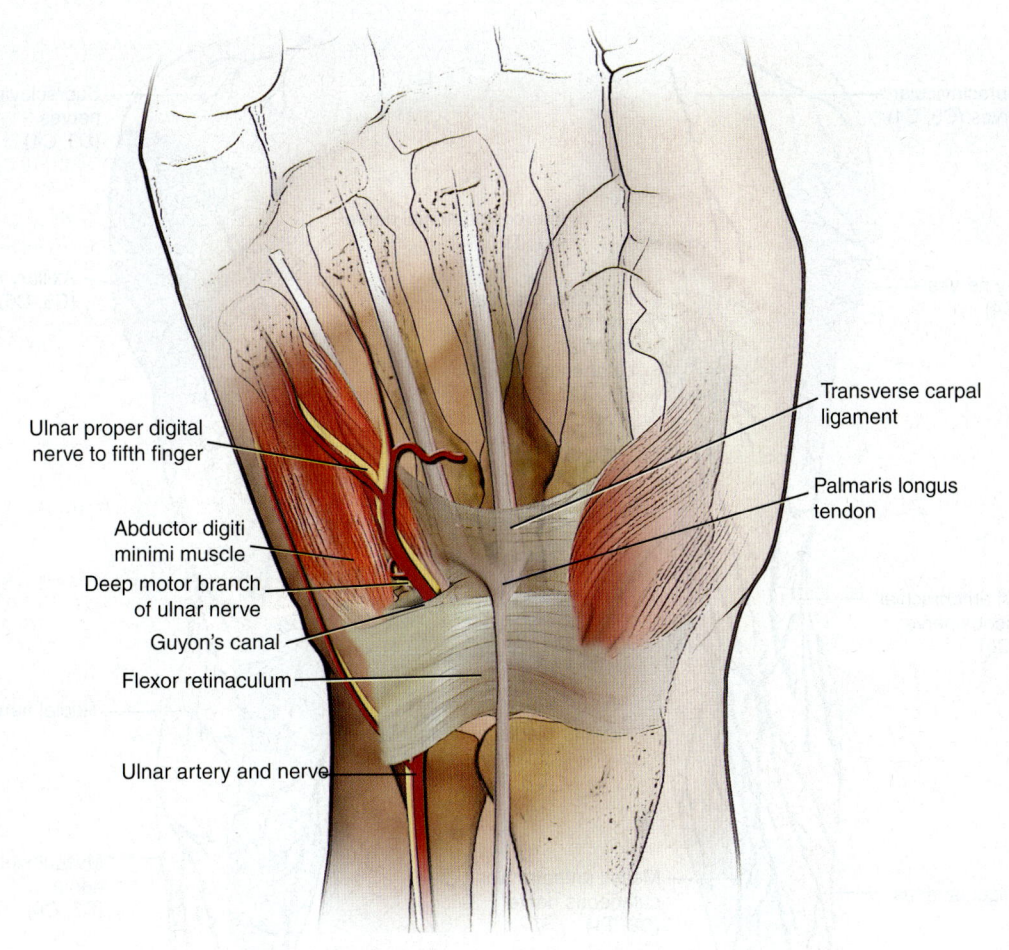

**FIGURE 65.5.** The ulnar nerve lies on the ulnar side of the ulnar artery as it passes through Guyon canal.

aid in the identification of the ulnar artery so it can be avoided when performing out-of-plane needle placement (Fig. 65.11). After the ulnar artery is identified, the skin overlying the area beneath the ultrasound transducer is then prepped with antiseptic solution. A sterile syringe containing 2.0 mL of 0.25% preservative-free bupivacaine and 40 mg of methylprednisolone is attached to a 1½-inch, 22-gauge needle using strict aseptic technique. The needle is placed through the skin just above the proximal aspect of the transversely oriented ultrasound transducer where the ulnar nerve was previously identified and is advanced using an out-of-plane approach beneath the transducer with the needle trajectory adjusted under real-time ultrasound guidance so that the needle tip ultimately rests in proximity to the ulnar nerve as it lies adjacent to the ulnar artery (Fig. 65.12). When the tip of needle is thought to be in satisfactory position, after careful aspiration, a small amount of local anesthetic and steroid is injected under real-time ultrasound guidance to confirm that the needle tip is in the proper position. After proper needle tip placement is confirmed, the remainder of the contents of the syringe are slowly injected. There should be minimal resistance to injection and no paresthesias should be elicited.

# COMPLICATIONS

The major complications of ultrasound-guided injection of ultrasound-guided ulnar nerve block at the wrist are related to improper needle placement with the possibility of inadvertent intravascular injection and/or persistent paresthesia secondary to needle trauma to the ulnar nerve. Although rare, infection may occur. Ecchymosis and hematoma formation following this procedure may also occur. These complications can be decreased if manual pressure is applied to the area of the block immediately after injection. Application of cold packs for 20-minute periods after the block will also decrease the amount of postprocedure pain and bleeding the patient may experience.

Approximately 25% of patients complain of a transient increase in pain after this injection technique; the patient should be warned of this.

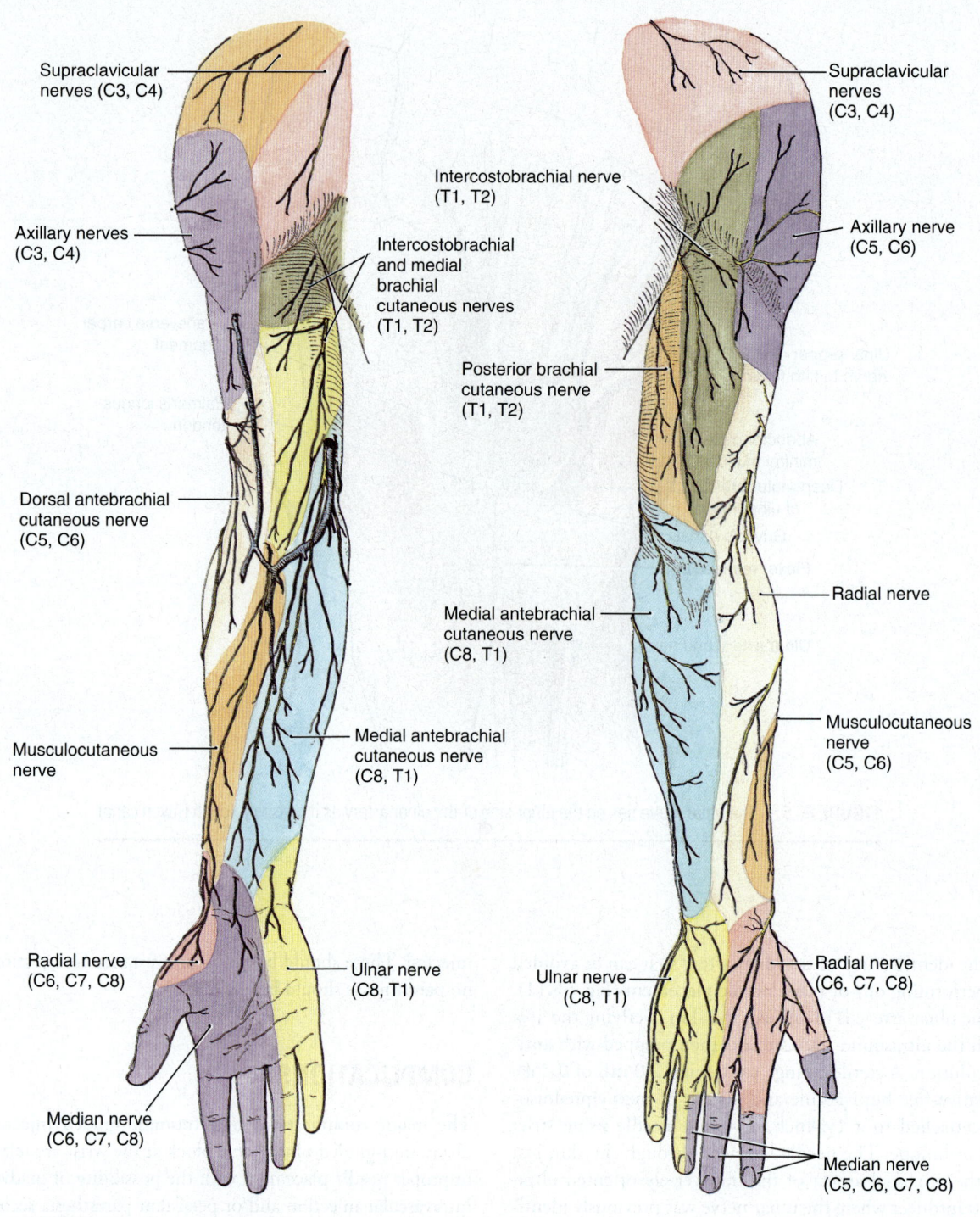

**FIGURE 65.6.** The sensory distribution of the ulnar nerve.

CHAPTER 65 ULTRASOUND-GUIDED ULNAR NERVE BLOCK AT THE WRIST 443

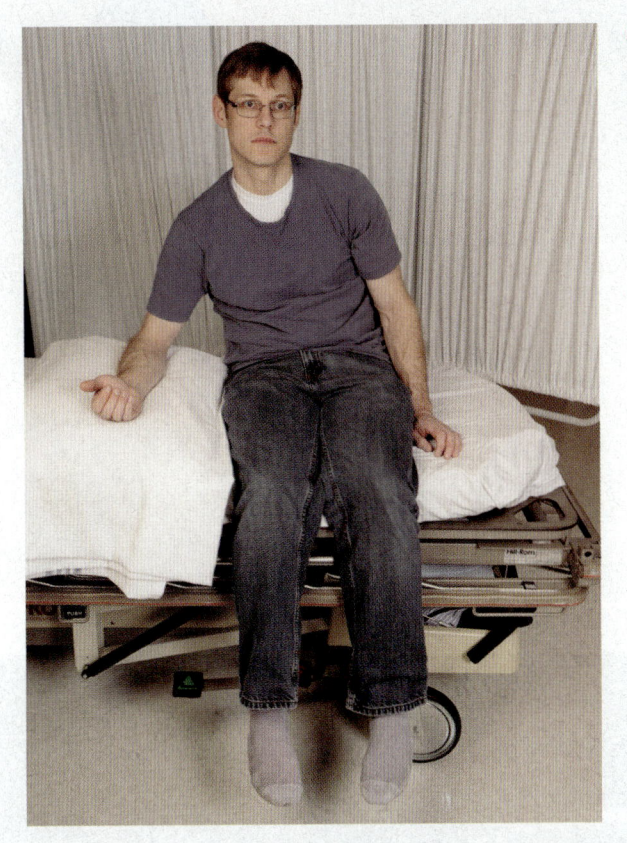

**FIGURE 65.7.** To perform ultrasound-guided injection of the ulnar nerve at the wrist, the patient is then placed in the sitting position with the elbow flexed to about 100 degrees and the forearm resting comfortably palm up on a padded bedside table with the fingers slightly flexed, which will relax the flexor tendons.

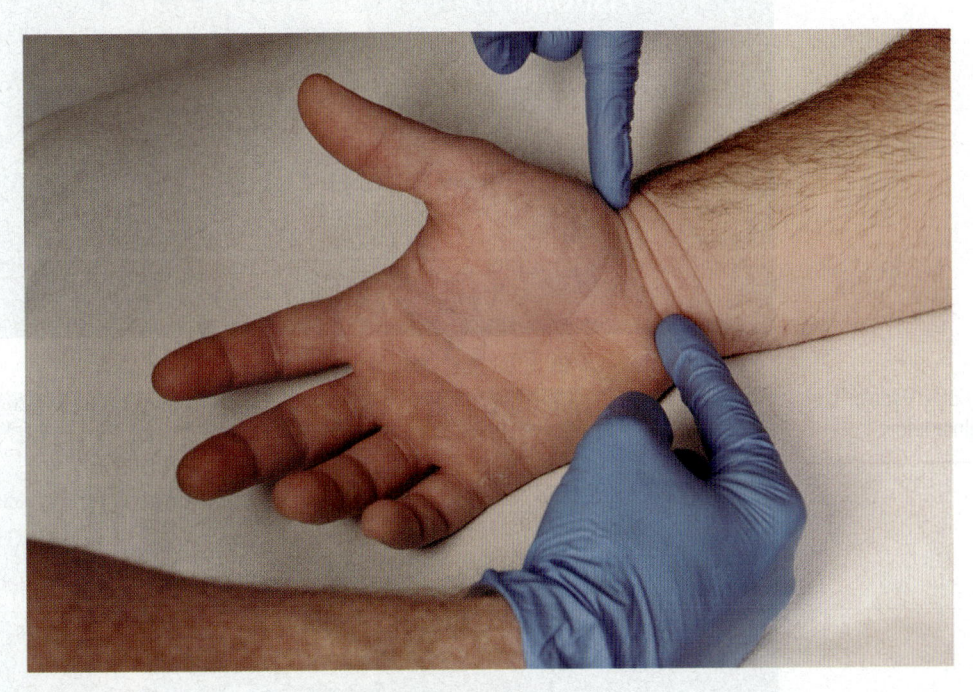

**FIGURE 65.8.** Identification of the distal crease of the wrist.

**FIGURE 65.9.** Proper transverse position for the linear high-frequency ultrasound transducer to perform ultrasound-guided ulnar nerve block at the wrist.

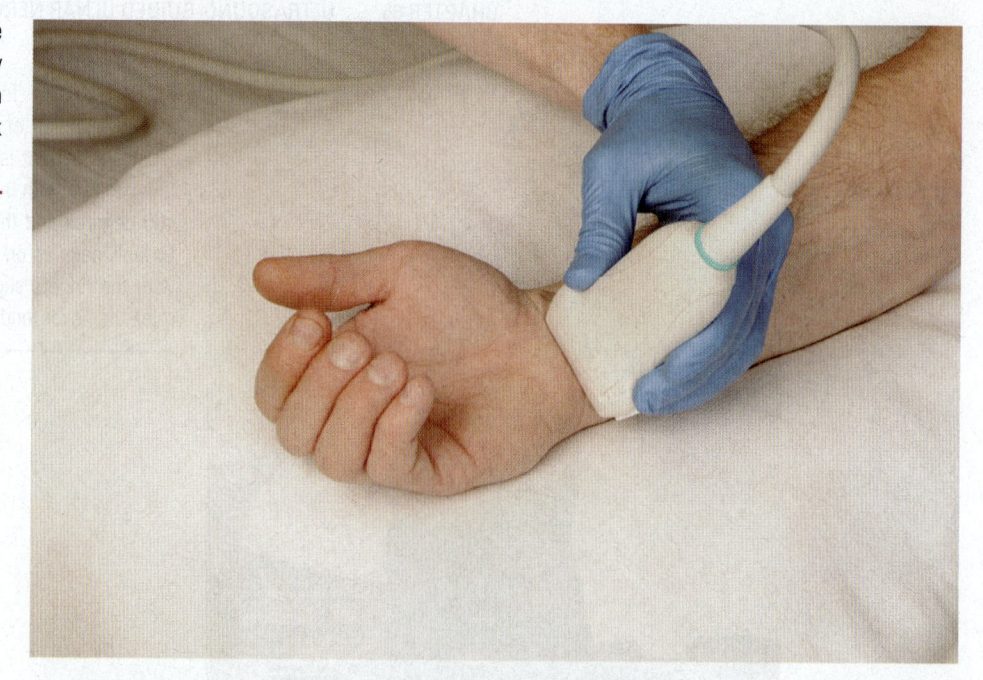

**FIGURE 65.10.** Transverse ultrasound image demonstrating the ulnar nerve lying on the ulnar side of the ulnar artery.

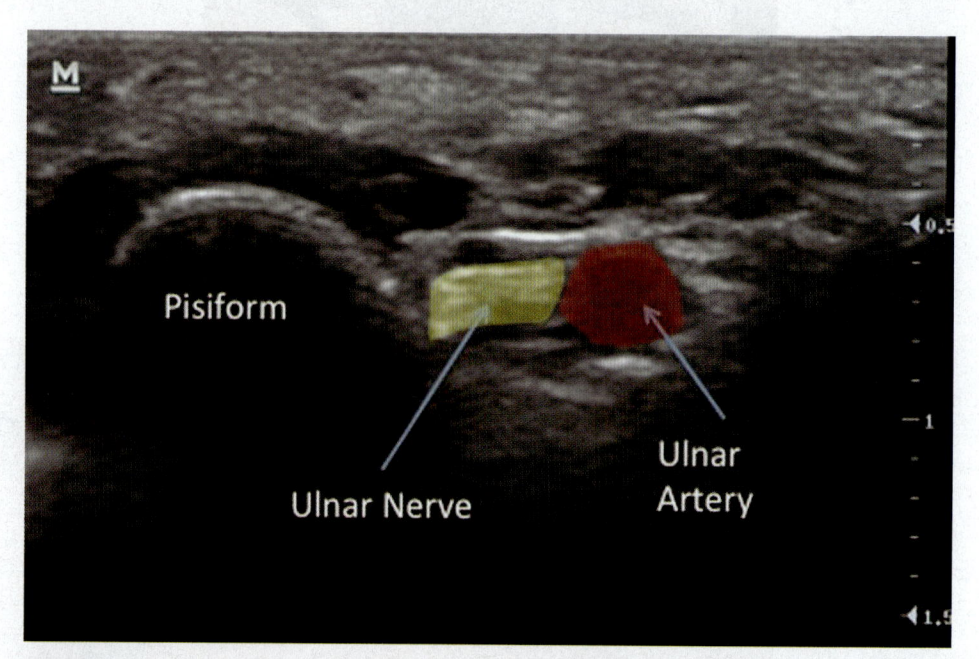

**FIGURE 65.11.** Color Doppler can help identify the ulnar artery.

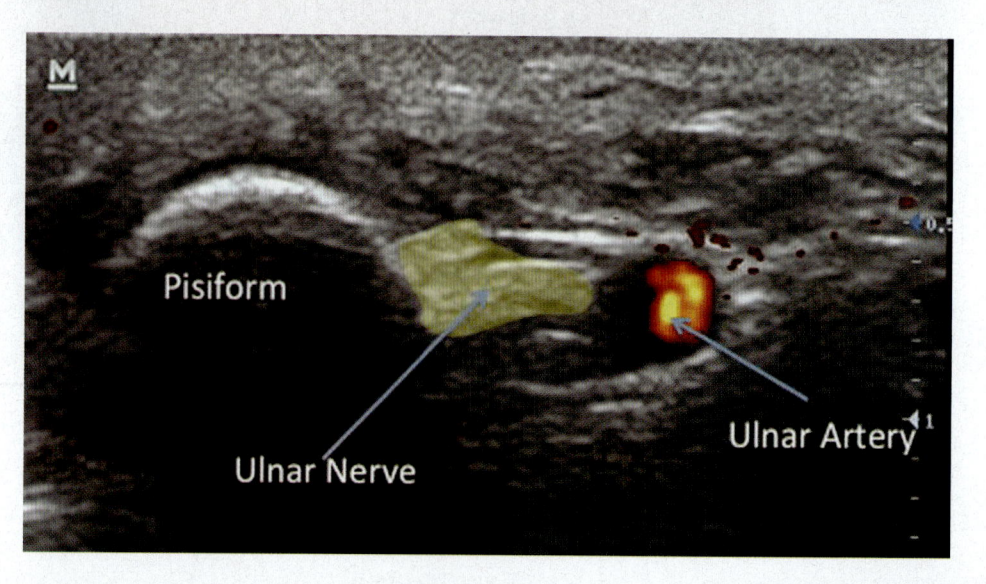

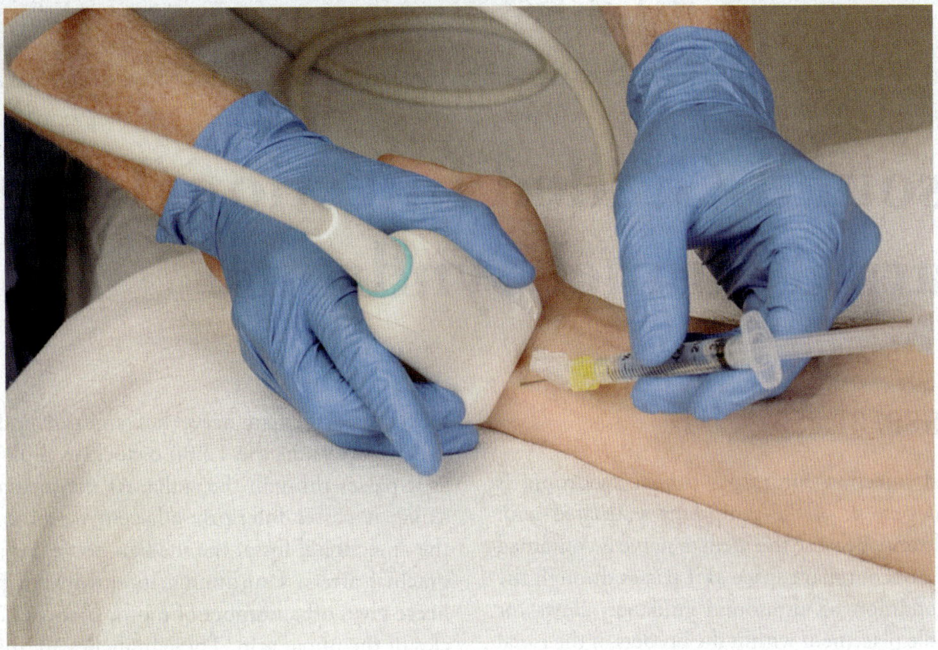

**FIGURE 65.12.** Proper needle placement for ultrasound-guided ulnar nerve block at the wrist.

## CLINICAL PEARLS

Ultrasound-guided ulnar nerve block at the wrist is a straightforward and relatively safe technique if attention is paid to the clinically relevant anatomy. It is useful as an adjunct to surgical anesthesia and has recently been used with increasing frequency in the treatment of ulnar tunnel syndrome. Careful neurologic examination to identify preexisting neurologic deficits that may later be attributed to the nerve block should be performed on all patients before beginning ulnar nerve block at the wrist, especially those suffering from ulnar tunnel syndrome.

## SUGGESTED READINGS

Waldman SD. Ulnar tunnel syndrome. In: *Atlas of Uncommon Pain Syndromes*. 2nd ed. Philadelphia, PA: WB Saunders; 2008:111–113.

Waldman SD. The ulnar nerve. In: *Pain Review*. Philadelphia, PA: Saunders Elsevier; 2009:76–77.

Waldman SD. The ulnar nerve. In: *Pain Review*. Philadelphia, PA: Saunders Elsevier; 2009:77–78.

Waldman SD. Ulnar nerve block at the wrist. In: *Atlas of Interventional Pain Management Injection Techniques*. 3rd ed. Philadelphia, PA: WB Saunders; 2009:239–243.

Waldman SD. The spread sign for ulnar tunnel syndrome. In: *Physical Diagnosis of Pain: An Atlas of Signs and Symptoms*. 2nd ed. Philadelphia, PA: WB Saunders; 2010:170–171.

# CHAPTER 66

# Ultrasound-Guided Injection Technique for Carpal Tunnel Syndrome

## CLINICAL PERSPECTIVES

Ultrasound-guided injection for carpal tunnel syndrome is useful in the management of the symptoms associated with carpal tunnel syndrome. Because the median nerve is contained within a relatively noncompliant space as it passes through the carpal canal, the addition of ultrasound guidance allows for more accurate needle placement within the borders of the canal while at the same time avoiding needle-induced trauma to the median nerve. Furthermore, the ability to observe the actual flow of the injectate within this closed space utilizing real-time ultrasound imaging allows the clinician to identify any further compression of the nerve as the injection proceeds.

Entrapment neuropathy of the median nerve at the wrist is known as carpal tunnel syndrome and is the most common entrapment neuropathy encountered in clinical practice (Fig. 66.1). While the clinical presentation of carpal tunnel syndrome is consistent, this entrapment neuropathy has many causes and is associated with many pathologic conditions (Table 66.1). Carpal tunnel syndrome presents as pain and dysesthesias with associated numbness and weakness in the hand and wrist that radiate to the thumb, index finger, middle finger, and radial half of the ring finger. These symptoms may also radiate proximal to the level of nerve entrapment into the distal forearm.

Physical findings associated with carpal tunnel syndrome include a positive Tinel sign over the median nerve at the site of injury (Fig. 66.2). Decreased sensation in the distribution of the median nerve of the thumb, index finger, middle finger, and radial half of the ring finger is often present as weakness of thumb opposition. A positive Phalen test is highly suggestive of the diagnosis of carpal tunnel syndrome. Phalen test is performed by having the patient place the wrists in complete unforced flexion for at least 30 seconds (Fig. 66.3). The test is considered positive if this maneuver elicits dysesthesia, pain, or numbness in the distribution of the median nerve.

## CLINICALLY RELEVANT ANATOMY

Arising from fibers from the ventral roots of C5 and C6 of the lateral cord and C8 and T1 of the medial cord of the brachial plexus, the median nerve lies anterior and superior to the axillary artery in the 12:00 o'clock to 3:00 o'clock quadrant as it passes through the axilla. As the median nerve exits the axilla, it passes inferiorly adjacent to the brachial artery. At the antecubital fossa, the median nerve lies just medial to the brachial artery. Continuing its downward path, the median nerve gives off a number of motor branches to the flexor muscles of the upper arm. These branches are susceptible to nerve entrapment by aberrant ligaments, muscle hypertrophy, and direct trauma. As the median nerve approaches the wrist, it overlies the radius where it is susceptible to trauma from radial fractures and lacerations. The nerve lies deep to and between the tendons of the palmaris longus muscle and the flexor carpi radialis muscle at the wrist. It is susceptible to entrapment as it passes through the carpal tunnel (Fig. 66.4). The terminal branches of the median nerve provide sensory innervation to a portion of the palmar surface of the hand as well as the palmar surface of the thumb, index and middle fingers, and the radial portion of the ring finger. The median nerve also provides sensory innervation to the distal dorsal surface of the index and middle fingers and the radial portion of the ring finger (Fig. 66.5).

## ULTRASOUND-GUIDED TECHNIQUE

The benefits, risks, and alternative treatments are explained to the patient and informed consent is obtained. The patient is then placed in the sitting position with the elbow flexed to about 100 degrees and the forearm resting comfortably palm up on a padded bedside table with the fingers slightly flexed, which will relax the flexor tendons (Fig. 66.6). With the patient in the above position, the distal crease of the wrist is identified (Fig. 66.7). A high-frequency linear ultrasound transducer is placed in a transverse position over the distal crease of the wrist, and an ultrasound survey scan is taken (Fig. 66.8). The median nerve will appear as a bundle of hyperechoic nerve fibers surrounded by a slightly more hyperechoic neural sheath lying beneath the flexor retinaculum and above the superficial flexor tendons (Fig. 66.9). The median nerve can be distinguished from the flexor tendons by simply having the patient flex and extend their fingers and observing the movement for

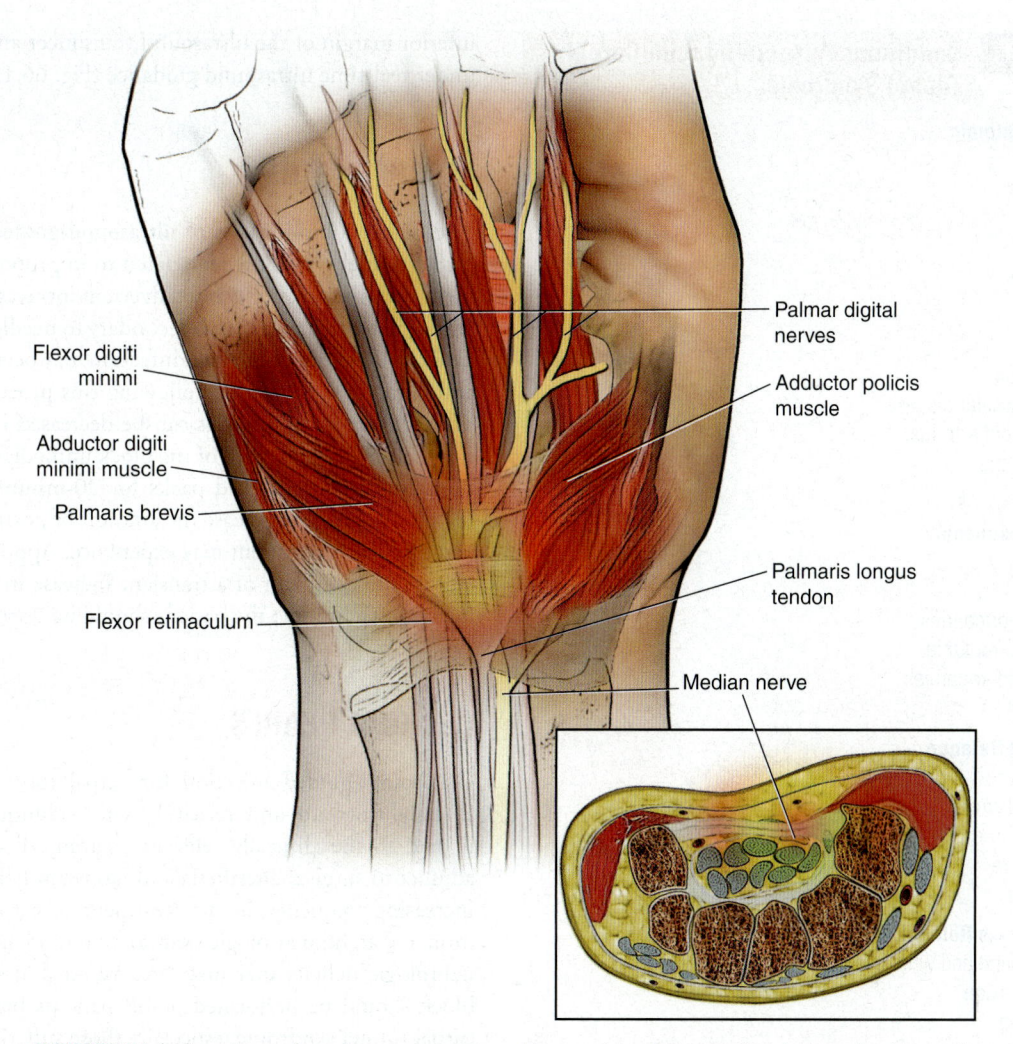

**FIGURE 66.1.** Carpal tunnel syndrome can be caused by a variety of structural and anatomic abnormalities and is associated with a number of pathologic conditions.

the tendons. The flexor tendons will also exhibit the property of anisotropy with the tipping of the ultrasound transducer back and forth over the tendons. The ulnar artery is then identified on the ulnar side of the wrist (Fig. 66.10). Color Doppler may aid in the identification of the ulnar artery so it can be avoided when performing in-plane needle placement (Fig. 66.11). After the ulnar artery is identified, the ultrasound transducer is slowly moved medially until the median nerve is again easily identifiable in the transverse ultrasound image. The skin overlying the area beneath the ultrasound transducer is then prepped with antiseptic solution. A sterile syringe containing 2.0 mL of 0.25% preservative-free bupivacaine and 40 mg of methylprednisolone is attached to a 1½-inch, 22-gauge needle using strict aseptic technique. The needle is placed through the skin just above the level of where the ulnar artery was previously identified and is advanced using an in-plane approach beneath the ulnar border of the ultrasound transducer with the needle trajectory adjusted under real-time ultrasound guidance so that the needle tip ultimately rests in proximity to the median nerve as it lies within the carpal tunnel beneath the flexor retinaculum (Fig. 66.12). When the tip of needle is thought to be in satisfactory position, after careful aspiration, a small amount of local anesthetic and steroid is injected under real-time ultrasound guidance to confirm that the needle tip is in the proper position. After proper needle tip placement is confirmed, the remainder of the contents of the syringe are slowly injected. There should be minimal resistance to injection, and no paresthesias should be elicited. Alternatively, this injection may be performed utilizing an out-of-plane technique by introducing the needle from the

| TABLE 66.1 | Conditions Associated with Carpal Tunnel Syndrome |
|---|---|

**Structural/Anatomic**
- Lipoma
- Ganglion
- Neuroma
- Aneurysm
- Acromegaly
- Fracture

**Inflammatory**
- Tenosynovitis
- Collagen vascular disease
    - Rheumatoid arthritis
    - Scleroderma
- Gout

**Neuropathic/Ischemic**
- Diabetes
- Alcoholism
- Vitamin abnormalities
- Ischemic neuropathies
- Peripheral neuropathies
- Amyloidosis

**Shifts in Fluid Balance**
- Pregnancy
- Hypothyroidism
- Obesity
- Kidney failure
- Menopause

**Repetitive Stress Related**
- Abnormal hand and wrist position
- Excessive flexion
- Microtrauma
- Vibration

inferior margin of the ultrasound transducer and advancing it under real-time ultrasound guidance (Fig. 66.13).

## COMPLICATIONS

The major complications of ultrasound-guided injection for carpal tunnel syndrome are related to improper needle placement with the possibility of inadvertent intravascular injection and/or persistent paresthesia secondary to needle trauma to the median nerve. Although rare, infection may occur. Ecchymosis and hematoma formation following this procedure may also occur. These complications can be decreased if manual pressure is applied to the area of the block immediately after injection. Application of cold packs for 20-minute periods after the block will also decrease the amount of postprocedure pain and bleeding the patient may experience. Approximately 25% of patients complain of a transient increase in pain after this injection technique; the patient should be warned of this.

## CLINICAL PEARLS

Ultrasound-guided injection for carpal tunnel syndrome is a straightforward and relatively safe technique if attention is paid to the clinically relevant anatomy. It is useful as an adjunct to surgical anesthesia and has recently been used with increasing frequency in the treatment of carpal tunnel syndrome. Careful neurologic examination to identify preexisting neurologic deficits that may later be attributed to the nerve block should be performed on all patients before beginning carpal tunnel syndrome, especially those suffering from carpal tunnel syndrome.

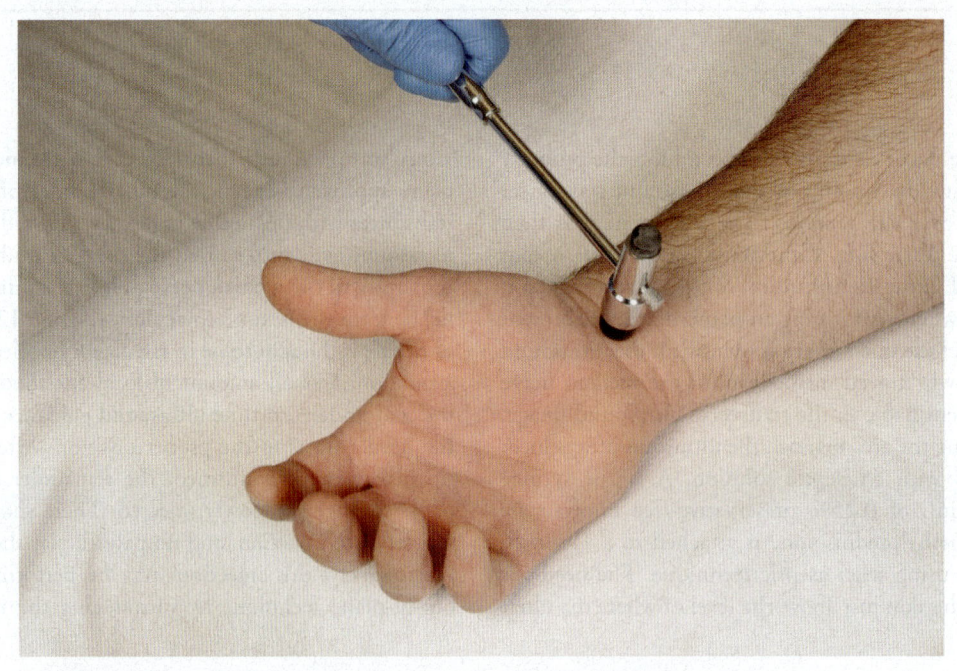

**FIGURE 66.2.** Patients suffering from carpal tunnel syndrome will exhibit a positive Tinel sign over the superficial median nerve.

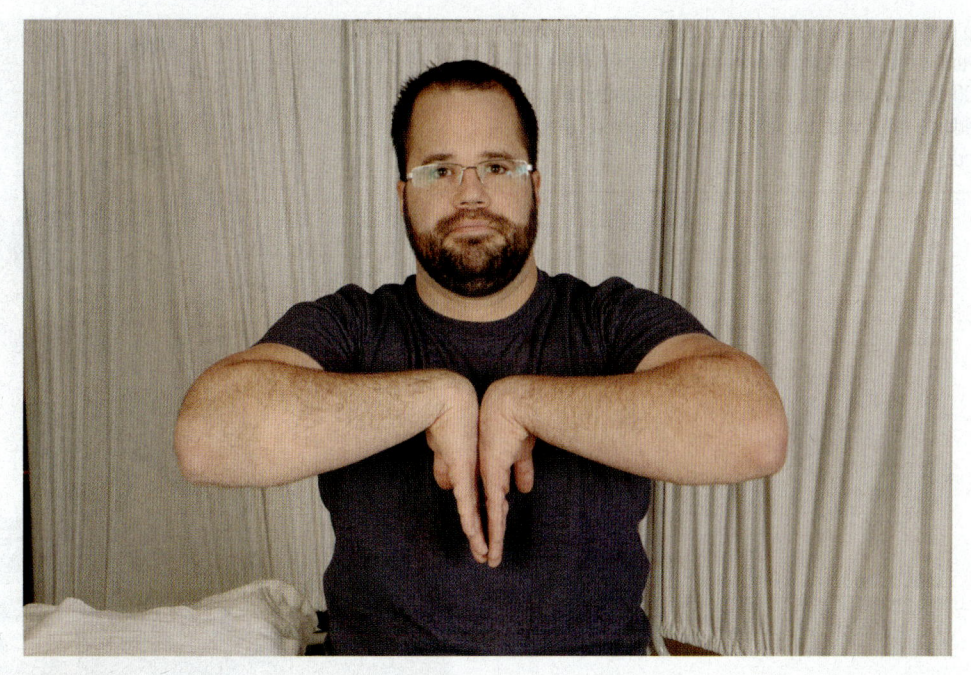

**FIGURE 66.3.** The Phalen test for carpal tunnel syndrome is performed by having the patient place their wrists in complete unforced flexion for at least 30 seconds. The test is considered positive if this maneuver elicits dysesthesia, pain, or numbness in the distribution of the median nerve.

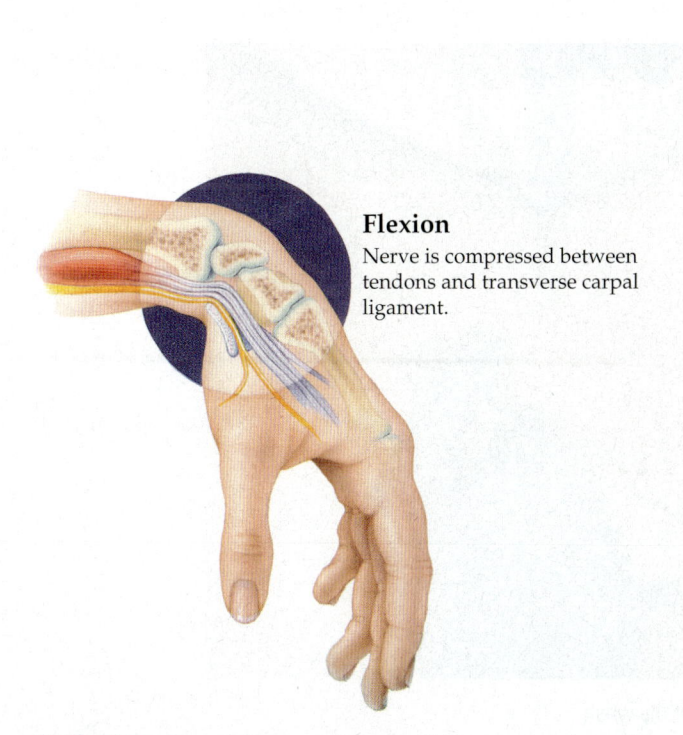

**Flexion**
Nerve is compressed between tendons and transverse carpal ligament.

**FIGURE 66.4.** The median nerve is susceptible to compression as it passes through the carpal tunnel. (Reused from The Anatomical Chart Company.)

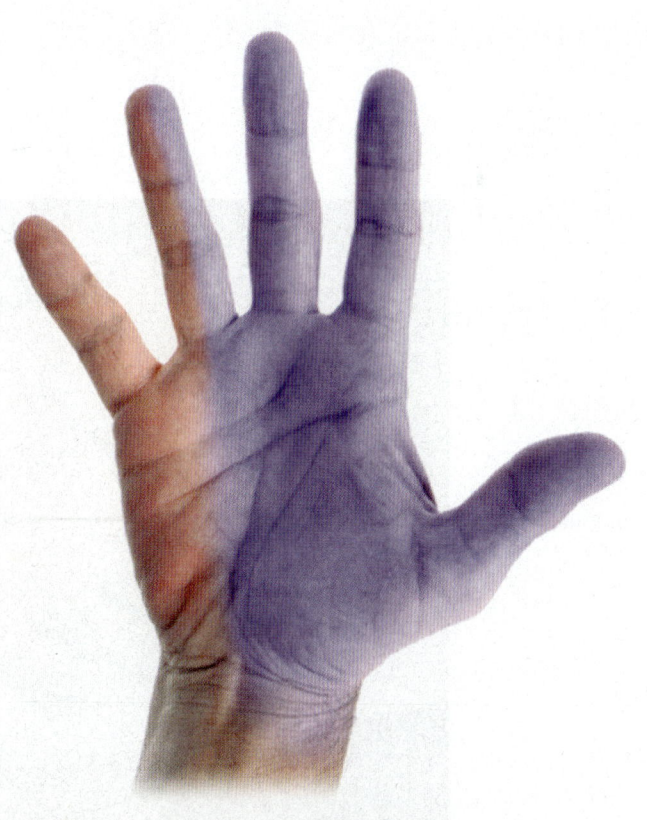

**FIGURE 66.5.** The sensory distribution of the median nerve, which is affected by carpal tunnel syndrome. (Reused from Clay JH, Pounds DM. *Basic Clinical Massage Therapy: Integrating Anatomy and Treatment*. 2nd ed. Philadelphia, PA: Lippincott Williams & Wilkins; 2008, with permission.)

**FIGURE 66.6.** To perform ultrasound-guided injection for carpal tunnel syndrome, the patient is then placed in the sitting position with the elbow flexed to about 100 degrees and the forearm resting comfortably palm up on a padded bedside table with the fingers slightly flexed, which will relax the flexor tendons.

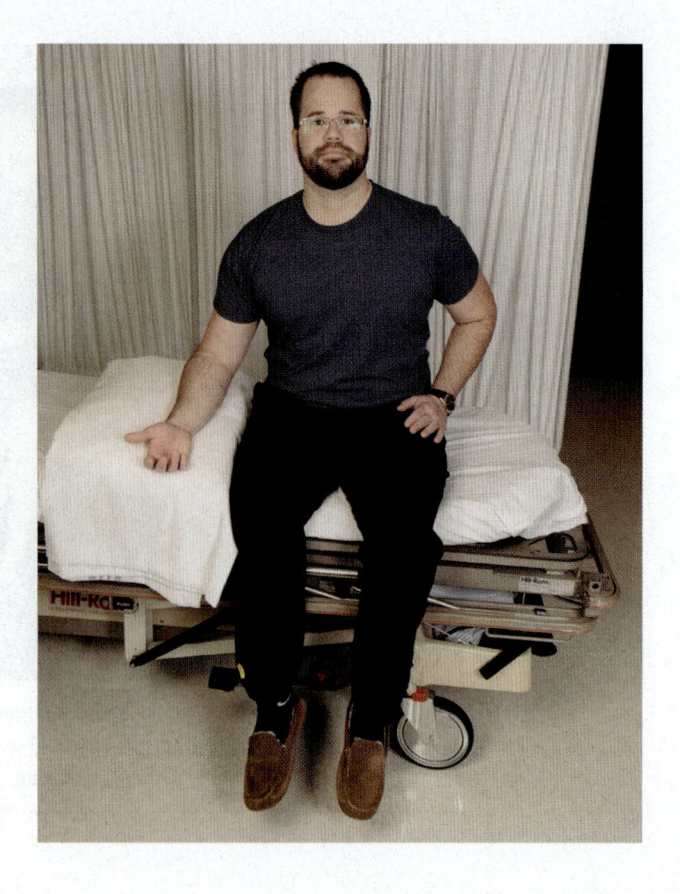

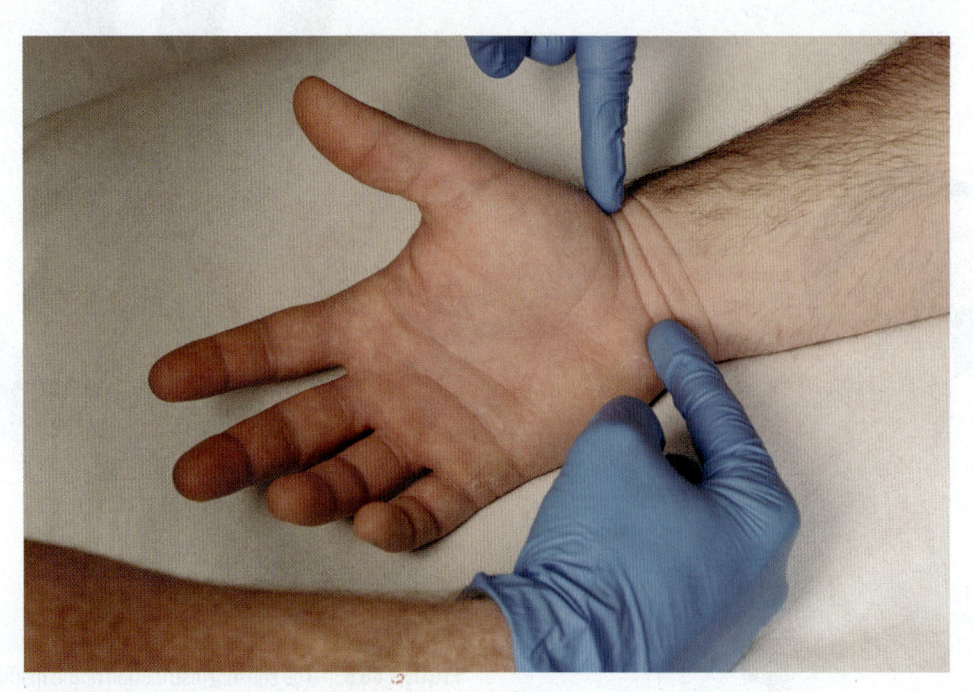

**FIGURE 66.7.** Identification of the distal crease of the wrist.

CHAPTER 66 ULTRASOUND-GUIDED INJECTION TECHNIQUE FOR CARPAL TUNNEL SYNDROME 451

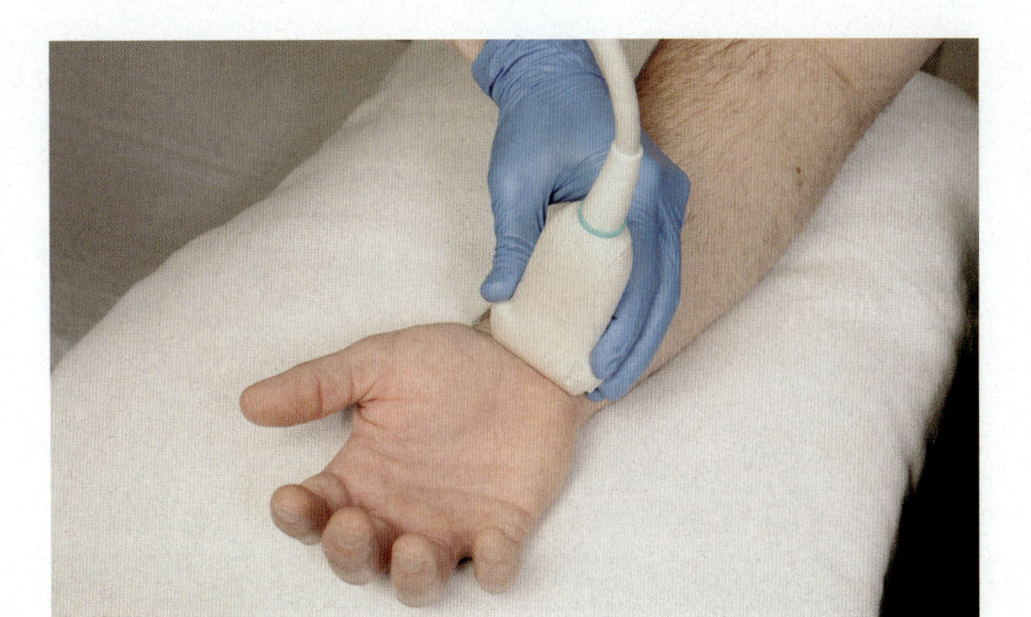

**FIGURE 66.8.** Proper transverse position for the linear high-frequency ultrasound transducer to perform ultrasound-guided injection for carpal tunnel syndrome.

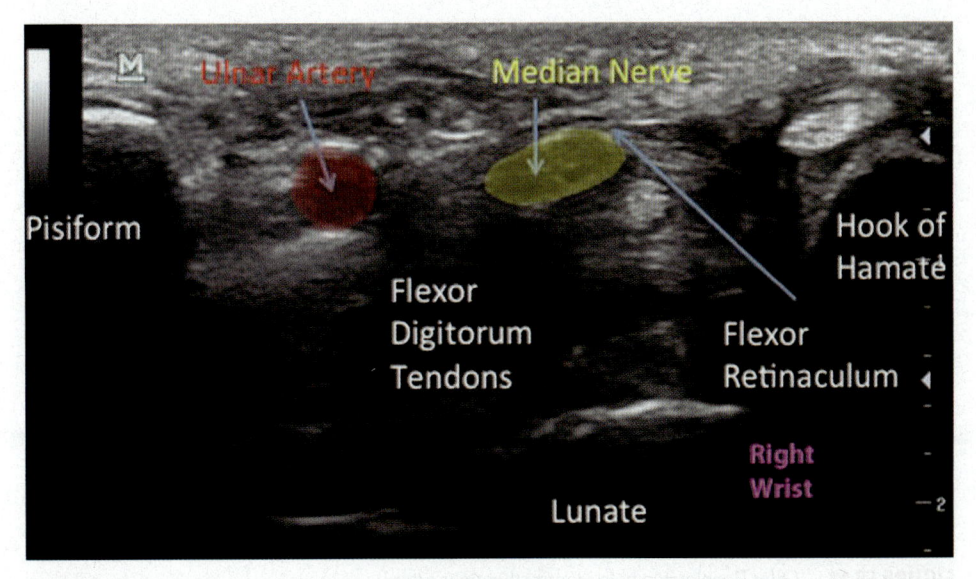

**FIGURE 66.9.** Transverse ultrasound image demonstrating the median nerve lying above the superficial flexor tendons.

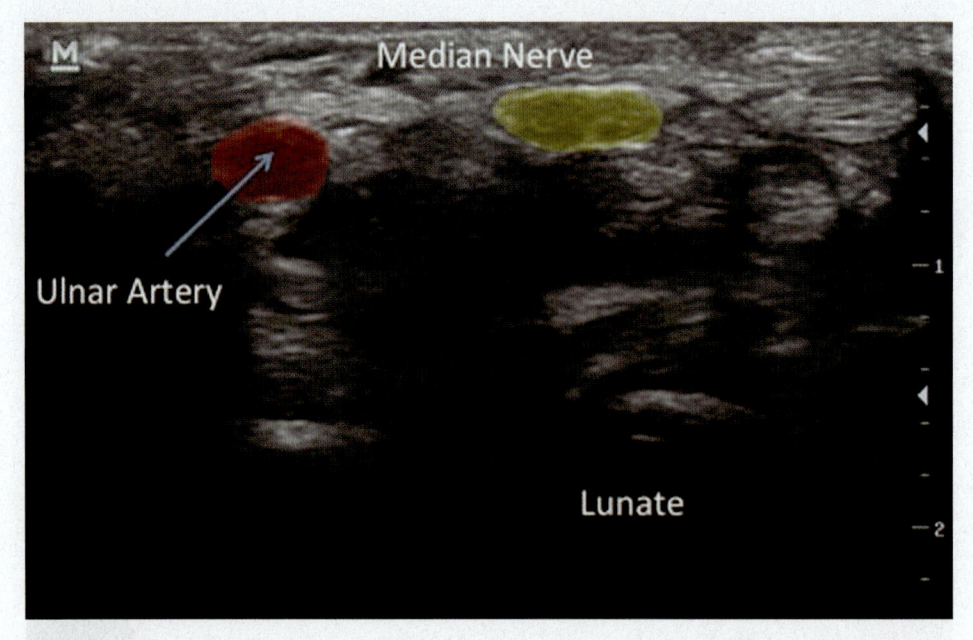

**FIGURE 66.10.** The ulnar artery is identified on transverse ultrasound scan so it can be avoided during needle placement when injecting the median nerve at the wrist.

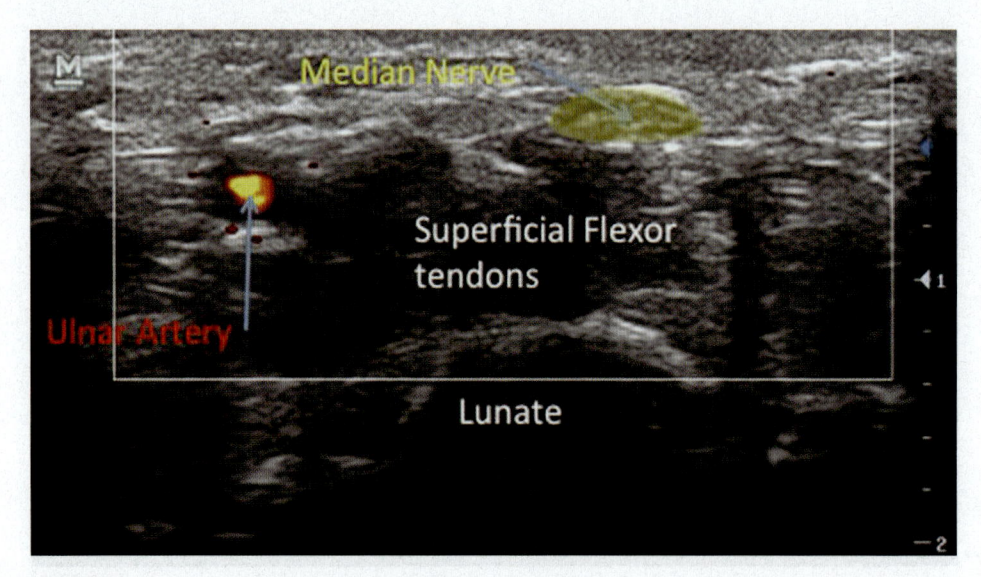

**FIGURE 66.11.** Color Doppler can help identify the ulnar artery.

CHAPTER 66    ULTRASOUND-GUIDED INJECTION TECHNIQUE FOR CARPAL TUNNEL SYNDROME    453

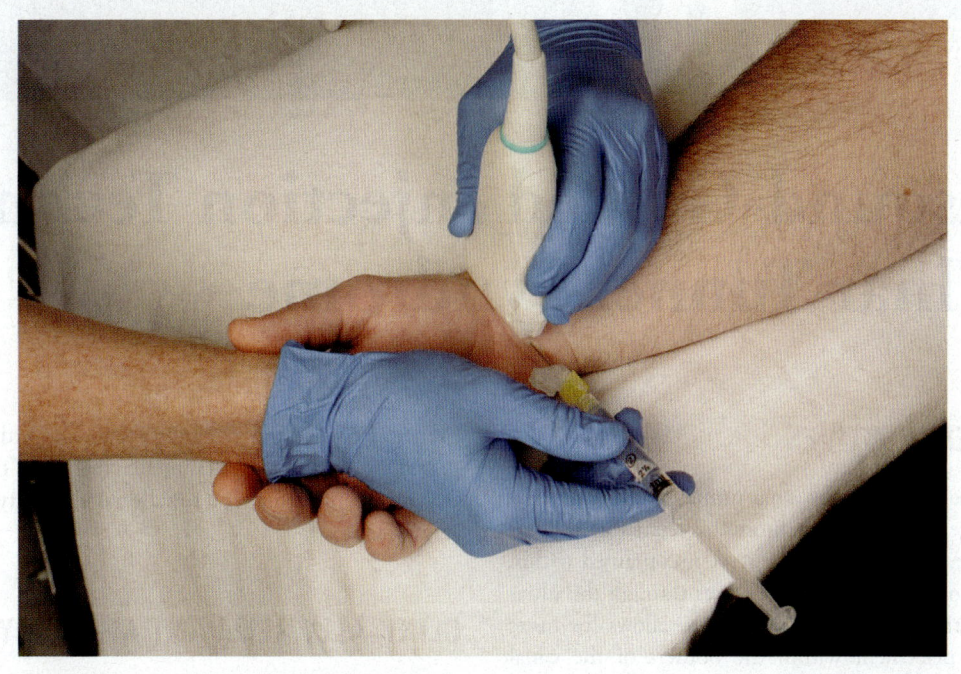

**FIGURE 66.12.** Proper needle placement for in-plane ultrasound-guided injection for carpal tunnel syndrome.

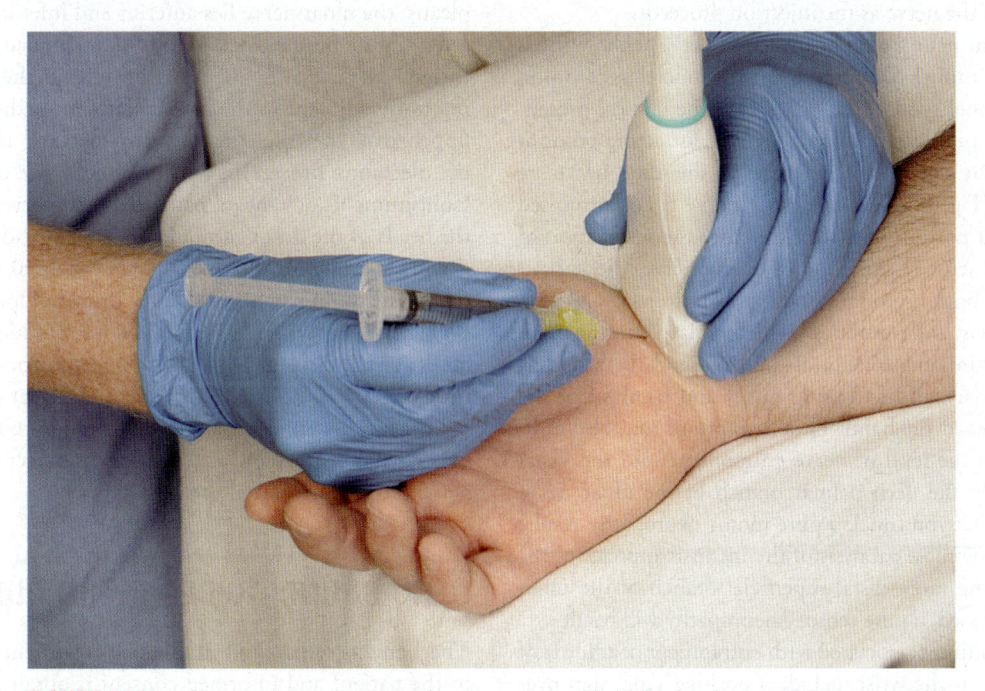

**FIGURE 66.13.** Proper needle placement for ultrasound-guided injection for carpal tunnel syndrome utilizing an out-of-plane approach at the wrist.

## SUGGESTED READINGS

Waldman SD. Carpal tunnel syndrome. In: *Atlas of Interventional Pain Management Injection Techniques*. 3rd ed. Philadelphia, PA: WB Saunders; 2009:239–243.

Waldman SD. The median nerve. In: *Pain Review*. Philadelphia, PA: Saunders Elsevier; 2009:77–78.

Waldman SD. Phalen's test. In: *Physical Diagnosis of Pain: An Atlas of Signs and Symptoms*. 2nd ed. Philadelphia, PA: Saunders Elsevier; 2010:165.

Waldman SD, Campbell RSD. Carpal tunnel syndrome. In: *Imaging of Pain*. Philadelphia, PA: Saunders Elsevier; 2011:319–320.

Waldman SD. Carpal tunnel syndrome. In: *Atlas of Common Pain Syndromes*. 3rd ed. Philadelphia, PA: Saunders Elsevier; 2013:160–163.

# CHAPTER 67

# Ultrasound-Guided Injection Technique for Ulnar Tunnel Syndrome

## CLINICAL PERSPECTIVES

Ultrasound-guided injection for ulnar tunnel syndrome is useful in the management of the symptoms associated with ulnar tunnel syndrome. Because the ulnar nerve is contained within a relatively noncompliant space as it passes through the ulnar tunnel, the addition of ultrasound guidance allows for more accurate needle placement within the borders of the canal while at the same time avoiding needle-induced trauma to the ulnar nerve. Furthermore, the ability to observe the actual flow of the injectate within this closed space utilizing real-time ultrasound imaging allows the clinician to identify any further compression of the nerve as the injection proceeds.

Entrapment neuropathy of the ulnar nerve at the wrist is known as ulnar tunnel syndrome and is the much less common than carpal tunnel syndrome (Fig. 67.1). The clinical presentation of ulnar tunnel syndrome is dependent at the point at which the motor and sensory branches of the ulnar nerve are compromised (Fig. 67.2). If the ulnar nerve is compromised in the proximal portion of the canal before the bifurcation of the motor and sensory components of the nerve, the patient will experience both motor and sensory symptomatology with pain, dysesthesias, and numbness, which radiate into the ulnar aspect of the palm and dorsum of the hand and the little finger and the ulnar half of the ring finger and paralysis of the intrinsic muscles of the hand. These symptoms may also radiate proximal to the level of nerve entrapment into the distal forearm. If only the deep palmar branch of the ulnar nerve passes through Guyon canal, a pure motor neuropathy results manifesting as painless paralysis of the intrinsic muscles of the hand. If only the more distal superficial branch of the ulnar nerve is compressed, a pure sensory neuropathy will result.

Physical findings associated with entrapment or trauma of the ulnar nerve at the wrist include a positive Tinel sign over the ulnar nerve at the site of injury. Decreased sensation in the distribution of the ulnar nerve of the palm and dorsum of the hand and the little finger and the ulnar half of the ring finger is common. A positive spread sign test is highly suggestive of the diagnosis of ulnar tunnel syndrome. The spread sign test is performed by having the patient relax the hand on the examination table and then spread his or her fingers as far apart as possible. The sign is considered positive if the patient is unable to spread two or more fingers apart. The little finger is often spared (see Fig. 65.3). A failure to treat ulnar tunnel syndrome can result in permanent functional disability and deformity (Fig. 67.3).

## CLINICALLY RELEVANT ANATOMY

The key landmark when performing ultrasound-guided ulnar nerve block at the elbow is ulnar artery at the wrist, which lies in proximity to the ulnar nerve (Fig. 67.4). Arising from fibers from the C8–T1 nerve roots of the medial cord of the brachial plexus, the ulnar nerve lies anterior and inferior to the axillary artery in the 3:00 o'clock to 6:00 o'clock quadrant as it passes through the axilla. As the ulnar nerve exits the axilla, it passes inferiorly adjacent to the brachial artery. At the middle of the upper arm, the ulnar nerve turns medially to pass between the olecranon process and medial epicondyle of the humerus. Continuing its downward path, the ulnar nerve passes between the heads of the flexor carpi ulnaris moving radially along with the ulnar artery. At a point ~1 inch proximal to the crease of the wrist, the ulnar nerve divides into the dorsal and palmar branches. The dorsal branch provides sensation to the ulnar aspect of the dorsum of the hand and the dorsal aspect of the little finger and the ulnar half of the ring finger (Fig. 67.5). The palmar branch provides sensory innervation to the ulnar aspect of the palm of the hand and the palmar aspect of the little finger and the ulnar half of the ring finger.

## ULTRASOUND-GUIDED TECHNIQUE

The benefits, risks, and alternative treatments are explained to the patient and informed consent is obtained. The patient is then placed in the sitting position with the elbow flexed to about 100 degrees and the forearm resting comfortably palm up on a padded bedside table with the fingers slightly flexed, which will relax the flexor tendons (Fig. 67.6). With the patient in the above position, the distal crease of the wrist is identified (Fig. 67.7). A high-frequency linear ultrasound transducer is placed in a transverse position over the ulnar side of the distal crease of the wrist, and an ultrasound survey scan

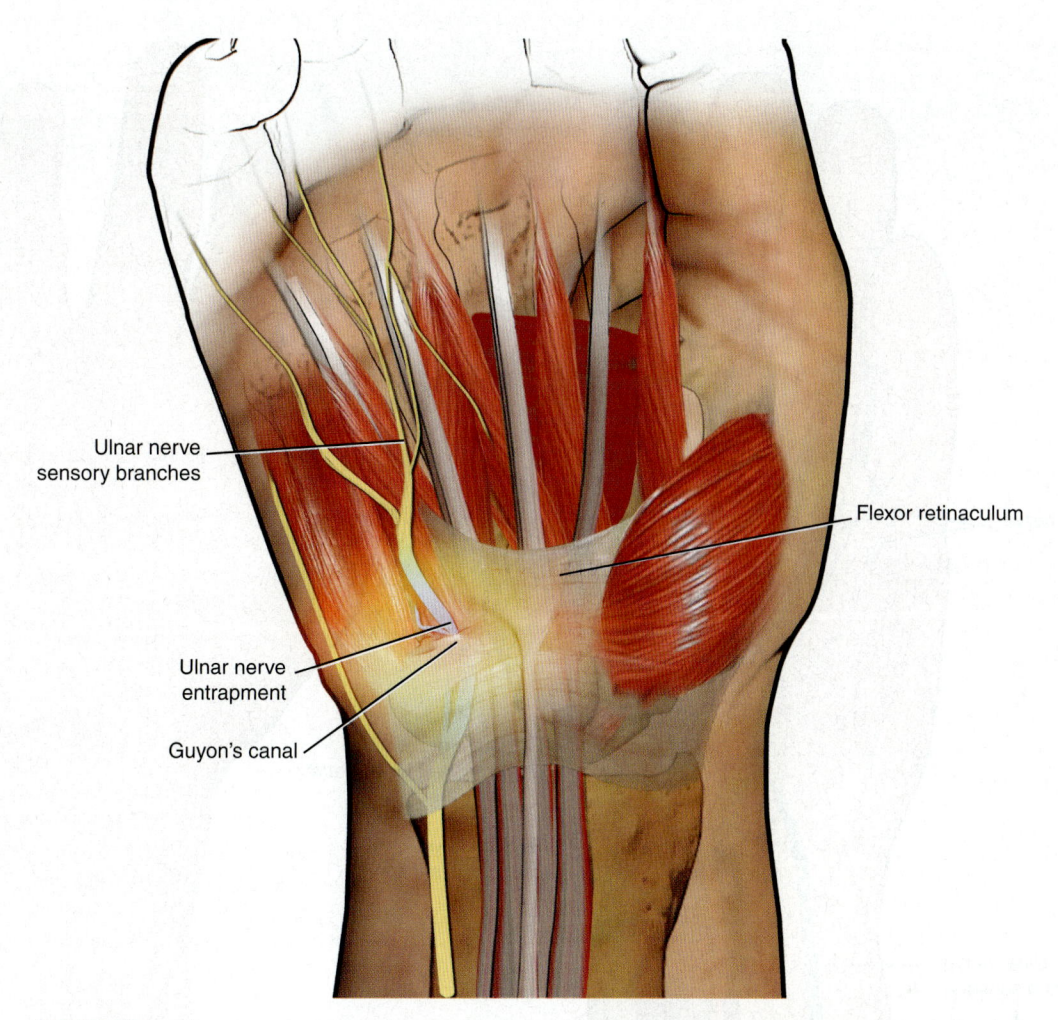

**FIGURE 67.1.** Ulnar tunnel syndrome is caused by entrapment of the ulnar nerve as it passes through the ulnar tunnel or Guyon canal and is caused by a variety of structural and anatomic abnormalities.

is taken (Fig. 67.8). The ulnar nerve will appear as a bundle of hyperechoic nerve fibers surrounded by a slightly more hyperechoic neural sheath lying on the ulnar side of the ulnar artery (Fig. 67.9). The ulnar nerve can be distinguished from the flexor tendons by simply having the patient flex and extend their fingers and observing the movement for the tendons. The flexor tendons will also exhibit the property of anisotropy with the tipping of the ultrasound transducer back and forth over the tendons. The ulnar artery is then identified on the ulnar side of the wrist (see Fig. 67.9). Color Doppler may aid in the identification of the ulnar artery so it can be avoided when performing out-of-plane needle placement (Fig. 67.10). After the ulnar artery is identified, the skin overlying the area beneath the ultrasound transducer is then prepped with antiseptic solution. A sterile syringe containing 2.0 mL of 0.25% preservative-free bupivacaine and 40 mg of methylprednisolone is attached to a 1½-inch, 22-gauge needle using strict aseptic technique. The needle is placed through the skin just above the proximal aspect of the ultrasound transducer at which the ulnar nerve was previously identified and is advanced using an out-of-plane approach beneath the with the needle trajectory adjusted under real-time ultrasound guidance so that the needle tip ultimately rests in proximity to the ulnar nerve as it lies adjacent to the ulnar artery (Fig. 67.11). When the tip of needle is thought to be in satisfactory position, after careful aspiration, a small amount of local anesthetic and steroid is injected under real-time ultrasound guidance to confirm that the needle tip is in the proper position. After proper needle tip placement is confirmed, the remainder of the contents of the syringe are slowly injected. There should be minimal resistance to injection and no paresthesias should be elicited.

## COMPLICATIONS

The major complications of ultrasound-guided injection of ultrasound-guided ulnar tunnel syndrome are related to improper needle placement with the possibility of inadvertent

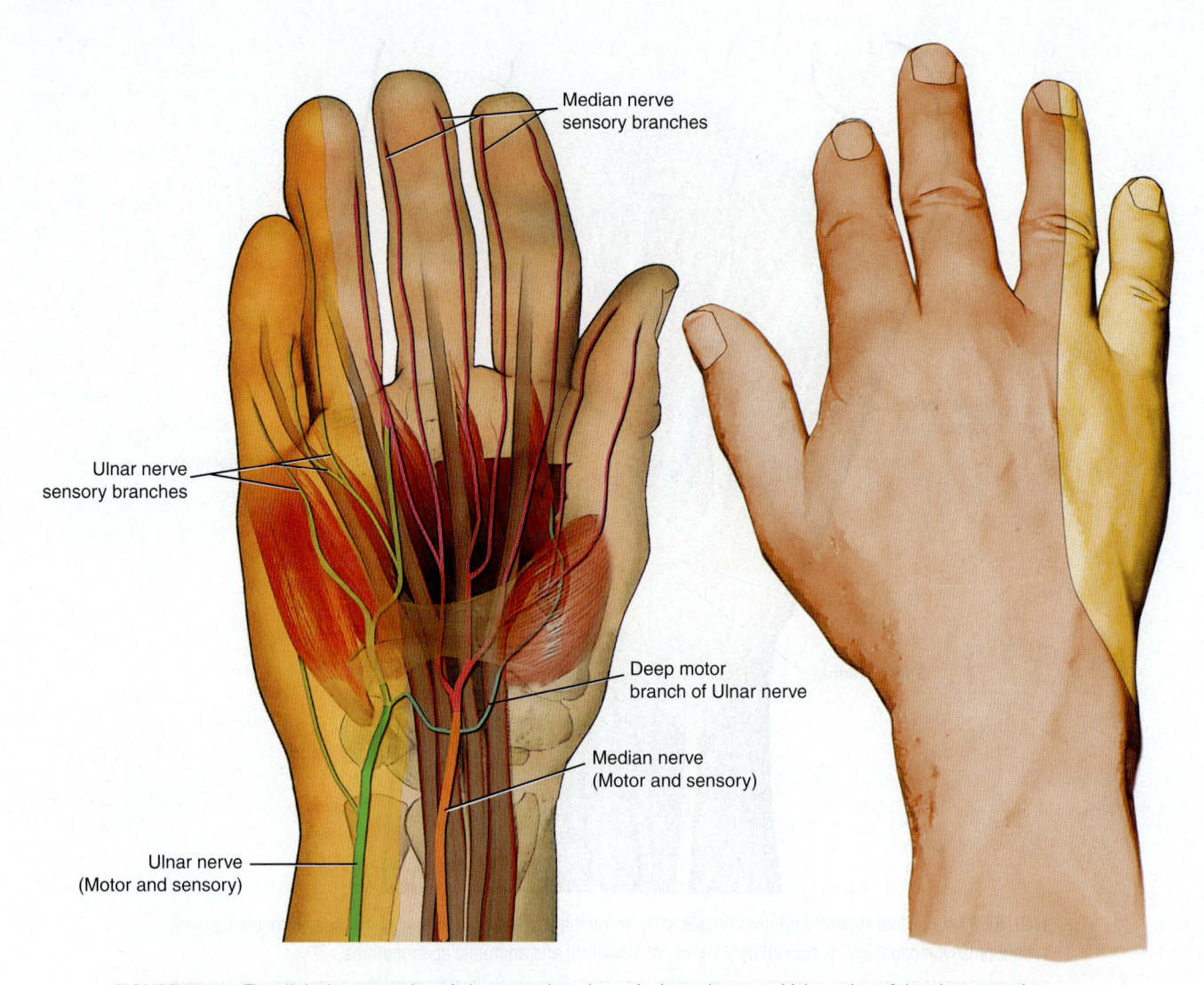

**FIGURE 67.2.** The clinical presentation of ulnar tunnel syndrome is dependent on which portion of the ulnar nerve is compromised as it passes through the ulnar tunnel.

**FIGURE 67.3.** Failure to treat ulnar tunnel syndrome can result in permanent functional disability and deformity. This photo demonstrates a typical claw hand deformity as a result of ulnar nerve compromise. (Reused from Strickland JW, Graham TJ. *Master Techniques in Orthopaedic Surgery: The Hand.* 2nd ed. Philadelphia, PA: Lippincott Williams & Wilkins; 2005, with permission.)

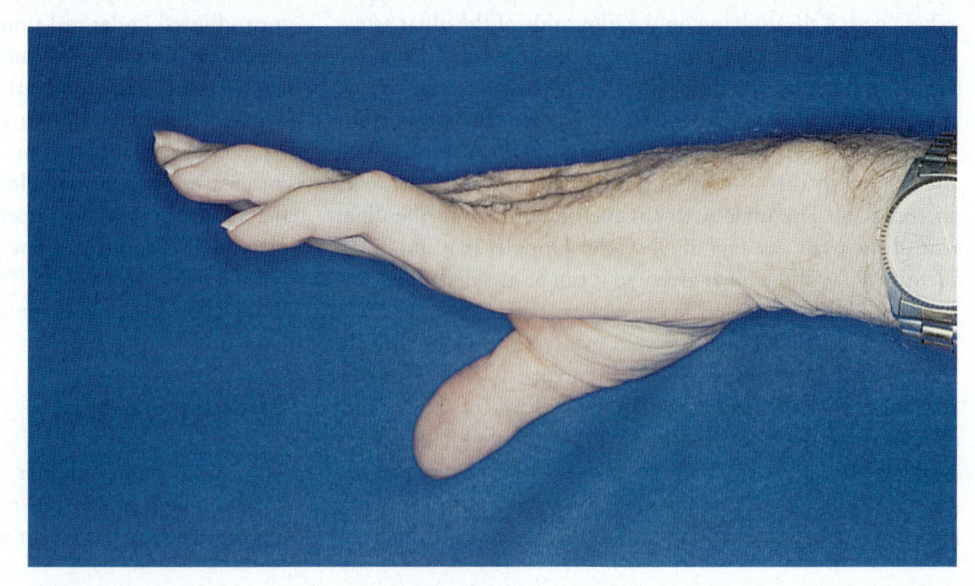

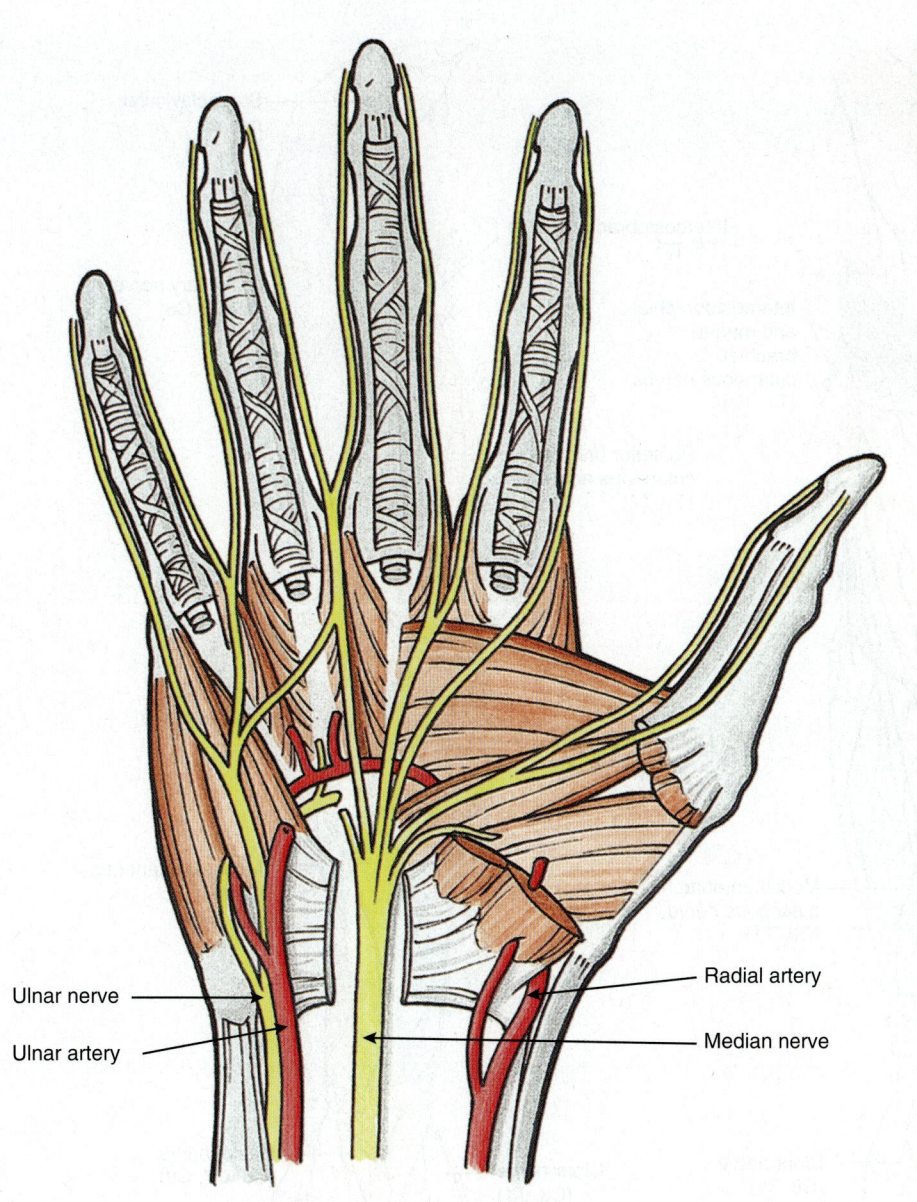

**FIGURE 67.4.** The ulnar nerve lies on the ulnar side of the ulnar artery as it passes through Guyon canal. (From Moore KL, Agur A. *Essential Clinical Anatomy*. 2nd ed. Philadelphia, PA: Lippincott Williams & Wilkins; 2002, with permission.)

intravascular injection and/or persistent paresthesia secondary to needle trauma to the ulnar nerve. Although rare, infection may occur. Ecchymosis and hematoma formation following this procedure may also occur. These complications can be decreased if manual pressure is applied to the area of the block immediately after injection. Application of cold packs for 20-minute periods after the block will also decrease the amount of postprocedure pain and bleeding the patient may experience.

Approximately 25% of patients complain of a transient increase in pain after this injection technique; the patient should be warned of this.

## CLINICAL PEARLS

Ultrasound-guided injection for ulnar tunnel syndrome is a straightforward and relatively safe technique if attention is paid to the clinically relevant anatomy. It is useful as an adjunct to surgical anesthesia and has recently been used with increasing frequency in the treatment of ulnar tunnel syndrome. Careful neurologic examination to identify preexisting neurologic deficits that may later be attributed to the nerve block should be performed on all patients before beginning ulnar nerve block at the wrist, especially those suffering from ulnar tunnel syndrome.

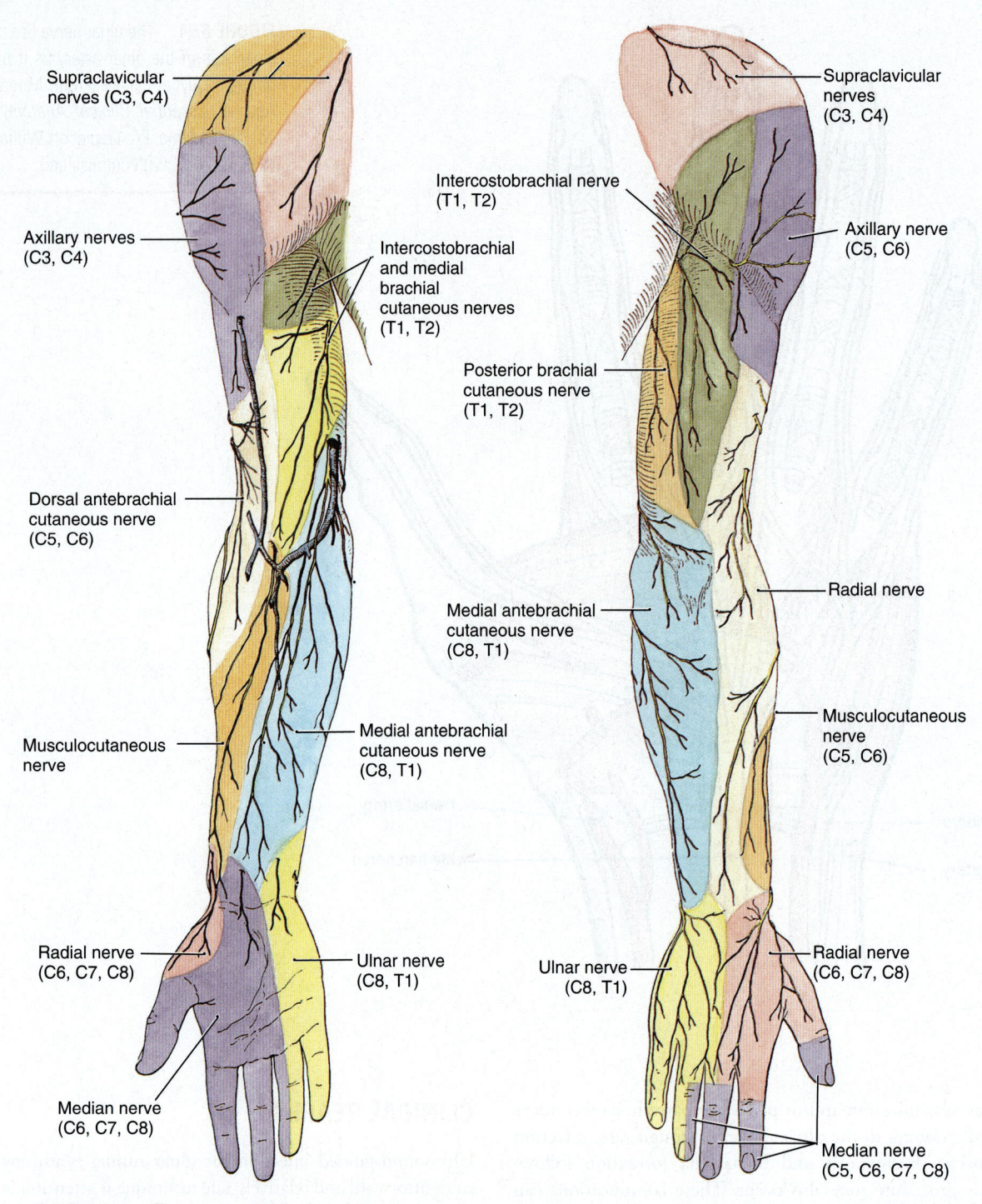

**FIGURE 67.5.** The sensory distribution of the ulnar nerve.

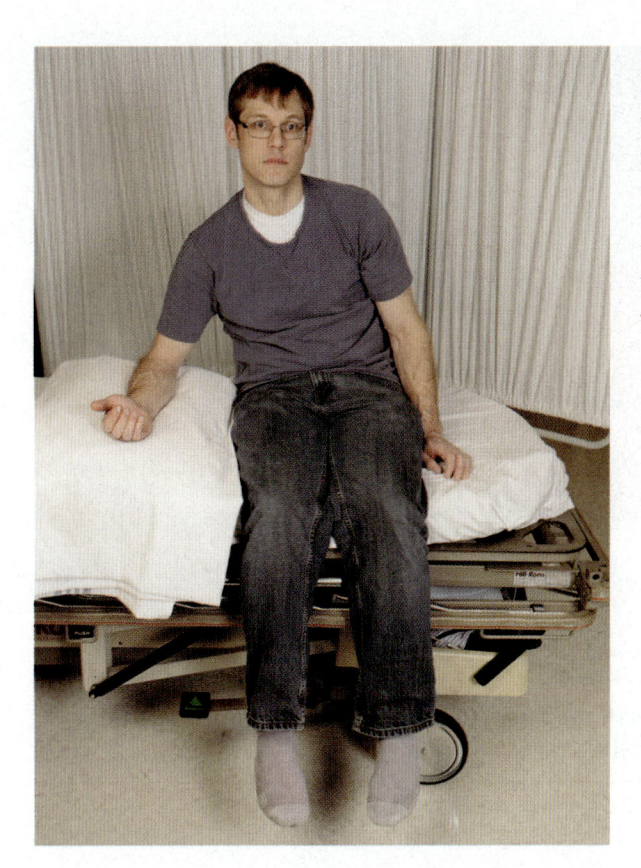

**FIGURE 67.6.** To perform ultrasound-guided injection for ulnar tunnel syndrome, the patient is then placed in the sitting position with the elbow flexed to about 100 degrees and the forearm resting comfortably palm up on a padded bedside table with the fingers slightly flexed, which will relax the flexor tendons.

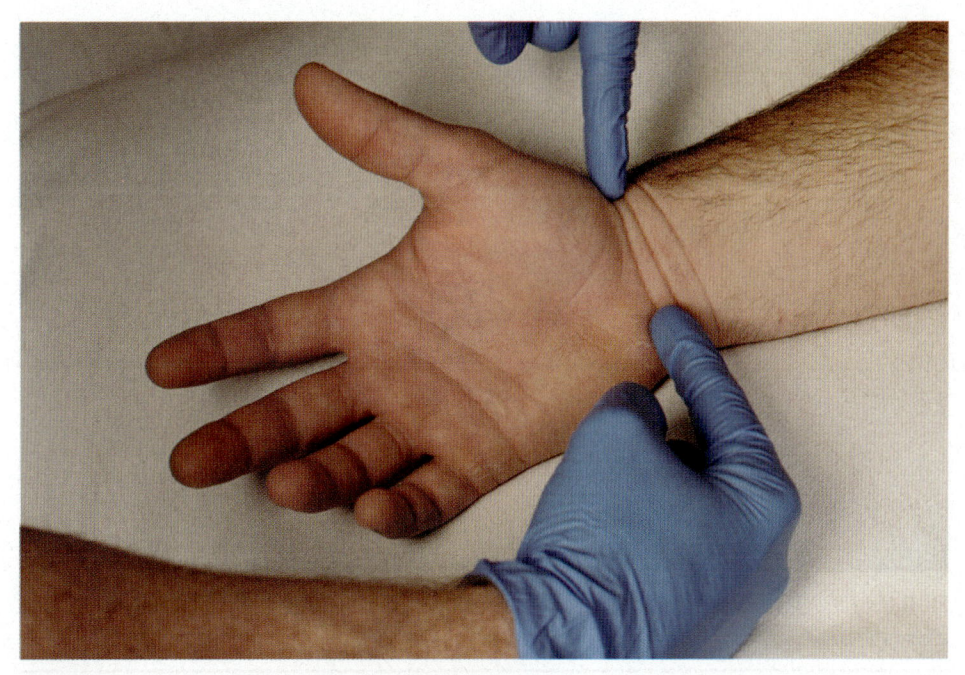

**FIGURE 67.7.** Identification of the distal crease of the wrist.

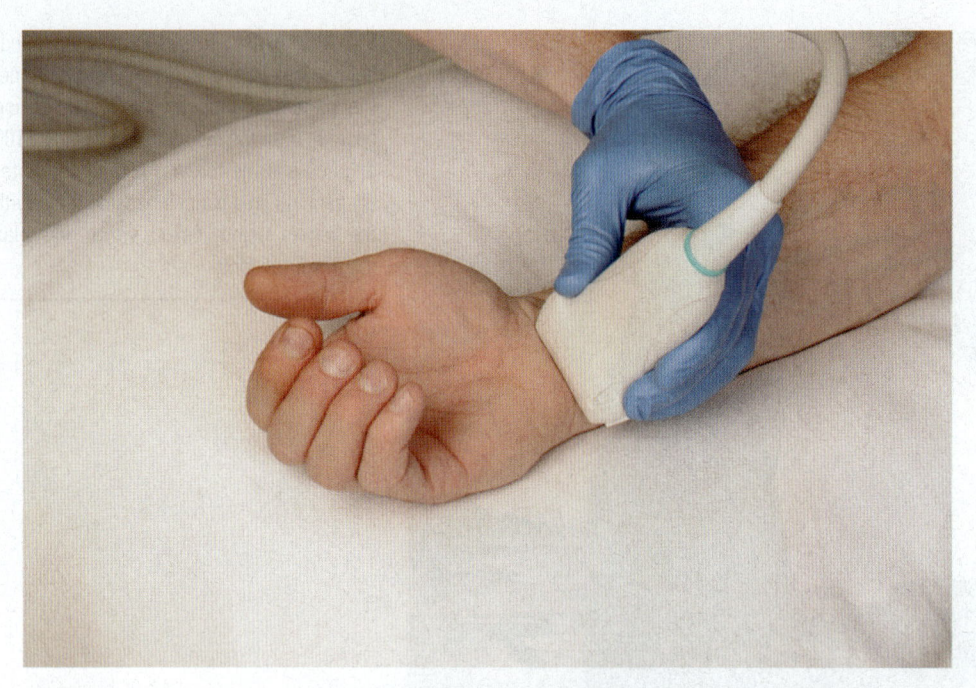

**FIGURE 67.8.** Proper transverse position for the linear high-frequency ultrasound transducer to perform ultrasound-guided injection for ulnar tunnel syndrome.

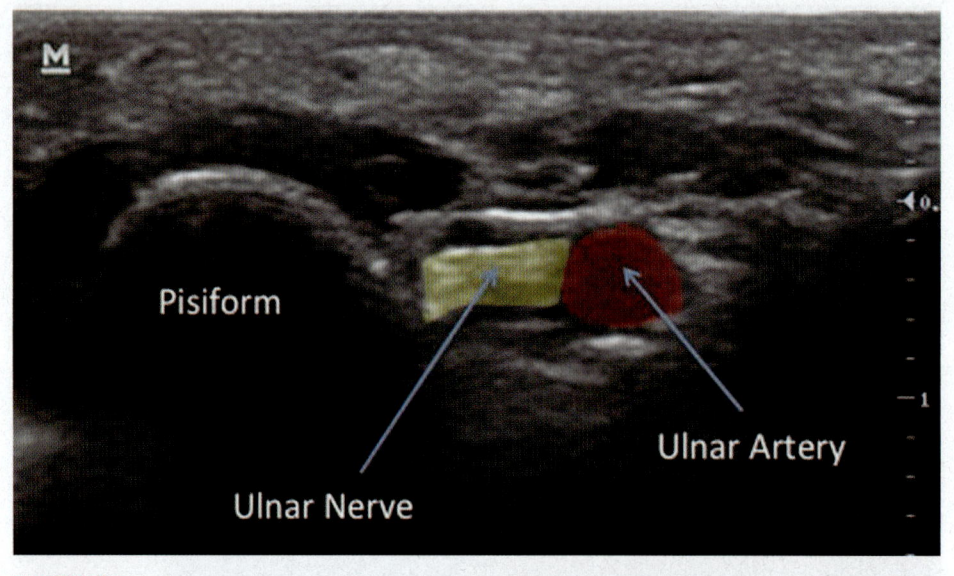

**FIGURE 67.9.** Transverse ultrasound image demonstrating the ulnar nerve lying on the ulnar side of the ulnar artery.

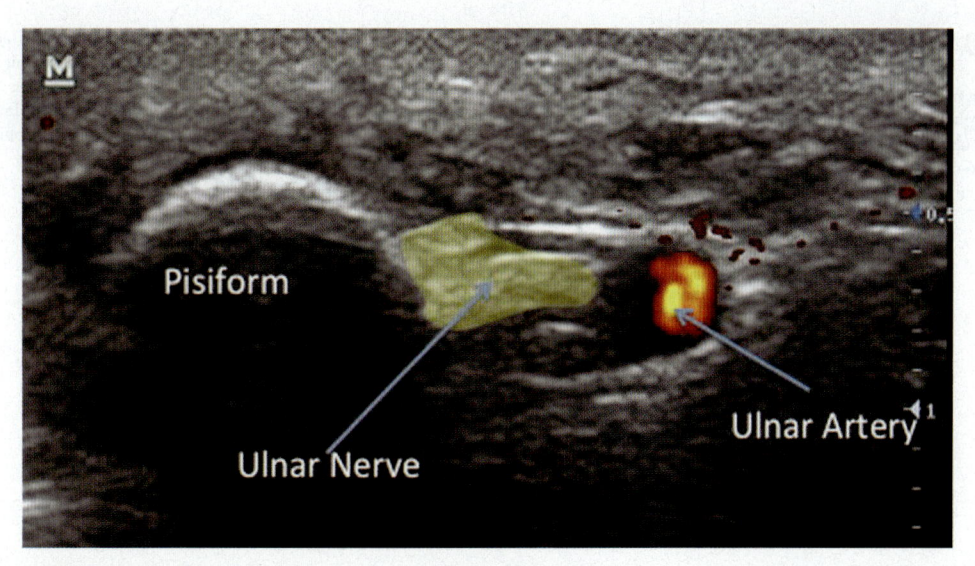

**FIGURE 67.10.** Color Doppler can help identify the ulnar artery.

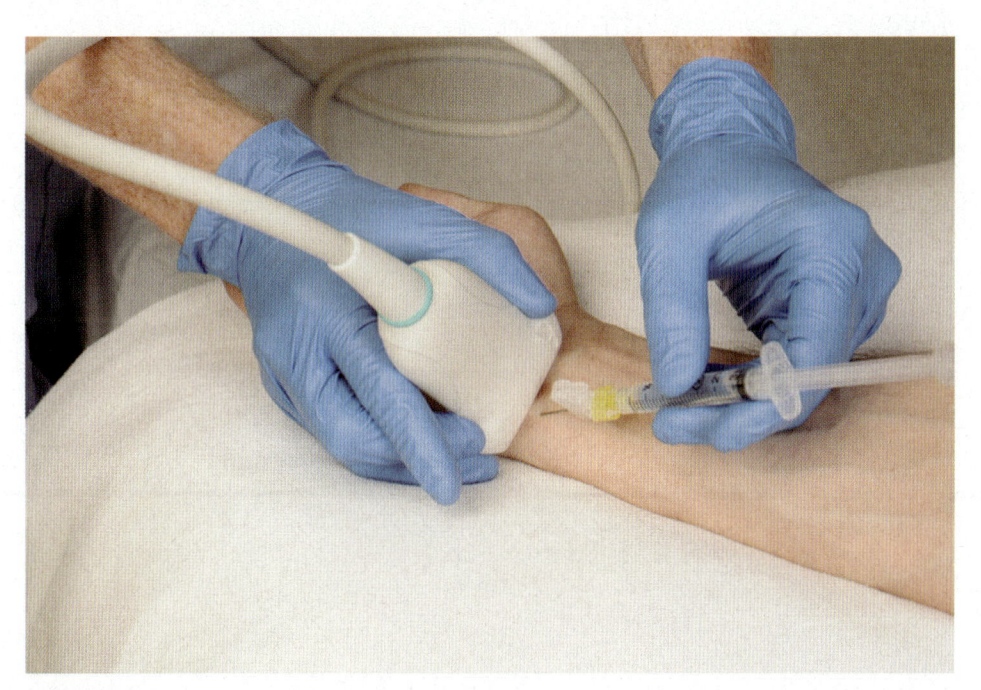

**FIGURE 67.11.** Proper out-of-plane needle placement for ultrasound-guided injection for ulnar tunnel syndrome.

## SUGGESTED READINGS

Waldman SD. Ulnar tunnel syndrome. In: *Atlas of Uncommon Pain Syndromes*. 2nd ed. Philadelphia, PA: WB Saunders; 2008:111–113.

Waldman SD. The ulnar nerve. In: *Pain Review*. Philadelphia, PA: Saunders Elsevier; 2009:76–77.

Waldman SD. The ulnar nerve. In: *Pain Review*. Philadelphia, PA: Saunders Elsevier; 2009:77–78.

Waldman SD. Ulnar nerve block at the wrist. In: *Atlas of Interventional Pain Management Injection Techniques*. 3rd ed. Philadelphia, PA: WB Saunders; 2009:239–243.

Waldman SD. The spread sign for ulnar tunnel syndrome. In: *Physical Diagnosis of Pain: An Atlas of Signs and Symptoms*. 2nd ed. Philadelphia, PA: WB Saunders; 2010:170–171.

# CHAPTER 68

# Ultrasound-Guided Injection Technique for Flexor Carpi Radialis Tendonitis

## CLINICAL PERSPECTIVES

The distal musculotendinous unit of the flexor carpi radialis muscle is subjected to an amazing variation of stresses as it performs its function of flexing and abducting the hand. The relatively poor blood supply of the distal musculotendinous unit limits the ability of the muscle and tendon to heal when traumatized. Over time, muscle tears and tendinopathy develop, further weakening the musculotendinous unit and making it susceptible to additional damage and ultimately complete rupture.

The flexor carpi radialis tendon of the hand may develop tendonitis after overuse or misuse, especially when performing activities that require repeated flexion and abduction of the hand. Acute flexor carpi radialis tendonitis has been seen in clinical practice with increasing frequency due to the increasing popularity of sports such as tennis and golf. Improper stretching of flexor carpi radialis muscle and flexor carpi radialis tendon before exercise has also been implicated in the development of flexor carpi radialis tendonitis as well as acute tendon rupture. Injuries ranging from partial to complete tears of the tendon can occur when the distal tendon sustains direct trauma while it is fully flexed under load or when the wrist is forcibly flexed while the hand is full ulnar deviation.

The pain of flexor carpi radialis tendonitis is constant and severe and is localized to the dorsoradial aspect of the wrist. The patient suffering from flexor carpi radialis tendonitis often complains of sleep disturbance due to pain. Patients with flexor carpi radialis tendonitis exhibit pain with active resisted flexion of the hand and with ulnar deviation of the wrist. In an effort to decrease pain, patients suffering from flexor carpi radialis tendonitis often splint the inflamed tendon by limiting hand flexion and ulnar deviation of the wrist to remove tension from the inflamed tendon. If untreated, patients suffering from flexor carpi radialis tendonitis may experience difficulty in performing any task that requires flexion and abduction of the wrist and hand such as using a hammer. Over time, if the tendonitis is not treated, muscle atrophy and calcific tendonitis may result, or the distal musculotendinous unit may suddenly rupture. Patients who experience complete rupture of the flexor carpi radialis tendon will not be able to fully and forcefully flex the hand or fully abduct the wrist.

Plain radiographs are indicated in all patients who present with wrist and hand pain. Based on the patient's clinical presentation, additional testing may be indicated, including complete blood cell count, sedimentation rate, and antinuclear antibody testing. Magnetic resonance imaging or ultrasound imaging of the wrist and hand is indicated if flexor carpi radialis tendinopathy or tear is suspected (Fig. 68.1). Magnetic resonance imaging or ultrasound evaluation of the affected area may also help delineate the presence of calcific tendonitis or other hand pathology.

## CLINICALLY RELEVANT ANATOMY

Located in the forearm, the flexor carpi radialis muscle serves to flex and abduct (radially deviate) the hand (Fig. 68.2). The flexor carpi radialis muscle finds its origin on the medial epicondyle of the humerus and finds its insertion on the bases of the second and third metacarpals, with a secondary insertion on the base of the trapezium (see Fig. 68.2). The flexor carpi radialis muscle is innervated by the median nerve and receives its blood supply from the ulnar artery. It is at its points of insertion and at the point at which the distal flexor carpi radialis musculotendinous unit passes beneath the flexor retinaculum that it is susceptible to the development of tendonitis, tears, and rupture (Fig. 68.3).

## ULTRASOUND-GUIDED TECHNIQUE

The benefits, risks, and alternative treatments are explained to the patient and informed consent is obtained. The patient is then placed in the sitting position with the elbow flexed to about 100 degrees and the forearm resting comfortably palm up on a padded bedside table with the fingers slightly flexed, which will relax the flexor tendons (Fig. 68.4). With the patient in the above position, the distal crease of the wrist is identified, and the patient is asked to forcibly flex his or her hand against resistance (Fig. 68.5). The tendon of the flexor carpi radialis tendon will be evident closest to the thumb (see Fig. 68.5).

463

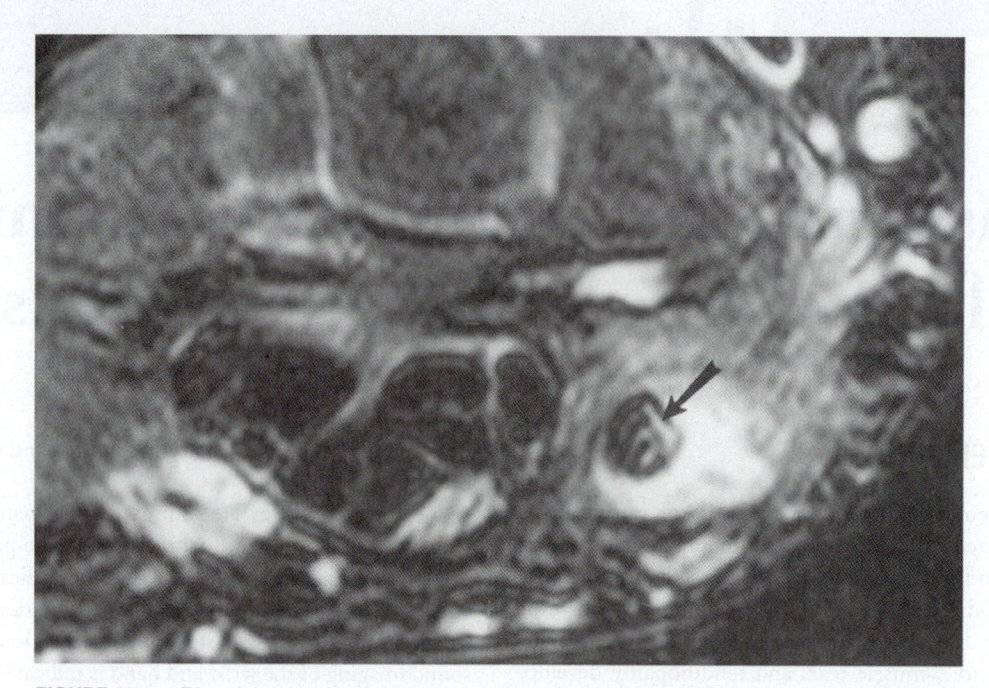

**FIGURE 68.1.** T2-weighted magnetic resonance image of a partial tear of the flexor carpi radialis tendon. Note the fluid surrounding the tendon and tendinopathy (*arrow*). (Reused from Berquist TH. *MRI of the Musculoskeletal System*. 6th ed. Philadelphia, PA: Lippincott Williams & Wilkins; 2012:830, with permission.)

A high-frequency linear ultrasound transducer is placed in a transverse position over the tendon, and an ultrasound survey scan is taken (Fig. 68.6). The tendon should appear just radial to the median nerve, which appears as a bundle of hyperechoic nerve fibers surrounded by a slightly more hyperechoic neural sheath lying beneath the flexor retinaculum (Fig. 68.7). The median nerve can be distinguished from the flexor tendons by simply having the patient flex and extend their fingers and observing the movement for the tendons. The flexor tendons will also exhibit the property of anisotropy with the tipping of the ultrasound transducer back and forth over the tendons. The flexor carpi radialis will be the most radial and superficial of the superficial flexor tendons. There may be significant effusion surrounding the tendon, which will appear on transverse ultrasound imaging as a hypoechoic ring around the tendon. If there is a question as to whether the tendon is the flexor carpi radialis tendon, the ultrasound transducer can be turned to the longitudinal plane, and the tendon can be followed distally to its insertion on the trapezium (Fig. 68.8). Color Doppler may identify hyperemia of the musculotendinous unit. After the musculotendinous unit is identified as it passes under the flexor retinaculum, the skin overlying the area beneath the ultrasound transducer is then prepped with antiseptic solution. A sterile syringe containing 2.0 mL of 0.25% preservative-free bupivacaine and 40 mg of methylprednisolone is attached to a 1½-inch, 22-gauge needle using strict aseptic technique. The needle is placed through the skin just above the transverse ultrasound transducer and is advanced using an out-of-plane approach with the needle trajectory adjusted under real-time ultrasound guidance so that the needle tip ultimately rests in proximity to the tendon of the flexor carpi radialis as it lies within the carpal tunnel beneath the flexor retinaculum (Fig. 68.9). When the tip of needle is thought to be in satisfactory position, after careful aspiration, a small amount of local anesthetic and steroid is injected under real-time ultrasound guidance to confirm that the needle tip is in the proper position. After proper needle tip placement is confirmed, the remainder of the contents of the syringe are slowly injected. There should be minimal resistance to injection and no paresthesias should be elicited. If calcific tendonitis is present, a two-needle ultrasound-guided lavage and aspiration technique may be beneficial.

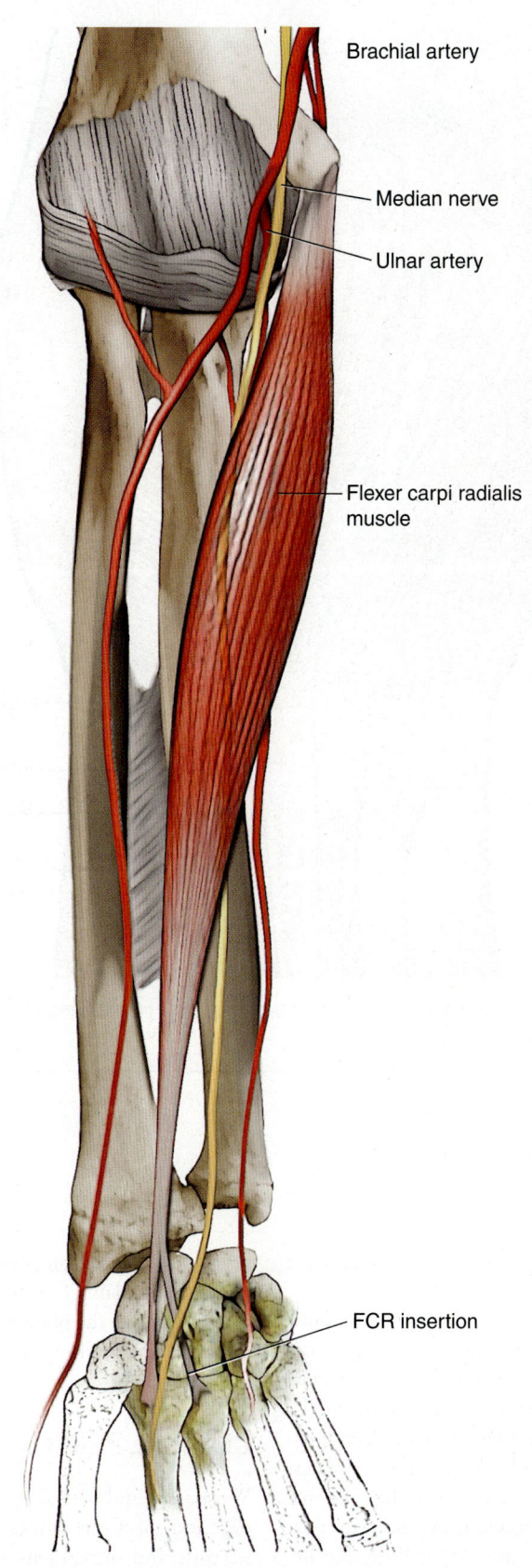

**FIGURE 68.2.** The anatomy of the flexor carpi radialis muscle and its distal tendinous insertion.

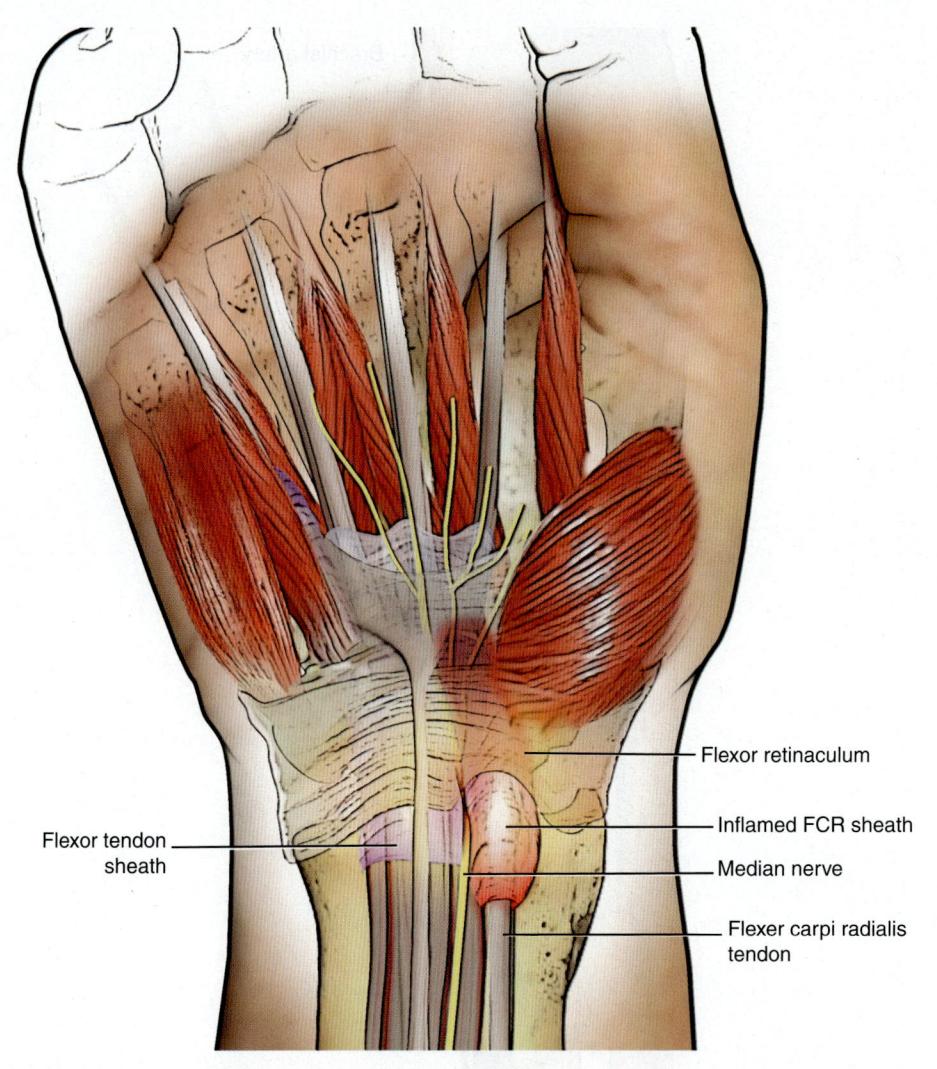

**FIGURE 68.3.** The flexor carpi radialis tendon is subject to tendonitis as it passes beneath the flexor retinaculum. Note the relationship of the tendon to the median nerve.

## COMPLICATIONS

The possibility of trauma to the flexor carpi radialis tendon from this injection technique itself remains an ever-present possibility, although the risk of this is decreased if care is taken to place the needle outside the tendon and the injection is performed under real-time ultrasound visualization. Tendons that are highly inflamed or previously damaged are subject to rupture if substances are injected directly into the tendon. This complication can be greatly decreased if the clinician uses gentle technique and stops injecting immediately if significant resistance to injection is encountered. Approximately 25% of patients complain of a transient increase in pain after this injection technique; the patient should be warned of this. Infection, although uncommon, can occur.

## CLINICAL PEARLS

Wrist and hand pathology including osteophytes of the scaphoid and pisiform bones, bursitis, osteoarthritis, avascular necrosis, and entrapment neuropathies including carpal tunnel

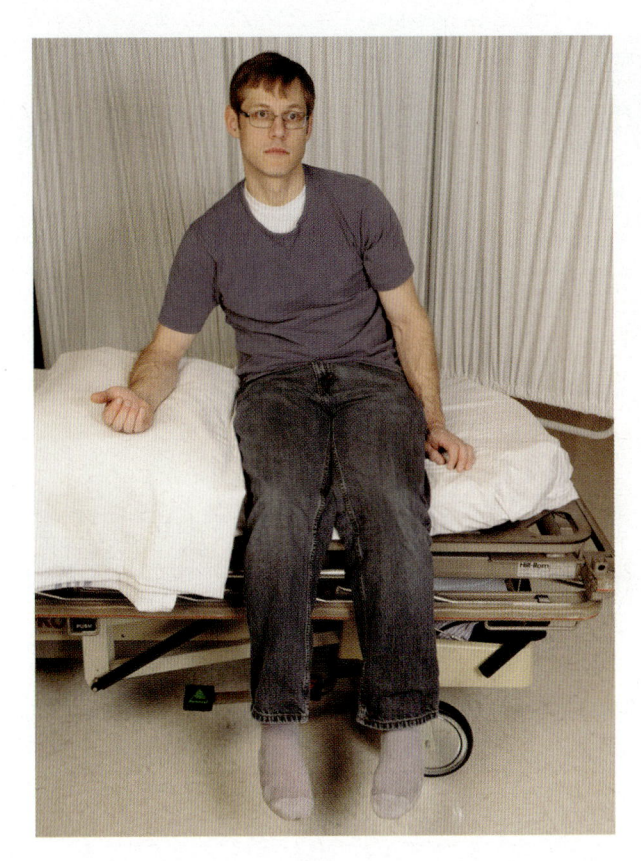

**FIGURE 68.4.** To perform ultrasound-guided injection for flexor carpi radialis tendonitis, the patient is then placed in the sitting position with the elbow flexed to about 100 degrees and the forearm resting comfortably palm up on a padded bedside table with the fingers slightly flexed, which will relax the flexor tendons.

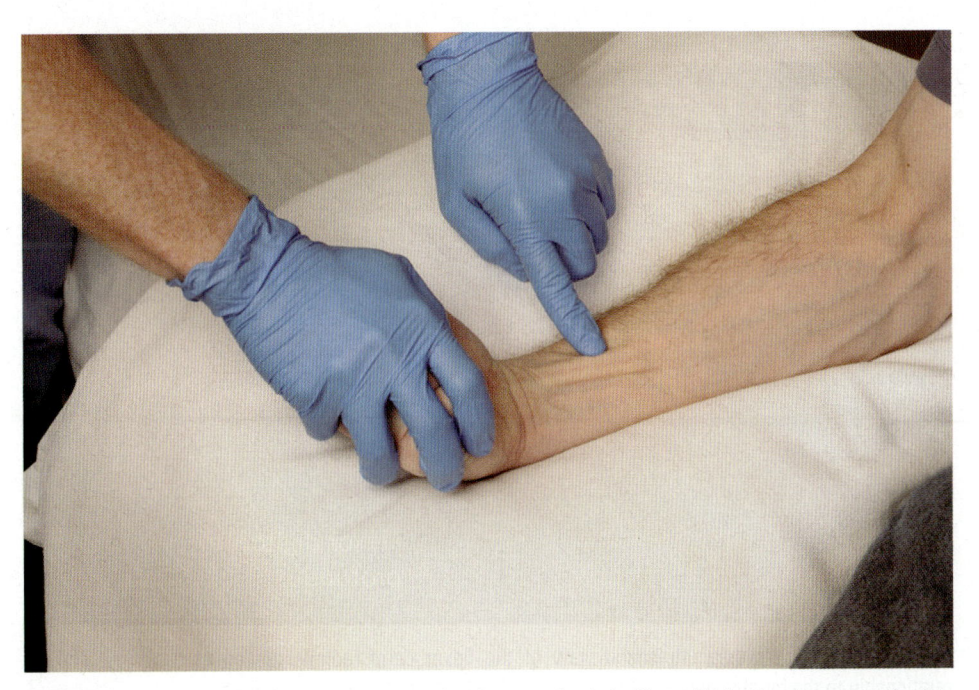

**FIGURE 68.5.** Identification of the flexor carpi radialis tendon is facilitated by having the patient forcibly flex his or her wrist.

**FIGURE 68.6.** Proper ultrasound transducer placement for ultrasound-guided injection for flexor carpi radialis tendonitis.

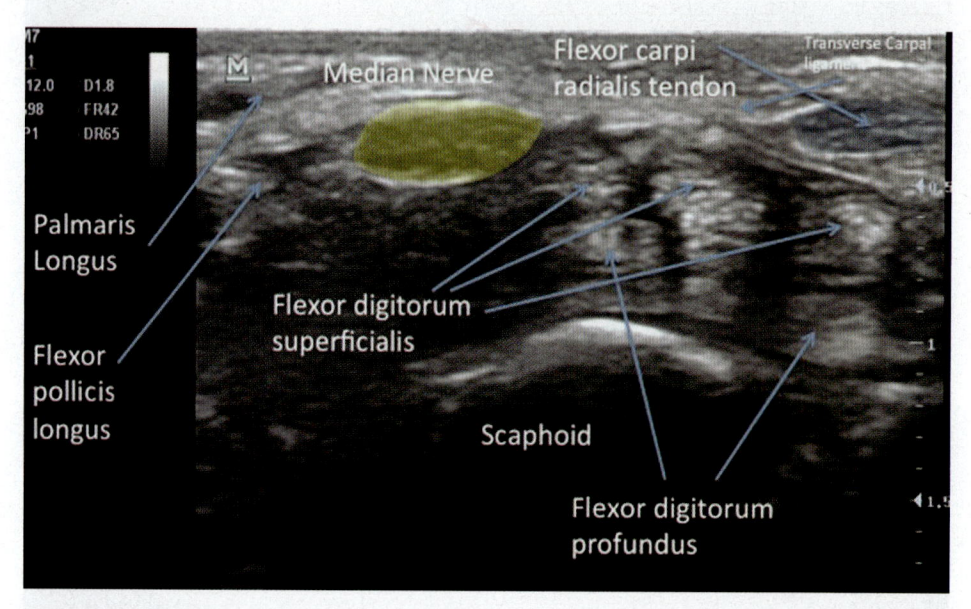

**FIGURE 68.7.** Transverse ultrasound view of the flexor carpi radialis tendon at the wrist and its relationship to the median nerve.

CHAPTER 68    ULTRASOUND-GUIDED INJECTION TECHNIQUE FOR FLEXOR CARPI RADIALIS TENDONITIS    469

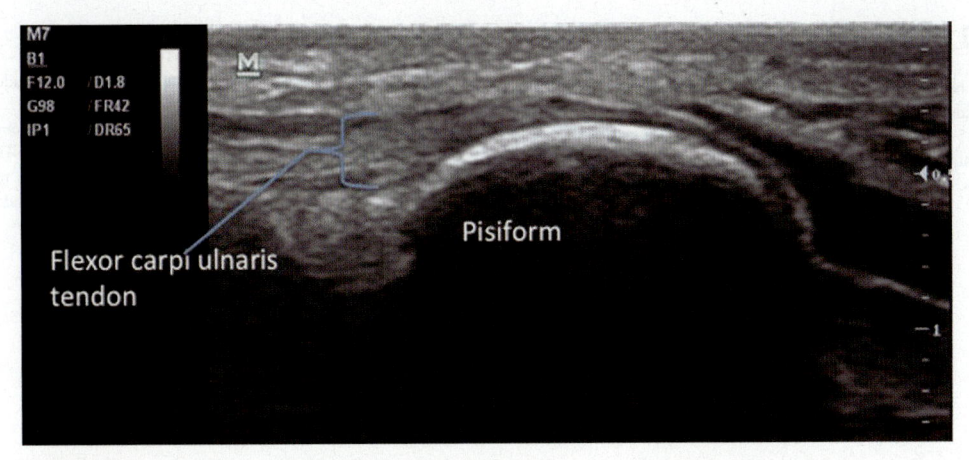

**FIGURE 68.8.** Longitudinal ultrasound view of the flexor carpi radialis tendon demonstrating its insertion on the trapezium.

syndrome may coexist with flexor carpi radialis tendonitis and may contribute to the patient's pain symptomatology. Universal precautions should always be observed to protect the operator, and strict adherence to sterile technique must be used to avoid infection. Gentle physical therapy and local heat should be introduced following ultrasound-guided injection of flexor carpi radialis tendonitis to reduce pain and improve function. Simple analgesics and nonsteroidal anti-inflammatory agents or COX-2 inhibitors may be used concurrently with this injection technique.

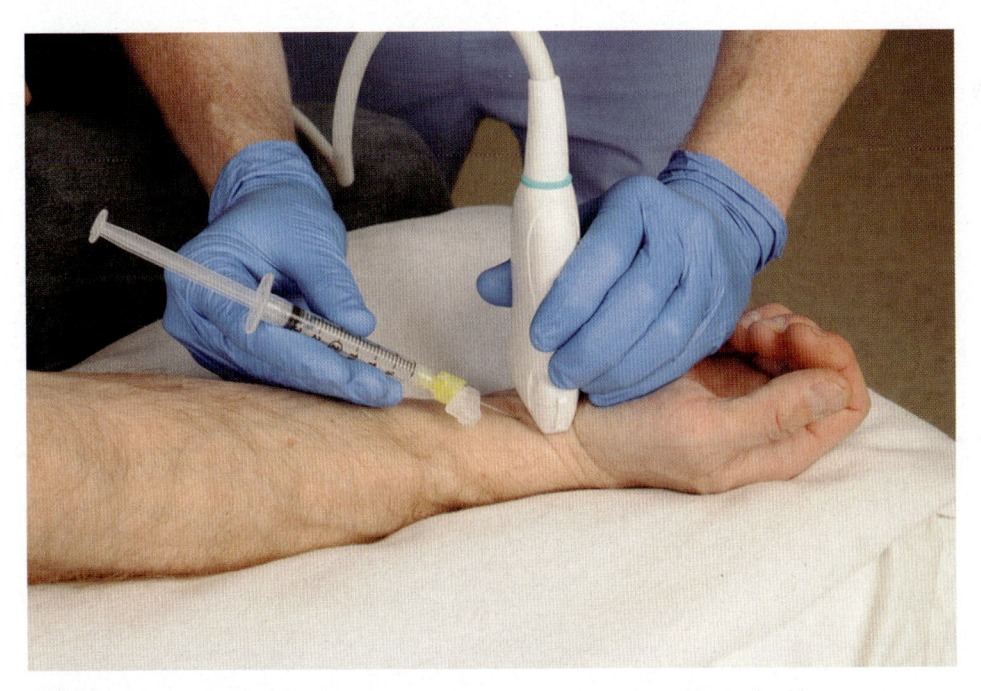

**FIGURE 68.9.** Injection of the distal flexor carpi radialis tendon under ultrasound guidance.

## SUGGESTED READINGS

Soejima O, Iida H, Naito M. Flexor carpi radialis tendinitis caused by malunited trapezial ridge fracture in a professional baseball player. *J Orthop Sci* 2002;7(1):151–153.

Waldman SD. Carpal tunnel syndrome. In: *Atlas of interventional pain management injection techniques*. 3rd ed. Philadelphia, PA: Saunders Elsevier; 2009:239–243.

Waldman SD. Functional anatomy of the wrist joint. In: *Pain Review*. Philadelphia, PA: Saunders Elsevier; 2009:101–102.

Waldman SD. The median nerve. In: *Pain Review*. Philadelphia, PA: Saunders Elsevier; 2009:77–78.

Waldman SD. Carpal tunnel syndrome. In: *Atlas of Common Pain Syndromes*. 3rd ed. Philadelphia, PA: Saunders Elsevier; 2013:160–163.

Waldman SD. Injection technique for flexor carpi radialis tendinitis. In: *Atlas of Pain Management Injection Techniques*. 3rd ed. Philadelphia, PA: Saunders Elsevier; 2013:193–194.

CHAPTER 69

# Ultrasound-Guided Injection Technique for Flexor Carpi Ulnaris Tendonitis

## CLINICAL PERSPECTIVES

The distal musculotendinous unit of the flexor carpi ulnaris muscle is subjected to an amazing variation of stresses as it performs its function of flexing and adducting the hand. The relatively poor blood supply of the distal musculotendinous unit limits the ability of the muscle and tendon to heal when traumatized. Over time, muscle tears and tendinopathy develop, further weakening the musculotendinous unit and making it susceptible to additional damage and ultimately complete rupture.

The flexor carpi ulnaris tendon of the hand may develop tendonitis after overuse or misuse, especially when performing activities that require repeated flexion and adduction of the hand. Acute flexor carpi ulnaris tendonitis has been seen in clinical practice with increasing frequency due to the increasing popularity of both racquet sports such as tennis and golf. Improper stretching of flexor carpi ulnaris muscle and flexor carpi ulnaris tendon before exercise has also been implicated in the development of flexor carpi ulnaris tendonitis as well as acute tendon rupture. Injuries ranging from partial to complete tears of the tendon can occur when the distal tendon sustains direct trauma while it is fully flexed under load or when the wrist is forcibly flexed while the hand is in full radial deviation.

The pain of flexor carpi ulnaris tendonitis is constant and severe and is localized to the dorso-ulnar aspect of the wrist. The patient suffering from flexor carpi ulnaris tendonitis often complains of sleep disturbance due to pain. Patients with flexor carpi ulnaris tendonitis exhibit pain with active resisted flexion of the hand and with radial deviation of the wrist. In an effort to decrease pain, patients suffering from flexor carpi ulnaris tendonitis often splint the inflamed tendon by limiting hand flexion and radial deviation of the wrist to remove tension from the inflamed tendon. If untreated, patients suffering from flexor carpi ulnaris tendonitis may experience difficulty in performing any task that requires flexion and adduction of the wrist and hand such as using a hammer or lifting a heavy coffee mug. Over time, if the tendonitis is not treated, muscle atrophy and calcific tendonitis may result, or the distal musculotendinous unit may suddenly rupture. Patients who experience complete rupture of the flexor carpi ulnaris tendon will not be able to fully and forcefully flex the hand or fully adduct the wrist.

Plain radiographs are indicated in all patients who present with wrist and hand pain. Based on the patient's clinical presentation, additional testing may be indicated, including complete blood cell count, sedimentation rate, and antinuclear antibody testing. Magnetic resonance imaging or ultrasound imaging of the wrist and hand is indicated if flexor carpi ulnaris tendinopathy or tear is suspected. Magnetic resonance imaging or ultrasound evaluation of the affected area may also help delineate the presence of calcific tendonitis or other hand pathology (Fig. 69.1).

## CLINICALLY RELEVANT ANATOMY

The key anatomic landmarks when performing ultrasound-guided injection for flexor carpi ulnaris tendonitis are the ulnar nerve and artery, which lie adjacent to the tendon at the level of the pisiform bone. Located in the forearm, the flexor carpi ulnaris muscle serves as to flex and adduct (radially deviate) the hand (Fig. 69.2). The flexor carpi ulnaris muscle has two heads, which find their origin on the medial epicondyle of the humerus and the medial margin of the olecranon process of the ulna. The muscle finds its insertion on the pisiform bone with a secondary insertion via ligaments to the hamate, the third and fifth metacarpals, and the tuberosity of the trapezium (see Fig. 69.2). The flexor carpi ulnaris muscle is innervated by the median nerve and receives its blood supply from the ulnar artery. It is at its points of insertion and at the point at which the distal flexor carpi ulnaris musculotendinous unit passes beneath the flexor retinaculum that it is susceptible to the development of tendonitis, tears, and rupture.

## ULTRASOUND-GUIDED TECHNIQUE

The benefits, risks, and alternative treatments are explained to the patient, and informed consent is obtained. The patient is then placed in the sitting position with the elbow flexed to about 100 degrees and the forearm resting comfortably palm up on a padded bedside table with the fingers slightly flexed, which will relax the flexor tendons (Fig. 69.3). With the patient in the above position, the distal crease of the wrist is identified, and the patient is asked to forcibly flex his or her hand against

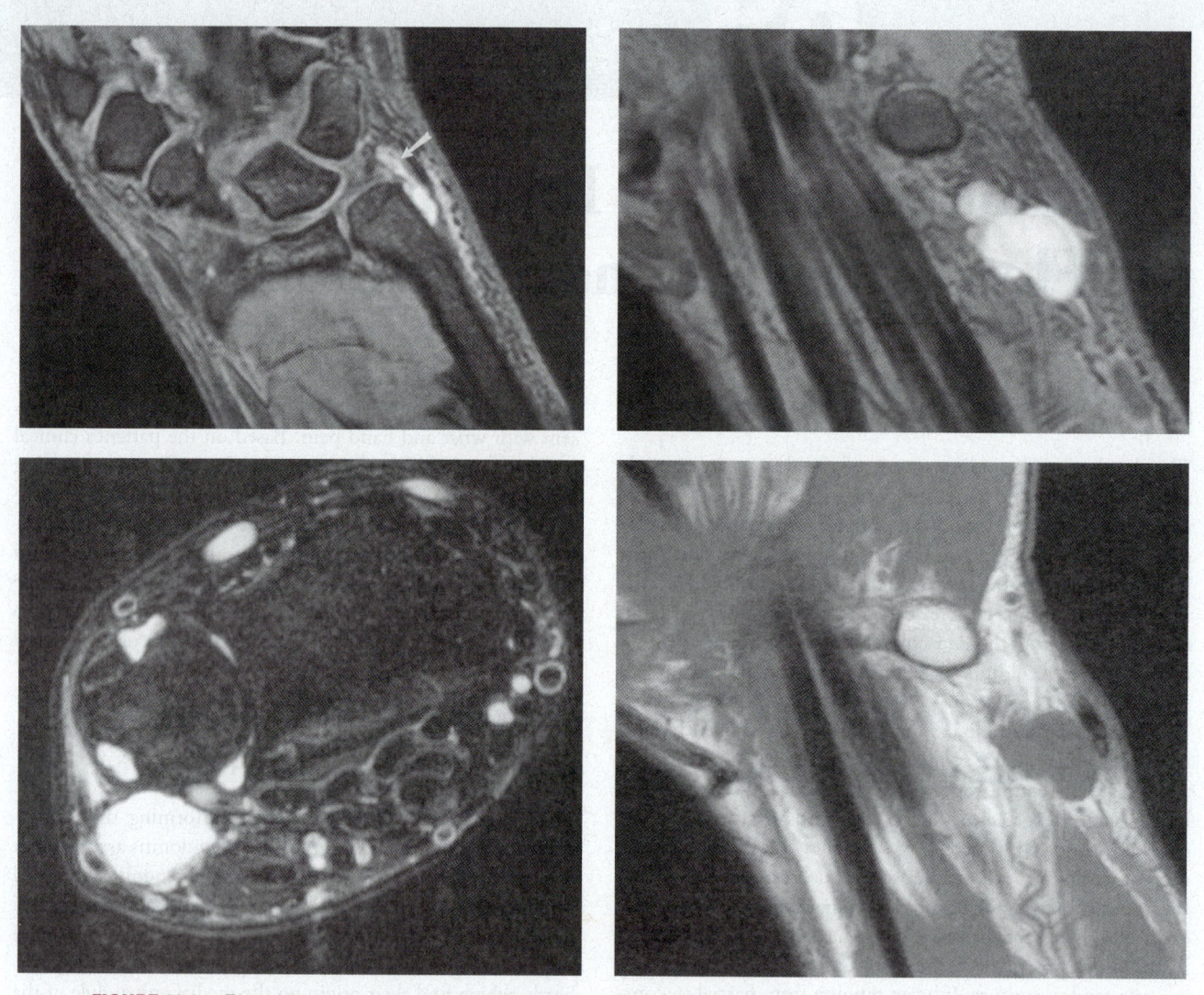

**FIGURE 69.1.** T2-weighted magnetic resonance image demonstrating a ganglion cyst arising from the triangular fibrocartilage complex causing ulnar-sided wrist pain (*arrow*). (Reused from Berquist TH. *MRI of the Musculoskeletal System.* 6th ed. Philadelphia, PA: Lippincott Williams & Wilkins; 2012:842, with permission.)

resistance (Fig. 69.4). The tendon of the flexor carpi ulnaris tendon will be evident closest to the little finger (see Fig. 69.4). A high-frequency linear ultrasound transducer is placed in a transverse position over the tendon, and an ultrasound survey scan is taken (Fig. 69.5). The tendon of the flexor carpi ulnaris tendon should appear on the ulnar side of the ulnar nerve and the ulnar artery. The ulnar nerve appears as a bundle of hyperechoic nerve fibers surrounded by a slightly more hyperechoic neural sheath lying beneath the flexor retinaculum with the ulnar artery just radial to it (Fig. 69.6). The median nerve can be distinguished from the flexor tendons by simply having the patient flex and extend their fingers and observing the movement for the tendons. The flexor tendons will also exhibit the property of anisotropy with the tipping of the ultrasound transducer back and forth over the tendons. The flexor carpi ulnaris will be the most ulnar and superficial of the superficial flexor tendons and can be seen to lie just above the dome-shaped pisiform (see Fig. 69.6). There may be significant effusion surrounding the tendon, which will appear on transverse ultrasound imaging as a hypoechoic ring around the tendon. If there is a question as to whether the tendon is the flexor carpi ulnaris tendon, the ultrasound transducer can be turned to the longitudinal plane, and the tendon can be followed distally to its insertion on the pisiform (Fig. 69.7). Color Doppler may identify hyperemia of the musculotendinous unit and may also be useful in helping identify the ulnar artery if the anatomy is not clear (Fig. 69.8). After the musculotendinous unit is identified as it passes under the flexor retinaculum, the skin overlying the area beneath the ultrasound transducer is then prepped with antiseptic solution. A sterile syringe containing 2.0 mL of 0.25% preservative-free bupivacaine and 40 mg of methylprednisolone is attached to a 1½-inch, 22-gauge needle using strict aseptic technique. The needle is placed through the skin just above the transverse ultrasound transducer and

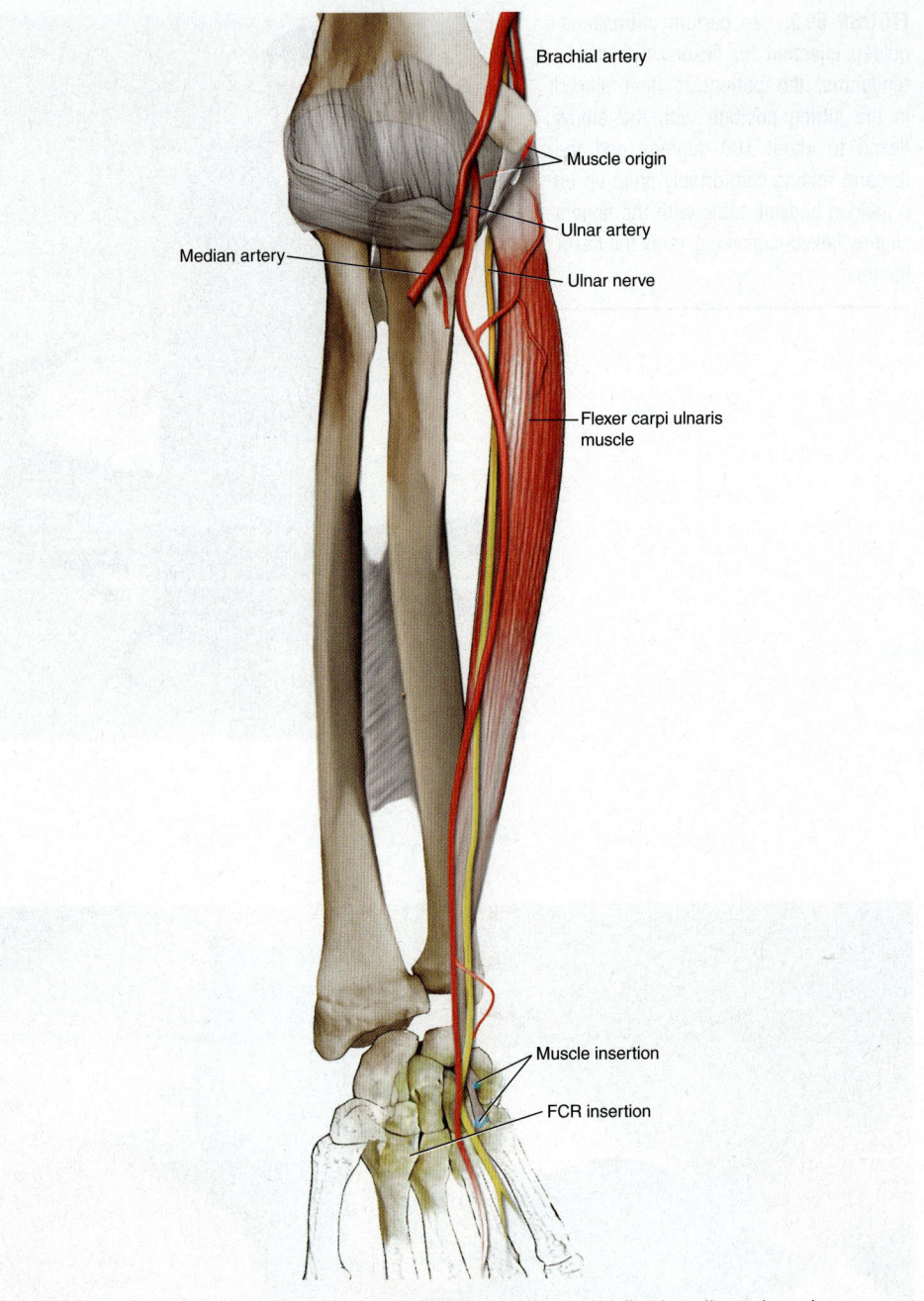

**FIGURE 69.2.** The anatomy of the flexor carpi ulnaris muscle and its distal tendinous insertion.

is advanced using an out-of-plane approach with the needle trajectory adjusted under real-time ultrasound guidance so that the needle tip ultimately rests in proximity to the tendon of the flexor carpi ulnaris as it lies within the carpal tunnel beneath the flexor retinaculum (Fig. 69.9). When the tip of needle is thought to be in satisfactory position, after careful aspiration, a small amount of local anesthetic and steroid is injected under real-time ultrasound guidance to confirm that the needle tip is in the proper position. After proper needle tip placement is confirmed, the remainder of the contents of the syringe are slowly injected. There should be minimal resistance to injection and no paresthesias should be elicited. If calcific tendonitis is present, a two-needle ultrasound-guided lavage and aspiration technique may be beneficial.

## COMPLICATIONS

The possibility of trauma to the flexor carpi ulnaris tendon from this injection technique itself remains an ever-present possibility, although the risk of this is decreased if care is taken to place the needle outside the tendon and the injection is performed under real-time ultrasound visualization. Tendons that are highly inflamed or previously damaged are subject to rupture if substances are

**FIGURE 69.3.** To perform ultrasound-guided injection for flexor carpi ulnaris tendonitis, the patient is then placed in the sitting position with the elbow flexed to about 100 degrees and the forearm resting comfortably palm up on a padded bedside table with the fingers slightly flexed, which will relax the flexor tendons.

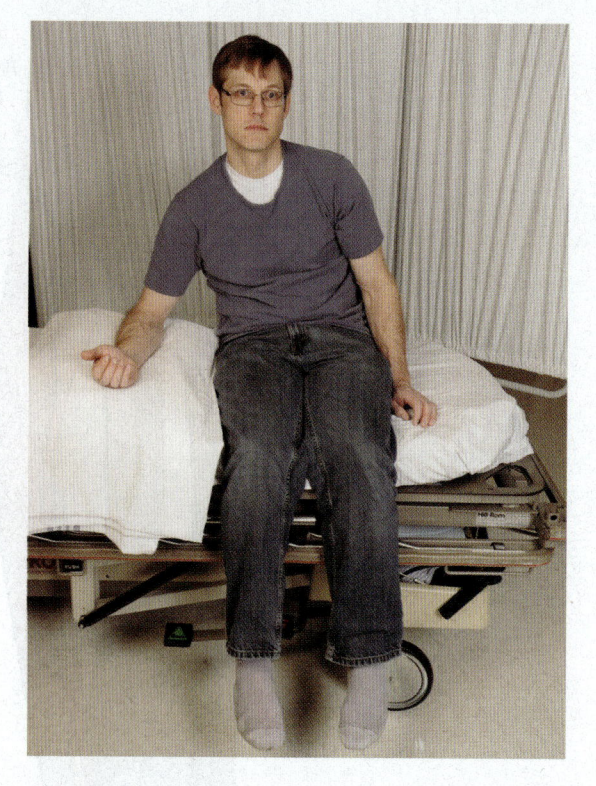

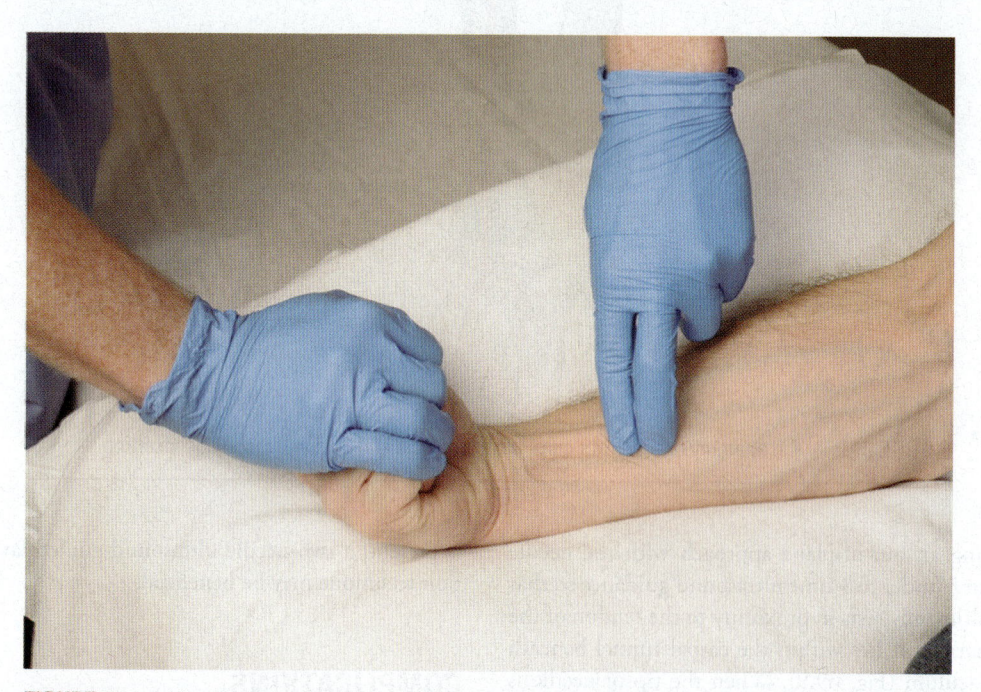

**FIGURE 69.4.** Identification of the flexor carpi ulnaris tendon is facilitated by having the patient forcibly flex his or her wrist.

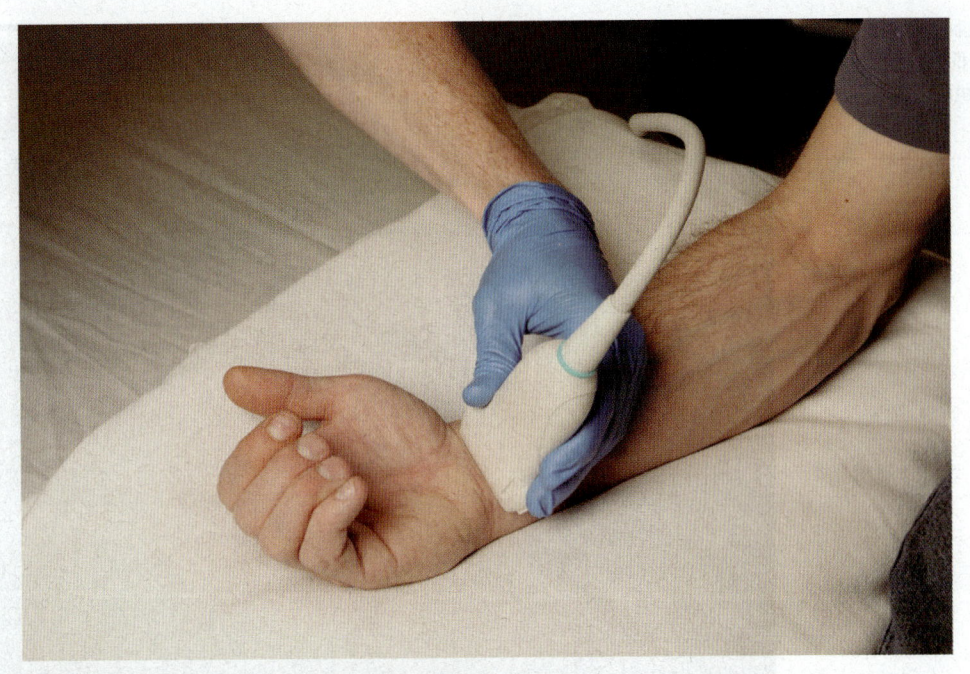

**FIGURE 69.5.** Proper ultrasound transducer placement for ultrasound-guided injection for flexor carpi ulnaris tendonitis.

injected directly into the tendon. This complication can be greatly decreased if the clinician uses gentle technique and stops injecting immediately if significant resistance to injection is encountered. Approximately 25% of patients complain of a transient increase in pain after this injection technique; the patient should be warned of this. Infection, although uncommon, can occur.

## CLINICAL PEARLS

Wrist and pathology including osteophytes of the scaphoid and pisiform bones, bursitis, osteoarthritis, avascular necrosis, and entrapment neuropathies including carpal tunnel syndrome may coexist with flexor carpi ulnaris tendonitis and may contribute to

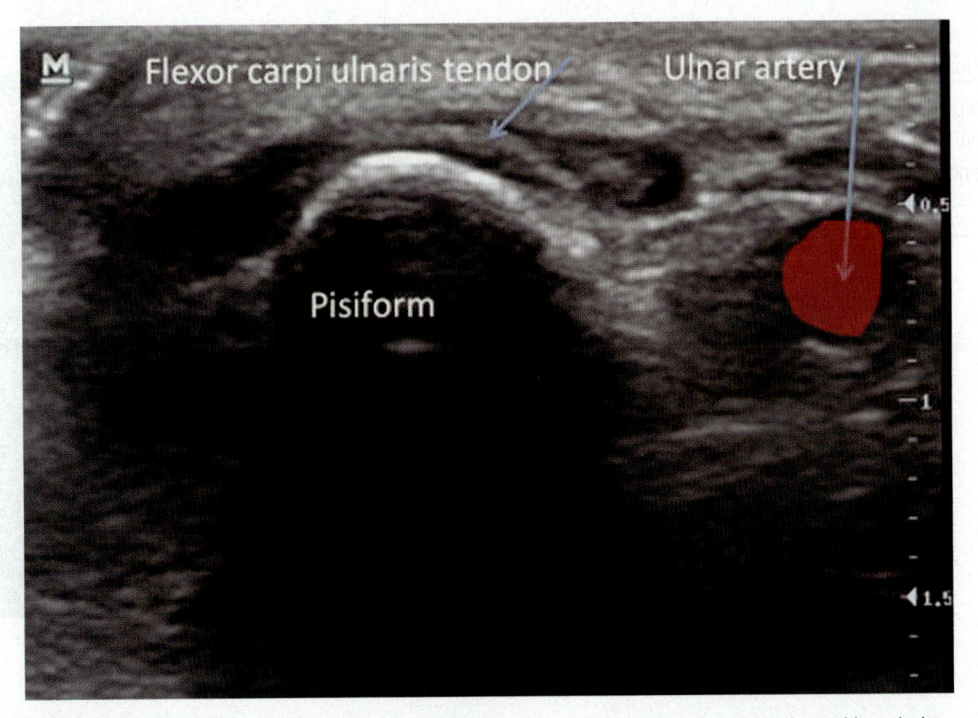

**FIGURE 69.6.** Transverse ultrasound view of the flexor carpi ulnaris tendon at the wrist and its relationship to the ulnar nerve and artery.

**FIGURE 69.7.** Longitudinal ultrasound view of the flexor carpi ulnaris tendon demonstrating its insertion on the trapezium.

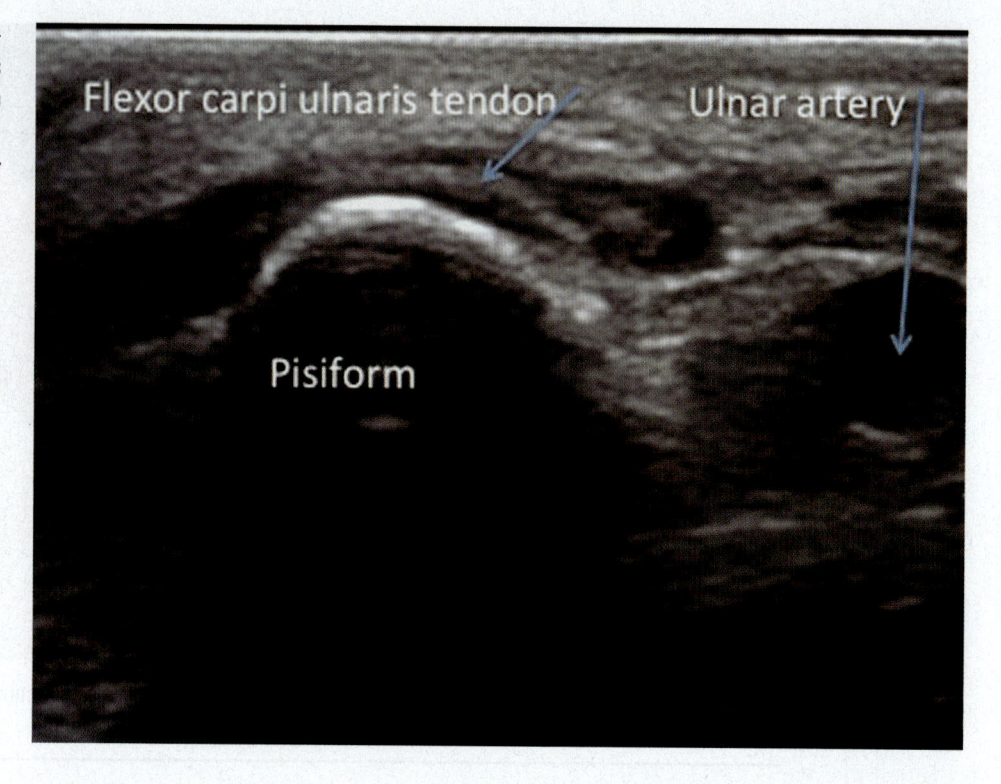

the patient's pain symptomatology. Universal precautions should always be observed to protect the operator, and strict adherence to sterile technique must be used to avoid infection. Gentle physical therapy and local heat should be introduced following ultrasound-guided injection of flexor carpi ulnaris tendonitis to reduce pain and improve function. Simple analgesics and non-steroidal anti-inflammatory agents or COX-2 inhibitors may be used concurrently with this injection technique.

**FIGURE 69.8.** Color Doppler can be useful in helping identify the ulnar artery, which lies just radial to the ulnar nerve and the flexor carpi ulnaris tendon.

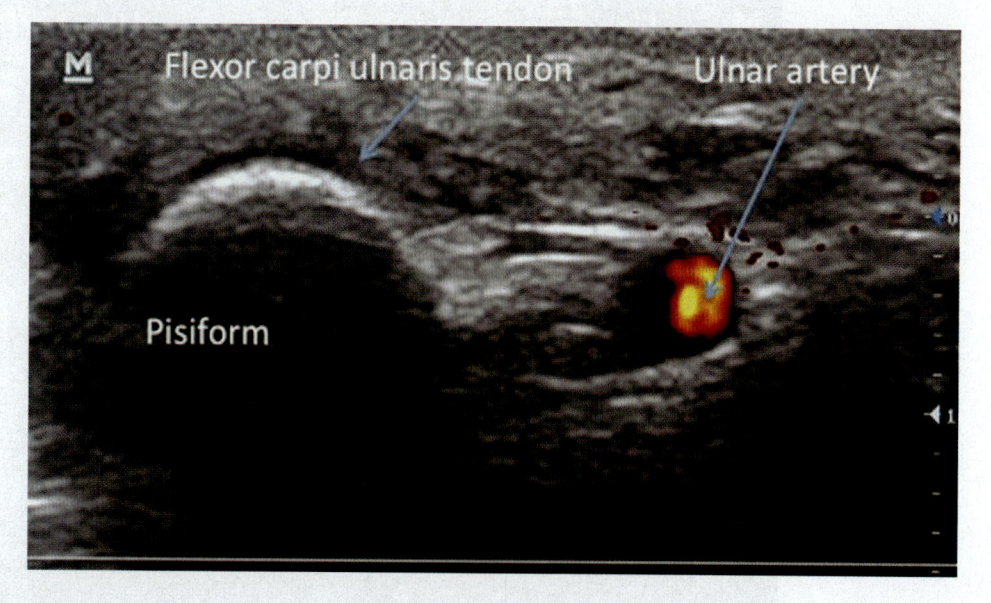

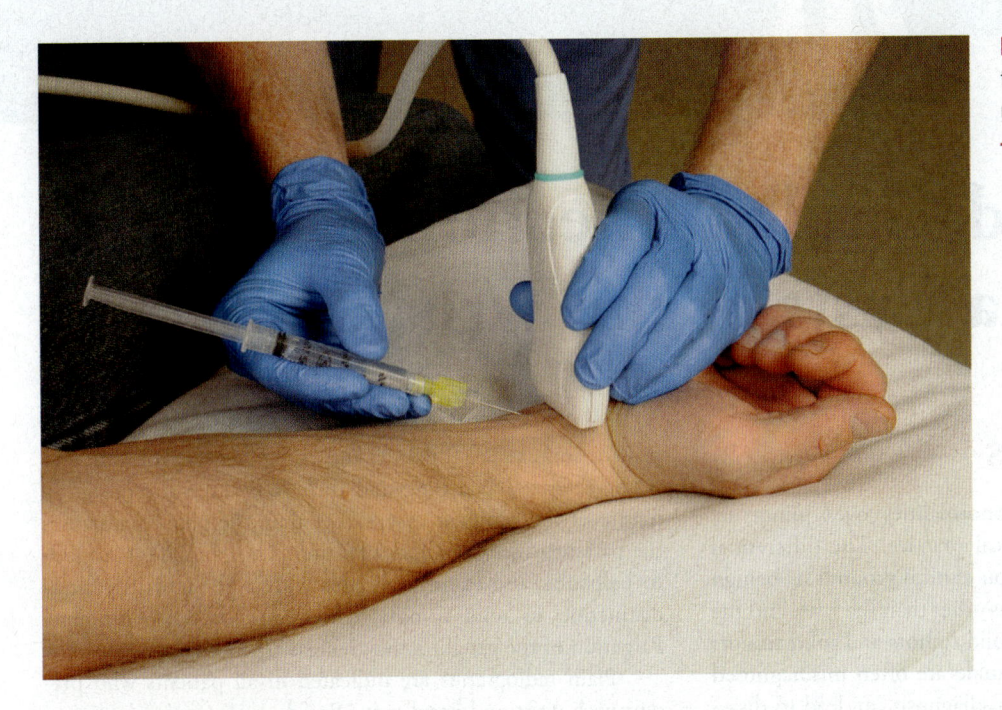

**FIGURE 69.9.** Injection of the distal flexor carpi ulnaris tendon under ultrasound guidance.

## SUGGESTED READINGS

Waldman SD. Ulnar tunnel syndrome. In: *Atlas of Uncommon Pain Syndromes*. 2nd ed. Philadelphia, PA: WB Saunders; 2008:111–113.

Waldman SD. Carpal tunnel syndrome. In: *Atlas of Interventional Pain Management Injection Techniques*. 3rd ed. Philadelphia, PA: WB Saunders; 2009:239–243.

Waldman SD. Functional anatomy of the wrist joint. In: *Pain Review*. Philadelphia, PA: WB Saunders; 2009:101–102.

Waldman SD. The median nerve. In: *Pain Review*. Philadelphia, PA: Saunders Elsevier; 2009:77–78.

Waldman SD. The ulnar nerve. In: *Pain Review*. Philadelphia, PA: Saunders Elsevier; 2009:76–77.

Waldman SD. The ulnar nerve. In: *Pain Review*. Philadelphia, PA: Saunders Elsevier; 2009:77–78.

Waldman SD. Ulnar nerve block at the wrist. In: *Atlas of Interventional Pain Management Injection Techniques*. 3rd ed. Philadelphia, PA: WB Saunders; 2009:239–243.

Waldman SD. Carpal tunnel syndrome. In: *Atlas of Common Pain Syndromes*. 3rd ed. Philadelphia, PA: WB Saunders; 2013:160–163.

Waldman SD. Injection technique for flexor carpi ulnaris tendinitis. In: *Atlas of Pain Management Injection Techniques*. 3rd ed. Philadelphia, PA: WB Saunders; 2013:195–196.

# CHAPTER 70

# Ultrasound-Guided Injection Technique for Ganglia Cysts of the Wrist and Hand

## CLINICAL PERSPECTIVES

Painless palpable soft tissue abnormalities over joints are commonly encountered in clinical practice. The differential diagnosis can be difficult solely on clinical grounds as benign ganglion cysts that present in areas other than the wrist and the ankle or often misdiagnosed as solid tumors and solid tumors that appear over the wrist and ankle are often misdiagnosed as benign ganglion cysts. Such misdiagnosis can lead to disastrous consequences if a malignant solid tumor is erroneously diagnosed as a benign ganglion cyst (Fig. 70.1). Ultrasound imaging of painless palpable soft tissue masses provides the clinician with immediate help with the solid tumor versus cystic mass differential diagnosis, and its increasing clinical use represents a great advance in the treatment of these sometimes confusing soft tissue abnormalities (Fig. 70.2). Ultrasound also allows the differentiation of simple versus complex multiloculated ganglion cysts that may require more involved treatment (Fig. 70.3). Ultrasound guidance also allows identification of adjacent structures that may be traumatized during injections, drainage, or surgical treatment of otherwise benign ganglion cysts (Fig. 70.4).

Ganglion cysts are thought to be the result of a mechanical pressure phenomenon that results in herniation of synovial-containing tissues from joint capsules, tendon sheaths, and other connective tissue structures such as the triangular fibrocartilage complex. As this ectopic connective tissue becomes chronically inflamed, its synovial components may begin producing increased amounts of synovial fluid, which can pool in cyst-like cavities overlying the tendons and joint space (Fig. 70.5). A one-way valve phenomenon may cause these cyst-like cavities to expand because the fluid cannot flow freely back into the synovial cavity. These cyst-like cavities can develop as simple thin-walled cysts or can become complex multiloculated structures that can be difficult to treat (see Figs. 70.2 and 70.3). Ganglion cysts can form anywhere where these structures exist with the dorsum of the wrist as the most common site of the development of ganglion cysts. Ganglion cysts may also occur on the volar aspect of the wrist.

Ganglion cysts tend to be painless soft tissue swellings, but extreme flexion and extension of the wrist can cause pain secondary to compression of adjacent structures (Fig. 70.6). Rest of the affected part and the application of local heat may provide some relief. If pain occurs, it tends to be constant and is characterized as aching and dull. It is often the unsightly nature of the ganglion cyst, rather than the pain, that causes the patient to seek medical attention. The ganglion is smooth to palpation and transilluminates with a penlight in contradistinction to solid tumors, which do not transilluminate. Palpation of the ganglion may increase the pain.

Plain radiographs are indicated in all patients who present with wrist and hand pain. Based on the patient's clinical presentation, additional testing may be indicated, including complete blood cell count, sedimentation rate, and antinuclear antibody testing. Magnetic resonance imaging or ultrasound imaging of the wrist and hand is indicated to confirm that the palpable soft tissue mass is in fact a ganglion cyst and not a solid tumor that may be malignant (Fig. 70.7).

## CLINICALLY RELEVANT ANATOMY

Ganglion cysts can occur almost anywhere in the body but most commonly develop on the dorsum of the wrist in the area overlying the extensor tendons or the various joint space. Statistically, there is a predilection for ganglion cyst development over the dorsal scapholunate interval (Fig. 70.8).

## ULTRASOUND-GUIDED TECHNIQUE

The benefits, risks, and alternative treatments are explained to the patient, and informed consent is obtained. The patient is then placed in the sitting position with the elbow flexed to about 100 degrees and the forearm resting comfortably palm down on a padded bedside table with the fingers slightly extended, which will relax the extensor tendons (Fig. 70.9). With the patient in the above position, the dorsal ganglion of the wrist is identified, a high-frequency linear ultrasound transducer is placed in a longitudinal position over the cyst, and an ultrasound survey scan is taken. The ganglion cyst will appear most commonly as a thin-walled anechoic cystic structure, although hypoechoic and hyperechoic presentations are not that rare, especially in more complex multiloculated cysts (see Figs. 70.2 and 70.3). Often posterior acoustic enhancement is seen (see Fig. 70.4). In general, the larger the

# CHAPTER 70 ULTRASOUND-GUIDED INJECTION TECHNIQUE FOR GANGLIA CYSTS OF THE WRIST AND HAND

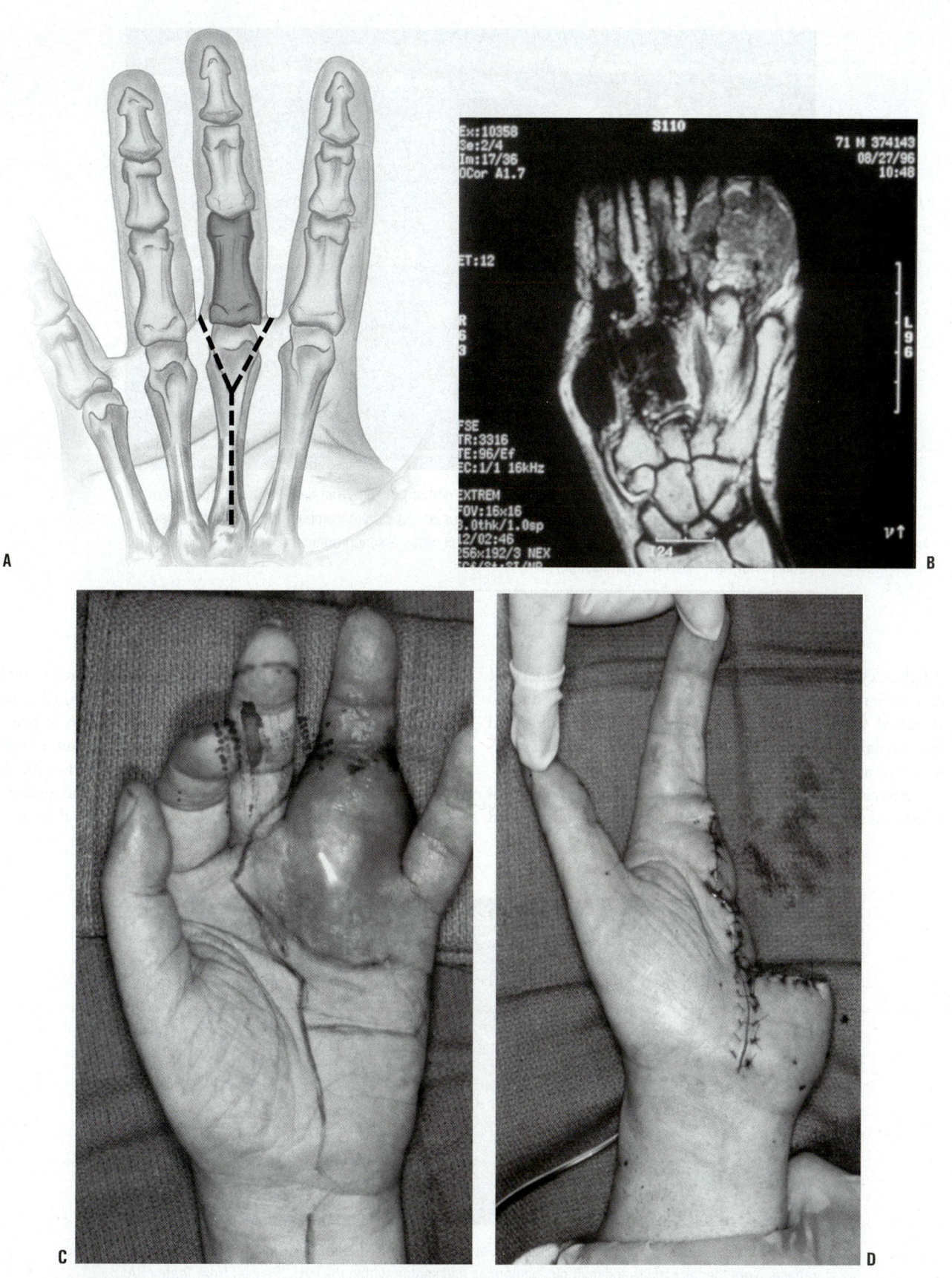

**FIGURE 70.1.** Malignant proximal phalanx lesions usually require single **(A)** or multiple ray amputation **(B–D)** as in this case of osteogenic sarcoma. (Reused from Berger RA, Weiss APC. *Hand Surgery*. Philadelphia, PA: Lippincott Williams & Wilkins; 2004, with permission.)

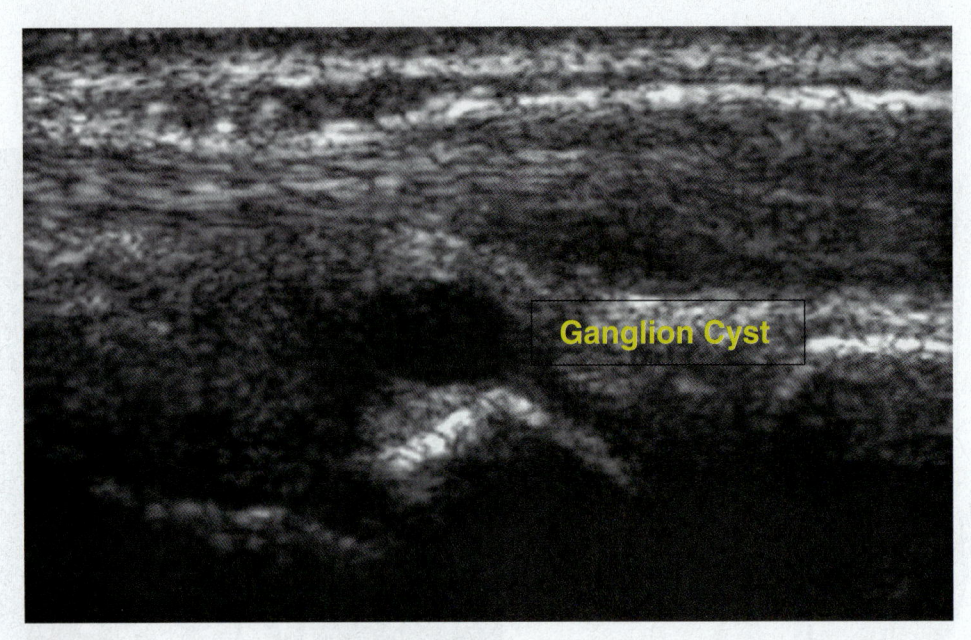

**FIGURE 70.2.** Simple anechoic ganglion cyst of the dorsum of the wrist seen on a longitudinal ultrasound image at the scapholunate interval. Note posterior acoustic enhancement. (Reused from Teefey SA, Dahiya N, Middleton WD, et al. Ganglia of the hand and wrist: a sonographic analysis. *Am J Roentgenol* 2008;191(3):716–720, with permission.)

ganglion cyst, the more likely it is that it will appear anechoic and present with posterior acoustic enhancement due to increased sound transmission through the large fluid-filled cyst. Ganglion cysts are usually noncompressible by the ultrasound transducer.

After the ganglion cyst and adjacent structures are identified, the skin overlying the area beneath the ultrasound transducer is then prepped with antiseptic solution. A sterile 10-mL syringe containing is attached to a 1½-inch, 22-gauge needle using strict aseptic technique. The needle is placed through the skin just above the transverse ultrasound transducer and is advanced using an in-plane approach with the needle trajectory adjusted under real-time ultrasound guidance so that the needle tip ultimately rests within the fluid-filled

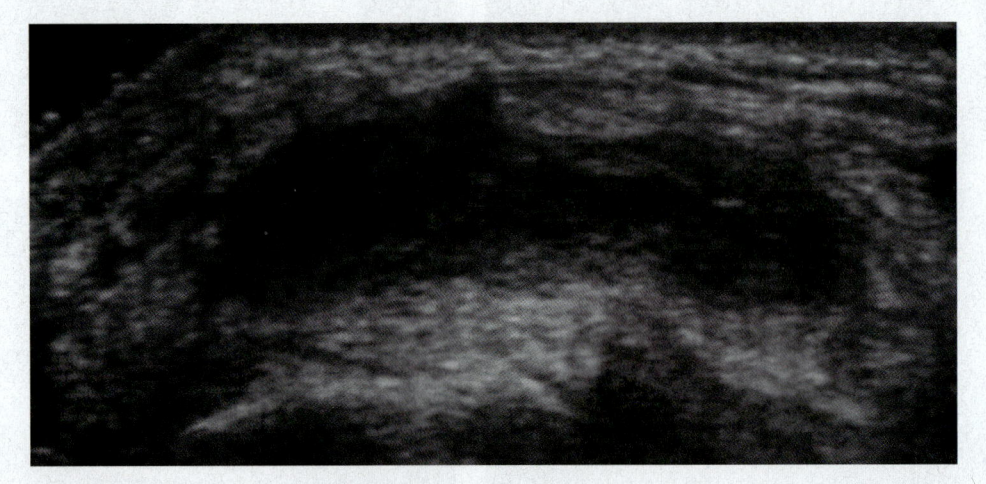

**FIGURE 70.3.** Complex ganglion cyst of the dorsum of the wrist seen on a longitudinal ultrasound image. Note the thick walls and multiple loculations and septae within the cyst. (Reused from Teefey SA, Dahiya N, Middleton WD, et al. Ganglia of the hand and wrist: a sonographic analysis. *Am J Roentgenol* 2008;191(3):716–720, with permission.)

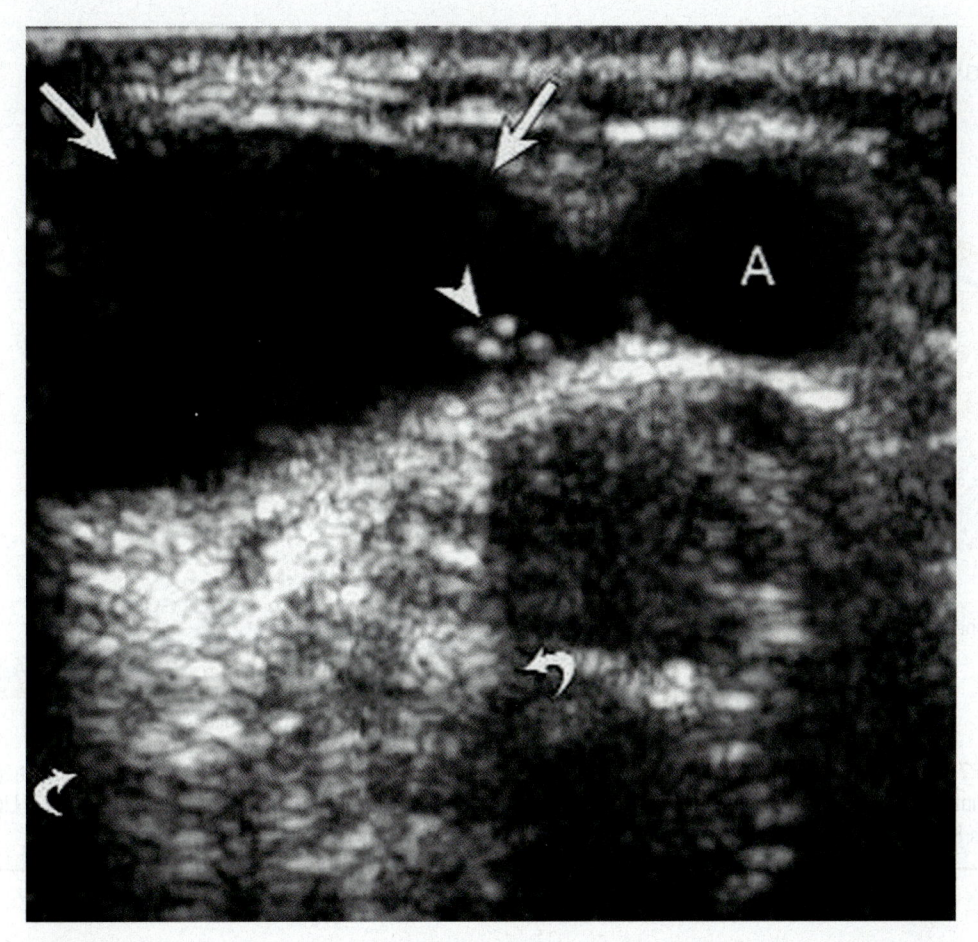

**FIGURE 70.4.** Large ganglion cyst (*arrows*) impinging on the radial artery (*A*). Note the posterior acoustic enhancement (*curved arrows*) and internal hyperechoic structures consistent with mucin (*arrowhead*). (Reused from Wang G, Jacobson JA, Feng FY, et al. Sonography of wrist ganglion cysts. Variable and noncystic appearances. *J Ultrasound Med* 2007;26:1323–1328, with permission.)

cyst. When the tip of needle is thought to be in satisfactory position, careful aspiration of the cyst is carried out. If loculations are present, the needle tip is repositioned under real-time ultrasound guidance, and the process is repeated. After aspiration of the ganglion cyst is completed, 1.0 mL of 0.25% preservative-free bupivacaine and 40 mg of methylprednisolone is injected into the residual cyst cavity under real-time ultrasound guidance. There should be minimal resistance to injection, and no paresthesias should be elicited. Some clinicians recommend placement of a pressure dressing over the site of the ganglion cyst to discourage refilling of the cyst with synovial fluid.

## COMPLICATIONS

The possibility of trauma to nerves and arteries that lie adjacent to the ganglion cyst of the flexor carpi remains an ever-present possibility, although the risk of this is decreased if care is taken to place the needle and perform the injection under real-time ultrasound visualization. It should be remembered that tendons that are associated with the ganglion cyst that are highly inflamed or previously damaged by compression and irritation from the ganglion cyst are subject to rupture if substances are injected directly into the tendon. This complication can be greatly decreased if the clinician uses gentle technique and stops injecting immediately if significant resistance to injection is encountered. Approximately 25% of patients complain of a transient increase in pain after this injection technique; the patient should be warned of this. Infection, although uncommon, can occur.

## CLINICAL PEARLS

Wrist and hand pathology may coexist with ganglion cyst and may contribute to the patient's pain symptomatology. Ultrasound imaging of the ganglion cyst and adjacent areas will help with the diagnosis of this occult wrist and hand pathology. Universal precautions should always be observed to protect the

**482** SECTION V　WRIST AND HAND

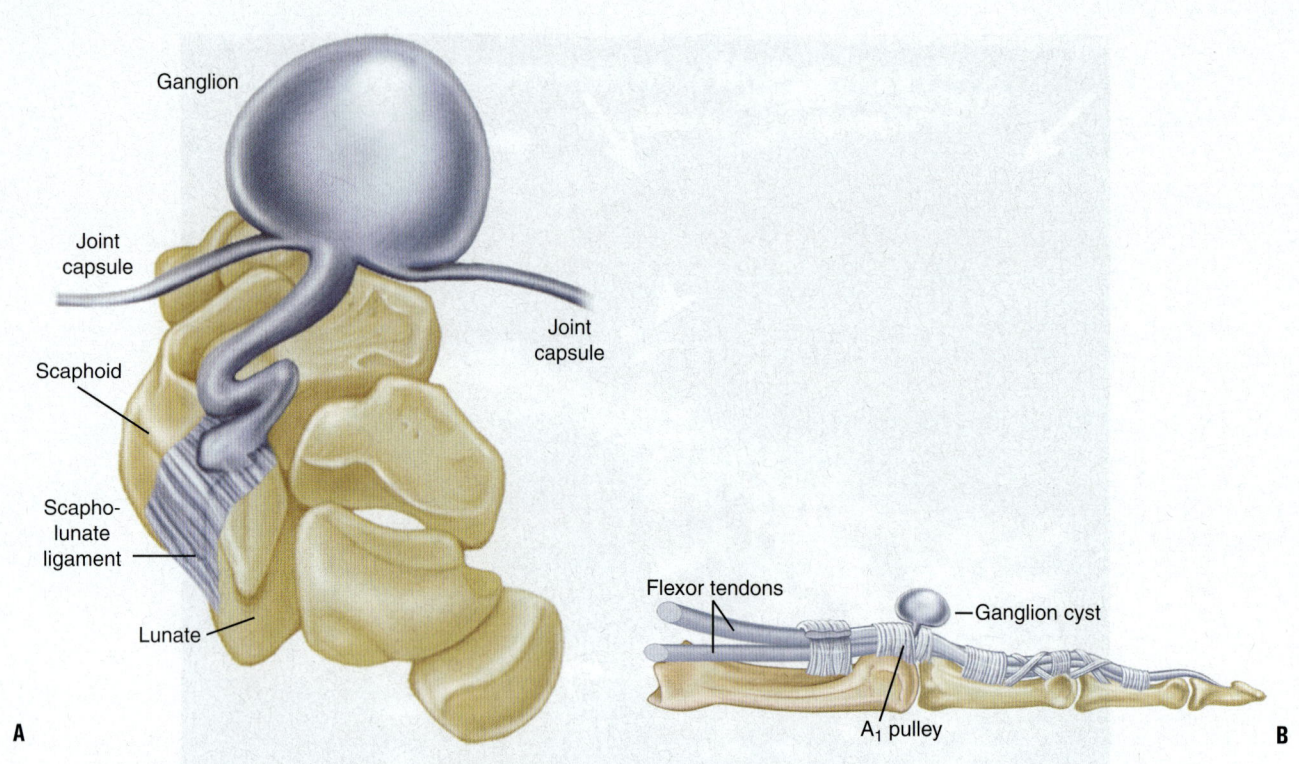

**FIGURE 70.5.** **A:** Ganglion cyst arising from dorsal scapholunate joint. **B:** Ganglion cyst arising from flexor sheath. (Reused from: Hunt TR, Flynn JM, Wiesel SW. *Operative Techniques in Hand, Wrist, and Forearm Surgery.* Philadelphia, PA: Lippincott Williams & Wilkins; 2011, with permission.)

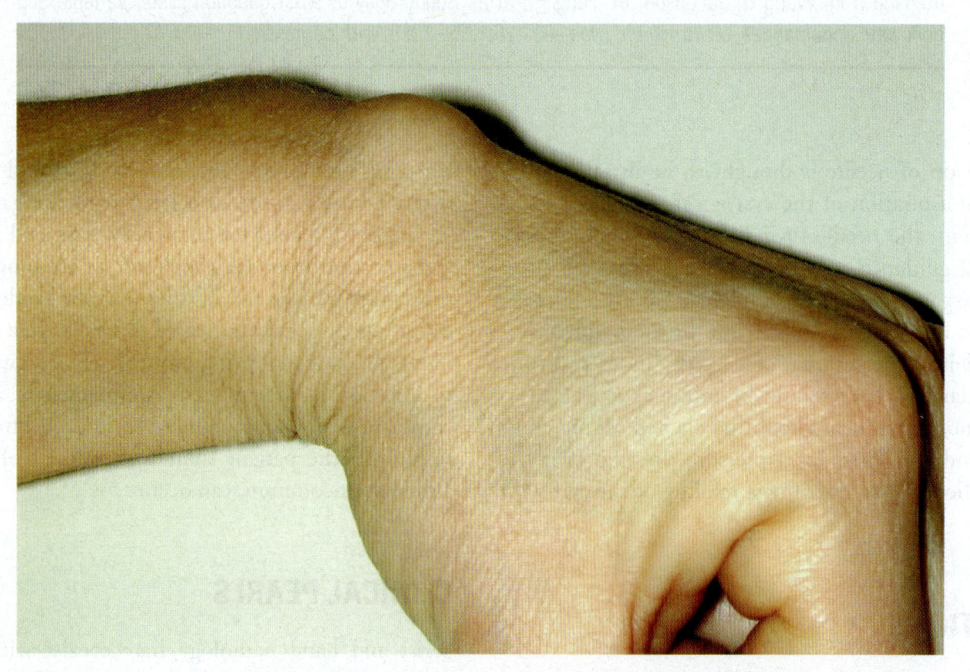

**FIGURE 70.6.** Photo of classic dorsal ganglion cyst in a 20-year-old female arising from the scapholunate interval. (Reused from Lotke PA, Abboud JA, Ende J. *Lippincott's Primary Care: Orthopaedics.* Philadelphia, PA: Lippincott Williams & Wilkins; 2008, with permission.)

CHAPTER 70　ULTRASOUND-GUIDED INJECTION TECHNIQUE FOR GANGLIA CYSTS OF THE WRIST AND HAND　483

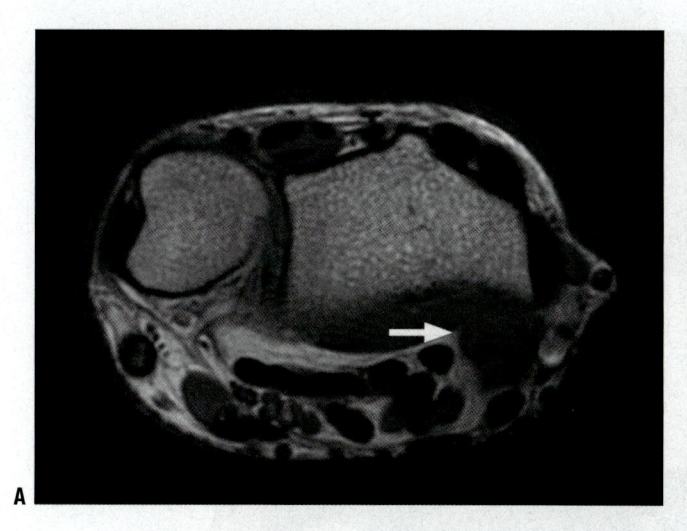

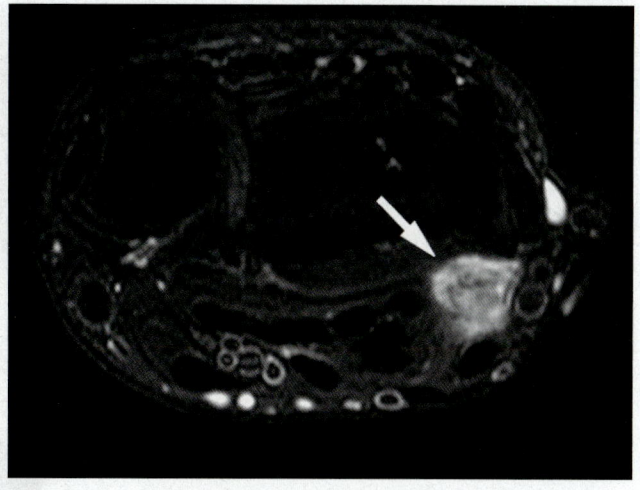

**FIGURE 70.7.** Synovial sarcoma. Axial T1-weighted **(A)** and fat-suppressed T2-weighted images **(B)** show an ill-defined nonspecific mass on the T1 image and heterogeneously bright mass on the T2 image (*arrow*). (Reused from Chung CB, Steinbach LS. *MRI of the Upper Extremity: Shoulder, Elbow, Wrist, and Hand*. Philadelphia, PA: Lippincott Williams & Wilkins; 2010, with permission.)

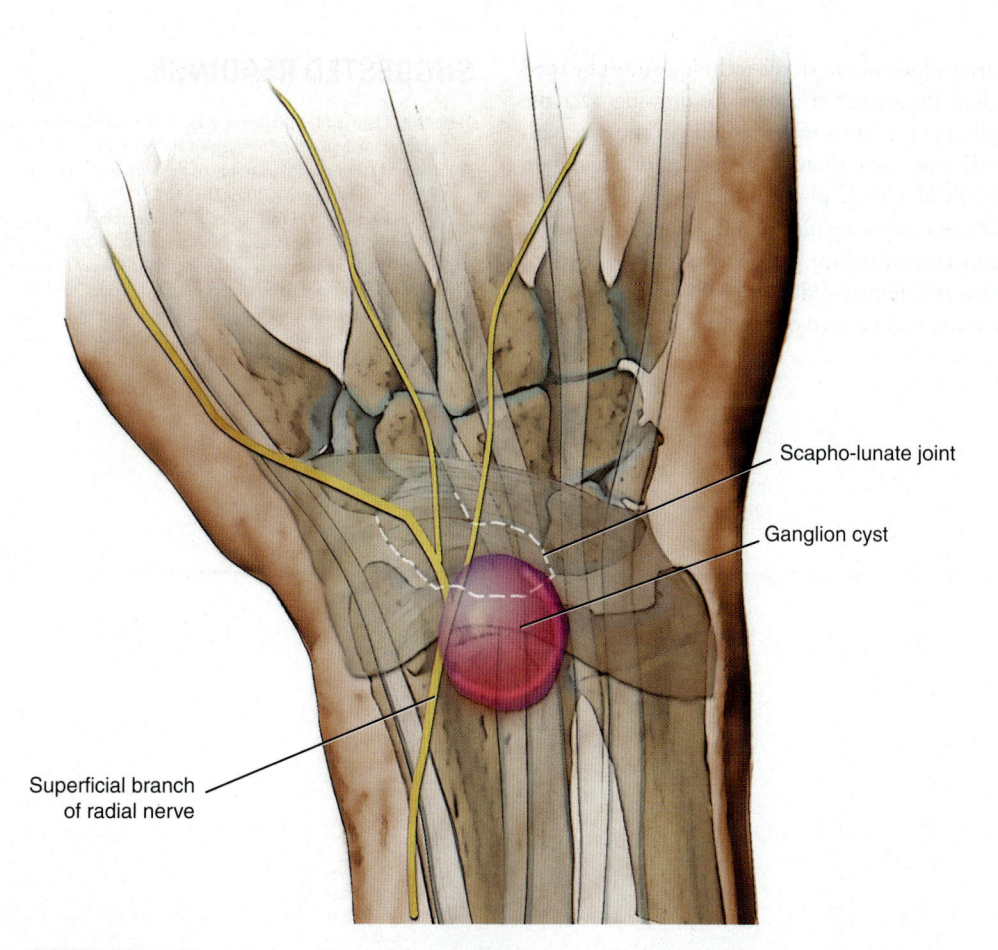

**FIGURE 70.8.** There is a predilection for ganglion cyst development over the dorsal scapholunate interval.

**FIGURE 70.9.** To perform ultrasound-guided injection for ganglion cyst injection, the patient is then placed in the sitting position with the elbow flexed to about 100 degrees and the forearm resting comfortably palm down on a padded bedside table with the fingers slightly extended, which will relax the extensor tendons.

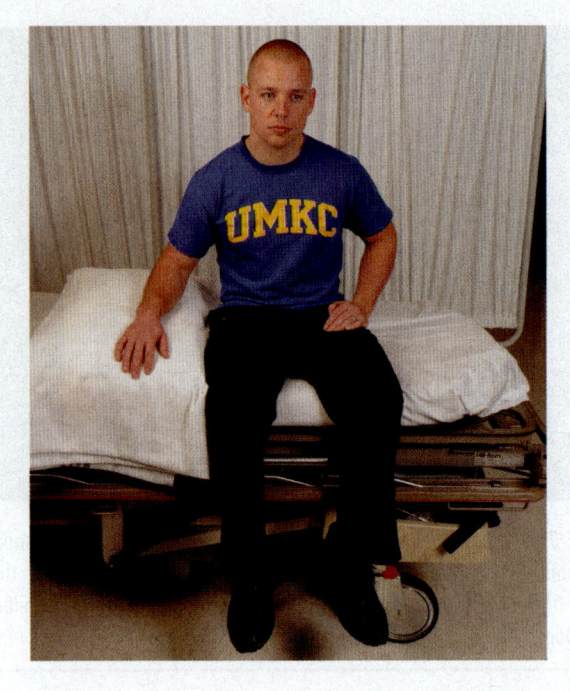

operator, and strict adherence to sterile technique must be used to avoid infection. Placement of a pressure dressing over the site of the ganglion cyst to discourage refilling of the cyst with synovial fluid following aspiration and injection of a ganglion cyst may be beneficial. Gentle physical therapy and local heat should be introduced following ultrasound-guided injection of a dorsal ganglion cyst to reduce pain and improve function. Simple analgesics and nonsteroidal anti-inflammatory agents or COX-2 inhibitors may be used concurrently with this injection technique.

## SUGGESTED READINGS

Teefey SA, Dahiya N, Middleton WD, et al. Ganglia of the hand and wrist: a sonographic analysis. *Am J Roentgenol* 2008;191(3):716–720.

Waldman SD. Functional anatomy of the wrist joint. In: *Pain Review*. Philadelphia, PA: Saunders Elsevier; 2009:101–102.

Wang G, Jacobson JA, Feng FY, et al. Sonography of wrist ganglion cysts: variable and noncystic appearances. *J Ultrasound Med* 2007;26(10):1323–1328.

Waldman SD. Ganglion cysts of the wrist. In: *Atlas of Common Pain Syndromes*. 3rd ed. Philadelphia, PA: Saunders Elsevier; 2013:170–174.

Waldman SD. Injection technique for ganglion cyst. In: *Atlas of Pain Management Injection Techniques*. 3rd ed. Philadelphia, PA: Saunders Elsevier; 2013:244–246.

# Ultrasound-Guided Injection Technique for de Quervain's Tenosynovitis

## CLINICAL PERSPECTIVES

De Quervain tenosynovitis is a common cause of radial-sided wrist pain encountered in clinical practice. This painful condition is named for Swiss surgeon Fritz de Quervain who first described this constellation of symptoms and their cause in 1895. As a result of repetitive high torque twisting motions of the wrist and occasionally as a result of direct trauma to the tendons of the abductor pollicis longus and extensor pollicis brevis at the level of the radial styloid process, de Quervain tenosynovitis can cause significant pain and functional disability if not promptly treated. On rare occasions, de Quervain tenosynovitis can develop without antecedent trauma, especially in the parturient, and this setting is often referred to as mommy's thumb or wrist. The symptoms of de Quervain tenosynovitis are the result of inflammation and edema of the tendons and tendon sheath of the abductor pollicis longus and extensor pollicis brevis muscles at the level of the radial styloid process (Fig. 71.1). If untreated, a thickening of the tendons and tendon sheath may occur with a constrictive tenosynovitis resulting (Fig. 71.2). In some patients, a triggering phenomenon of the thumb may occur as a result of the thickened tendon locking or catching in the constricted tendon sheath. Arthritis and gout of the first metacarpal joint also may coexist with and exacerbate the pain and disability of de Quervain tenosynovitis.

Activities associated with the development of de Quervain tenosynovitis include repetitive hand shaking, scooping ice cream, or using a screwdriver. The pain of de Quervain tenosynovitis is sharp and constant and is exacerbated by any activities requiring active pinching of the thumb or ulnar deviation of the wrist. The pain is localized to the area over the radial styloid process and is associated with increasing functional disability if the inflammatory process remains untreated.

On physical examination, there is tenderness and swelling over the tendons and tendon sheaths along the distal radius, with point tenderness over the radial styloid. A creaking tendon sign may be noted with flexion and extension of the thumb, and triggering of the thumb may occur. Patients with de Quervain tenosynovitis demonstrate a positive Finkelstein test (Fig. 71.3). The Finkelstein test is performed by stabilizing the patient's forearm, having the patient fully flex his or her thumb into the palm, and then actively forcing the wrist toward the ulna. Sudden severe pain is highly suggestive of de Quervain tenosynovitis.

Plain radiographs of the wrist are indicated in all patients suspected of suffering from de Quervain tenosynovitis to rule out occult bony pathology and to identify calcific tendonitis. Based on the patient's clinical presentation, additional testing may be indicated, including complete blood cell count, uric acid, sedimentation rate, and antinuclear antibody testing. Magnetic resonance imaging and ultrasound imaging of the wrist are indicated to assess the status of the abductor pollicis longus and extensor pollicis brevis tendons and tendon sheath

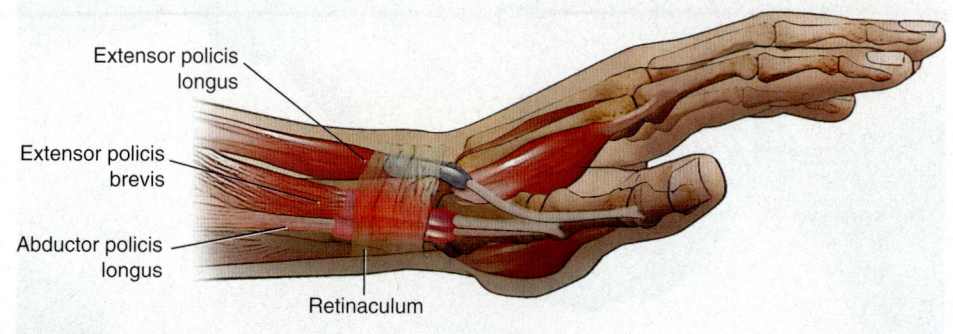

**FIGURE 71.1.** de Quervain tenosynovitis, which is also known as mommy's thumb or wrist, is caused by inflammation of the tendons and tendon sheath of the abductor pollicis longus and extensor pollicis brevis muscles.

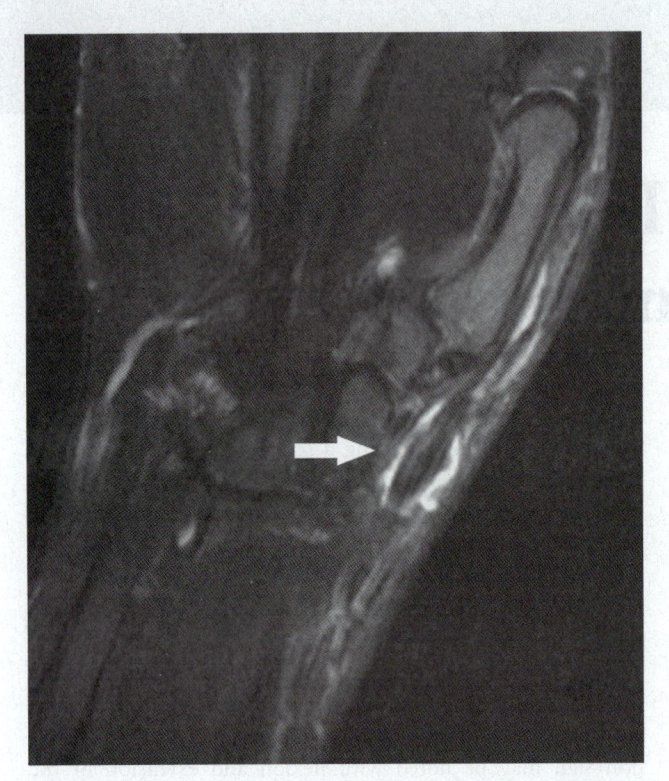

**FIGURE 71.2.** de Quervain disease. Coronal fat-suppressed T2-weighted image shows intermediate to high signal intensity within, and enlargement of, the first-compartment tendons (*arrow*) compatible with tendinosis. Fluid surrounding the tendon is compatible with tenosynovitis. (Reused from Chung CB, Steinbach LS. *MRI of the Upper Extremity*. Philadelphia, PA: Lippincott Williams & Wilkins; 2009:587, with permission.)

as well as to identify other occult pathology including arthritis and gout involving the first metacarpal joint (Fig. 71.4).

## CLINICALLY RELEVANT ANATOMY

The key landmarks when performing ultrasound-guided injection for de Quervain tenosynovitis are the radial styloid process and the abductor pollicis longus and extensor pollicis brevis tendons and tendon sheath (Fig. 71.5). The function of the abductor pollicis longus and extensor pollicis brevis muscles is radial abduction of the thumb. The radial artery and the superficial branch of the radial nerve are in proximity to the injection site for de Quervain tenosynovitis and may be traumatized if the needle is placed too medially.

## ULTRASOUND-GUIDED TECHNIQUE

The benefits, risks, and alternative treatments are explained to the patient, and informed consent is obtained. The patient is then placed in the sitting position with the elbow flexed to about 100 degrees and the forearm resting comfortably with the hand in neutral position and the little finger against a padded bedside table (Fig. 71.6). With the patient in the above position, the radial styloid process and the abductor pollicis longus and extensor pollicis brevis tendons at that level are identified by palpation. Identification of the tendons is facilitated by having the patient radial deviate the wrist against examiner resistance (Fig. 71.7). At the level of the radial styloid, a high-frequency linear ultrasound transducer is placed in a transverse position

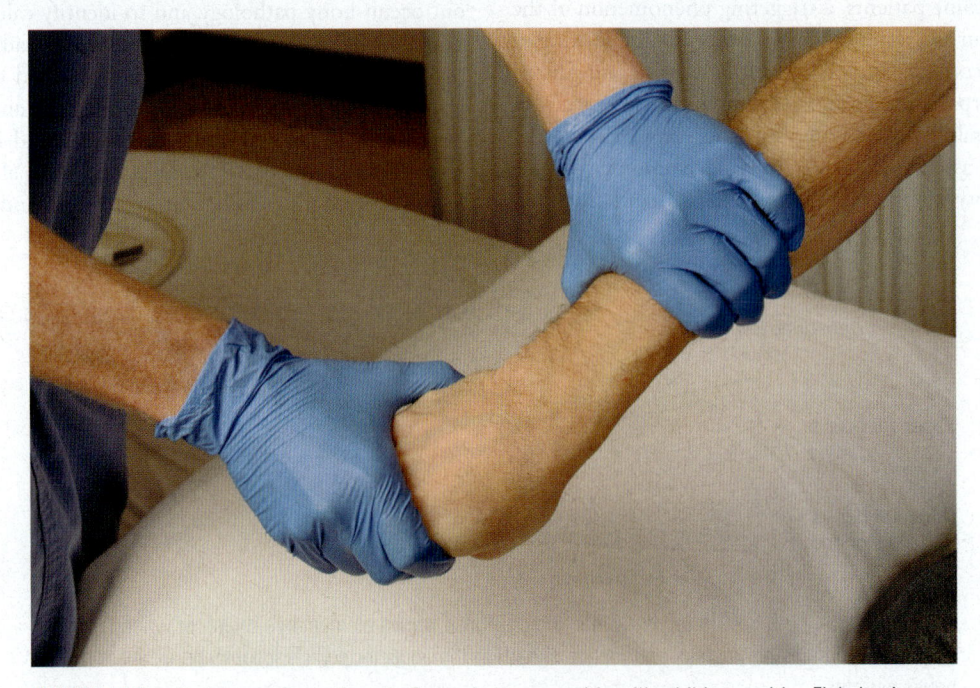

**FIGURE 71.3.** Patients suffering from de Quervain tenosynovitis will exhibit a positive Finkelstein test.

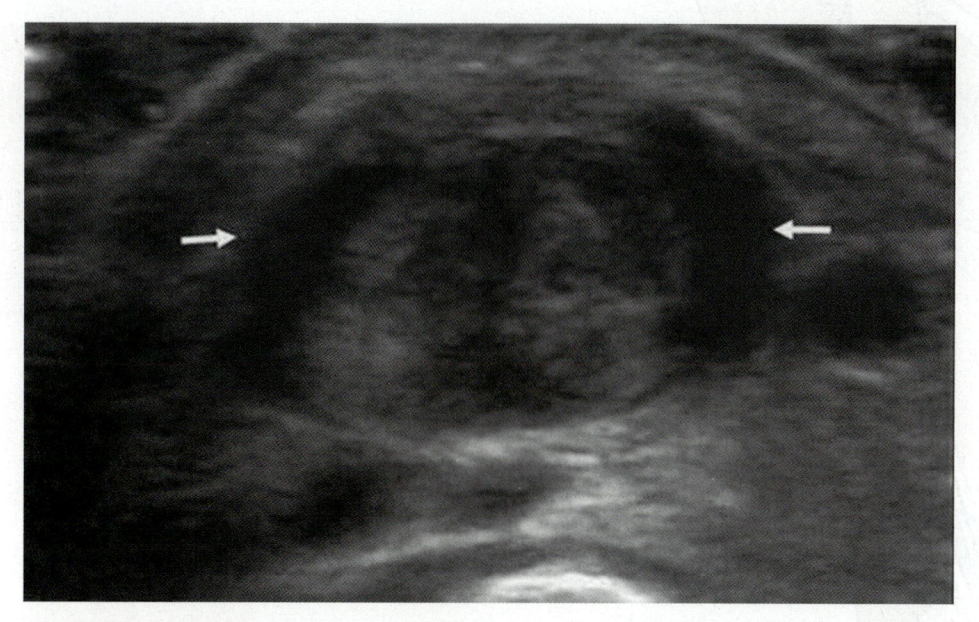

**FIGURE 71.4.** Transverse ultrasound image of the first dorsal compartment tendons (abductor pollicis longus and extensor pollicis brevis) showing tenosynovitis (*arrows*). (Reused from Jeyapalan K, Choudhary S. Ultrasound-guided injection of triamcinolone and bupivacaine in the management of De Quervain's disease. *Skeletal Radiol* 2009;38(11):1099–1103, with permission.)

over the abductor pollicis longus and extensor pollicis brevis tendons, and an ultrasound survey scan is taken (Figs. 71.8 and 71.9). Color Doppler may aid in identification of the radial artery and help separate it with the superficial radial nerve, which lies just radial to the radial artery (Fig. 71.10). The tendons will appear as the hyperechoic "hole" in the hypoechoic tendon sheath. In most patients, the tendons will be seen to pass through a single sheath (see Fig. 71.4). However, in a small number of patients, the tendon sheath will appear to travel through separate subcompartments divided by a subcompartmental septum (Fig. 71.11). An effusion surrounding the affected tendons can often be identified with ultrasound imaging (Fig. 71.12). When the tendon sheath is identified, the skin overlying the area beneath the ultrasound transducer is then prepped with antiseptic solution. A sterile syringe containing 1.0 mL of 0.25% preservative-free bupivacaine and 40 mg of methylprednisolone is attached to a 1½-inch, 22-gauge needle using strict aseptic technique. The needle is placed through the skin just above the superior border of the transducer and is then advanced using an out-of-plane approach with the needle trajectory adjusted under real-time ultrasound guidance so that the needle tip ultimately rests within the tendon sheath but outside the substance of the tendons themselves (Figs. 71.13 and 71.14). When the tip of needle is thought to be in satisfactory position, after careful aspiration, a small amount of local anesthetic and steroid is injected under real-time ultrasound guidance to confirm that the needle tip is in the proper position. After proper needle tip placement is confirmed, the remainder of the contents of the syringe are slowly injected. There should be minimal resistance to injection. If subcompartments are identified within the tendon sheath, repositioning of the needle to inject both compartments may be required.

## COMPLICATIONS

The possibility of trauma to the abductor pollicis longus and extensor pollicis brevis tendons from this injection technique itself remains an ever-present possibility, although the risk of this is decreased if care is taken to place the needle outside the tendon and the injection is performed under real-time ultrasound visualization. Tendons that are highly inflamed or previously damaged are subject to rupture if substances are injected directly into the tendon. This complication can be greatly decreased if the clinician uses gentle technique and stops injecting immediately if significant resistance to injection is encountered. Approximately 25% of patients complain of a transient increase in pain after this injection technique; the patient should be warned of this. Infection, although uncommon, can occur. Ecchymosis and hematoma formation following this procedure may also occur. These complications can be decreased if manual pressure is applied to the area of the block immediately after injection. Application of cold packs for 20-minute periods after the block will also decrease the amount of postprocedure pain and bleeding the patient may experience.

## CLINICAL PEARLS

Ultrasound-guided injection for de Quervain tenosynovitis is a straightforward and relatively safe technique if attention is paid to the clinically relevant anatomy. Cheiralgia paresthetica can mimic de Quervain tenosynovitis as both syndromes cause pain when the patient ulnar deviates the wrist. However, de Quervain tenosynovitis pain is more common with activity, while the pain and numbness associated with cheiralgia

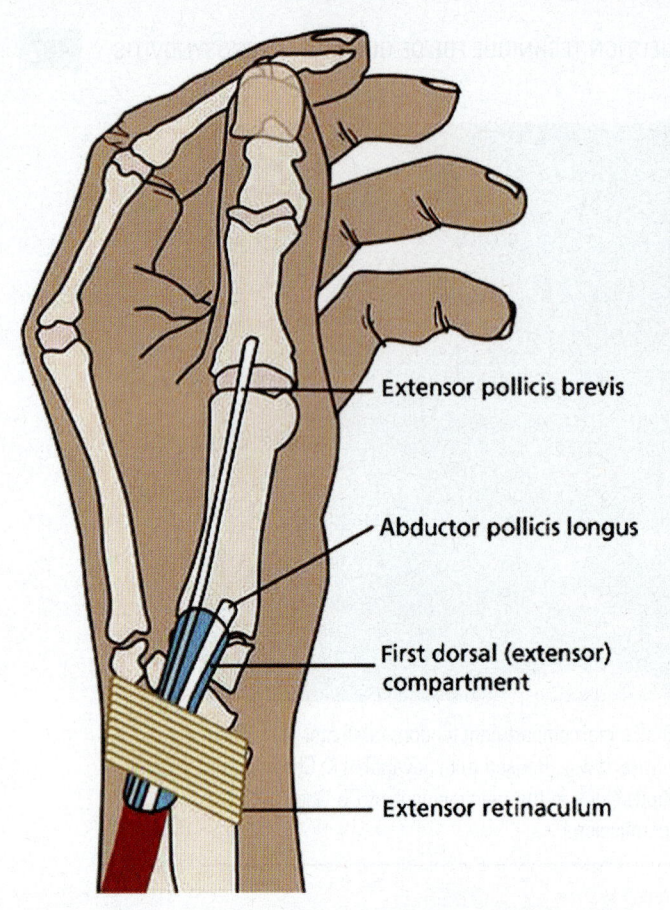

**FIGURE 71.5.** Anatomy of the first extensor compartment illustrating the relationship between the extensor pollicis brevis and abductor pollicis longus tendons as they pass beneath the extensor retinaculum within their tendon sheath at the level of the radial styloid. (Reused from Jeyapalan K, Choudhary S. Ultrasound-guided injection of triamcinolone and bupivacaine in the management of De Quervain's disease. *Skeletal Radiol* 2009;38(11):1099–1103, with permission.)

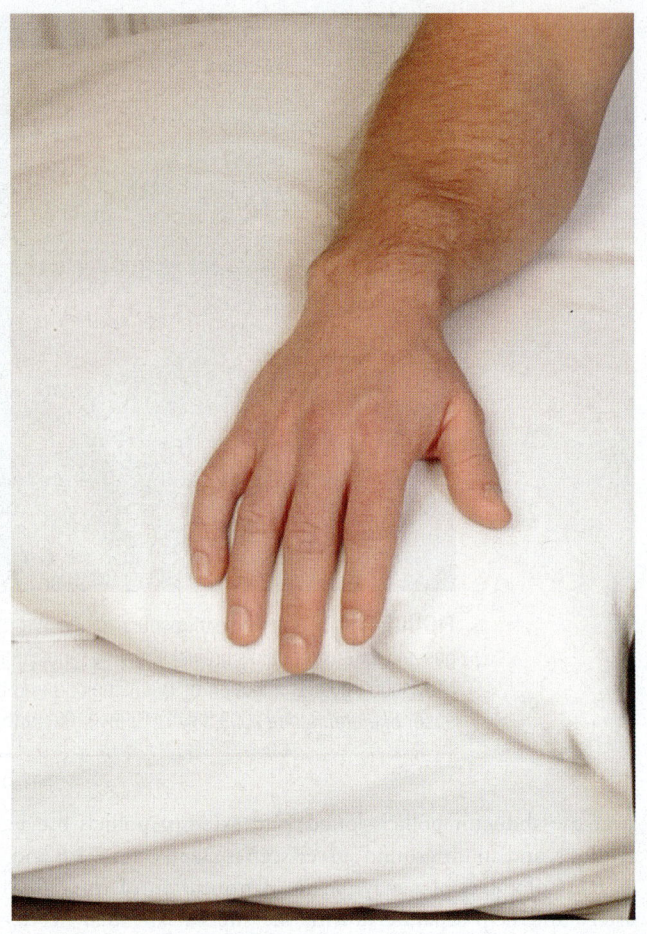

**FIGURE 71.6.** Proper patient position for ultrasound-guided injection for de Quervain tenosynovitis.

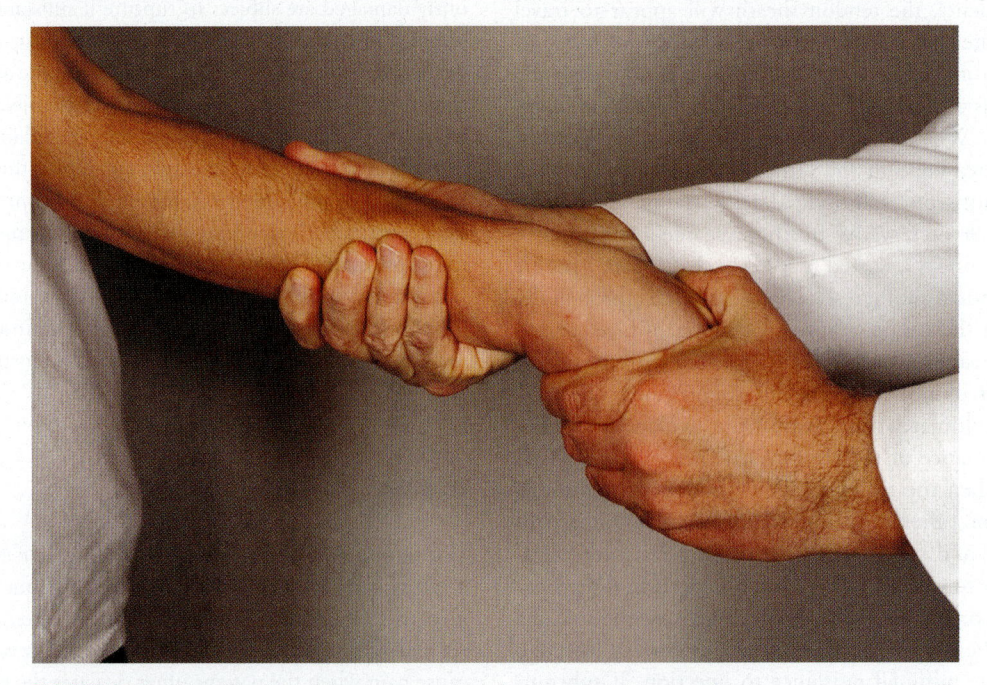

**FIGURE 71.7.** Identification of the extensor pollicis brevis and abductor pollicis longus tendons is facilitated by having the patient radial deviate the wrist against examiner resistance.

CHAPTER 71   ULTRASOUND-GUIDED INJECTION TECHNIQUE FOR DE QUERVAIN'S TENOSYNOVITIS

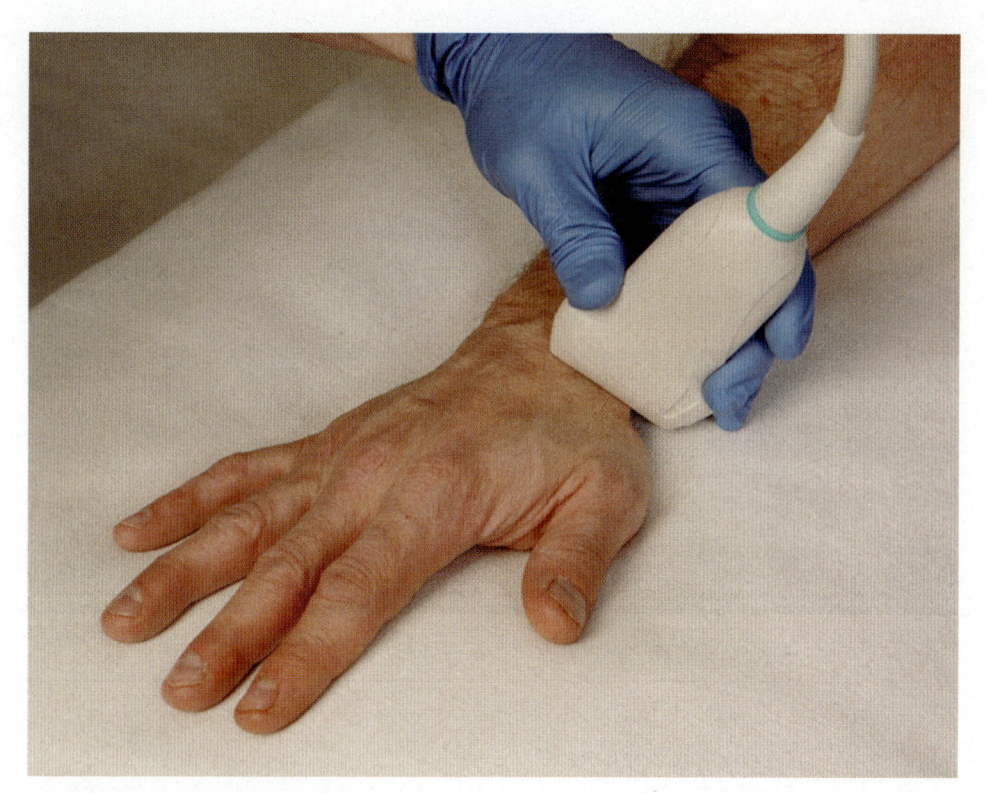

**FIGURE 71.8.** Proper transverse position for the linear high-frequency ultrasound transducer to perform ultrasound-guided de Quervain tenosynovitis.

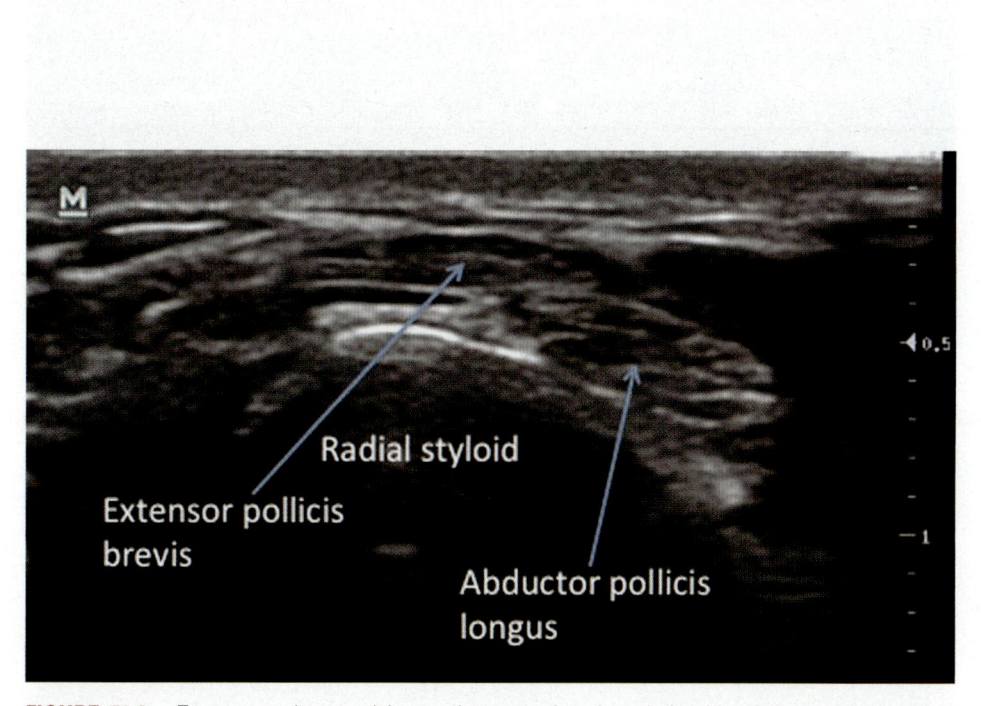

**FIGURE 71.9.** Transverse ultrasound image demonstrating the relationship of the extensor pollicis brevis and abductor pollicis longus tendons within their tendon sheath at the level of the radial styloid.

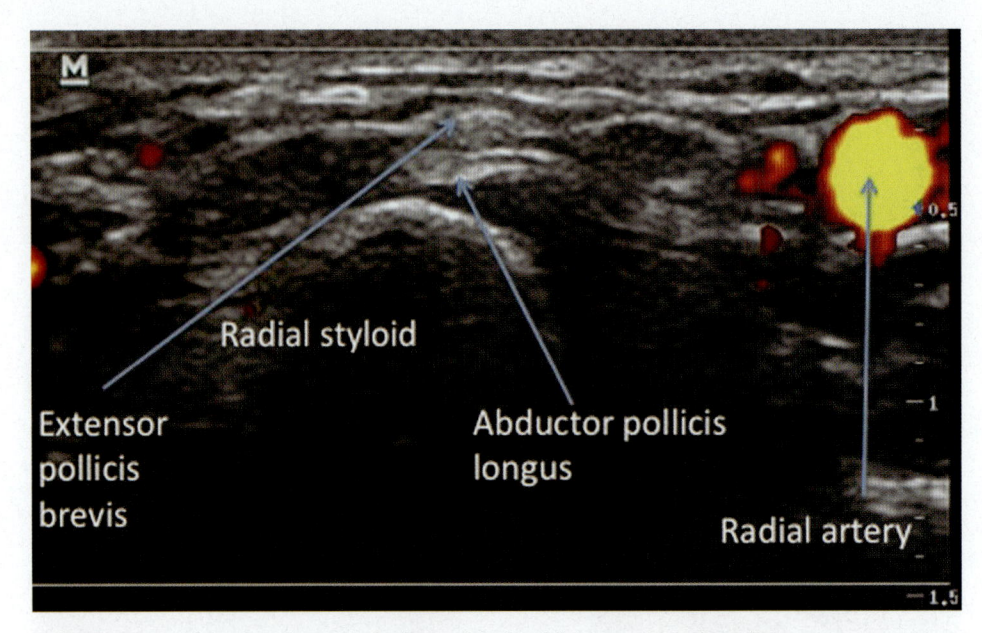

**FIGURE 71.10.** Color Doppler can help distinguish the radial artery from the radial nerve.

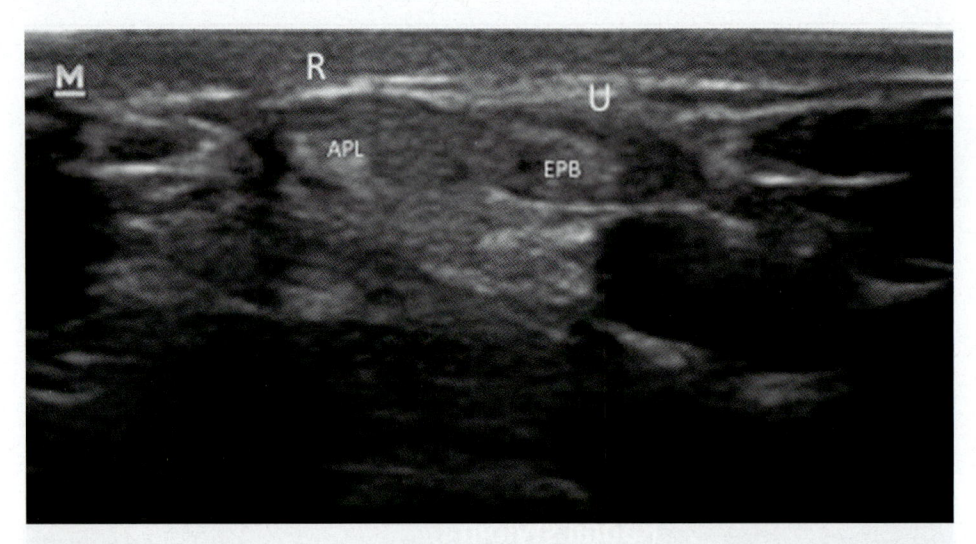

**FIGURE 71.11.** Transverse ultrasound image of the first dorsal compartment shows two subcompartments containing the extensor pollicis brevis and abductor pollicis longus tendons within. (APL, abductor pollicis longus; EPB, extensor pollicis brevis; R, radial; U, ulnar.)

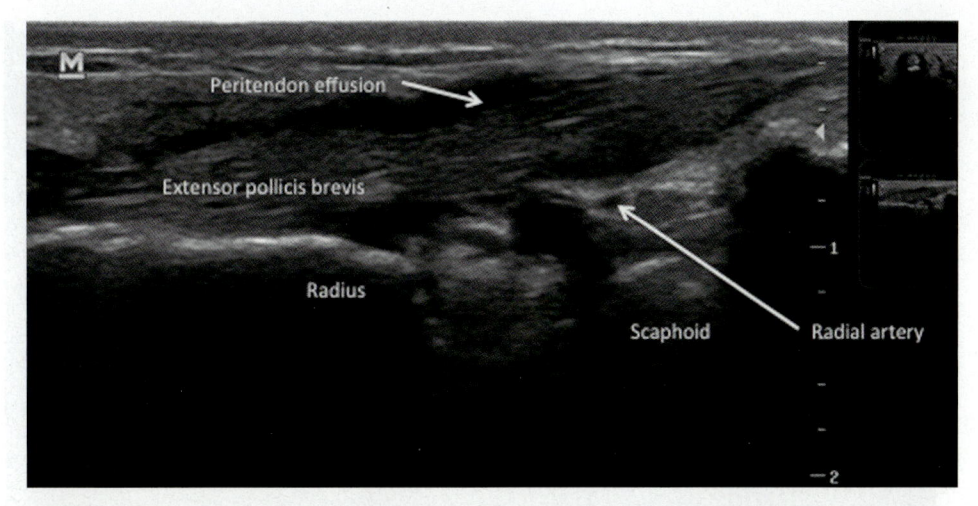

**FIGURE 71.12.** Longitudinal ultrasound view demonstrating effusion around the extensor pollicis brevis tendon.

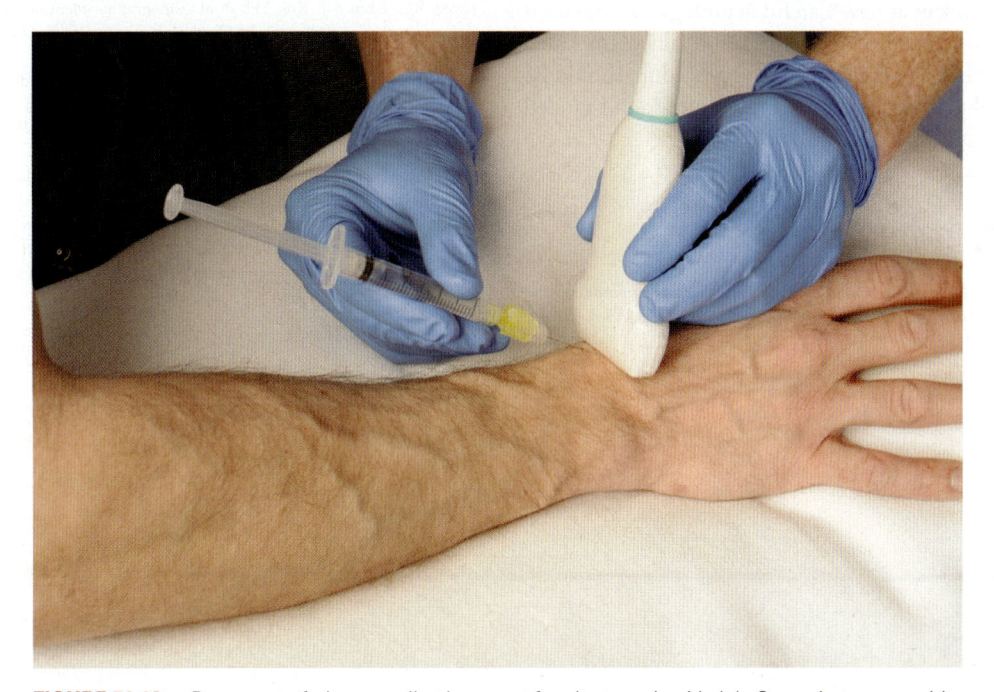

**FIGURE 71.13.** Proper out-of-plane needle placement for ultrasound-guided de Quervain tenosynovitis.

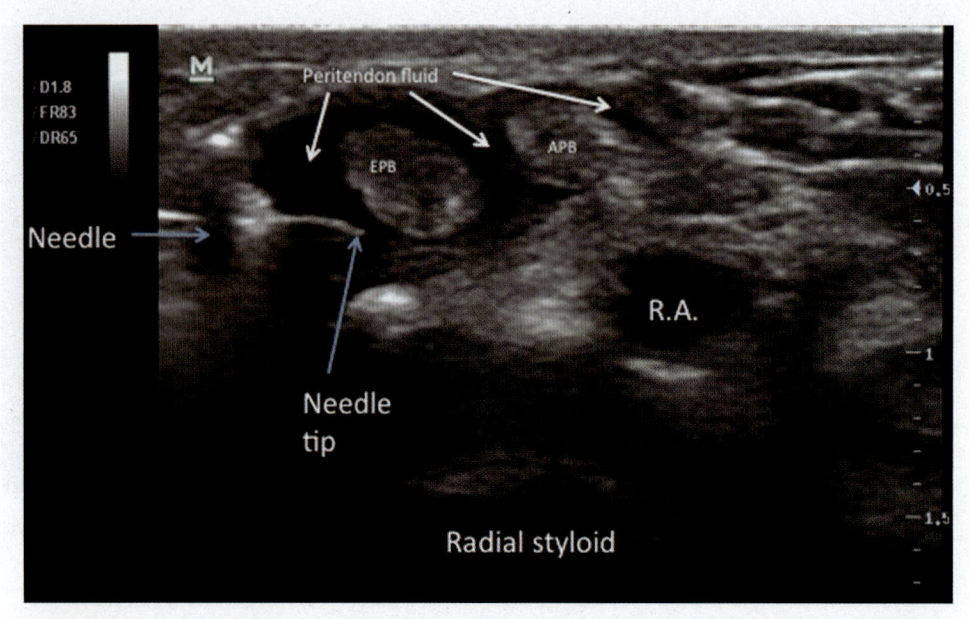

**FIGURE 71.14.** Transverse ultrasound view showing proper needle trajectory. Note peritendinous effusion. (APB, abductor pollicis brevis; EPB, extensor pollicis brevis; R.A., radial artery.)

paresthetica are present at rest. Careful neurologic examination to identify preexisting neurologic deficits especially of the radial nerve that may later be attributed to the procedure should be performed on all patients before beginning ultrasound-guided injection for de Quervain tenosynovitis.

## SUGGESTED READINGS

Jeyapalan K, Choudhary S. Ultrasound-guided injection of triamcinolone and bupivacaine in the management of De Quervain's disease. *Skeletal Radiol* 2009;38(11):1099–1103.

Kwon BC, Choi S-J, Koh SH, et al. Sonographic identification of the intracompartmental septum in de Quervain's disease. *Clin Orthop Relat Res* 2010;468(8):2129–2134.

McDermott JD, Ilyas AM, Nazarian LN, et al. Ultrasound-guided injections for de Quervain's tenosynovitis. *Clin Orthopaed Rel Res* 2012;470(7):1925–31.

Waldman SD. Cheiralgia paresthetica. In: *Atlas of Common Pain Syndromes*. 3rd ed. Philadelphia, PA: Saunders Elsevier; 2012:164–167.

Waldman SD. Cheiralgia paresthetica. In: *Pain Review*. Philadelphia, PA: Saunders Elsevier; 2009:275–276.

Waldman SD. De Quervain's tenosynovitis. In: *Atlas of Pain Management Injection Techniques*. 3rd ed. Philadelphia, PA: Saunders Elsevier; 2012:201–203.

Waldman SD. The radial nerve. In: *Pain Review*. Philadelphia, PA: Saunders Elsevier; 2009:76–77.

# CHAPTER 72

# Ultrasound-Guided Injection Technique for Intersection Syndrome

## CLINICAL PERSPECTIVES

The anatomy of the wrist is among the most complex in the human body. A large number of flexor and extensor tendons pass from the forearm across the wrist to the hand. In order to help delineate the myriad extensor tendons within this anatomic region, anatomists have organized them into six compartments (Table 72.1). It is at the intersection of the first and second extensor compartments, which contain the extensor carpi radialis longus, the extensor carpi radialis brevis, the extensor pollicis brevis, and the abductor pollicis longus tendons and associated muscles, that a painful tenosynovitis known as intersection syndrome can occur (Fig. 72.1). The inflammation responsible for the pain and functional disability associated with intersection syndrome is due to repetitive flexion and extension of the wrist when performing activities such as cross-country skiing, sculling, rowing, and weight lifting. Often confused with other radial-sided wrist pain syndromes including de Quervain tenosynovitis, cheiralgia paresthetica (Wartenberg syndrome), and arthritis of the first metacarpal joint, intersection syndrome tends to occur more dorsally and proximally than these other conditions (Table 72.2).

The pain of intersection syndrome will be exacerbated by flexion or extension of the affected wrist. Palpation at the site of tendon intersection may reveal tenderness, color, and swelling. A positive creaking tendon sign is often present if there is significant inflammation (Fig. 72.2). The examiner may appreciate what has been named "wet leather" crepitus with flexion and extension of the wrist.

Plain radiographs of the wrist are indicated in all patients suspected of suffering from intersection syndrome to rule out occult bony pathology and to identify calcific tendonitis. Based on the patient's clinical presentation, additional testing may be indicated, including complete blood cell count, uric acid, sedimentation rate, and antinuclear antibody testing. Magnetic resonance imaging and ultrasound imaging of the wrist are indicated to assess the status of the extensor carpi radialis longus, the extensor carpi radialis brevis, the extensor pollicis brevis, and the abductor pollicis longus tendons and tendon sheaths as well as to identify other occult pathology including coexistent bursitis, arthritis, and gout involving the first metacarpal joint, cheiralgia paresthetica, and/or de Quervain tenosynovitis (Fig. 72.3).

## CLINICALLY RELEVANT ANATOMY

The key landmarks when performing ultrasound-guided injection for intersection syndrome are Lister tubercle and the intersection of the extensor carpi radialis longus, the extensor carpi radialis brevis, the extensor pollicis brevis, and the abductor pollicis longus tendons and tendon sheaths (Fig. 72.4). Passing obliquely over the extensor carpi radialis brevis and extensor carpi radialis longus tendons of the second compartment, the abductor pollicis longus and extensor pollicis brevis of the first compartment intersect at their musculotendinous junctions. This intersection is just proximal to the extensor retinaculum, which serves to tether down the tendons and may contribute to the evolution of intersection syndrome (see Fig. 72.4).

## ULTRASOUND-GUIDED TECHNIQUE

The benefits, risks, and alternative treatments are explained to the patient, and informed consent is obtained. The patient is then placed in the sitting position with the elbow flexed to about 100 degrees and the forearm resting comfortably with the hand in neutral position palm down against a padded bedside table (Fig. 72.5). With the patient in the above position, the Lister tubercle of the radius is identified by palpation (Fig. 72.6). Identification of the affected tendons is facilitated by having the patient extend the wrist against examiner resistance. At the level of Lister tubercle, a high-frequency linear ultrasound transducer is placed in a transverse position over the intersection of the extensor carpi radialis longus, the extensor carpi radialis brevis, the extensor pollicis brevis, and the abductor pollicis longus tendons (Figs. 72.7 and 72.8). The tendons will appear as the hyperechoic "hole" in the hypoechoic tendon sheath. The ultrasound transducer may be turned into the longitudinal axis to further delineate

### TABLE 72.1 The Extensor Tendon Compartments of the Wrist

**Compartment 1**
Contains the abductor pollicis longus and the extensor pollicis brevis tendons as they pass along the radial border of the anatomic snuff box

**Compartment 2**
Contains the extensor carpi radialis longus and extensor carpi radialis brevis tendons

**Compartment 3**
Contains the extensor pollicis longus tendon, which passes medial to the dorsal tubercle of the radius. The extensor pollicis longus tendon deviates around the tubercle on its path to the base of the distal phalanx of the thumb.

**Compartment 4**
Contains the extensor digitorum and extensor indicis tendons to the hand. Proximally the four tendons of the extensor digitorum join the tendon of the extensor indicis to pass deep to the extensor retinaculum through the tendinous sheath of the extensor digitorum and extensor indicis. Then, on the dorsum of the hand, the tendons spread out as they run toward the fingers.

**Compartment 5**
Contains the extensor digiti minimi tendon posterior to the distal radioulnar joint

**Compartment 6**
Contains the extensor carpi ulnaris tendon, which runs in the groove between the ulnar head and its styloid process

---

the point of intersection (Fig. 72.9). When the point of intersection is identified, the skin overlying the area beneath the ultrasound transducer is then prepped with antiseptic solution. A sterile syringe containing 1.0 mL of 0.25% preservative-free bupivacaine and 40 mg of methylprednisolone is attached to a 1½-inch, 22-gauge needle using strict aseptic technique. The needle is placed through the skin just above the superior border of the transversely placed transducer and is then advanced using an out-of-plane approach with the needle trajectory adjusted under real-time ultrasound

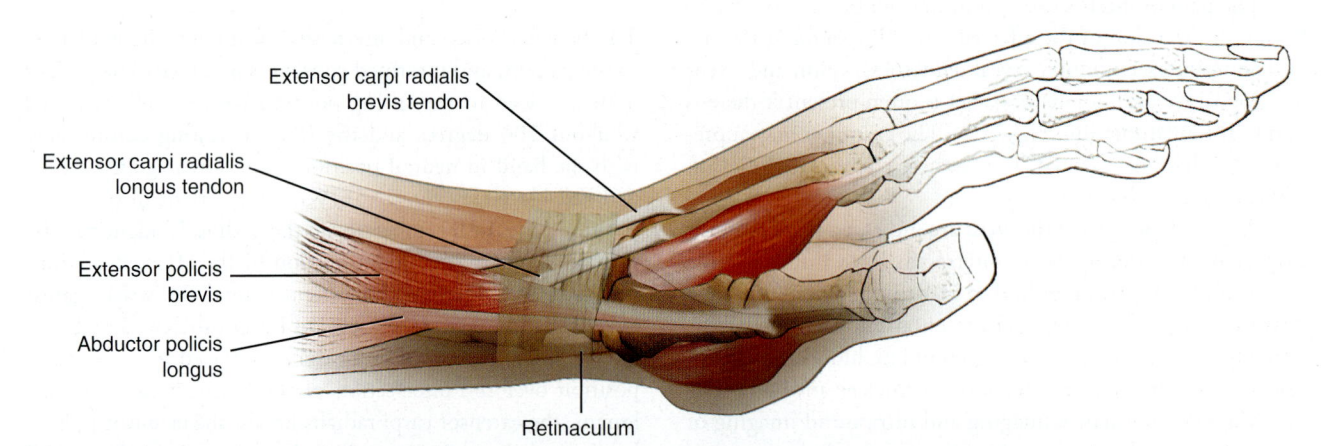

**FIGURE 72.1.** Intersection syndrome is caused by inflammation of the tendons and tendon sheaths of the extensor carpi radialis longus, the extensor carpi radialis brevis, the extensor pollicis brevis, and the abductor pollicis longus muscles.

| TABLE 72.2 | Comparison of Intersection Syndrome with de Quervain Tenosynovitis | |
|---|---|---|
| | **Intersection syndrome** | **de Quervain tenosynovitis** |
| **Tendons involved** | • Extensor carpi radialis longus<br>• Extensor carpi radialis brevis<br>• Extensor pollicis brevis<br>• Abductor pollicis longus | • Abductor pollicis longus<br>• Extensor pollicis brevis |
| **Alternate names** | Washerwoman's wrist<br>Bugaboo forearm | Oarsman's wrist<br>Mommy's wrist |
| **Clinical signs** | Creaking tendon sign<br>Wet leather crepitus | Finkelstein sign |
| **Location of pain** | 5–7 cm above radial styloid around Lister tubercle | At the radial styloid |
| **Site of injection** | At Lister tubercle at the point of maximal tenderness | At the radial styloid |
| **Frequency** | Rare | Common |

guidance so that the needle tip ultimately rests in proximity to the point of intersection but outside the substance of the tendons themselves (Fig. 72.10). When the tip of needle is thought to be in satisfactory position, after careful aspiration, a small amount of local anesthetic and steroid is injected under real-time ultrasound guidance to confirm that the needle tip is in the proper position. After proper needle tip placement is confirmed, the remainder of the contents of the syringe are slowly injected. There should be minimal resistance to injection.

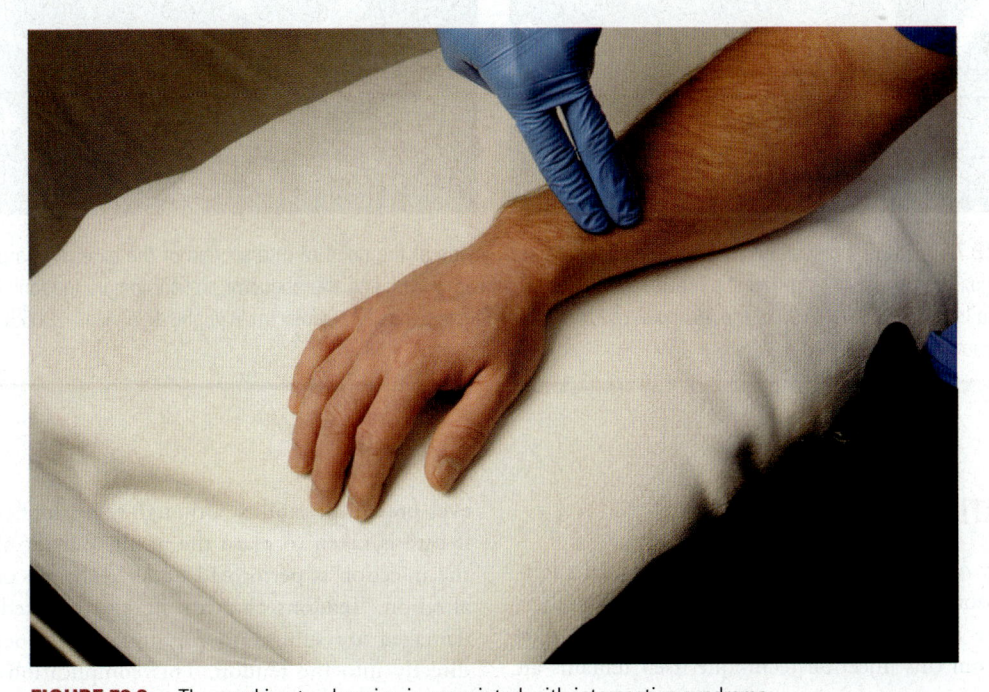

**FIGURE 72.2.** The creaking tendon sign is associated with intersection syndrome.

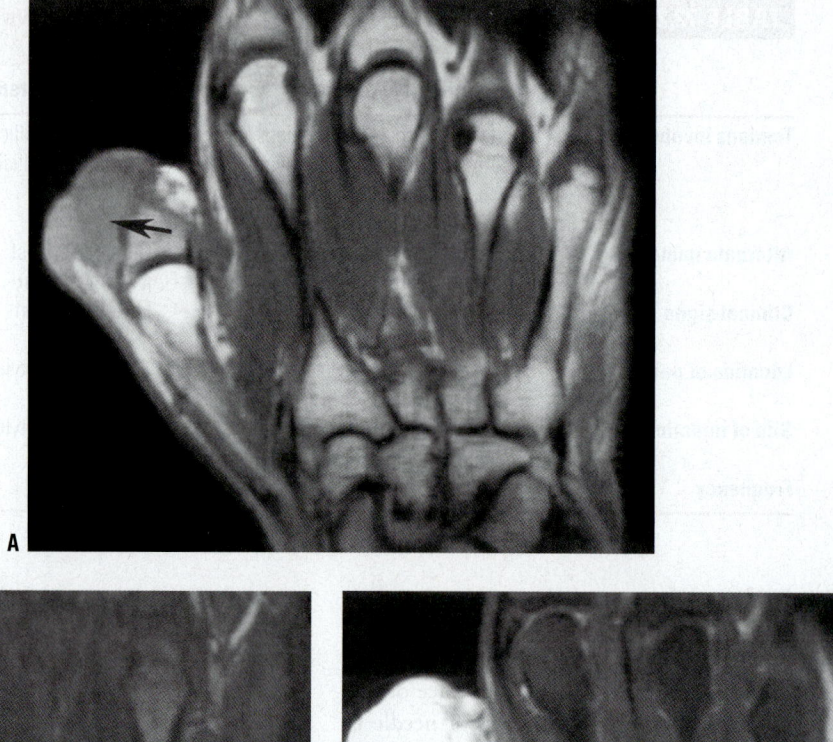

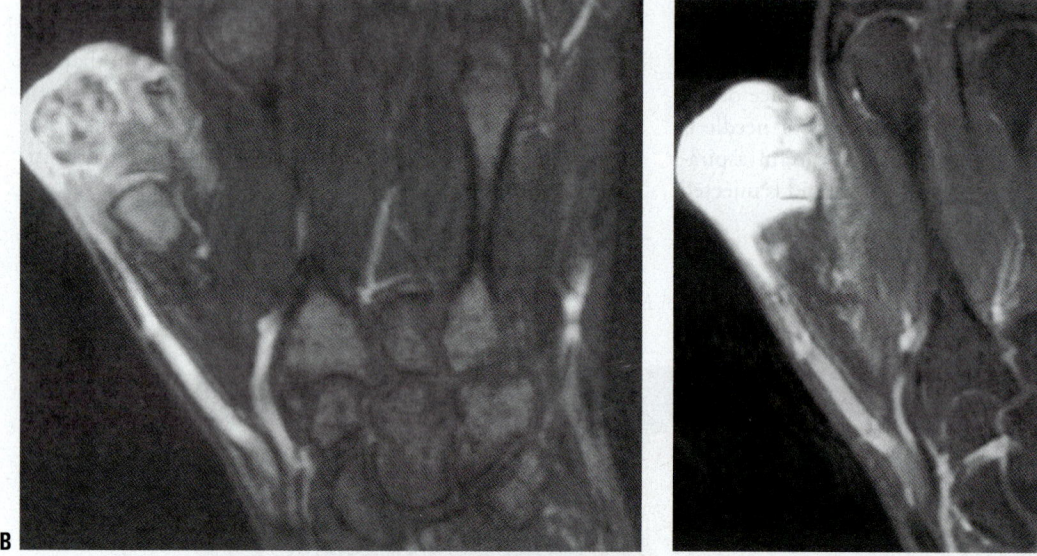

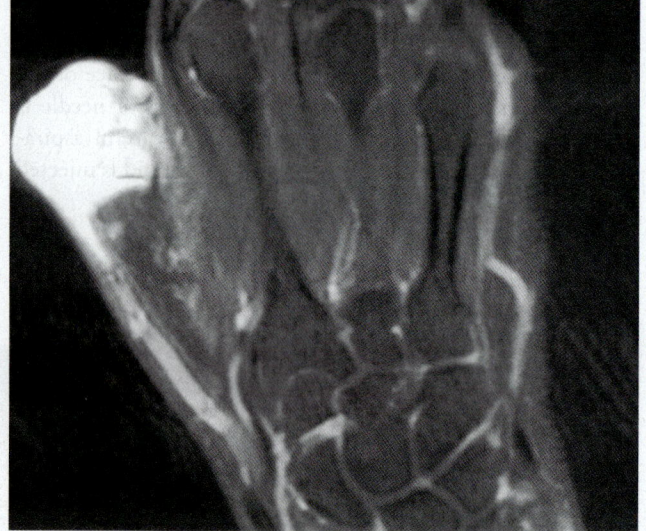

**FIGURE 72.3.** MRI images demonstrating tendonitis and synovitis at the point of intersection of the extensor carpi radialis longus, the extensor carpi radialis brevis, the extensor pollicis brevis, and the abductor pollicis longus tendons (*arrow*). (Reused from Berquist TH. *MRI of the Musculoskeletal System*. Philadelphia, PA: Lippincott Williams & Wilkins; 2005:836, with permission.)

## COMPLICATIONS

The possibility of trauma to the extensor carpi radialis longus, the extensor carpi radialis brevis, the extensor pollicis brevis, and the abductor pollicis longus tendons and tendon sheaths from this injection technique itself remains an ever-present possibility, although the risk of this is decreased if care is taken to place the needle outside the tendon and the injection is performed under real-time ultrasound visualization. Tendons that are highly inflamed or previously damaged are subject to rupture if substances are injected directly into the tendon. This complication can be greatly

CHAPTER 72  ULTRASOUND-GUIDED INJECTION TECHNIQUE FOR INTERSECTION SYNDROME

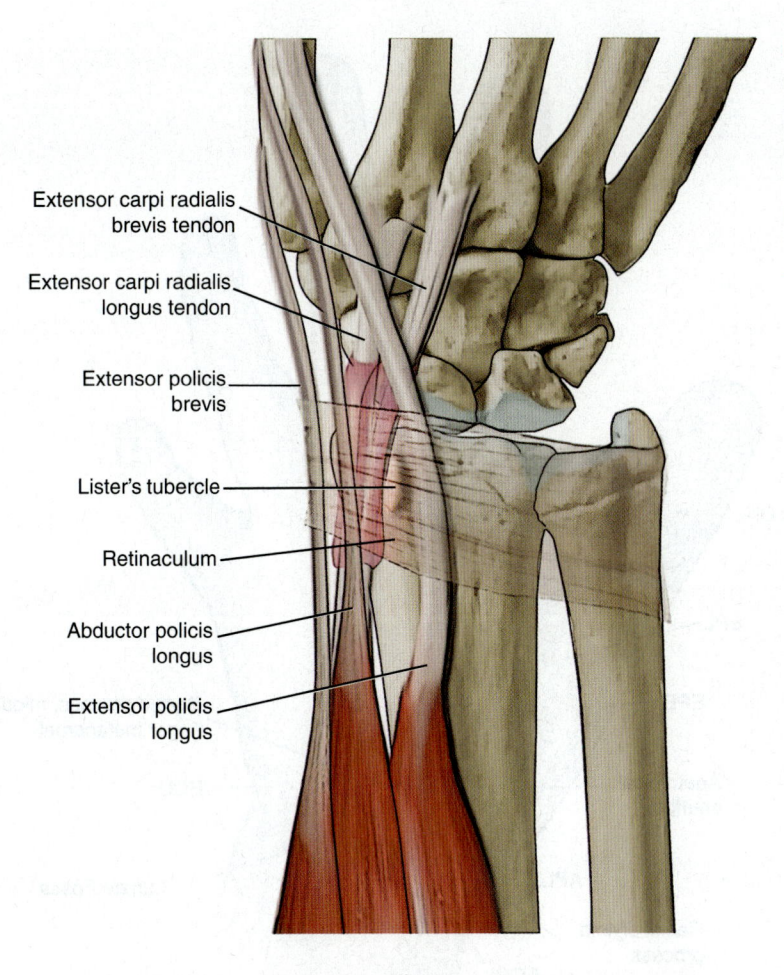

**FIGURE 72.4.** The key landmarks when performing ultrasound-guided injection for intersection syndrome are Lister tubercle and the intersection of the extensor carpi radialis longus, the extensor carpi radialis brevis, the extensor pollicis brevis, and the abductor pollicis longus tendons and tendon sheaths.

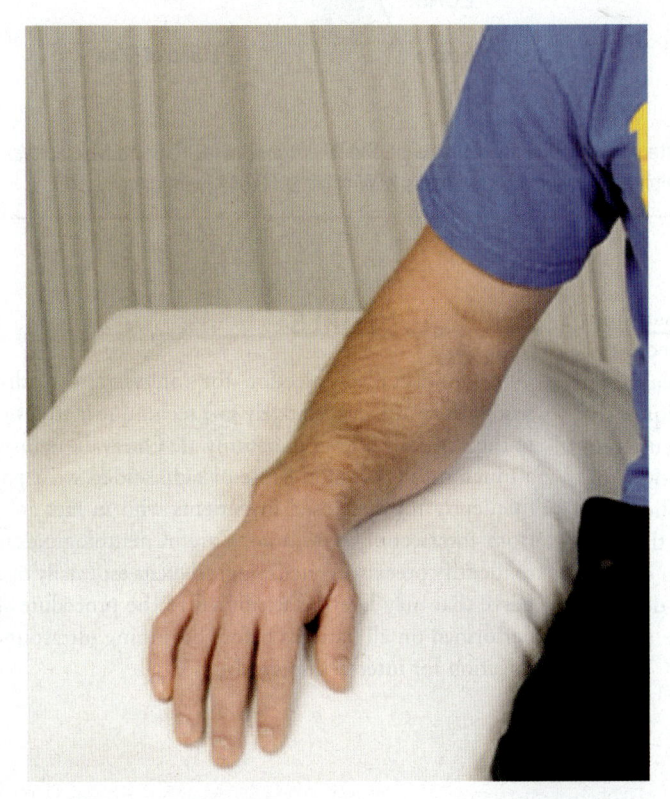

**FIGURE 72.5.** Proper patient position for ultrasound-guided injection for intersection syndrome.

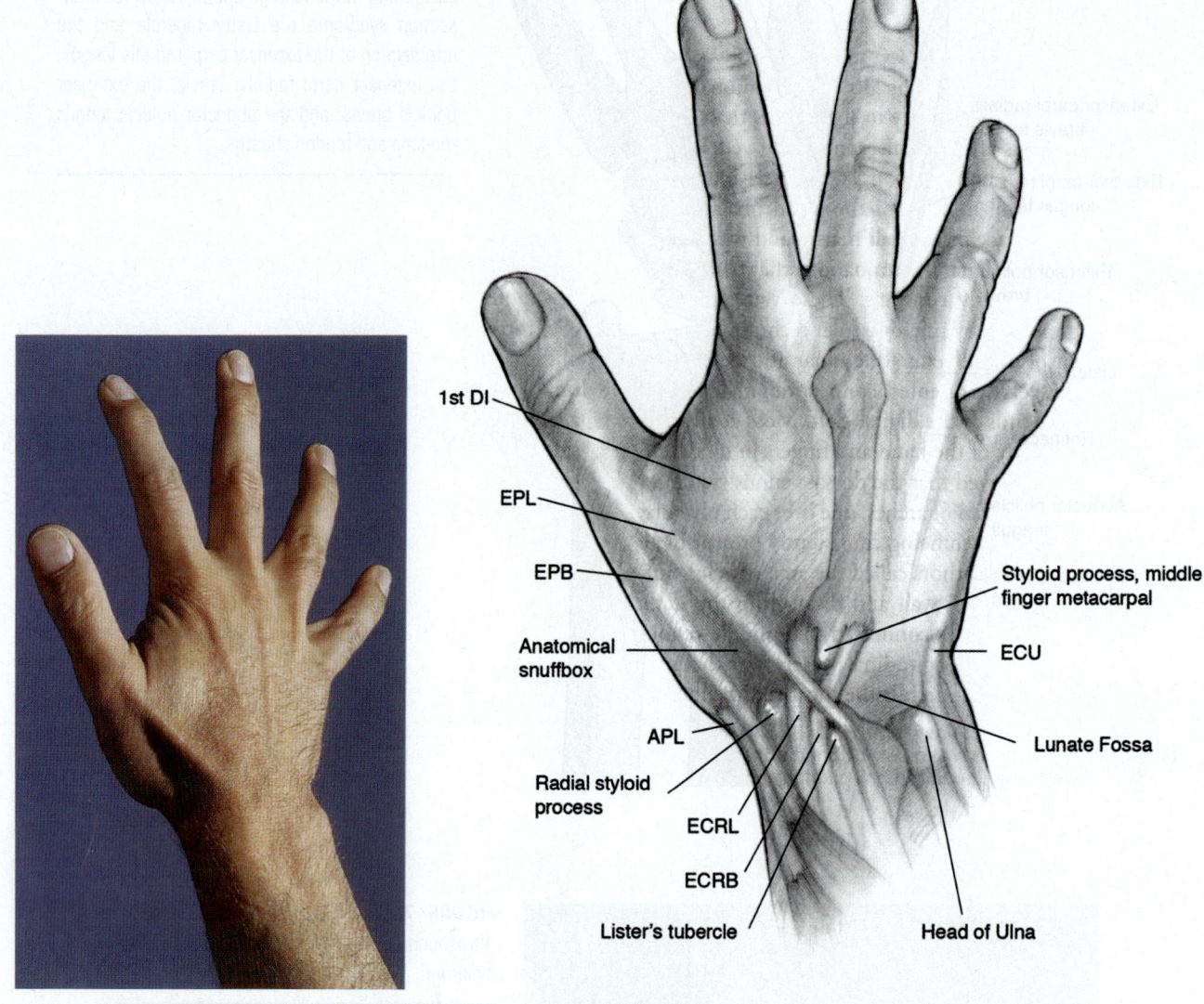

**FIGURE 72.6.** Lister tubercle lies beneath the extensor retinaculum of the wrist. (Reused from Doyle JR, Botte MJ. *Surgical Anatomy of the Hand and Upper Extremity.* Philadelphia, PA: Lippincott Williams & Wilkins; 2003:643, with permission.)

decreased if the clinician uses gentle technique and stops injecting immediately if significant resistance to injection is encountered. Approximately 25% of patients complain of a transient increase in pain after this injection technique; the patient should be warned of this. Infection, although uncommon, can occur. Ecchymosis and hematoma formation following this procedure may also occur. These complications can be decreased if manual pressure is applied to the area of the block immediately after injection. Application of cold packs for 20-minute periods after the block will also decrease the amount of postprocedure pain and bleeding the patient may experience.

## CLINICAL PEARLS

Ultrasound-guided injection for intersection syndrome is a straightforward and relatively safe technique if attention is paid to the clinically relevant anatomy. de Quervain tenosynovitis is a much more common cause of radial-sided wrist pain and is frequently misdiagnosed in patients who in fact are suffering from intersection syndrome. Careful neurologic examination to identify preexisting neurologic deficits especially of the radial nerve that may later be attributed to the procedure should be performed on all patients before beginning ultrasound-guided injection for intersection syndrome.

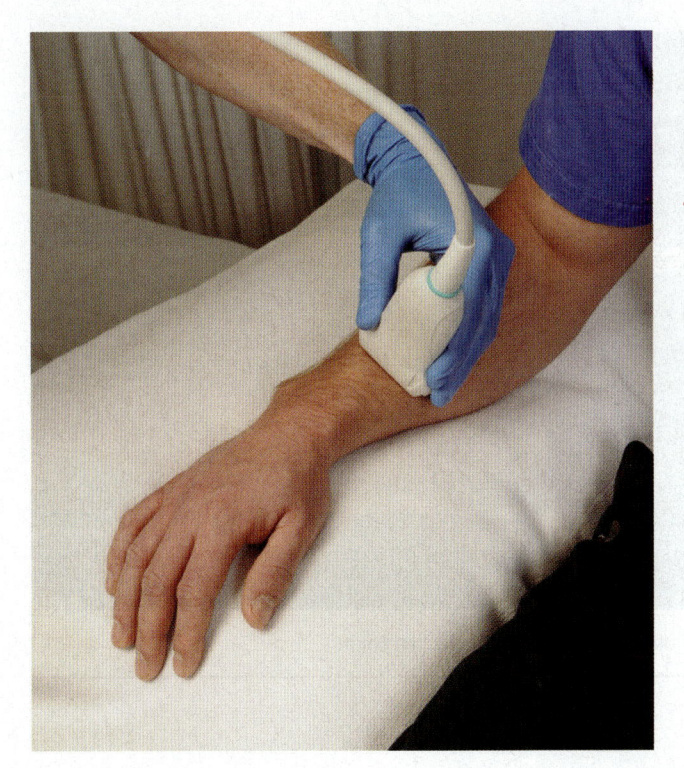

**FIGURE 72.7.** Proper transverse position for the linear high-frequency ultrasound transducer to perform ultrasound-guided intersection syndrome.

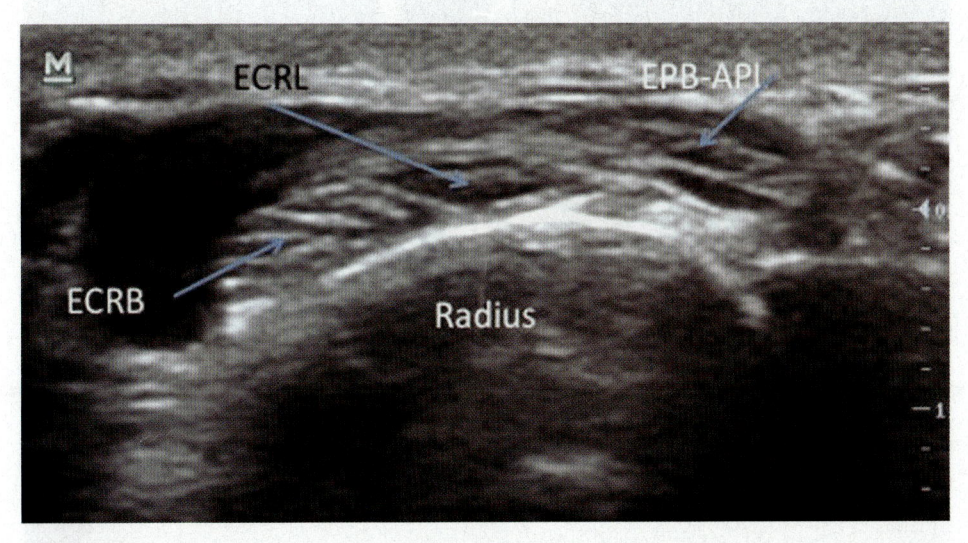

**FIGURE 72.8.** Transverse ultrasound image demonstrating the relationship of the tendon and tendon sheaths of the first and second extensor compartments and their point of intersection.

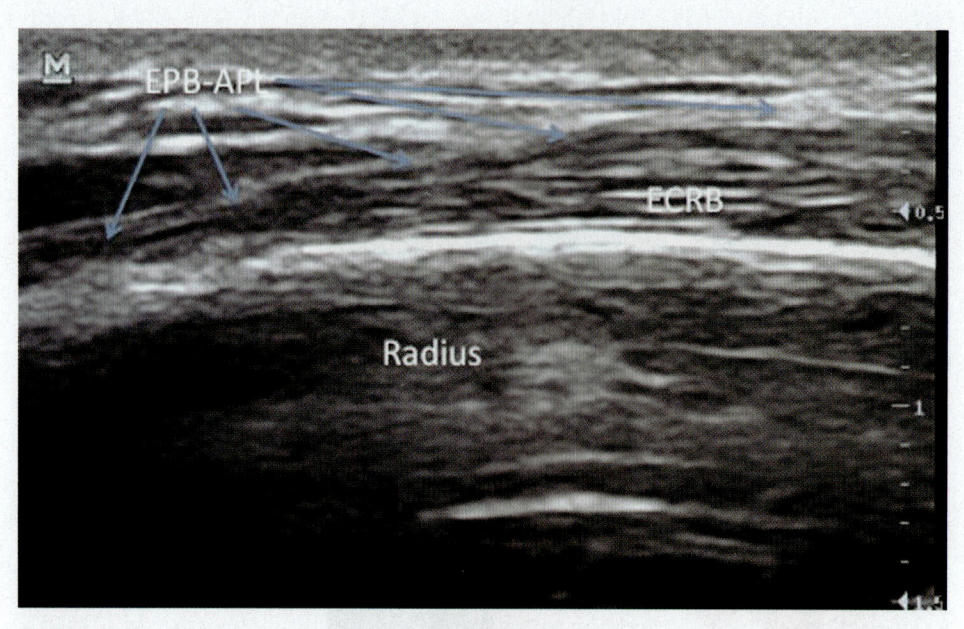

**FIGURE 72.9.** Longitudinal ultrasound view of the intersection point.

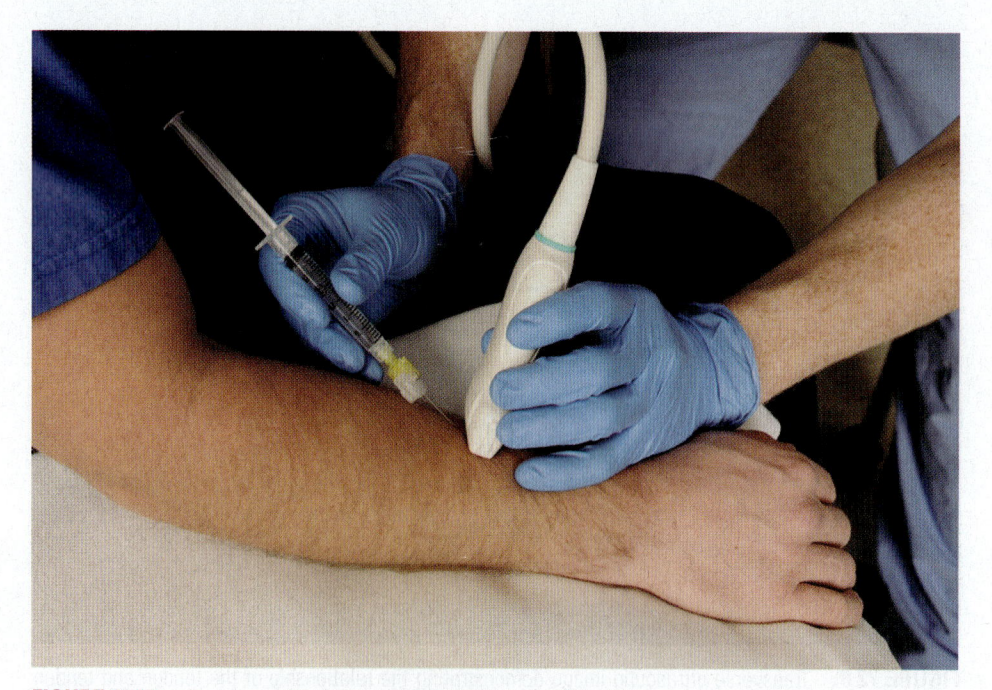

**FIGURE 72.10.** Proper needle placement for ultrasound-guided intersection syndrome.

## SUGGESTED READINGS

Waldman SD. The radial nerve. In: *Pain Review*. Philadelphia, PA: Saunders Elsevier; 2009:76–77.

Waldman SD. Cheiralgia paresthetica. In: *Atlas of Common Pain Syndromes*. 3rd ed. Philadelphia, PA: WB Saunders; 2012:164–167.

Waldman SD. Intersection syndrome. In: *Atlas of Pain Management Injection Techniques*. 3rd ed. Philadelphia, PA: WB Saunders; 2012:204–207.

# CHAPTER 73

# Ultrasound-Guided Intra-articular Injection of the First Carpometacarpal Joint

## CLINICAL PERSPECTIVES

The first carpometacarpal or trapeziometacarpal joint is a synovium-lined saddle-type joint formed by the articular surface of the trapezium proximally and the base of the first metacarpal (thumb) distally (Fig. 73.1). The primary function of the first carpometacarpal joint is to aid in orientation of the thumb to allow pinching movements as well as flexion and extension in the plane of the palm of the hand, abduction and adduction in a plane at right angles to the palm, circumduction, and opposition (Fig. 73.2). The joint's articular cartilage is susceptible to damage, which, if left untreated, will result in arthritis with its associated pain and functional disability. Osteoarthritis of the joint is the most common form of arthritis that results in first carpometacarpal joint pain and functional disability, with rheumatoid arthritis, posttraumatic arthritis, and crystal arthropathy also causing arthritis of the first carpometacarpal joint. Less common causes of arthritis-induced first carpometacarpal joint pain include the collagen vascular diseases, infection, villonodular synovitis, and Lyme disease. Acute infectious arthritis of the first carpometacarpal joint is best treated with early diagnosis, with culture and sensitivity of the synovial fluid, and with prompt initiation of antibiotic therapy. The collagen vascular diseases generally manifest as a polyarthropathy rather than a monoarthropathy limited to the first carpometacarpal joint, although first carpometacarpal pain secondary to the collagen vascular diseases responds exceedingly well to ultrasound-guided intra-articular injection of the first carpometacarpal joint. Interestingly, osteoarthritis of the thumb occurs over twenty times more frequently in elderly females when compared with elderly males. This is thought to be due to sexual dimorphism in the shape of the joint with the female joint having a significantly smaller trapezial articular surface when compared with males of the same age.

Patients with first carpometacarpal joint pain secondary to arthritis, gout, synovitis, and collagen vascular disease related joint pain complain of pain that is localized to the base of the thumb. Activity, including pinching and gripping motions, makes the pain worse, with rest and heat providing some relief. The pain is constant and characterized as aching in nature. Sleep disturbance is common with awakening when patients roll over onto the affected upper extremity. Some patients complain of a grating, catching, or popping sensation with range of motion of the joint, and crepitus may be appreciated on physical examination. Watson stress test is positive in patients who suffer from inflammation and arthritis of the carpometacarpal joint of the thumb. Watson test is performed by having the patient place the dorsum of the hand against a table with the fingers fully extended and then pushing the thumb back toward the table (Fig. 73.3). The test is positive if the patient's pain is reproduced.

Functional disability often accompanies the pain of many pathologic conditions of the first carpometacarpal joint. Patients will often notice increasing difficulty in performing their activities of daily living and tasks that require gripping or pinching objects such as writing with a pen or pencil or opening a jar. If the pathologic process responsible for the first carpometacarpal pain is not adequately treated, the patient's functional disability may worsen, and muscle wasting and ultimately a frozen first carpometacarpal joint may occur.

Plain radiographs are indicated in all patients who present with first carpometacarpal joint pain (Fig. 73.4). Based on the patient's clinical presentation, additional testing may be indicated, including complete blood cell count, sedimentation rate, and antinuclear antibody testing. Magnetic resonance imaging or ultrasound of the first carpometacarpal joint is indicated if fracture, effusion, tendinopathy, crystal arthropathy, joint mice, synovitis, bursitis, or ligamentous injury is suspected.

## CLINICALLY RELEVANT ANATOMY

The first carpometacarpal or trapeziometacarpal joint is a synovial-lined saddle-type joint formed by the articular surface of the trapezium proximally and the base of the first metacarpal (thumb) distally (see Fig. 73.1). The primary function of the first carpometacarpal joint is to aid in orientation of the thumb to allow pinching movements as well as flexion and extension in the plane of the palm of the hand, abduction and adduction in a plane at right angles to the palm, circumduction, and

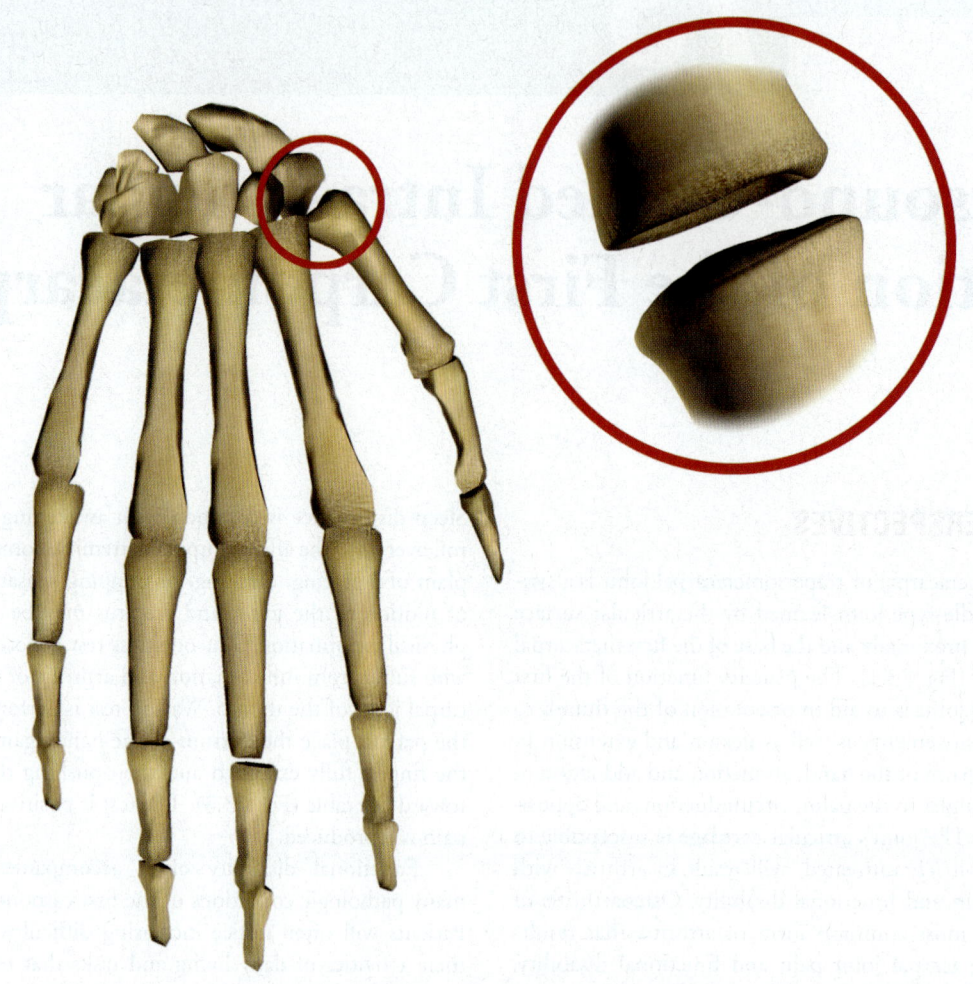

**FIGURE 73.1.** The first carpometacarpal (trapeziometacarpal) joint is a saddle joint that allows a variety of motions of the thumb. (Reused from LifeART, Lippincott Williams & Wilkins.)

Abduction        Adduction        Extension        Flexion        Opposition        Reposition

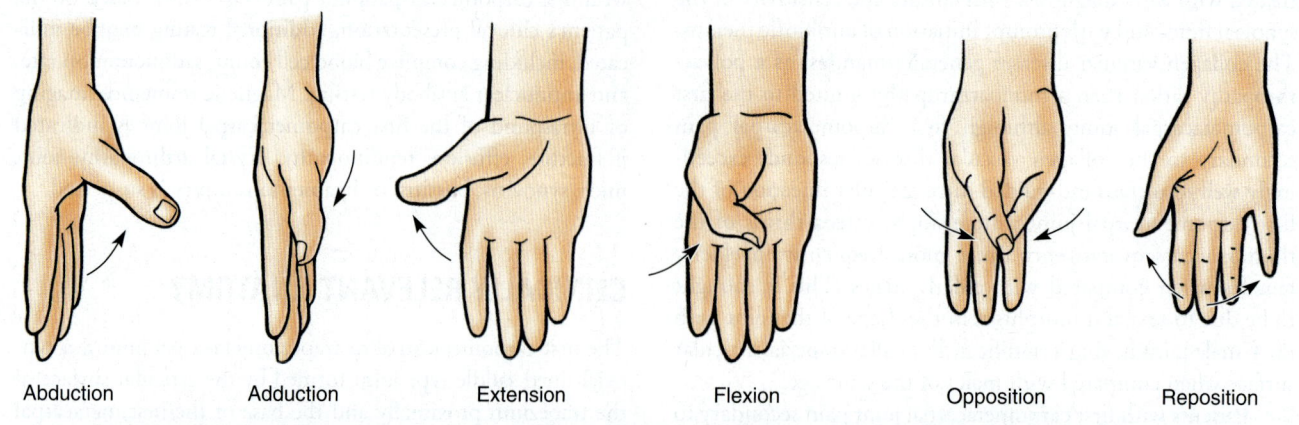

**FIGURE 73.2.** Movements of the *thumb*. Opposition, the action bringing the tip of the *thumb* in contact with the pads of the other fingers (e.g., with the little finger), is the most complex movement. The components of opposition are medial rotation at the carpometacarpal joint and abduction and flexion of the metacarpophalangeal joint. (Reused from Moore KL, Dalley AF. *Clinical Oriented Anatomy*. 4th ed. Baltimore, MD: Lippincott Williams & Wilkins; 1999, with permission.)

CHAPTER 73   ULTRASOUND-GUIDED INTRA-ARTICULAR INJECTION OF THE FIRST CARPOMETACARPAL JOINT   503

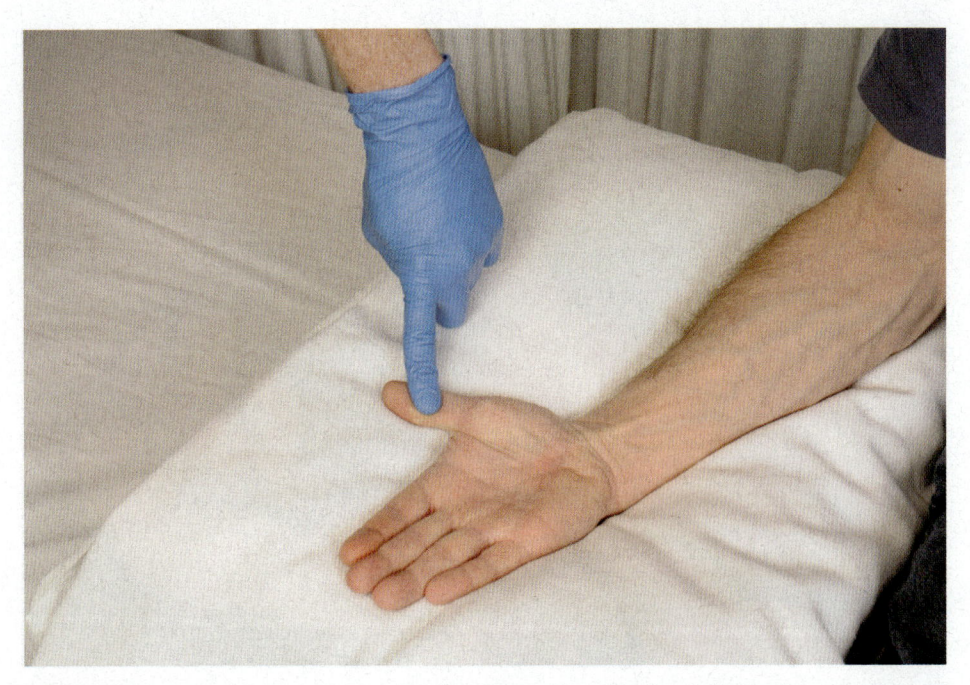

**FIGURE 73.3.** Watson stress test is positive in patients who suffer from inflammation and arthritis of the carpometacarpal joint of the thumb. Watson test is performed by having the patient place the dorsum of the hand against a table with the fingers fully extended and then pushing the thumb back toward the table. The test is positive if the patient's pain is reproduced.

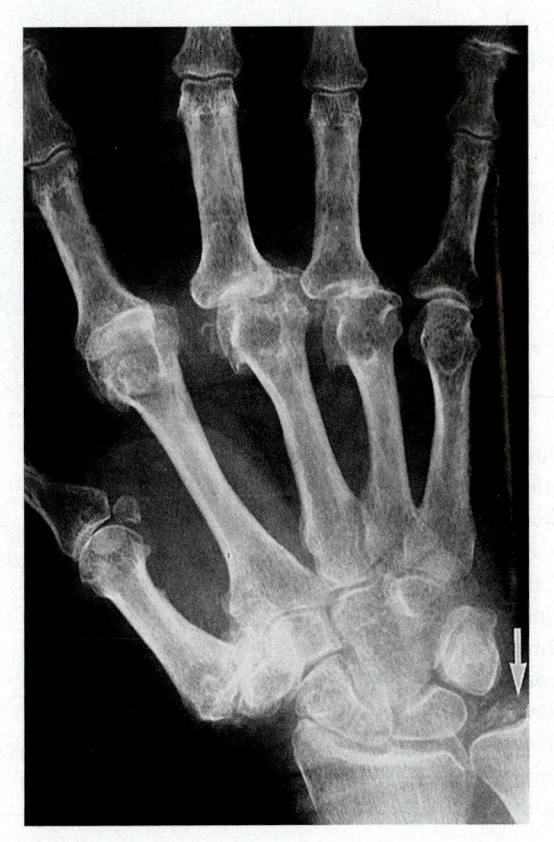

**FIGURE 73.4.** Calcium pyrophosphate dihydrate crystal deposition disease involving the joints of the wrist and hand. Note the articular changes at the metacarpophalangeal joints. Calcification of the triangular cartilage is evident in the ulnar compartment of the wrist (*arrow*). Also noted is exuberant degenerative change in the first carpometacarpal joint, secondary to crystal deposition. (Reused from Yochum TR, Rowe LJ. *Yochum and Rowe's Essentials of Skeletal Radiology.* 3rd ed. Philadelphia, PA: Lippincott Williams & Wilkins; 2004, with permission.)

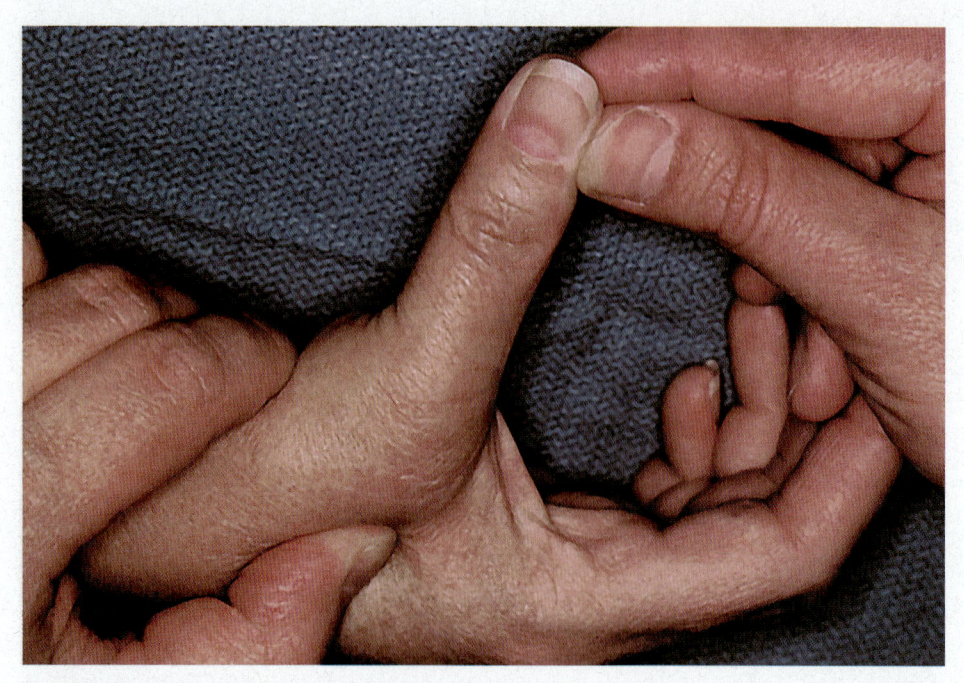

**FIGURE 73.5.** The ulnar aspect of the first carpometacarpal joint opens ~35 degrees with radially directed stress, which is strongly suggestive of a complete tear of the ulnar collateral ligament. (Reused from Strickland JW, Graham TJ. *Master Techniques in Orthopaedic Surgery: The Hand.* 2nd ed. Philadelphia, PA: Lippincott Williams & Wilkins; 2005, with permission.)

opposition. The joint is lined with synovium, and the ample synovial space allows for intra-articular placement of needles for injection and aspiration. Due to the extensive and diverse range of motion of the first carpometacarpal joint combined with a relatively weak and slack joint capsule, the joint is especially susceptible to trauma including subluxation and fractures of the base of the metacarpal through the articular surface, which can result in the development of arthritis (Fig. 73.5). The joint is also susceptible to overuse and misuse with resultant inflammation and arthritis. Much of the joints strength is derived from the three intracapsular and two extracapsular ligaments and the surrounding tendons.

## ULTRASOUND-GUIDED TECHNIQUE

The benefits, risks, and alternative treatments are explained to the patient, and informed consent is obtained. The patient is then placed in the sitting position with the elbow flexed and the forearm and hand resting comfortably palm up and thumb in neutral position on a pillow or padded bedside table (Fig. 73.6). The skin overlying the first carpometacarpal joint is then prepped with antiseptic solution. A sterile syringe containing 1.0 mL of 0.25% preservative-free bupivacaine and 40 mg of methylprednisolone is attached to a 1½-inch, 22-gauge needle using strict aseptic technique. A small linear high-frequency ultrasound transducer is placed in a longitudinal parallel axis over the base of the first metacarpal lying against

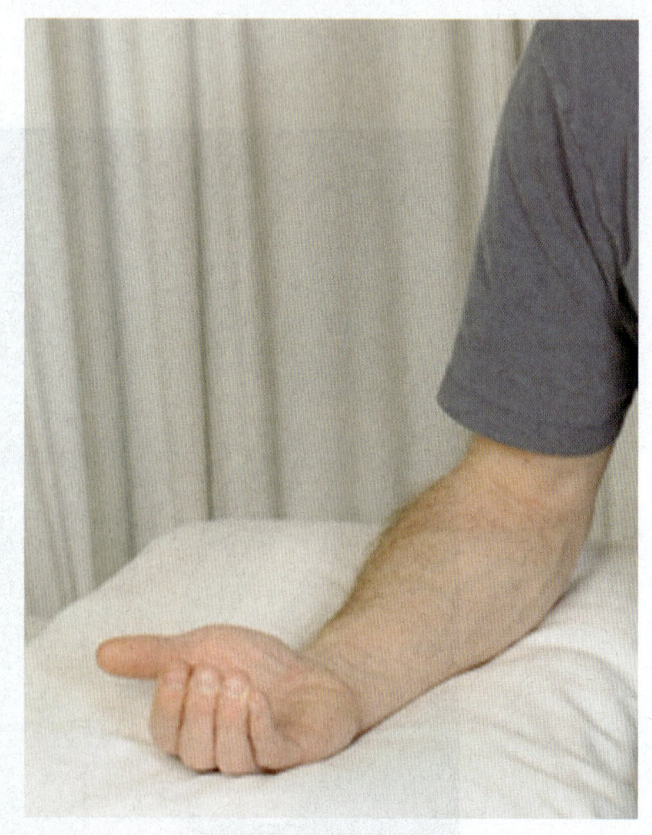

**FIGURE 73.6.** Correct patient position for ultrasound-guided intra-articular injection of the first carpometacarpal joint.

# CHAPTER 73  ULTRASOUND-GUIDED INTRA-ARTICULAR INJECTION OF THE FIRST CARPOMETACARPAL JOINT

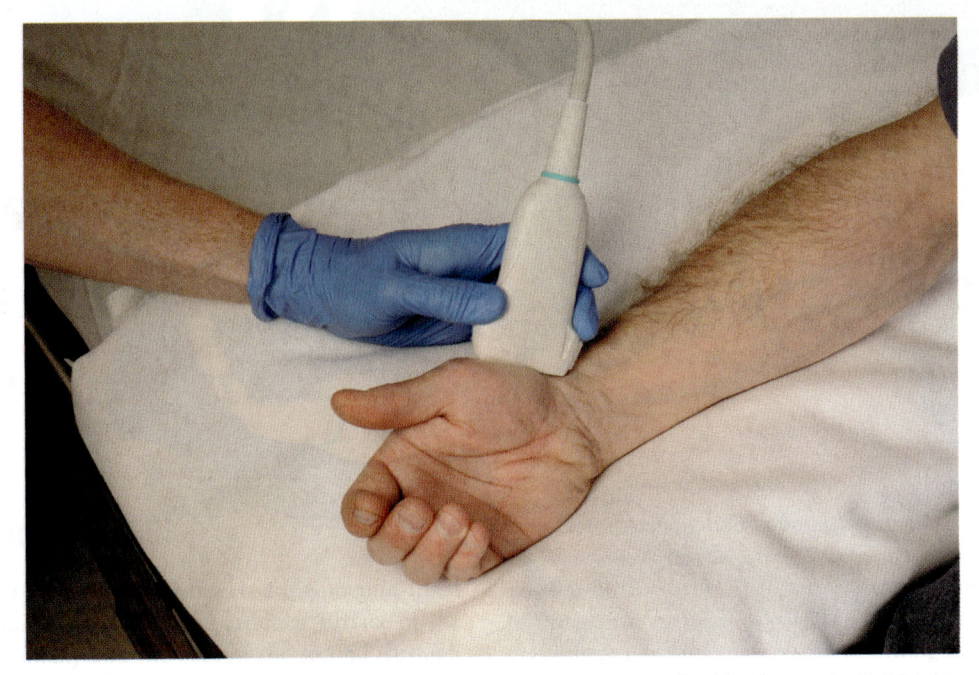

**FIGURE 73.7.** Correct position for ultrasound transducer for ultrasound-guided intra-articular injection of the first carpometacarpal joint.

the volar radial aspect of the thumb, and a survey scan is taken (Fig. 73.7). The transducer is slowly moved proximally along the volar radial aspect of the thumb until the hypoechoic cleft between the base of the thumb and the distal articular surface of the trapezium is in the center of the image (Fig. 73.8). The needle is placed through the skin ~0.5 cm below the center of the distal aspect of the ultrasound transducer and is then advanced using an out-of-plane approach with the needle trajectory adjusted between 30 and 40 degrees under real-time ultrasound guidance to enter the first carpometacarpal joint (Fig. 73.9). A pop is often appreciated as the needle tip enters the joint. When the tip of needle is thought to be within the joint, a small amount of local anesthetic and steroid is injected under real-time ultrasound guidance to confirm intra-articular placement by the characteristic spreading swirl of hyperechoic injectate within the joint. After intra-articular needle tip placement is confirmed, the remainder of the contents of the syringe are slowly injected. There should be minimal resistance

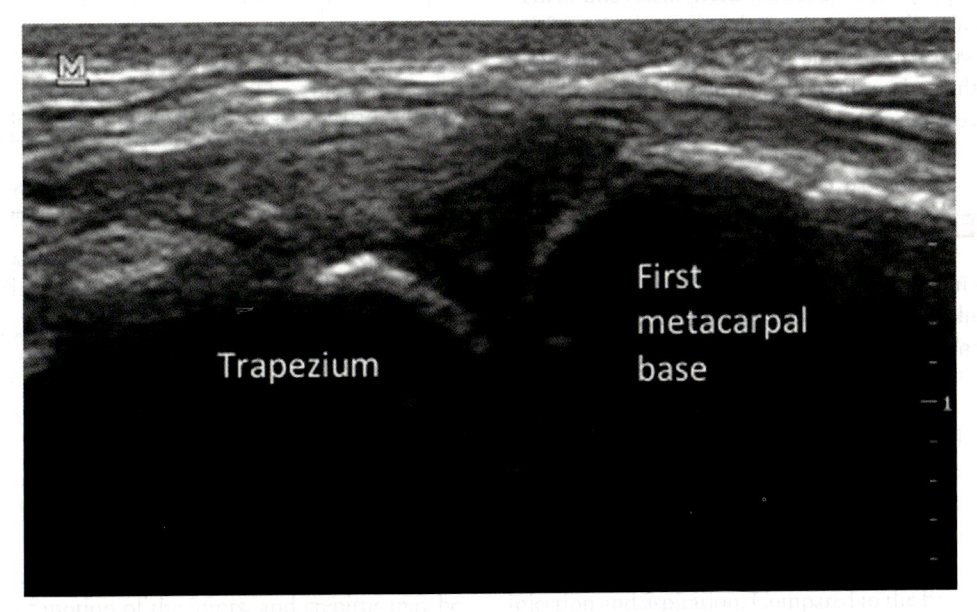

**FIGURE 73.8.** Longitudinal parallel axis ultrasound view of the carpometacarpal joint space.

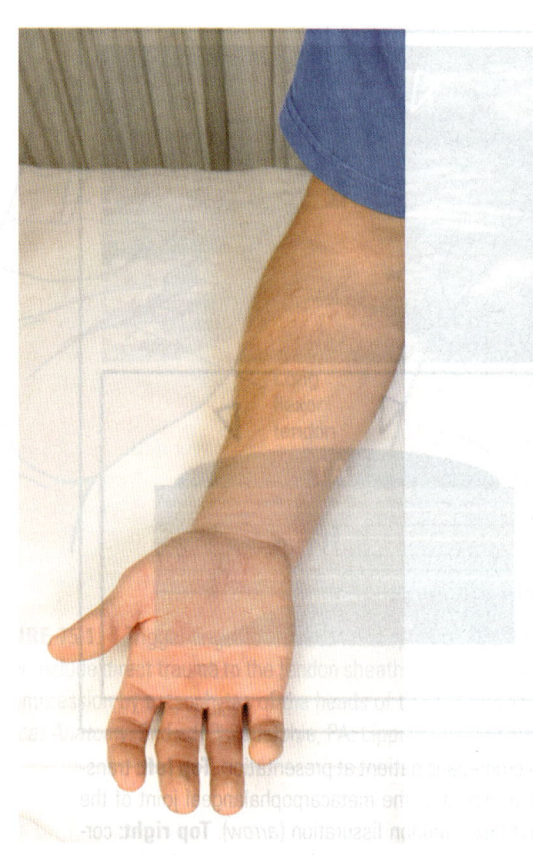

**FIGURE 75.5.** Proper patient position for ultrasound-guided injection for trigger finger.

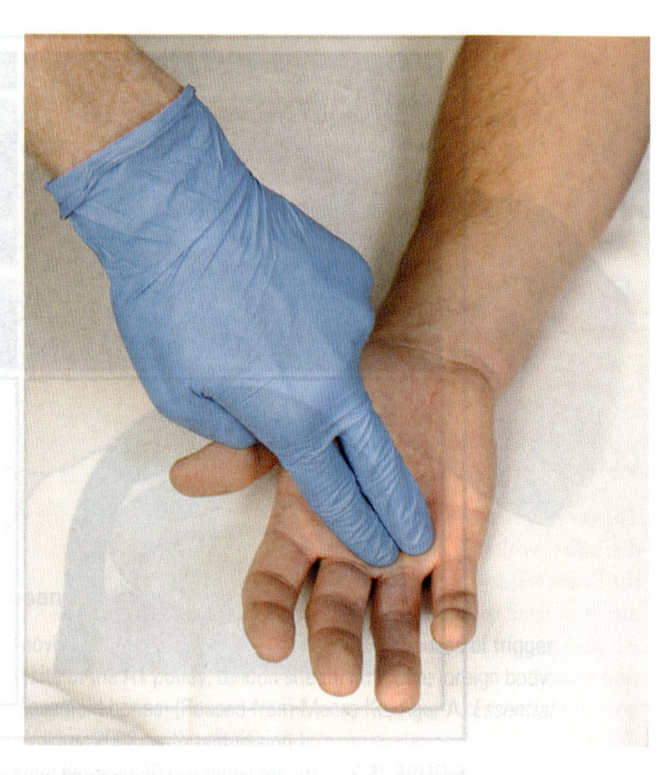

**FIGURE 75.6.** Identification of the metacarpophalangeal joint by palpation.

**FIGURE 75.7.** Proper transverse position for the linear high-frequency ultrasound transducer to perform ultrasound-guided trigger finger injection.

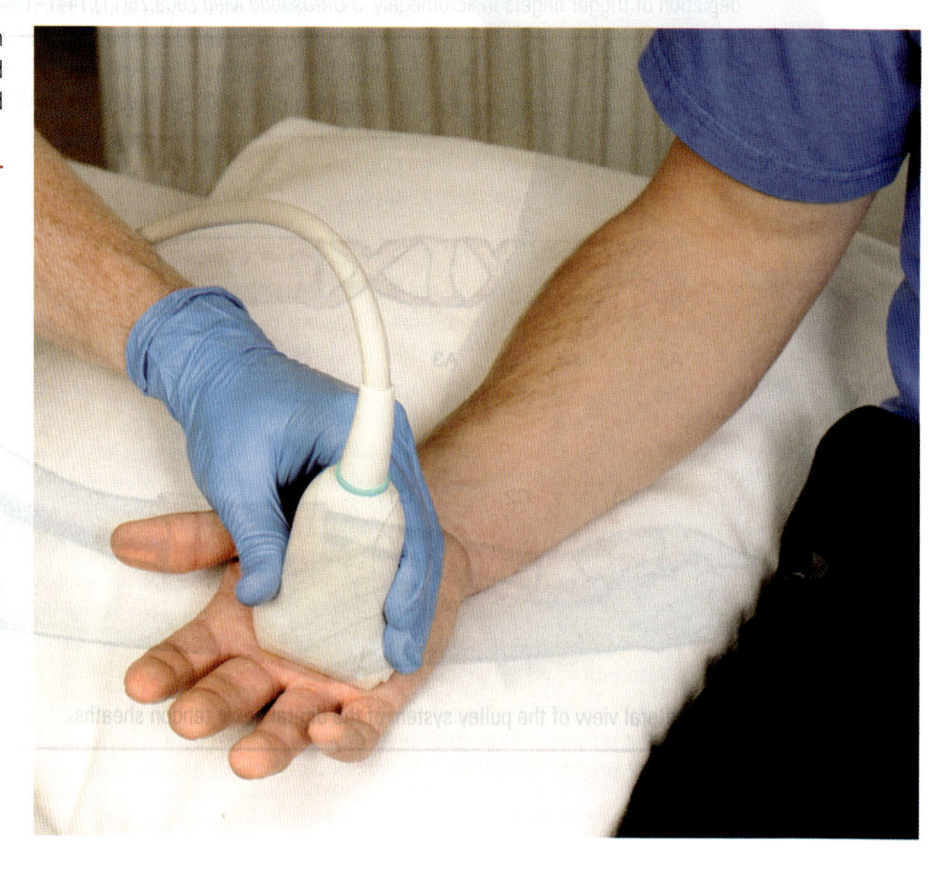

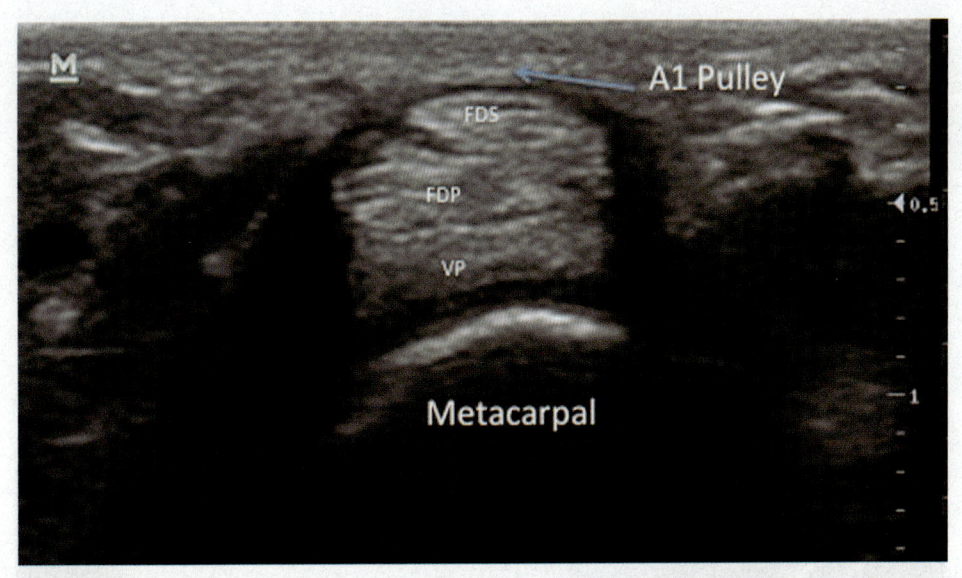

**FIGURE 75.8.** Transverse ultrasound image demonstrating the relationship of the A1 pulley, the tendons of the flexor digitorum superficialis and profundus, the volar plate, and the metacarpal.

visualize the pulley's lateral expansions by slightly inclining the transverse-oriented probe to eliminate the anisotropic artifact that may cause these expansions to appear hypoechoic if the probe remains at a right angle to the expansions (Fig. 75.8). When the A1 pulley is identified, the patient is asked to flex and extend the finger under real-time ultrasound imaging in both the transverse and longitudinal planes, and the tendons are observed for tendinosis, defect, swelling, nodules, and a triggering phenomenon. After assessment of the tendon is completed, the skin overlying the area beneath the ultrasound transducer is then prepped with antiseptic solution. A sterile syringe containing 1.0 mL of 0.25% preservative-free bupivacaine and 40 mg of methylprednisolone is attached to a 1½-inch, 22-gauge needle using strict aseptic technique. The needle is placed through the skin just below the inferior border of the transducer and is then advanced using an out-of-plane approach with the needle trajectory adjusted under real-time ultrasound guidance so that the needle tip ultimately rests in

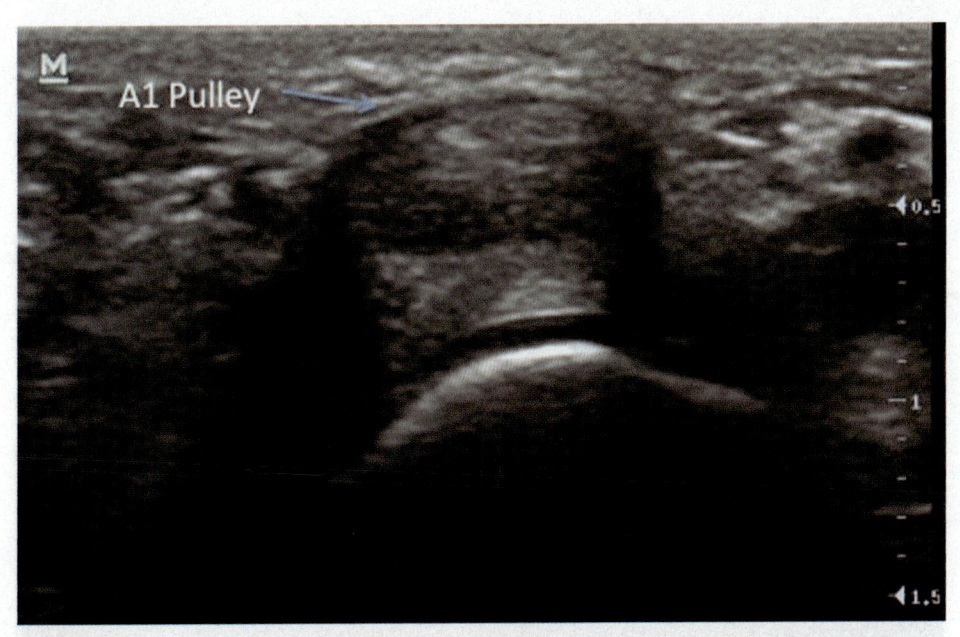

**FIGURE 75.9.** Inclining the transversely placed transducer may aid in identifying the A1 pulley and its expansions.

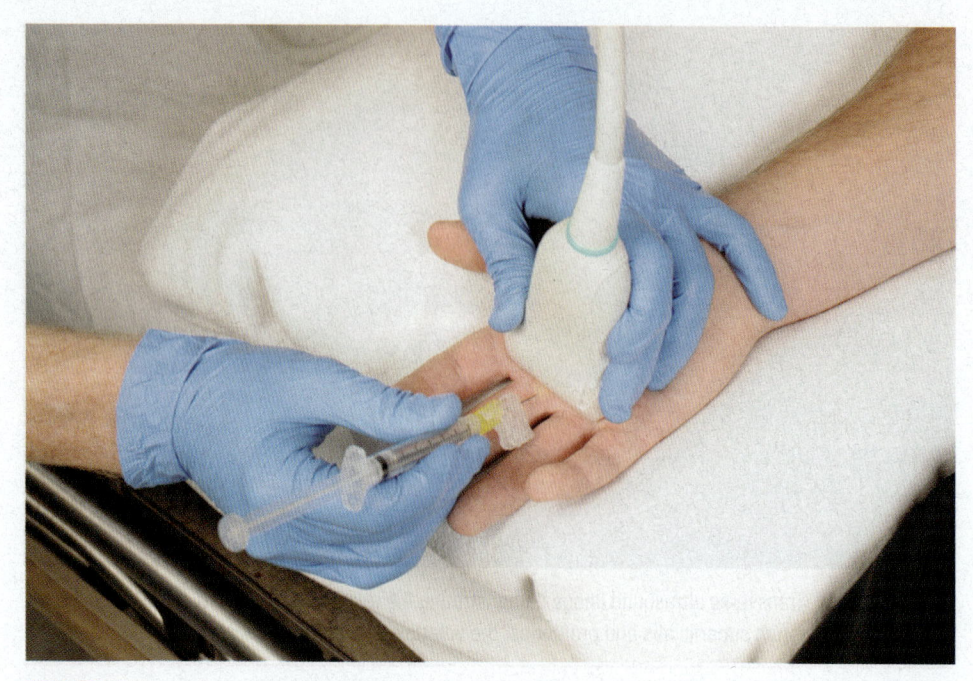

**FIGURE 75.10.** Proper needle placement for ultrasound-guided trigger finger injection.

the hypotenuse of the triangle formed by the A1, the flexor digitorum superficialis and profundus tendons and associated volar plate, and the palmar surface of the distal metacarpal bone (Figs. 75.10 and 75.11). When the tip of needle is thought to be in satisfactory position, after careful aspiration, a small amount of local anesthetic and steroid is injected under real-time ultrasound guidance to confirm that the needle tip is in the proper position. After proper needle tip placement is confirmed, the remainder of the contents of the syringe are slowly injected. There should be minimal resistance to injection.

## COMPLICATIONS

The possibility of trauma to the flexor digitorum superficialis and profundus tendons from this injection technique itself remains an ever-present possibility, although the risk of this is

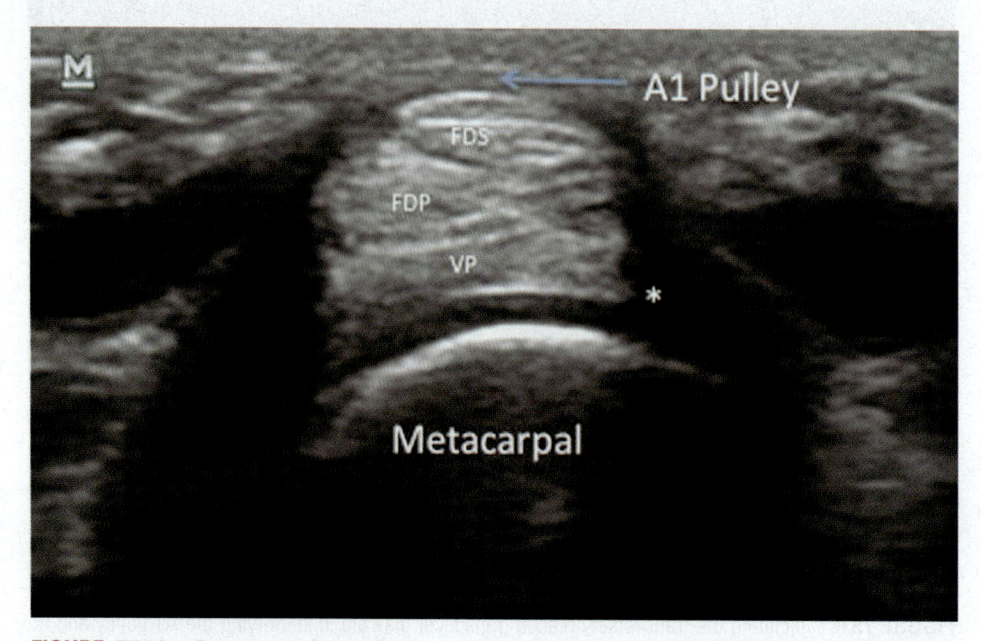

**FIGURE 75.11.** Transverse ultrasound image demonstrating the triangular needle tip target for ultrasound-guided trigger finger injection.

decreased if care is taken to place the needle outside the tendon and the injection is performed under real-time ultrasound visualization. Tendons that are highly inflamed or previously damaged are subject to rupture if substances are injected directly into the tendon. This complication can be greatly decreased if the clinician uses gentle technique and stops injecting immediately if significant resistance to injection is encountered. Approximately 25% of patients complain of a transient increase in pain after this injection technique; the patient should be warned of this. Infection, although uncommon, can occur. Ecchymosis and hematoma formation following this procedure may also occur. These complications can be decreased if manual pressure is applied to the area of the block immediately after injection. Application of cold packs for 20-minute periods after the block will also decrease the amount of postprocedure pain and bleeding the patient may experience.

## CLINICAL PEARLS

Ultrasound-guided injection for trigger finger is a straightforward and relatively safe technique if attention is paid to the clinically relevant anatomy. The use of physical modalities, including local heat and gentle range-of-motion exercises, should be introduced several days after the patient undergoes this injection technique. A hand splint at nighttime to protect the fingers also may help relieve the symptoms of trigger finger. Vigorous exercise should be avoided because it may exacerbate the patient's symptomatology. Simple analgesics and nonsteroidal anti-inflammatory agents may be used concurrently with this injection technique. Careful examination to identify preexisting tendon ruptures that may later be attributed to the procedure should be performed on all patients before beginning ultrasound-guided injection for trigger finger.

## SUGGESTED READINGS

Bodor M, Fullerton B. Ultrasonography of the hand, wrist, and elbow. *Phys Med Rehabil Clin N Am* 2010;21(3):509–531.
Brito JL, Rozental TD. Corticosteroid injection for idiopathic trigger finger. *J Hand Surg* 2010;35(5):831–833.
Ragheb D, Stanley A, Gentili A, et al. MR imaging of the finger tendons: normal anatomy and commonly encountered pathology. *Eur J Radiol* 2005;56(3):296–306.
Ryzewicz M, Wolf JM. Trigger digits: principles, management, and complications. *J Hand Surg* 2006;31(1):135–146.
Sbernardori MC, Bandiera P. Histopathology of the A1 pulley in adult trigger fingers. *J Hand Surg* 2007;32(5):556–559.
Waldman SD. Trigger finger. In: *Atlas of Pain Management Injection Techniques*. 3rd ed. Philadelphia, PA: WB Saunders; 2012:215–217.
Wang AA, Hutchinson DT. The effect of corticosteroid injection for trigger finger on blood glucose level in diabetic patients. *J Hand Surg* 2006;31(6):979–981.

# CHAPTER 76

# Ultrasound-Guided Injection Technique for Dupuytren Contracture

## CLINICAL PERSPECTIVES

Dupuytren contracture is a common cause of hand pain and functional disability, which is most commonly caused by a progressive fibrosis of the palmar fascia, which was first described by Baron Guillaume Dupuytren in 1831. Early symptoms of Dupuytren contracture are tender fibrotic nodules along the course of the flexor tendons of the hand, although the nodules actually arise from the palmar fascia rather than the flexor tendons themselves. Although the ring and little fingers are most often affected, all fingers can develop the disease. As the disease progresses, these isolated nodules begin to coalesce and surround the flexor tendons, which draws the affected fingers into a characteristic posture of flexion (Fig. 76.1). Left untreated, the disease will progress until the affected fingers develop permanent flexion contractures, which cause significant functional disability. The pain of Dupuytren contracture tends to burn itself out as the disease progresses.

The exact cause of Dupuytren contracture remains unknown although the disease seems to have a genetic basis with an autosomal dominant inheritance pattern with variable penetrance. A biochemical pathogenesis has been hypothesized, which suggests that excess deposition of type I collagen combined with abnormal myofibroblast formation and increased levels of beta-catenin responsible for the disease. Dupuytren contracture occurs most commonly in males of northern European descent with a gender predilection approaching 10 males for every female affected. The disease rarely occurs before the fourth decade. Diabetes, smoking, cirrhosis of the liver, chronic barbiturate use, trauma to the palmar fascia, and alcoholism are risk factors.

Frequently, the painful, fibrotic nodules of the palmar surface that are seen early in the course of the disease are misdiagnosed as warts or ganglion cysts. As the disease progresses, taut, fibrous bands that may cross the metacarpophalangeal joint and ultimately the proximal interphalangeal joint are noted on physical examination, clarifying the diagnosis. These fibrous bands are not painful to palpation. As the functional disability associated with limitation of finger extension progresses, the patient will seek medical attention due to difficulty on putting on gloves or reaching into their pockets. Ultimately, permanent flexion contracture of the affected fingers results (Fig. 76.2).

Plain radiographs of the hand are indicated in all patients suspected of suffering from Dupuytren contracture to rule out occult bony pathology and to identify calcific tendinitis. Based on the patient's clinical presentation, additional testing may be indicated, including complete blood cell count, uric acid, sedimentation rate, and antinuclear antibody testing. Magnetic resonance imaging or ultrasound imaging of the hand is indicated to assess the status of the affected tendons and tendon sheath as well as to identify other occult pathology including arthritis, sesamoiditis, and synovitis (Fig. 76.3).

## CLINICALLY RELEVANT ANATOMY

Dupuytren contracture is the result of the thickening of the palmar fascia and ultimately the effect this thickening has on the flexor tendons (see Fig. 76.1). The primary function of the palmar fascia, which is also known as the palmar aponeurosis, is to provide firm support to the overlying skin to aid the hand in gripping as well as to protect the underlying tendons.

## ULTRASOUND-GUIDED TECHNIQUE

The benefits, risks, and alternative treatments are explained to the patient and informed consent is obtained. The patient is then placed in the sitting position with the elbow flexed to about 100 degrees and the forearm resting comfortably against a padded bedside table with the hand in neutral position palm up (Fig. 76.4). With the patient in the above position, the fibrous cords of the affected fingers are identified by palpation on the palmar surface just proximal to the metacarpophalangeal joint of the affected finger. A high-frequency linear ultrasound transducer is then placed in a longitudinal position just proximal to the metacarpophalangeal joint of the affected finger, and an ultrasound survey scan is taken (Figs. 76.5 and 76.6). The affected flexor digitorum superficialis and profundus tendons and the surrounding fibrous plaques are identified. After the affected tendons are identified, the skin overlying the area beneath the ultrasound transducer is then prepped with antiseptic solution. A sterile syringe containing 1.0 mL of 0.25% preservative-free bupivacaine and 40 mg of methylprednisolone is attached to a 1½-inch,

CHAPTER 76   ULTRASOUND-GUIDED INJECTION TECHNIQUE FOR DUPUYTREN CONTRACTURE

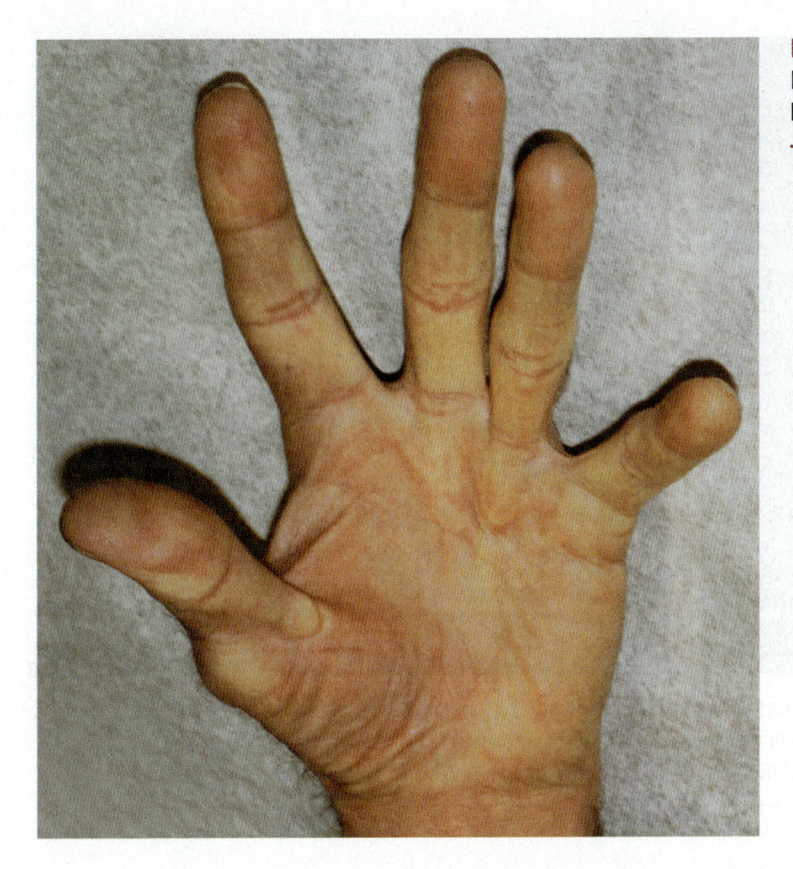

**FIGURE 76.1.** Dupuytren contracture. (Reused from Berg D, Worzala K. *Atlas of Adult Physical Diagnosis*. Philadelphia, PA: Lippincott Williams & Wilkins; 2006, with permission.)

22-gauge needle using strict aseptic technique. The needle is placed through the skin just below the distal border of the transducer and is then advanced using an in-plane approach with the needle trajectory adjusted under real-time ultrasound guidance so that the needle tip ultimately rests in proximity to the tendon sheath of the affected tendons, but not within the tendon substance itself (Fig. 76.7). When the tip of needle is thought to be in satisfactory position, after careful aspiration, a small amount of local anesthetic and steroid is injected under real-time ultrasound guidance to confirm that the needle tip is in the proper position. After proper needle tip placement is confirmed, the remainder of the contents

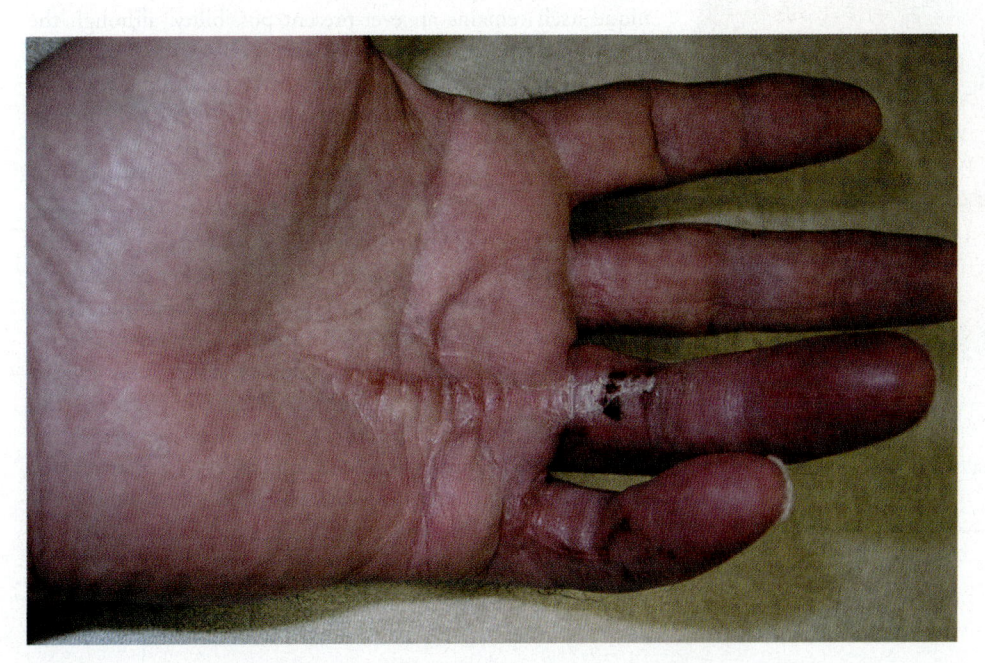

**FIGURE 76.2.** The characteristic flexion contracture of the fourth and fifth digits of Dupuytren contracture. (Reused from *Stedman's Medical Dictionary*. Philadelphia, PA: Lippincott Williams & Wilkins; with permission.)

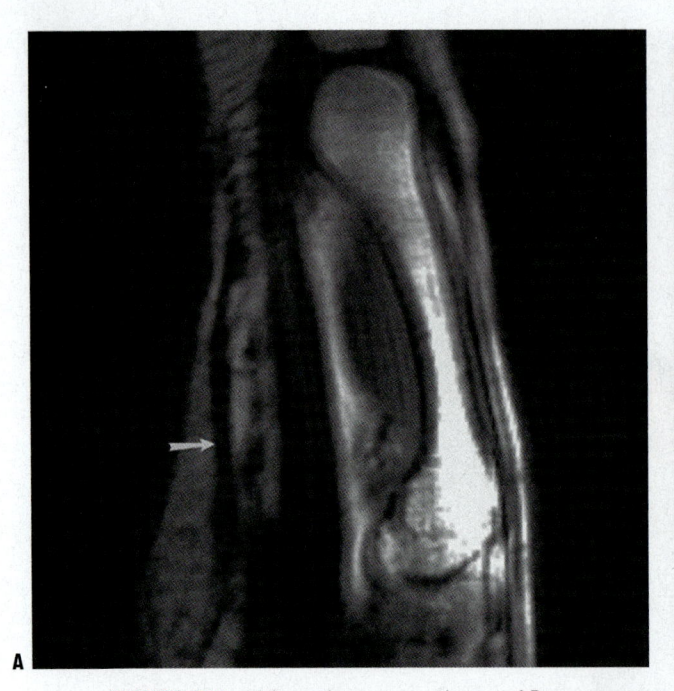

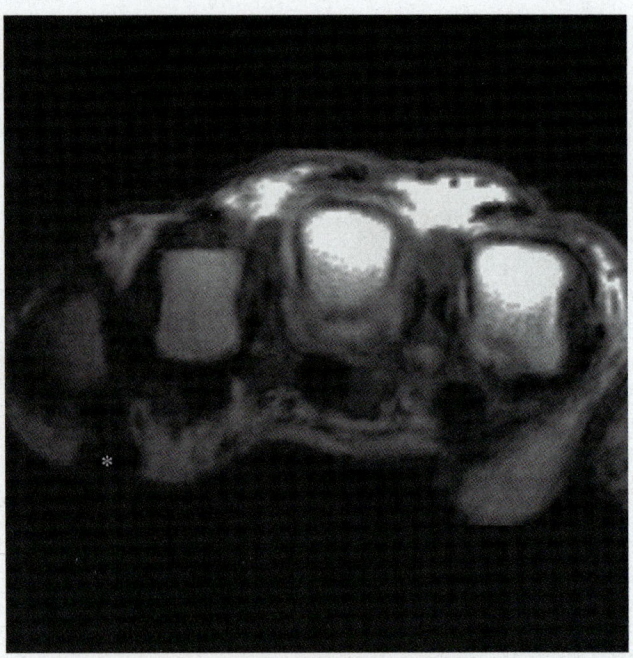

**FIGURE 76.3.** Magnetic resonance image of Dupuytren contracture. **A:** Sagittal T1-weighted image of the fifth metacarpal showing low-intensity cord (*arrow*). **B:** Axial T1-weighted image shows a classic subcutaneous nodule. (Reused from Berquist TH. *MRI of the Musculoskeletal System.* 5th ed. Philadelphia, PA: Lippincott Williams & Wilkins; 2006:920, with permission.)

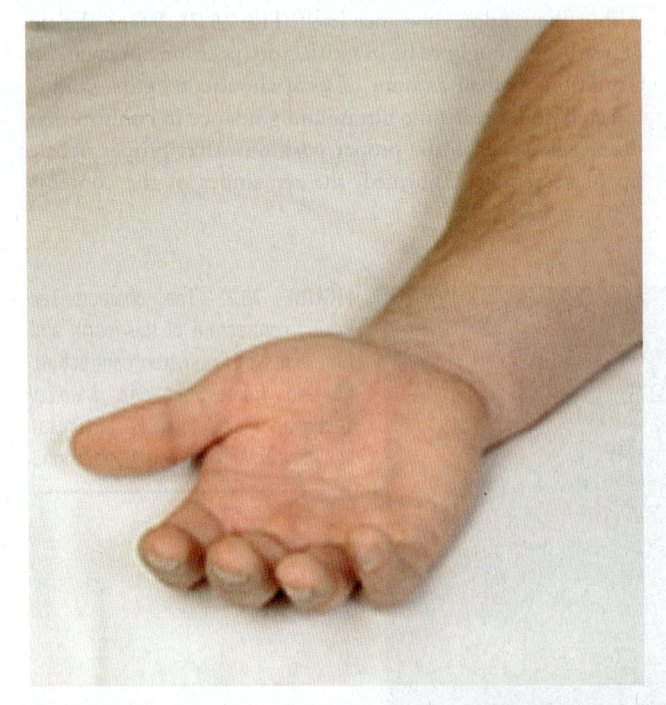

**FIGURE 76.4.** Proper patient positioning for ultrasound-guided injection for Dupuytren contracture.

of the syringe are slowly injected. There should be minimal resistance to injection.

## COMPLICATIONS

The possibility of trauma to the affected flexor digitorum superficialis and profundus tendons from this injection technique itself remains an ever-present possibility, although the risk of this is decreased if care is taken to place the needle outside the tendon and the injection is performed under real-time ultrasound visualization. Tendons that are highly inflamed or previously damaged are subject to rupture if substances are injected directly into the tendon. This complication can be greatly decreased if the clinician uses gentle technique and stops injecting immediately if significant resistance to injection is encountered. Approximately 25% of patients complain of a transient increase in pain after this injection technique; the patient should be warned of this. Infection, although uncommon, can occur. Ecchymosis and hematoma formation following this procedure may also occur. These complications can be decreased if manual pressure is applied to the area of the block immediately after injection. Application of cold packs for 20-minute periods after the block will also decrease the amount of postprocedure pain and bleeding the patient may experience.

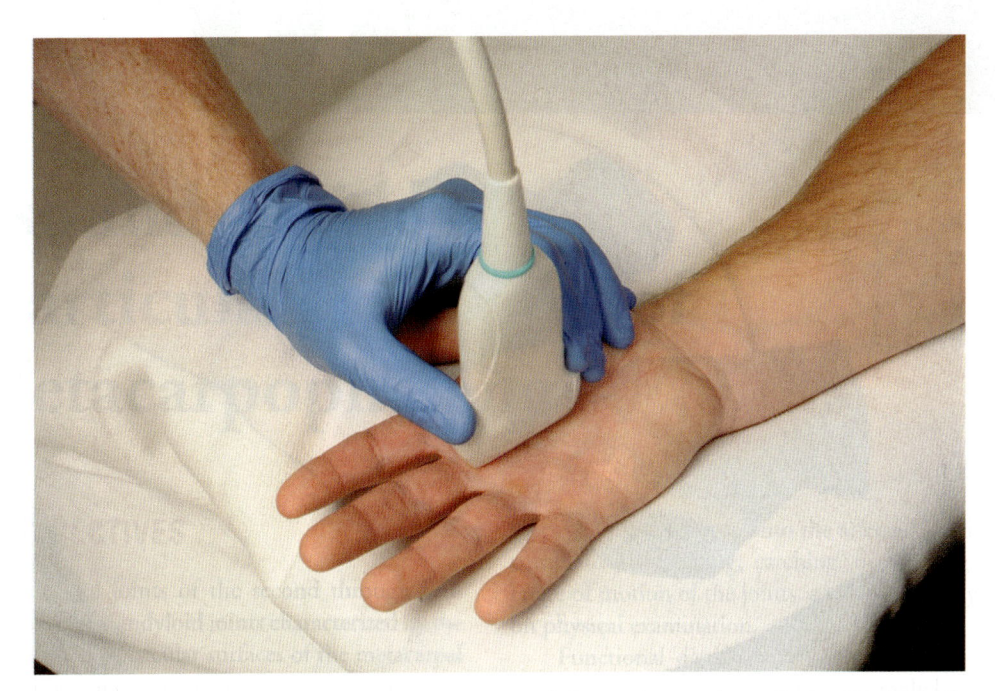

**FIGURE 76.5.** Proper longitudinal position of the small linear ultrasound transducer over the flexor tendons just proximal to the metacarpophalangeal joint.

## CLINICAL PEARLS

Ultrasound-guided injection for Dupuytren contracture is a straightforward and relatively safe technique if attention is paid to the clinically relevant anatomy. Recently, the use of collagenase *Clostridium histolyticum* injection has been advocated in the nonsurgical treatment of Dupuytren contracture.

The use of physical modalities, including local heat and gentle range-of-motion exercises, should be introduced several days after the patient undergoes this injection technique. Vigorous exercise should be avoided because it may exacerbate the patient's symptomatology. Simple analgesics and nonsteroidal anti-inflammatory agents may be used concurrently with this injection technique. Careful examination to identify

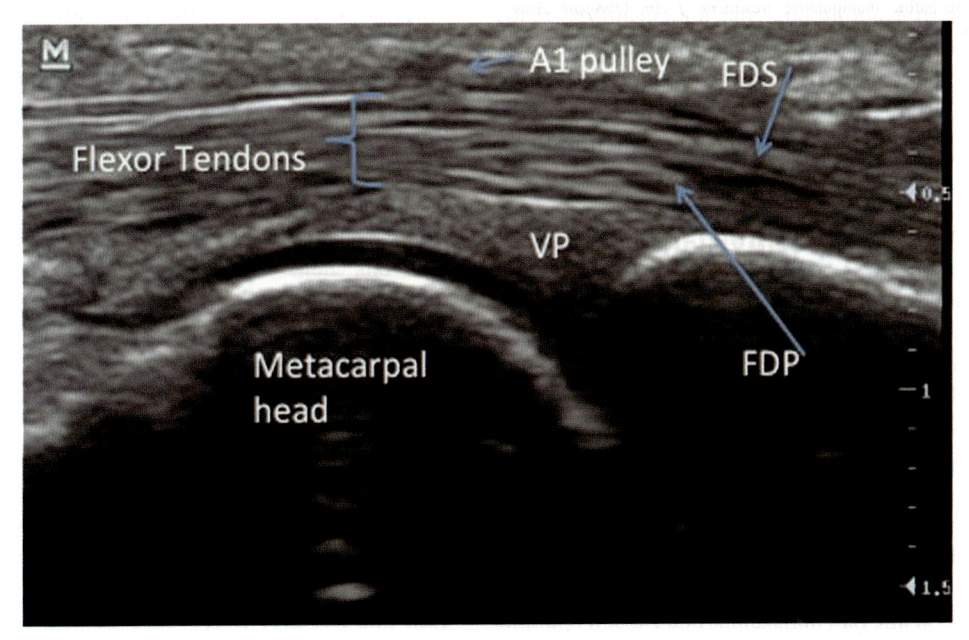

**FIGURE 76.6.** Longitudinal ultrasound image demonstrating the relationship of the A1 pulley, the tendons of the flexor digitorum superficialis and profundus, the volar plate, and the metacarpal.

**528** SECTION V WRIST AND HAND

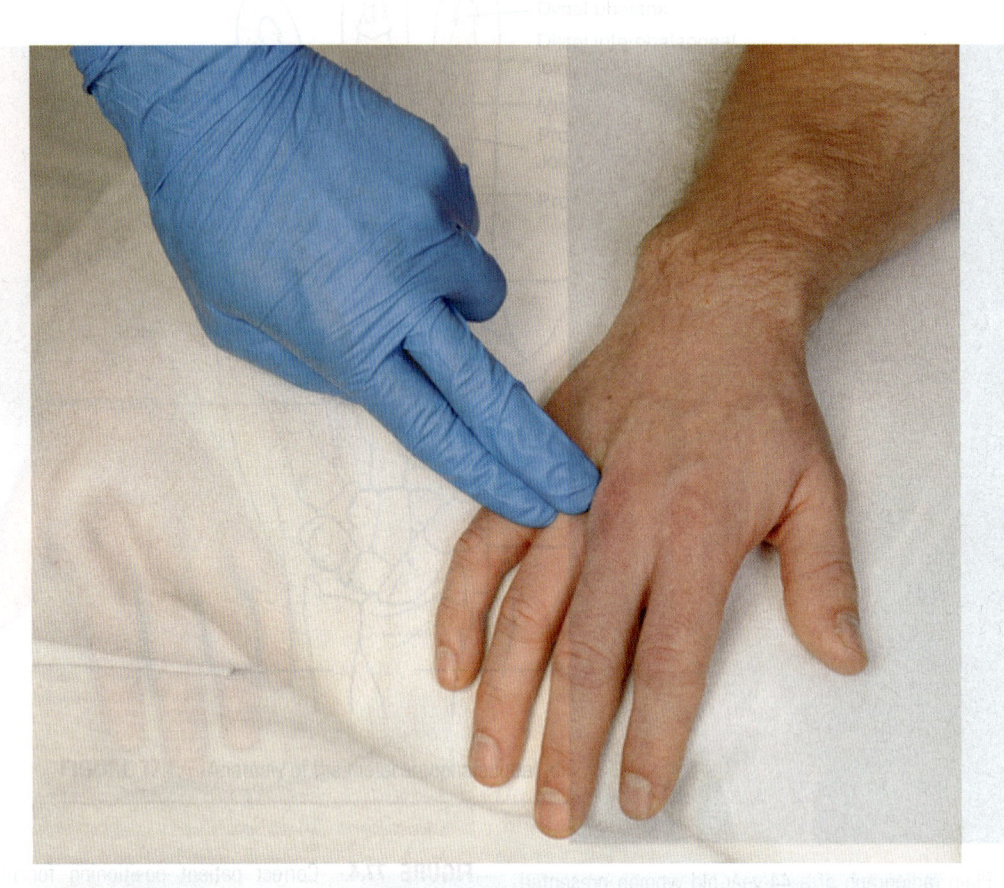

**FIGURE 77.5.** Palpation of the metacarpophalangeal joint.

**FIGURE 77.6.** Correct longitudinal position for ultrasound transducer for ultrasound-guided intra-articular injection of the metacarpophalangeal joints of the fingers joint.

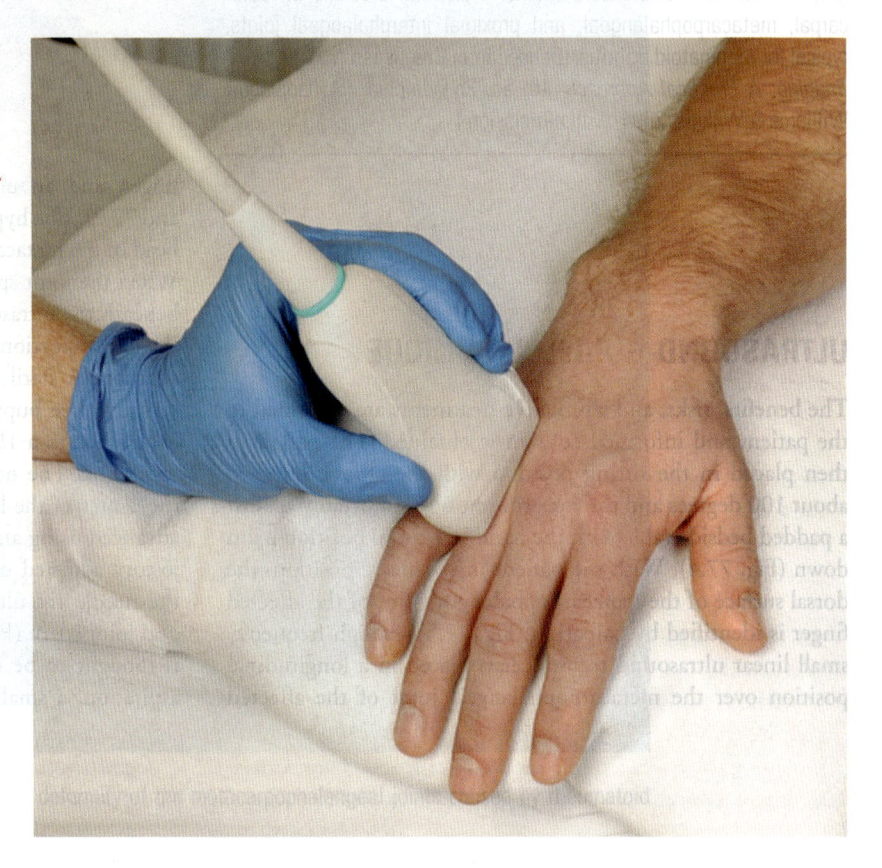

CHAPTER 77 ULTRASOUND-GUIDED INTRA-ARTICULAR INJECTION OF THE METACARPOPHALANGEAL JOINTS 529

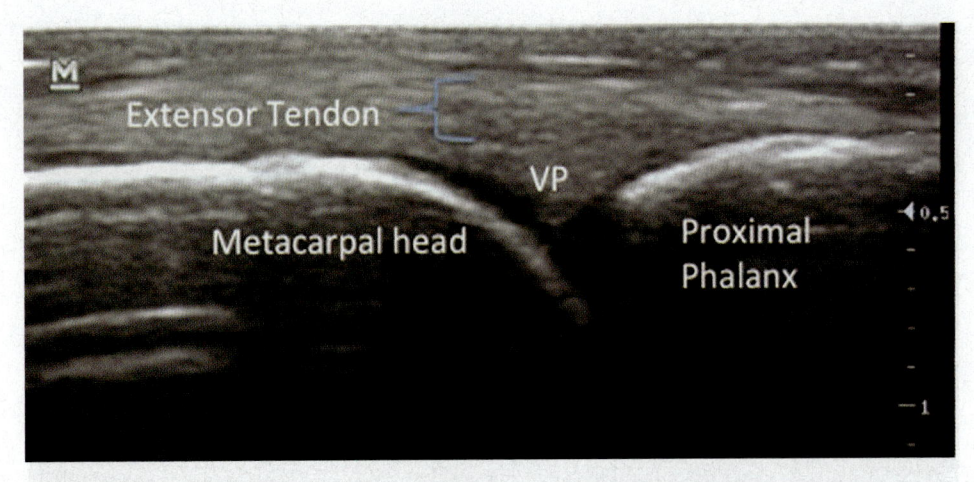

**FIGURE 77.7.** Longitudinal ultrasound view of the metacarpophalangeal joint space. (VP, volar plate.)

injected under real-time ultrasound guidance to confirm that the needle tip is in the proper position. After proper needle tip placement is confirmed, the remainder of the contents of the syringe are slowly injected. There should be minimal resistance to injection.

## COMPLICATIONS

The major complication of ultrasound-guided injection of the metacarpophalangeal joints of the fingers is infection. Ecchymosis and hematoma formation may also occur. A

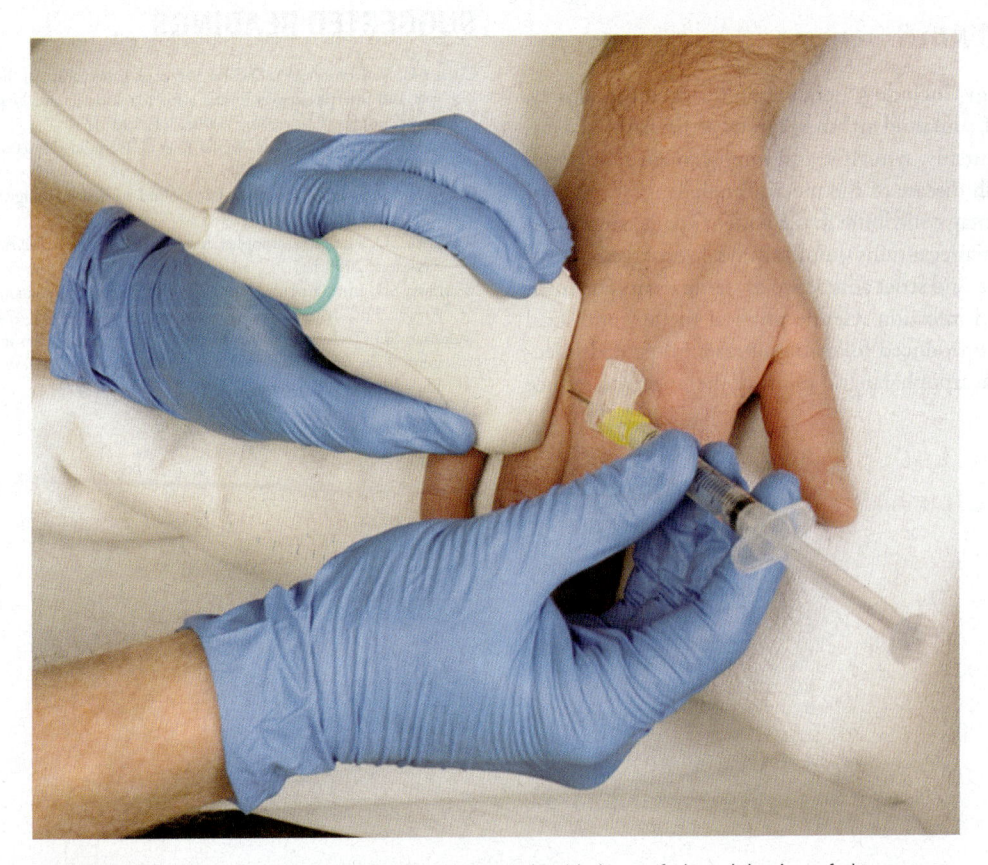

**FIGURE 77.8.** Proper needle position for ultrasound-guided out-of-plane injection of the metacarpophalangeal joint.

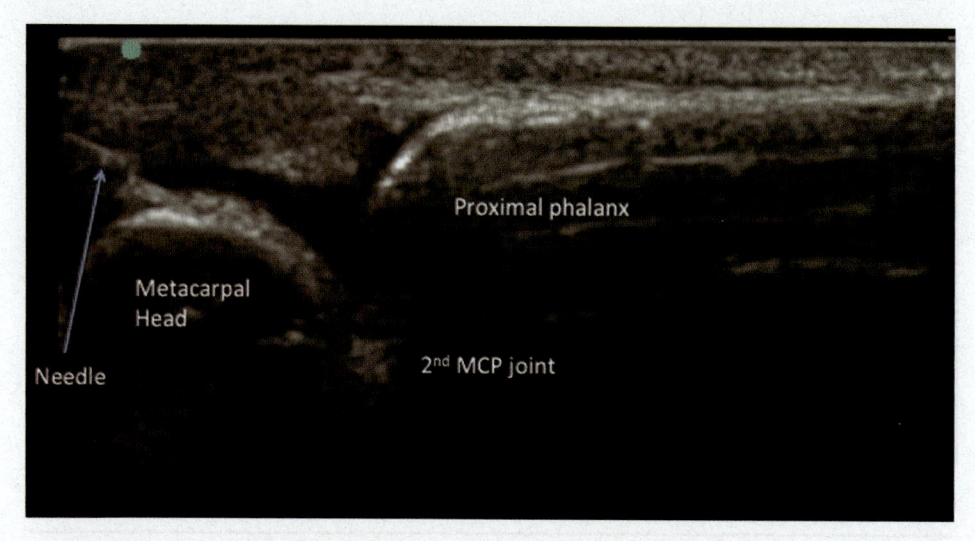

**FIGURE 77.9.** Ultrasound image of injection of the second metacarpophalangeal joint.

transient exacerbation of the patient's pain occurs ~25% of the time following this injection technique, and the patient should be warned of this possibility prior to the procedure.

## CLINICAL PEARLS

Finger pathology including tendinopathy, occult fractures, osteoarthritis, rheumatoid arthritis, crystal arthropathies, avascular necrosis bursitis, synovitis, and impingement syndromes may coexist with disease of the metacarpophalangeal joints of the fingers and may contribute to the patient's pain symptomatology. Universal precautions should always be observed to protect the operator, and strict adherence to sterile technique must be used to avoid infection. Gentle physical therapy and local heat should be introduced following ultrasound-guided injection of the metacarpophalangeal joints of the fingers to reduce pain and improve function. Simple analgesics and nonsteroidal anti-inflammatory agents or COX-2 inhibitors may be used concurrently with this injection technique.

## SUGGESTED READINGS

Chen Y-G, McClinton MA, DaSilva MF, et al. Innervation of the metacarpophalangeal and interphalangeal joints: a microanatomic and histologic study of the nerve endings. *J Hand Surg* 2000;25(1):128–133.

DeZordo T, Mur E, Bellmann-Weiler R, et al. US guided injections in arthritis. *Eur J Radiol* 2009;71(2):197–203.

Grassi W, Salaffi F, Filippucci E. Ultrasound in rheumatology. *Best Pract Res Clin Rheumatol* 2005;19(3):467–485.

Waldman SD. The metacarpophalangeal joints. In: *Pain Review*. Philadelphia, PA: Saunders; 2009:107.

Waldman SD. Intra-articular injection of the metacarpophalangeal joints. In: *Pain Review*. Philadelphia, PA: Saunders Elsevier; 2009:473–474.

Waldman SD. Technique for intra-articular injection of the metacarpophalangeal joint of the fingers. In: *Atlas of Pain Management Injection Techniques*. 3rd ed. Philadelphia, PA: Saunders Elsevier; 2013:224–225.

# CHAPTER 78

# Ultrasound-Guided Intra-articular Injection of the Interphalangeal Joints

## CLINICAL PERSPECTIVES

The interphalangeal joints are hinge-type joints between the phalanges that allow flexion and extension of the fingers (Fig. 78.1). The primary function of the interphalangeal joints of the fingers is to aid in the gripping and pinching functions of the hand. The articular cartilage of the interphalangeal joints of the fingers is susceptible to damage, which, if left untreated, will result in arthritis with its associated pain and functional disability. Osteoarthritis is most common cause of arthritis in the interphalangeal joints. Less common causes of arthritis-induced pain of the interphalangeal joints of the fingers include the collagen vascular diseases, infection, posttraumatic arthritis, villonodular synovitis, and Lyme disease (Fig. 78.2). Acute infectious arthritis of the interphalangeal joints of the fingers joint is best treated with early diagnosis, with culture and sensitivity of the synovial fluid and prompt initiation of antibiotic therapy. The collagen vascular diseases generally manifest as a polyarthropathy rather than a monoarthropathy limited to the interphalangeal joints of the fingers, although pain of the interphalangeal joints of the fingers secondary to the collagen vascular diseases responds exceedingly well to ultrasound-guided intra-articular injection.

Patients with pain of the interphalangeal joints of the fingers secondary to arthritis, gout, synovitis, and collagen vascular disease–related joint pain complain of pain that is localized to the head of the metacarpals. Activity, including grasping and pinching motions, makes the pain worse, with rest and heat providing some relief. The pain is constant and characterized as aching in nature. Sleep disturbance is common with awakening when patients roll over onto the affected hand. Some patients complain of a grating, catching, or popping sensation with range of motion of the joints, and crepitus may be appreciated on physical examination. Swelling of the joints commonly occurs with enlargement of the distal interphalangeal joints (called Heberden nodes) and enlargement of the proximal interphalangeal joints (called Bouchard nodes) (Figs. 78.3 and 78.4).

Plain radiographs are indicated in all patients who present with pain of the interphalangeal joints of the fingers (see Fig. 78.4). Based on the patient's clinical presentation, additional testing may be indicated, including complete blood cell count, sedimentation rate, and antinuclear antibody testing. Magnetic resonance imaging or ultrasound of the interphalangeal joints of the fingers joint is indicated if fracture, effusion, tendinopathy, crystal arthropathy, joint mice, synovitis, bursitis, or ligamentous injury is suspected.

## CLINICALLY RELEVANT ANATOMY

The interphalangeal joints of the fingers are hinge-type joints that provide articulation between the phalanges and allow ~100 degrees of flexion at the proximal interphalangeal joint and 80 degrees of flexion at the distal interphalangeal joint (Fig. 78.5). Hyperextension is limited by the volar and collateral ligaments, which, along with a dense joint capsule and surrounding tendons, help strengthen the interphalangeal joints and protect against subluxation.

## ULTRASOUND-GUIDED TECHNIQUE

The benefits, risks, and alternative treatments are explained to the patient, and informed consent is obtained. The patient is then placed in the sitting position with the elbow flexed to about 100 degrees and the forearm resting comfortably against a padded bedside table with the hand in neutral position palm down (Fig. 78.6). With the patient in the above position, the dorsal surface of the affected interphalangeal joint is identified by palpation. A high-frequency small linear ultrasound transducer is placed in a longitudinal position over the dorsal surface of the affected interphalangeal joint, and an ultrasound survey scan is taken (Figs. 78.7 and 78.8). The hypoechoic joint space is identified between the head of the metacarpal and the base of the proximal phalanges. When the joint space is identified, the skin overlying the area beneath the ultrasound transducer as well as the skin covering the lateral portion of the joint is then prepped with antiseptic solution. A sterile syringe containing 1.0 mL of 0.25% preservative-free bupivacaine

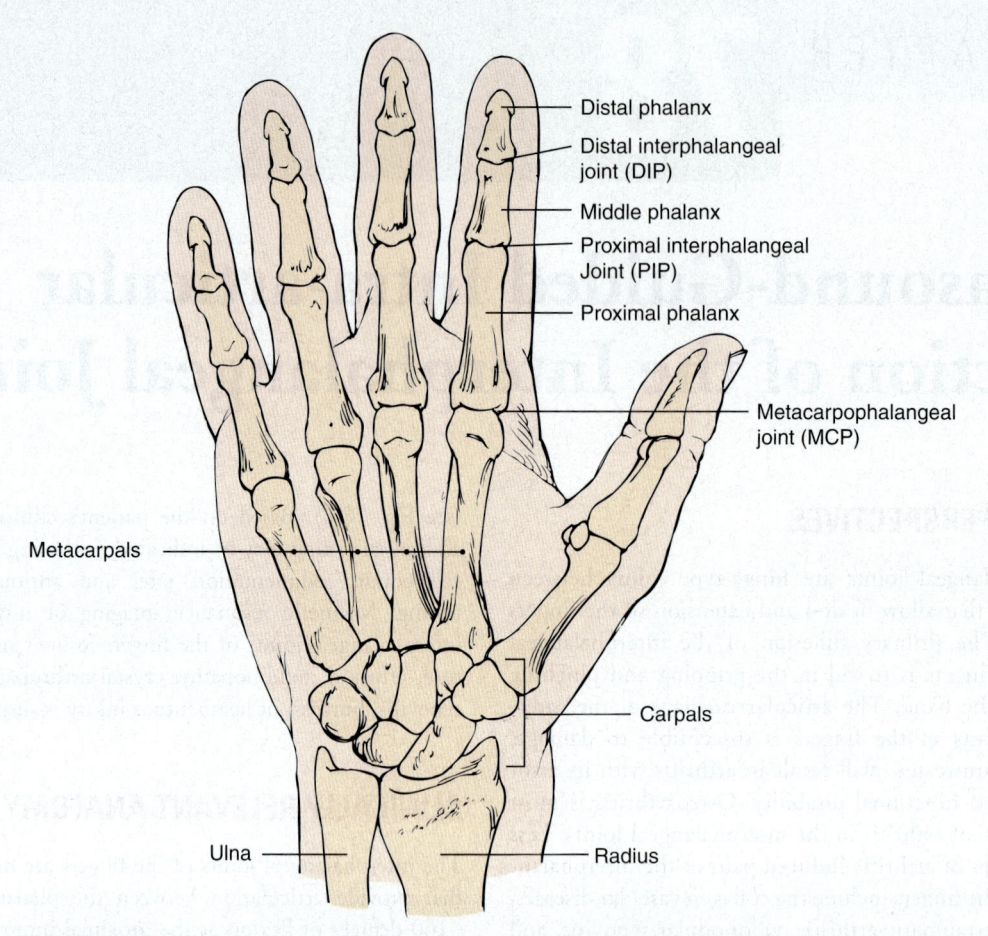

**FIGURE 78.1.** Anatomy of the interphalangeal joints. (Reused from Weber J, Kelley J. *Health Assessment in Nursing.* 2nd ed. Philadelphia, PA: Lippincott Williams & Wilkins; 2003, with permission.)

**FIGURE 78.2.** The characteristic deformity of the interphalangeal joints known as sausage finger caused by psoriatic arthritis. (Reused from Goodheart HP. *Goodheart's Photoguide of Common Skin Disorders.* 2nd ed. Philadelphia, PA: Lippincott Williams & Wilkins; 2003, with permission.)

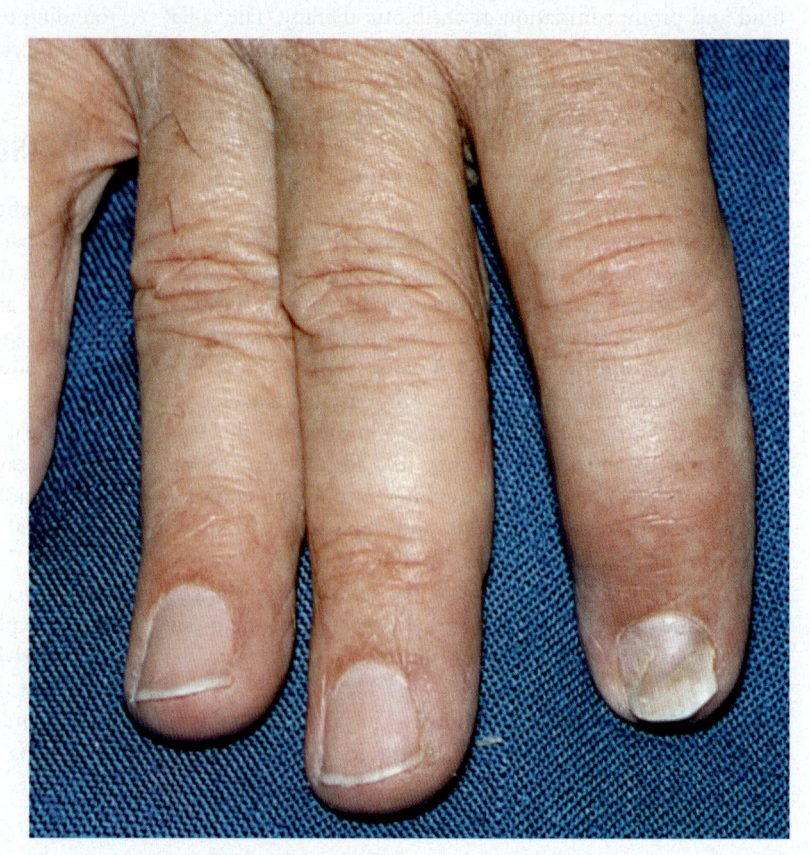

CHAPTER 78 ULTRASOUND-GUIDED INTRA-ARTICULAR INJECTION OF THE INTERPHALANGEAL JOINTS  533

and 40 mg of methylprednisolone is attached to a 1½-inch, 25-gauge needle using strict aseptic technique. The needle is placed through the skin just below the center of the longitudinally placed transducer and is then advanced using an out-of-plane approach with the needle trajectory adjusted under real-time ultrasound guidance so that the needle tip ultimately rests within the interphalangeal joint space (Fig. 78.9). When the tip of needle is thought to be in satisfactory position, after careful gentle aspiration, a small amount of local anesthetic and steroid is injected under real-time ultrasound guidance to confirm that the needle tip is in the proper position. After proper needle tip placement is confirmed, the remainder of the contents of the syringe are slowly injected. There should be minimal resistance to injection. The technique can be repeated for the distal interphalangeal joints (Fig. 78.10).

## COMPLICATIONS

The major complication of ultrasound-guided injection of the interphalangeal joints of the fingers is infection. Ecchymosis and hematoma formation may also occur. A transient exacerbation of the patient's pain occurs ~25% of the time following

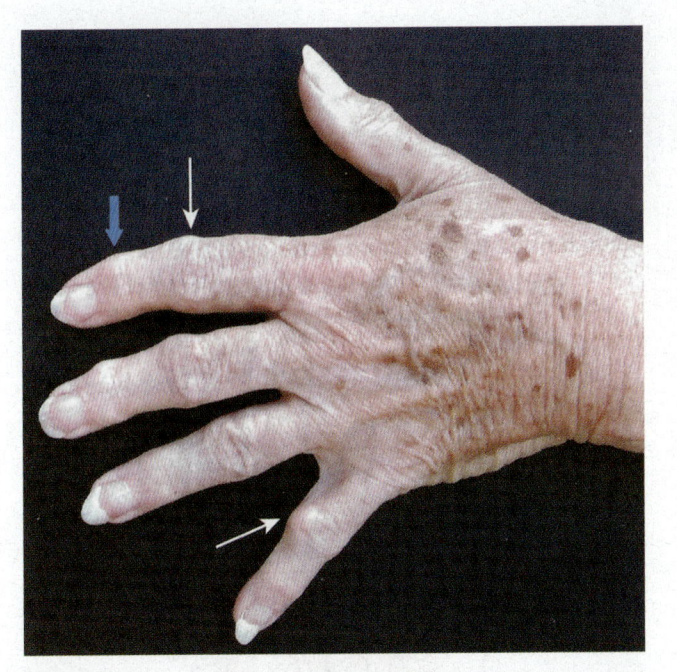

**FIGURE 78.3.** Heberden (*blue arrow*) and Bouchard (*white arrows*) nodes are characteristic findings of osteoarthritis of the interphalangeal joints.

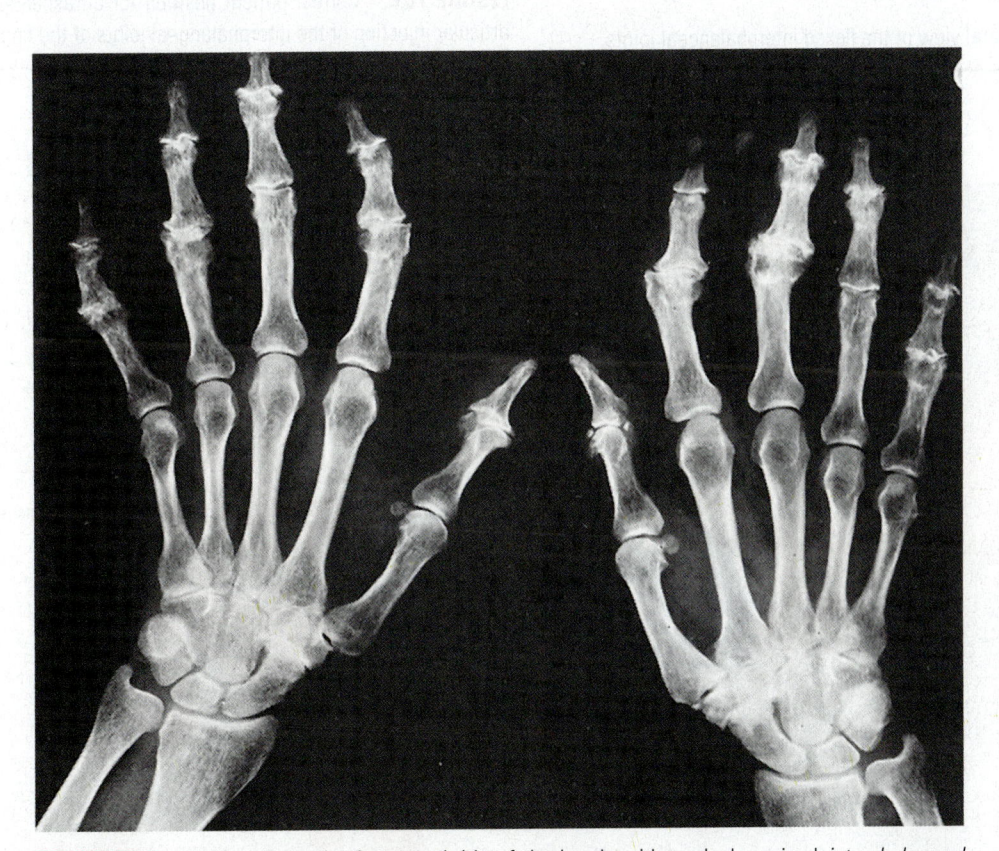

**FIGURE 78.4.** Plain radiograph of osteoarthritis of the hands with marked proximal *interphalangeal joint* involvement (Bouchard nodes) as well as distal *interphalangeal joint* involvement (Heberden nodes). (Reused from Koopman WJ, Moreland LW. *Arthritis and Allied Conditions: A Textbook of Rheumatology.* 15th ed. Philadelphia, PA: Lippincott Williams & Wilkins; 2005, with permission.)

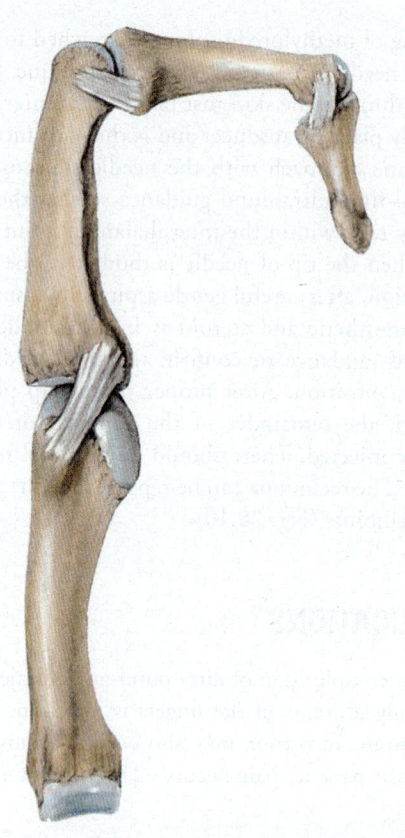

**FIGURE 78.5.** Lateral view of the flexed interphalangeal joints.

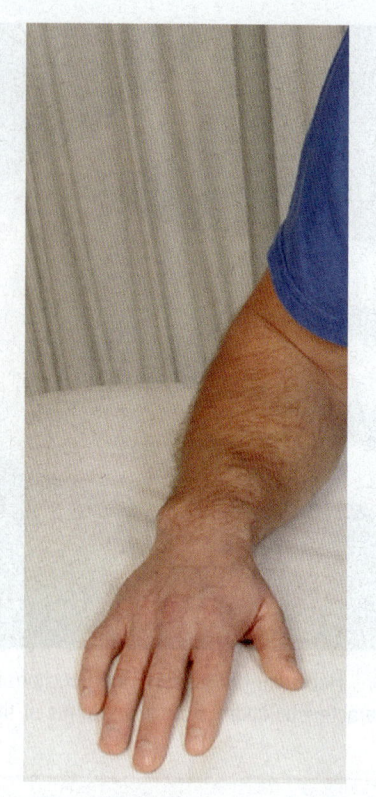

**FIGURE 78.6.** Correct patient position for ultrasound-guided intra-articular injection of the interphalangeal joints of the fingers joint.

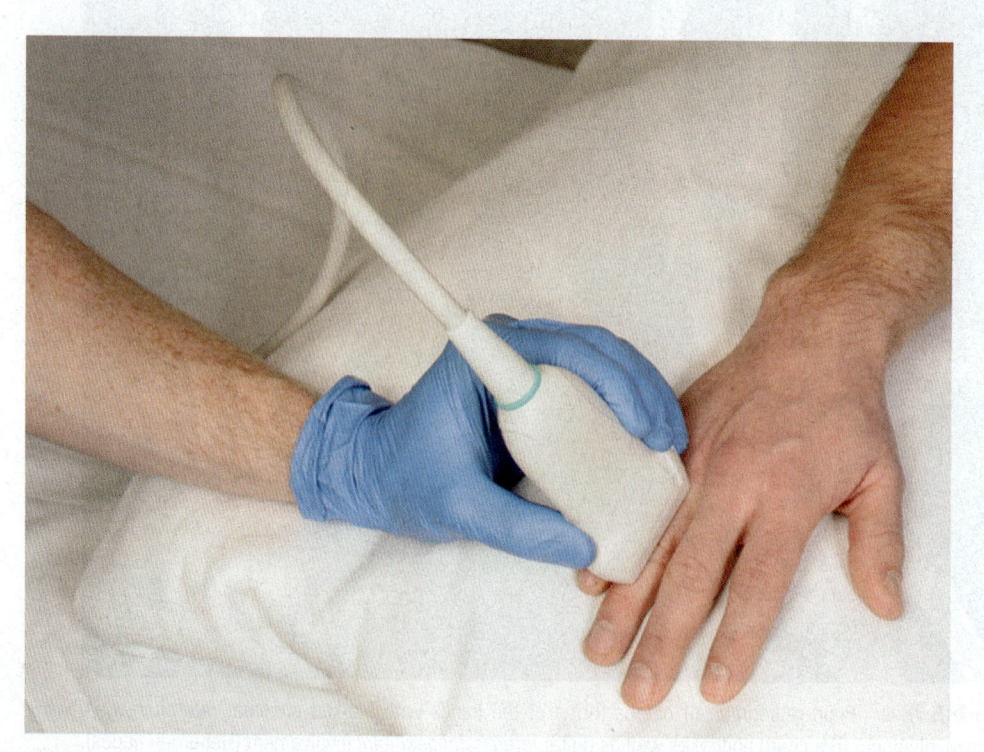

**FIGURE 78.7.** Correct longitudinal position for ultrasound transducer for ultrasound-guided intra-articular injection of the interphalangeal joints of the fingers joint.

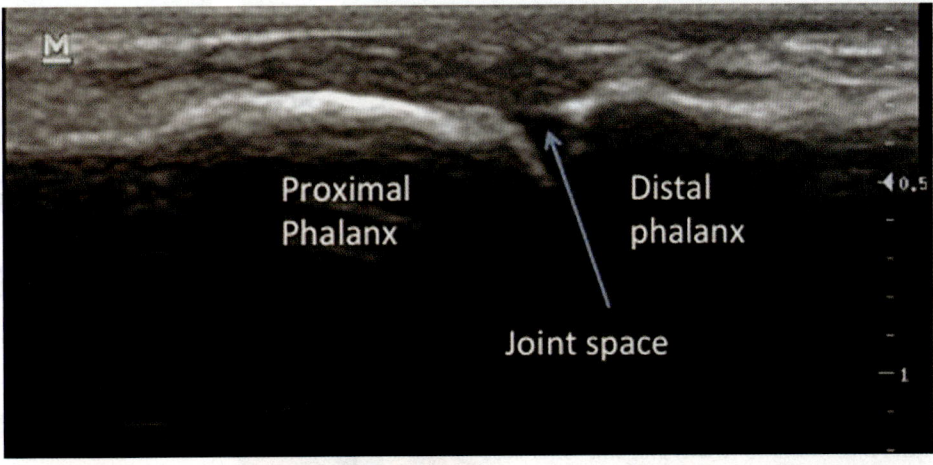

**FIGURE 78.8.** Longitudinal ultrasound view of the interphalangeal joint space.

this injection technique, and the patient should be warned of this possibility prior to the procedure.

## CLINICAL PEARLS

Finger pathology including tendinopathy, occult fractures, osteoarthritis, rheumatoid arthritis, crystal arthropathies, avascular necrosis bursitis, synovitis, and impingement syndromes may coexist with disease of the interphalangeal joints of the fingers and may contribute to the patient's pain symptomatology. Universal precautions should always be observed to protect the operator, and strict adherence to sterile technique must be used to avoid infection. Gentle physical therapy and local heat should be introduced following ultrasound-guided injection of the interphalangeal joints of the fingers to reduce pain and improve function. Simple analgesics and nonsteroidal anti-inflammatory agents or COX-2 inhibitors may be used concurrently with this injection technique.

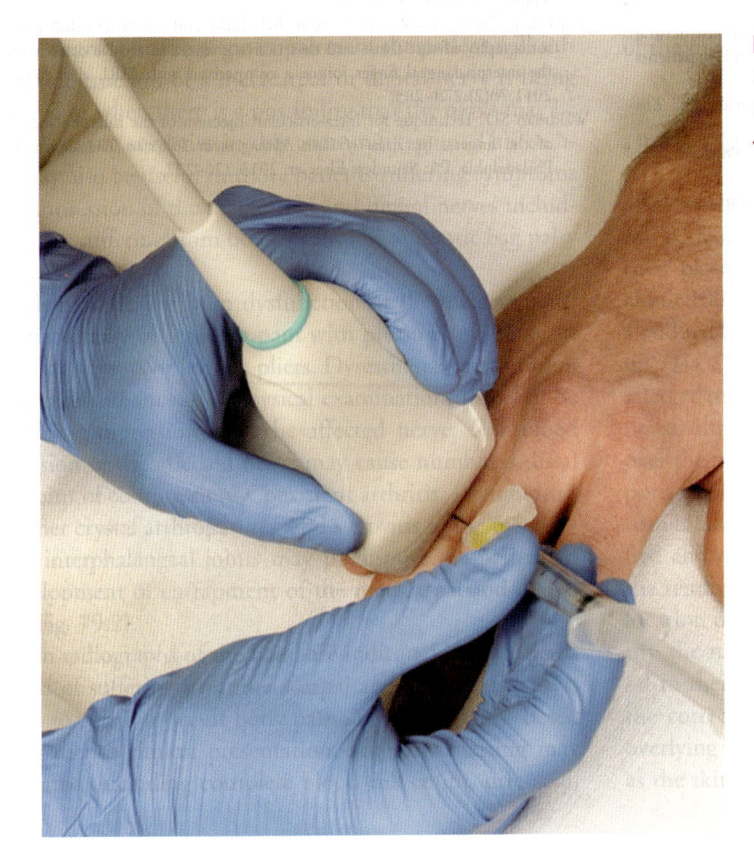

**FIGURE 78.9.** Proper needle position for ultrasound-guided out-of-plane injection of the proximal interphalangeal joint.

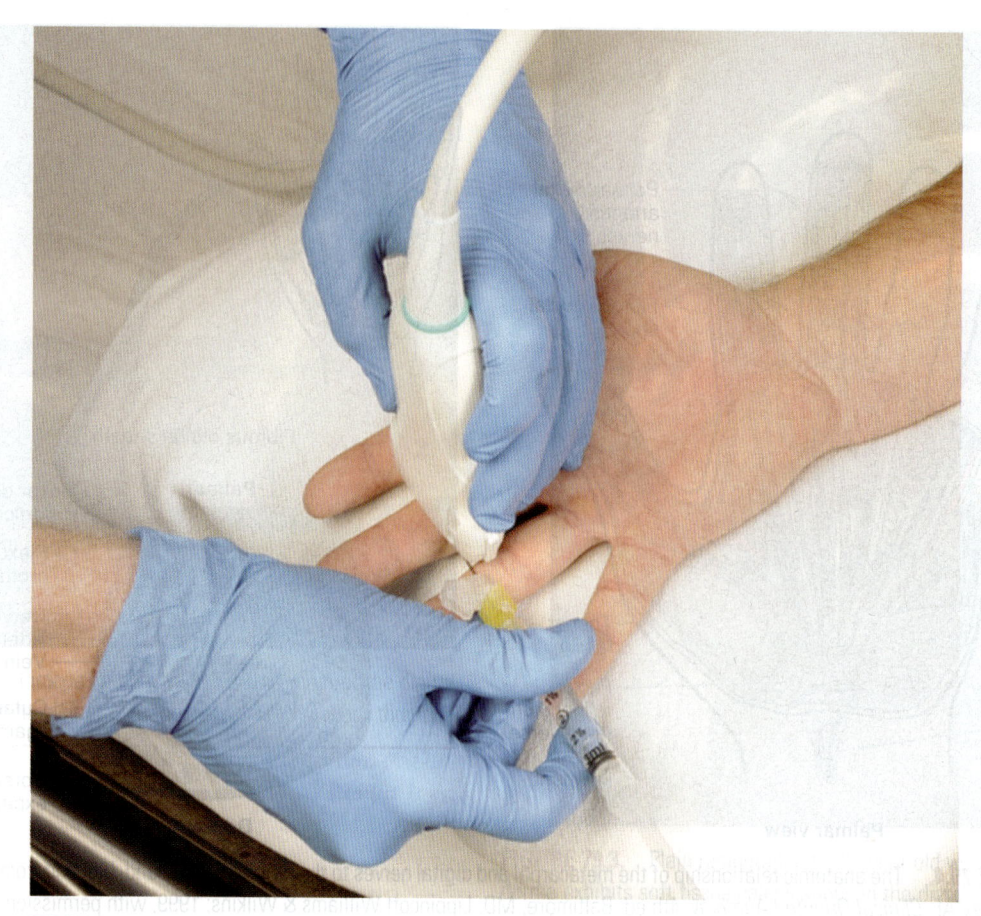

**FIGURE 79.6.** Proper transverse position for the linear high-frequency ultrasound transducer to perform ultrasound-guided metacarpal and digital nerves injection.

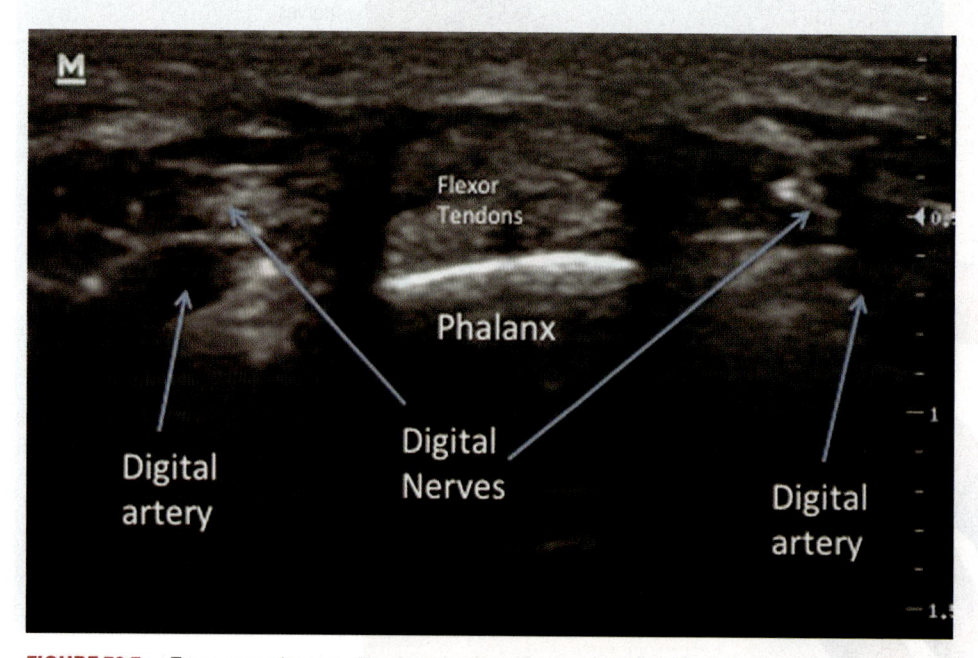

**FIGURE 79.7.** Transverse ultrasound image demonstrating the relationship of the flexor tendons and the artery and nerve at the level of the distal metacarpal.

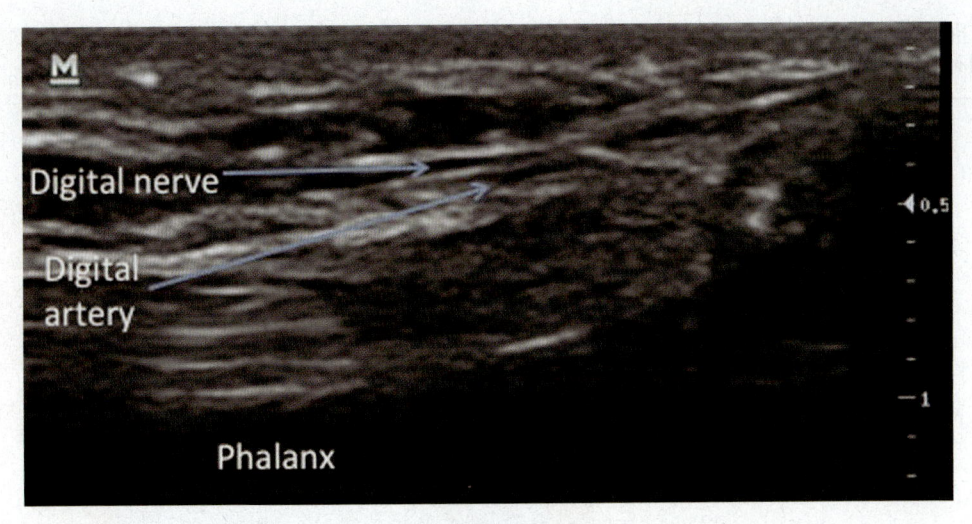

**FIGURE 79.8.** Longitudinal ultrasound view of the digital nerve of the index finger.

prepped with antiseptic solution. A sterile syringe containing 1.0 mL of 0.25% preservative-free bupivacaine and 40 mg of methylprednisolone is attached to a 1½-inch, 25-gauge needle using strict aseptic technique. The needle is placed through the skin just below the inferior border of the transducer and is then advanced using an out-of-plane approach with the needle trajectory adjusted under real-time ultrasound guidance so that the needle tip ultimately rests in proximity to the digital nerve (Fig. 79.10). When the tip of needle is thought to be in satisfactory position, after careful aspiration, a small amount of local anesthetic and steroid is injected under real-time ultrasound guidance to confirm that the needle tip is in the proper position. After proper needle tip placement is confirmed, the remainder of the contents of the syringe are slowly injected. There should be minimal resistance to injection.

## COMPLICATIONS

The possibility of trauma to the flexor digitorum superficialis and profundus tendons, the metacarpal or digital nerves, and their corresponding arteries from this injection technique remains an ever-present possibility, although the risk of this is decreased if care is taken to place the needle outside the tendon and nerve and the injection is performed under real-time ultrasound visualization. Tendons that are highly inflamed or previously damaged are subject to rupture if substances are injected directly into the tendon. This complication can be greatly decreased if the clinician uses gentle technique and stops injecting immediately if significant resistance to injection is encountered. Approximately 25% of patients complain of a transient increase in pain after this injection technique; the

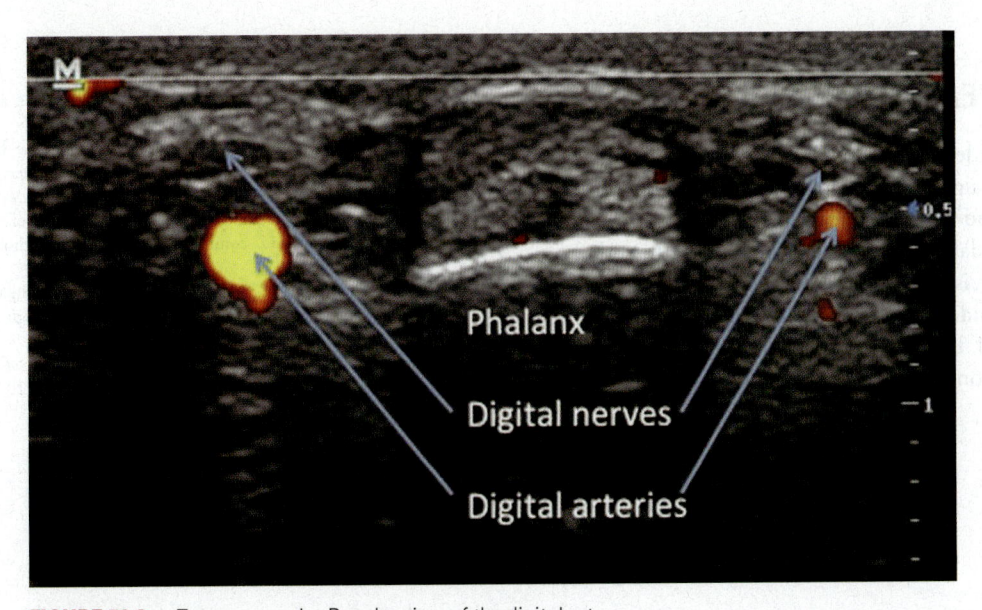

**FIGURE 79.9.** Transverse color Doppler view of the digital artery.

**FIGURE 79.10.** Proper in-plane needle placement for ultrasound-guided injection of the digital nerve.

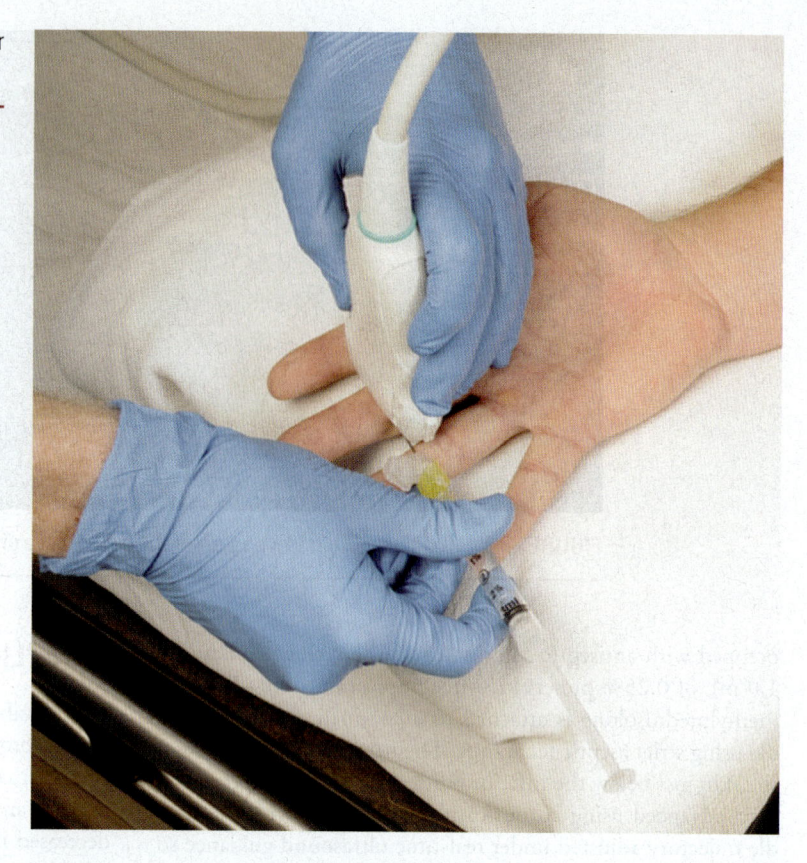

patient should be warned of this. Infection, although uncommon, can occur. Ecchymosis and hematoma formation following this procedure may also occur. These complications can be decreased if manual pressure is applied to the area of the block immediately after injection. Application of cold packs for 20-minute periods after the block will also decrease the amount of postprocedure pain and bleeding the patient may experience.

## CLINICAL PEARLS

Ultrasound-guided injection of the metacarpal and digital nerves is a straightforward and relatively safe technique if attention is paid to the clinically relevant anatomy. The use of physical modalities, including local heat and gentle range-of-motion exercises, should be introduced several days after the patient undergoes this injection technique. Vigorous exercise should be avoided because it may exacerbate the patient's symptomatology. Simple analgesics and nonsteroidal anti-inflammatory agents may be used concurrently with this injection technique. Careful neurologic examination to identify preexisting nerve compromise that may later be attributed to the procedure should be performed on all patients before beginning ultrasound-guided injection for metacarpal and digital nerves.

## SUGGESTED READINGS

Bodor M, Fullerton B. Ultrasonography of the hand, wrist, and elbow. *Phys Med Rehabil Clin N Am* 2010;21(3):509–531.

Mohan PP. Towards evidence based emergency medicine: best BETs from the Manchester Royal Infirmary. Epinephrine in digital nerve block. *Emerg Med J* 2007;24(11):789–790.

Ragheb D, Stanley A, Gentili A, et al. MR imaging of the finger tendons: normal anatomy and commonly encountered pathology. *Eur J Radiol* 2005;56(3):296–306.

Thomson CJ, Lalonde DH. Randomized double-blind comparison of duration of anesthesia among three commonly used agents in digital nerve block. *Plast Reconstr Surg* 2006;118(2):429–432.

Waldman SD. Metacarpal and digital nerves. In: *Atlas of Interventional Pain Management*. 3rd ed. Philadelphia, PA: WB Saunders; 2009:248–250.

# SECTION VI

# Chest Wall, Trunk, and Abdomen

# CHAPTER 80

# Ultrasound-Guided Injection Technique for Sternoclavicular Joint Pain

## CLINICAL PERSPECTIVES

The sternoclavicular (SC) joint is susceptible to injury from acute blunt trauma from motor vehicle accidents and contact sports such as football and rugby as well as repetitive microtrauma from activities that require repeated thrusting of the arm forward to grab objects off an assembly line or shrugging of the shoulder when reaching overhead in close quarters. Left untreated, the acute inflammation associated with the injury may result in arthritis with its associated pain and functional disability. Patients suffering from SC joint dysfunction or inflammation will complain of a marked exacerbation of pain when they perform activities that require thrusting the arm forward and retracting or shrugging the shoulder. A grating or grinding sensation with joint movement is often noted, and the patient frequently is unable to sleep on the affected side. Patients with SC joint dysfunction and inflammation will exhibit pain on active protraction or retraction of the shoulder as well as with raising of the arm high above the head. Palpation of the SC joint often reveals swelling or enlargement of the joint secondary to joint effusion. If there is disruption of the ligaments that surround and support the SC joint, joint instability and a cosmetic defect may be evident on physical examination (Fig. 80.1).

Plain radiographs and computerized tomography are indicated in patients suffering from SC joint pain. They may reveal narrowing or sclerosis of the joint consistent with osteoarthritis or widening of the joint consistent with ligamentous injury (Fig. 80.2). They may also reveal occult fractures or primary or metastatic tumors as the joint is subject to invasion from malignant thymomas. If joint instability, infection, or tumor is suspected or detected on physical examination, magnetic resonance imaging, computerized tomography, and/or ultrasound scanning is a reasonable next step. Ultrasound-guided SC joint injection can aid the clinician in both the diagnosis and treatment of SC joint pain and dysfunction (Fig. 80.3).

## CLINICALLY RELEVANT ANATOMY

The SC joint is a double gliding saddle-type synovial joint with an intra-articular disc separating the medial end of the clavicle and manubrium of the sternum (Fig. 80.4). Articulation occurs between the sternal end of the clavicle, the sternal manubrium, and the cartilage of the first rib with only ~50% of the medial end of the clavicle actually articulating with the manubrium of the sternum. Because of this the joint is inherently unstable, with the inferior portion of the joint most subject to subluxation or dislocation. The joint is reinforced in front and back by the SC ligaments. Additional support is provided by the costoclavicular ligament, which runs from the junction of the first rib and its costal cartilage to the inferior surface of the clavicle. Additional strength is provided by the joint capsule. The joint is dually innervated by both the supraclavicular nerve and the nerve supplying the subclavius muscle. Behind the SC joint are a number of large arteries and veins, including the left common carotid and brachiocephalic vein and, on the right, the brachiocephalic artery. These vessels are susceptible to needle-induced trauma if the needle is placed too deeply or trauma from the elements of the joint should the joint be dislocated posteriorly due to blunt trauma to the anterior chest. The serratus anterior muscle produces forward movement of the clavicle at the SC joint, with backward movement at the joint produced by the rhomboid and trapezius muscles. Elevation of the clavicle at the SC joint is produced by the sternocleidomastoid, rhomboid, and levator scapulae. Depression of the clavicle at the joint is produced by the pectoralis minor and subclavius muscle. On palpation of the joint, a small indentation can be felt where the medial clavicle abuts the manubrium. The volume of the SC joint space is small, and care must be taken not to disrupt the joint by forcefully injecting large volumes of local anesthetic and corticosteroid into the intra-articular space when performing this injection technique.

## ULTRASOUND-GUIDED TECHNIQUE

The benefits, risks, and alternative treatments are explained to the patient and informed consent is obtained. The patient is then placed in the supine position with the shoulders relaxed and the arms resting comfortably at the patient's side (Fig. 80.5). The SC joint is then identified by palpation (Fig. 80.6). The skin overlying the SC joint is then prepped with antiseptic solution. A sterile syringe containing 1.0 mL of 0.25% preservative-free bupivacaine and 40 mg of methylprednisolone is attached to a 1½-inch, 22-gauge needle using

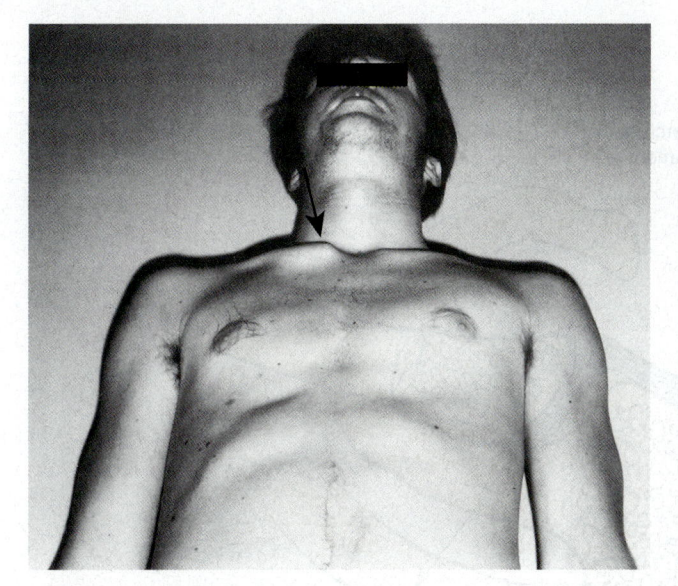

**FIGURE 80.1.** Patient with an anterior dislocation of the right *sternoclavicular joint* (*arrow*). (Reused from Bucholz RW, Heckman JD. *Rockwood and Green's Fractures in Adults*. 5th ed. Philadelphia, PA: Lippincott Williams & Wilkins; 2001, with permission.)

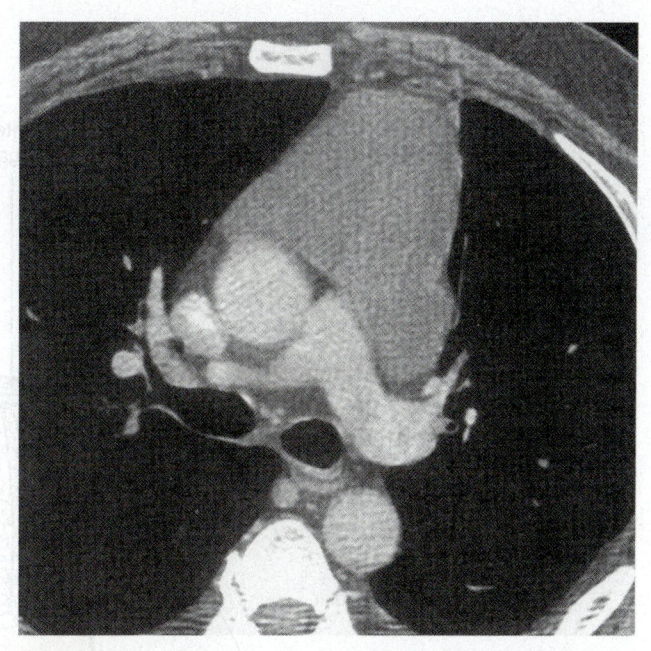

**FIGURE 80.2.** Computerized tomography (CT) demonstrating a cystic thymoma invading the anterior chest wall and SC joint. (Reused from Eisenberg RL. *Clinical Imaging*. 5th ed. Philadelphia, PA: Lippincott Williams & Wilkins; 2010, with permission.)

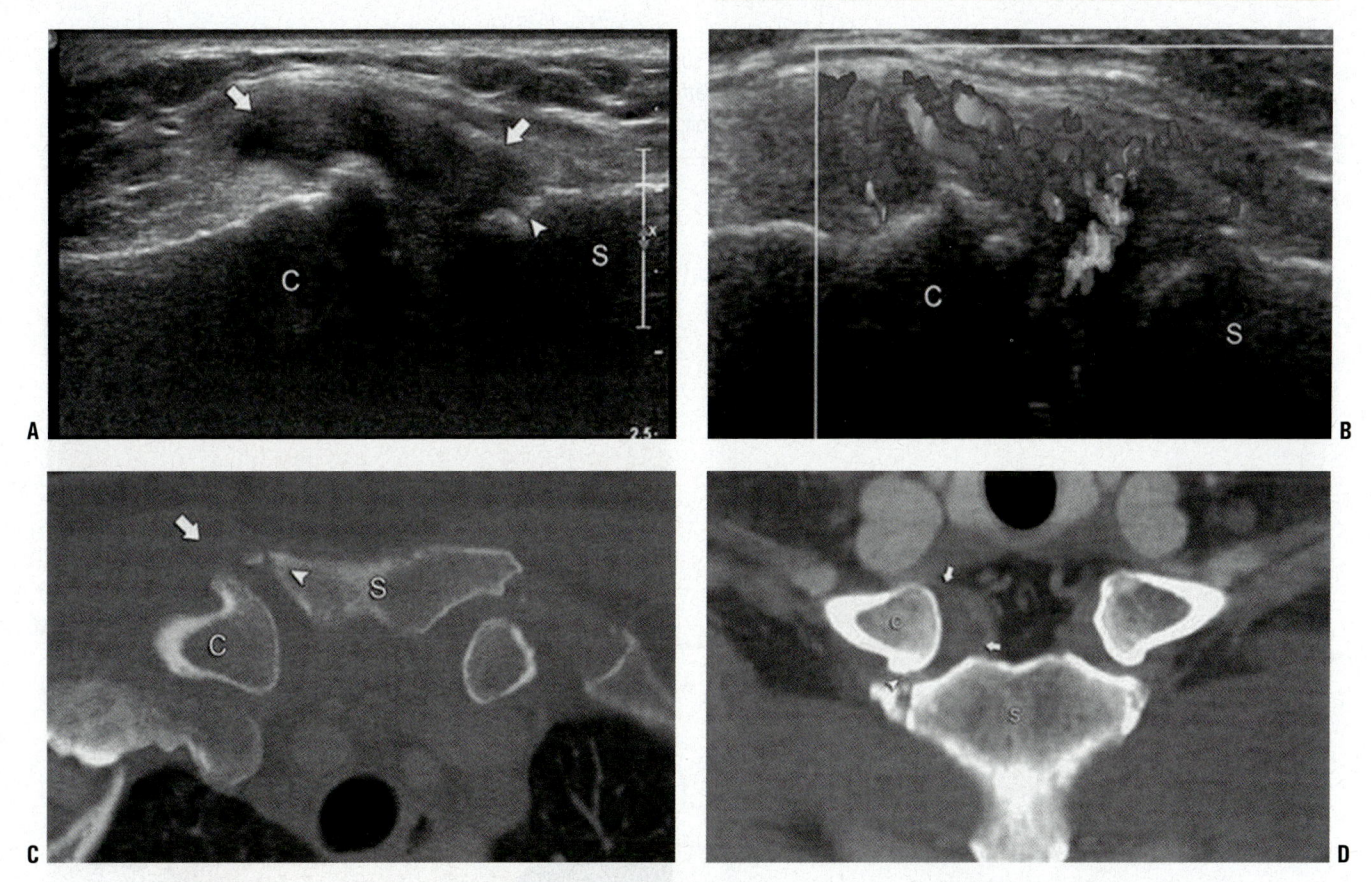

**FIGURE 80.3.** A 53-year-old woman with a degenerative right SC joint (history of mass and pain). **(A)** Coronal–oblique ultrasound image and **(B)** coronal–oblique color Doppler ultrasound image. **(C)** Axial noncontrast CT image and **(D)** coronal multiplanar reformatted CT image after intravenous administration of contrast agent show distention of the SC joint (*arrows*) (8 mm) that extends over the clavicle (C), which is predominately hypoechoic on ultrasound (A) and soft tissue attenuation on CT (C). Note bone irregularity from osteophytes (*arrowheads*), and hyperemia on color Doppler ultrasound (B). After intravenous administration of contrast medium (D) there is peripheral enhancement of the joint. (Reused from Johnson MC, Jacobson JA, Fessell DP, et al. The sternoclavicular joint: can imaging differentiate infection from degenerative change? *Skeletal Radiol* 2010;39(6):551–558, with permission.)

**546** SECTION VI CHEST WALL, TRUNK, AND ABDOMEN

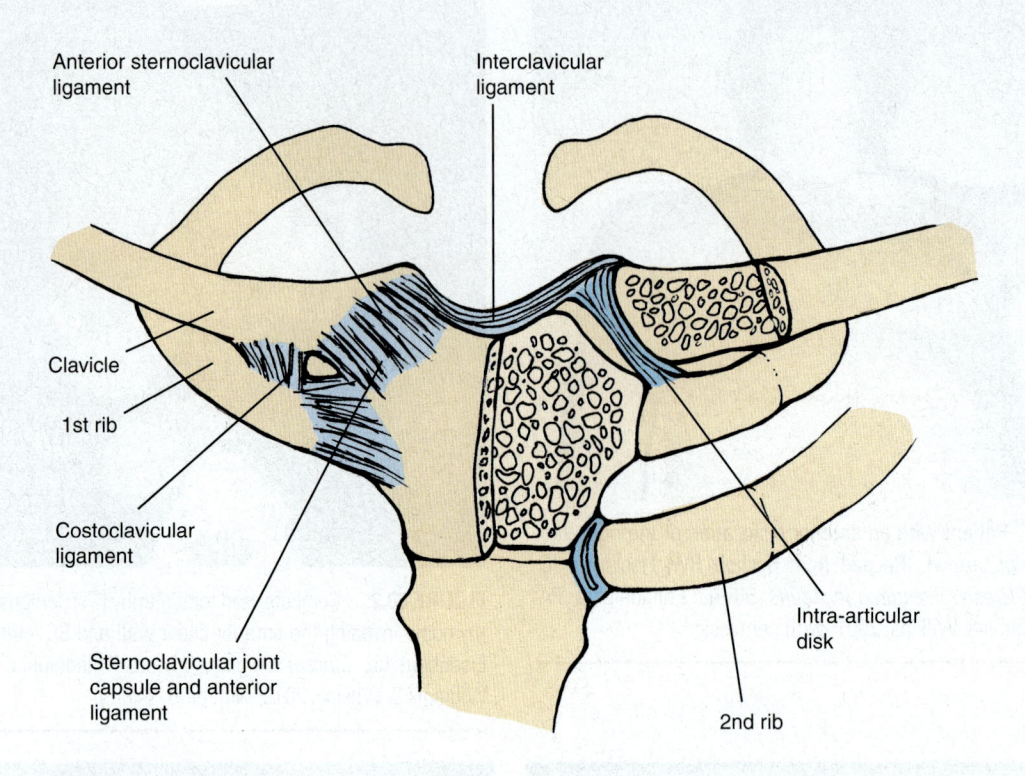

**FIGURE 80.4.** Anatomy of the SC joint. Note the supporting ligaments and intra-articular disc. (Reused from Oatis CA. *Kinesiology: The Mechanics and Pathomechanics of Human Movement.* Baltimore, MD: Lippincott Williams & Wilkins; 2003, with permission.)

**FIGURE 80.5.** Proper supine position for ultrasound-guided injection of the SC joint.

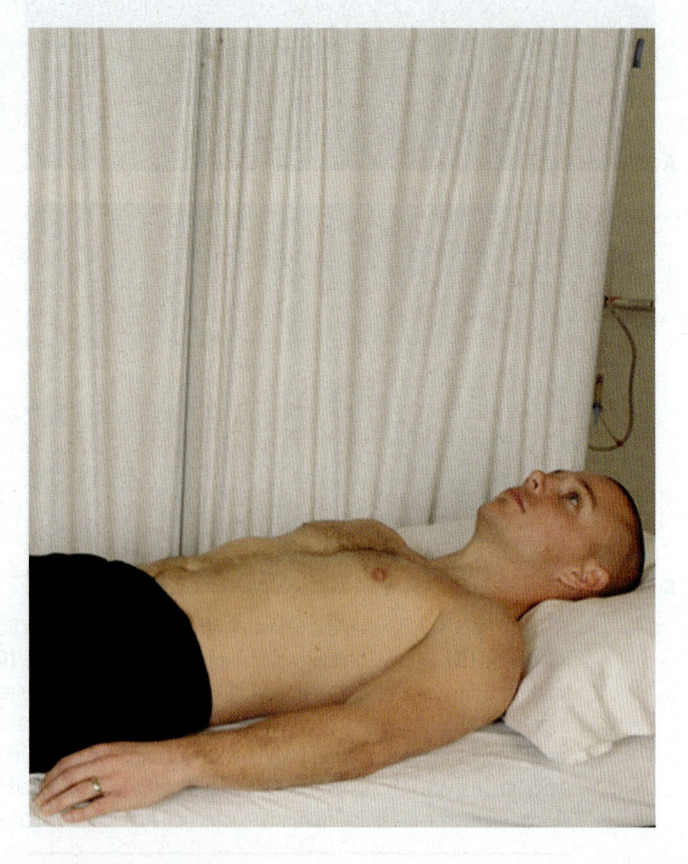

# CHAPTER 80  ULTRASOUND-GUIDED INJECTION TECHNIQUE FOR STERNOCLAVICULAR JOINT PAIN

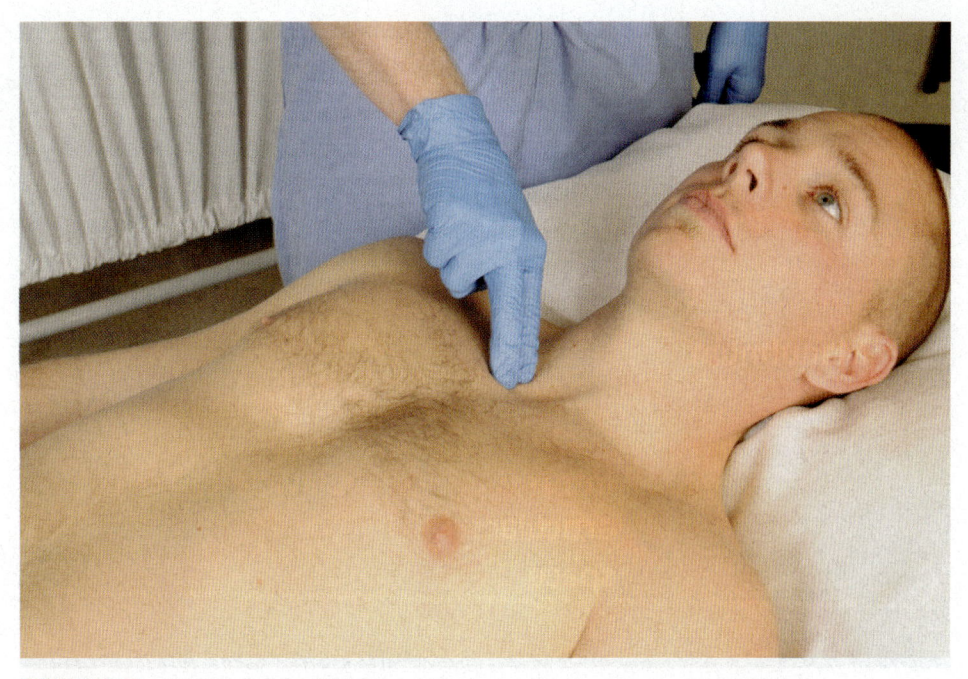

**FIGURE 80.6.** Palpation of the SC joint.

strict aseptic technique. A linear high-frequency ultrasound transducer is placed in the transverse plane across the SC joint in the coronal plane (Fig. 80.7). Slowly move the ultrasound transducer to identify the manubrium and the medial end of the clavicle and the SC joint in between (Fig. 80.8). To facilitate needle placement, position the ultrasound transducer so the center of the V-shaped hypoechoic joint is in the center of the image between the hyperechoic margins of the manubrium of the sternum and medial end of the clavicle. In some patients, a hyperechoic intra-articular disc can be identified, and if a significant joint effusion is present, bulging of the joint capsule may be apparent. After the joint space is identified, the needle is placed through the skin just below the middle of the ultrasound transducer and is then advanced using an

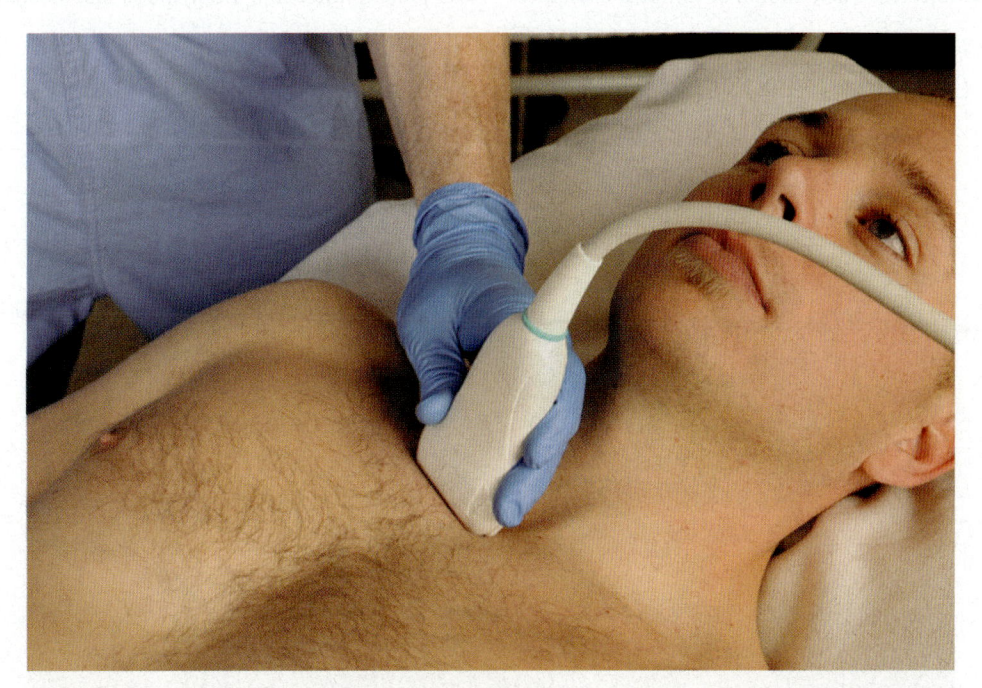

**FIGURE 80.7.** Proper transverse placement of the high-frequency linear ultrasound probe for ultrasound-guided SC joint injection.

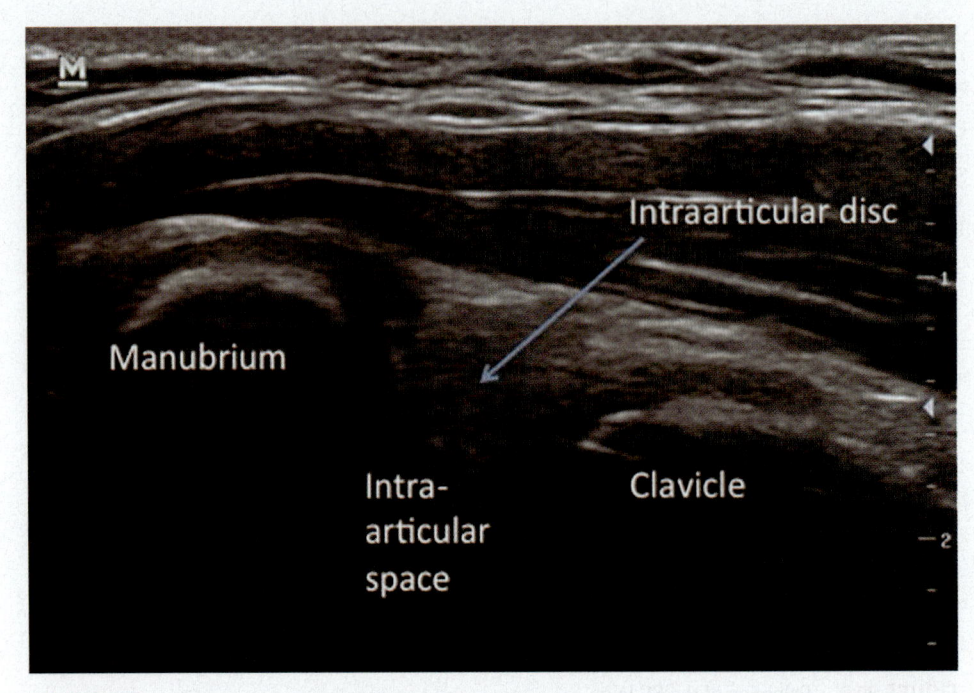

**FIGURE 80.8.** Transverse ultrasound image of the SC joint.

out-of-plane approach with the needle trajectory adjusted under real-time ultrasound guidance to enter the center of the SC joint (Fig. 80.9). When the tip of needle is thought to be within the joint space, a small amount of local anesthetic and steroid is injected under real-time ultrasound guidance to confirm intra-articular placement. After intra-articular needle tip placement is confirmed, the remainder of the contents of the syringe are slowly injected. There should be minimal resistance to injection. The needle is then removed, and a sterile pressure dressing and ice pack are placed at the injection site.

## COMPLICATIONS

The major complication of ultrasound-guided injection of the SC joint is infection. Ecchymosis and hematoma formation

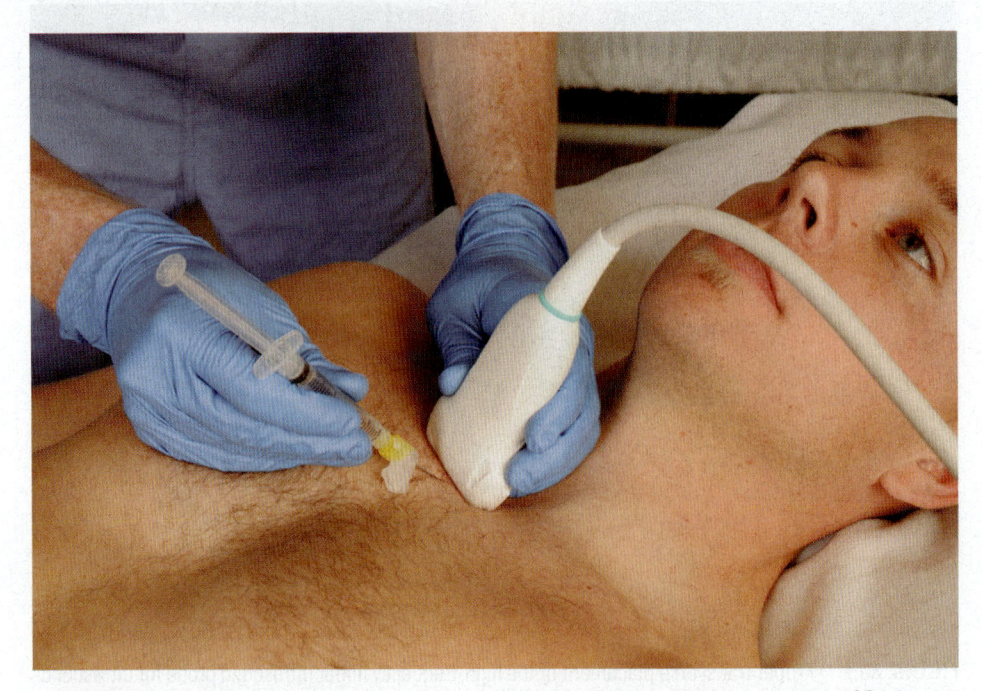

**FIGURE 80.9.** Proper needle placement for out-of-plane ultrasound-guided injection of the SC joint.

may also occur. A transient exacerbation of the patient's pain occurs ~25% of the time following this injection technique, and the patient should be warned of this possibility prior to the procedure. If the needle is placed too deeply, needle-induced trauma of great vessels is a distinct possibility.

## CLINICAL PEARLS

Pain emanating from the SC joint is often attributed to a cardiac source with many patients rushing to the emergency from believing they are suffering a heart attack. Reassurance often is required, although it should be remembered that this musculoskeletal pain syndrome and coronary artery disease can coexist as can diseases of the superior mediastinum. Universal precautions should always be observed to protect the operator, and strict adherence to sterile technique must be used to avoid infection. Gentle physical therapy and local heat should be introduced following ultrasound-guided injection of the SC joint to reduce pain and improve function. Simple analgesics and nonsteroidal anti-inflammatory agents or COX-2 inhibitors may be used in conjunction with this injection technique.

## SUGGESTED READINGS

Ferrera PC, Wheeling HM. Sternoclavicular joint injuries. *Am J Emerg Med* 2000;18(1):58–61.

Johnson MC, Jacobson JA, Fessell DP, et al. The sternoclavicular joint: can imaging differentiate infection from degenerative change? *Skeletal Radiol* 2010;39(6):551–558.

Narouze SN. Ultrasound-guided shoulder joint and bursa injections. In: *Atlas of Ultrasound Guided Procedures in Pain Management*. New York, NY: Springer; 2010:304–306.

Waldman SD. Manubriosternal joint injection. In: *Atlas of Pain Management Injection Techniques*. 3rd ed. Philadelphia, PA: WB Saunders; 2013:266–268.

Waterman J, Emery R. The diagnosis and treatment of disorders of the sternoclavicular joint. *Curr Orthop* 2002;16(5):368–373.

Wisniewski SJ, Smith J. Synovitis of the sternoclavicular joint: the role of ultrasound. *Am J Phys Med Rehabil* 2007;86(4):322–323.

# CHAPTER 81

# Ultrasound-Guided Injection Technique for Costosternal Joint Pain

## CLINICAL PERSPECTIVES

The costosternal joint is susceptible to injury from acute blunt trauma from motor vehicle accidents and contact sports such as football and rugby as well as repetitive microtrauma from chronic coughing and activities that require active protraction and retraction of the shoulders. Left untreated, the acute inflammation associated with the injury may result in arthritis with its associated pain and functional disability. Acute onset of severe costosternal pain and swelling, especially of the second and third costal cartilages that is associated with acute upper respiratory tract infection, is known as Tietze syndrome. Tietze syndrome was first described in 1921 and most commonly occurs in the second and third decade of life.

Patients suffering from costosternal joint dysfunction or inflammation will complain of a marked exacerbation of pain when they perform activities that require thrusting the arm forward and retracting or shrugging the shoulder and with deep inspiration. A clicking sensation with joint movement is often noted, and the patient frequently is unable to sleep on the affected side. Patients with costosternal joint dysfunction and inflammation will exhibit pain on active protraction or retraction of the shoulder as well as with raising of the arm high above the head. Palpation of the costosternal joint often reveals swelling or enlargement of the joint secondary to joint inflammation. If there is disruption of the ligaments that surround and support the costosternal joint, joint instability and a cosmetic defect may be evident on physical examination.

Plain radiographs are indicated in patients suffering from costosternal joint pain. They may reveal psoriatic arthritis, ankylosing spondylitis, costochondritis, and Tietze syndrome or widening of the joint consistent with ligamentous injury (Fig. 81.1). They may also reveal occult fractures or primary or metastatic tumors of the joint. If joint instability, infection, or tumor is suspected or detected on physical examination, magnetic resonance imaging, computerized tomography, and/or ultrasound scanning is a reasonable next step. Ultrasound-guided costosternal joint injection can aid the clinician in both the diagnosis and treatment of costosternal joint pain and dysfunction.

## CLINICALLY RELEVANT ANATOMY

The costosternal joints are the articulations between the cartilage of the true ribs and the sternum (Fig. 81.2). The cartilage of the first rib articulates directly with the manubrium of the sternum and is a synarthrodial joint that allows a limited gliding movement. The cartilage of the second through sixth ribs articulates with the body of the sternum and are true arthrodial joints. The costosternal joints are surrounded by a thin articular capsule. The costosternal joints are strengthened by ligaments but can be subluxed or dislocated by blunt trauma to the anterior chest wall. Posterior to the costosternal joint are the structures of the mediastinum. These structures are susceptible to needle-induced trauma if the needle is placed too deeply. The pleural space may be entered if the needle is placed too deeply and laterally, pneumothorax may result.

## ULTRASOUND-GUIDED TECHNIQUE

The benefits, risks, and alternative treatments are explained to the patient and informed consent is obtained. The patient is then placed in the supine position with the shoulder relaxed and the arms resting comfortably by the patient's sides (Fig. 81.3). The costosternal joint is then identified by palpation (Fig. 81.4). The skin overlying the costosternal joint is then prepped with antiseptic solution. A sterile syringe containing 1.0 mL of 0.25% preservative-free bupivacaine and 40 mg of methylprednisolone is attached to a 1½-inch, 22-gauge needle using strict aseptic technique. A linear high-frequency ultrasound transducer is placed in the transverse plane across the affected costosternal joint in the coronal plane (Fig. 81.5). Slowly move the ultrasound transducer to identify the manubrium and the proximal end of the cartilage and the costosternal joint in between (Fig. 81.6). To facilitate needle placement, position the ultrasound transducer so the center of the hypoechoic joint is in the center of the image between the hyperechoic articular margins of the sternum and medial end of the clavicle. In some patients, significant joint swelling is present. After the joint space is identified, the needle is placed through the skin just below

CHAPTER 81 ULTRASOUND-GUIDED INJECTION TECHNIQUE FOR COSTOSTERNAL JOINT PAIN 551

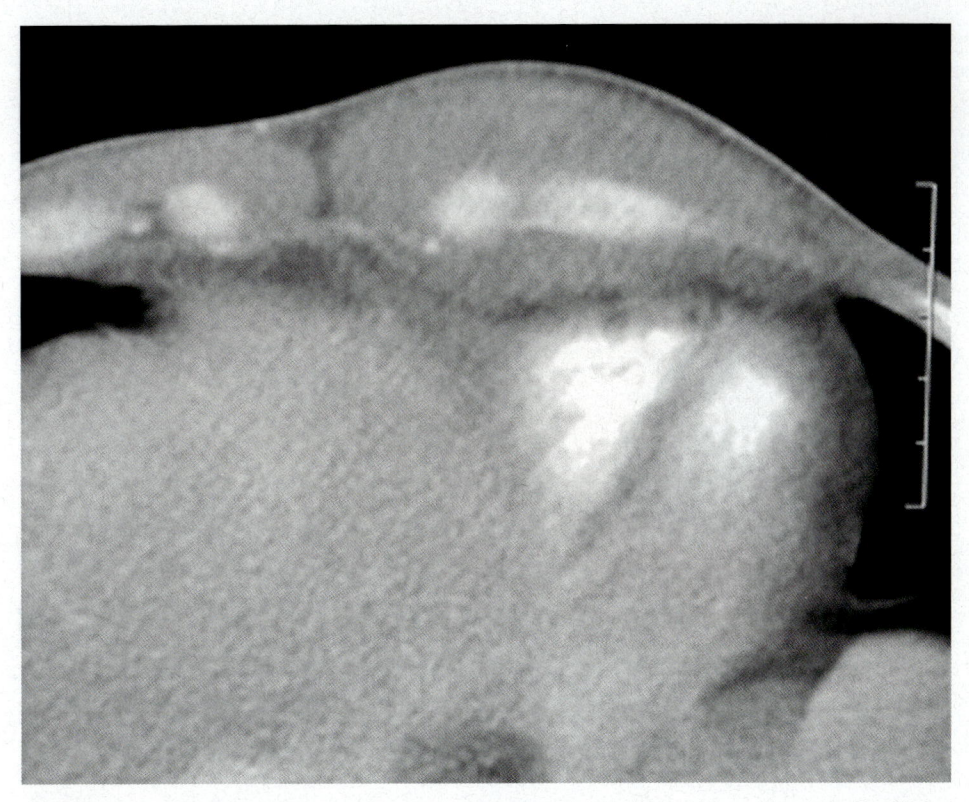

**FIGURE 81.1.** Costochondritis of left lower costochondral joints. (Reused from Eisenberg RL. *Clinical Imaging: An Atlas of Differential Diagnosis*. Philadelphia, PA: Lippincott Williams & Wilkins; 2010:309, with permission.)

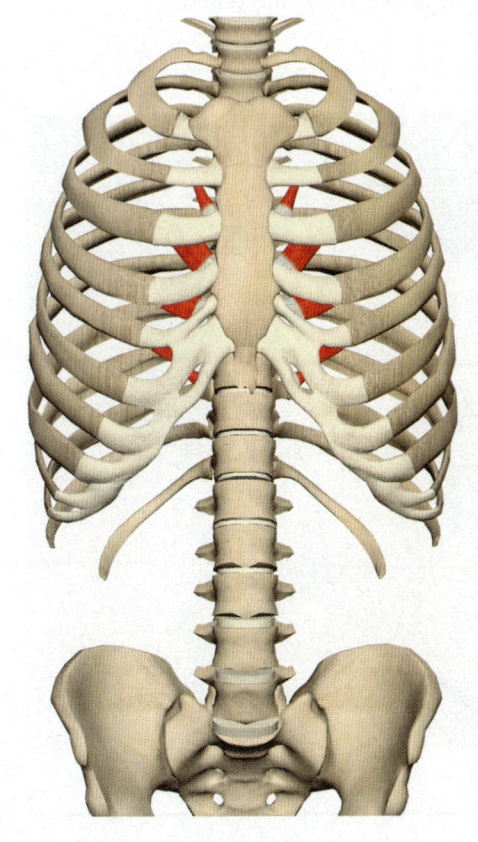

**FIGURE 81.2.** The anatomy of the costochondral joints. (Reused from LifeART Image 2013. Lippincott Williams & Wilkins.)

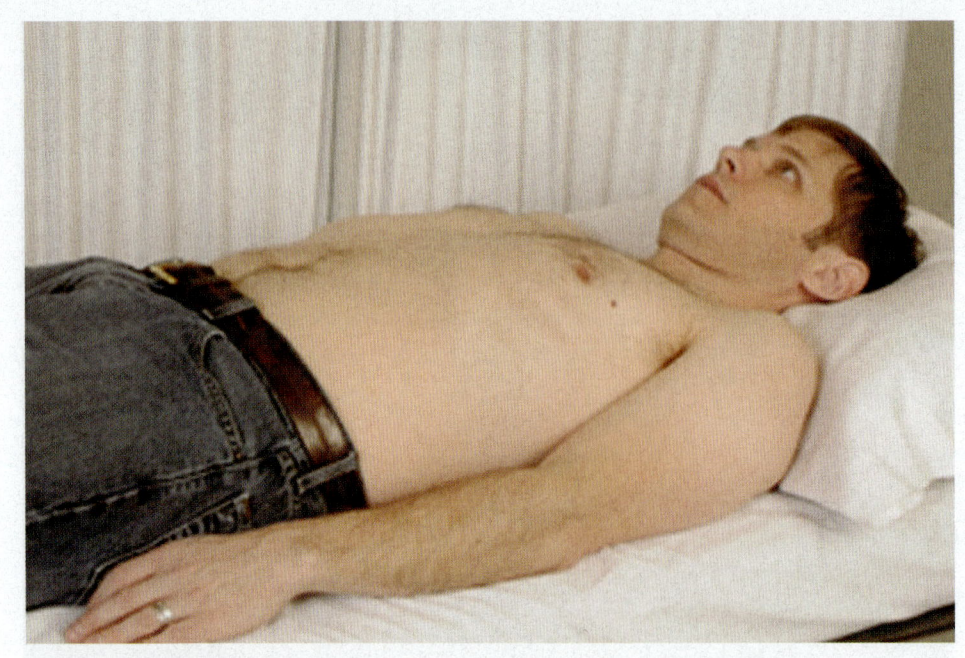

FIGURE 81.3. Proper positioning for ultrasound-guided injection of the costosternal joint.

the middle of the ultrasound transducer and is then advanced using an out-of-plane approach with the needle trajectory adjusted under real-time ultrasound guidance to enter the center of the costosternal joint (Fig. 81.7). When the tip of needle is thought to be within the joint space, a small amount of local anesthetic and steroid is injected under real-time ultrasound guidance to confirm intra-articular placement. After intra-articular needle tip placement is confirmed, the remainder of the contents of the syringe are slowly injected. There should be minimal resistance to injection. The needle is then removed, and a sterile pressure dressing and ice pack are placed at the injection site.

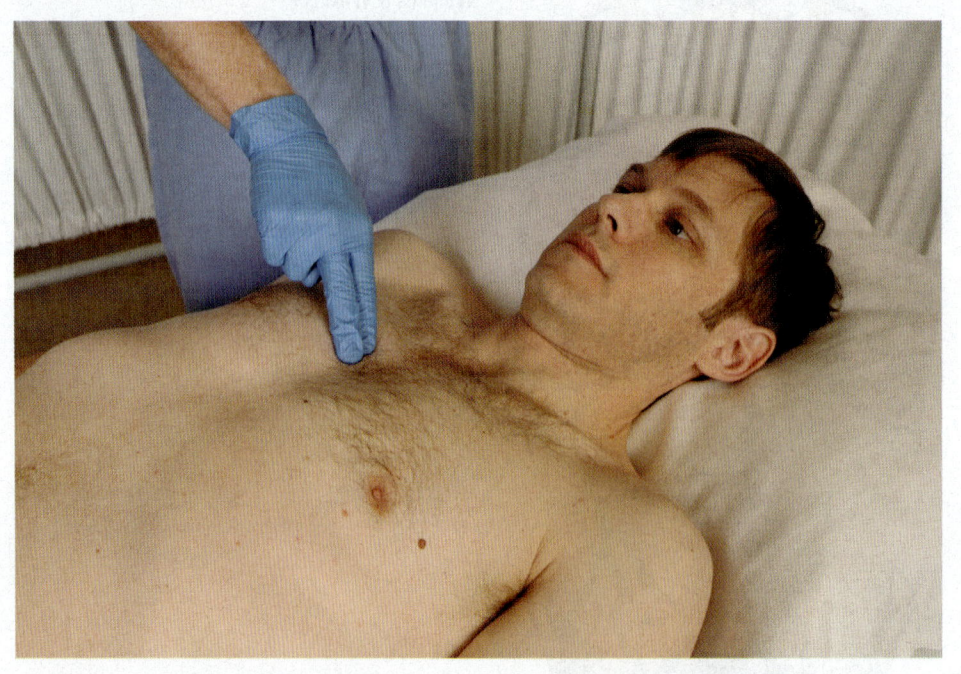

FIGURE 81.4. Palpation of the costosternal joint.

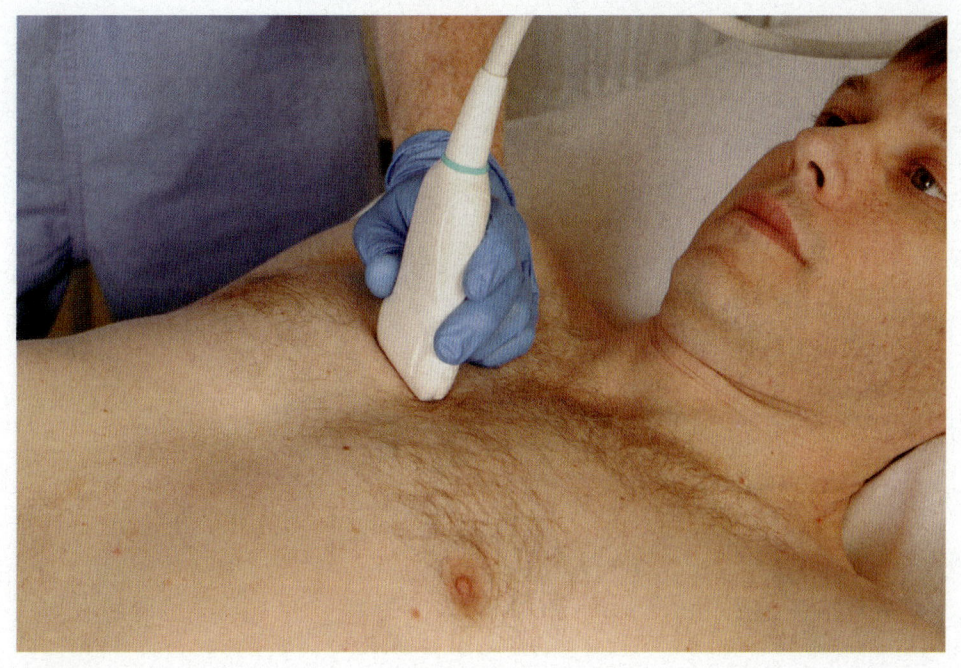

**FIGURE 81.5.** Proper placement of the high-frequency linear ultrasound probe for ultrasound-guided costosternal joint injection.

## COMPLICATIONS

The major complication of ultrasound-guided injection of the costosternal joint is infection. Ecchymosis and hematoma formation may also occur. A transient exacerbation of the patient's pain occurs ~25% of the time following this injection technique, and the patient should be warned of this possibility prior to the procedure. If the needle is placed too deeply, needle-induced trauma to the structures of the mediastinum is a distinct possibility.

## CLINICAL PEARLS

Pain emanating from the costosternal joint is often attributed to a cardiac source with many patients rushing to the emergency room believing they are suffering a heart attack. Reassurance often is required, although it should be remembered that this musculoskeletal pain syndromes and coronary artery disease can coexist as can diseases of the superior mediastinum. Universal precautions should

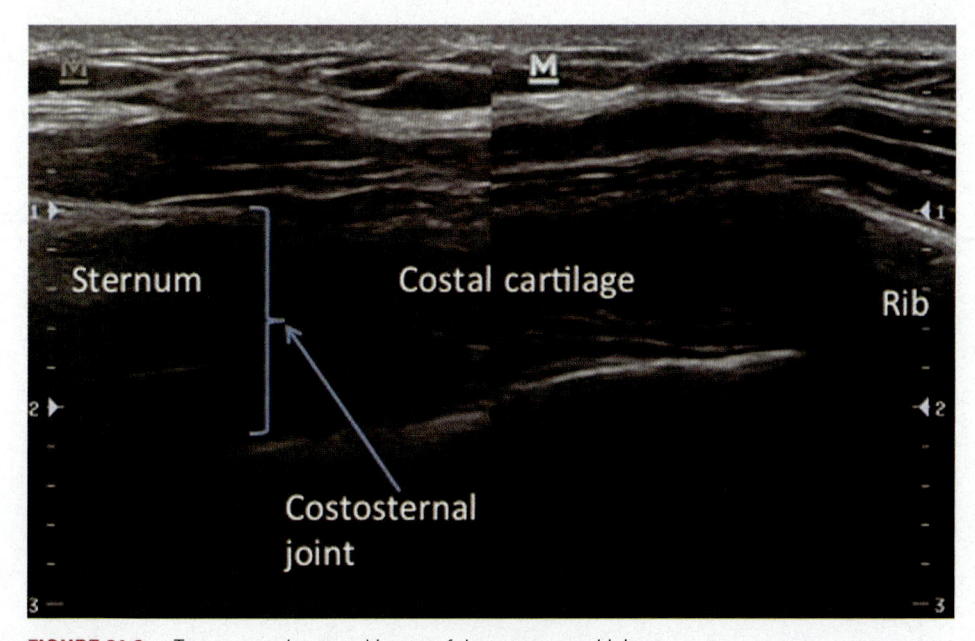

**FIGURE 81.6.** Transverse ultrasound image of the costosternal joint.

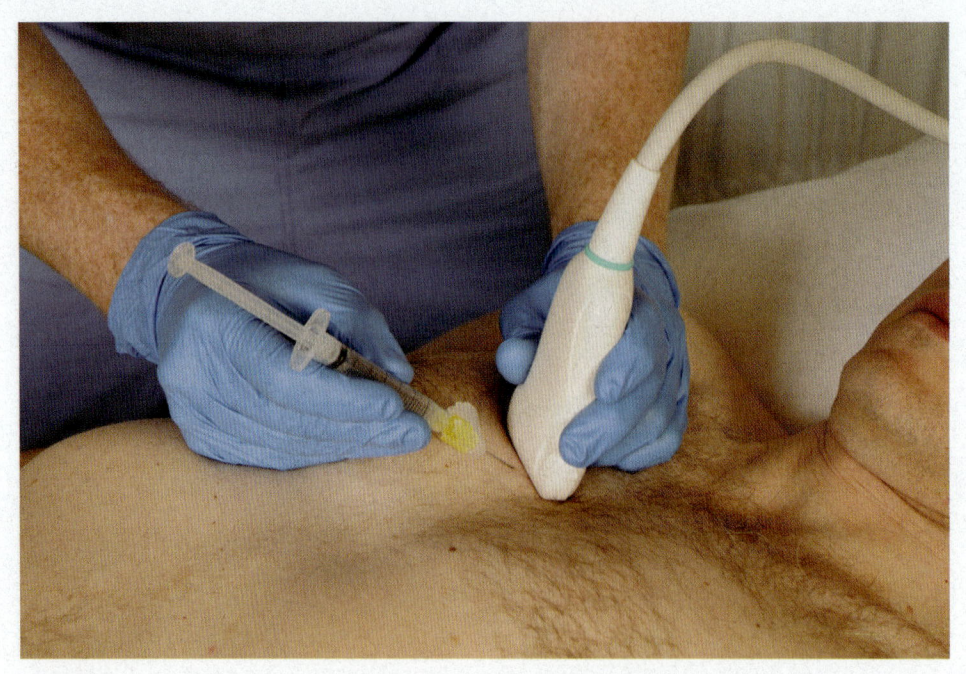

**FIGURE 81.7.** Proper needle placement for ultrasound-guided injection of the costosternal joint.

always be observed to protect the operator, and strict adherence to sterile technique must be used to avoid infection. Gentle physical therapy and local heat should be introduced following ultrasound-guided injection of the costosternal joint to reduce pain and improve function. Simple analgesics and nonsteroidal anti-inflammatory agents or COX-2 inhibitors may be used in conjunction with this injection technique.

## SUGGESTED READINGS

Baldor RA. Costochondritis. In: Domino FJ, ed. *5-Minute Clinical Consult 2009*. 17th ed. Philadelphia, PA: Lippincott Williams & Wilkins; 2008.

Kulig J, Neinstein LS. Chest pain. In: Neinstein LS, ed. *Adolescent Health Care: A Practical Guide*. 5th ed. Philadelphia, PA: Lippincott Williams & Wilkins; 2008:517–521.

Waldman SD. Tietze's syndrome. In: *Pain Review*. Philadelphia, PA: Saunders Elsevier; 2009:282.

Waldman SD. Manubriosternal joint injection. In: *Atlas of Pain Management Injection Techniques*. 3rd ed. Philadelphia, PA: Saunders Elsevier; 2013:266–268.

# CHAPTER 82

# Ultrasound-Guided Injection Technique for Manubriosternal Joint Pain

## CLINICAL PERSPECTIVES

The manubriosternal joint is susceptible to injury from acute blunt trauma from motor vehicle accidents and contact sports such as football and rugby as well as repetitive microtrauma from chronic coughing and activities that require active protraction and retraction of the shoulders. Left untreated, the acute inflammation associated with the injury may result in arthritis with its associated pain and functional disability.

Patients suffering from manubriosternal joint dysfunction or inflammation will complain of a marked exacerbation of pain when they perform activities that require thrusting the arm forward and retracting or shrugging the shoulder and with deep inspiration. A clicking sensation with joint movement is often noted, and the patient frequently is unable to sleep on the abdomen or side. Patients with manubriosternal joint dysfunction and inflammation will exhibit pain on active protraction or retraction of the shoulder as well as with raising of the arm high above the head. Palpation of the manubriosternal joint often reveals swelling or enlargement of the joint secondary to joint inflammation. If there is disruption of the joint, it may sublux or dislocate, and joint instability and a cosmetic defect may be evident on physical examination.

Plain radiographs are indicated in patients suffering from manubriosternal joint pain. They may reveal psoriatic arthritis, ankylosing spondylitis, Reiter syndrome, or widening of the joint consistent with joint injury (Fig. 82.1). They may also reveal occult fractures or primary or metastatic tumors of the joint as the joint is susceptible to invasion by tumors of the mediastinum including thymoma. If joint instability, infection, or tumor is suspected or detected on physical examination, magnetic resonance imaging, computerized tomography, and/or ultrasound scanning is a reasonable next step (Fig. 82.2). Ultrasound-guided manubriosternal joint injection can aid the clinician in both the diagnosis and treatment of manubriosternal joint pain and dysfunction.

## CLINICALLY RELEVANT ANATOMY

The manubriosternal joint is the fibrocartilaginous articulation between the manubrium and body of the sternum (Fig. 82.3). The joint articulates at an angle called the angle of Louis (which was named after 19th century French physician Pierre Charles Louis), which allows for easy identification by palpation. The joint lies at the level of the second costal cartilage. Posterior to the manubriosternal joint are the structures of the mediastinum including the arch of the aorta. These structures are susceptible to needle-induced trauma if the needle is placed too deeply. The manubriosternal joint allows protraction and retraction of the thorax. Above, the manubrium articulates with the sternal end of the clavicle and the cartilage of the first rib. Below, the body of the sternum articulates with the xiphoid process. Posterior to the manubriosternal joint are the structures of the mediastinum including the arch of the aorta.

## ULTRASOUND-GUIDED TECHNIQUE

The benefits, risks, and alternative treatments are explained to the patient and informed consent is obtained. The patient is then placed in the supine position with the shoulder relaxed and the arms resting comfortably by the patient's side (Fig. 82.4). The manubriosternal joint is then identified by palpation (Fig. 82.5). The skin overlying the manubriosternal joint is then prepped with antiseptic solution. A sterile syringe containing 1.0 mL of 0.25% preservative-free bupivacaine and 40 mg of methylprednisolone is attached to a 1½-inch, 22-gauge needle using strict aseptic technique. A linear high-frequency ultrasound transducer is placed in the longitudinal plane across the manubriosternal joint (Fig. 82.6). Slowly move the ultrasound transducer to identify the manubriosternal joint (Fig. 82.7). To facilitate needle placement, position the ultrasound transducer so the center of the hypoechoic joint is in the center of the image between the hyperechoic articular margins of the sternum and medial end of the clavicle. In some patients, significant joint swelling is present. After the joint space is identified, the needle is placed through the skin at the middle of the ultrasound transducer and is then advanced using an out-of-plane approach with the needle trajectory adjusted under real-time ultrasound guidance to enter the center of the manubriosternal joint (Fig. 82.8). When the tip of needle is thought to be within the joint space, a small amount of local anesthetic and steroid is injected under

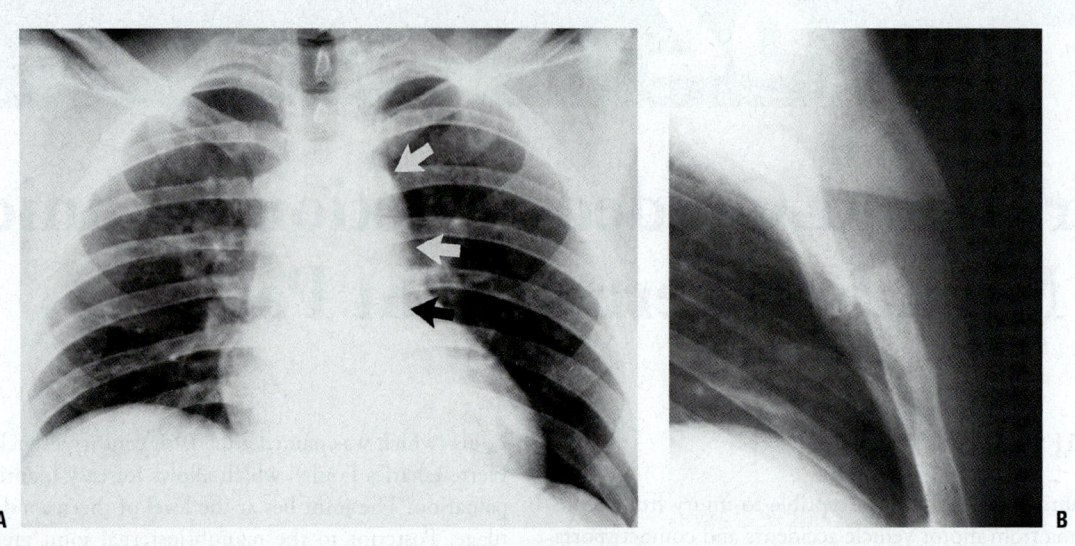

**FIGURE 82.1.** Plain radiograph of patient who sustained blunt chest wall trauma. **A:** *Arrows* indicated a widened mediastinum. **B:** lateral radiograph reveals complete posterior dislocation of the body of the sternum at the manubriosternal joint. Note the anterior chest wall soft tissue swelling. (Reused from Pope TL, Harris JH Jr. *Harris & Harris' The Radiology of Emergency Medicine*. 5th ed. Philadelphia, PA: Lippincott Williams & Wilkins; 2013:505, with permission.)

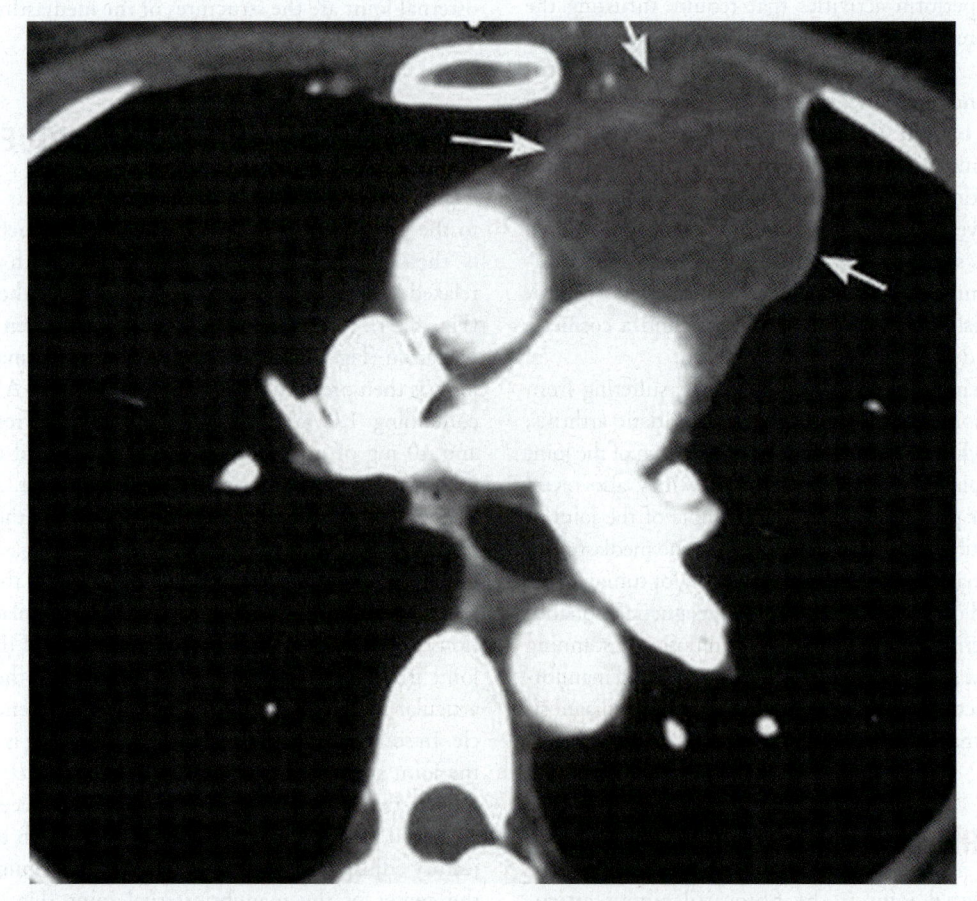

**FIGURE 82.2.** Tumors of the mediastinum can mimic pain emanating from the manubriosternal joint. Example of an invasive thymoma, which is invading the anterior chest wall (*arrows*).

CHAPTER 82   ULTRASOUND-GUIDED INJECTION TECHNIQUE FOR MANUBRIOSTERNAL JOINT PAIN   557

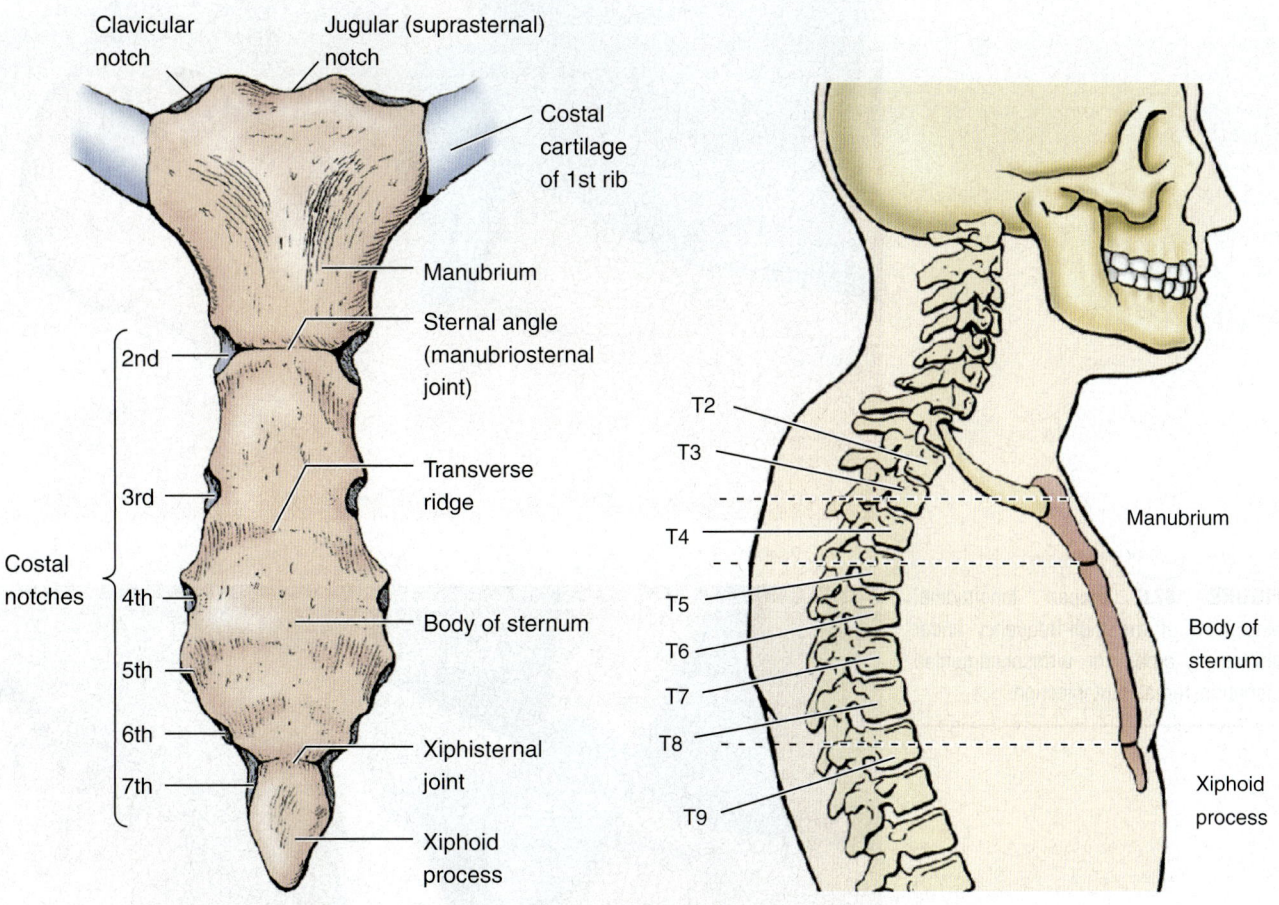

**FIGURE 82.3.** Anatomy of the manubriosternal joint. (Reused from Moore KL, Agur A. *Essential Clinical Anatomy*. 2nd ed. Philadelphia, PA: Lippincott Williams & Wilkins; 2002, with permission.)

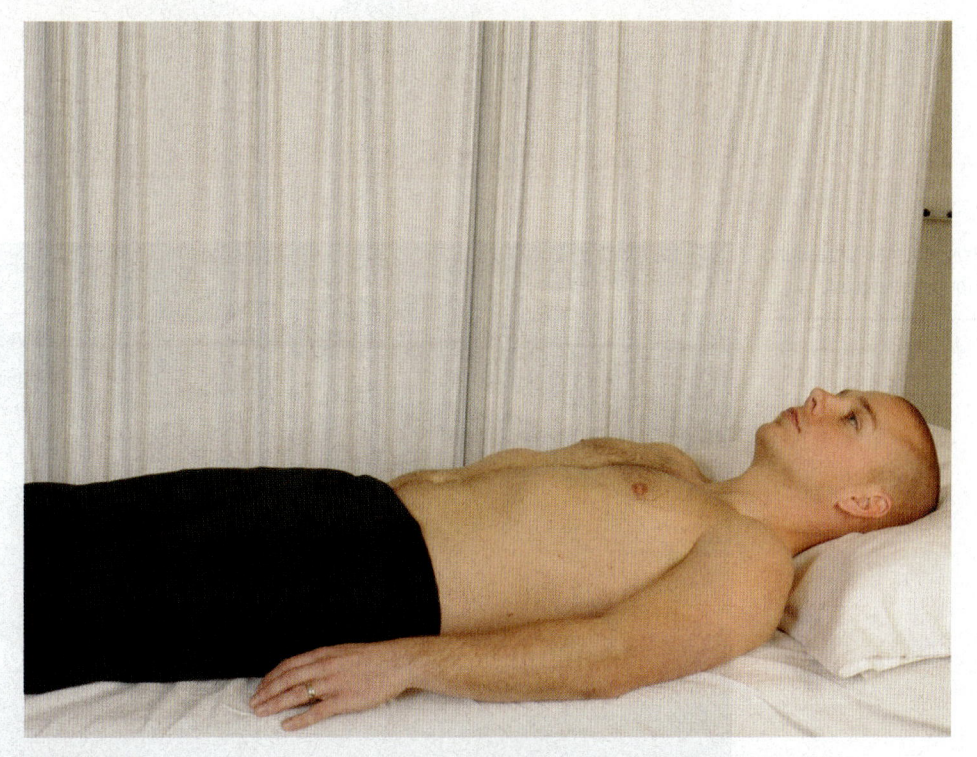

**FIGURE 82.4.** Proper positioning for ultrasound-guided injection of the manubriosternal joint.

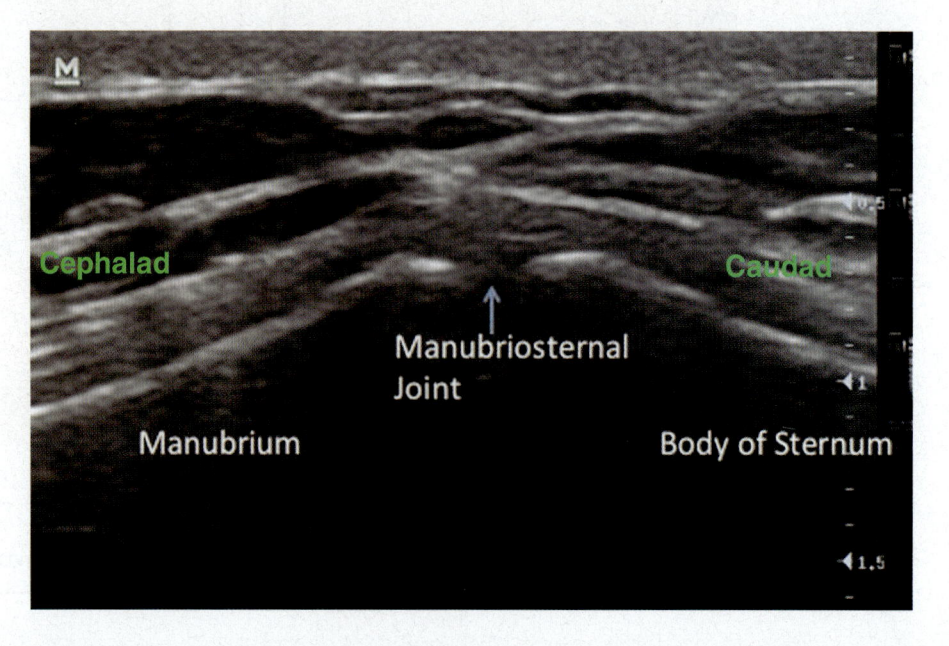

**FIGURE 82.5.** Palpation of the manubriosternal joint.

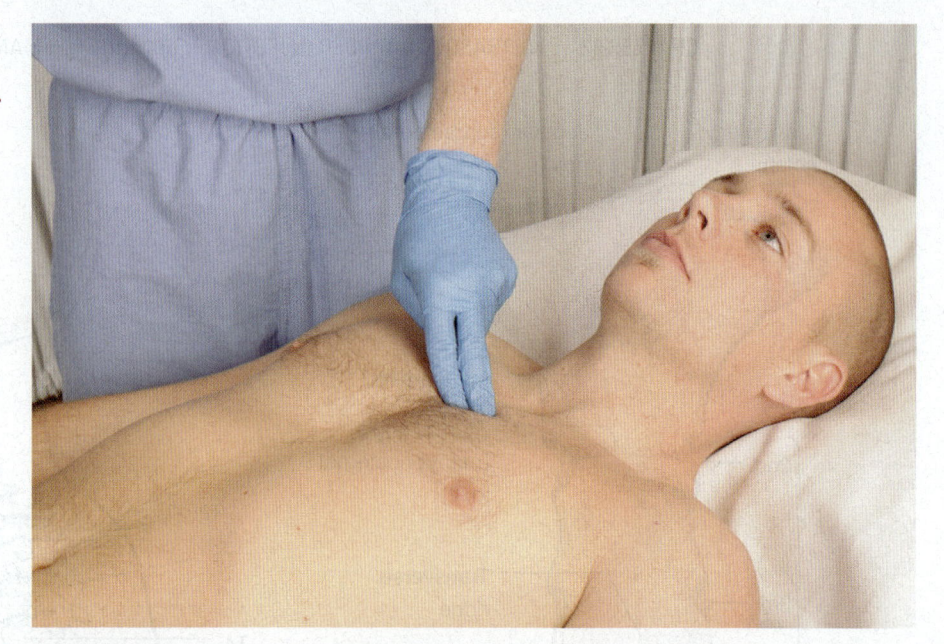

**FIGURE 82.6.** Proper longitudinal placement of the high-frequency linear ultrasound probe for ultrasound-guided manubriosternal joint injection.

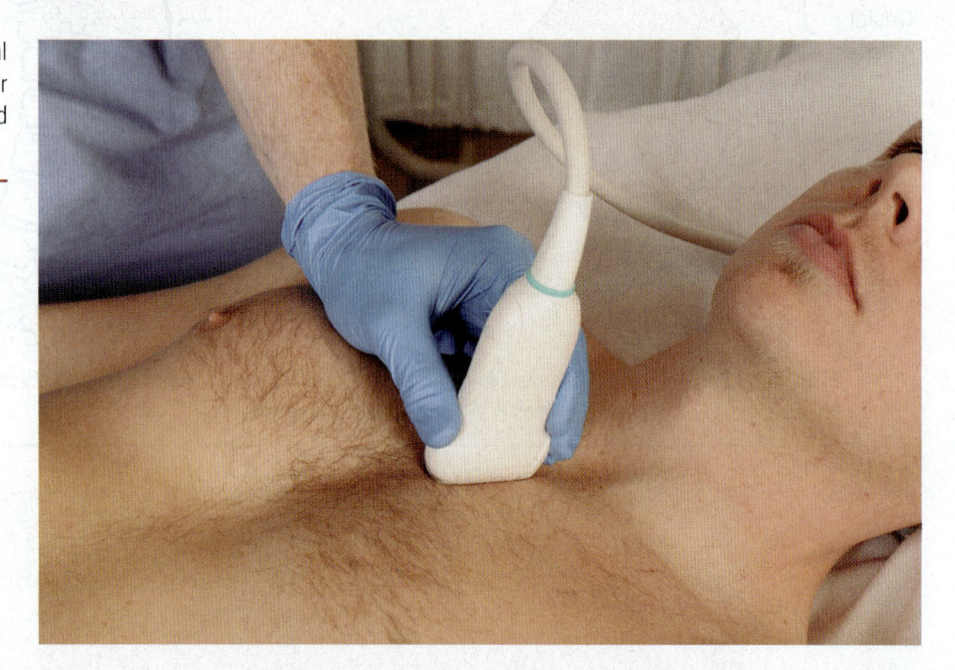

**FIGURE 82.7.** Longitudinal ultrasound image of the manubriosternal joint.

# CHAPTER 82 ULTRASOUND-GUIDED INJECTION TECHNIQUE FOR MANUBRIOSTERNAL JOINT PAIN

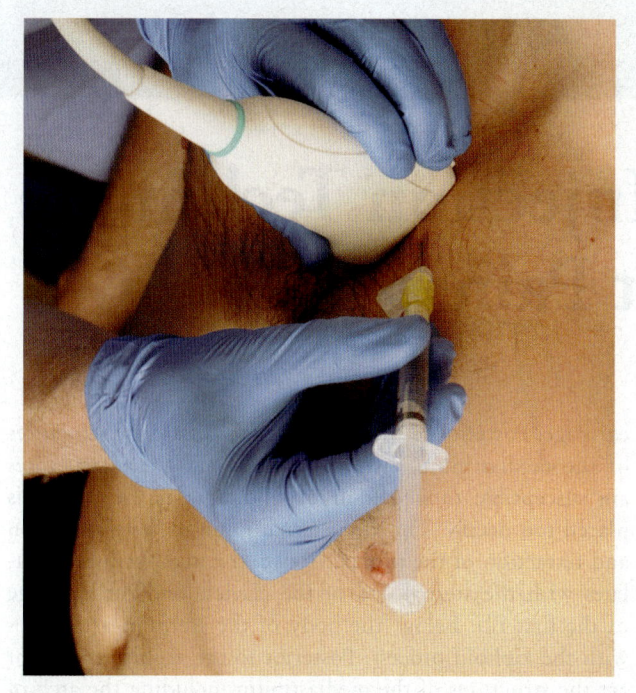

**FIGURE 82.8.** Proper needle placement for out-of-plane ultrasound-guided injection of the manubriosternal joint.

real-time ultrasound guidance to confirm intra-articular placement. After intra-articular needle tip placement is confirmed, the remainder of the contents of the syringe are slowly injected. There should be minimal resistance to injection. The needle is then removed, and a sterile pressure dressing and ice pack are placed at the injection site.

## COMPLICATIONS

The major complication of ultrasound-guided injection of the manubriosternal joint is infection. Ecchymosis and hematoma formation may also occur. A transient exacerbation of the patient's pain occurs ~25% of the time following this injection technique, and the patient should be warned of this possibility prior to the procedure. If the needle is placed too deeply, needle-induced trauma to the structures of the mediastinum is a distinct possibility.

## CLINICAL PEARLS

Pain emanating from the manubriosternal joint is often attributed to a cardiac source with many patients rushing to the emergency room believing they are suffering a heart attack. Reassurance is often required, although it should be remembered that this musculoskeletal pain syndromes and coronary artery disease can coexist as can occult diseases of the superior mediastinum. Universal precautions should always be observed to protect the operator, and strict adherence to sterile technique must be used to avoid infection. Gentle physical therapy and local heat should be introduced following ultrasound-guided injection of the manubriosternal joint to reduce pain and improve function. Simple analgesics and nonsteroidal anti-inflammatory agents or COX-2 inhibitors may be used in conjunction with this injection technique.

## SUGGESTED READINGS

Brims FJH, Davies HE, Gary YC. Respiratory chest pain: diagnosis and treatment. *Med Clin North Am* 2010;94(2):217–232.
Costochondritis. In: Domino FJ, ed. *5-Minute Clinical Consult 2009*. 17th ed. Philadelphia, PA: Lippincott Williams & Wilkins; 2008.
Stochkendahl MJ, Christensen HW. Chest pain in focal musculoskeletal disorders. *Med Clin North Am* 2010;94(2):259–273.
Waldman SD. Tietze's syndrome. In: *Pain Review*. Philadelphia, PA: Saunders Elsevier; 2009:282.
Waldman SD. Manubriosternal injection technique for Tietze's syndrome. In: *Atlas of Pain Management Injection Techniques*. 3rd ed. Philadelphia, PA: WB Saunders; 2013:284–285.

# CHAPTER 83

# Ultrasound-Guided Injection Technique for Xiphisternal Joint Pain

## CLINICAL PERSPECTIVES

The xiphisternal joint is susceptible to injury from acute blunt trauma from motor vehicle accidents and contact sports such as football and rugby as well as repetitive microtrauma from chronic coughing and activities that require repeated stooping. Left untreated, the acute inflammation associated with the injury may result in arthritis with its associated pain and functional disability.

Patients suffering from xiphisternal joint dysfunction or inflammation will complain of a pain when overeating, stooping, bending inspiring deeply, or coughing. A clicking sensation with joint movement is often noted, and the patient frequently is unable to sleep on the abdomen or side. Patients with xiphisternal joint dysfunction and inflammation will exhibit pain with any movement of the xiphisternal joint. Palpation of the xiphisternal joint often reveals swelling or enlargement of the joint secondary to joint inflammation. If there is disruption of the supporting ligaments of the joint, it may sublux or dislocate and joint instability and a cosmetic defect may be evident on physical examination (Fig. 83.1).

Plain radiographs are indicated in patients suffering from xiphisternal joint pain. They may reveal psoriatic arthritis, ankylosing spondylitis, Reiter syndrome, or widening of the joint consistent with joint injury (Fig. 83.2). They may also reveal occult fractures or primary or metastatic tumors of the joint as the joint is susceptible to invasion by tumors of the mediastinum including thymoma. If joint instability, infection, or tumor is suspected or detected on physical examination, magnetic resonance imaging, computerized tomography, and/or ultrasound scanning is a reasonable next step (Fig. 83.3). Ultrasound-guided xiphisternal joint injection can aid the clinician in both the diagnosis and treatment of xiphisternal joint pain and dysfunction.

## CLINICALLY RELEVANT ANATOMY

The xiphisternal joint is the fibrocartilaginous articulation at the apex of the infrasternal angle between the body of the sternum and the xiphoid (Fig. 83.4). The joint lies at the level of the T9 vertebral body and is easily identifiable by palpation. The joint lies at the level of the second costal cartilage. Posterior to the xiphisternal joint are the structures of the mediastinum including the heart. These structures are susceptible to needle-induced trauma if the needle is placed too deeply. The xiphisternal joint allows protraction and retraction of the thorax. Above, the manubrium articulates with the sternal end of the clavicle and the cartilage of the first rib. Below, the body of the sternum articulates with the xiphoid process. Posterior to the xiphisternal joint are the structures of the mediastinum including the arch of the aorta. The xiphisternal joint is strengthened by ligaments but can be subluxed or dislocated by blunt trauma to the anterior chest. The xiphisternal joint is innervated by the T4–T7 intercostal nerves as well as by the phrenic nerve. It is thought that this innervation by the phrenic nerve is responsible for the referred pain associated with xiphodynia syndrome.

## ULTRASOUND-GUIDED TECHNIQUE

The benefits, risks, and alternative treatments are explained to the patient and informed consent is obtained. The patient is then placed in the supine position with the shoulder relaxed and the arms resting comfortably by the patient's side (Fig. 83.5). The xiphisternal joint is then identified by palpation (Fig. 83.6). The skin overlying the xiphisternal joint is then prepped with antiseptic solution. A sterile syringe containing 1.0 mL of 0.25% preservative-free bupivacaine and 40 mg of methylprednisolone is attached to a 1½-inch, 22-gauge needle using strict aseptic technique. A linear high-frequency ultrasound transducer is placed in the longitudinal plane across the xiphisternal joint (Fig. 83.7). The ultrasound transducer is then slowly moved in a cephalad and caudad direction to identify the xiphisternal joint, and an ultrasound survey scan is taken (Fig. 83.8). To facilitate needle placement, position the ultrasound transducer so the center of the hypoechoic joint is in the center of the image between the hyperechoic articular margins of the sternum and medial end of the clavicle. In some patients, significant joint swelling is present. After the joint space is identified, the needle is placed through the skin at the middle of the longitudinally placed ultrasound transducer and is then advanced using an out-of-plane approach with the needle trajectory adjusted

CHAPTER 83   ULTRASOUND-GUIDED INJECTION TECHNIQUE FOR XIPHISTERNAL JOINT PAIN

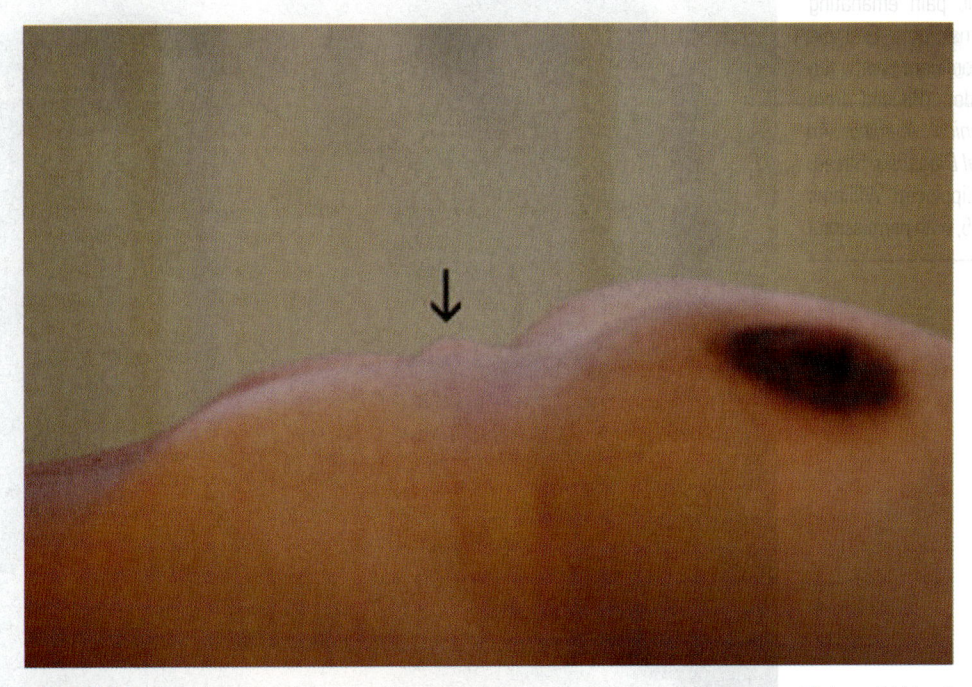

**FIGURE 83.1.** Subluxation of the xiphoid can result in cosmetic defect. (Reused from Maigne JY, Vareli M, Rousset P, et al. Xiphodynia and prominence of the xyphoid process. Value of xiphosternal angle measurement: three case reports. *Joint Bone Spine* 2010;77(5):474–476, with permission.)

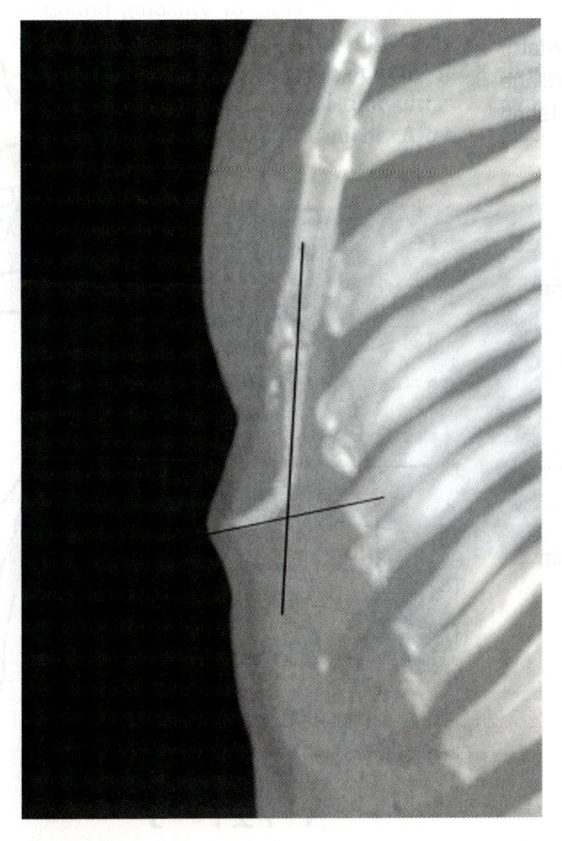

**FIGURE 83.2.** Plain radiograph of patient with subluxation of the xiphoid. (Reused from Maigne JY, Vareli M, Rousset P, et al. Xiphodynia and prominence of the xyphoid process. Value of xiphosternal angle measurement: three case reports. *Joint Bone Spine* 2010;77(5):474–476, with permission.)

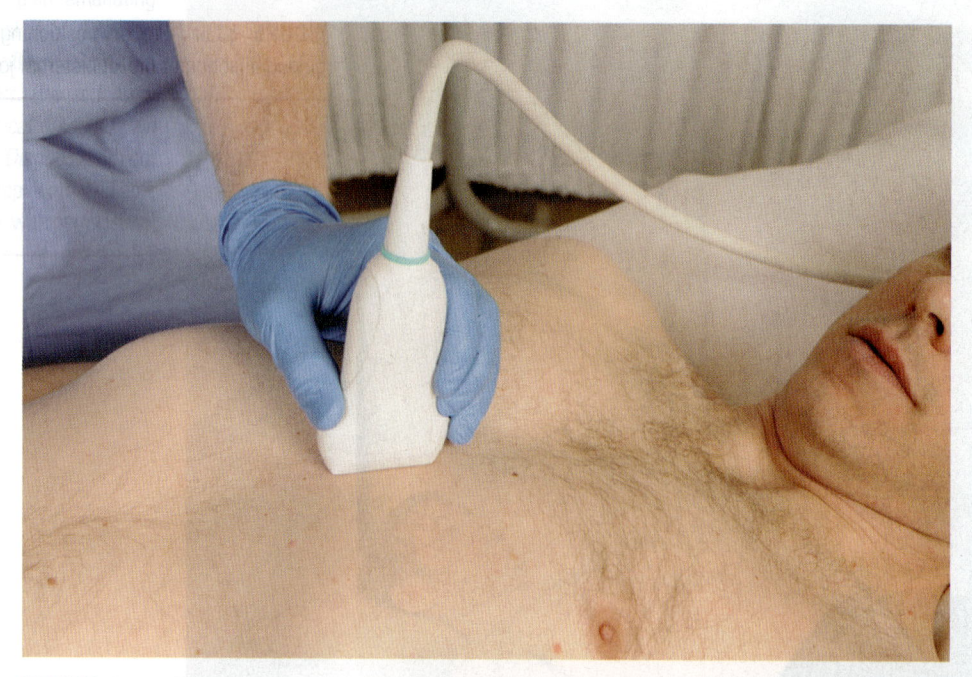

**FIGURE 83.7.** Proper longitudinal placement of the high-frequency linear ultrasound probe for ultrasound-guided xiphisternal joint injection.

## COMPLICATIONS

The major complication of ultrasound-guided injection of the xiphisternal joint is infection. Ecchymosis and hematoma formation may also occur. A transient exacerbation of the patient's pain occurs ~25% of the time following this injection technique, and the patient should be warned of this possibility prior to the procedure. If the needle is placed too deeply, needle-induced trauma to the structures of the mediastinum is a distinct possibility.

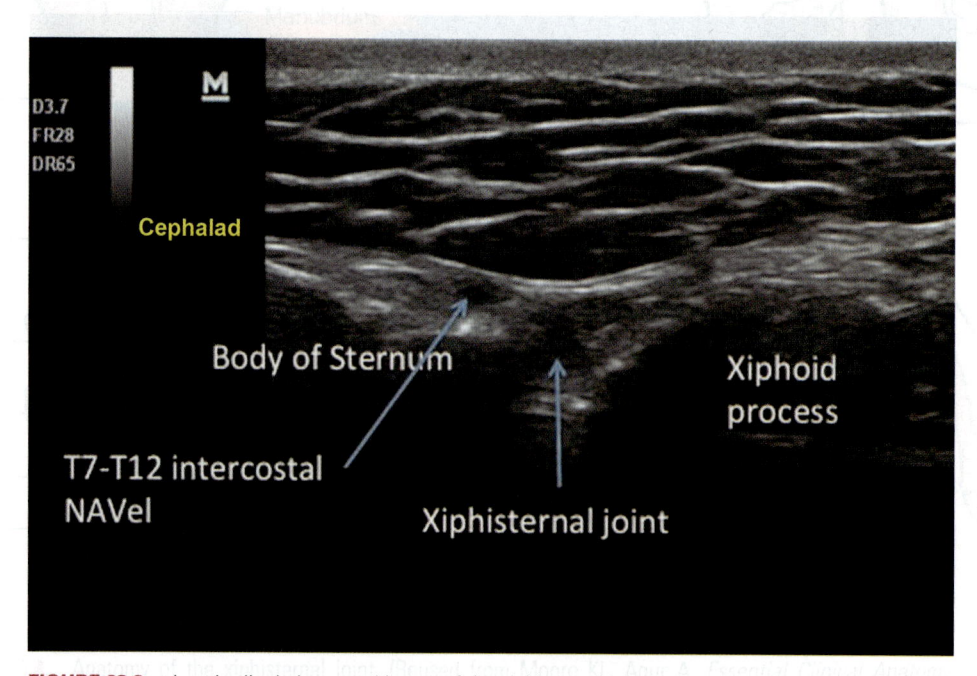

**FIGURE 83.8.** Longitudinal ultrasound image of the xiphisternal joint.

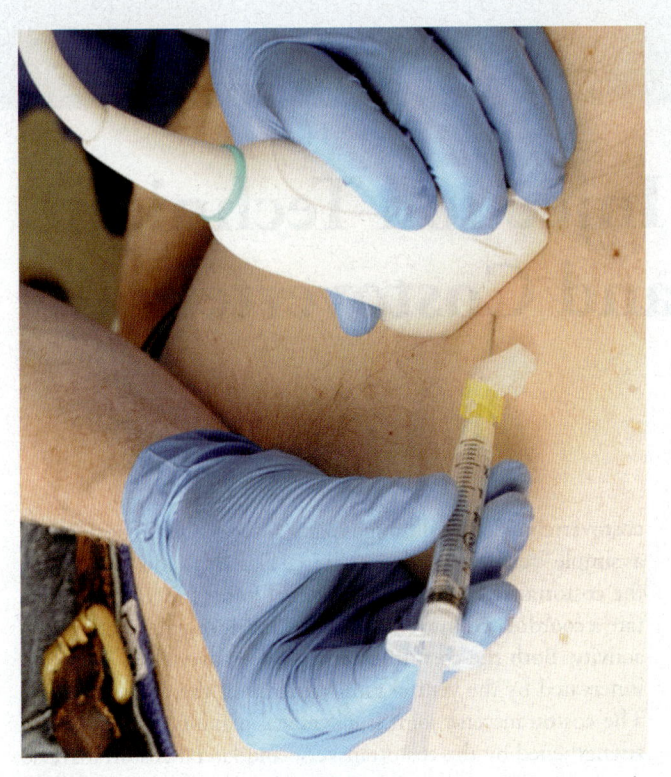

**FIGURE 83.9.** Proper needle placement for out-of-plane ultrasound-guided injection of the xiphisternal joint.

## CLINICAL PEARLS

Pain emanating from the xiphisternal joint is often attributed to a cardiac source or ulcer disease with many patients rushing to the emergency room believing they are suffering a heart attack or a bleeding ulcer. Reassurance is often is required, although it should be remembered that this musculoskeletal pain syndromes and coronary artery disease can coexist as can occult diseases of the superior mediastinum. Tietze syndrome has been reported to affect this joint in addition to the costosternal joint. Universal precautions should always be observed to protect the operator, and strict adherence to sterile technique must be used to avoid infection. Gentle physical therapy and local heat should be introduced following ultrasound-guided injection of the xiphisternal joint to reduce pain and improve function. Simple analgesics and nonsteroidal anti-inflammatory agents or COX-2 inhibitors may be used in conjunction with this injection technique.

## SUGGESTED READINGS

Brims FJH, Davies HE, Gary YC. Respiratory chest pain: diagnosis and treatment. *Med Clin North Am* 2010;94(2):217–232.
Stochkendahl MJ, Christensen HW. Chest pain in focal musculoskeletal disorders. *Med Clin North Am* 2010;94(2):259–273.
Waldman SD. Tietze's syndrome. In: *Pain Review*. Philadelphia, PA: Saunders Elsevier; 2009:283.
Waldman SD. Xiphisternal joint injection. In: *Atlas of Pain Management Injection Techniques*. 3rd ed. Philadelphia, PA: WB Saunders; 2013:271–273.

# Ultrasound-Guided Injection Technique for Costotransverse and Costovertebral Joint Pain

## CLINICAL PERSPECTIVES

The costotransverse and costovertebral joints are susceptible to injury from acute blunt trauma of both the anterior chest wall and the dorsal spine from motor vehicle accidents and contact sports such as football and rugby as well as repetitive microtrauma from chronic coughing and activities that require repeated flexion, extension, and lateral bending. Left untreated, the acute inflammation associated with the injury may result in arthritis with its associated pain and functional disability.

Patients suffering from costotransverse and costovertebral joint dysfunction or inflammation will complain of a pain when flexing, extending, or lateral bending of the dorsal spine. The patient will often attempt to splint the painful area by retracting the scapula. Sleep disturbance is common with the patient awakening when rolling from side to side. Palpation of the area of the affected costovertebral joint will often elicit pain and paraspinous muscle spasm.

Plain radiographs are indicated for all patients who present with pain thought to be emanating from the costotransverse or costovertebral joints to rule out occult bony pathology, including tumor. Based on the patient's clinical presentation, additional testing may be indicated, including complete blood cell count, prostate-specific antigen, sedimentation rate, and antinuclear antibody testing. Magnetic resonance, computerized tomographic, and/or ultrasonographic imaging of the joint is indicated if primary joint pathology is suspected (Fig. 84.1). The injection technique presented below serves as both a diagnostic and a therapeutic maneuver.

## CLINICALLY RELEVANT ANATOMY

The first through tenth ribs articulate with the thoracic vertebra at two places. The first is the point at which the facet of the tubercle of the rib articulates with the transverse process of the vertebral body. This articulation is known as the costotransverse joint (Figs. 84.2 and 84.3). The second, more proximal articulation of the rib is the point at which the head of the rib articulates with the vertebral body and is known as the costovertebral joint (although many authors refer to both joints as simple "costovertebral joints") (see Figs. 84.2 and 84.3). Both the costotransverse and costovertebral joints function to facilitate a coordinated movement of the ribs during respiration and activity. Both the costotransverse and costovertebral joints are innervated by the ventral rami rather than the medial branch. The costotransverse joint is a synovial plane-type joint and is strengthened by the costotransverse and lateral costotransverse ligaments. The costovertebral joint is a trochoid joint and is reinforced by the superficial radiate and radiate ligaments. The 11th and 12th ribs lack a true costotransverse joint, and both have a larger single articulation at the head of the rib.

## ULTRASOUND-GUIDED TECHNIQUE

The benefits, risks, and alternative treatments are explained to the patient and informed consent is obtained. The patient is then placed in the sitting position with the forehead resting comfortably on a padded bedside table and the arms resting comfortably on the patient's lap (Fig. 84.4). The area of the affected costotransverse and costovertebral joint is then identified by palpation (Fig. 84.5). The skin overlying the affected joint is then prepped with antiseptic solution. A sterile syringe containing 3.0 mL of 0.25% preservative-free bupivacaine and 40 mg of methylprednisolone is attached to a 3½-inch, 22-gauge needle using strict aseptic technique. A linear high-frequency ultrasound transducer is placed in the transverse plane over the spinous process of the vertebral body at the level of the affected joint, and an ultrasound survey scan is obtained (Fig. 84.6). The hyperechoic margin of the transverse process is then followed laterally until the gap of the costotransverse joint is seen where the tubercle of the rib lies adjacent to the transverse process (Fig. 84.7). To facilitate needle placement into the costotransverse joint, the ultrasound transducer is then slowly moved in a lateral and medial direction and angled in a cephalad and caudad manner until the view of the costotransverse joint is optimized (Fig. 84.8). To facilitate needle placement, position the ultrasound transducer so the gap that represents the costotransverse joint lies in the lateral portion of the ultrasound view. After the joint space is identified and

CHAPTER 84  ULTRASOUND-GUIDED INJECTION TECHNIQUE FOR COSTOTRANSVERSE AND COSTOVERTEBRAL JOINT PAIN    567

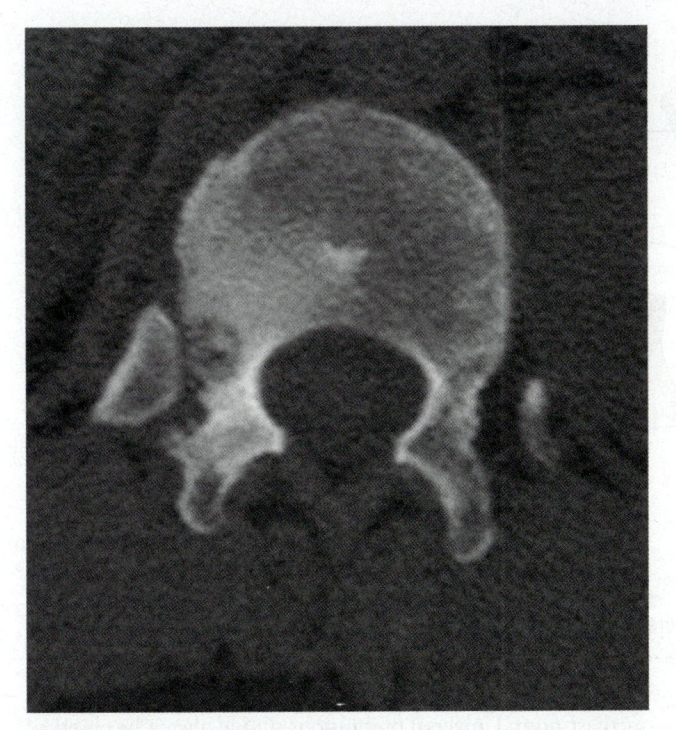

**FIGURE 84.1.** Computed tomography image through T12 shows a 1-cm rounded lesion within the right lateral portion of the vertebral body adjacent to the costovertebral joint consistent with an osteoid osteoma. (From Chew FS, Roberts CC. *Musculoskeletal Imaging: A Teaching File.* 2nd ed. Philadelphia, PA: Lippincott Williams & Wilkins; 2006, with permission.)

positioned to optimize injection, the needle is placed through the skin at the lateral margin of the ultrasound transducer closest to the costotransverse joint and is then advanced using an in-plane approach with the needle trajectory adjusted under real-time ultrasound guidance to enter the center of the costotransverse joint (Fig. 84.9). When the tip of needle is thought to be within the joint space, a small amount of local anesthetic and steroid is injected under real-time ultrasound guidance to confirm intra-articular placement. After intra-articular needle tip placement is confirmed, the remainder of the contents of the syringe are slowly injected. There should be minimal resistance to injection. The needle is then removed, and a sterile pressure dressing and ice pack are placed at the injection site.

## COMPLICATIONS

The major complication of ultrasound-guided injection of the costovertebral and costovertebral joint is infection. Given the proximity to the neuroaxis and exiting nerve roots, care must be taken to keep the needle within the confines between the tubercle of the rib and the costotransverse space. Furthermore, if the needle is placed through the intercostal space and pleura is pierced, pneumothorax could result. Ecchymosis and hematoma formation may also occur. A transient exacerbation of the patient's pain occurs ~25% of the time following this injection technique, and the patient should be warned of this possibility prior to the procedure. If the needle is placed too deeply, needle-induced trauma to the structures of the mediastinum is a distinct possibility.

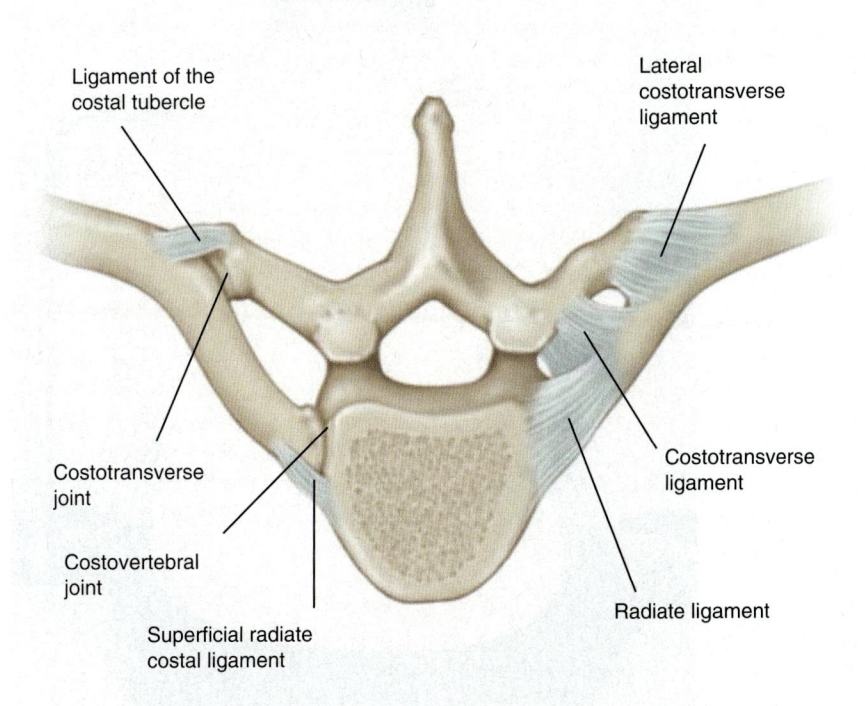

**FIGURE 84.2.** Anatomy of the costovertebral joint. (Reused from Premkumar K. *The Massage Connection Anatomy and Physiology.* Baltimore, MD: Lippincott Williams & Wilkins; 2004, with permission.)

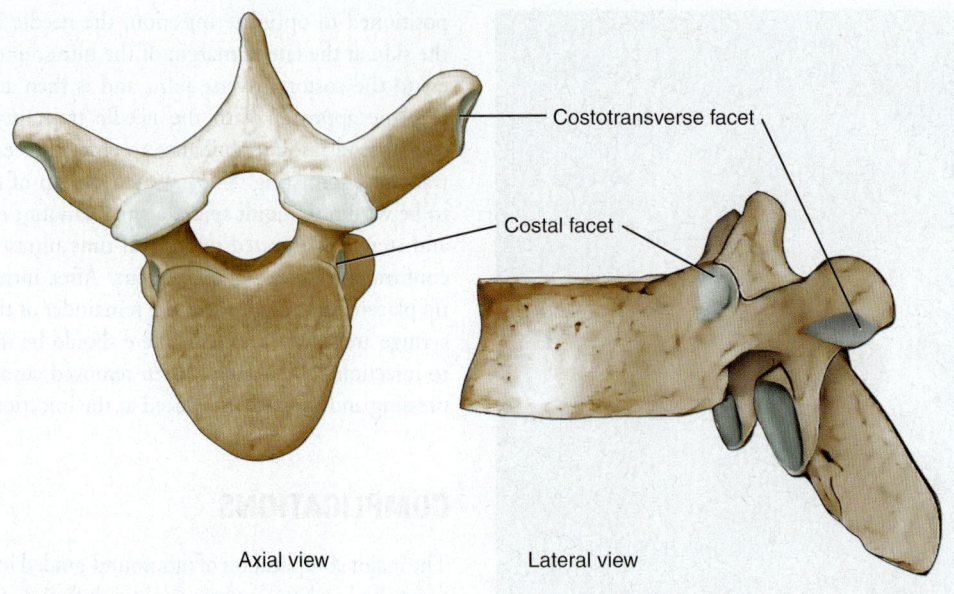

**FIGURE 84.3.** The articulations of the costotransverse and costovertebral joints.

## CLINICAL PEARLS

Pain emanating from the costotransverse and costovertebral joints is often attributed to a kidney stone with many patients rushing to the emergency room for evaluation and treatment. Reassurance is often is required, although it should be remembered that this musculoskeletal pain syndromes and renal or ureteral calculi can coexist as can occult diseases of the superior mediastinum. Universal precautions should always be observed to protect the operator, and strict adherence to sterile technique must be used to avoid infection. Gentle physical therapy and local heat should be introduced following ultrasound-guided injection of the costovertebral joint to reduce pain and improve function. Simple analgesics and nonsteroidal anti-inflammatory agents or COX-2 inhibitors may be used in conjunction with this injection technique.

**FIGURE 84.4.** Proper positioning for ultrasound-guided injection of the costovertebral joint.

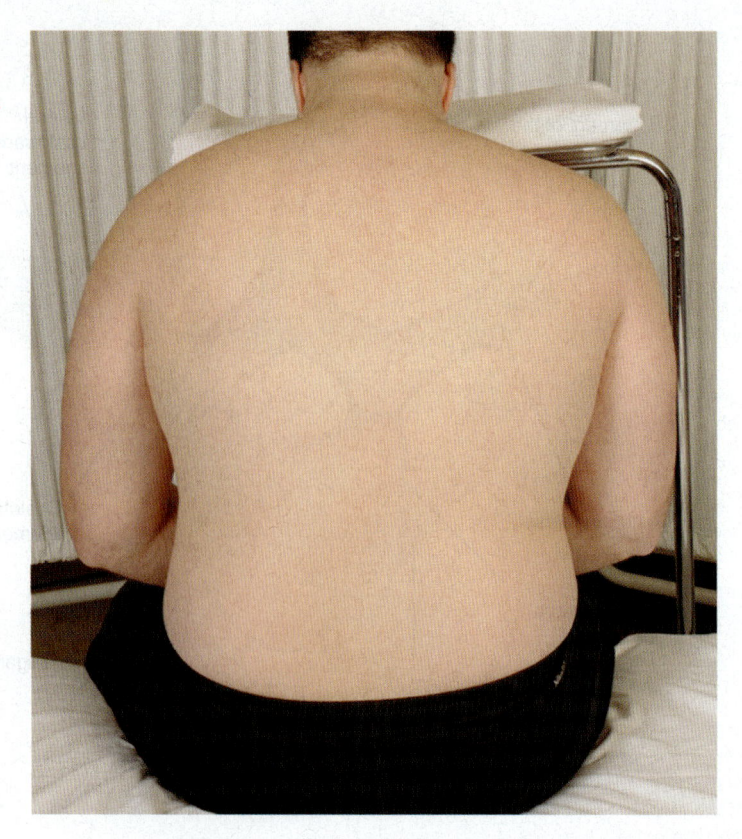

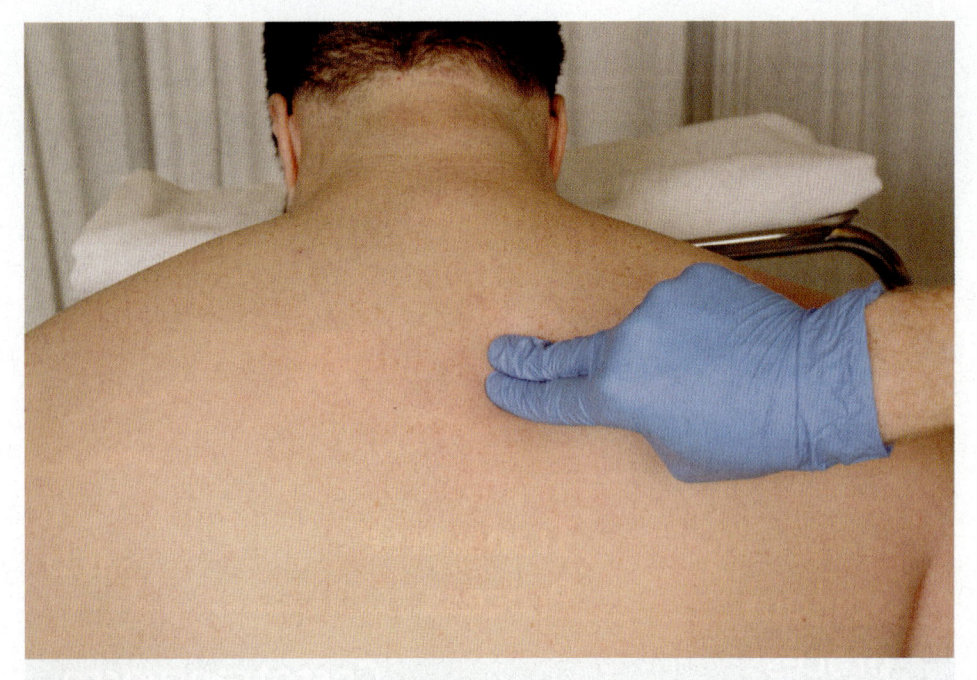

**FIGURE 84.5.** Palpation of the costovertebral joint.

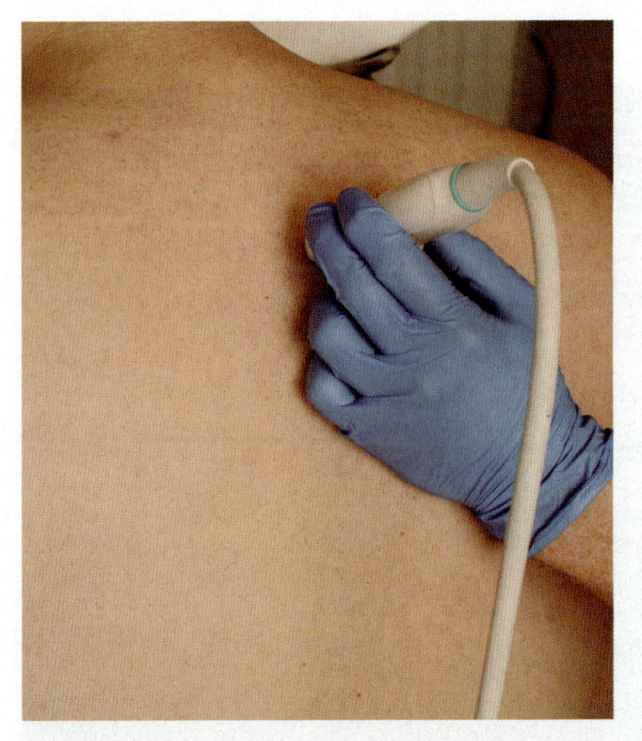

**FIGURE 84.6.** Proper placement of the high-frequency linear ultrasound probe for ultrasound-guided costovertebral joint injection.

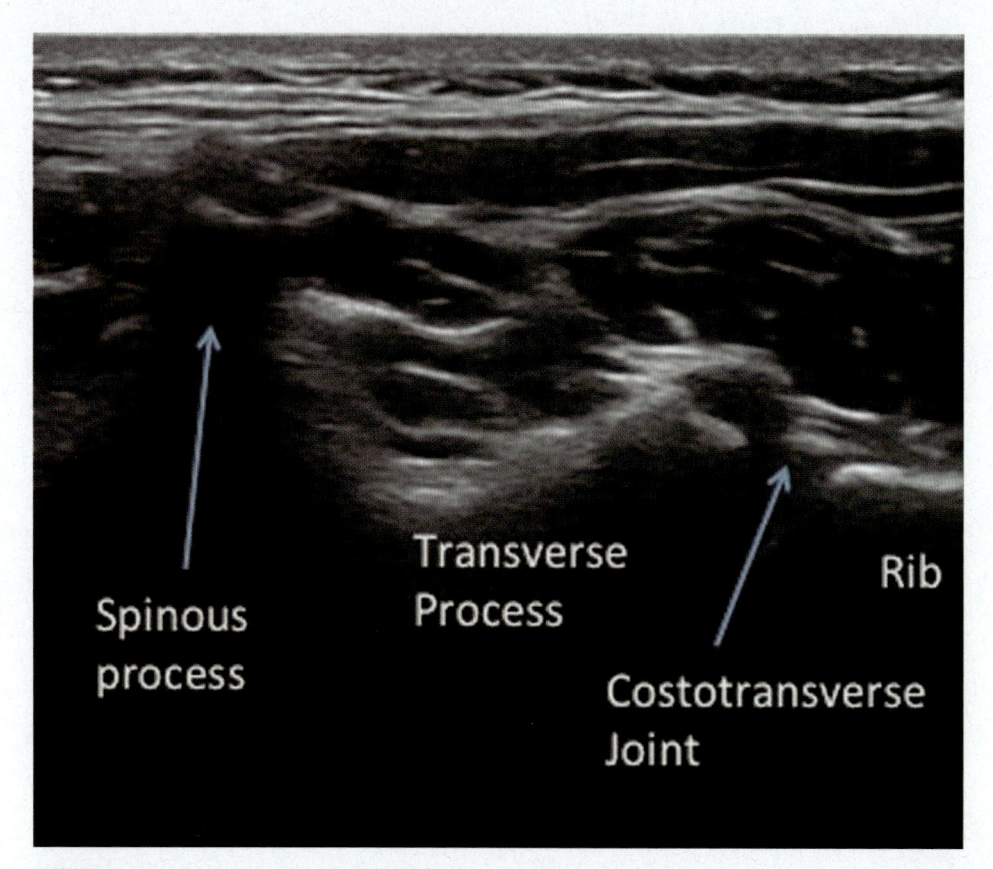

**FIGURE 84.7.** Transverse ultrasound image of the costotransverse joint.

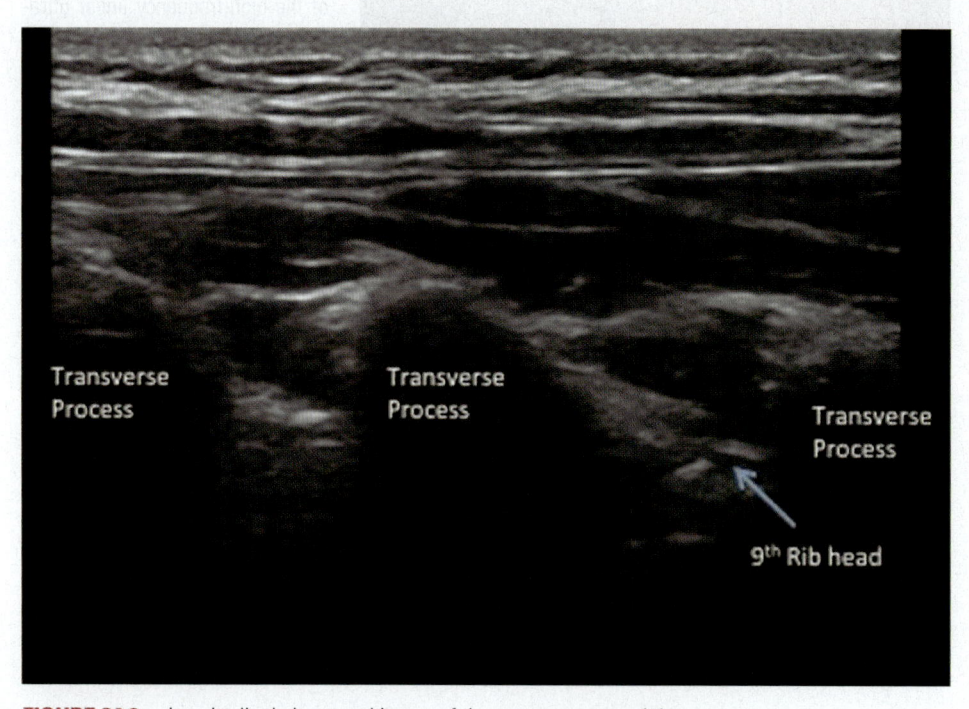

**FIGURE 84.8.** Longitudinal ultrasound image of the costotransverse joint.

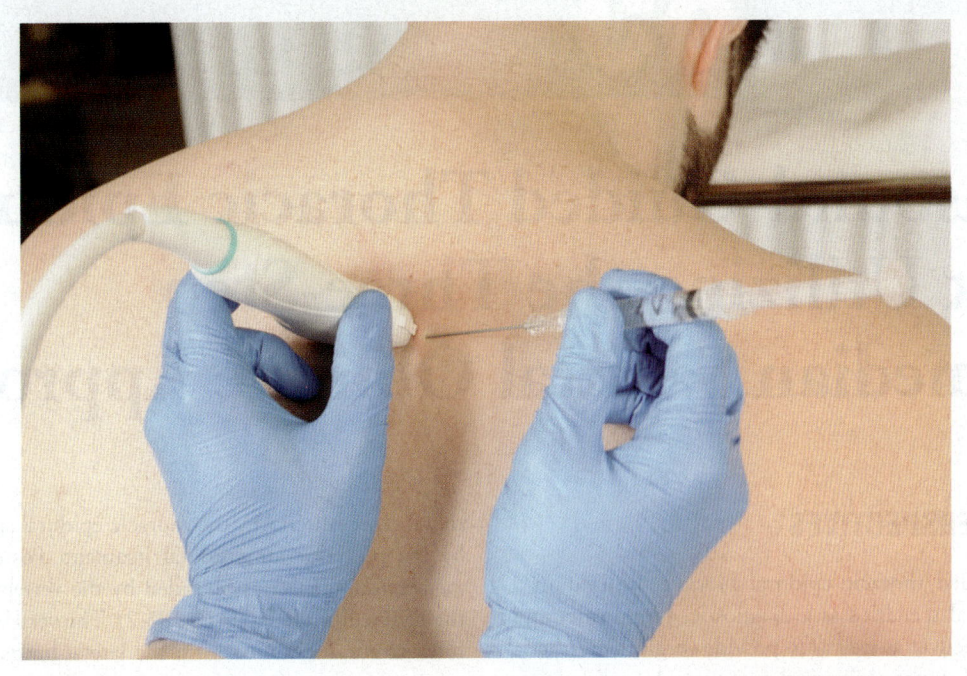

**FIGURE 84.9.** Proper in-plane needle placement for ultrasound-guided injection of the costovertebral oint.

## SUGGESTED READINGS

Erwin WM, Jackson PC, Homonko DA. Innervation of the human costovertebral joint: implications for clinical back pain syndromes. *J Manipulative Physiol Ther* 2000;23(6):395–403.

Malmivaara A, Videman T, Kuosma E, et al. Facet joint orientation, facet and costovertebral joint osteoarthrosis, disc degeneration, vertebral body osteophytosis and Schmorl's nodes in the thoracolumbar junctional region of cadaveric spines. *Spine* 1987;12:458–463.

Waldman SD, Campbell RSD. *Costovertebral Joint Abnormalities. Imaging of Pain.* Philadelphia, PA: Saunders Elsevier; 2011:81–82.

Waldman SD. Costovertebral joint injection. In: *Atlas of Pain Management Injection Techniques.* 3rd ed. Philadelphia, PA: WB Saunders; 2013:261–263.

Wang CC. Pseudomonas aeruginosa costovertebral arthritis in association with spontaneous cervical spondylodiscitis and epidural abscesses in the elderly. *J Clin Gerontol Geriatr* 2012;3(2):82–86.

# Ultrasound-Guided Thoracic Epidural Block Utilizing the Three-Step Paramedian Sagittal Oblique Approach

## CLINICAL PERSPECTIVES

Ultrasound-guided thoracic epidural block is utilized in a variety of clinical scenarios as a diagnostic, prognostic, and therapeutic maneuver as well as to provide surgical anesthesia for thoracic and upper abdominal surgeries. As a diagnostic tool, ultrasound-guided thoracic epidural block allows accurate placement of the epidural needle tip within a specific area of the epidural space when performing differential neural blockade on an anatomic basis in the evaluation of chest wall and intra-abdominal pain. As a prognostic tool, ultrasound-guided thoracic epidural block can be utilized as a prognostic indicator of the degree of motor and sensory impairment that the patient may experience if thoracic nerve roots are going to be destroyed in an effort to palliate intractable pain in patients too sick to undergo neurosurgical destructive procedures. In the acute pain setting, ultrasound-guided thoracic epidural block with local anesthetics and/or opioids may be used to palliate acute pain emergencies while waiting for pharmacologic, surgical, and/or antiblastic methods to become effective. This technique has great clinical utility in both children and adults when managing acute postoperative and posttrauma pain. Sympathetically mediated pain syndromes including the pain of acute herpes zoster of the thoracic dermatomes, intractable angina, phantom breast syndrome, and the pain of acute pancreatitis can also be effectively managed with epidurally administered local anesthetics, steroids, and/or opioids. Pain of malignant origin of the chest wall, flank, and abdomen as well as spinal metastatic disease (especially from breast and prostate primary cancers) is also amenable to treatment with epidurally administered local anesthetics, steroids, and/or opioids (Fig. 85.1).

## CLINICAL RELEVANT ANATOMY

The cephalad boundary of the epidural space is the fused periosteal and spinal layers of dura at the level of the foramen magnum. The caudad border of the epidural space is the fused layers of connective tissue that make up the sacrococcygeal membrane. Anteriorly, the thoracic epidural space is bounded by the posterior longitudinal ligament. Posteriorly the thoracic epidural space is bounded by the vertebral laminae and the ligamentum flavum (Fig. 85.2). The vertebral pedicles and intervertebral foramina form the lateral limits of the epidural space. The thoracic epidural space is 3 to 4 mm at the C7–T1 interspace with the cervical spine flexed and ~5 mm at the T11–T12 interspace. The thoracic epidural space contains fat, veins, arteries, lymphatics, and connective tissue.

From the standpoint of performing ultrasound-guided epidural blocks, the upper thoracic vertebral interspaces from T1–T2 and the lower thoracic vertebral interspaces from T10–T12 are functionally equivalent insofar as the technique of epidural block is concerned, being most analogous to performing a lumbar epidural block. The thoracic vertebral interspaces between T3 and T9 are morphologically and functionally unique when compared with the T1–T2 and T10–T12 segments because of the acute downward angle of the spinous processes (Fig. 85.3). Blockade of these middle thoracic interspaces requires use of the paramedian oblique or transforaminal approach to the thoracic epidural space, and the close proximity of the spinous processes limits the size of the acoustic window, thus decreasing the utility of ultrasound guidance.

## ULTRASOUND-GUIDED TECHNIQUE

Ultrasound-guided thoracic epidural block can be carried out by placing the patient in the sitting position with the head resting comfortably on a padded bedside table and the arms resting comfortably on the patient's lap (Fig. 85.4). A total of 5 to 7 mL of local anesthetic is drawn up in a 10-mL sterile syringe. If the painful condition being treated is thought to have an inflammatory component, 40 to 80 mg of depot steroid is added to the local anesthetic. If performing ultrasound-guided epidural block in the upper thoracic or lower thoracic levels, the technique is more analogous to that used for ultrasound cervical or thoracic epidural block, and a transverse interlaminar ultrasound view is easily obtained. Because of the more sharply angled spinous processes of the midthoracic spine, a clinically usable interlaminar

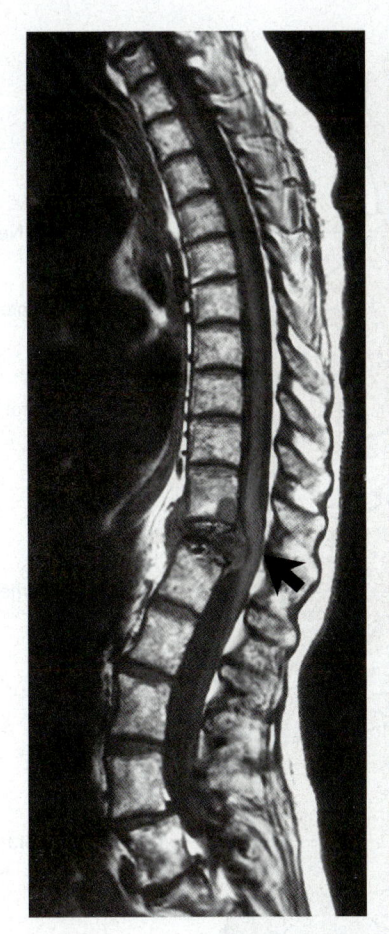

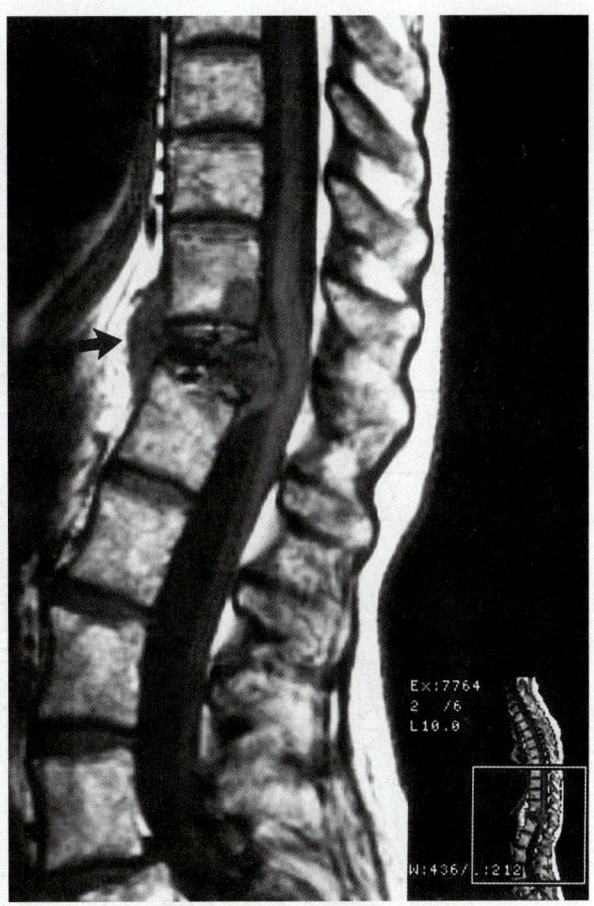

**FIGURE 85.1.** T1-weighted MRI image demonstrating metastasis to the thoracic spine with cord compression from breast cancer. (Reused from Berquist TH. *MRI of the Musculoskeletal System.* 6th ed. Philadelphia, PA: Lippincott Williams & Wilkins; 2013:167, with permission.)

view is more elusive. In the midthoracic region, a parasagittal oblique view will offer the greatest clinical utility.

To perform ultrasound-guided thoracic epidural block, a three-step process is used. Although this may seem cumbersome, the three-step process allows the clinician to quickly identify critical anatomic structures while at the same time maintaining a transducer position that allows a safe and easy placement of needles into the thoracic epidural space.

## Step One: Obtain the Paramedian Sagittal Transverse Process View

Step one is to obtain a paramedian sagittal transverse process view by placing the 2- to 5-MHz low-frequency curvilinear probe in the longitudinal plane 3 to 4 cm lateral to the right side of the middle of the spinous processes at the level to be blocked for the right-handed clinician and 3 to 4 cm to the lateral to the left side of the middle of the spinous processes at the level to be blocked for the left-handed clinician (Figs. 85.5 and 85.6). An initial depth setting of 7 to 8 cm will work for most patients. An ultrasound survey is taken and the transducer is slowly moved medially and laterally until successive transverse processes are visualized. The transverse processes of the thoracic spine will appear as hyperechoic domes with sausage-like acoustic shadows beneath them (Fig. 85.7). This classic appearance of successive transverse processes viewed in the longitudinal plane has been named the "trident sign" after Neptune's trident (Fig. 85.8).

## Step Two: Obtain the Paramedian Sagittal Articular Process View

After the transverse processes are identified in the paramedian sagittal transverse process view, the ultrasound transducer is slowly slid toward the midline until the superior and inferior articular facets are visualized (Step Two) (Figs. 85.9 and 85.10). In longitudinal paramedian ultrasound articular process view, the superior and inferior articular facets will appear

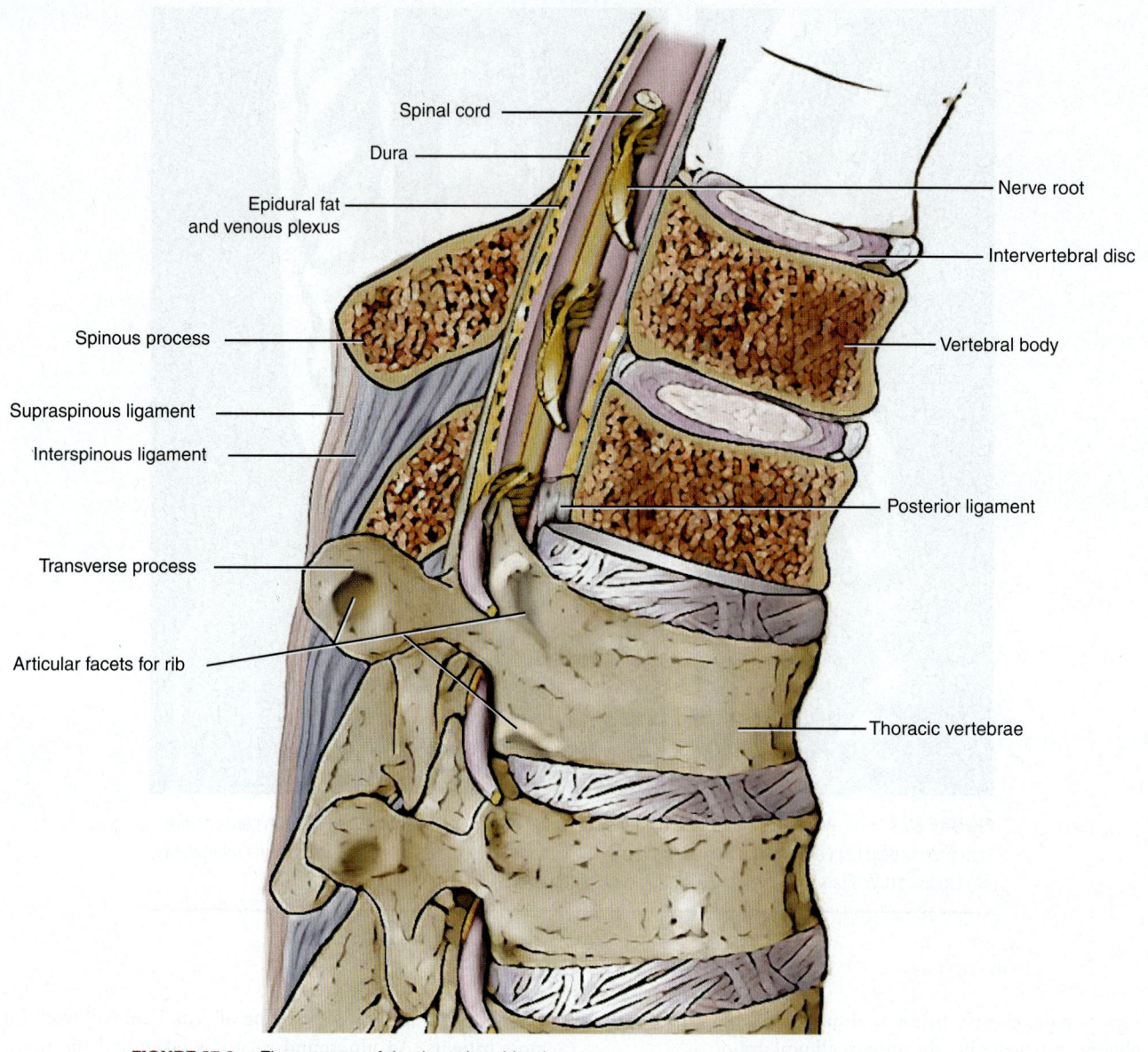

**FIGURE 85.2.** The anatomy of the thoracic epidural space.

as successive hyperechoic hills and valleys, with each hill representing a facet joint (Fig. 85.11).

## Step Three: Obtain the Paramedian Sagittal Oblique View

After the articular processes are identified using the paramedian sagittal articular process view the longitudinally oriented ultrasound transducer is then slowly tilted to angle the ultrasound beam in a lateral to medial oblique trajectory toward the midline (Figs. 85.12 and 85.13) (Step Three). The lamina of successive thoracic vertebrae will appear as a series of hyperechoic curvilinear lines with an acoustic shadow beneath each one (Fig. 85.14). The interlaminar space will appear as gaps between each successive vertebra providing an acoustic window that will allow visualization of the ligamentum flavum, epidural space, and posterior dura. By making minor adjustments to the position of the ultrasound transducer, in some patients, the ligamentum flavum and posterior dura can be distinguished as two distinct hyperechoic linear structures with a hyperechoic epidural space in between (Fig. 85.15). In other patients, these structures simply appear as a single hyperechoic line, which is known as the posterior complex (Fig. 85.16).

CHAPTER 85 ULTRASOUND-GUIDED THORACIC EPIDURAL BLOCK 575

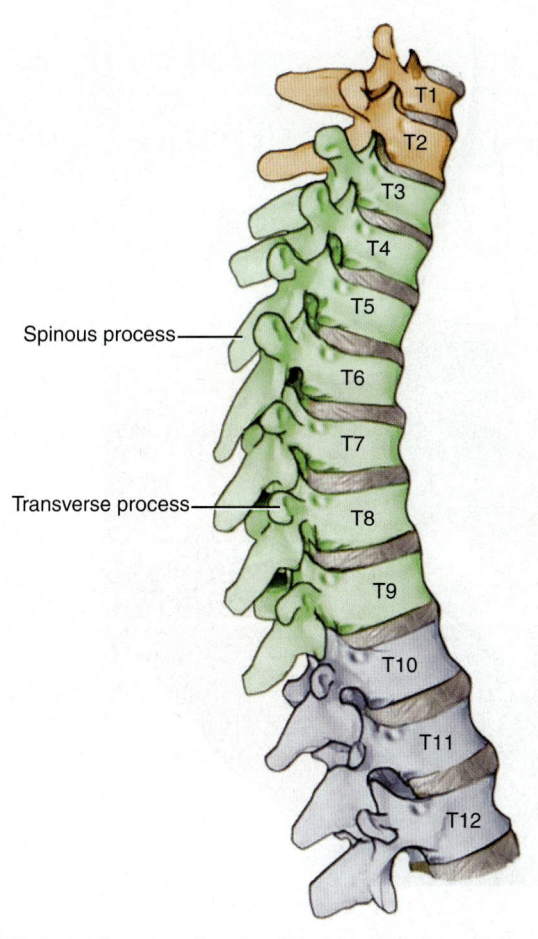

**FIGURE 85.3.** The thoracic spine. Note the similarities of the upper and lower thoracic segments and the sharp downward angles of the spinous processes of the midthoracic vertebra.

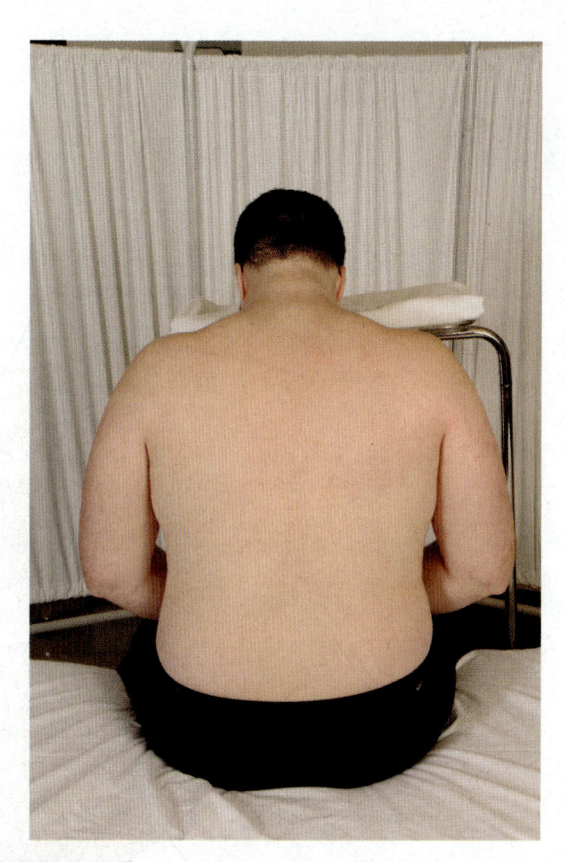

**FIGURE 85.4.** Proper patient positioning for ultrasound-guided thoracic epidural block.

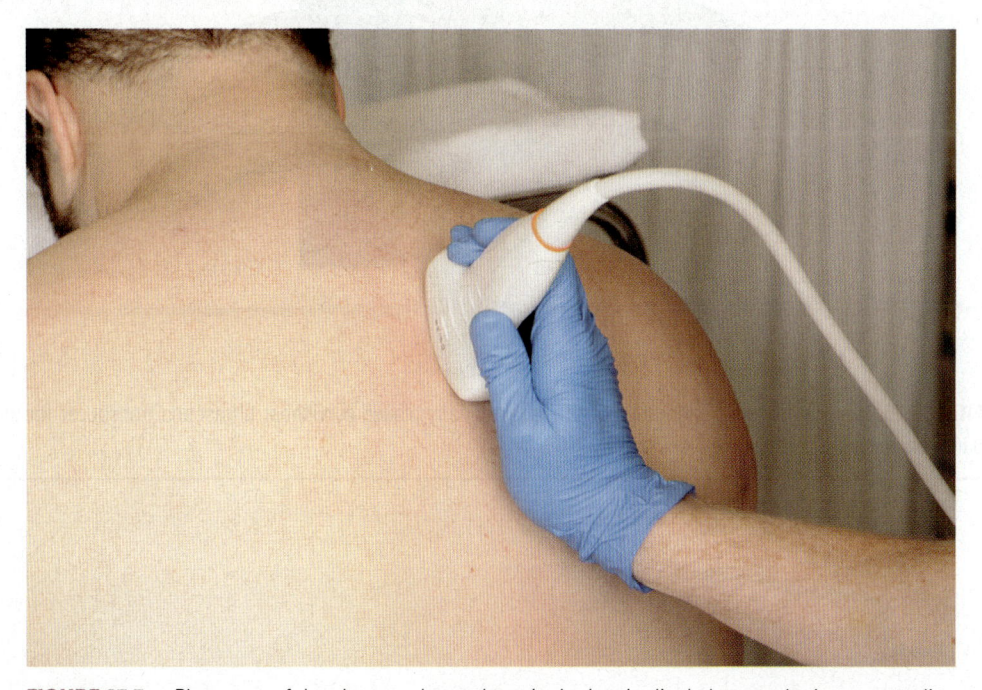

**FIGURE 85.5.** Placement of the ultrasound transducer in the longitudinal plane to obtain a paramedian sagittal transverse process view (Step One).

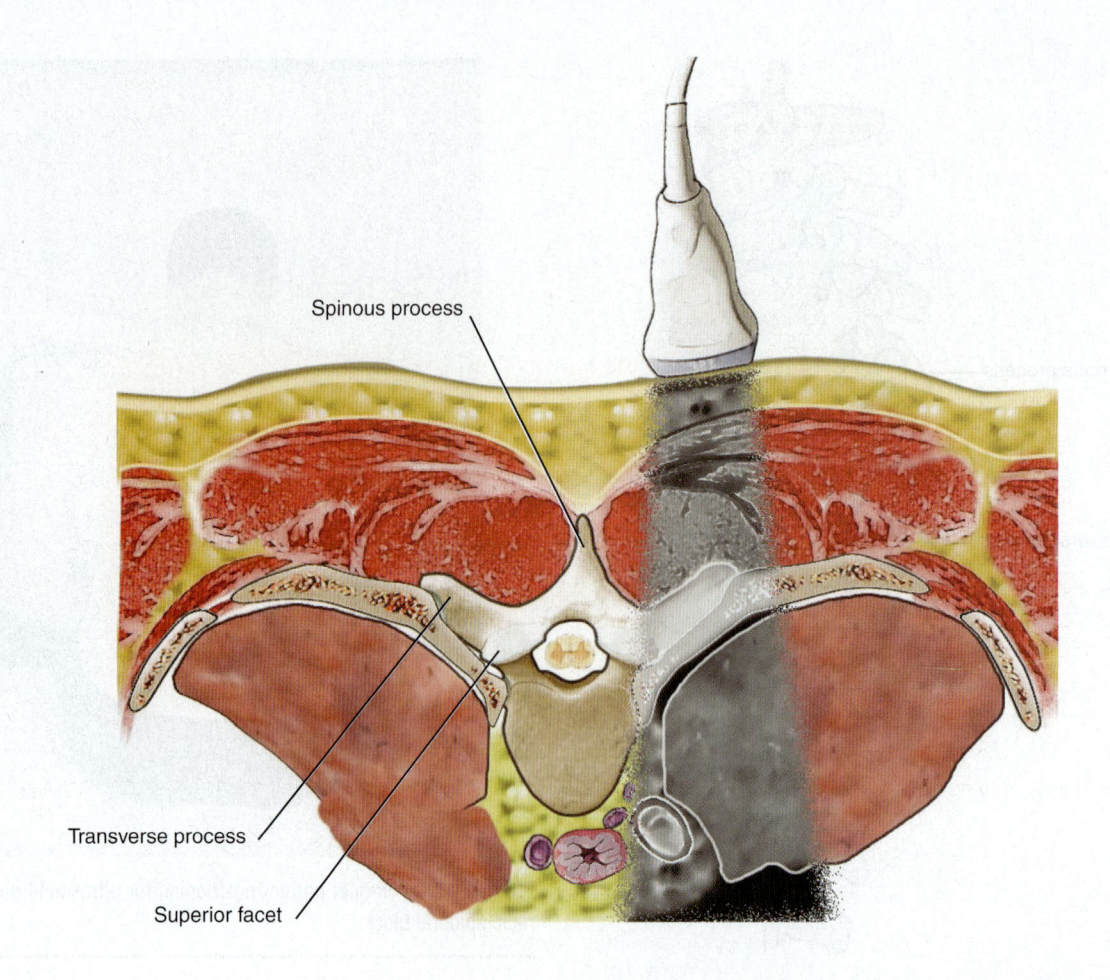

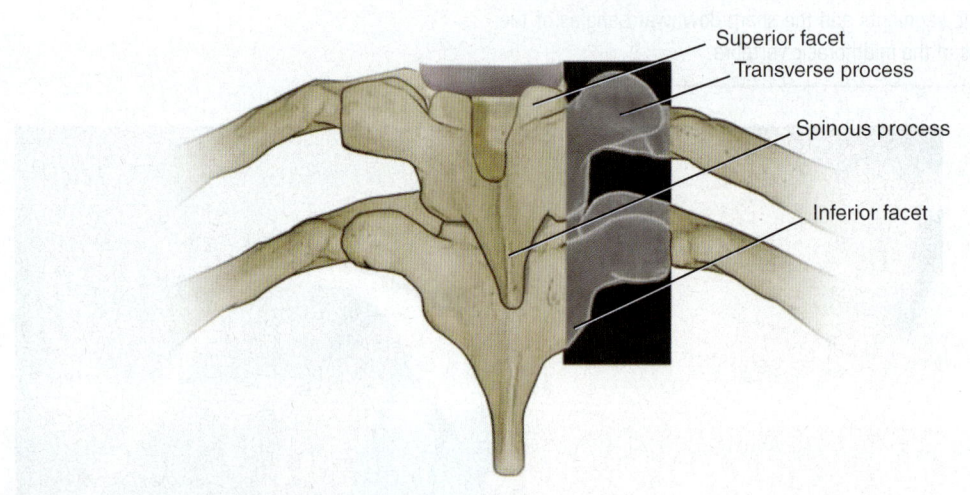

**FIGURE 85.6.** The anatomic orientation of the longitudinally placed curvilinear ultrasound transducer for the paramedian sagittal transverse process view (Step One).

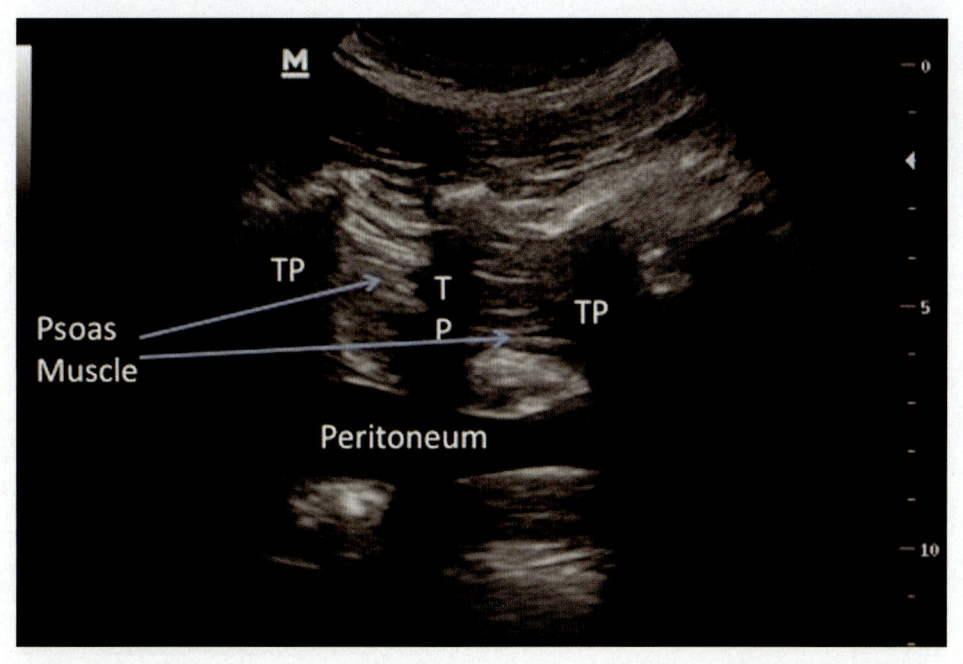

**FIGURE 85.7.** Longitudinal ultrasound image demonstrating successive transverse processes when performing the paramedian sagittal transverse process view (Step One). This classic image is named the "trident sign."

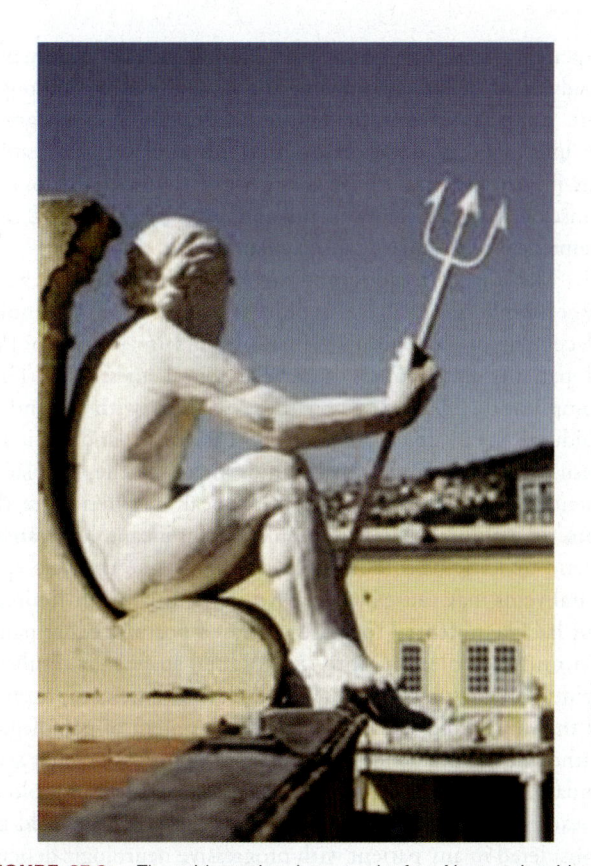

**FIGURE 85.8.** The trident sign is named after Neptune's trident, which according to Roman mythology had the power to conjure water and cause tsunamis and earthquakes.

After interlaminar space is identified, the skin is prepped with antiseptic solution, and a 22-gauge, 3½-inch needle suitable for epidural use is inserted through the skin at the middle of the lateral aspect of the longitudinally placed ultrasound transducer utilizing an out-of-plane approach (Fig. 85.17). While an assistant holds and adjusts the ultrasound transducer, the clinician advances the needle under real-time ultrasound guidance in an oblique lateral to medial trajectory using a loss of resistance technique until the needle tip rests within the epidural space. After gentle aspiration, 5 to 7 mL of solution is injected. The needle is removed and pressure is placed on the injection site to avoid hematoma formation.

## COMPLICATIONS

Because of potential hematogenous spread via the valveless epidural veins of the thoracic epidural space, sepsis and local infection at the injection site represent absolute contraindications to ultrasound-guided thoracic epidural block as do anticoagulation and coagulopathy. The epidural space is in close proximity to the subarachnoid space and spinal cord as well as the exiting spinal nerve roots, which suggests that this procedure should only be performed by those well versed in the regional anatomy and skilled at ultrasound-guided interventional pain management procedures. Trauma to the exiting thoracic nerve roots and spinal cord can be avoided if careful attention is paid to the regional anatomy and if the clinician immediately stops advancing the needle should the patient

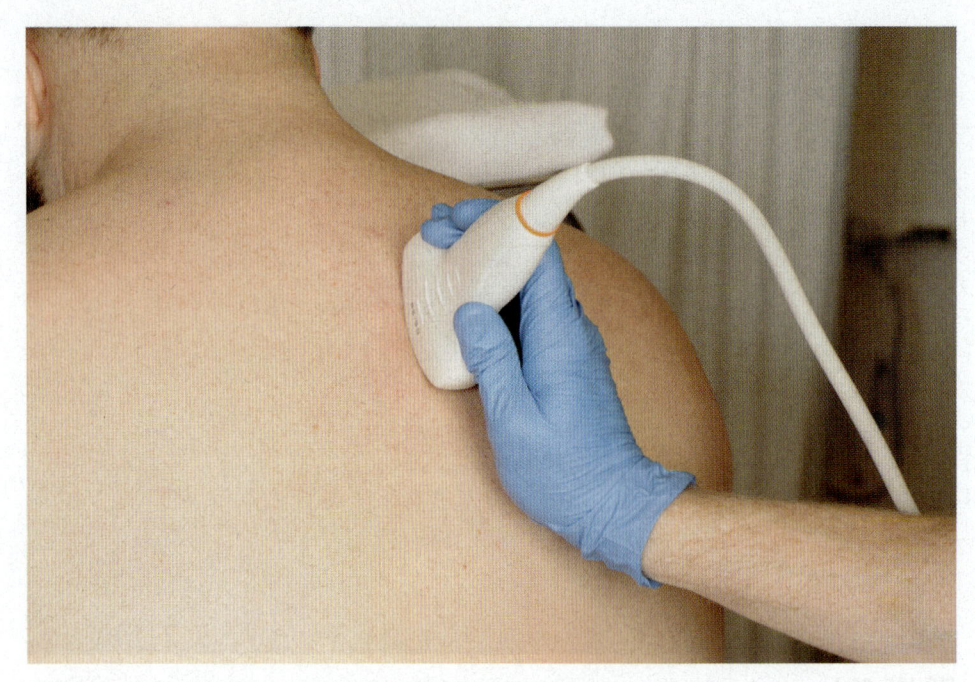

**FIGURE 85.9.** Proper longitudinal ultrasound transducer placement to obtain paramedian sagittal articular view (Step Two).

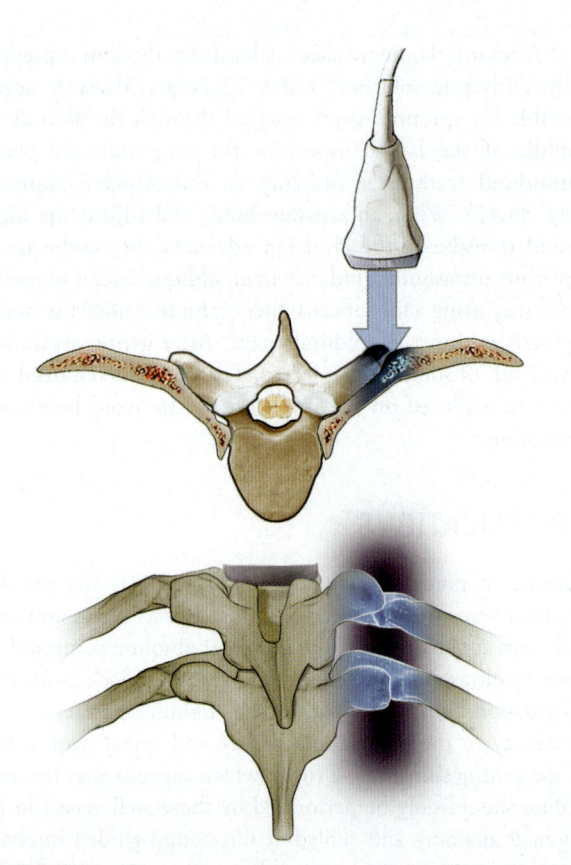

**FIGURE 85.10.** The anatomic orientation of the longitudinally placed curvilinear ultrasound transducer for the paramedian sagittal articular view (Step Three).

experience any significant pain during needle placement. Inadvertent subarachnoid and subdural injection, although rare, can occur even in the best of hands. Failure to recognize an unintentional dural or subdural injection with its resultant immediate total spinal anesthesia with associated loss of consciousness, hypotension, and apnea can be disastrous if not immediately recognized and treated.

The thoracic epidural space is highly vascular with large numbers of valveless epidural veins. The intravenous placement of the epidural needle occurs in ~0.5% to 1% of patients undergoing thoracic epidural anesthesia. This complication is increased in those patients with distended epidural veins, for example, the parturient and patients with large intra-abdominal tumor mass. If the misplacement is unrecognized, injection of local anesthetic directly into an epidural vein will result in significant local anesthetic toxicity. Needle-induced trauma to the thoracic epidural veins may cause bleeding, which is usually self-limited, but has the potential to cause increased postprocedure pain. Uncontrolled bleeding into the epidural space may result in epidural hematoma formation, which can cause compression of the spinal cord with the rapid development of paraplegia. Although the incidence of significant neurologic deficit secondary to epidural hematoma after thoracic epidural block is exceedingly rare, this devastating complication should be considered in any patient with progressive neurologic deficits following this procedure.

Although uncommon, infection in the thoracic epidural space remains an ever-present possibility, especially in the

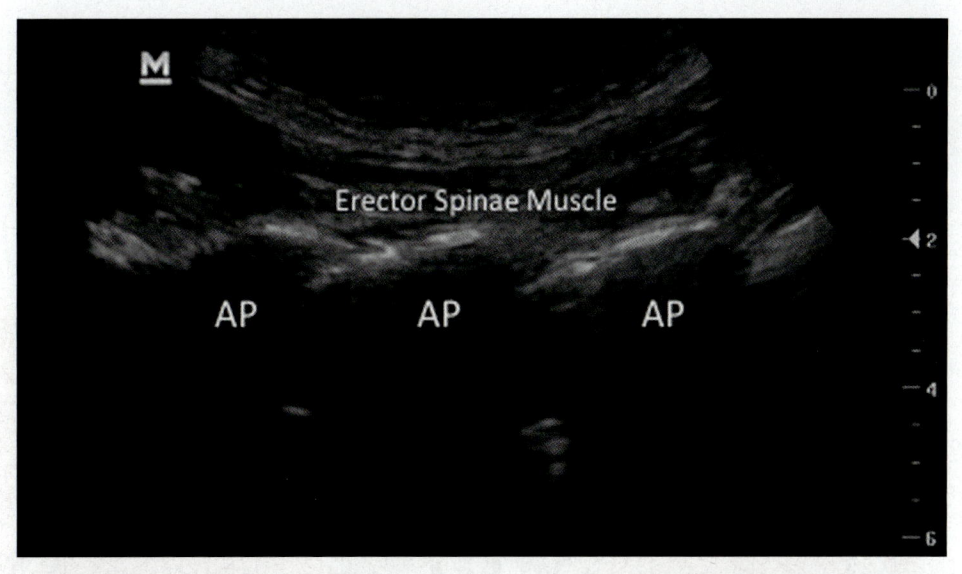

**FIGURE 85.11.** Longitudinal ultrasound image of the paramedian sagittal articular process view demonstrating the articular processes (Step Two).

immunocompromised AIDS or cancer patient, and should be considered in any patient with fever and the onset of neurologic symptomatology after undergoing an epidural block. Early detection and treatment of epidural infection is crucial to avoid potentially life-threatening sequelae, and urgent computerized tomography and/or magnetic resonance imaging (MRI) should be obtained in any patient suspected of having an epidural abscess. Emergent surgical drainage to avoid spinal cord compression and irreversible neurologic deficit is often required.

## CLINICAL PEARLS

The key to performing successful ultrasound cervical neuraxial blocks is the proper identification of the sonographic anatomy.

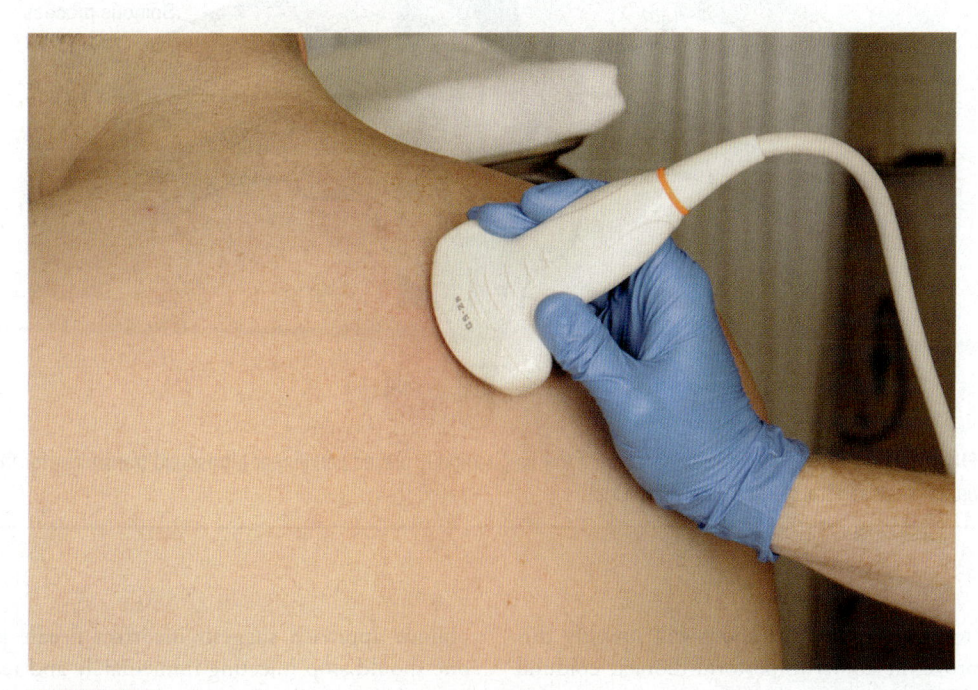

**FIGURE 85.12.** Proper longitudinal ultrasound transducer placement to obtain paramedian sagittal oblique view (Step Three).

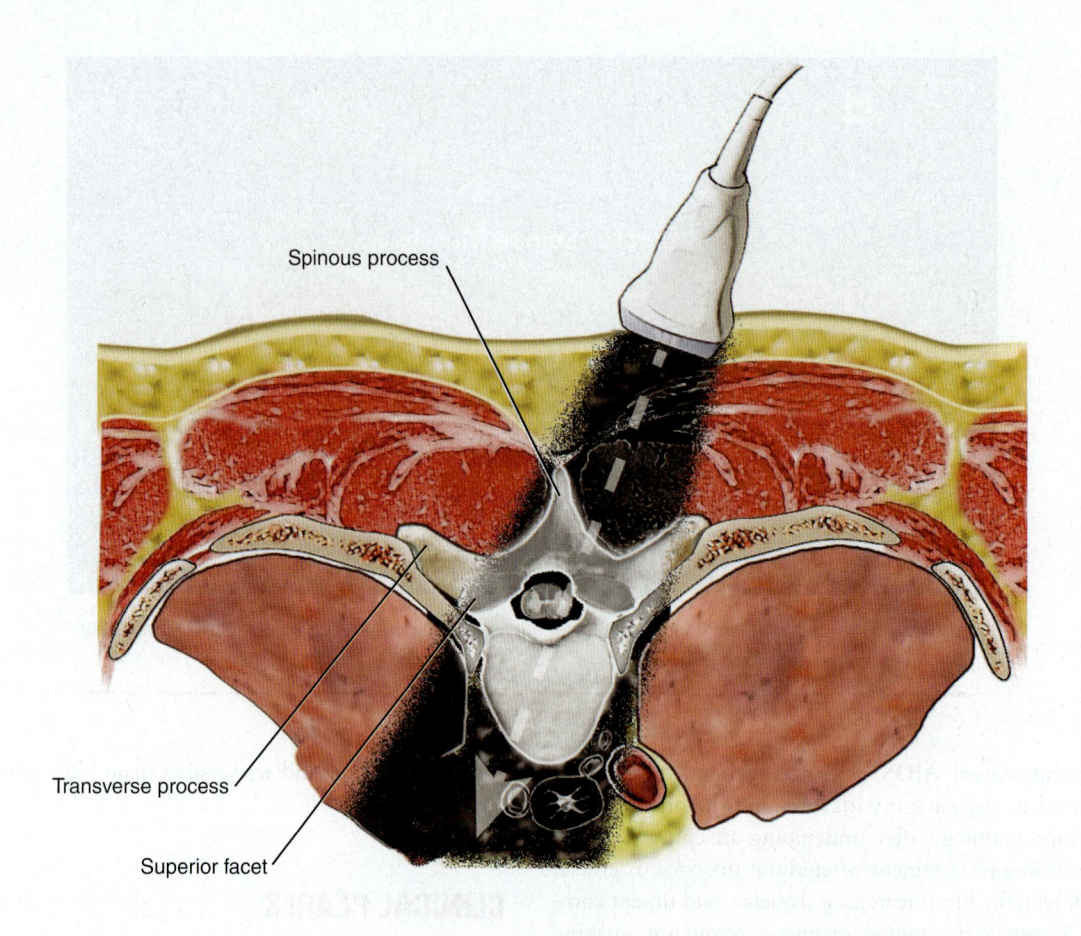

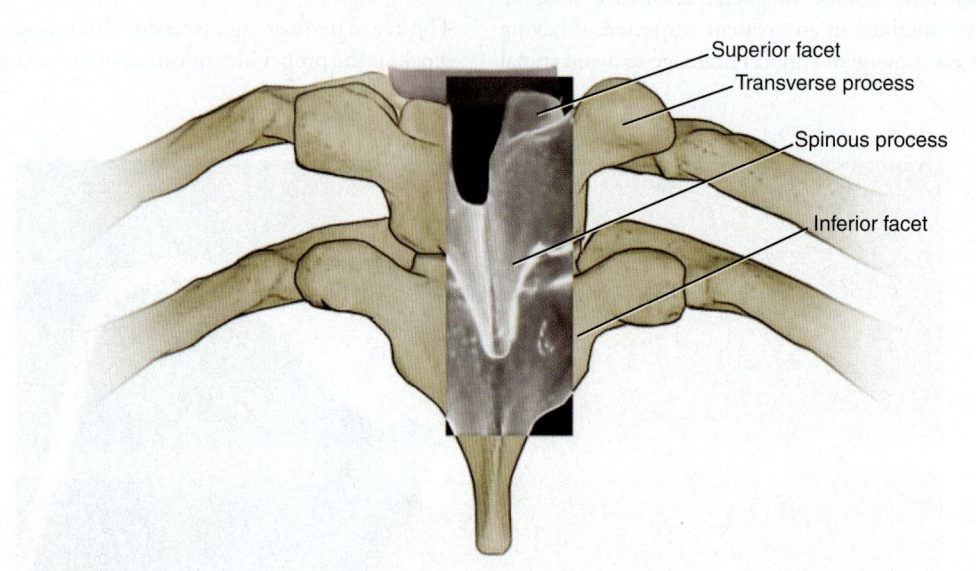

**FIGURE 85.13.** The anatomic orientation of the longitudinally placed curvilinear ultrasound transducer for the paramedian sagittal oblique view (Step One).

The three-step technique presented above will simplify this process and improve the ability to perform thoracic epidural block. Any significant pain or sudden increase in resistance during injection when performing ultrasound-guided thoracic epidural block utilizing the three-step paramedian sagittal oblique approach suggests incorrect needle placement, and one should stop injecting immediately and reassess the position of the needle. Because pain is an important indication of improper needle placement, the practitioner should avoid the use of excessive sedation when performing this technique.

CHAPTER 85    ULTRASOUND-GUIDED THORACIC EPIDURAL BLOCK    581

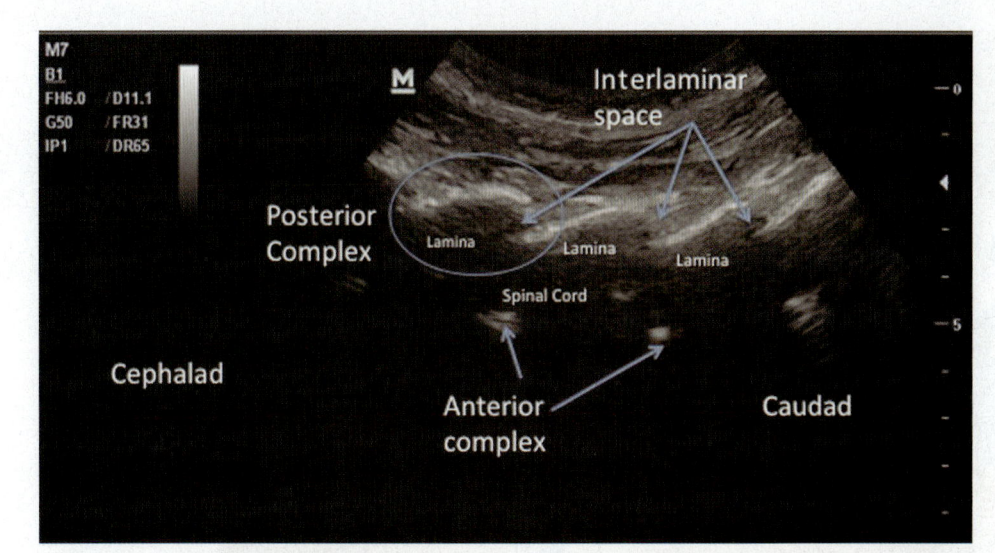

**FIGURE 85.14.** Longitudinal ultrasound image of the paramedian sagittal oblique view demonstrating the interlaminar space and posterior complex made of the ligamentum flavum, posterior epidural space, and posterior dura (Step Three).

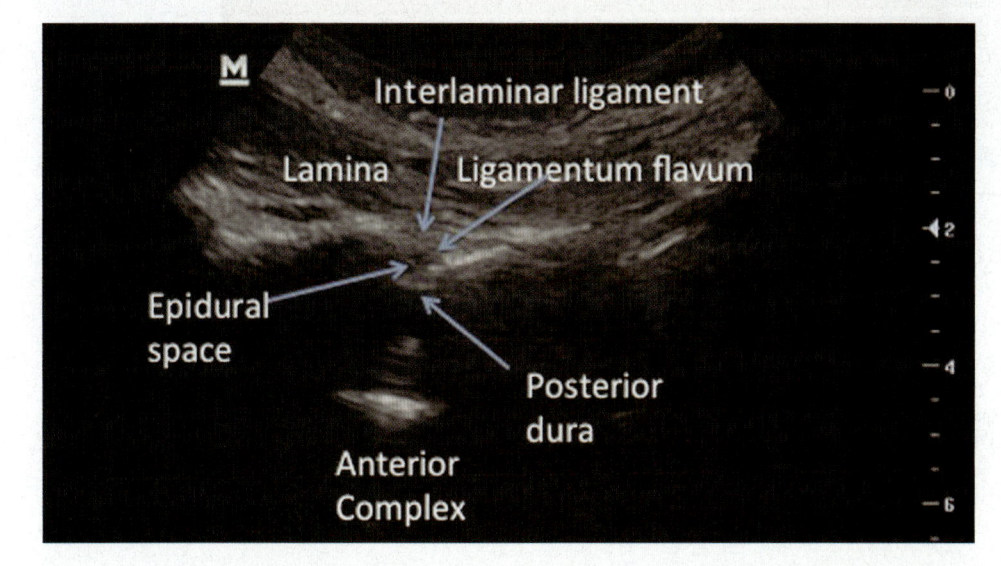

**FIGURE 85.15.** Longitudinal ultrasound image of the paramedian sagittal oblique view demonstrating the interlaminar space and posterior complex made of the ligamentum flavum, posterior epidural space, and posterior dura.

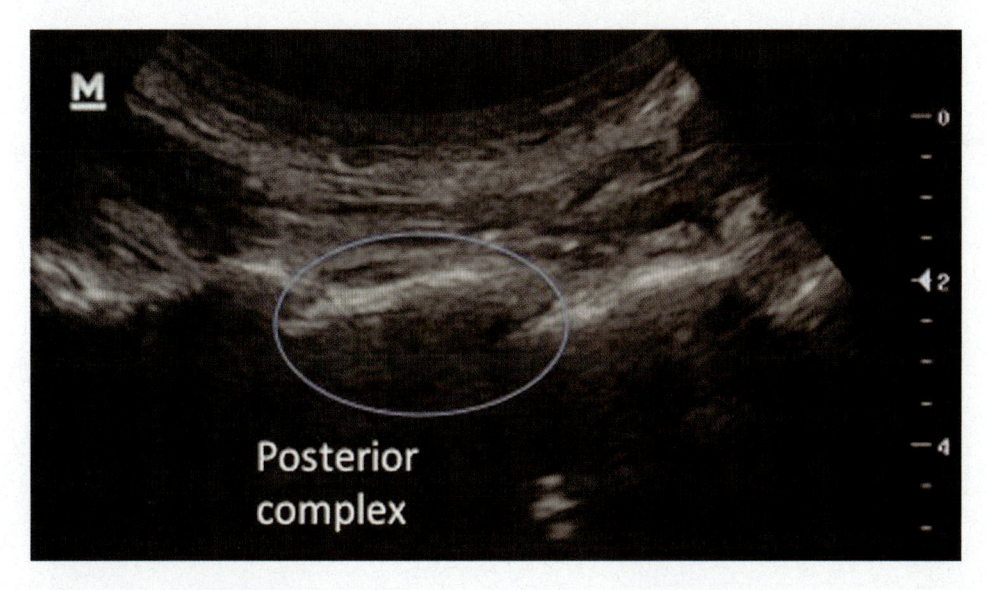

**FIGURE 85.16.** Longitudinal ultrasound image of the paramedian sagittal oblique view demonstrating the interlaminar space and posterior complex.

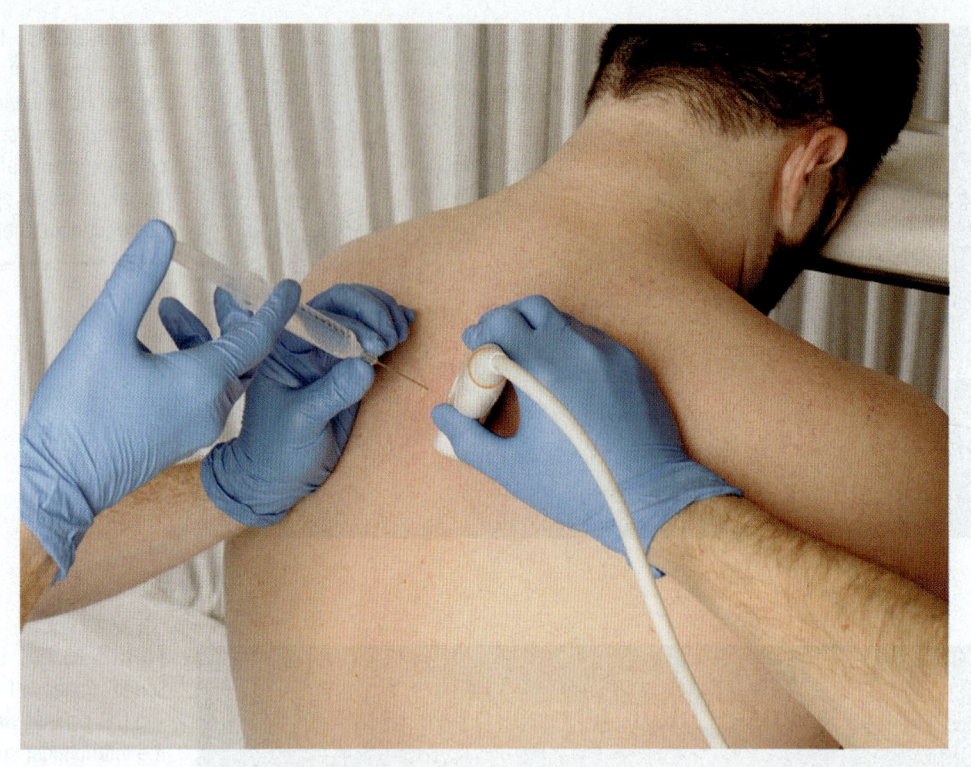

**FIGURE 85.17.** Proper needle position for performing ultrasound-guided thoracic epidural block.

## SUGGESTED READINGS

Shankar H, Zainer CM. Ultrasound guidance for epidural steroid injections. *Tech Reg Anesth Pain Manag* 2009;13(4):229–235.

Waldman SD, Campbell RSD. Anatomy: special imaging considerations of the thoracic spine. In: *Imaging of Pain*. Philadelphia, PA: Saunders Elsevier; 2009:67–68.

Waldman SD. Thoracic epidural block. In: *Pain Review*. Philadelphia, PA: Saunders Elsevier; 2009:476–480.

Waldman SD. Thoracic epidural nerve block: paramedian approach. In: *Atlas of Interventional Pain Management*. 3rd ed. Philadelphia, PA: Saunders Elsevier; 2011:264–268.

Yamauchi M. Ultrasound-guided neuraxial block. *Trends Anaesth Crit Care* 2012;2(5):234–243.

# CHAPTER 86

# Ultrasound-Guided Thoracic Paravertebral Nerve Block

## CLINICAL PERSPECTIVES

Ultrasound-guided thoracic paravertebral nerve block is utilized in a variety of clinical scenarios as a diagnostic, prognostic, and therapeutic maneuver as well as to provide surgical anesthesia for thoracic and upper abdominal surgeries. As a diagnostic tool, ultrasound-guided thoracic paravertebral block allows accurate placement of the needle tip within the thoracic paravertebral space when performing differential neural blockade on an anatomic basis in the evaluation of chest wall and intra-abdominal pain. As a prognostic tool, ultrasound-guided thoracic paravertebral block can be utilized as a prognostic indicator of the degree of motor and sensory impairment that the patient may experience if thoracic nerve roots are going to be destroyed in an effort to palliate intractable pain in patients too sick to undergo neurosurgical destructive procedures. In the acute pain setting, ultrasound-guided thoracic paravertebral block with local anesthetics may be used to palliate acute pain emergencies while waiting for pharmacologic, surgical, and/or antiblastic methods to become effective. This technique has great clinical utility in both children and adults when managing acute postoperative and posttrauma pain. Sympathetically mediated pain syndromes including the pain of acute herpes zoster of the thoracic dermatomes, intractable angina, phantom breast syndrome, and the pain of acute pancreatitis can also be effectively managed with local anesthetics and or steroids administered into the thoracic paravertebral space (Fig. 86.1). Pain of malignant origin of the chest wall, flank, and abdomen as well as spinal metastatic disease (especially from breast and prostate primary cancers) is also amenable to treatment with local anesthetics and/or steroids and neurolytic agents such as phenol administered into the thoracic paravertebral space.

## CLINICALLY RELEVANT ANATOMY

The boundaries of the triangular-shaped thoracic paravertebral space are the parietal pleura anterolaterally, the superior costotransverse ligament posteriorly, and the vertebral elements including the posterolateral surface of the vertebral body, intervertebral disc, and the intervertebral foramen (Fig. 86.2). Exiting their respective intervertebral foramen and passing just below the transverse process are the thoracic paravertebral nerves. After exiting the intervertebral foramen, the thoracic paravertebral nerve gives off a recurrent branch that loops back through the foramen to provide innervation to the spinal ligaments, meninges, and its respective vertebra and can be an important contributor to spinal pain. The thoracic paravertebral nerve also provides fibers to the sympathetic nervous system and the thoracic sympathetic chain via the myelinated preganglionic fibers of the white rami communicantes as well as the unmyelinated postganglionic fibers of the gray rami communicantes. The thoracic paravertebral nerve then divides into a posterior and an anterior primary division (see Fig. 86.2). The posterior division courses posteriorly and, along with its branches, provides innervation to the facet joints and the muscles and skin of the back. The larger, anterior division courses laterally to pass into the subcostal groove beneath the rib to become the respective intercostal nerves. The 12th thoracic nerve courses beneath the 12th rib and is called the subcostal nerve. The intercostal and subcostal nerves provide the innervation to the skin, muscles, ribs, and the parietal pleura and parietal peritoneum. Because blockade of the thoracic paravertebral nerve is performed at the point at which the nerve is beginning to give off its various branches, it is possible to block the anterior division and the posterior division as well as the recurrent and sympathetic components of each respective thoracic paravertebral nerve (see Fig. 86.2). Since the thoracic paravertebral space is not a closed space, drugs injected into this space not only block the paravertebral nerve at the level of needle placement, but if the volume of injectate is large enough, the injectate may spread to block adjacent thoracic paravertebral nerves as well as spread into the epidural space medially.

## ULTRASOUND-GUIDED TECHNIQUE

Ultrasound-guided thoracic paravertebral block can be carried out by placing the patient in the sitting position with the patient's head resting comfortably on a padded bedside table and the arms resting comfortably on the patient's lap (Fig. 86.3).

**FIGURE 86.1.** Acute herpes zoster of the thoracic dermatomes is amenable to treatment with ultrasound-guided thoracic paravertebral block. (Reused from Weber J, Kelley J. *Health Assessment in Nursing*. 2nd ed. Philadelphia, PA: Lippincott Williams & Wilkins, 2003, with permission.)

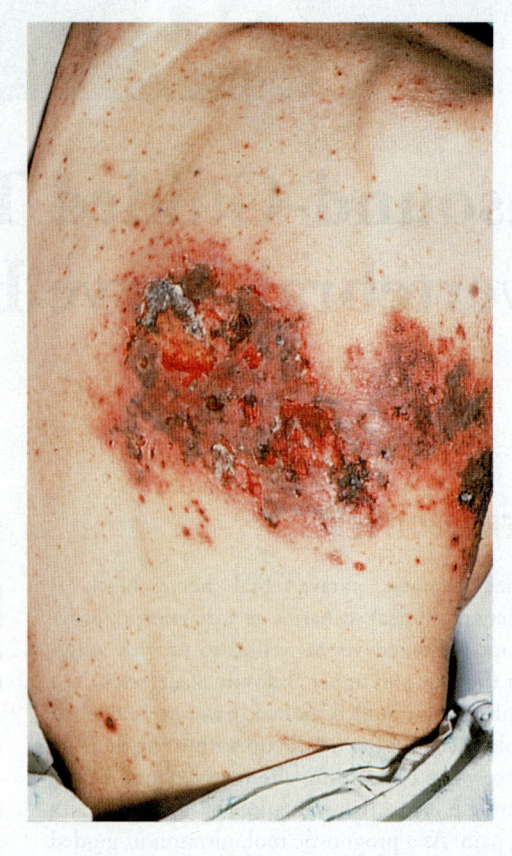

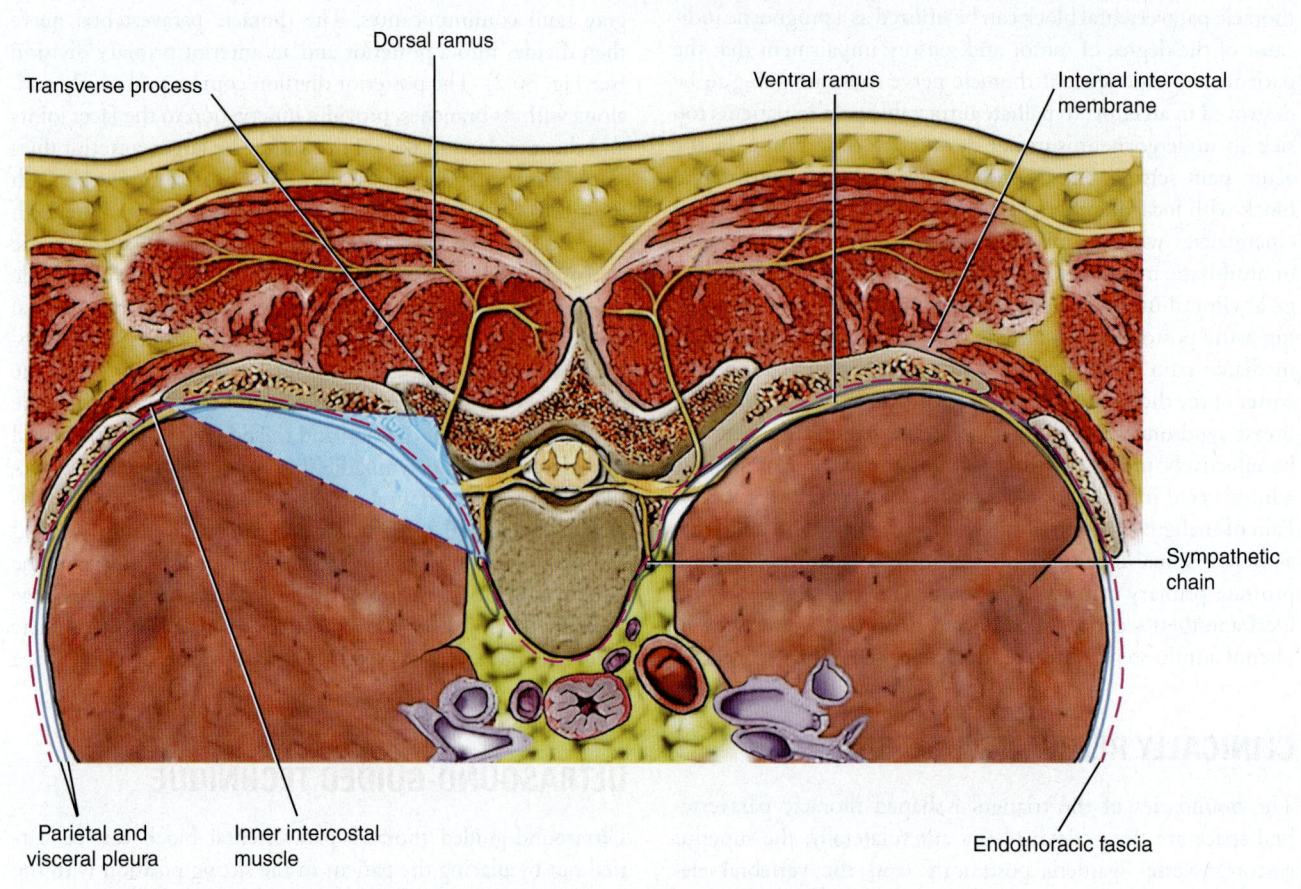

**FIGURE 86.2.** Cross-sectional view of the thoracic paravertebral space. Note the relationship of the transverse process, the exiting paravertebral nerve, and the pleura and lung beneath it.

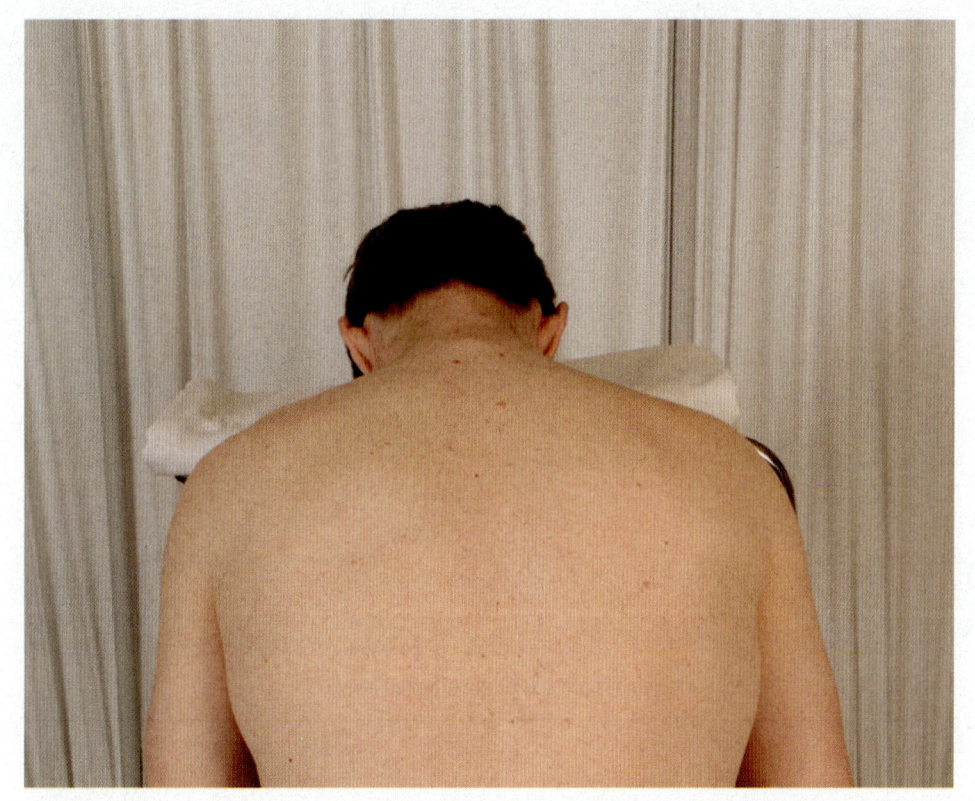

**FIGURE 86.3.** Proper patient position for ultrasound-guided thoracic paravertebral block.

A total of 5 mL of local anesthetic is drawn up in a 10-mL sterile syringe. If the painful condition being treated is thought to have an inflammatory component, 40 to 80 mg of depot steroid is added to the local anesthetic. The spinous process of the level to be blocked is then identified by palpation (Fig. 86.4). A linear high-frequency ultrasound transducer is then placed in the transverse plane with its medial border just lateral to the previously identified spinous process of the vertebral body at the level of the affected joint, and an ultrasound survey scan is obtained (Fig. 86.5). The transverse process is visualized as a bright hyperechoic line with an acoustic shadow, which obscures the paravertebral space beneath it. Once the transverse process is identified, the transducer is slowly moved superiorly or inferiorly until the space between two adjacent transverse processes is identified. This space between adjacent transverse processes provides an excellent acoustic window, which allows identification of the thoracic paravertebral space (Fig. 86.6). The clinician should first identify the pleura that appears as a bright hyperechoic downward curving line, which can be seen to slide back and forth with respiration (see Fig. 86.6). The pleura and the lung beneath it have been described as having the appearance of "waves on a sandy beach" (see Fig. 86.6). Just above the hyperechoic pleural line as it curves down as it moves medially toward the vertebral body is the triangular-shaped thoracic paravertebral space (see Fig. 86.6). Just above the paravertebral space is the linear hyperechoic internal intercostal membrane. The depth of the posterior border of the paravertebral space is noted. When these anatomic structures are clearly identified on transverse ultrasound scan, the skin is prepped with anesthetic solution, and a 3½-inch styletted needle is advanced from the middle of the inferior border of the ultrasound transducer using an out-of-plane approach with the trajectory being adjusted under real-time ultrasound guidance until the needle tip is at the previously identified depth of the posterior border of the paravertebral space (Fig. 86.7). After careful aspiration, a small amount of solution can be injected to aid in identification of the position of the needle tip. The needle is then advanced slowly with attention paid to the relative location of the bight hyperechoic pleura line until the needle tip is seen to be within the paravertebral space. After careful aspiration, the remainder of the solution is slowly injected. There should be minimal resistance to injection. The needle is then removed, and a sterile pressure dressing and ice pack are placed at the injection site.

## COMPLICATIONS

The thoracic paravertebral nerve is in close proximity to the spinal cord and pleural space, and this procedure should be performed only by those well versed in the regional anatomy and skilled at ultrasound-guided interventional pain management procedures. Trauma to the exiting thoracic paravertebral nerves as well as inadvertent subarachnoid, subdural, and/or

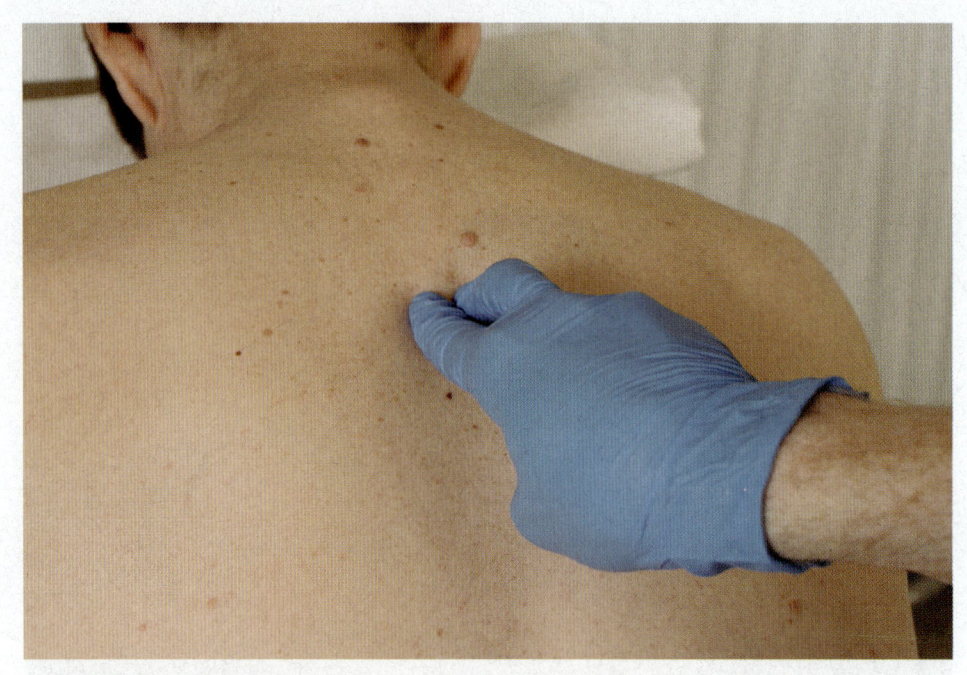

**FIGURE 86.4.** Palpation of the spinous process at the affected level.

epidural injection can occur even in the best of hands. Failure to recognize an unintentional dural or subdural injection can result in immediate total spinal anesthesia with associated loss of consciousness, hypotension, and apnea. This can be disastrous if not immediately recognized. The proximity to the pleural space makes the potential for pneumothorax an ever-present possibility. Should a pneumothorax occur, the "waves on a sandy beach" appearance of the normal pleural lung interface will be replaced with a more chaotic "ripples on a pond" appearance.

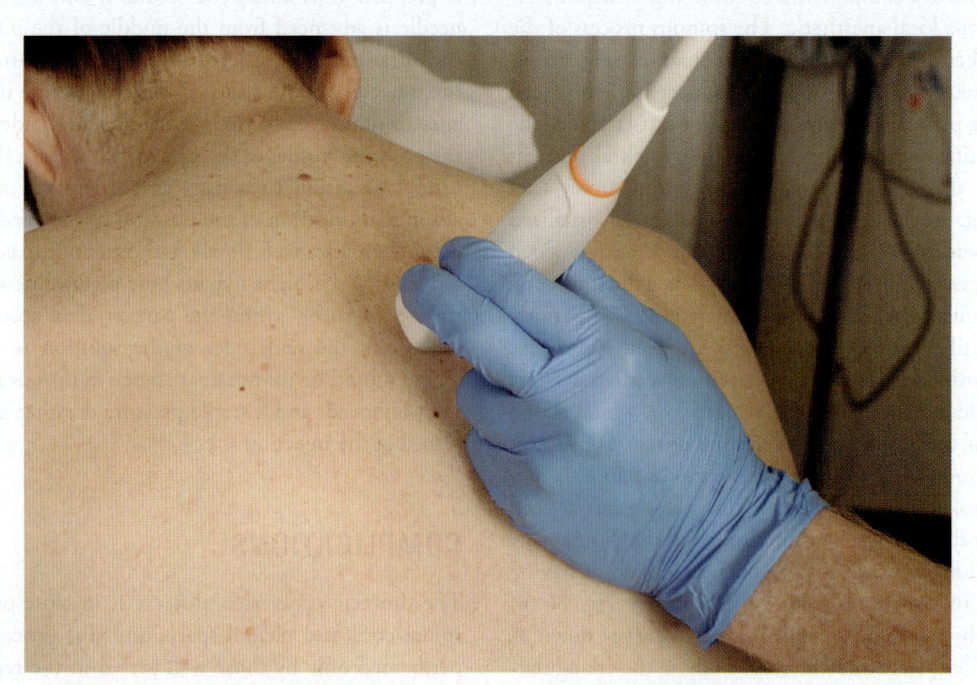

**FIGURE 86.5.** Placement of the ultrasound transducer in the transverse plane with the medial border of the transducer over the spinous process.

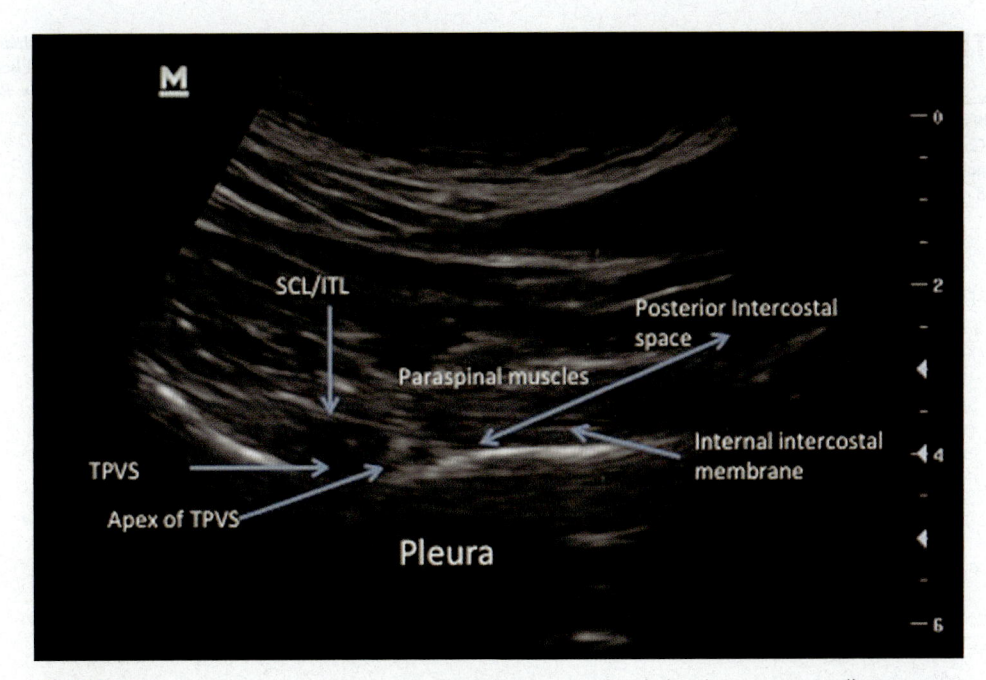

**FIGURE 86.6.** Transverse ultrasound view through the acoustic window between two adjacent transverse processes demonstrating triangular paravertebral space. SCL, superior costotransverse ligament; TPVS, thoracic paravertebral space.

## CLINICAL PEARLS

The key to performing successful ultrasound thoracic paravertebral block is the proper identification of the sonographic anatomy and in particular the ability to properly identify the pleura. This should not be a problem if the above technique is used. Any significant pain or sudden increase in resistance during injection when performing ultrasound-guided selective thoracic nerve root block suggests incorrect needle placement, and one should stop injecting immediately and reassess the position of the needle. Because pain is an important indication of improper needle placement, the practitioner should avoid the use of excessive sedation during ultrasound-guided paravertebral block.

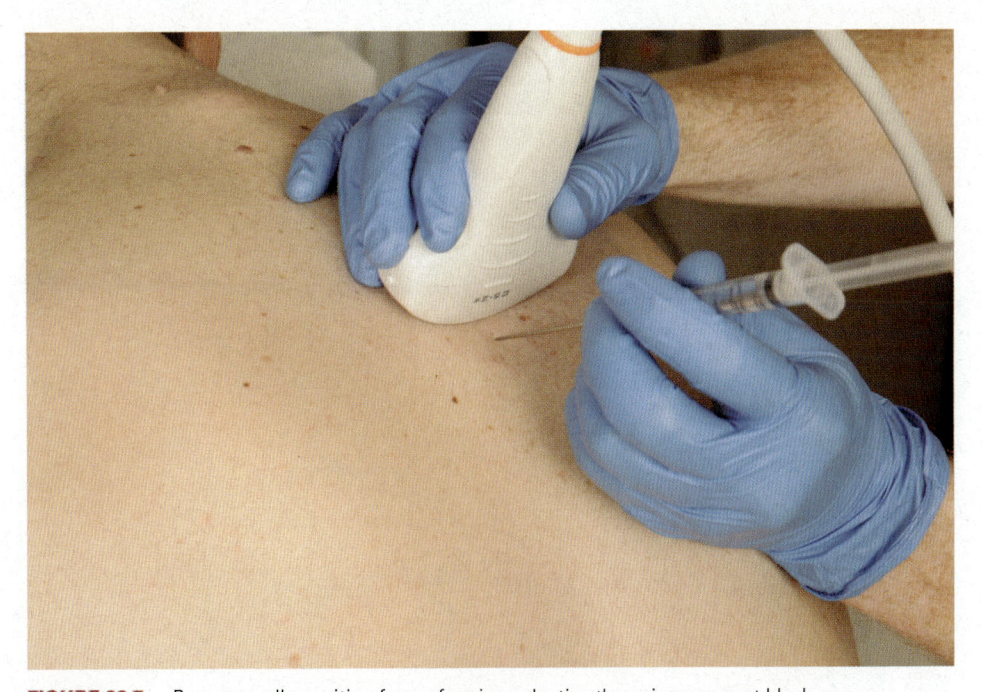

**FIGURE 86.7.** Proper needle position for performing selective thoracic nerve root block.

## SUGGESTED READINGS

Vogt A. Review about ultrasounds in paravertebral blocks. *Eur J Pain* 2011; 5(2):489–494.

Waldman SD, Campbell RSD. Anatomy: special imaging considerations of the thoracic spine. In: *Imaging of Pain*. Philadelphia, PA: Saunders Elsevier, 2009:67–68.

Waldman SD. Thoracic paravertebral block. In: *Atlas of Interventional Pain Management*. 3rd ed. Philadelphia, PA: Saunders Elsevier, 2009:276–278.

Waldman SD. Thoracic paravertebral block. In: *Pain Review*. Philadelphia, PA: Saunders Elsevier, 2009:481–482.

# Ultrasound-Guided Thoracic Facet Block: Intra-articular Technique

## CLINICAL PERSPECTIVES

Ultrasound-guided thoracic intra-articular facet block is utilized in a variety of clinical scenarios as a diagnostic and therapeutic maneuver in painful conditions involving the thoracic facet joint. As a diagnostic tool, ultrasound-guided thoracic intra-articular facet block allows accurate placement of the needle tip within a specific facet joint that is believed to be the source of the patient's pain. In the acute pain setting, ultrasound-guided thoracic intra-articular facet block with local anesthetics and/or steroids may be used to palliate acute thoracic spine pain emergencies while waiting for pharmacologic methods to become effective. This technique has great clinical utility when managing acute post-trauma pain. This technique is also useful in the treatment arthritis-related facet joint pain (Fig. 87.1). Clinically, pain emanating from the thoracic facet joints is perceived in the paraspinous region and radiates anteriorly in a nondermatomal pattern.

## CLINICALLY RELEVANT ANATOMY

The thoracic facet joints are formed by the articulations of the superior and inferior articular facets of adjacent thoracic vertebrae (Fig. 87.2). The thoracic facet joints are lined with synovium and possess a dense joint capsule. The joint capsule is richly innervated and explains why the facet joint can serve as a nidus for thoracic pain when it becomes damaged or inflamed. The thoracic joint is susceptible to degenerative arthritis and is frequently affected by the collagen vascular diseases. The joint is frequently injured in acceleration/deceleration injuries resulting in intra-articular hemorrhage with subsequent inflammation and development of adhesions.

Each thoracic facet joint receives innervation from two spinal levels, receiving fibers from the dorsal ramus at the same level as the vertebra as well as fibers from the dorsal ramus of the vertebra above (Fig. 87.3). This fact has clinical import in that it provides an explanation for the ill-defined nature of facet-mediated pain and explains why the dorsal nerve from the vertebra above the offending level must often also be blocked to provide the patient with complete pain relief.

## ULTRASOUND-GUIDED TECHNIQUE

Ultrasound-guided thoracic intra-articular facet block can be carried out by placing the patient in the sitting position with the patient's head resting comfortably on a padded bedside table and the arms resting comfortably on the patient's lap (Fig. 87.4). A total of 1 mL of local anesthetic is drawn up in a 5-mL sterile syringe. If the painful condition being treated is thought to have an inflammatory component, 40 to 80 mg of depot steroid is added to the local anesthetic.

To perform ultrasound-guided thoracic intra-articular facet block, a two-step process is used. This two-step process allows the clinician to quickly identify critical anatomic structures while at the same time maintaining a transducer position that allows a safe and easy placement of needles into the selected thoracic facet joint.

### Step One: Obtain the Paramedian Sagittal Transverse Process View

Step One is to obtain a paramedian sagittal transverse process view by placing the 2- to 5-MHz low-frequency curvilinear probe in the longitudinal plane 3 to 4 cm lateral to the right side of the middle of the spinous processes at the level to be blocked for the right-handed clinician and 3 to 4 cm lateral to the left side of the middle of the spinous processes at the level to be blocked for the left-handed clinician (Figs. 87.5 and 87.6). An initial depth setting of 7 to 8 cm will work for most patients. An ultrasound survey is taken and the transducer is slowly moved medially and laterally until successive transverse processes are visualized. The transverse processes of the thoracic spine will appear as hyperechoic domes with sausage-like acoustic shadows beneath them (Fig. 87.7). This classic appearance of successive transverse processes viewed in the longitudinal plane has been named the "trident sign" after Neptune's trident (Fig. 87.8).

### Step Two: Obtain the Paramedian Sagittal Articular Process View

After the transverse processes are identified in the paramedian sagittal transverse process view, the ultrasound transducer is slowly slid toward the midline until the superior and inferior

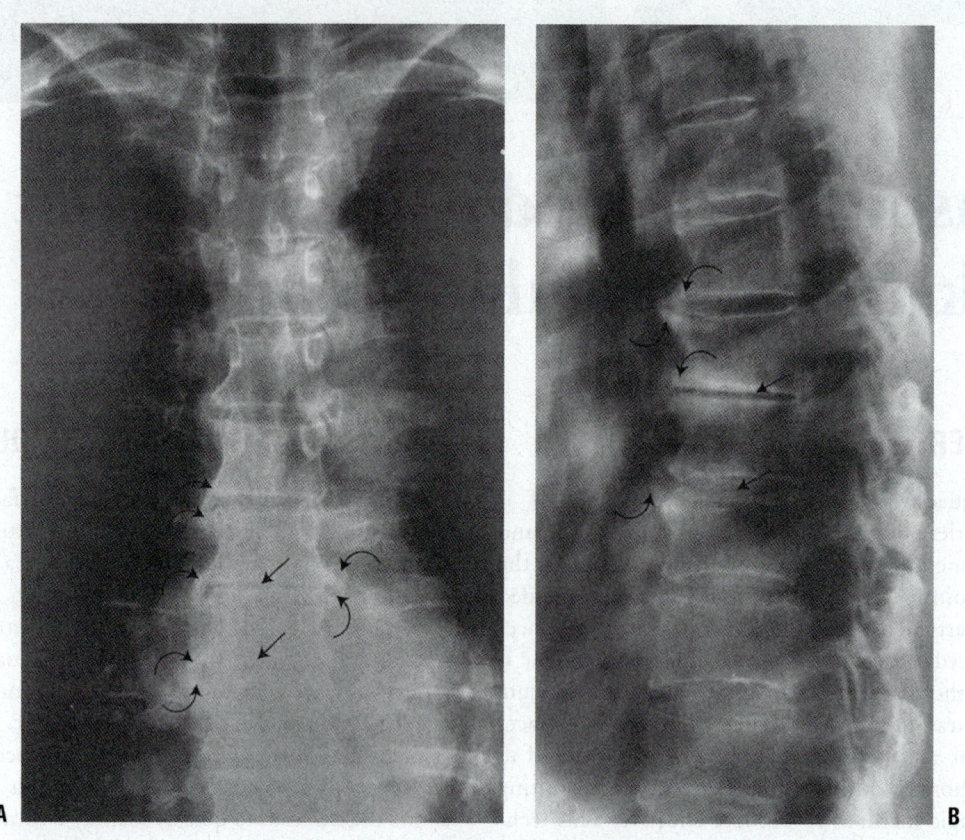

**FIGURE 87.1.** Plain radiographs of the thoracic spine demonstrating osteoarthritis. Note multiple osteophytes (*curved arrows*) are present and multiple disc spaces are narrowed (*straight arrows*) secondary to degenerative disc disease. (Reused from Erkonen WE, Smith WL. *Radiology 101: The Basics and Fundamentals of Imaging*. 2nd ed. Philadelphia, PA: Lippincott Williams & Wilkins; 2005, with permission.)

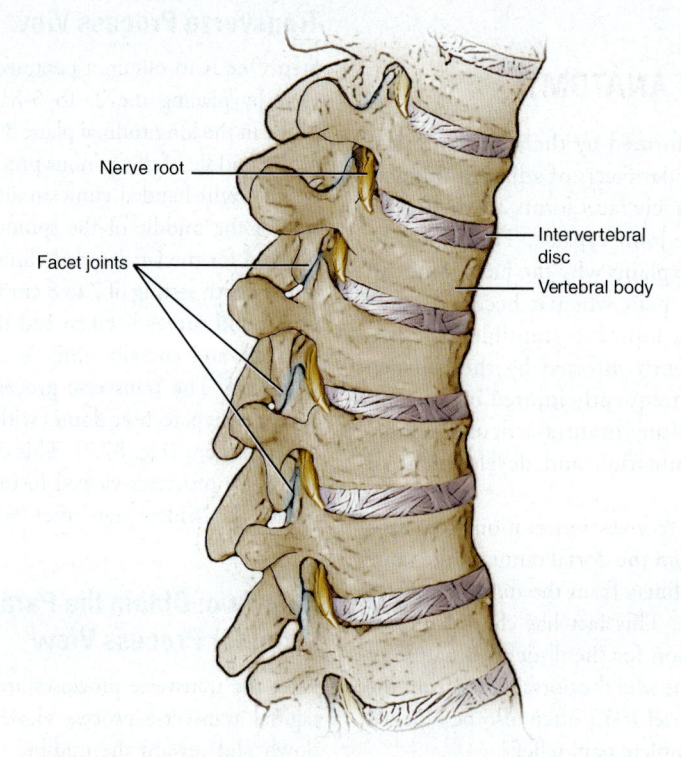

**FIGURE 87.2.** The anatomy of the thoracic facet joint.

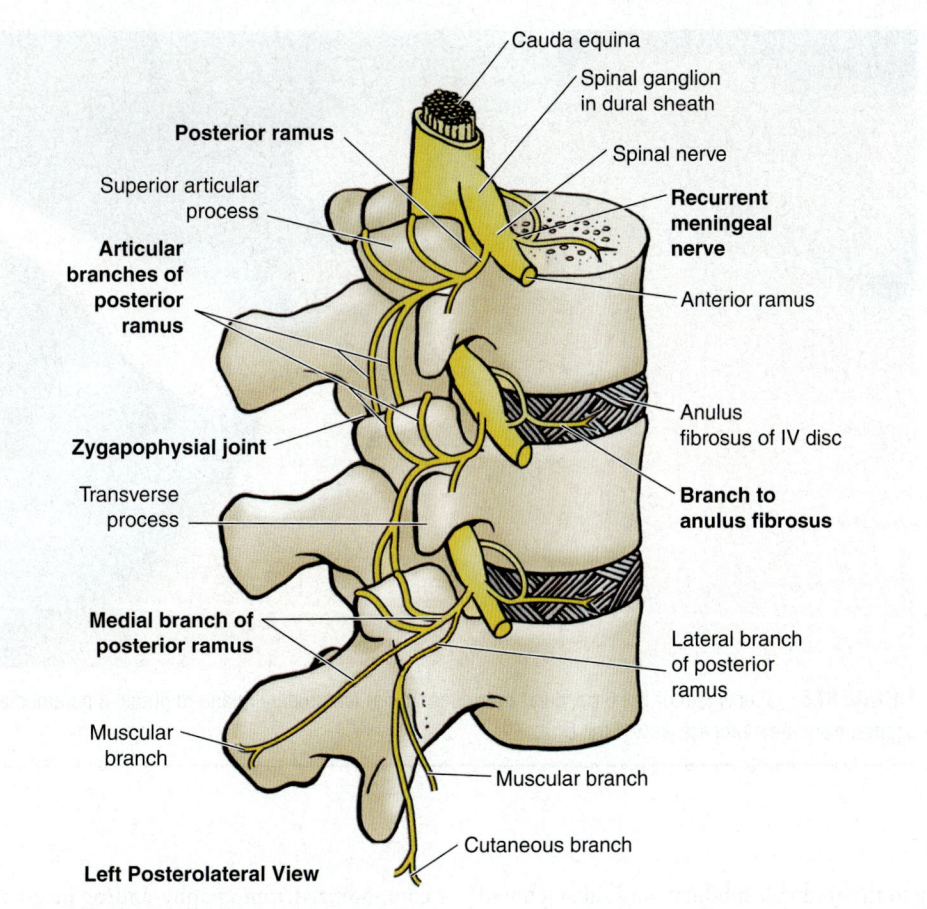

**FIGURE 87.3.** Innervation of the facet joints.

articular facets are visualized (Step Two) (Figs. 87.9 and 87.10). In longitudinal paramedian ultrasound articular process view, the superior and inferior articular facets will appear as successive hyperechoic hills and valleys, with the space within the center each hill representing a facet joint (Figs. 87.11 and 87.12). When the facet joint of interest is identified, the skin beneath and below the ultrasound transducer is prepped with antiseptic solution, and a 22-gauge, 3½-inch styletted needle is inserted through the skin just below the inferior aspect of the longitudinally placed ultrasound transducer utilizing an in-plane approach (Fig. 87.13). The clinician then advances the needle under real-time ultrasound guidance in inferior to superior trajectory until the needle tip rests within the joint space. After gentle aspiration, 1 mL of solution is injected. The needle is removed and pressure is placed on the injection site to avoid hematoma formation.

## COMPLICATIONS

Because of potential hematogenous spread via the valveless epidural veins of the thoracic epidural space, sepsis and local infection at the injection site represent absolute contraindications to ultrasound-guided thoracic intra-articular facet block as do anticoagulation and coagulopathy. The thoracic facet joints are

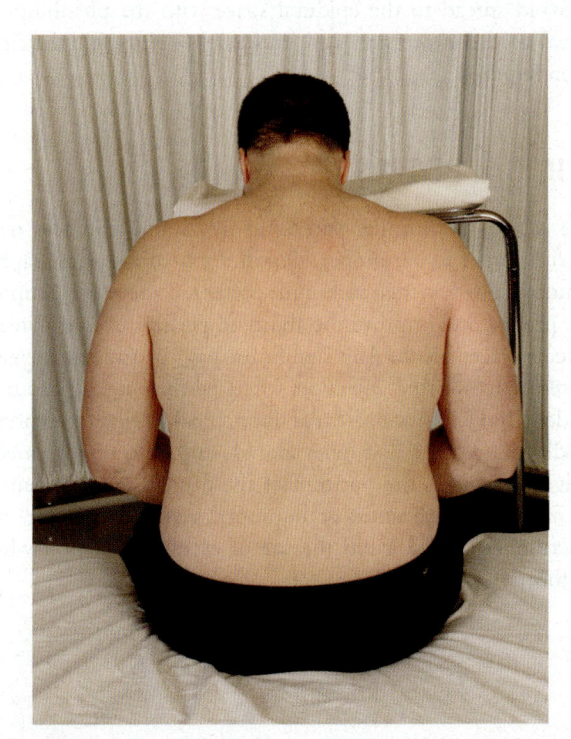

**FIGURE 87.4.** Proper patient position for ultrasound-guided thoracic intra-articular facet block.

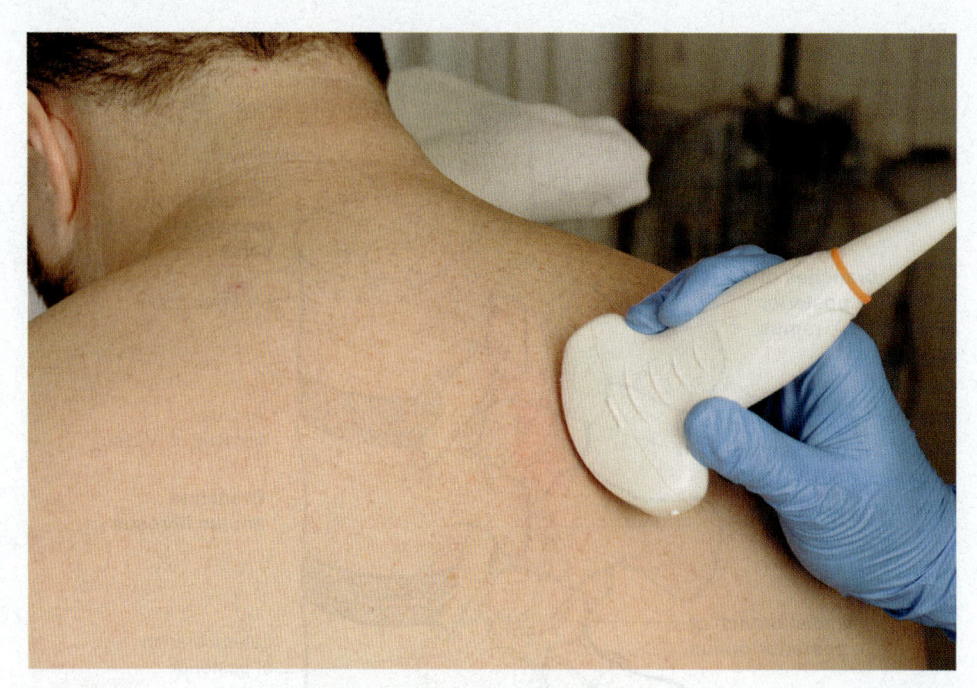

**FIGURE 87.5.** Placement of the ultrasound transducer in the longitudinal plane to obtain a paramedian sagittal transverse process view (Step One).

in close proximity to the epidural, subdural, and subarachnoid space and spinal cord as well as the exiting spinal nerve roots, which suggests that this procedure should only be performed by those well versed in the regional anatomy and skilled at ultrasound-guided interventional pain management procedures. Trauma to the exiting thoracic nerve roots and spinal cord can be avoided if careful attention is paid to the regional anatomy and if the clinician immediately stops advancing the needle should the patient experience any significant pain during needle placement. Inadvertent subarachnoid and subdural injection, although rare, can occur even in the best of hands. Failure to recognize an unintentional dural or subdural injection with its resultant immediate total spinal anesthesia with associated loss of consciousness, hypotension, and apnea can be disastrous if not immediately recognized and treated.

Although uncommon, infection in the thoracic neuroaxis remains an ever-present possibility, especially in the immunocompromised AIDS or cancer patient, and should be considered in any patient with fever and the onset of neurologic symptomatology after undergoing an intra-articular facet block. Early detection and treatment of infection is crucial to avoid potentially life-threatening sequelae, and urgent computerized tomography and/or magnetic resonance imaging should be obtained in any patient suspected of having an infection in this anatomic region. Emergent surgical drainage to avoid spread to the epidural space with the possibility of spinal cord compression and irreversible neurologic deficit is often required.

## CLINICAL PEARLS

The key to performing successful ultrasound thoracic neuroaxial blocks is the proper identification of the sonographic anatomy. The two-step technique presented above will simplify this process and improve the ability to perform thoracic intra-articular facet block. Any significant pain or sudden increase in resistance during injection when performing ultrasound-guided thoracic intra-articular facet block suggests incorrect needle placement, and one should stop injecting immediately and reassess the position of the needle. Because pain is an important indication of improper needle placement, the practitioner should avoid the use of excessive sedation when performing this technique.

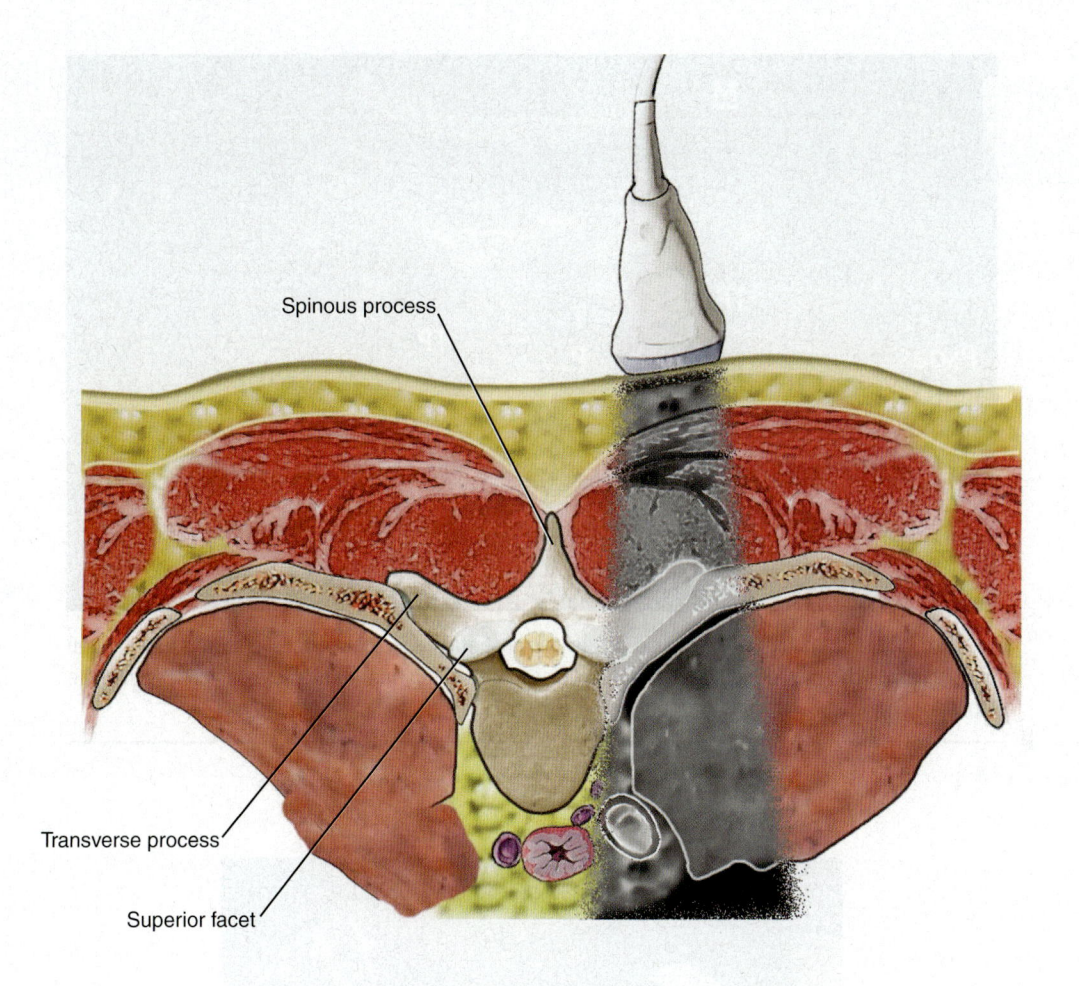

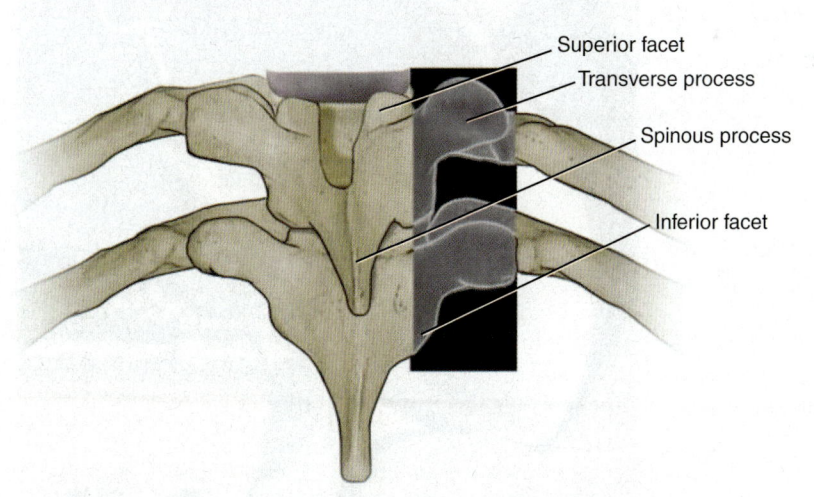

**FIGURE 87.6.** The anatomic orientation of the longitudinally placed curvilinear ultrasound transducer for the paramedian sagittal transverse process view (Step One).

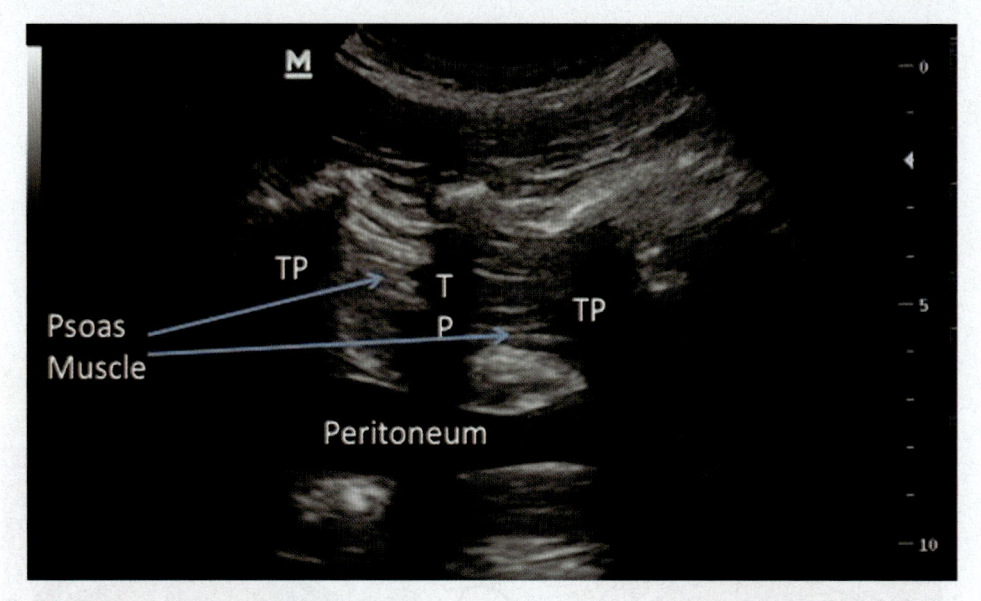

**FIGURE 87.7.** Longitudinal ultrasound image demonstrating successive transverse processes when performing the paramedian sagittal transverse process view (Step One). This classic image is named the "trident sign."

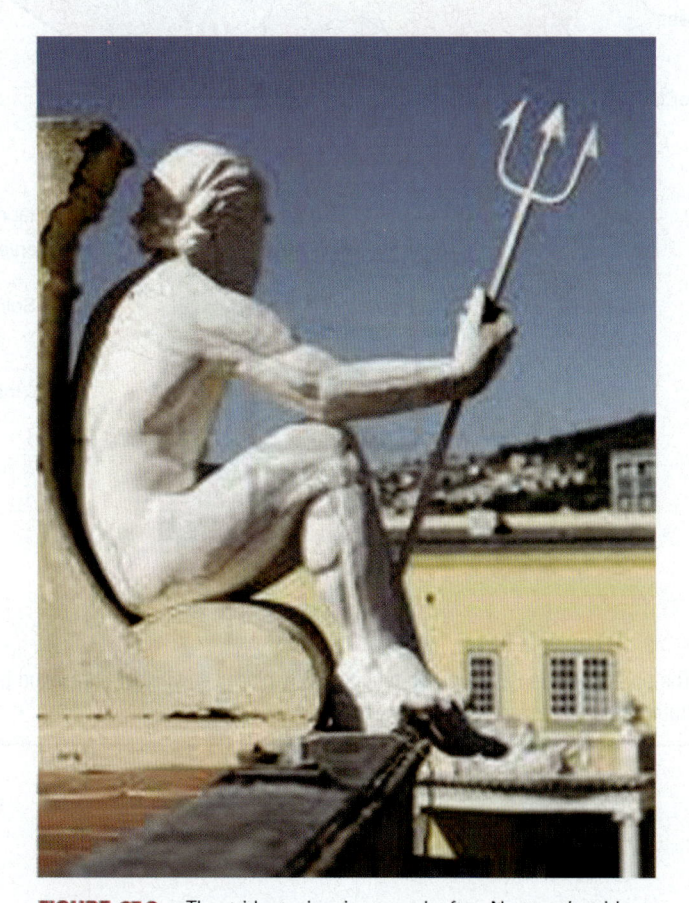

**FIGURE 87.8.** The trident sign is named after Neptune's trident, which according to Roman mythology had the power to conjure water and cause tsunamis and earthquakes.

CHAPTER 87    ULTRASOUND-GUIDED THORACIC FACET BLOCK: INTRA-ARTICULAR TECHNIQUE    595

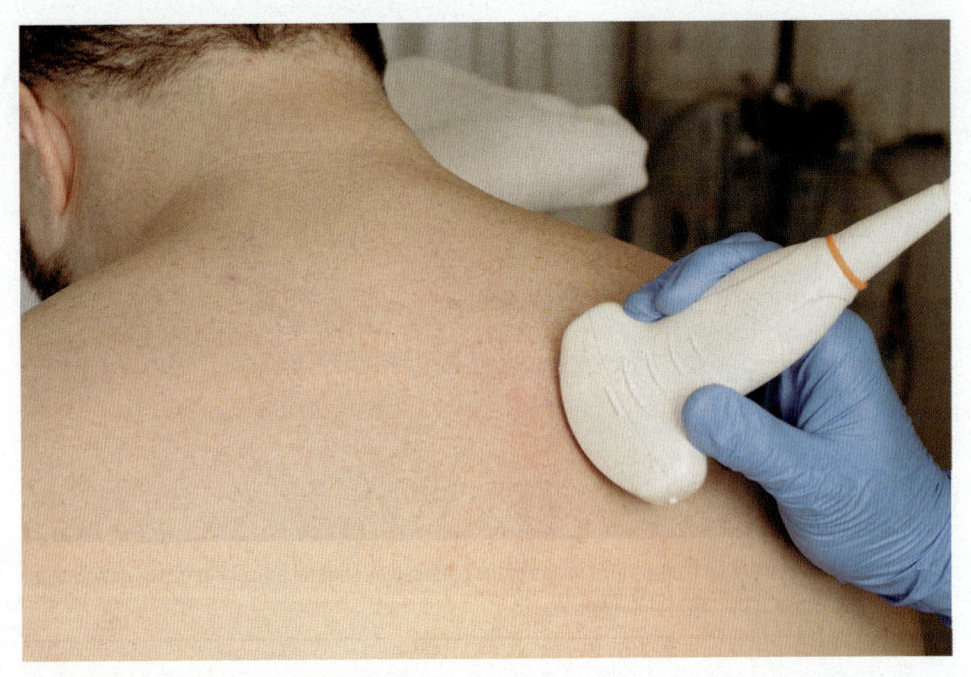

**FIGURE 87.9.** Proper longitudinal ultrasound transducer placement to obtain paramedian sagittal articular view (Step Two).

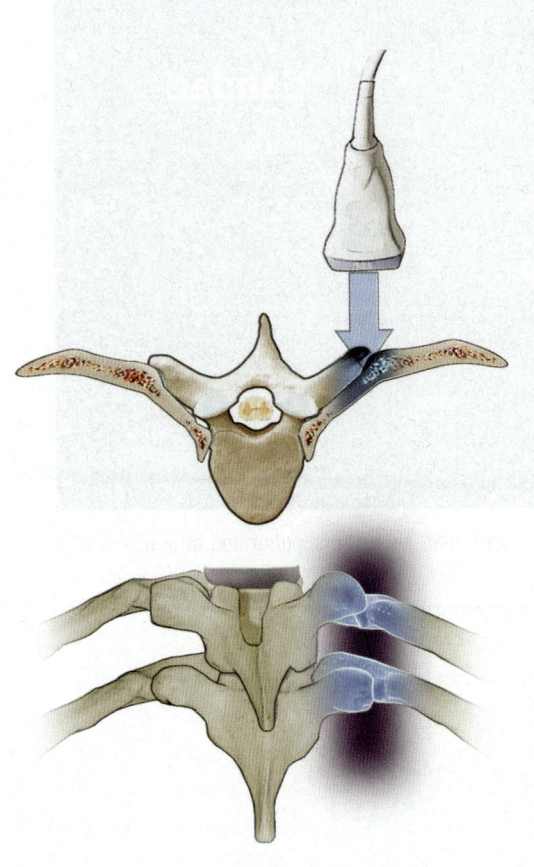

**FIGURE 87.10.** The anatomic orientation of the longitudinally placed curvilinear ultrasound transducer for the paramedian sagittal articular view (Step Two).

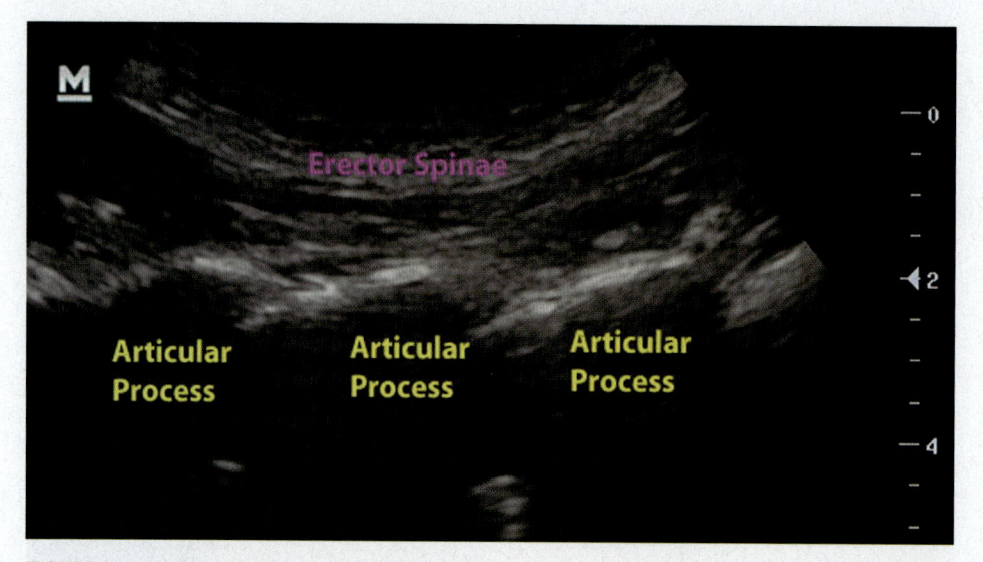

**FIGURE 87.11.** Longitudinal ultrasound image of the paramedian sagittal articular process view demonstrating the articular processes (Step Two).

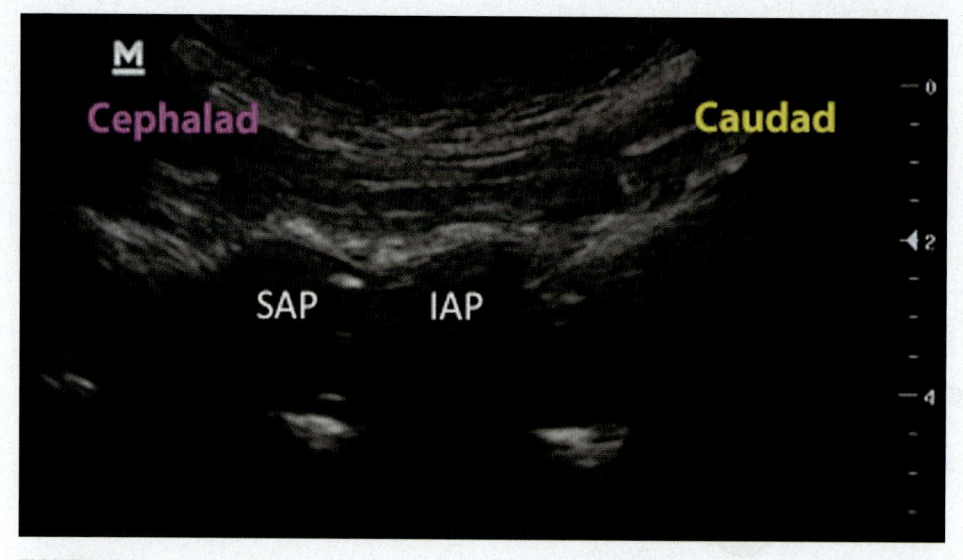

**FIGURE 87.12.** Longitudinal view of the thoracic facet joint. Note the superior and inferior articular processes.

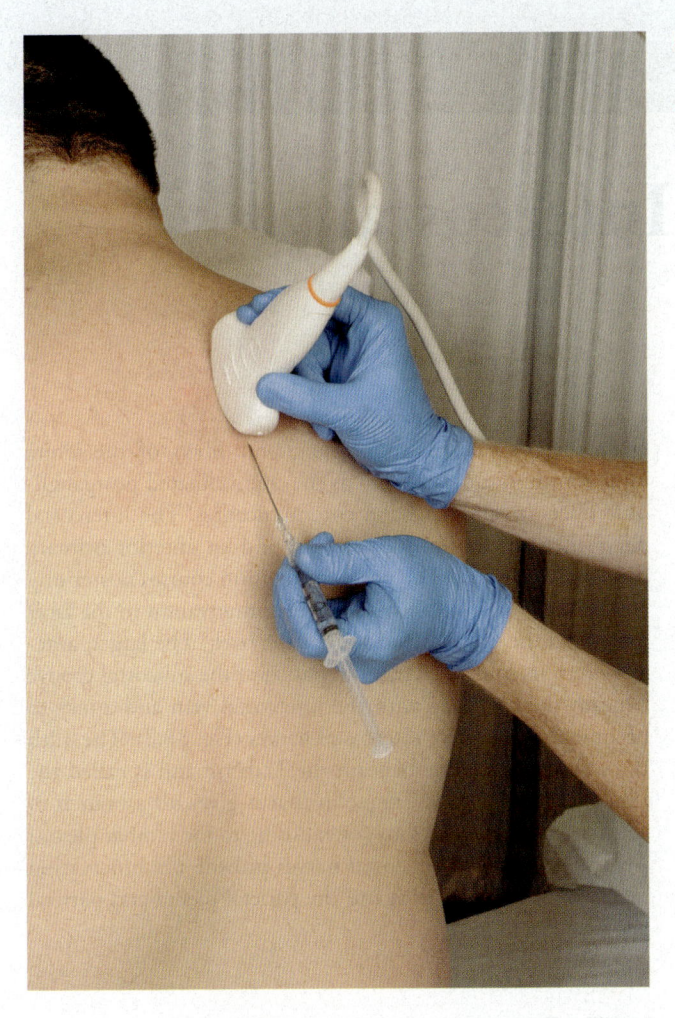

**FIGURE 87.13.** Proper needle position for ultrasound thoracic intra-articular facet injection.

## SUGGESTED READINGS

Stulc SM, Hurdle MFB, Pingree MJ. Ultrasound-guided thoracic facet injections: description of a technique. *J Ultrasound Med* 2011;30(3):357–362.

Waldman SD, Campbell RSD. Anatomy: special imaging considerations of the thoracic spine. In: *Imaging of Pain*. Philadelphia, PA: Saunders Elsevier; 2009:67–68.

Waldman SD. Thoracic facet block. In: *Pain Review*. Philadelphia, PA: Saunders Elsevier; 2009:382–385.

Waldman SD. Thoracic facet block: intra-articular approach. In: *Atlas of Interventional Pain Management*. 3rd ed. Philadelphia, PA: Saunders Elsevier; 2011:287–291.

Yamauchi M. Ultrasound-guided neuraxial block. *Trends Anaesth Crit Care* 2012;2(5):234–243.

# CHAPTER 88

# Ultrasound-Guided Intercostal Nerve Block

## CLINICAL PERSPECTIVES

Ultrasound-guided intercostal nerve block is utilized in a variety of clinical scenarios as a diagnostic, prognostic, and therapeutic maneuver as well as to provide surgical anesthesia for thoracic and upper abdominal surgeries. As a diagnostic tool, ultrasound-guided intercostal block allows accurate placement of the needle tip within the intercostal space when performing differential neural blockade on an anatomic basis in the evaluation of chest wall and upper intra-abdominal pain. As a prognostic tool, ultrasound-guided intercostal block can be utilized as a prognostic indicator of the degree of motor and sensory impairment that the patient may experience if intercostal nerves are going to be destroyed in an effort to palliate intractable pain in patients too sick to undergo neurosurgical neurodestructive procedures. In the acute pain setting, ultrasound-guided intercostal block with local anesthetics may be used to palliate acute pain emergencies while waiting for pharmacologic, surgical, and/or antiblastic methods to become effective. This technique has great clinical utility in both children and adults when managing acute postoperative and posttrauma pain including fractured ribs and flail chest and to provide anesthesia for placement of chest and nephrostomy tubes (Fig. 88.1). Pain of malignant origin of the chest wall, flank, and upper abdomen as well as liver and lung tumors that involve the pleura and peritoneum is also amenable to treatment with local anesthetics and/or steroids and neurolytic agents such as phenol administered into the intercostal space.

## CLINICAL RELEVANT ANATOMY

Exiting their respective intervertebral foramen and passing just below the transverse process are the paravertebral nerves. After exiting the intervertebral foramen, the intercostal nerve gives off a recurrent branch that loops back through the foramen to provide innervation to the spinal ligaments, meninges, and its respective vertebra and can be an important contributor to spinal pain. The paravertebral nerve also provides fibers to the sympathetic nervous system and the thoracic sympathetic chain via the myelinated preganglionic fibers of the white rami communicantes as well as the unmyelinated postganglionic fibers of the gray rami communicantes. The intercostal nerve then divides into a posterior and an anterior primary division (Fig. 88.2). The posterior division courses posteriorly and, along with its branches, provides innervation to the facet joints and the muscles and skin of the back. The larger, anterior division courses laterally to pass into the subcostal groove beneath the rib along with the intercostal vein and artery to become the respective intercostal nerves (Fig. 88.3). The 12th thoracic nerve courses beneath the 12th rib and is called the subcostal nerve and is unique in that it gives off a branch to the first lumbar nerve, thus contributing to the lumbar plexus. The intercostal and subcostal nerves provide the innervation to the skin, muscles, ribs, and the parietal pleura and parietal peritoneum.

## ULTRASOUND-GUIDED TECHNIQUE

Ultrasound-guided intercostal block can be carried out by placing the patient in the sitting position with the patient's head resting comfortably on a padded bedside table and the arms resting comfortably on the patient's lap (Fig. 88.4). A total of 5 mL of local anesthetic is drawn up in a 10-mL sterile syringe. If the painful condition being treated is thought to have an inflammatory component, 40 to 80 mg of depot steroid is added to the local anesthetic. The rib at the level to be blocked is then identified by palpation and then traced posteriorly to the posterior angulation of the affected rib (Fig. 88.5). A linear high-frequency ultrasound transducer is then placed in the longitudinal plane with the superior aspect of the ultrasound transducer rotated ~15 degrees laterally over the affected rib at the posterior angulation of the ribs, and an ultrasound survey scan is obtained (Figs. 88.6 and 88.7). The rib will be identified as a hyperechoic curvilinear line with an acoustic shadow beneath it. The three layers of intercostal muscle, the external, internal, and innermost, will be identified in the intercostal space between the adjacent ribs (Fig. 88.8). Color Doppler will help identify beneath the adjacent intercostal artery and vein (Fig. 88.9). This space between adjacent

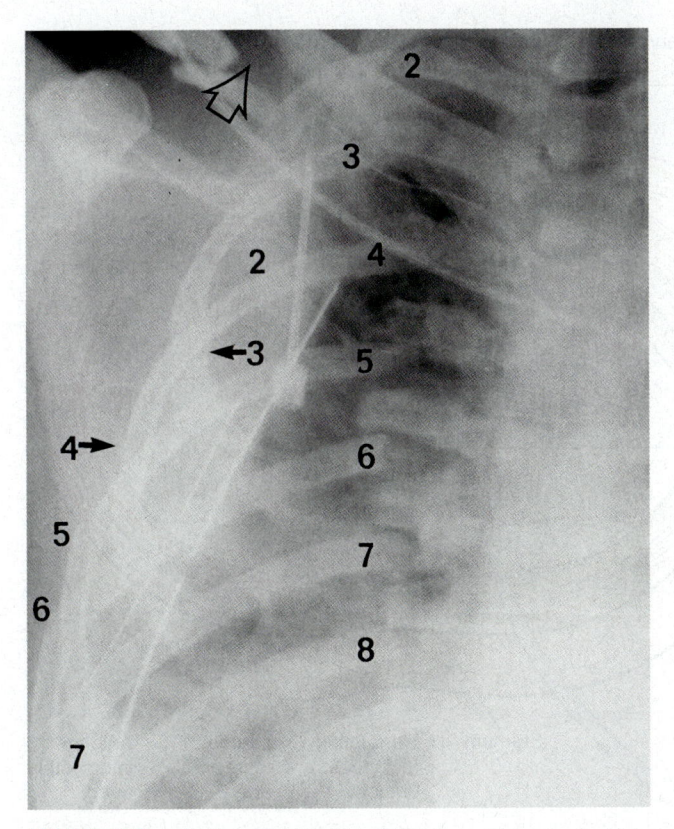

**FIGURE 88.1.** Flail chest involving ribs 2 to 7 (*arrows*). Note comminuted and displaced clavicular fracture (*open arrow*). (Reused from Pope T, Harris J. *Harris & Harris' Radiology of Emergency Medicine*. 5th ed. Philadelphia, PA: Lippincott Williams & Wilkins; 2012:510, with permission.)

ribs provides an excellent acoustic window, which allows easy identification of the intercostal space and the pleura beneath it. Adjacent ribs with the intercostal space in between have been described as having the appearance of a "flying bat" (Fig. 88.10A and B). The clinician should then identify the pleura that appears as a bright hyperechoic line having the appearance of a bright sunset on the ocean beneath the innermost intercostal muscle, which can be seen to slide back and forth with respiration (see Fig. 88.7). The pleura and the lung beneath it have been described as having the appearance of "waves on a sandy beach" (Fig. 88.11A and B). The depth of the pleura is noted. When these anatomic structures are clearly identified on transverse ultrasound scan, the skin is prepped with anesthetic solution, and a 1½-inch, 22-gauge needle is advanced from the inferior border of the ultrasound transducer using an in-plane approach with the trajectory being adjusted under real-time ultrasound guidance until the needle tip is resting within the internal layer of intercostal muscle (Fig. 88.12). At that point, after careful aspiration, a small amount of solution is injected under real-time ultrasound imaging to utilize hydrodissection to reconfirm the position of the needle tip (Fig. 88.13). Once the position of the needle tip is reconfirmed, the needle is carefully advanced into the innermost layer of intercostal muscle just short of the previously identified depth of the pleura. After careful aspiration, a small amount of solution is again injected to aid in identification of the position of the needle tip with attention paid to the relative location of the bright hyperechoic pleural line. After careful aspiration, the remainder of the solution is slowly injected. There should be minimal resistance to injection. The needle is then removed, and a sterile pressure dressing and ice pack are placed at the injection site.

## COMPLICATIONS

The intercostal nerves are in close proximity to the spinal cord and pleural space, and this procedure should be performed only by those well versed in the regional anatomy and skilled at ultrasound-guided interventional pain management procedures. Trauma to the intercostal nerves, arteries, and veins as well as inadvertent subarachnoid, subdural, and/or epidural injection can occur even in the best of hands. Failure to recognize an unintentional dural or subdural injection can result in immediate total spinal anesthesia with associated loss of consciousness, hypotension, and apnea. This can be disastrous if not immediately recognized. The proximity to the pleural space makes the potential for pneumothorax an ever-present possibility. Should a pneumothorax occur, the "waves on a sandy beach" appearance of the normal pleural lung interface will be replaced with a more chaotic "ripples on a pond" appearance.

## CLINICAL PEARLS

The key to performing successful ultrasound intercostal block is the proper identification of the sonographic anatomy and in particular the ability to properly identify the pleura. This should not be a problem if the above technique is used. Any significant pain or sudden increase in resistance during injection when performing ultrasound-guided intercostal nerve block suggests incorrect needle placement, and one should stop injecting immediately and reassess the position of the needle. Because pain is an important indication of improper needle placement, the practitioner should avoid the use of excessive sedation during ultrasound-guided intercostal block.

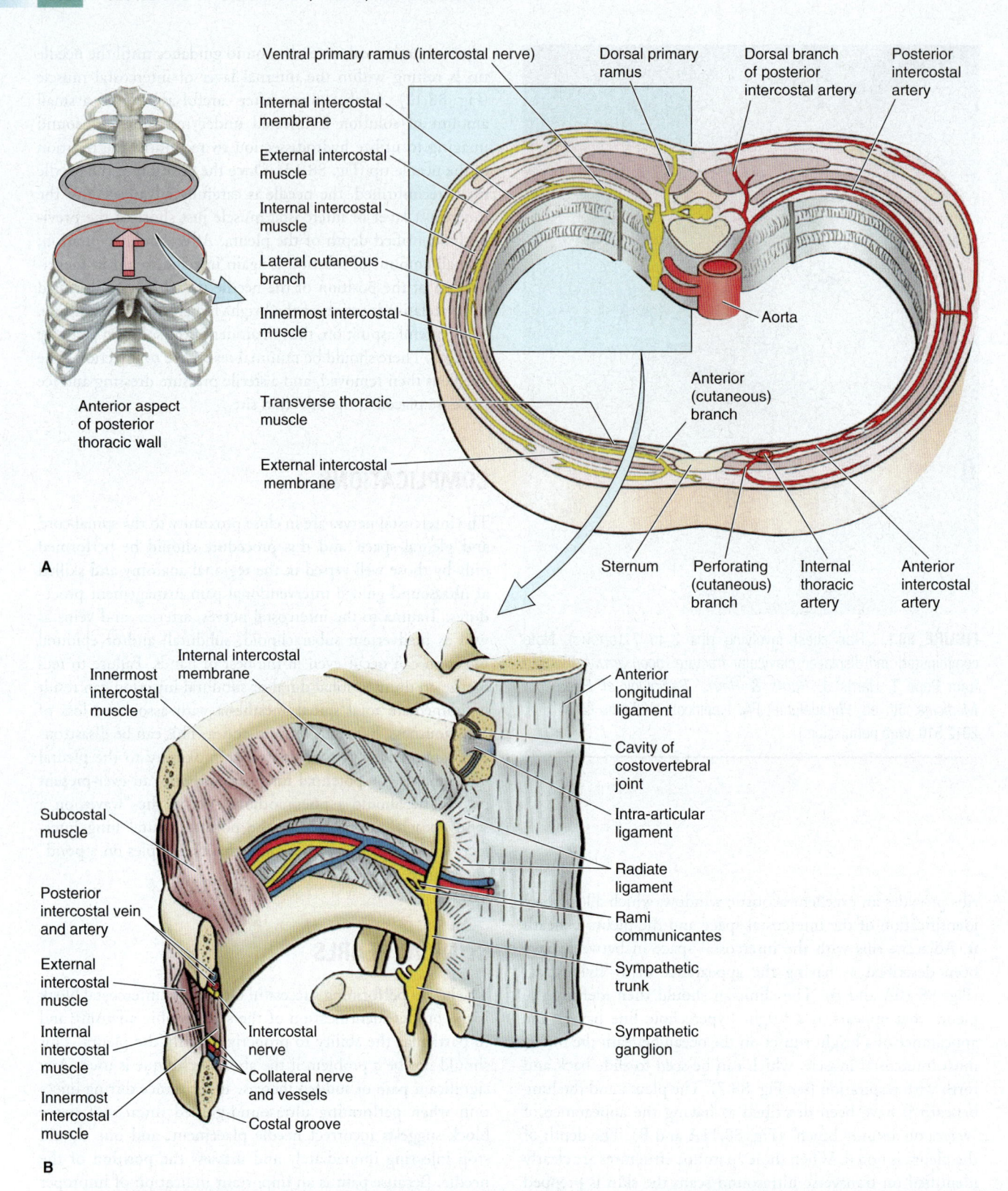

**FIGURE 88.2.** **A,B:** The anatomy of the intercostal nerve. (Reused from Moore KL, Dalley AF. *Clinical Oriented Anatomy*. 4th ed. Baltimore, MD: Lippincott Williams & Wilkins; 1999, with permission.)

CHAPTER 88   ULTRASOUND-GUIDED INTERCOSTAL NERVE BLOCK   **601**

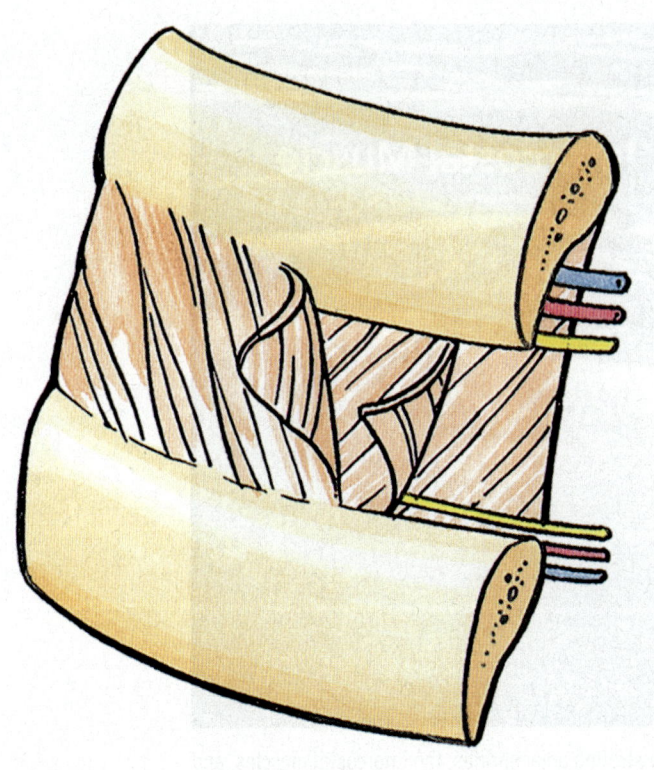

**FIGURE 88.3.** The relationship of the intercostal vein, artery, and nerve within the intercostal space. (Reused from Moore KL, Agur A. *Essential Clinical Anatomy*. 2nd ed. Philadelphia, PA: Lippincott Williams & Wilkins; 2002, with permission.)

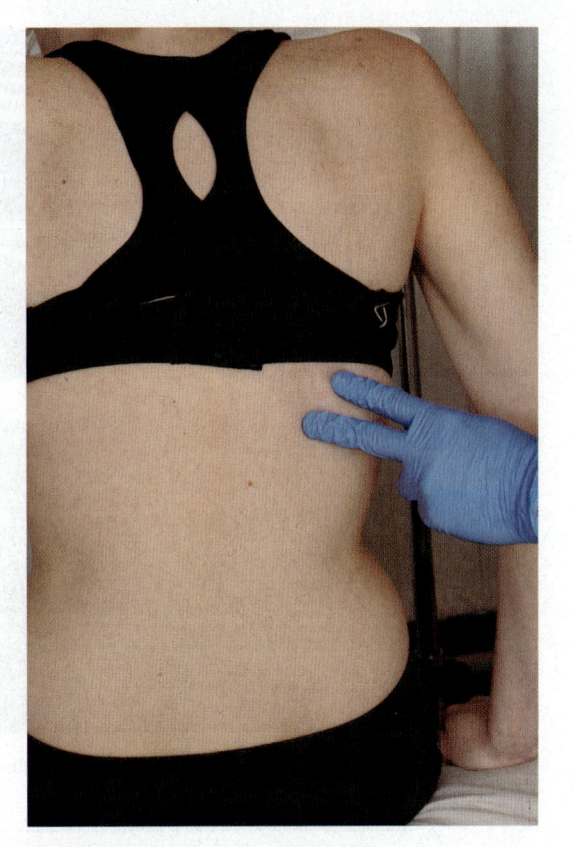

**FIGURE 88.5.** Palpation of the affected rib.

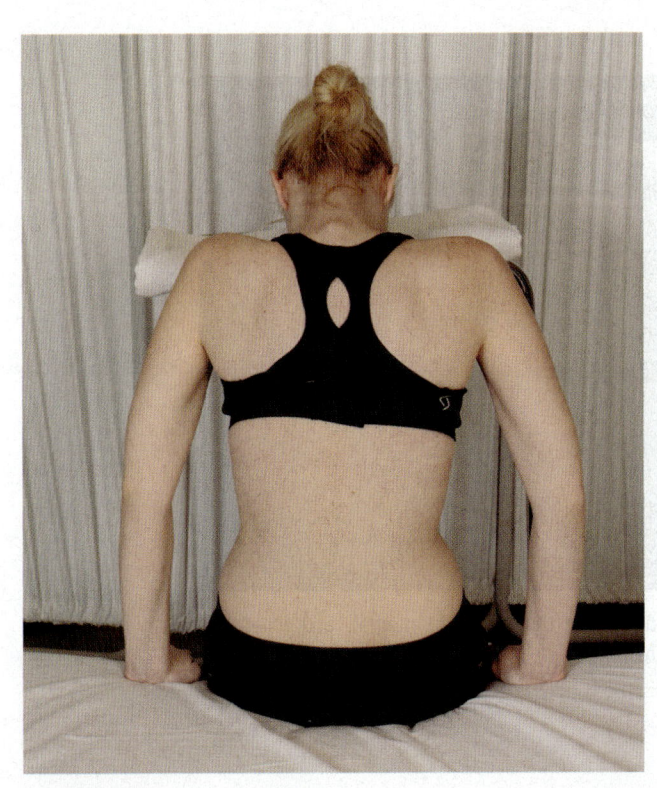

**FIGURE 88.4.** Proper patient position for ultrasound-guided intercostal block.

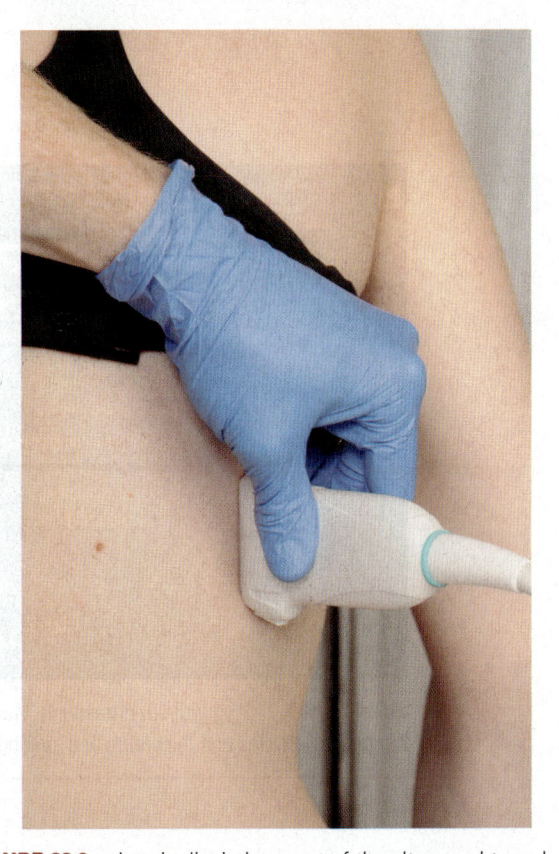

**FIGURE 88.6.** Longitudinal placement of the ultrasound transducer at the posterior angle of the ribs with the superior aspect of the transducer rotated ~15 degrees.

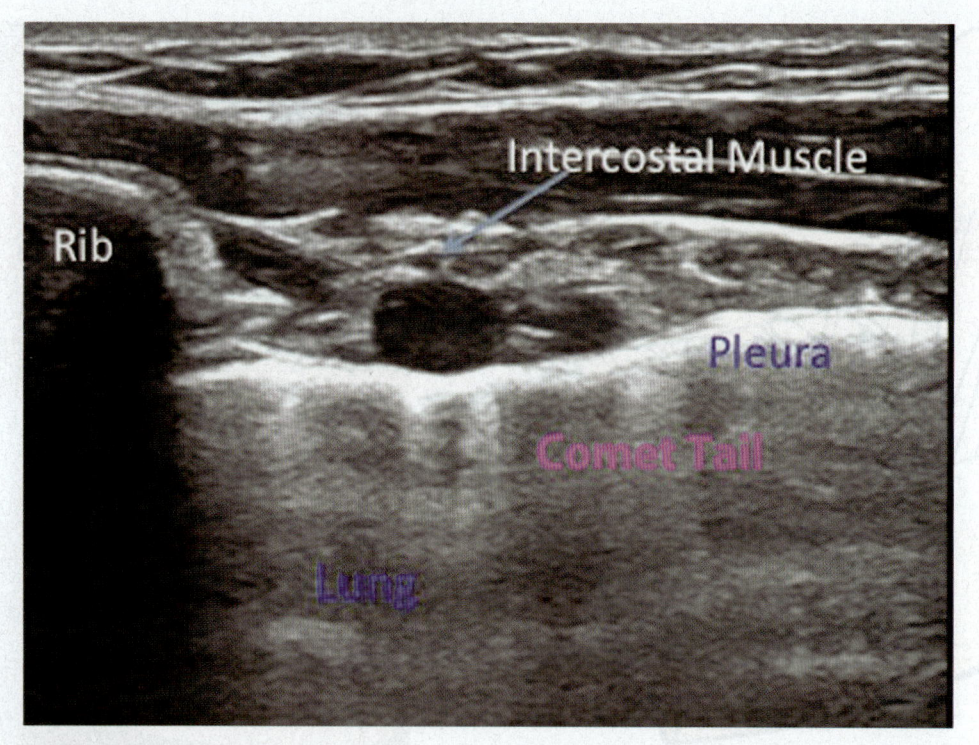

**FIGURE 88.7.** Longitudinal ultrasound image demonstrating adjacent ribs, the intercostal muscles, and pleura with the lung beneath.

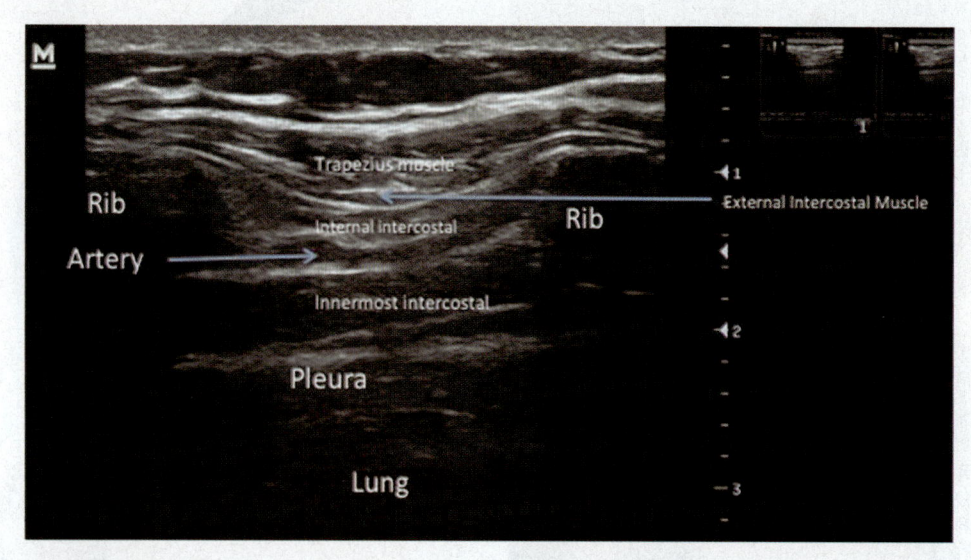

**FIGURE 88.8.** Longitudinal ultrasound view demonstrating the external, internal, and innermost intercostal muscles and the pleura and lung beneath them.

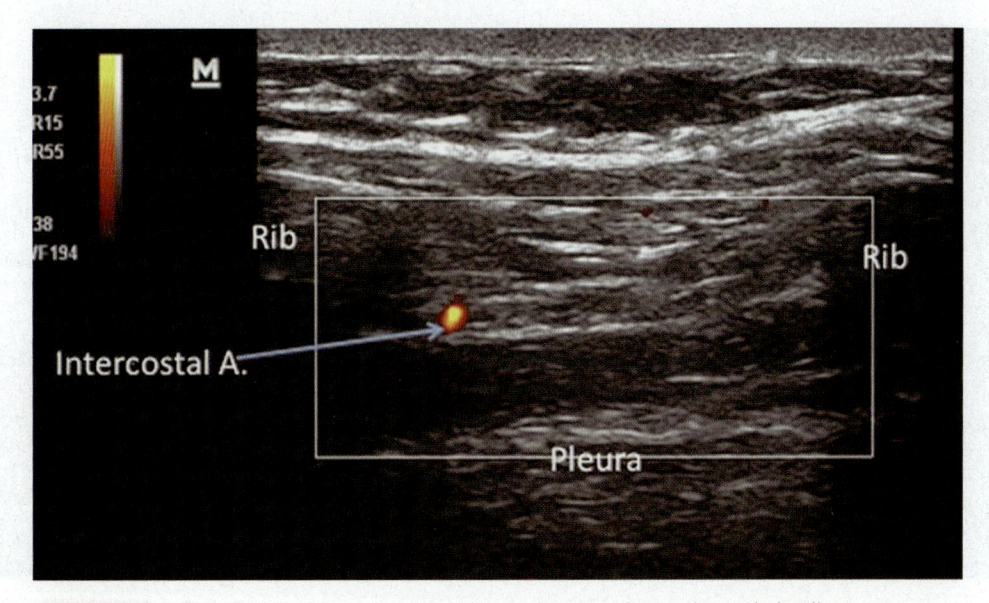

**FIGURE 88.9.** Color Doppler image demonstrating the intercostal artery beneath the rib.

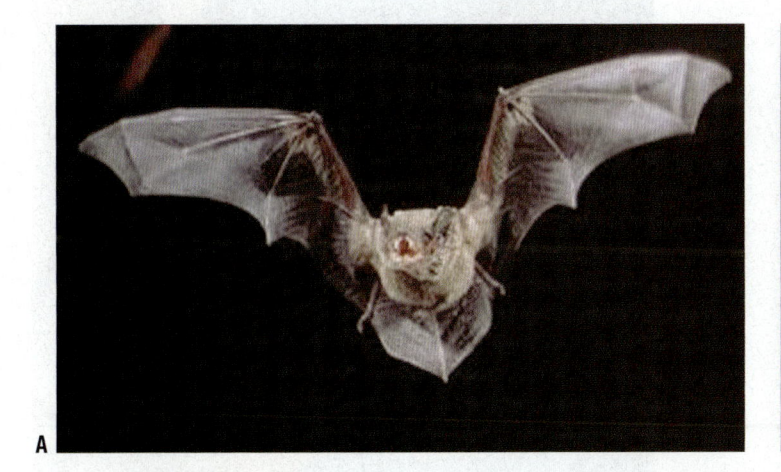

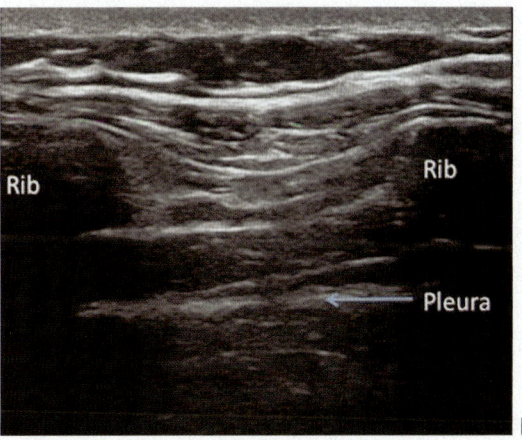

**FIGURE 88.10.** The ultrasound appearance of adjacent ribs and intercostal space in between **(B)** has been described as having the appearance of a "flying bat" **(A)**.

**604** SECTION VI CHEST WALL, TRUNK, AND ABDOMEN

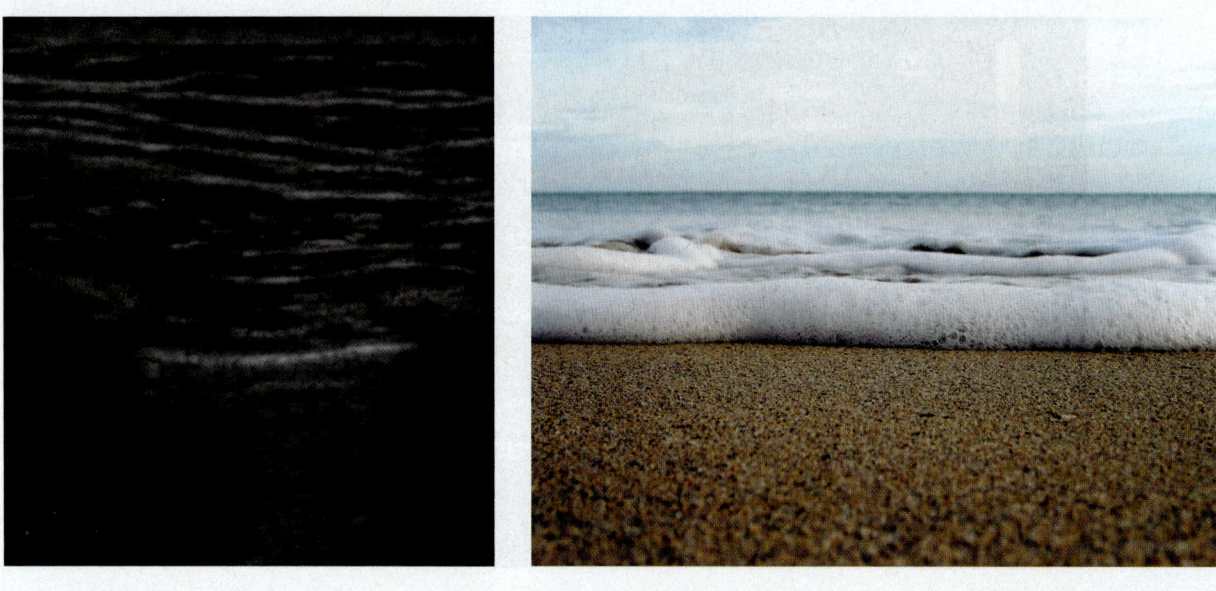

**FIGURE 88.11.** **A,B:** The ultrasound appearance of the pleura and lung has been described as having the appearance of waves on a sandy beach.

**FIGURE 88.12.** Proper needle position for performing intercostal nerve block.

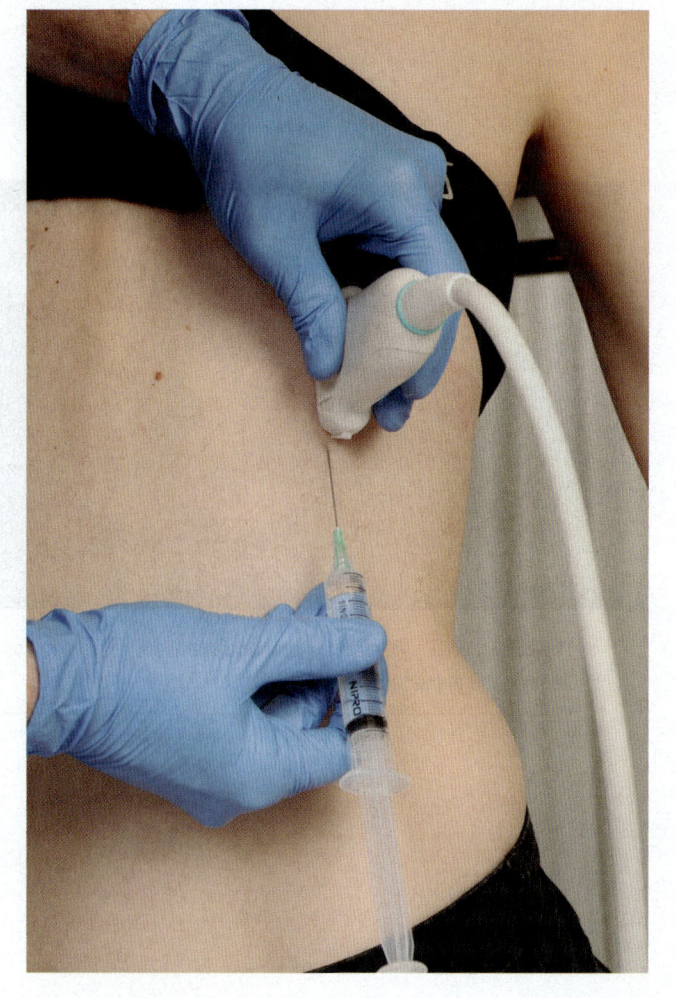

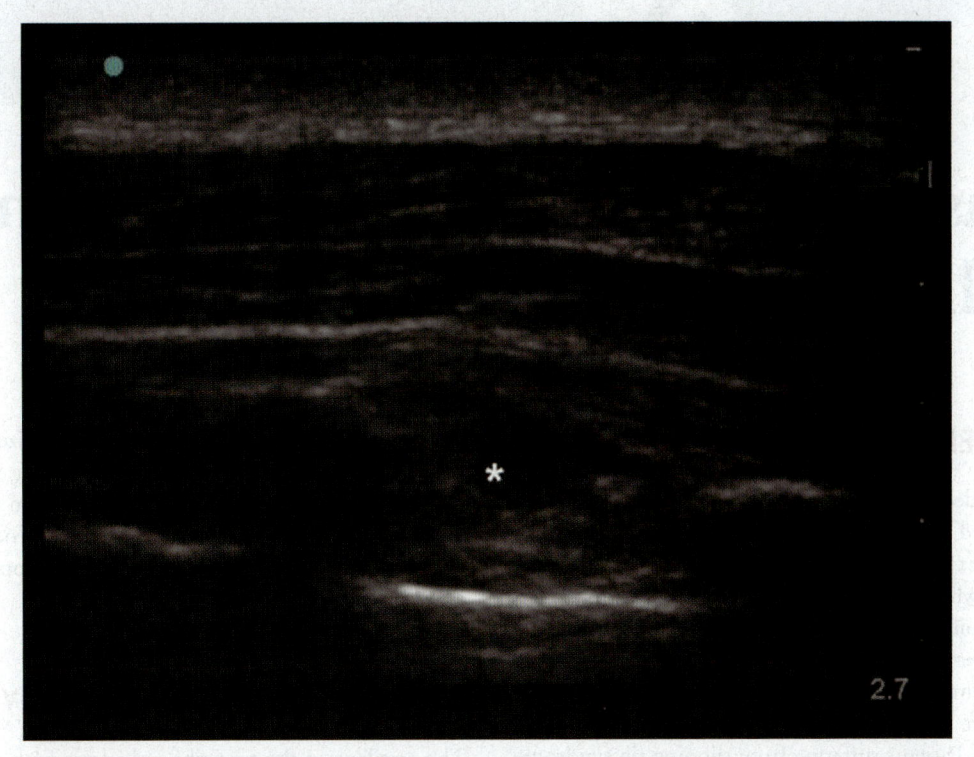

**FIGURE 88.13.** Local anesthetic (*asterisk*) visualized as it spreads within the intercostal space. (Reused from Stone MB, Carnell J, Fischer JWJ, et al. Ultrasound-guided intercostal nerve block for traumatic pneumothorax requiring tube thoracostomy. *Am J Emerg Med* 2011;29(6):697.e1–697.e2, with permission.)

## SUGGESTED READINGS

Narouze S. Intercostal block. In: *Atlas of Ultrasound Guided Procedures in Interventional Pain Management*. New York, NY: Springer; 2011:287–289.

Stone MB, Carnell J, Fischer JWJ, et al. Ultrasound-guided intercostal nerve block for traumatic pneumothorax requiring tube thoracostomy. *Am J Emerg Med* 2011;29(6):697.

Waldman SD. Intercostal block. In: *Atlas of Interventional Pain Management*. 3rd ed. Philadelphia, PA: Saunders Elsevier; 2009:295–297.

Waldman SD. Intercostal block. In: *Pain Review*. Philadelphia, PA: Saunders Elsevier; 2009:487–488.

# CHAPTER 89

# Ultrasound-Guided Injection Technique for Slipping Rib Syndrome

## CLINICAL PERSPECTIVES

Ultrasound-guided injection technique for slipping rib syndrome is utilized to help diagnose and treat this uncommon cause of anterior chest wall and upper abdominal pain. Slipping rib syndrome, which is also known as rib tip syndrome, is a painful condition due to hypermobility of the anterior portion of the lower costal cartilages. Most often involving the 10th rib, and sometimes the 8th and 9th ribs, slipping rib syndrome is almost always the result of trauma to the anterior costal cartilages. Patients suffering from slipping rib syndrome complain of sharp, knife-like pain with any movement of the lower anterior cartilages. The patient may also note a clicking, snapping, or catching sensation with movement of the anterior costal cartilages or with deep inspiration.

On physical exam, the patient suffering from slipping rib syndrome will often exhibit splinting of the affected cartilages by forward flexing the thoracolumbar spine. Palpation of the affected anterior costal cartilages will cause pain as will the hooking maneuver test (Fig. 89.1). The hooking maneuver test is performed by having the patient lie in the supine position with the abdominal muscles relaxed while the clinician hooks his or her fingers under the lower rib cage and pulls gently outward. Pain and a clicking or snapping sensation of the affected ribs and cartilage indicate a positive test. Patients suffering from slipping rib syndrome will also exhibit a positive ultrasound slipping rib test on transverse ultrasound imaging of the affected rib. The ultrasound slipping rib test is performed by imaging the rib and associated anterior costal cartilage suspected of slipping with the patient's abdominal wall completely relaxed and then having the patient perform a vigorous Valsalva maneuver. The test is positive if the affected rib moves cranially and overlaps the rib above it (Fig. 89.2A–F). If the anterior costal cartilage and adjacent ribs are intact, under ultrasound imaging, with vigorous Valsalva maneuver, the adjacent ribs will be seen to move in concert downward (Fig. 89.3A–F).

Plain radiographs are indicated for all patients who present with pain thought to be emanating from the lower costal cartilage and ribs to rule out occult bony pathology, including rib fracture and tumor. Based on the patient's clinical presentation, additional testing may be indicated, including complete blood cell count, prostate-specific antigen, sedimentation rate, and antinuclear antibody testing. Computerized tomographic, magnetic resonance, or ultrasound imaging of the affected ribs and cartilage is indicated to help confirm the diagnosis of slipping rib syndrome and to help identify occult mass and/or lower intrathoracic or upper intra-abdominal or tumor (see Figs. 89.2 and 89.4).

## CLINICALLY RELEVANT ANATOMY

The cartilage of the true ribs articulates with the sternum via the costosternal joints (Fig. 89.5). The cartilage of the first rib articulates directly with the manubrium of the sternum and is a synarthrodial joint that allows a limited gliding movement. The cartilage of the 2nd through 6th ribs articulates with the body of the sternum via true arthrodial joints. These joints are surrounded by a thin articular capsule. The costosternal joints are strengthened by ligaments. The 8th, 9th, and 10th ribs attach to the costal cartilage of the rib directly above. The cartilages of the 11th and 12th ribs are called floating ribs because they end in the abdominal musculature (see Fig. 89.5). The pleural space and peritoneal cavity may be entered when performing the following injection technique, and if the needle is placed too deeply and laterally, pneumothorax or damage to the abdominal viscera may result.

## ULTRASOUND-GUIDED TECHNIQUE

Ultrasound-guided injection technique for slipping rib syndrome can be carried out by placing the patient in the supine position with the patient's arms resting comfortably at the patient's side (Fig. 89.6). A total of 5 mL of local anesthetic is drawn up in a 10-mL sterile syringe. If the painful condition being treated is thought to have an inflammatory component, 40 to 80 mg of depot steroid is added to the local anesthetic. The anterior costal cartilage and associated ribs at the level to be blocked are then identified by palpation (Fig. 89.7). A linear high-frequency ultrasound transducer is then placed in the transverse plane with the superior aspect of the ultrasound transducer rotated ~15 degrees laterally over the affected costal cartilage and rib, and an ultrasound survey scan is obtained (Figs. 89.8 and 89.9). The rib will be identified as a slightly

CHAPTER 89  ULTRASOUND-GUIDED INJECTION TECHNIQUE FOR SLIPPING RIB SYNDROME    607

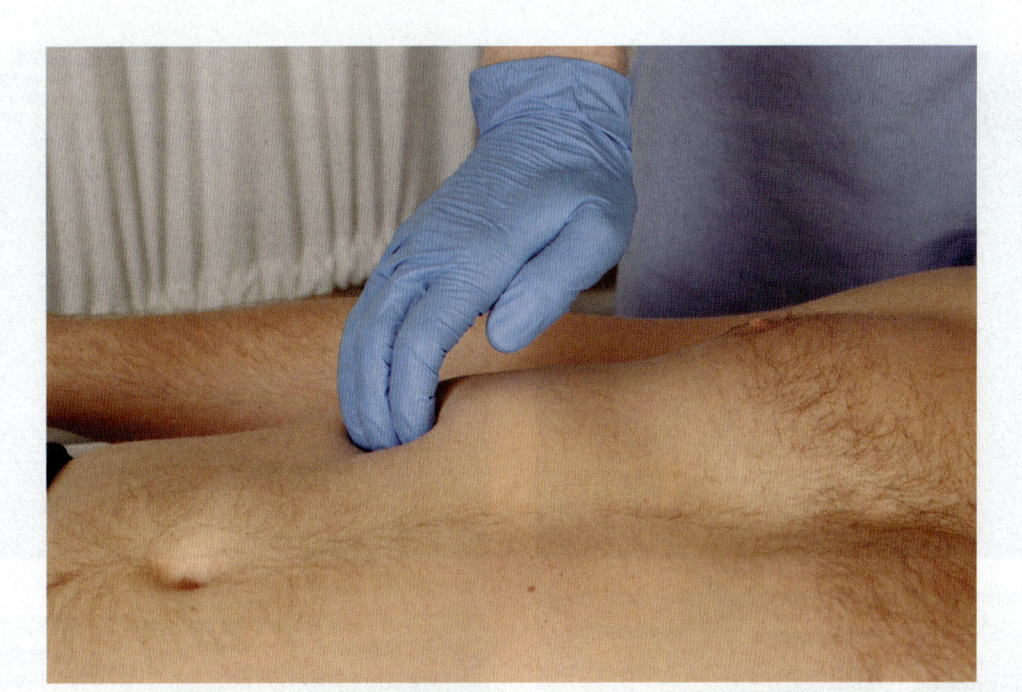

**FIGURE 89.1.** The hooking maneuver test for slipping rib syndrome is performed by having the patient lie in the supine position with the abdominal muscles relaxed while the clinician hooks his or her fingers under the lower rib cage and pulls gently outward. Pain and a clicking or snapping sensation of the affected ribs and cartilage indicate a positive test.

hyperechoic ovoid structure with a hypoechoic center. The rectus muscle will be seen just caudad to the ribs. The affected costal cartilages and associated ribs are then identified by the ultrasound slipping rib test (see Figs. 89.2 and 89.3).

When the affected costal cartilages and associated ribs are clearly identified by the ultrasound slipping rib test, the skin beneath and adjacent to the transversely placed ultrasound transducer is prepped with anesthetic solution, and a 1½-inch, 22-gauge needle is advanced from the medial aspect of the ultrasound transducer using an in-plane approach with the trajectory being adjusted under real-time ultrasound guidance until the needle tip is resting in proximity to the affected costal cartilage

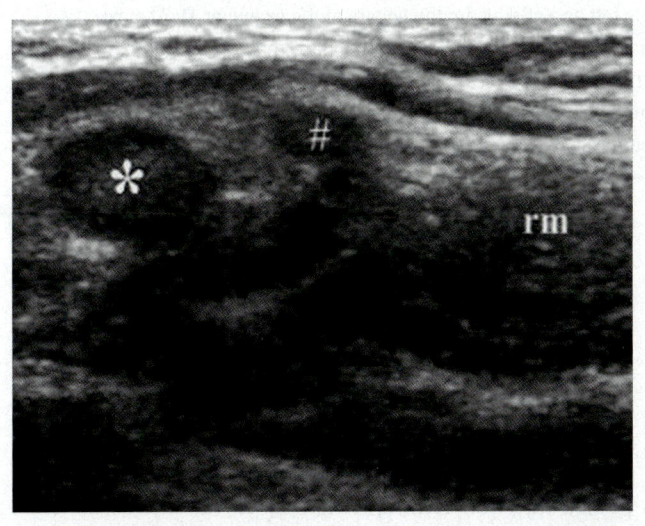

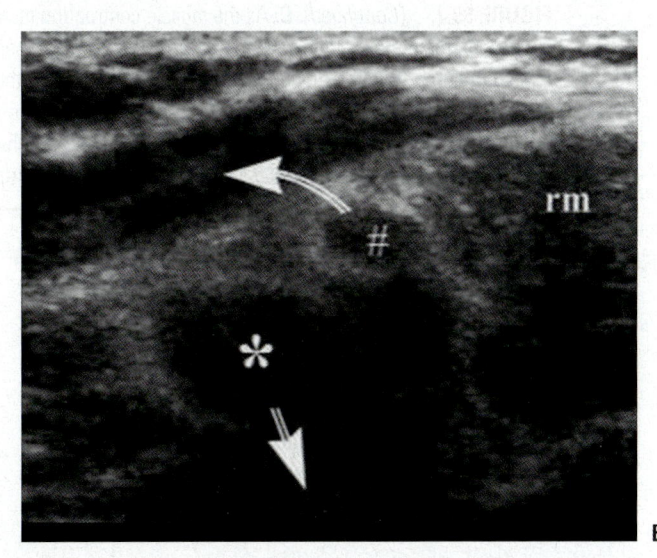

**FIGURE 89.2.** High-resolution sonographic longitudinal views of the lower right thoracic wall in a patient with slipping rib syndrome, with transverse sections of the seventh (*) and eighth (#) ribs, which appear as hypoechoic rounded structures. The *arrows* depict the movements of the ribs. **A:** At rest, the two cartilages lie at about the same level. **B:** When rectus muscle (rm) contraction is initiated, the eighth rib moves cranially and overlaps the seventh rib (*curved arrow*).

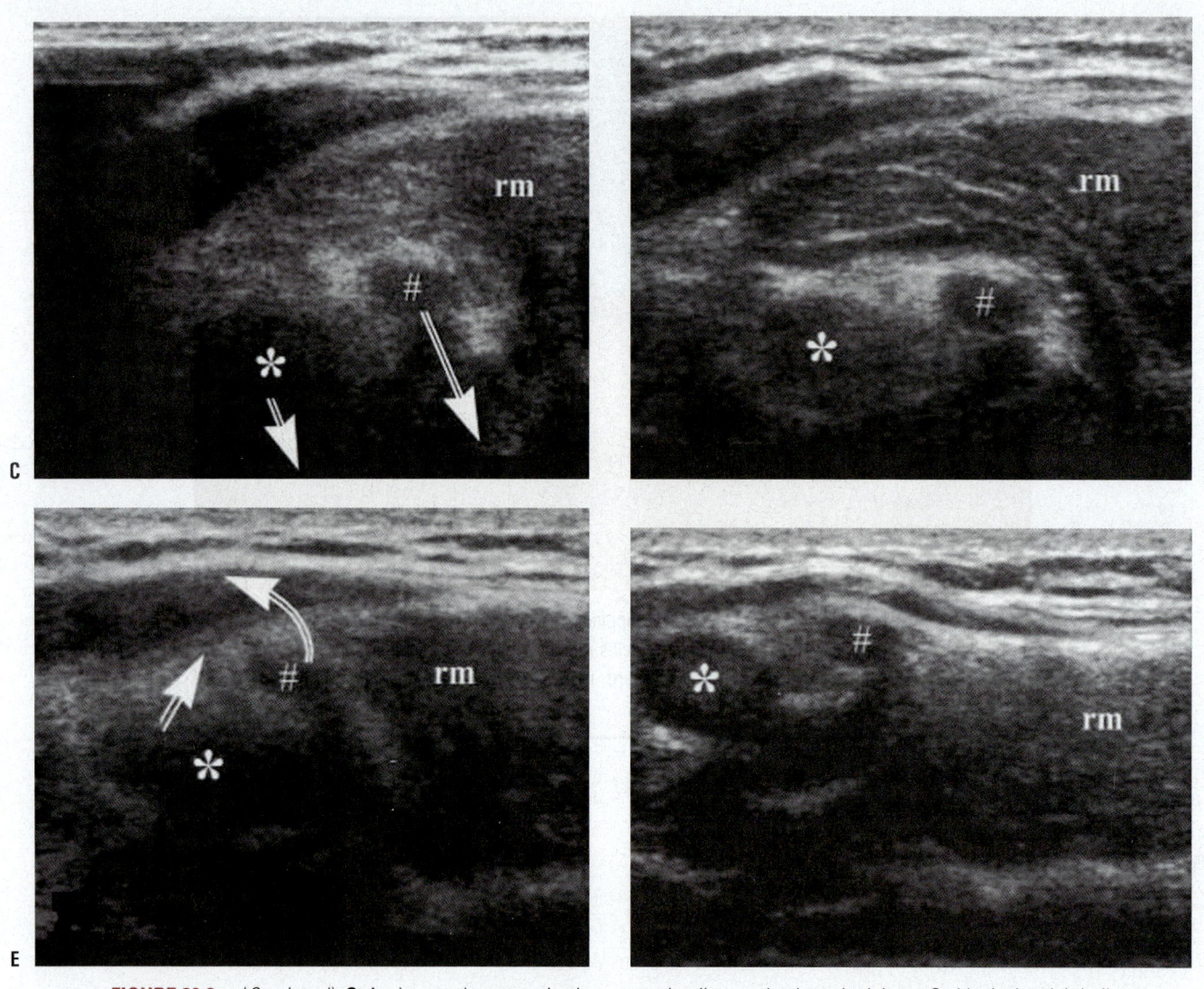

**FIGURE 89.2.** (Continued). **C:** As the muscle contraction increases, the ribs are slowly pushed down. Suddenly the eighth rib slips along the margin of the seventh rib (*arrow*). This movement is felt as a click under the fingers of the examiner. **D:** At maximal contraction, the two ribs are at the same depth, below the rectus muscle. **E:** As the contraction decreases, the eighth rib jumps away from the seventh rib (*arrow*). **F:** At rest, the ribs return to their initial locations. (Reused from Meuwly J-Y, Wicky S, Schnyder P, et al. Slipping rib syndrome: a place for sonography in the diagnosis of a frequently overlooked cause of abdominal or low thoracic pain. *J Ultrasound Med* 2002;21:339–343, with permission.)

and associated rib. At that point, after careful aspiration, a small amount of solution is injected under real-time ultrasound imaging to utilize hydrodissection to confirm the position of the needle tip (Fig. 89.10). Once the position of the needle tip is confirmed, after careful aspiration the remainder of the solution is slowly injected. There should be minimal resistance to injection. The needle is then removed, and a sterile pressure dressing and ice pack are placed at the injection site.

## COMPLICATIONS

The proximity of the pleura, lung, and the abdominal viscera to the anterior costal cartilage and associated ribs means that if the needle is placed too medially or deeply and invades the pleural space or peritoneal cavity, pneumothorax or damage to the abdominal viscera can occur. Infection, although uncommon, can occur if strict aseptic technique is not followed or if the needle is placed too deeply and it pierces the bowel and becomes contaminated. These complications can be greatly decreased with the use of ultrasound guidance to optimize accurate needle placement. Because this ultrasound-guided injection technique may block the intercostal nerve corresponding to the rib injected, the patient should be warned to expect some transient numbness of the chest and abdominal wall, as well as bulging of the abdomen in the subcostal region due to blockade of the motor innervation to these muscles.

## CLINICAL PEARLS

The proximity to the pleural space makes the potential for pneumothorax an ever-present possibility. Should a pneumothorax occur, the "waves on a sandy beach" ultrasound appearance of the normal pleural lung interface will be replaced with a more chaotic "ripples on a pond" appearance (see Fig. 88.11). Patients who suffer from pain emanating from slipping rib often attribute their pain symptomatology to a gallbladder attack or ulcer disease. Reassurance is required, although it should be remembered that this musculoskeletal pain syndrome and intra-abdominal pathology can coexist. Care must be taken to use sterile technique to avoid infection; universal precautions should be used to avoid risk to the operator. The incidence of ecchymosis and hematoma formation can be decreased if pressure is placed on the injection site immediately after injection. The use of physical modalities, including local heat and gentle range-of-motion exercises, should be introduced several days after the patient undergoes this injection technique for slipping rib syndrome. Vigorous exercise should be avoided because it exacerbates the patient's symptomatology. Simple analgesics and nonsteroidal anti-inflammatory agents may be used concurrently with this injection technique. Laboratory evaluation for collagen vascular disease is indicated for patients who suffer from costal cartilage pain with other joints involved.

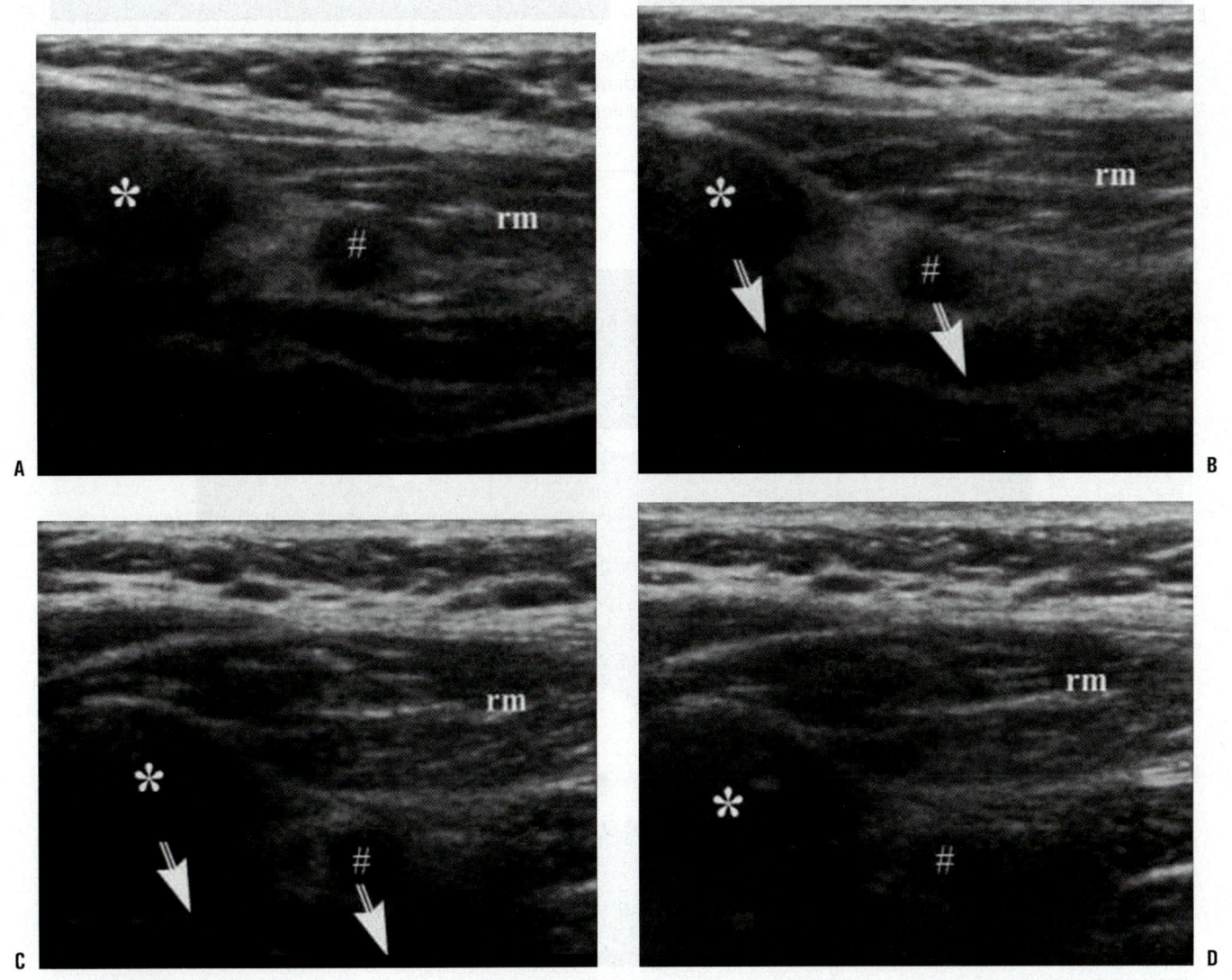

**FIGURE 89.3.** High-resolution sonographic longitudinal views of the lower right thoracic wall in a healthy volunteer, with transverse sections of the seventh (*) and eighth (#) ribs. The *arrows* depict the movements of the ribs. **A:** At rest, the two cartilages lie at the same level. **B:** When rectus muscle (rm) contraction is initiated, the seventh and eighth ribs move down jointly (*arrows*). **C:** As the muscle contraction increased, the ribs continue to be pushed down together (*arrows*). **D:** At maximal contraction, the two ribs are at the same depth, below the rectus muscle.

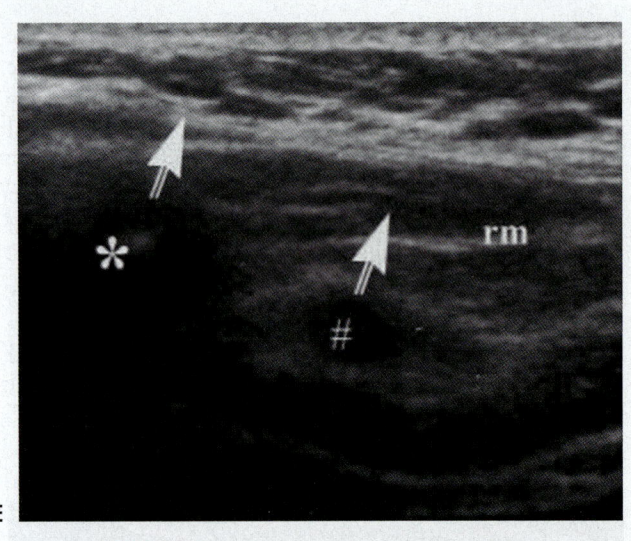

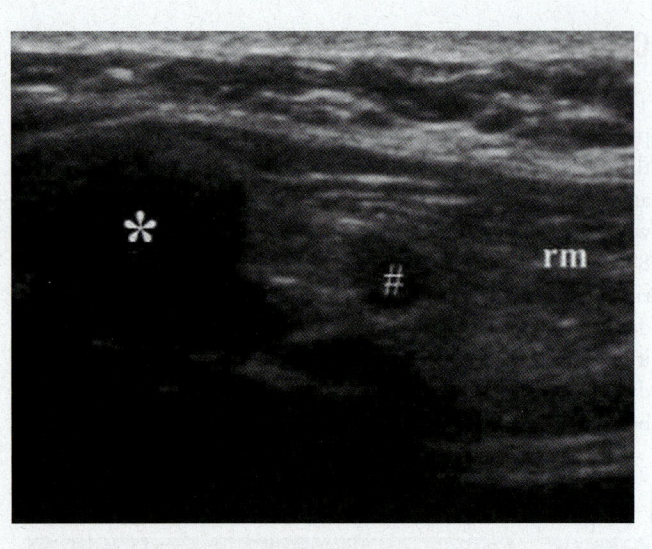

**FIGURE 89.3.** *(Continued)* **E:** As the contraction decreases, the two ribs move up jointly (*arrow*). **F:** At rest, the ribs return to their initial locations. (Reused from Meuwly J-Y, Wicky S, Schnyder P, et al. Slipping rib syndrome: a place for sonography in the diagnosis of a frequently overlooked cause of abdominal or low thoracic pain. *J Ultrasound Med* 2002;21:339–343, with permission.)

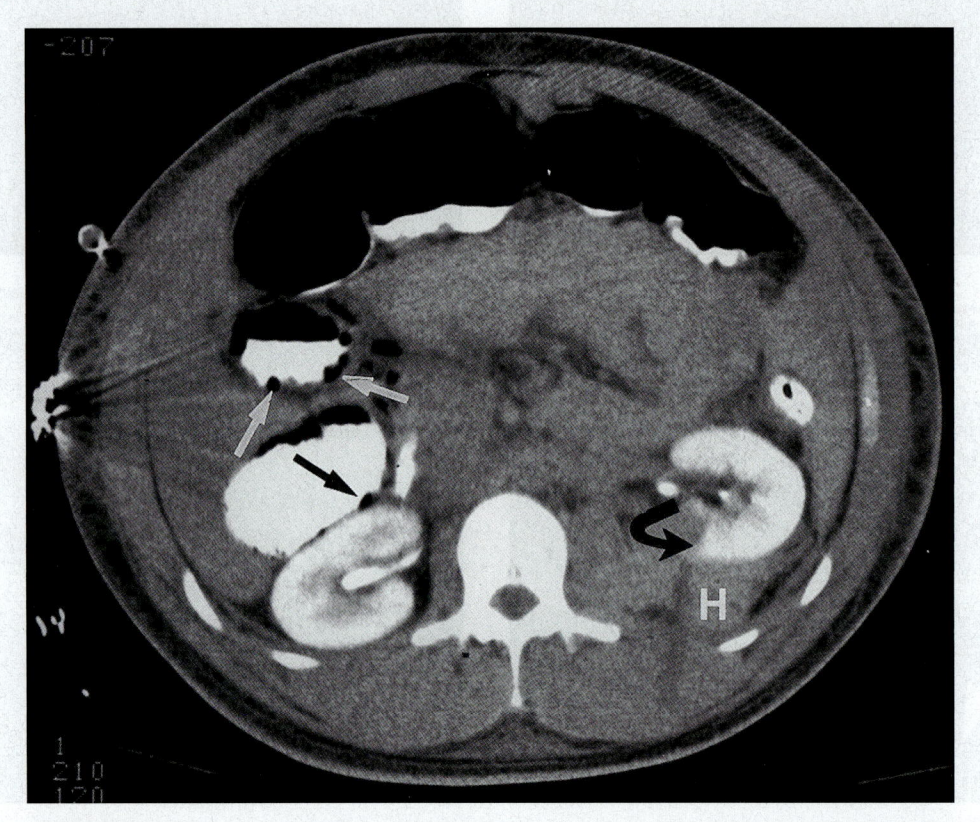

**FIGURE 89.4.** Computed tomography demonstrating infarction of the hepatic flexure of the colon secondary to avulsion of the mesenteric artery following blunt upper abdominal trauma. *Straight arrows* indicate gas bubbles in the colon wall. *Curved arrows* indicate a left perinephric hematoma. (Reused from Pope T, Harris J. *Harris & Harris' Radiology of Emergency Medicine*. 5th ed. Philadelphia, PA: Lippincott Williams & Wilkins; 2012, with permission.)

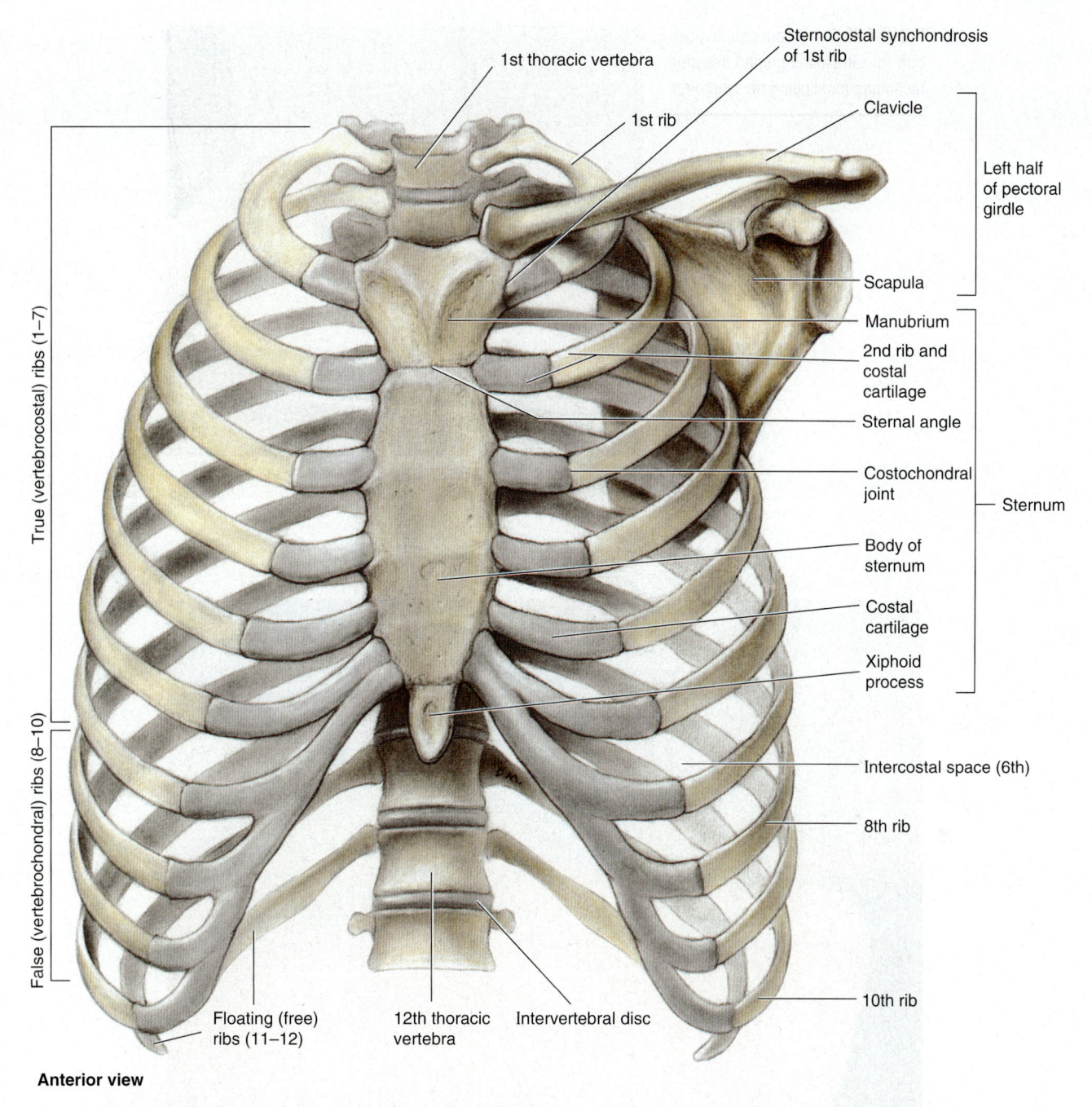

**FIGURE 89.5.** The anatomy of the anterior costal cartilage and associated ribs. (Reused from Moore KL, Dalley AF. *Clinical Oriented Anatomy*. 4th ed. Baltimore, MD: Lippincott Williams & Wilkins; 1999, with permission.)

**FIGURE 89.6.** Proper patient position for ultrasound-guided injection technique for slipping rib syndrome.

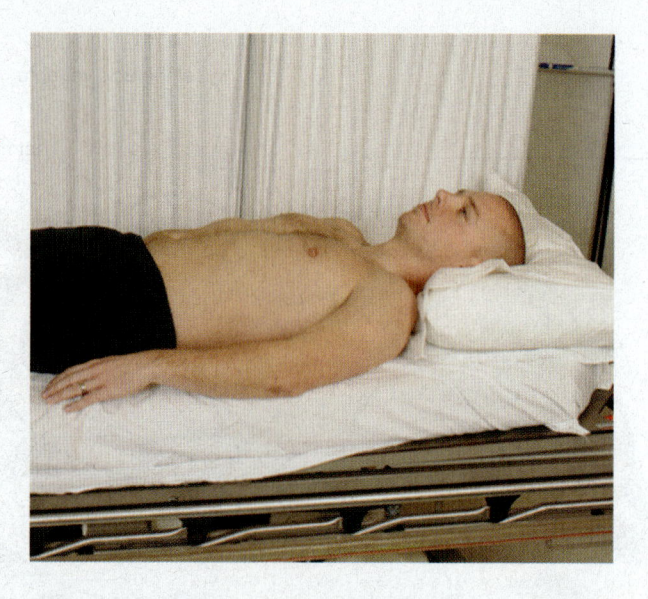

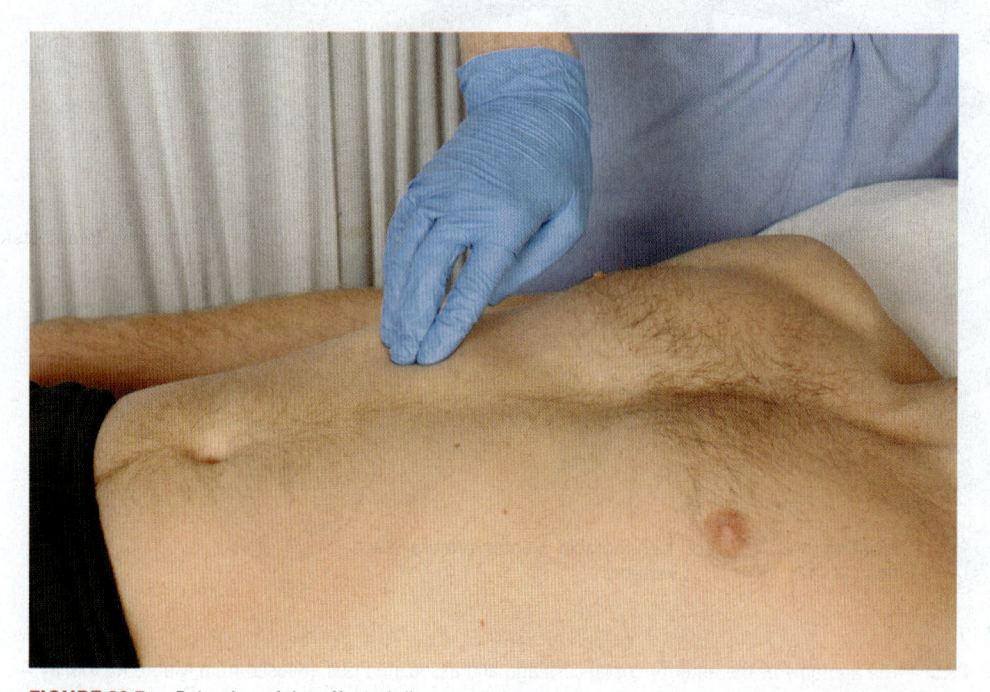

**FIGURE 89.7.** Palpation of the affected rib.

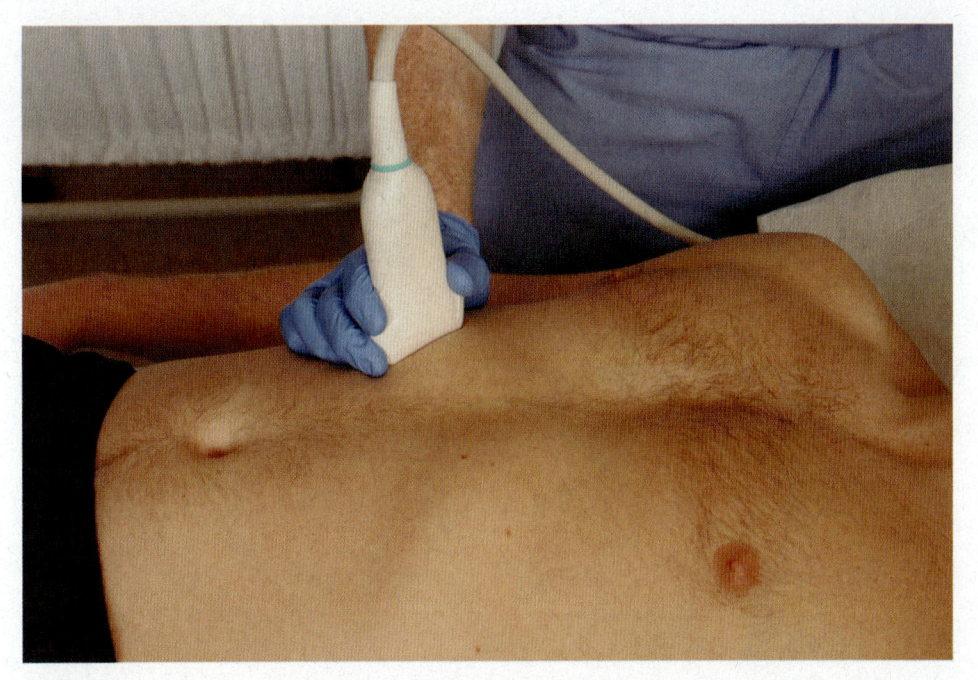

**FIGURE 89.8.** Longitudinal placement of the ultrasound transducer over the anterior costal cartilage and associated ribs with the superior aspect of the transducer rotated laterally ~15 degrees.

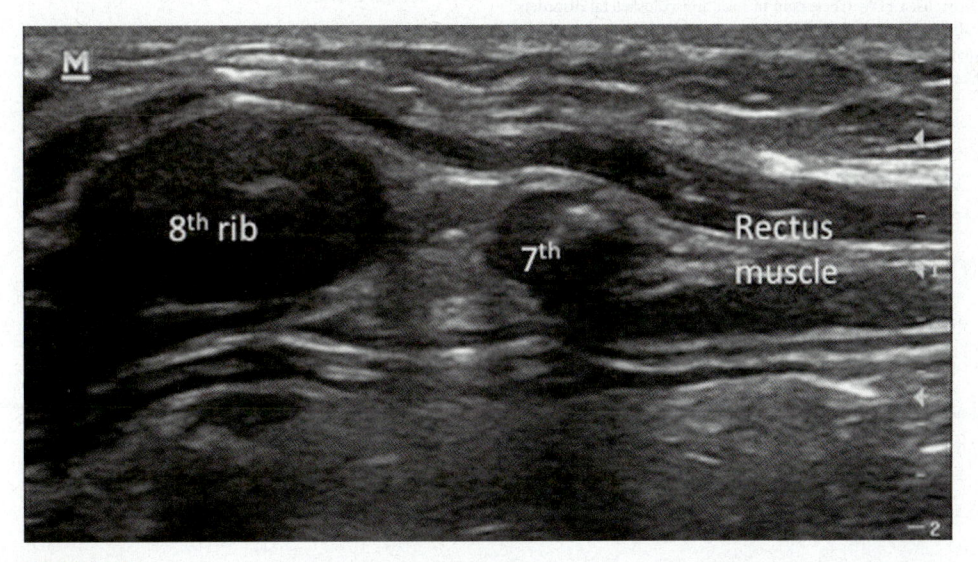

**FIGURE 89.9.** Longitudinal ultrasound image demonstrating adjacent ribs and the rectus muscles.

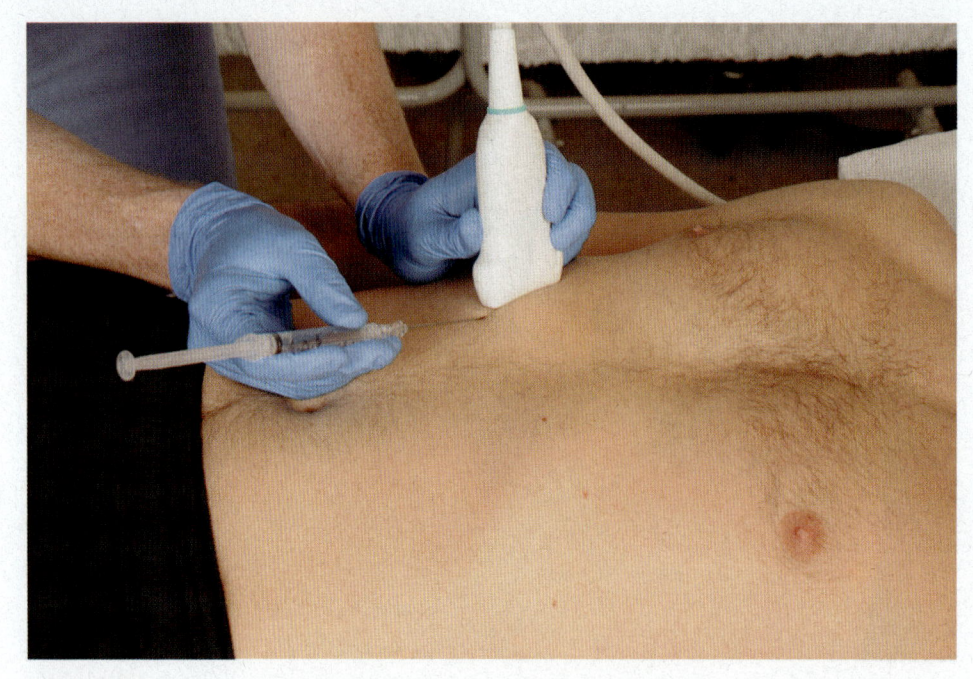

**FIGURE 89.10.** Proper needle position for performing ultrasound-guided injection for slipping rib.

## SUGGESTED READINGS

Meuwly J-Y, Wicky S, Schnyder P, et al. Slipping rib syndrome: a place for sonography in the diagnosis of a frequently overlooked cause of abdominal or low thoracic pain. *J Ultrasound Med* 2002;21:339–343.

Stochkendahl MJ, Christensen HW. Chest pain in focal musculoskeletal disorders. *Med Clin North Am* 2010;94(2):259–273.

Udermann BE, Cavanaugh DG, Gibson MH. Slipping rib syndrome in a collegiate swimmer: a case report. *J Athl Train* 2005;40(2):120–122.

Waldman SD. Hooking maneuver test for slipping rib syndrome. In: *Physical Diagnosis of Pain: An Atlas of Signs and Symptoms*. Philadelphia, PA: Saunders Elsevier; 2010:198.

Waldman SD. Injection technique for slipping rib syndrome. In: *Atlas of Pain Management Injection Techniques*. 3rd ed. Philadelphia, PA: Saunders Elsevier; 2012:274–275.

# CHAPTER 90

# Ultrasound-Guided Transversus Abdominis Plane Block

## CLINICAL PERSPECTIVES

Ultrasound-guided transversus abdominis plane block is utilized in a variety of clinical scenarios as a diagnostic and therapeutic maneuver as well as to provide surgical anesthesia for abdominal surgeries below the umbilicus. As a diagnostic tool, ultrasound-guided transversus abdominis plane block aids in the differential diagnosis of abdominal pain helping distinguish abdominal wall pain from pain of intraperitoneal origin. This technique has great clinical utility in both children and adults when managing acute postoperative and posttrauma pain including post–cesarean section pain that emanates from the abdominal wall below the umbilicus. This technique has recently been utilized to provide surgical anesthesia for laparoscopy. Pain of malignant origin involving the anterior abdominal wall has been successfully managed by the placement of a catheter for continuous infusions of local anesthetics utilizing this ultrasound-guided technique.

## CLINICALLY RELEVANT ANATOMY

Exiting their respective intervertebral foramen and passing just below the transverse process are the paravertebral nerves. After exiting the intervertebral foramen, the intercostal nerve gives off a recurrent branch that loops back through the foramen to provide innervation to the spinal ligaments, meninges, and its respective vertebra and can be an important contributor to spinal pain. The paravertebral nerve also provides fibers to the sympathetic nervous system and the thoracic sympathetic chain via the myelinated preganglionic fibers of the white rami communicantes as well as the unmyelinated postganglionic fibers of the gray rami communicantes. The intercostal nerve then divides into a posterior and an anterior primary division (Fig. 90.1). The posterior division courses posteriorly and, along with its branches, provides innervation to the facet joints and the muscles and skin of the back. The larger, anterior division courses laterally to pass into the subcostal groove beneath the rib along with the intercostal vein and artery to become the respective intercostal nerves. The 12th thoracic nerve courses beneath the 12th rib and is called the subcostal nerve and is unique in that it gives off a branch to the first lumbar nerve, thus contributing to the lumbar plexus. The intercostal and subcostal nerves provide the innervation to the skin, muscles, ribs, and the parietal pleura and parietal peritoneum. The anatomic basis of the transversus abdominis plane block is the fact that the innervation of the anterolateral abdominal wall is provided by the lower six intercostal nerves and the first lumbar nerve. The anterior branches of these nerves pass within a fascial plane between the internal oblique muscle and the transversus abdominis muscle making them easily assessable for blockade with local anesthetic by placing a needle into this fascial plane (Fig. 90.2). Within this fascial plane there are many interconnections between the various intercostal nerves, and it is thought that these interconnections form a "pseudoplexus" contributing to the efficacy of this block.

## ULTRASOUND-GUIDED TECHNIQUE

Ultrasound-guided transversus abdominis plane block can be carried out by placing the patient in the supine position with the arms resting comfortably by the patient's side (Fig. 90.3). A total of 20 mL of local anesthetic is drawn up in a 20-mL sterile syringe. If the painful condition being treated is thought to have an inflammatory component, 40 to 80 mg of depot steroid is added to the local anesthetic. The iliac crest at the level of the midaxillary line is identified by palpation (Fig. 90.4). A curvilinear low-frequency ultrasound transducer is then placed in the transverse plane just above the iliac crest at the midaxillary line with the medial aspect of the ultrasound transducer pointed toward the patient's umbilicus, and an ultrasound survey scan is taken (Figs. 90.5 and 90.6). The three layers of muscle, the external oblique, the internal oblique, and the transversus abdominis muscles, are identified as well with the fascial plane between the internal oblique muscle and the transversus abdominis muscle (see Fig. 90.6). When these anatomic structures are clearly identified on transverse ultrasound scan, the skin is prepped with anesthetic solution, and a 1½-inch, 22-gauge needle is advanced from the superior border of the ultrasound transducer using an in-plane approach in a medial to lateral direction with the trajectory being adjusted under real-time ultrasound guidance until the needle tip is resting within internal oblique muscle. At that point, after careful aspiration, a small amount of solution is injected under real-time ultrasound imaging to utilize

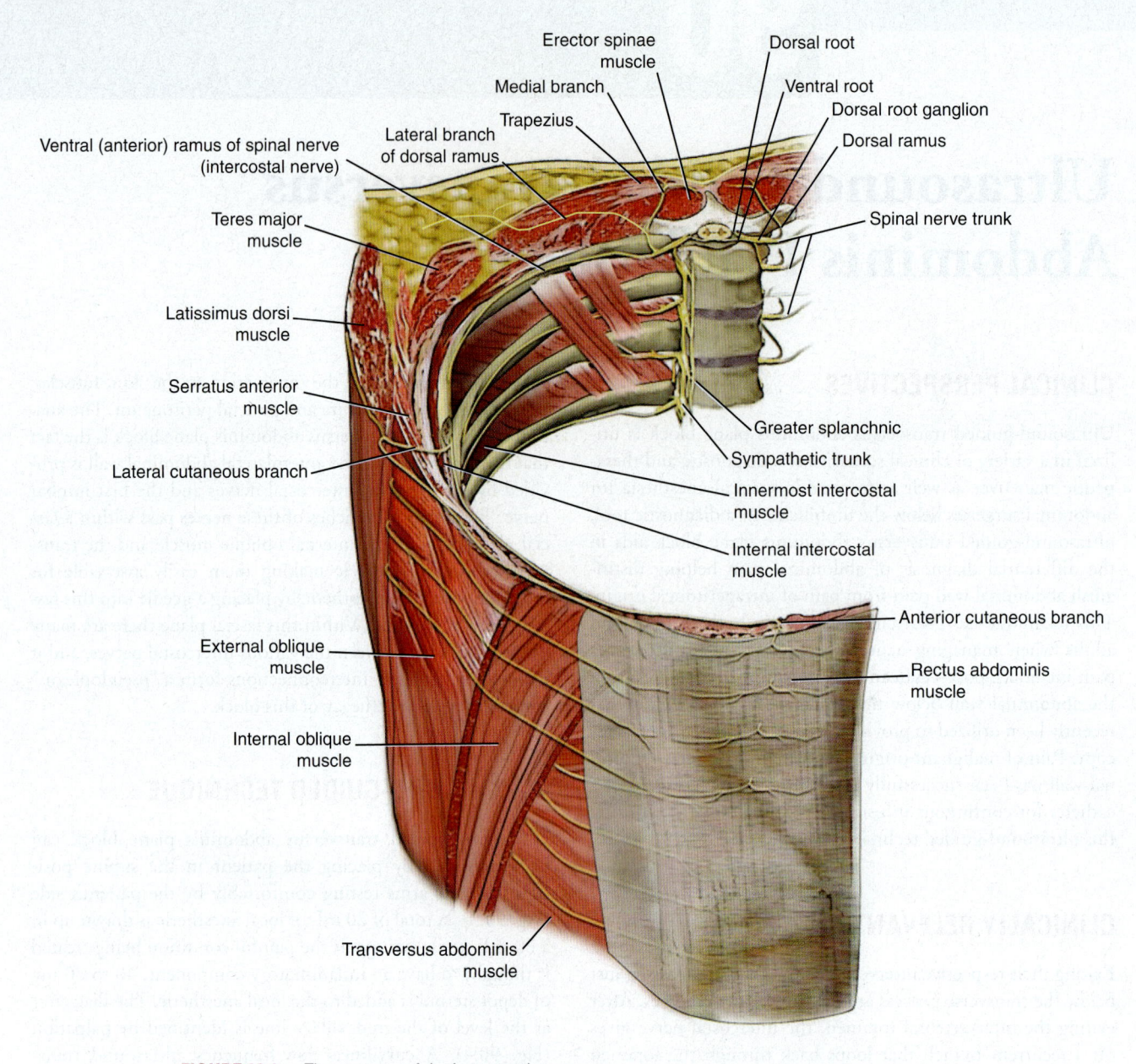

**FIGURE 90.1.** The anatomy of the intercostal nerve.

hydrodissection to reconfirm the position of the needle tip. Once the position of the needle tip is reconfirmed, the needle is carefully advanced through the deep fascia of the internal oblique muscle into the fascial plane between the internal oblique muscle and the transversus abdominis muscle. After careful aspiration, a small amount of solution is again injected to aid in identification of the exact position of the needle tip.

After careful aspiration, the remainder of the solution is slowly injected under ultrasound guidance, which will demonstrate a bowing downward of the superficial fascia of the transversus abdominis muscle by the injectate (Fig. 90.7). There should be minimal resistance to injection. The needle is then removed, and a sterile pressure dressing and ice pack are placed at the injection site.

CHAPTER 90  ULTRASOUND-GUIDED TRANSVERSUS ABDOMINIS PLANE BLOCK  **617**

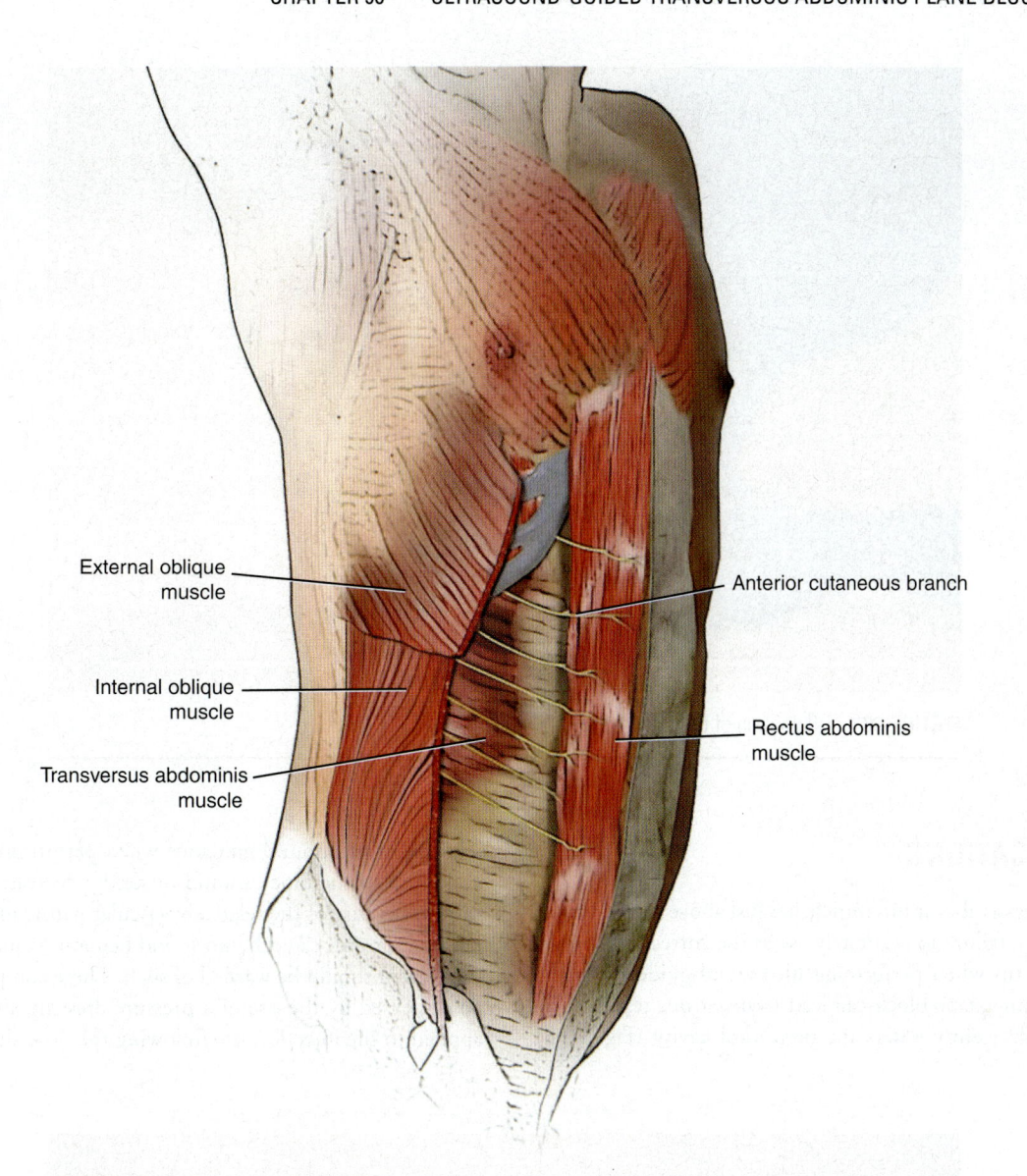

**FIGURE 90.2.** The intercostal nerves travel within a fascial plane that lies between the internal oblique and the transversus abdominis muscle.

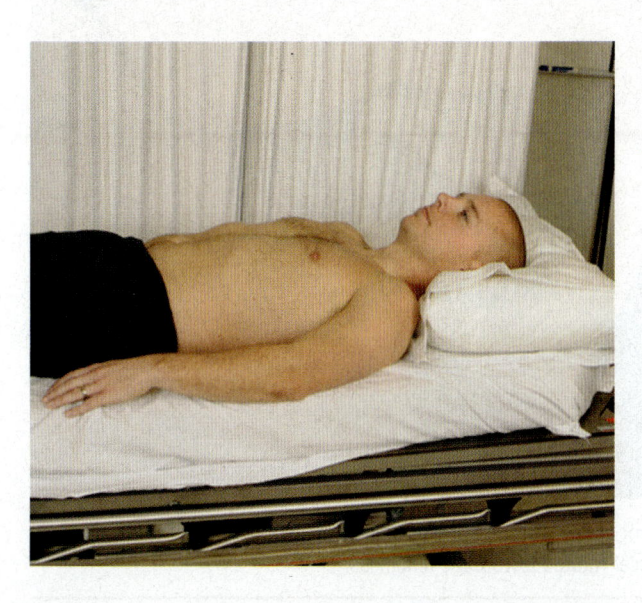

**FIGURE 90.3.** Proper patient position for ultrasound-guided transversus abdominis plane block.

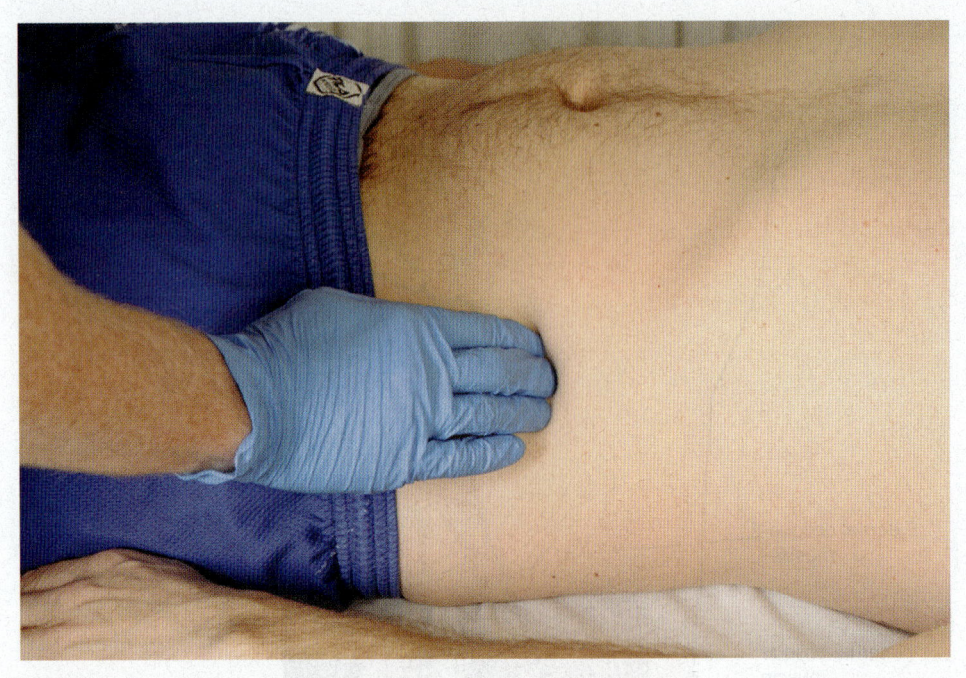

**FIGURE 90.4.** Palpation of the affected rib.

## COMPLICATIONS

The transversus abdominis muscle lies just above the peritoneal cavity, and a failure to accurately assess the correct position of the needle tip when performing ultrasound-guided transversus abdominis plane block can lead to disastrous results if the needle inadvertently enters the peritoneal cavity (Fig. 90.8). The use of ultrasound guidance when performing transversus abdominis plane block should markedly decrease this complication. Because of the relatively vascular nature of the abdominal wall, postblock ecchymosis and hematoma may occur, and the patient should be warned of such. These complications can be decreased by the use of a pressure dressing and cold packs applied to the injection site following the procedure.

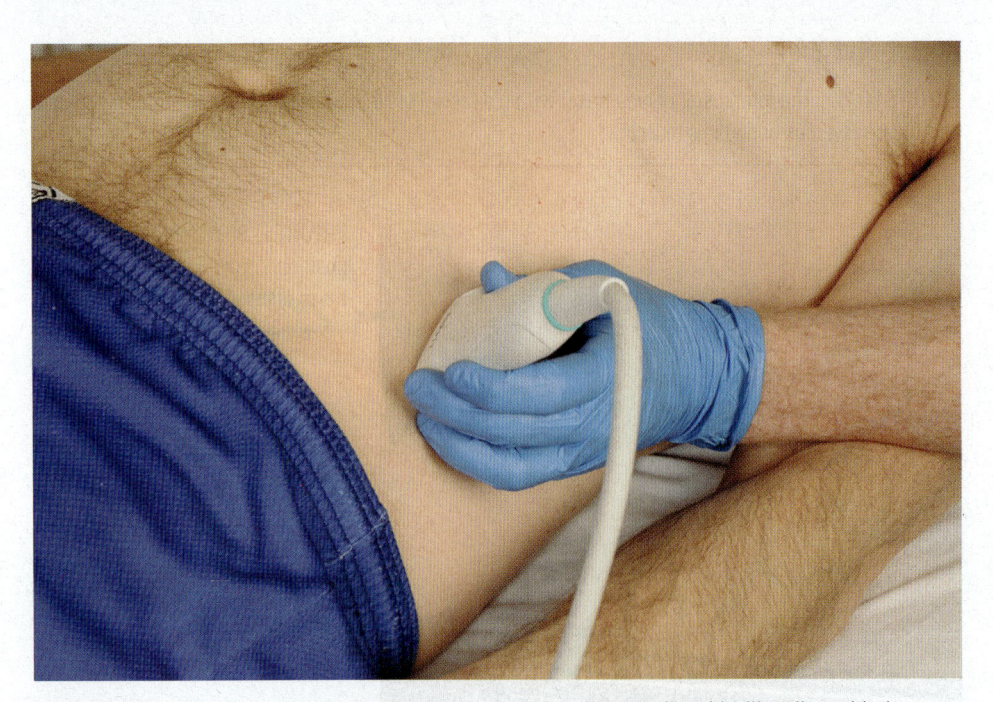

**FIGURE 90.5.** Transverse placement of the ultrasound transducer at the midaxillary line with the superior aspect of the ultrasound transducer rotated toward the umbilicus.

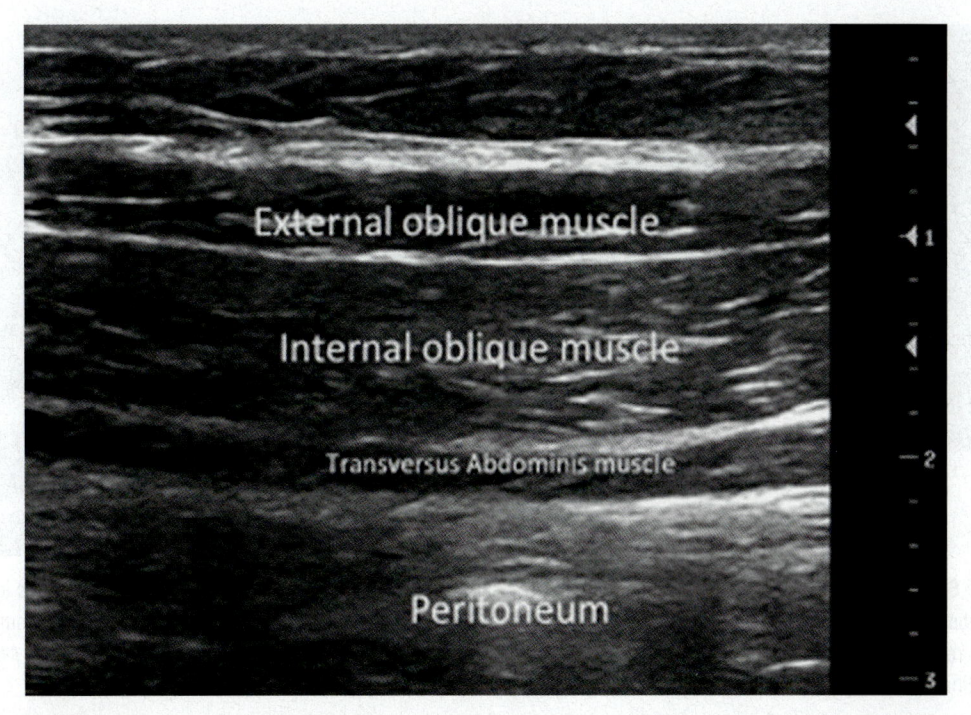

**FIGURE 90.6.** Longitudinal ultrasound image demonstrating external, internal, and transversus abdominis muscles; the fascial plane between the internal and transversus abdominis muscles; and the peritoneal cavity.

## CLINICAL PEARLS

The key to performing successful ultrasound-guided transversus abdominis plane block is the proper identification of the sonographic anatomy and in particular the ability to properly identify the layers of muscle that comprise the abdominal wall at the midaxillary line. This should not be a problem if the above technique is used. Any significant pain or sudden increase in resistance during injection when performing ultrasound-guided suggests incorrect needle placement, and one should stop injecting immediately and reassess the position of the needle.

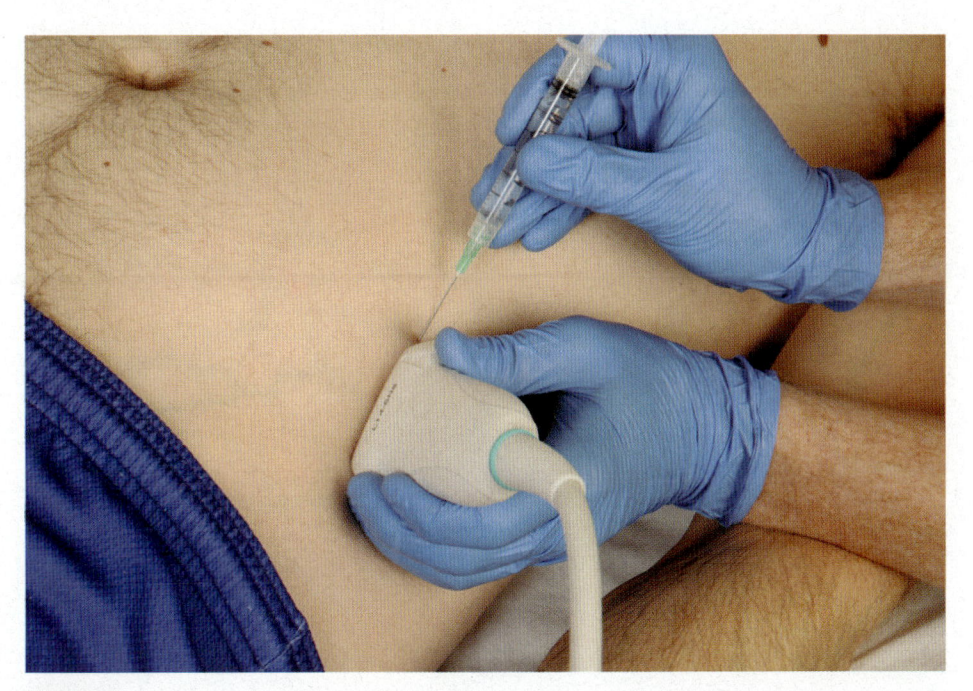

**FIGURE 90.7.** Proper needle position for performing transversus abdominis plane block.

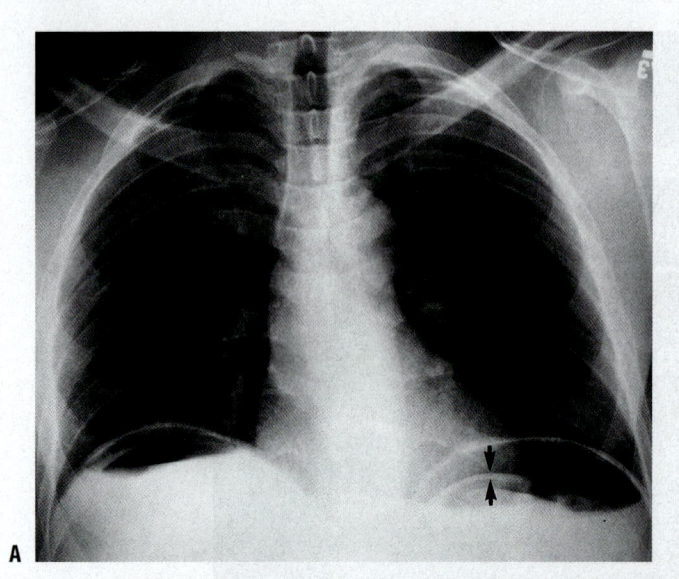

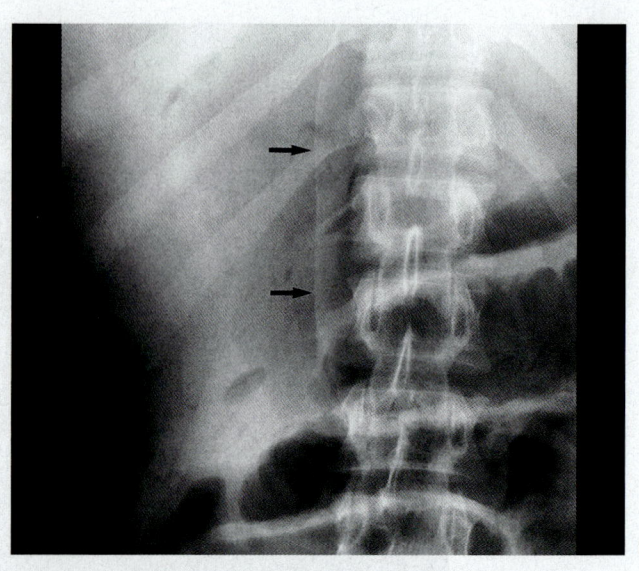

**FIGURE 90.8.** Pneumoperitoneum in standing chest x-ray showing free air beneath the hemidiaphragm. *Arrows* in image (**A**) demonstrate air outlining the stomach. *Arrows* in image (**B**) demonstrate free air outlining the falciform ligament. These findings represent a surgical emergency. (Reused from Pope T, Harris J. *Harris & Harris Radiology of Emergency Medicine.* 5th ed. Philadelphia, PA: Lippincott Williams & Wilkins; 2013:592, with permission.)

## SUGGESTED READINGS

Allcock E, Spencer E, Frazer R, et al. Continuous transversus abdominis plane (TAP) block catheters in a combat surgical environment. *Pain Med* 2010;11(9):1426–1429.

Kanazi GE, Aouad MT, Abdallah FW, et al. The analgesic efficacy of subarachnoid morphine in comparison with ultrasound-guided transversus abdominis plane block after cesarean delivery: a randomized controlled trial. *Anesth Analg* 2010;111(2):475–481.

Narouze S. Transversus abdominis plane block. In: *Atlas of Ultrasound Guided Procedures in Interventional Pain Management.* New York, NY: Springer; 2011:193–197.

Singh M, Chin KJ, Chan V. Ultrasound-guided transversus abdominis plane (TAP) block: a useful adjunct in the management of postoperative respiratory failure. *J Clin Anesth* 2011;23(4):303–306.

# CHAPTER 91

# Ultrasound-Guided Injection Technique for Anterior Cutaneous Nerve Entrapment Syndrome

## CLINICAL PERSPECTIVES

Ultrasound-guided anterior cutaneous nerve block is utilized as a diagnostic and therapeutic maneuver in the evaluation and treatment of anterior cutaneous nerve entrapment syndrome. This commonly overlooked cause of abdominal pain presents with a constellation of symptoms including severe, knife-like anterior abdominal wall pain that is associated with point tenderness over the affected anterior cutaneous nerve. The pain of anterior cutaneous nerve entrapment syndrome radiates medially to the linea alba and rarely crossed the midline. This entrapment syndrome occurs most commonly in young females and is often attributed to ovarian pain or mittelschmerz. Often the patient can accurately localize the site of nerve entrapment, which can be confirmed by the clinician by palpating the spot the patient identifies with a straightened index finger. If the patient confirms that the point being palpated is the nidus of the patient's pain symptomatology, the patient is then asked to contract the abdominal muscles, which should further exacerbate the pain if the cause is anterior cutaneous nerve entrapment. This increase in pain is thought to be caused by the herniation of small amounts of fat into the fascial ring, which contains the anterior cutaneous nerve as it turns anteriorly along with the epigastric artery and vein to provide sensory innervation to the anterior abdominal wall (Fig. 91.1). Patients suffering from anterior cutaneous nerve entrapment will often attempt to avoid eliciting anterior abdominal wall pain by splinting the affected nerve by keeping the thoracolumbar spine slightly flexed to avoid increasing tension on the abdominal musculature.

Plain radiographs are indicated for all patients who present with pain thought to be emanating from the lower costal cartilage and ribs to rule out occult bony pathology, including rib fracture and tumor. Radiographic evaluation of the gallbladder is indicated if cholelithiasis is suspected (Fig. 91.2). Based on the patient's clinical presentation, additional testing may be indicated, including complete blood cell count, rectal examination with stool guaiac, sedimentation rate, and antinuclear antibody testing. Computed tomography of the abdomen is indicated if intra-abdominal pathology or an occult mass is suspected.

## CLINICALLY RELEVANT ANATOMY

Exiting their respective intervertebral foramen and passing just below the transverse process are the paravertebral nerves. After exiting the intervertebral foramen, the intercostal nerve gives off a recurrent branch that loops back through the foramen to provide innervation to the spinal ligaments, meninges, and its respective vertebra and can be an important contributor to spinal pain. The paravertebral nerve also provides fibers to the sympathetic nervous system and the thoracic sympathetic chain via the myelinated preganglionic fibers of the white rami communicantes as well as the unmyelinated postganglionic fibers of the gray rami communicantes. The intercostal nerve then divides into a posterior and an anterior primary division (Fig. 91.3). The posterior division courses posteriorly and, along with its branches, provides innervation to the facet joints and the muscles and skin of the back. The larger, anterior division courses laterally to pass into the subcostal groove beneath the rib along with the intercostal vein and artery to become the respective intercostal nerves. The 12th thoracic nerve courses beneath the 12th rib and is called the subcostal nerve and is unique in that it gives off a branch to the first lumbar nerve, thus contributing to the lumbar plexus. The intercostal and subcostal nerves provide the innervation to the skin, muscles, ribs, and the parietal pleura and parietal peritoneum. The anatomic basis of the anterior cutaneous nerve block is the fact that the innervation of the anterolateral abdominal wall is provided by the lower six intercostal nerves and the first lumbar nerve. The anterior branches of these nerves pass within a fascial plane between the internal oblique muscle and the transversus abdominis muscle making them easily assessable for blockade with local anesthetic by placing a needle into this fascial plane (see Chapter 90). The anterior cutaneous branch then pierces the fascia of the abdominal wall at the lateral border of the rectus abdominis muscle (see Fig. 91.3). The nerve turns sharply in an anterior direction to provide innervation to the anterior wall (Fig. 91.4). The nerve passes through a firm fibrous ring as it pierces the fascia, and it is at this point that the nerve is

**622** SECTION VI CHEST WALL, TRUNK, AND ABDOMEN

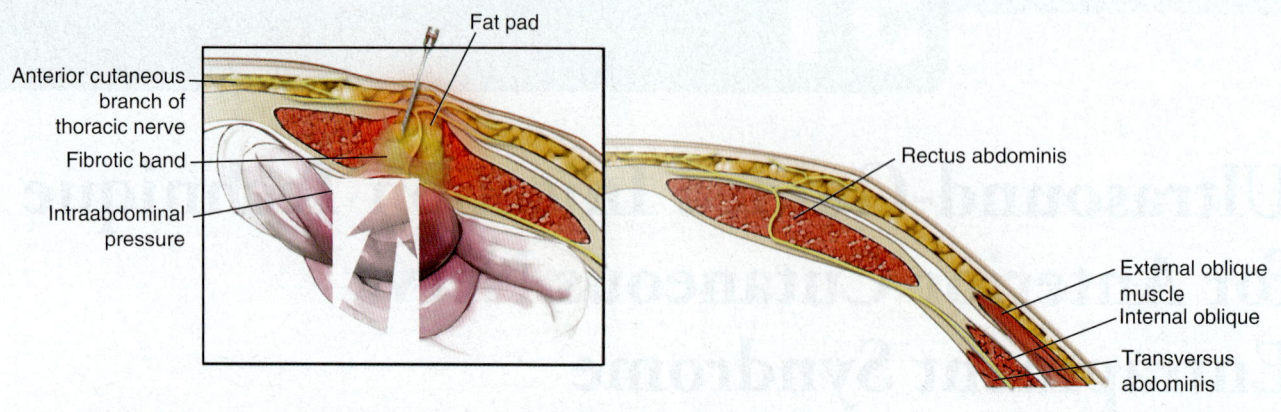

**FIGURE 91.1.** The mechanism of anterior cutaneous nerve entrapment.

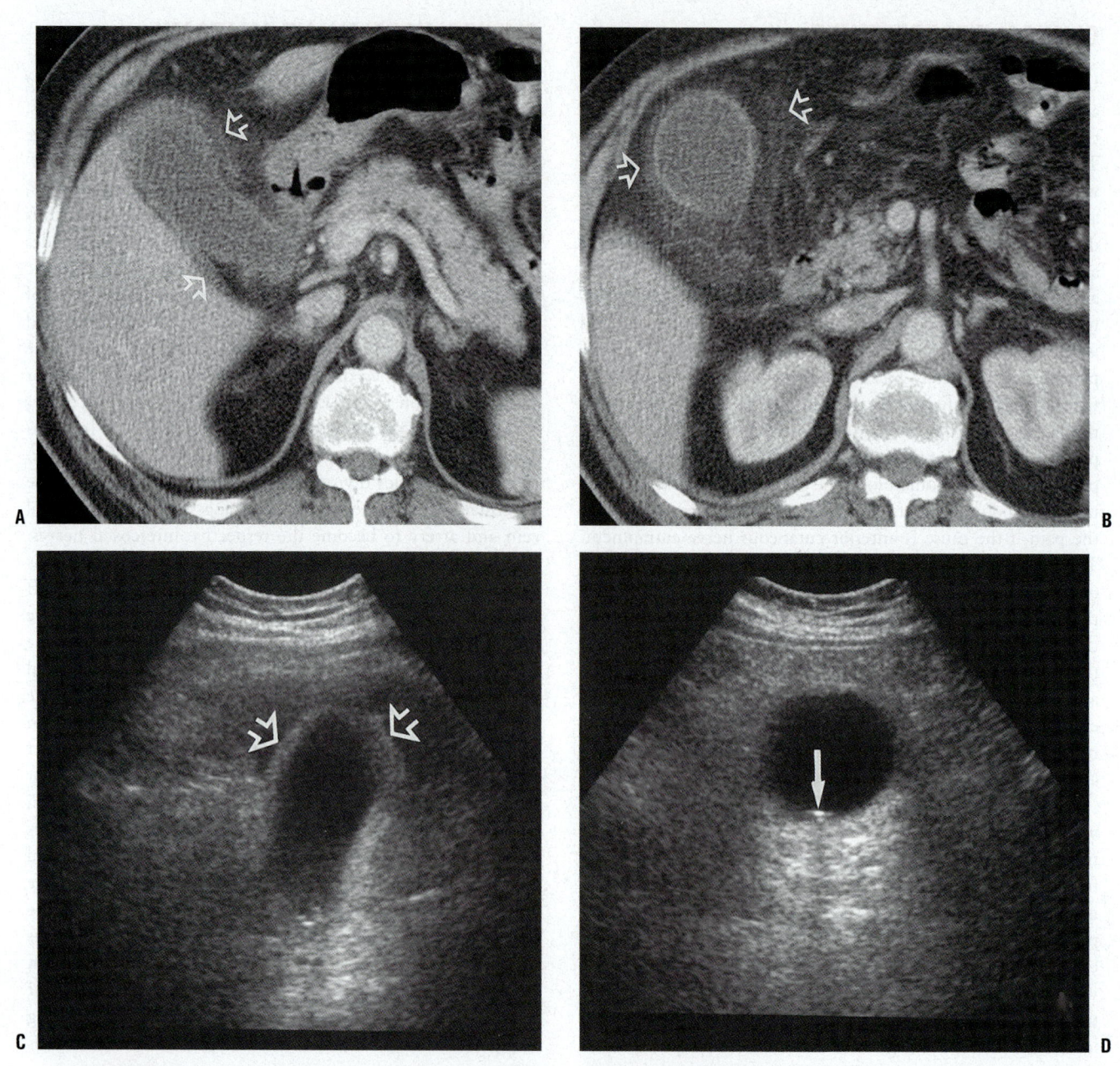

**FIGURE 91.2.** Acute cholecystitis. (Reused from Pope TL Jr, Harris JH Jr. *Harris & Harris' The Radiology of Emergency Medicine.* 5th ed. Philadelphia, PA: Lippincott Williams & Wilkins; 2013:605, with permission.)

CHAPTER 91 ULTRASOUND-GUIDED INJECTION TECHNIQUE FOR ANTERIOR CUTANEOUS NERVE ENTRAPMENT SYNDROME 623

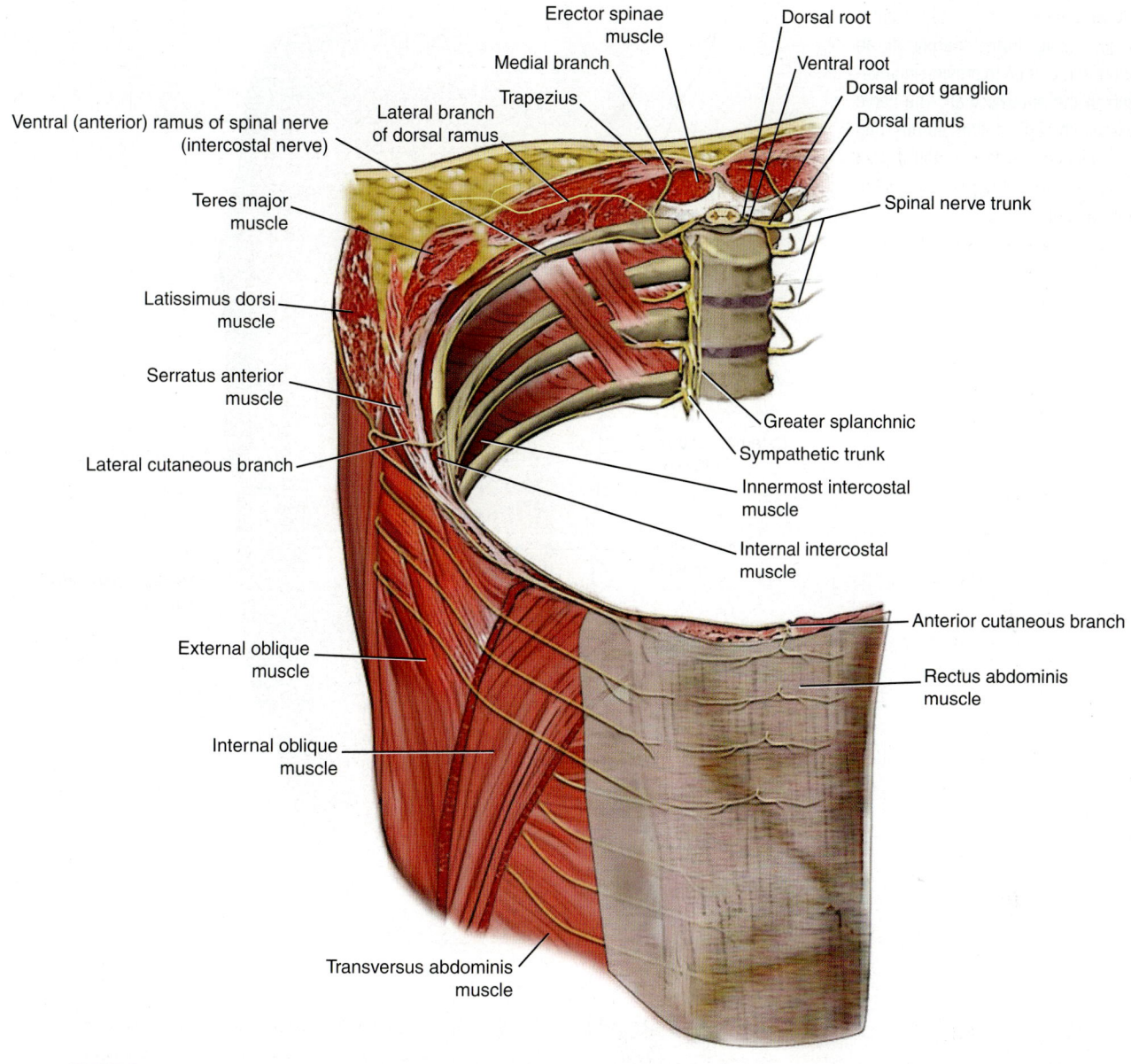

**FIGURE 91.3.** The anatomy of the anterior cutaneous nerve.

subject to entrapment. The nerve is accompanied through the fascia by an epigastric artery and vein. Occasionally, the terminal branches of a given intercostal nerve may actually cross the midline to provide sensory innervation to the contralateral chest and abdominal wall.

## ULTRASOUND-GUIDED TECHNIQUE

Ultrasound-guided anterior cutaneous nerve block can be carried out by placing the patient in the supine position with the arms resting comfortably by the patient's side (Fig. 91.5). A total of 3 mL of local anesthetic for each anterior cutaneous nerve to be blocked is drawn up in a 20-mL sterile syringe. If the painful condition being treated is thought to have an inflammatory component, 40 to 80 mg of depot steroid is added to the local anesthetic. The patient is asked to identify the painful point that is thought to be the source of the pain. After the clinician confirms by palpation that in fact this is the site of the patient's abdominal wall pain, the skin overlying the point is prepped with antiseptic solution (Fig. 91.6). A curvilinear low-frequency ultrasound transducer is then placed in the transverse plane just above the previously identified point of nerve entrapment, and an ultrasound survey scan is taken (Fig. 91.7). The skin, subcutaneous tissue, and rectus abdominis muscles as well as the anterior cutaneous nerve are identified (Fig. 91.8). Color Doppler can be utilized to help identify the epigastric artery and vein as they turn upward accompanying the anterior cutaneous nerve as it passes anteriorly (Fig. 91.9). When these anatomic structures are clearly identified on transverse ultrasound scan,

**FIGURE 91.4.** The anterior cutaneous nerve turns sharply in an anterior direction to provide innervation to the anterior wall. The nerve passes through a firm fibrous ring as it pierces the fascia, and it is at this point that the nerve is subject to entrapment.

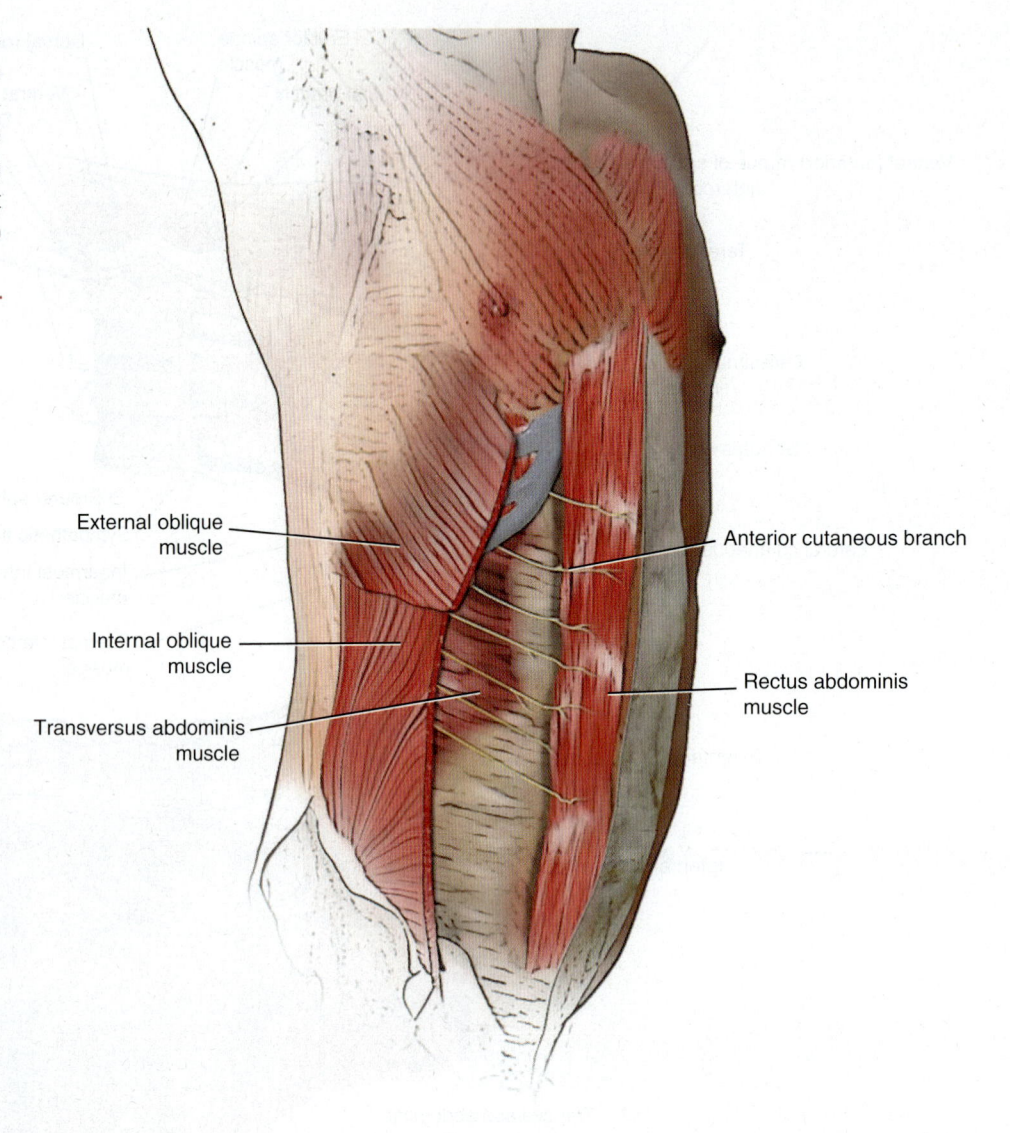

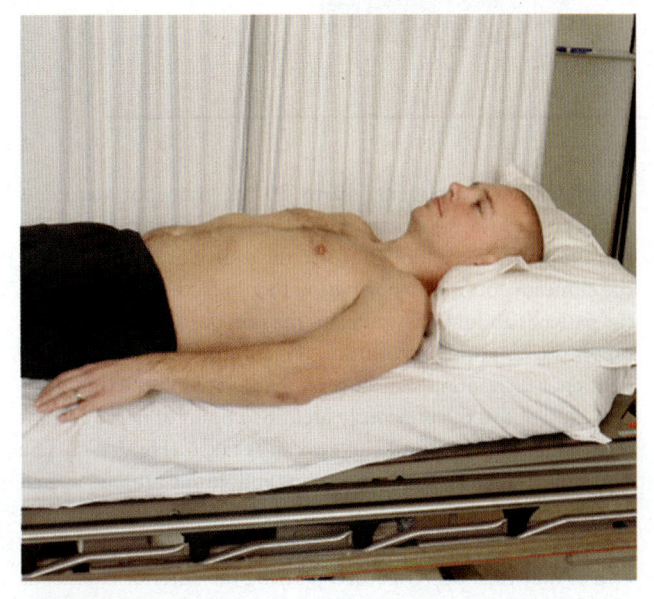

**FIGURE 91.5.** Proper patient position for ultrasound-guided anterior cutaneous nerve block.

the skin is prepped with anesthetic solution, and a 1½-inch, 22-gauge needle is advanced from the medial border of the ultrasound transducer using an in-plane approach in a medial to lateral direction with the trajectory being adjusted under real-time ultrasound guidance until the needle tip is resting within proximity to the anterior cutaneous nerve (Fig. 91.10). At that point, after careful aspiration, a small amount of solution is injected under real-time ultrasound imaging to utilize hydrodissection to reconfirm the position of the needle tip. Once the position of the needle tip is reconfirmed, after careful aspiration, the remainder of the solution is slowly injected under ultrasound guidance. There should be minimal resistance to injection. The needle is then removed, and a sterile pressure dressing and ice pack are placed at the injection site.

## COMPLICATIONS

The transverse abdominis muscle lies just above the peritoneal cavity, and a failure to accurately assess the correct position of the needle tip when performing ultrasound-guided

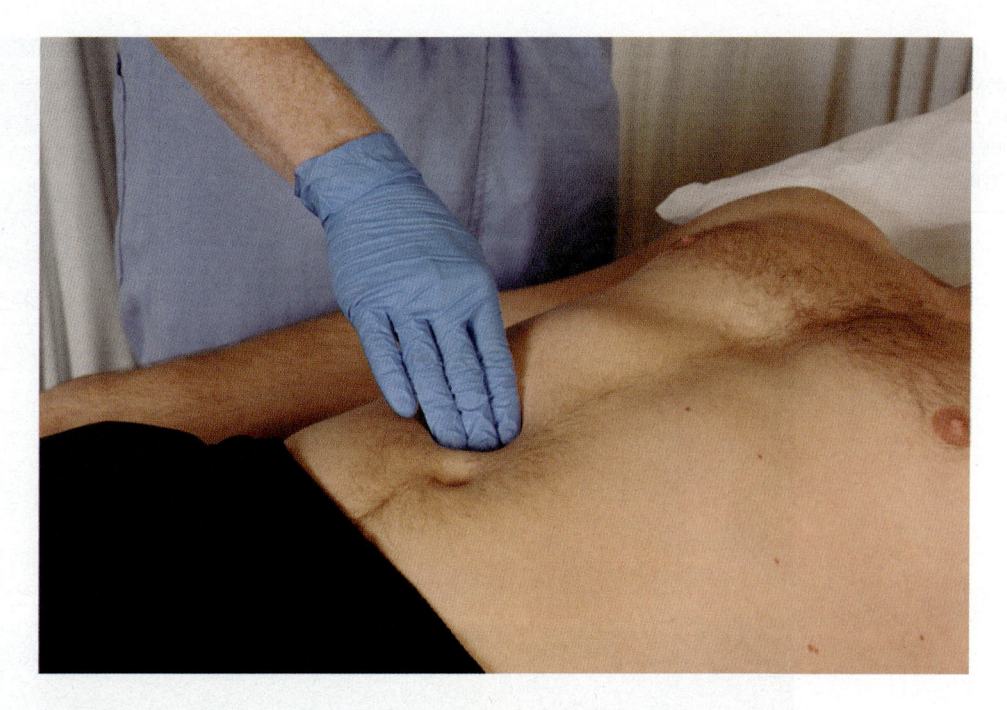

**CHAPTER 91** ULTRASOUND-GUIDED INJECTION TECHNIQUE FOR ANTERIOR CUTANEOUS NERVE ENTRAPMENT SYNDROME

**FIGURE 91.6.** Palpation of the point of maximal pain as identified by the patient.

anterior cutaneous nerve block can lead to disastrous results if the needle inadvertently enters the peritoneal cavity and traumatizing the underlying viscera (Fig. 91.11). Because of the relatively vascular nature of the abdominal wall, postblock ecchymosis and hematoma may occur, and the patient should be warned of such. These complications can be decreased by the use of a pressure dressing and cold packs applied to the injection site following the procedure.

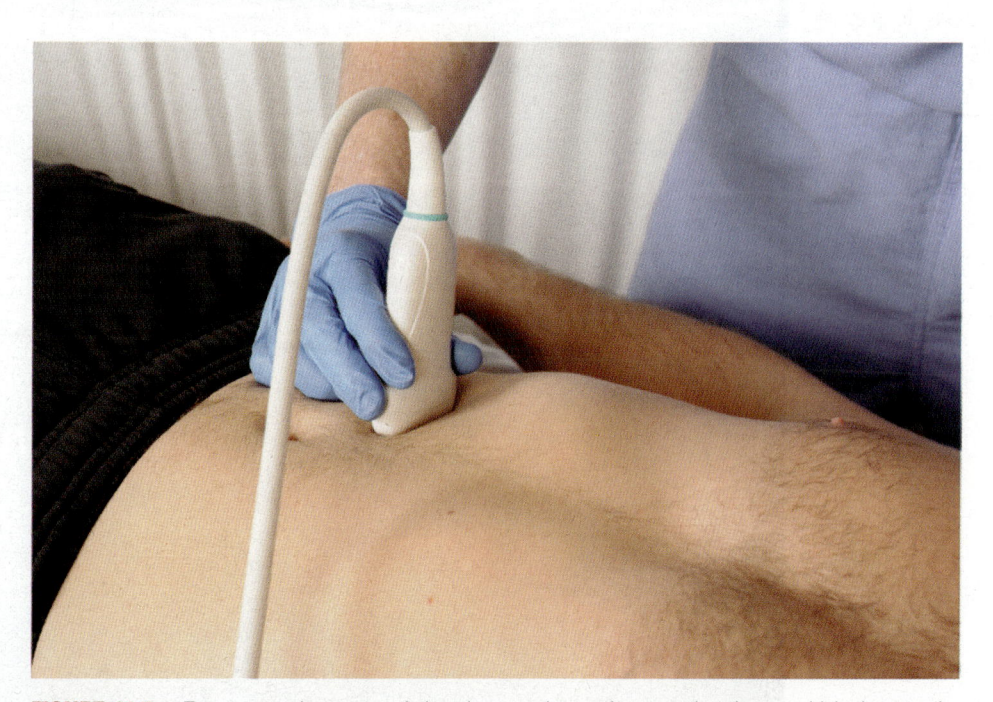

**FIGURE 91.7.** Transverse placement of the ultrasound transducer at the site at which the anterior cutaneous nerve pierces the abdominal wall.

**FIGURE 91.8.** Transverse ultrasound image demonstrating external rectus muscle, peritoneal cavity, skin, subcutaneous tissue, and anterior cutaneous nerve.

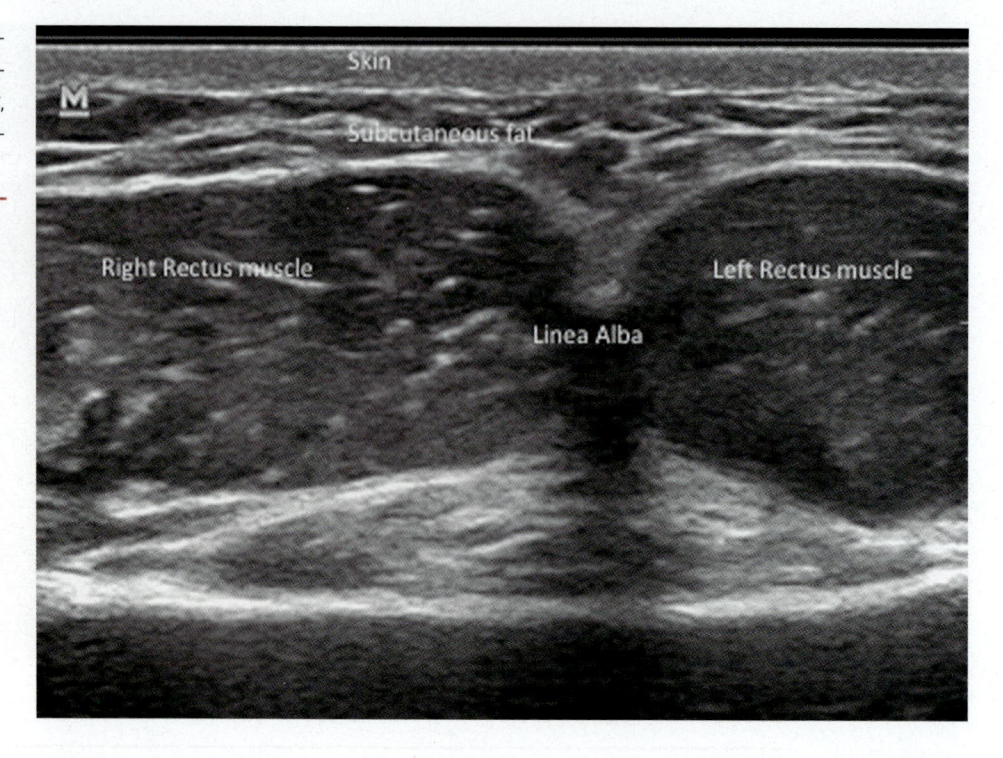

**FIGURE 91.9.** The use of color Doppler can aid in identification of the epigastric artery, which accompanies the anterior cutaneous nerve as it passes anteriorly to provide sensory innervation to the anterior abdominal wall.

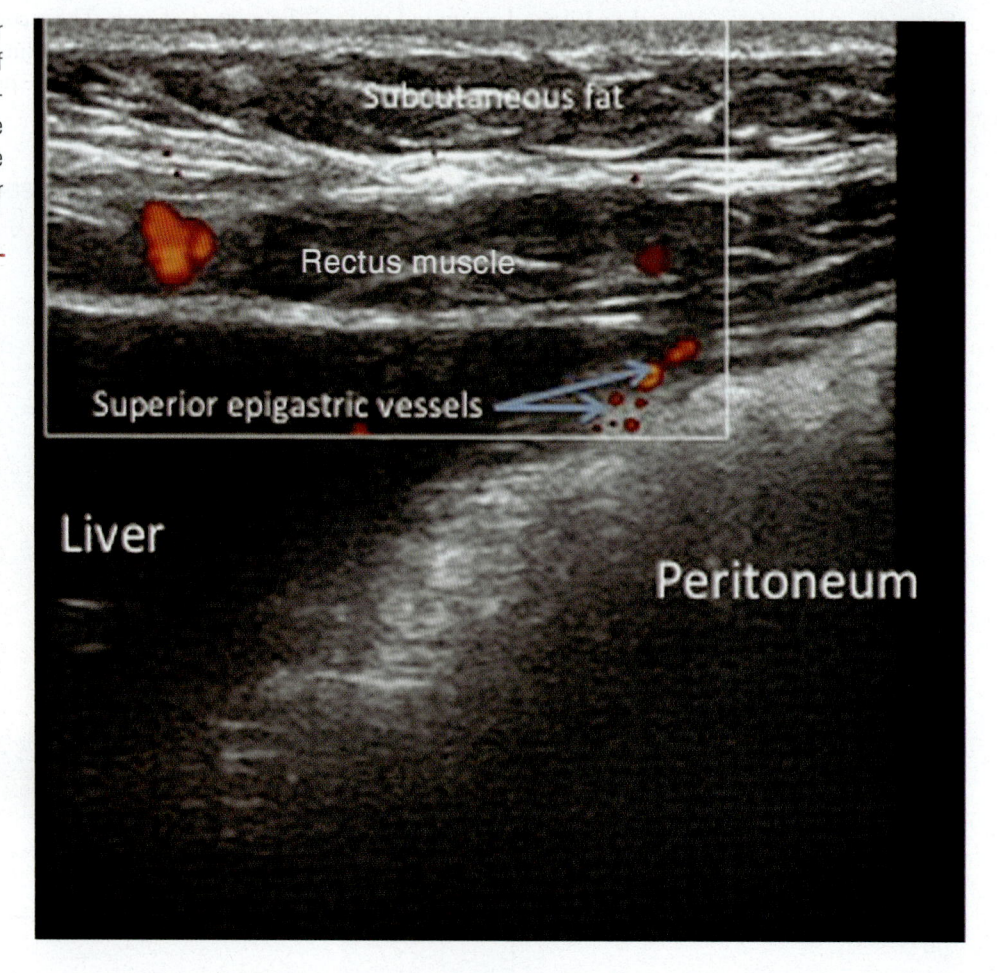

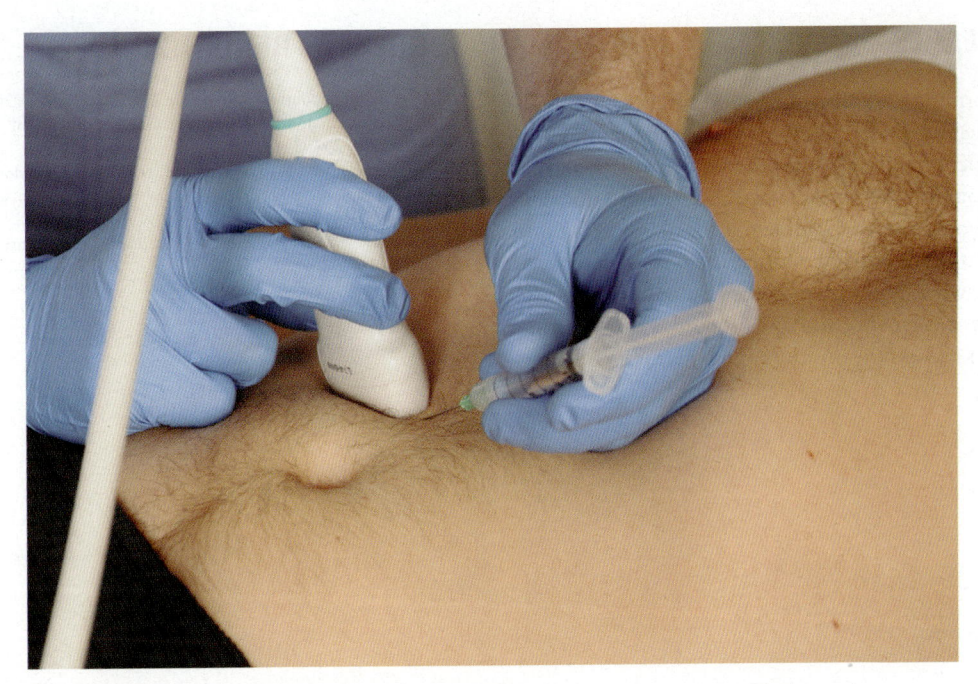

CHAPTER 91 ULTRASOUND-GUIDED INJECTION TECHNIQUE FOR ANTERIOR CUTANEOUS NERVE ENTRAPMENT SYNDROME 627

**FIGURE 91.10.** Proper needle position for performing anterior cutaneous nerve block.

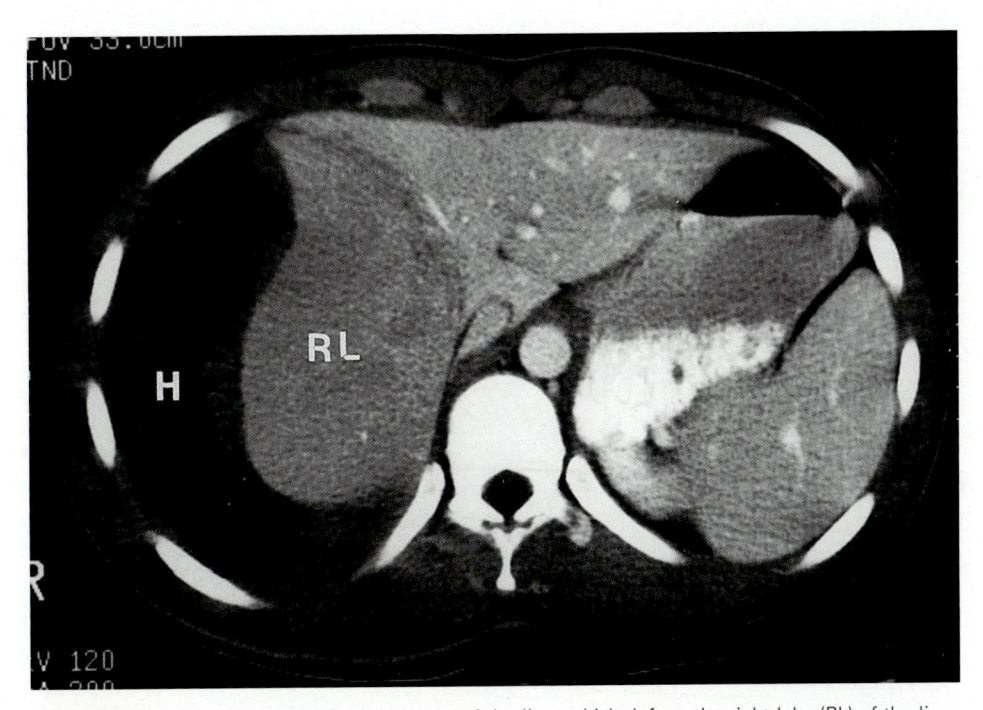

**FIGURE 91.11.** Large subcapsular hematoma of the liver which deform the right lobe (RL) of the liver. (Reused from Pope TL Jr, Harris JH Jr. *Harris & Harris' The Radiology of Emergency Medicine.* 5th ed. Philadelphia, PA: Lippincott Williams & Wilkins; 2013:673, with permission.)

## CLINICAL PEARLS

The key to performing successful ultrasound anterior cutaneous nerve block is the proper identification of the sonographic anatomy and in particular the ability to properly identify the layers of muscle that comprise the abdominal wall at the anterior axillary line. This should not be a problem if the above technique is used. Any significant pain or sudden increase in resistance during injection when performing ultrasound-guided suggests incorrect needle placement, and one should stop injecting immediately and reassess the position of the needle.

## SUGGESTED READINGS

Ellis H. Anterior abdominal wall. *Anesth Intensive Care Med* 2006;7(2):36–37.

Mahadevan V. Anatomy of the anterior abdominal wall and groin. *Surgery* 2009;27(6):251–254.

Rahn DD, Phelan JN, Roshanravan SM, et al. Anterior abdominal wall nerve and vessel anatomy: clinical implications for gynecologic surgery. *Am J Obstet Gynecol* 2010;202(3):234.

Waldman SD. *Anterior Cutaneous Nerve Block*. Philadelphia, PA: WB Saunders; 2009:497–498.

# CHAPTER 92

# Ultrasound-Guided Celiac Plexus Block: Anterior Approach

## CLINICAL PERSPECTIVES

Ultrasound-guided anterior celiac plexus block is utilized in a variety of clinical scenarios as a diagnostic and therapeutic maneuver. As a diagnostic tool, ultrasound-guided anterior celiac plexus block aids in the differential diagnosis of abdominal pain helping determine whether flank, retroperitoneal, or upper abdominal pain is sympathetically mediated via the celiac plexus. Prognostically, this technique may be used to determine if celiac plexus neurolysis will in fact provide pain relief for pain thought to be mediated via the celiac plexus. Early use of ultrasound-guided anterior celiac plexus block to deliver local anesthetic and steroid is not only efficacious in the relief of pain secondary to acute pancreatitis but can markedly reduce the morbidity and mortality associated with this disease. This technique also has utility in the management of abdominal angina and may aid in bowel preservation in patients suffering from ischemic bowel. Ultrasound-guided anterior celiac plexus block can also be utilized to provide acute pain management for arterial embolization of the liver procedures to treat liver tumors. Destruction of the celiac plexus with alcohol and phenol using ultrasound-guided anterior celiac plexus block is a mainstay of cancer pain management when treating pain secondary to malignancies of the retroperitoneum including pancreatic cancer and can be utilized in selected patients suffering from chronic nonmalignant abdominal pain syndromes including chronic pancreatitis (Fig. 92.1).

Advantages of the ultrasound-guided anterior approach to celiac plexus block over traditional posterior approaches include its ease and speed of performance; the lack of radiation associated with fluoroscopic or computed tomography (CT) techniques; the ability to perform the procedure with the patient in the supine position, sparing the patient the need to remain in the prone position for prolonged periods of time or to lie on colostomies or ileostomies; the lack of periprocedure pain due to the fact that the needle does not have to pass through the major muscles of posture; and the fact that the needle is placed in the precrural space, avoiding the possibility of trauma to exiting nerve roots or inadvertent injection of the epidural, subdural, or subarachnoid space due to retrocrural spread of injectate (Table 92.1).

## CLINICALLY RELEVANT ANATOMY

The sympathetic innervation of the abdominal viscera originates in the anterolateral horn of the spinal cord (Fig. 92.2). Preganglionic fibers from T5–T12 exit the spinal cord in conjunction with the ventral roots to join the white communicating rami on their way to the sympathetic chain. Rather than synapsing with the sympathetic chain, these preganglionic fibers pass through it to ultimately synapse on the celiac ganglia. The greater, lesser, and least splanchnic nerves provide the major preganglionic contribution to the celiac plexus. The greater splanchnic nerve has its origin from the T5–T10 spinal roots. The nerve travels along the thoracic paravertebral border through the crus of the diaphragm into the abdominal cavity, ending on the celiac ganglion of its respective side. The lesser splanchnic nerve arises from the T10–T11 roots and passes with the greater nerve to end at the celiac ganglion. The least splanchnic nerve arises from the T11–T12 spinal roots and passes through the diaphragm to the celiac ganglion.

There is significant interpatient anatomic variability of the celiac ganglia with the number of ganglia varying from one to five and ranging in diameter from 0.5 to 4.5 cm. The ganglia lie anterior and anterolateral to the aorta at the level of the celiac trunk (Fig. 92.3). In most patients, the ganglia located on the left are uniformly more inferior than their right-sided counterparts by as much as a vertebral level, but both groups of ganglia usually lie approximately at the level of the upper first lumbar vertebra.

Postganglionic fibers radiate from the celiac ganglia to follow the course of the blood vessels to innervate the abdominal viscera. These organs include much of the distal esophagus, stomach, duodenum, small intestine, ascending and proximal transverse colon, adrenal glands, pancreas, spleen, liver, and biliary system. It is these postganglionic fibers, the fibers arising from the preganglionic splanchnic nerves, and the celiac ganglion that make up the celiac plexus. The diaphragm separates the thorax from the abdominal cavity while still permitting the passage of the thoracoabdominal structures, including the aorta, vena cava, and splanchnic nerves. The diaphragmatic crura are bilateral structures that arise from the anterolateral surfaces of the upper two or three lumbar vertebrae and discs. The crura of the diaphragm serve as a barrier to effectively

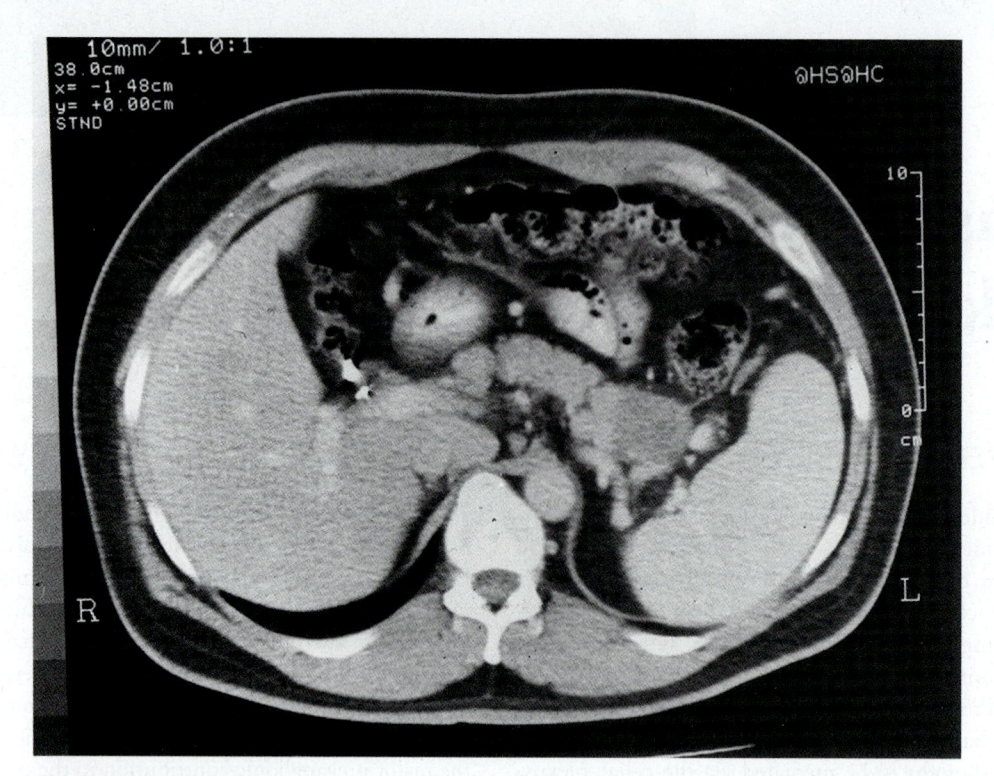

**FIGURE 92.1.** Computed tomography scan demonstrating pancreatic cancer with liver metastases. (Reused from Kelsen DP, Daly JM, Kern SE, et al. *Gastrointestinal Oncology: Principles and Practice.* Philadelphia, PA: Lippincott Williams & Wilkins; 2002, with permission.)

separate the splanchnic nerves from the celiac ganglia and plexus below.

The celiac plexus is anterior (precrural) to the crus of the diaphragm. The plexus extends in front of and around the aorta, with the greatest concentration of fibers anterior to the aorta at the level of the celiac truck, which along with the aorta provides the clinician with an easily identifiable sonographic landmark when performing this technique (Fig. 92.4). With the ultrasound-guided anterior approach to celiac plexus block, the needle is placed close to this concentration of plexus fibers. The relationship of the celiac plexus to the surrounding structures is as follows: The aorta lies anterior and slightly to the left of the anterior margin of the vertebral body (Fig. 92.5). The inferior vena cava lies to the right, with the kidneys posterolateral to the great vessels. The pancreas lies anterior to the celiac plexus. All of these structures lie within the retroperitoneal space. With the anterior approach, the needle may traverse the liver, stomach, intestine, vessels, and pancreas.

## ULTRASOUND-GUIDED TECHNIQUE

Patients that are to undergo ultrasound-guided anterior approach to celiac plexus block should be well hydrated and should receive appropriate prophylactic antibiotics prior to undergoing this procedure. Ultrasound-guided anterior celiac plexus block can be carried out by placing the patient in the supine position with the arms resting comfortably by the patient's side (Fig. 92.6). For diagnostic or prognostic blocks, a total of 12 to 15 mL of local anesthetic is drawn up in a 20-mL sterile syringe. If the painful condition being treated is thought to have an inflammatory component, 40 to 80 mg of depot steroid is added to the local anesthetic. For neurolytic blocks, the same volume of aqueous phenol or absolute alcohol is utilized. A separate 20-mL syringe should also be filled with sterile saline to aid in accurate placement of the needle tip in proximity to the celiac trunk.

**TABLE 92.1  Advantages of the Ultrasound-Guided Anterior Approach to Celiac Plexus Block When Compared to the Posterior Approach**

- Ease of performance
- Speed of performance
- Performed with patient in supine position obviating need for patient to lie prone
- Can be performed at bedside in critically ill patients
- No radiation
- Less perioperative pain
- Precrural needle placement avoiding potential for nerve root trauma or inadvertent epidural, subdural, or subarachnoid injection

# CHAPTER 92 ULTRASOUND-GUIDED CELIAC PLEXUS BLOCK: ANTERIOR APPROACH

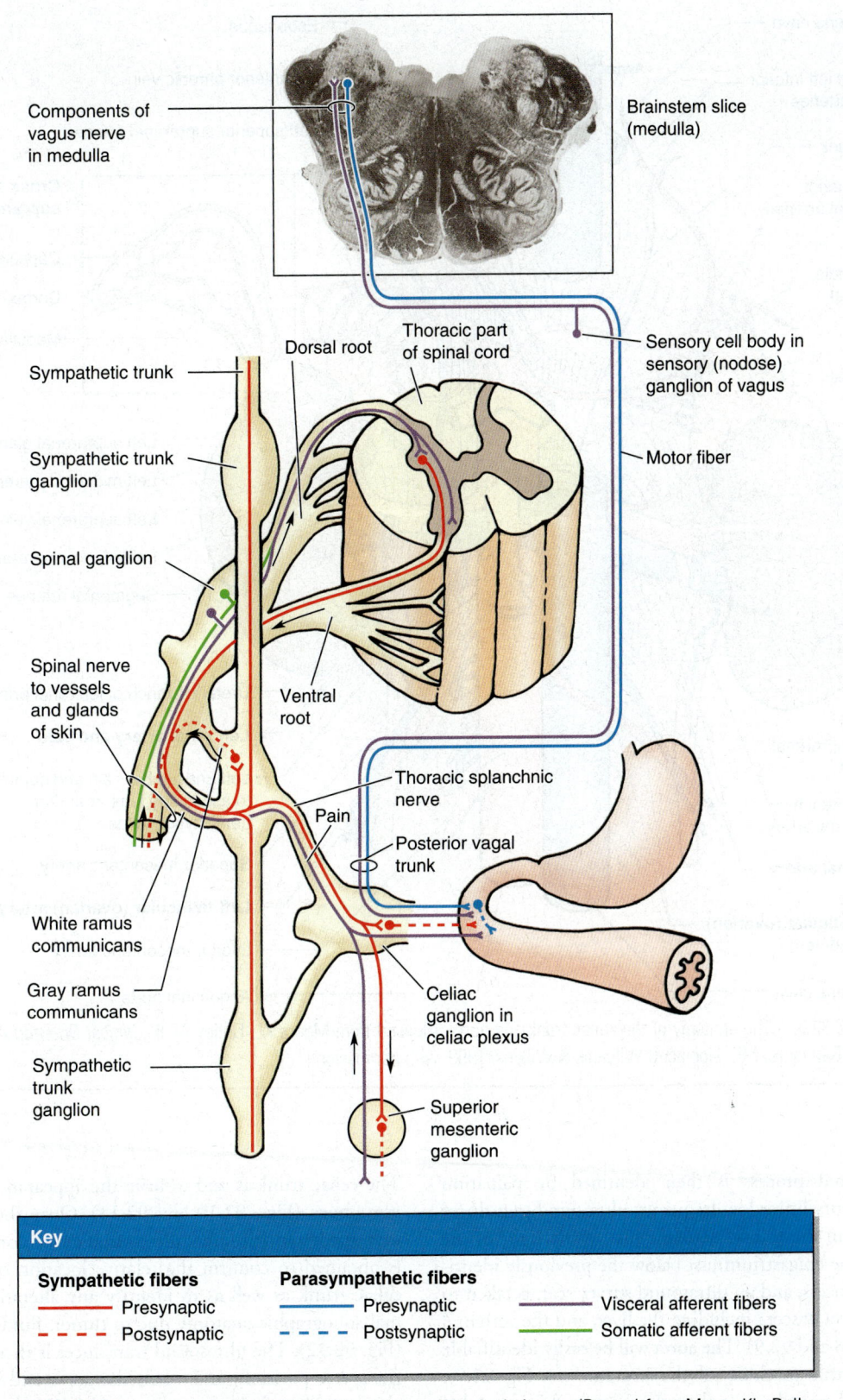

**FIGURE 92.2.** The sympathetic innervation of the abdominal viscera. (Reused from Moore KL, Dalley AF II. *Clinical Oriented Anatomy.* 4th ed. Baltimore, MD: Lippincott Williams & Wilkins; 1999, with permission.)

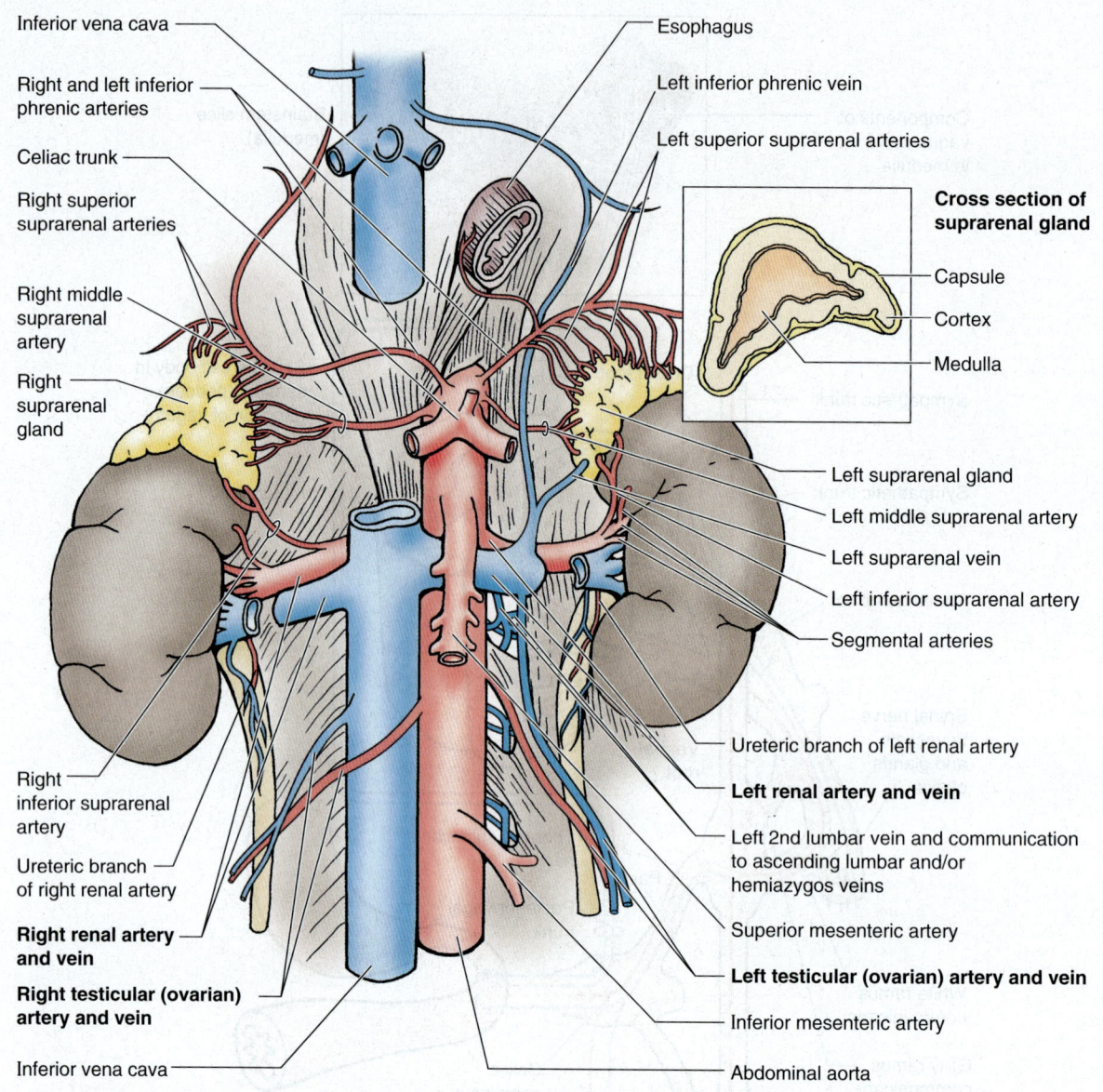

**FIGURE 92.3.** The anatomy of the celiac trunk and aorta. (Reused from Moore KL, Dalley AF II. *Clinical Oriented Anatomy*. 4th ed. Baltimore, MD: Lippincott Williams & Wilkins; 1999, with permission.)

The xiphoid process is then identified by palpation (Fig. 92.7). A curvilinear low-frequency ultrasound transducer is then placed in the transverse plane just to the right of the midline over the epigastrium just below the previously identified xiphoid process, and an ultrasound survey scan is taken to identify the aorta, viscera including the liver, and the vertebral body (Figs. 92.8 and 92.9). The aorta will be easily identifiable as a large, pulsatile anechoic tubular structure (see Fig. 92.9). The ultrasound transducer is then slowly moved in a caudad direction until the celiac trunk is identified (see Fig. 92.9). In some patients, the ultrasound transducer may have to be tilted in a slightly cephalad direction to avoid the diaphragm. Color Doppler can aid in the identification of the celiac trunk, which is the first artery arising from the aorta below the diaphragm.

The celiac trunk is said to have the appearance of a shofar or ram's horn (Figs. 92.10 and 92.11). Once the celiac trunk is identified, a longitudinal ultrasound and color Doppler image is obtained to confirm the relative location of the aorta and celiac trunk as well as to identify any alterations of the normal sonographic anatomy due to tumor, fluid, or adenopathy (Fig. 92.12). The ultrasound transducer is then returned to its transverse position, and when the aorta and celiac trunk are clearly reidentified on transverse ultrasound scan, the skin is prepped with anesthetic solution and a 13-cm, 22-gauge Chiba needle is advanced from the lateral border of the ultrasound transducer using an in-plane approach in a lateral to medial direction with the trajectory being adjusted under real-time ultrasound guidance until the needle tip is resting just cephalad

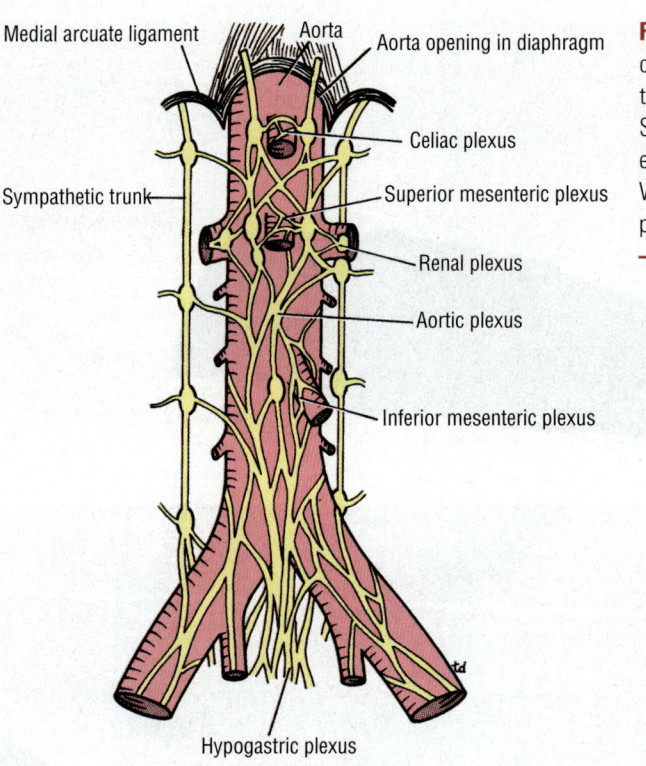

**FIGURE 92.4.** The relationship of the celiac plexus to the celiac trunk and aorta. (Reused from Snell RS. *Clinical Anatomy*. 7th ed. Philadelphia, PA: Lippincott Williams & Wilkins; 2003, with permission.)

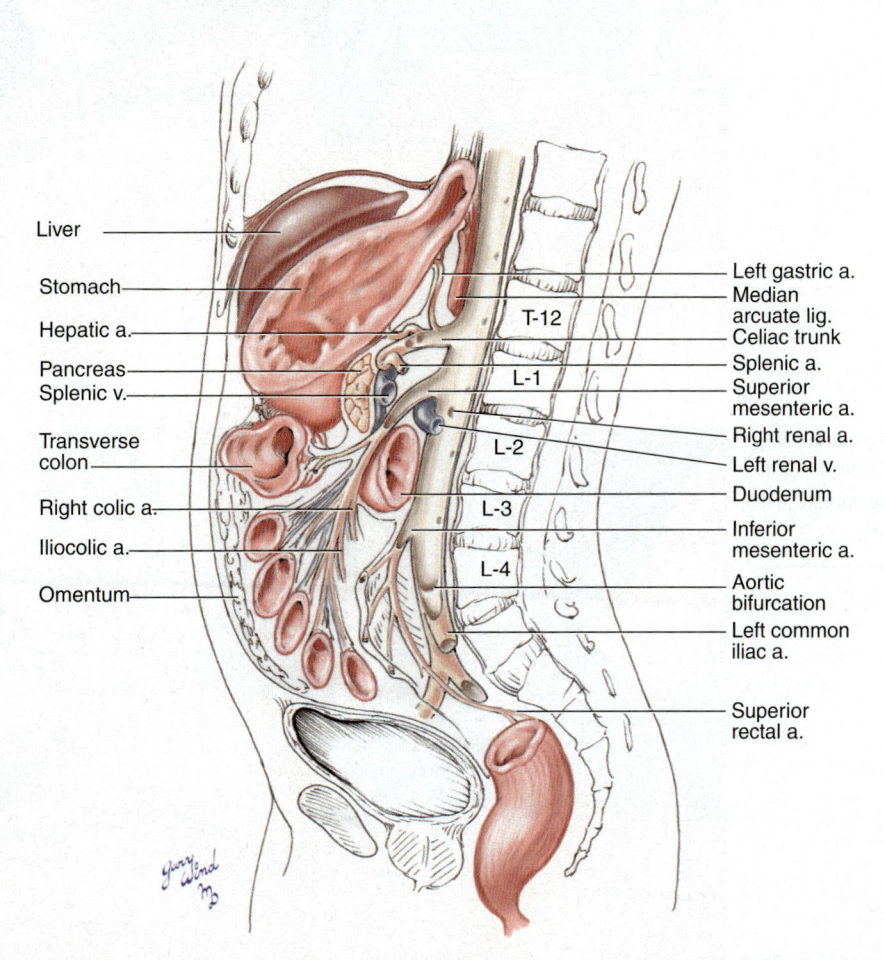

**FIGURE 92.5.** The cross-sectional anatomy of the celiac trunk. Note the anatomic relationship of the crura of the diaphragm, the vertebral body, the aorta, and the celiac trunk. (Reused from Wind GG, Valentine RJ. *Anatomic Exposures in Vascular Surgery*. 3rd ed. Philadelphia, PA: Lippincott Williams & Wilkins; 2013.)

**SECTION VI     CHEST WALL, TRUNK, AND ABDOMEN**

**FIGURE 92.6.** Proper patient position for ultrasound-guided anterior celiac plexus block.

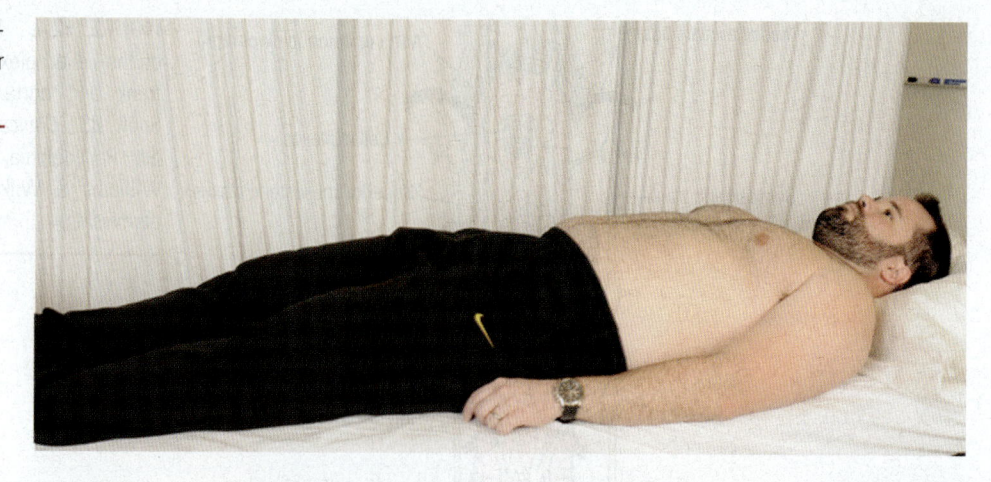

**FIGURE 92.7.** Palpation of the xiphoid process.

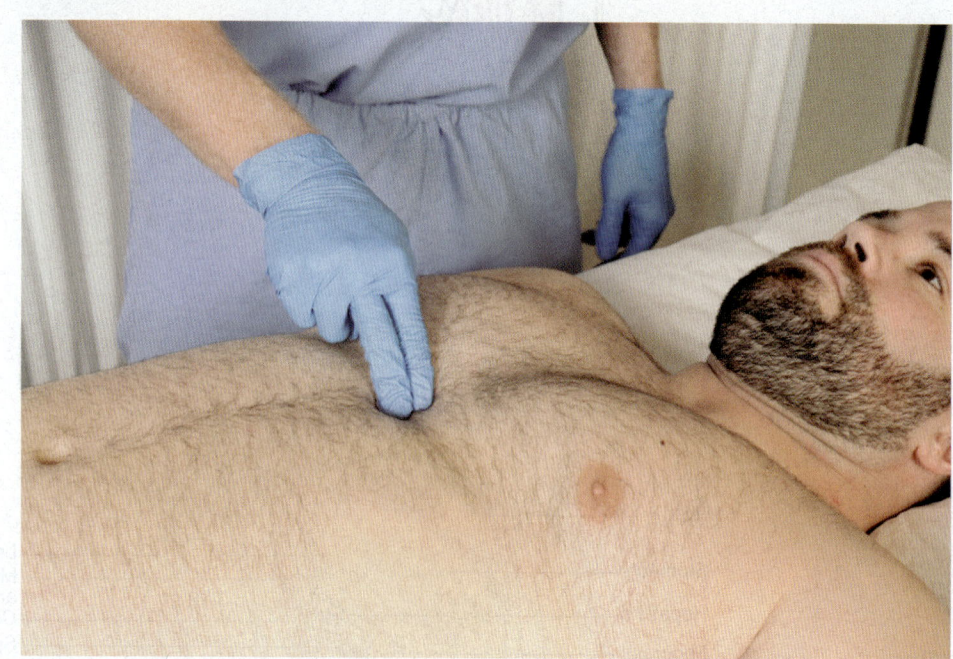

**FIGURE 92.8.** Transverse placement of the ultrasound transducer in the midline of the epigastrium just below the xiphoid process.

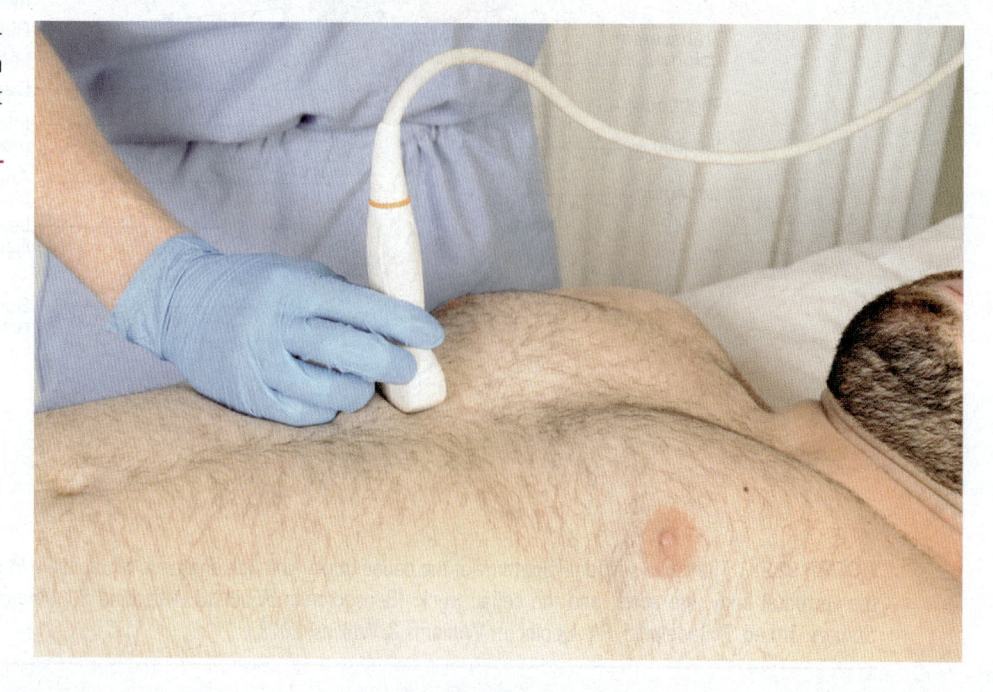

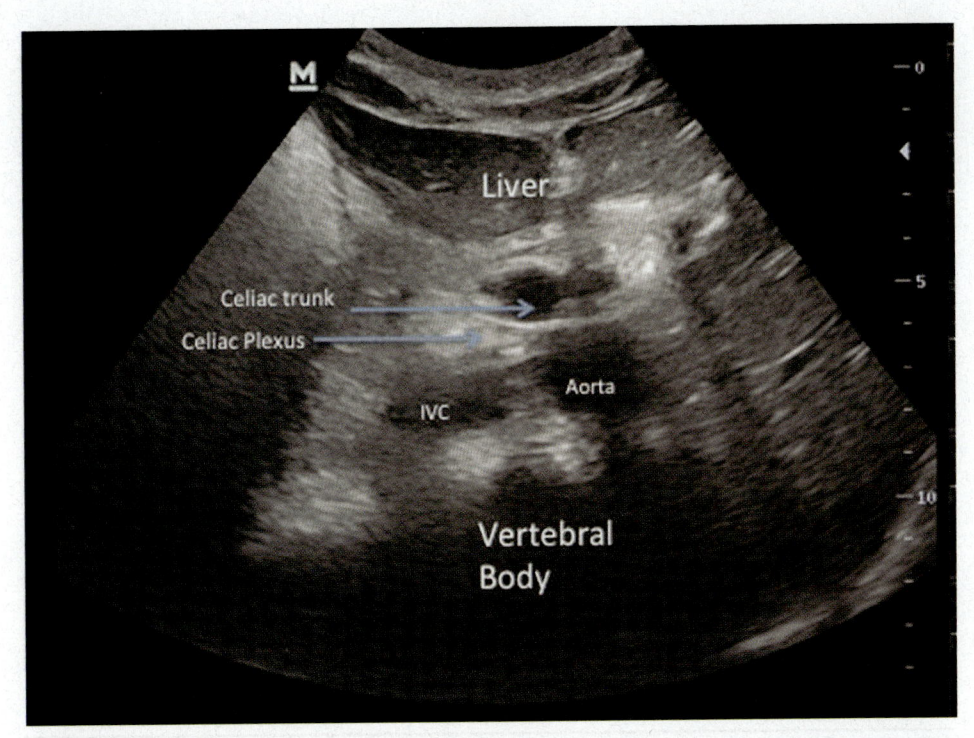

**FIGURE 92.9.** Transverse ultrasound image demonstrating the vertebral body, aorta, celiac truck, celiac plexus, inferior vena cava, liver, and stomach.

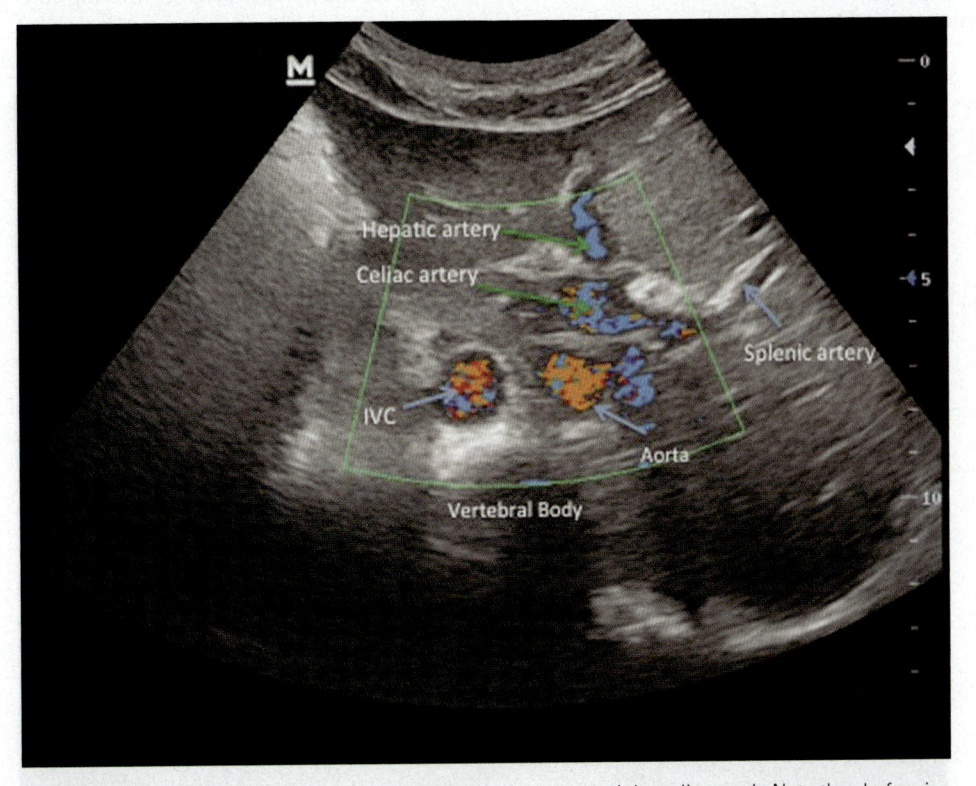

**FIGURE 92.10.** Color Doppler image demonstrating the aorta and the celiac trunk. Note the shofar sign indicating the celiac trunk.

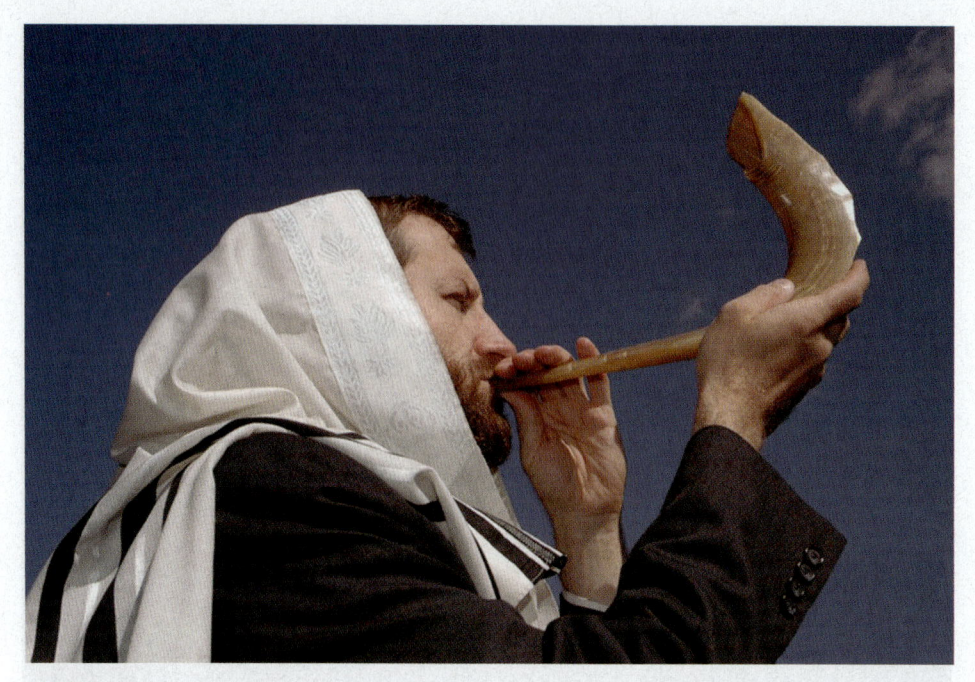

**FIGURE 92.11.** The shofar or ram's horn.

to the celiac trunk (Fig. 92.13). At that point, after careful aspiration, a small amount of sterile saline is injected under real-time ultrasound imaging to reconfirm the position of the needle tip prior to the injection of local anesthetic and/or steroids or neurolytic agents. Once the satisfactory placement of the needle tip is confirmed, after careful aspiration, the chosen solution is slowly injected under ultrasound guidance. There should be minimal resistance to injection. The needle is then removed, and a sterile pressure dressing and ice pack are placed at the injection site.

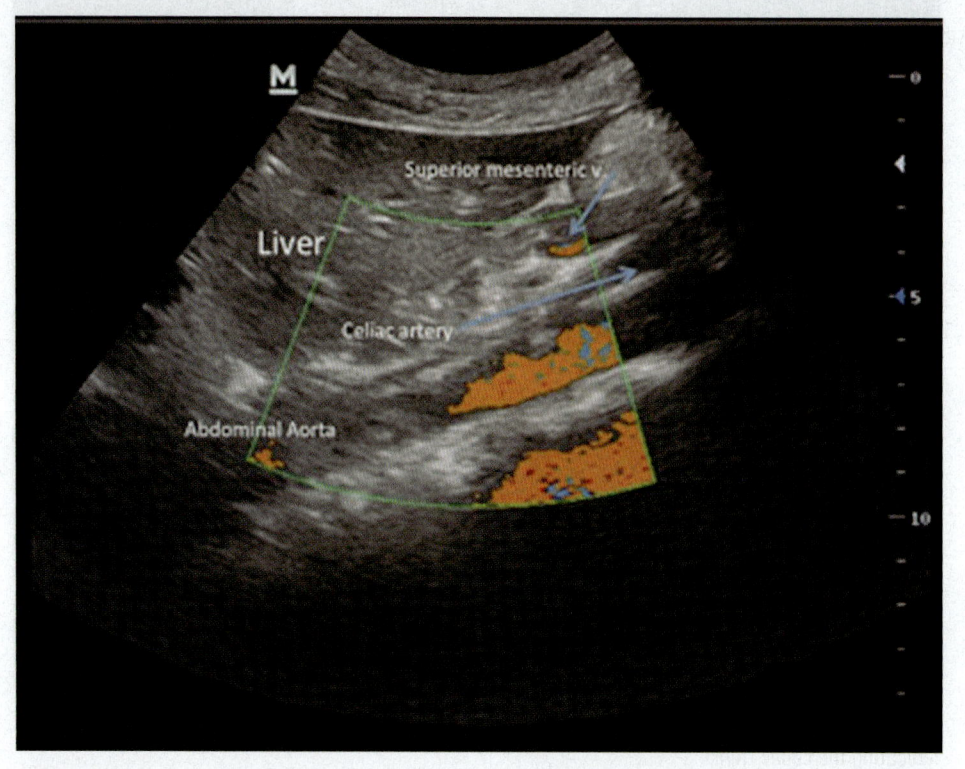

**FIGURE 92.12.** Longitudinal color Doppler image demonstrating the aorta, celiac trunk, and superior mesenteric artery.

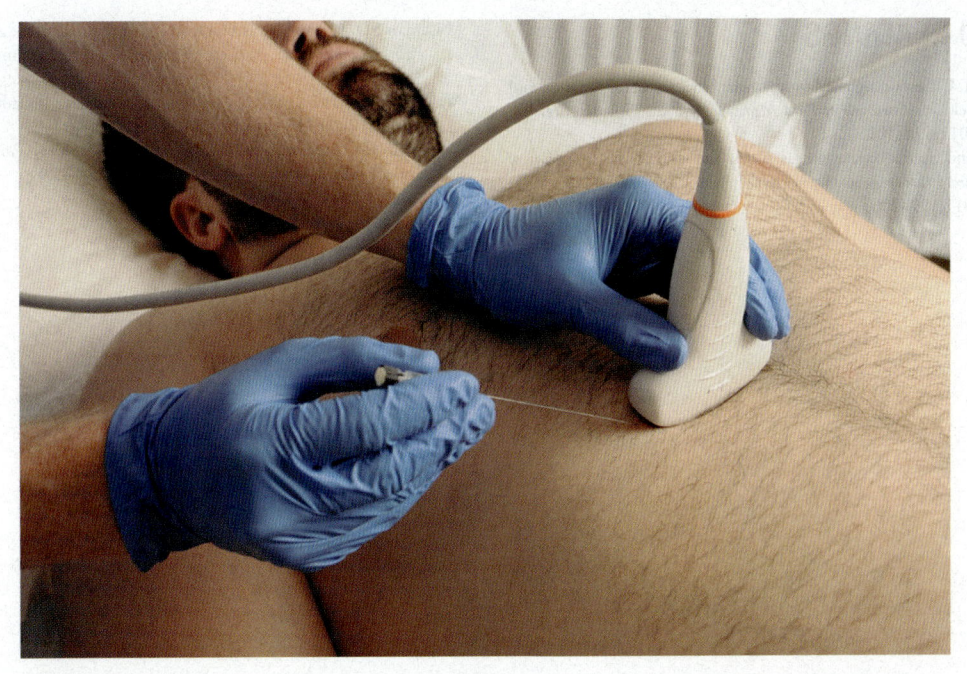

**FIGURE 92.13.** Proper in-plane needle position for performing ultrasound-guided anterior celiac plexus block.

## COMPLICATIONS

The ultrasound-guided anterior approach to celiac plexus block has many advantages when compared with more traditional posterior approaches, but the anterior placement of the needle necessitates the passage of a fine needle through the liver, stomach, intestine, vessels, and pancreas and presents the possibility of needle-induced trauma to the aorta, gastric artery, celiac trunk, superior mesenteric, and renal arteries. This presents the possibility of needle-induced trauma to all of these structures, even in the best of hands. Fortunately, the incidence of serious complications is very low. It should be remembered that many patients suffering from cancer pain may suffer from coagulopathy and thrombocytopenia caused by antiblastic treatments or liver abnormalities. Because the needle is placed through the abdominal viscera, peritonitis and intraabdominal abscess remain a distinct possibility. These problems with infection are decreased by the use of prophylactic antibiotics.

Because blockade of the celiac plexus results in increased bowel motility, this technique should be avoided in patients with bowel obstruction. Postblock diarrhea occurs in ~50% of patients. Celiac plexus block should be deferred in patients who suffer from chronic abdominal pain, who are chemically dependent, or who exhibit drug-seeking behavior until these issues have been adequately addressed. Alcohol should not be used as a neurolytic agent in patients on disulfiram therapy for alcohol abuse.

The proximity to the spinal cord, exiting nerve roots, pleural space, and viscera makes it imperative that this procedure be performed only by those well versed in the regional anatomy and experienced in interventional pain management techniques. Needle placement that is too posterior may result in epidural, subdural, or subarachnoid injections or trauma to the spinal cord and exiting nerve roots. Such incorrect needle placement can result in severe neurologic deficits, including paraplegia. Medial needle placement may also result in intradiscal placement and resultant discitis. Because the needle terminus is precrural with the single-needle anterior approach to celiac plexus, there is a decreased incidence of neurologic complications, including neurolysis of the lumbar nerve roots with resultant hip flexor weakness and lower extremity numbness compared with the classic two-needle approach to celiac plexus block.

Given the proximity of the pleural space, pneumothorax after celiac plexus block may occur if the needle is placed too cephalad. Trauma to the thoracic duct with resultant chylothorax may also occur. If the needle is placed too laterally, trauma to the spleen, liver, kidneys, and ureters is a distinct possibility.

## CLINICAL PEARLS

The key to performing successful ultrasound anterior celiac plexus block is the proper identification of the sonographic anatomy and in particular the ability to properly identify the celiac trunk. Any significant pain or sudden increase in resistance during injection when performing ultrasound-guided suggests incorrect needle placement, and one should stop injecting immediately and reassess the position of the needle.

## SUGGESTED READINGS

Gofeld M, Shankar H. Ultrasound-guided sympathetic blocks: stellate ganglion and celiac plexus block. In: *Essentials of Pain Medicine*. 3rd ed. Philadelphia, PA: WB Saunders; 2011:494–501.

Narouze S. Ultrasound guided celiac plexus block and neurolysis. In: *Atlas of Ultrasound Guided Procedures in Interventional Pain Management*. New York, NY: Springer; 2011:199–206.

Waldman SD. Celiac plexus block: anterior approach. In: *Atlas of Interventional Pain Management*. 3rd ed. Philadelphia, PA: Saunders Elsevier; 2009:355–358.

Waldman SD. The celiac plexus. In: *Pain Review*. Philadelphia, PA: Saunders Elsevier; 2009:113–114.

Waldman SD. Acute pancreatitis. In: *Atlas of Common Pain Syndromes*. 3rd ed. Philadelphia, PA: Saunders Elsevier; 2011:227–229.

# CHAPTER 93

# Ultrasound-Guided Ilioinguinal Nerve Block

## CLINICAL PERSPECTIVES

Ultrasound-guided ilioinguinal nerve block is utilized as a diagnostic and therapeutic maneuver in the evaluation and treatment of groin pain thought to be mediated via the ilioinguinal nerve. The most common pain syndrome mediated via the ilioinguinal nerve is the entrapment neuropathy, ilioinguinal neuralgia. The patient suffering from ilioinguinal neuralgia will complain of burning pain, paresthesias, and numbness over the lower abdomen that radiates into the scrotum or labia and occasionally into the upper inner thigh, but never below the knee. Extension of the lumbar spine exacerbated the pain of ilioinguinal neuralgia, and the patient will often assume the novice skier's position to relieve pressure on the affected nerve (Fig. 93.1). Untreated, the symptoms of ilioinguinal neuralgia often worsen with the motor impairment causing a bulging of the anterior abdominal wall, which may be misdiagnosed as an inguinal hernia. A Tinel sign may be elicited by tapping over the ilioinguinal nerve at the point where it pierces the transversus abdominis muscle.

Ultrasound-guided ilioinguinal nerve block can also be utilized to provide surgical anesthesia for groin surgery, including inguinal herniorrhaphy when combined with ultrasound-guided iliohypogastric and genitofemoral nerve block. Ultrasound-guided ilioinguinal nerve block with local anesthetics can be employed as a diagnostic maneuver when performing differential neural blockade on an anatomic basis to determine if the patient's lower abdominal and groin pain are subserved by the ilioinguinal nerve. If destruction of the ilioinguinal nerve is being contemplated, ultrasound-guided ilioinguinal nerve block with local anesthetic can provide prognostic information as to the extent of motor and sensory deficit the patient will experience following nerve destruction.

Ultrasound-guided ilioinguinal nerve block with local anesthetic may also be used to provide postoperative pain relief following lower abdominal and groin surgeries and is useful in the treatment of persistent postoperative neuropathic pain following inguinal hernia surgery.

Electromyography can distinguish ilioinguinal nerve entrapment from lumbar plexopathy, lumbar radiculopathy, and diabetic polyneuropathy. Plain radiographs of the hip and pelvis are indicated in all patients who present with ilioinguinal neuralgia to rule out occult bony pathology. Based on the patient's clinical presentation, additional testing may be warranted, including a complete blood count, uric acid level, erythrocyte sedimentation rate, and antinuclear antibody testing. Magnetic resonance imaging of the lumbar plexus and retroperitoneum is indicated if tumor or hematoma is suspected (Fig. 93.2). The injection technique described later serves as both a diagnostic and a therapeutic maneuver.

## CLINICALLY RELEVANT ANATOMY

The ilioinguinal nerve is derived from the L1 nerve root with a contribution from T12 in some patients. The nerve exits the lateral border of the psoas muscle to follow a curvilinear course that takes it from its origin of the L1 and occasionally T12 somatic nerves to inside the concavity of the ilium (Fig. 93.3). The ilioinguinal nerve continues in an anterior trajectory as it runs between the layers of the internal oblique and transversus abdominis muscles. It is at this point that the nerve can consistently be identified with ultrasound scanning and is amenable to ultrasound-guided nerve block. The ilioinguinal nerve then perforates the transverse abdominis muscle at the level of the anterior superior iliac spine, and its terminal branches provide sensory innervation to the skin over the inferior portion of the rectus abdominis muscle. The ilioinguinal nerve may interconnect with the iliohypogastric nerve as it continues to pass along its course medially and inferiorly, where it accompanies the genital branch of the genitofemoral nerve as well as the spermatic cord in men and the round ligament in women through the inguinal ring and into the inguinal canal. The distribution of the sensory innervation of the ilioinguinal nerves varies from patient to patient due to considerable overlap with the iliohypogastric nerve. In most patients, the ilioinguinal nerve provides sensory innervation to the upper portion of the skin of the inner thigh and the root of the penis and upper scrotum in men or the mons pubis and lateral labia in women (Fig. 93.4).

## ULTRASOUND-GUIDED TECHNIQUE

Ultrasound-guided ilioinguinal nerve block can be carried out by placing the patient in the supine position with the arms resting comfortably by the patient's side (Fig. 93.5). A total of 7 mL of local anesthetic is drawn up in a 12-mL sterile syringe. If the

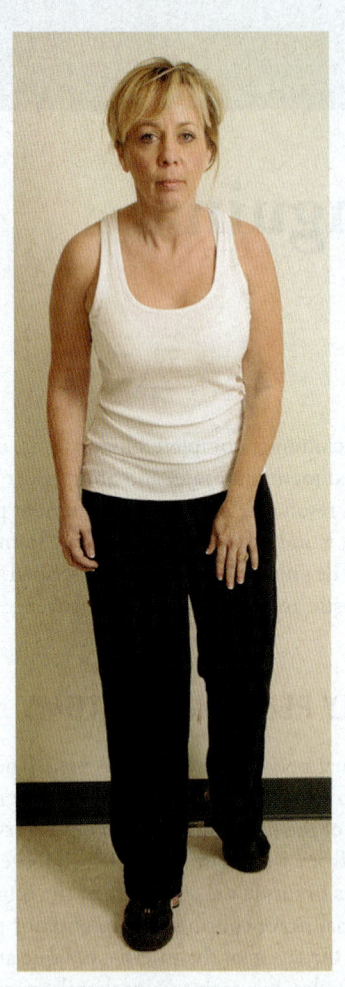

**FIGURE 93.1.** The patient suffering from ilioinguinal neuralgia will often assume the novice skier position.

painful condition being treated is thought to have an inflammatory component, 40 to 80 mg of depot steroid is added to the local anesthetic. The umbilicus, anterior superior iliac spine, and inguinal ligament are identified by visual inspection and palpation, and an imaginary line is drawn between the anterior superior iliac spine and the umbilicus (Fig. 93.6). A linear high-frequency ultrasound transducer is placed in a plane perpendicular with the inguinal ligament with the inferior aspect of the transducer lying over the anterior superior iliac spine and the superior aspect of the transducer pointed directly at the umbilicus, and an ultrasound survey scan is obtained (Fig. 93.7). The hyperechoic anterior superior iliac spine and its acoustic shadow is identified as are the external oblique, internal oblique, and transversus abdominis muscles, which extend outward from it (Fig. 93.8). The fascial plane between the internal oblique and transversus abdominis muscles is then identified, and the ilioinguinal nerve should be easily identifiable as an ovoid hypoechoic structure highlighted by a hyperechoic epineurium lying close to the anterior superior iliac spine (Fig. 93.9). The iliohypogastric nerve may also be seen lying medial to the ilioinguinal nerve in the same fascial plane (Fig. 93.10). Color Doppler may be used to aid in identifying the fascial plane between the internal oblique and transversus abdominis muscles as this plane is also shared with the deep circumflex iliac artery (Fig. 93.11). When these anatomic structures are clearly identified on oblique ultrasound scan, the skin is prepped with anesthetic solution, and a 1½- inch, 22-gauge needle is advanced from the inferior border of the ultrasound transducer and advanced utilizing an in-plane approach with the trajectory being adjusted under real-time ultrasound guidance until the needle tip is resting within the internal oblique muscle (Fig. 93.12). At that point, after careful aspiration, a small amount of solution is injected under real-time ultrasound imaging to utilize hydrodissection to reconfirm the position of the needle tip. Once the position of the needle tip is reconfirmed, the needle is carefully advanced through the deep fascia of the internal oblique muscle into the fascial plane between the internal oblique muscle and the transversus abdominis muscle in proximity to the previously identified ilioinguinal nerve. After careful aspiration, a small amount of solution is again injected to aid in identification of the exact position of the needle tip. After careful aspiration, the remainder of the solution is slowly injected under ultrasound guidance, which will demonstrate a bowing downward of the superficial fascia of the transversus abdominis muscle by the injectate. There should be minimal resistance to injection. The needle is then removed, and a sterile pressure dressing and ice pack are placed at the injection site.

## COMPLICATIONS

The transversus abdominis muscle lies just above the peritoneal cavity, and a failure to accurately assess the correct position of the needle tip when performing ultrasound-guided ilioinguinal nerve block can lead to disastrous results if the needle inadvertently enters the peritoneal cavity and traumatizes the underlying viscera. The use of ultrasound guidance when performing ilioinguinal nerve block should markedly decrease this complication. Because of the relatively vascular nature of the abdominal wall and the proximity of the deep circumflex iliac artery, postblock ecchymosis and hematoma may occur, and the patient should be warned of such. These complications can be decreased by the use of a pressure dressing and cold packs applied to the injection site following the procedure.

## CLINICAL PEARLS

The key to performing successful ultrasound-guided ilioinguinal nerve block is the proper identification of the sonographic anatomy and in particular the ability to properly identify the layers of muscle that comprise the abdominal wall at the anterior axillary line. This should not be a problem if the above technique is used. Any significant pain or sudden increase in resistance during injection when performing this ultrasound-guided technique suggests incorrect needle placement, and one should stop injecting immediately and reassess the position of the needle.

CHAPTER 93  ULTRASOUND-GUIDED ILIOINGUINAL NERVE BLOCK   641

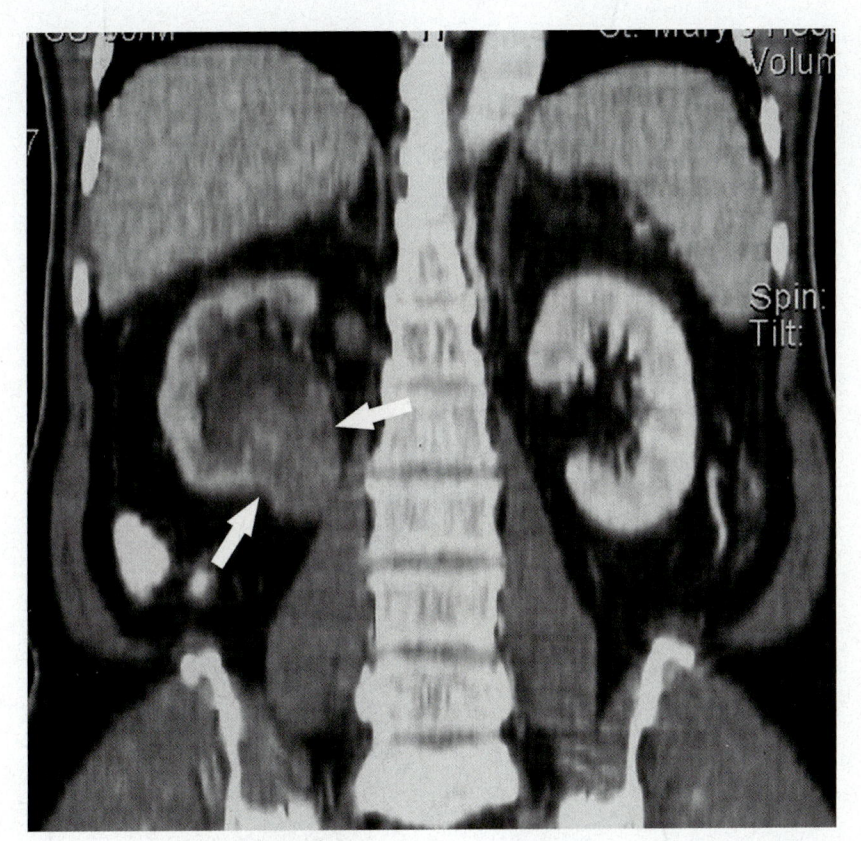

**FIGURE 93.2.** Coronal computed tomography (CT) scan of a large retroperitoneal liposarcoma (*arrows*) invading the kidney. (Reused from Eisenberg RL. *Clinical Imaging: An Atlas of Differential Diagnosis*. 5th ed. Philadelphia, PA: Lippincott Williams & Wilkins; 2010:883, with permission.)

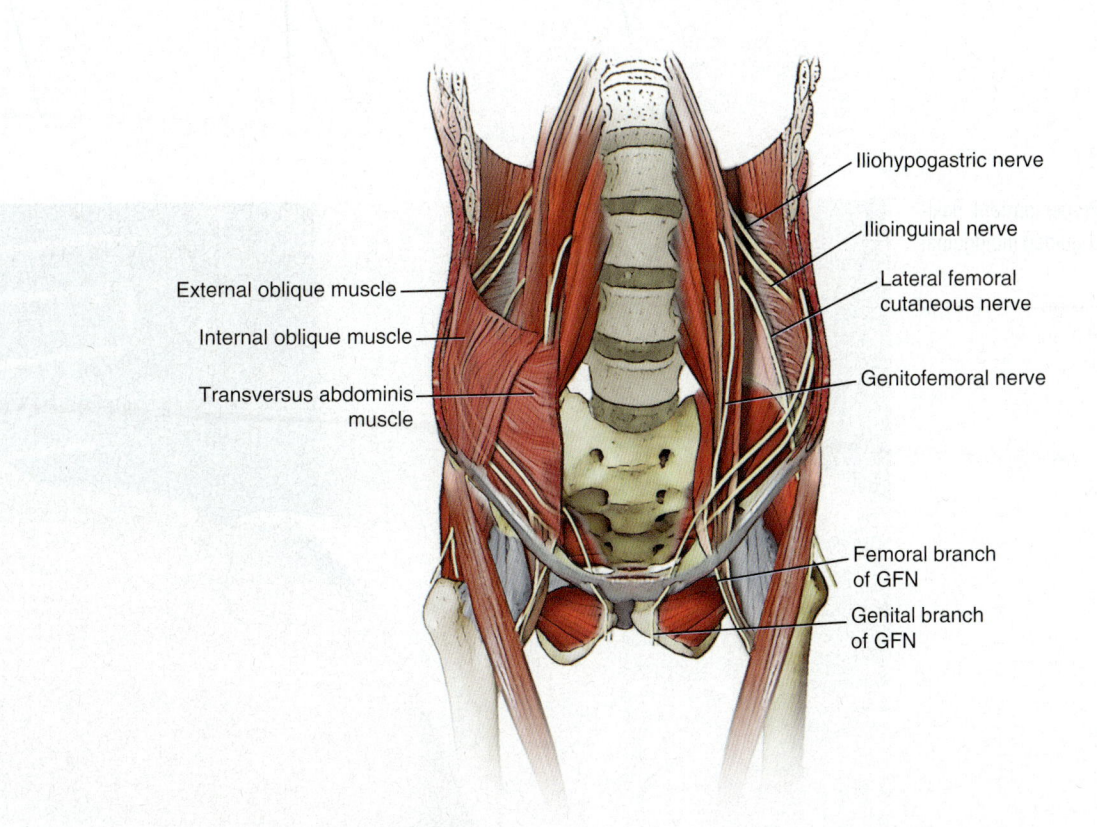

**FIGURE 93.3.** The anatomy of the ilioinguinal nerve.

**FIGURE 93.4.** The sensory distribution of the ilioinguinal nerve.

Iliohypogastric nerve

Ilioinguinal nerve

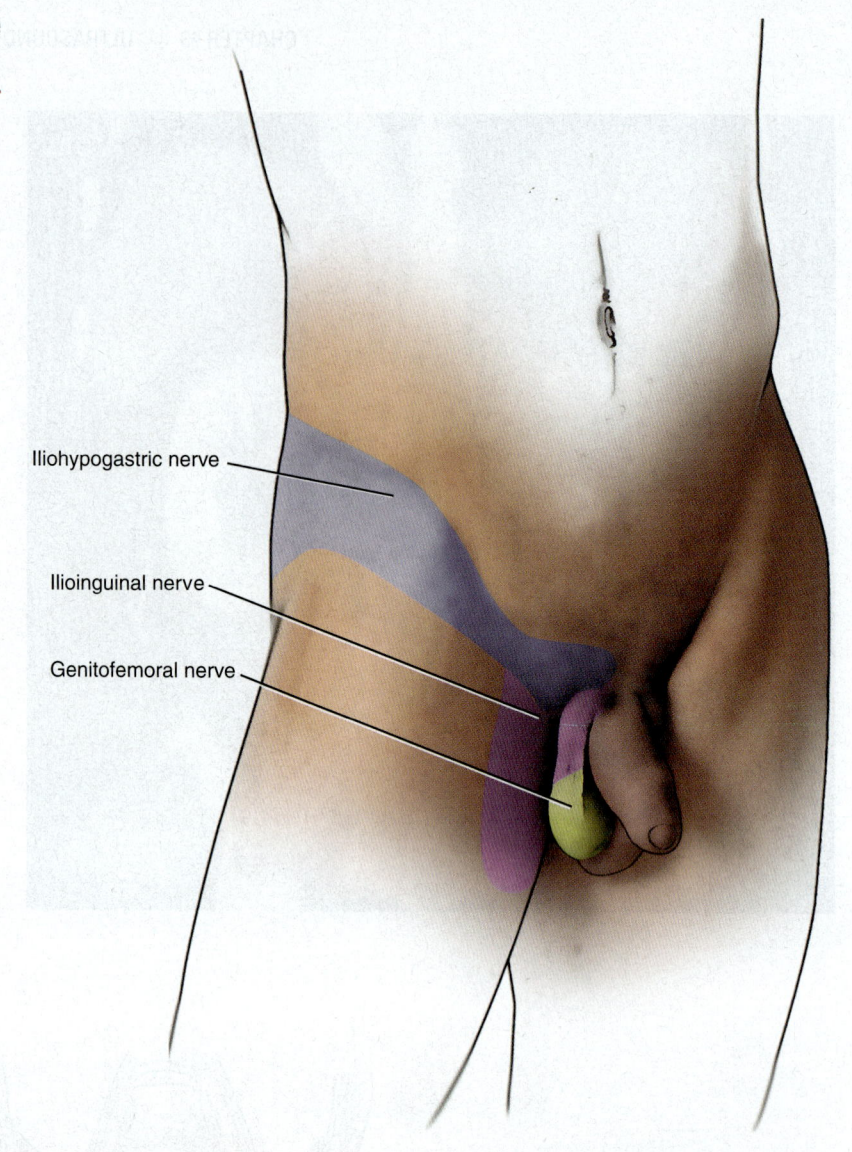

Genitofemoral nerve

**FIGURE 93.5.** Proper patient position for ultrasound-guided ilioinguinal nerve block.

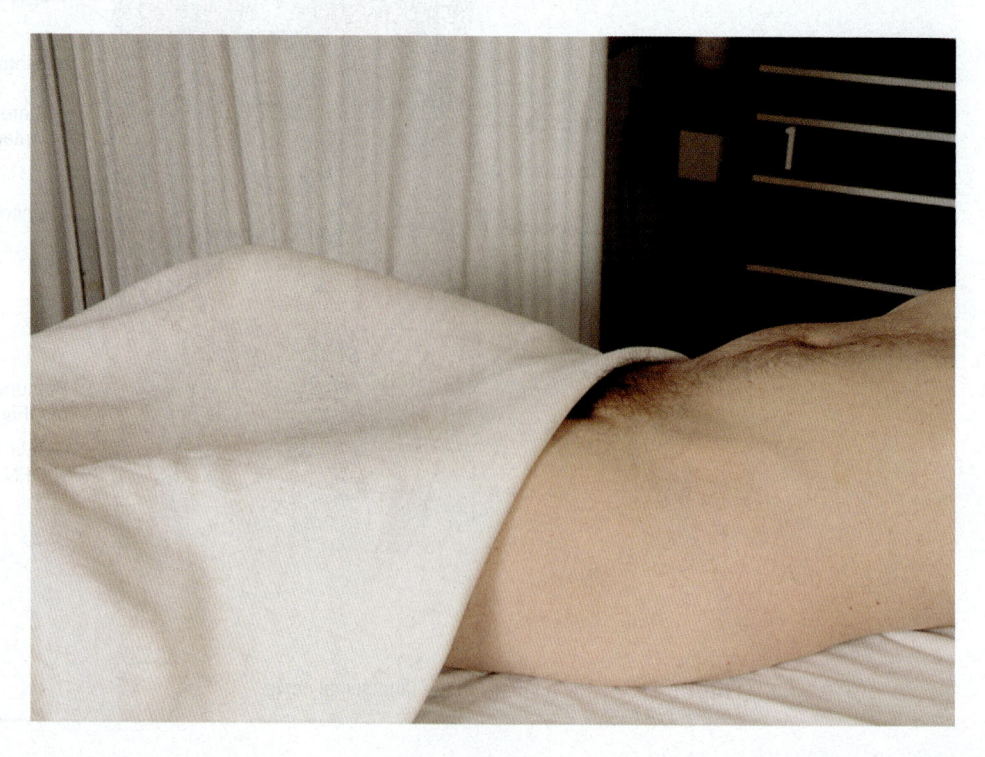

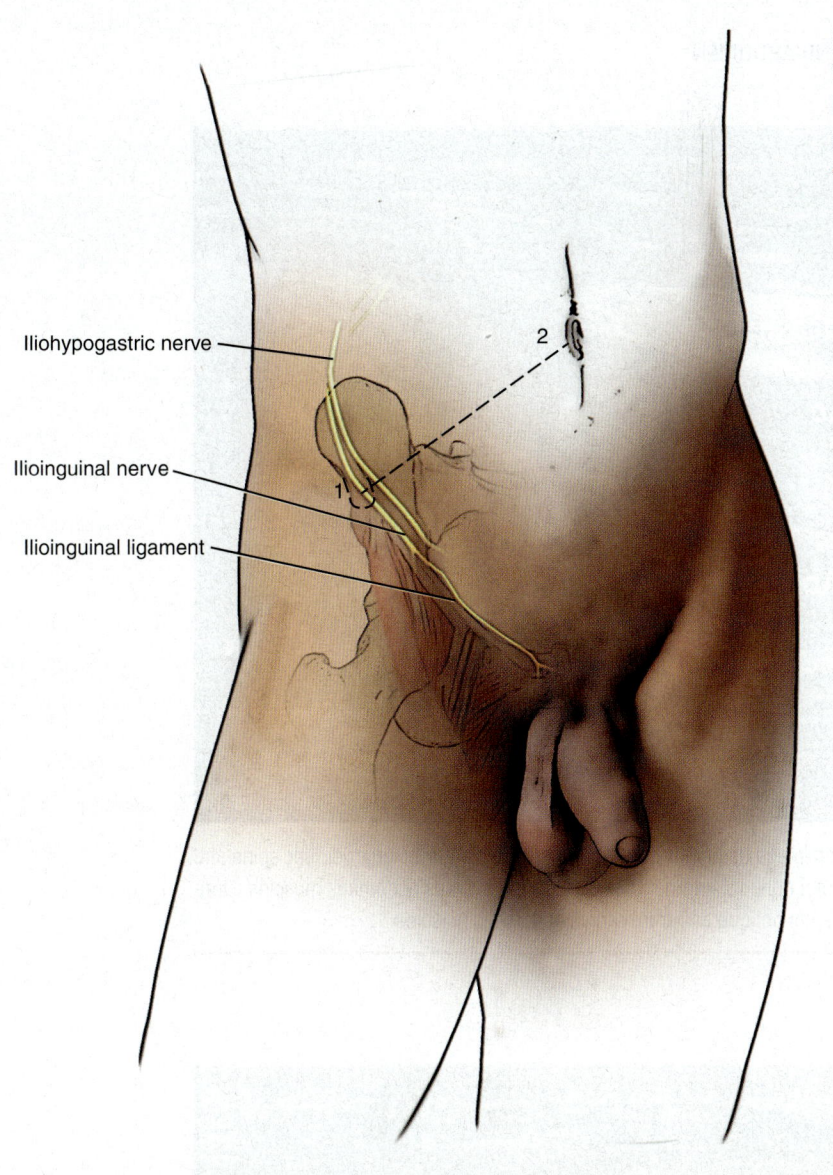

**FIGURE 93.6.** To perform ultrasound-guided ilioinguinal nerve block, an imaginary line is drawn between the anterior superior iliac spine and the patient's umbilicus.

- Iliohypogastric nerve
- Ilioinguinal nerve
- Ilioinguinal ligament

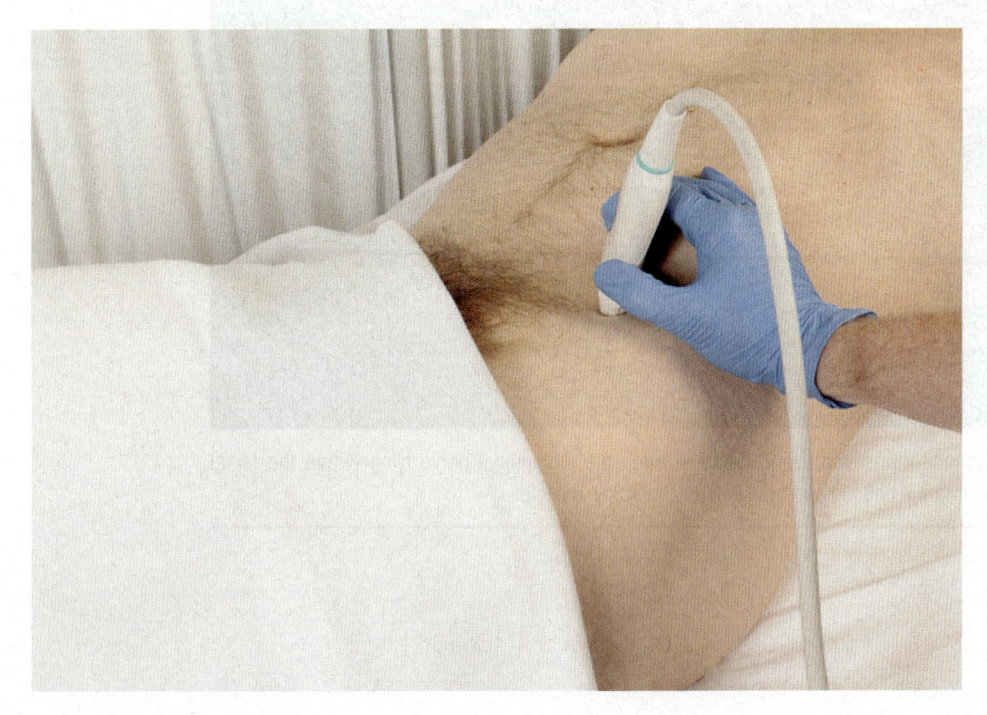

**FIGURE 93.7.** Oblique placement of the ultrasound transducer placed in a plane perpendicular with the inguinal ligament with the inferior aspect of the transducer lying over the anterior superior iliac spine and the superior aspect of the transducer pointed directly at the umbilicus.

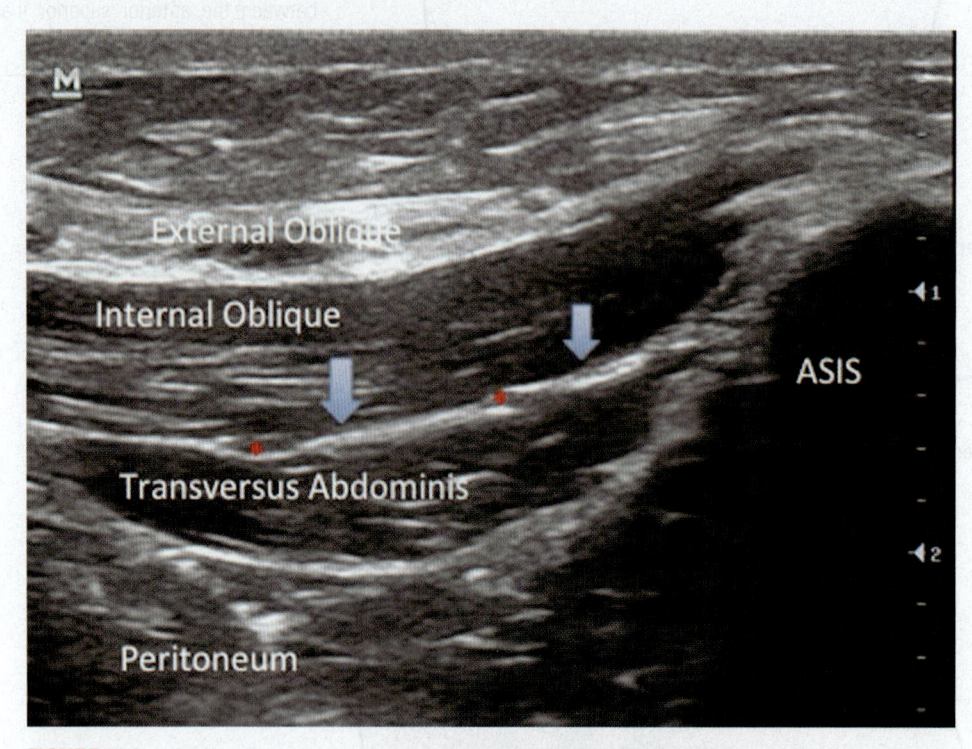

**FIGURE 93.8.** Oblique ultrasound image demonstrating the hyperechoic anterior superior iliac spine and its acoustic shadow and the external oblique, internal oblique, and transversus abdominis muscles. Note the fascial plane between the internal oblique and transversus abdominis muscles.

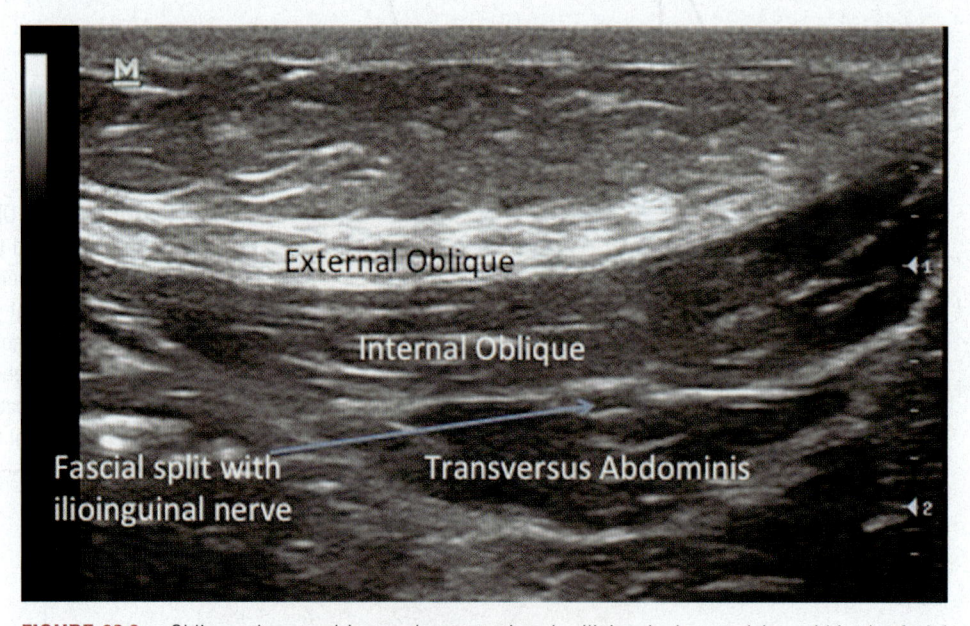

**FIGURE 93.9.** Oblique ultrasound image demonstrating the ilioinguinal nerve lying within the facial plane between the internal oblique and transversus abdominis muscles.

CHAPTER 93  ULTRASOUND-GUIDED ILIOINGUINAL NERVE BLOCK  645

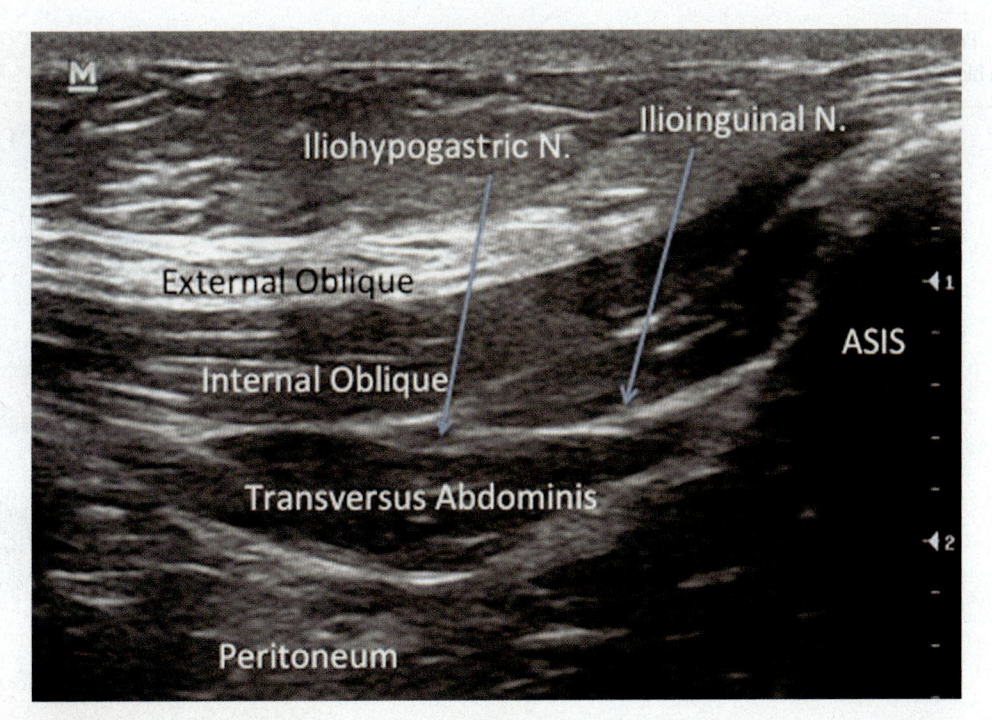

**FIGURE 93.10.** The ilioinguinal nerve and iliohypogastric nerve both lie in the fascial plane between the internal oblique and transversus abdominis muscles. Note that the ilioinguinal nerve is closest to the anterior superior iliac spine.

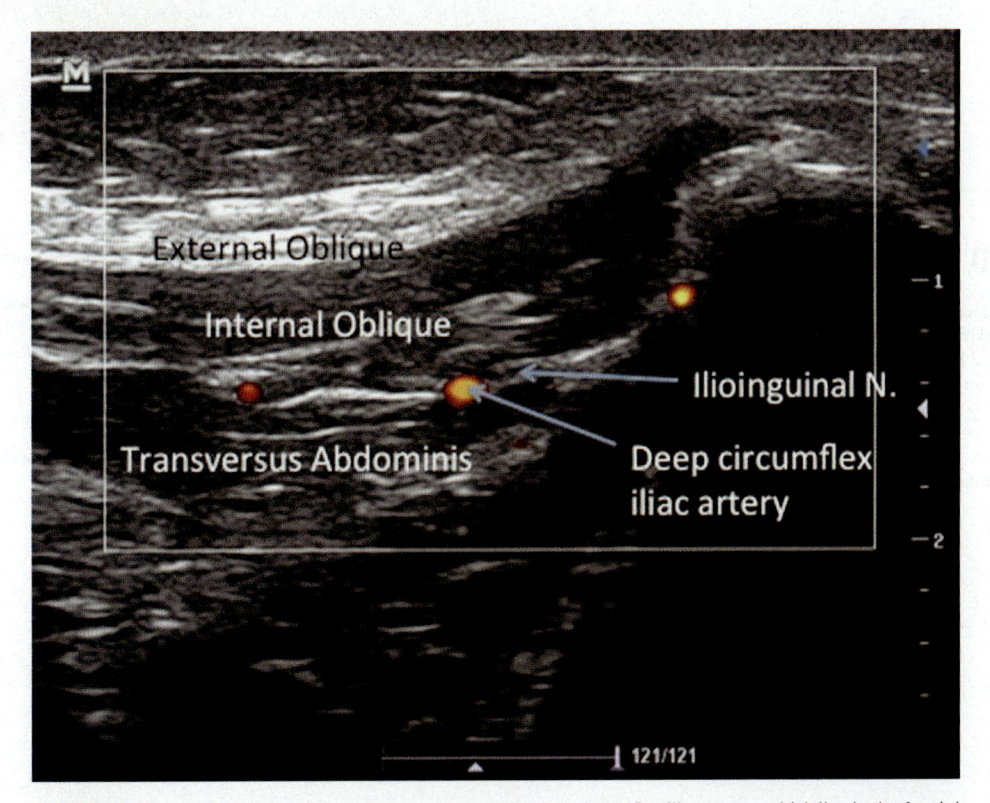

**FIGURE 93.11.** Color Doppler image demonstrating the deep circumflex iliac artery, which lies in the fascial plane between the internal oblique and transversus abdominis muscles adjacent to the ilioinguinal nerve.

**FIGURE 93.12.** Proper in-plane needle position for performing ilioinguinal nerve block.

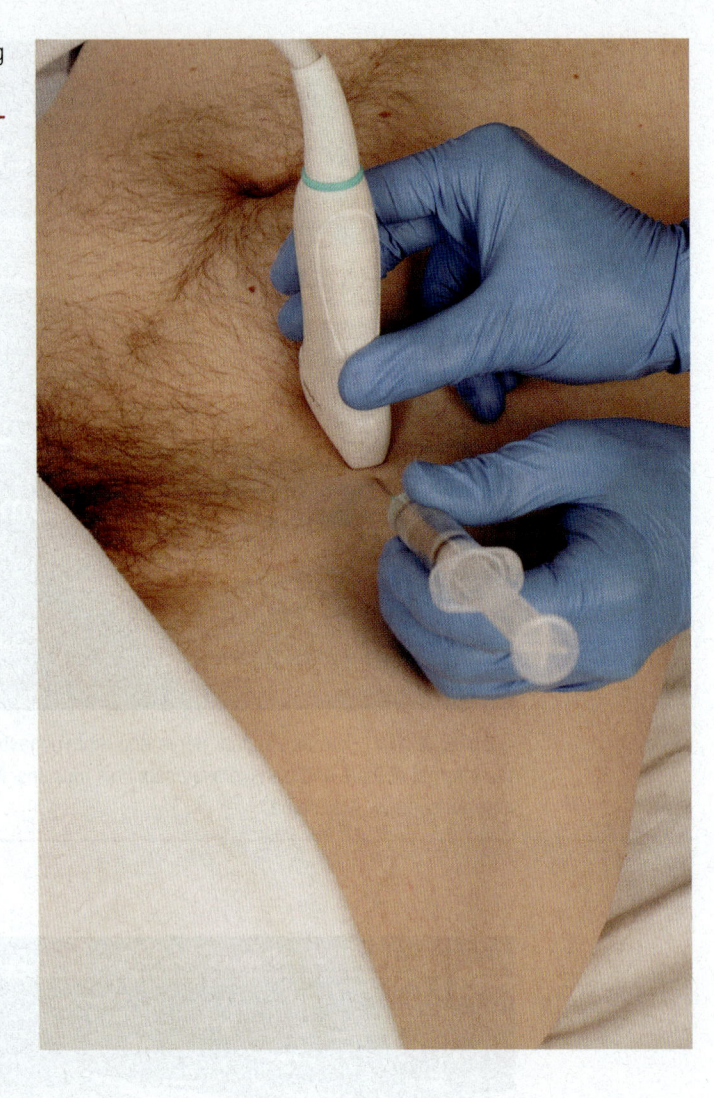

## SUGGESTED READINGS

Ellis H. Anterior abdominal wall. *Anaesth Intensive Care Med* 2006;7(2):36–37.
Gofeld M, Christakis M. Sonographically guided ilioinguinal nerve block. *J Ultrasound Med* 2006;25:1571–1575.
Mahadevan V. Anatomy of the anterior abdominal wall and groin. *Surgery* 2009;27(6):251–254.
Waldman SD. Ilioinguinal nerve. In: *Pain Review*. Philadelphia, PA: Saunders Elsevier; 2009:124–125.
Waldman SD. Ilioinguinal nerve block. In: *Atlas of Interventional Pain Management*. 3rd ed. Philadelphia, PA: Saunders Elsevier; 2009:359–361.
Waldman SD. Ilioinguinal neuralgia. In: *Atlas of Common Pain Syndromes*. 3rd ed. Philadelphia, PA: Saunders Elsevier; 2011:233–234.

# CHAPTER 94

# Ultrasound-Guided Iliohypogastric Nerve Block

## CLINICAL PERSPECTIVES

Ultrasound-guided iliohypogastric nerve block is utilized as a diagnostic and therapeutic maneuver in the evaluation and treatment of groin pain thought to be mediated via the iliohypogastric nerve. The most common pain syndrome mediated via the iliohypogastric nerve is postoperative neuropathy secondary to surgical injuries to the iliohypogastric nerve during appendectomies and inguinal hernia repairs. Less commonly, iliohypogastric neuralgia can be seen in patients in their third trimester of pregnancy when a rapidly expanding abdomen causes a traction neuropathy of the nerve. The symptoms associated with iliohypogastric neuralgia depend on whether the main trunk of the nerve is damaged or if the injury is isolated to the anterior or the lateral branch of the nerve (Fig. 94.1). If the injury is isolated to the anterior branch of the iliohypogastric nerve, the patient will complain of burning pain, paresthesias, and numbness in the skin overlying the pubis. If the lateral branch is damaged, the patient will complain of burning pain, paresthesias, and numbness in the skin overlying the posterior lateral gluteal region. A Tinel sign may be elicited by tapping over the iliohypogastric nerve at the point where it pierces the transversus abdominis muscle.

Ultrasound-guided iliohypogastric nerve block can also be utilized to provide surgical anesthesia for groin surgery, including inguinal herniorrhaphy when combined with ultrasound-guided ilioinguinal and genitofemoral nerve block. Ultrasound-guided iliohypogastric nerve block with local anesthetics can be employed as a diagnostic maneuver when performing differential neural blockade on an anatomic basis to determine if the patient's lower abdominal and groin pain are subserved by the iliohypogastric nerve. If destruction of the iliohypogastric nerve is being contemplated, ultrasound-guided iliohypogastric nerve block with local anesthetic can provide prognostic information as to the extent of motor and sensory deficit the patient will experience following nerve destruction.

Ultrasound-guided iliohypogastric nerve block with local anesthetic may also be used to provide postoperative pain relief following lower abdominal and groin surgeries and is useful in the treatment of persistent postoperative neuropathic pain following inguinal hernia surgery. Electromyography can distinguish iliohypogastric nerve entrapment from lumbar plexopathy, lumbar radiculopathy, and diabetic polyneuropathy. Plain radiographs of the hip and pelvis are indicated in all patients who present with iliohypogastric neuralgia to rule out occult bony pathology. Based on the patient's clinical presentation, additional testing may be warranted, including a complete blood count, uric acid level, erythrocyte sedimentation rate, and antinuclear antibody testing. Magnetic resonance imaging of the lumbar plexus and retroperitoneum is indicated if tumor or hematoma is suspected (Fig. 94.2). The injection technique described later serves as both a diagnostic and a therapeutic maneuver.

## CLINICALLY RELEVANT ANATOMY

The iliohypogastric nerve is derived from the L1 nerve root with a contribution from T12 in some patients. The nerve exits the lateral border of the psoas muscle to follow a curvilinear course that takes it from its origin of the L1 and occasionally T12 somatic nerves to inside the concavity of the ilium (Fig. 94.3). The iliohypogastric nerve continues in an anterior trajectory as it runs between the layers of the internal oblique and transversus abdominis muscles along with the ilioinguinal nerve and deep circumflex iliac artery (Fig. 94.4). It is at this point that the nerve can consistently be identified with ultrasound scanning and is amenable to ultrasound-guided nerve block. Within the fascial plane between the internal oblique and transversus abdominis muscles, the iliohypogastric nerve divides into an anterior and a lateral branch. The lateral branch provides cutaneous sensory innervation to the posterolateral gluteal region. The anterior branch pierces the external oblique muscle just beyond the anterior superior iliac spine to provide cutaneous sensory innervation to the abdominal skin above the pubis. The distribution of the sensory innervation of the iliohypogastric nerves varies from patient to patient due to considerable overlap with the ilioinguinal nerve. In most patients, the anterior branch of the iliohypogastric nerve provides sensory innervation to the skin overlying the pubis, with the lateral branch providing sensory innervation to the skin overlying posterolateral gluteal region (see Fig. 94.1).

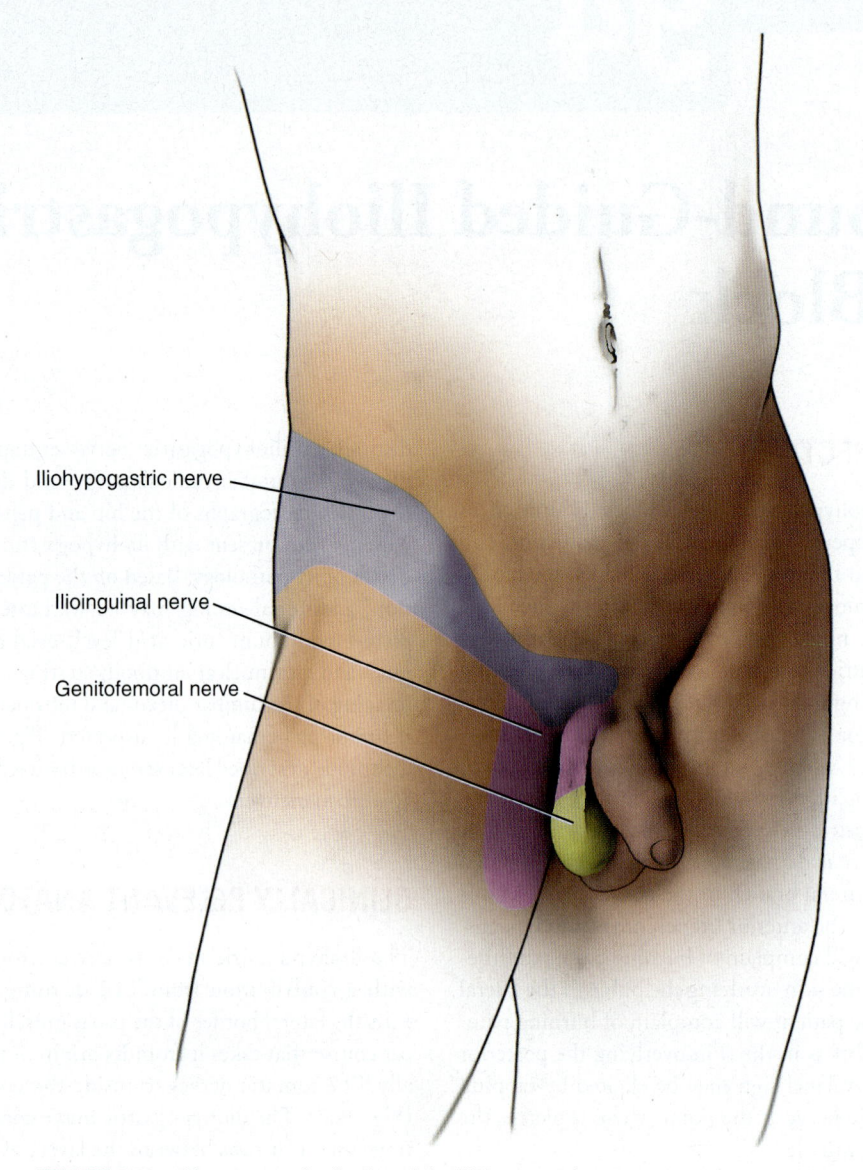

**FIGURE 94.1.** The sensory distribution of the iliohypogastric nerve.

## ULTRASOUND-GUIDED TECHNIQUE

Ultrasound-guided iliohypogastric nerve block can be carried out by placing the patient in the supine position with the arms resting comfortably by the patient's side (Fig. 94.5). A total of 7 mL of local anesthetic is drawn up in a 12-mL sterile syringe. If the painful condition being treated is thought to have an inflammatory component, 40 to 80 mg of depot steroid is added to the local anesthetic. The umbilicus, anterior superior iliac spine, and inguinal ligament are identified by visual inspection and palpation, and an imaginary line is drawn between the anterior superior iliac spine and the umbilicus (Fig. 94.6). A linear high-frequency ultrasound transducer is placed in a plane perpendicular with the inguinal ligament with the inferior aspect of the transducer lying over the anterior superior iliac spine and the superior aspect of the transducer pointed directly at the umbilicus, and an ultrasound survey scan is obtained (Fig. 94.7). The hyperechoic anterior superior iliac spine and its acoustic shadow is identified as are the external oblique, internal oblique, and transversus abdominis muscles, which extend outward from it (Fig. 94.8). The fascial plane between the internal oblique and transversus abdominis muscles is then identified, and the iliohypogastric nerve should be easily identifiable as an ovoid hypoechoic structure highlighted by a hyperechoic epineurium lying more medial in relation to the anterior superior iliac spine as compared to the ilioinguinal nerve, which lies closer to the anterior superior iliac spine (Figs. 94.9 and 94.10). In larger patients, it is sometimes necessary to slowly move the ultrasound transducer toward the umbilicus to visualize the more medial lying iliohypogastric nerve. Color Doppler identification of the deep circumflex artery may be used to aid in identifying the fascial

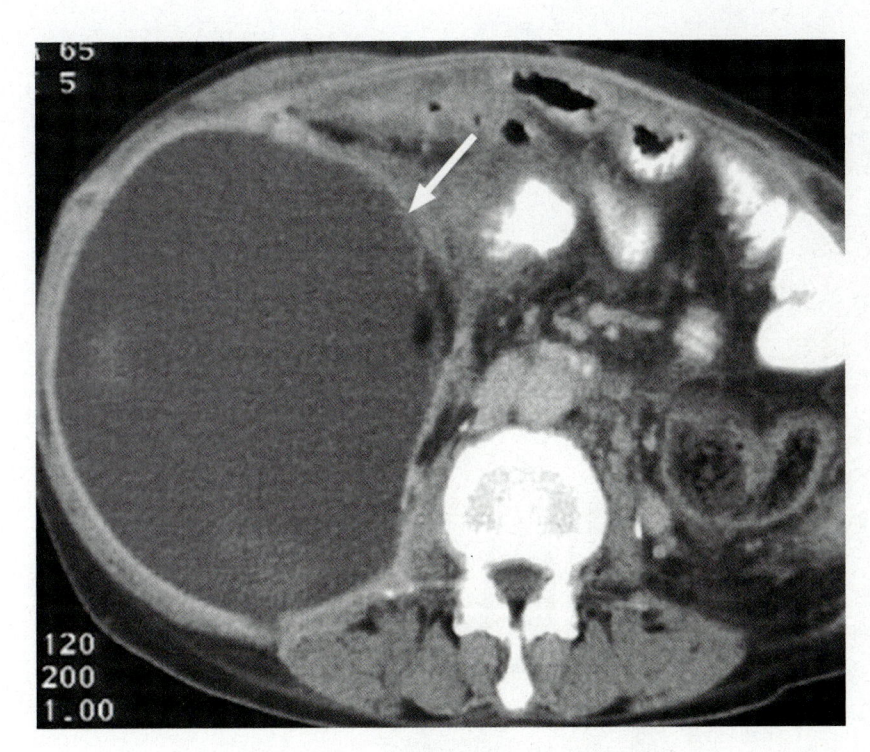

**FIGURE 94.2.** Coronal computed tomography scan of a large retroperitoneal lymphoma (*arrow*). (Reused from Eisenberg RL. *Clinical Imaging: An Atlas of Differential Diagnosis*. 5th ed. Philadelphia, PA: Lippincott Williams & Wilkins; 2010:921, with permission.)

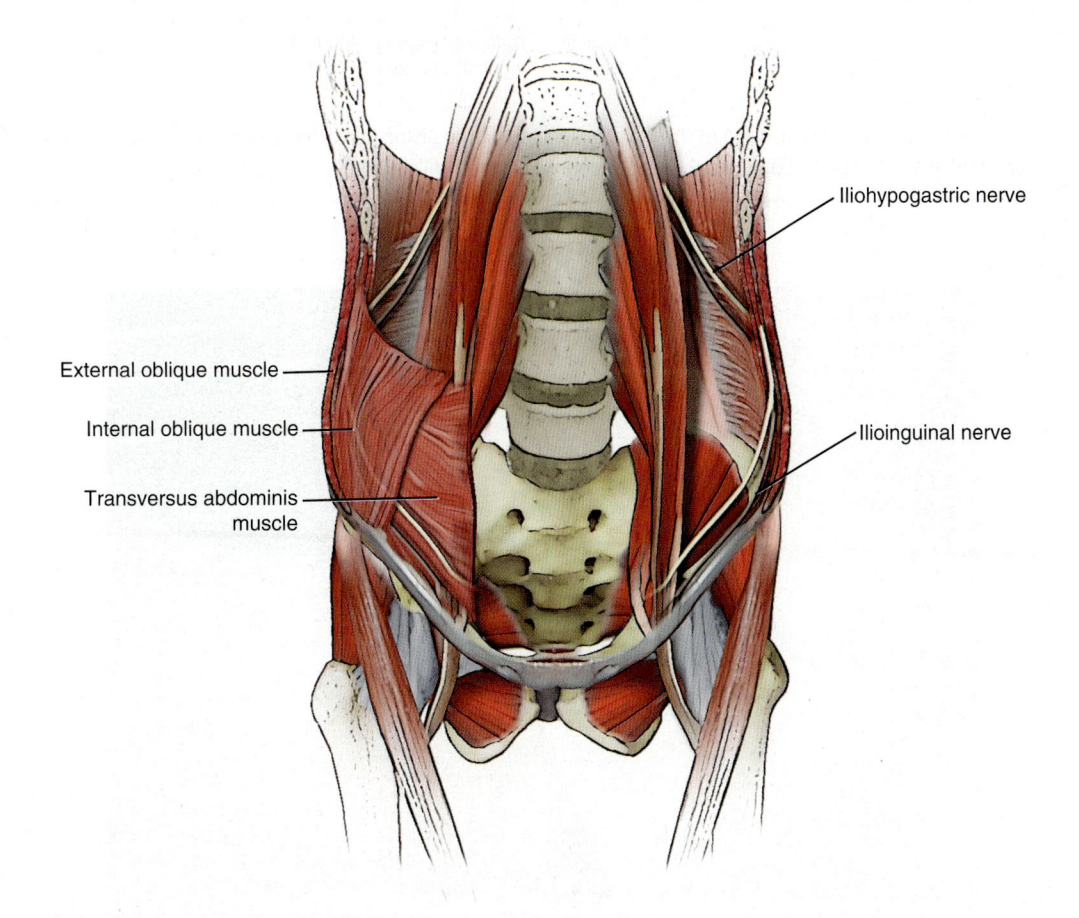

**FIGURE 94.3.** The anatomy of the iliohypogastric nerve.

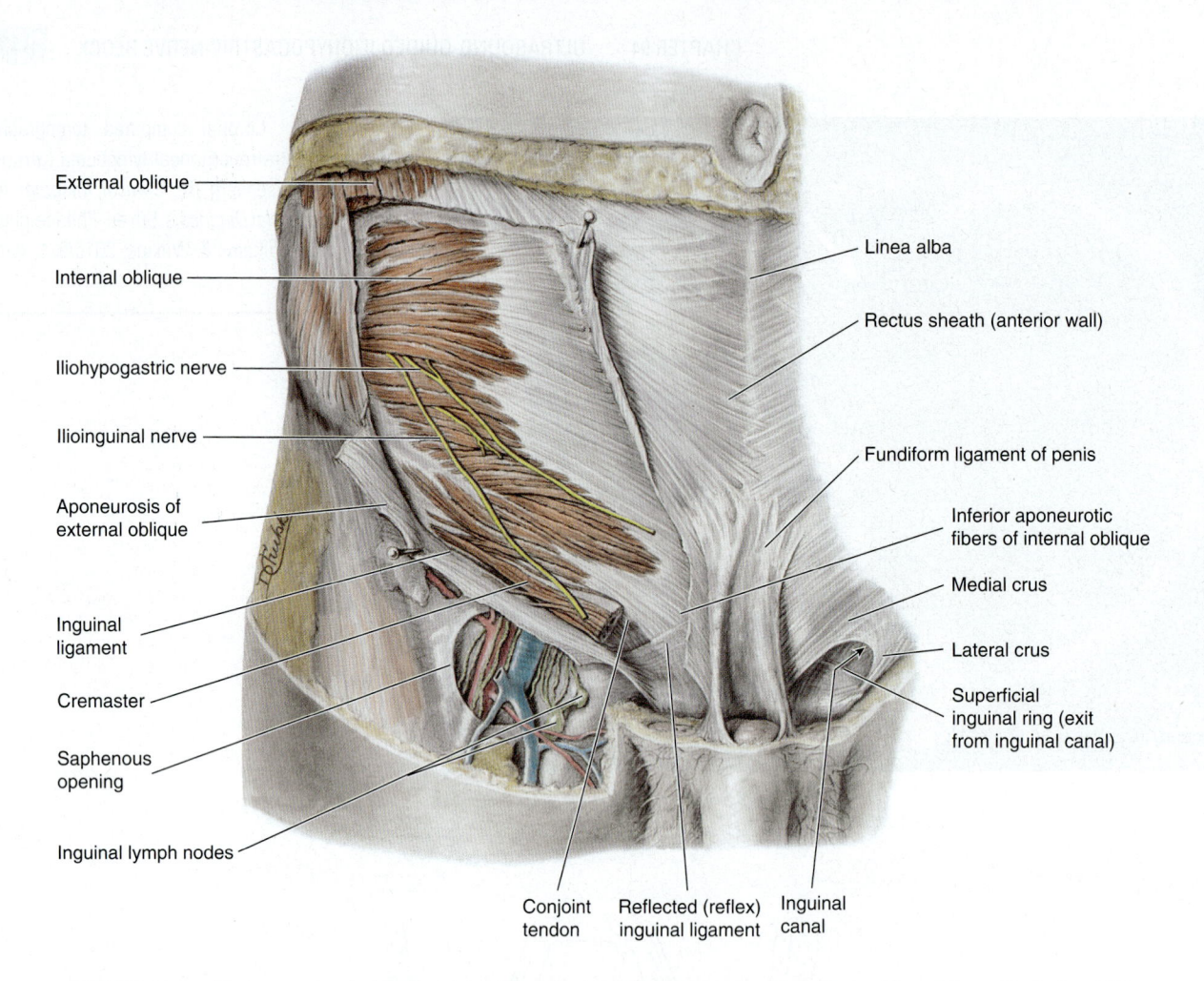

**FIGURE 94.4.** The anatomic relationship of the ilioinguinal and iliohypogastric nerve. (Reused from Moore KL, Dalley AF II. *Clinical Oriented Anatomy.* 4th ed. Baltimore, MD: Lippincott Williams & Wilkins; 1999, with permission.)

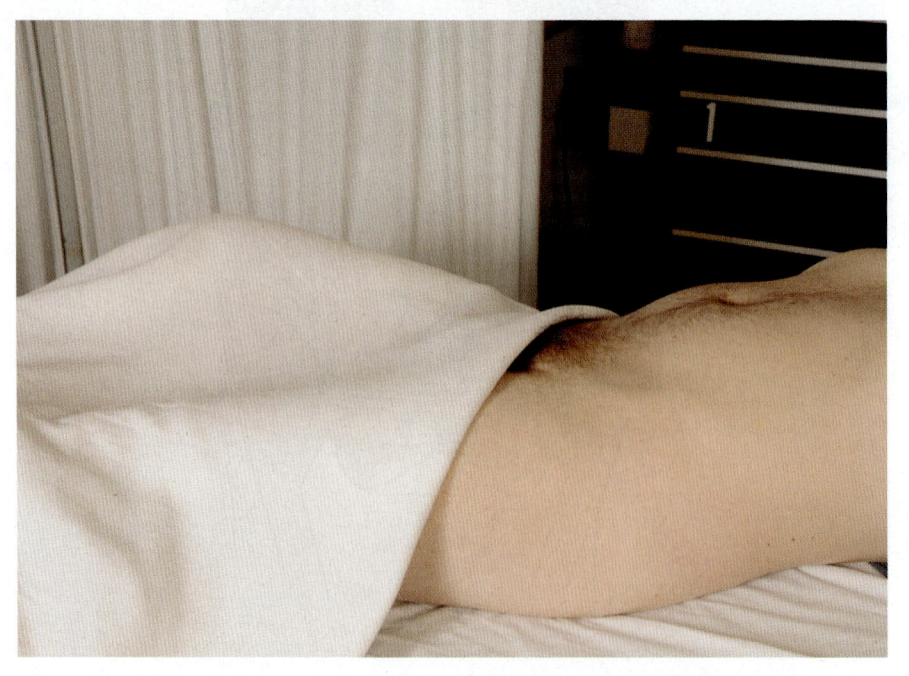

**FIGURE 94.5.** Proper patient position for ultrasound-guided iliohypogastric nerve block.

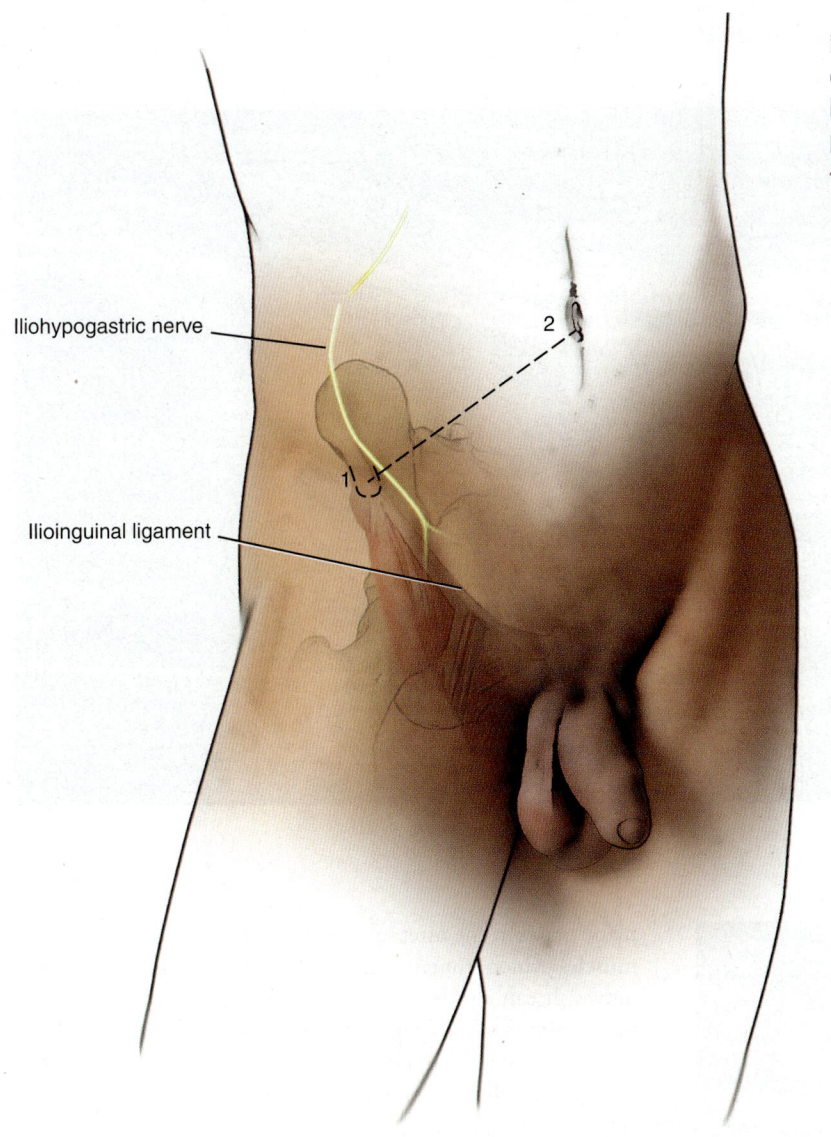

**FIGURE 94.6.** To perform ultrasound-guided iliohypogastric nerve block, an imaginary line is drawn between the anterior superior iliac spine and the patient's umbilicus.

Iliohypogastric nerve

Ilioinguinal ligament

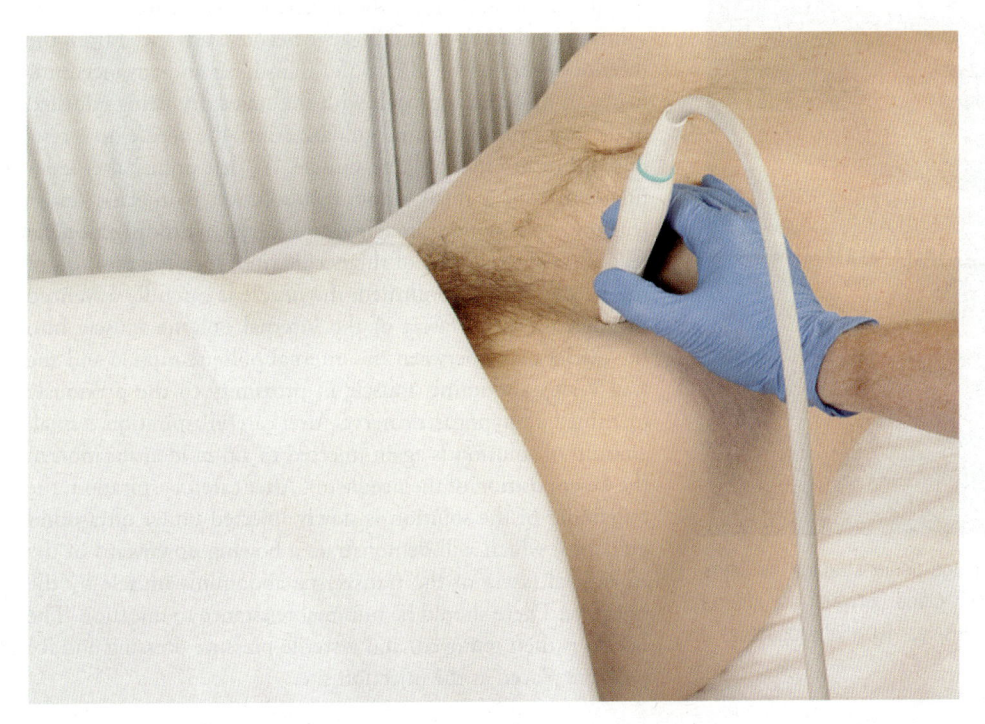

**FIGURE 94.7.** Oblique placement of the ultrasound transducer placed in a plane perpendicular with the inguinal ligament with the inferior aspect of the transducer lying over the anterior superior iliac spine and the superior aspect of the transducer pointed directly at the umbilicus.

**FIGURE 94.8.** Oblique ultrasound image demonstrating the hyperechoic anterior superior iliac spine and its acoustic shadow and the external oblique, internal oblique, and transversus abdominis muscles. Note the fascial plane between the internal oblique and transversus abdominis muscles. *Asterisk* (*) marks the ideal sites of injection between the muscular layers, adjacent to the nerves.

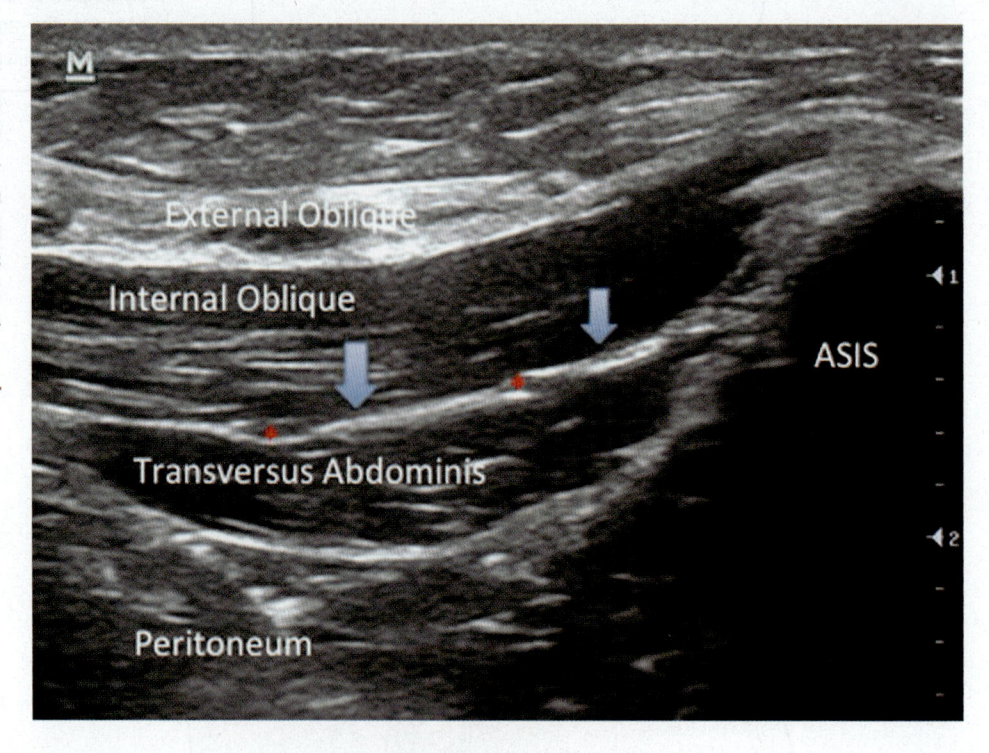

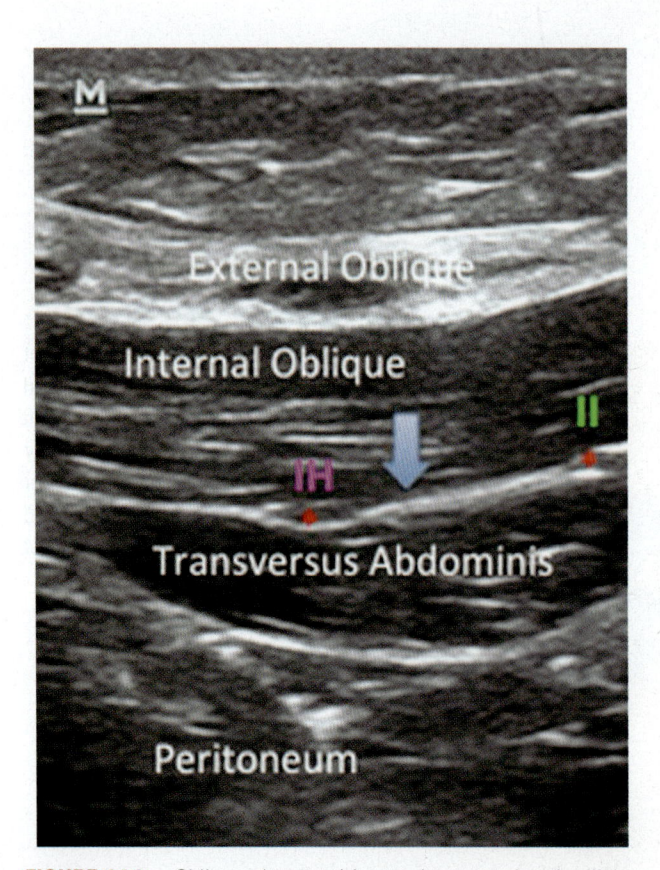

**FIGURE 94.9.** Oblique ultrasound image demonstrating the iliohypogastric nerve lying within the fascial plane between the internal oblique and transversus abdominis muscles. IH, iliohypogastric; II, ilioinguinal.

plane between the internal oblique and transversus abdominis muscles which contains the iliohypogastric and ilioinguinal nerves. It can also be used to help distinguish the ilioinguinal nerve from the iliohypogastric nerve as the artery runs between the ilioinguinal and iliohypogastric nerve, with the ilioinguinal nerve lying closer to the anterior superior iliac spine (Figs. 94.11 and 94.12).

When these anatomic structures are clearly identified on oblique ultrasound scan, the skin is prepped with anesthetic solution, and a 1½-inch, 22-gauge needle is advanced from the inferior border of the ultrasound transducer and advanced utilizing an in-plane approach with the trajectory being adjusted under real-time ultrasound guidance until the needle tip is resting within internal oblique muscle. At that point, after careful aspiration, a small amount of solution is injected under real-time ultrasound imaging to utilize hydrodissection to reconfirm the position of the needle tip. Once the position of the needle tip is reconfirmed, the needle is carefully advanced through the deep fascia of the internal oblique muscle into the fascial plane between the internal oblique muscle and the transversus abdominis muscle in proximity to the previously identified iliohypogastric nerve. After careful aspiration, a small amount of solution is again injected to aid in identification of the exact position of the needle tip. After careful aspiration, the remainder of the solution is slowly injected under ultrasound guidance, which will demonstrate a bowing downward of the superficial fascia of the transversus abdominis muscle by the injectate. There should be minimal resistance to injection. The needle is then removed, and a sterile pressure dressing and ice pack are placed at the injection site.

CHAPTER 94    ULTRASOUND-GUIDED ILIOHYPOGASTRIC NERVE BLOCK    653

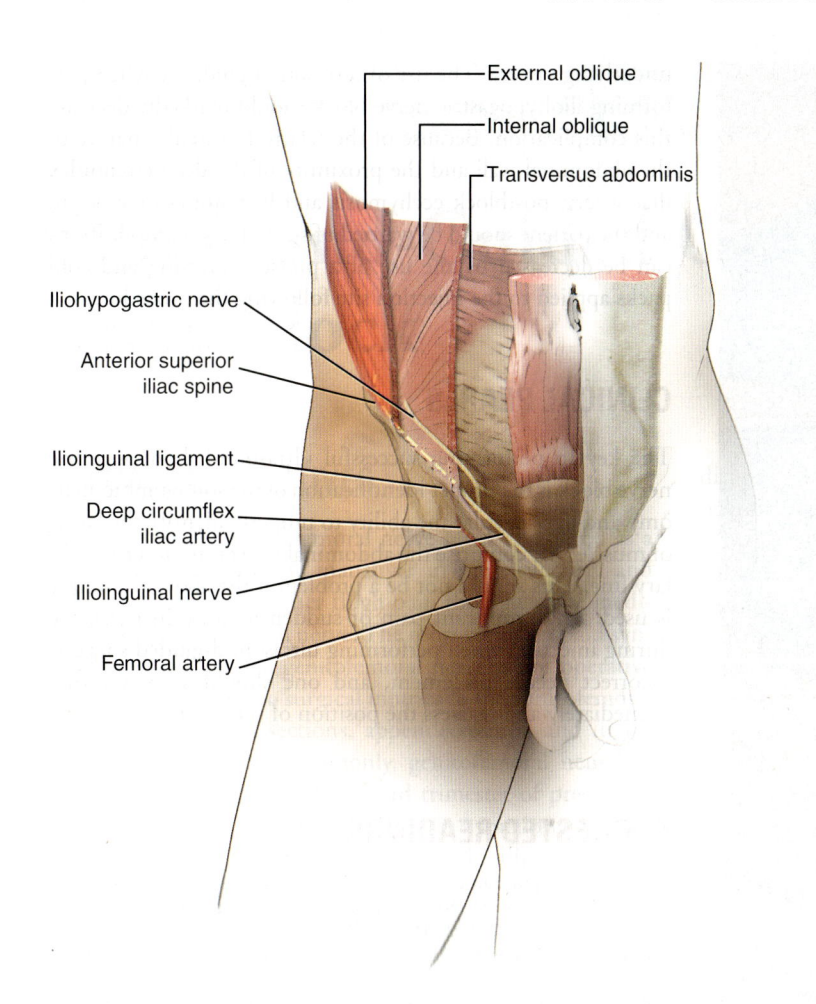

**FIGURE 94.10.** The iliohypogastric nerve and iliohypogastric nerve both lie in the fascial plane between the internal oblique and transversus abdominis muscles. Note that the ilioinguinal nerve is closest to the anterior superior iliac spine.

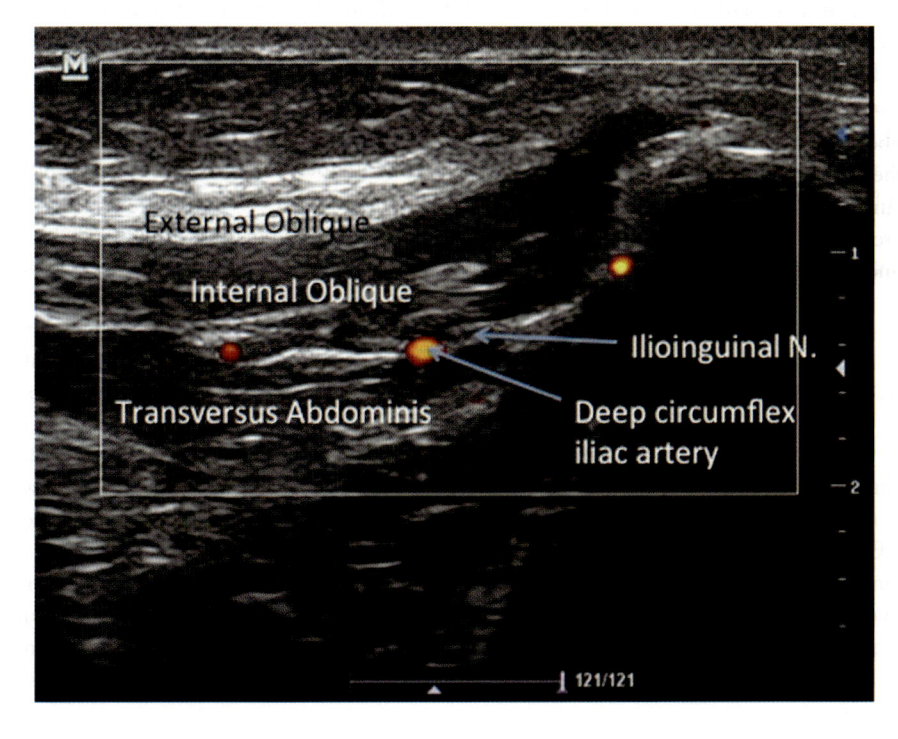

**FIGURE 94.11.** Color Doppler image demonstrating the deep circumflex iliac artery, which lies in the fascial plane between the internal oblique and transversus abdominis muscles. The artery runs between the ilioinguinal and the iliohypogastric nerve.

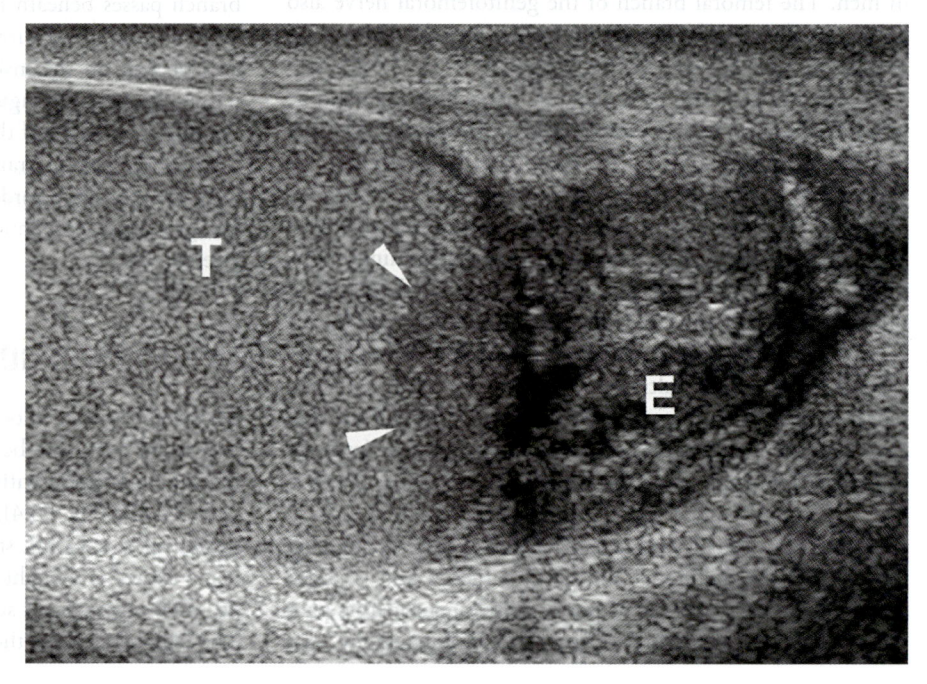

**FIGURE 95.1.** The sensory distribution of the genitofemoral nerve.

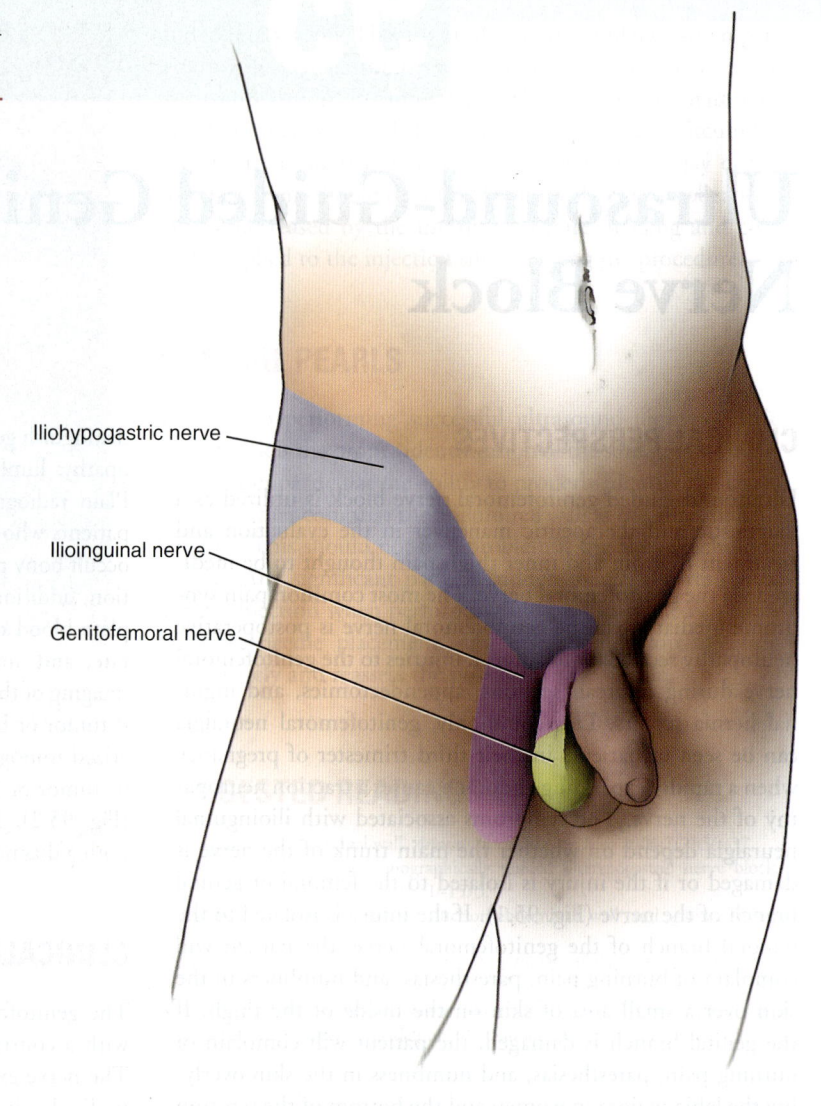

**FIGURE 95.2.** Orchitis. *Acute focal epididymo-orchitis.* Longitudinal sonogram shows an enlarged left testis (*T*) containing a small hypoechoic area (*arrowheads*) posteriorly, which represents focal *orchitis*. The epididymal tail (*E*) is hypoechoic relative to the testis. (Reused from Siegel MJ, Coley B. *Core Curriculum: Pediatric Imaging.* Philadelphia, PA: Lippincott Williams & Wilkins; 2006, with permission.)

CHAPTER 95  ULTRASOUND-GUIDED GENITOFEMORAL NERVE BLOCK  657

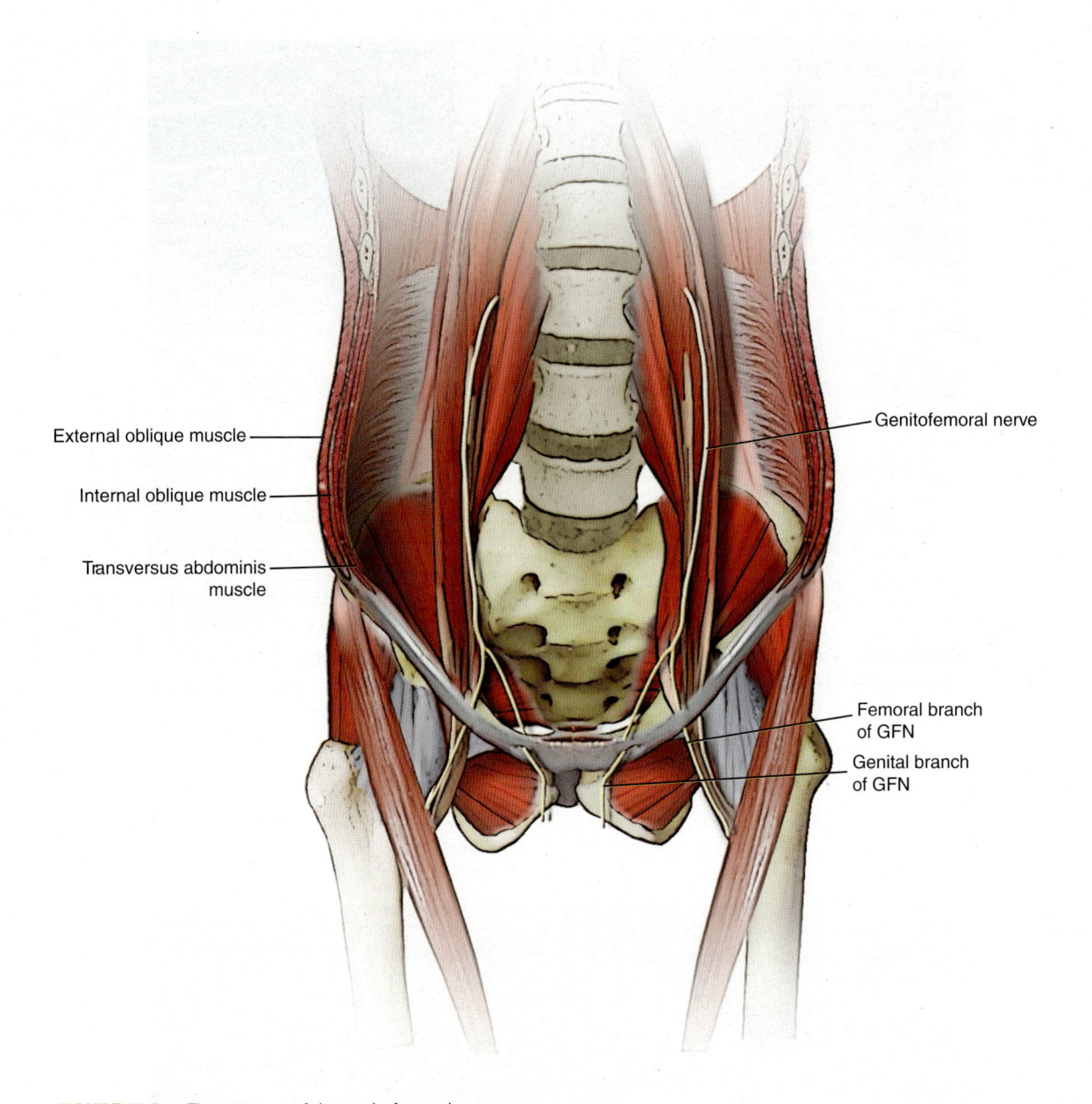

**FIGURE 95.3.** The anatomy of the genitofemoral nerve.

A linear high-frequency ultrasound transducer is placed in long axis over the previously identified femoral artery, and an ultrasound survey scan is obtained (Figs. 95.6 and 95.7). The ultrasound transducer is then slowly moved in a cephalad trajectory following the femoral artery until it begins to descend beneath the inguinal ligament into the abdominal cavity as it becomes the external iliac artery (Figs. 95.8 and 95.9). Color Doppler may be utilized to aid in the identification of this point of transition between the femoral and external iliac arteries (Fig. 95.10). When this point of transition is identified, the inguinal canal should be visible just above the external iliac artery, appearing as an ovoid structure containing tubular structures including the spermatic cord in males and the round ligament in women (Figs. 95.11 and 95.12). When the inguinal canal and its contents are identified on ultrasound imaging, the skin is prepped with anesthetic solution, and a 3½-inch, 22-gauge needle is advanced from the lateral border of the ultrasound transducer and advanced utilizing an out-of-plane approach with the trajectory being adjusted under real-time ultrasound guidance until the needle tip is resting within the inguinal canal (Fig. 95.13). In women, after careful aspiration, the contents of the syringe are injected around the round ligament. In men, after careful aspiration, 4 mL of solution is injected within the spermatic cord while avoiding the testicular artery. Then after withdrawing the needle from the spermatic cord, after careful aspiration, 4 mL of solution are outside the

**SECTION VI**     CHEST WALL, TRUNK, AND ABDOMEN

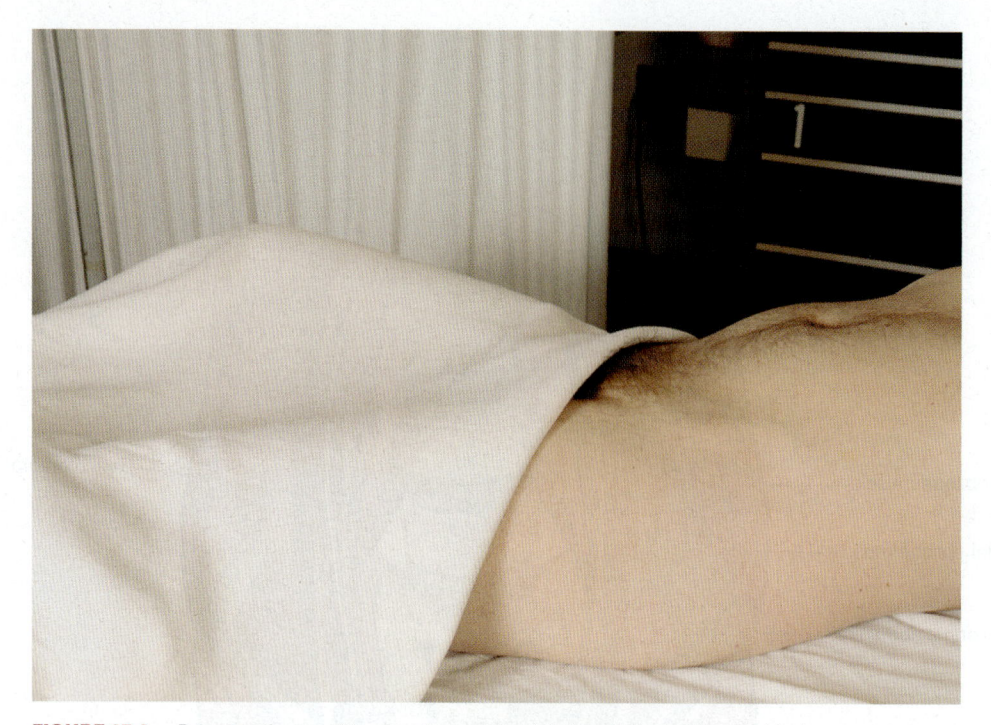

**FIGURE 95.4.** Proper patient position for ultrasound-guided genitofemoral nerve block.

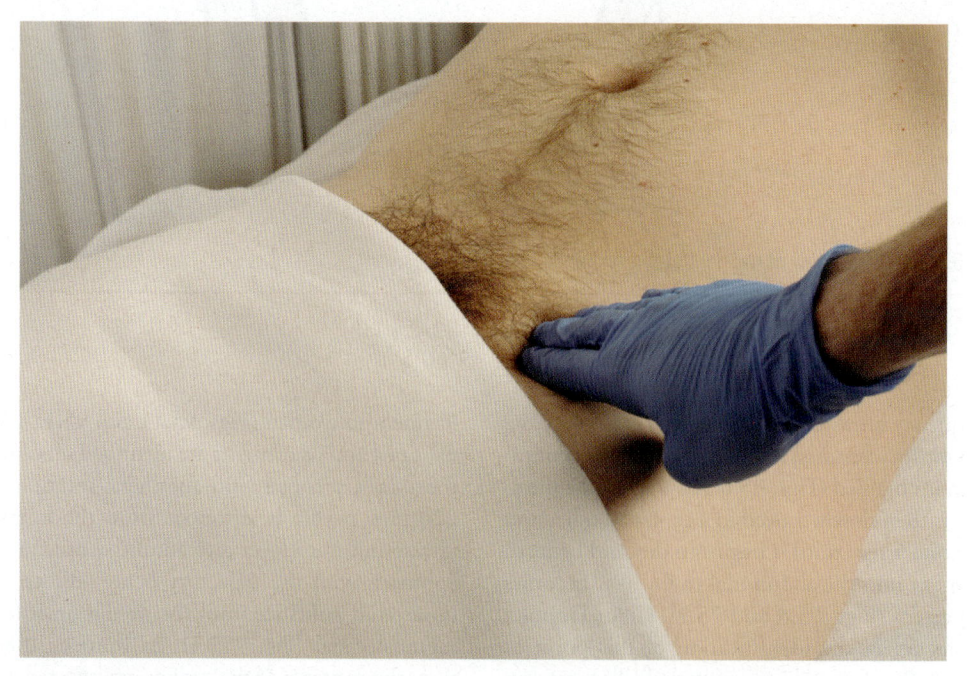

**FIGURE 95.5.** The femoral artery is then identified by palpation.

CHAPTER 95 ULTRASOUND-GUIDED GENITOFEMORAL NERVE BLOCK 659

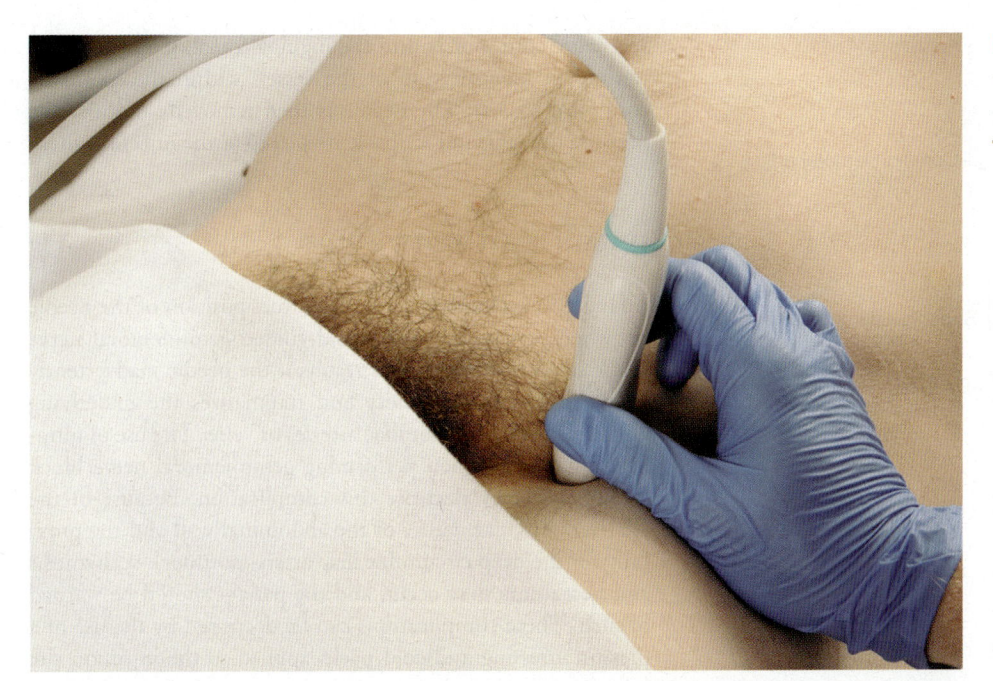

**FIGURE 95.6.** Placement of the ultrasound transducer over the long axis of the femoral artery.

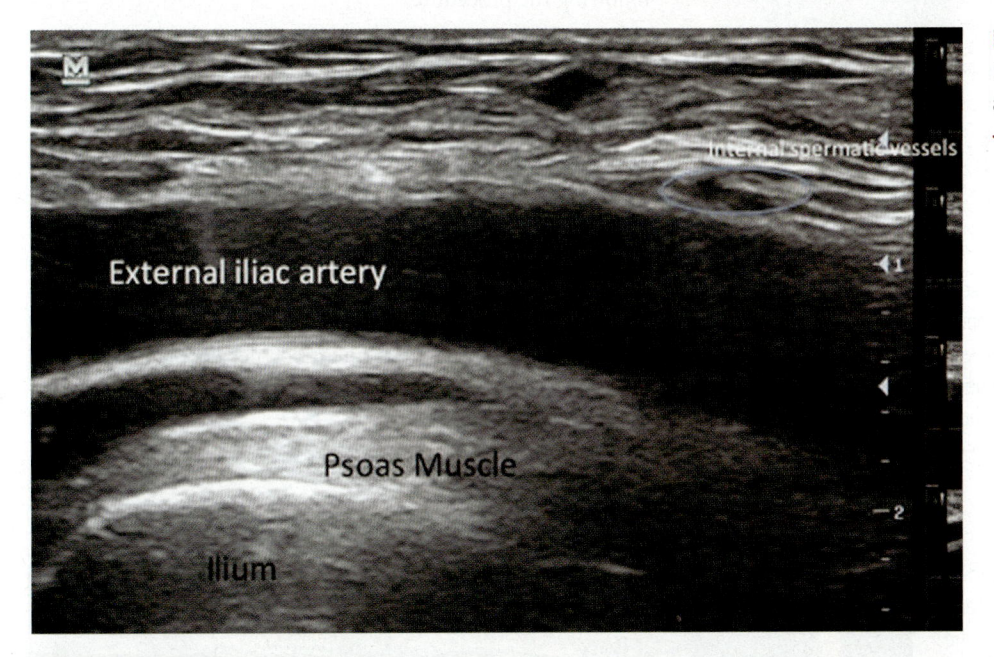

**FIGURE 95.7.** Long axis ultrasound image demonstrating the femoral and external iliac artery.

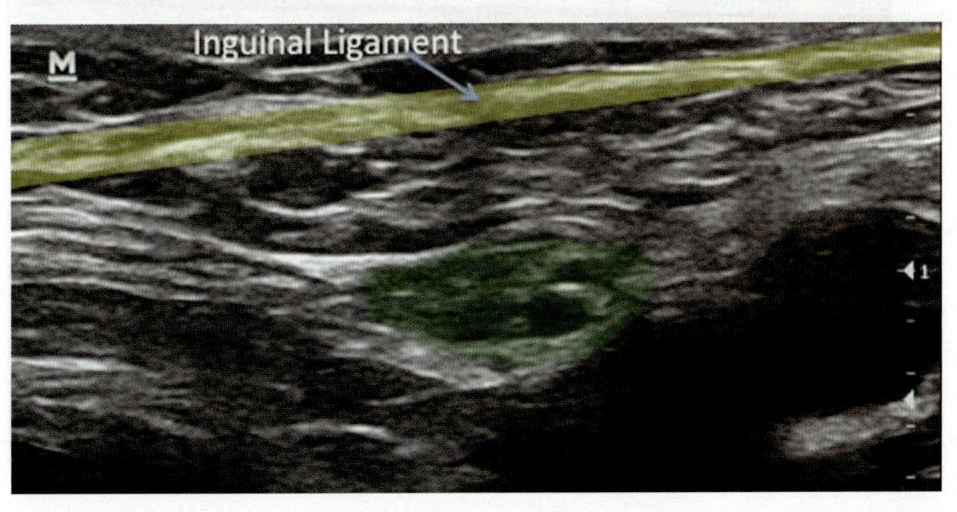

**FIGURE 95.8.** Long axis ultrasound image demonstrating the femoral artery as it begins to descend beneath the inguinal ligament into the abdominal cavity as it becomes the external iliac artery.

spermatic cord, but within the inguinal canal. Color Doppler can aid in identification of the vessels within the spermatic cord (Fig. 95.14). The needle is then removed, and a sterile pressure dressing and ice pack are placed at the injection site.

## COMPLICATIONS

A failure to accurately assess the correct position of the needle tip when performing ultrasound-guided genitofemoral nerve block can lead to disastrous results if the needle inadvertently enters the peritoneal cavity and traumatizes the underlying viscera or the femoral or iliac arteries or veins. The use of ultrasound guidance when performing genitofemoral nerve block should markedly decrease this complication. Because of the relatively vascular nature of the abdominal wall and the proximity of the deep circumflex iliac artery, postblock ecchymosis and hematoma may occur, and the patient should be warned of such. These complications can be decreased by the use of a pressure dressing and cold packs applied to the injection site following the procedure.

## CLINICAL PEARLS

The key to performing successful ultrasound genitofemoral nerve block is the proper identification of the sonographic anatomy and in particular the ability to properly identify the femoral and external iliac arteries. This should not be a problem if the above technique is used. Any significant pain or sudden increase in resistance during injection when performing ultrasound-guided suggests incorrect needle placement, and one should stop injecting immediately and reassess the position of the needle.

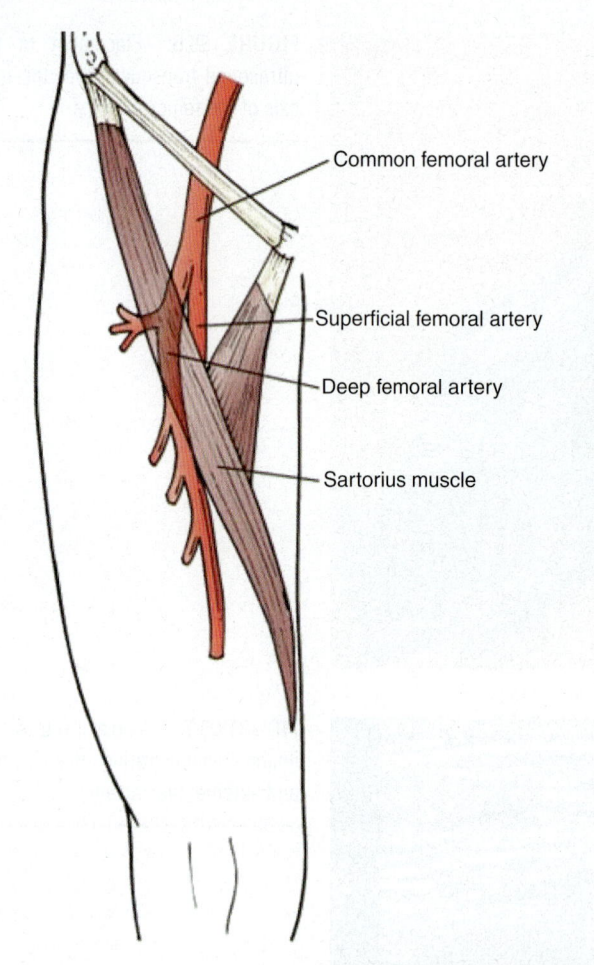

**FIGURE 95.9.** The femoral artery descends beneath the inguinal ligament into the abdominal cavity as it becomes the external iliac artery. (From Mills JL Sr, Lucas LC. Reversed vein bypass grafts to popliteal, tibial, and peroneal arteries. In: Fischer JE, ed. *Fischer's Mastery of Surgery*. 6th ed. Philadelphia, PA: Lippincott Williams & Wilkins; 2012.)

**FIGURE 95.10.** Color Doppler image of the femoral artery as it begins to descend beneath the inguinal ligament into the abdominal cavity as it becomes the external iliac artery.

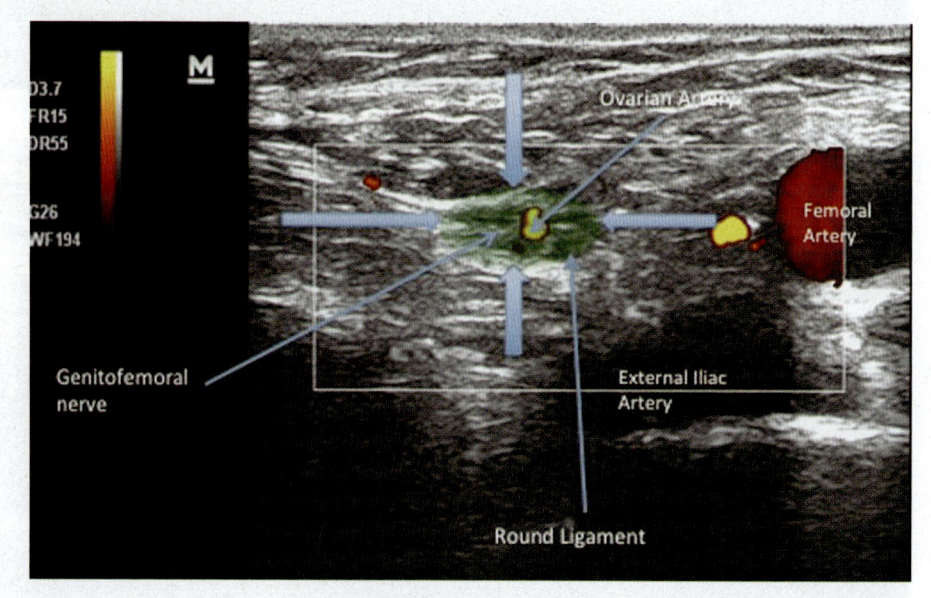

CHAPTER 95 ULTRASOUND-GUIDED GENITOFEMORAL NERVE BLOCK 661

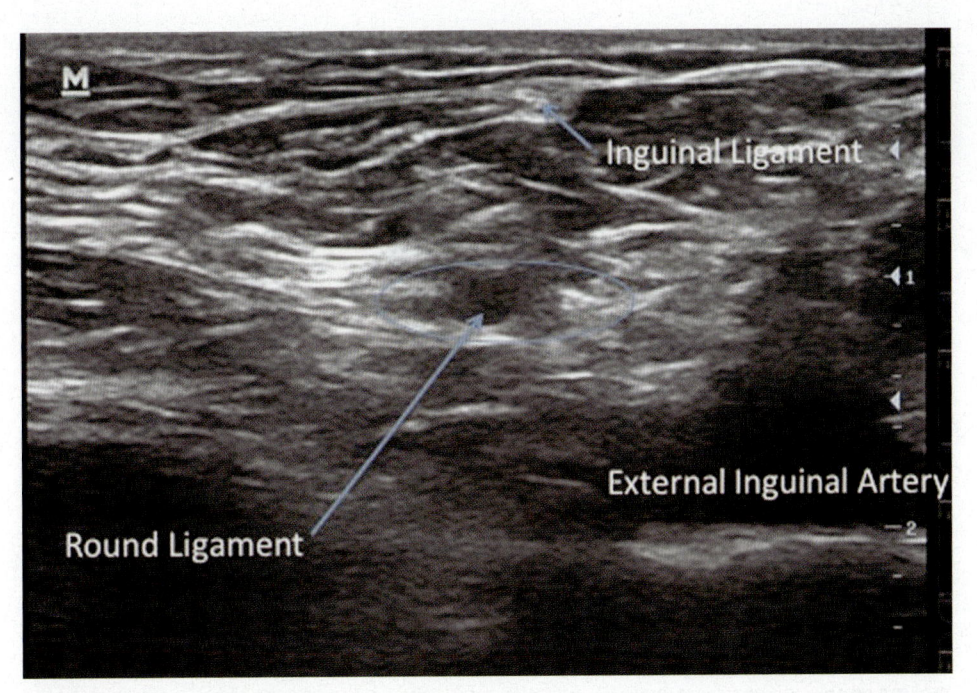

**FIGURE 95.11.** Long axis view of inguinal canal and spermatic cord within. Note relationship of the inguinal canal to the transition point of the femoral artery to the external iliac artery.

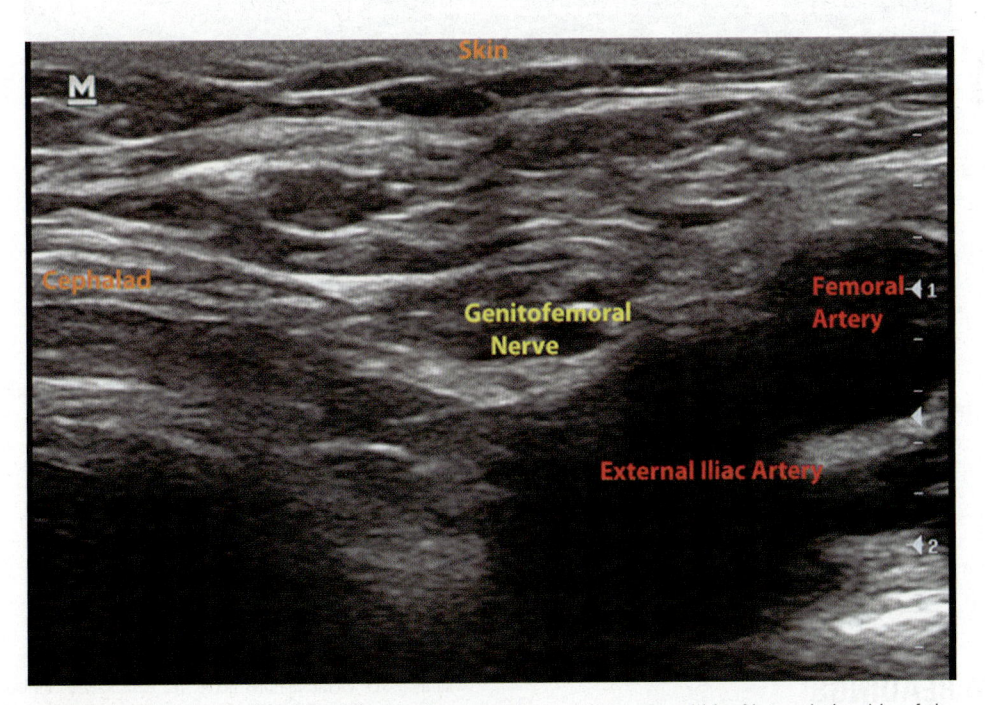

**FIGURE 95.12.** Long axis view of inguinal canal and round ligament within. Note relationship of the inguinal canal to the transition point of the femoral artery to the external iliac artery.

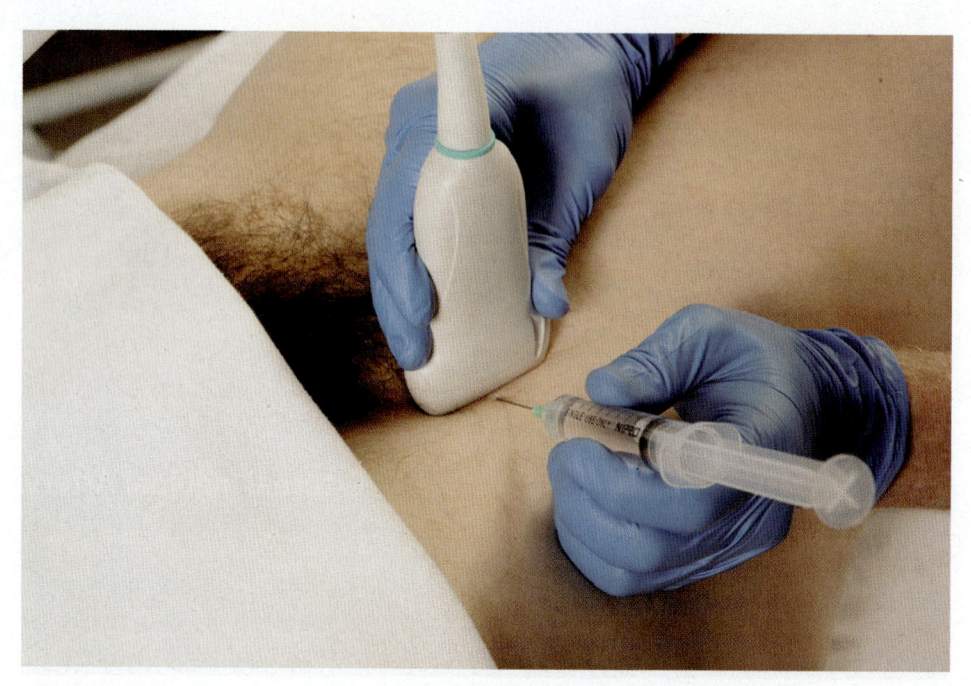

**FIGURE 95.13.** Proper out-of-plane needle position for performing genitofemoral nerve block.

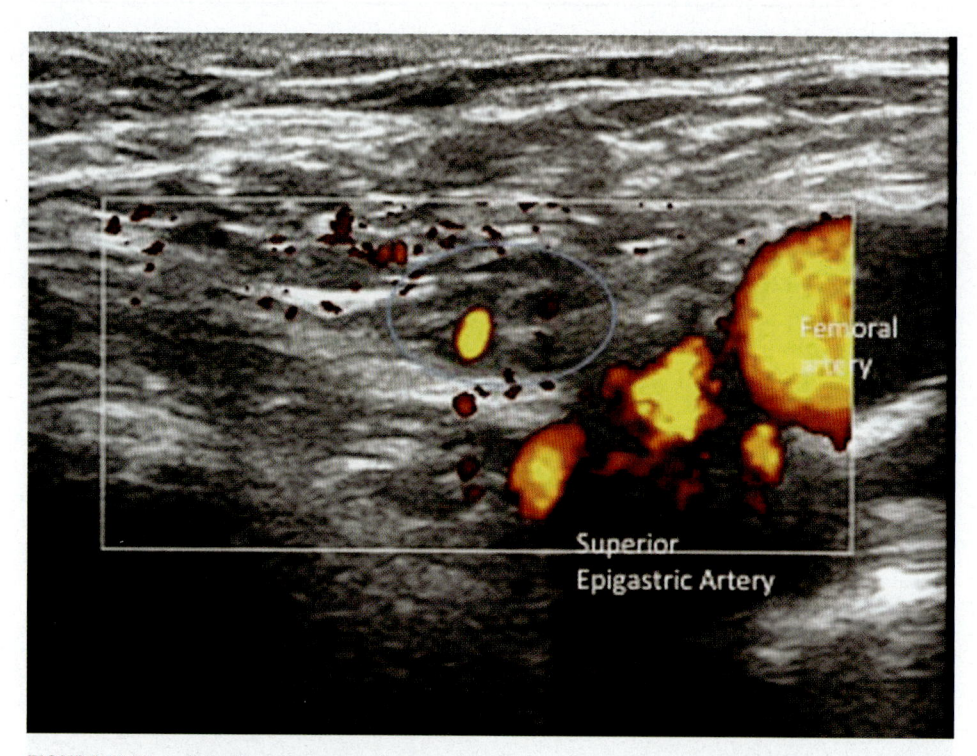

**FIGURE 95.14.** Color Doppler image of spermatic cord.

## SUGGESTED READINGS

Bellingham GA, Peng PWH. Ultrasound-guided interventional procedures for chronic pelvic pain. *Tech Reg Anesth Pain Manag* 2009;13(3):171–178.

Ellis H. Anterior abdominal wall. *Anaesth Intensive Care Med* 2006;7(2):36–37.

Mahadevan V. Anatomy of the anterior abdominal wall and groin. *Surgery* 2009; 27(6):251–254.

Waldman SD. Genitofemoral nerve. In: *Pain Review*. Philadelphia, PA: Saunders Elsevier; 2009:127–128.

Waldman SD. Genitofemoral nerve block. In: *Atlas of Interventional Pain Management*. 3rd ed. Philadelphia, PA: Saunders Elsevier; 2009:366–368.

SECTION VII

# Low Back

# CHAPTER 96

# Ultrasound-Guided Lumbar Facet Block: Medial Branch Technique

## CLINICAL PERSPECTIVES

Ultrasound-guided lumbar medial branch block is utilized in a variety of clinical scenarios as a diagnostic and therapeutic maneuver in painful conditions involving the lumbar facet joint. As a diagnostic tool, ultrasound-guided lumbar medial branch block allows accurate placement of the needle tip to determine if a specific pair of medial branch nerves is in fact subserving the patient's pain. In the acute pain setting, ultrasound-guided lumbar medial branch block with local anesthetics and/or steroids may be used to palliate acute low back pain emergencies while waiting for pharmacologic methods to become effective. This technique has great clinical utility when managing acute posttrauma pain. This technique is also useful in the treatment of arthritis-related facet joint pain (Fig. 96.1). Clinically, pain emanating from the lumbar facet joints is perceived in the paraspinous region and radiates in a nondermatomal pattern (Fig. 96.2).

## CLINICALLY RELEVANT ANATOMY

The lumbar facet joints are formed by the articulations of the superior and inferior articular facets of adjacent lumbar vertebrae (Fig. 96.3). The lumbar facet joints are lined with synovium and possess a dense joint capsule. The joint capsule is richly innervated and explains why the facet joint can serve as a nidus for lumbar pain when it becomes damaged or inflamed. The lumbar joint is susceptible to degenerative arthritis and is frequently affected by the collagen vascular diseases. The joint is frequently injured in acceleration/deceleration injuries resulting in intra-articular hemorrhage with subsequent inflammation and development of adhesions.

Each lumbar facet joint receives innervation from two spinal levels, receiving fibers from the dorsal ramus at the same level as the vertebra as well as fibers from the dorsal ramus of the vertebra above (see Fig. 96.3). This fact has clinical import in that it provides an explanation for the ill-defined nature of facet-mediated pain and explains why the dorsal nerve from the vertebra above the offending level must often also be blocked to provide the patient with complete pain relief.

## ULTRASOUND-GUIDED TECHNIQUE

Ultrasound-guided lumbar medial branch block can be carried out by placing the patient in the prone position with a thin pillow placed beneath the abdomen to slightly flex the lumbar spine (Fig. 96.4). A total of 1 mL of local anesthetic is drawn up in a 5-mL sterile syringe for each medial branch to be blocked. If the painful condition being treated is thought to have an inflammatory component, 40 to 80 mg of depot steroid is added to the local anesthetic.

To perform ultrasound-guided lumbar medial branch block, a two-step process is used. This two-step process allows the clinician to quickly identify critical anatomic structures while at the same time maintaining a transducer position that allows a safe and easy placement of needles in proximity to the affected lumbar medial branch nerves.

### Step One: Obtain the Paramedian Sagittal Transverse Process View

Step One is to obtain a paramedian sagittal transverse process view by placing the 2- to 5-MHz low-frequency curvilinear probe in the longitudinal plane 3 to 4 cm lateral to the right side of the middle of the spinous processes at the level to be blocked for blockade of the right lumbar medial branch nerves and 3 to 4 cm lateral to the left side of the middle of the spinous processes at the level to be blocked for left-sided medial branch nerves (Figs. 96.5 and 96.6). An initial depth setting of 7 to 8 cm will work for most patients. An ultrasound survey is taken and the transducer is slowly moved medially and laterally until successive transverse processes are visualized. The transverse processes of the lumbar spine will appear as hyperechoic domes with sausage-like acoustic shadows beneath them (Fig. 96.7). This classic appearance of successive transverse processes viewed in the longitudinal plane has been named the "trident sign" after Neptune's trident (Fig. 96.8).

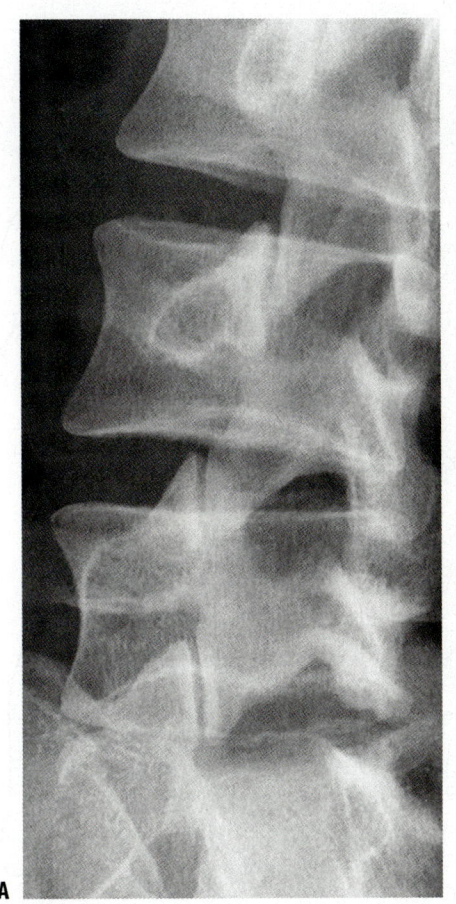

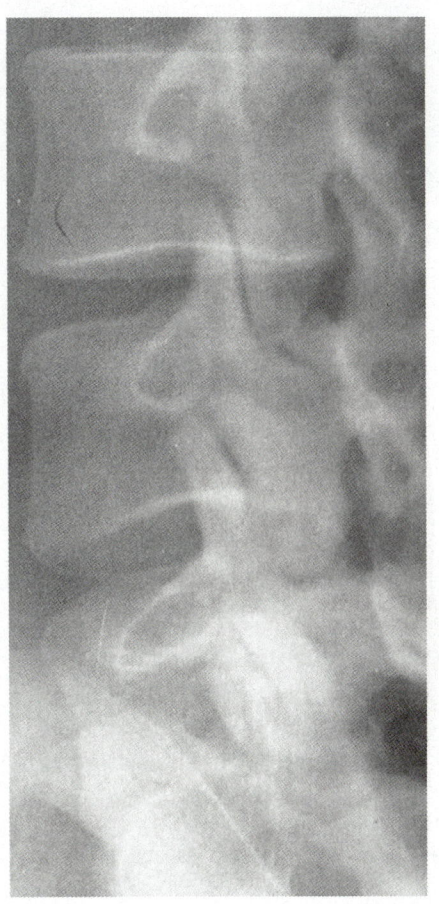

**FIGURE 96.1.** Facet arthrosis: oblique lumbar. **A:** Normal lumbar facets. Note that the joint spaces are smooth and uniform; the articular processes are of a triangular shape. **B:** Lumbar facet arthrosis. Observe that the joint spaces are narrowed and the articular processes sclerotic and altered in shape owing to osteophytes. (Reused from Yochum TR, Rowe LJ. *Essentials of Skeletal Radiology*. 3rd ed. Philadelphia, PA: Lippincott Williams & Wilkins; 2005:971, with permission.)

### Step Two: Obtain the Paramedian Sagittal Articular Process View

After the transverse processes are identified in the paramedian sagittal transverse process view, the ultrasound transducer is slowly slid toward the midline until the superior and inferior articular facets are visualized (Step Two) (Figs. 96.9 and 96.10). In longitudinal paramedian ultrasound articular process view, the superior and inferior articular facets will appear as successive hyperechoic hills and valleys, with the space within the center each hill representing a facet joint (Figs. 96.11 and 96.12). The junction between the superior articular facet and the transverse process is then identified as the target for needle tip placement (see Fig. 96.11). When the junction between the superior articular facet and the transverse process of interest is identified, the skin beneath and below the ultrasound transducer is prepped with antiseptic solution, and a 3½ inch, 22-gauge styletted needle is inserted through the skin just below the inferior aspect of the longitudinally placed ultrasound transducer utilizing an in-plane approach (Fig. 96.13). While an assistant holds and adjusts the ultrasound transducer, the clinician advances the needle under real-time ultrasound guidance in inferior to superior trajectory until the needle tip rests next to the junction between the superior articular facet and the transverse process. After gentle aspiration, 1 mL of solution is injected. The needle is removed and pressure is placed on the injection site to avoid hematoma formation.

## COMPLICATIONS

Because of potential hematogenous spread via the valveless epidural veins of the lumbar epidural space, sepsis and local infection at the injection site represent absolute contraindications to ultrasound-guided lumbar medial branch block as do anticoagulation and coagulopathy. The lumbar facet joints are in close proximity to the epidural, subdural, and subarachnoid space and spinal cord as well as the exiting spinal

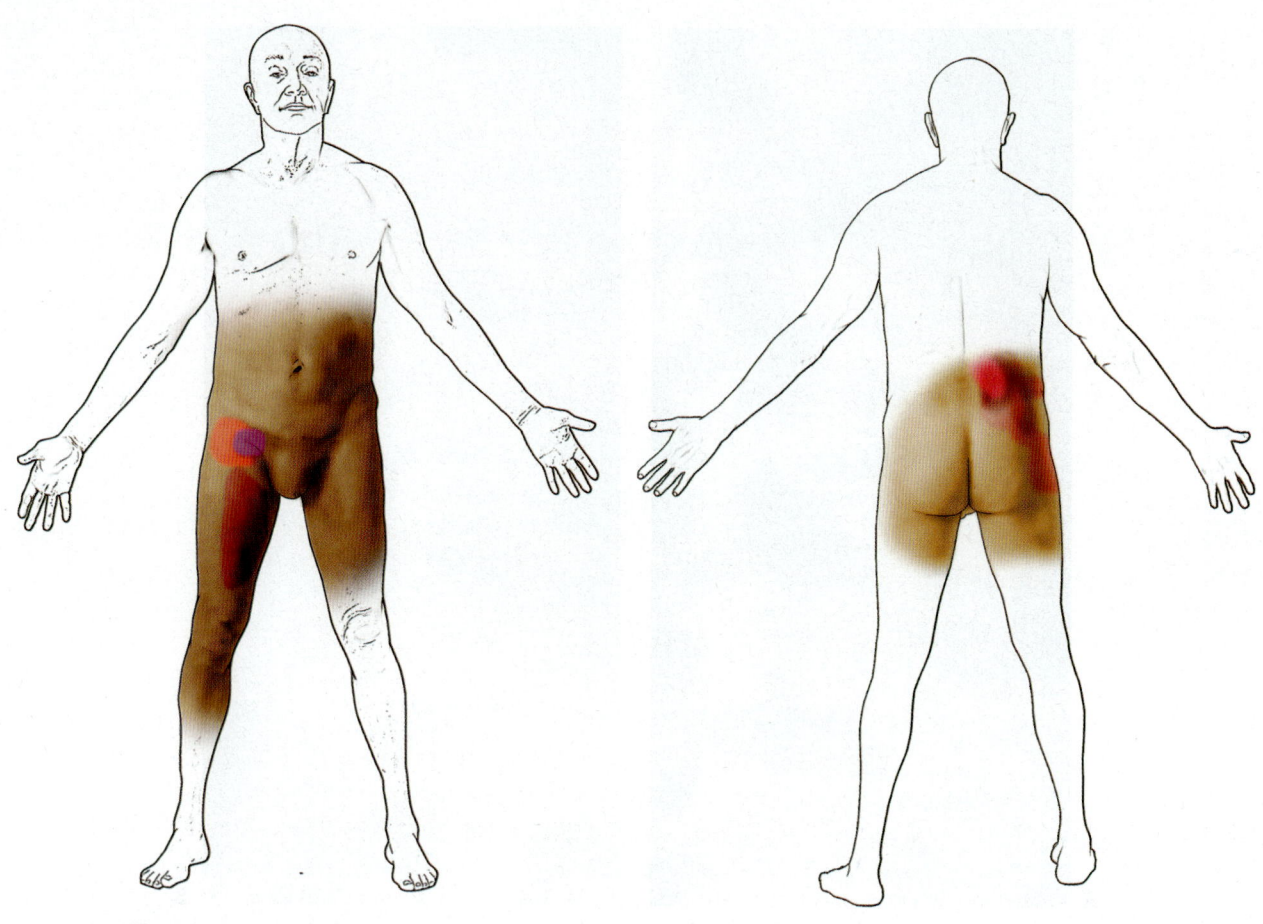

**FIGURE 96.2.** Distribution of pain emanating from the lumbar facet joints.

nerve roots, which suggests that this procedure should only be performed by those well versed in the regional anatomy and skilled at ultrasound-guided interventional pain management procedures. Trauma to the exiting lumbar nerve roots and spinal cord can be avoided if careful attention is paid to the regional anatomy and if the clinician immediately stops advancing the needle should the patient experience any significant pain during needle placement. Inadvertent subarachnoid and subdural injection, although rare, can occur even in the best of hands. Failure to recognize an unintentional dural or subdural injection with its resultant immediate total spinal anesthesia with associated loss of consciousness, hypotension, and apnea can be disastrous if not immediately recognized and treated.

Although uncommon, infection in the lumbar neuroaxis remains an ever-present possibility, especially in the immunocompromised acquired immune deficiency syndrome or cancer patient, and should be considered in any patient with fever and the onset of neurologic symptomatology after undergoing an intra-articular facet block. Early detection and treatment of infection is crucial to avoid potentially life-threatening sequelae, and urgent computerized tomography and/or magnetic resonance imaging should be obtained in any patient suspected of having an infection in this anatomic region. Emergent surgical drainage to avoid spread to the epidural space with the possibility of spinal cord compression and irreversible neurologic deficit is often required.

## CLINICAL PEARLS

The key to performing successful ultrasound-guided cervical neuraxial blocks is the proper identification of the sonographic anatomy. The two-step technique presented above will simplify this process and improve the ability to perform lumbar medial branch block. Any significant pain or sudden increase in resistance during injection when performing ultrasound-guided lumbar medial branch block suggests incorrect needle placement, and one should stop injecting immediately and reassess the position of the needle. Because pain is an important indication of improper needle placement, the practitioner should avoid the use of excessive sedation when performing this technique.

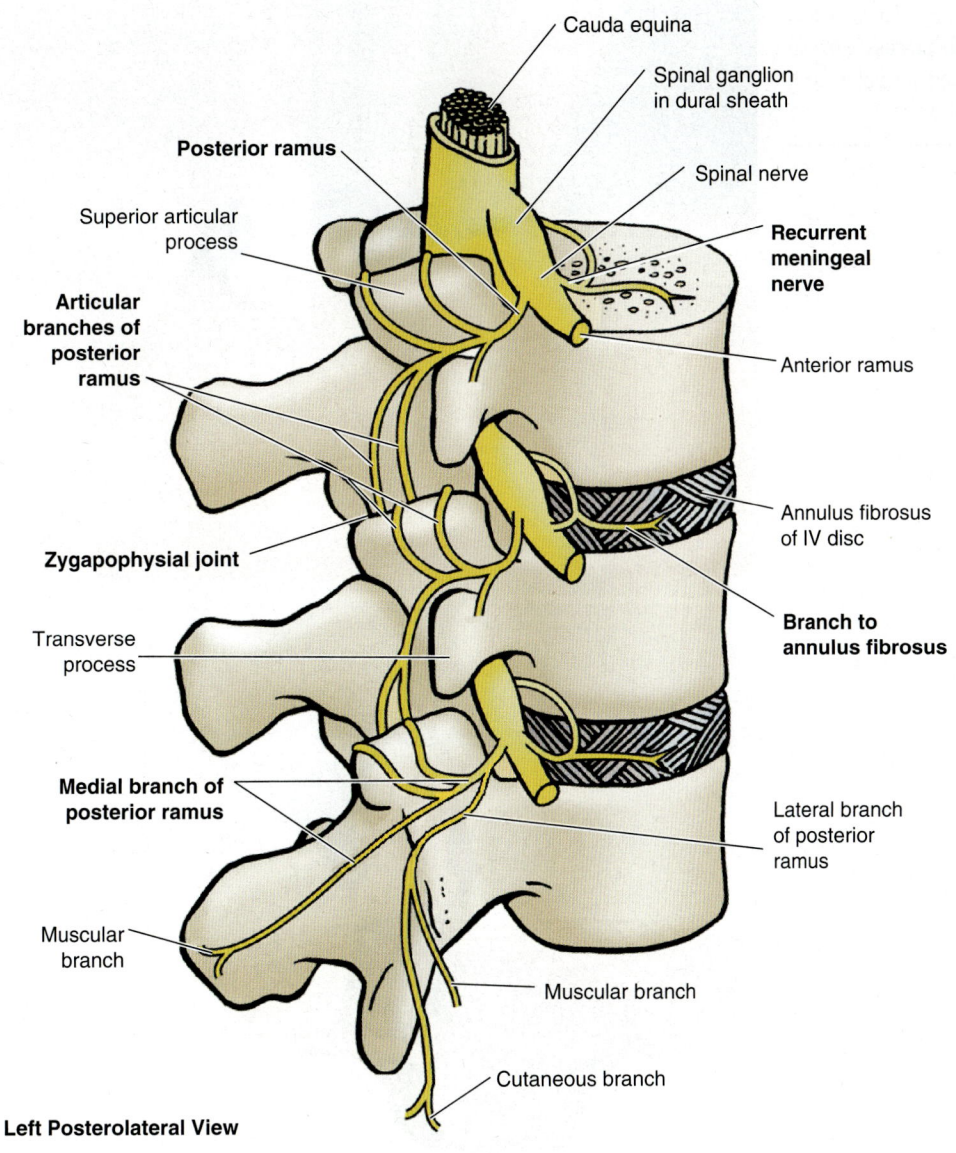

**FIGURE 96.3.** The anatomy and innervation of the lumbar facet joints.

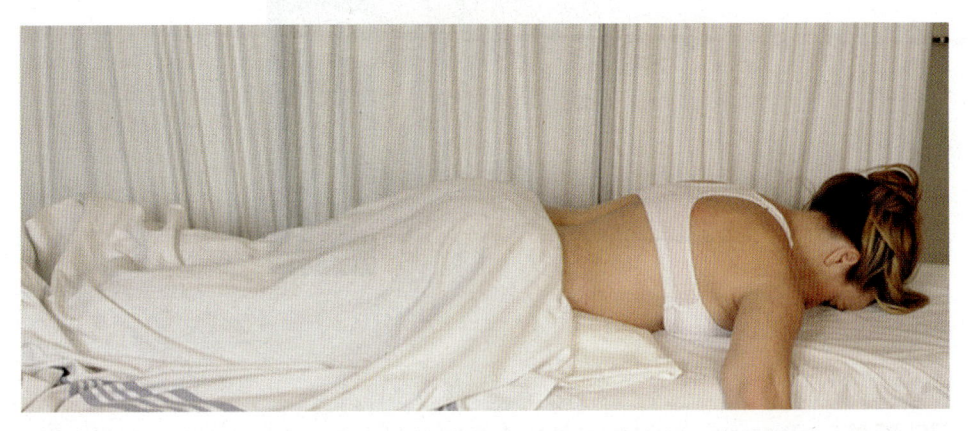

**FIGURE 96.4.** Proper patient position for ultrasound-guided lumbar medial branch block.

**FIGURE 96.5.** Placement of the ultrasound transducer in the longitudinal plane to obtain a paramedian sagittal transverse process view to block the left-sided medial branch nerves (Step One).

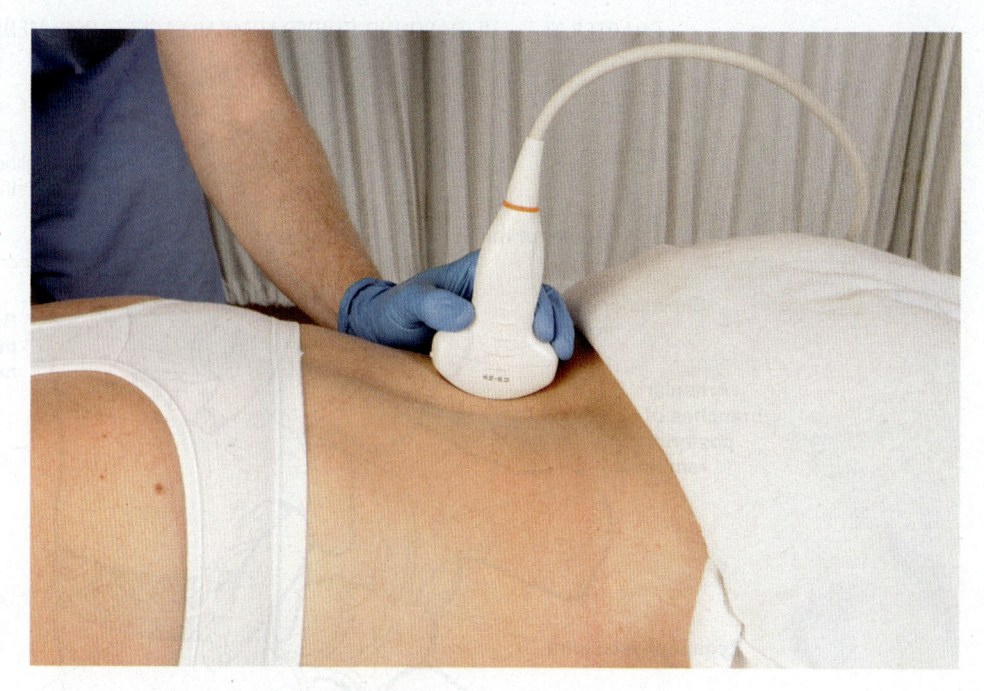

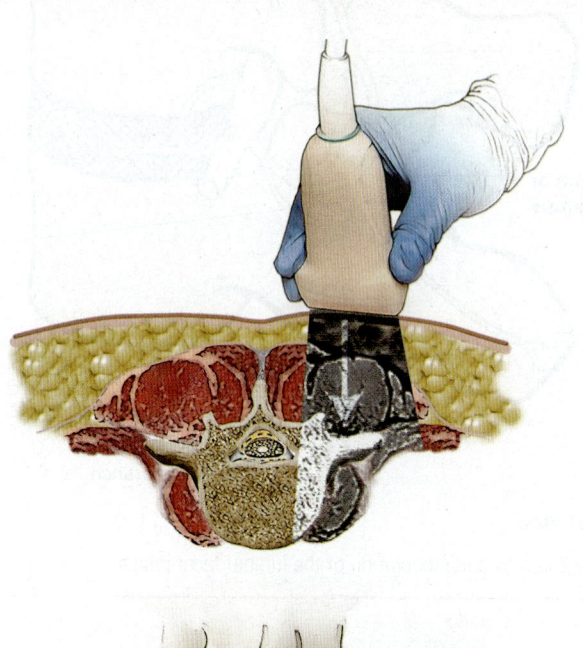

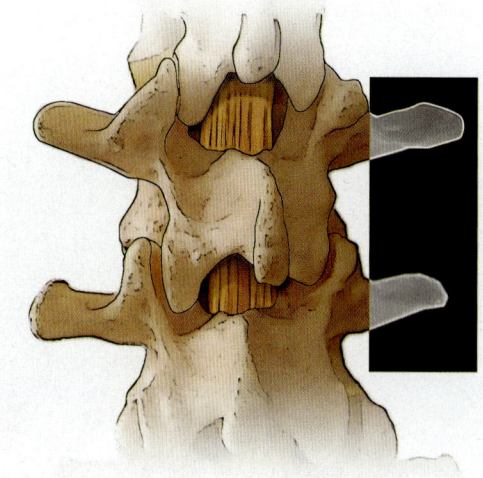

**FIGURE 96.6.** The anatomic orientation of the longitudinally placed curvilinear ultrasound transducer for the paramedian sagittal transverse process view (Step One).

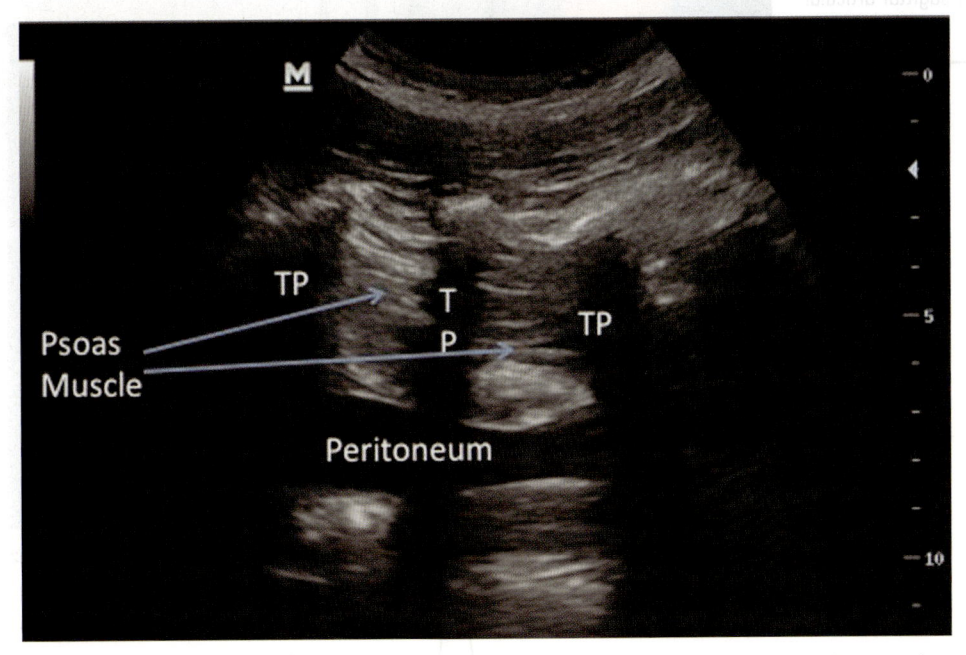

**FIGURE 96.7.** Longitudinal ultrasound image demonstrating successive transverse processes when performing the paramedian sagittal transverse process view (Step One). This classic image is named the "trident sign."

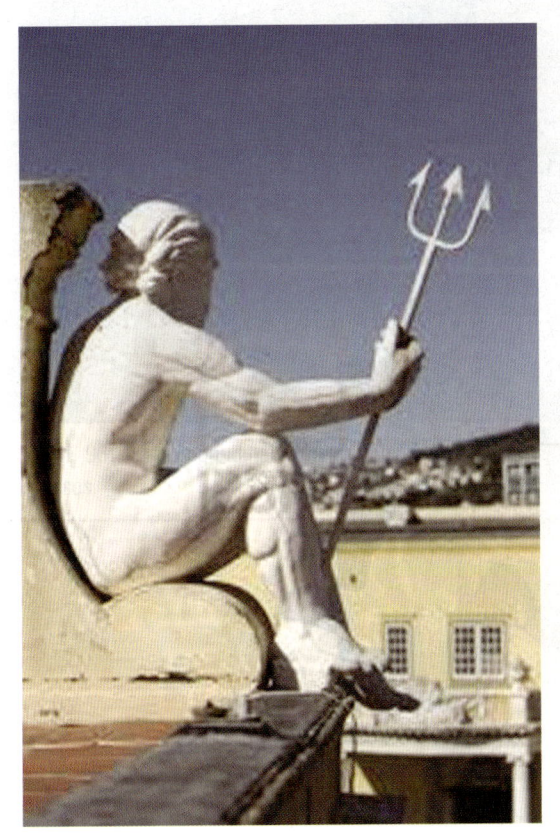

**FIGURE 96.8.** The trident sign is named after Neptune's trident, which according to Roman mythology had the power to conjure water and cause tsunamis and earthquakes.

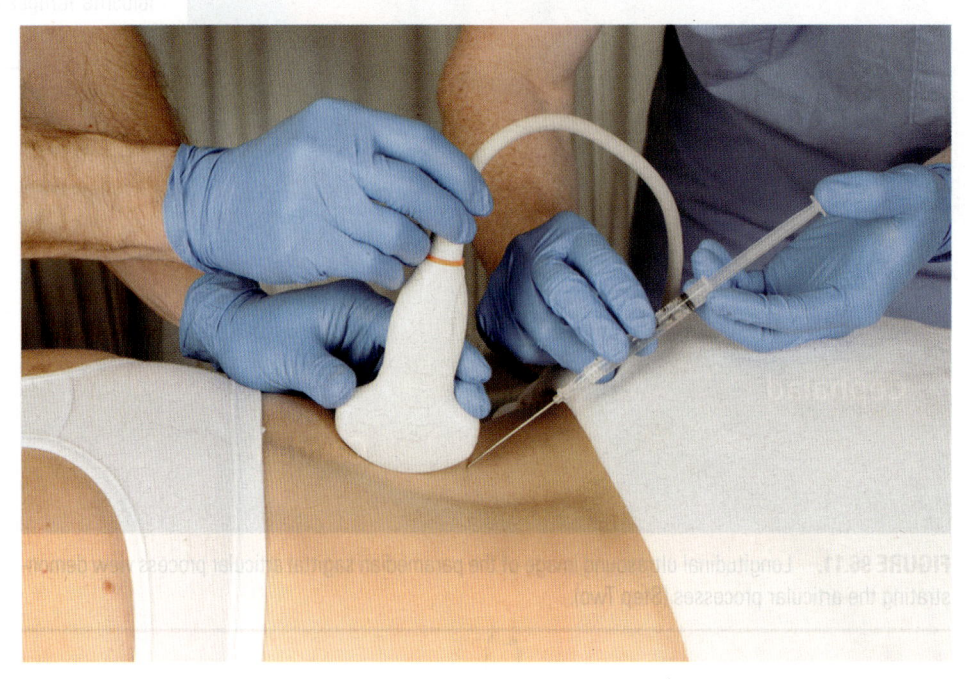

**FIGURE 96.13.** Proper in-plane needle position for ultrasound lumbar intra-articular facet injection.

## SUGGESTED READINGS

Siegenthaler A, Curatolo M. Ultrasound guided spinal procedures. *Eur J Pain* 2011;5(2):495–497.

Waldman SD. Lumbar facet block: medial branch approach. In: *Atlas of Interventional Pain Management*. 3rd ed. Philadelphia, PA: Saunders Elsevier; 2011:383–389.

Waldman SD, Campbell R. Anatomy: special imaging considerations of the lumbar spine. In: *Imaging of Pain*. Philadelphia, PA: Saunders Elsevier; 2009:109–110.

Waldman SD. Lumbar facet block. In: *Pain Review*. Philadelphia, PA: Saunders Elsevier; 2009:520–522.

Yamauchi M. Ultrasound-guided neuraxial block. *Trends Anaesth Crit Care* 2012;2(5):234–243.

# CHAPTER 97

# Ultrasound-Guided Lumbar Facet Block: Intra-articular Technique

## CLINICAL PERSPECTIVES

Ultrasound-guided lumbar intra-articular facet block is utilized in a variety of clinical scenarios as a diagnostic and therapeutic maneuver in painful conditions involving the lumbar facet joint. As a diagnostic tool, ultrasound-guided lumbar intra-articular facet block allows accurate placement of the needle tip to determine if a specific facet joint is in fact subserving the patient's pain. In the acute pain setting, ultrasound-guided lumbar intra-articular facet block with local anesthetics and/or steroids may be used to palliate acute low back pain emergencies while waiting for pharmacologic methods to become effective. This technique has great clinical utility when managing acute posttrauma pain. This technique is also useful in the treatment arthritis-related facet joint pain (Fig. 97.1). Clinically, pain emanating from the lumbar facet joints is perceived in the paraspinous region and radiates in a nondermatomal pattern (Fig. 97.2).

## CLINICALLY RELEVANT ANATOMY

The lumbar facet joints are formed by the articulations of the superior and inferior articular facets of adjacent lumbar vertebrae (Fig. 97.3). The lumbar facet joints are lined with synovium and possess a dense joint capsule. The joint capsule is richly innervated and explains why the facet joint can serve as a nidus for lumbar pain when it becomes damaged or inflamed. The lumbar joint is susceptible to degenerative arthritis and is frequently affected by the collagen vascular diseases. The joint is frequently injured in acceleration/deceleration injuries resulting in intra-articular hemorrhage with subsequent inflammation and development of adhesions.

Each lumbar facet joint receives innervation from two spinal levels, receiving fibers from the dorsal ramus at the same level as the vertebra as well as fibers from the dorsal ramus of the vertebra above (see Fig. 97.3). This fact has clinical import in that it provides an explanation for the ill-defined nature of facet-mediated pain and explains why the dorsal nerve from the vertebra above the offending level must often also be blocked to provide the patient with complete pain relief.

## ULTRASOUND-GUIDED TECHNIQUE

Ultrasound-guided lumbar intra-articular facet block can be carried out by placing the patient in the prone position with a thin pillow placed beneath the abdomen to slightly flex the lumbar spine (Fig. 97.4). A total of 1 mL of local anesthetic is drawn up in a 5-mL sterile syringe for each medial branch to be blocked. If the painful condition being treated is thought to have an inflammatory component, 40 to 80 mg of depot steroid is added to the local anesthetic.

To perform ultrasound-guided lumbar intra-articular facet, a two-step process is used. This two-step process allows the clinician to quickly identify critical anatomic structures while at the same time maintaining a transducer position that allows a safe and easy placement of needles in proximity to the affected lumbar medial branch nerves.

### Step One: Obtain the Paramedian Sagittal Transverse Process View

Step One is to obtain a paramedian sagittal transverse process view by placing the 2- to 5-MHz low-frequency curvilinear probe in the longitudinal plane 3 to 4 cm lateral to the right side of the middle of the spinous processes at the level to be blocked for blockade of the right lumbar medial branch nerves and 3 to 4 cm lateral to the left side of the middle of the spinous processes at the level to be blocked for left-sided medial branch nerves (Figs. 97.5 and 97.6). An initial depth setting of 7 to 8 cm will work for most patients. An ultrasound survey is taken, and the transducer is slowly moved medially and laterally until successive transverse processes are visualized. The transverse processes of the lumbar spine will appear as hyperechoic domes with sausage-like acoustic shadows beneath them (Fig. 97.7). This classic appearance of successive transverse processes viewed in the longitudinal plane has been named the "trident sign" after Neptune's trident (Fig. 97.8).

### Step Two: Obtain the Paramedian Sagittal Articular Process View

After the transverse processes are identified in the paramedian sagittal transverse process view, the ultrasound transducer is slowly slid toward the midline until the superior and

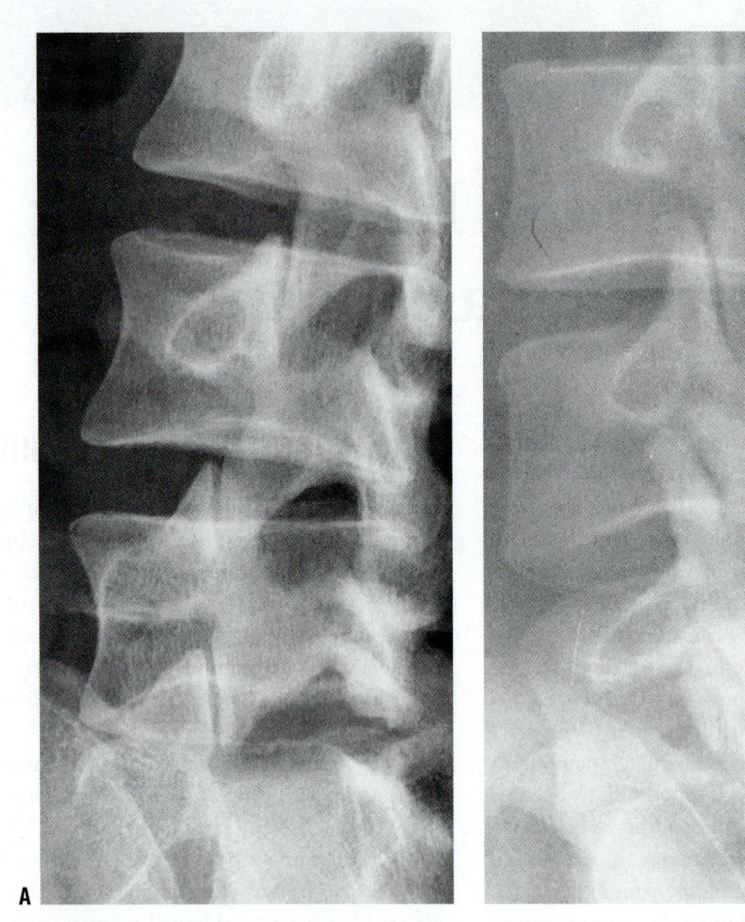

**FIGURE 97.1.** Facet arthrosis: Oblique lumbar. **A:** Normal lumbar facets. Note that the joint spaces are smooth and uniform; the articular processes are of a triangular shape. **B:** Lumbar facet arthrosis. Observe that the joint spaces are narrowed and the articular processes sclerotic and altered in shape owing to osteophytes. (Reused from Yochum TR, Rowe LJ. *Essentials of Skeletal Radiology*. 3rd ed. Philadelphia, PA: Lippincott Williams & Wilkins; 2005:971, with permission.)

inferior articular facets are visualized (Step Two) (Figs. 97.9 and 97.10). In longitudinal paramedian ultrasound articular process view, the superior and inferior articular facets will appear as successive hyperechoic hills and valleys, with the space within the center in each hill representing a facet joint (Figs. 97.11 and 97.12). The junction between the superior articular facet and the transverse process is then identified as the target for needle tip placement (see Fig. 97.11). When the junction between the superior articular facet and the transverse process of interest is identified, the skin beneath and below the ultrasound transducer is prepped with antiseptic solution, and a 3½-inch, 22-gauge styletted needle is inserted through the skin just below the inferior aspect of the longitudinally placed ultrasound transducer utilizing an in-plane approach (Fig. 97.13). While an assistant holds and adjusts the ultrasound transducer, the clinician advances the needle under real-time ultrasound guidance in inferior to superior trajectory until the needle tip rests within the joint space. After gentle aspiration, 1 mL of solution is injected. The needle is removed and pressure is placed on the injection site to avoid hematoma formation.

## COMPLICATIONS

Because of potential hematogenous spread via the valveless epidural veins of the lumbar epidural space, sepsis and local infection at the injection site represent absolute contraindications to ultrasound-guided lumbar intra-articular facet block as do anticoagulation and coagulopathy. The lumbar facet joints are in close proximity to the epidural, subdural, and subarachnoid space and spinal cord as well as the exiting spinal nerve roots, which suggests that this procedure should only be performed by those well versed in the regional

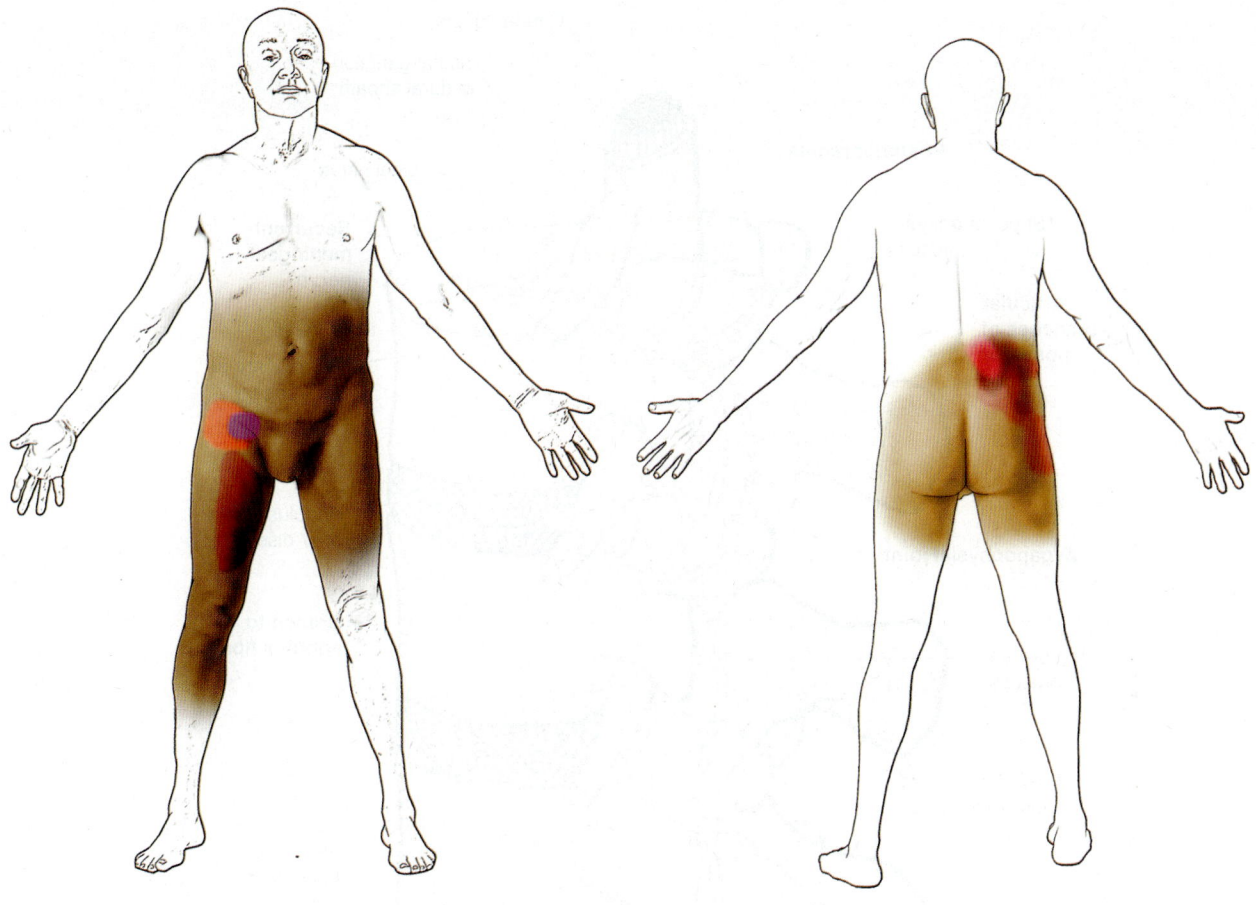

**FIGURE 97.2.** Distribution of pain emanating from the lumbar facet joints.

anatomy and skilled at ultrasound-guided interventional pain management procedures. Trauma to the exiting lumbar nerve roots and spinal cord can be avoided if careful attention is paid to the regional anatomy and if the clinician immediately stops advancing the needle should the patient experience any significant pain during needle placement. Inadvertent subarachnoid and subdural injection, although rare, can occur even in the best of hands. Failure to recognize an unintentional dural or subdural injection with its resultant immediate total spinal anesthesia with associated loss of consciousness, hypotension, and apnea can be disastrous if not immediately recognized and treated.

Although uncommon, infection in the lumbar neuraxis remains an ever-present possibility, especially in the immunocompromised AIDS or cancer patient, and should be considered in any patient with fever and the onset of neurologic symptomatology after undergoing an intra-articular facet block. Early detection and treatment of infection is crucial to avoid potentially life-threatening sequelae, and urgent computerized tomography and/or magnetic resonance imaging should be obtained in any patient suspected of having an infection in this anatomic region. Emergent surgical drainage to avoid spread to the epidural space with the possibility of spinal cord compression and irreversible neurologic deficit is often required.

## CLINICAL PEARLS

The key to performing successful ultrasound-guided cervical neuraxial blocks is the proper identification of the sonographic anatomy. The two-step technique presented above will simplify this process and improve the ability to perform lumbar intra-articular facet. Any significant pain or sudden increase in resistance during injection when performing ultrasound-guided lumbar intra-articular facet block suggests incorrect needle placement, and one should stop injecting immediately and reassess the position of the needle. Because pain is an important indication of improper needle placement, the practitioner should avoid the use of excessive sedation when performing this technique.

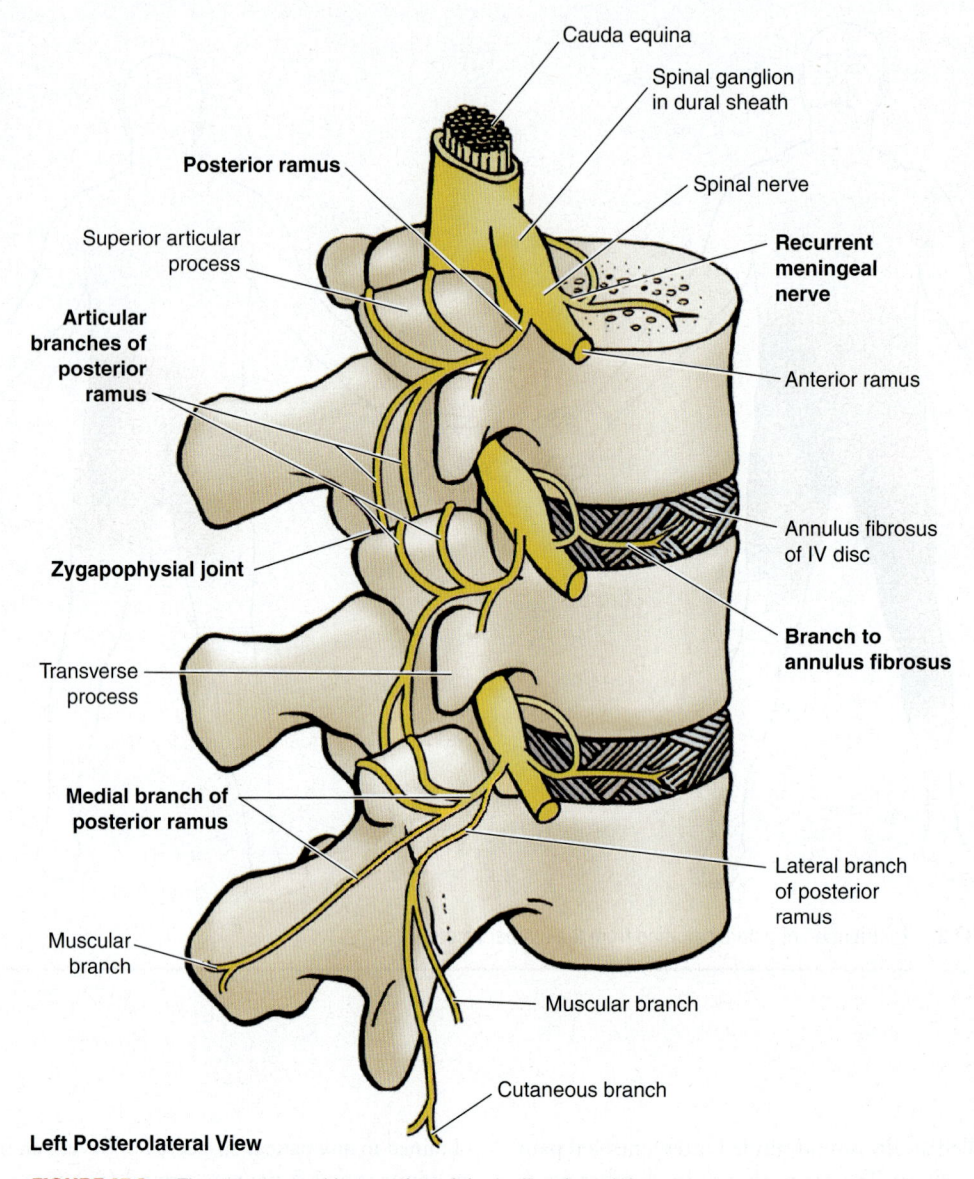

**FIGURE 97.3.** The anatomy and innervation of the lumbar facet joints.

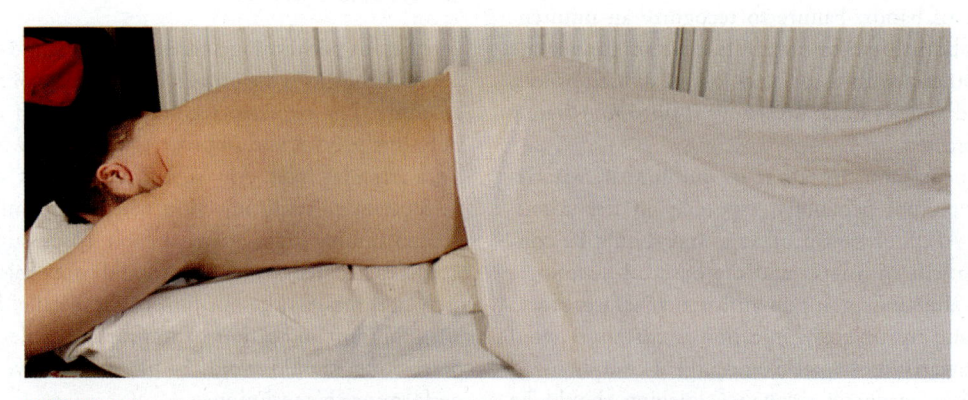

**FIGURE 97.4.** Proper patient position for ultrasound-guided lumbar intra-articular facet.

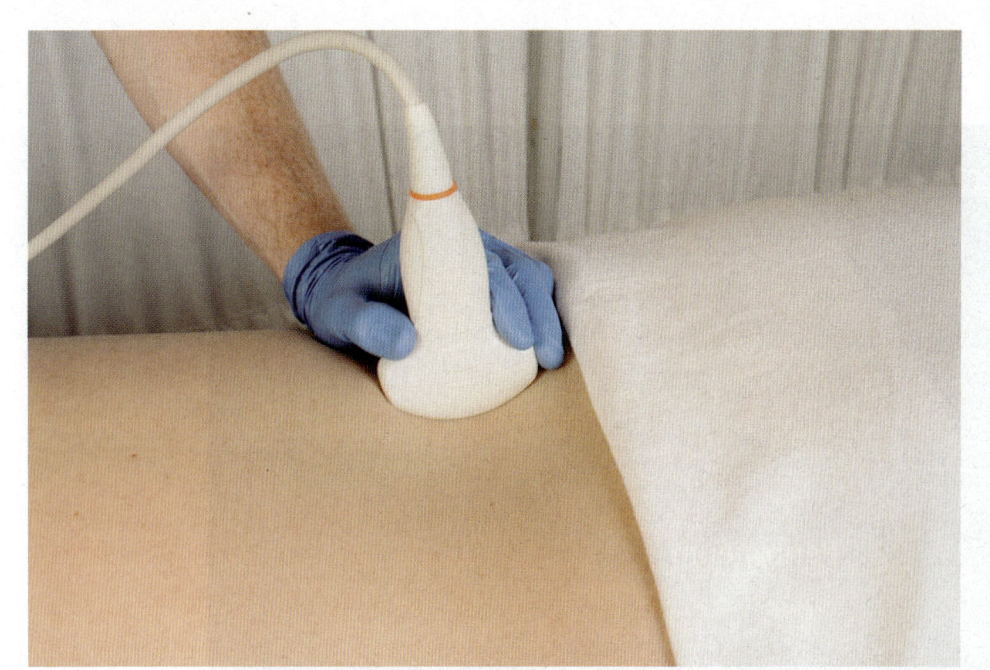

**FIGURE 97.5.** Placement of the ultrasound transducer in the longitudinal plane to obtain a paramedian sagittal transverse process view to perform intra-articular facet joint block (Step One).

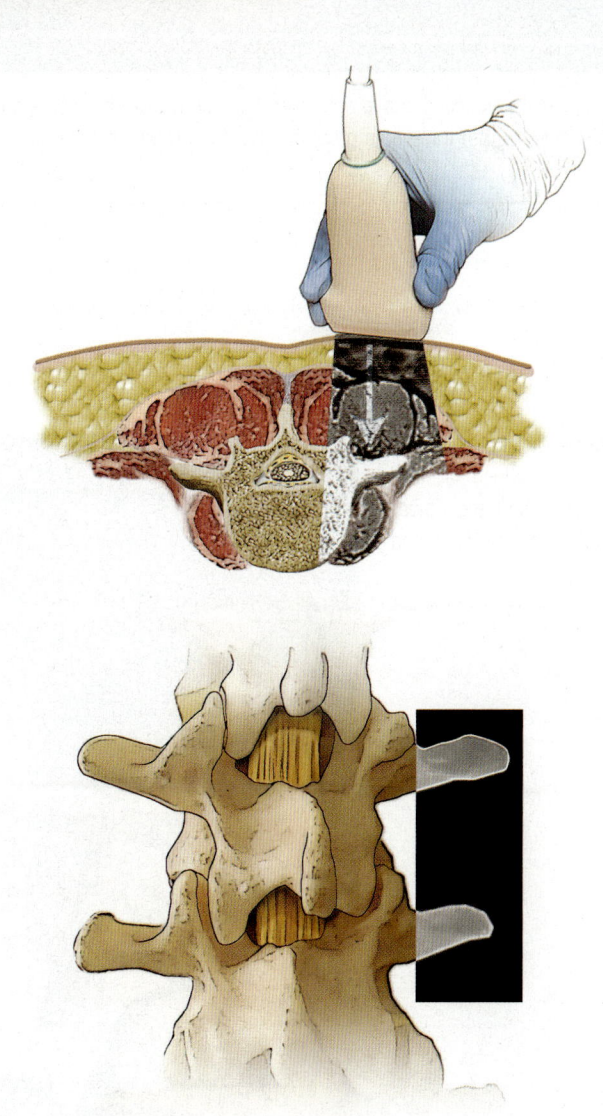

**FIGURE 97.6.** The anatomic orientation of the longitudinally placed curvilinear ultrasound transducer for the paramedian sagittal transverse process view (Step One).

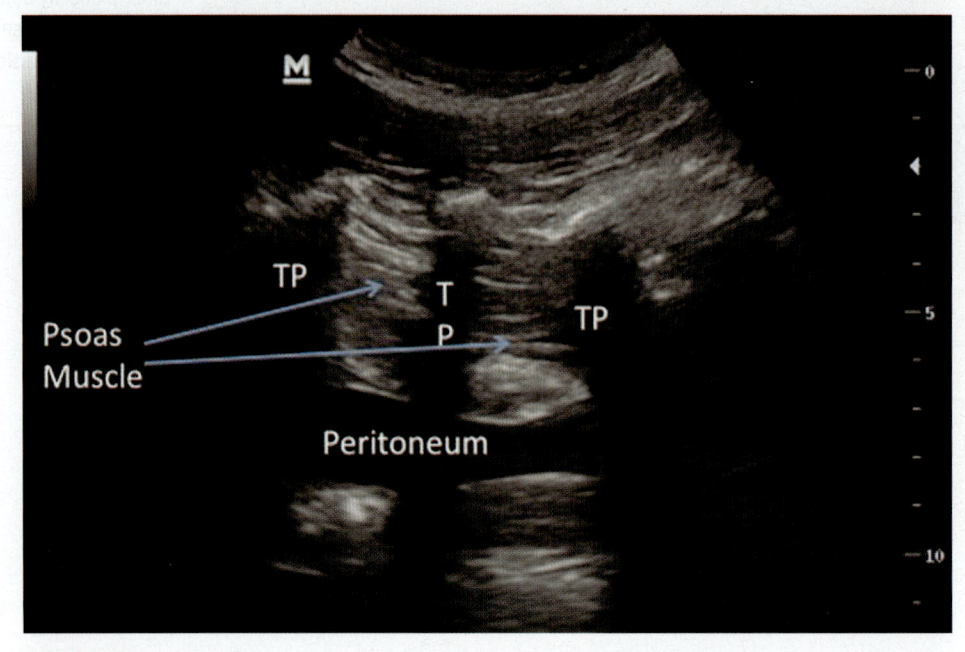

**FIGURE 97.7.** Longitudinal ultrasound image demonstrating successive transverse processes (TP) when performing the paramedian sagittal transverse process view (Step One). This classic image is named the "trident sign."

**FIGURE 97.8.** The trident sign is named after Neptune's trident, which according to Roman mythology had the power to conjure water and cause tsunamis and earthquakes.

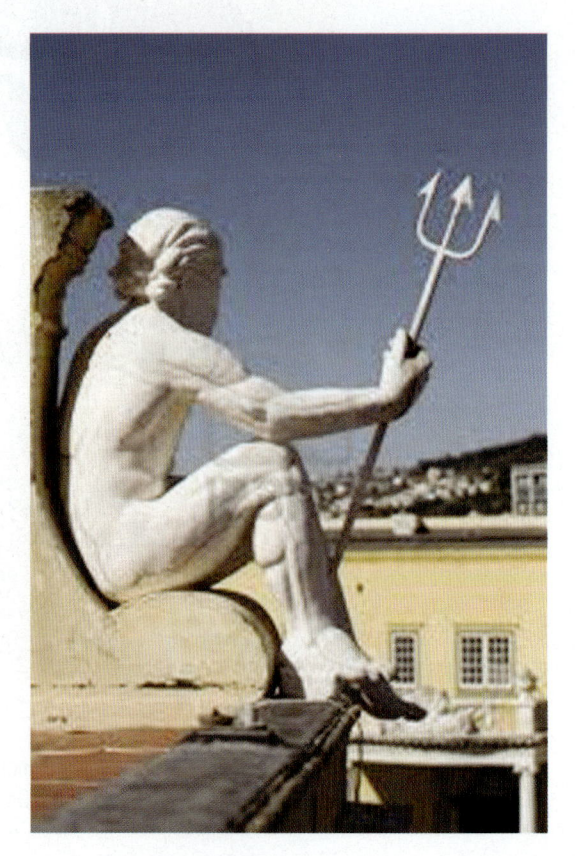

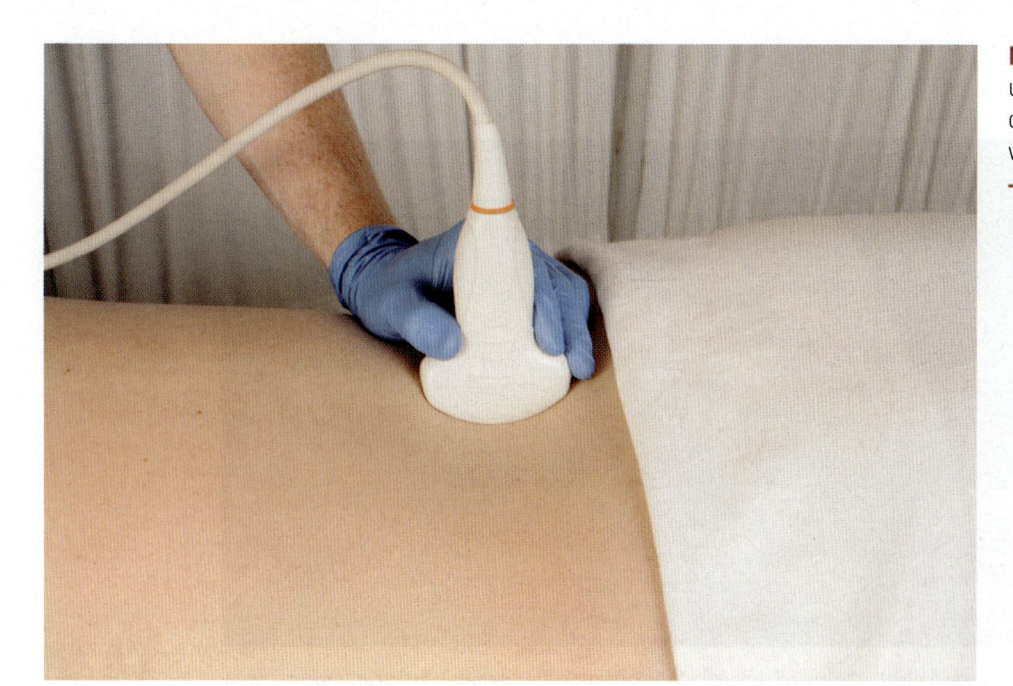

**FIGURE 97.9.** Proper longitudinal ultrasound transducer placement to obtain paramedian sagittal articular view (Step Two).

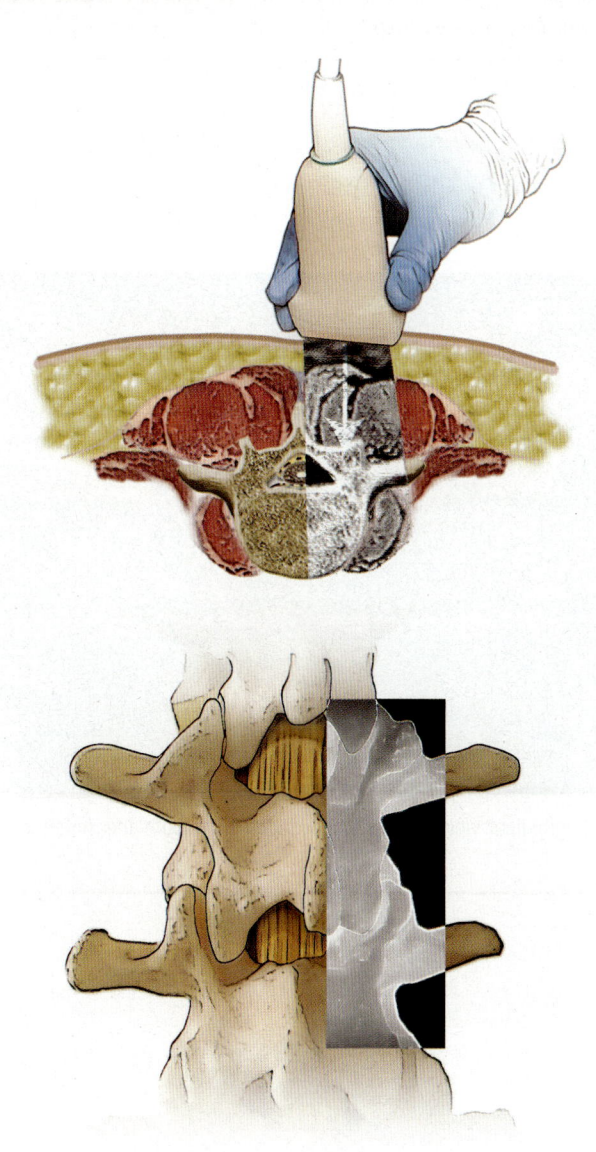

**FIGURE 97.10.** The anatomic orientation of the longitudinally placed curvilinear ultrasound transducer for the paramedian sagittal articular view (Step Two).

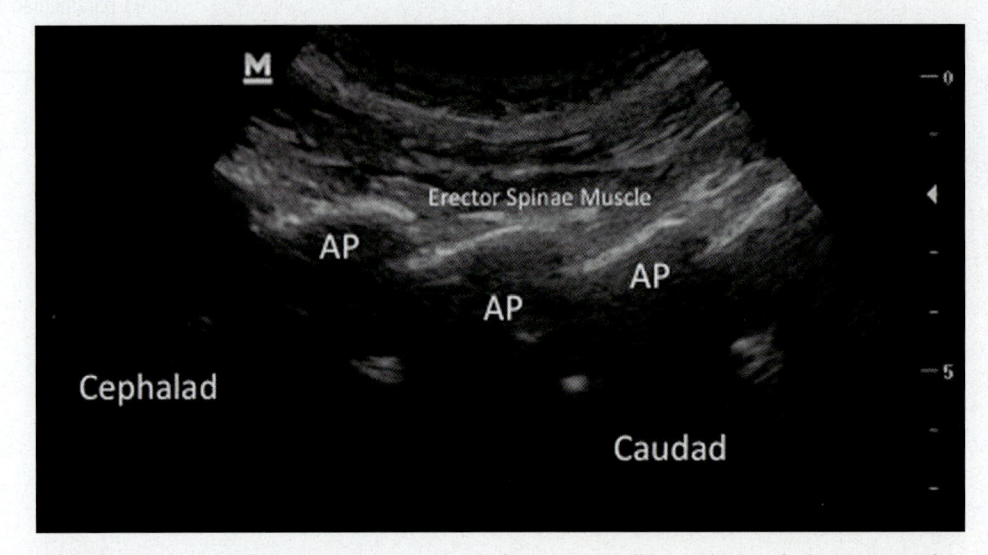

**FIGURE 97.11.** Longitudinal ultrasound image of the paramedian sagittal articular process view demonstrating the articular processes (Step Two).

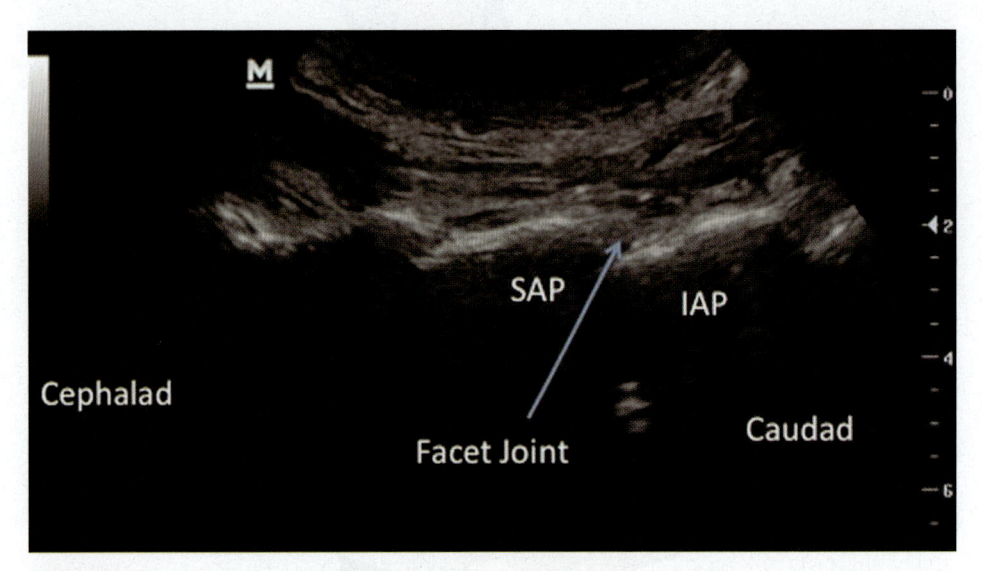

**FIGURE 97.12.** Longitudinal view of the lumbar facet joint. Note the superior and inferior articular processes.

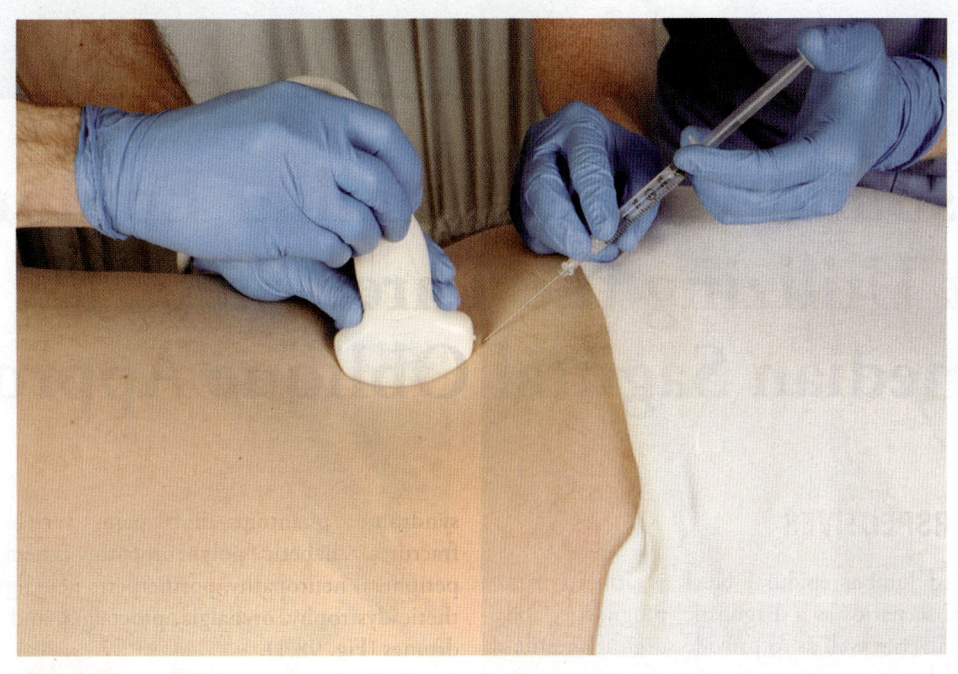

**FIGURE 97.13.** Proper in-plane needle position for ultrasound lumbar intra-articular facet block injection.

## SUGGESTED READINGS

Siegenthaler A, Curatolo M. Ultrasound guided spinal procedures. *Eur J Pain* 2011;5(2):495–497.

Waldman SD, Campbell R. Anatomy: special imaging considerations of the lumbar spine. In: *Imaging of Pain*. Philadelphia, PA: Saunders Elsevier; 2009:109–110.

Waldman SD. Lumbar facet block. In: *Pain Review*. Philadelphia, PA: Saunders Elsevier; 2009:520–522.

Waldman SD. Lumbar facet block: Intra-articular approach. In: *Atlas of Interventional Pain Management*. 3rd ed. Philadelphia, PA: Saunders Elsevier; 2011:395–396.

Yamauchi M. Ultrasound-guided neuraxial block. *Trends Anaesth Crit Care* 2012;2(5):234–243.

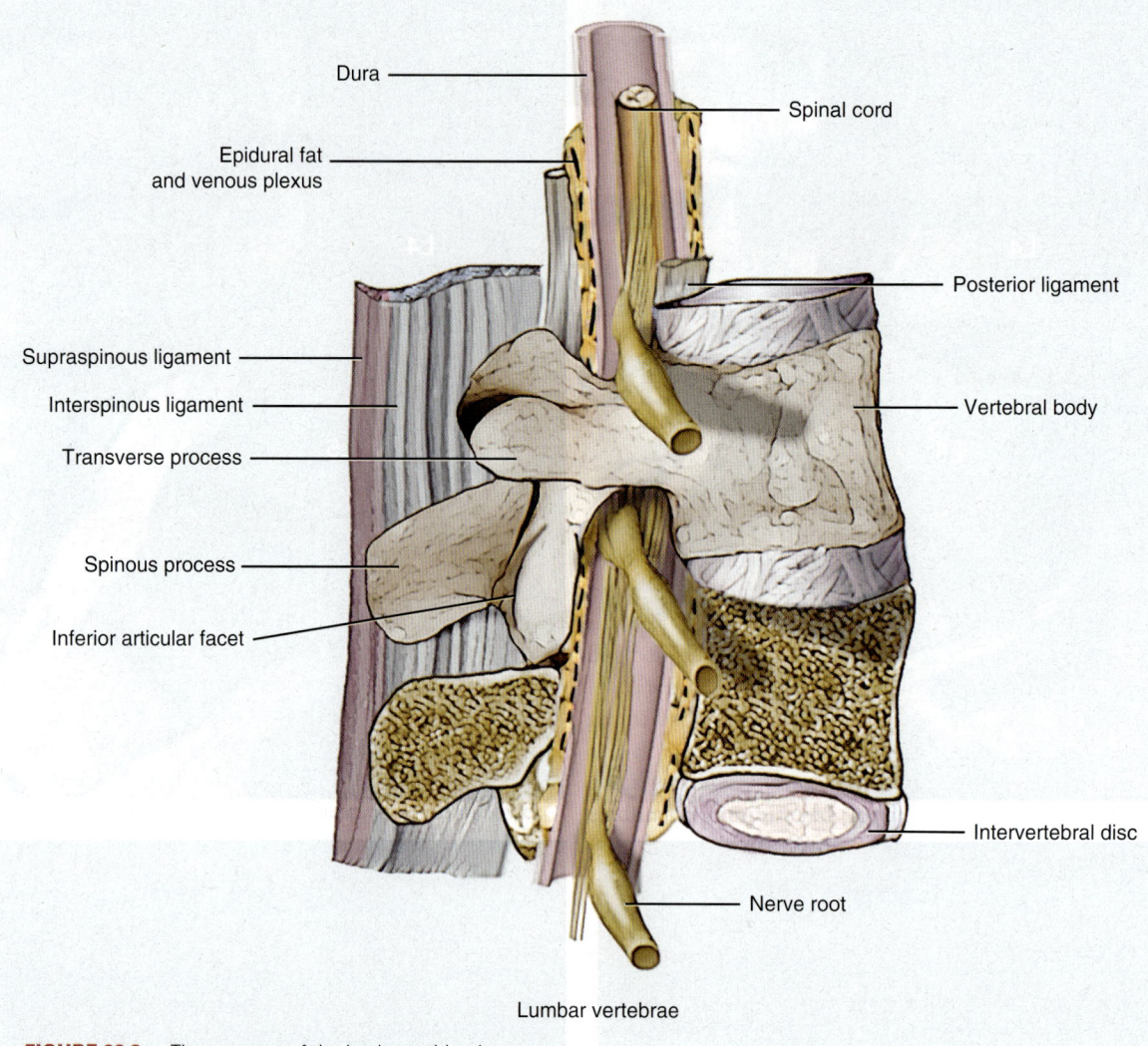

**FIGURE 98.2.** The anatomy of the lumbar epidural space.

anesthetic. To perform ultrasound-guided lumbar epidural block, a three-step process is used. Although this may seem cumbersome, the three-step process allows the clinician to quickly identify critical anatomic structures while at the same time maintaining a transducer position that allows a safe and easy placement of needles into the lumbar epidural space.

## Step One: Obtain the Paramedian Sagittal Transverse Process View

Step One is to obtain a paramedian sagittal transverse process view by placing the 2- to 5-MHz low-frequency curvilinear probe in the longitudinal plane 3 to 4 cm lateral to the right side of the middle of the spinous processes at the level to be blocked for the right-handed clinician and 3 to 4 cm to the later to the left side of the middle of the spinous processes at the level to be blocked for the left-handed clinician (Figs. 98.5 and 98.6). An ultrasound survey is taken and the transducer is slowly moved medially and laterally until successive transverse processes are visualized. The transverse processes of the lumbar spine will appear as hyperechoic domes with sausage-like acoustic shadows beneath them (Fig. 98.7). This classic appearance of successive transverse processes viewed in the longitudinal plane has been named the "trident sign" after Neptune's trident (Fig. 98.8).

## Step Two: Obtain the Paramedian Sagittal Articular Process View

After the transverse processes are identified in the paramedian sagittal transverse process view, the ultrasound transducer is slowly slid toward the midline until the superior and inferior articular facets are visualized (Step Two) (Figs. 98.9 and 98.10).

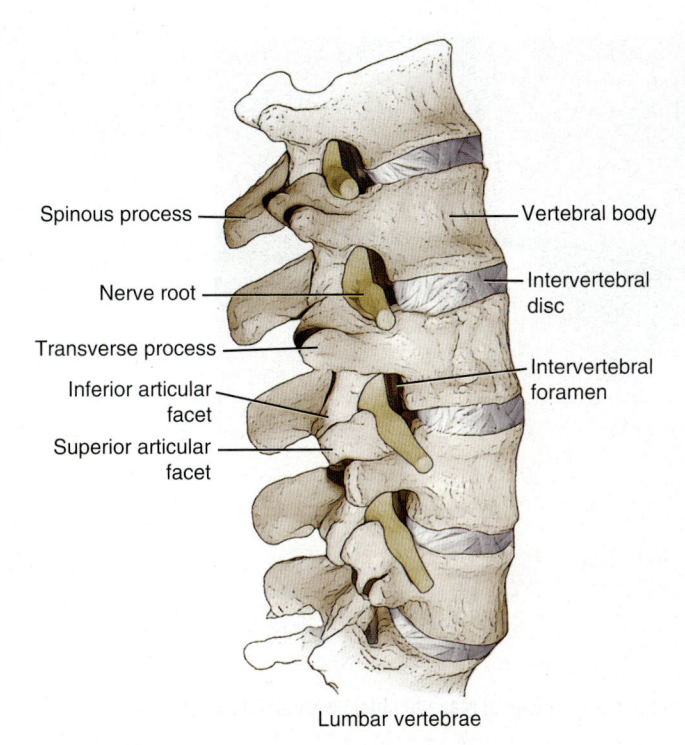

**FIGURE 98.3.** The lumbar spine, lateral view. (Reused from LifeART image. ©2013, Lippincott Williams & Wilkins. All rights reserved.)

In longitudinal paramedian ultrasound articular process view, the superior and inferior articular facets will appear as successive hyperechoic hills and valleys, with the gap in the center of each hill representing a facet joint (Fig. 98.11).

### Step Three: Obtain the Paramedian Sagittal Oblique View

After the articular processes are identified using the paramedian sagittal articular process view (Step Three), the longitudinally oriented ultrasound transducer is then slowly tilted to angle the ultrasound beam in a lateral to medial oblique trajectory toward the midline (Figs. 98.12 and 98.13). The lamina of successive lumbar vertebrae will appear as a series of hyperechoic curvilinear lines with an acoustic shadow beneath each one (Fig. 98.14). The interlaminar space will appear as gaps between each successive vertebra providing an acoustic window that will allow visualization of the ligamentum flavum, epidural space, and posterior dura. By making minor adjustments to the position of the ultrasound transducer, in some patients, the ligamentum flavum and posterior dura can be distinguished as two distinct hyperechoic linear structures with a hyperechoic epidural space in between (Fig. 98.15). In other patients, these structures simply appear as a single hyperechoic line, which is known as the posterior complex (Fig. 98.16).

After interlaminar space is identified, the skin is prepped with antiseptic solution, and a 3½-inch, 22-gauge needle suitable for epidural use is inserted through the skin at the middle of the lateral aspect of the longitudinally placed ultrasound transducer utilizing an out-of-plane approach (Fig. 98.17). While an assistant holds and adjusts the ultrasound transducer, the clinician advances the needle under real-time ultrasound guidance in an oblique lateral to medial trajectory using a loss of resistance technique until the needle tip rests within the epidural space. After gentle aspiration, 5 to 7 mL of solution is injected. The needle is removed and pressure is placed on the injection site to avoid hematoma formation.

## COMPLICATIONS

Because of potential hematogenous spread via the valveless epidural veins of the lumbar epidural space, sepsis and local infection at the injection site represent absolute contraindications to ultrasound-guided lumbar epidural block as do anticoagulation and coagulopathy. The epidural space is in close proximity to the subarachnoid space and spinal cord as well as the exiting spinal nerve roots, which suggests that this procedure should only be performed by those well versed in the regional anatomy and skilled at ultrasound-guided interventional pain

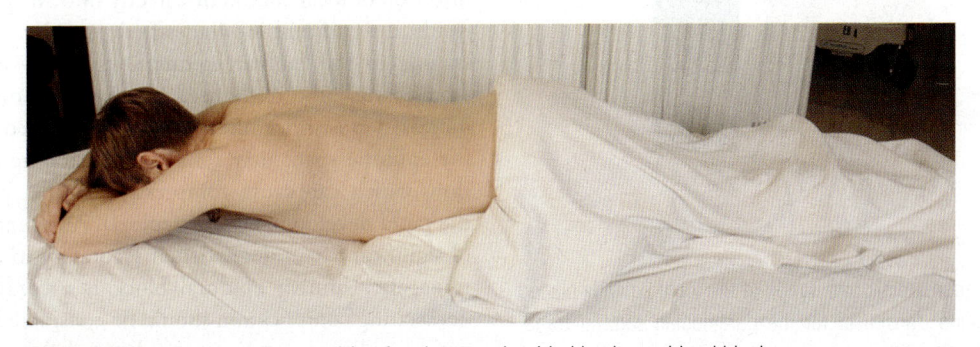

**FIGURE 98.4.** Proper patient position for ultrasound-guided lumbar epidural block.

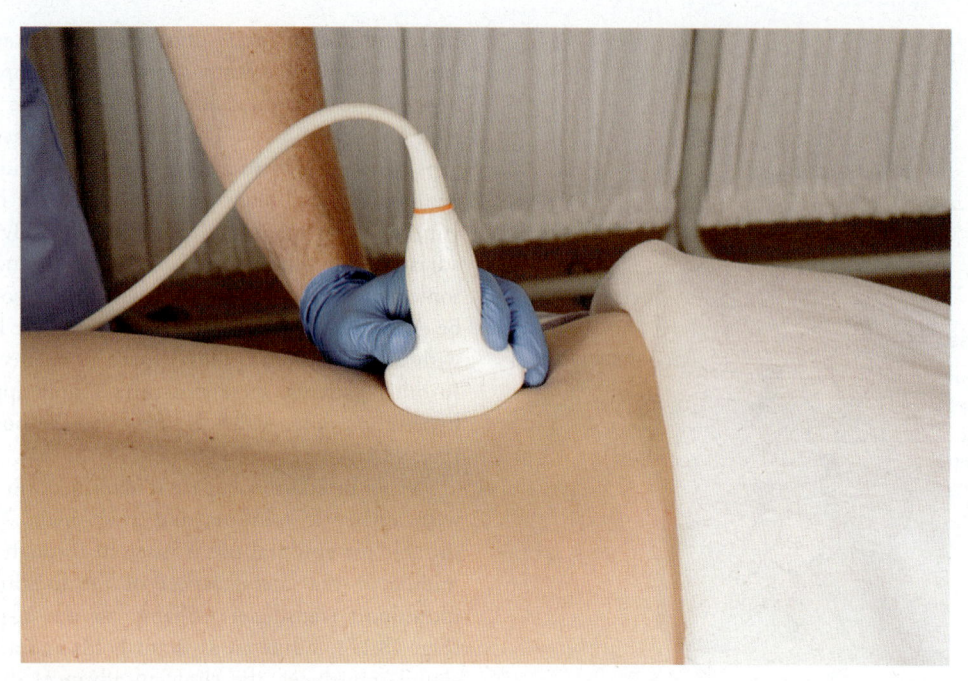

**FIGURE 98.5.** Placement of the ultrasound transducer in the longitudinal plane to obtain a paramedian sagittal transverse process view (Step One).

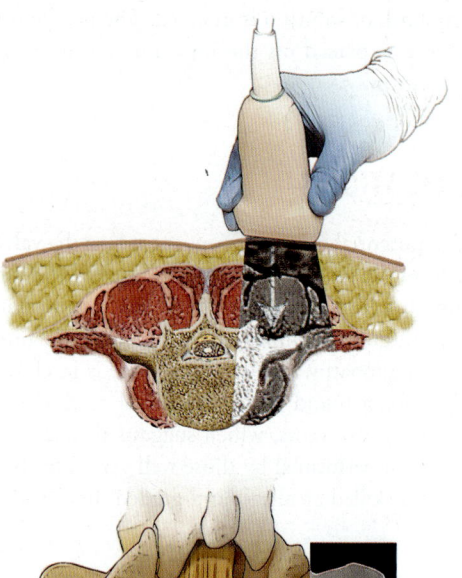

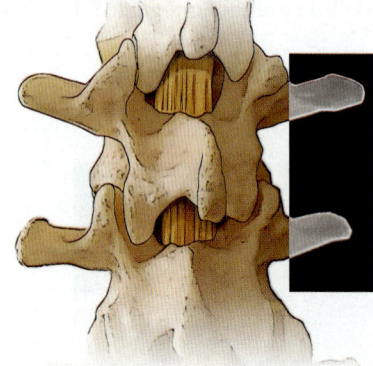

**FIGURE 98.6.** The anatomic orientation of the longitudinally placed curvilinear ultrasound transducer for the paramedian sagittal transverse process view (Step One).

management procedures. Trauma to the exiting lumbar nerve roots and spinal cord can be avoided if careful attention is paid to the regional anatomy and if the clinician immediately stops advancing the needle should the patient experience any significant pain during needle placement. Inadvertent subarachnoid and subdural injection, although rare, can occur even in the best of hands. Failure to recognize an unintentional dural or subdural injection with its resultant immediate total spinal anesthesia with associated loss of consciousness, hypotension, and apnea can be disastrous if not immediately recognized and treated.

The lumbar epidural space is highly vascular with large numbers of valveless epidural veins. The intravenous placement of the epidural needle occurs in ~0.5% to 1% of patients undergoing lumbar epidural anesthesia. This complication is increased in those patients with distended epidural veins, for example, the parturient and patients with large intra-abdominal tumor mass. If the misplacement is unrecognized, injection of local anesthetic directly into an epidural vein will result in significant local anesthetic toxicity. Needle-induced trauma to the lumbar epidural veins may cause bleeding, which is usually self-limited but has the potential to cause increased postprocedure pain. Uncontrolled bleeding into the epidural space may result in epidural hematoma formation, which can cause compression of the spinal cord with the rapid development of paraplegia. Although the incidence of significant neurologic deficit secondary to epidural hematoma after lumbar epidural block is exceedingly rare, this devastating complication should be considered in any patient with rapidly progressive neurologic deficits following this technique.

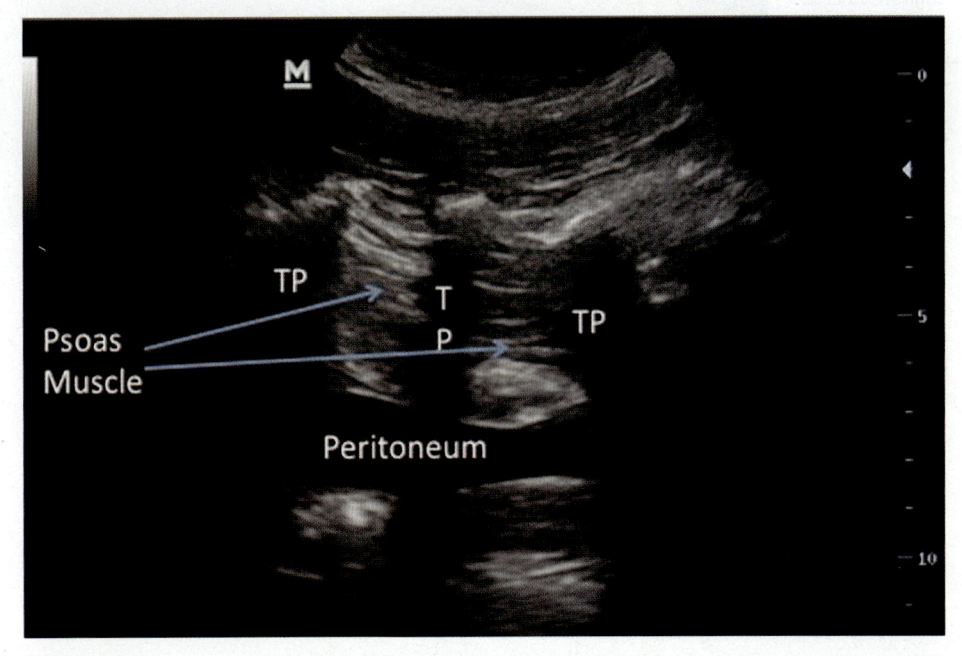

**FIGURE 98.7.** Longitudinal ultrasound image demonstrating successive transverse processes (TP) when performing the paramedian sagittal transverse process view (Step One). This classic image is named the "trident sign."

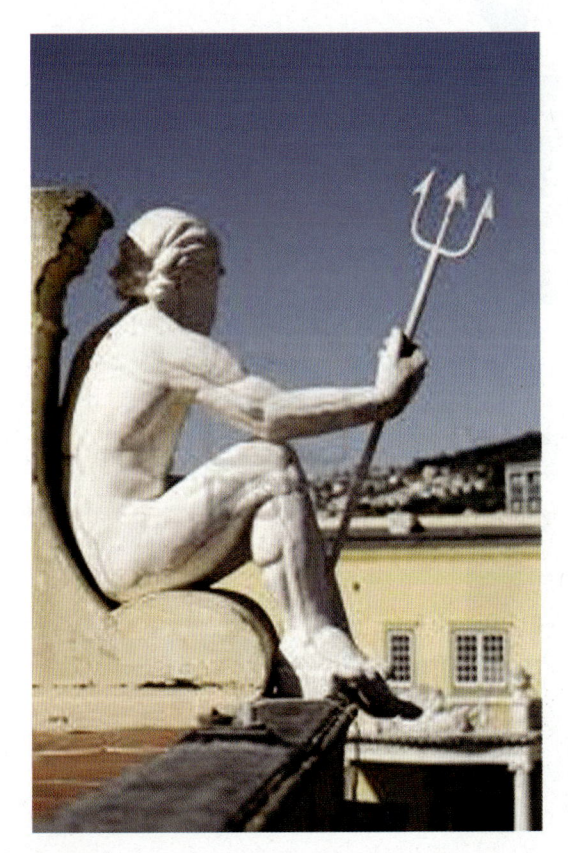

**FIGURE 98.8.** The trident sign is named after Neptune's trident, which according to Roman mythology had the power to conjure water and cause tsunamis and earthquakes.

Although uncommon, infection in the lumbar epidural space remains an ever-present possibility, especially in the immunocompromised AIDS or cancer patient, and should be considered in any patient with fever and the onset of neurologic symptomatology after undergoing an epidural block. Early detection and treatment of epidural infection is crucial to avoid potentially life-threatening sequelae, and urgent computerized tomography and/or magnetic resonance imaging should be obtained in any patient suspected of having an epidural abscess. Emergent surgical drainage to avoid spinal cord compression and irreversible neurologic deficit is often required.

## CLINICAL PEARLS

The key to performing successful ultrasound-guided lumbar neuraxial blocks is the proper identification of the sonographic anatomy. The three-step technique presented above will simplify this process and improve the ability to perform lumbar epidural block. Any significant pain or sudden increase in resistance during injection when performing ultrasound-guided lumbar epidural block utilizing the three-step paramedian sagittal oblique approach suggests incorrect needle placement, and one should stop injecting immediately and reassess the position of the needle. Because pain is an important indication of improper needle placement, the practitioner should avoid the use of excessive sedation when performing this technique.

**FIGURE 98.9.** Proper longitudinal ultrasound transducer placement to obtain paramedian sagittal articular view (Step Two).

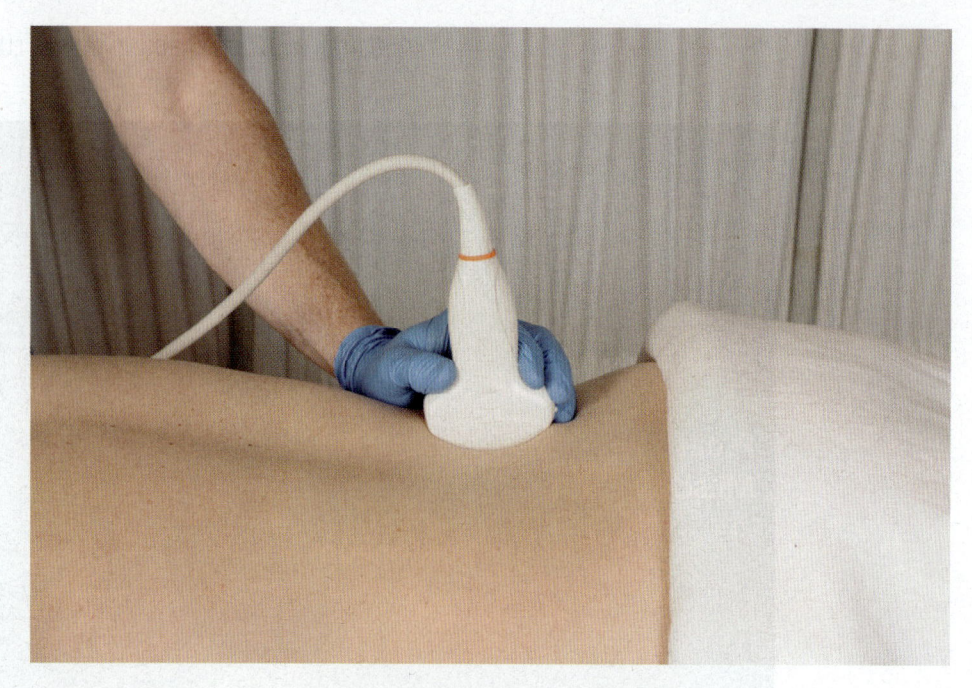

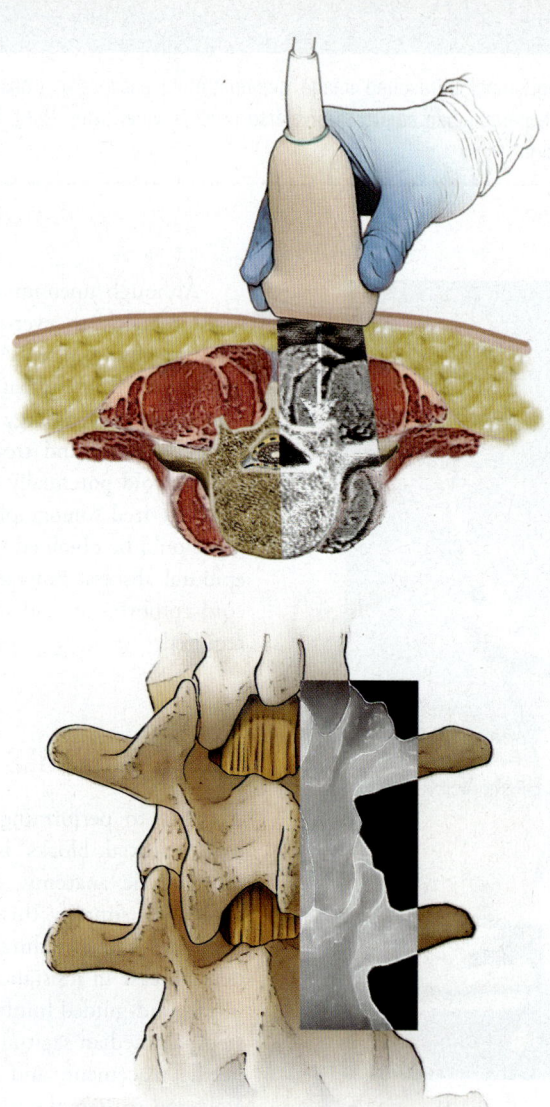

**FIGURE 98.10.** The anatomic orientation of the longitudinally placed curvilinear ultrasound transducer for the paramedian sagittal articular view (Step Two).

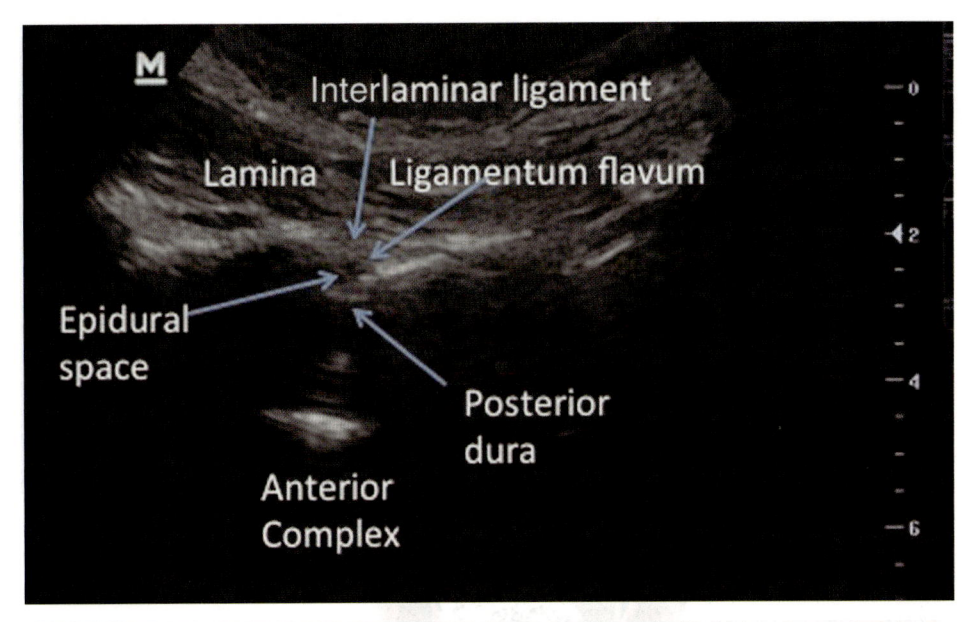

**FIGURE 98.11.** Longitudinal ultrasound image of the paramedian sagittal articular process view demonstrating the articular processes (Step Two).

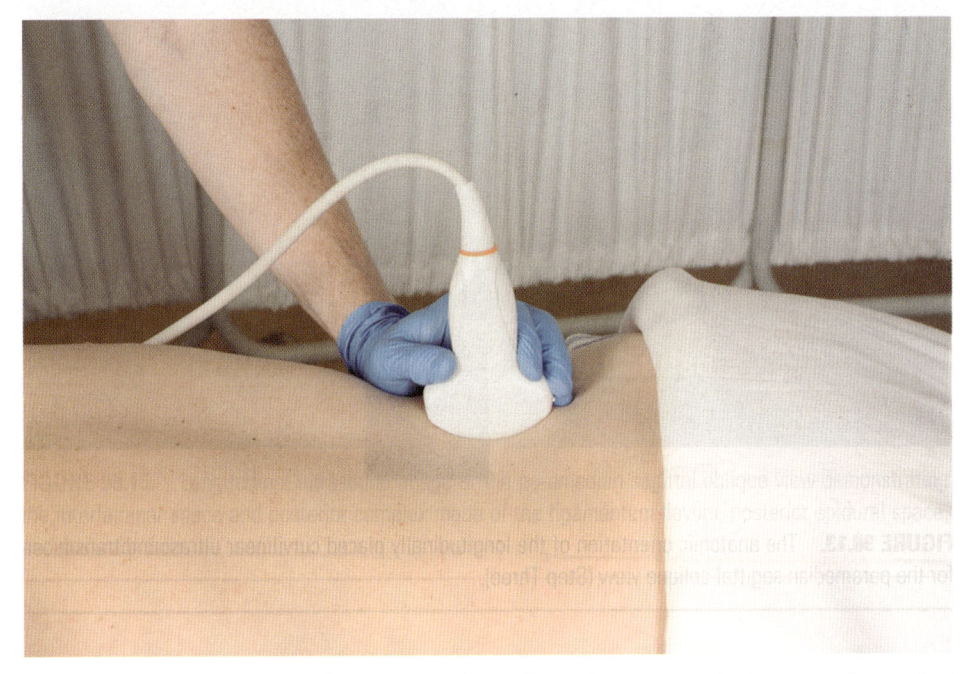

**FIGURE 98.12.** Proper longitudinal ultrasound transducer placement to obtain paramedian sagittal oblique view (Step Three).

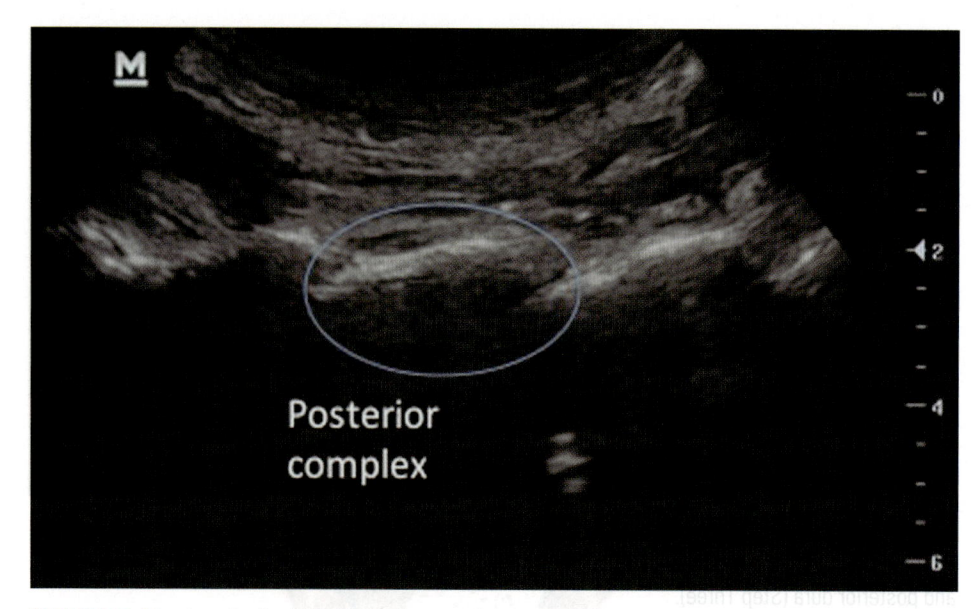

**FIGURE 98.16.** Longitudinal ultrasound image of the paramedian sagittal oblique view demonstrating the interlaminar space and posterior complex.

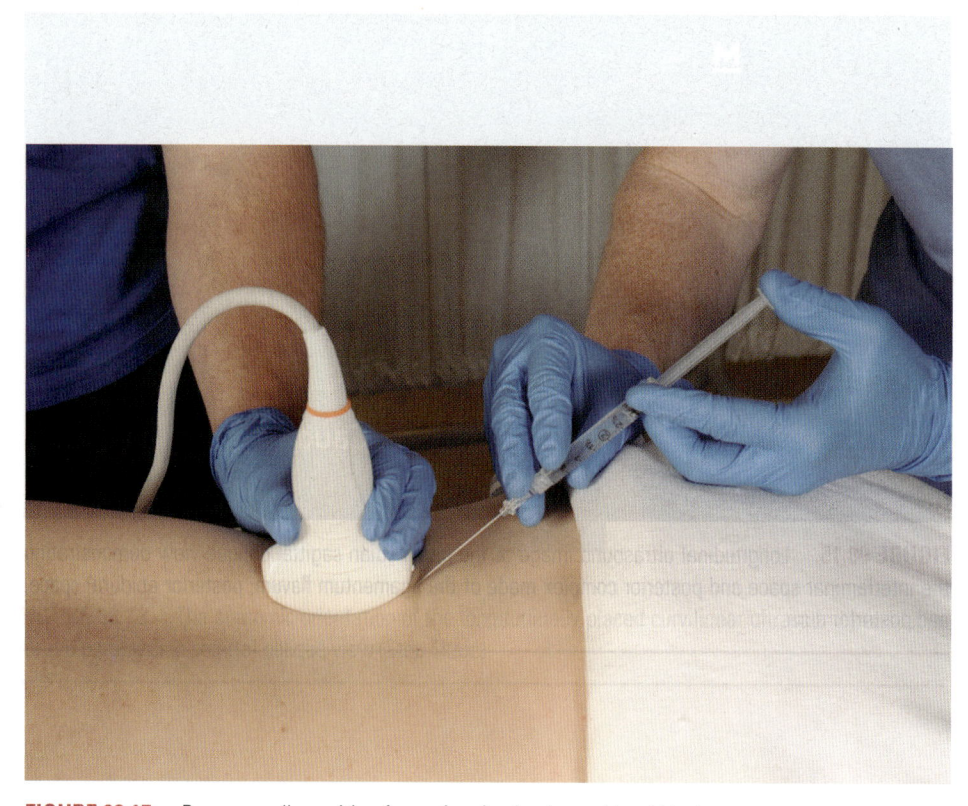

**FIGURE 98.17.** Proper needle position for performing lumbar epidural block.

## SUGGESTED READINGS

Shankar H, Zainer CM. Ultrasound guidance for epidural steroid injections. *Tech Reg Anesth Pain Manag* 2009;13(4):229–235.

Waldman SD. Lumbar epidural block. In: *Pain Review*. Philadelphia, PA: Saunders Elsevier; 2009:476–480.

Waldman SD. Lumbar epidural nerve block: paramedian approach. In: *Atlas of Interventional Pain Management*. 3rd ed. Philadelphia, PA: Saunders Elsevier; 2011:264–268.

Waldman SD, Campbell R. Anatomy: special imaging considerations of the lumbar spine. In: *Imaging of Pain*. Philadelphia, PA: Saunders Elsevier; 2009:67–68.

Yamauchi M. Ultrasound-guided neuraxial block. *Trends Anaesth Crit Care* 2012;2(5):234–243.

# CHAPTER 99

# Ultrasound-Guided Lumbar Selective Nerve Root Block

## CLINICAL PERSPECTIVES

Ultrasound-guided lumbar selective nerve root block is utilized most frequently as a diagnostic maneuver to confirm that a specific nerve root is in fact subserving a patient's pain symptomatology. In order for this technique to provide the clinician with accurate diagnostic information, the needle tip must be placed just outside the neural foramen adjacent to the target nerve root *without* entering the epidural, subdural, or subarachnoid space. If these conditions are met, selective spinal nerve root block is diagnostic to the specific targeted root. However, if the needle enters the neural foramen and local anesthetic is injected, then not only is the targeted nerve root blocked but there is also the potential for the sinuvertebral, medial branch, and ramus communicans nerves to be blocked. In this situation, if the local anesthetic does not enter the epidural, subdural, or subarachnoid space, the diagnostic block can be considered to be specific to that spinal segment and nerve root. However, if the local anesthetic also enters the epidural, subdural, or subarachnoid space, the diagnostic block cannot be said to be specific to a given nerve root or segment and may be simply called a diagnostic neuraxial block. Although these distinctions may seem minor, the implications of failing to distinguish these subtle differences relative to technique could lead to surgical interventions that fail to benefit the patient. Ultrasound-guided blockade of the lumbar nerve root block is also useful as a therapeutic maneuver when treating radiculitis or radiculopathy involving a single nerve root.

## CLINICALLY RELEVANT ANATOMY

The superior boundary of the lumbar epidural space is the fusion of the periosteal and spinal layers of dura at the foramen magnum. The epidural space continues inferiorly to the sacrococcygeal membrane. The lumbar epidural space is bounded anteriorly by the posterior longitudinal ligament and posteriorly by the vertebral laminae and the ligamentum flavum. The vertebral pedicles and intervertebral foramina form the lateral limits of the epidural space. The lumbar epidural space is 5 to 6 mm at L5-3 and widens at the S-S1 level with the lumbar spine flexed. The lumbar epidural space contains a small amount of fat, veins, arteries, lymphatics, and connective tissue. The five lumbar nerve roots exit their respective neural foramina and move anteriorly and inferiorly away from the lumbar spine (Fig. 99.1).

When performing selective nerve root block of the lumbar nerve roots, the goal is to place the needle just outside the neural foramen of the affected nerve root with precise application of local anesthetic. As mentioned above, placement of the needle within the neural foramina may change how the information obtained from this diagnostic maneuver should be interpreted.

## ULTRASOUND-GUIDED TECHNIQUE

Ultrasound-guided lumbar selective nerve root block can be carried out by placing the patient in the prone position with a thin pillow placed under the abdomen to slightly flex the lumbar spine (Fig. 99.2). A total of 0.25 to 0.5 mL of local anesthetic is drawn up in a 10-mL sterile syringe for each lumbar nerve root to be blocked. If the painful condition being treated is thought to have an inflammatory component, 40 to 80 mg of depot steroid is added to the local anesthetic.

After preparation of the skin with antiseptic solution, a curvilinear low-frequency ultrasound transducer is placed in the longitudinal plane over the spinous processes to identify the affected spinal level, and an ultrasound survey scan is obtained (Figs. 99.3 and 99.4). Once the affected level is identified, the transducer is rotated 90 degrees and a transverse ultrasound view is obtained. The spinous process is reidentified and its image is traced anteriorly to the lamina (Fig. 99.5). Once the lamina is identified, the ultrasound transducer is slowly moved inferiorly to identify the inferior border of the lamina (Figs. 99.6 and 99.7). The ultrasound transducer is then moved laterally until the facet joint is visualized (Fig. 99.8). Once the facet joint at the affected level is identified, a 3½-inch, 22-gauge blunt needle is inserted utilizing an in-plane approach and is advanced from a posterior to anterior trajectory until the needle tip is in proximity to the nerve root, which is resting just inferior and slightly lateral and anterior to the facet joint (Fig. 99.9). After gentle aspiration, 0.25 to 0.5 mL of solution is injected. The needle is removed and pressure is placed on the injection site to avoid hematoma formation.

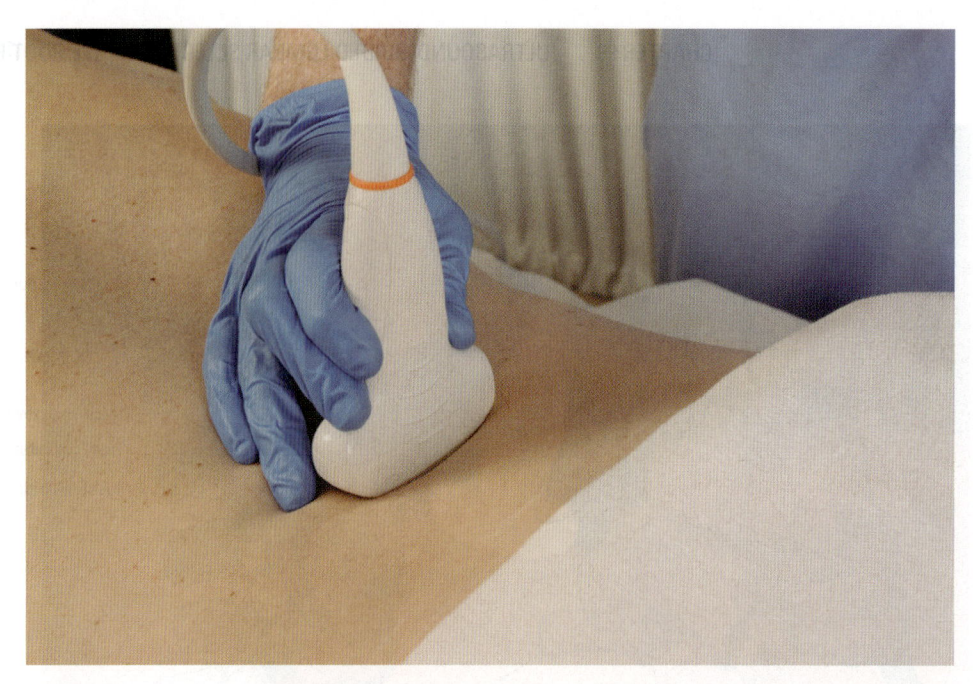

**FIGURE 99.5.** Once the affected level is identified on the longitudinal ultrasound scan, the transducer is rotated 90 degrees and a transverse ultrasound view is obtained. The spinous process is reidentified and its image is traced anteriorly to the lamina.

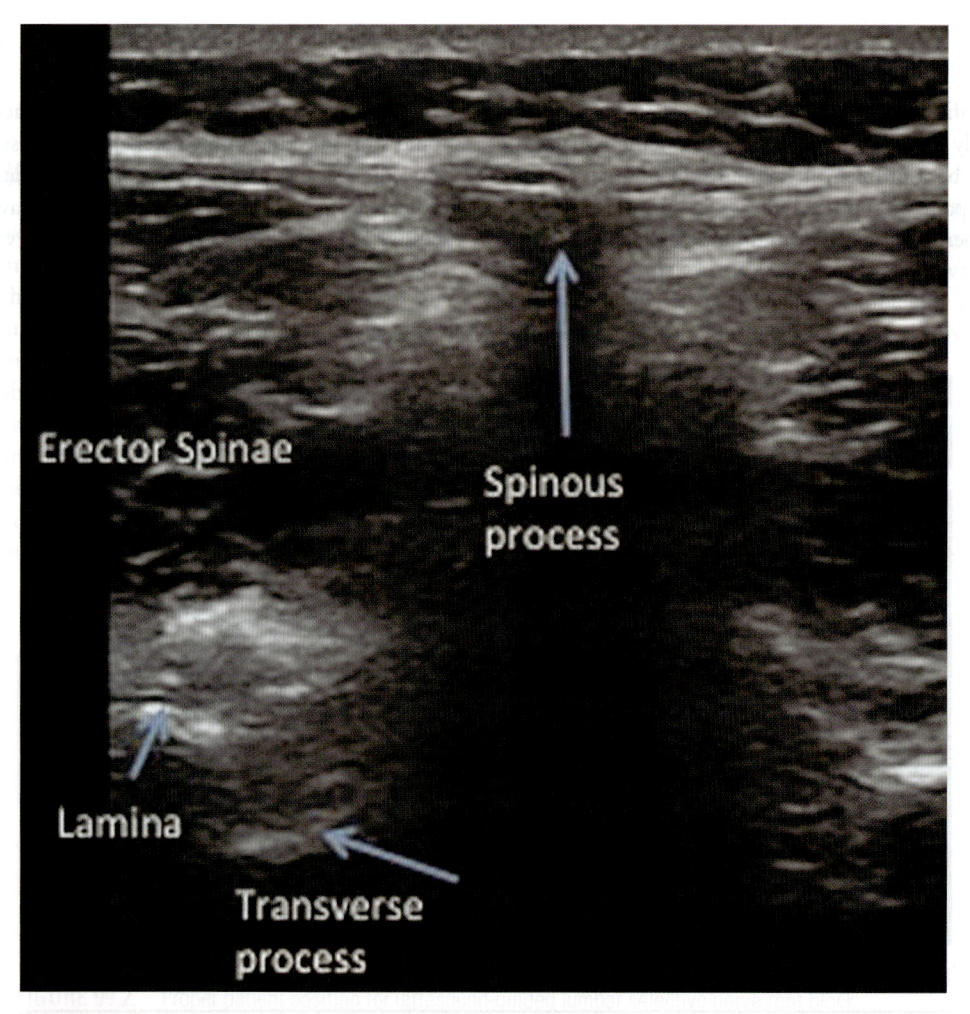

**FIGURE 99.6.** Transverse ultrasound view of the L5 vertebra.

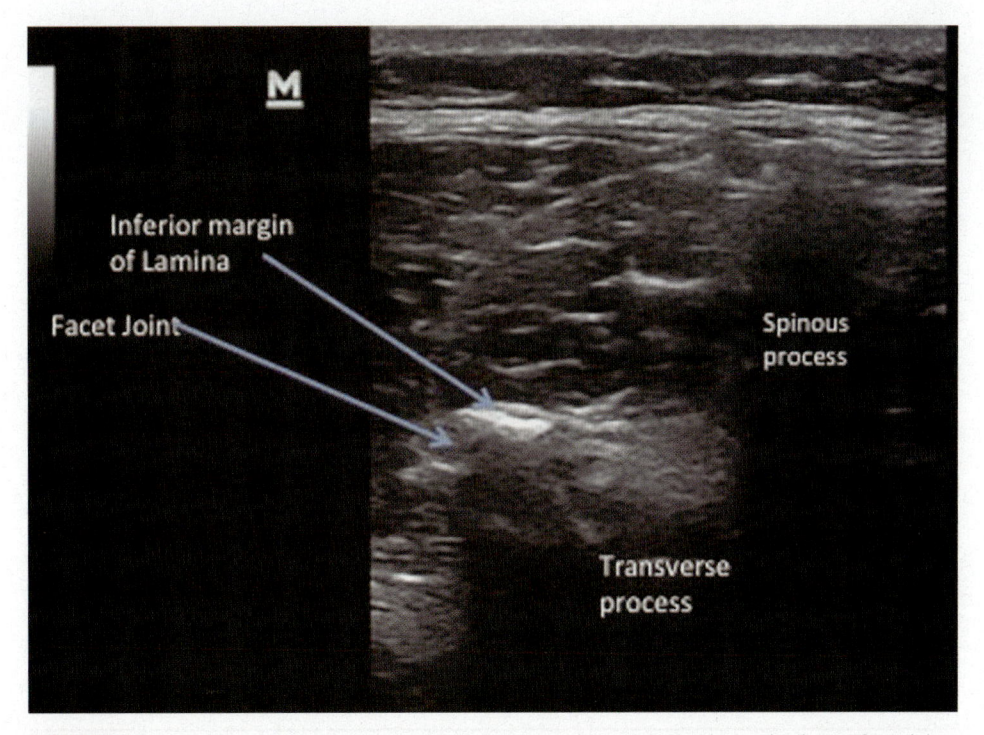

**FIGURE 99.7.** Transverse ultrasound view of the inferior margin of the lamina and adjacent facet joint.

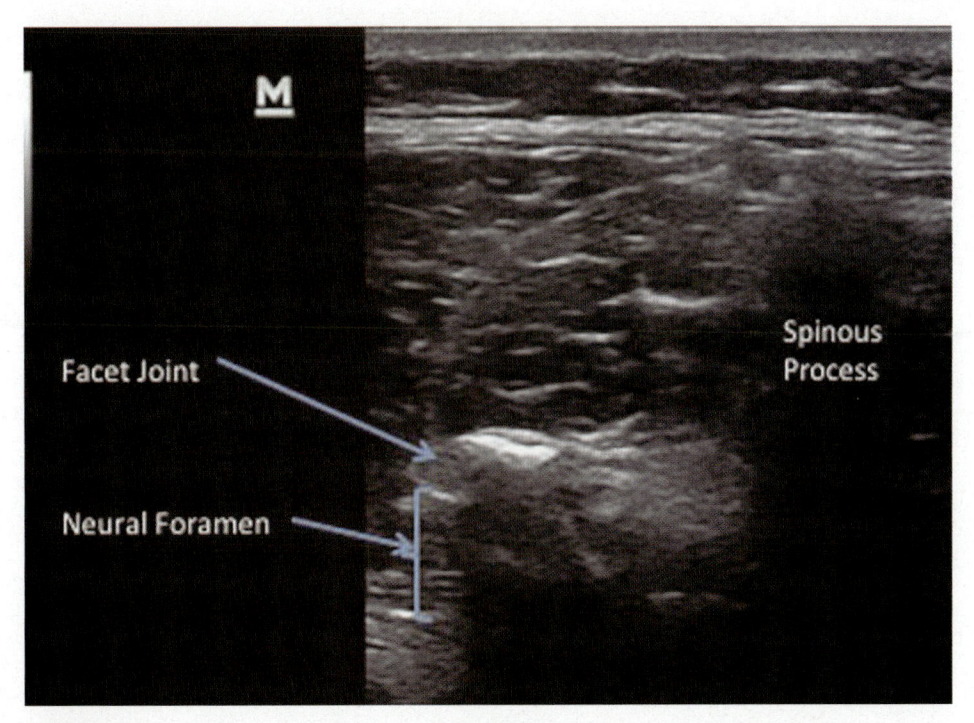

**FIGURE 99.8.** Transverse ultrasound view of the facet joint and intervertebral foramen.

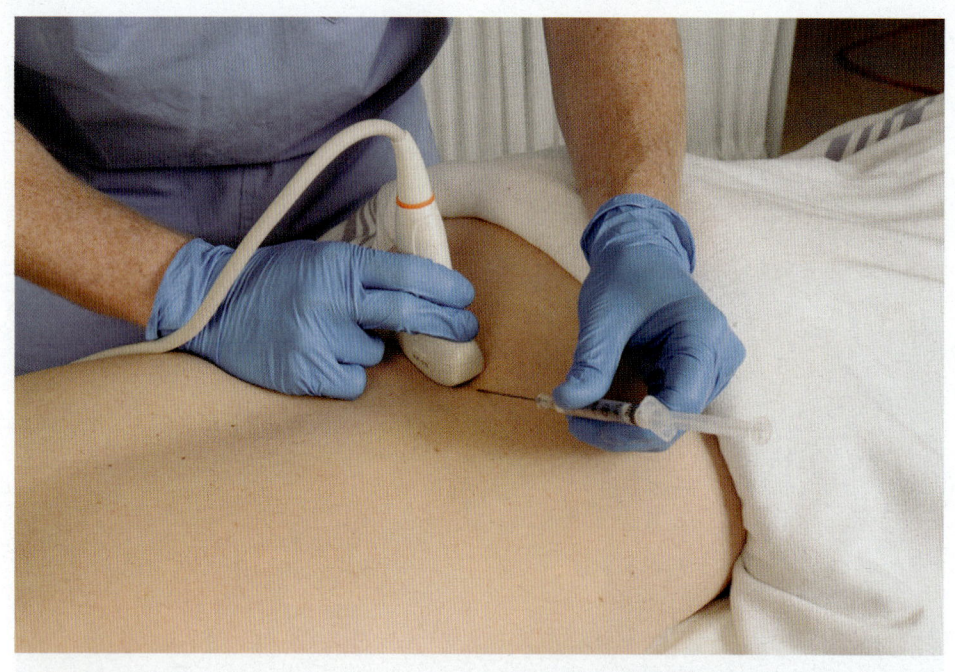

**FIGURE 99.9.** Proper needle position for performing selective lumbar nerve root block.

## SUGGESTED READINGS

Galiano K, Obwegeser AA, Bale R, et al. Ultrasound-guided and CT-navigation-assisted periradicular and facet joint injections in the lumbar and cervical spine: a new teaching tool to recognize the sonoanatomic pattern. *Reg Anesth Pain Med* 2007;32(3):254–257.

Galiano K, Obwegeser AA, Gruber H. Ultrasound guidance for periradicular injections in the lumbar spine: a review article. *Tech Reg Anesth Pain Manag* 2009;13(3):154–156.

Waldman SD. Lumbar selective nerve root block. In: *Atlas of Interventional Pain Management*. 3rd ed. Philadelphia, PA: Saunders Elsevier; 2009:413–417.

Waldman SD. Functional anatomy of the lumbar spine. In: *Pain Review*. Philadelphia, PA: Saunders Elsevier; 2009:65–67.

# CHAPTER 100

# Ultrasound-Guided Lumbar Subarachnoid Block Utilizing the Three-Step Paramedian Sagittal Oblique Approach

## CLINICAL PERSPECTIVES

Ultrasound-guided lumbar subarachnoid block is utilized in a variety of clinical scenarios as a diagnostic, prognostic, and therapeutic maneuver as well as to provide surgical anesthesia for pelvic and lower extremity surgeries. As a diagnostic tool, ultrasound-guided lumbar subarachnoid block allows accurate placement of the needle tip within the subarachnoid space to perform differential spinal block on a pharmacologic basis to determine if the patient's lower abdominal, back, groin, pelvic, bladder, perineal, genital, rectal, anal, and lower extremity pain are somatic, sympathetic, or central in origin. As a prognostic tool, ultrasound-guided lumbar subarachnoid block can be utilized as a prognostic indicator of the degree of motor and sensory impairment that the patient may experience if neurodestructive procedures of the spinal cord are being contemplated in an effort to palliate intractable pain in patients too sick to undergo neurosurgical destructive procedures. This technique also provides important prognostic information regarding the side effects of drugs administered into the subarachnoid space for the treatment of pain or spasticity when an implantable drug delivery system is being considered.

In the acute pain setting, ultrasound-guided lumbar subarachnoid block with local anesthetics and/or opioids may be used to palliate acute pain emergencies while waiting for pharmacologic, surgical, and/or antiblastic methods to become effective. This technique has great clinical utility in both children and adults when managing acute postoperative and posttrauma pain when the local anesthetics and/or opioids are administered via a catheter placed into the subarachnoid space. This paramedian oblique approach to the subarachnoid space has an advantage over the midline approach to the subarachnoid space as the paramedian oblique approach allows the catheter to enter the subarachnoid space at a less acute angle than with the midline approach. This results in less catheter kinking and breakage. Lumbar subarachnoid block is used primarily for surgical and obstetric anesthesia.

It is unique among regional anesthesia techniques in that the small amounts of drugs used to perform a successful lumbar subarachnoid nerve block exert essentially no systemic pharmacologic effects.

The lumbar subarachnoid administration of local anesthetic in combination with opioids is useful in the palliation of cancer-related lower abdominal, groin, back, pelvic, perineal, and rectal pain. The long-term subarachnoid administration of opioids via implantable drug delivery systems has become a mainstay in the palliation of cancer-related pain. The role of chronic subarachnoid opioid administration in the management of chronic benign pain syndromes remains controversial.

## CLINICALLY RELEVANT ANATOMY

The spinal cord ends at approximately L2 in the majority of adults and at approximately L4 in most infants (Fig. 100.1). Therefore, in most settings, lumbar subarachnoid nerve block should be performed below these levels to avoid the potential for trauma to the spinal cord. The spinal cord is surrounded by three layers of protective connective tissue: the dura, the arachnoid, and the pia mater (Fig. 100.2). The dura is the outermost layer and is composed of tough fibroelastic fibers that form a mechanical barrier to protect the spinal cord. The next layer is the arachnoid. The arachnoid is separated from the dura by only a small potential space, which is filled with serous fluid. The arachnoid is a barrier to the diffusion of substances and effectively serves to limit the spread of drugs administered into the epidural space from diffusing into the spinal fluid. The innermost layer is the pia, a vascular structure that helps provide lateral support to the spinal cord.

To reach the subarachnoid space, a needle placed via the paramedian approach at the L3–L4 interspace will pass through the skin, subcutaneous tissues, the inner margin of the interspinous ligament, the ligamentum flavum, the epidural space, dura, the subdural space, and arachnoid (Fig. 100.3). Drugs administered into the subarachnoid space are placed between

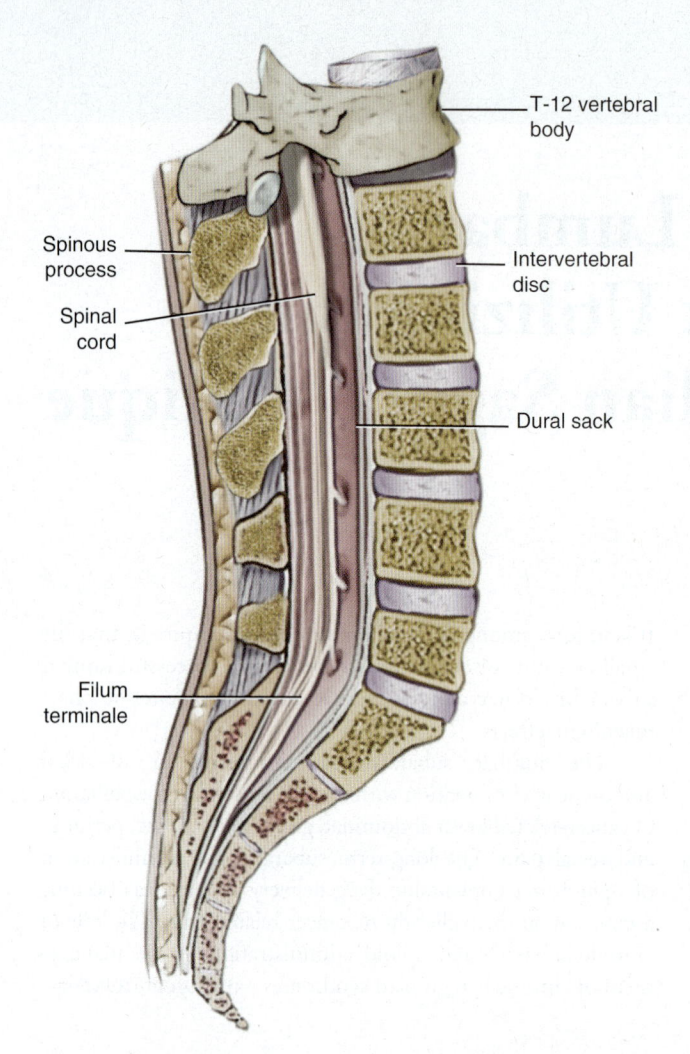

**FIGURE 100.1.** The spinal cord ends at approximately L2 in adults and L4 in newborns.

the arachnoid and pia, although inadvertent subdural injection is possible. Subdural injection of local anesthetic is characterized by a spotty, incomplete block.

## ULTRASOUND-GUIDED TECHNIQUE

Ultrasound-guided lumbar subarachnoid block can be carried out by placing the patient in sitting position (Fig. 100.4). If the painful condition being treated is thought to have an inflammatory component, 40 to 80 mg of depot steroid is added to the local anesthetic. To perform ultrasound-guided lumbar subarachnoid block, a three-step process is used. Although this may seem cumbersome, the three-step process allows the clinician to quickly identify critical anatomic structures while at the same time maintaining a transducer position that allows a safe and easy placement of needles into the lumbar subarachnoid space.

### Step One: Obtain the Paramedian Sagittal Transverse Process View

Step One is to obtain a paramedian sagittal transverse process view by placing the 2- to 5-MHz low-frequency curvilinear probe in the longitudinal plane 3 to 4 cm lateral to the right side of the middle of the spinous processes at the level to be blocked for the right-handed clinician and 3 to 4 cm to the later to the left side of the middle of the spinous processes at the level to be blocked for the left-handed clinician (Figs. 100.5 and 100.6). An ultrasound survey is taken and the transducer is slowly moved medially and laterally until successive transverse processes are visualized. The transverse processes of the lumbar spine will appear as hyperechoic domes with sausage-like acoustic shadows beneath them (Fig. 100.7). This classic appearance of successive transverse processes viewed in the longitudinal plane has been named the "trident sign" after Neptune's trident (Fig. 100.8).

### Step Two: Obtain the Paramedian Sagittal Articular Process View

After the transverse processes are identified in the paramedian sagittal transverse process view, the ultrasound transducer is slowly slid toward the midline until the superior and inferior articular facets are visualized (Step Two) (Figs. 100.9 and 100.10). In longitudinal paramedian ultrasound articular process view, the superior and inferior articular facets will appear as successive hyperechoic hills and valleys, with the gap in the center of each hill representing a facet joint (Fig. 100.11).

### Step Three: Obtain the Paramedian Sagittal Oblique View

After the articular processes are identified using the paramedian sagittal articular process view (Step Three), the longitudinally oriented ultrasound transducer is then slowly tilted to angle the ultrasound beam in a lateral to medial oblique trajectory toward the midline (Figs. 100.12 and 100.13). The lamina of successive lumbar vertebrae will appear as a series of hyperechoic curvilinear lines with an acoustic shadow beneath each one (Fig. 100.14). The interlaminar space will appear as gaps between each successive vertebra providing an acoustic window that will allow visualization of the ligamentum flavum, subarachnoid space, and posterior dura. By making minor adjustments to the position of the ultrasound transducer, in some patients, the ligamentum flavum and posterior dura can be distinguished as two distinct hyperechoic linear structures with a hyperechoic subarachnoid space in between (Fig. 100.15). In other patients, these structures simply appear as a single hyperechoic line, which is known as the posterior complex (Fig. 100.16).

After interlaminar space is identified, the skin is prepped with antiseptic solution, and a 3½-inch, 22-gauge styletted

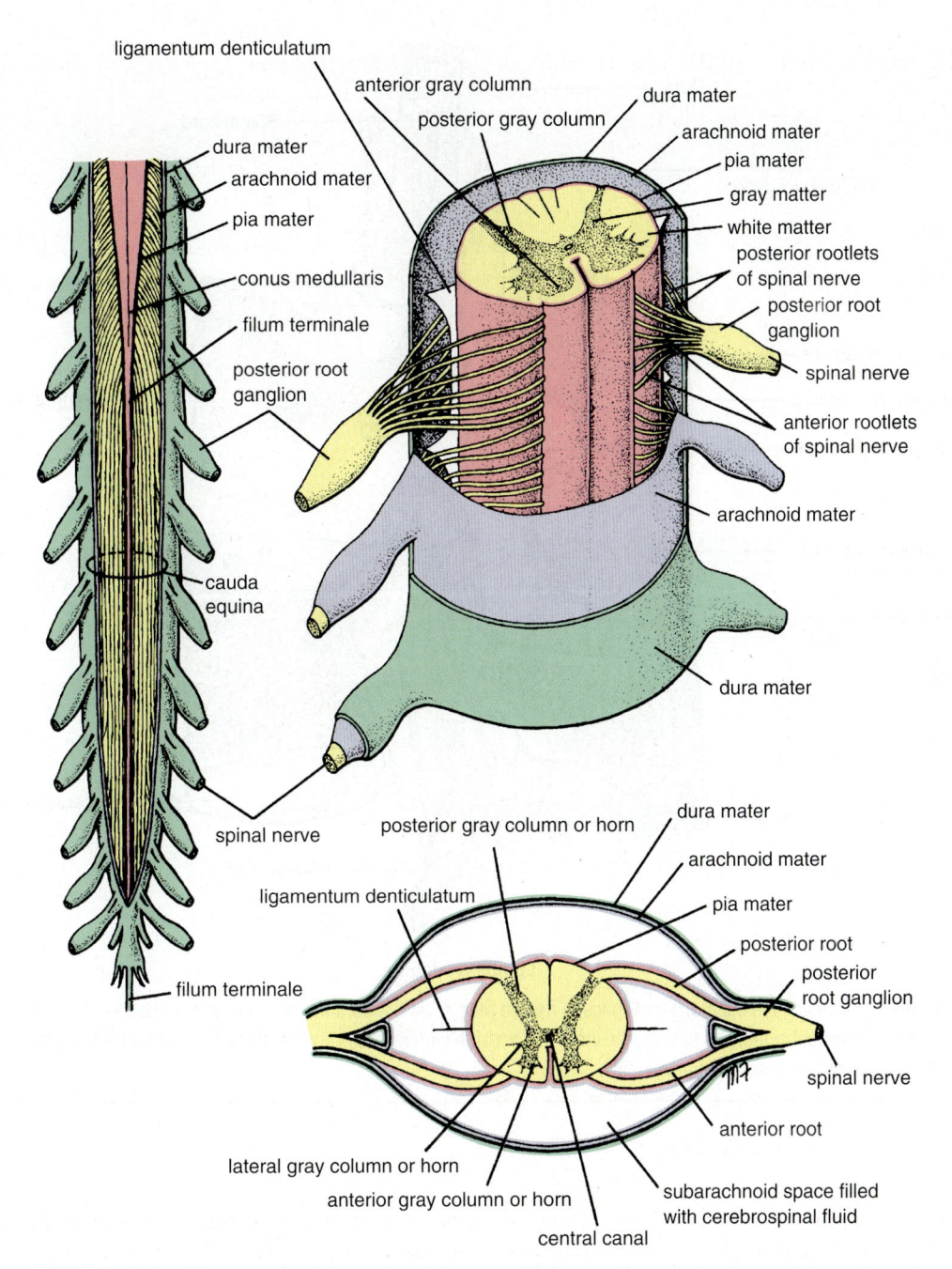

**FIGURE 100.2.** The anatomy of the lumbar subarachnoid space and surrounding layers of dura. (Reused from Snell. *Clinical Anatomy*. 7th ed. Philadelphia, PA: Lippincott Williams & Wilkins; 2003, with permission.)

needle suitable for subarachnoid use is inserted through the skin at the middle of the lateral aspect of the longitudinally placed ultrasound transducer utilizing an out-of-plane approach (Fig. 100.17). The clinician then advances the needle under real-time ultrasound guidance in an oblique lateral to medial trajectory toward the posterior complex until the needle tip rests within the subarachnoid space. Often, the clinician will appreciate a "pop" as the needle tip pierces the dura. The needle is then slowly advanced an additional 1 mm, and the stylet is removed. A free flow of spinal fluid should be observed, or if a smaller spinal needle has been used, cerebrospinal fluid should appear in the hub. If no spinal fluid is observed, the stylet is replaced and the needle is advanced slightly and then rotated 90 degrees. The stylet is again removed, and the hub is again observed for spinal fluid. If no spinal fluid appears, the needle should be removed and the midline reidentified before

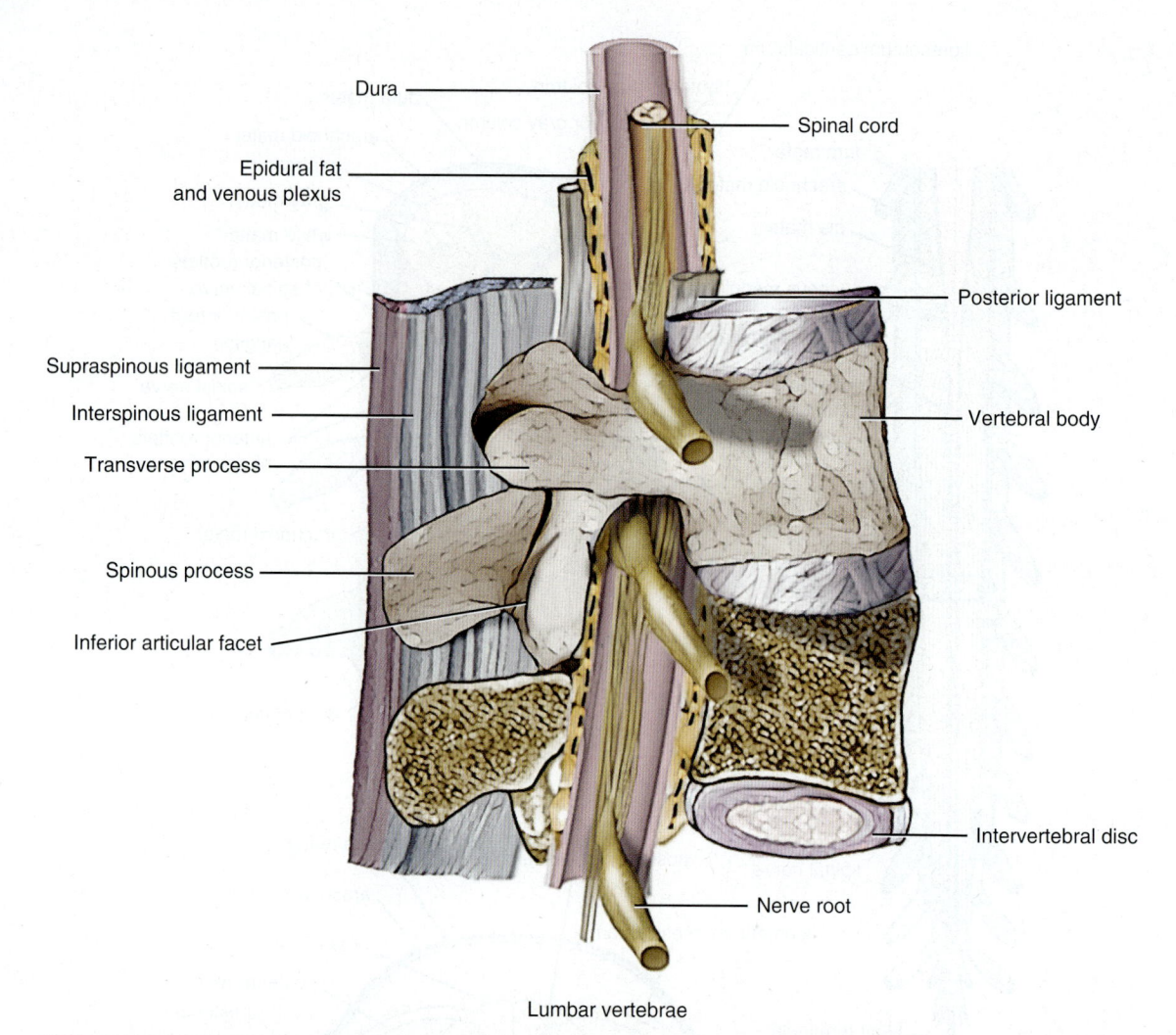

**FIGURE 100.3.** To reach the subarachnoid space, a needle placed via the paramedian approach at the L3–L4 interspace will pass through the skin, subcutaneous tissues, the inner margin of the interspinous ligament, the ligamentum flavum, the epidural space, dura, the subdural space, and arachnoid.

attempting to repeat the previous technique. After spinal fluid is observed, the needle is fixed in position by the operator placing his or her hand against the patient's back. A drug suitable for subarachnoid administration is chosen, and the solution is slowly injected, with the injection immediately being discontinued if the patient reports any pain. The needle is then removed and pressure is placed on the injection site to avoid hematoma formation.

## COMPLICATIONS

Because of potential hematogenous spread via the valveless epidural veins of Batson plexus within the lumbar epidural space, sepsis and local infection at the injection site represent absolute contraindications to ultrasound-guided lumbar subarachnoid block as do anticoagulation and coagulopathy. The subarachnoid space is in close proximity to the cord as well as the exiting spinal nerve roots, which suggests that this procedure should only be performed by those well versed in the regional anatomy and skilled at ultrasound-guided interventional pain management procedures. Trauma to the exiting lumbar nerve roots and spinal cord can be avoided if careful attention is paid to the regional anatomy and if the clinician immediately stops advancing the needle should the patient experience any significant pain during needle placement. Inadvertent epidural and/or subdural injection, although rare, can occur even in the best of hands.

Hypotension secondary to profound sympathetic blockade is a common side effect of lumbar subarachnoid nerve block with local anesthetics. Prophylactic intramuscular or intravenous administration of vasopressors and fluid loading may help avoid this potentially serious side effect of lumbar

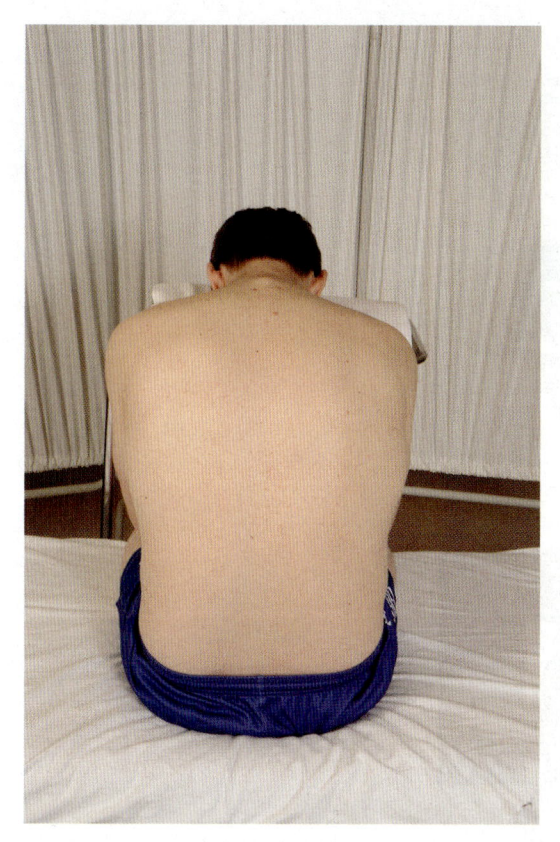

**FIGURE 100.4.** Proper patient position for ultrasound-guided lumbar subarachnoid block.

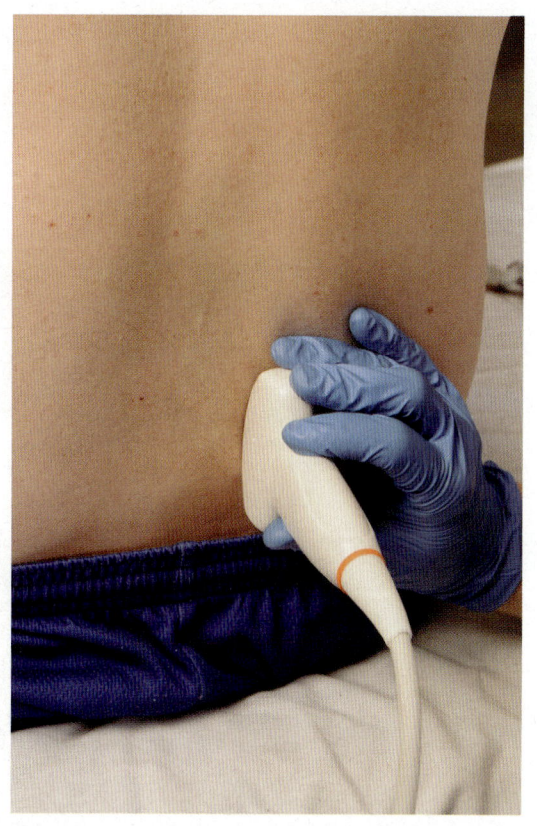

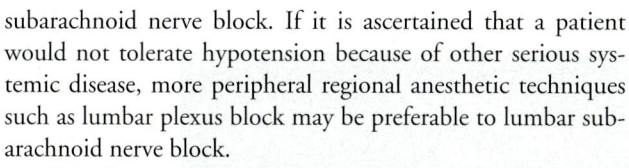

**FIGURE 100.5.** Placement of the ultrasound transducer in the longitudinal plane to obtain a paramedian sagittal transverse process view (Step One).

subarachnoid nerve block. If it is ascertained that a patient would not tolerate hypotension because of other serious systemic disease, more peripheral regional anesthetic techniques such as lumbar plexus block may be preferable to lumbar subarachnoid nerve block.

It is also possible to inadvertently place a needle or catheter intended for the subarachnoid space into the subdural space. If subdural placement is unrecognized, the resulting block will be spotty. This problem can be avoided if the operator advances the needle slightly after perceiving the pop of the needle as it pierces the dura and observing a free flow of spinal fluid.

Neurologic complications after lumbar subarachnoid nerve block are uncommon if proper technique is used. Direct trauma to the spinal cord and/or nerve roots is usually accompanied by pain. If significant pain occurs during placement of the spinal needle or catheter or during injection, the physician should immediately stop and ascertain the cause of the pain to avoid the possibility of additional neural trauma. Delayed neurologic complications due to chemical irritation of the coverings of the spinal cord, nerves, and the spinal cord have been reported. Most severe complications have been attributed to contaminants to the local anesthetic, although the addition of steroids and vasopressors and the use of concentrated hyperbaric solutions have also been implicated.

Although uncommon, infection in the subarachnoid space remains an ever-present possibility, especially in the immunocompromised AIDS or cancer patient. If epidural abscess occurs, emergent surgical drainage to avoid spinal cord compression and irreversible neurologic deficit is usually required. Meningitis occurring after lumbar subarachnoid nerve block may require subarachnoid administration of antibiotics. Early detection and treatment of infection is crucial to avoid potentially life-threatening sequelae.

## CLINICAL PEARLS

The key to performing successful ultrasound-guided lumbar neuraxial blocks is the proper identification of the sonographic anatomy. The three-step technique presented above will simplify this process and improve the ability to perform lumbar subarachnoid block. Any significant pain or sudden increase in resistance during injection when performing ultrasound-guided lumbar subarachnoid block utilizing the three-step paramedian sagittal oblique approach suggests incorrect needle placement, and one should stop injecting immediately and reassess the position of the needle. Because pain is an important indication of improper needle placement, the practitioner should avoid the use of excessive sedation when performing this technique.

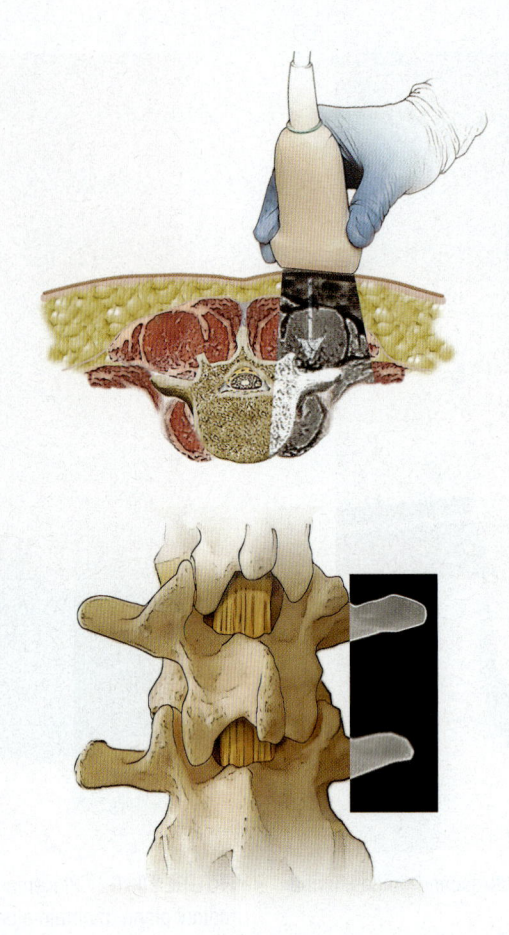

**FIGURE 100.6.** The anatomic orientation of the longitudinally placed curvilinear ultrasound transducer for the paramedian sagittal transverse process view (Step One).

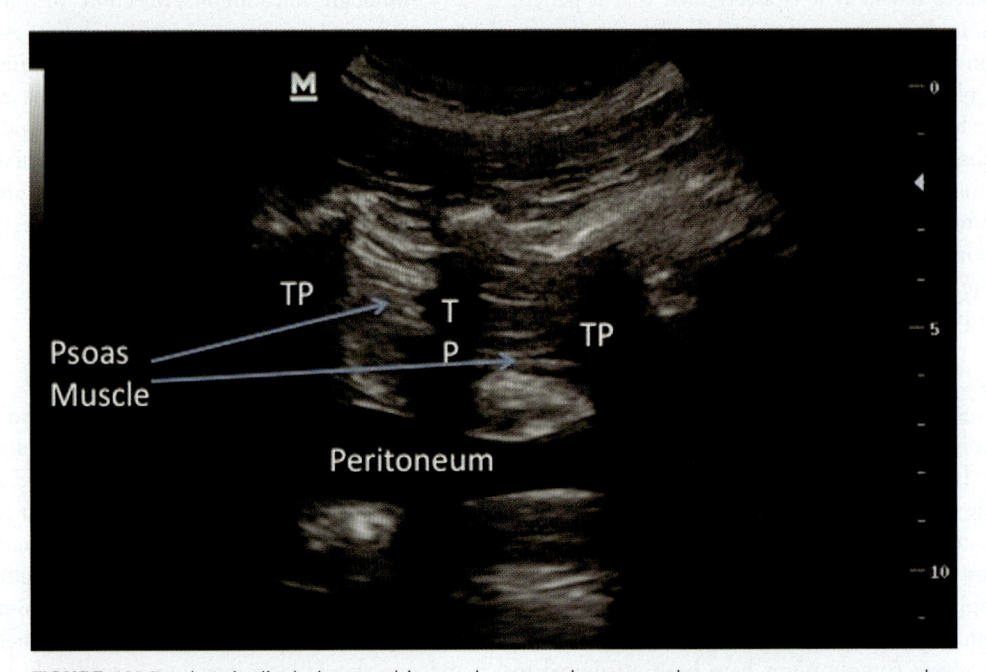

**FIGURE 100.7.** Longitudinal ultrasound image demonstrating successive transverse processes when performing the paramedian sagittal transverse process view (Step One). This classic image is named the "trident sign."

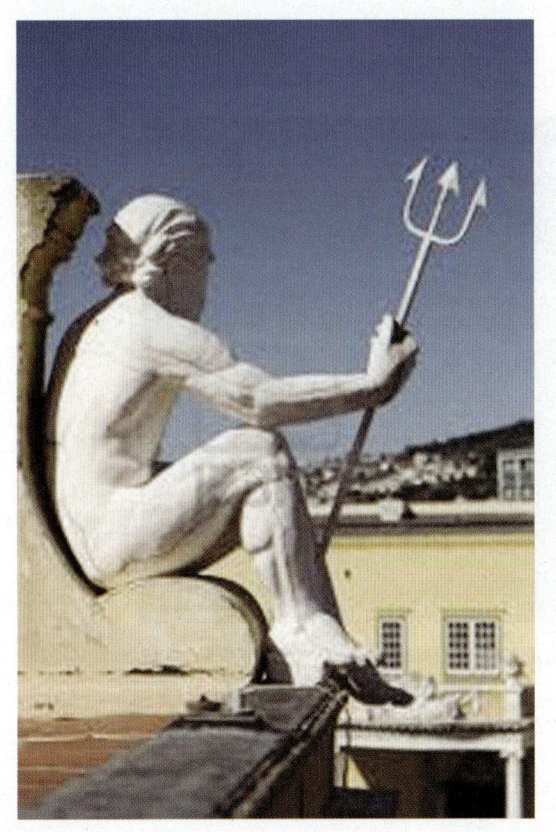

**FIGURE 100.8.** The trident sign is named after Neptune's trident, which according to Roman mythology had the power to conjure water and cause tsunamis and earthquakes.

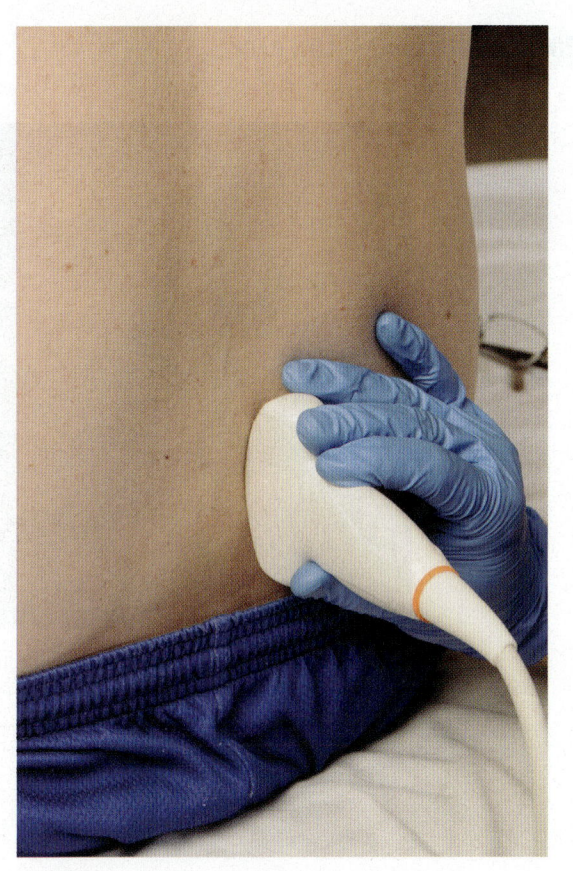

**FIGURE 100.9.** Proper longitudinal ultrasound transducer placement to obtain paramedian sagittal articular view (Step Two).

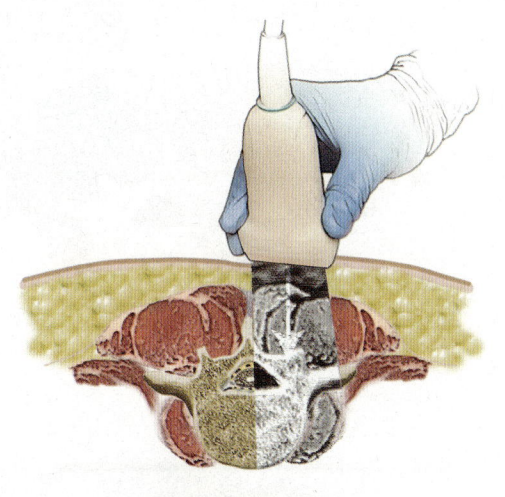

**FIGURE 100.10.** The anatomic orientation of the longitudinally placed curvilinear ultrasound transducer for the paramedian sagittal articular view (Step Two).

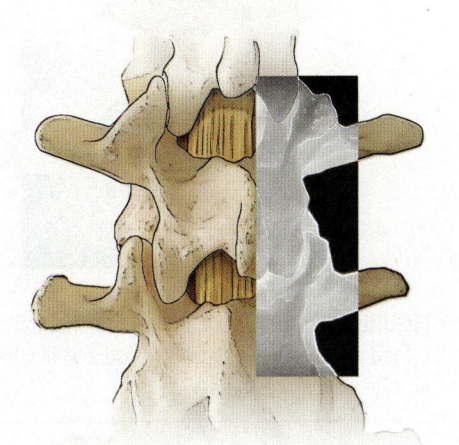

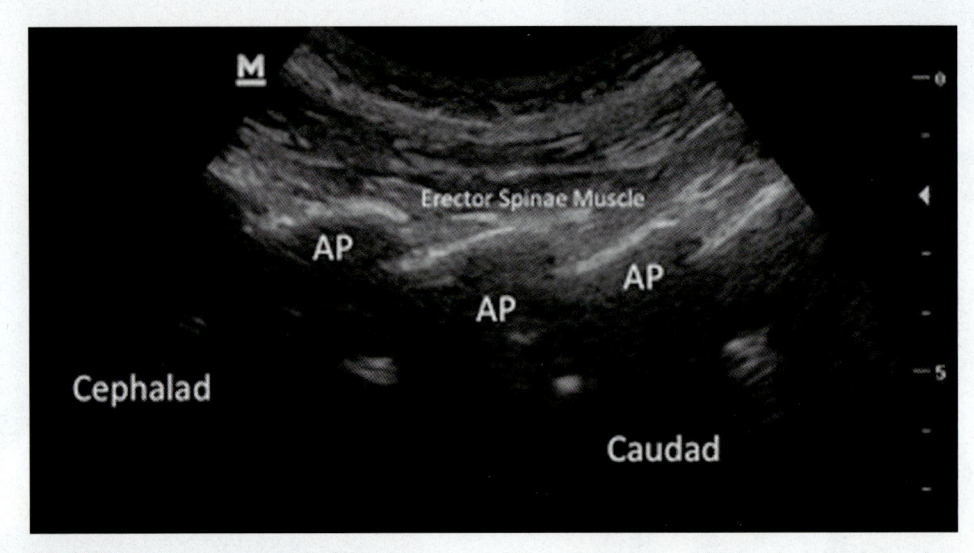

**FIGURE 100.11.** Longitudinal ultrasound image of the paramedian sagittal articular process view demonstrating the articular processes (Step Two).

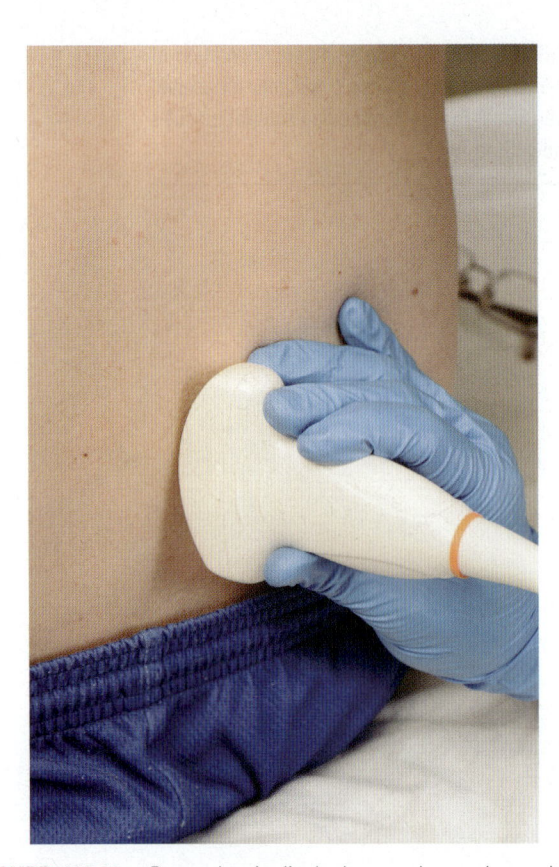

**FIGURE 100.12.** Proper longitudinal ultrasound transducer placement to obtain paramedian sagittal oblique view (Step Three).

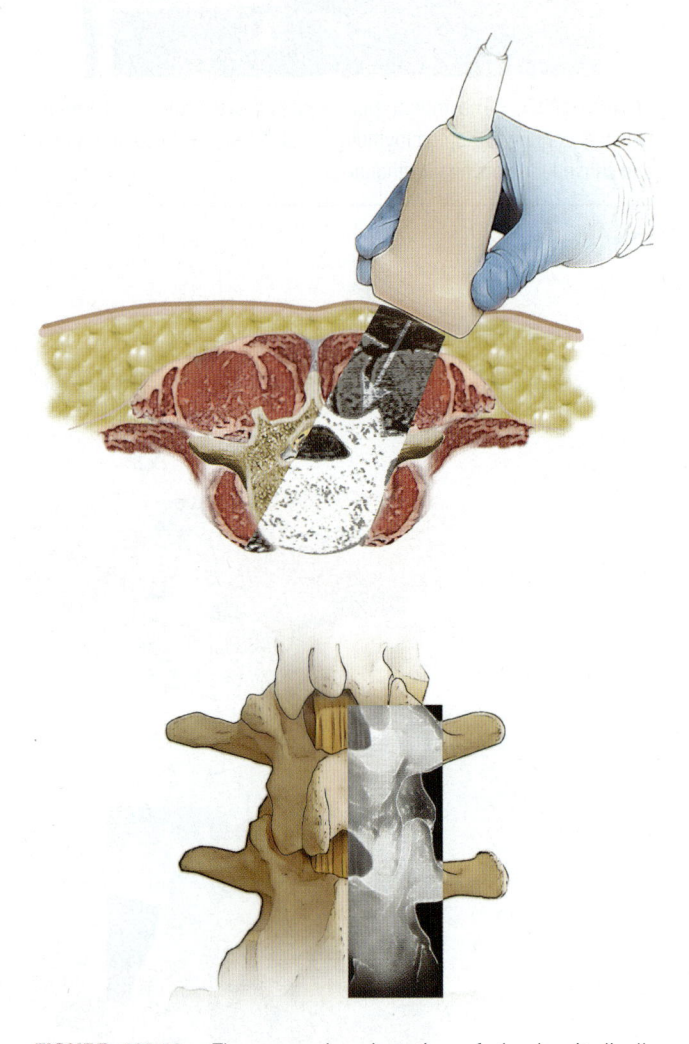

**FIGURE 100.13.** The anatomic orientation of the longitudinally placed curvilinear ultrasound transducer for the paramedian sagittal oblique view (Step Three).

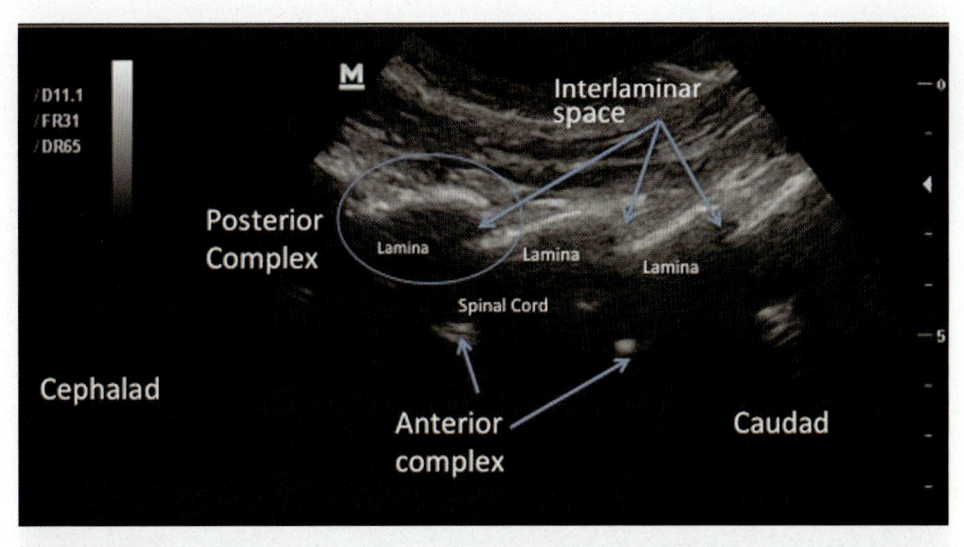

**FIGURE 100.14.** Longitudinal ultrasound image of the paramedian sagittal oblique view demonstrating the interlaminar space and posterior complex made of the ligamentum flavum, posterior subarachnoid space, and posterior dura (Step Three).

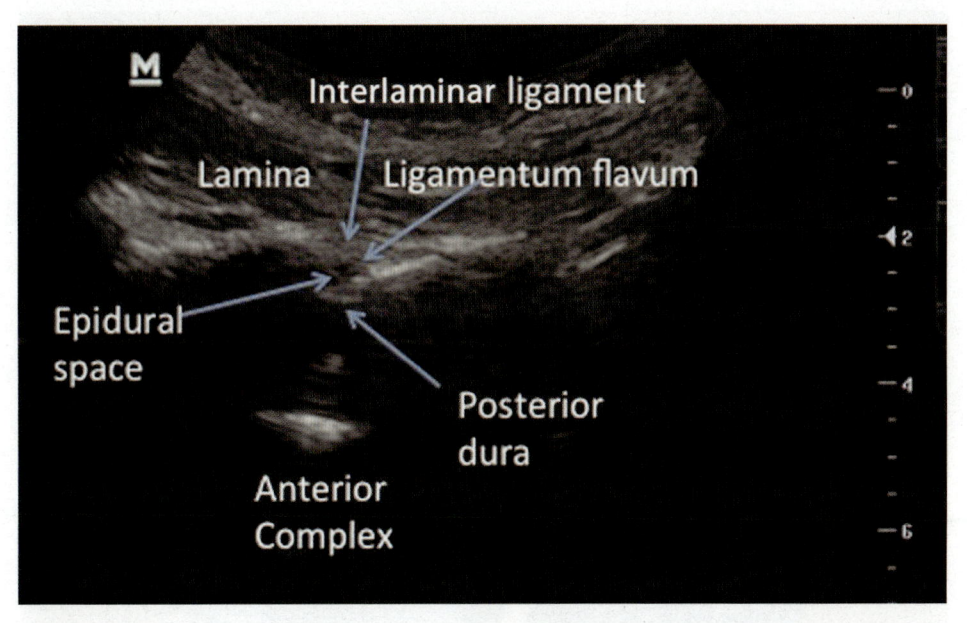

**FIGURE 100.15.** Longitudinal ultrasound image of the paramedian sagittal oblique view demonstrating the interlaminar space and posterior complex made of the ligamentum flavum, posterior subarachnoid space, and posterior dura.

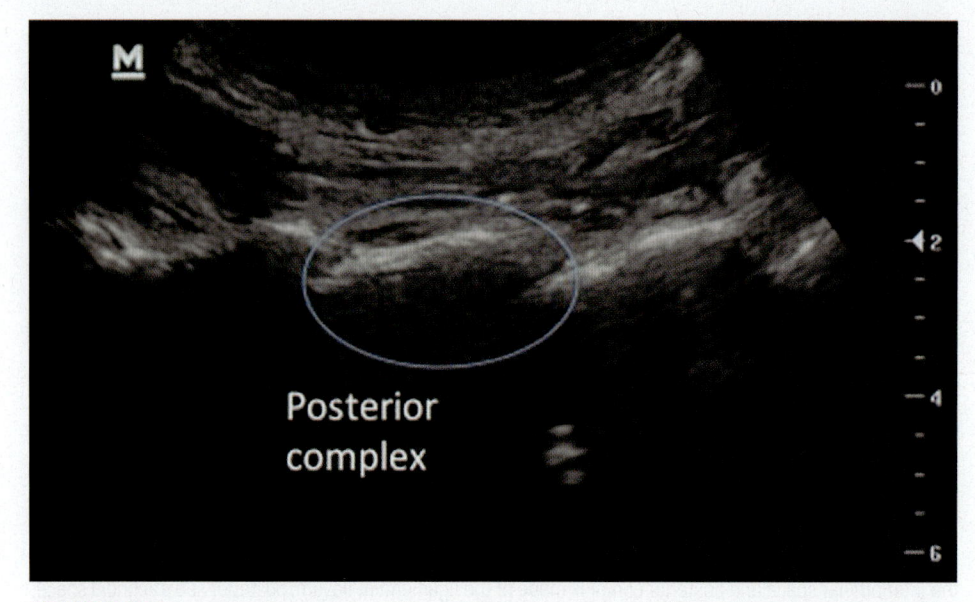

**FIGURE 100.16.** Longitudinal ultrasound image of the paramedian sagittal oblique view demonstrating the interlaminar space and posterior complex.

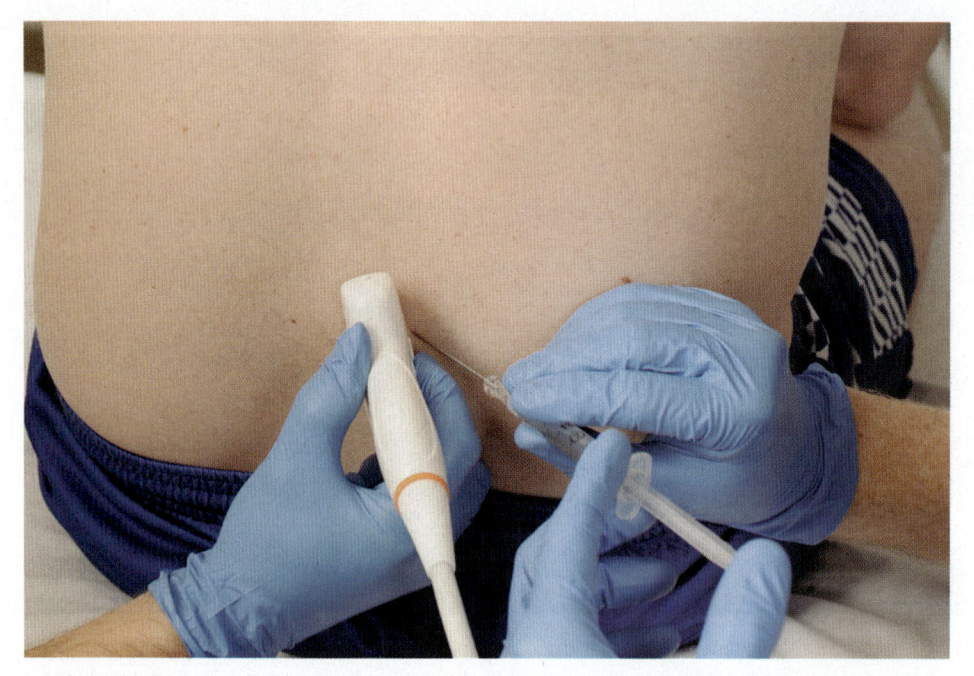

**FIGURE 100.17.** Proper out-of-plane needle position for performing lumbar subarachnoid block.

## SUGGESTED READINGS

Strony R. Ultrasound-assisted lumbar puncture in obese patients. *Crit Care Clin* 2010;26(4):661–664.

Waldman SD. Lumbar subarachnoid nerve block: paramedian approach. In: *Atlas of Interventional Pain Management*. 3rd ed. Philadelphia, PA: Saunders Elsevier; 2009:422–423.

Waldman SD, Campbell R. Anatomy: special imaging considerations of the lumbar spine. In: *Imaging of Pain*. Philadelphia, PA: Saunders Elsevier; 2009:67–68.

Yamauchi M. Ultrasound-guided neuraxial block. *Trends Anaesth Crit Care* 2012;2(5):234–243.

# CHAPTER 101

# Ultrasound-Guided Caudal Epidural Block

## CLINICAL PERSPECTIVES

Ultrasound-guided caudal epidural block is utilized in a variety of clinical scenarios as a diagnostic, prognostic, and therapeutic maneuver as well as to provide surgical anesthesia for pelvic and lower extremity surgeries. As a diagnostic tool, ultrasound-guided caudal epidural block allows accurate placement of the needle tip within the epidural space when performing differential neural blockade on an anatomic basis in the evaluation of back, groin, pelvic, bladder, perineal, genital, rectal, anal, and lower extremity pain. As a prognostic tool, ultrasound-guided caudal epidural block can be utilized as a prognostic indicator of the degree of motor and sensory impairment that the patient may experience if lower lumbar and/or sacral nerve roots are going to be destroyed in an effort to palliate intractable pain in patients too sick to undergo neurosurgical destructive procedures. In the acute pain setting, ultrasound-guided caudal epidural block with local anesthetics and/or opioids may be used to palliate acute pain emergencies while waiting for pharmacologic, surgical, and/or antiblastic methods to become effective. This technique has great clinical utility in both children and adults when managing acute postoperative and posttrauma pain. Sympathetically mediated pain syndromes including the pain of acute herpes zoster of the lumbosacral dermatomes and the pain of urethral calculi can also be effectively managed with epidurally administered local anesthetics, steroids, and/or opioids. Additionally, this technique is of value in patients suffering from acute vascular insufficiency of the lower extremities secondary to vasospastic and vasoocclusive disease, including frostbite and ergotamine toxicity (Fig. 101.1). There is increasing evidence that the prophylactic or preemptive use of caudal epidural nerve blocks in patients scheduled to undergo lower extremity amputations for ischemia will result in a decreased incidence of phantom limb pain. The administration of local anesthetic and/or steroids via the ultrasound-guided caudal approach to the epidural space is useful in the treatment of a variety of chronic benign pain syndromes, including lumbar radiculopathy, low back syndrome, spinal stenosis, postlaminectomy syndrome, phantom limb pain, vertebral compression fractures, diabetic polyneuropathy, chemotherapy-related peripheral neuropathy, postherpetic neuralgia, reflex sympathetic dystrophy, orchalgia, proctalgia, and pelvic pain syndromes.

Pain of malignant origin involving the groin, back, pelvis, perineum, rectum, and lower extremities as well as spinal metastatic disease (especially from breast and prostate primary cancers) is also amenable to treatment with caudally administered local anesthetics, steroids, and/or opioids.

## CLINICALLY RELEVANT ANATOMY

The five sacral vertebrae are fused together to form the triangular-shaped sacrum (Fig. 101.2). The dorsally convex sacrum inserts in a wedge-like manner between the two iliac bones with superior articulations with the fifth lumbar vertebra and caudad articulations with the coccyx. On the anterior concave surface, there are four pairs of unsealed anterior sacral foramina that allow passage of the anterior rami of the upper four sacral nerves. The posterior sacral foramina are smaller than their anterior counterparts. Leakage of drugs injected into the sacral canal is effectively prevented by the sacrospinal and multifidus muscles. The vestigial bony remnants that are the result of the incomplete fusion of the inferior articular processes of the lower half of the S4 and all of the S5 vertebrae project downward on each side of the sacral hiatus (see Fig. 101.2). These bony projections are called the sacral cornua and represent important clinical landmarks when performing ultrasound-guided caudal epidural nerve block. The U-shaped sacral hiatus is covered posteriorly by the sacrococcygeal ligament, which is also an important clinical landmark when performing ultrasound-guided caudal epidural nerve block (Fig. 101.3). Penetration of the sacrococcygeal ligament provides direct access to the epidural space of the sacral canal. Although there are gender- and race-determined differences in the shape of the sacrum, they are of little importance relative to the ultimate ability to successfully perform caudal epidural nerve block on a given patient.

## ULTRASOUND-GUIDED TECHNIQUE

Ultrasound-guided caudal epidural block can be carried out by placing the patient in the prone position with the patient's abdomen resting on a thin pillow (Fig. 101.4). To relax the gluteal muscles, the patient is asked to turn his or her heels

CHAPTER 101 ULTRASOUND-GUIDED CAUDAL EPIDURAL BLOCK 711

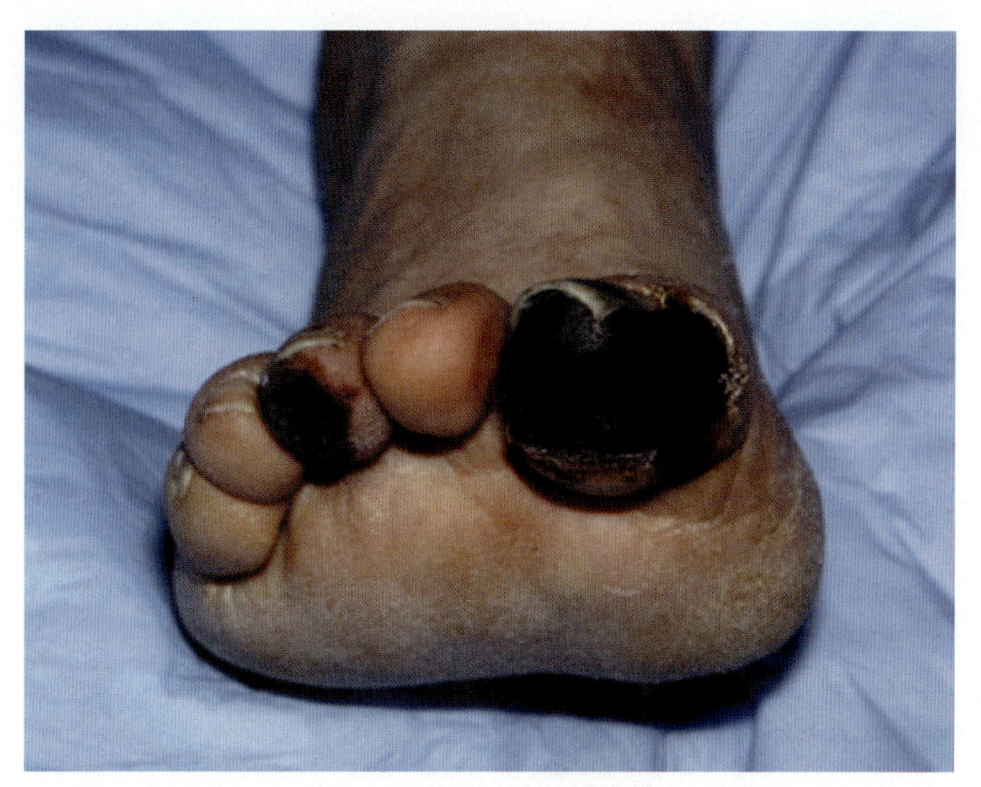

**FIGURE 101.1.** Ultrasound-guided caudal epidural block is useful in the management of the pain of acute vaso-occlusive disease of the lower extremity. (Reused from Topol EJ, Califf RM, et al. *Textbook of Cardiovascular Medicine*. 3rd ed. Philadelphia, PA: Lippincott Williams & Wilkins; 2006, with permission.)

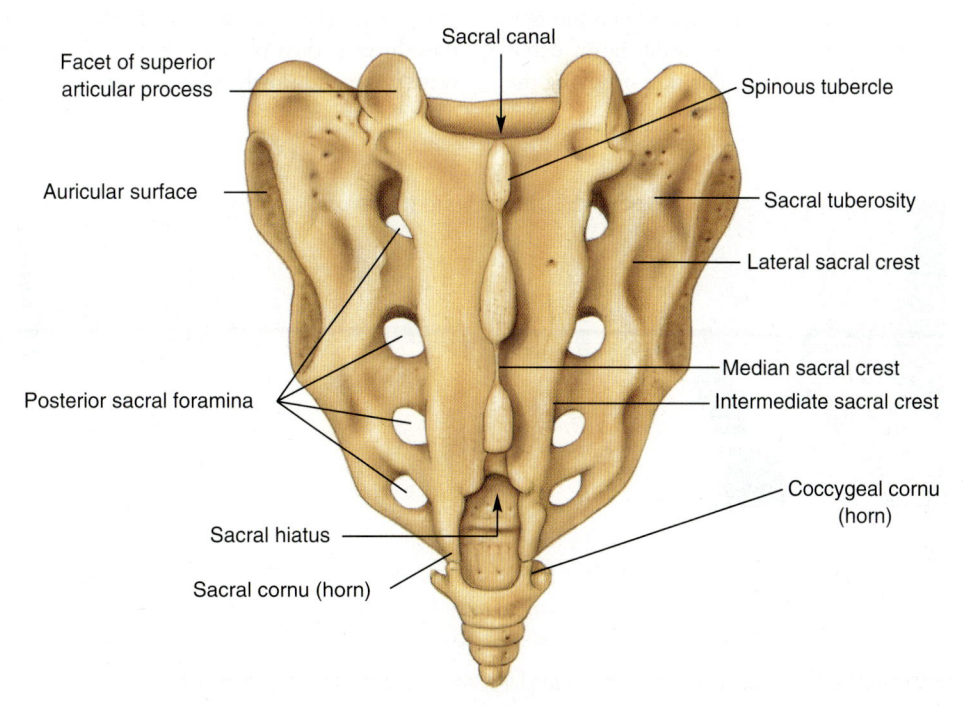

**FIGURE 101.2.** The anatomy of the sacrum. Note the relationship of the sacral cornua and sacral hiatus. (Reused from Anatomical Chart Company, Lippincott Williams & Wilkins; 2013.)

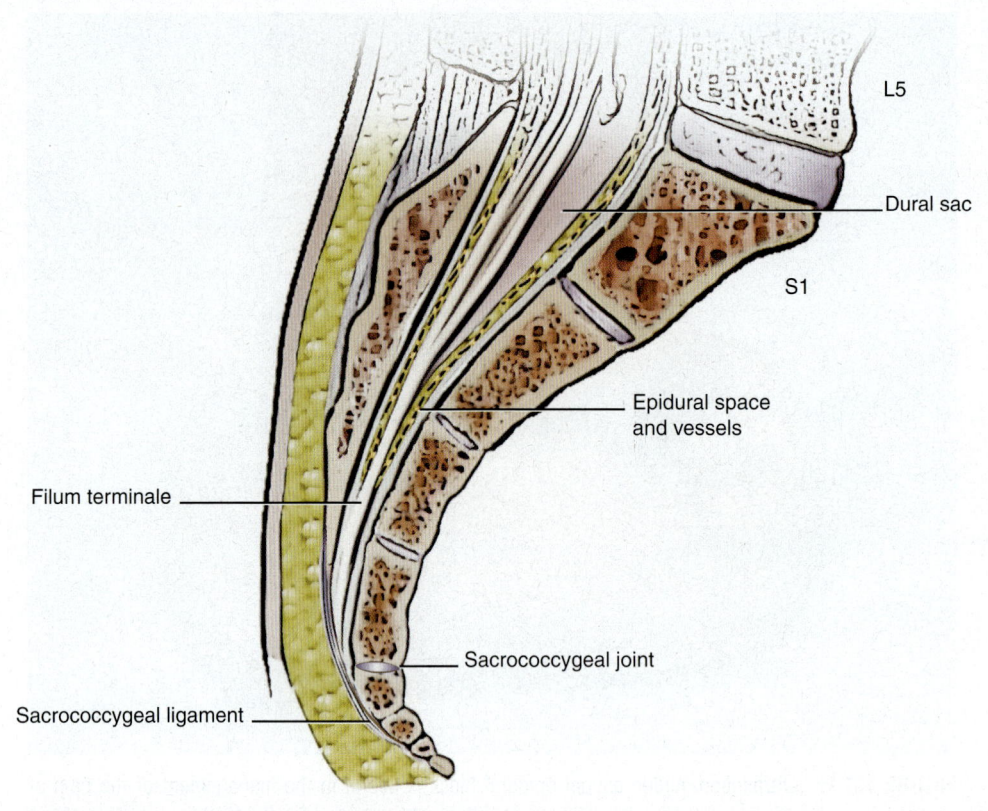

**FIGURE 101.3.** The sacrococcygeal ligament and caudal canal.

outward (Fig. 101.5). A total of 12 mL of local anesthetic suitable for epidural administration is drawn up in a 20-mL sterile syringe. If the painful condition being treated is thought to have an inflammatory component, 40 to 80 mg of depot steroid is added to the local anesthetic. The skin overlying the sacrum and sacral hiatus is then prepped with antiseptic solution, and the sacral hiatus and cornua are palpated using a rocking motion (Fig. 101.6). A high-frequency linear ultrasound transducer is then placed over the lower sacrum in the transverse plane and slowly moved caudally until the sacral cornua

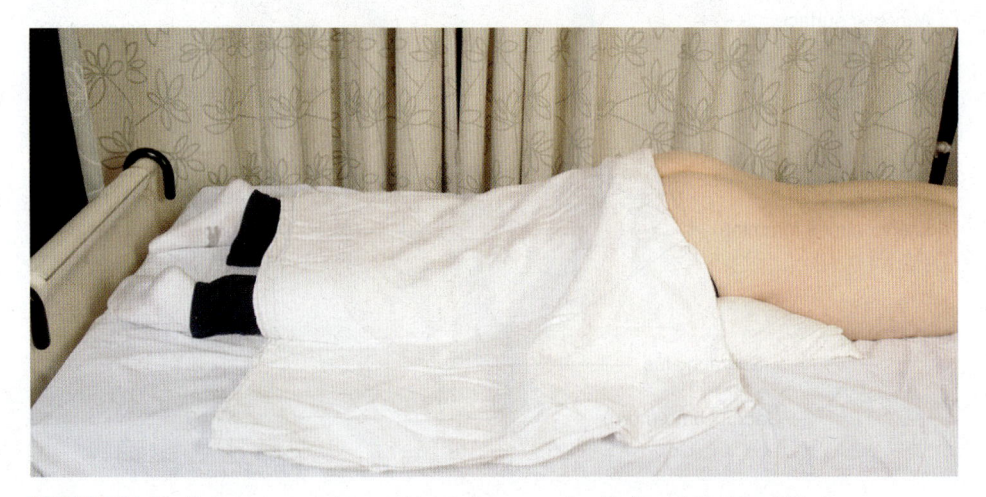

**FIGURE 101.4.** Proper prone patient position for ultrasound-guided caudal epidural block.

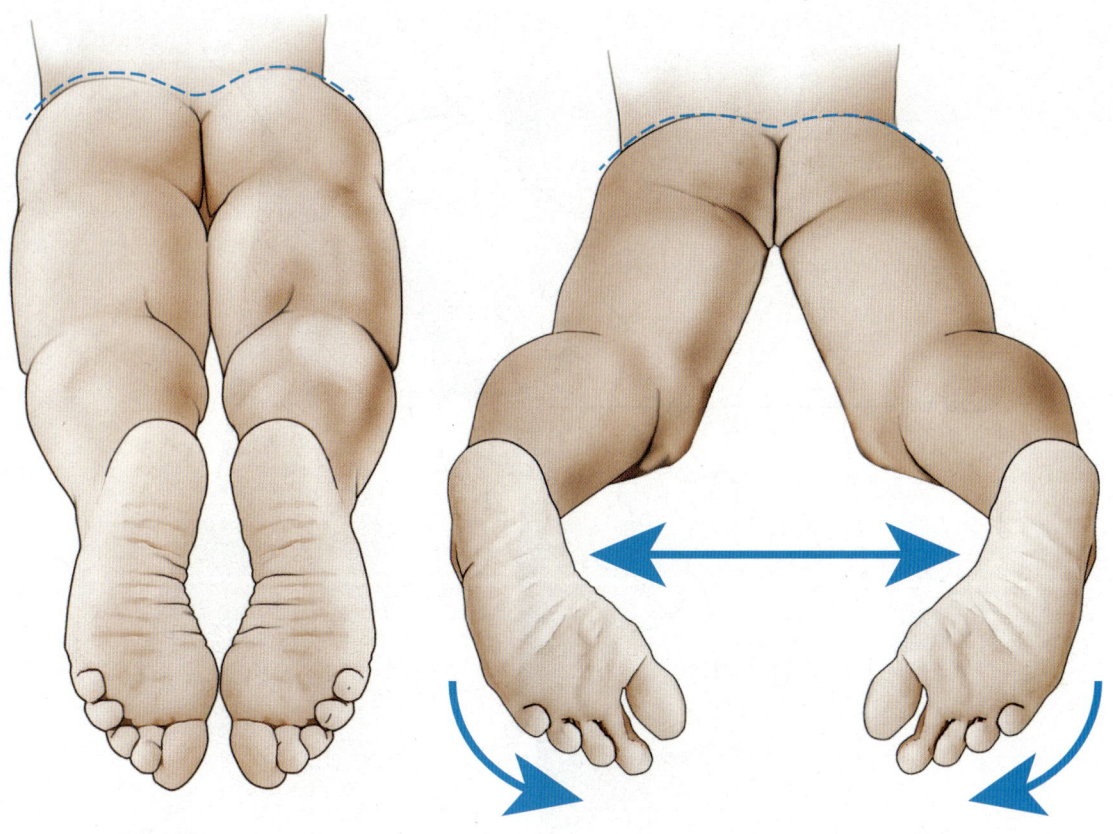

**FIGURE 101.5.** The patient is asked to turn his or her heels outward to relax the gluteal muscles.

are visualized (Figs. 101.7 and 101.8). The classic ultrasound appearance of the sacral cornua and their acoustic shadow is reminiscent of two nuns walking down the street (Fig. 101.9). Lying between the two nuns is the sacral hiatus, which provides access to the epidural space (see Fig. 101.8). Between the necks of the two is the sacrococcygeal ligament, which appears as a hyperechoic band–like structure (Fig. 101.10). Lying just beneath the sacrococcygeal ligament is the hypoechoic caudal canal (see Fig. 101.10). The floor of the caudal canal will appear as a bright hyperechoic line (see Fig. 101.10).

After the sacral cornua, sacral hiatus, and sacrococcygeal ligament are identified, the ultrasound transducer is turned to the longitudinal position and moved slowly cephalad until the inferior portion of the ultrasound transducer lies toward the top of the sacral hiatus (Figs. 101.11 and 101.12). After the sacral hiatus, sacrococcygeal ligament, and caudal canal are reidentified, a 22- or 25-gauge, 2-inch needle is inserted through the skin ~1 cm below the inferior border of the transducer utilizing an in-plane approach and advanced with a 45-degree angle to the skin through the sacrococcygeal ligament into the caudal canal under real-time ultrasound guidance until the entire needle tip rests just beyond sacrococcygeal ligament within the caudal canal (Fig. 101.13). As the sacrococcygeal ligament is penetrated, a "pop" will be felt. If contact with the interior bony wall of the sacral canal occurs, the needle should be withdrawn slightly. This will disengage the needle tip from the periosteum. The needle is then advanced ~0.5 cm into the canal. This is to ensure that the entire needle bevel is beyond the sacrococcygeal ligament to avoid injection into the ligament.

After gentle aspiration is negative for cerebrospinal fluid and blood, 12 mL of solution is injected. The needle is removed and pressure is placed on the injection site to avoid hematoma formation.

## COMPLICATIONS

Because of potential hematogenous spread via the valveless epidural veins of the caudal epidural space, sepsis and local infection at the injection site represent absolute contraindications to ultrasound-guided caudal epidural block. Although rare, inadvertent dural puncture can occur, and careful observation for spinal fluid must be carried out.

The lumbar epidural space is highly vascular with large numbers of valveless epidural veins. The intravenous placement of the epidural needle occurs in ~0.5% to 1% of patients undergoing lumbar epidural anesthesia. This complication

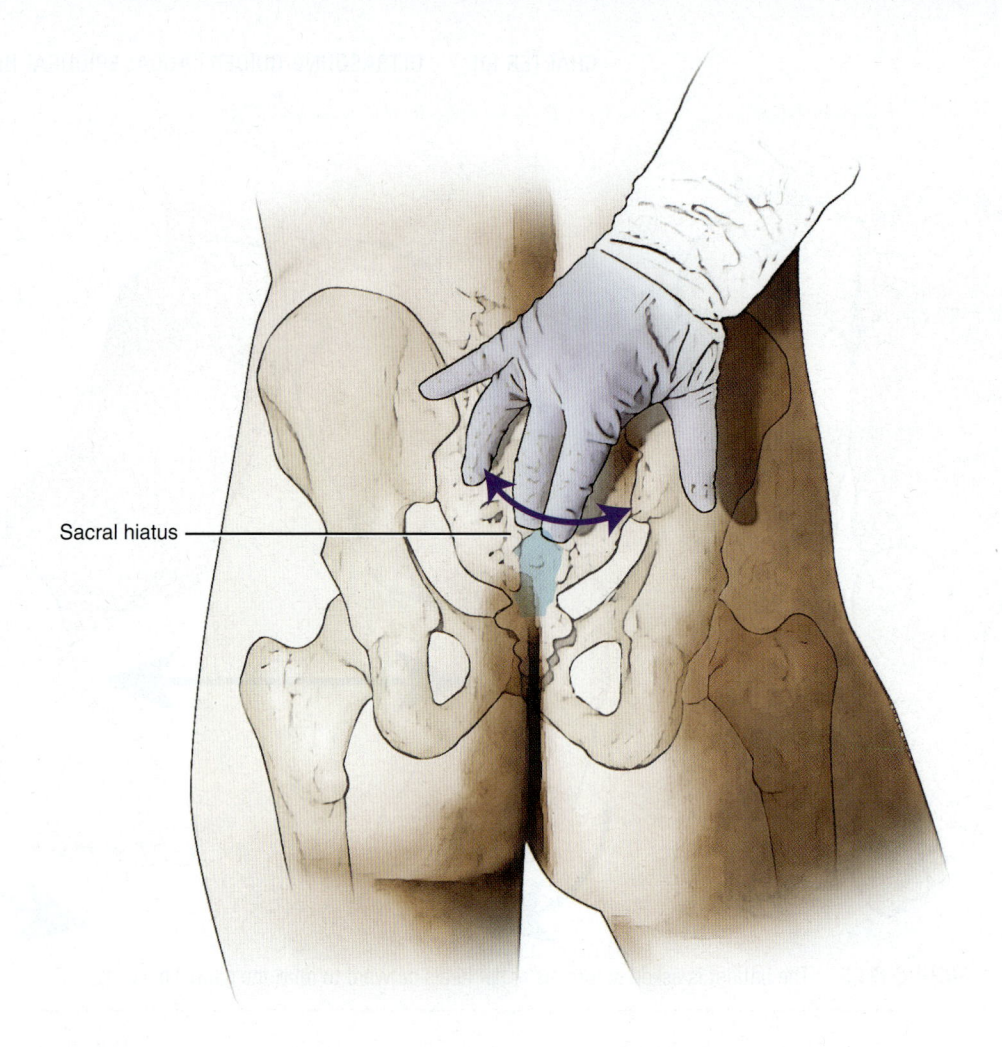

**FIGURE 101.6.** The sacral hiatus is identified by palpating with a lateral rocking motion.

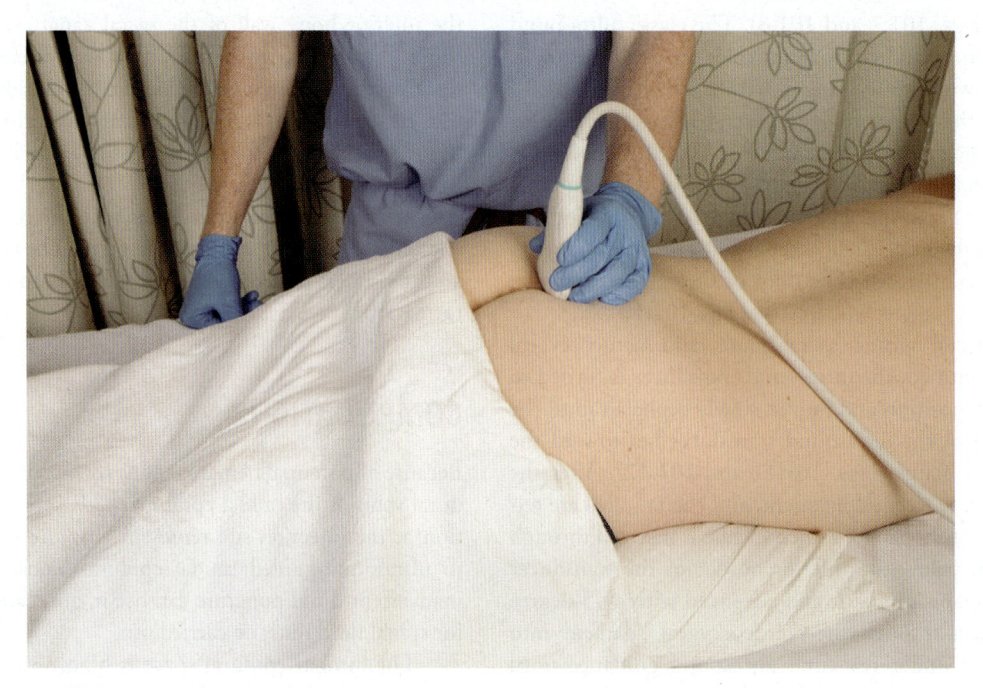

**FIGURE 101.7.** Placement of the ultrasound transducer in the transverse plane across the sacrum to obtain a paramedian sagittal transverse process view.

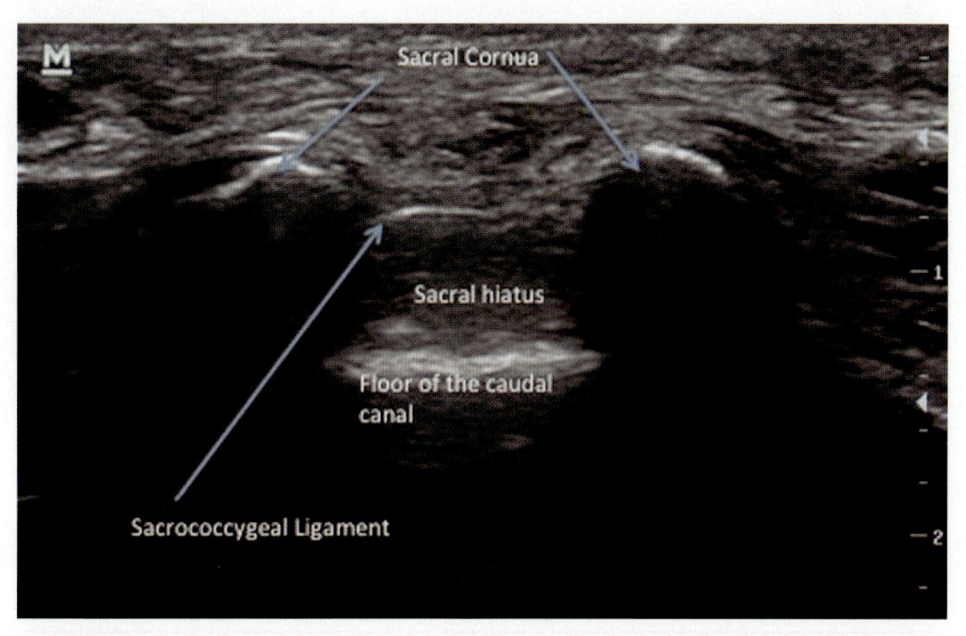

**FIGURE 101.8.** Transverse ultrasound image demonstrating the sacrum and top of sacral hiatus.

is increased in those patients with distended epidural veins, for example, the parturient and patients with large intra-abdominal tumor mass. If the misplacement is unrecognized, injection of local anesthetic directly into an epidural vein will result in significant local anesthetic toxicity. Needle-induced trauma to the lumbar epidural veins may cause bleeding, which is usually self-limited but has the potential to cause increased postprocedure pain. Uncontrolled bleeding into the epidural space may result in epidural hematoma formation, which can cause compression of the spinal cord with the rapid development of paraplegia. Although the incidence of significant neurologic deficit secondary to epidural hematoma after caudal epidural block is exceedingly rare, this devastating complication should be considered in any patient with rapidly progressive neurologic deficits following this technique.

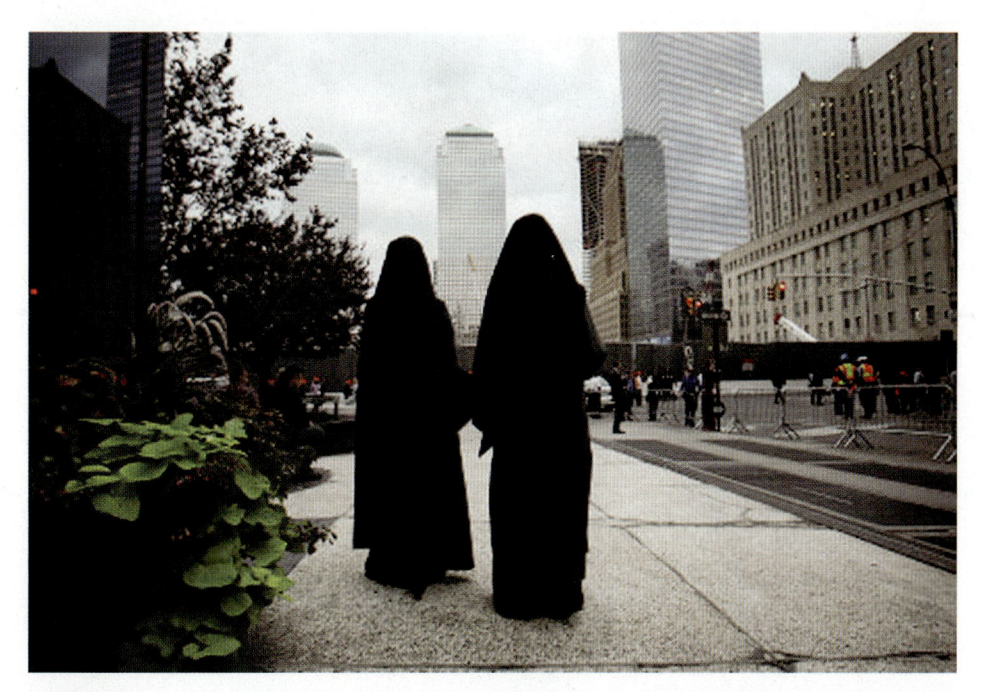

**FIGURE 101.9.** The sacral cornua and their acoustic shadow are reminiscent of two nuns walking down the street.

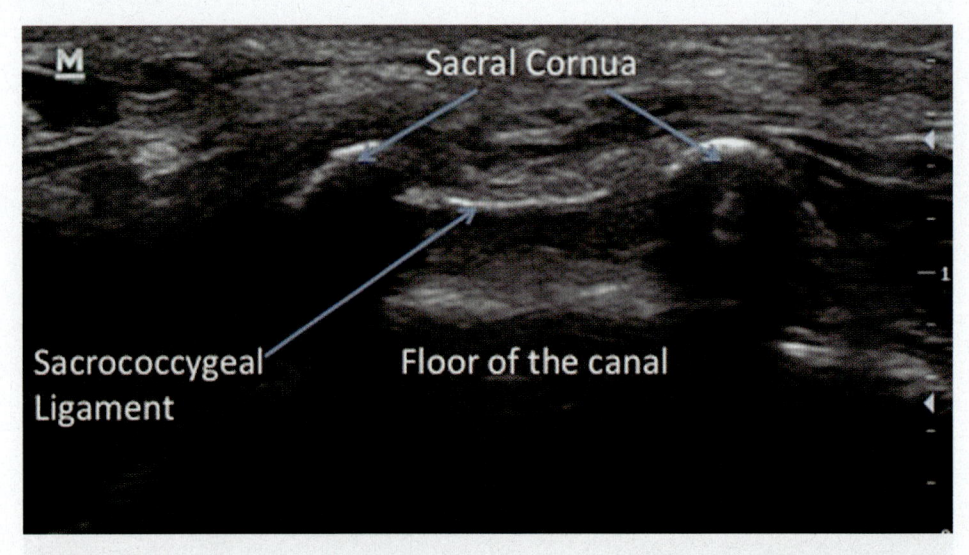

**FIGURE 101.10.** Transverse ultrasound view of sacral hiatus, sacrococcygeal ligament, and caudal canal.

When performing ultrasound-guided caudal block, should the aspiration test be positive for either spinal fluid or blood, the needle must be repositioned and the aspiration test repeated. If the test is negative, subsequent injections of 0.5-mL increments of local anesthetic are undertaken. Careful observation for signs of local anesthetic toxicity or subarachnoid spread of local anesthetic during the injection and after the procedure is indicated. Clinical experience has led to the use of smaller volumes of local anesthetic without sacrificing the clinical efficacy of caudal steroid epidural blocks. The use of smaller volumes of local anesthetic has markedly decreased the number of local anesthetic–related side effects.

Although uncommon, infection in the lumbar epidural space remains an ever-present possibility, especially in the immunocompromised AIDS or cancer patient, and should be considered in any patient with fever and the onset of neurologic symptomatology after undergoing an epidural block. Early detection and treatment of epidural infection is crucial

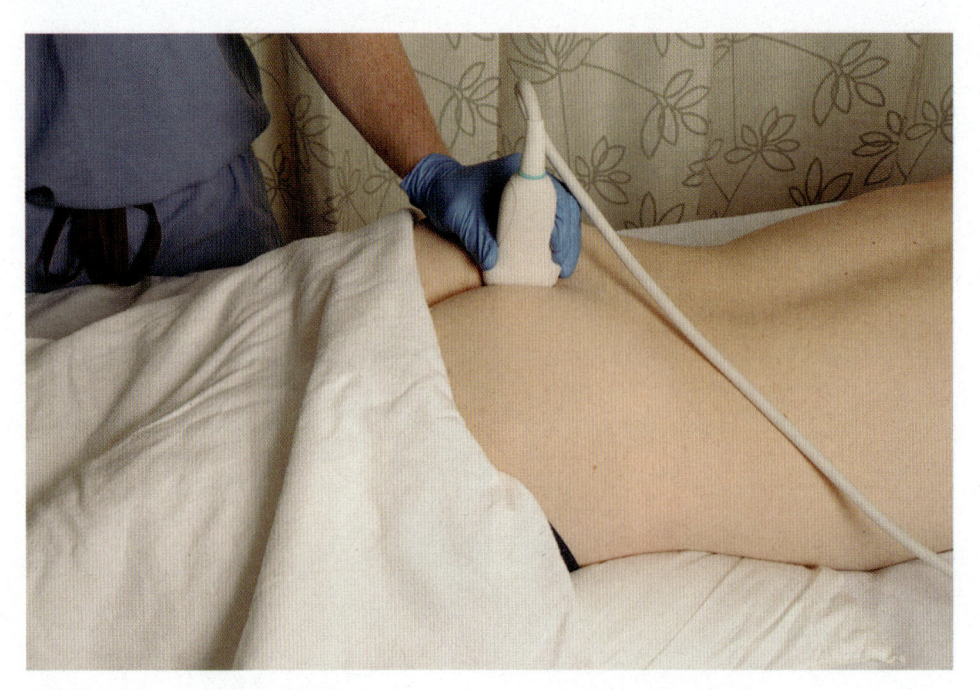

**FIGURE 101.11.** Proper longitudinal ultrasound transducer placement to visualize the sacrococcygeal ligament and caudal canal.

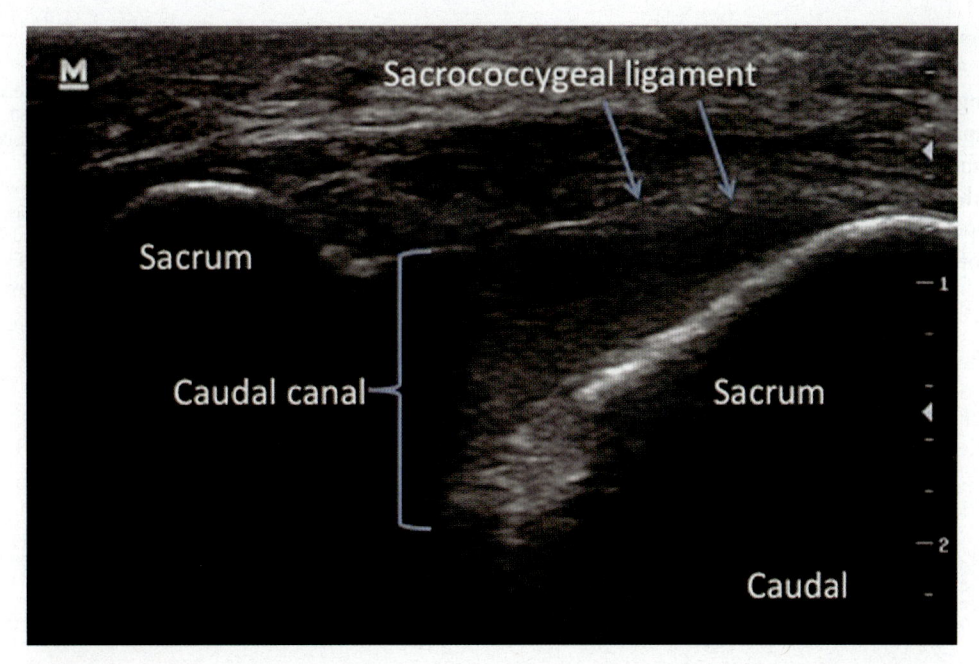

**FIGURE 101.12.** Longitudinal ultrasound image of the sacral hiatus, sacrococcygeal ligament, and caudal canal.

to avoid potentially life-threatening sequelae, and urgent computerized tomography and/or magnetic resonance imaging should be obtained in any patient suspected of having an epidural abscess. Emergent surgical drainage to avoid spinal cord compression and irreversible neurologic deficit is often required.

## CLINICAL PEARLS

The key to performing successful ultrasound neuraxial blocks is the proper identification of the sonographic anatomy. Ultrasound-guided caudal block is a much simpler technique than ultrasound-guided lumbar epidural block and,

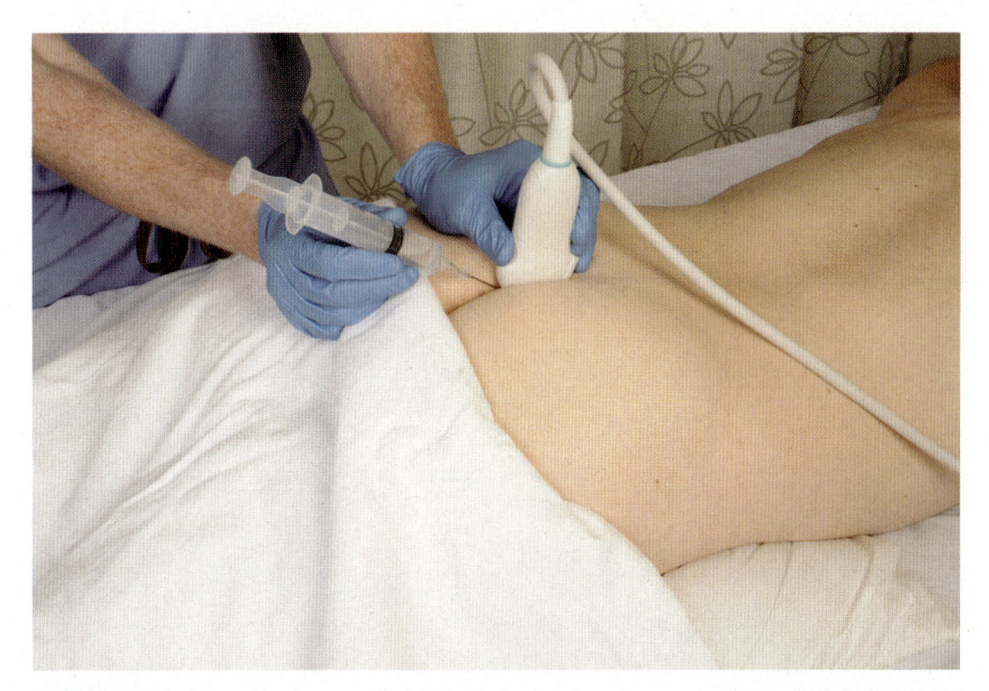

**FIGURE 101.13.** Proper in-plane needle position for performing ultrasound-guided caudal epidural block.

in many centers, is the preferred approach to the lower epidural space. Any significant pain or sudden increase in resistance during injection when performing ultrasound-guided caudal epidural block suggests incorrect needle placement, and one should stop injecting immediately and reassess the position of the needle. Because pain is an important indication of improper needle placement, the practitioner should avoid the use of excessive sedation when performing this technique.

## SUGGESTED READINGS

Vydyanathan A, Narouze S. Ultrasound-guided caudal and sacroiliac joint injections. *Tech Reg Anesth Pain Manag* 2009;13(3):157–160.

Waldman SD. Caudal epidural block. In: *Pain Review*. Philadelphia, PA: Saunders Elsevier; 2009:530–533.

Waldman SD. Caudal epidural nerve block. In: *Atlas of Interventional Pain Management*. 3rd ed. Philadelphia, PA: Saunders Elsevier; 2009:441–448.

Waldman SD, Campbell R. Anatomy: special imaging considerations of the lumbar spine. In: *Imaging of Pain*. Philadelphia, PA: Saunders Elsevier; 2009:67–68.

Yamauchi M. Ultrasound-guided neuraxial block. *Trends Anaesth Crit Care* 2012;2(5):234–243.

# CHAPTER 102

# Ultrasound-Guided Lumbar Plexus Nerve Block

## CLINICAL PERSPECTIVES

Ultrasound-guided lumbar plexus block is utilized most frequently for surgical anesthesia of the lower extremity. This technique is occasionally utilized as a diagnostic maneuver when performing differential neural blockade on an anatomic basis in the evaluation of groin and lower extremity pain. The technique may be utilized in a prognostic manner if destruction of the lumbar plexus is being contemplated to demonstrate the degree of motor and sensory impairment that the patient may experience. Ultrasound-guided blockade of the lumbar plexus is also useful as a therapeutic maneuver when treating inflammatory conditions involving the lumbar plexus including idiopathic, diabetic, and viral plexitis. The technique is also used to palliate acute pain emergencies, including groin and lower extremity trauma or fracture, acute herpes zoster, and cancer pain including tumor invasion of the lumbar plexus while waiting for pharmacologic, surgical, and antiblastic therapies to become effective. Destruction of the lumbar plexus is indicated for the palliation of cancer pain, including invasive tumors of the lumbar plexus and the tissues that the plexus innervates. More selective techniques such as radiofrequency lesioning of specific lumbar paravertebral nerve roots may cause less morbidity than lumbar plexus neurolysis.

## CLINICALLY RELEVANT ANATOMY

The lumbar plexus is comprised of fibers from the ventral roots of the first four lumbar nerves and, in most patients, a contribution from the 12th thoracic nerve (Fig. 102.1). The lumbar plexus lies within the posterior substance of the psoas muscle where it is amenable to ultrasound-guided neural blockade (Fig. 102.2). The nerves lie in front of the transverse processes of their respective vertebrae, and as they course inferolaterally, they divide into a number of peripheral nerves. The ilioinguinal and iliohypogastric nerves are branches of the L1 nerves, with an occasional contribution of fibers from T12. The genitofemoral nerve is made up of fibers from L1 and L2. The lateral femoral cutaneous nerve is derived from fibers of L2 and L3. The obturator nerve receives fibers from L2–L4, and the femoral nerve is made up of fibers from L2–L4. The lumbar plexus also provides interconnecting branches to the sacral plexus via the lumbosacral trunk (see Fig. 102.1).

## ULTRASOUND-GUIDED TECHNIQUE

Ultrasound-guided lumbar plexus block can be carried out by placing the patient in the lateral decubitus position (Fig. 102.3). A total of 20 to 25 mL of local anesthetic is drawn up in a sterile syringe. Given the large volume of local anesthetic required for this technique, the clinician must carefully calculate the total milligram dosage of local anesthetic to be injected to avoid local anesthetic toxicity. If the painful condition being treated is thought to have an inflammatory component, 40 to 80 mg of depot steroid is added to the local anesthetic. The midline of the lumbar spine is identified by palpation as is the iliac crest, and a line is drawn from each of these anatomic landmarks (see Fig. 102.3).

After preparation of the skin with antiseptic solution, a curvilinear low-frequency ultrasound transducer is placed in the transverse plane ~3 cm laterally from the midline along the line drawn from the iliac crest, and an ultrasound survey is taken (Figs. 102.4 and 102.5). This should place the transducer at the L2–L3 level. Note that the transverse process blocks ultrasound visualization of the lumbar plexus (Fig. 102.6). Once the transverse process is identified, the ultrasound transducer is slowly moved in a cephalad direction to identify the acoustic window between two adjacent transverse processes (Fig. 102.7). Once the acoustic window between the adjacent transverse processes is identified, the lateral aspect of the ultrasound transducer is rocked anteriorly to identify the intervertebral foramen and the lateral margin of the vertebral body (Figs. 102.8 and 102.9). The lumbar plexus can then be seen within the psoas muscle, which is just lateral to the vertebral body and intervertebral foramen (see Figs. 102.9 and 102.10). A color Doppler image is then obtained to identify adjacent vasculature to avoid inadvertent intravascular injection (Fig. 102.11).

Once the lumbar plexus is identified within the psoas muscle, a 13-cm stimulating needle is advanced under real-time ultrasound guidance utilizing an in-plane approach from the lateral aspect of the transversely placed ultrasound transducer until the needle is in proximity to the lumbar plexus (Fig. 102.12).

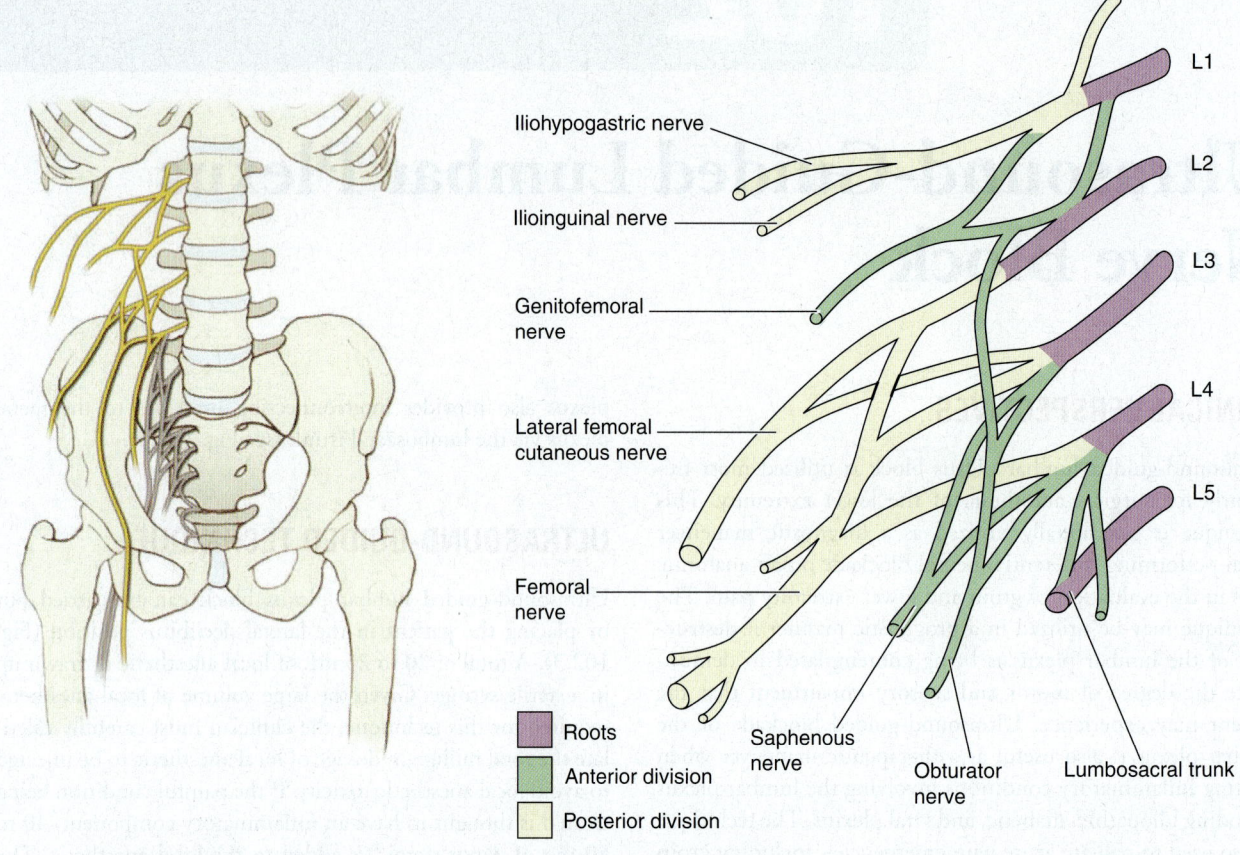

**FIGURE 102.1.** The anatomy of the lumbar plexus. (Reused from Premkumar K. *The Massage Connection Anatomy and Physiology.* Baltimore, MD: Lippincott Williams & Wilkins; 2004, with permission.)

**FIGURE 102.2.** The lumbar plexus travels through the posterior portion of the psoas muscle. The psoas muscle on the right has been removed to demonstrate the proximity of the lumbar plexus to the lateral aspect of the vertebral body.

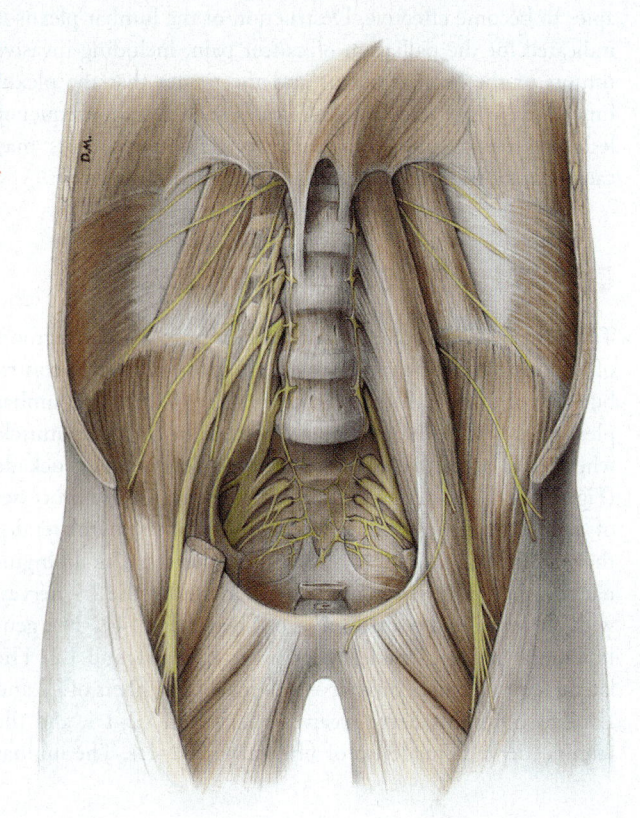

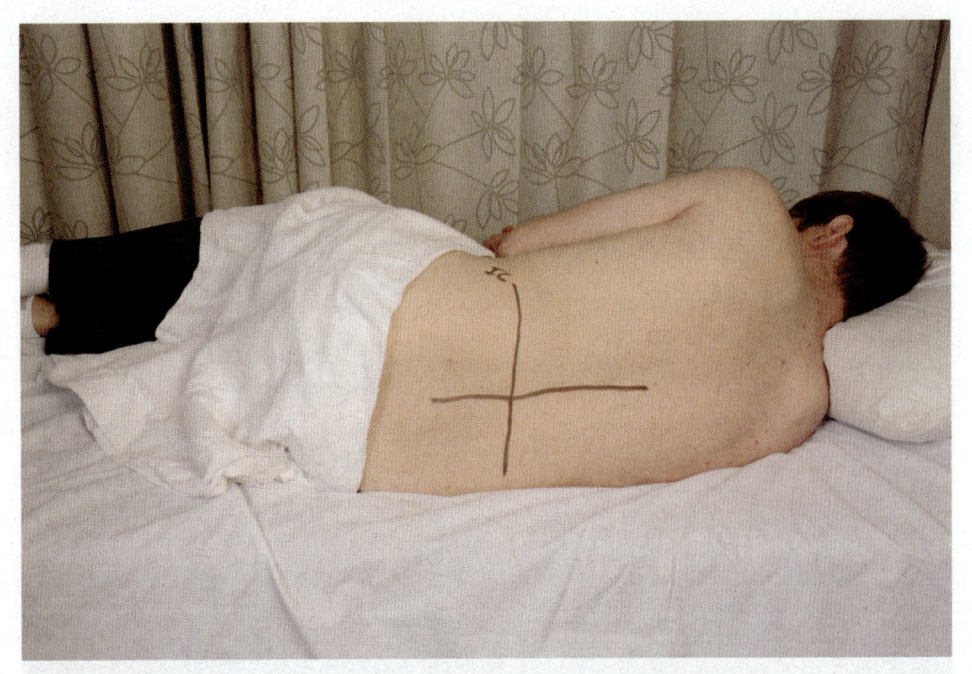

**FIGURE 102.3.** Proper lateral decubitus patient position for ultrasound-guided lumbar plexus block. (IC, iliac crest.)

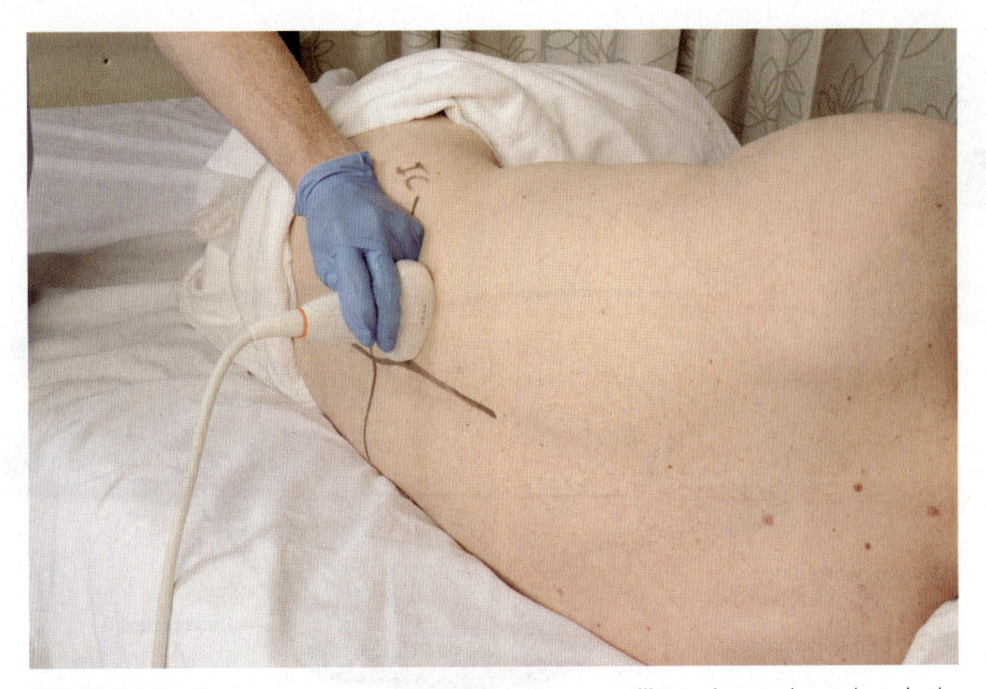

**FIGURE 102.4.** Transverse placement of the low-frequency curvilinear ultrasound transducer in the transverse plane 3 cm lateral to midline at level of iliac crest (L2–L3).

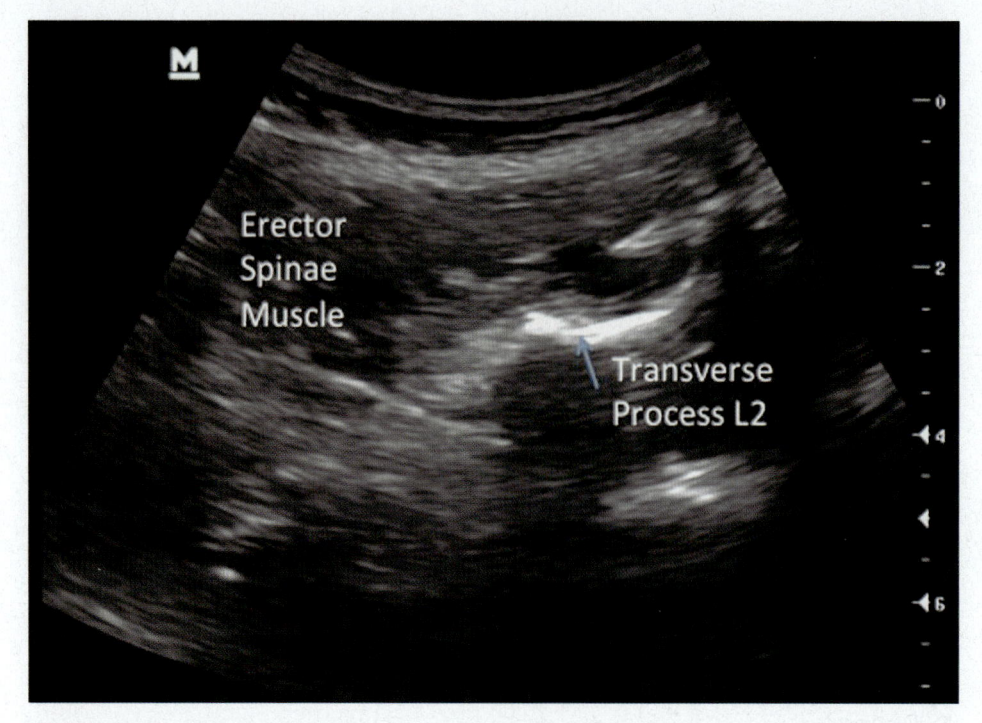

**FIGURE 102.5.** Transverse ultrasound view demonstrating transverse process.

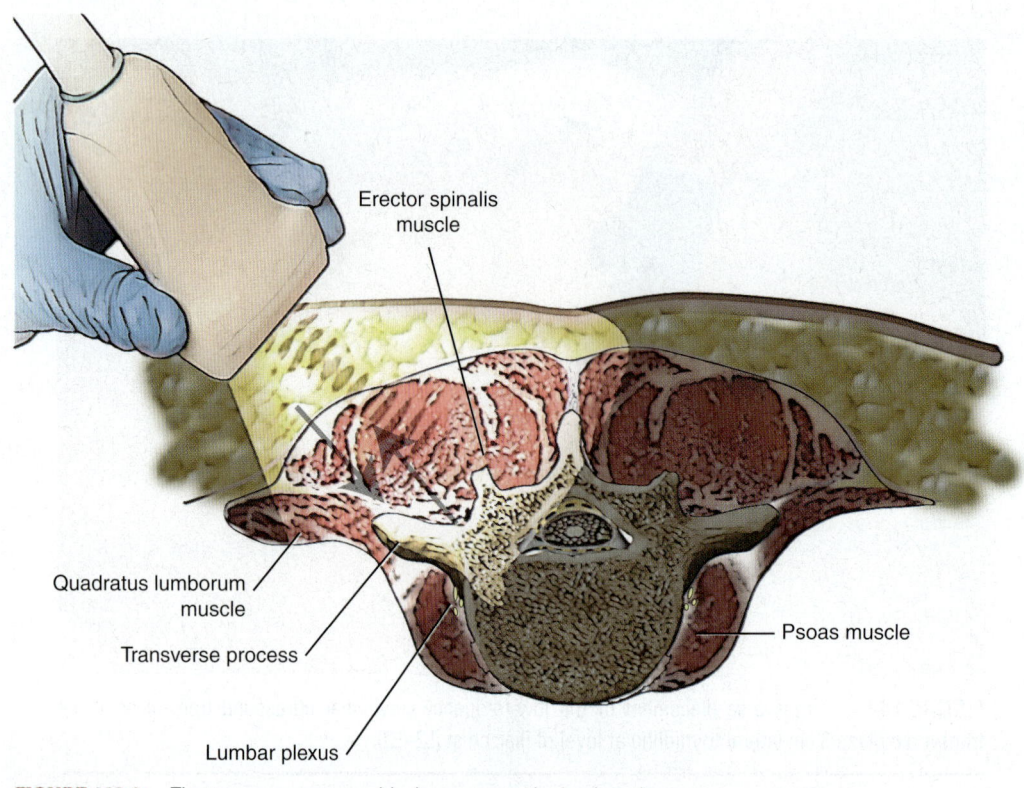

**FIGURE 102.6.** The transverse process blocks access to the lumbar plexus.

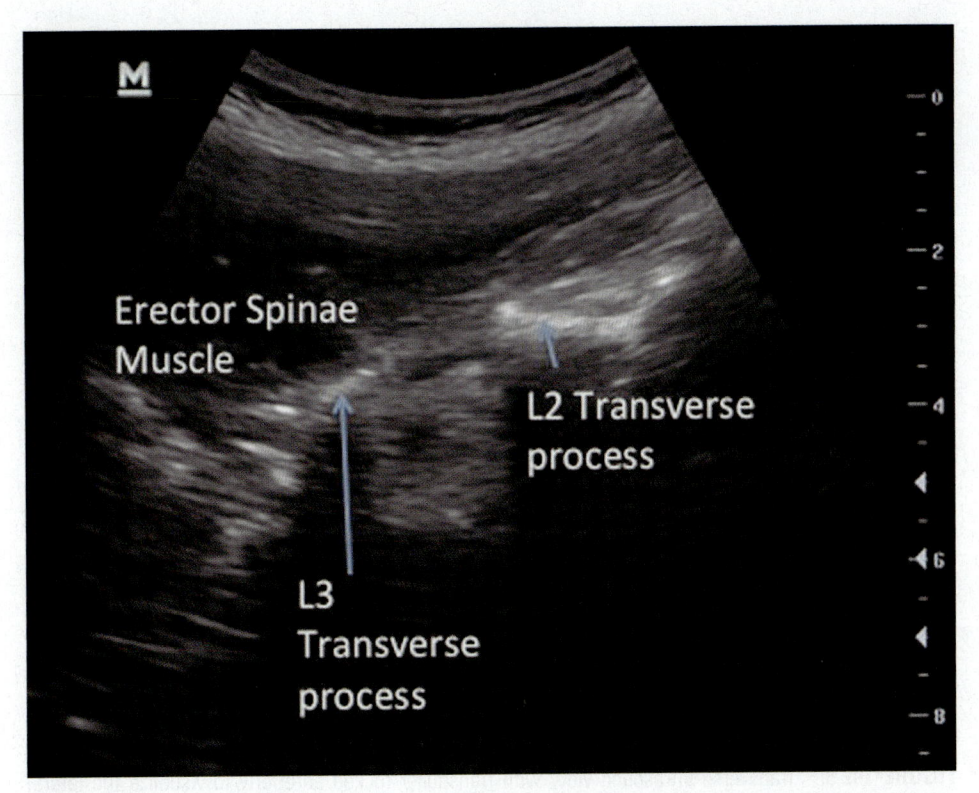

**FIGURE 102.7.** Transverse ultrasound image demonstrating acoustic window between two adjacent transverse processes.

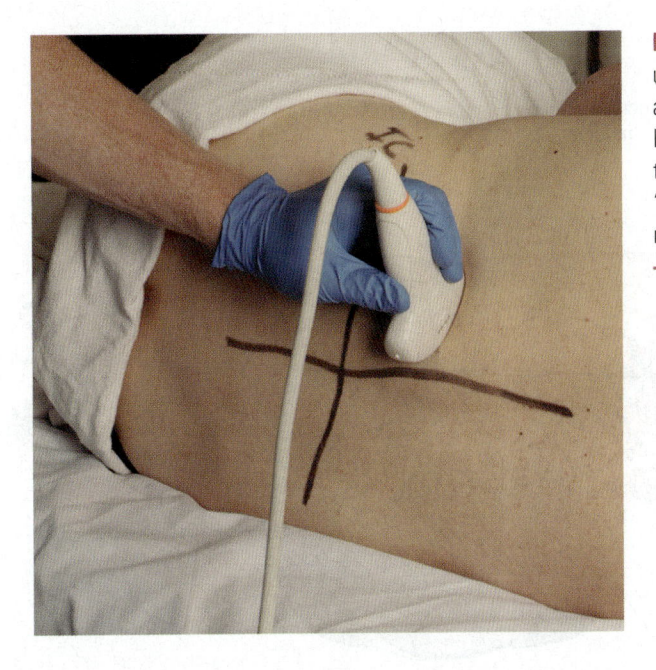

**FIGURE 102.8.** To obtain an ultrasound image of the lateral aspect of the vertebral body, the lateral aspect of the ultrasound transducer is rocked anteriorly to "see" around the posterior elements of the vertebra.

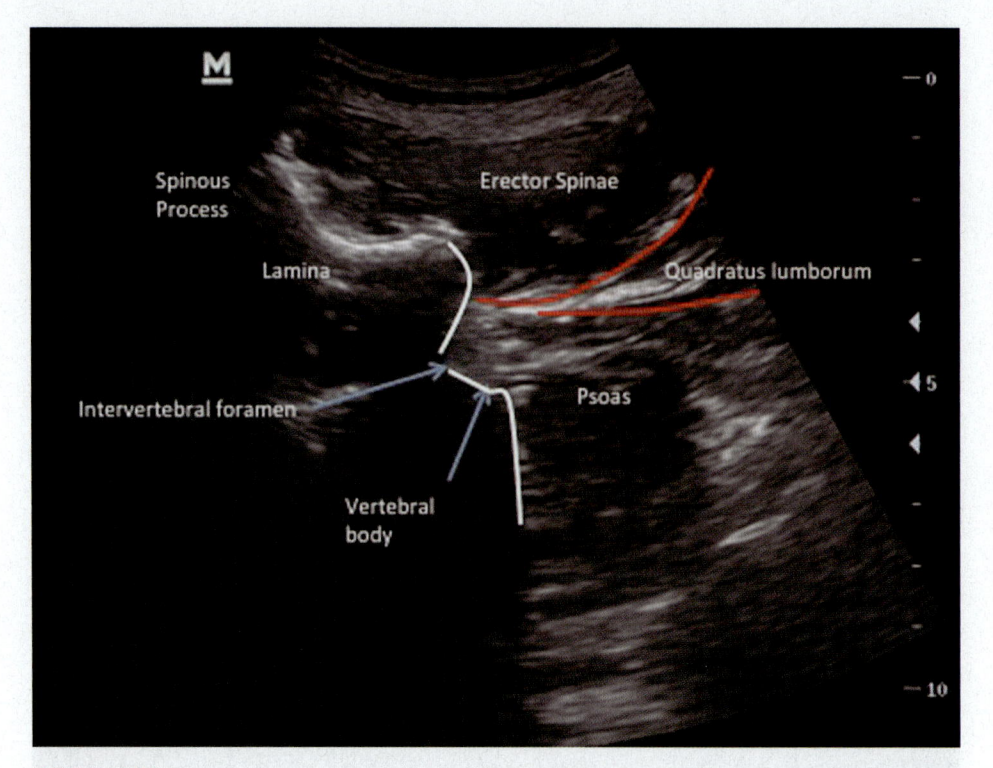

**FIGURE 102.9.** Transverse ultrasound view with transducer rocked anteriorly to visualize the lateral margin of the vertebral body and the lumbar plexus lying adjacent to it embedded in the psoas muscle.

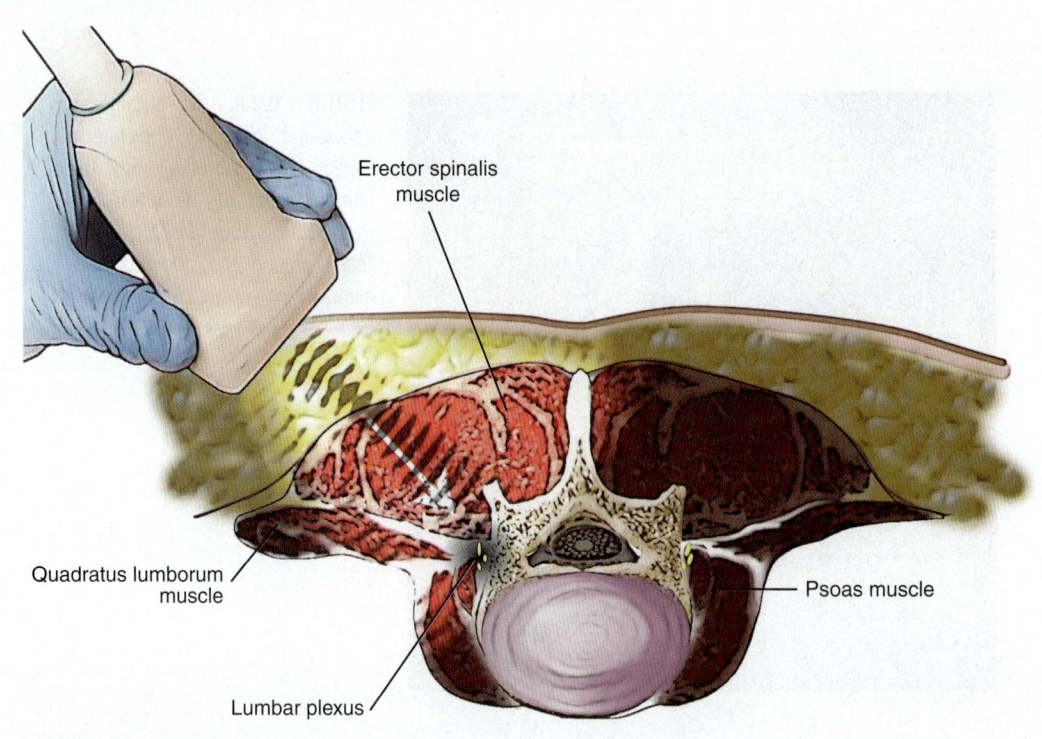

**FIGURE 102.10.** The lumbar plexus lies within the psoas muscle just lateral to the lateral margin of the vertebral body.

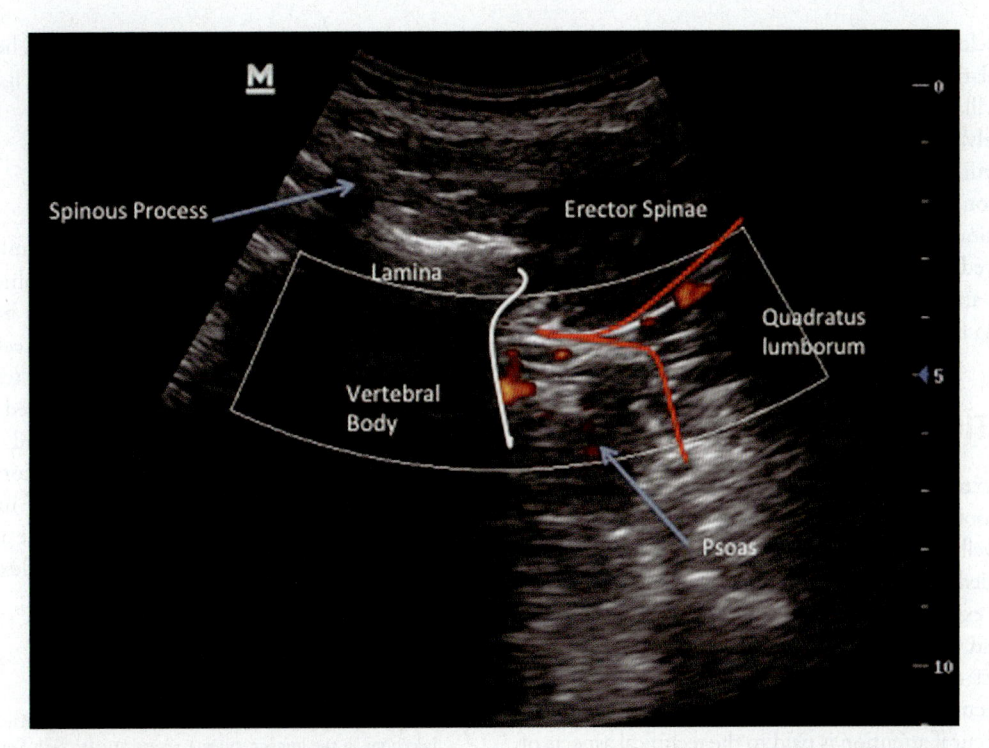

**FIGURE 102.11.** Transverse color Doppler image demonstrating vasculature in proximity to the lumbar plexus.

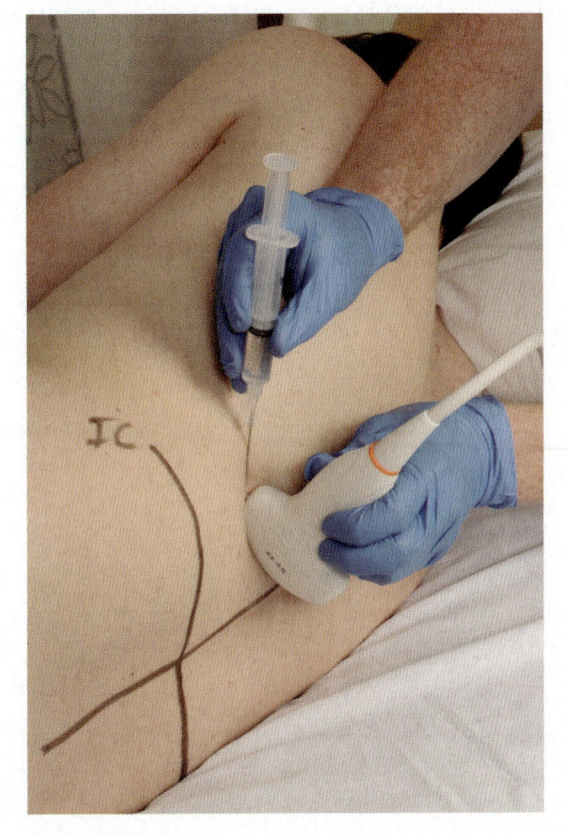

**FIGURE 102.12.** Proper in-plane needle position for performing selective lumbar nerve root block.

Intrapsoas muscle needle tip placement can be confirmed by electrical stimulation of the psoas muscle. Contraction of the psoas muscle will be readily apparent under ultrasound imaging. Alternatively, injection of a small amount of solution to demonstrate hydrodissection is also a suitable way to identify the exact location of the needle tip. After gentle aspiration for blood, the solution is injected in small aliquots while the patient is closely observed for signs of local anesthetic toxicity. The needle is removed and pressure is placed on the injection site to avoid hematoma formation.

## COMPLICATIONS

The lumbar plexus is in close proximity to the spinal cord and exiting nerve roots, and this procedure should be performed only by those well versed in the regional anatomy and skilled at ultrasound-guided interventional pain management procedures. Trauma to the exiting lumbar nerve roots as well as inadvertent subarachnoid, subdural, and/or epidural injection can occur even in the best of hands. Inadvertent dural puncture occurring during selective nerve root block of the lumbar nerve roots should rarely occur if attention is paid to the technical aspects of this procedure. However, failure to recognize an unintentional dural or subdural injection can result in immediate total spinal anesthesia with associated loss of consciousness, hypotension, and apnea. This can be disastrous if not immediately recognized. The vascular nature of this anatomic region makes the potential for intravascular injection high although the use of color Doppler to identify vascular structures should help the clinician avoid this potentially fatal complication (see Fig. 102.12).

## CLINICAL PEARLS

The key to performing successful ultrasound-guided blocks is the proper identification of the sonographic anatomy and the ability to properly identify the anatomy being visualized. This should not be a problem if the above technique is used. Any significant pain or sudden increase in resistance during injection when performing ultrasound-guided lumbar plexus block suggests incorrect needle placement, and one should stop injecting immediately and reassess the position of the needle. Because pain is an important indication of improper needle placement, the practitioner should avoid the use of excessive sedation during ultrasound-guided lumbar plexus block.

## SUGGESTED READINGS

Galiano K, Obwegeser AA, Gruber H. Ultrasound guidance for periradicular injections in the lumbar spine: a review article. *Tech Reg Anesth Pain Manag* 2009;13(3):154–156.

Gray AT, Collins AB, Schafhalter-Zoppoth I. An introduction to femoral nerve and associated lumbar plexus nerve blocks under ultrasonic guidance. *Tech Reg Anesth Pain Manag* 2004;8(4):155–163.

Waldman SD. Functional anatomy of the lumbar spine. In: *Pain Review*. Philadelphia, PA: Saunders Elsevier; 2009:65–67.

Waldman SD. Lumbar plexus block. In: *Atlas of Interventional Pain Management*. 3rd ed. Philadelphia, PA: Saunders Elsevier; 2009:513–516.

# CHAPTER 103

# Ultrasound-Guided Injection Technique for Lumbar Myofascial Pain Syndrome

## CLINICAL PERSPECTIVES

The muscles of the back often develop myofascial pain following repeated microtrauma from overuse including improper lifting and bending or from chronic deconditioning of the agonist and antagonist muscle unit. The sine qua non of myofascial pain syndrome on physical examination is the identification of myofascial trigger points. The end result of repetitive microtrauma to a muscle or group of muscles is the trigger point, which is a localized point of exquisite tenderness in the affected muscle or muscle groups. The trigger point is identified by mechanical stimulation of the painful area by palpation (Fig. 103.1). The result of trigger point stimulation is localized pain, referred pain, and an involuntary withdrawal of the stimulated muscle that is known as a "jump sign." The referred pain associated with myofascial pain syndrome is often misdiagnosed or attributed to other organ systems, leading to extensive evaluations and ineffective treatment. Patients with myofascial pain syndrome involving the muscles of the low back often have referred pain into the hips, sacroiliac joint, and buttocks (Fig. 103.2).

In addition to muscle trauma, a variety of other factors seem to predispose the patient to develop myofascial pain syndrome. The weekend athlete who subjects his or her body to unaccustomed physical activity often develops myofascial pain syndrome. Poor posture while sitting at a computer keyboard or while watching television also has been implicated as a predisposing factor to the development of myofascial pain syndrome. Previous injuries may result in abnormal muscle function and predispose to the subsequent development of myofascial pain syndrome. All of these predisposing factors may be intensified if the patient also suffers from poor nutritional status or coexisting psychological or behavioral abnormalities, including chronic stress and depression. The muscles of the low back seem to be particularly susceptible to stress-induced myofascial pain syndrome.

Stiffness and fatigue often coexist with the pain of myofascial pain syndrome, increasing the functional disability associated with this disease and complicating its treatment. Myofascial pain syndrome may occur as a primary disease state or in conjunction with other painful conditions, including radiculopathy and chronic regional pain syndromes. Sleep disturbance is common. Psychological or behavioral abnormalities, including depression, frequently coexist with the muscle abnormalities associated with myofascial pain syndrome. Treatment of these psychological and behavioral abnormalities must be an integral part of any successful treatment plan for myofascial pain syndrome.

## CLINICALLY RELEVANT ANATOMY

The muscles of the back work together as a functional unit to stabilize and allow coordinated movement of the low back and allow one to maintain an upright position. Trauma to an individual muscle can result in dysfunction of the entire functional unit. The rhomboids, latissimus dorsi, iliocostalis lumborum, multifidus, psoas, and quadratus lumborum muscles are frequent sites of myofascial pain syndrome (Figs. 103.3 and 103.4). The points of origin and attachments of these muscles as well as the muscles themselves are particularly susceptible to trauma and the subsequent development of myofascial trigger points. Injection of these trigger points serves as both a diagnostic and a therapeutic maneuver.

## ULTRASOUND-GUIDED TECHNIQUE

Ultrasound-guided injection for lumbar myofascial pain syndrome can be carried out by placing the patient in the lateral decubitus position (Fig. 103.5). A syringe containing 10 mL of 0.25% preservative-free bupivacaine and 40 mg of methylprednisolone is attached to a 25-gauge needle of a length adequate to reach the trigger point. For the deeper muscles of posture in the low back, a 3½-inch needle is required. A volume of 0.5 to 1.0 mL of solution is then injected into each trigger point. A series of two to five treatment sessions may be required to completely abolish the trigger point; the patient should be informed of this. The midline of the lumbar spine is identified by palpation as is the iliac crest, and a line is drawn from each of these anatomic landmarks (see Fig. 103.6).

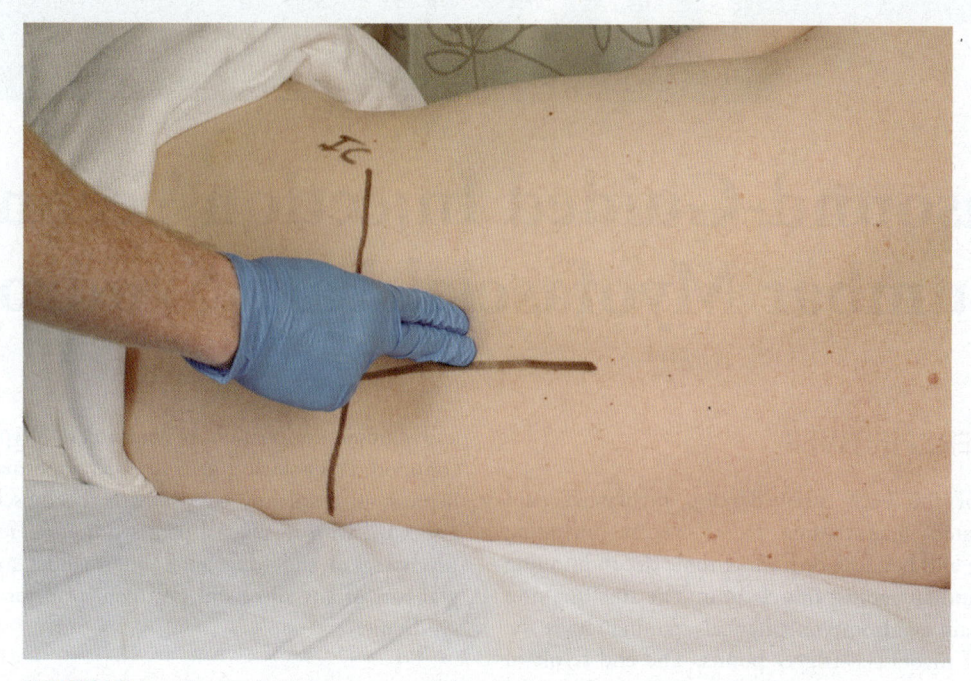

**FIGURE 103.1.** The myofascial trigger point is identified by palpation of the affected muscle.

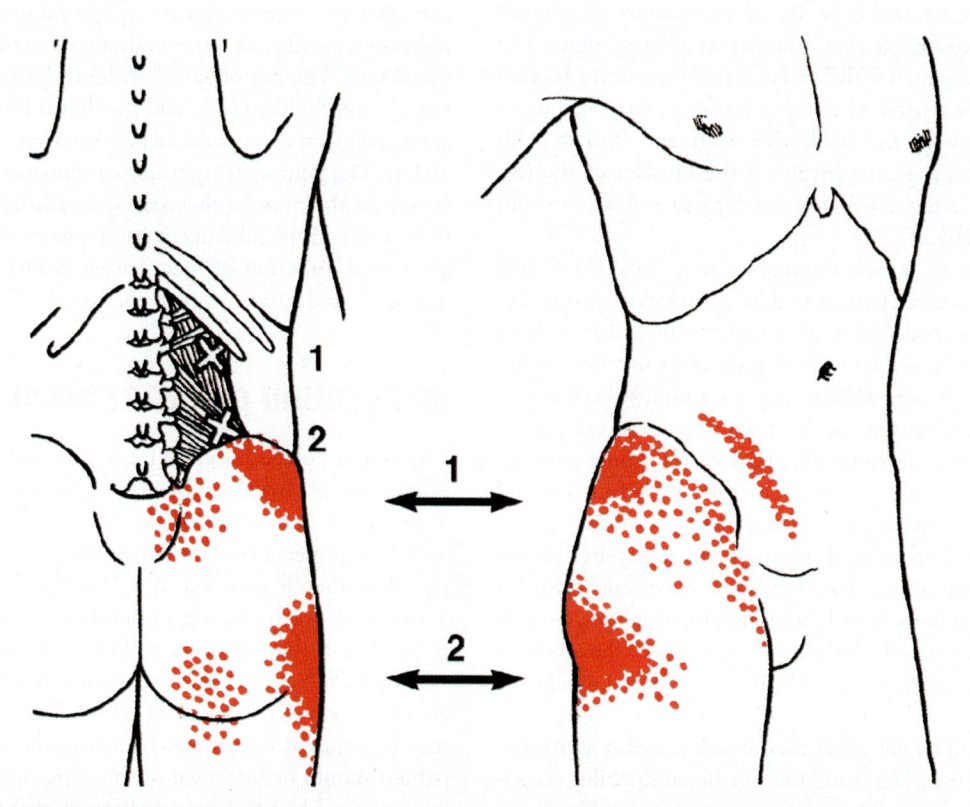

**FIGURE 103.2.** The pain of myofascial pain of the lumbar muscles is not only localized to the affected muscle but is often referred into the hip and buttocks. This figure demonstrates the local and referred pain patterns of myofascial pain involving the quadratus lumborum muscle. (MediClip ©2003, Lippincott Williams & Wilkins. All Rights Reserved.)

**Anterior view**

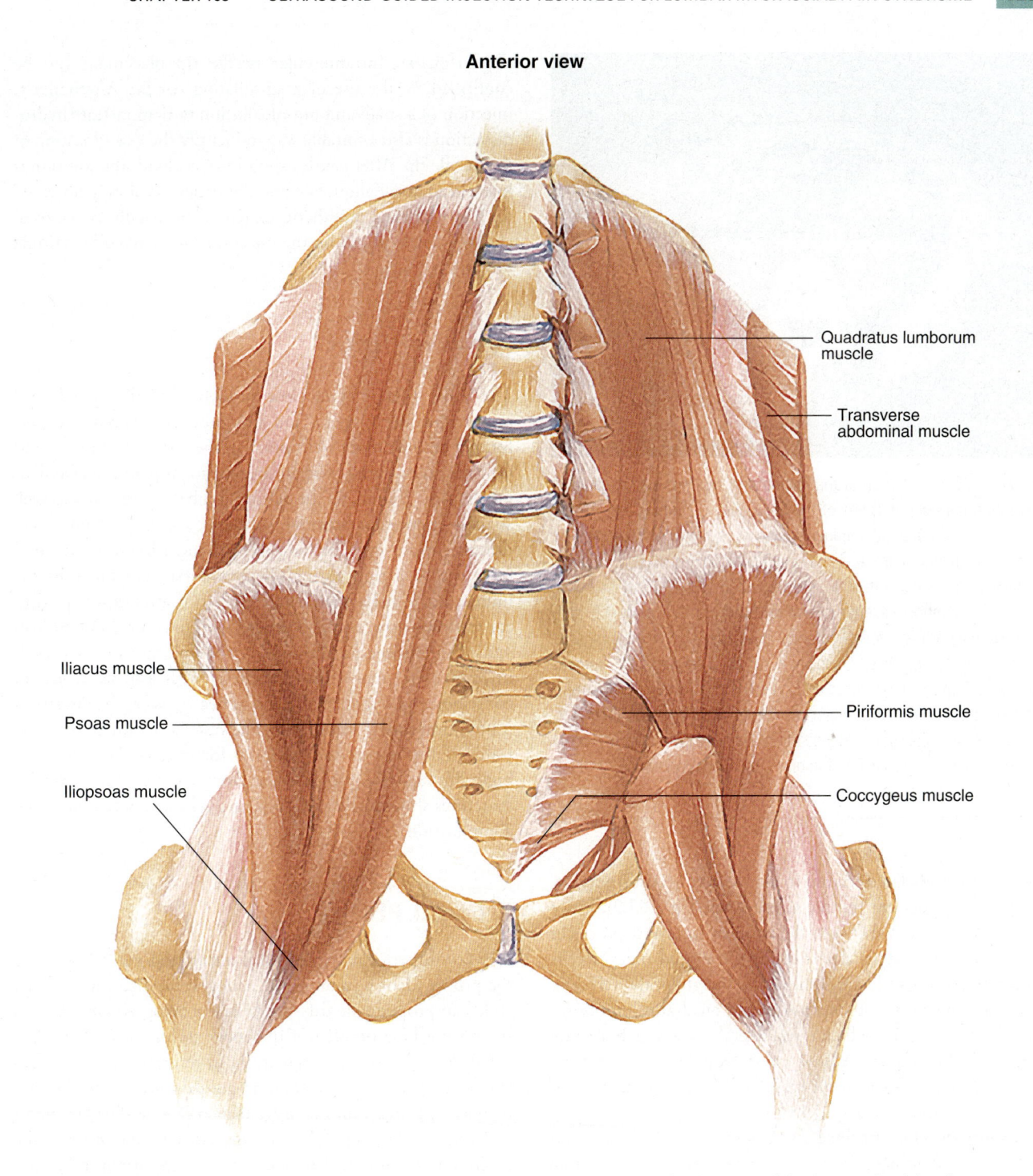

Labels: Quadratus lumborum muscle; Transverse abdominal muscle; Iliacus muscle; Psoas muscle; Iliopsoas muscle; Piriformis muscle; Coccygeus muscle

**FIGURE 103.3.** The deep muscles of the low back are susceptible to the development of lumbar myofascial pain. (From Anatomical Chart Company, 2013.)

After preparation of the skin with antiseptic solution, a curvilinear low-frequency ultrasound transducer is placed in the transverse plane ~3 cm laterally from the midline along the line drawn from the iliac crest, and an ultrasound survey is taken (Figs. 103.7 and 103.8). This should place the transducer at the L2–L3 level. Note that the transverse process blocks ultrasound visualization of the lumbar plexus (Fig. 103.8). Once the transverse process is identified, the ultrasound transducer is slowly

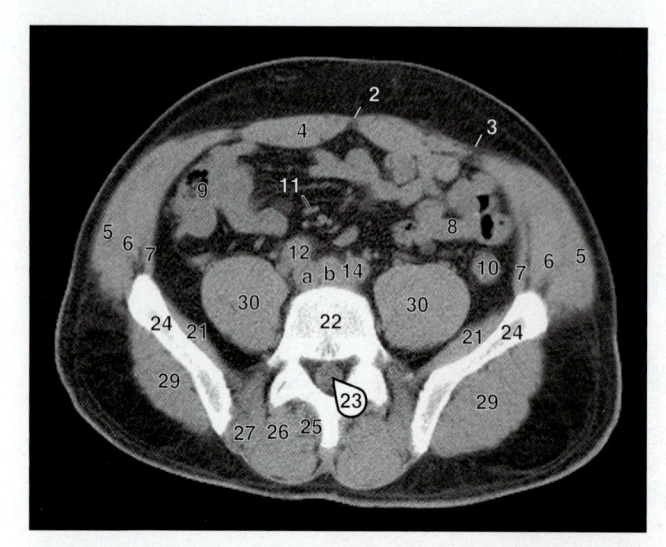

**FIGURE 103.4.** CT scan at the level of the superior iliac crest demonstrating the deep muscles of the back. (Key: *2*, linea alba; *3*, linea semilunaris; *4*, rectus abdominis muscle; *5*, external oblique muscle; *6*, internal oblique muscle; *7*, transversus abdominis muscle; *8*, ileum portion of the small intestine; *9*, ascending colon; *10*, descending colon; *11*, superior mesenteric arterial branches to ileum; *12*, right common iliac artery; *14*, left common iliac artery; *21*, iliacus muscle; *22*, fifth lumbar vertebra; *23*, spinal cord; *24*, iliac blade; *25*, spinalis muscle; *26*, longissimus muscle; *27*, iliocostalis muscle; *29*, gluteus medius muscle; *30*, psoas major muscle; *a*, right common iliac vein; *b*, Left common iliac vein.) (Reused from Dean D, Herbener TE. Cross-sectional human anatomy. Baltimore: Lippincott Williams & Wilkins, 2000, with permission.)

moved in a cephalad direction to identify the acoustic window between two adjacent transverse processes (Fig. 103.9). Once the acoustic window between the adjacent transverse processes is identified, the lateral aspect of the ultrasound transducer is rocked anteriorly to identify the lateral margin of the vertebral body and the erector spinae, psoas, and quadratus lumborum muscles (Fig. 103.10) which is just lateral to the vertebral body (Figs. 103.11 and 103.12). A color Doppler image is then obtained to identify adjacent vasculature to avoid inadvertent intravascular injection (Fig. 103.13).

Once the erector spinae, psoas, and quadratus lumborum muscles are identified, the needle is advanced under real-time ultrasound guidance utilizing an in-plane approach from the lateral aspect of the transversely placed ultrasound transducer until the needle is within the body of the muscle to be injected (Fig. 103.14). Intramuscular needle tip placement can be confirmed by the use of a stimulating needle. Alternatively, injection of a small amount of solution to demonstrate hydrodissection is also a suitable way to identify the exact location of the needle tip. After gentle aspiration for blood, the solution is injected in small aliquots while the patient is closely observed for signs of local anesthetic toxicity. The needle is removed and pressure is placed on the injection site to avoid hematoma formation.

## COMPLICATIONS

The psoas muscle is in close proximity to the spinal cord and exiting nerve roots, and this procedure should be performed only by those well versed in the regional anatomy and skilled at ultrasound-guided interventional pain management procedures. Trauma to the exiting lumbar nerve roots as well as inadvertent subarachnoid, subdural, and/or epidural injection can occur even in the best of hands. Inadvertent dural puncture occurring during selective nerve root block of the lumbar nerve roots should rarely occur if attention is paid to the technical aspects of this procedure. However, failure to recognize an unintentional dural or subdural injection can result in immediate total spinal anesthesia with associated loss of consciousness, hypotension, and apnea. This can be disastrous if not immediately recognized. The vascular nature of this anatomic region makes the potential for intravascular injection high although the use of color Doppler to identify vascular structures should help the clinician avoid this potentially fatal complication.

## CLINICAL PEARLS

The key to performing successful ultrasound-guided blocks is the proper identification of the sonographic anatomy and the ability to properly identify the anatomy being visualized. This should not be a problem if the above technique is used. Any significant pain or sudden increase in resistance during injection when performing ultrasound-guided injection for lumbar myofascial pain syndrome suggests incorrect needle placement, and one should stop injecting immediately and reassess the position of the needle. Because pain is an important indication of improper needle placement, the practitioner should avoid the use of excessive sedation during ultrasound-guided injection for lumbar myofascial pain syndrome.

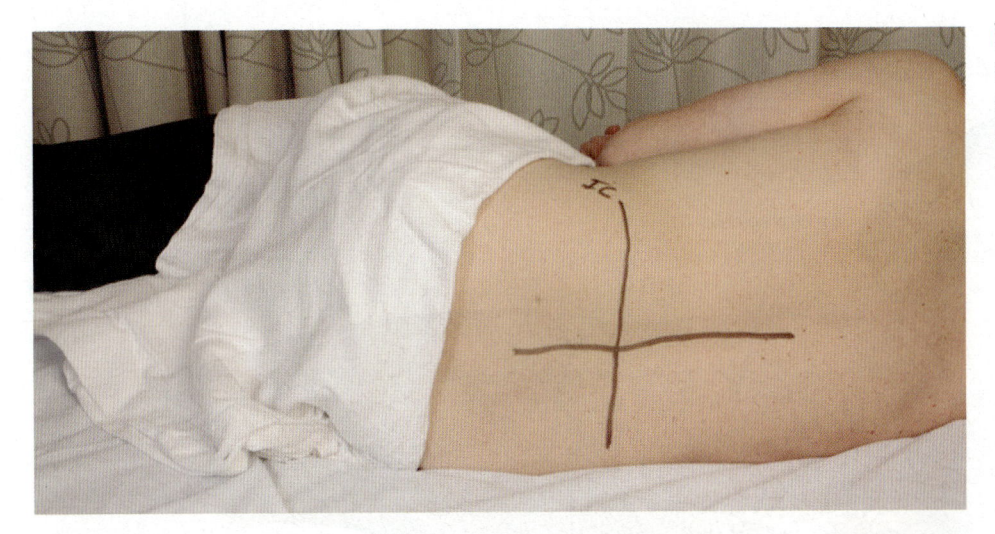

**FIGURE 103.5.** Proper lateral decubitus patient position for ultrasound-guided lumbar myofascial pain syndrome.

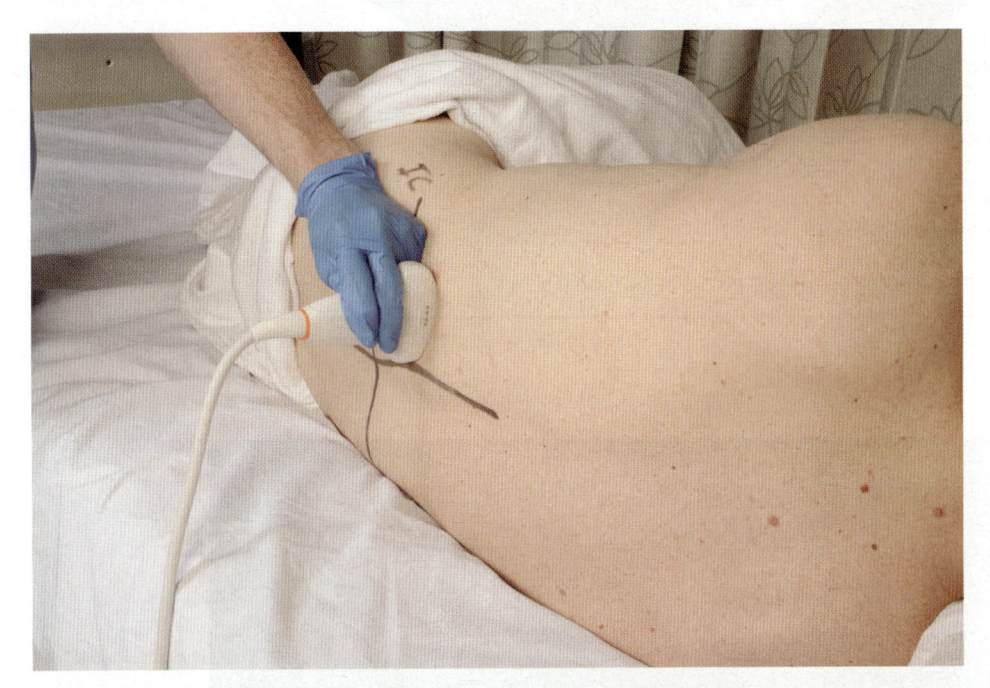

**FIGURE 103.6.** Transverse placement of the low-frequency curvilinear ultrasound transducer in the transverse plane 3 cm lateral to midline at level of iliac crest (L2–L3).

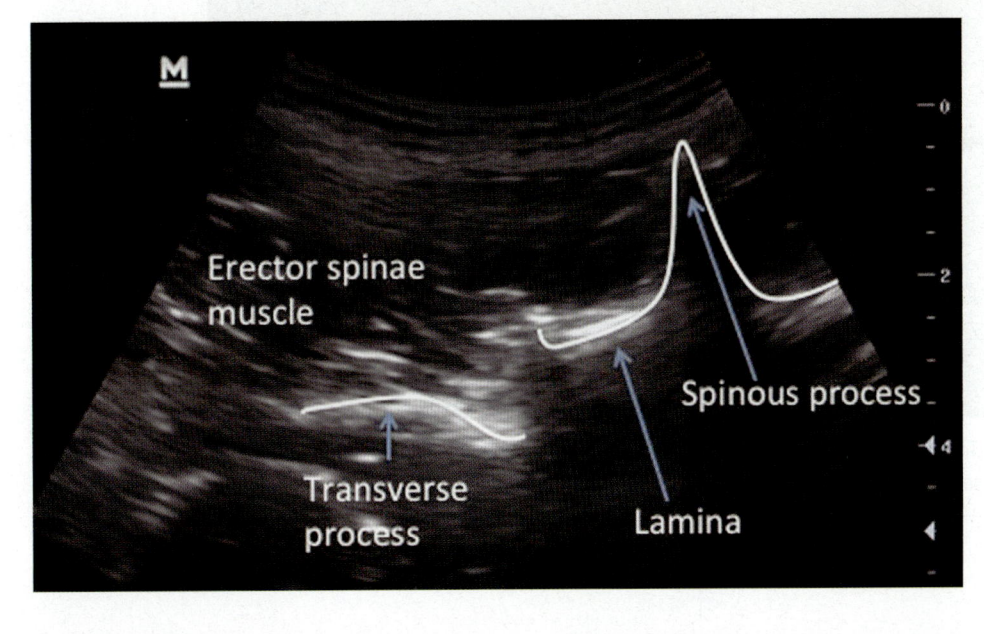

**FIGURE 103.7.** Transverse ultrasound view demonstrating transverse process.

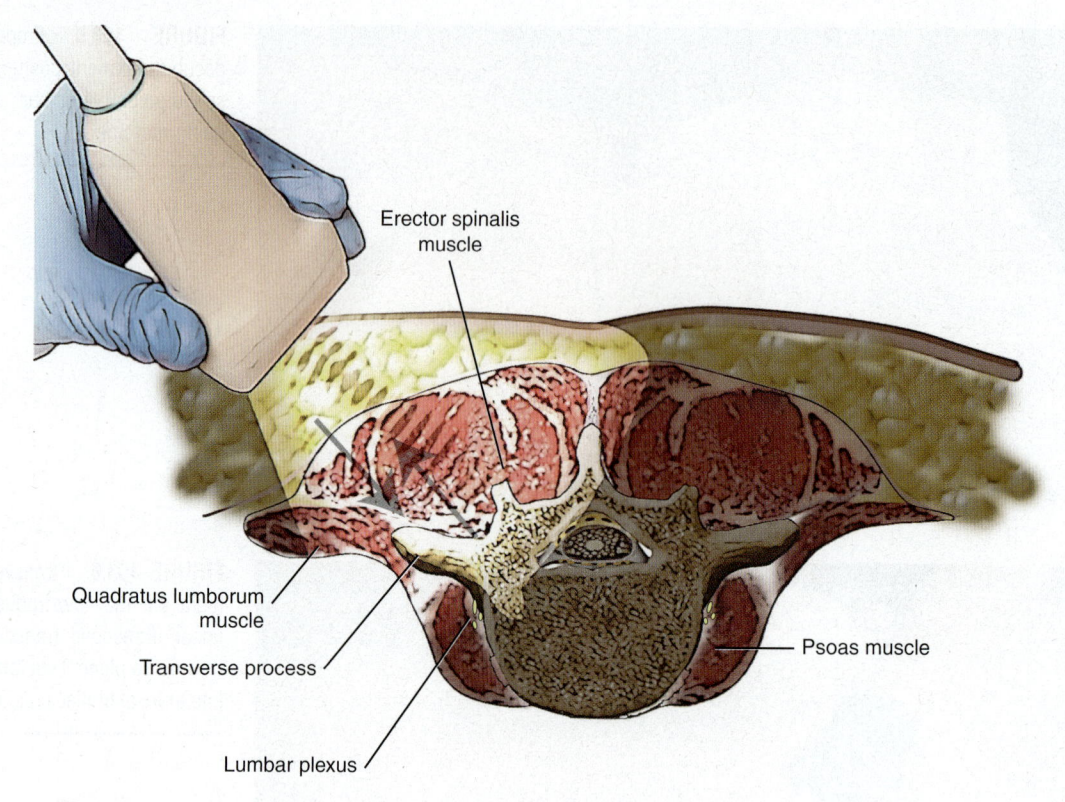

**FIGURE 103.8.** The transverse process blocks access to the lumbar plexus.

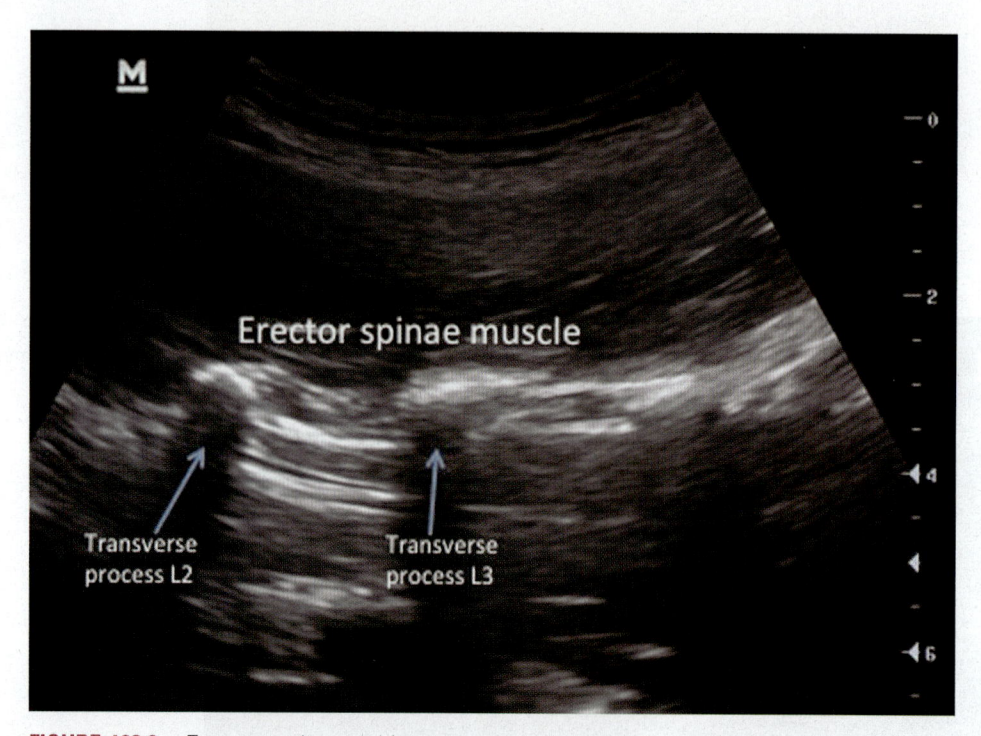

**FIGURE 103.9.** Transverse ultrasound image demonstrating acoustic window between two adjacent transverse processes.

CHAPTER 103 ULTRASOUND-GUIDED INJECTION TECHNIQUE FOR LUMBAR MYOFASCIAL PAIN SYNDROME 733

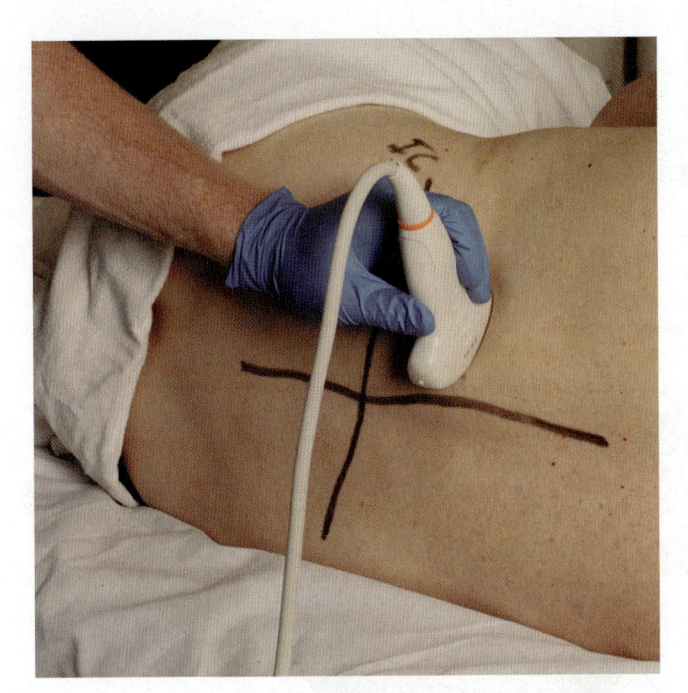

**FIGURE 103.10.** To obtain an ultrasound image of the lateral aspect of the vertebral body, the lateral aspect of the ultrasound transducer is rocked anteriorly to "see" around the posterior elements of the vertebra.

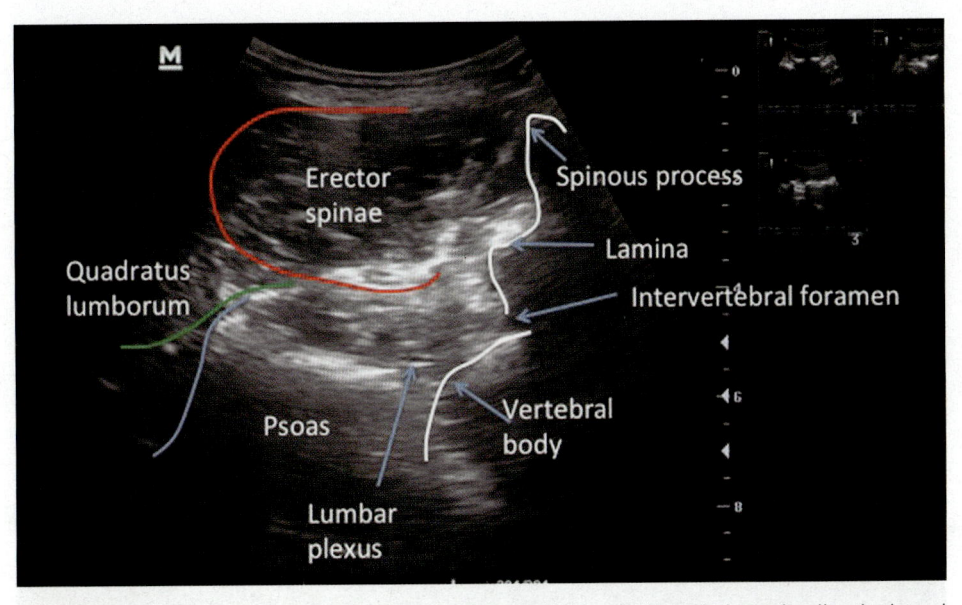

**FIGURE 103.11.** Transverse ultrasound view with transducer rocked anteriorly to visualize the lateral margin of the vertebral body and the lumbar plexus lying adjacent to it embedded in the psoas muscle.

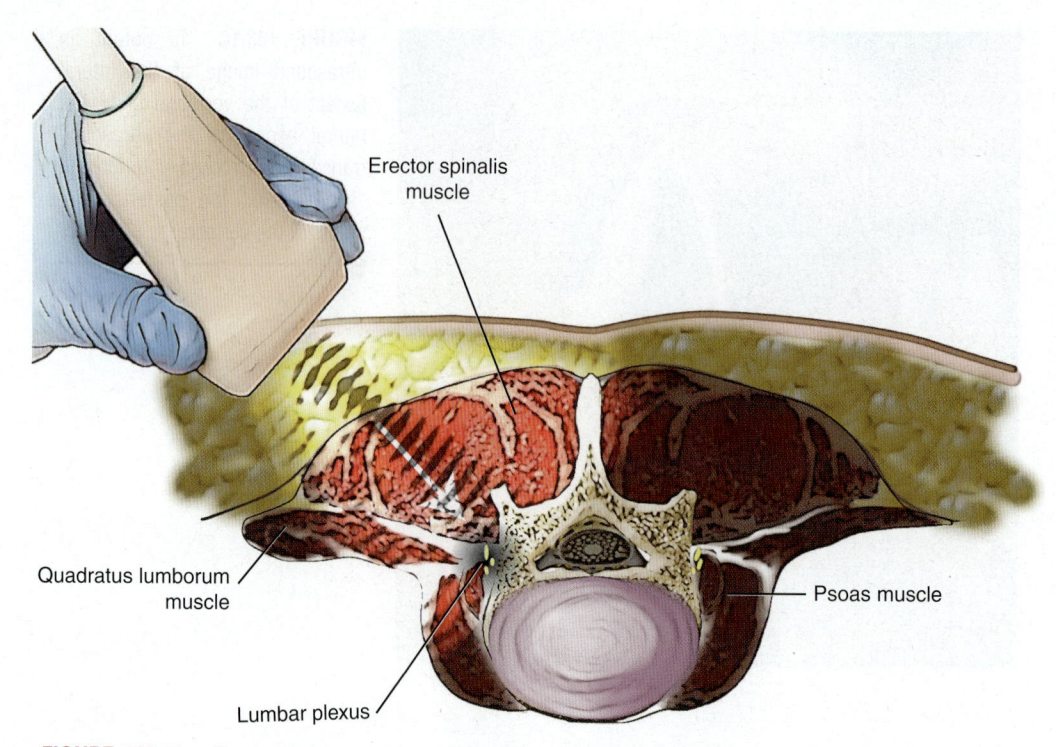

**FIGURE 103.12.** The lumbar plexus lies within the psoas muscle just lateral to the lateral margin of the vertebral body.

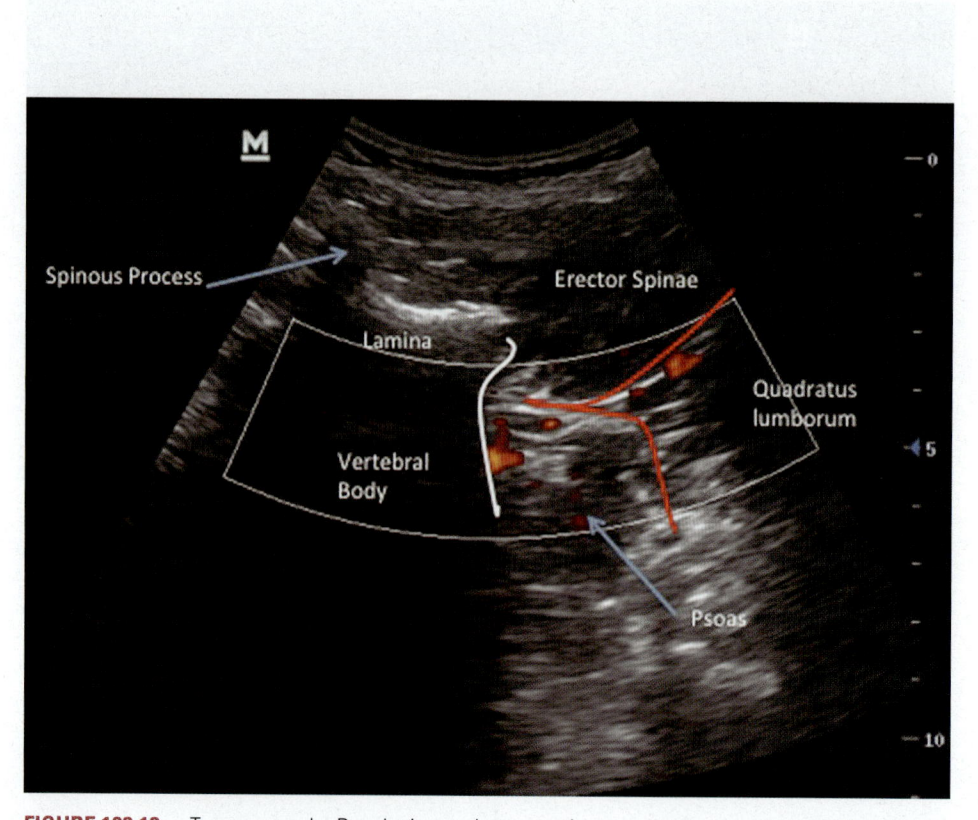

**FIGURE 103.13.** Transverse color Doppler image demonstrating vasculature in proximity to the injection site.

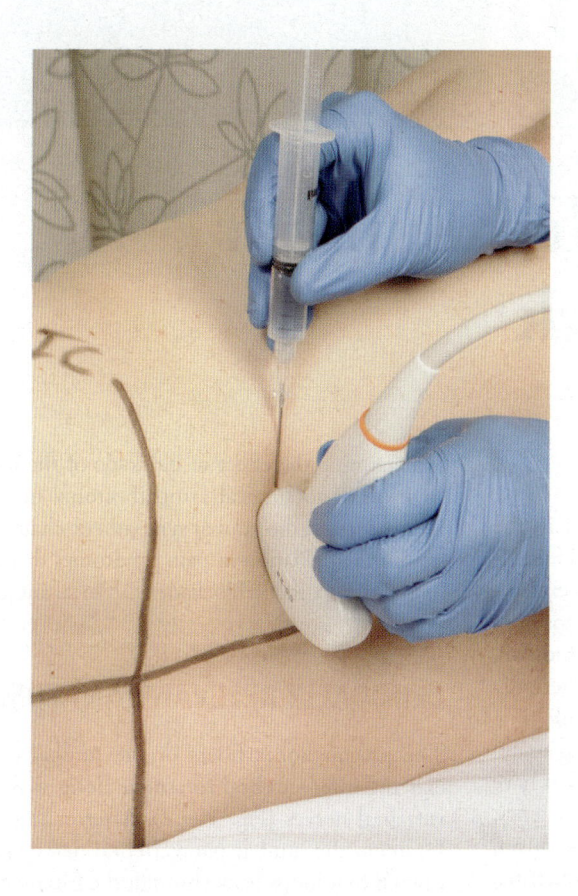

**FIGURE 103.14.** Proper in-plane needle position for performing selective lumbar nerve root block.

## SUGGESTED READINGS

Cummings M, Baldry P. Regional myofascial pain: diagnosis and management. *Best Pract Res Clin Rheumatol* 2007;21(2):367–387.

Malanga GA, Cruz EJ. Colon, myofascial low back pain: a review. *Phys Med Rehabil Clin N Am* 2010;21(4):711–724.

Waldman SD. Lumbar myofascial pain syndrome. In: *Atlas of Pain Management Injection Techniques*. 3rd ed. Philadelphia, PA: Saunders Elsevier; 2012:280–281.

Waldman SD. Functional anatomy of the lumbar spine. In: *Pain Review*. Philadelphia, PA: Saunders Elsevier; 2009:65–67.

# Ultrasound-Guided Lumbar Sympathetic Block

## CLINICAL PERSPECTIVES

Ultrasound-guided lumbar sympathetic block is useful in the diagnosis and treatment of a variety of painful conditions including reflex sympathetic dystrophy of the pelvis and lower extremity, causalgia involving the lower extremity, acute herpes zoster in the distribution of the lumbosacral dermatomes, hyperhidrosis, phantom limb pain, peripheral neuropathies, sympathetically mediated pain of malignant origin, and ureteral calculi (Fig. 104.1). Ultrasound-guided lumbar sympathetic block is useful in the diagnosis and treatment of a number of diseases that have in common their ability to cause acute vascular insufficiency. These diseases include acute frostbite, acute angina, ergotism, obliterative vascular disease, Raynaud disease, scleroderma, vasospastic disorders, posttraumatic vascular insufficiency, and embolic phenomenon (Table 104.1). Ultrasound-guided stellate ganglion block can also be used in a prognostic manner to determine the effect of blockade of the lumbar sympathetic chain prior to surgical sympathectomy in the lumbar region. Destruction of the lumbar sympathetic chain is a reasonable next step in the palliation of pain syndromes that have responded to lumbar sympathetic blockade with local anesthetic.

## CLINICALLY RELEVANT ANATOMY

The preganglionic fibers of the lumbar sympathetic nerves exit the intervertebral foramina along with the lumbar paravertebral nerves (Fig. 104.2). After exiting the intervertebral foramen, the lumbar paravertebral nerve gives off a recurrent branch that loops back through the foramen to provide innervation to the spinal ligaments, meninges, and its respective vertebra. The upper lumbar paravertebral nerve also interfaces with the lumbar sympathetic chain via the myelinated preganglionic fibers of the white rami communicantes. All five of the lumbar nerves interface with the unmyelinated postganglionic

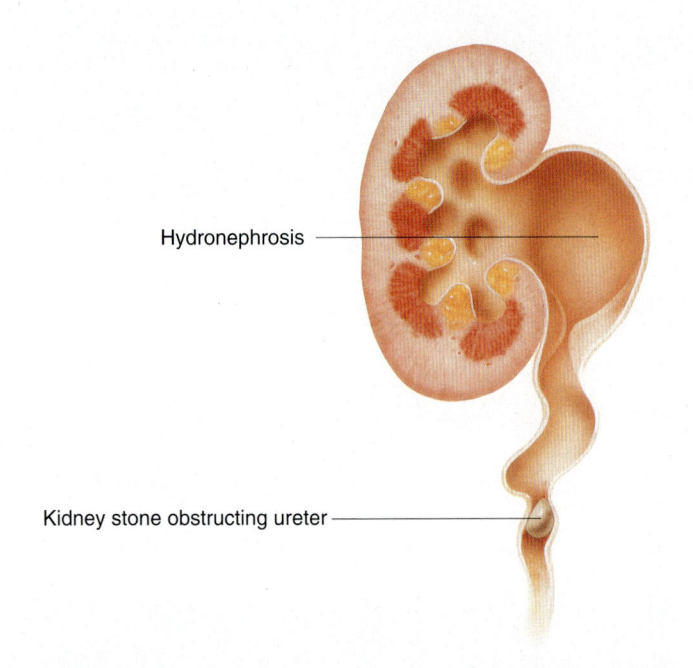

**FIGURE 104.1.** Ultrasound-guided lumbar sympathetic block is useful in the management of the pain of ureteral calculi. (From Anatomical Chart Company, 2013.)

**TABLE 104.1  Indications for Ultrasound-Guided Lumbar Sympathetic Block**

**Painful Conditions**
- Reflex sympathetic dystrophy of the pelvis and lower extremity
- Causalgia involving the lower extremity
- Acute herpes zoster in the distribution of the lumbosacral dermatomes
- Hyperhidrosis
- Phantom limb pain
- Ureteral calculi
- Sympathetically mediated pain of malignant origin

**Acute Vascular Insufficiency**
- Acute frostbite
- Ergotism
- Obliterative vascular disease
- Raynaud disease
- Scleroderma
- Vasospastic disorders
- Posttraumatic vascular insufficiency
- Embolic phenomenon
- Prognostic lumbar sympathetic block prior to surgical sympathectomy

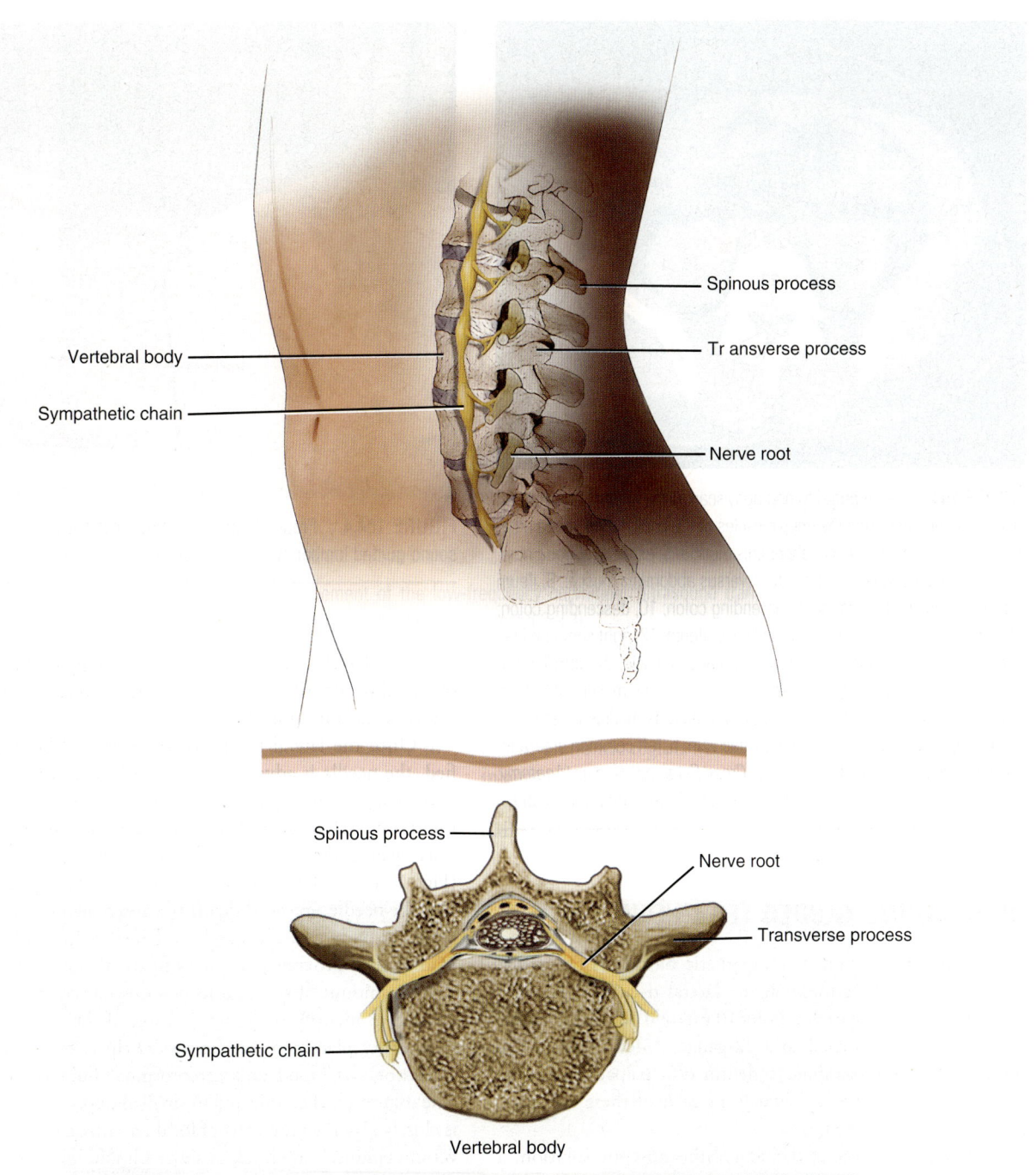

**FIGURE 104.2.** The anatomy of the lumbar sympathetic chain. Note the relationship of the lumbar sympathetic chain to the anterolateral margin of the vertebral body.

fibers of the gray rami communicantes. At the level of the lumbar sympathetic ganglia, preganglionic and postganglionic fibers synapse. Additionally, some of the postganglionic fibers return to their respective somatic nerves via the gray rami communicantes. Other lumbar sympathetic postganglionic fibers travel to the aortic and hypogastric plexus and course up and down the sympathetic trunk to terminate in distant ganglia.

In many patients, the first and second lumbar ganglia are fused. These ganglia and the remainder of the lumbar chain and ganglia lie at the anterolateral margin of the lumbar vertebral bodies (see Figs. 104.2 and 104.3). The peritoneal cavity lies lateral and anterior to the lumbar sympathetic chain. Given the proximity of the lumbar somatic nerves to the lumbar sympathetic chain, the potential exists for both neural pathways to be blocked when performing blockade of the lumbar sympathetic ganglion.

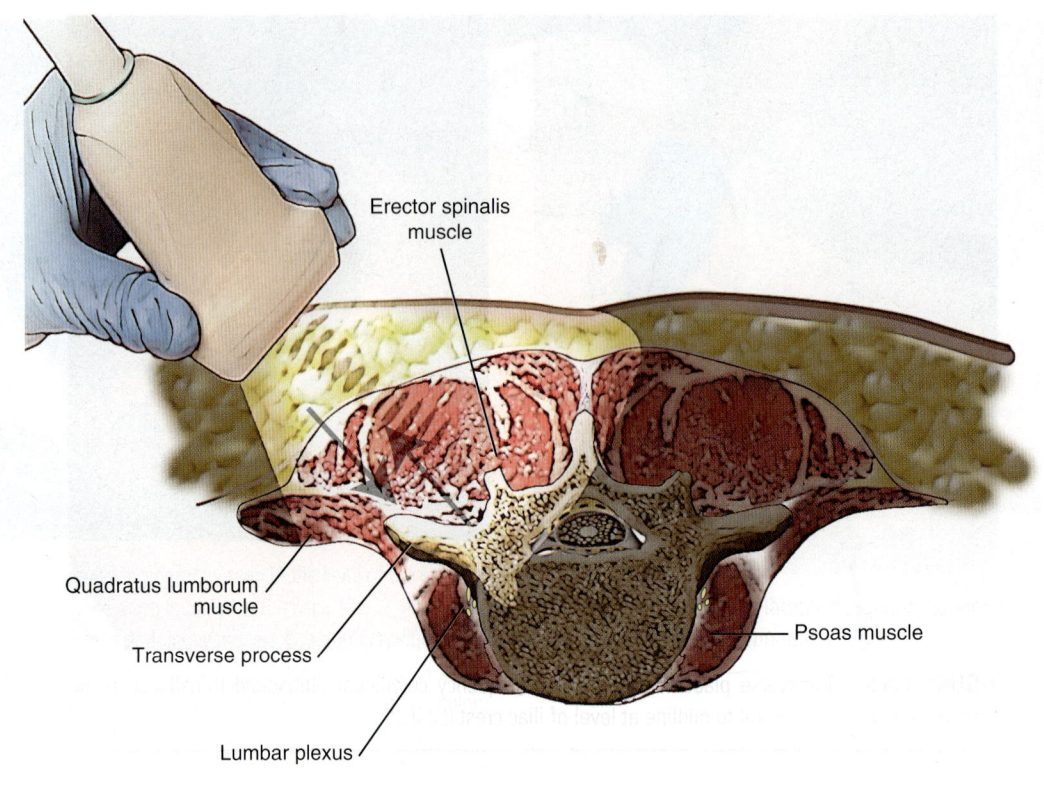

**FIGURE 104.7.** The transverse process blocks access to the lumbar sympathetic chain.

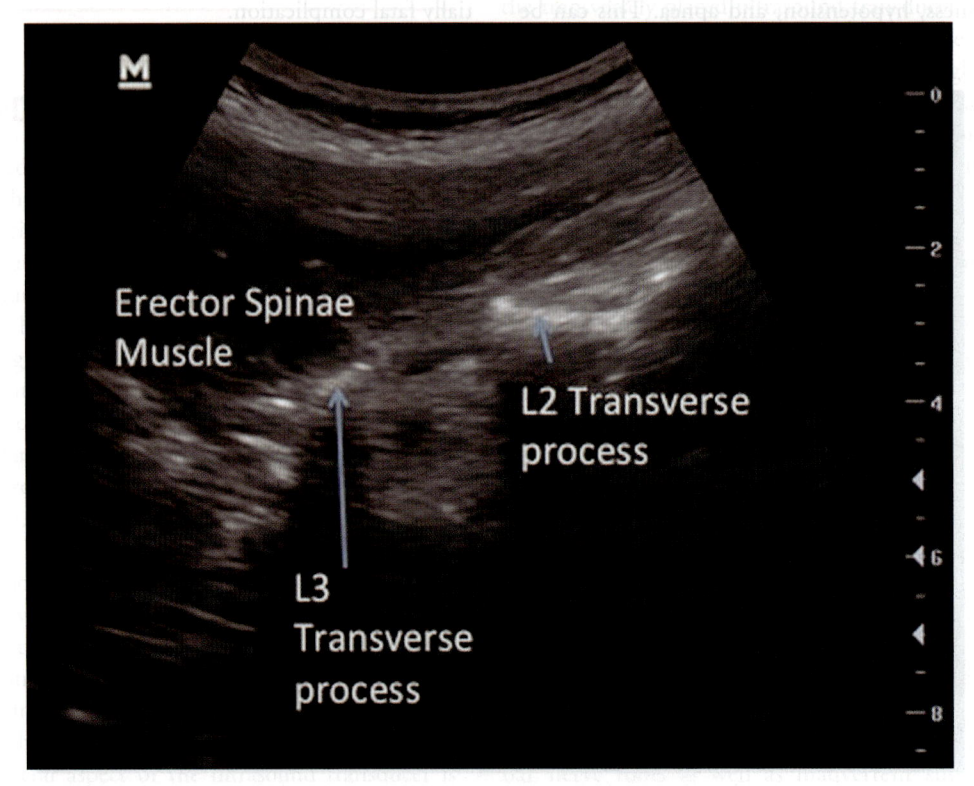

**FIGURE 104.8.** Transverse ultrasound image demonstrating acoustic window between two adjacent transverse processes.

CHAPTER 104    ULTRASOUND-GUIDED LUMBAR SYMPATHETIC BLOCK    741

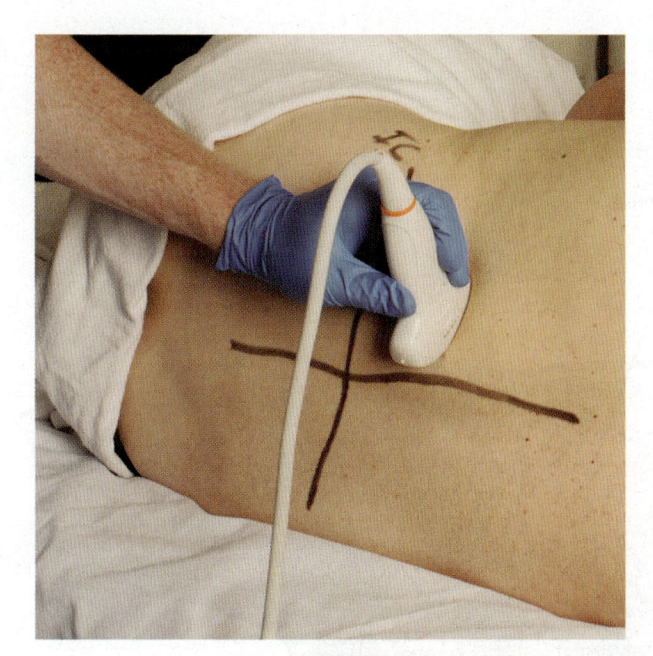

**FIGURE 104.9.** To obtain an ultrasound image of the lateral aspect of the vertebral body, the lateral aspect of the ultrasound transducer is rocked anteriorly to "see" around the posterior elements of the vertebra.

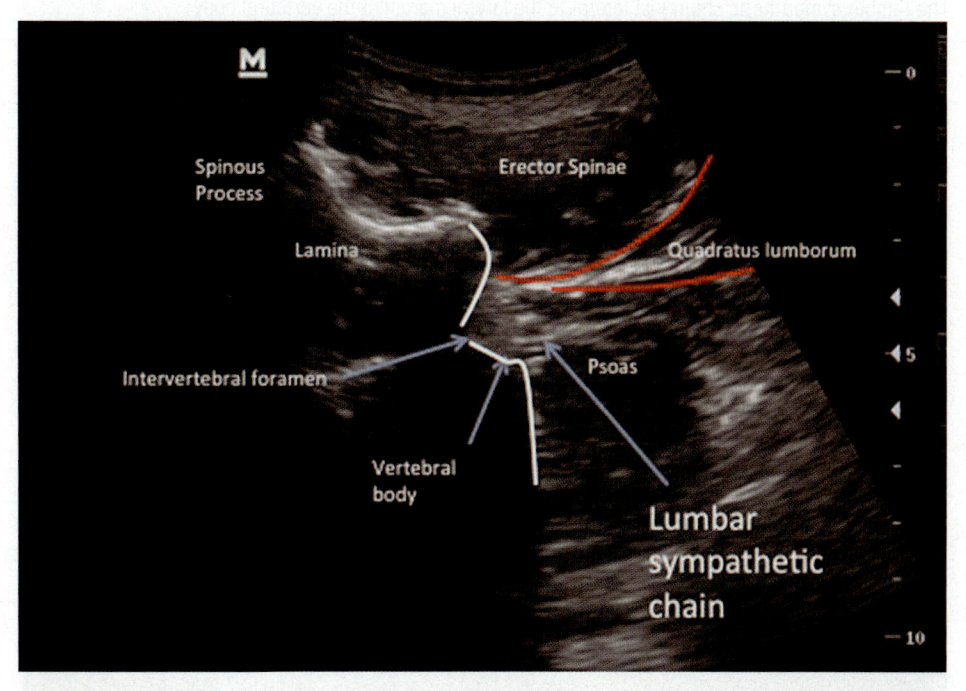

**FIGURE 104.10.** Transverse ultrasound view with transducer rocked anteriorly to visualize the lateral margin of the vertebral body and the lumbar sympathetic chain lying adjacent to it embedded in the psoas muscle.

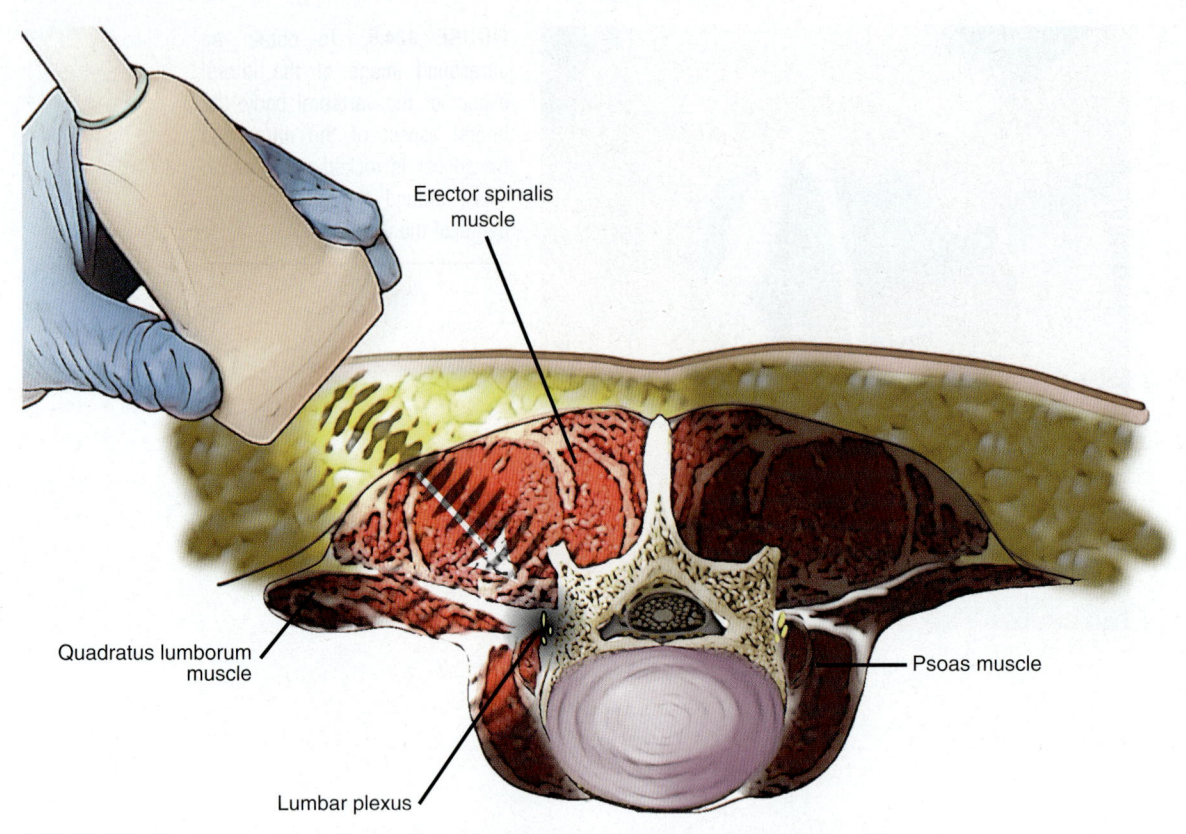

**FIGURE 104.11.** The lumbar sympathetic chain just lateral to the lateral margin of the vertebral body.

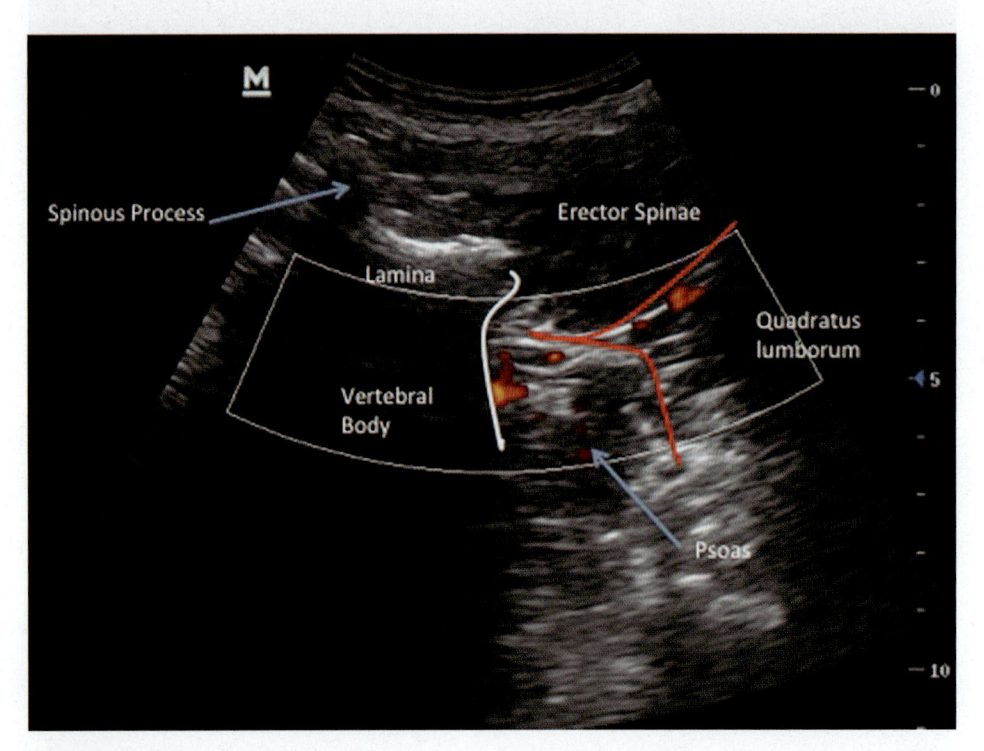

**FIGURE 104.12.** Transverse color Doppler image demonstrating vasculature in proximity to the lumbar sympathetic block.

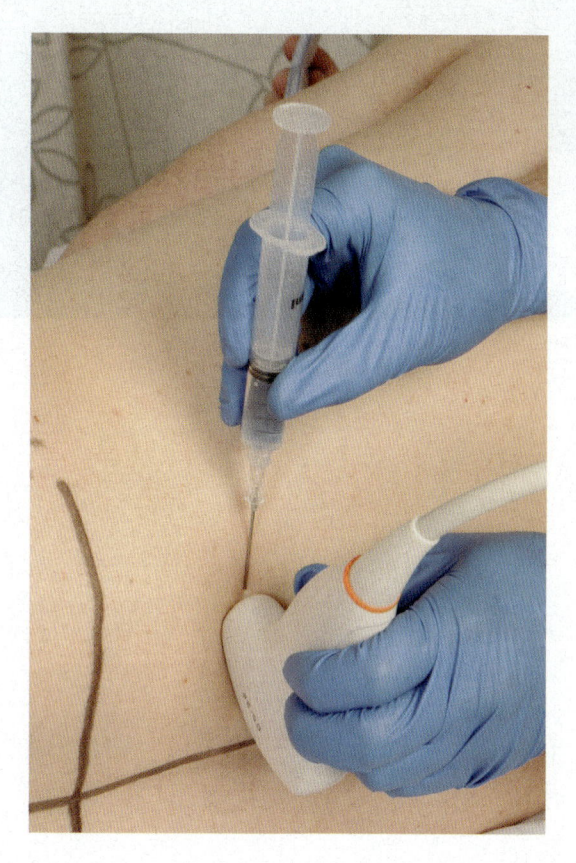

**FIGURE 104.13.** Proper in-plane needle position for performing sympathetic lumbar block.

## CLINICAL PEARLS

The key to performing successful ultrasound-guided nerve blocks is the ability to properly identify the clinically relevant sonographic anatomy. This should not be a problem if the above technique is used. Any significant pain or sudden increase in resistance during injection when performing ultrasound-guided suggests incorrect needle placement, and one should stop injecting immediately and reassess the position of the needle. Because pain is an important indication of improper needle placement, the practitioner should avoid the use of excessive sedation during ultrasound-guided lumbar sympathetic block.

## SUGGESTED READINGS

Plancarte-Sánchez R, Guajardo-Rosas J, Guillen-Nuñez R. Sympathetic block: thoracic and lumbar. *Tech Reg Anesth Pain Manag* 2005;9(2):91–96.
Waldman SD. Lumbar sympathetic block. In: *Atlas of Interventional Pain Management*. 3rd ed. Philadelphia, PA: Saunders Elsevier; 2009:371–374.
Waldman SD. Lumbar sympathetic neurolysis. In: *Atlas of Interventional Pain Management*. 3rd ed. Philadelphia, PA: Saunders Elsevier; 2009:374–377.
Waldman SD. Lumbar sympathetic block. In: *Pain Review*. Philadelphia, PA: Saunders Elsevier; 2009:514–516.

# SECTION VIII

# Hip and Pelvis

# CHAPTER 105

# Ultrasound-Guided Intra-articular Injection of the Hip Joint

## CLINICAL PERSPECTIVES

The hip joint is a synovial joint that provides the interface between the axial skeleton and pelvis weightbearing lower extremities. The joint is comprised of the articulation between the spheroid head of the femur and the socket-like acetabulum (Fig. 105.1). The joint's articular cartilage is susceptible to damage, which, if left untreated, will result in arthritis with its associated pain and functional disability. Osteoarthritis of the joint is the most common form of arthritis that results in hip joint pain and functional disability, with rheumatoid arthritis and posttraumatic arthritis also causing arthritis of the hip joint (Fig. 105.1). Less common causes of arthritis-induced hip joint pain include the collagen vascular diseases, infection, villonodular synovitis, and Lyme disease. Acute infectious arthritis of the hip joint is best treated with early diagnosis, with culture and sensitivity of the synovial fluid, and with prompt initiation of antibiotic therapy. The collagen vascular diseases generally manifest as a polyarthropathy rather than a monoarthropathy limited to the hip joint, although hip pain secondary to the collagen vascular diseases responds exceedingly well to ultrasound-guided intra-articular injection of the hip joint.

Patients with hip joint pain secondary to arthritis, tears of the fibrocartilaginous labrum, and collagen vascular disease–related joint pain complain of pain that is localized to the hip and proximal lower extremity. Activity makes the pain worse, with rest and heat providing some relief. The pain is constant and characterized as aching. Sleep disturbance is common with awakening when the patient rolls over onto the affected hip. Some patients complain of a grating, catching, or popping sensation with range of motion of the joint, and crepitus may be appreciated on physical examination.

Functional disability often accompanies the pain associated with many pathologic conditions of the hip joint. Patients will often notice increasing difficulty in performing their activities of daily living, and tasks that require walking, climbing stairs, and getting in and out of cars are particularly problematic. If the pathologic process responsible for the patient's pain symptomatology is not adequately treated, the patient's functional disability may worsen, and muscle wasting and ultimately a frozen hip may occur.

Plain radiographs are indicated in all patients who present with hip pain as not only intrinsic hip disease as well as other regional pathology may be perceived as hip pain by the patient (Fig. 105.2). Based on the patient's clinical presentation, additional testing may be indicated, including complete blood cell count, sedimentation rate, and antinuclear antibody testing. MRI or ultrasound of the hip is indicated if avascular necrosis or labral tear is suspected.

## CLINICALLY RELEVANT ANATOMY

The hip joint is comprised of the articulation between the spheroid head of the femur and the cup-shaped acetabulum of the hip (see Fig. 105.1). The articular surface of the hip joint is covered with hyaline cartilage, which is susceptible to arthritis from a variety of causes. Because the vascular supply to the articular cartilage is tenuous, the hip joint is especially susceptible to avascular necrosis (Fig. 105.3). Approximately 50% of the head of the femur rests within the acetabulum with a fibrocartilaginous layer called the acetabular labrum adding additional stability to the joint (see Fig. 105.1). The labrum is susceptible to degenerative changes as well as trauma should the femur be subluxed or dislocated. The hip joint is surrounded by a dense capsule that allows the wide range of motion of the hip joint while preventing subluxation. The joint capsule is lined with a synovial membrane that attaches to the articular cartilage. This membrane gives rise to synovial tendon sheaths and bursae that are subject to inflammation. The hip joint is innervated by the femoral, obturator, and sciatic nerves. The major ligaments of the hip joint include the iliofemoral, pubofemoral, ischiofemoral, and transverse acetabular, which along with the labrum and joint capsule provide strength to the hip joint (Fig. 105.4). The muscles of the hip and their attaching tendons are susceptible to trauma and to wear and tear from overuse and misuse.

## ULTRASOUND-GUIDED TECHNIQUE

The benefits, risks, and alternative treatments are explained to the patient and informed consent is obtained. The patient is then placed in the supine position with the lower

**Lateral View
(Opened)**

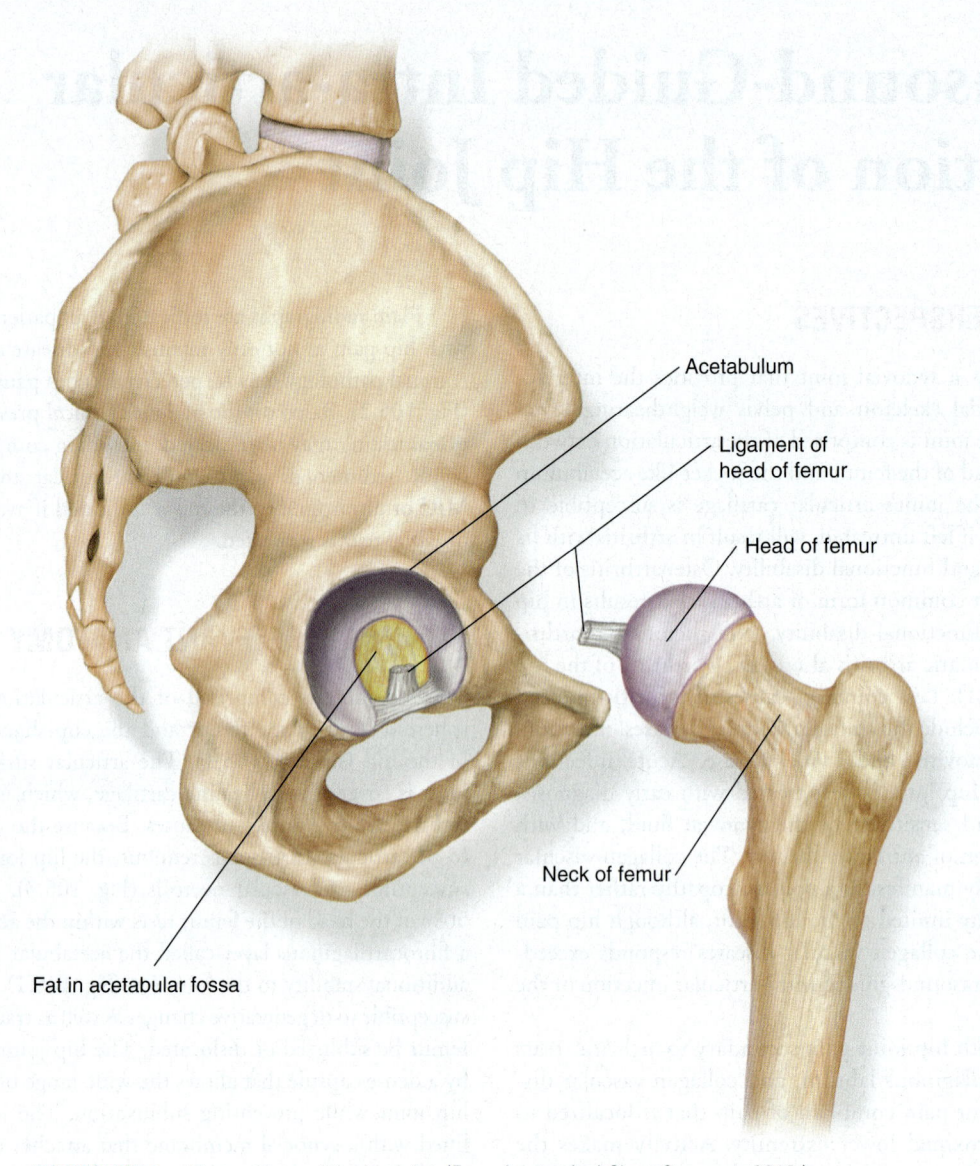

**FIGURE 105.1.** The anatomy of the hip joint. (From Anatomical Chart Company, 2013.)

extremity slightly externally rotated (Fig. 105.5). The skin overlying the hip joint is then prepped with antiseptic solution. A sterile syringe containing 2.0 mL of 0.25% preservative-free bupivacaine and 40 mg of methylprednisolone is attached to a 3½-inch, 22-gauge needle using strict aseptic technique. A curvilinear low-frequency ultrasound transducer is placed over the proximal femur in the longitudinal plane with the transducer parallel to the femur (Fig. 105.6). A survey scan is taken, which demonstrates the femur as a linear hyperechoic structure (Fig. 105.7). The medial margin of the femur is identified. The ultrasound transducer is then slowly moved toward the head of the femur following the medial margin of the femur until hyperechoic margin of the femur swings sharply upward at the junction of the femoral neck and the femoral head (Fig. 105.8). At the junction of the medial margin of the femoral neck and femoral head is the joint space, which is amenable to injection (Fig. 105.9). The hip joint is then identified as a hypoechoic fluid-containing structure at the "V" of the junction of the femoral neck and head. After the joint space is identified, the needle is placed through the skin ~1 cm below the inferior end of the transducer and is then advanced using an in-plane

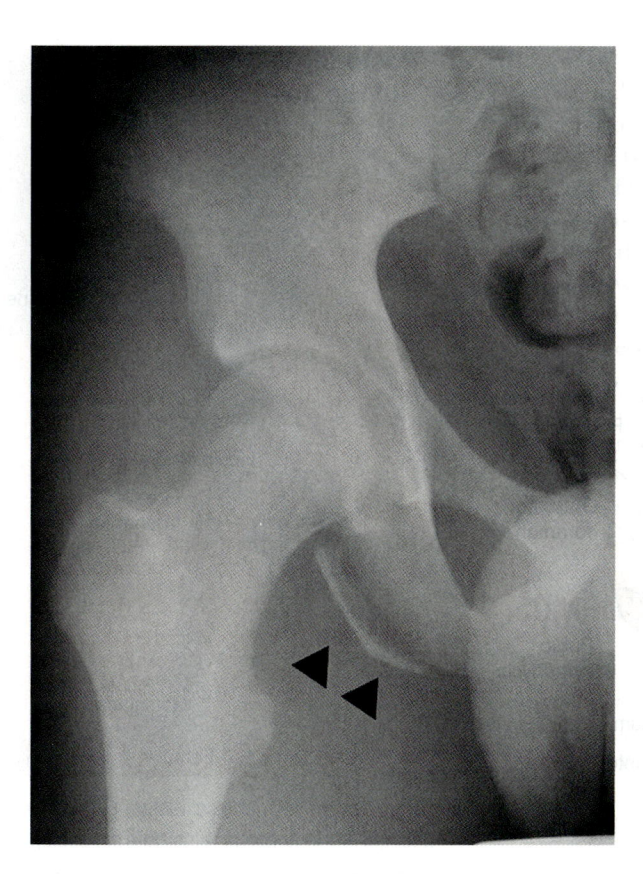

CHAPTER 105  ULTRASOUND-GUIDED INTRA-ARTICULAR INJECTION OF THE HIP JOINT    747

**FIGURE 105.2.** Avulsion fracture (*arrowhead*) of the ischial tuberosity in patient presenting with hip pain. (Reused from Fleisher GR, Ludwig S, Baskin MN. *Atlas of Pediatric Emergency Medicine*. Philadelphia, PA: Lippincott Williams & Wilkins; 2004, with permission.)

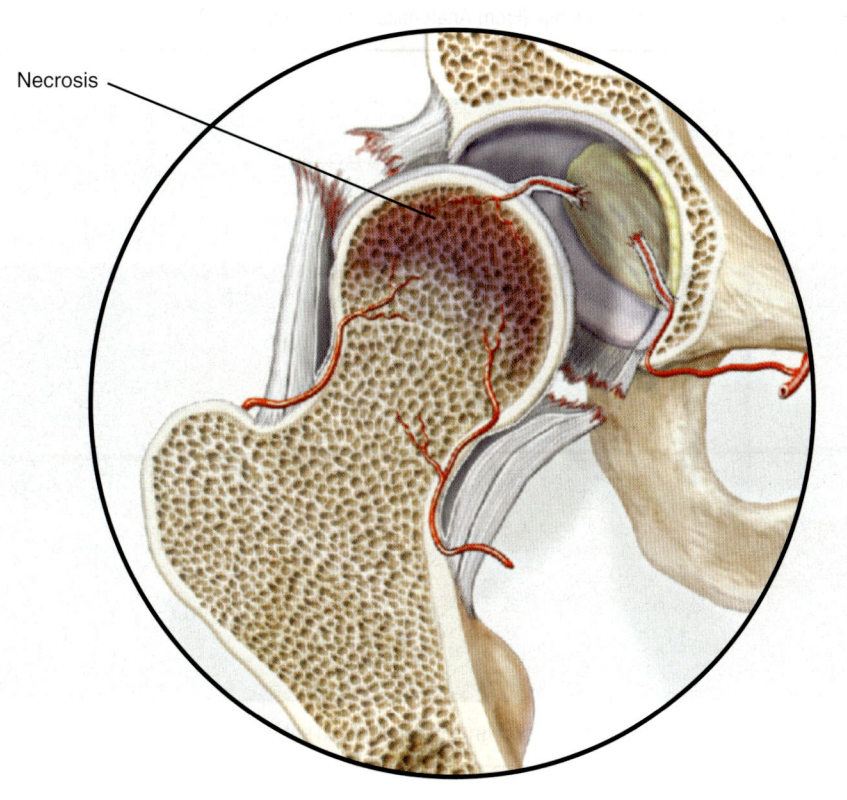

**FIGURE 105.3.** The hip joint is susceptible to the development of avascular necrosis due to the tenuous blood supply to the articular cartilage. (From Anatomical Chart Company, 2013.)

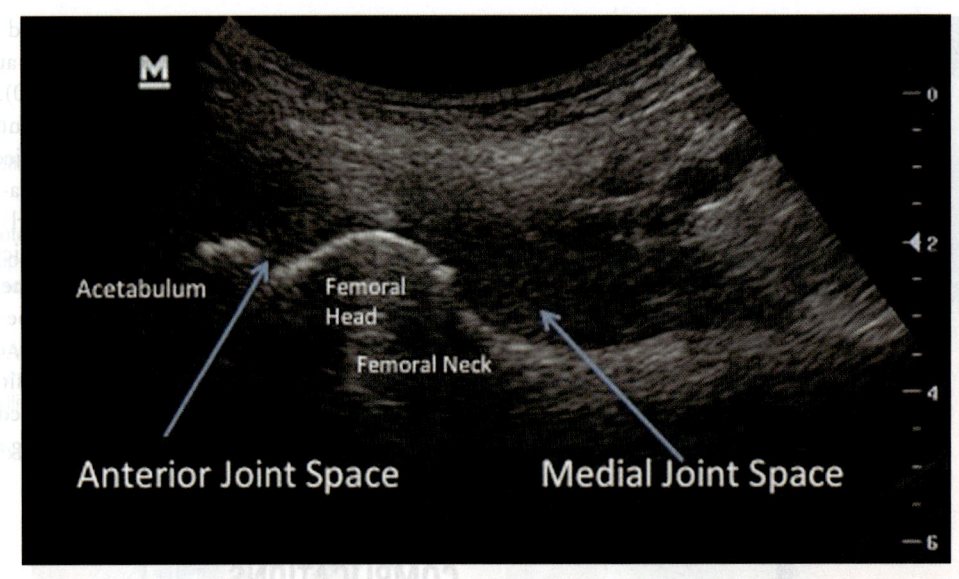

**FIGURE 105.8.** Longitudinal ultrasound image of the junction between the femoral neck and femoral head.

## CLINICAL PEARLS

Care must be taken not to place the needle too medially or trauma to the femoral artery, vein, and/or nerve may result. Bursitis, labral tears, tendinopathy, osteoarthritis, synovitis, and avascular necrosis of the femoral head and impingement syndromes may coexist with hip joint disease and may contribute to the patient's pain symptomatology (Fig. 105.11).

Universal precautions should always be observed to protect the operator, and strict adherence to sterile technique must be used to avoid infection. Gentle physical therapy and local heat should be introduced following ultrasound-guided injection of the hip joint to reduce pain and improve function. Simple analgesics and nonsteroidal anti-inflammatory agents or COX-2 inhibitors may be used concurrently with this injection technique.

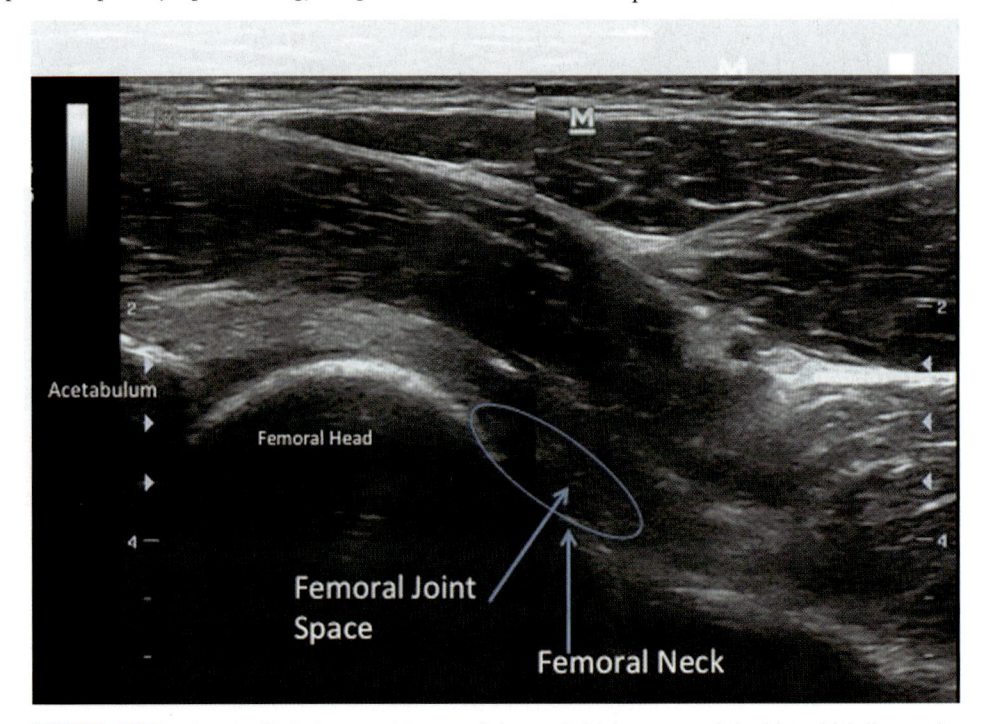

**FIGURE 105.9.** Longitudinal ultrasound image of the medial joint space of the hip, which lies at the junction between the femoral neck and femoral head.

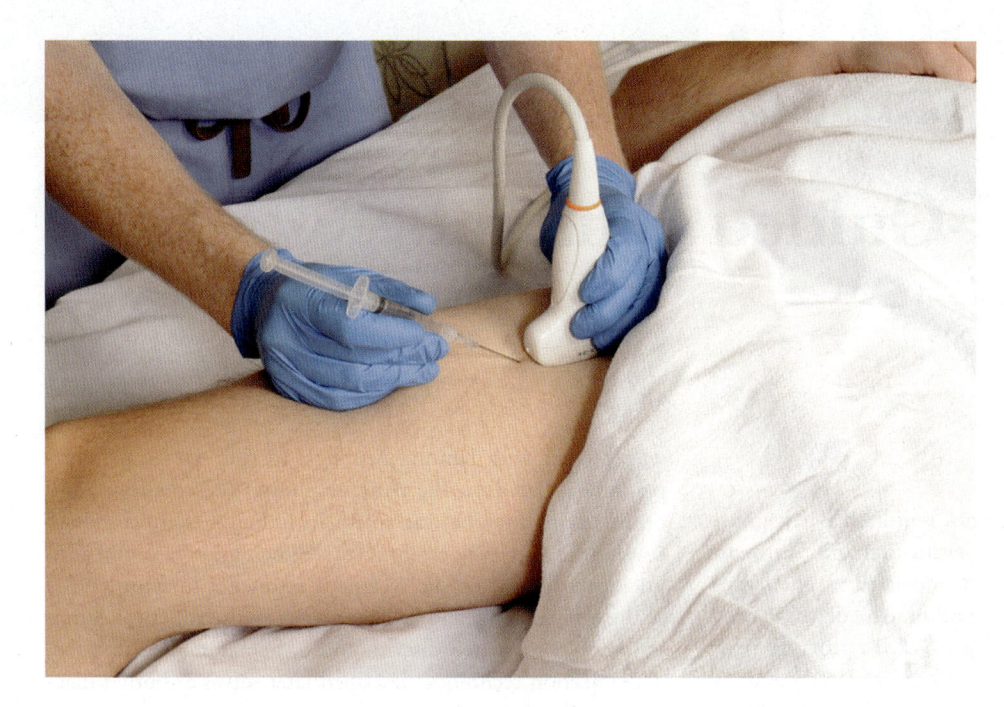

**FIGURE 105.10.** Correct in-plane needle placement for ultrasound-guided hip joint injection.

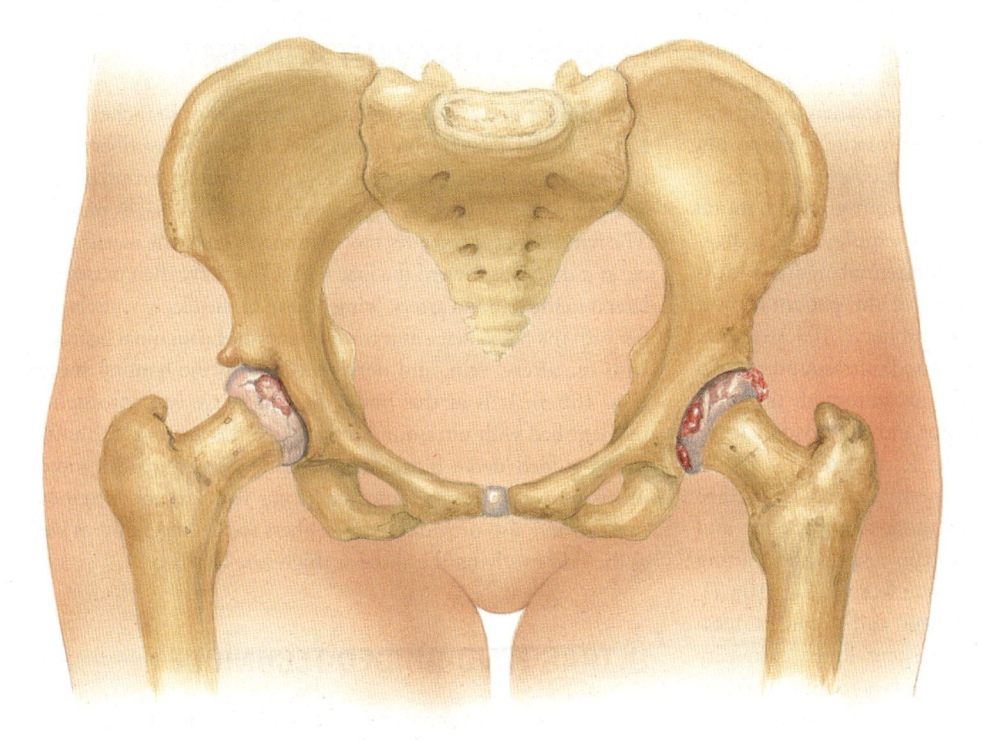

**FIGURE 105.11.** Advanced osteoarthritis of the hip joint with osteophytes, joint space narrowing, and denuded chondral surfaces. (From Anatomical Chart Company, 2013.)

## SUGGESTED READINGS

Cheng PH, Kim HJ, Ottestad E, et al. Ultrasound-guided injections of the knee and hip joints. *Tech Reg Anesth Pain Manag* 2009;13(3):191–197.

Nallamshetty L, Buchowski JM, Nazarian LA, et al. Septic arthritis of the hip following cortisone injection: case report and review of the literature. *Clin Imaging* 2003;27(4):225–228.

Waldman SD. Intra-articular injection of the hip joint. In: *Pain Review*. Philadelphia, PA: Saunders Elsevier; 2009:546–547.

Waldman SD. Intra-articular injection of the hip joint. In: *Atlas of Pain Management Injection Techniques*. 3rd ed. Philadelphia, PA: Saunders Elsevier; 2012:282–284.

Waldman SD, Campbell RSD. Anatomy, special imaging considerations of pelvis, hip, and lower extremity pain syndromes. In: *Imaging of Pain*. Philadelphia, PA: Saunders Elsevier; 2011:335–336.

Waldman SD, Campbell RSD. Osteoarthritis of the hip. In: *Imaging of Pain*. Philadelphia, PA: Saunders Elsevier; 2011:351–352.

# CHAPTER 106

# Ultrasound-Guided Femoral Nerve Block

## CLINICAL PERSPECTIVES

Ultrasound-guided femoral nerve block is utilized as a diagnostic and therapeutic maneuver in the evaluation and treatment of lower extremity pain thought to be mediated via the femoral nerve. The most common pain syndrome mediated via the femoral nerve is diabetic amyotrophy, which is a proximal neuropathy commonly seen in diabetic patients, which presents as neuropathic burning pain in the hip and thigh and weakness and wasting of quadriceps muscles.

Ultrasound-guided femoral nerve block can also be utilized to provide surgical anesthesia for the hip and lower extremity when combined with lateral femoral cutaneous, sciatic, and obturator nerve block or lumbar plexus block when the patient would not tolerate general anesthesia and/or the hypotension secondary to the blockade of the sympathetic nerves associated with spinal or epidural anesthesia. Ultrasound-guided femoral nerve block with local anesthetics can be employed as a diagnostic maneuver when performing differential neural blockade on an anatomic basis to determine if the patient's lower extremity pain is subserved by the femoral nerve. If destruction of the femoral nerve is being contemplated, ultrasound-guided femoral nerve block with local anesthetic can provide prognostic information as to the extent of motor and sensory deficit the patient will experience following nerve destruction.

Femoral nerve block with local anesthetic may be used to palliate acute pain emergencies, including femoral neck and shaft fractures, and for postoperative pain relief while waiting for pharmacologic methods to become effective (Fig. 106.1). Femoral nerve block with local anesthetic and steroid is occasionally used in the treatment of persistent lower extremity pain when the pain is thought to be secondary to inflammation or when entrapment of the femoral nerve as it passes under the inguinal ligament is suspected. Femoral nerve block with local anesthetic and steroid is also indicated in the palliation of pain and motor dysfunction associated with diabetic femoral amyotrophy. Destruction of the femoral nerve is occasionally used in the palliation of persistent lower extremity pain secondary to invasive tumor that is mediated by the femoral nerve and has not responded to more conservative measures.

Electromyography can distinguish femoral nerve entrapment from lumbar plexopathy and lumbar radiculopathy. Plain radiographs of the hip and pelvis are indicated in all patients who present with femoral neuralgia to rule out occult bony pathology. Based on the patient's clinical presentation, additional testing may be warranted, including a complete blood count, uric acid level, erythrocyte sedimentation rate, and antinuclear antibody testing. Magnetic resonance imaging (MRI) of the lumbar spine and lumbar plexus and retroperitoneum is indicated if herniated disc, tumor, or hematoma is suspected. The injection technique described later serves as both a diagnostic and a therapeutic maneuver.

## CLINICALLY RELEVANT ANATOMY

The femoral nerve is derived from the posterior branches of the L2, L3, and L4 nerve roots (Fig. 106.2). The nerve fibers enter the psoas muscle where they fuse together within the muscle body and then descend laterally between the psoas and iliacus muscles. The femoral nerve provides motor innervation to the iliacus muscle as it descends toward the iliac fossa. The nerve then passes just lateral to the femoral artery, lying on top of the iliacus muscle and beneath the fascia iliaca as it travels beneath the inguinal ligament with the artery, vein, and nerve enclosed in the femoral sheath (Fig. 106.3). It is at this point that the nerve can consistently be identified with ultrasound scanning and is amenable to ultrasound-guided nerve block. The femoral nerve provides motor innervation to the sartorius, quadriceps femoris, and pectineus muscles and also provides sensory fibers to the knee joint as well as the skin overlying the anterior thigh (see Fig. 106.2).

## ULTRASOUND-GUIDED TECHNIQUE

Ultrasound-guided femoral nerve block can be carried out by placing the patient in the supine position with the arms resting comfortably across the patient's chest (Fig. 106.4). A total of 7 mL of local anesthetic is drawn up in a 12-mL sterile syringe. If the painful condition being treated is thought to have an inflammatory component, 40 to 80 mg of depot steroid is added to the local anesthetic. The inguinal creased on the affected side is identified, and a linear high-frequency ultrasound transducer is placed in an oblique plane perpendicular with the inguinal ligament. An ultrasound survey scan is obtained (Fig. 106.5). The iliacus muscle is identified with the femoral

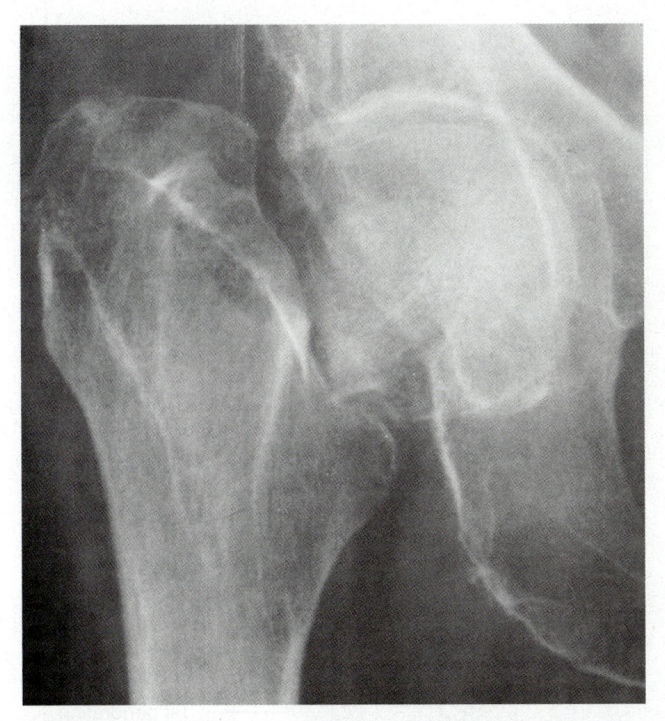

**FIGURE 106.1.** Plain radiograph demonstrating a transcervical fracture of the femoral neck resulting in varus deformity and external rotation. (Reused from Pope TL Jr, Harris JH Jr. *Harris & Harris' The Radiology of Emergency Medicine*. 5th ed. Philadelphia, PA: Lippincott Williams & Wilkins; 2013:845, with permission.)

nerve lying between the muscle and the pulsatile femoral artery (Fig. 106.6). The femoral vein lies medial to the femoral artery and is easily compressible by pressure from the ultrasound transducer (Fig. 106.7). Color Doppler can be utilized to aid in the identification of the femoral artery and vein (Fig. 106.8). When these anatomic structures are clearly identified on oblique ultrasound scan, the skin is prepped with anesthetic solution, and a 3½-inch, 22-gauge needle is advanced from the lateral border of the ultrasound transducer and advanced utilizing an in-plane approach with the trajectory being adjusted under real-time ultrasound guidance so that the needle passes just on top of the iliacus muscle until the needle tip is resting beneath the fascia iliaca in proximity to the femoral nerve (Fig. 106.9). At that point, after careful aspiration, a small amount of solution is injected under real-time ultrasound imaging to utilize hydrodissection to reconfirm the position of the needle tip. Once the position of the needle tip is reconfirmed, after careful aspiration, the remainder of the solution is slowly injected under ultrasound guidance. There should be minimal resistance to injection. The needle is then removed, and a sterile pressure dressing and ice pack are placed at the injection site.

## COMPLICATIONS

Needle-induced trauma to the femoral nerve can result in persistent paresthesias. The use of ultrasound guidance when

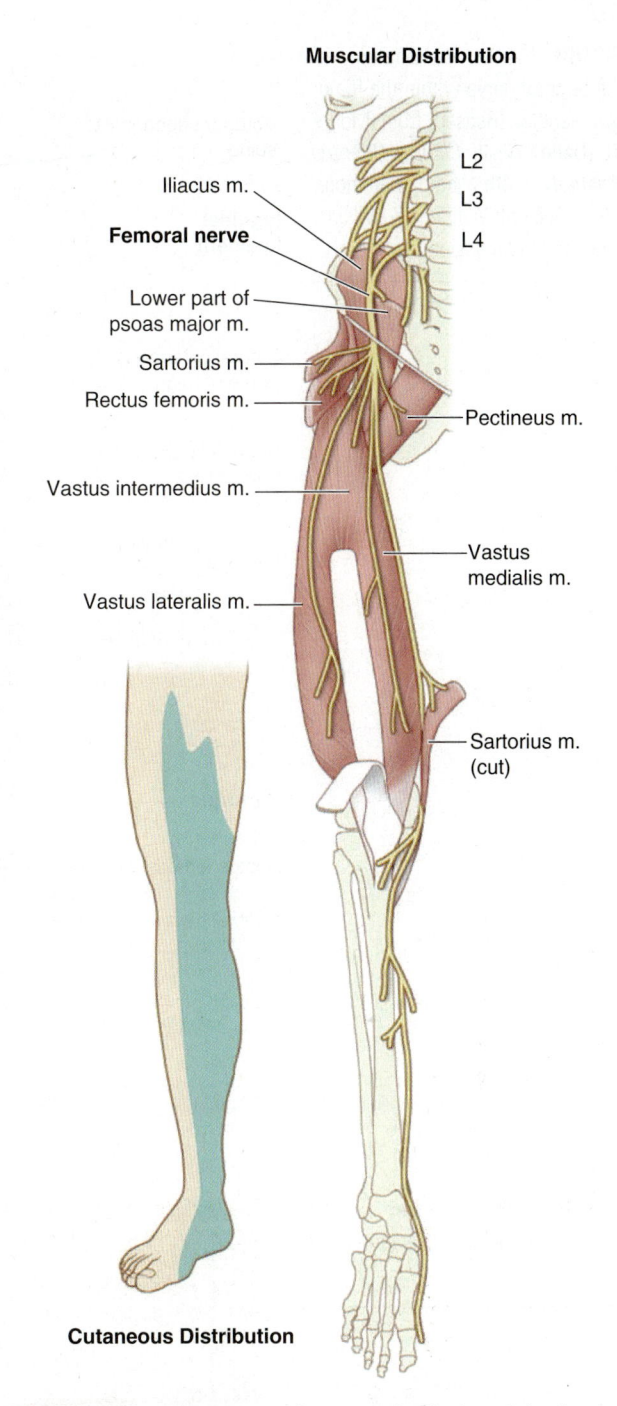

**FIGURE 106.2.** The motor and sensory distribution of the femoral nerve. (Reused from Premkumar K. *The Massage Connection: Anatomy and Physiology.* Baltimore, MD: Lippincott Williams & Wilkins; 2004, with permission.)

performing femoral nerve block should markedly decrease this complication. Because of the relatively vascular nature of the lower abdominal wall and the proximity of the femoral artery and vein, postblock ecchymosis and hematoma may occur, and the patient should be warned of such. These complications can be decreased by the use of a pressure dressing and cold packs applied to the injection site following the procedure.

**FIGURE 106.3.** The anatomy of the femoral nerve within the femoral triangle. (Reused from Moore KL, Dalley AF II. *Clinical Oriented Anatomy*. 4th ed. Baltimore, MD: Lippincott Williams & Wilkins; 1999, with permission.)

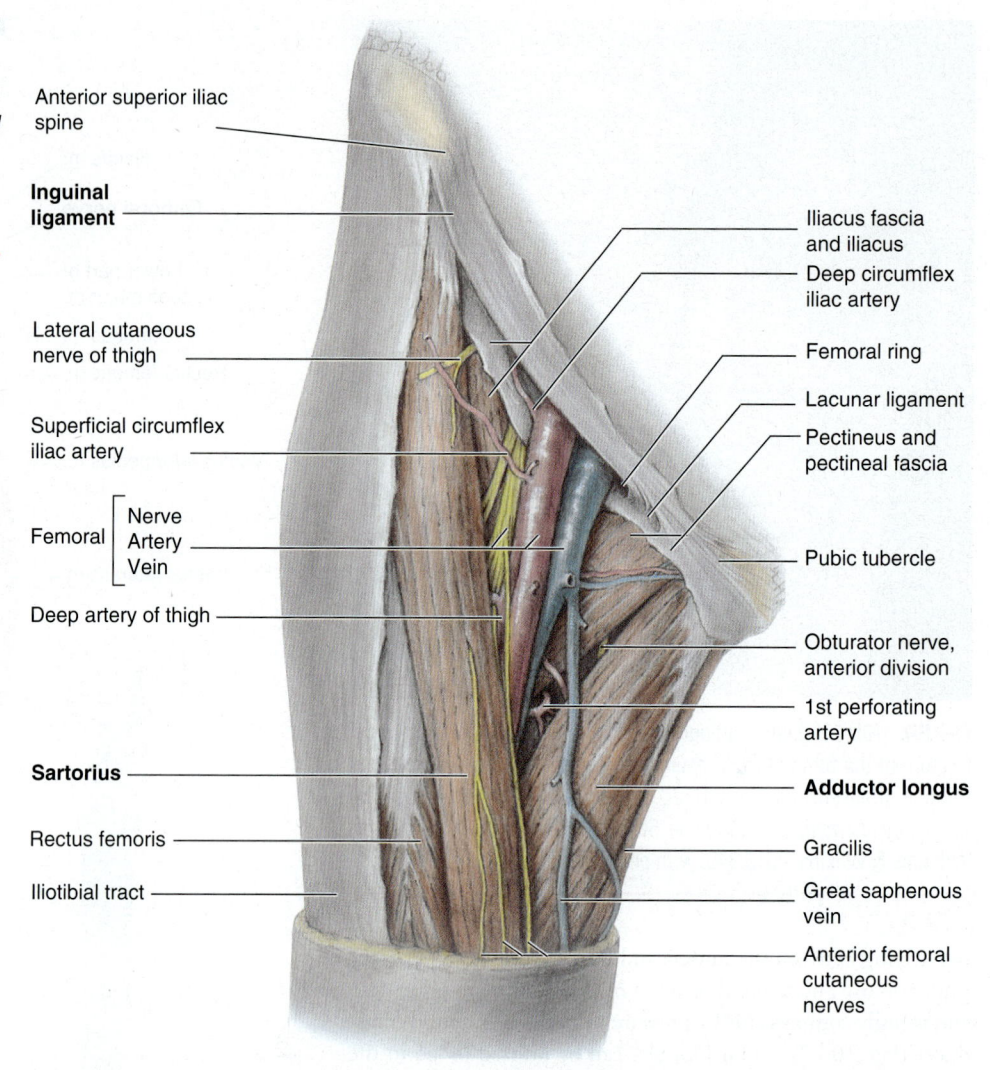

**FIGURE 106.4.** Proper supine patient positioning for femoral nerve block.

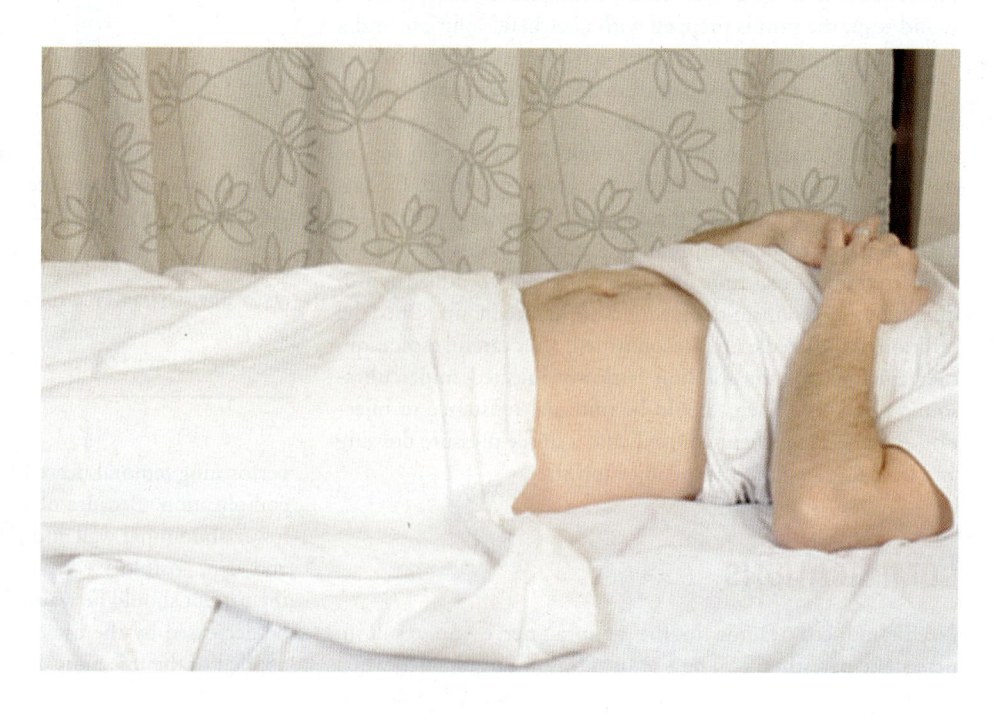

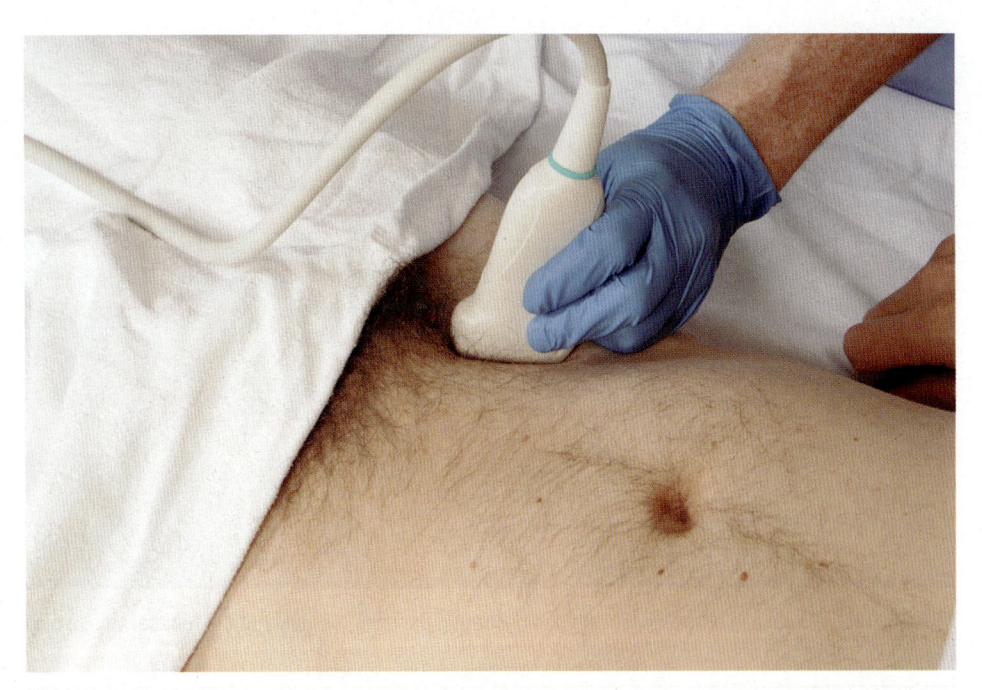

**FIGURE 106.5.** Oblique placement of the ultrasound transducer placed in a plane perpendicular with the inguinal ligament with the inferior aspect of the transducer lying over the anterior superior iliac spine and the superior aspect of the transducer pointed directly at the umbilicus.

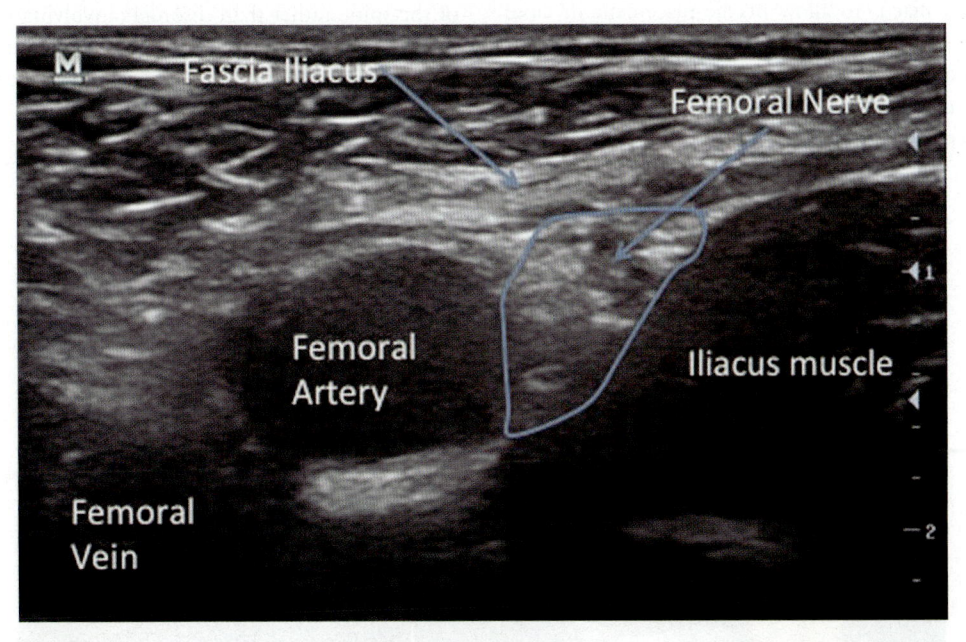

**FIGURE 106.6.** Oblique ultrasound image demonstrating the iliacus muscle, the fascia iliacus, the femoral nerve, artery, and vein.

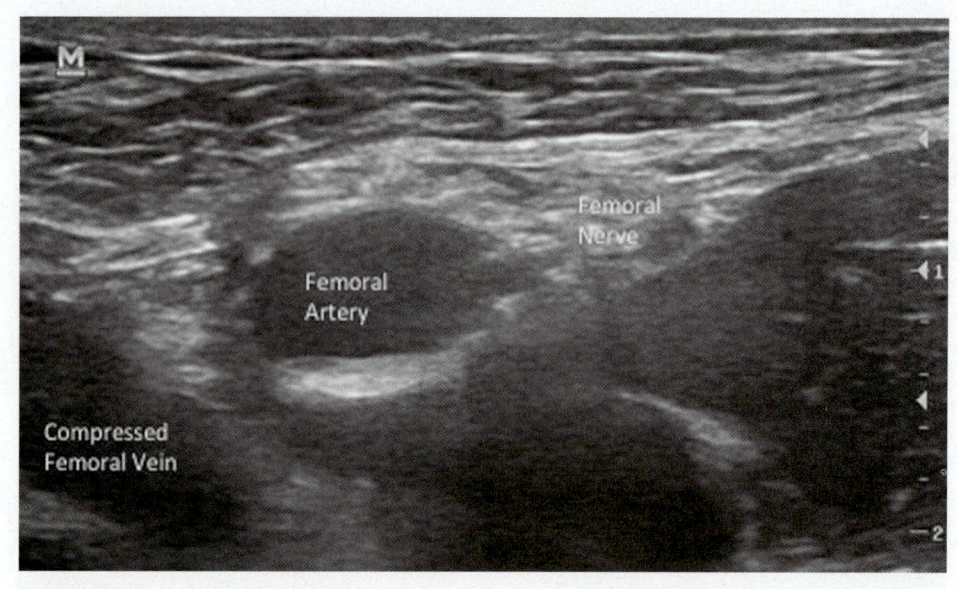

**FIGURE 106.7.** Oblique ultrasound image demonstrating the compressibility of the femoral vein, which lies medial to the pulsatile femoral artery.

## CLINICAL PEARLS

The key to performing successful ultrasound femoral nerve block is the proper identification of the sonographic anatomy and in particular the ability to properly identify the iliacus muscle and fascia iliacus to allow needle placement in close proximity to the femoral nerve. This should not be a problem if the above technique is used. Any significant pain or sudden increase in resistance during injection when performing ultrasound-guided femoral nerve block suggests incorrect needle placement, and one should stop injecting immediately and reassess the position of the needle.

It should be remembered that the most common cause of pain radiating into the lower extremity is a herniated lumbar disc or nerve impingement secondary to degenerative arthritis of the spine rather than disorders involving the femoral nerve per se. Electromyography and MRI of the lumbar spine, combined with the clinical history and physical examination, help sort out the etiology of pain thought to be mediated via the femoral nerve.

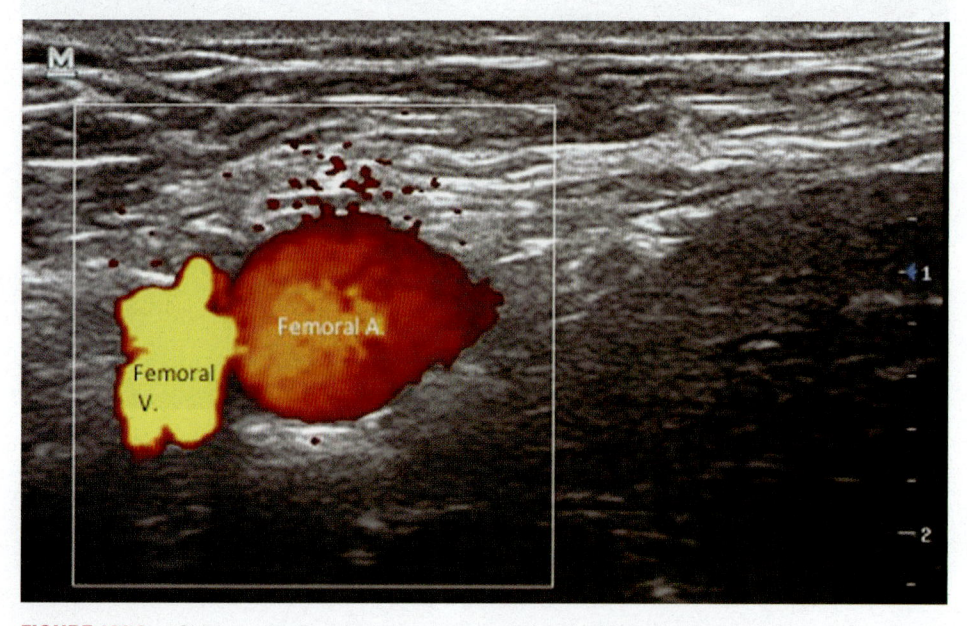

**FIGURE 106.8.** Oblique color Doppler image demonstrating the femoral artery and vein.

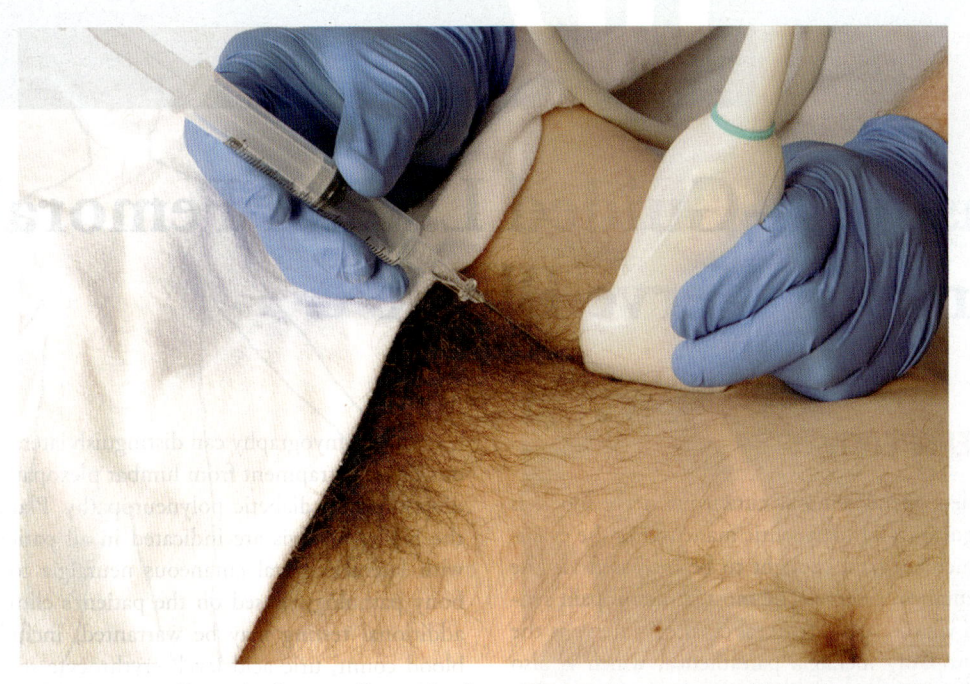

**FIGURE 106.9.** Proper in-plane needle position for performing ultrasound-guided femoral nerve block.

## SUGGESTED READINGS

Beaudoin FL, Nagdev A, Merchant RC, et al. Ultrasound-guided femoral nerve blocks in elderly patients with hip fractures. *Am J Emerg Med* 2010;28(1):76–81.

Mahadevan V. Anatomy of the anterior abdominal wall and groin. *Surgery* 2009;27(6):251–254.

Waldman SD. Femoral neuralgia. In: *Atlas of Uncommon Pain Syndromes*. 2nd ed. Philadelphia, PA: Saunders Elsevier; 2008:245–247.

Waldman SD. Femoral nerve block. In: *Atlas of Interventional Pain Management*. 3rd ed. Philadelphia, PA: Saunders Elsevier; 2009:517–521.

Waldman SD. The femoral nerve. In: *Pain Review*. Philadelphia, PA: Saunders Elsevier; 2009:121–122.

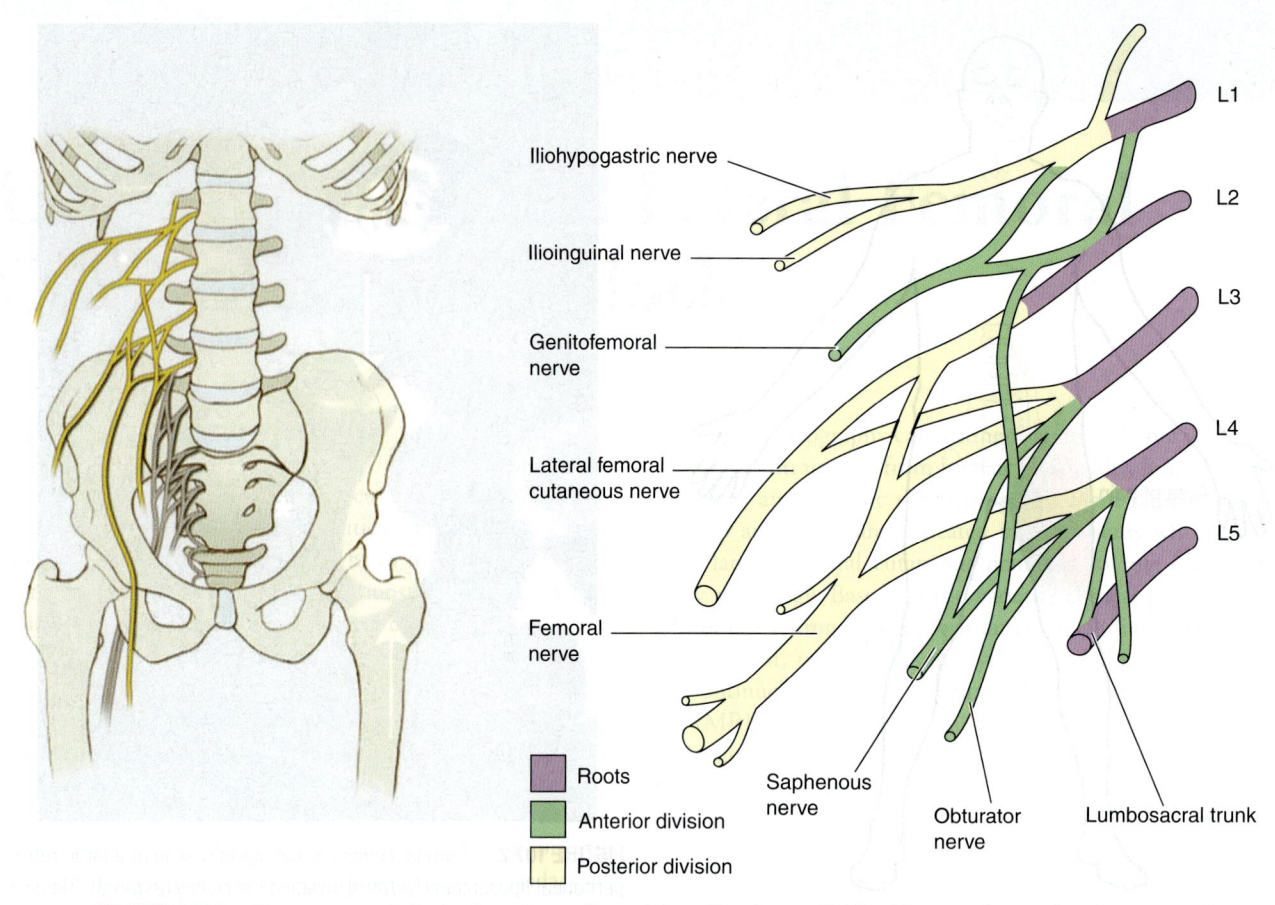

**FIGURE 107.3.** The anatomy of the lumbar plexus. (Reused from Premkumar K. *The Massage Connection Anatomy and Physiology.* Baltimore, MD: Lippincott Williams & Wilkins; 2004, with permission.)

## COMPLICATIONS

Needle-induced trauma to the lateral femoral cutaneous nerve and the adjacent femoral nerve can result in persistent paresthesias. The use of ultrasound guidance when performing lateral femoral nerve block should markedly decrease this complication. Because of the relatively vascular nature of the lower abdominal wall and the proximity of the femoral artery and vein, postblock ecchymosis and hematoma may occur, and the patient should be warned of such. These complications can be decreased by the use of a pressure dressing and cold packs applied to the injection site following the procedure.

## CLINICAL PEARLS

The key to performing successful ultrasound lateral femoral nerve block is the proper identification of the sonographic anatomy and in particular the ability to properly identify the classic honeycombed sonographic signature of the lateral femoral cutaneous nerve as it lies just beneath the fascia lata. This should not be a problem if the above technique is used. Any significant pain or sudden increase in resistance during injection when performing this ultrasound-guided technique suggests incorrect needle placement, and one should stop injecting immediately and reassess the position of the needle.

It should be remembered that the most common cause of pain radiating into the lower extremity is a herniated lumbar disc or nerve impingement secondary to degenerative arthritis of the spine rather than disorders involving the lateral femoral cutaneous nerve per se. Electromyography and MRI of the lumbar spine, combined with the clinical history and physical examination, help sort out the etiology of pain thought to be mediated via the femoral nerve.

Because of the relatively vascular nature of the lower abdominal wall and the proximity of the femoral artery and vein, postblock ecchymosis and hematoma may occur, and the patient should be warned of such. These complications can be decreased by the use of a pressure dressing and cold packs applied to the injection site following the procedure.

Ultrasound-guided lateral femoral cutaneous nerve block is a straightforward technique that is quite effective in treating the symptoms of meralgia paresthetica. Destruction of the lateral femoral cutaneous nerve can be carried out using this technique by injecting small amounts of aqueous phenol or performing radiofrequency lesioning.

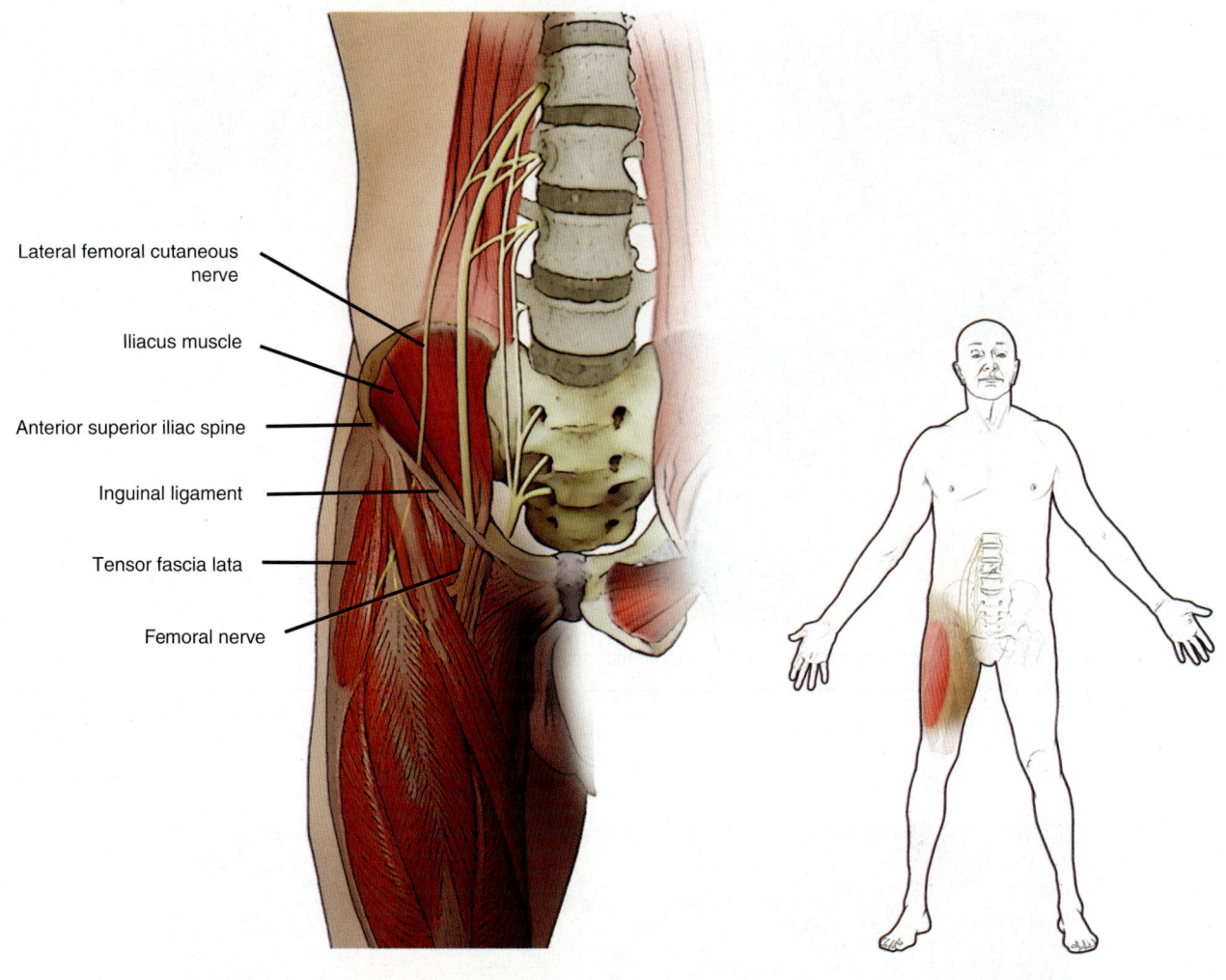

**FIGURE 107.4.** The course of the lateral femoral cutaneous nerve.

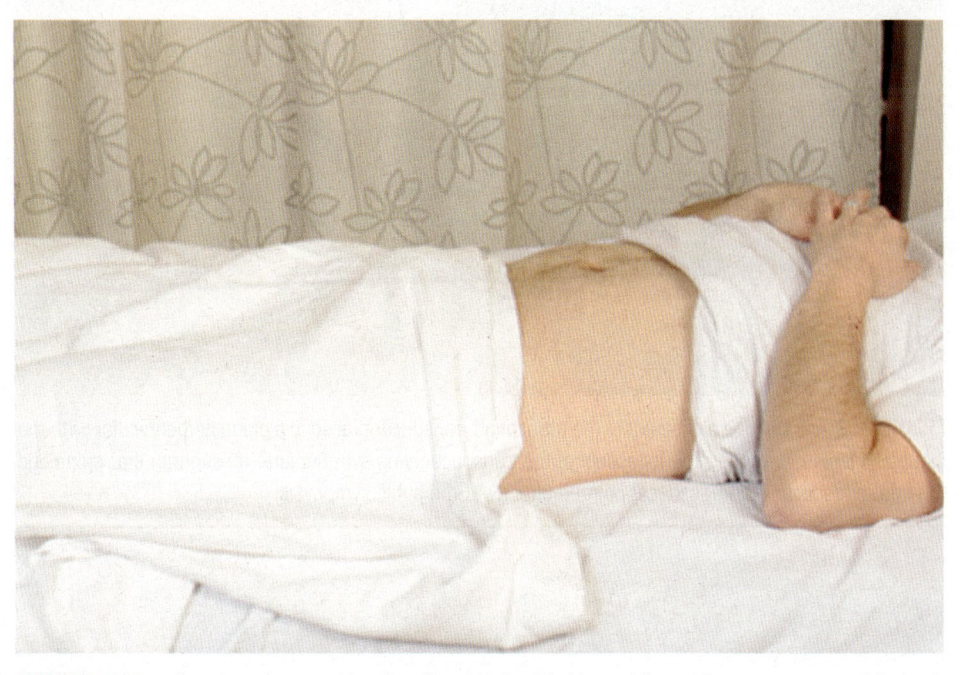

**FIGURE 107.5.** Proper patient position for ultrasound-guided lateral femoral cutaneous nerve block.

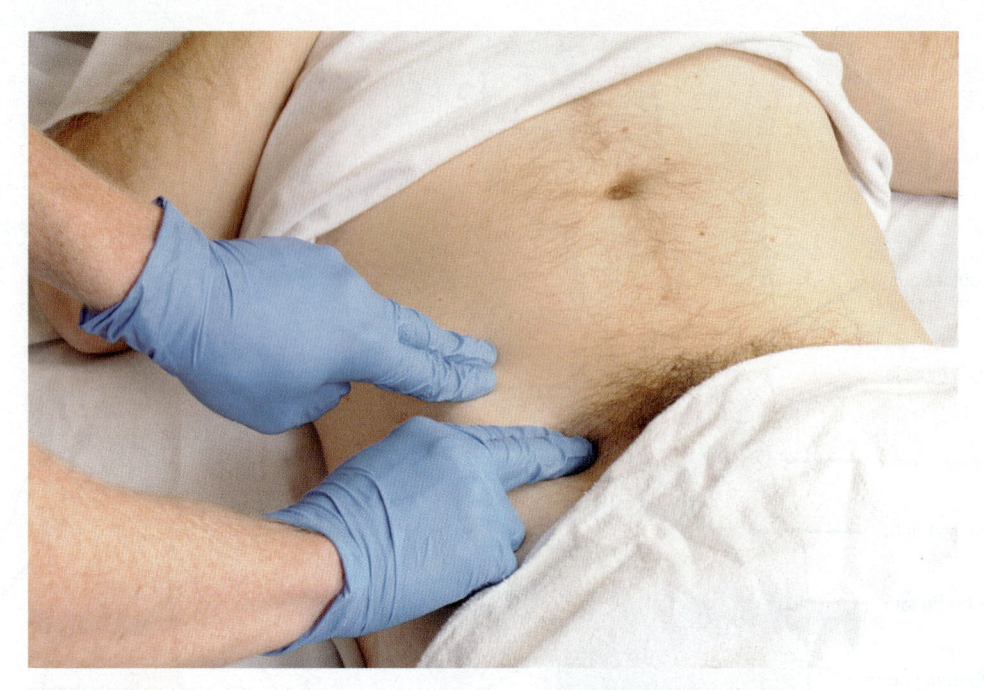

**FIGURE 107.6.** Palpation of the anterior superior iliac spine and inguinal ligament.

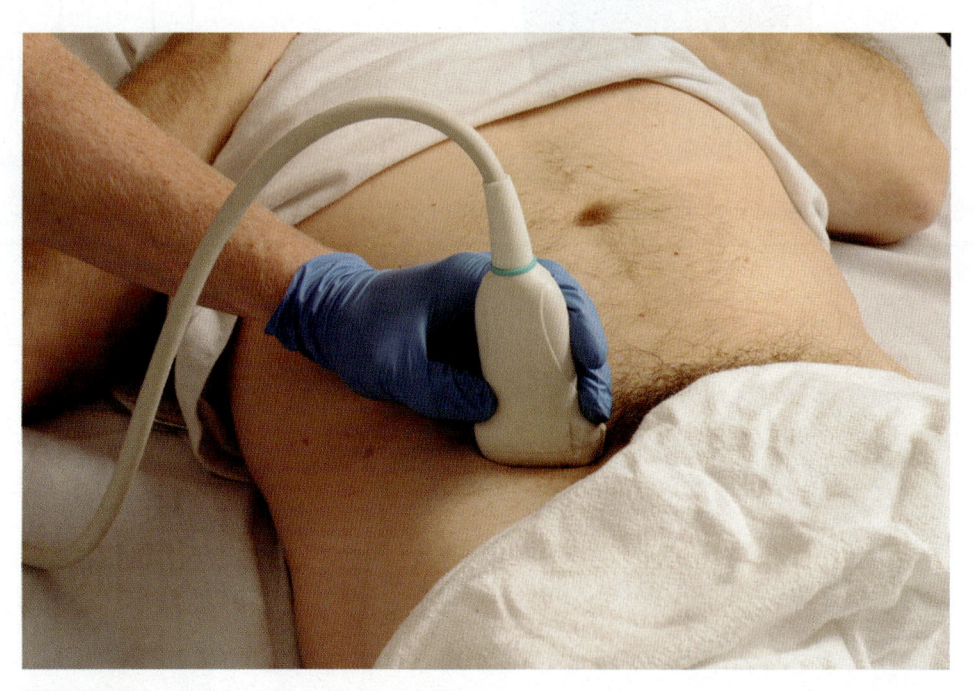

**FIGURE 107.7.** Oblique placement of the ultrasound transducer placed in a plane perpendicular with the inguinal ligament with the superior aspect of the transducer lying over the anterior superior iliac spine and the inferior aspect of the transducer pointed directly at the pubic symphysis.

CHAPTER 107   ULTRASOUND-GUIDED LATERAL FEMORAL CUTANEOUS NERVE BLOCK   **763**

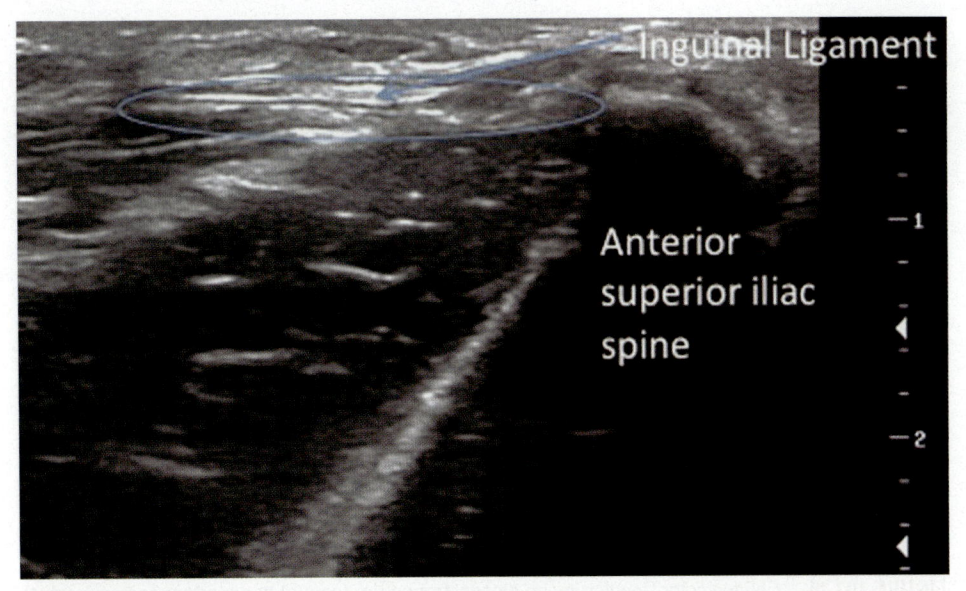

**FIGURE 107.8.**   Oblique ultrasound image demonstrating the hyperechoic anterior superior iliac spine and its acoustic shadow and the inguinal ligament.

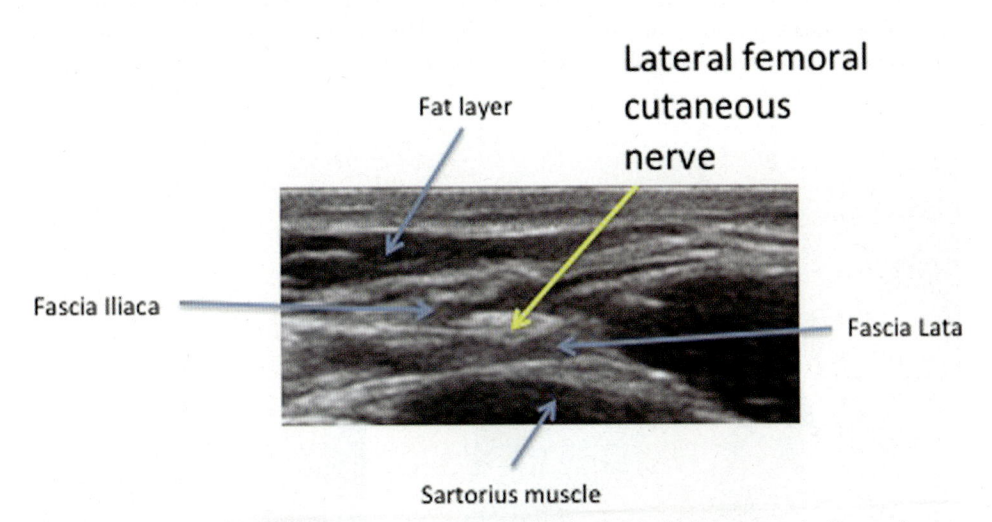

**FIGURE 107.9.**   Oblique ultrasound image demonstrating the hyperechoic honeycombed-appearing lateral femoral cutaneous nerve that appears lying beneath the fascia lata and on top of the sartorius muscle.

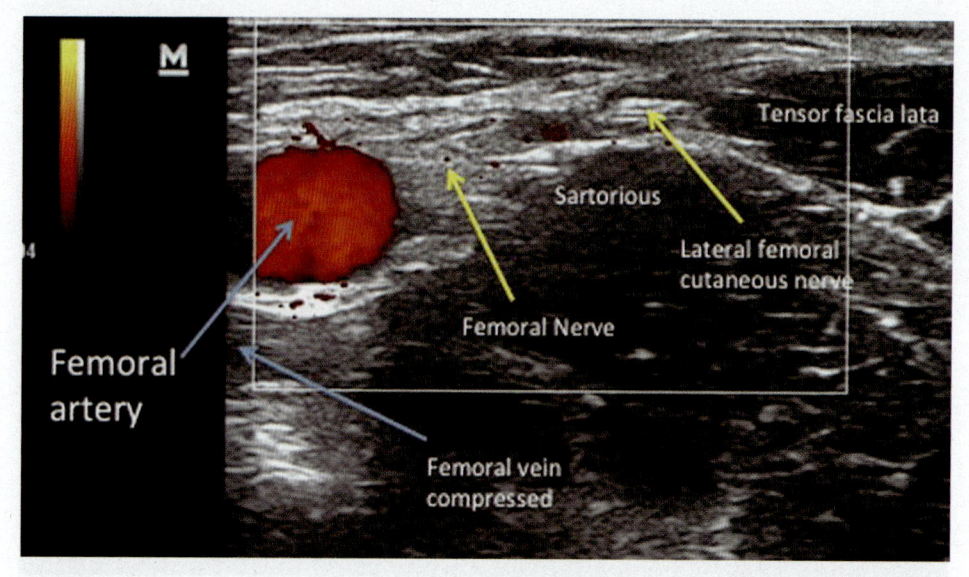

**FIGURE 107.10.** Oblique color Doppler image demonstrating the femoral nerve artery and vein, which lie medial to the lateral femoral cutaneous nerve.

Lateral femoral cutaneous neuralgia is often misdiagnosed as either trochanteric bursitis or lumbar radiculopathy. Electromyography can help confirm the diagnosis. Therapeutic lateral femoral cutaneous nerve blocks with local anesthetic and steroid are extremely beneficial when treating meralgia paresthetica. However, if a patient presents with pain suggestive of meralgia paresthetica and lateral femoral cutaneous nerve blocks are ineffectual, a diagnosis of lesions more proximal in the lumbar plexus or L2–L3 radiculopathy should be considered. Electromyography and MRI of the lumbar plexus are indicated in this patient population to help rule out other causes of lateral femoral cutaneous pain, including malignancy invading the lumbar plexus or epidural or vertebral metastatic disease at L2–L3.

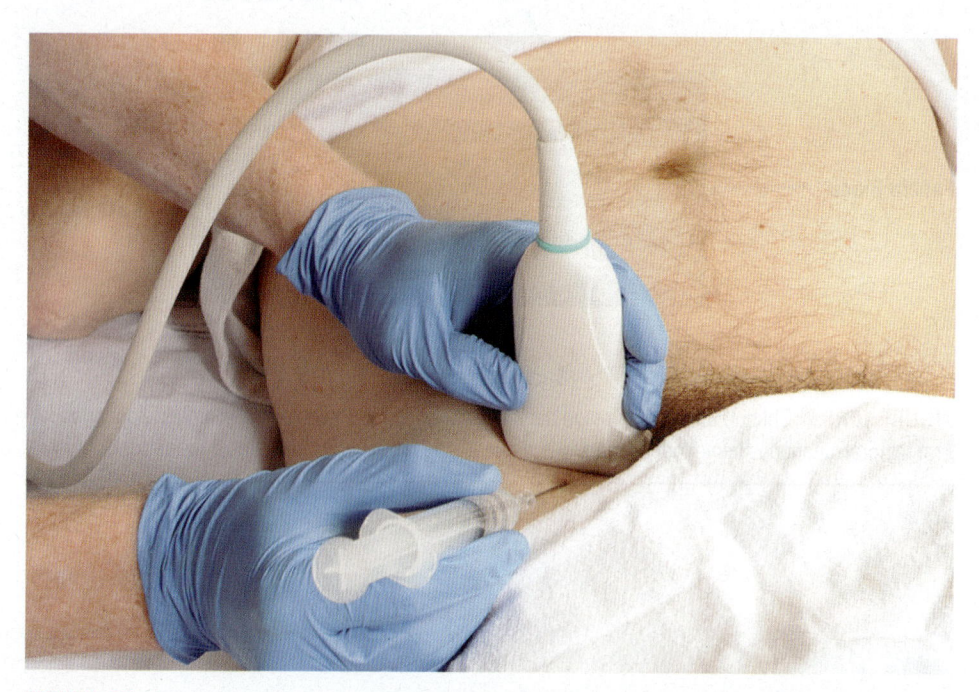

**FIGURE 107.11.** Proper in-plane needle position for performing lateral femoral cutaneous nerve block.

## SUGGESTED READINGS

Mahadevan V. Anatomy of the anterior abdominal wall and groin. *Surgery* 2009;27(6):251–254.

Moucharafieh R, Wehbe J, Maalouf G. Meralgia paresthetica: a result of tight new trendy low cut trousers ('taille basse'). *Int J Surg* 2008;6(2):164–168.

Trummer M, Flaschka G, Unger F, et al. Lumbar disc herniation mimicking meralgia paresthetica: case report. *Surg Neurol* 2000;54(1):80–81.

Waldman SD. Meralgia paresthetica. In: *Pain Review*. Philadelphia, PA: Saunders Elsevier; 2009:301.

Waldman SD. Injection technique for meralgia paresthetica. In: *Pain Review*. Philadelphia, PA: Saunders Elsevier; 2009:556–557.

Waldman SD. Meralgia paresthetica. In: *Atlas of Common Pain Syndromes*. 3rd ed. Philadelphia, PA: Saunders Elsevier; 2012:291–293.

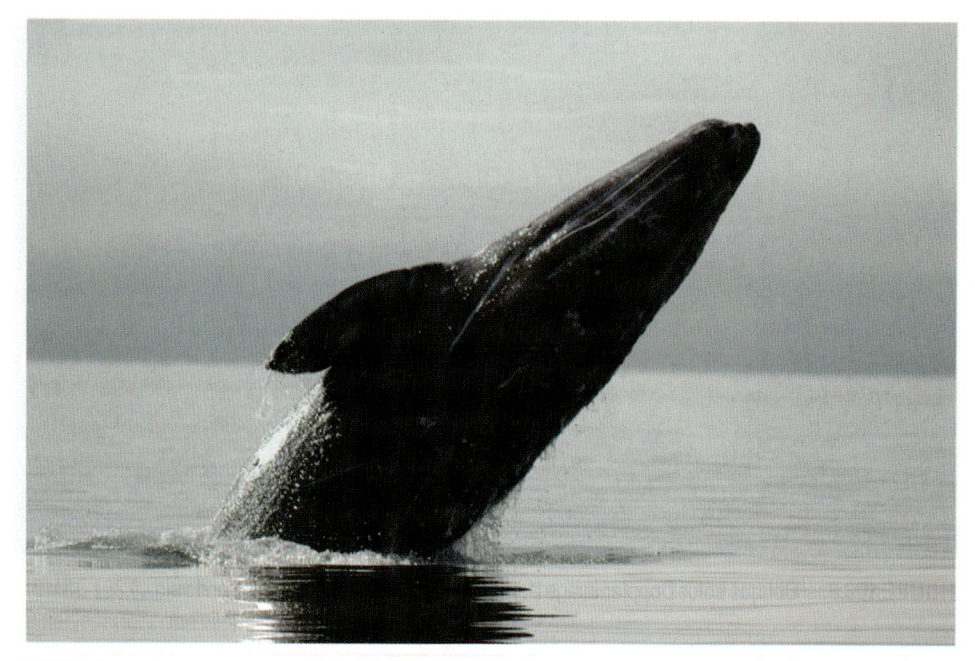

**FIGURE 108.10.** The pectineus muscle looks like a breaching whale.

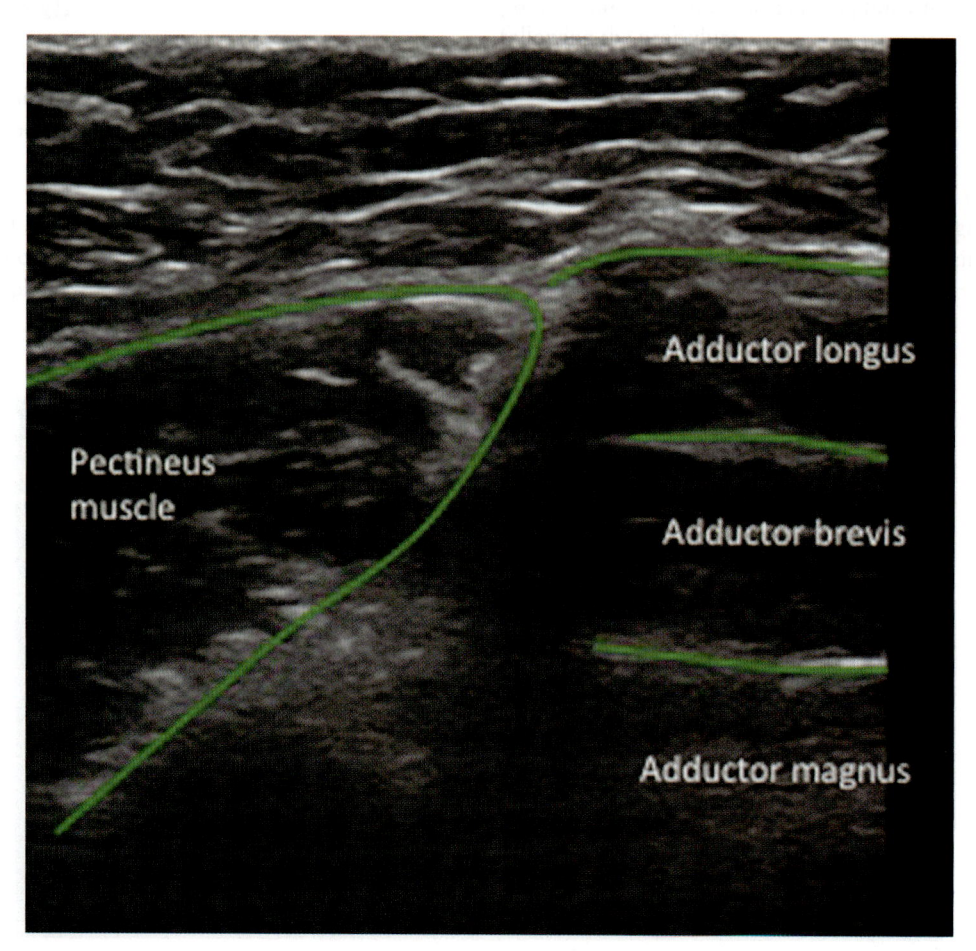

**FIGURE 108.11.** Just medial to the medial border of the pectineus muscle lie the adductor longus, brevis, and magnus muscles, which are stacked on top of one another like a double-decker sandwich.

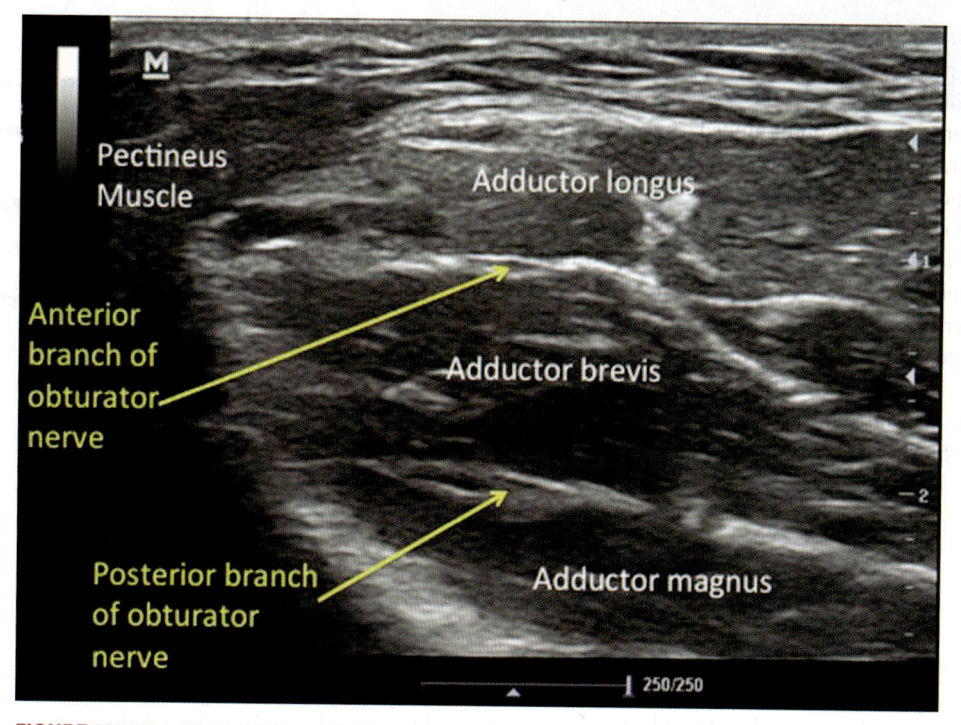

**FIGURE 108.12.** The anterior branch of the obturator nerve lies in the fascial cleft between the adductor longus and brevis muscles, and the posterior branch of the obturator nerve lies between the fascial cleft between the adductor brevis and magnus muscles.

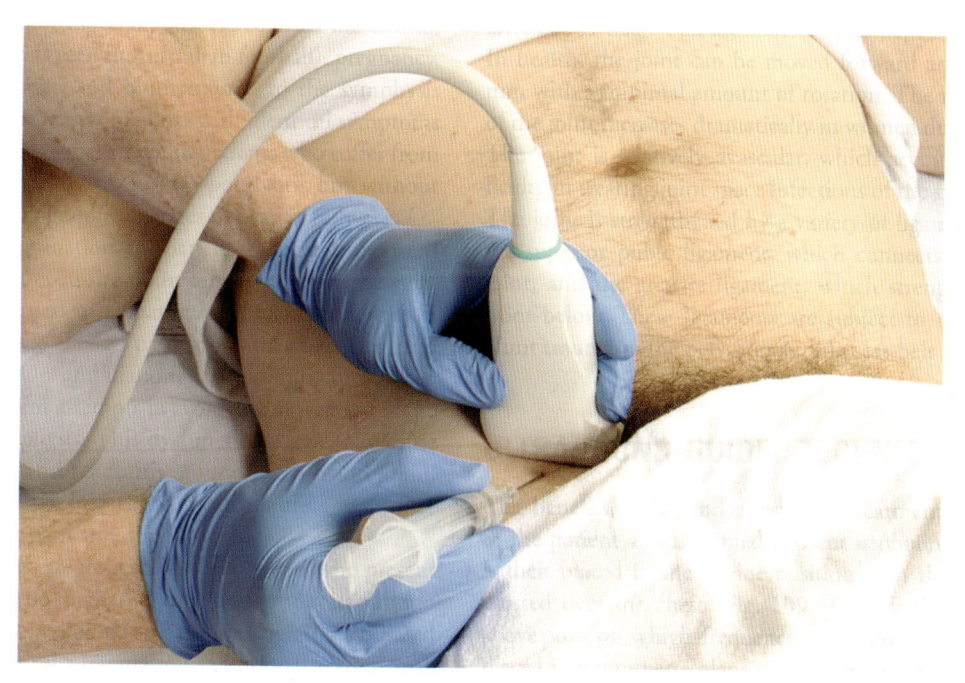

**FIGURE 108.13.** Proper out-of-plane needle position for performing ultrasound-guided obturator nerve block.

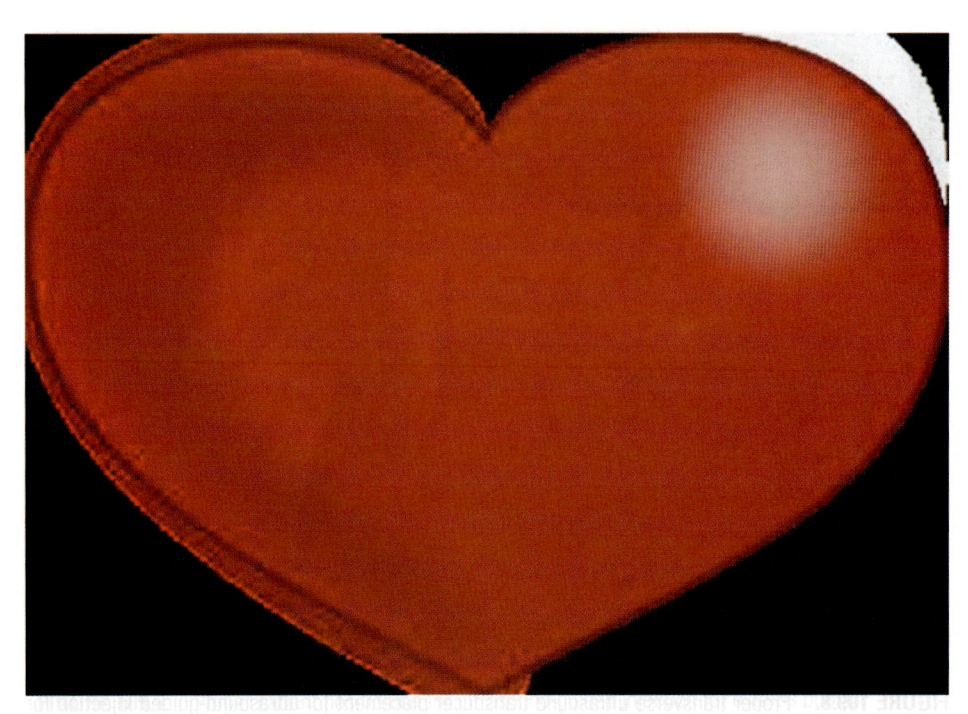

**FIGURE 109.10.** The asymmetrical shape of the interpubic fibroelastic cartilage that gives the joint space and its adjacent pubic bodies their characteristic heart-shaped appearance on transverse ultrasound scan.

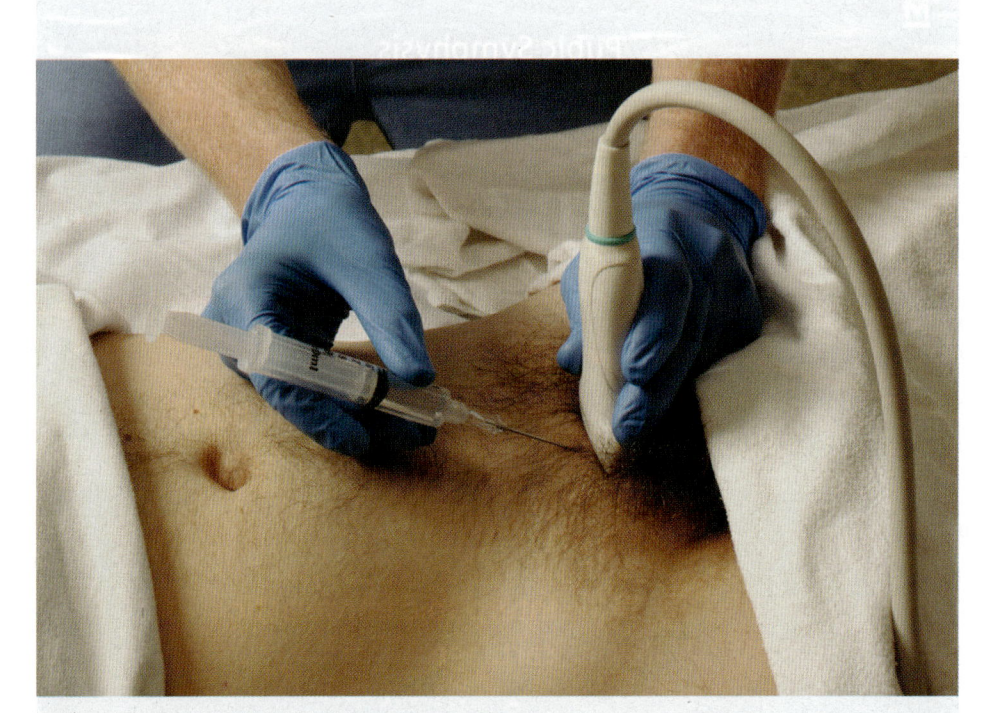

**FIGURE 109.11.** Proper needle placement for an ultrasound-guided out-of-plane injection for osteitis pubis.

Cutting

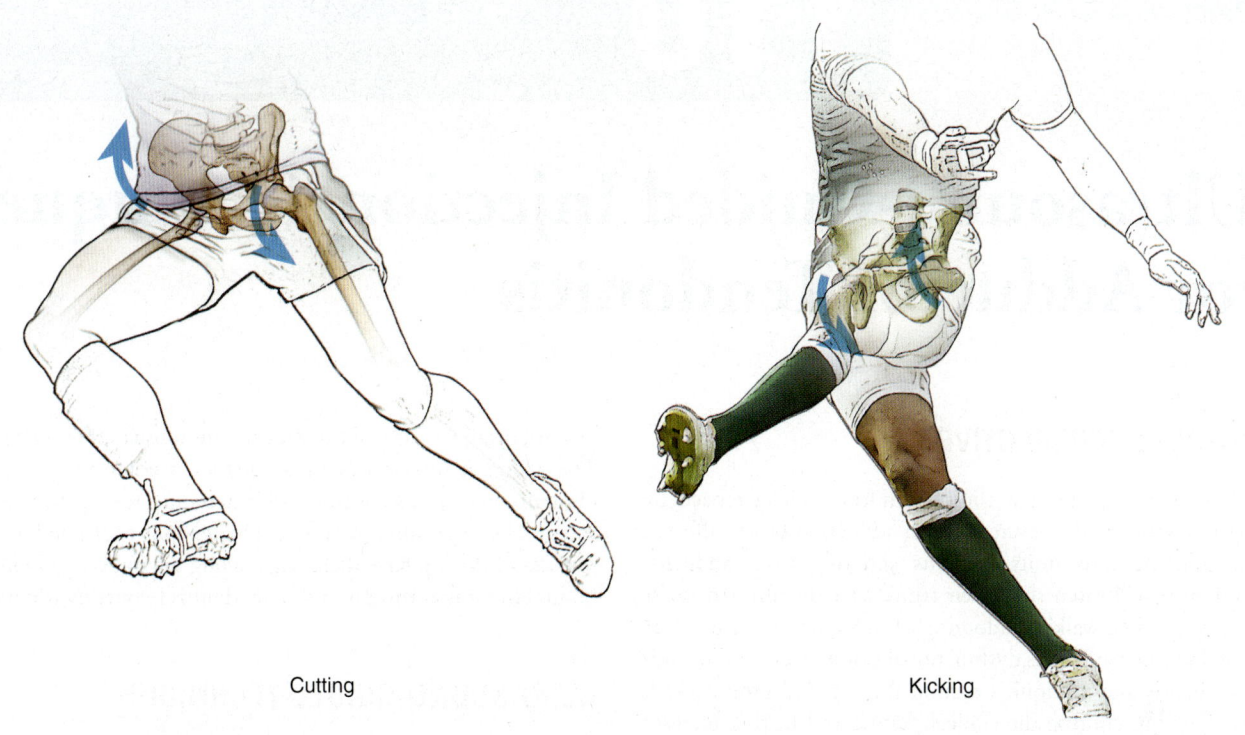

Kicking

**FIGURE 109.12.** The stresses placed on the pubic symphysis during cutting and kick maneuvers in Australian football players.

## COMPLICATIONS

The major complication of ultrasound-guided injection of the symphysis pubis is infection. Ecchymosis and hematoma formation following this procedure may also occur. The possibility of trauma to the already compromised joint from the injection itself remains an ever-present possibility, although the risk of this is decreased if the clinician uses gentle technique and stops injecting immediately if significant resistance to injection is encountered. Approximately 25% of patients complain of a transient increase in pain after this injection technique; the patient should be warned of this.

## CLINICAL PEARLS

The stresses placed on the relatively immobile pubic symphysis during activity are significant. The recent increase in the occurrence of osteitis pubis in Australian football players had led to an examination of these forces, especially during cutting and kicking maneuvers (Fig. 109.12). Bursitis and tendinitis of the hip and groin may coexist with osteitis pubis and may contribute to the patient's pain symptomatology. Universal precautions should always be observed to protect the operator, and strict adherence to sterile technique must be used to avoid infection. Gentle physical therapy and local heat should be introduced following ultrasound-guided injection of the symphysis pubis to reduce pain and improve function. Simple analgesics and nonsteroidal anti-inflammatory agents or COX-2 inhibitors may be used concurrently with this injection technique.

## SUGGESTED READINGS

Garcia-Porrua C, Picallo JA, Gonzalez-Gay MA. Osteitis pubis after Marshall–Marchetti–Krantz urethropexy. *Joint Bone Spine* 2003;70(1):61–63.
Kai B, Lee KD, Andrews G, et al. Puck to pubalgia: imaging of groin pain in professional hockey players. *Can Assoc Radiol J* 2010;61(2):74–79.
MacMahon PJ, Hogan BA, Shelly MJ, et al. Imaging of groin pain. *Magn Reson Imaging Clin N Am* 2009;17(4):655–666.
Morelli V, Espinoza L. Groin injuries and groin pain in athletes: part 2. *Prim Care* 2005;32(1):185–200.
Waldman SD. Osteitis pubis. In: *Pain Review*. Philadelphia, PA: Saunders Elsevier; 2009:309.
Waldman SD. Injection technique for osteitis pubis. In: *Atlas of Pain Management Injection Techniques*. 3rd ed. Philadelphia, PA: Saunders Elsevier; 2013:333–337.
Waldman SD, Campbell RSD. Osteitis pubis. In: *Imaging of Pain*. Philadelphia, PA: Saunders Elsevier; 2011:207–208.
Waldman SD, Campbell RSD. Osteitis pubis. In: *Atlas of Common Pain Syndromes*. 3rd ed. Philadelphia, PA: Saunders Elsevier; 2013:260–262.

# CHAPTER 110

# Ultrasound-Guided Injection Technique for Adductor Tendonitis

## CLINICAL PERSPECTIVES

Adductor tendonitis is a clinical syndrome characterized by sharp, constant, and severe pain on adduction of the affected musculotendinous units. Patients suffering from adductor tendonitis will often shift their trunk over the affected lower extremity when walking, adopting a lurch type gait in an effort to reduce the pain. This dysfunctional gait may cause a secondary bursitis and tendonitis around the hip and groin, which may serve to confuse the clinical picture and further increase the patient's pain and disability. Pain on palpation of the insertions of the adductor tendon is a consistent finding in patients with adductor tendonitis as is exacerbation of pain with active resisted abduction. Patients suffering from adductor tendonitis will also exhibit a positive Waldman knee squeeze test. This test is performed by having the patient sit on the edge of the examination table. The examiner places a tennis ball between the patient's knees and asks the patient to gently hold it there with gentle pressure from the knees (Fig. 110.1A). The patient is then instructed to quickly squeeze the ball between the knees as hard as possible. Patients suffering from adductor tendonitis will reflexly abduct the affected extremity due to the pain of forced adduction, thereby causing the ball to drop to the floor (see Fig. 110.1B). Untreated, adductor tendonitis will result in increasing pain and functional disability with patients complaining of an inability to get in and out of a car.

Plain radiographs of the hip and pelvis are indicated in all patients who present with pain thought to be secondary to adductor tendonitis (Fig. 110.2). Based on the patient's clinical presentation, additional testing may be indicated, including complete blood cell count, prostate-specific antigen, sedimentation rate, and antinuclear antibody testing. Magnetic resonance imaging of the pelvis is indicated if occult mass or tumor is suggested as well as to confirm the diagnosis. Radionuclide bone scanning may be useful in ruling out pelvic stress fractures not seen on plain radiographs. Ultrasound-guided injection of adductor tendonitis serves as both a diagnostic and a therapeutic maneuver.

## CLINICALLY RELEVANT ANATOMY

The adductor muscles of the hip include the adductor longus, adductor brevis, and adductor magnus muscles as well as the gracilis, pectineus, and obturator externus muscles (Fig. 110.3). The adductor function of these muscles is innervated by the obturator nerve, which is susceptible to trauma from pelvic fractures and compression by tumor. The tendons of the adductor muscles of the hip have their origin along the pubis and ischial ramus, and it is at this point that tendonitis frequently occurs.

## ULTRASOUND-GUIDED TECHNIQUE

The benefits, risks, and alternative treatments are explained to the patient and informed consent is obtained. The patient is then placed in the supine position with the patient's arms crossed over the chest (Fig. 110.4). With the patient in the above position, a high-frequency linear ultrasound transducer is placed in a transverse plane over the pubic prominence, which lies just above the penis in males and the clitoris in females, and an ultrasound survey scan is taken (Figs. 110.5 and 110.6). The bright hyperechoic pubic bodies are identified with the hypoechoic interpubic fibroelastic cartilage in between (Fig. 110.7). The interpubic fibroelastic cartilage is wider anteriorly, narrowing toward the back of the joint space (see Fig. 109.1). It is this asymmetrical shape that gives the joint space and its adjacent pubic bodies their characteristic heart-shaped appearance on transverse ultrasound scan (see Fig. 110.7). After the pubic symphysis is identified, the transversely placed ultrasound transducer is slowly moved laterally following the superior pubic ramus until the insertions of the adductor muscles are identified (Fig. 110.8). When the insertions of the adductor muscles are identified, the skin overlying the area above the ultrasound transducer is prepped with antiseptic solution. A sterile syringe containing 3.0 mL of 0.25% preservative-free bupivacaine and 40 mg of methylprednisolone is attached to a 3½-inch, 22-gauge needle using strict aseptic technique. The needle is placed through the skin ~1 cm above the superior border of the ultrasound transducer and is then advanced using an out-of-plane approach with the needle trajectory adjusted under real-time ultrasound guidance so that the needle tip rests against the site of tendinous insertion (Fig. 110.9). When the tip of needle is thought to be in satisfactory position, after careful aspiration, the contents of the syringe are slowly injected. There should be minimal resistance to injection. The patient may note an exacerbation of his or her pain during the injection.

CHAPTER 110 ULTRASOUND-GUIDED INJECTION TECHNIQUE FOR ADDUCTOR TENDONITIS 783

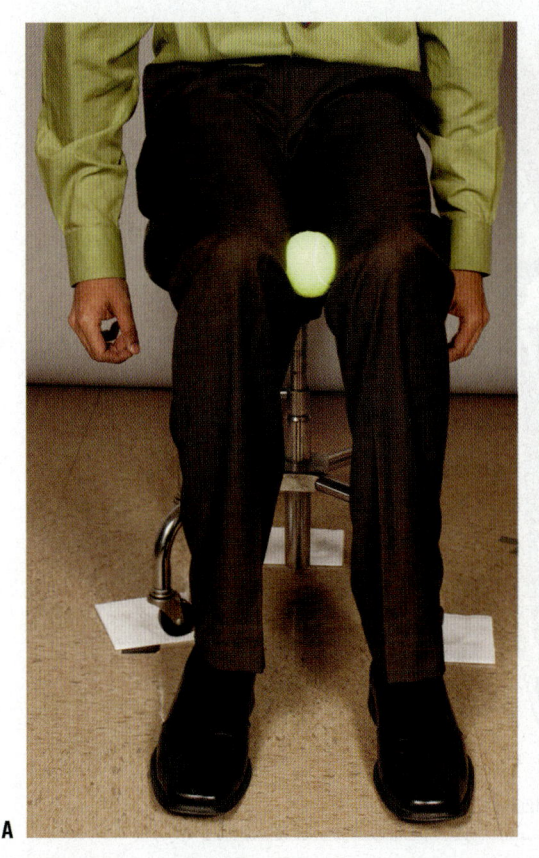

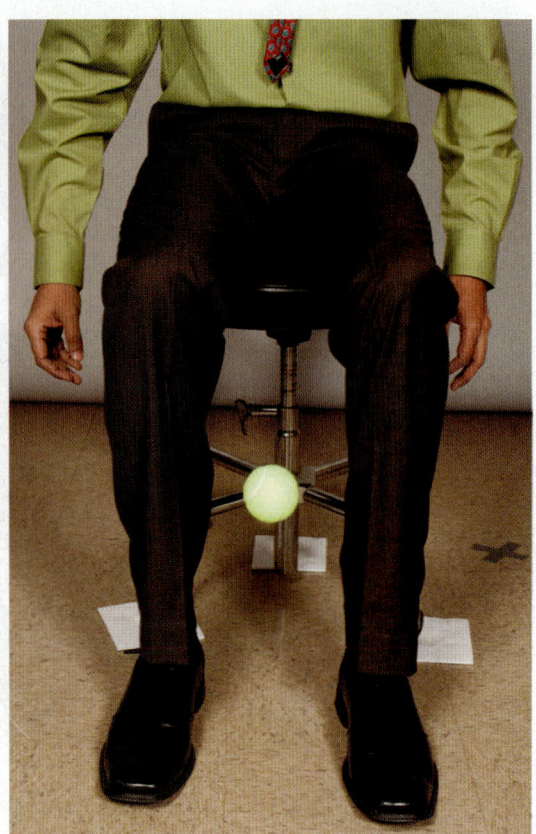

**FIGURE 110.1.** **A:** The Waldman knee squeeze test for adductor tendonitis. The examiner places a tennis ball between the patient's knees and asks the patient to gently hold it there with gentle pressure from the knees. The patient is then instructed to quickly squeeze the ball between the knees as hard as possible. **B:** The Waldman knee squeeze test for adductor tendonitis. Patients suffering from adductor tendonitis will reflexly abduct the affected extremity due to the pain of quickly forced adduction, thereby causing the ball to drop to the floor.

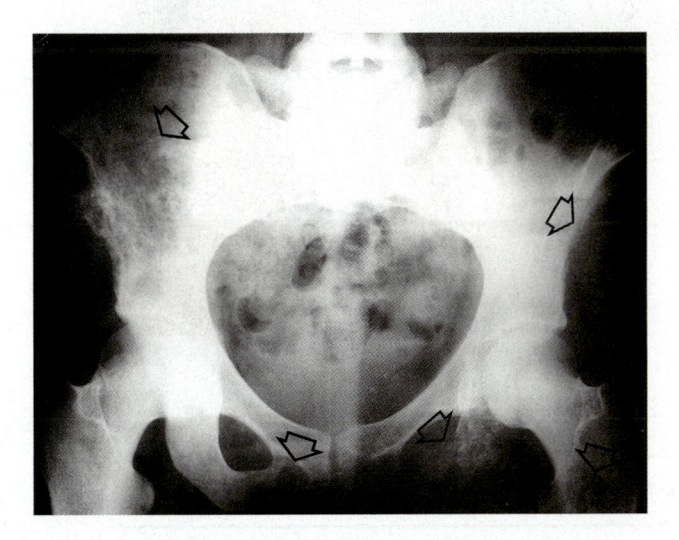

**FIGURE 110.2.** Plain radiograph demonstrating osteolytic metastasis from primary breast carcinoma (*open arrows*). (Reused from Pope TL Jr, Harris JH Jr. *Harris & Harris' the Radiology of Emergency Medicine.* 5th ed. Philadelphia, PA: Lippincott Williams & Wilkins; 2013, with permission.)

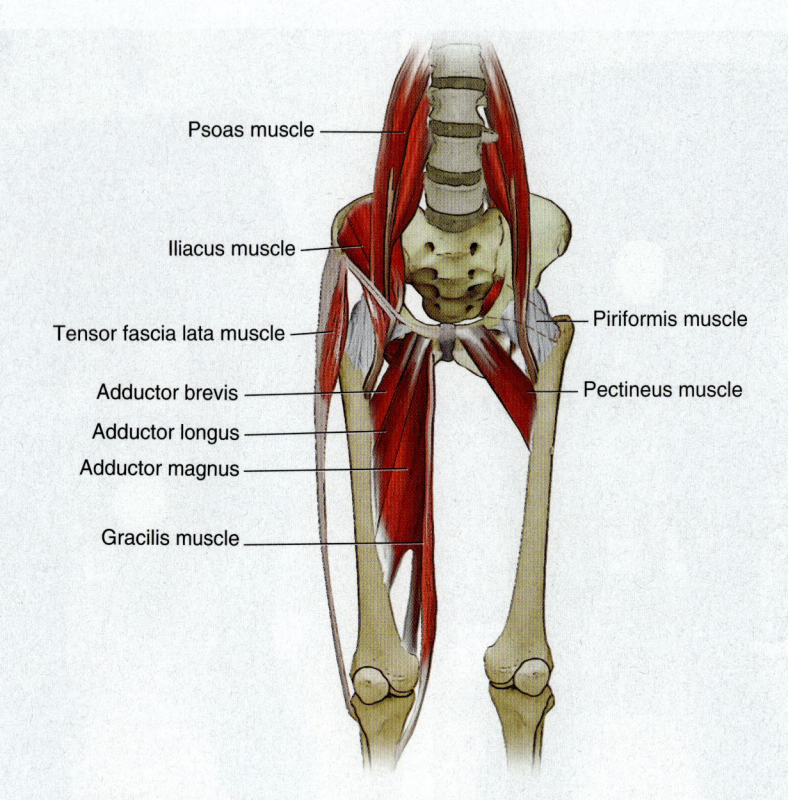

**FIGURE 110.3.** Anatomy of the hip adductors.

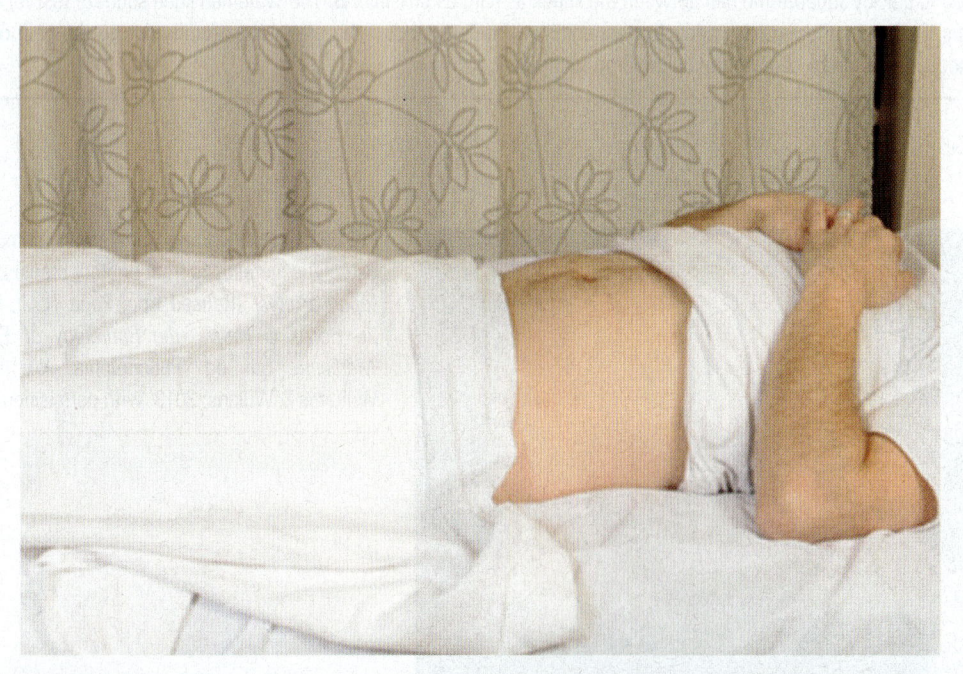

**FIGURE 110.4.** Proper patient positioning for ultrasound-guided injection for adductor tendonitis.

CHAPTER 110   ULTRASOUND-GUIDED INJECTION TECHNIQUE FOR ADDUCTOR TENDONITIS   785

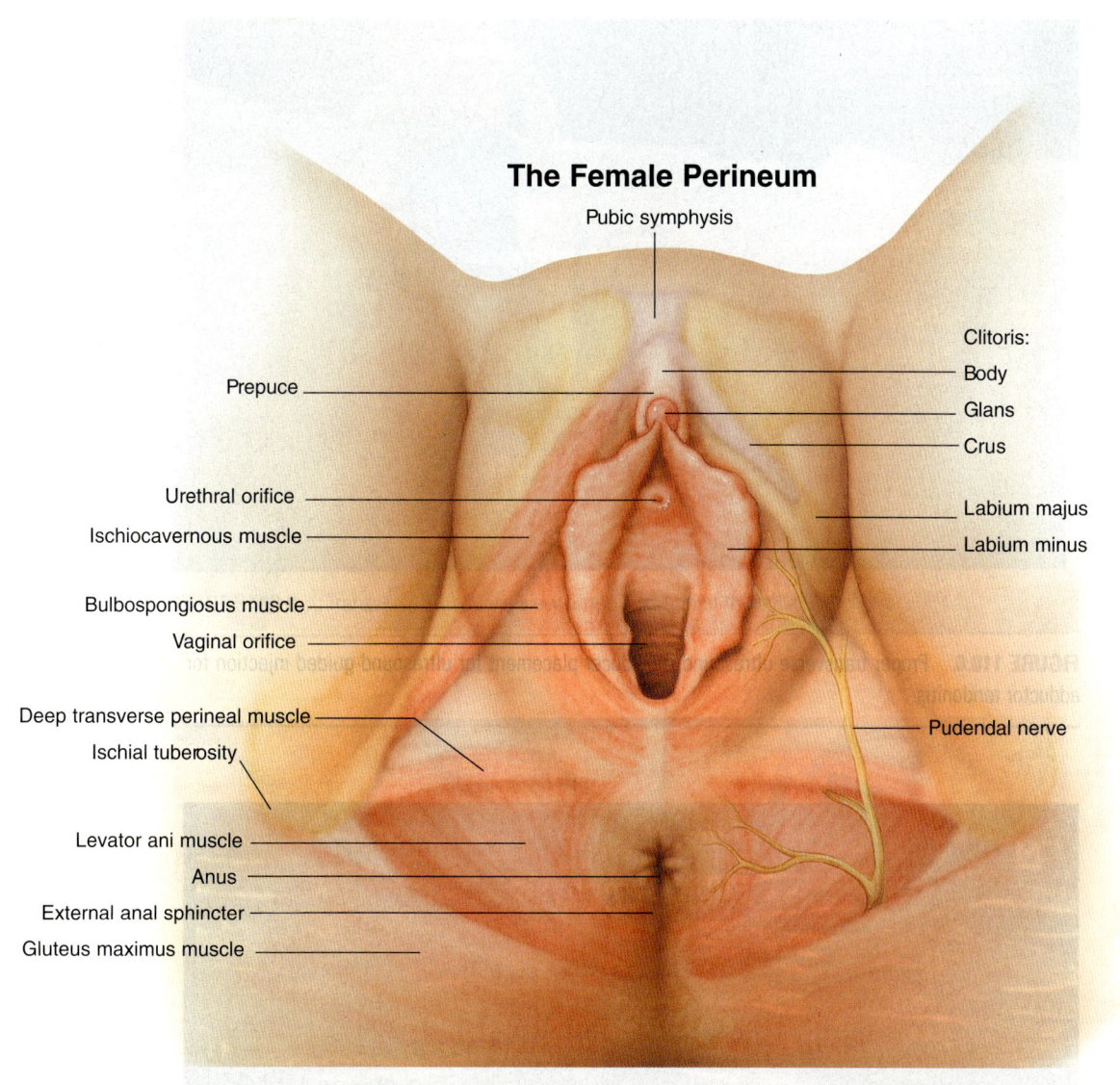

**FIGURE 110.5.** The pubic symphysis is located just above the clitoris in females. (Anatomic Chart Company, 2013.)

## COMPLICATIONS

The major complication of this ultrasound-guided injection technique is infection. Ecchymosis and hematoma formation following this procedure may also occur. The possibility of trauma to the already compromised tendons from the injection itself remains an ever-present possibility, although the risk of this is decreased if the clinician uses gentle technique and stops injecting immediately if significant resistance to injection is encountered. Approximately 25% of patients complain of a transient increase in pain after this injection technique; the patient should be warned of this.

## CLINICAL PEARLS

Bursitis and tendonitis of the hip and groin may coexist with adductor tendonitis and may contribute to the patient's pain symptomatology. Universal precautions should always be observed to protect the operator, and strict adherence to sterile technique must be used to avoid infection. Gentle physical therapy and local heat should be introduced following ultrasound-guided injection of adductor tendonitis to reduce pain and improve function. Simple analgesics and nonsteroidal anti-inflammatory agents or COX-2 inhibitors may be used concurrently with this injection technique.

# Ultrasound-Guided Injection Technique for Ischial Bursitis Pain

## CLINICAL PERSPECTIVES

Ischial bursitis is a common cause of posterior hip and buttocks pain. The ischial bursa lies between the gluteus maximus muscle and the ischial tuberosity (Fig. 111.1). The bursa serves to cushion and facilitate sliding of the musculotendinous unit of the gluteus maximus muscle over the bony ischial tuberosity. The bursa is subject to inflammation from a variety of causes with acute trauma to the buttocks and repetitive microtrauma being the most common. Acute injuries to the bursa can occur from direct trauma such as when falling on the ice onto the buttocks, from prolonged bicycle or horse riding, or being tackled when playing football or checked when playing ice hockey. Direct pressure forcing the ischial bursa against the ischial tuberosity from prolonged sitting on hard surfaces has also been implicated in the development of ischial bursitis. If the inflammation of the bursa is not treated and the condition becomes chronic, calcification of the bursa with further functional disability may occur. Gout and other crystal arthropathies may also precipitate acute ischial bursitis as may bacterial, tubercular, or fungal infections (Fig. 111.2).

The patient suffering from ischial bursitis, which is also known as weaver's bottom (due to its prevalence in weavers that have to sit on the edge of their seat to operate their loom), most frequently presents with the complaint of severe pain with any pressure on the gluteus maximus muscle and ischial bursa (Fig. 111.3). Flexion of the spine to maintain a sitting position such as when riding a horse or sitting on a stool will exacerbate the pain. Physical examination of the patient suffering from ischial bursitis will reveal point tenderness over the ischial tuberosity (Fig. 111.4). The patient may also exhibit a positive hip extension test when the patient is asked to actively extend his or her hip against resistance while in the prone position (Fig. 111.5). If there is significant inflammation, rubor and color may be present and the entire area may feel boggy or edematous to palpation. Swelling, which at times can be quite dramatic, is often present. Passive flexion of the hip may exacerbate the pain of ischial bursitis. If calcification or gouty tophi of the bursa and surrounding tendons are present, the examiner may appreciate crepitus with active flexion of the trunk and/or hip, especially in the sitting position (see Fig. 111.2).

Plain radiographs are indicated in all patients who present with hip pain to rule out occult bony pathology. Based on the patient's clinical presentation, additional testing may be indicated, including complete blood cell count, sedimentation rate, and antinuclear antibody testing. Magnetic resonance imaging (MRI) or ultrasound imaging of the affected area may also help delineate the presence of other hip bursitis, calcific tendinitis, tendinopathy, triceps tendinitis, or other hip pathology. MRI or ultrasound imaging of the affected area may also help delineate the presence of calcific tendinitis or other hip pathology. Rarely, the inflamed bursa may become infected, and failure to diagnose and treat the acute infection can lead to dire consequences (Fig. 111.6).

## CLINICALLY RELEVANT ANATOMY

The ischial bursa lies between the gluteus maximus muscle and the ischial tuberosity. It is superior and medial to the insertion of the hamstring muscle onto the ischium (see Fig. 111.1). The action of the gluteus maximus muscle includes the flexion of trunk on thigh when maintaining a sitting position as when riding a horse. This action can irritate the ischial bursa, as can repeated pressure against the bursa that forces it against the ischial tuberosity. The hamstring muscles find a common origin at the ischial tuberosity and can also be irritated from overuse or misuse. The action of the hamstrings includes flexion of the lower extremity at the knee. Running on soft or uneven surfaces can cause a tendinitis at the origin of the hamstring muscles.

## ULTRASOUND-GUIDED TECHNIQUE

The benefits, risks, and alternative treatments are explained to the patient and informed consent is obtained. The patient is then placed in the modified Sims position (Fig. 111.7). With the patient in the above position, the posterior superior iliac spine and the ischial tuberosity are identified, and an imaginary line is drawn between the two points (Fig. 111.8). At the level of the patient's coccyx, a high-frequency linear ultrasound

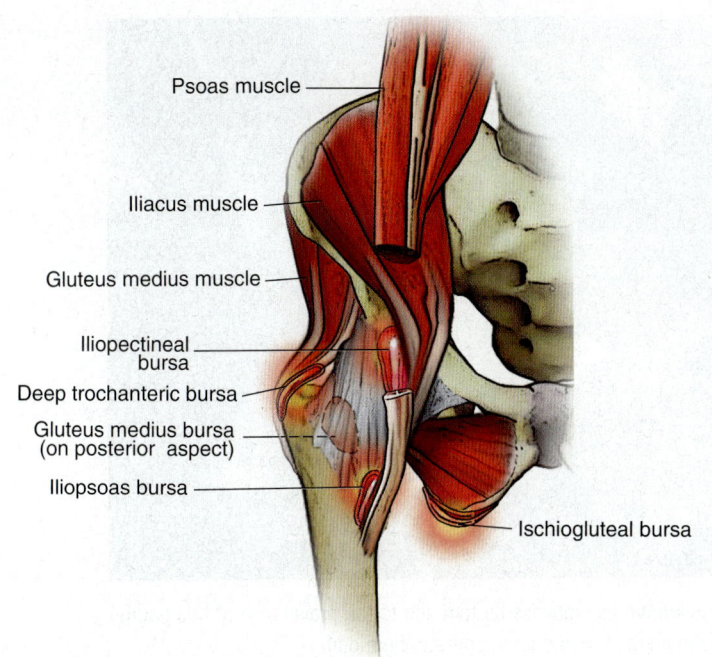

**FIGURE 111.1.** The anatomy of the bursae of the hip.

transducer is placed on the line in a transverse plane, and an ultrasound survey scan is taken (Fig. 111.9). The sacrum is identified as a curved hyperechoic structure. The ischial bursa lies just anterior to the ischium and beneath the gluteus maximus muscle (Fig. 111.10). In health, the ischial bursa may appear as a thin, hypoechoic space between the gluteus maximus muscle and the ischial tuberosity. If the bursa is inflamed, it will appear as a large, sometimes, loculated fluid-filled sac (Fig. 111.11). After the bursa is identified, the skin overlying the area beneath the ultrasound transducer is prepped with antiseptic solution. A sterile syringe containing 3.0 mL of 0.25% preservative-free bupivacaine and 40 mg of methylprednisolone is attached to a 3½-inch, 22-gauge needle using strict aseptic technique. The needle is placed through the skin ~1cm above the superior edge of the transducer and is then advanced using an in-plane approach with the needle trajectory adjusted under real-time ultrasound guidance so that the needle tip rests within the bursa sac (Fig. 111.12). When the tip of needle is thought to be in satisfactory position, after careful aspiration, a small amount of local anesthetic and steroid is injected under real-time ultrasound guidance to confirm that the needle tip is not within the substance of the tendon. After proper needle tip placement is confirmed, the remainder of the contents of the syringe are slowly injected. There should be minimal resistance to injection. If loculations or calcifications are present, the needle may have to be repositioned several times to fully treat and/or aspirate the bursa.

## COMPLICATIONS

The major complication of ultrasound-guided injection of the ischial bursa is infection. Ecchymosis and hematoma formation may also occur. A transient exacerbation of the patient's pain occurs ~25% of the time following this injection technique, and the patient should be warned of this possibility prior to the procedure.

**FIGURE 111.2.** Hydroxyapatite deposition causing ischial bursitis.

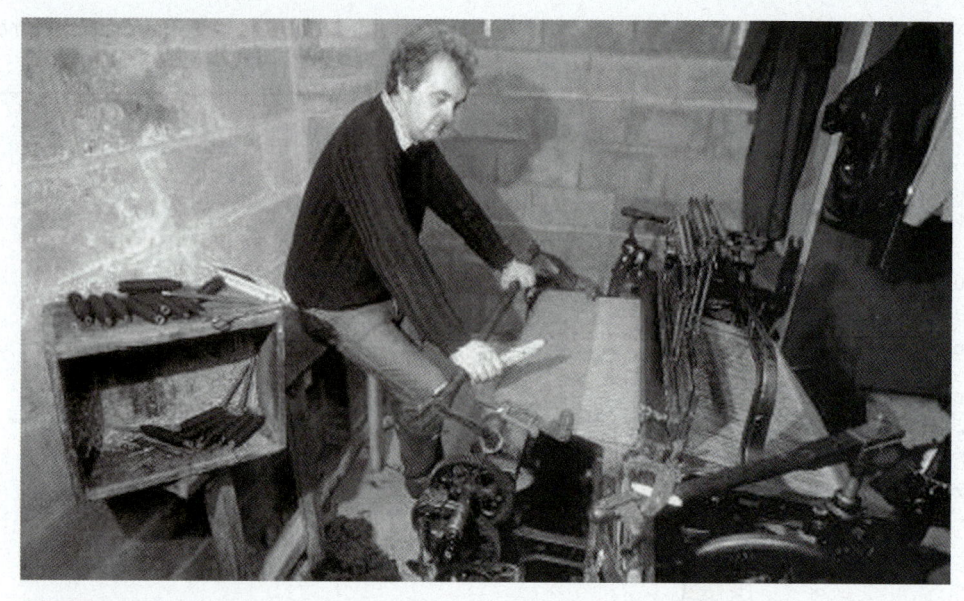

**FIGURE 111.3.** Ischial bursitis is also known as weaver's bottom due to the prevalence of this painful condition in weavers who must sit on the edge of their seat to operate their loom.

## CLINICAL PEARLS

Hip pathology including bursitis of the other bursa of the hip, medial and lateral epicondylitis, tendinopathy, osteoarthritis, avascular necrosis, and entrapment neuropathies may coexist with ischial bursitis and may contribute to the patient's pain symptomatology. Universal precautions should always be observed to protect the operator, and strict adherence to sterile technique must be used to avoid infection. Gentle physical therapy and local heat should be introduced following ultrasound-guided injection of the ischial bursa to reduce pain and improve function. Simple analgesics and nonsteroidal anti-inflammatory agents or COX-2 inhibitors may be used concurrently with this injection technique.

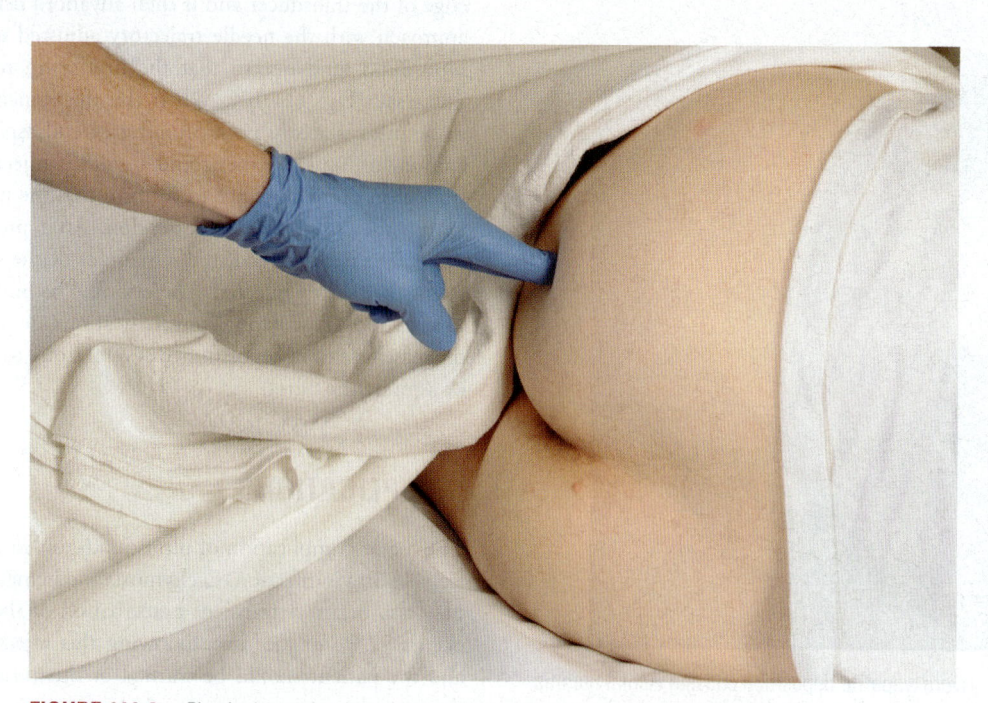

**FIGURE 111.4.** Physical examination of the patient suffering from ischial bursitis will reveal point tenderness over the ischial tuberosity.

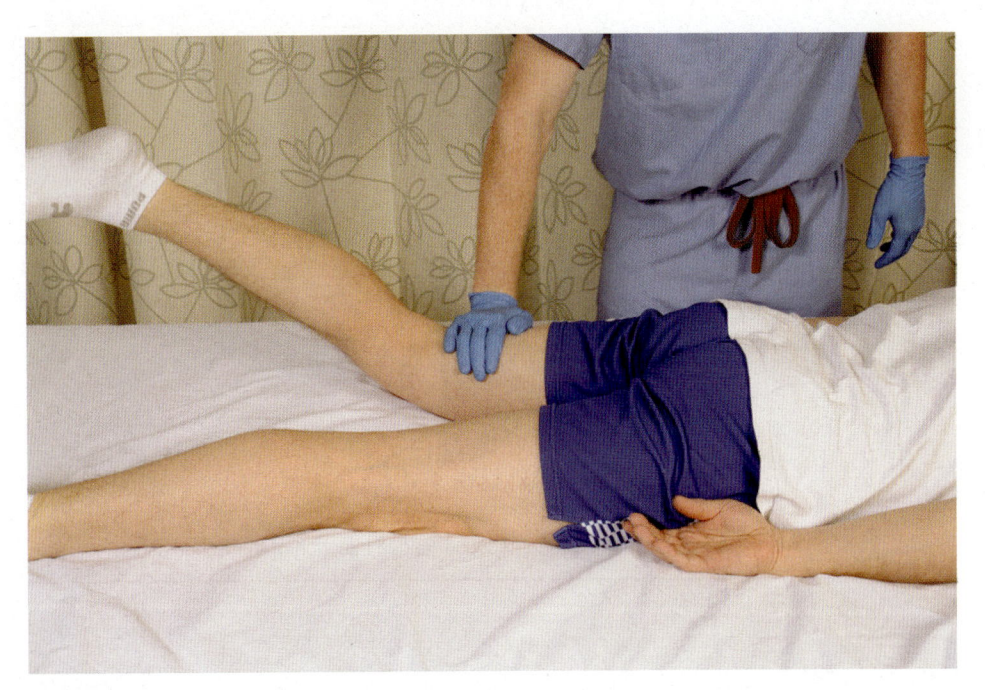

**FIGURE 111.5.** Patients suffering from ischial bursitis will exhibit a positive resisted hip extension test. The resisted hip extension test is performed by placing the patient in a prone position and having the patient perform vigorous hip extension against resistance.

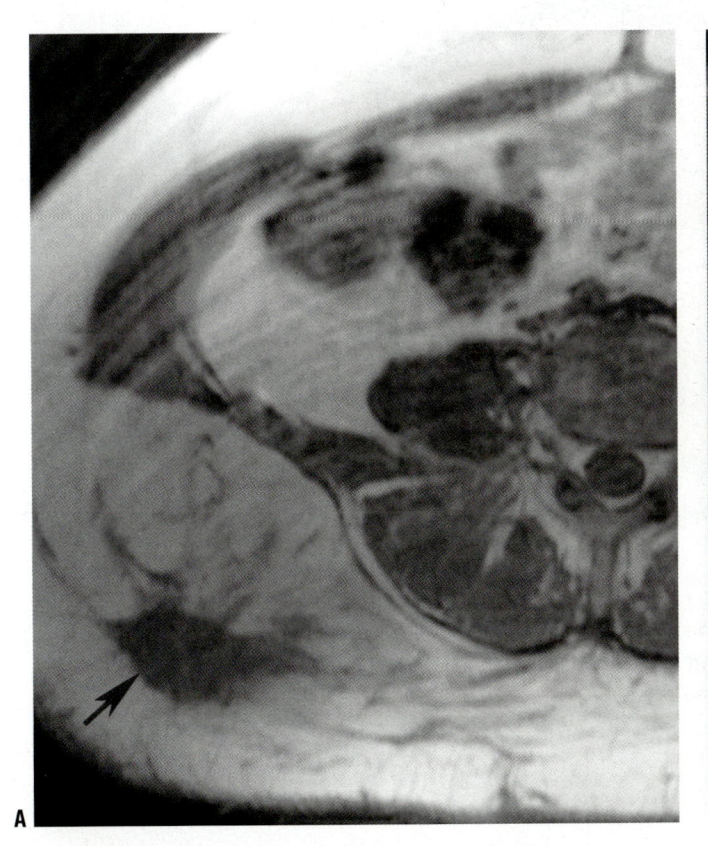

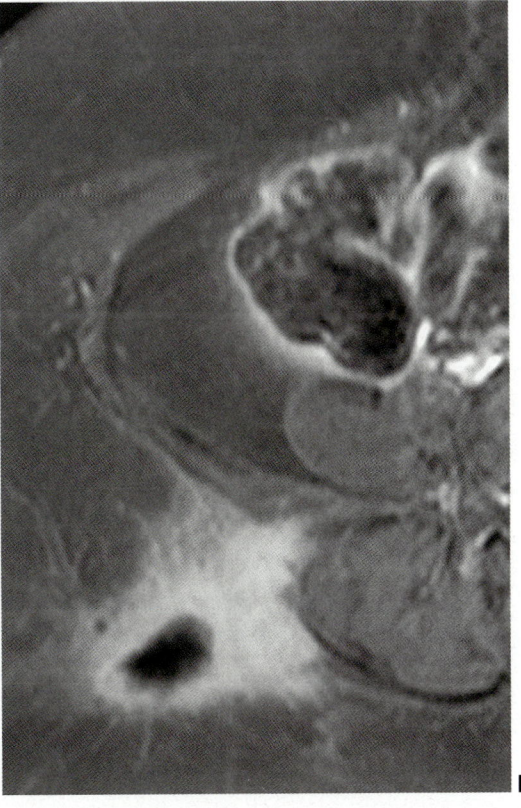

**FIGURE 111.6.** Pre– and post–gadolinium MRI images in a patient with a soft tissue abscess in the gluteal region. **A:** T1-weighted image demonstrates an irregular low-intensity lesion in the soft tissues. **B:** Postcontrast fat-suppressed T1-weighted image demonstrates an abscess with no central enhancement and surrounding inflammation. (Reused from Berquist TH. *MRI of the Musculoskeletal System*. 5th ed. Philadelphia, PA: Lippincott Williams & Wilkins; 2013, with permission.)

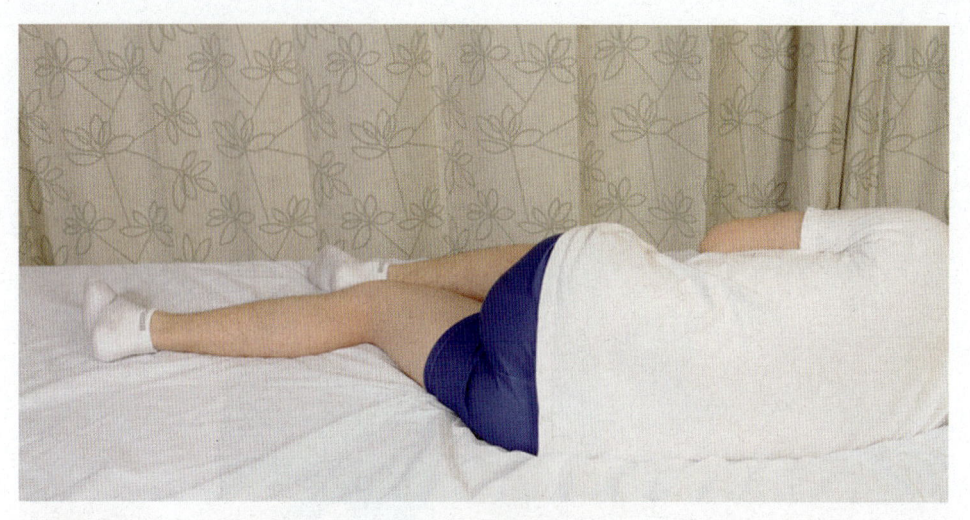

**FIGURE 111.7.** Proper patient positioning for ultrasound-guided injection of the ischial bursa.

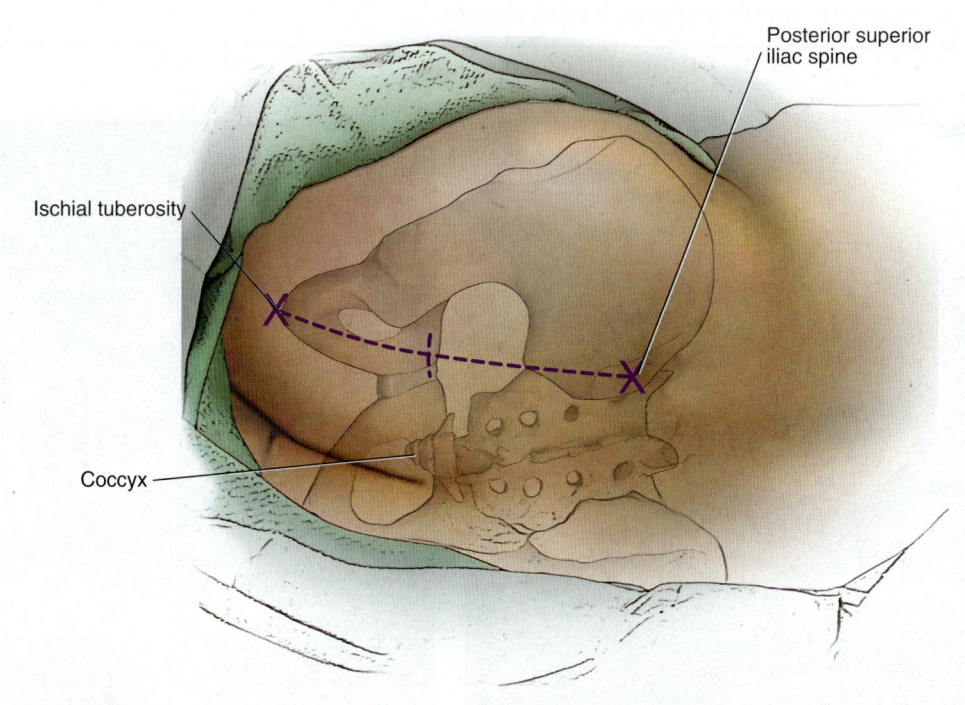

**FIGURE 111.8.** With the patient in the modified Sims position, the posterosuperior iliac spine and the ischial tuberosity are identified, and an imaginary line is drawn between the two points.

CHAPTER 111  ULTRASOUND-GUIDED INJECTION TECHNIQUE FOR ISCHIAL BURSITIS   793

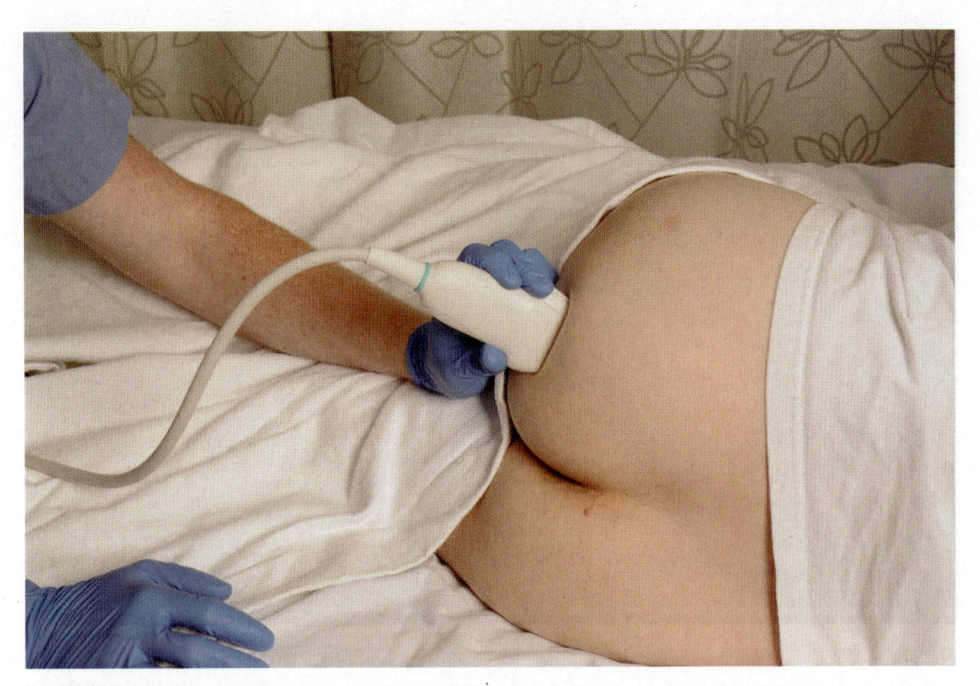

**FIGURE 111.9.** Proper transverse placement of the high-frequency ultrasound transducer for ultrasound-guided injection of ischial bursitis.

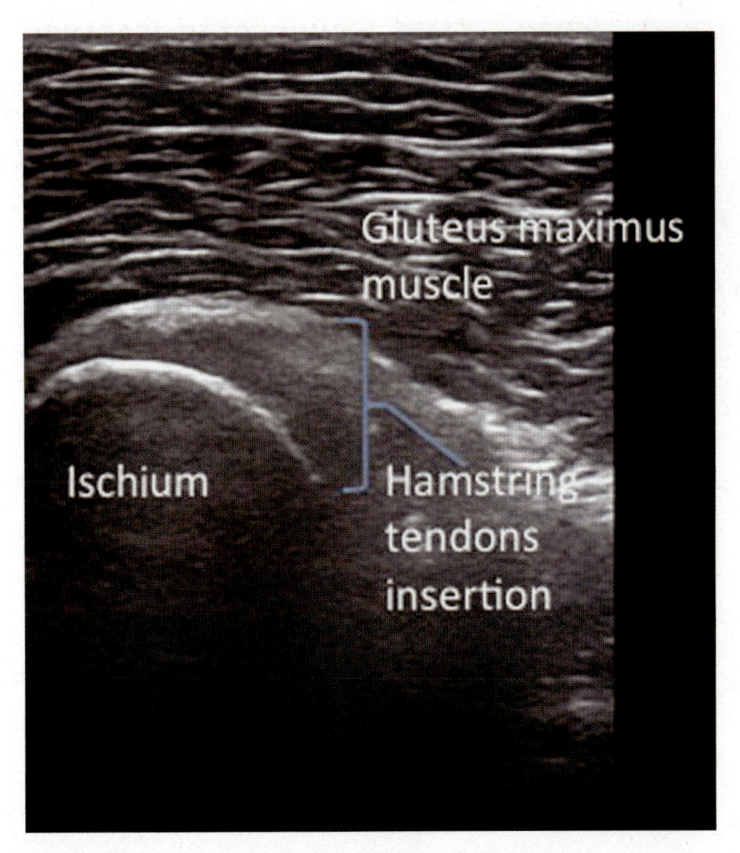

**FIGURE 111.10.** Transverse ultrasound view of the ischium, ischial bursa, gluteus maximus muscle, and insertion of the hamstrings on ischium.

**FIGURE 111.11.** Transverse ultrasound image of ischial bursitis (*asterisk*). (From Kim SM, Shin MJ, Kim KS, et al. Imaging features of ischial bursitis with an emphasis on ultrasound. *Skeletal Radiol* 2002;31(11):631–636, with permission.)

## SUGGESTED READINGS

Hodnett PA, Shelly MJ, MacMahon PJ, et al. MR Imaging of overuse injuries of the hip. *Magn Reson Imaging Clin N Am* 2009;17(4):667–679.

Ramamurthy S, Alanmanou E, Rogers JN. Bursitis: lower extremities. In: *Decision Making in Pain Management*. 2nd ed. Philadelphia, PA: Saunders Elsevier; 2006:210–211.

Waldman SD. The ischial bursa. In: *Pain Review*. Philadelphia, PA: Saunders Elsevier; 2009:138–139.

Waldman SD. Injection technique for ischial bursitis. In: *Pain Review*. Philadelphia, PA: Saunders Elsevier; 2009:547–549.

Waldman SD. Ischial bursitis. In: *Imaging of Pain*. Philadelphia, PA: Saunders Elsevier; 2011:349–350.

Waldman SD. Injection technique for ischial bursitis. In: *Atlas of Pain Management Injection Techniques*. 3rd ed. Philadelphia, PA: Saunders Elsevier; 2013:289–291.

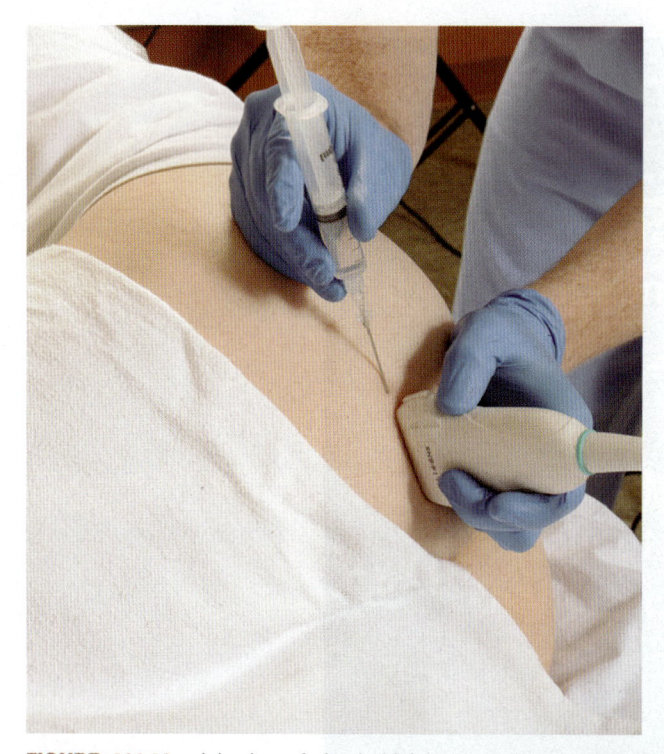

**FIGURE 111.12.** Injection of the ischial bursa under ultrasound guidance.

# CHAPTER 112

# Ultrasound-Guided Injection Technique for Iliopsoas Bursitis Pain

## CLINICAL PERSPECTIVES

Iliopsoas bursitis is a common cause of anterior hip pain. The iliopsoas bursa is one of the largest bursa in the body and lies within the medial femoral triangle between the insertional tendon of the iliopsoas muscle and the hip joint (Fig. 112.1). The bursa serves to cushion and facilitate sliding of the musculotendinous unit of the iliopsoas muscle over the bony hip joint (Fig. 112.2). The bursa is subject to inflammation from a variety of causes with acute trauma to the hip and repetitive microtrauma being the most common. Acute injuries to the bursa can occur from direct trauma from seat belt during motor vehicle accidents as well as from overuse injuries that required repeated hip flexion, such as javelin throwing and ballet. Direct pressure that forces the iliopsoas bursa against the hip joint when sitting while leaning forward for prolonged periods has also been implicated in the development of iliopsoas bursitis. If the inflammation of the bursa is not treated and the condition becomes chronic, calcification of the bursa with further functional disability may occur. Gout and other crystal arthropathies may also precipitate acute iliopsoas bursitis as may bacterial, tubercular, or fungal infections.

The patient suffering from iliopsoas bursitis most frequently presents with the complaint of severe pain with any pressure on the area overlying the anterior hip joint and inflamed iliopsoas bursa. Extension and rotation of the hip will exacerbate the pain, and the patient may alter their gait by taking shorter "baby steps" with the affected extremity to avoid extending the leg. Physical examination of the patient suffering from iliopsoas bursitis will reveal point tenderness over the medial anterior hip. The pain may radiate into the anterior thigh. If there is significant inflammation, rubor and color may be present and the entire area may feel boggy or edematous to palpation. Swelling, which at times can be quite dramatic, is often present and may actually compress adjacent nerves causing numbness, which can confuse the clinical picture (Fig. 112.3). Often, the swelling of iliopsoas bursitis is misdiagnosed as an inguinal hernia. If calcification or gouty tophi of the bursa and surrounding tendons are present, the examiner may appreciate crepitus with active extension and rotation of the hip, especially in the sitting position. Often, the patient will not be able to sleep on the affected side.

Plain radiographs are indicated in all patients who present with hip pain to rule out occult bony pathology. Based on the patient's clinical presentation, additional testing may be indicated, including complete blood cell count, sedimentation rate, and antinuclear antibody testing. Magnetic resonance imaging (MRI) or ultrasound imaging of the affected area may also confirm the diagnosis and help delineate the presence of other hip bursitis, calcific tendonitis, tendinopathy, triceps tendonitis, or other hip pathology (Fig. 112.4). MRI or ultrasound imaging of the affected area may also help delineate the presence of calcific tendonitis or other hip pathology. Rarely, the inflamed bursa may become infected and failure to diagnose and treat the acute infection can lead to dire consequences.

## CLINICALLY RELEVANT ANATOMY

The psoas bursa lies between the psoas tendon and the anterior aspect of the femoral neck (Fig. 112.5). The bursa lies deep to the femoral artery, vein, and nerve. The psoas muscle arises from the transverse processes, vertebral bodies, and intervertebral disks of the T12–L5 vertebrae and inserts into the lesser trochanter of the femur. The psoas muscle flexes the thigh on the trunk or, if the thigh is fixed, flexes the trunk on the thigh, as when moving from a supine to sitting position. This action can irritate the psoas bursa, as can repeated trauma from repetitive activity, including running up stairs or overuse of exercise equipment for lower extremity strengthening. The psoas muscle is innervated by the lumbar plexus.

## ULTRASOUND-GUIDED TECHNIQUE

The benefits, risks, and alternative treatments are explained to the patient and informed consent is obtained. The patient is then placed in the supine position with the lower extremity slightly externally rotated (Fig. 112.6). The skin overlying the hip joint is then prepped with antiseptic solution. A sterile syringe containing 2.0 mL of 0.25% preservative-free bupivacaine and 40 mg of methylprednisolone is attached to a 3½-inch, 22-gauge needle using strict aseptic technique. A

**FIGURE 112.1.** The bursa of the hip region.

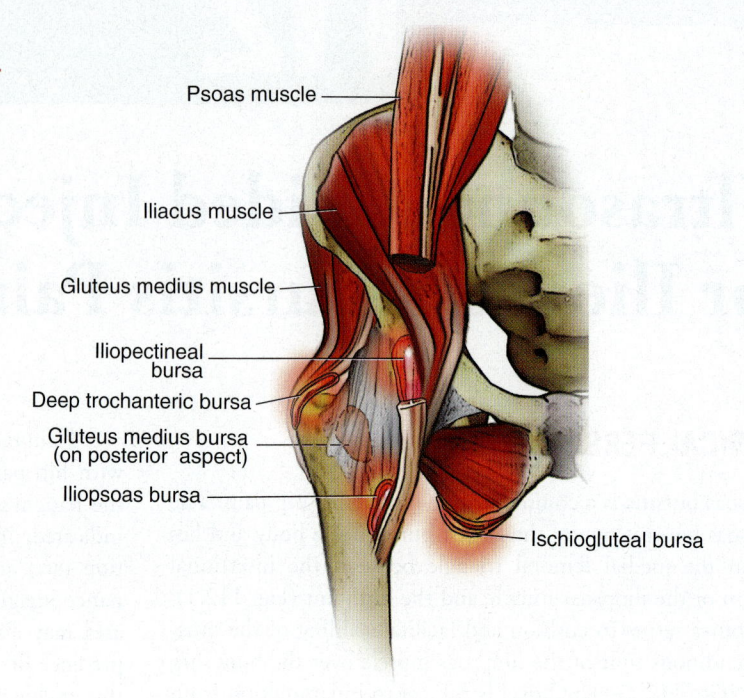

curvilinear low-frequency ultrasound transducer is placed over the proximal femur in the longitudinal plane with the transducer parallel to the femur (Fig. 112.7). A survey scan is taken, which demonstrates the femur as a linear hyperechoic structure (Fig. 112.8). The medial margin of the femur is identified. The ultrasound transducer is then slowly moved toward the head of the femur following the medial border of the femur until hyperechoic border of the femur swings sharply upward at the junction of the femoral neck and the femoral head (Fig. 112.9). Overlying the medial aspect of the femoral head lies the hyperechoic iliopsoas tendon with the iliopsoas bursa beneath it (see Figs. 112.4 and 112.10).

After the iliopsoas tendon and bursa beneath it are identified, the needle is placed through the skin ~1 cm below the inferior end of the transducer and is then advanced using an in-plane approach with the needle trajectory adjusted under

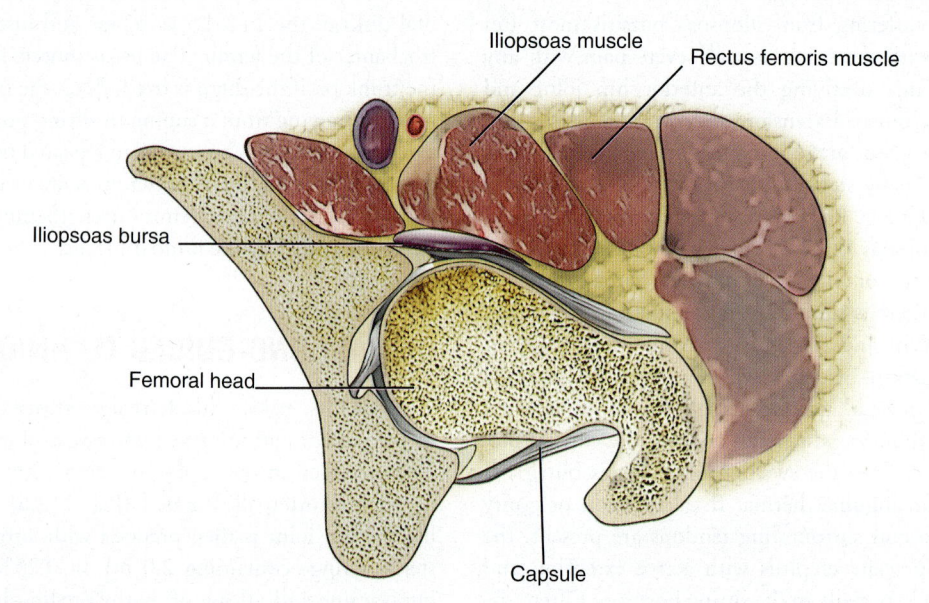

**FIGURE 112.2.** The iliopsoas bursa serves to cushion and facilitate sliding of the musculotendinous unit of the iliopsoas muscle over the bony hip joint.

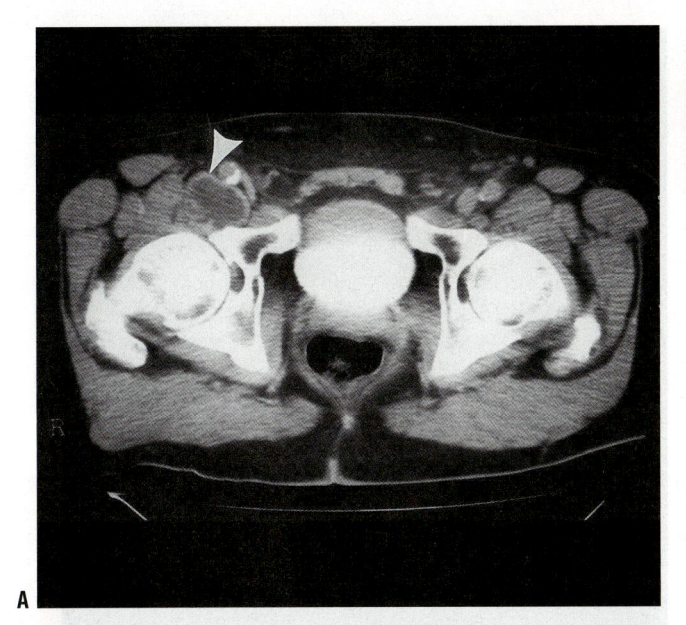

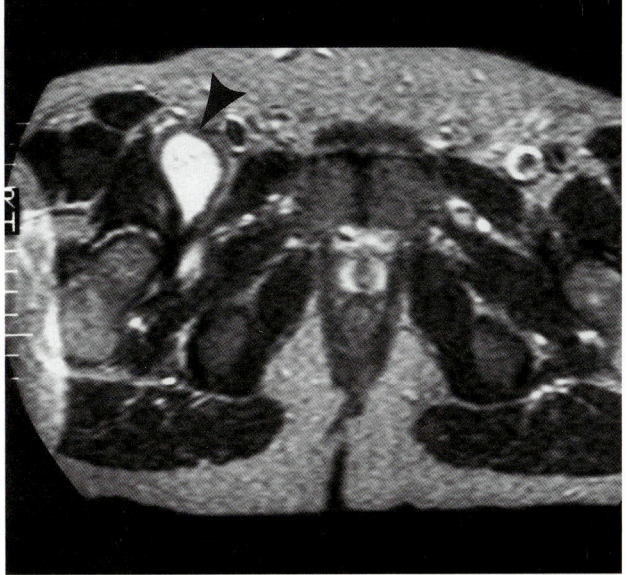

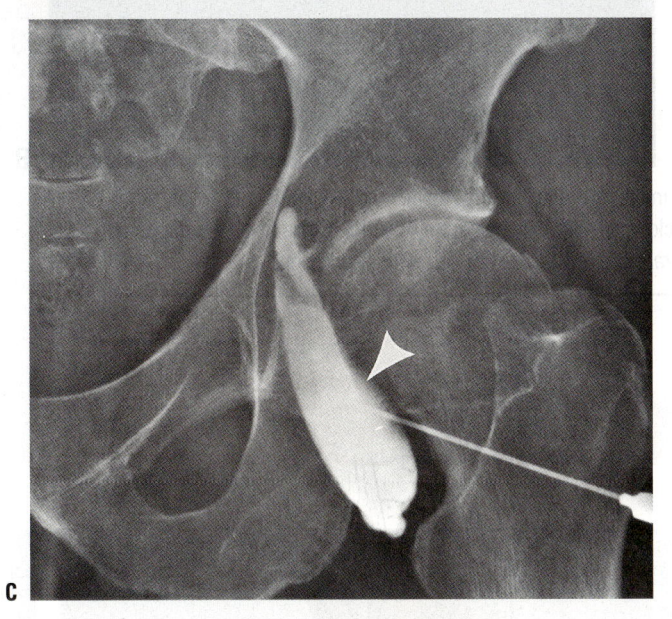

**FIGURE 112.3.** Enlarged iliopsoas bursa. **A:** Computed tomography (CT) demonstrating mass anterior to the hip joint (*white arrow*). **B:** T2-weighted MRI demonstrating characteristic appearance of fluid-filled enlarged iliopsoas bursa. **C:** Contrast injection of enlarged iliopsoas bursa. (Reused from Berquist TH. *MRI of the Musculoskeletal System*. 6th ed. Philadelphia, PA: Lippincott Williams & Wilkins; 2013:235.)

real-time ultrasound guidance to pass through the substance of the iliopsoas tendon to place the needle tip between the tendon and the hip joint (Fig. 112.11). When the tip of needle is thought to be within the space between the iliopsoas tendon and the hip joint, a small amount of local anesthetic and steroid is injected under real-time ultrasound guidance to confirm proper placement of the needle tip by hydrodissection. After proper positioning of the needle tip placement is confirmed, the remainder of the contents of the syringe are slowly injected. There should be minimal resistance to injection. If synechiae, loculations, or calcifications are present, the needle may have to be repositioned to ensure that the entire bursa is treated. The needle is then removed, and a sterile pressure dressing and ice pack are placed at the injection site.

## COMPLICATIONS

The major complication of ultrasound-guided injection of the iliopsoas bursa is infection. Ecchymosis and hematoma formation may also occur. A transient exacerbation of the patient's pain occurs ~25% of the time following this injection technique, and the patient should be warned of this possibility prior to the procedure.

**FIGURE 112.9.** Longitudinal ultrasound image of the junction between the femoral neck and femoral head.

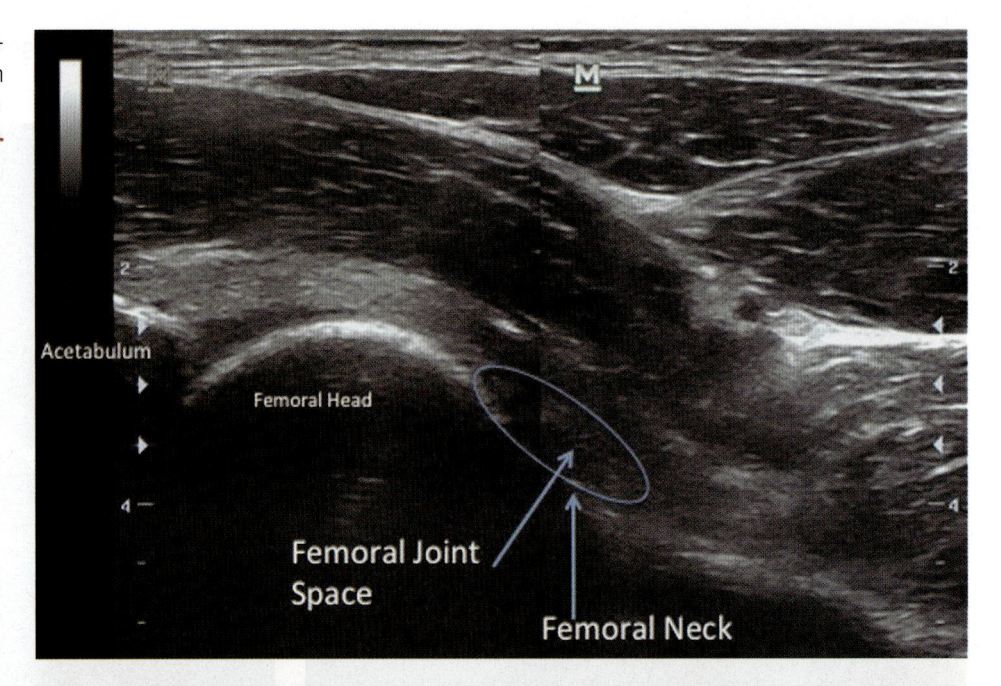

**FIGURE 112.10.** Longitudinal ultrasound image demonstrating the relationship of the iliopsoas tendon, bursa, and the femoral head and acetabulum.

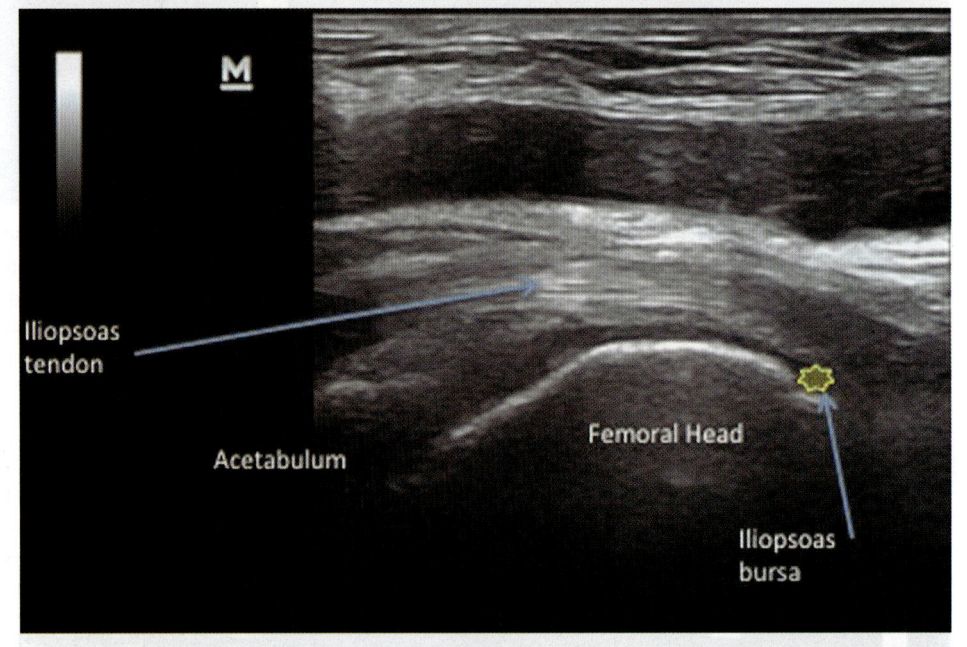

**FIGURE 112.11.** Correct in-plane needle placement for ultrasound-guided hip joint injection.

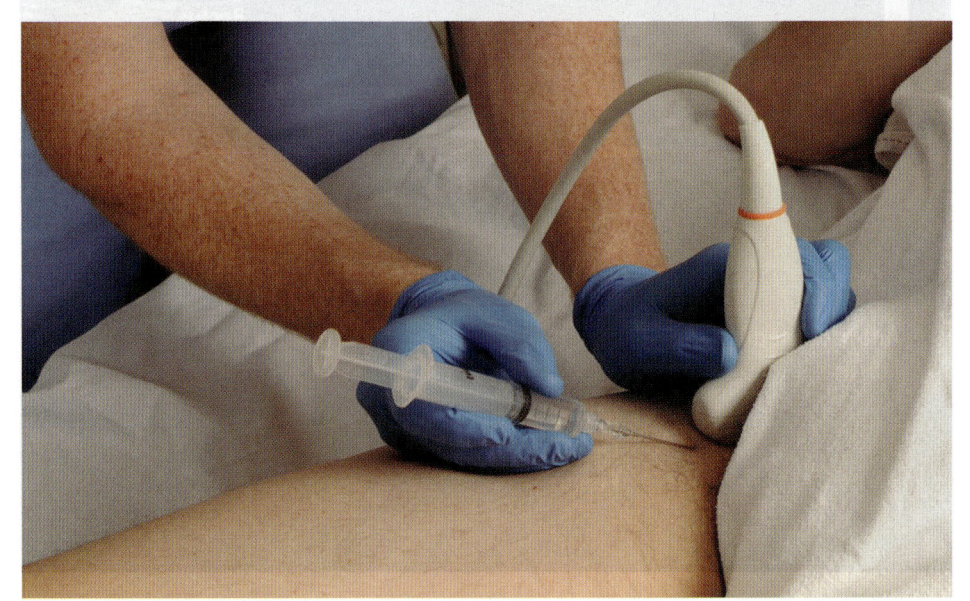

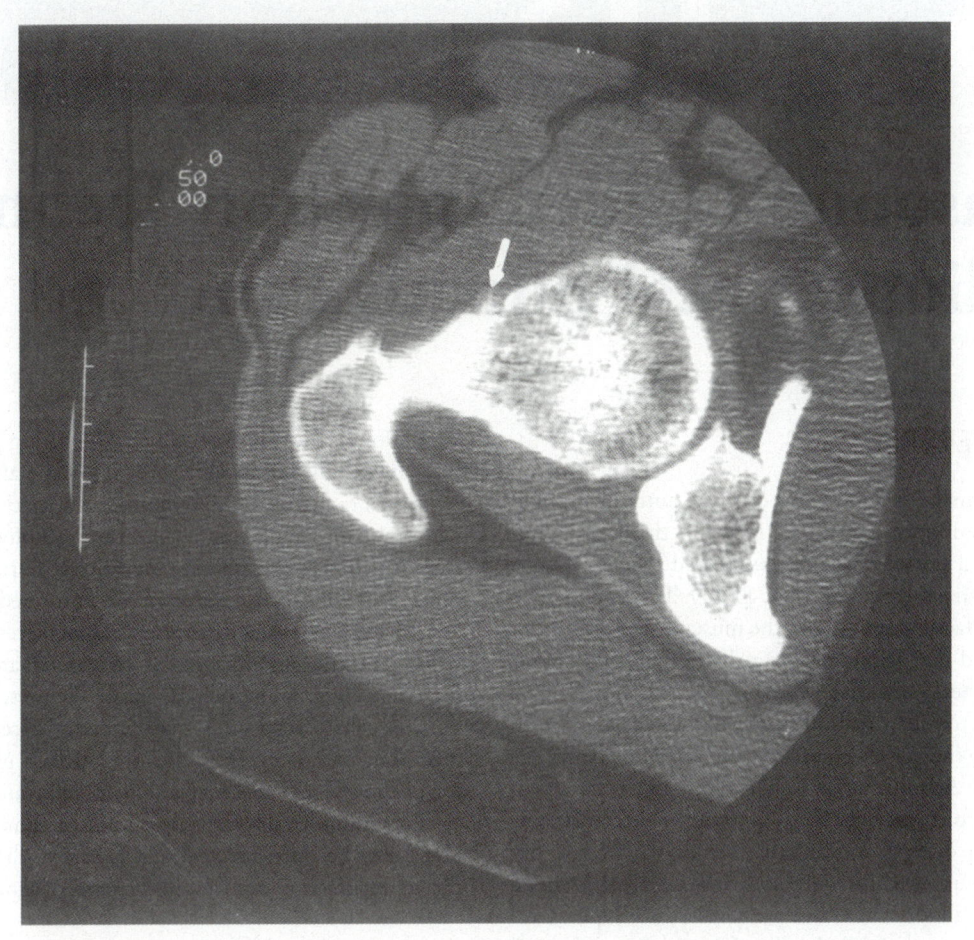

**FIGURE 112.12.** CT of the hip demonstrating an intracapsular osteoid osteoma. (Reused from Berquist TH. *MRI of the Musculoskeletal System.* 6th ed. Philadelphia, PA: Lippincott Williams & Wilkins; 2013:303.)

## CLINICAL PEARLS

Care must be taken not to place the needle too medially, or trauma to the femoral artery, vein, and/or nerve may result. Bursitis, labral tears, tendinopathy, osteoarthritis, synovitis, nerve compression, avascular necrosis of the femoral head, and impingement syndromes may coexist with other hip joint disease and may contribute to the patient's pain symptomatology (Fig. 112.12). Universal precautions should always be observed to protect the operator, and strict adherence to sterile technique must be used to avoid infection. Gentle physical therapy and local heat should be introduced following ultrasound-guided injection of the elbow joint to reduce pain and improve function. Simple analgesics and nonsteroidal anti-inflammatory agents or COX-2 inhibitors may be used concurrently with this injection technique.

## SUGGESTED READINGS

Hochman MG, Ramappa AJ, Newman JS, et al. Imaging of tendons and bursae. In: Weissman BNW, ed. *Imaging of Arthritis and Metabolic Bone Disease.* Philadelphia, PA: Saunders Elsevier; 2009:196–238.

MacMahon PJ, Hogan BA, Shelly MJ, et al. Imaging of groin pain. *Magn Reson Imaging Clin N Am* 2009;17(4):655–666.

Shabshin N, Rosenberg ZS, Calvalcanti CFA. MR imaging of iliopsoas musculotendinous injuries. *Magn Reson Imaging Clin N Am* 2005;13(4):705–716.

Waldman SD. Injection technique for psoas bursitis. In: *Pain Review.* Philadelphia, PA: Saunders; 2009:551–552.

Waldman SD. Psoas bursa injection. In: *Atlas of Pain Management Injection Techniques.* 3rd ed. Philadelphia, PA: Saunders Elsevier; 2012:294–296.

Waldman SD, Campbell RSD. Anatomy, special imaging considerations of pelvis, hip, and lower extremity pain syndromes. In: *Imaging of Pain.* Philadelphia, PA: Saunders Elsevier; 2011:335–336.

# CHAPTER 113

# Ultrasound-Guided Injection Technique for Iliopectineal Bursitis Pain

## CLINICAL PERSPECTIVES

Iliopectineal bursitis is a common cause of anterior hip and groin pain. The iliopectineal bursa is one of the larger bursa in the body and lies between the psoas and iliacus muscles and the iliopectineal eminence (Fig. 113.1). The bursa serves to cushion and facilitate sliding of the musculotendinous unit of the psoas and iliacus muscles over the bony protuberance of the iliopectineal eminence (Fig. 113.2). The iliopectineal bursa is subject to inflammation from a variety of causes with acute trauma to the hip and repetitive microtrauma being the most common. Acute injuries to the bursa can occur from direct trauma from seat belts during motor vehicle accidents as well as from overuse injuries that required repeated hip flexion, such as javelin throwing and ballet. Direct pressure that forces the iliopectineal bursa against the iliopectineal eminence when sitting while leaning forward for prolonged periods has also been implicated in the development of iliopectineal bursitis. If the inflammation of the bursa is not treated and the condition becomes chronic, calcification of the bursa with further functional disability may occur. Gout and other crystal arthropathies may also precipitate acute iliopectineal bursitis as may bacterial, tubercular, or fungal infections.

The patient suffering from iliopectineal bursitis most frequently presents with the complaint of severe anterior hip and groin pain with any pressure on the area overlying the anterior hip joint and inflamed iliopectineal bursa. Flexion and rotation of the hip will exacerbate the pain. Physical examination of the patient suffering from iliopectineal bursitis will reveal point tenderness over the medial anterior hip. The pain may radiate into the anterior thigh and pelvis. If there is significant inflammation, rubor and color may be present and the entire area may feel boggy or edematous to palpation. Swelling, which at times can be quite dramatic, is often present and may actually compress adjacent nerves causing numbness, which can confuse the clinical picture (Fig. 113.3). Often, the swelling of iliopectineal bursitis is misdiagnosed as an inguinal hernia. If calcification or gouty tophi of the bursa and surrounding tendons are present, the examiner may appreciate crepitus with active flexion and adduction of the hip, especially in the sitting position. Often, the patient will not be able to sleep on the affected side.

Plain radiographs are indicated in all patients who present with hip pain to rule out occult bony pathology. Based on the patient's clinical presentation, additional testing may be indicated, including complete blood cell count, sedimentation rate, and antinuclear antibody testing. Magnetic resonance imaging (MRI) or ultrasound imaging of the affected area may also confirm the diagnosis and help delineate the presence of other hip bursitis, calcific tendonitis, tendinopathy, triceps tendonitis, or other hip pathology (Fig. 113.4). MRI or ultrasound imaging of the affected area may also help delineate the presence of calcific tendonitis or other hip pathology. Rarely, the inflamed bursa may become infected, and failure to diagnose and treat the acute infection can lead to dire consequences.

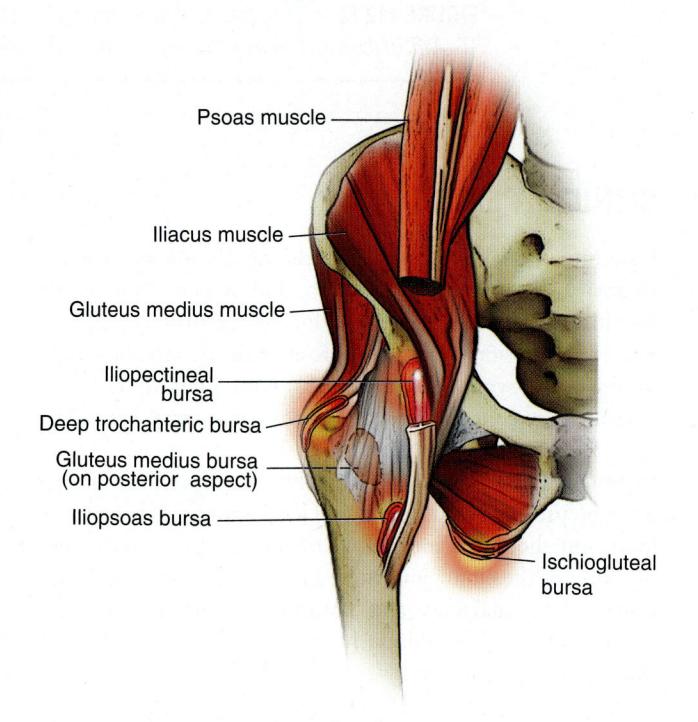

**FIGURE 113.1.** The bursa of the hip region.

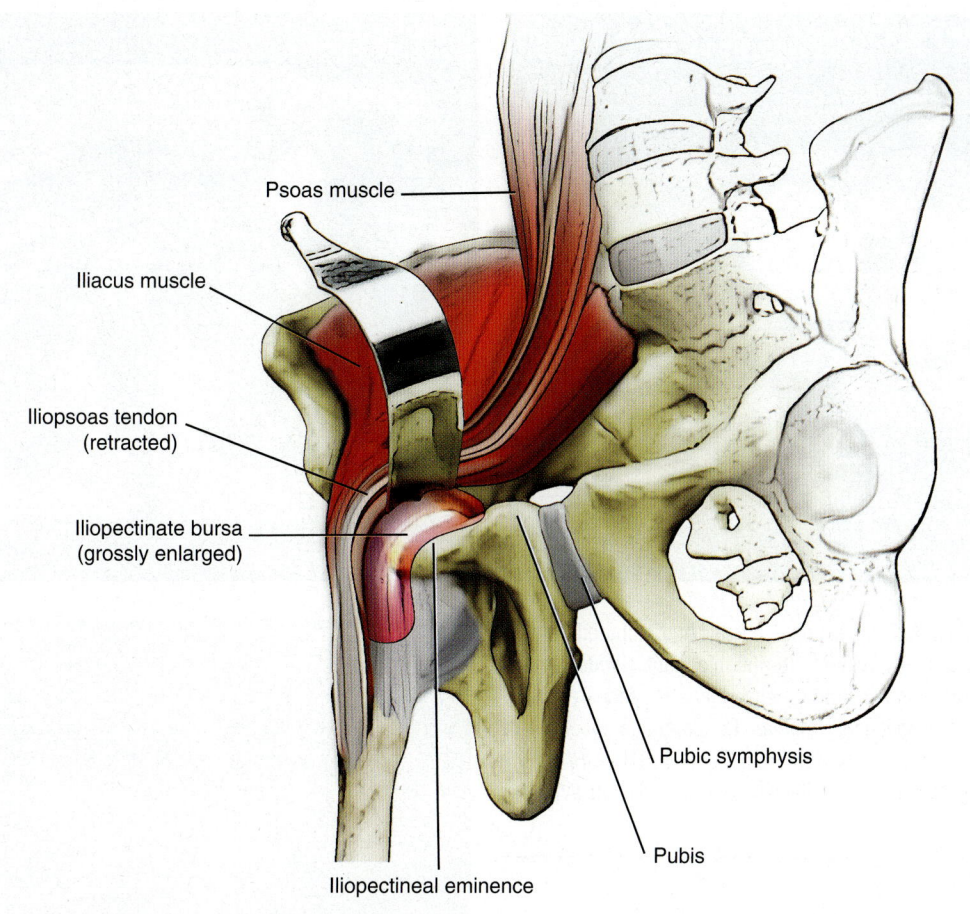

CHAPTER 113 ULTRASOUND-GUIDED INJECTION TECHNIQUE FOR ILIOPECTINEAL BURSITIS PAIN

**FIGURE 113.2.** The iliopectineal bursa serves to cushion and facilitate sliding of the musculotendinous unit of the iliacus and psoas over the iliopectineal eminence.

## CLINICALLY RELEVANT ANATOMY

The iliopectineal bursa lies between the psoas and iliacus muscles and the iliopectineal eminence, the bony prominence at the point at which the ilium and the pubis bones fuse (see Figs. 113.2 and 113.5). The psoas and iliacus muscles join at the lateral side of the psoas, and the combined fibers are referred to as the iliopsoas muscle. Like the psoas, the iliacus flexes the thigh on the trunk or, if the thigh is fixed, flexes the trunk on the thigh, as when moving from a supine to sitting position. This action can cause inflammation of the iliopectineal bursa, as can repeated trauma from repetitive activity including sit-ups or overuse of exercise equipment for lower extremity strengthening. The iliacus muscle is innervated by the femoral nerve.

## ULTRASOUND-GUIDED TECHNIQUE

The benefits, risks, and alternative treatments are explained to the patient and informed consent is obtained. The patient is then placed in the supine position with the patient's arms crossed over the chest (Fig. 113.6). With the patient in the above position, a high-frequency linear ultrasound transducer is placed in a transverse plane over the pubic prominence, which lies just above the penis in males and the clitoris in females, and an ultrasound survey scan is taken (Figs. 113.7 and 113.8). The bright hyperechoic pubic bodies are identified with the hypoechoic interpubic fibroelastic cartilage in between (Fig. 113.9). After the interpubic fibroelastic cartilage is identified, the ultrasound transducer is slowly moved laterally toward the affected side while following the superior margin of the pubic bone as it curves upward to meet the ilium (Fig. 113.10). A iliopectineal eminence will appear as a protuberance on the otherwise smooth superior margin of the pubic bone (Fig. 113.11). When the iliopectineal eminence is identified, the skin overlying the area above the ultrasound transducer is prepped with antiseptic solution. A sterile syringe containing 7.0 mL of 0.25% preservative-free bupivacaine and 40 mg of methylprednisolone is attached to a 3½-inch, 22-gauge needle using strict aseptic technique. The needle is placed through the skin ~1 cm above the superior border of the ultrasound transducer and is then advanced using an out-of-plane approach with the needle trajectory adjusted

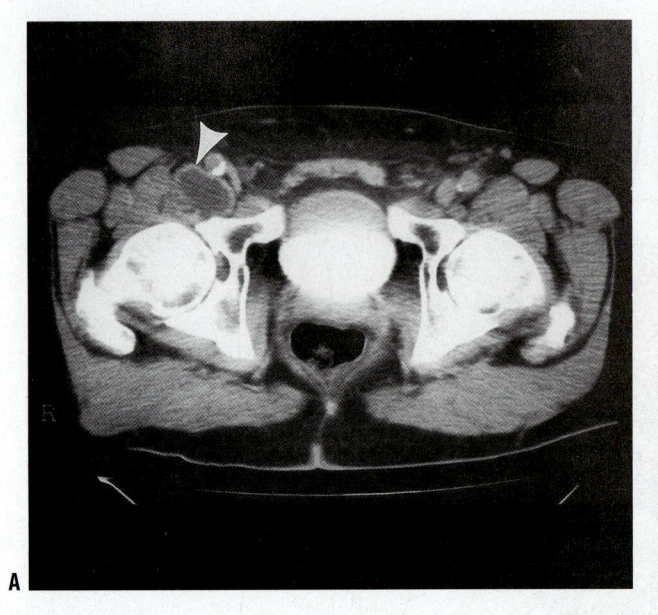

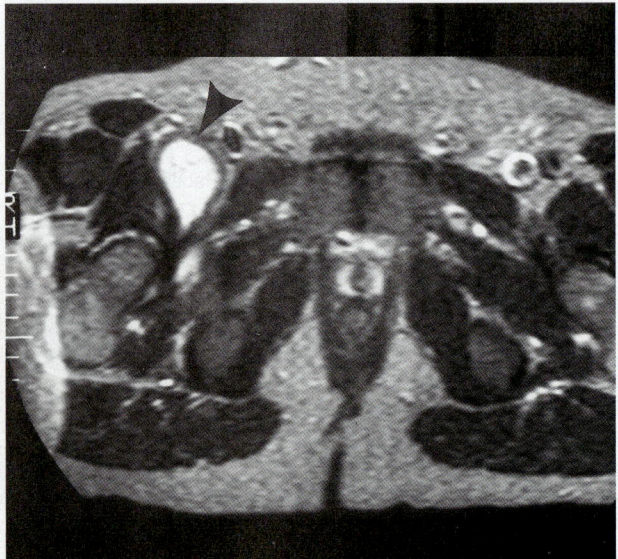

**FIGURE 113.3.** Enlarged iliopectineal bursa. **A:** Computed tomography demonstrating mass anterior to the hip joint (*white arrow*). **B:** T2-weighted MRI demonstrating characteristic appearance of fluid-filled enlarged iliopectineal bursa. **C:** Contrast injection of enlarged iliopectineal bursa. (Reused from Berquist TH. *MRI of the Musculoskeletal System*. 6th ed. Philadelphia, PA: Lippincott Williams & Wilkins; 2013:235.)

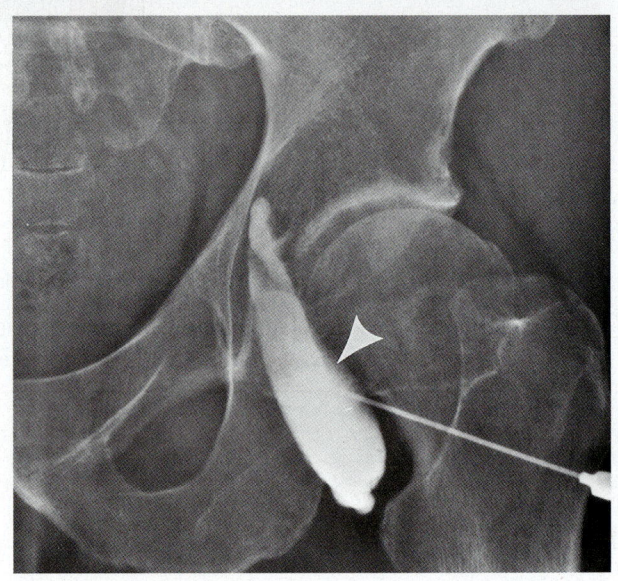

under real-time ultrasound guidance so that the needle tip rests against the iliopectineal prominence, which puts the needle tip in proximity to the iliopectineal bursa (Fig. 113.12). When the tip of needle is thought to be in satisfactory position, after careful aspiration, the contents of the syringe are slowly injected. There should be minimal resistance to injection.

## COMPLICATIONS

The major complication of ultrasound-guided injection of the iliopectineal bursa is infection. Ecchymosis and hematoma formation may also occur. A transient exacerbation of the patient's pain occurs ~25% of the time following this injection technique, and the patient should be warned of this possibility prior to the procedure.

## CLINICAL PEARLS

Care must be taken not to place the needle too medially, or trauma to the femoral artery, vein, and/or nerve may result. Bursitis, labral tears, tendinopathy, osteoarthritis, synovitis, nerve compression, avascular necrosis of the femoral head, and impingement syndromes may coexist with other hip joint disease and may contribute to the patient's pain symptomatology (Fig. 113.12). Universal precautions should always be observed to protect the operator, and strict adherence to sterile technique must be used to avoid infection. Gentle physical therapy and local heat should be introduced following ultrasound-guided injection of the iliopectineal bursa to reduce pain and improve function. Simple analgesics and nonsteroidal anti-inflammatory agents or COX-2 inhibitors may be used concurrently with this injection technique.

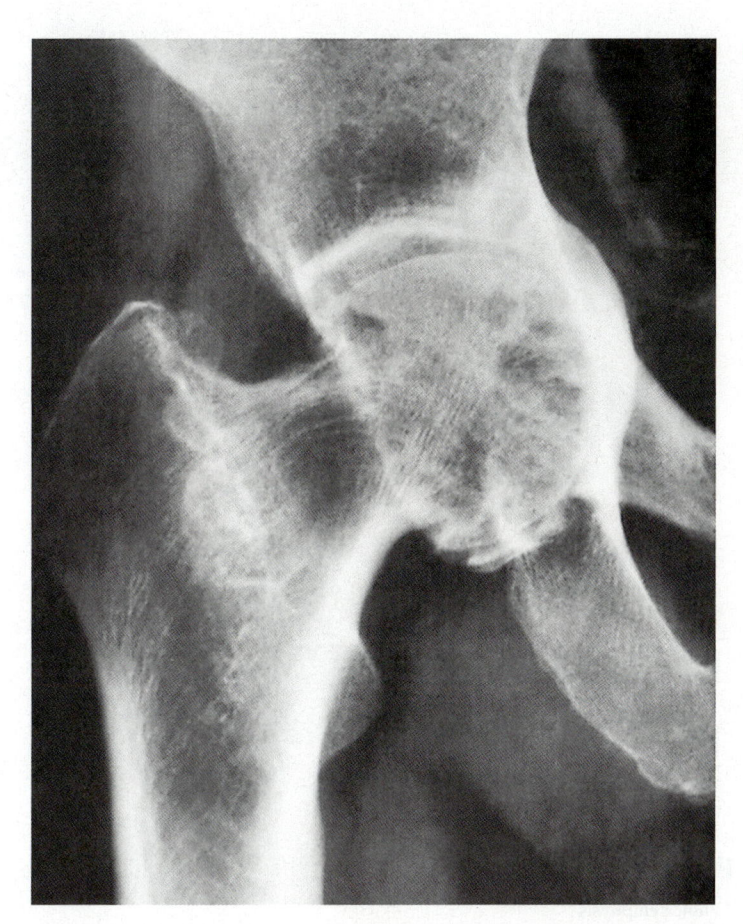

**FIGURE 113.4.** Plain radiograph of 42-year-old women demonstrating rheumatoid arthritis with superimposed osteoarthritis of the hip. (Greenspan A. *Orthopedic Imaging: A Practical Approach.* 5th ed. Philadelphia, PA: Lippincott Williams & Wilkins; 2011:465.)

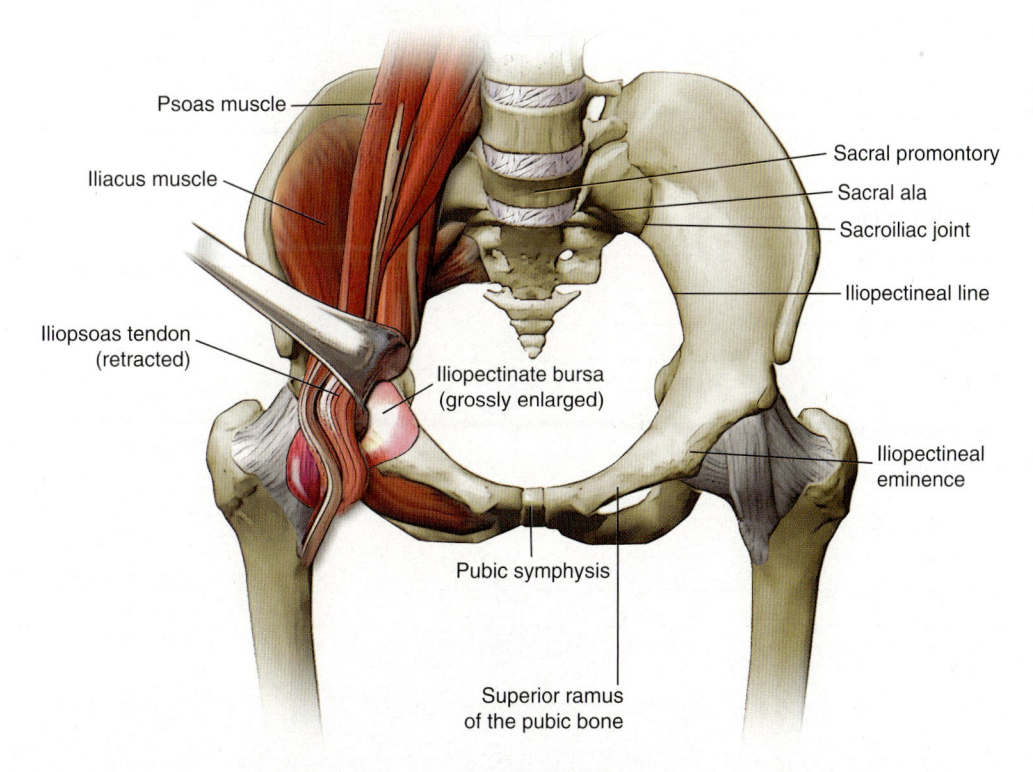

**FIGURE 113.5.** The iliopectineal eminence is the point of fusion between the pubic bone and ilium.

**FIGURE 113.6.** Proper patient positioning for ultrasound-guided injection of the iliopectineal bursa.

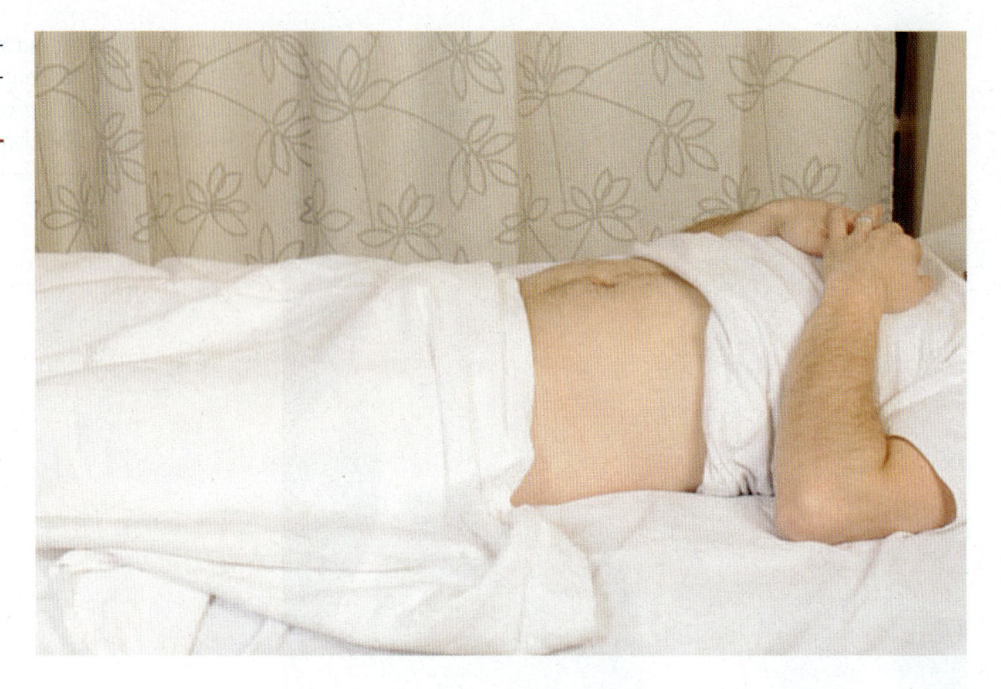

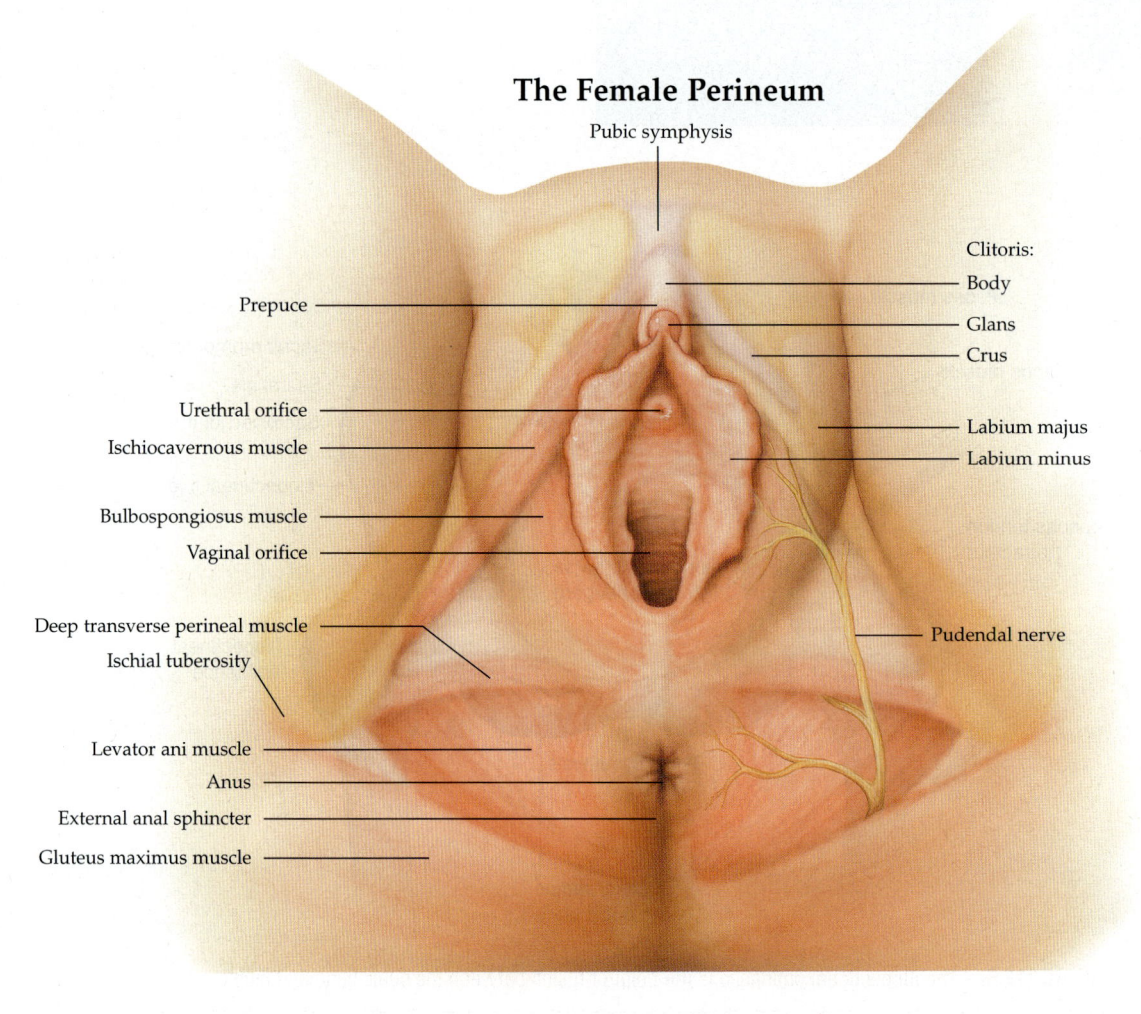

## The Female Perineum

Labels: Pubic symphysis; Clitoris: Body, Glans, Crus; Prepuce; Urethral orifice; Ischiocavernous muscle; Labium majus; Labium minus; Bulbospongiosus muscle; Vaginal orifice; Deep transverse perineal muscle; Ischial tuberosity; Pudendal nerve; Levator ani muscle; Anus; External anal sphincter; Gluteus maximus muscle

**FIGURE 113.7.** The pubic symphysis is located just above the clitoris in females. (Anatomical Chart Company, 2013.)

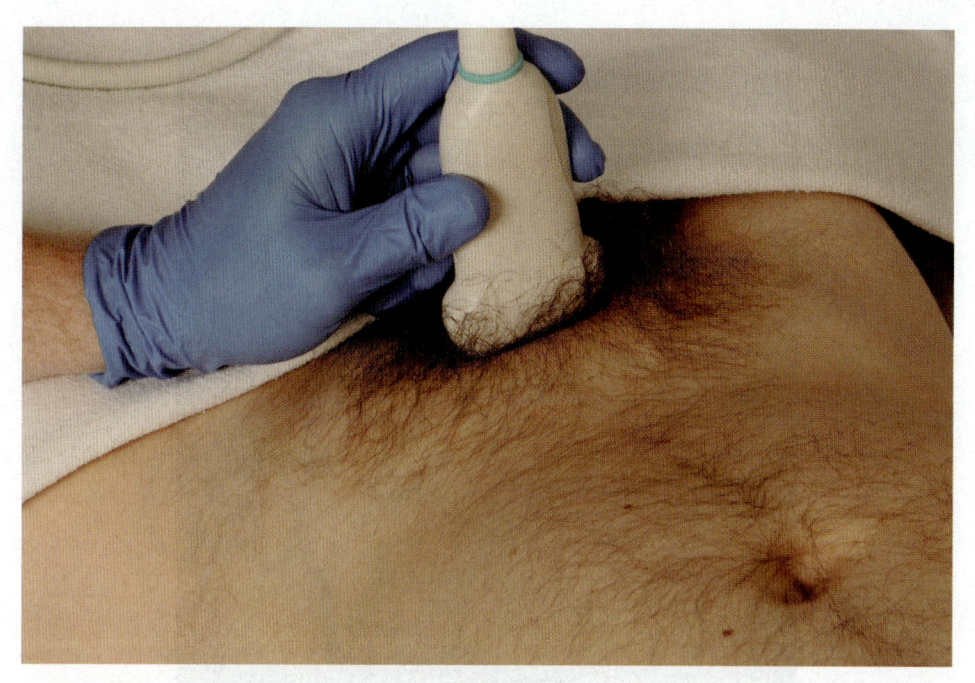

**FIGURE 113.8.** Proper transverse ultrasound transducer placement for ultrasound-guided injection for osteitis pubis.

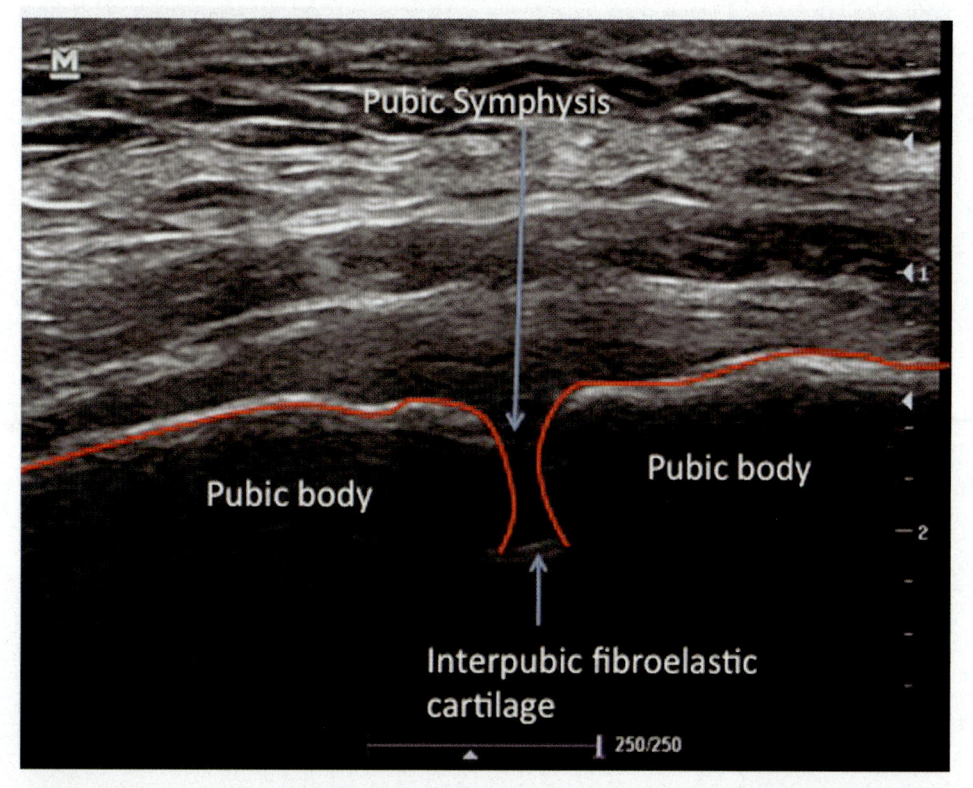

**FIGURE 113.9.** Transverse ultrasound view of the pubic symphysis and pubic bodies.

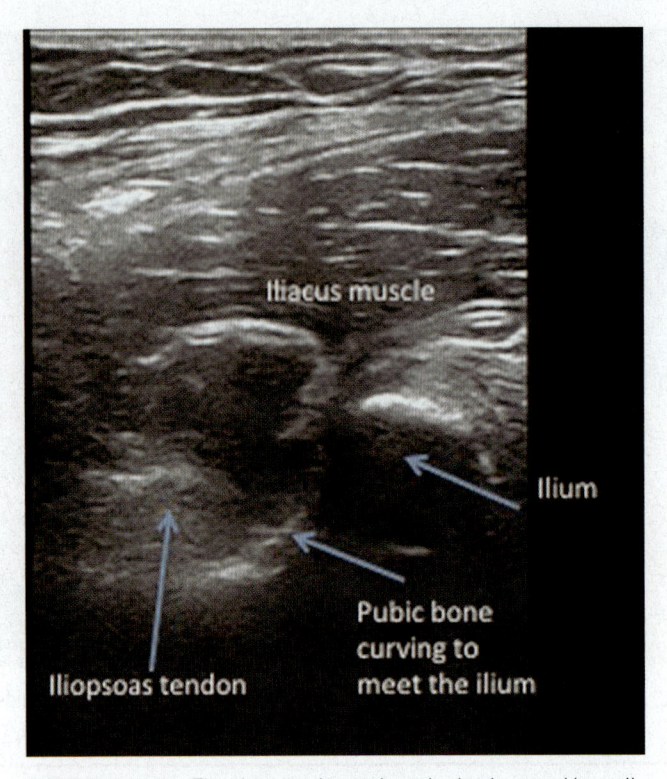

**FIGURE 113.10.** The ultrasound transducer is slowly moved laterally toward the affected side while following the superior margin of the pubic bone as it curves upward to meet the ilium.

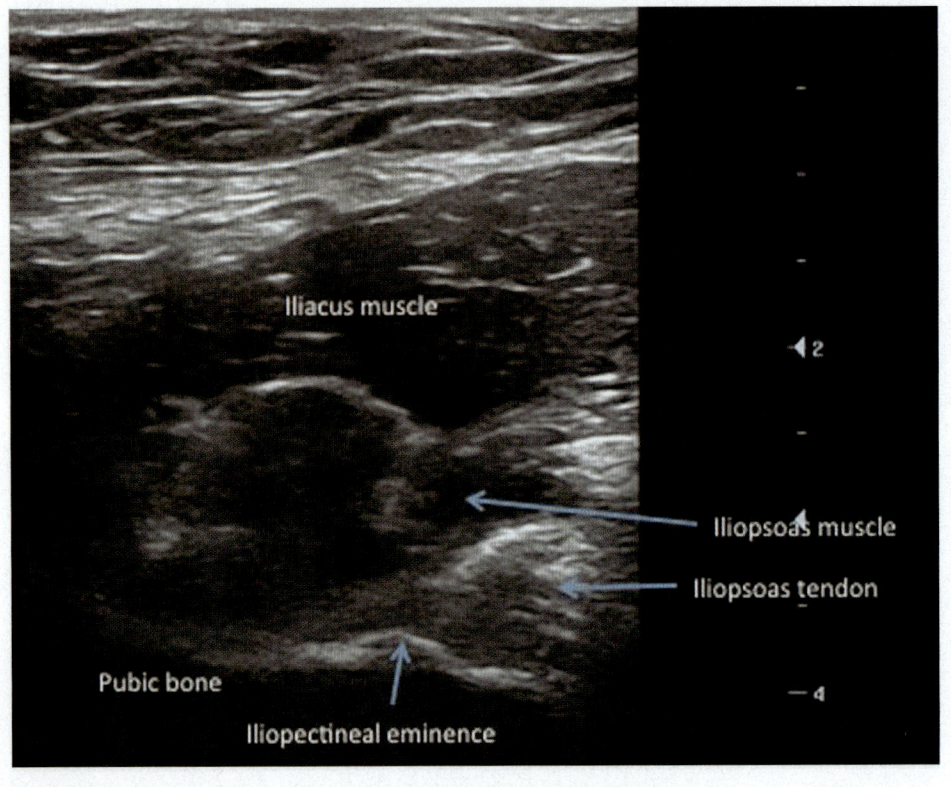

**FIGURE 113.11.** Transverse ultrasound view of iliopectineal eminence.

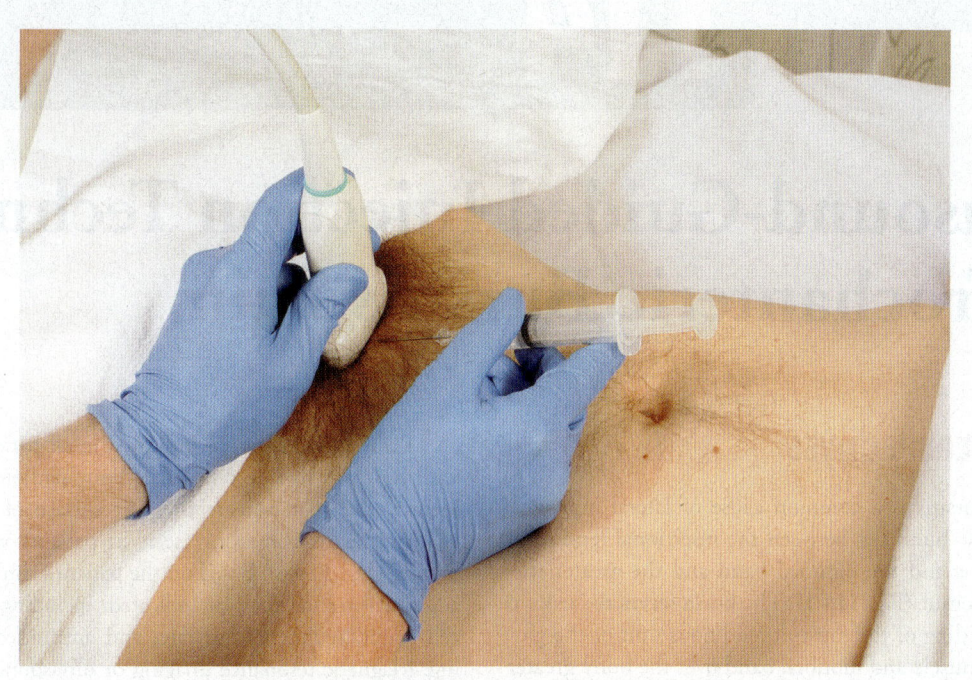

**FIGURE 113.12.** Proper needle placement for an ultrasound-guided out-of-plane injection for iliopectineal bursitis.

## SUGGESTED READINGS

MacMahon PJ, Hogan BA, Shelly MJ, et al. Imaging of groin pain. *Magn Reson Imaging Clin N Am* 2009;17(4):655–666.

Waldman SD. Injection technique for iliopectineal bursitis. In: *Pain Review*. Philadelphia, PA: Saunders Elsevier; 2009:354.

Waldman SD. Injection technique for iliopectineal bursitis. In: *Atlas of Pain Management Injection Techniques*. 3rd ed. Philadelphia, PA: Saunders Elsevier; 2013:287–298.

Waldman SD, Campbell RSD. Osteitis pubis. In: *Atlas of Uncommon Pain Syndromes*. 2nd ed. Philadelphia, PA: Saunders Elsevier; 2009:255–257.

Waldman SD, Campbell RSD. Osteitis pubis. In: *Imaging of Pain*. Philadelphia, PA: Saunders Elsevier; 2011:207–208.

# Ultrasound-Guided Injection Technique for Trochanteric Bursitis Pain

## CLINICAL PERSPECTIVES

Trochanteric bursitis is a common cause of lateral hip pain. The trochanteric bursa lies between the insertional tendon of gluteus maximus and the iliotibial band and the greater trochanter of the femur (Fig. 114.1). The bursa serves to cushion and facilitate sliding of the musculotendinous unit of the gluteus maximus muscle and iliotibial band over the bony greater trochanter (Fig. 114.2). The bursa is subject to inflammation from a variety of causes with acute trauma to the hip and repetitive microtrauma being the most common. Acute injuries to the bursa can occur from direct blunt trauma to the lateral hip as well as from overuse injuries including running on uneven or soft surfaces. If the inflammation of the bursa is not treated and the condition becomes chronic, calcification of the bursa with further functional disability may occur. Gout and other crystal arthropathies may also precipitate acute trochanteric bursitis as may bacterial, tubercular, or fungal infections.

The patient suffering from trochanteric bursitis most frequently presents with the complaint of lateral hip pain that can radiate down the leg with a significant increase in pain on any pressure on the area overlying the greater trochanter of the femur and the inflamed trochanteric bursa. The patient may find walking up stairs increasingly difficult. Physical examination of the patient suffering from trochanteric bursitis will reveal point tenderness over the greater trochanter. The pain may radiate into the lateral lower extremity. If there is significant inflammation, rubor and color may be present and the entire area may feel boggy or edematous to palpation. Swelling, which at times can be quite dramatic, is often present. Passive adduction and abduction, as well as active resisted abduction of the affected lower extremity, will reproduce the pain. Sudden release of resistance to abduction during the resisted abduction release test for trochanteric bursitis markedly increases the pain (Fig. 114.3). There should be no sensory deficit in the distribution of the lateral femoral cutaneous nerve, as is seen with meralgia paresthetica, which often is confused with trochanteric bursitis. If calcification or gouty tophi of the bursa and surrounding tendons are present, the examiner may appreciate crepitus with active abduction of the hip. Often, the patient will not be able to sleep on the affected side.

Plain radiographs are indicated in all patients who present with hip pain to rule out occult bony pathology as well as to identify the characteristic irregular surface of the greater trochanter that is commonly seen in patients with trochanteric bursitis (Fig. 114.4). Based on the patient's clinical presentation, additional testing may be indicated, including complete blood cell count, sedimentation rate, and antinuclear antibody testing. Magnetic resonance imaging or ultrasound imaging of the affected area may also confirm the diagnosis and help delineate the presence of other hip bursitis, calcific tendonitis, tendinopathy, triceps tendonitis, or other hip pathology (Fig. 114.5). Magnetic resonance imaging or ultrasound imaging of the affected area may also help delineate the presence of calcific tendonitis or other hip pathology. Rarely, the inflamed bursa may become infected, and failure to diagnose and treat the acute infection can lead to dire consequences. Electromyography helps distinguish trochanteric bursitis from meralgia paresthetica and sciatica.

## CLINICALLY RELEVANT ANATOMY

The trochanteric bursa is one of several bursae including the subgluteus medius and subgluteal minimus bursa that are situated around the hip joint to aid in hip movement (Fig. 114.6). The trochanteric bursa lies between the greater trochanter and the tendon of the gluteus medius and the iliotibial tract (see Fig. 114.2). The gluteus medius muscle has its origin from the outer surface of the ilium, and its fibers pass downward and laterally to attach on the lateral surface of the greater trochanter. The gluteus medius locks the pelvis in place when walking and running. This action can irritate the trochanteric bursa as can repeated trauma from repetitive activity, including jogging on soft or uneven surfaces or overuse of exercise equipment for lower extremity strengthening. The gluteus medius muscle is innervated by the superior gluteal nerve.

## ULTRASOUND-GUIDED TECHNIQUE

The benefits, risks, and alternative treatments are explained to the patient and informed consent is obtained. The patient is then placed in the modified Sims position (Fig. 114.7). The

# CHAPTER 114  ULTRASOUND-GUIDED INJECTION TECHNIQUE FOR TROCHANTERIC BURSITIS PAIN

**FIGURE 114.1.** The bursa of the hip region.

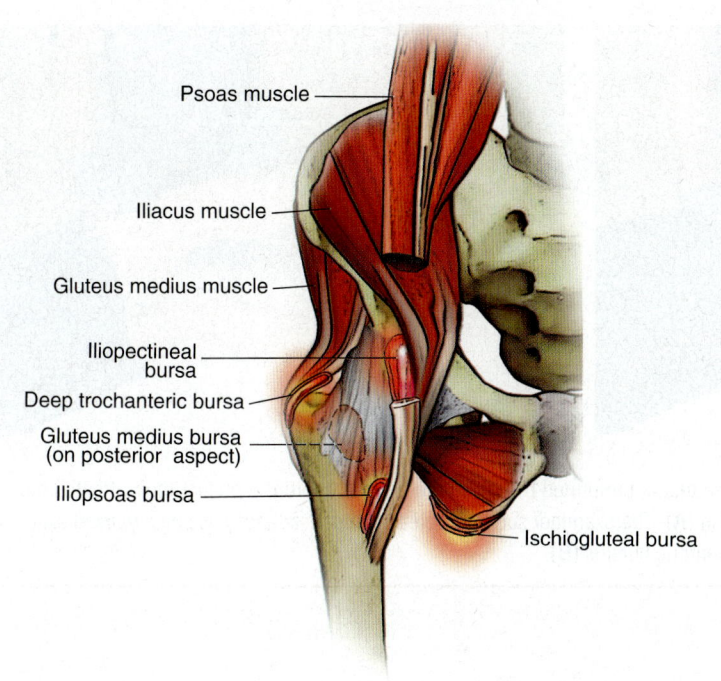

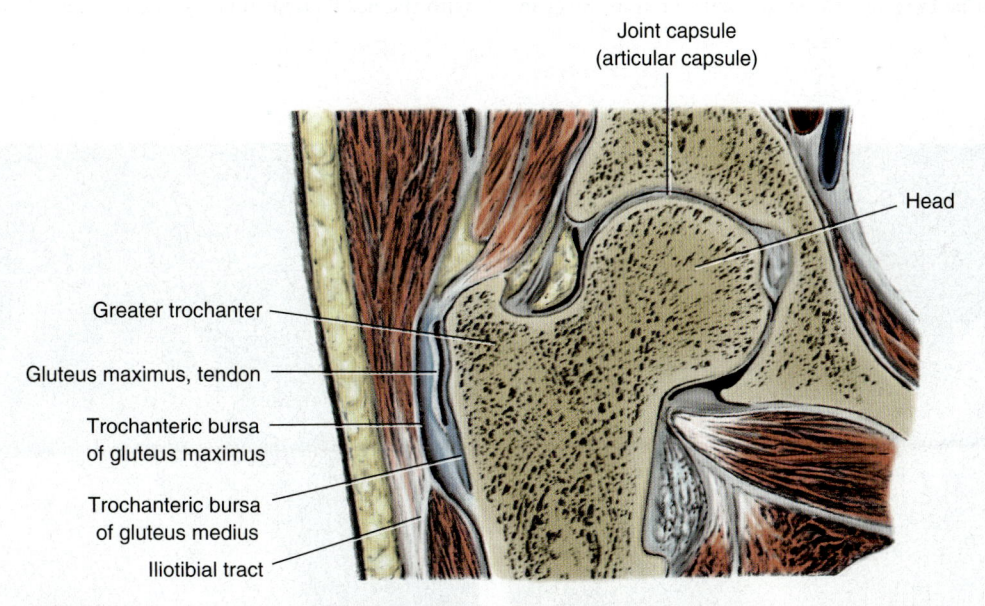

**FIGURE 114.2.** The trochanteric bursa serves to cushion and facilitate sliding of the musculotendinous unit of the gluteus maximus muscle over the greater trochanter of the femur. (Reused from McNabb JW. Trochanteric bursitis. In: *A Practical Guide to Joint and Soft Tissue Injection and Aspiration.* 1st ed. Philadelphia, PA: Lippincott Williams & Wilkins; 2005.)

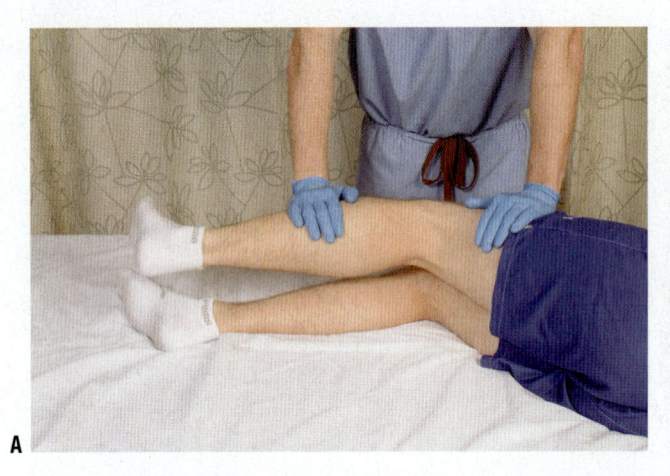

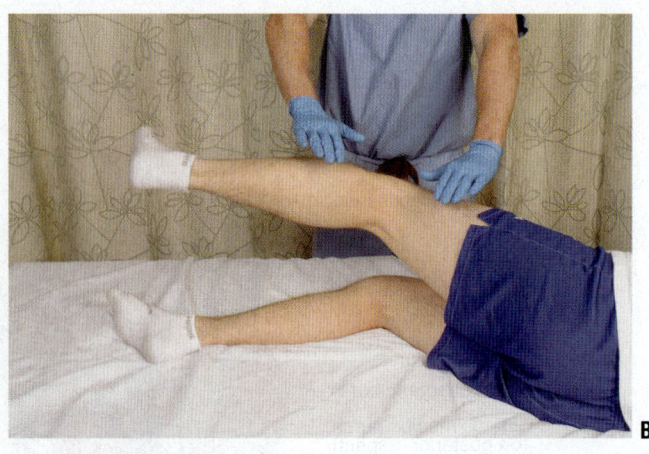

**FIGURE 114.3.** The resisted abduction release test is performed by having the patient vigorously abduct their affected hip against resistance, which will produce some pain **(A)**. The examiner suddenly releases the resistance causing a marked exacerbation of pain in patients suffering from trochanteric bursitis **(B)**.

skin overlying the greater trochanter of the femur is then prepped with antiseptic solution. The greater trochanter is then identified by using a grasping maneuver (Fig. 114.8). A sterile syringe containing 4.0 mL of 0.25% preservative-free bupivacaine and 40 mg of methylprednisolone is attached to a 1½-inch, 22-gauge needle using strict aseptic technique. A linear high-frequency ultrasound transducer is placed over the previously identified greater trochanter with the transducer in a transverse orientation (Fig. 114.9). A survey scan is taken, which demonstrates the irregular hyperechoic margin of the greater trochanter and the trochanteric bursa and tendon of the gluteus maximus muscle above it (Fig. 114.10). After the greater trochanter and bursa above it are identified, the needle is placed through the skin ~1 cm from the anterior end of the transducer and is then advanced using an in-plane approach with the needle trajectory adjusted under real-time ultrasound

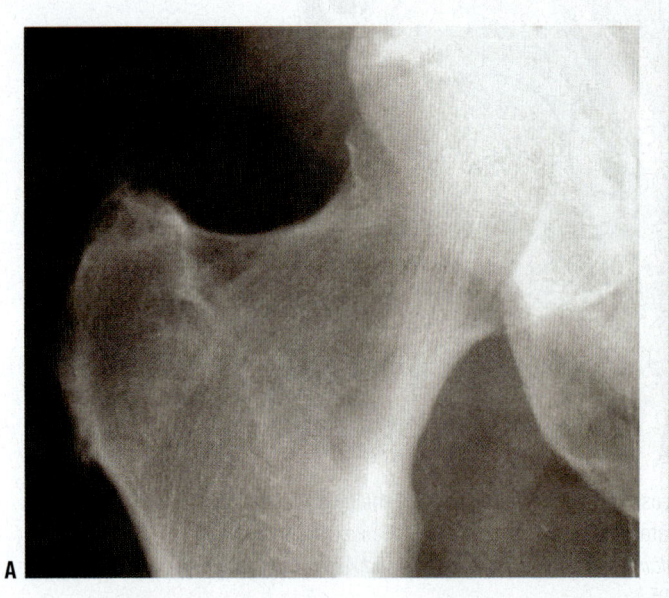

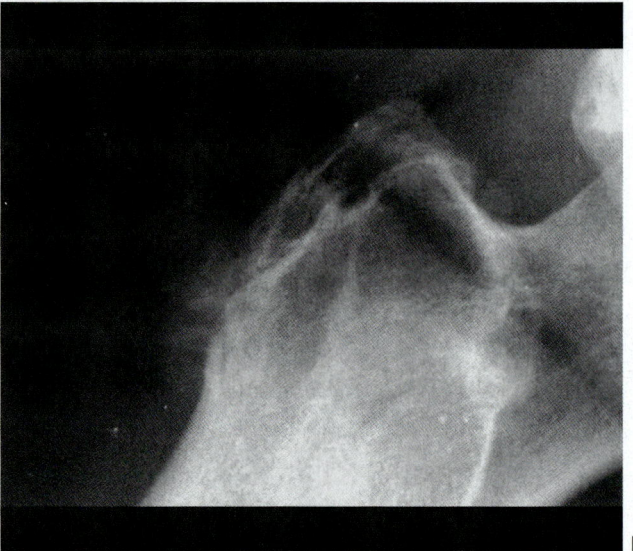

**FIGURE 114.4.** Plain anteroposterior **(A)** and lateral **(B)** radiographs of the greater trochanter demonstrating the characteristic irregularity of the bony surface seen in patients with trochanteric bursitis.

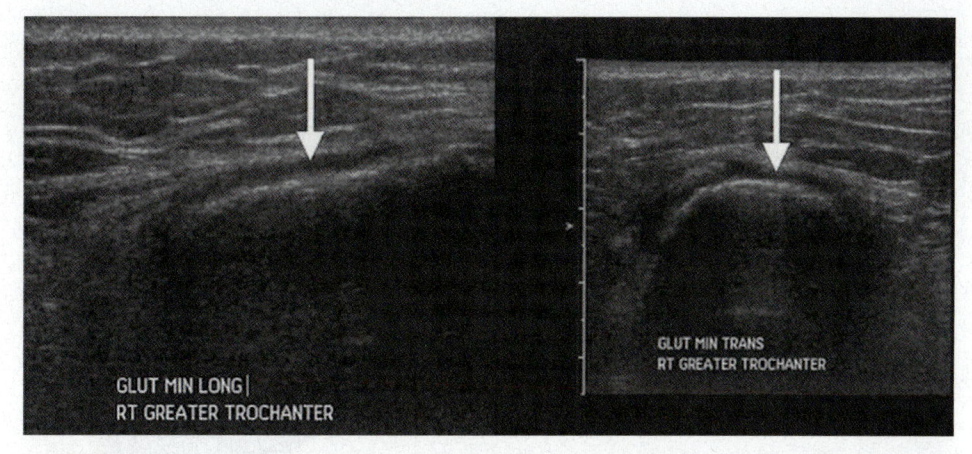

**FIGURE 114.5.** Ultrasound longitudinal and transverse. A "bald" greater trochanter appearance suggests absence of the gluteus minimus tendon signifying a complete tear (*arrow*). (Reused from Kong A, Van der Vliet A, Zadow S. MRI and US of gluteal tendinopathy in greater trochanteric pain syndrome. *Eur Radiol* 2007;17(7):1772–1783, with permission.)

guidance to pass through the substance of the gluteus maximus tendon to place the needle tip between the tendon and greater trochanter (Fig. 114.11). When the tip of needle is thought to be in satisfactory position in proximity to the trochanteric bursa, a small amount of local anesthetic and steroid is injected under real-time ultrasound guidance to confirm proper placement of the needle tip by hydrodissection. After proper positioning of the needle tip placement is confirmed, the remainder of the contents of the syringe are slowly injected. There should be minimal resistance to injection. If synechiae, loculations, or calcifications are present, the needle may have to be repositioned to ensure that the entire bursa is treated. The needle is then removed, and a sterile pressure dressing and ice pack are placed at the injection site.

## COMPLICATIONS

The major complication of ultrasound-guided injection of the trochanteric bursa is infection. Ecchymosis and hematoma formation may also occur. A transient exacerbation of the patient's pain occurs ~25% of the time following this injection technique, and the patient should be warned of this possibility prior to the procedure.

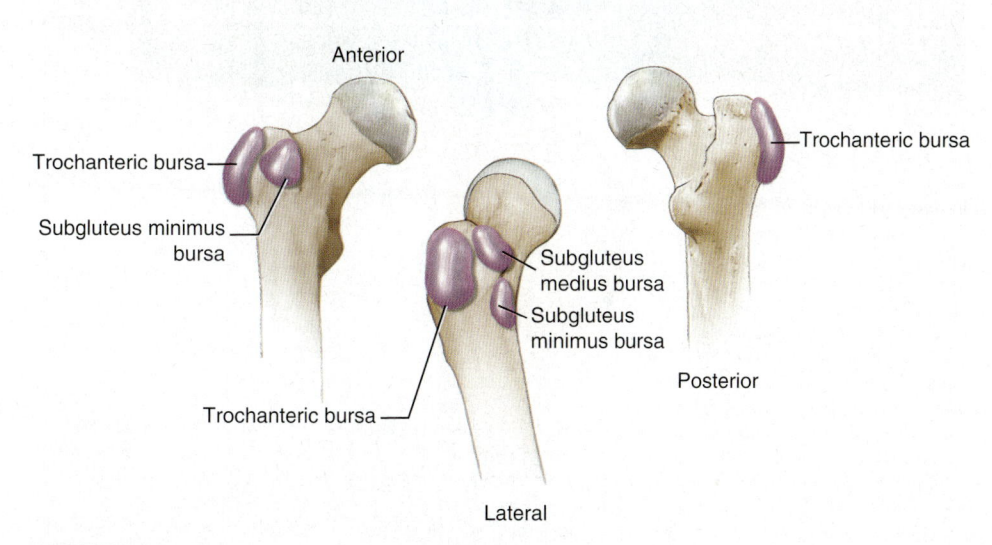

**FIGURE 114.6.** The bursa surrounding the greater trochanter.

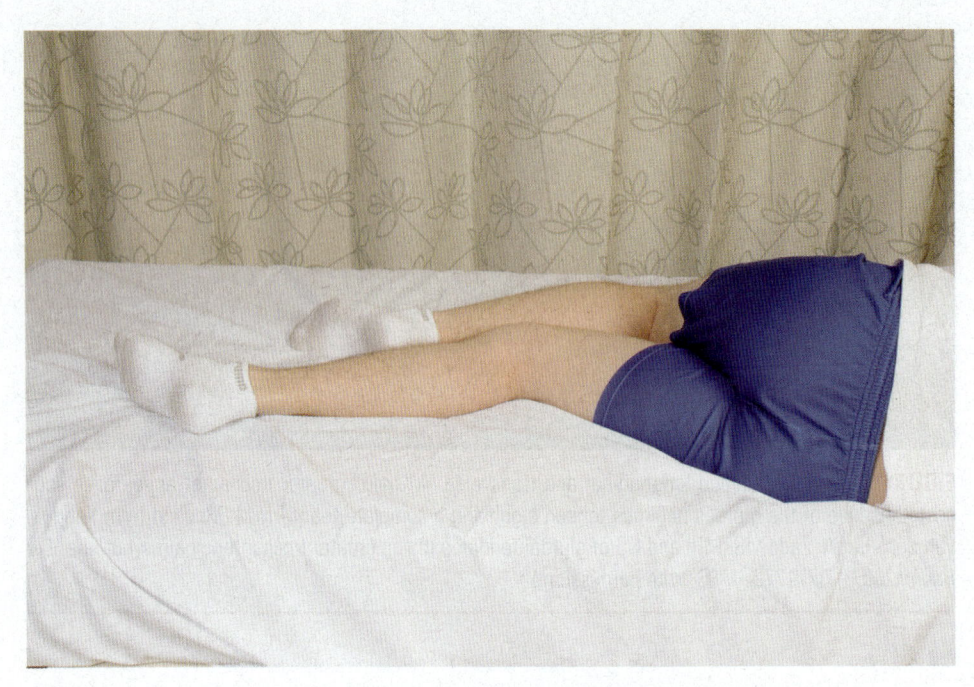

**FIGURE 114.7.** Proper patient position for ultrasound-guided injection of the trochanteric bursa.

## CLINICAL PEARLS

Bursitis, labral tears, tendinopathy, osteoarthritis, synovitis, nerve entrapment, avascular necrosis of the femoral head, and impingement syndromes may coexist with other hip joint disease and may contribute to the patient's pain symptomatology. Universal precautions should always be observed to protect the operator, and strict adherence to sterile technique must be used to avoid infection. Gentle physical therapy and local heat should be introduced following ultrasound-guided injection of the elbow joint to reduce pain and improve function. Simple analgesics and nonsteroidal anti-inflammatory agents or COX-2 inhibitors may be used concurrently with this injection technique.

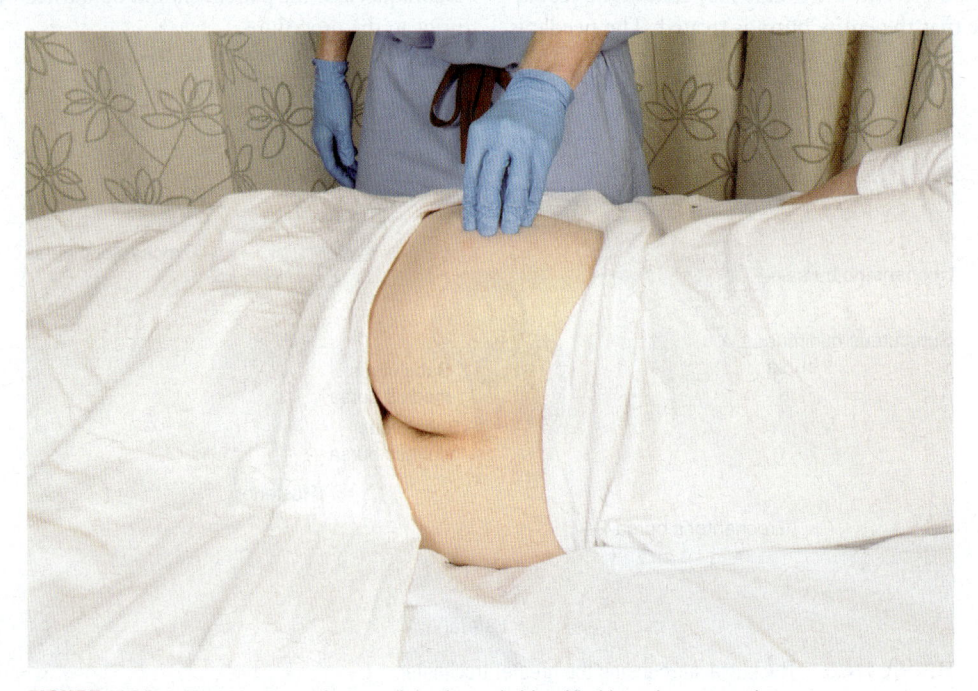

**FIGURE 114.8.** The greater trochanter of the femur is identified by using a grasping maneuver.

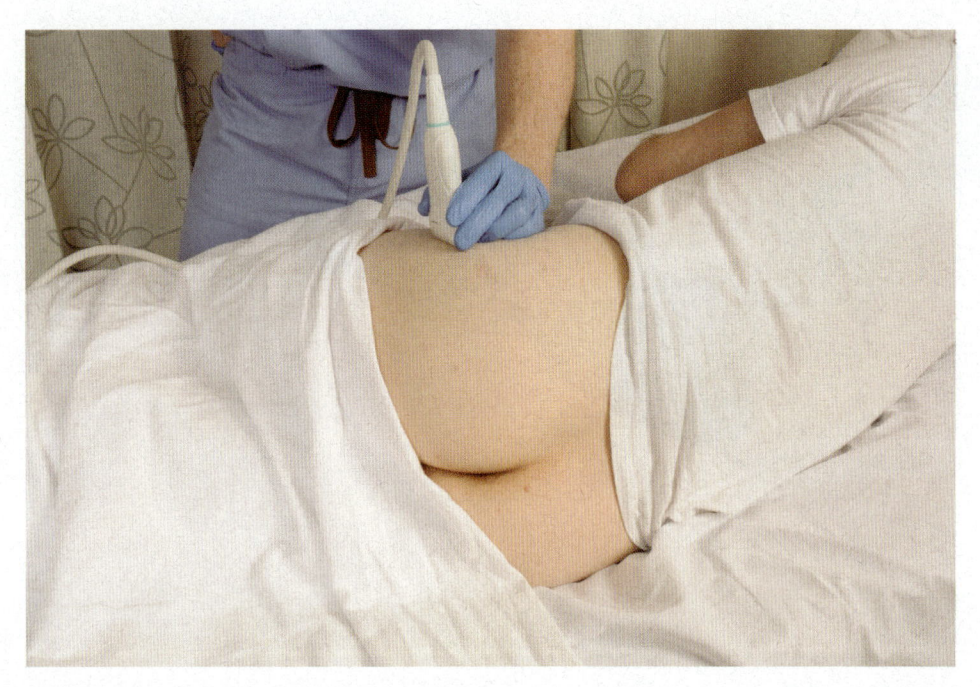

**FIGURE 114.9.** Correct transverse position for ultrasound transducer for ultrasound-guided injection of the trochanteric bursa.

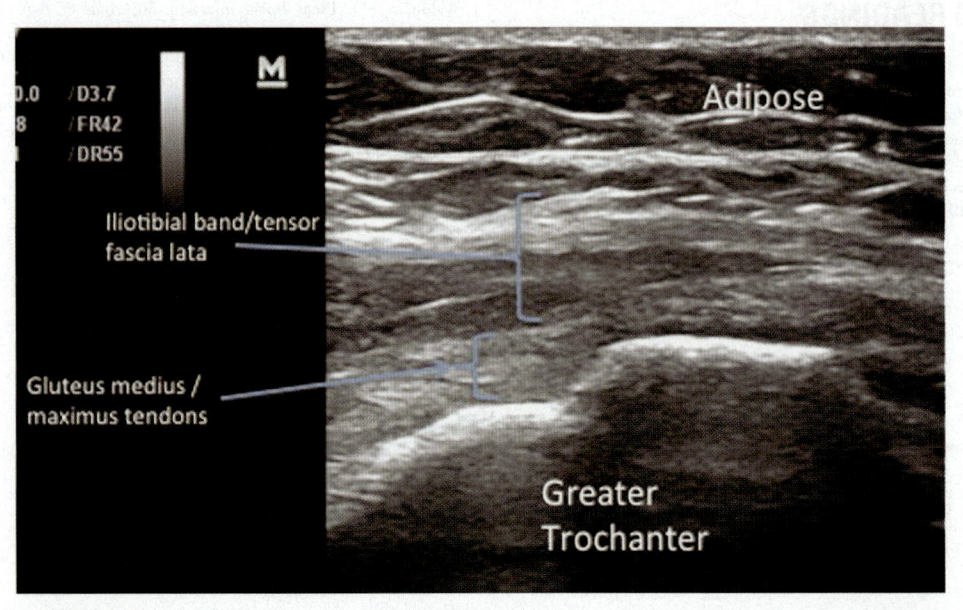

**FIGURE 114.10.** Ultrasound image of the hip joint demonstrating the medial border of the proximal femur.

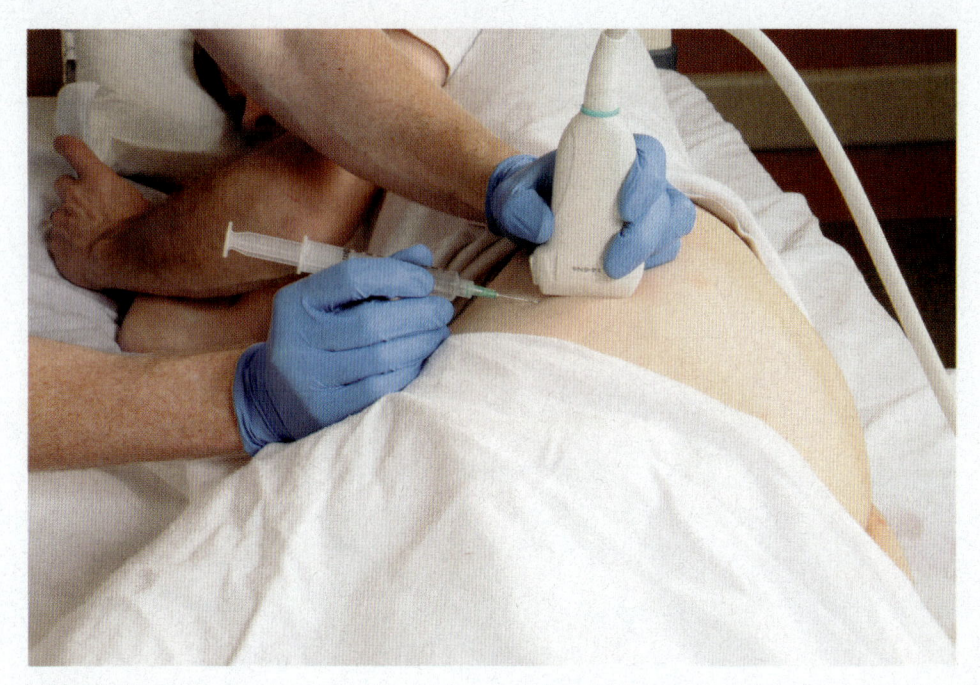

**FIGURE 114.11.** Correct in-plane needle placement for ultrasound-guided injection of the trochanteric bursa.

## SUGGESTED READINGS

Segal NA, Felson DT, Torner JC, et al.; Multicenter Osteoarthritis (MOST) Study Group. Greater trochanteric pain syndrome: epidemiology and associated factors. *Arch Phys Med Rehabil* 2007;88(8):988–992.

Waldman SD. Injection technique for trochanteric bursitis. In: *Pain Review*. Philadelphia, PA: Saunders Elsevier; 2009:554–555.

Waldman SD. The trochanteric bursa. In: *Pain Review*. Philadelphia, PA: Saunders Elsevier; 2009:140–141.

Waldman SD. Psoas bursa injection. In: *Atlas of Pain Management Injection Techniques*. 3rd ed. Philadelphia, PA: Saunders Elsevier; 2012:299–302.

Waldman SD. Trochanteric bursitis. In: *Atlas of Common Pain Syndromes*. 3rd ed. Philadelphia, PA: Saunders Elsevier; 2012:297–298.

Waldman SD, Campbell RSD. Anatomy, special imaging considerations of pelvis, hip, and lower extremity pain syndromes. In: *Imaging of Pain*. Philadelphia, PA: Saunders Elsevier; 2011:335–336.

# CHAPTER 115

# Ultrasound-Guided Injection Technique for Gluteus Medius Bursitis Pain

## CLINICAL PERSPECTIVES

Gluteus medius bursitis is a common cause of lateral hip and buttocks pain. The gluteus medius bursa lies between the distal insertional tendons of gluteus medius and gluteus minimus muscles (Fig. 115.1). The bursa serves to cushion and facilitate sliding of the musculotendinous units of the gluteus medius and minimus muscles over the bony greater trochanter. The bursa is subject to inflammation from a variety of causes with acute trauma to the hip and repetitive microtrauma being the most common. Acute injuries to the bursa can occur from direct blunt trauma to the lateral hip as well as from overuse injuries including running on uneven or soft surfaces. If the inflammation of the bursa is not treated and the condition becomes chronic, calcification of the bursa with further functional disability may occur. Gout and other crystal arthropathies may also precipitate acute gluteus medius bursitis as may bacterial, tubercular, or fungal infections.

The patient suffering from gluteus medius bursitis most frequently presents with the complaint of pain in the upper outer quadrant of the buttocks that can radiate down the leg and into the sciatic notch. The patient may find walking up stairs and getting in and out of the car increasingly difficult. Physical examination of the patient suffering from gluteus medius bursitis will reveal point tenderness over the upper outer quadrant of the buttocks. If there is significant inflammation, rubor and color may be present and the entire area may feel boggy or edematous to palpation. Active resisted abduction and extension of the affected lower extremity reproduce the pain. Sudden release of resistance to abduction during the resisted abduction release test for gluteus medius bursitis markedly increases the pain. There should be no sensory deficit in the distribution of the lateral femoral cutaneous nerve, as is seen with meralgia paresthetica, which often is confused with gluteus medius bursitis. If calcification or gouty tophi of the bursa and surrounding tendons are present, the examiner may appreciate crepitus with active abduction of the hip and the patient may complain of a catching sensation when moving the affected lower extremity, especially on awaking. Often, the patient will not be able to sleep on the affected side.

Plain radiographs are indicated in all patients who present with hip pain to rule out occult bony pathology (Fig. 115.2). Based on the patient's clinical presentation, additional testing may be indicated, including complete blood cell count, sedimentation rate, and antinuclear antibody testing. Magnetic resonance imaging or ultrasound imaging of the affected area may also confirm the diagnosis and help delineate the presence of other hip bursitis, calcific tendonitis, tendinopathy, triceps tendonitis, or other hip pathology. Magnetic resonance imaging or ultrasound imaging of the affected area may also help delineate the presence of calcific tendonitis or other hip pathology (Fig. 115.3). Rarely, the inflamed bursa may become infected, and failure to diagnose and treat the acute infection can lead to dire consequences. Electromyography helps distinguish gluteus medius bursitis from meralgia paresthetica and sciatica.

## CLINICALLY RELEVANT ANATOMY

There is significant intrapatient variability in the size, number, and location of the gluteal bursae. The gluteal medius bursa lies between the gluteal maximus and medius muscle (Fig. 115.4). The gluteus minimus bursa lies between the gluteus medius and minimus muscles (see Fig. 115.1). With the leg in anatomic position, the gluteus medius and gluteus minimus muscles work as a single functional unit to abduct the hip (Fig. 115.5). When ambulating, both muscles act principally to support the body on one leg and, in conjunction with the tensor fascia lata, prevent the pelvis from dropping to the opposite side. With the hip in flexed position, the gluteus medius and minimus muscles act to internally rotate the thigh. With the hip in extension, the gluteus medius and gluteus minimus muscles act to externally rotate the thigh.

## ULTRASOUND-GUIDED TECHNIQUE

The benefits, risks, and alternative treatments are explained to the patient and informed consent is obtained. The patient is then placed in the modified Sims position (Fig. 115.6). The skin overlying the greater trochanter of the femur is then prepped with antiseptic solution. The greater trochanter is then identified by using a grasping maneuver (Fig. 115.7). A sterile syringe containing 4.0 mL of 0.25% preservative-free bupivacaine and

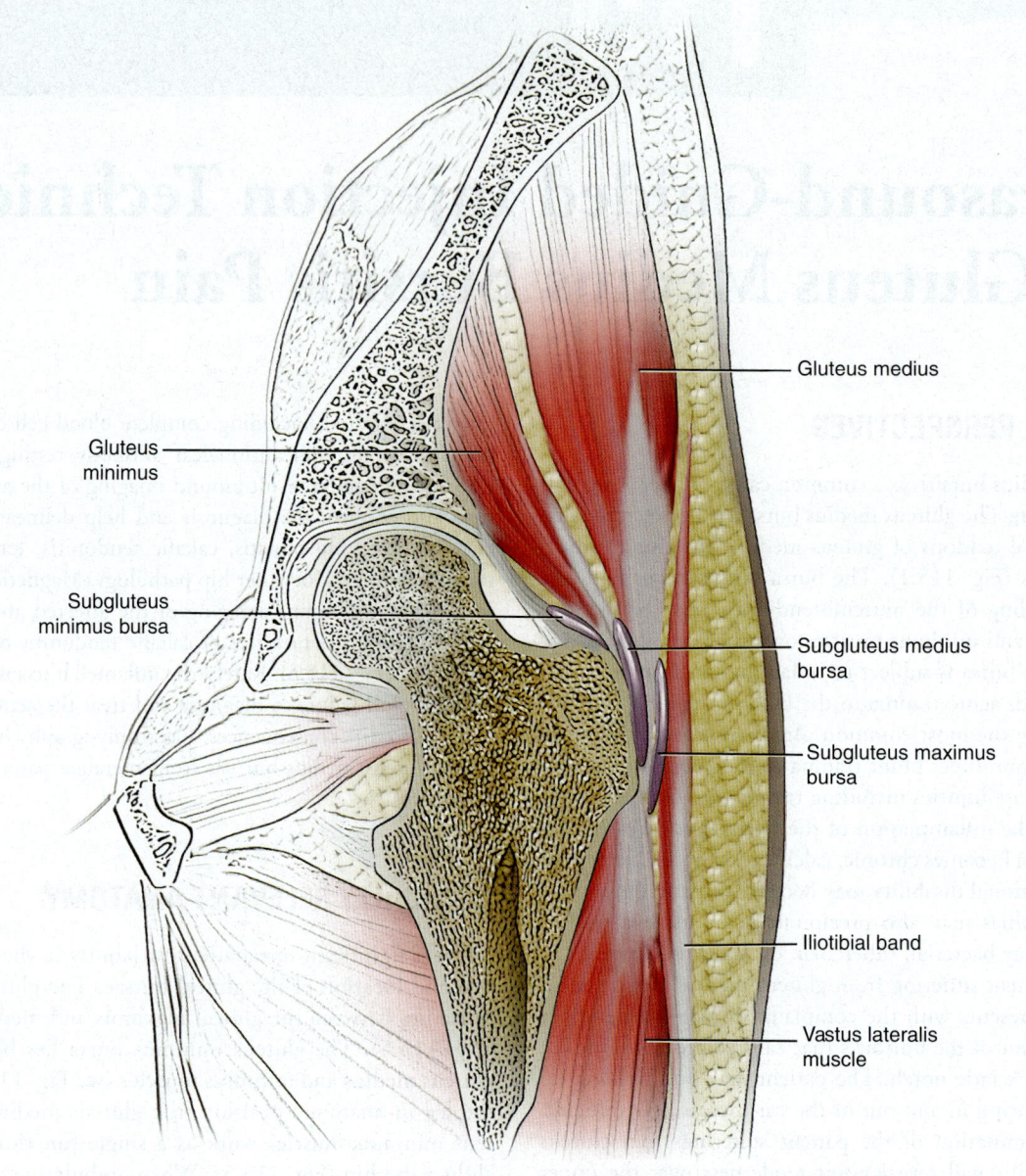

**FIGURE 115.1.** The gluteus medius bursa lies between the gluteus medius and minimus musculotendinous insertions.

40 mg of methylprednisolone is attached to a 1½-inch, 22-gauge needle using strict aseptic technique. A linear high-frequency ultrasound transducer is placed over the previously identified greater trochanter with the transducer in a transverse orientation (Fig. 115.8). A survey scan is taken, which demonstrates the hyperechoic margin of the greater trochanter, the trochanteric bursa, and tendon of the gluteus maximus muscle above it (Fig. 115.9). After the greater trochanter is identified, the transversely placed ultrasound transducer is then slowly moved superiorly until the superior margin of the greater trochanter of the femur and the insertion of the gluteus medius muscle is identified (Fig. 115.10). Just medial to the gluteus medius musculotendinous unit is the gluteus minimus musculotendinous unit (see Fig. 115.1 also for orientation, Fig. 115.11). The gluteus medius bursa lies between the two. When the fascial plane between the gluteus medius and gluteus minimus musculotendinous units are identified, a 3½-inch needle is placed through the skin ~1 cm from the anterior aspect of the transducer and is then advanced using an in-plane approach with the needle trajectory adjusted under real-time ultrasound guidance to place the needle tip into the fascial cleft between the musculotendinous units of the gluteus medius and gluteus minimus muscles (Fig. 115.12). When the tip of needle is thought to be in satisfactory position within the fascial cleft, a small amount of local anesthetic and steroid is injected under real-time ultrasound guidance to confirm proper placement of the needle tip by hydrodissection. After proper positioning of the needle tip placement is confirmed, the remainder of the contents of the syringe are slowly injected. There should be minimal resistance to injection. If synechiae, loculations, or

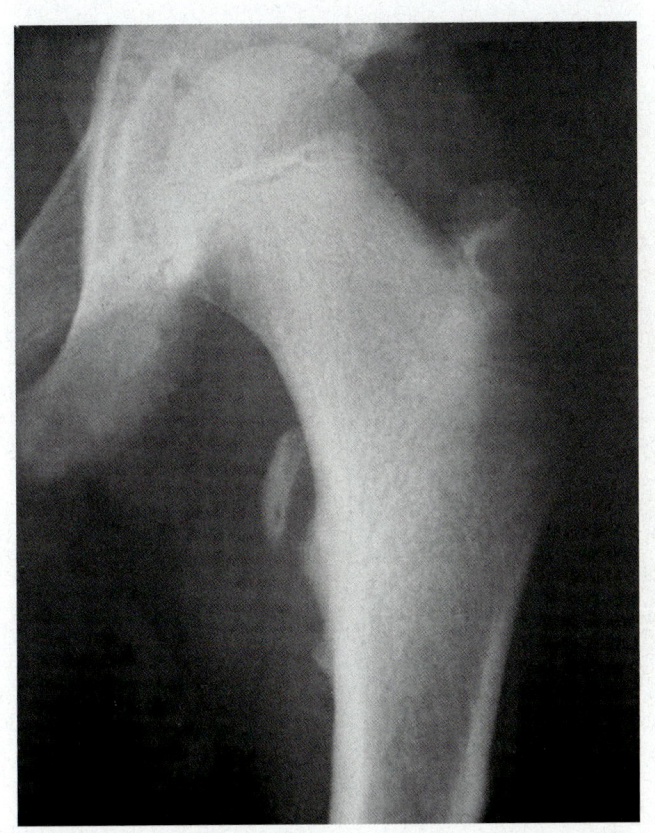

**FIGURE 115.2.** An avulsion fracture of the lesser trochanter. (Reused from Court-Brown C, Mcqueen M, Tornetta P. *Trauma*. Philadelphia, PA: Lippincott Williams & Wilkins; 2006, with permission.)

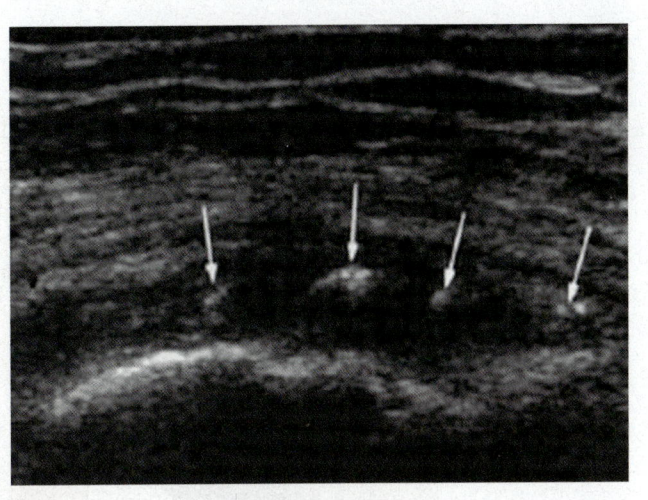

**FIGURE 115.3.** Calcific tendinosis. Ultrasound image longitudinal to the gluteus medius tendon shows intratendinous echogenic foci consistent with calcific tendinopathy (*arrows*). (Reused from Klauser AS, Martinoli C, Tagliafico A, et al. Greater trochanteric pain syndrome. *Semin Musculoskelet Radiol* 2013;17(1):43–48, with permission.)

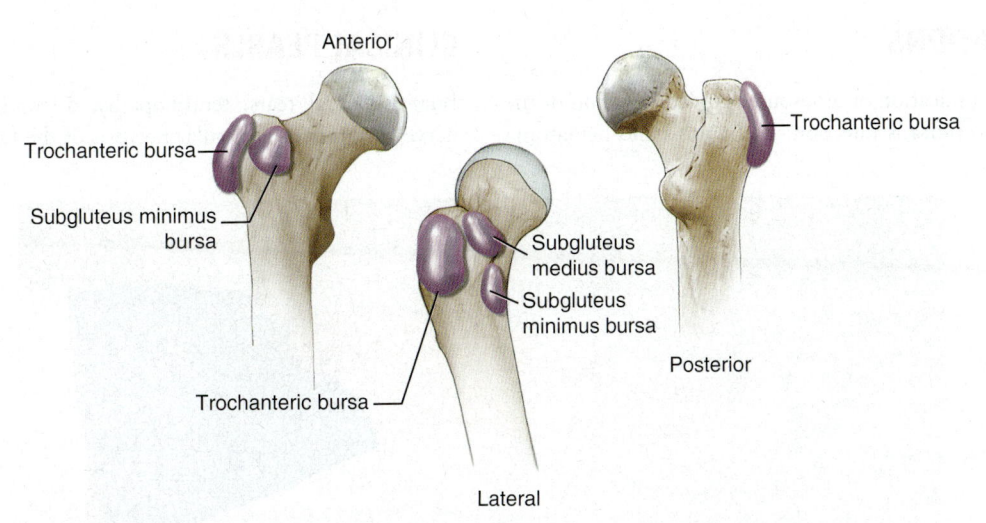

**FIGURE 115.4.** There is significant intrapatient variability in the size, number, and location of the gluteal bursae. The gluteal medius bursa lies between the gluteal maximus and medius muscle.

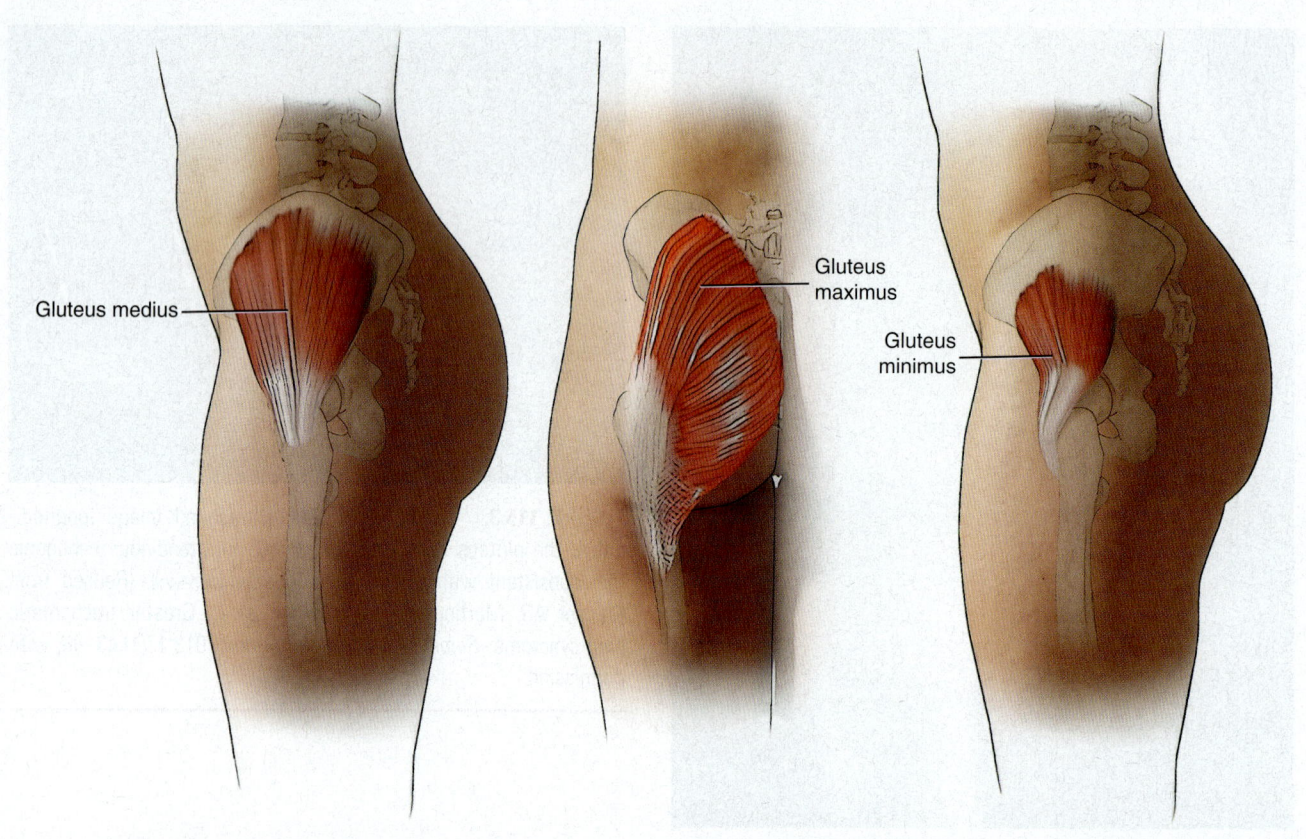

**FIGURE 115.5.** The gluteal muscles work together and independently to provide a wide range of motions at the hip.

calcifications are present, the needle may have to be repositioned to ensure that the entire bursa is treated. The needle is then removed, and a sterile pressure dressing and ice pack are placed at the injection site.

## COMPLICATIONS

The major complication of ultrasound-guided injection of the gluteus medius bursa is infection. Ecchymosis and hematoma formation may also occur. A transient exacerbation of the patient's pain occurs ~25% of the time following this injection technique, and the patient should be warned of this possibility prior to the procedure.

## CLINICAL PEARLS

Bursitis, labral tears, tendinopathy, osteoarthritis, synovitis, nerve entrapment, avascular necrosis of the femoral head, and

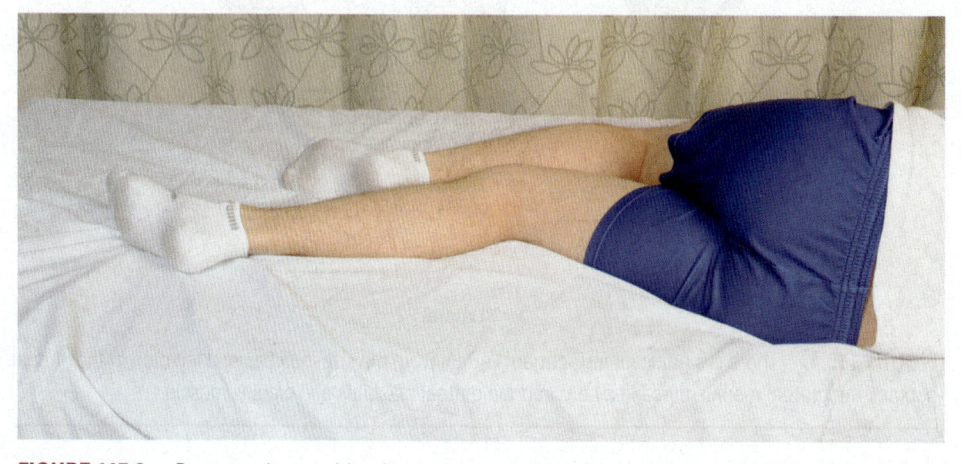

**FIGURE 115.6.** Proper patient position for ultrasound-guided injection of the gluteus medius bursa.

CHAPTER 115  ULTRASOUND-GUIDED INJECTION TECHNIQUE FOR GLUTEUS MEDIUS BURSITIS PAIN   821

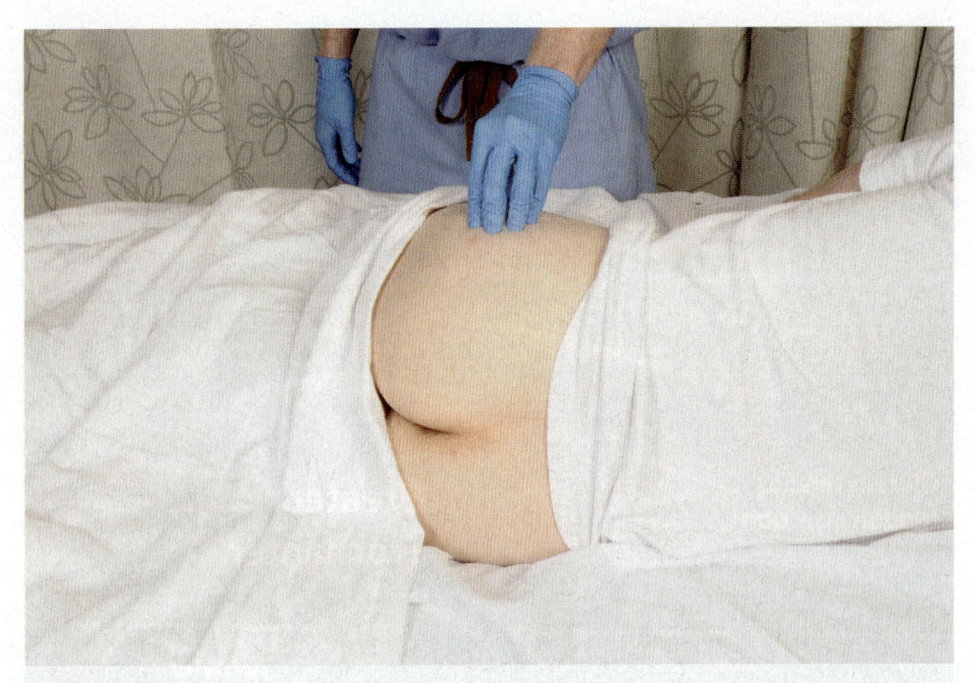

**FIGURE 115.7.** The greater trochanter of the femur is identified by using a grasping maneuver.

impingement syndromes may coexist with other hip joint disease and may contribute to the patient's pain symptomatology. Universal precautions should always be observed to protect the operator, and strict adherence to sterile technique must be used to avoid infection. Gentle physical therapy and local heat should be introduced following ultrasound-guided injection of the elbow joint to reduce pain and improve function. Simple analgesics and nonsteroidal anti-inflammatory agents or COX-2 inhibitors may be used concurrently with this injection technique.

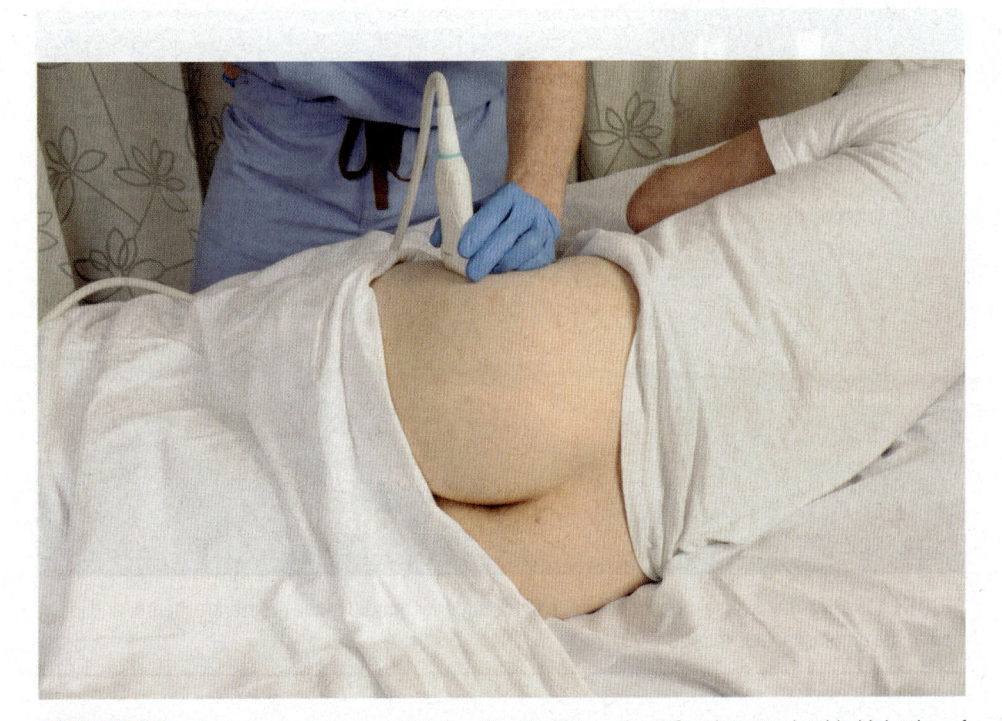

**FIGURE 115.8.** Correct transverse position for ultrasound transducer for ultrasound-guided injection of the gluteus medius bursa.

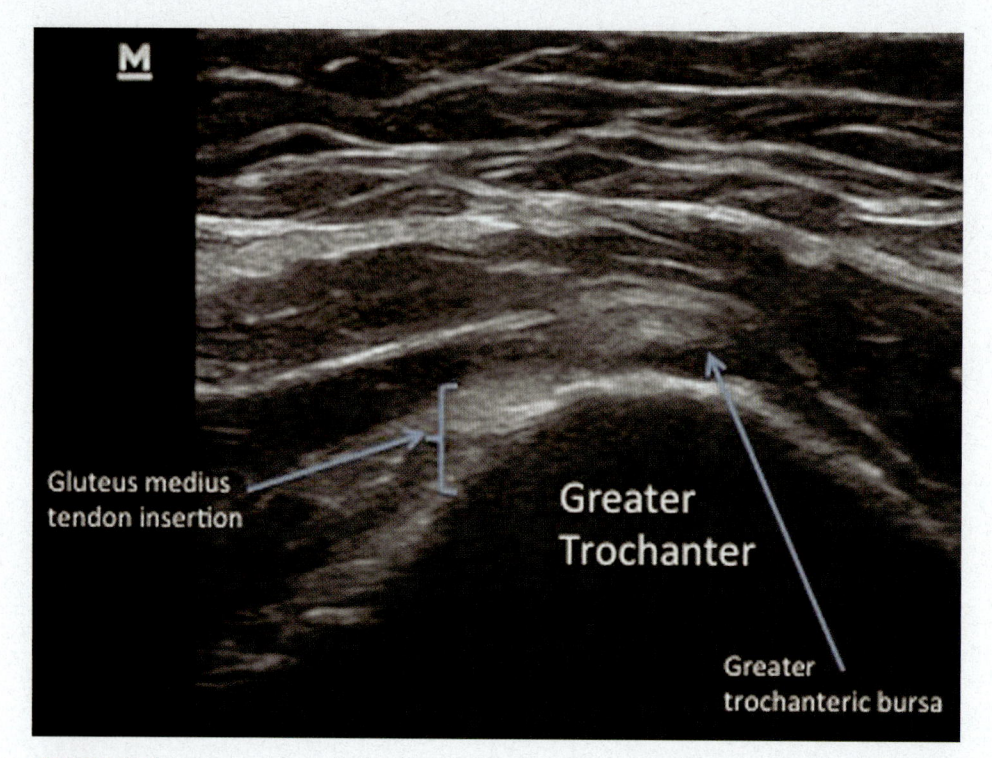

**FIGURE 115.9.** Ultrasound image of the hip joint demonstrating the greater trochanter and trochanteric bursa.

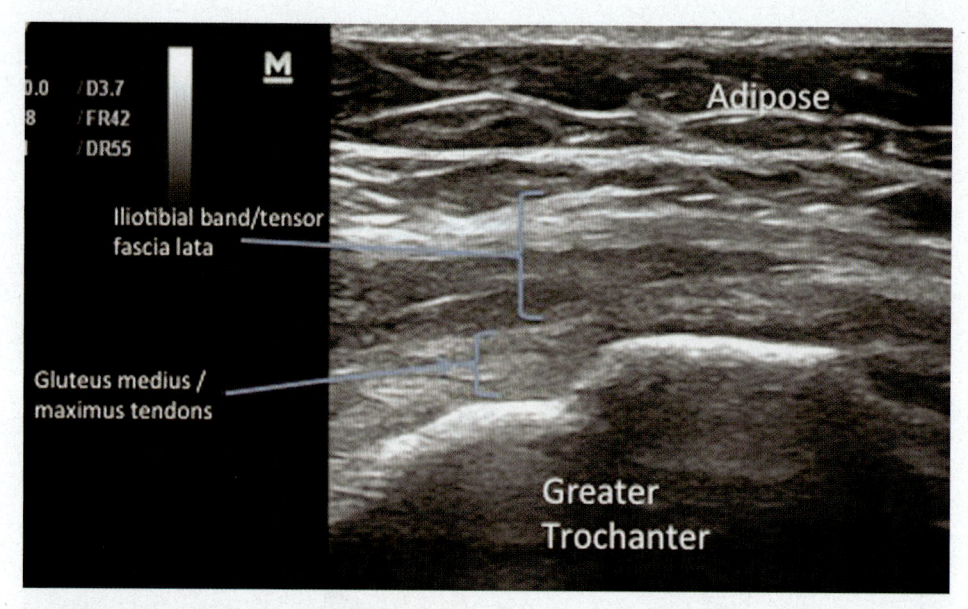

**FIGURE 115.10.** Transverse ultrasound image of the superior margin of the greater trochanter and insertion of the gluteus medius muscle.

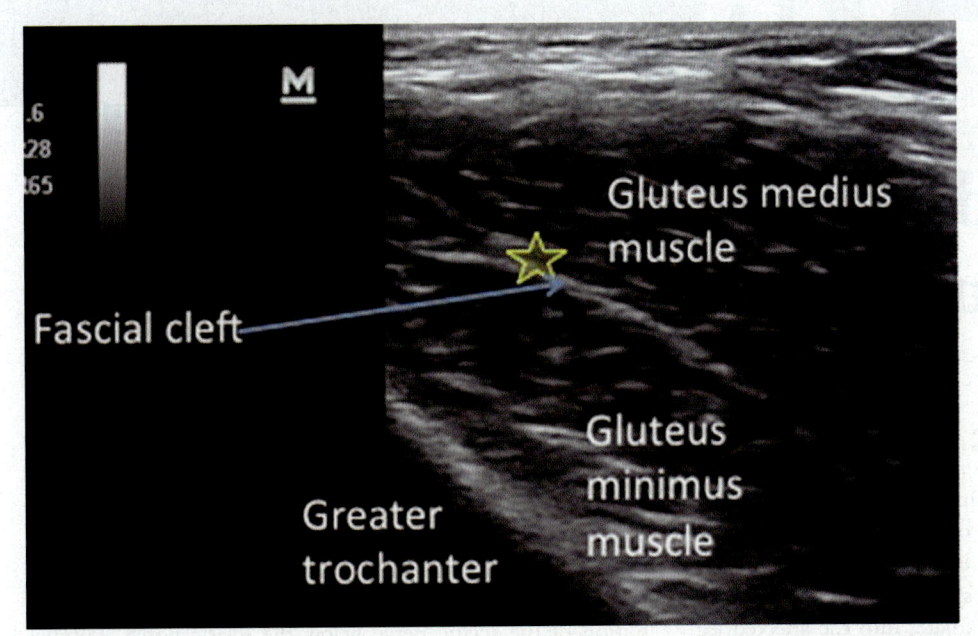

**FIGURE 115.11.** Transverse ultrasound image of the insertions of the musculotendinous units of the gluteus medius and gluteus minimus muscles. The gluteal medial bursa lies within the fascial plane between the muscles.

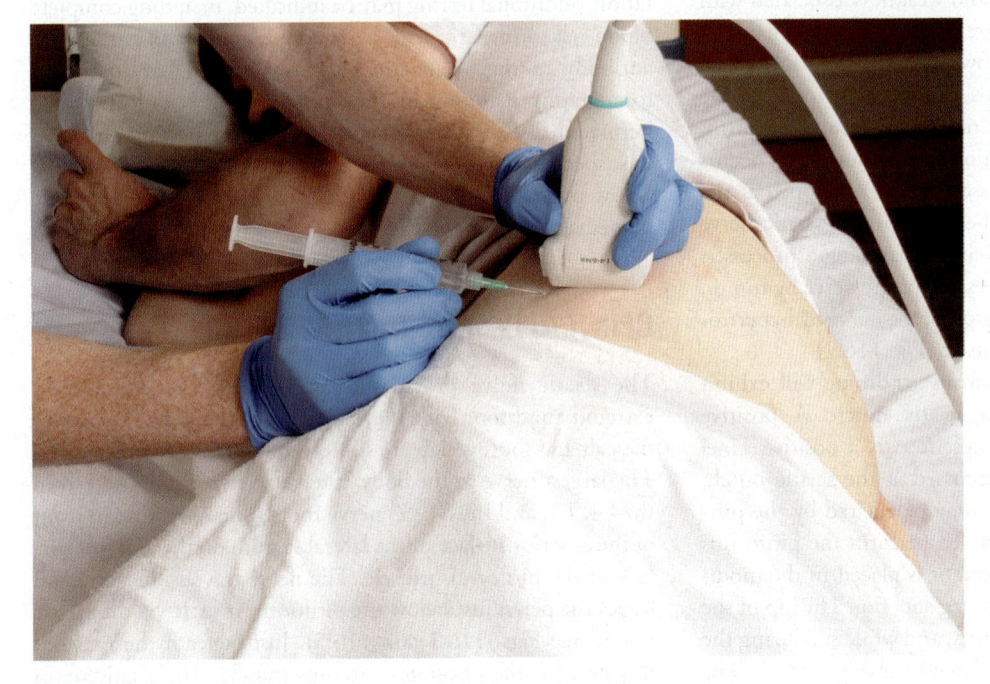

**FIGURE 115.12.** Correct in-plane needle placement for ultrasound-guided injection of the gluteus medius bursa.

## SUGGESTED READINGS

Arnold ML. Bursitis: lower extremities. In: Ramamurthy S, Alanmanou E, Rogers JN, eds. *Decision Making in Pain Management.* 2nd ed. Philadelphia, PA: Saunders Elsevier; 2006:210–211.

Hodnett PA, Shelly MJ, MacMahon PJ, et al. MR imaging of overuse injuries of the hip. *Magn Reson Imaging Clin N Am* 2009;17(4):667–679.

Waldman SD. Gluteal bursitis. In: *Atlas of Uncommon Pain Syndromes.* 2nd ed. Philadelphia, PA: Saunders Elsevier; 2009:230–232.

Waldman SD. Injection technique for gluteal bursitis. In: *Pain Review.* Philadelphia, PA: Saunders Elsevier; 2009:549–551.

Waldman SD. The gluteal bursa. In: *Pain Review.* Philadelphia, PA: Saunders Elsevier; 2009:139–140.

Waldman SD. Gluteal bursa injection. In: *Atlas of Pain Management Injection Techniques.* 3rd ed. Philadelphia, PA: Saunders Elsevier; 2012:292.

# Ultrasound-Guided Injection Technique for Piriformis Syndrome

## CLINICAL PERSPECTIVES

An uncommon cause of sciatica, piriformis syndrome is caused by entrapment and compression of the sciatic nerve by the piriformis muscle at the level of the sciatic notch (Fig. 116.1). Patients suffering from piriformis syndrome complain of pain that begins in the buttocks and radiates into the affected leg all the way to the foot. There is associated numbness and dysesthesias as well as weakness in the distribution of the sciatic nerve. As the syndrome progresses, the patient may experience altered gait as a result of the pain and weakness associated with the compromise of the sciatic nerve. This alteration of gait will often cause secondary sacroiliac, low back, and hip pain, which may serve to confuse the diagnosis. Untreated, atrophy of the muscles innervated by the sciatic nerve may result. Piriformis syndrome is the clinical constellation of symptoms that occurs when the sciatic nerve is compressed and/or entrapped at the level of the piriformis muscle. The cause of this sciatic nerve compromise can be from a variety of pathologic processes: direct trauma to the nerve; compression of the nerve by tumor, hematoma, or mass; and compression of the nerve by hypertrophied or anomalous piriformis muscle (Fig. 116.2).

Patients suffering from piriformis syndrome will exhibit tenderness on palpation of the sciatic notch. A positive straight-leg raising test is often present as is a positive Tinel sign when the sciatic nerve is percussed at the sciatic notch. The pain of piriformis syndrome may be elicited by the piriformis syndrome provocation test. To perform the piriformis syndrome provocation test, the patient is placed in the modified Sims position with the affected leg superior. The hip of the affected leg is then flexed ~50 degrees, and while stabilizing the pelvis, the affected leg is pushed downward (Fig. 116.3). The test is considered positive if the patient's pain symptomatology is reproduced. On palpation of the piriformis muscle, a swollen, indurated muscle belly may be appreciated. Weakness of the affected gluteal muscles and muscle wasting may be identified in more advanced cases of untreated piriformis syndrome.

Piriformis syndrome is frequently misdiagnosed as lumbar radiculopathy or is attributed to primary hip pathology leading to both diagnostic and therapeutic misadventures. Plain radiographs of the hip will help identify primary hip pathology, and electromyography will help distinguish the compromise of sciatic nerve function associated with piriformis syndrome from radiculopathy. Most patients who suffer from lumbar radiculopathy have back pain associated with reflex, motor, and sensory changes that are associated with back pain, whereas patients with piriformis syndrome have only secondary back pain and no reflex changes. Furthermore, the motor and sensory changes of piriformis syndrome are limited to the distribution of the sciatic nerve below the sciatic notch. Lumbar radiculopathy and sciatic nerve entrapment may coexist as the so-called "double crush" syndrome, and this can further confuse the clinical picture. Based on the patient's clinical presentation, additional testing may be indicated, including complete blood cell count, uric acid, sedimentation rate, and antinuclear antibody testing. Magnetic resonance imaging or computed tomography scanning of the lumbar spine is indicated if a herniated disc, a spinal stenosis, or a space-occupying lesion is suspected (Fig. 116.4). The injection technique described below can be utilized as both a diagnostic and a therapeutic maneuver.

## CLINICALLY RELEVANT ANATOMY

The sciatic nerve provides innervation to the distal lower extremity and foot with the exception of the medial aspect of the calf and foot, which are subserved by the saphenous nerve. The largest nerve in the body, the sciatic nerve is derived from the L4, L5, and the S1–S3 nerve roots. The roots fuse in front of the anterior surface of the lateral sacrum on the anterior surface of the piriformis muscle. The nerve travels inferiorly and leaves the pelvis just below the piriformis muscle via the sciatic notch (see Figs. 116.1 and 116.5). Just beneath the nerve at this point is the obturator internus muscle. The sciatic nerve lies anterior to the gluteus maximus muscle; at this muscle's lower border, the sciatic nerve lies halfway between the greater trochanter and the ischial tuberosity. The sciatic nerve courses downward past the lesser trochanter to lie posterior and medial to the femur (Fig. 116.6). In the midthigh, the nerve gives off branches to the hamstring muscles and the adductor magnus muscle. In most patients, the nerve divides to form the tibial and common peroneal nerves in the upper portion of the popliteal fossa, although in some patients these nerves can remain separate through their entire course. The tibial nerve continues downward to provide innervation to the distal lower

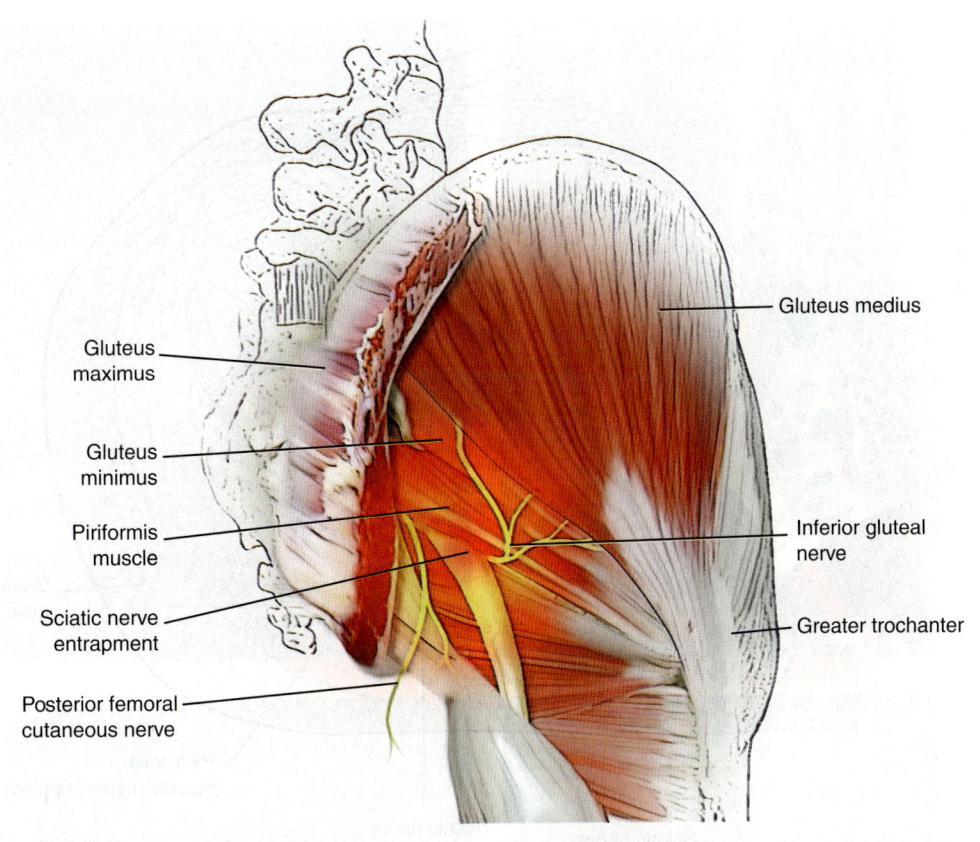

# CHAPTER 116 ULTRASOUND-GUIDED INJECTION TECHNIQUE FOR PIRIFORMIS SYNDROME

**FIGURE 116.1.** Piriformis syndrome is caused by entrapment of the sciatic nerve by the piriformis muscle.

extremity, whereas the common peroneal nerve travels laterally to innervate a portion of the knee joint and, via its lateral cutaneous branch, provide sensory innervation to the back and lateral side of the upper calf.

The piriformis muscle has its origin from the anterior sacrum. It passes laterally through the greater sciatic foramen to insert on the upper border of the greater trochanter of the femur (Fig. 116.7). The piriformis muscle's primary function is to externally rotate the femur at the hip joint. The piriformis muscle is innervated by the sacral plexus. With internal rotation of the femur, the tendinous insertion and belly of the muscle can compress the sciatic nerve and, if this persists, cause entrapment of the sciatic nerve.

## ULTRASOUND-GUIDED TECHNIQUE

The benefits, risks, and alternative treatments are explained to the patient, and informed consent is obtained. The patient is then placed in the prone position (Fig. 116.8). With the patient in the above position, the posterosuperior iliac spine is identified by palpation (Fig. 116.9). A curvilinear low-frequency linear ultrasound transducer is placed over posterosuperior iliac spine in the transverse position, and the ultrasound transducer is then slowly moved laterally until the ilium is visualized (Fig. 116.10). The ilium will appear as an S-shaped hyperechoic line ascending from the inferolateral position of the ultrasound image to meet the sacrum in the superomedial portion of the image (Fig. 116.11). Once the ilium is identified, the transversely placed ultrasound probe is rotated in a counterclockwise direction ~25 degrees to lie parallel to the path of the piriformis muscle as it extends from the anterior sacrum to extend through the sciatic notch to attach on the greater trochanter of the femur (see Fig. 116.7 for orientation, Fig. 116.12). The ultrasound probe is then slowly moved in a caudad direction until the sciatic notch is identified. The two layers of the gluteus maximus and piriformis muscles are then identified (Fig. 116.13). The exact location of the piriformis muscle is then confirmed by flexing the knee of the patient's affected lower extremity and rotating the hip externally and internally (Fig. 116.14). The piriformis muscle will be clearly seen to slide back and forth beneath the

**FIGURE 116.5.** The sciatic nerve passes beneath or through the piriformis muscle.

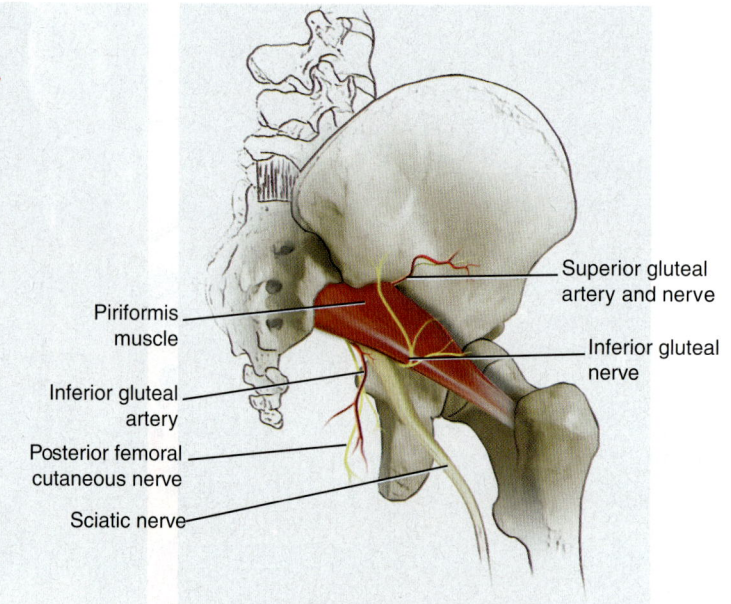

**FIGURE 116.6.** The path of the sciatic nerve. (From Bucci C. *Condition-specific Massage Therapy*. Baltimore, MD: Lippincott Williams & Wilkins; 2012.)

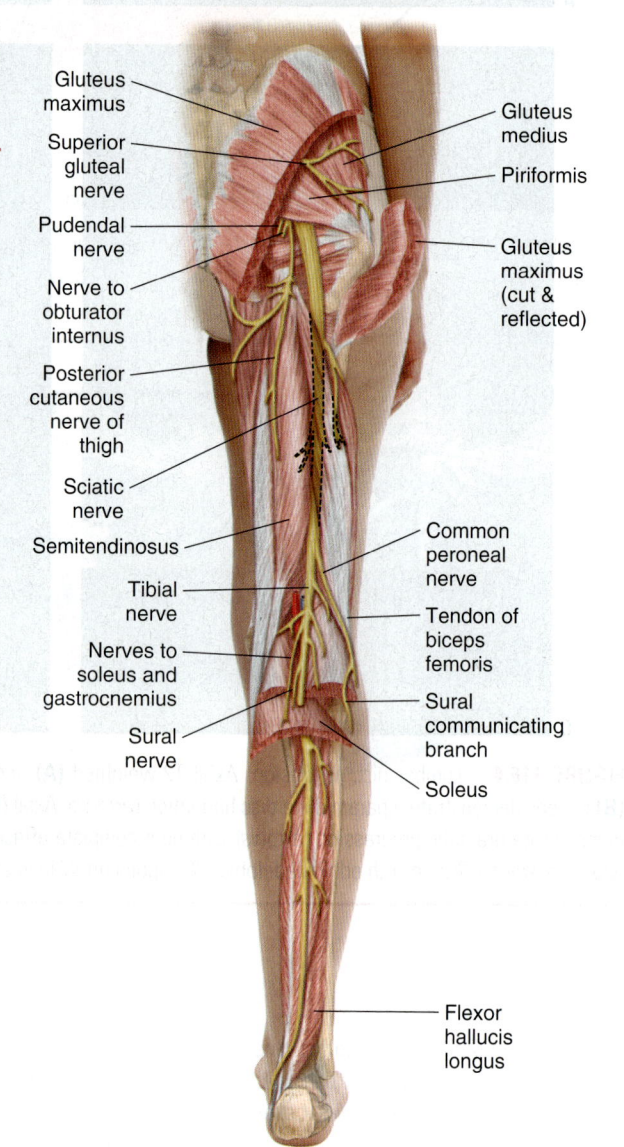

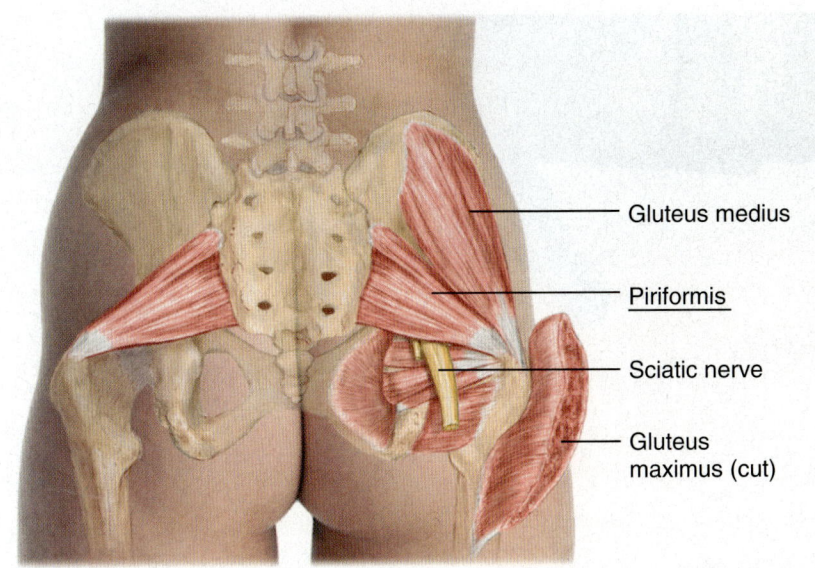

**FIGURE 116.7.** The piriformis muscle finds its origin on the anterior sacrum and passing through the sciatic notch inserts on the greater trochanter of the femur. (Adapted from Clay JH, Pounds DM. *Basic Clinical Massage Therapy: Integrating Anatomy and Treatment.* 2nd ed. Philadelphia, PA: Lippincott Williams & Wilkins; 2008.)

**PIRIFORMIS**

| | |
|---|---|
| Origin | Anterior surface of sacrum. |
| Insertion | Greater trochanter of the femur. |
| Action | Laterally rotate hip, abduct the flexed hip. |
| Nerve | L5–S2 nerve roots of sacral plexus. |

gluteus maximus muscle. The sciatic nerve, which will appear as a hyperechoic flattened structure, is then identified either within the substance of the piriformis muscle or lying in close proximity above or below it (Fig. 116.15). If the sciatic nerve is difficult to identify, color Doppler may be utilized in the pudendal artery, which should lie just medial to the sciatic nerve (Fig. 116.16). Once the sciatic nerve is identified, the skin overlying the area beneath the ultrasound transducer is prepped with antiseptic solution. A sterile syringe containing 3.0 mL of 0.25% preservative-free bupivacaine and 40 mg of methylprednisolone is attached to a 3½-inch, 22-gauge needle using strict aseptic technique. The needle is placed through the skin ~1 cm above the medial edge of the transducer and is then advanced using an in-plane approach with the needle trajectory adjusted under real-time ultrasound guidance to avoid the sciatic nerve and so that the needle tip rests within the belly of the piriformis muscle in proximity to the sciatic nerve (Fig. 116.17). When the tip of needle is thought to be

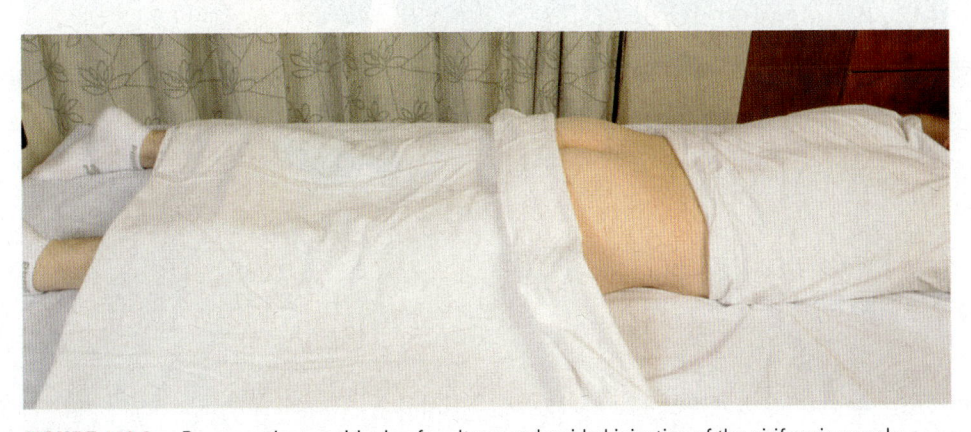

**FIGURE 116.8.** Proper patient positioning for ultrasound-guided injection of the piriformis muscle.

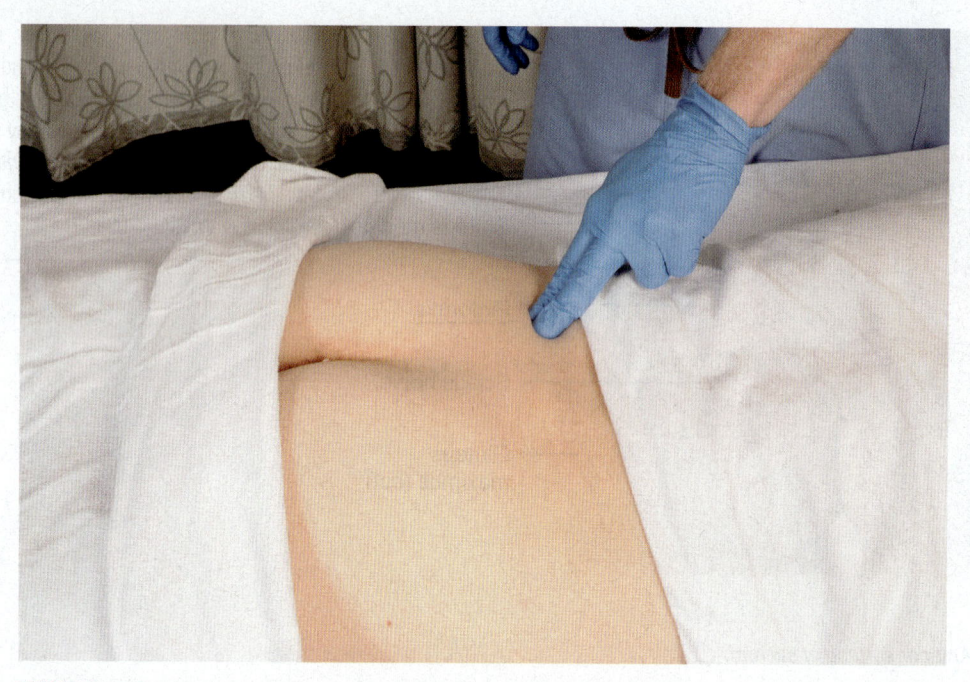

**FIGURE 116.9.** With the patient in the prone position, the posterior superior iliac spine is identified by palpation.

in satisfactory position, after careful aspiration, a small amount of local anesthetic and steroid is injected under real-time ultrasound guidance to confirm that the needle tip is not within the sciatic nerve. After proper needle tip placement is confirmed, the remainder of the contents of the syringe are slowly injected. There should be minimal resistance to injection.

## COMPLICATIONS

Given the proximity of the sciatic nerve to the injection target of the belly of the piriformis muscle, the possibility of needle-induced trauma remains an ever-present possibility. This potentially disastrous complication can be greatly decreased if attention

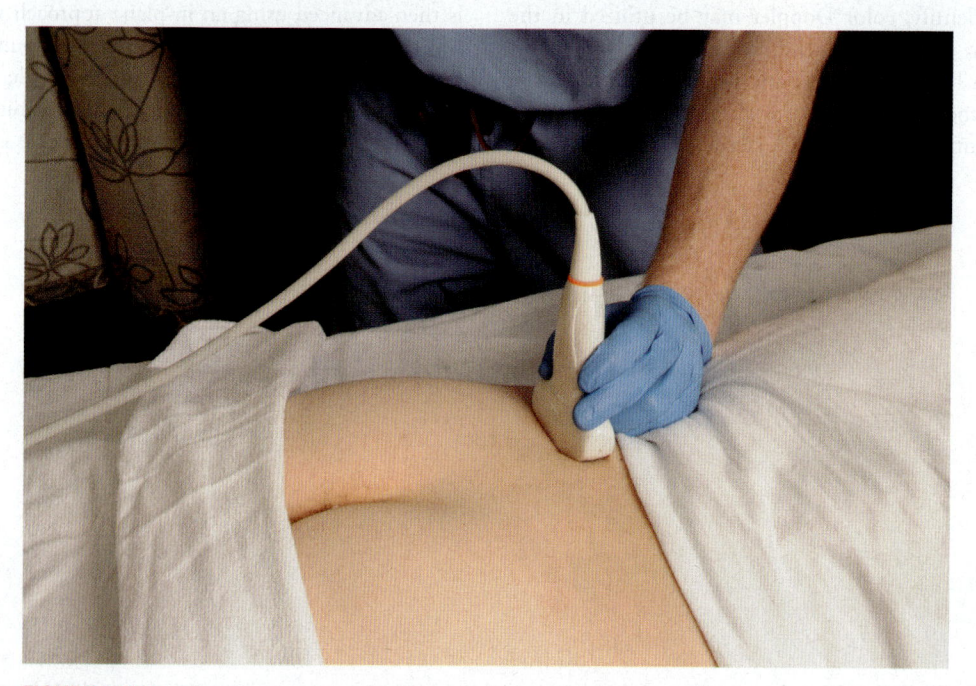

**FIGURE 116.10.** Proper transverse placement of the low-frequency curvilinear ultrasound transducer over the posterior superior iliac spine for ultrasound-guided injection of piriformis syndrome.

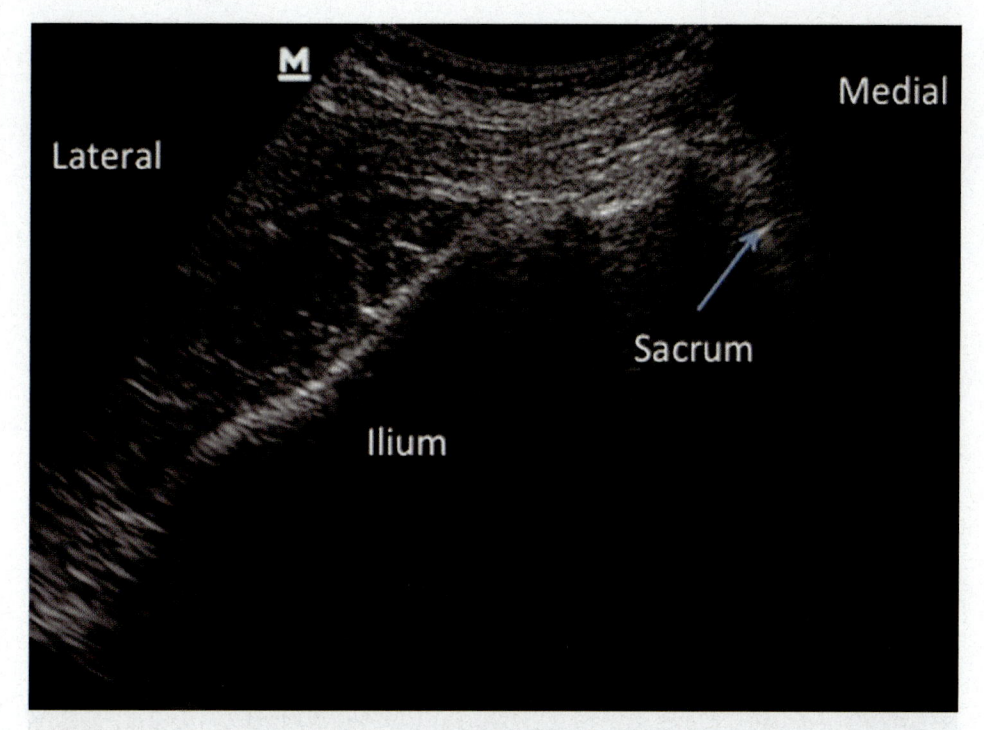

**FIGURE 116.11.** Transverse ultrasound view demonstrating the sacrum medially and S-shaped ilium laterally.

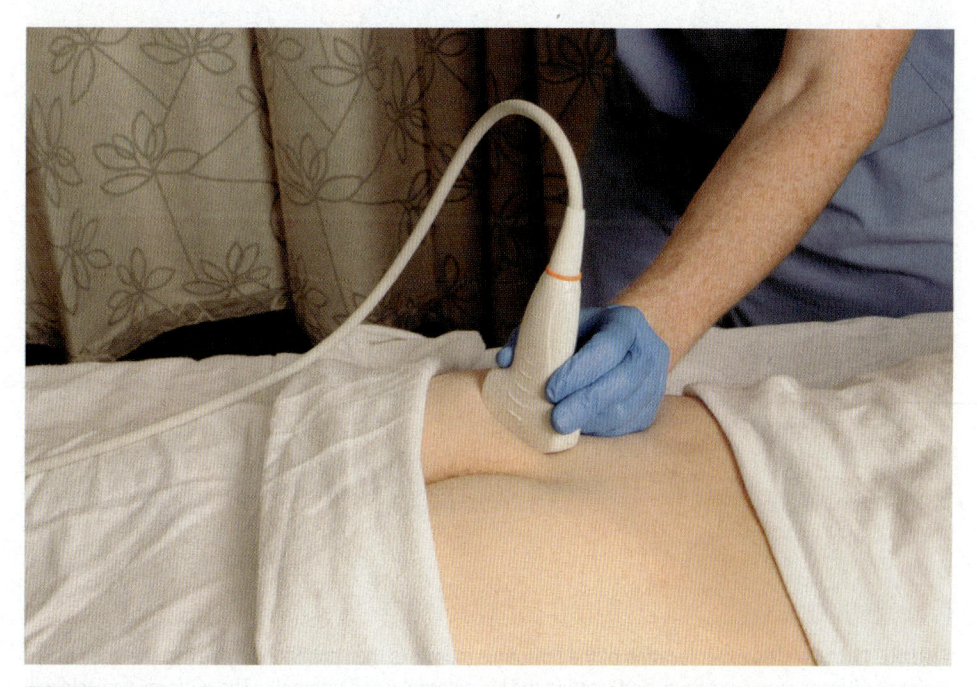

**FIGURE 116.12.** The low-frequency curvilinear ultrasound transducer is rotated counterclockwise 25 degrees to place the ultrasound beam parallel to the piriformis muscle.

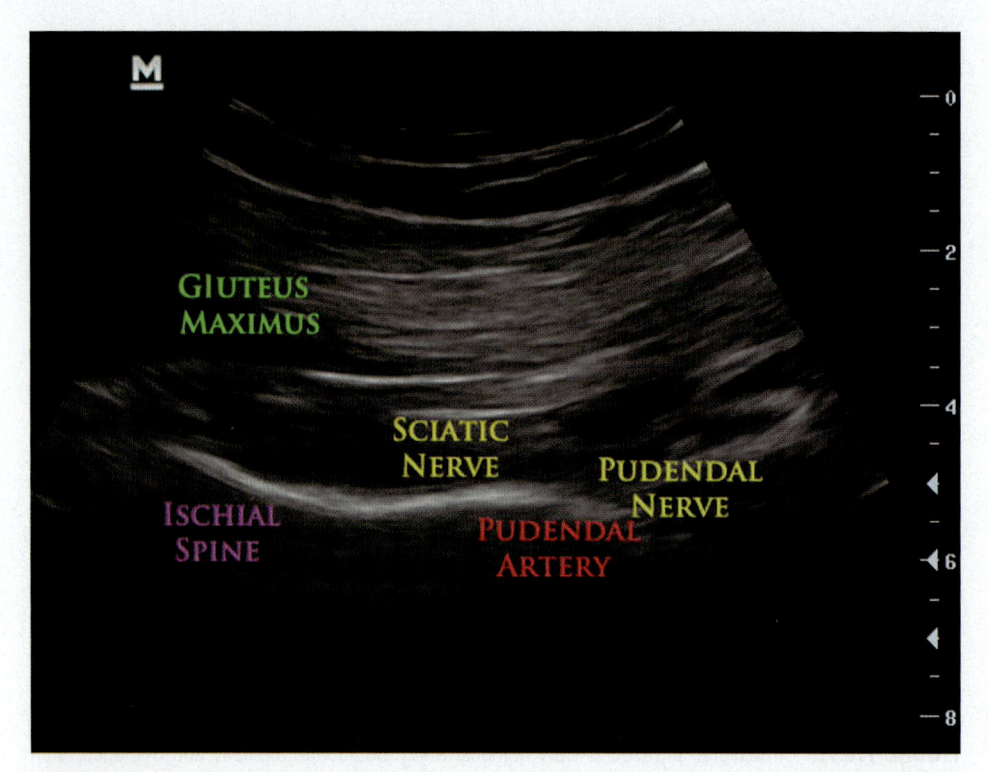

**FIGURE 116.13.** Transverse ultrasound image demonstrating the gluteus maximus muscle lying above the piriformis muscle.

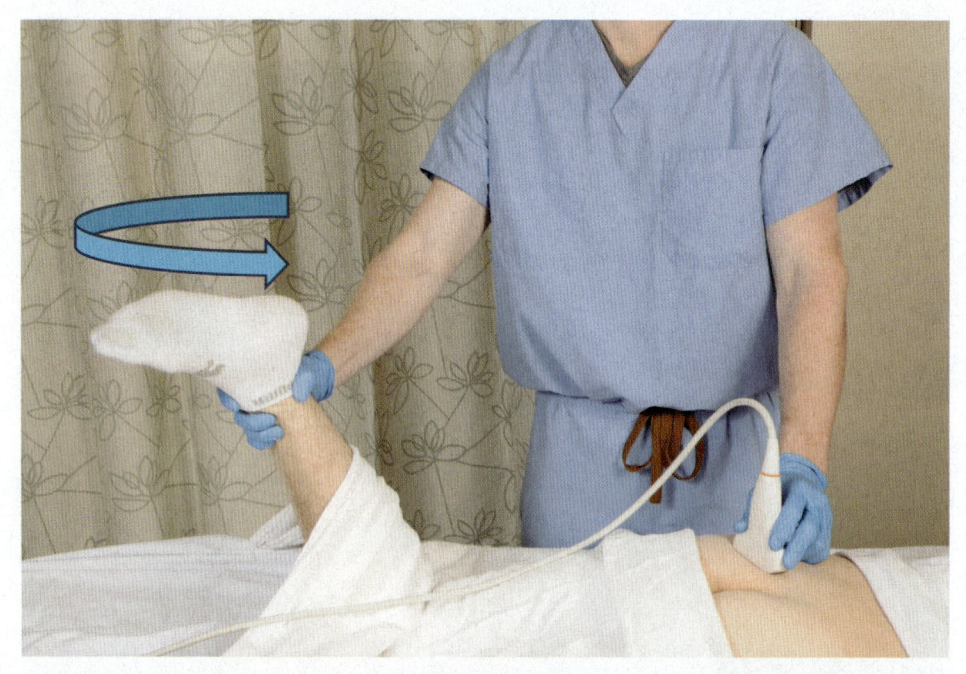

**FIGURE 116.14.** The exact location of the piriformis muscle is then confirmed by flexing the knee of the patient's affected lower extremity and rotating the hip externally and internally. The piriformis muscle will be clearly seen to slide back and forth beneath the gluteus maximus muscle.

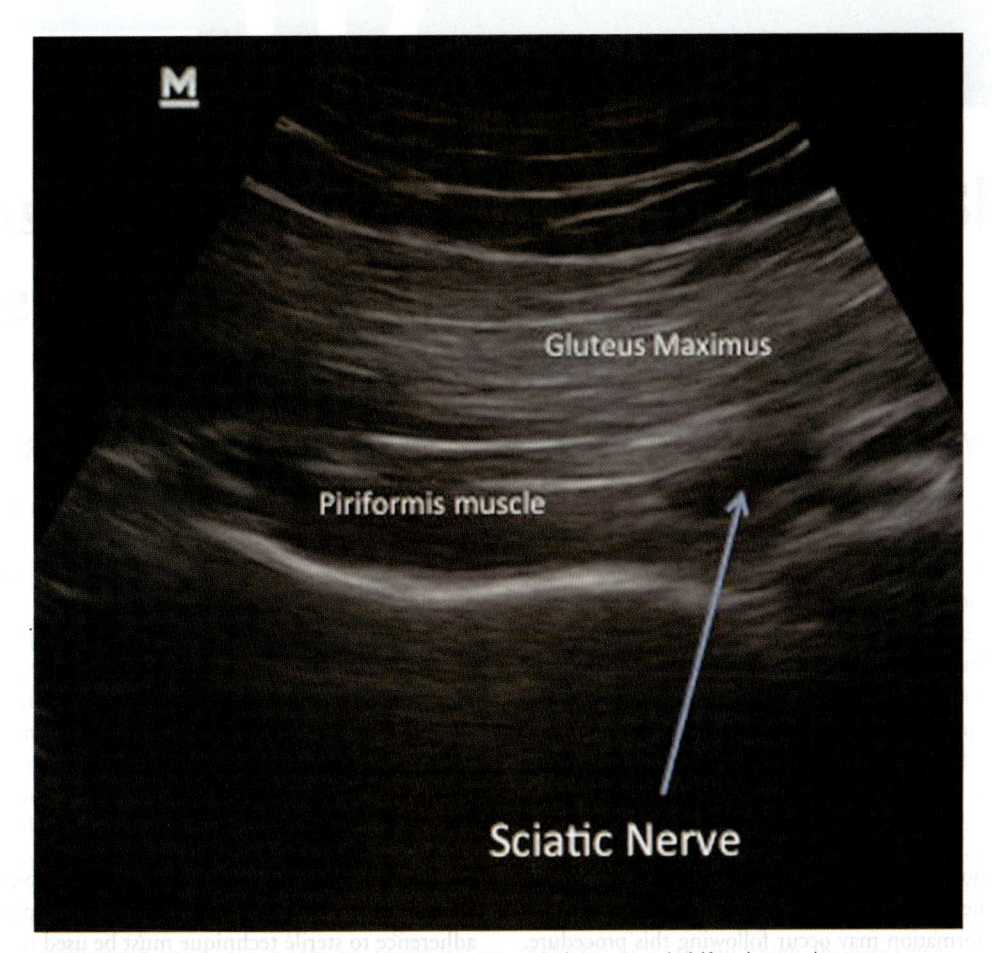

**FIGURE 116.15.** Transverse ultrasound image of the sciatic nerve and piriformis muscle.

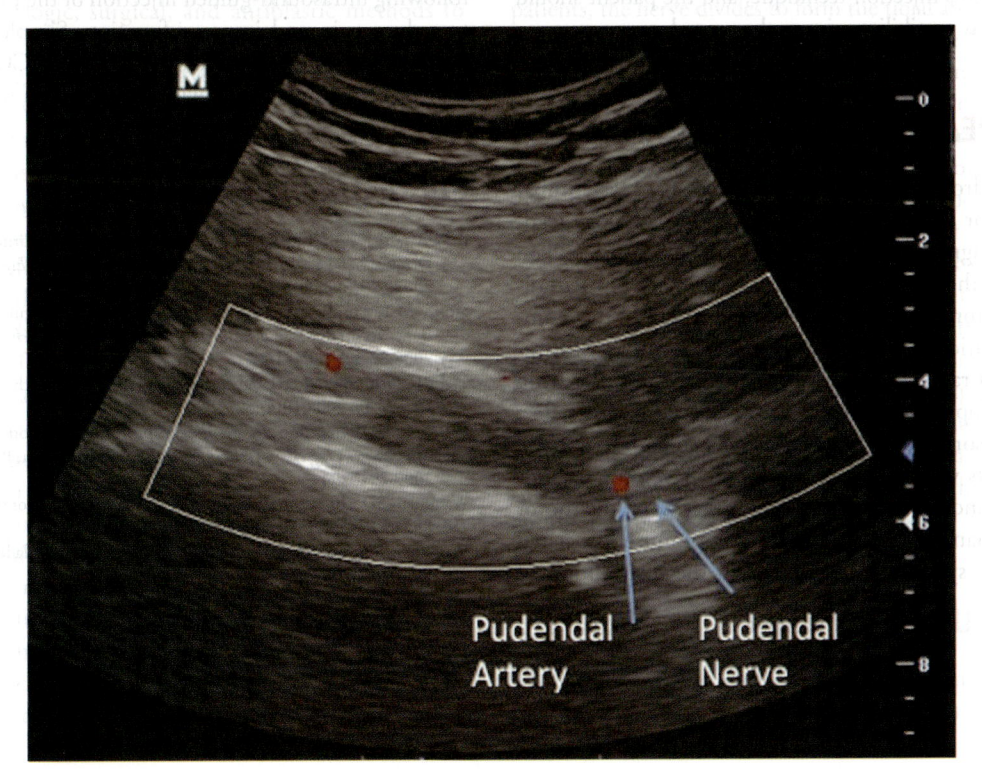

**FIGURE 116.16.** Transverse color Doppler image demonstrating the pudendal artery, which lies medial to the sciatic nerve.

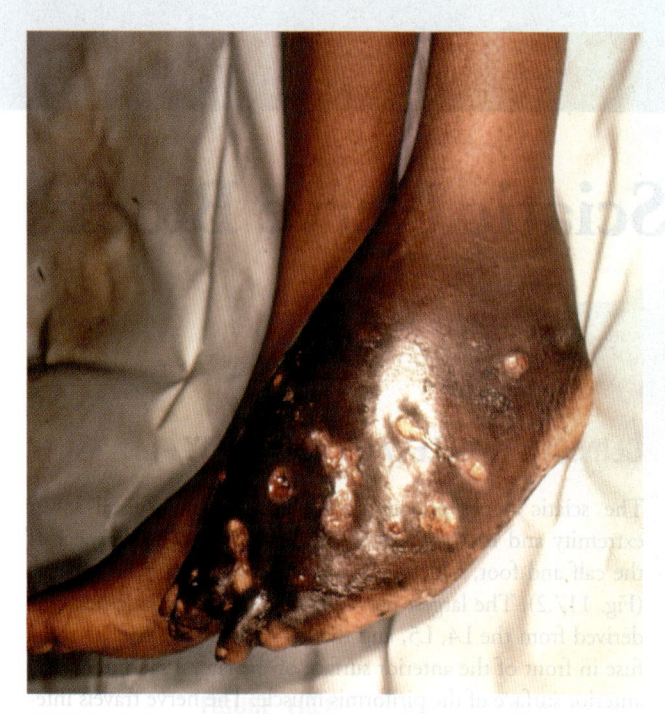

**FIGURE 117.1.** Mycetoma of the foot requiring amputation. (From Rubin E, Farber JL. *Pathology*. 3rd ed. Philadelphia, PA: Lippincott Williams & Wilkins; 1999, with permission.)

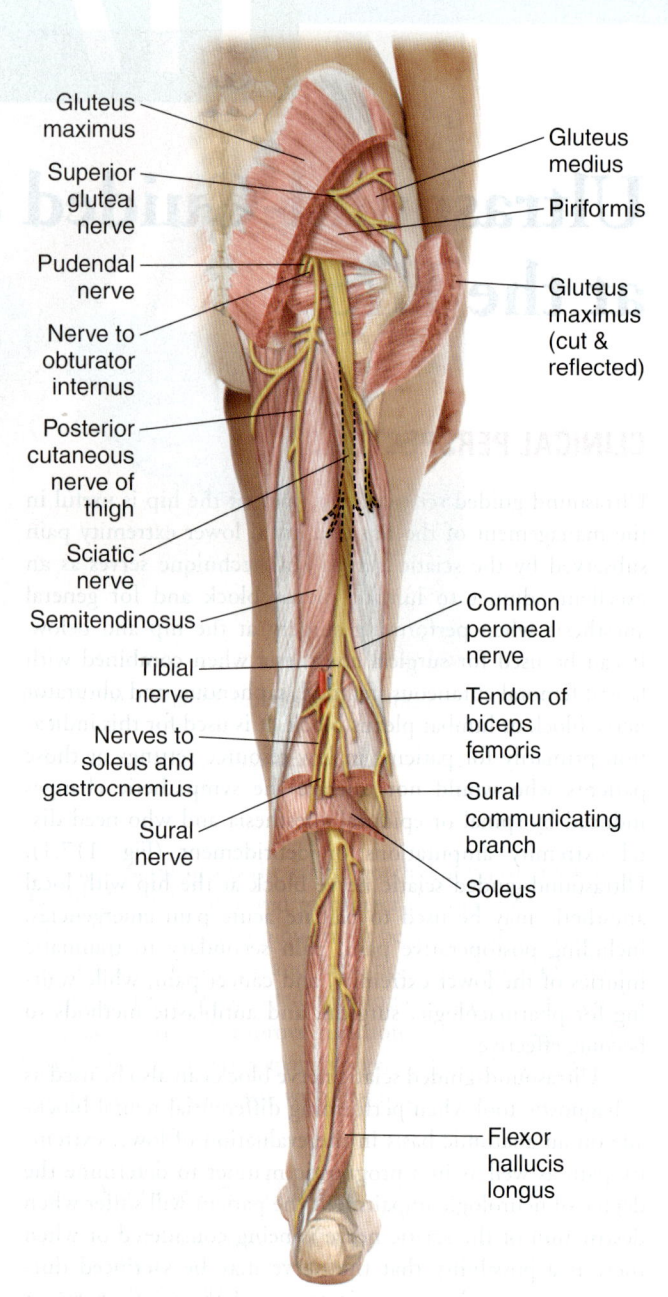

**FIGURE 117.2.** The anatomy of the sciatic nerve. (From Bucci C. *Condition-Specific Massage Therapy*. Baltimore, MD: Lippincott Williams & Wilkins; 2012, with permission.)

patient is then placed in the modified Sims position (Fig. 117.4). With the patient in the above position, the posterior superior iliac spine and the ischial tuberosity are identified, and an imaginary line is drawn between the two points (Fig. 117.5). At the level of the patient's coccyx, a high-frequency linear ultrasound transducer is placed on the line in a transverse plane, and an ultrasound survey scan is taken (Fig. 117.6). The sacrum and ischial bone are identified as a curved hyperechoic structures (Fig. 117.7). The sciatic nerve is visualized as a flattened hyperechoic structure lying between the hyperechoic curves of the sacrum and ilium (see Fig. 117.7). Color Doppler is then utilized to identify vessels including the inferior gluteal artery that are in proximity to the sciatic nerve (Fig. 117.8). After the sciatic nerve is identified, the skin overlying the area beneath the ultrasound transducer is prepped with antiseptic solution. A sterile syringe containing 10.0 mL of 0.25% preservative-free bupivacaine is attached to a 3½-inch, 22-gauge needle using strict aseptic technique. If the painful condition being treated is thought to have an inflammatory component, 40 to 80 mg of depot steroid is added to the local anesthetic. The needle is placed through the skin ~1 cm above the superior edge of the transducer and is then advanced using an in-plane approach with the needle trajectory adjusted under real-time ultrasound guidance so that the needle tip rests within proximity but outside the substance of the sciatic nerve (Fig. 117.9). When the tip of needle is thought to be in satisfactory position, after careful aspiration, a small amount of local anesthetic and steroid is injected under real-time ultrasound guidance to confirm that the needle tip is not within the substance of the nerve. After proper needle tip placement is confirmed, the remainder of the contents of the syringe are slowly injected. There should be minimal resistance to injection, and the clinician should stop injecting immediately if the patient experiences any increase in pain during the injection procedure.

CHAPTER 117    ULTRASOUND-GUIDED SCIATIC NERVE BLOCK AT THE HIP    837

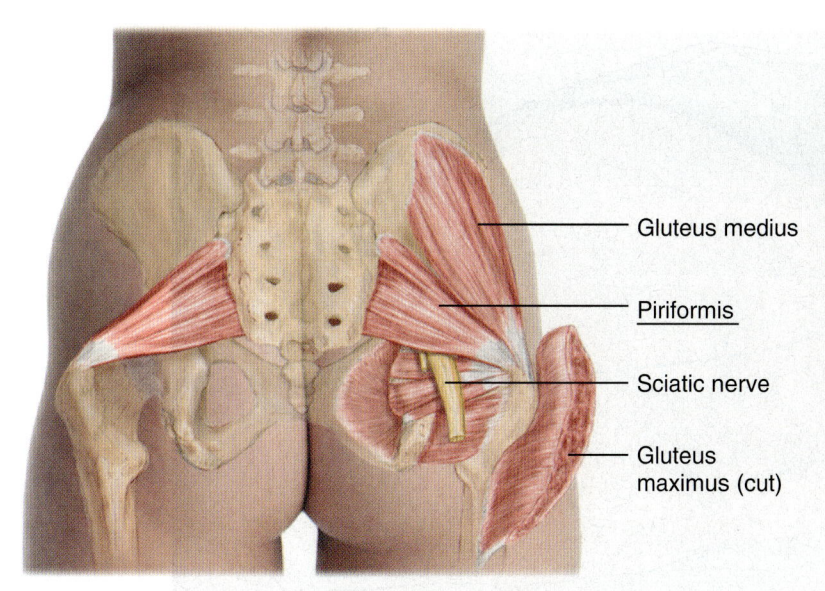

**FIGURE 117.3.** The sciatic nerve passes beneath or through the piriformis muscle where it is subject to compression or entrapment. (Adapted from Clay JH, Pounds DM. *Basic Clinical Massage Therapy: Integrating Anatomy and Treatment.* 2nd ed. Philadelphia, PA: Lippincott Williams & Wilkins; 2008, with permission.)

**PIRIFORMIS**

| | |
|---|---|
| Origin | Anterior surface of sacrum. |
| Insertion | Greater trochanter of the femur. |
| Action | Laterally rotate hip, abduct the flexed hip. |
| Nerve | L5–S2 nerve roots of sacral plexus. |

## COMPLICATIONS

Given the proximity of the sciatic nerve to the injection target of the belly of the piriformis muscle, the possibility of needle-induced trauma remains an ever-present possibility. This potentially disastrous complication can be greatly decreased if attention is paid to the sonographic anatomy and the needle is not placed until the sciatic nerve has been positively identified. Ecchymosis and hematoma formation may occur following this procedure. A transient exacerbation of the patient's pain occurs ~25% of the time following this injection technique, and the patient should be warned of this possibility prior to the procedure.

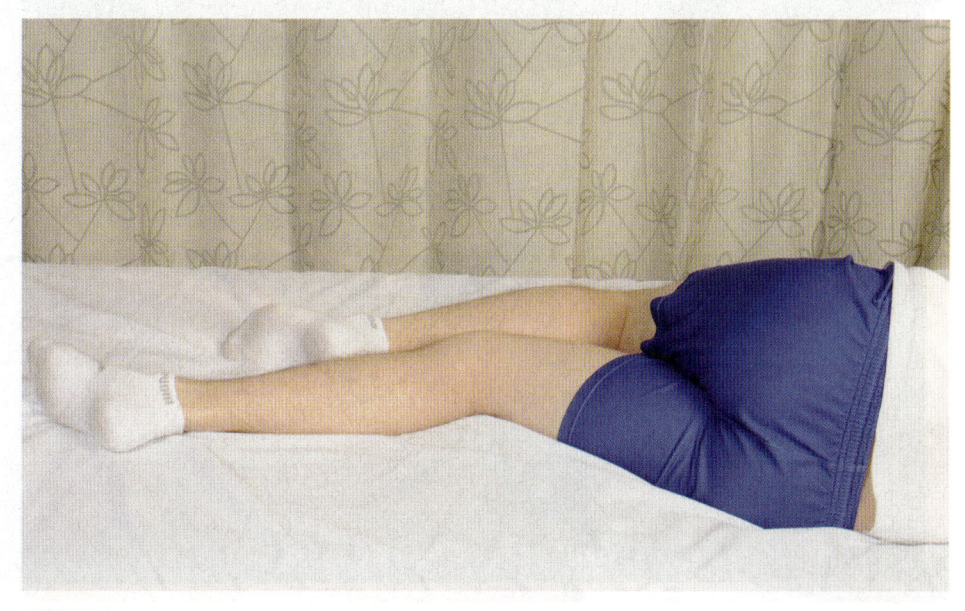

**FIGURE 117.4.** Proper patient positioning for ultrasound-guided injection of the sciatic nerve.

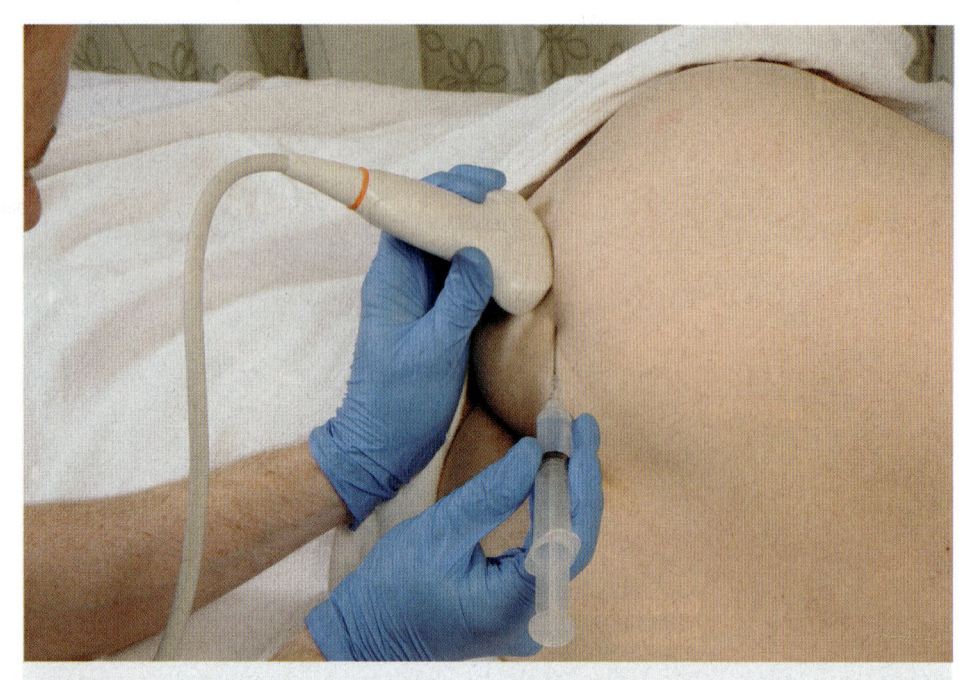

**FIGURE 117.9.** Proper needle placement for injection of the sciatic nerve at the hip under ultrasound guidance.

Furthermore, the motor and sensory changes associated with sciatic nerve compromise are limited to the distribution of the sciatic nerve below the sciatic notch. Universal precautions should always be observed to protect the operator, and strict adherence to sterile technique must be used to avoid infection. Gentle physical therapy and local heat should be introduced following ultrasound-guided injection of the sciatic nerve at the hip to reduce pain and improve function. Simple analgesics and nonsteroidal anti-inflammatory agents or COX-2 inhibitors may be used concurrently with this injection technique.

## SUGGESTED READINGS

Hodnett PA, Shelly MJ, MacMahon PJ, et al. MR imaging of overuse injuries of the hip. *Magn Reson Imag Clin N Am* 2009;17(4):667–679.

Waldman SD. Injection technique for sciatic nerve-posterior approach. In: *Atlas of Interventional Pain Management Techniques*. 3rd ed. Philadelphia, PA: Saunders Elsevier; 2009:534–538.

Waldman SD. Piriformis syndrome. In: *Pain Review*. Philadelphia, PA: Saunders Elsevier; 2009:310.

Waldman SD. The sciatic nerve. In: *Pain Review*. Philadelphia, PA: WB Saunders; 2009:138–139.

Waldman SD. Ischial bursitis. In: *Imaging of Pain*. Philadelphia, PA: WB Saunders; 2011:349–350.

CHAPTER 118

# Ultrasound-Guided Sacral Nerve Block

## CLINICAL PERSPECTIVES

Ultrasound-guided sacral nerve block is useful in the evaluation and management of radicular and perineal pain thought to be subserved by the sacral nerve. This technique serves as an excellent adjunct to caudal and epidural nerve block for surgical anesthesia. Ultrasound-guided sacral nerve block with local anesthetic may be used to palliate acute pain emergencies, including postoperative pain, pain secondary to traumatic injuries of the sacrum, and cancer pain, while waiting for pharmacologic, surgical, and antiblastic methods to become effective.

Ultrasound-guided sacral nerve block can also be used as a diagnostic tool when performing differential neural blockade on an anatomic basis in the evaluation of radicular or perineal pain as well as in a prognostic manner to determine the degree of neurologic impairment the patient will suffer when destruction of the sacral nerve or nerves is being considered or when there is a possibility that the nerve may be sacrificed during surgeries in the anatomic region of the sacral nerves. Ultrasound-guided sacral nerve block with local anesthetic and steroid is occasionally used in the treatment of sacral root or perineal pain when the pain is believed to be secondary to inflammation of the sacral nerve or when entrapment of the sacral nerve is suspected. Ultrasound-guided sacral nerve block with local anesthetic and steroid is also indicated in the palliation of pain associated with diabetic neuropathy and is useful in the treatment of bladder dysfunction after injury to the cauda equina. Destruction of the sacral nerves via this approach is occasionally used in the palliation of persistent perineal pain secondary to invasive tumor or bladder dysfunction that is mediated by the sacral nerves and has not responded to more conservative measures. The technique can also be utilized to identify the posterior sacral foramina for introduction of stimulating electrodes for bladder dysfunction.

Because of the potential for hematogenous spread via Batson plexus, local infection and sepsis represent absolute contraindications to ultrasound-guided sacral nerve block. Pilonidal cyst and congenital abnormalities of the dural sac and its contents also represent relative contraindications to this technique.

Plain radiographs of the sacrum and bony pelvis are indicated in all patients who present with sacral and perineal pain to identify occult bony pathology (Fig. 118.1). Based on the patient's clinical presentation, additional testing may be indicated, including complete blood cell count, sedimentation rate, and antinuclear antibody testing. Electrodiagnostic testing should be considered in all patients who suffer from sacral nerve dysfunction to provide both neuroanatomic and neurophysiologic information regarding nerve function. Magnetic resonance imaging and/or computerized tomographic scanning of the lumbar spine and the pelvis are also useful in determining the cause of sacral nerve compromise.

## CLINICALLY RELEVANT ANATOMY

The five sacral vertebrae are fused together to form the triangular-shaped sacrum (Fig. 118.2). The dorsally convex sacrum inserts in a wedge-like manner between the two iliac bones with superior articulations with the fifth lumbar vertebra and caudad articulations with the coccyx. On the anterior concave surface, there are four pairs of unsealed anterior sacral foramina that allow passage of the anterior rami of the upper four sacral nerves. The posterior sacral foramina are smaller than their anterior counterparts. Leakage of drugs injected into the sacral canal is effectively prevented by the sacrospinal and multifidus muscles. The vestigial bony remnants that are the result of the incomplete fusion of the inferior articular processes of the lower half of the S4 and all of the S5 vertebrae project downward on each side of the sacral hiatus (see Fig. 118.2). These bony projections are called the sacral cornua and represent important clinical landmarks when performing ultrasound-guided sacral nerve block. The U-shaped sacral hiatus is covered posteriorly by the sacrococcygeal ligament, which is also an important clinical landmark when performing ultrasound sacral nerve block. Penetration of the sacrococcygeal ligament provides direct access to the epidural space of the sacral canal. Although there are gender- and race-determined differences in the shape of the sacrum, they are of little importance relative to the ultimate ability to successfully perform sacral nerve block on a given patient.

841

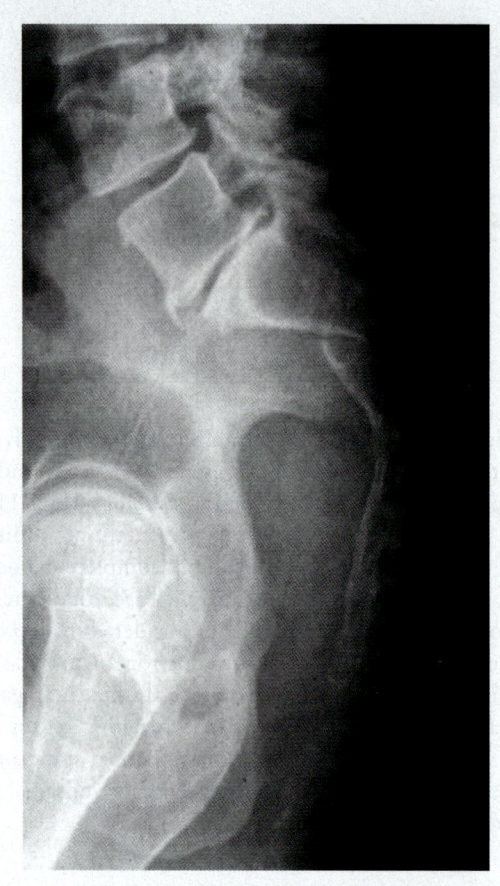

**FIGURE 118.1.** Lateral radiograph of a jumper's fracture of the sacrum. (Reused from Bucholz RW, Heckman JD. *Rockwood & Green's Fractures in Adults*. 5th ed. Philadelphia, PA: Lippincott Williams & Wilkins; 2001, with permission.)

## ULTRASOUND-GUIDED TECHNIQUE

The benefits, risks, and alternative treatments are explained to the patient and informed consent is obtained. Ultrasound-guided sacral nerve block can be carried out by placing the patient in the prone position with the patient's abdomen resting on a thin pillow (Fig. 118.3). To relax the gluteal muscles, the patient is asked to turn his or her heels outward (Fig. 118.4). A total of 16 mL of local anesthetic suitable for epidural administration is drawn up in a 20-mL sterile syringe. If the painful condition being treated is thought to have an inflammatory component, 40 to 80 mg of depot steroid is added to the local anesthetic. The skin overlying the sacrum is then prepped with antiseptic solution, and the medial sacral crest is palpated using a rocking motion (Fig. 118.5). A low-frequency curvilinear ultrasound transducer is then placed in the transverse plane over the superior medial sacral crest, and an ultrasound survey scan is taken (Fig. 118.6). The dorsal median sacral crest will be seen as a hyperechoic line that curves downward toward the sacral foramina in a shape reminiscent of baseball player Rollie Fingers' famous mustache (Figs. 118.7 and 118.8). After the median sacral crest is identified, the transversely placed ultrasound transducer is slowly moved caudally and laterally toward the affected side until the first dorsal sacral foramen is visualized (Fig. 118.9). The foramen will appear as a cone-shaped indentation of the dorsal surface of the sacrum. The ligament covering the foramina may be visible (see Fig. 118.9). Color Doppler may assist in identification of the sacral foramen by allowing identification of the foraminal branch of the lateral sacral artery, which exits the inferolateral aspect of each sacral foramina (Fig. 118.10).

After the first sacral foramen is identified, the transducer may be slowly moved caudally to identify the second to fourth dorsal foramina. Once the desired dorsal sacral foramen is identified, a 22- or 25-gauge, 3½-inch needle is inserted through the skin ~1 cm from the medial border of the transducer utilizing an in-plane approach and advanced into the medial portion of the dorsal sacral foramina under real-time ultrasound guidance until the entire needle tip rests just beyond the ligament within the caudal canal (Fig. 118.11). The medial portion of the foramina is preferable as the target of needle tip placement because the foraminal branch of the lateral sacral artery lies in the inferolateral aspect of each dorsal sacral foramina. As the ligamentous covering of the dorsal foramen is penetrated, a "pop" will be felt. If contact with the interior bony wall of the sacral canal occurs, the needle should be withdrawn slightly. This will disengage the needle tip from the periosteum. After gentle aspiration is negative for cerebrospinal fluid and blood, 2 mL of solution is injected. The needle is removed and pressure is placed on the injection site to avoid hematoma formation. The procedure can be repeated for each sacral nerve root to be injected.

## COMPLICATIONS

Because of potential hematogenous spread via the valveless venous plexus of the caudal space, sepsis and local infection at the injection site represent absolute contraindications to ultrasound-guided sacral nerve block. Although rare, inadvertent dural puncture can occur, and careful observation for spinal fluid must be carried out. Because the foraminal branch provided by the lateral sacral artery to each foramen entered the inferior lateral quadrant of each foramen, adjacent to the nerve root medially, the potential for intravascular injection remains ever present. This complication is increased in those patients with distended epidural veins, for example, the parturient and patients with large intra-abdominal tumor mass. If the misplacement is unrecognized, injection of local anesthetic directly into an epidural vein has the potential to result in local anesthetic toxicity. Needle-induced trauma to the foraminal branch of the lateral sacral artery may cause bleeding, which is usually

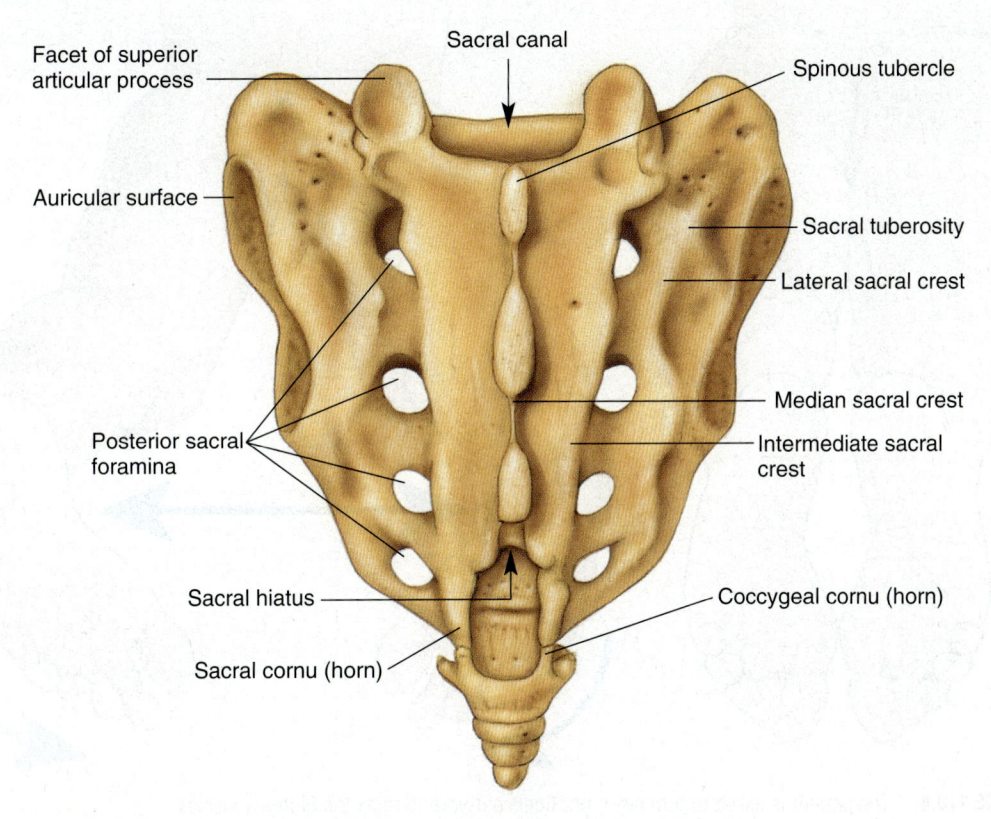

**FIGURE 118.2.** Dorsal anatomy of the sacrum. (Anatomical Chart Co., 2013.)

self-limited, but has the potential to cause increased postprocedure pain. Uncontrolled bleeding into the epidural space following sacral nerve block may result in epidural hematoma formation, which can cause compression of the spinal cord with the rapid development of paraplegia. Although the incidence of significant neurologic deficit secondary to epidural hematoma after sacral nerve block is exceedingly rare, this devastating complication should be considered in any patient with rapidly progressive neurologic deficits following this technique.

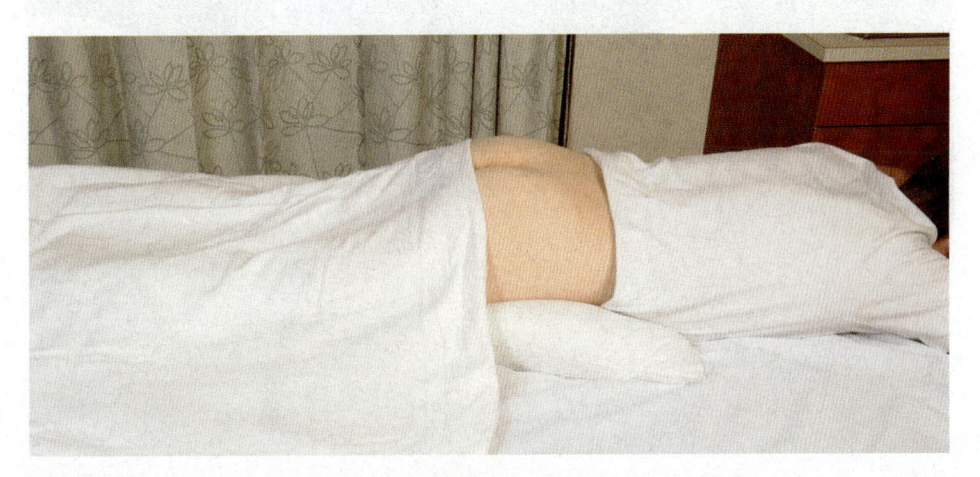

**FIGURE 118.3.** Proper patient position for ultrasound-guided sacral nerve block.

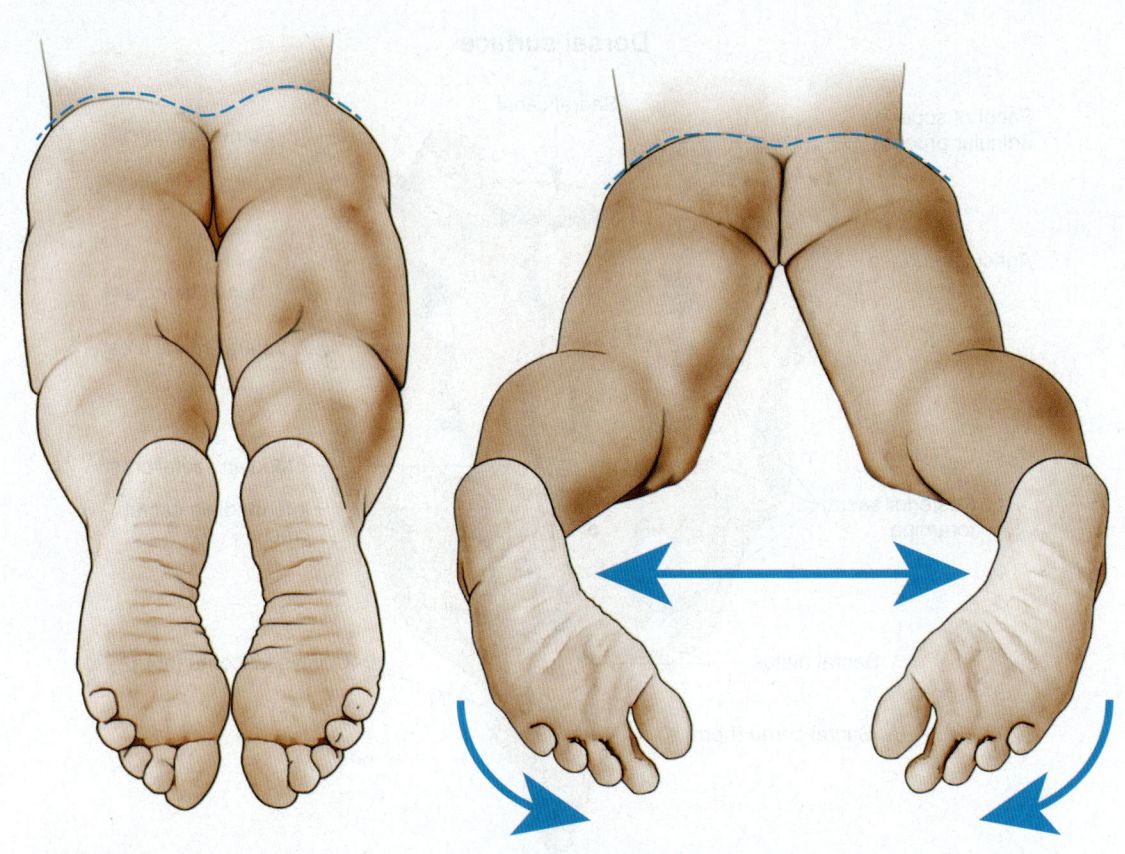

**FIGURE 118.4.** The patient is asked to turn his or her heels outward to relax the gluteal muscles.

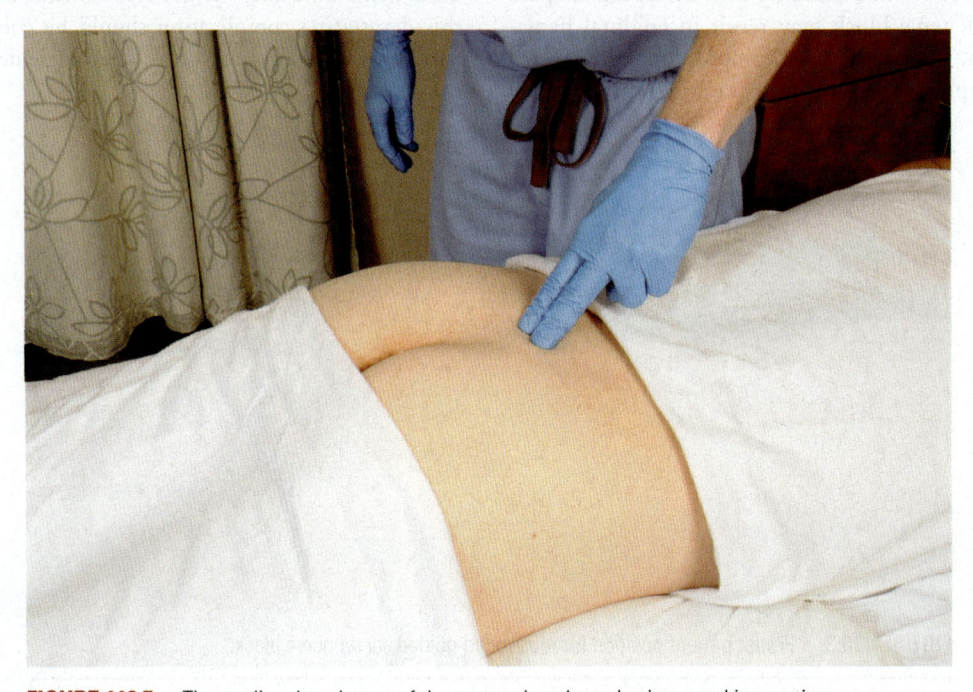

**FIGURE 118.5.** The median dorsal crest of the sacrum is palpated using a rocking motion.

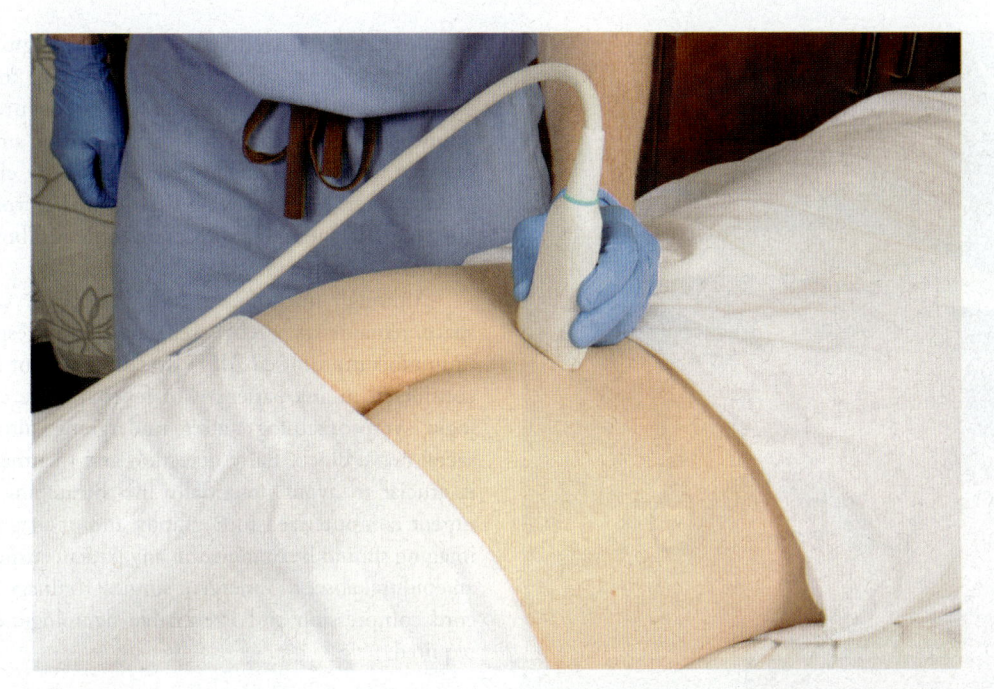

**FIGURE 118.6.** Proper transverse placement of the high-frequency ultrasound transducer for ultrasound-guided injection of the sacral nerve.

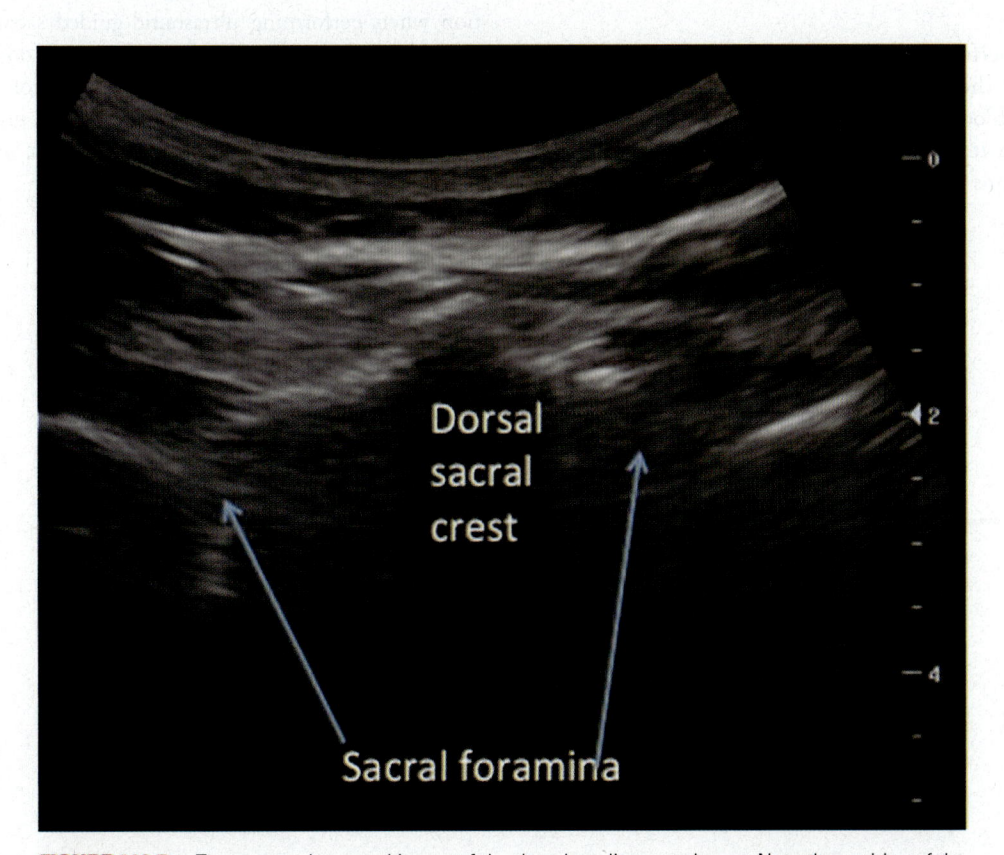

**FIGURE 118.7.** Transverse ultrasound image of the dorsal median sacral crest. Note the position of the sacral nerve between the sacrum and ilium.

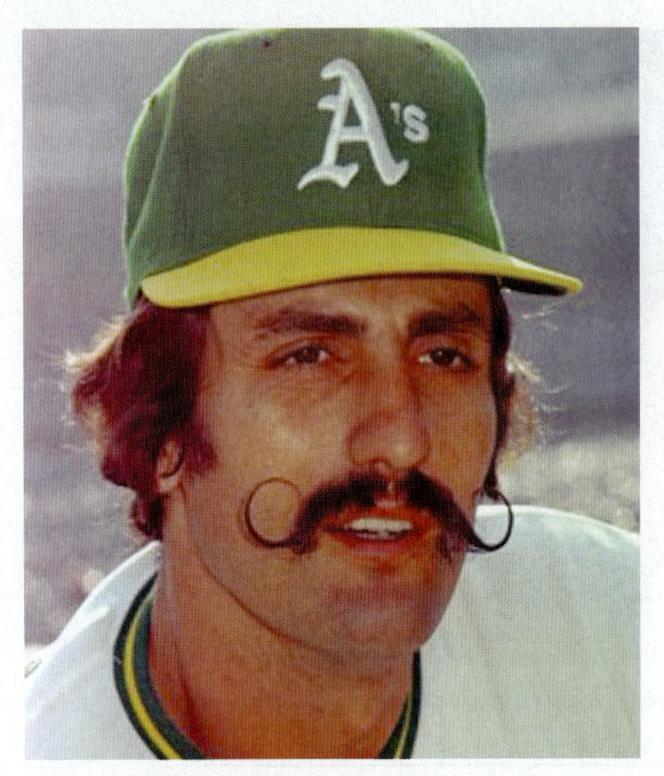

**FIGURE 118.8.** The hyperechoic curve of the dorsal median sacral crest is reminiscent of Rollie Fingers' famous mustache.

When performing ultrasound-guided sacral nerve block, should the aspiration test be positive for either spinal fluid or blood, the needle must be repositioned and the aspiration test repeated. If the test is negative, subsequent injections of 0.5-mL increments of local anesthetic are undertaken. Careful observation for signs of local anesthetic toxicity or subarachnoid spread of local anesthetic during the injection and after the procedure is indicated. Clinical experience has led to the use of smaller volumes of local anesthetic without sacrificing the clinical efficacy of sacral nerve blocks. The use of smaller volumes of local anesthetic has markedly decreased the number of local anesthetic related side effects.

Although uncommon, infection in the caudal epidural space remains an ever-present possibility, especially in the immunocompromised AIDS or cancer patient, and should be considered in any patient with fever and the onset of neurologic symptomatology after undergoing ultrasound-guided sacral nerve block. Early detection and treatment of infection is crucial to avoid potentially life-threatening sequelae, and urgent computerized tomography and/or magnetic resonance imaging should be obtained in any patient suspected of having an epidural abscess. Emergent surgical drainage to avoid spinal cord compression and irreversible neurologic deficit is often required.

## CLINICAL PEARLS

The key to performing successful ultrasound neuroaxial blocks is the proper identification of the sonographic anatomy. Any significant pain or sudden increase in resistance during injection when performing ultrasound-guided sacral nerve block suggests incorrect needle placement, and one should stop injecting immediately and reassess the position of the needle. Because pain is an important indication of improper needle placement, the practitioner should avoid the use of excessive sedation when performing this technique.

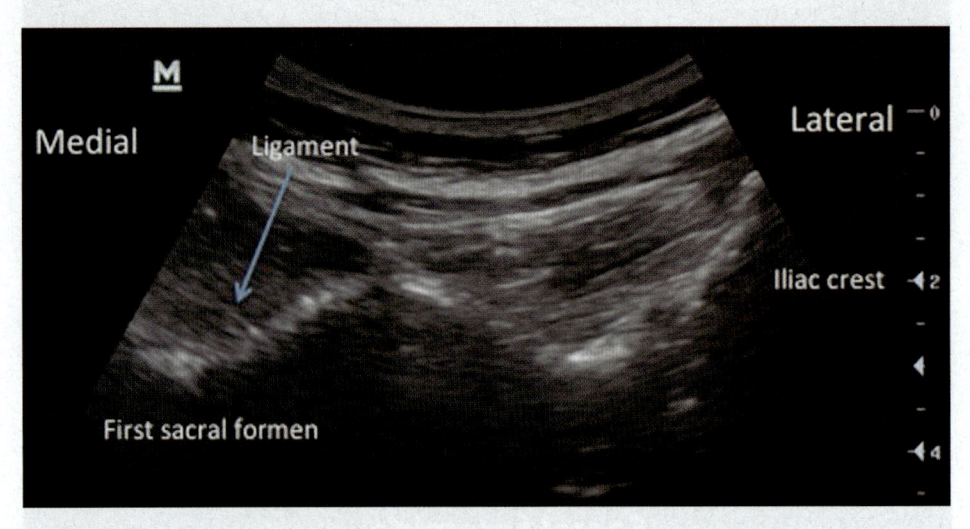

**FIGURE 118.9.** Transverse ultrasound view of the first sacral foramen.

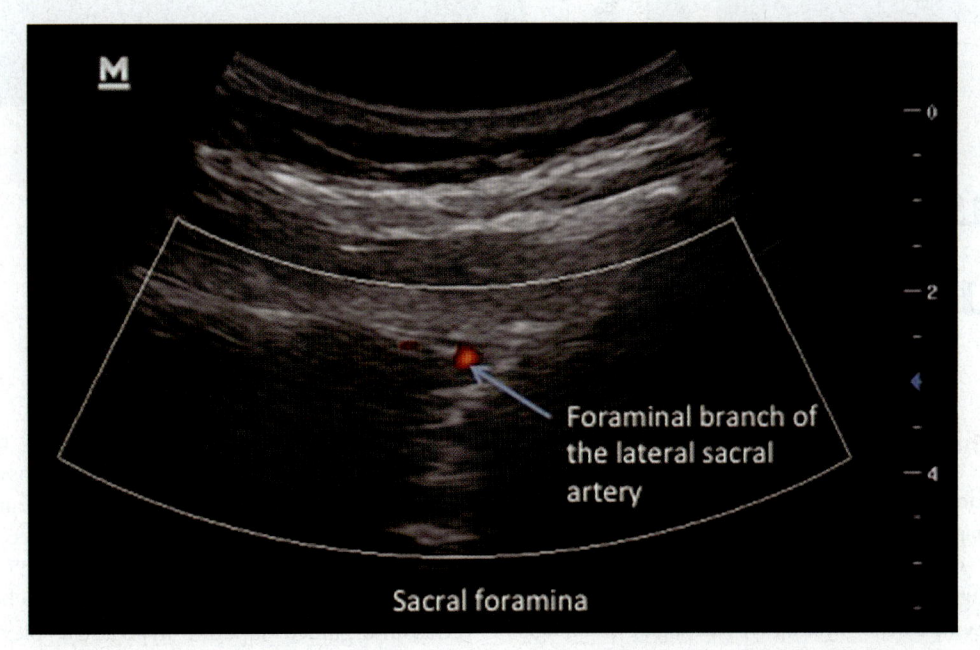

**FIGURE 118.10.** Transverse color Doppler image of the dorsal foraminal artery exiting the dorsal sacral foramen.

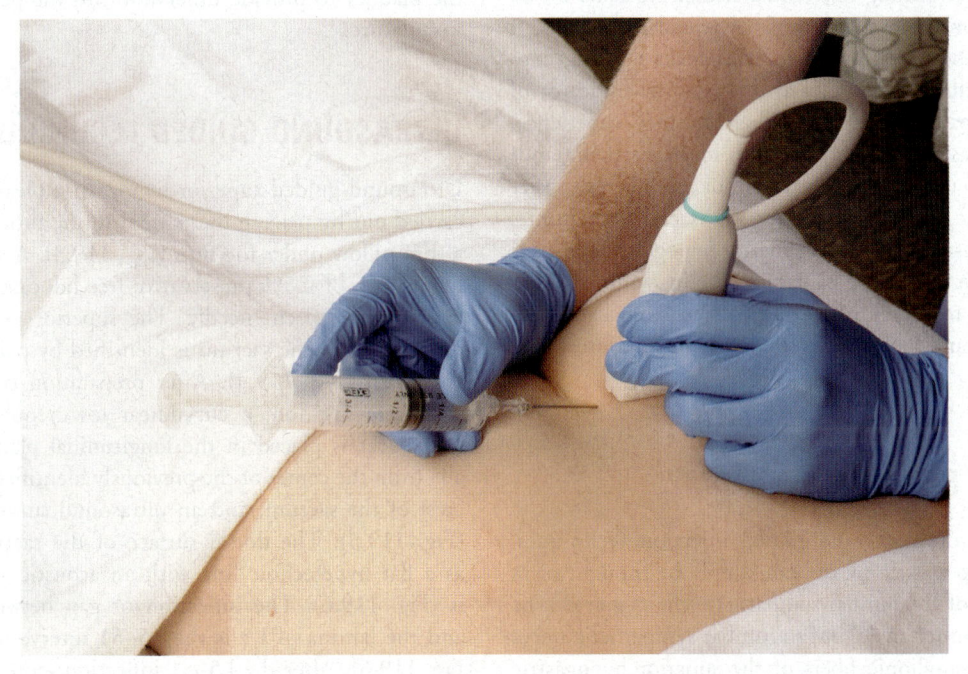

**FIGURE 118.11.** Proper needle position for injection of the sacral nerve under ultrasound guidance.

## SUGGESTED READINGS

McGrath MC, Jeffery R, Stringer MD. The dorsal sacral rami and branches: sonographic visualisation of their vascular signature. *Int J Osteopath Med* 2012;15(1):3–12.

Vydyanathan A, Narouze S. Ultrasound-guided caudal and sacroiliac joint injections. *Tech Reg Anesth Pain Manage* 2009;13(3):157–160.

Waldman SD. Injection technique for sacral nerve block: trans-sacral approach. In: *Atlas of Interventional Pain Management Techniques*. 3rd ed. Philadelphia, PA: Saunders Elsevier; 2009:462–466.

Waldman SD. Sacral nerve block. In: *Pain Review*. Philadelphia, PA: Saunders Elsevier; 2009:536–537.

# CHAPTER 119

# Ultrasound-Guided Hypogastric Plexus Block

## CLINICAL PERSPECTIVES

Ultrasound-guided superior hypogastric plexus block is useful in the diagnosis and treatment of a variety of painful sympathetically mediated painful conditions of the pelvic viscera including pain secondary to malignancy, endometriosis, reflex sympathetic dystrophy, causalgia, proctalgia fugax, and radiation enteritis. Superior hypogastric plexus block is also useful in the palliation of tenesmus secondary to radiation therapy to the rectum. Superior hypogastric plexus block with local anesthetic can be used as a diagnostic tool when performing differential neural blockade on an anatomic basis in the evaluation of pelvic and rectal pain. If destruction of the superior hypogastric plexus is being considered, this technique is useful as a prognostic indicator of the degree of pain relief that the patient may experience. Superior hypogastric plexus block with local anesthetic and/or steroid is also useful in the treatment of acute herpes zoster and postherpetic neuralgia involving the sacral dermatomes (Fig. 119.1). Destruction of the superior hypogastric plexus is a reasonable next step in the palliation of pain syndromes that have responded to superior hypogastric plexus blockade with local anesthetic and have not responded to more conservative measures.

## CLINICALLY RELEVANT ANATOMY

In the context of ultrasound-guided injection techniques, the superior hypogastric plexus can simply be thought of as a continuation of the lumbar sympathetic chain that can be blocked in a manner analogous to lumbar sympathetic nerve block. The preganglionic fibers of the superior hypogastric plexus find their origin primarily in the lower thoracic and upper lumbar region of the spinal cord. These preganglionic fibers interface with the lumbar sympathetic chain via the white communicantes. Postganglionic fibers exit the lumbar sympathetic chain and, together with fibers from the parasympathetic sacral ganglion, make up the superior superior hypogastric plexus. The superior hypogastric plexus lies in front of L4 as a coalescence of sympathetic nerve fibers. As these fibers descend, at a level of L5, they begin to divide into the hypogastric nerves following in close proximity the iliac vessels (Fig. 119.2). As the hypogastric nerves continue their lateral and inferior course, they are accessible for neural blockade as they pass in front of the L5–S1 interspace, which is the key sonographic landmark when performing ultrasound-guided superior hypogastric plexus block. The hypogastric nerves pass inferiorly from this point, following the concave curve of the sacrum and passing on each side of the rectum to form the inferior hypogastric plexus. These nerves continue their downward course along each side of the bladder to provide innervation to the pelvic viscera and vasculature.

## ULTRASOUND-GUIDED TECHNIQUE

Ultrasound-guided superior hypogastric plexus block can be carried out by placing the patient in the prone position with a thin pillow under the hips (Fig. 119.3). A syringe containing 18 mL of 0.5% preservative-free lidocaine is attached to a 22-gauge, 13-cm needle. The superior extent of median dorsal crest of the sacrum is identified by palpation as is the iliac crest (Fig. 119.4). After preparation of the skin with antiseptic solution, a curvilinear low-frequency ultrasound transducer is placed in the longitudinal plane ~3 cm laterally from the center of the previously identified median dorsal crest of the sacrum, and an ultrasound survey scan is taken (Fig. 119.5). The dorsal surface of the sacrum will appear as a flat hyperechoic line with an acoustic shadow beneath it (Fig. 119.6). The inflection or gap between the sacrum and the lamina of L5 is the L5–S1 intervertebral space (see Fig. 119.6). After the L5–S1 inflection representing the L5–S1 interspace is identified, the longitudinally placed transducer is slowly moved cephalad until the L4–L5 interspace is visualized (see Fig. 119.6). After satisfactory identification of the L4–L5 interspace, the ultrasound transducer is turned 90 degrees to the transverse plane, and another ultrasound survey scan is taken (Fig. 119.7). Note that the transverse processes block ultrasound visualization of the lateral margin of the vertebral body (Figs. 119.8 and 119.9). Once the transverse process is identified, the ultrasound transducer is slowly moved in a cephalad direction to identify the acoustic window between two adjacent transverse processes (Fig. 119.10). Once the acoustic window between the adjacent transverse processes is identified, the lateral aspect of the ultrasound transducer is rocked laterally to identify the lateral margin of the vertebral body and the adjacent psoas muscle (Figs. 119.11 to 119.13). A color Doppler image is then obtained to identify adjacent vasculature to avoid inadvertent intravascular injection (Fig. 119.14).

Once the lateral border of the vertebral body is identified, the needle is advanced under real-time ultrasound guidance utilizing an in-plane approach from the lateral aspect of the transversely placed ultrasound transducer until the needle rests against the anterolateral margin of the vertebral body (Fig. 119.15). The needle is redirected slightly laterally so that the needle tip can slide off the anterolateral margin of the vertebral body and ultimately rest just in front of this body landmark in proximity to the sympathetic chain. Injection of a small amount of solution to demonstrate hydrodissection is utilized to identify the exact location of the needle tip. After satisfactory placement of the needle tip is confirmed, gentle aspiration for blood and cerebrospinal fluid is carried out. The solution is then injected in small aliquots while the patient is closely observed for signs of local anesthetic toxicity or inadvertent epidural, subdural, or subarachnoid injection. The needle is removed and pressure is placed on the injection site to avoid hematoma formation. In patients who have not undergone previous abdominopelvic surgery or radiation, placement of a single needle is often adequate as the injectate will flow to the contralateral side of the presacral space. If pain relief is not complete on the contralateral side, this technique can be repeated on the side contralateral to the one that was previously blocked.

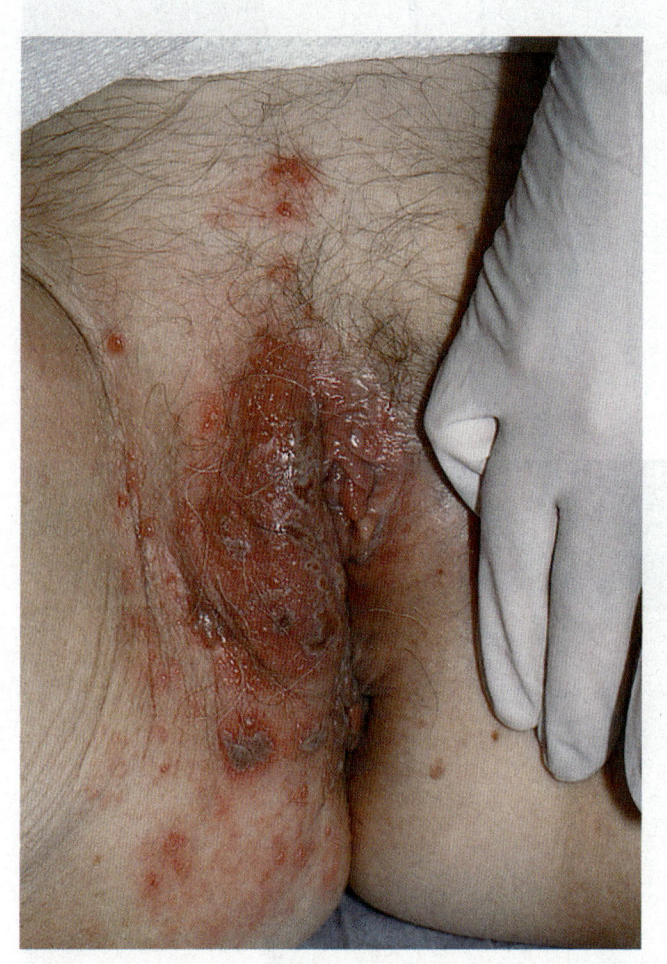

**FIGURE 119.1.** Ultrasound-guided superior superior hypogastric plexus block is useful in the management of the pain of acute herpes zoster involving the sacral dermatomes. (Reused from Goodheart HP. *Goodheart's Photoguide of Common Skin Disorders*. 2nd ed. Philadelphia, PA: Lippincott Williams & Wilkins; 2003, with permission.)

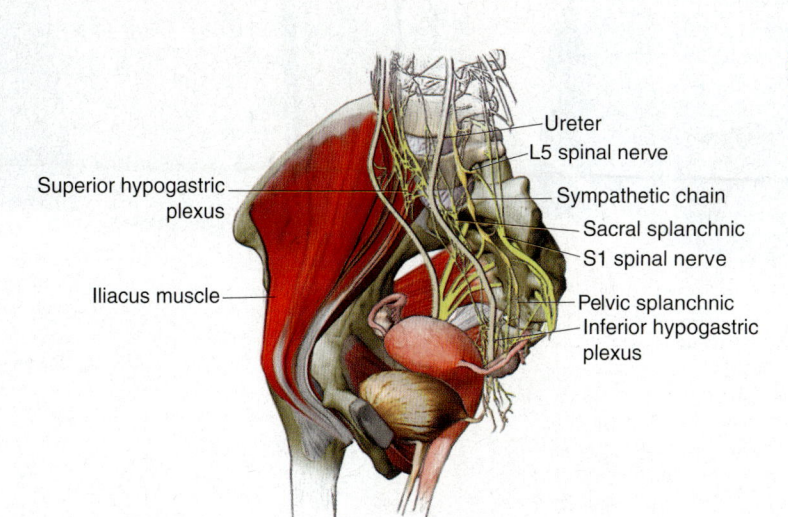

**FIGURE 119.2.** The superior superior hypogastric plexus lies in front of the L5–S1 interspace.

**FIGURE 119.3.** Proper prone patient position for ultrasound-guided superior hypogastric plexus block.

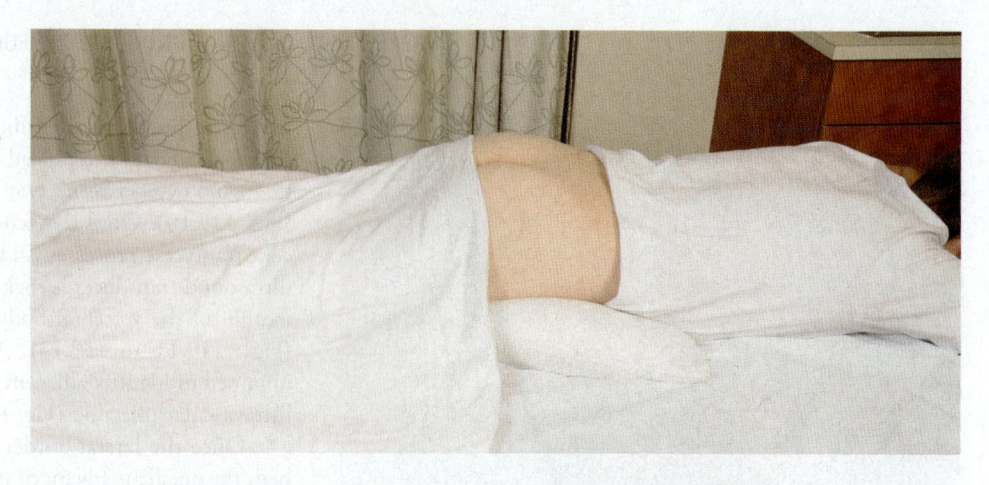

**FIGURE 119.4.** Palpation of the superior extent of the dorsal median sacral crest.

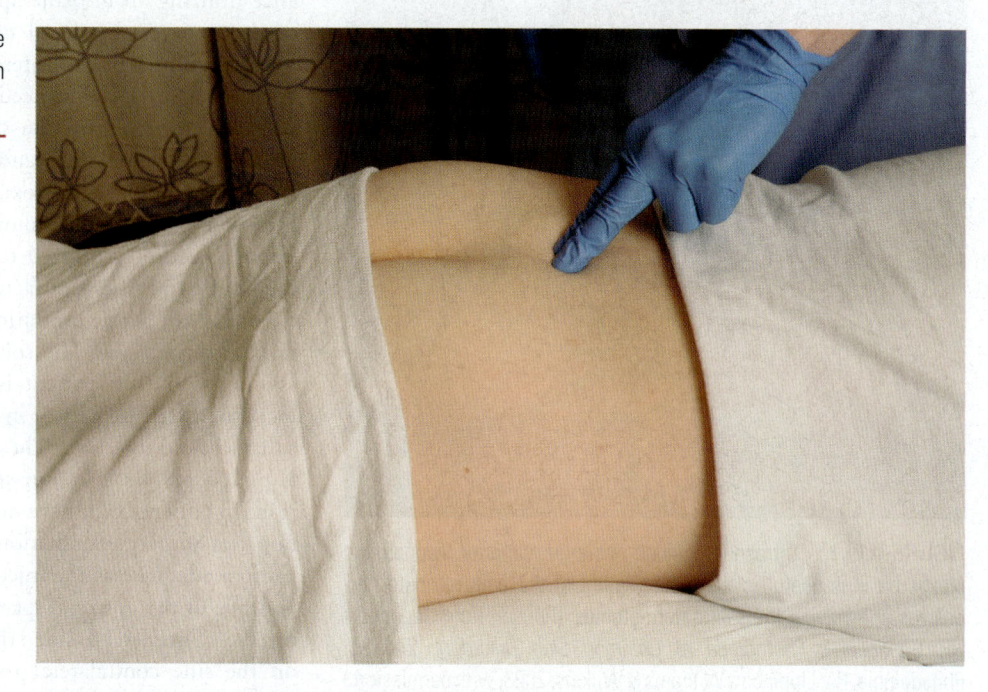

**FIGURE 119.5.** Longitudinal placement of the low-frequency curvilinear ultrasound transducer plane 3 cm lateral to midline at level of the superior extent dorsal median crest.

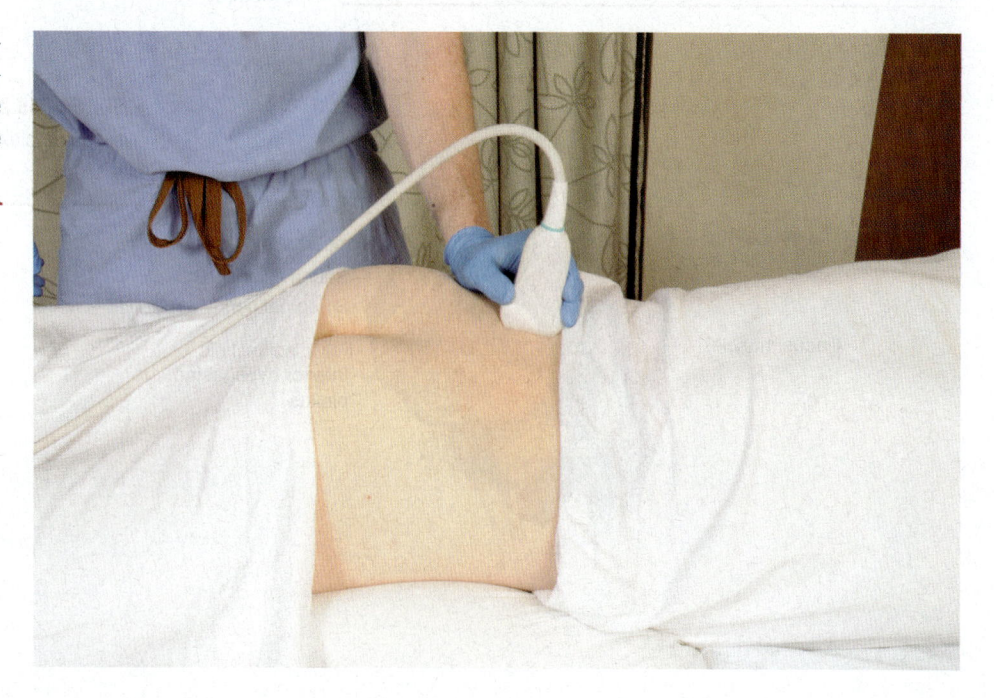

**FIGURE 119.6.** Longitudinal ultrasound image demonstrating the dorsal surface of the sacrum, which appears as a flat hyperechoic line with an acoustic shadow beneath it. The inflection or gap between the sacrum and the lamina of L5 is the L5–S1 intervertebral space.

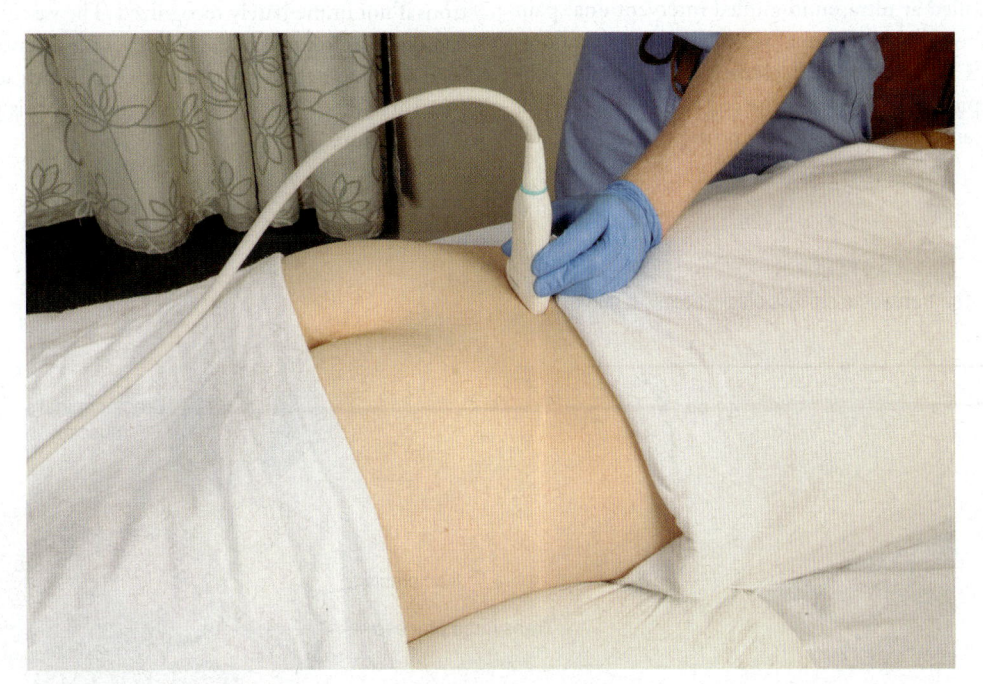

**FIGURE 119.7.** Proper paramedian transverse placement of the ultrasound transducer to visualize the L4–L5 interspace.

**FIGURE 119.8.** Transverse ultrasound view demonstrating transverse process.

## COMPLICATIONS

The superior hypogastric plexus chain is in close proximity to the cauda equine and exiting nerve roots, and this procedure should be performed only by those well versed in the regional anatomy and skilled at ultrasound-guided interventional pain management procedures. Trauma to the exiting lumbosacral nerve roots as well as inadvertent subarachnoid, subdural, and/or epidural injection can occur even in the best of hands. Inadvertent dural puncture occurring during superior hypogastric plexus block should rarely occur if attention is paid to the technical aspects of this procedure. However, failure to recognize an unintentional dural or subdural injection can result in immediate total spinal anesthesia with associated loss of consciousness, hypotension, and apnea. This can be disastrous if not immediately recognized. The vascular nature of this anatomic region makes the potential for intravascular injection high although the use of color Doppler to identify vascular structures should help the clinician avoid this potentially fatal complication.

**FIGURE 119.9.** The transverse process blocks access to the lumbar plexus.

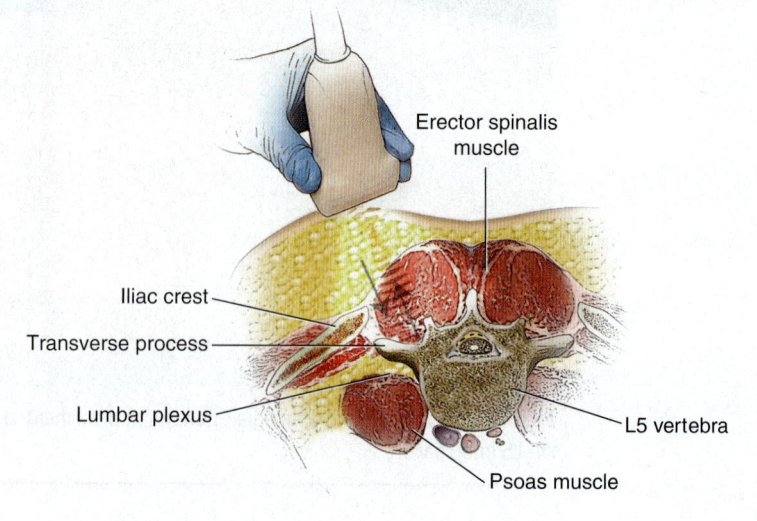

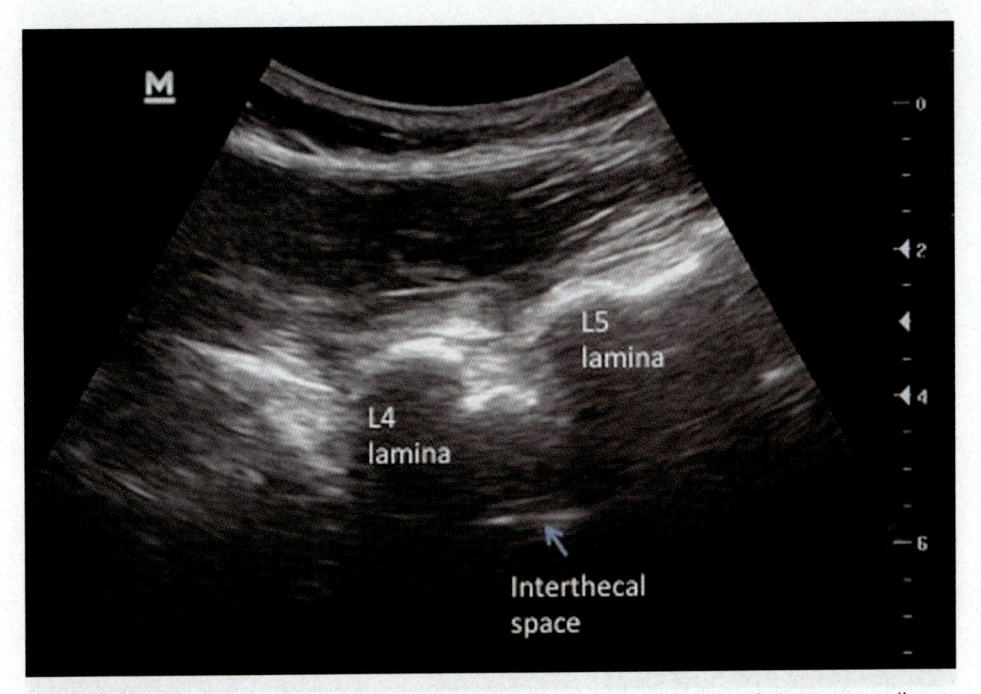

**FIGURE 119.10.** Transverse ultrasound image demonstrating acoustic window between two adjacent transverse processes.

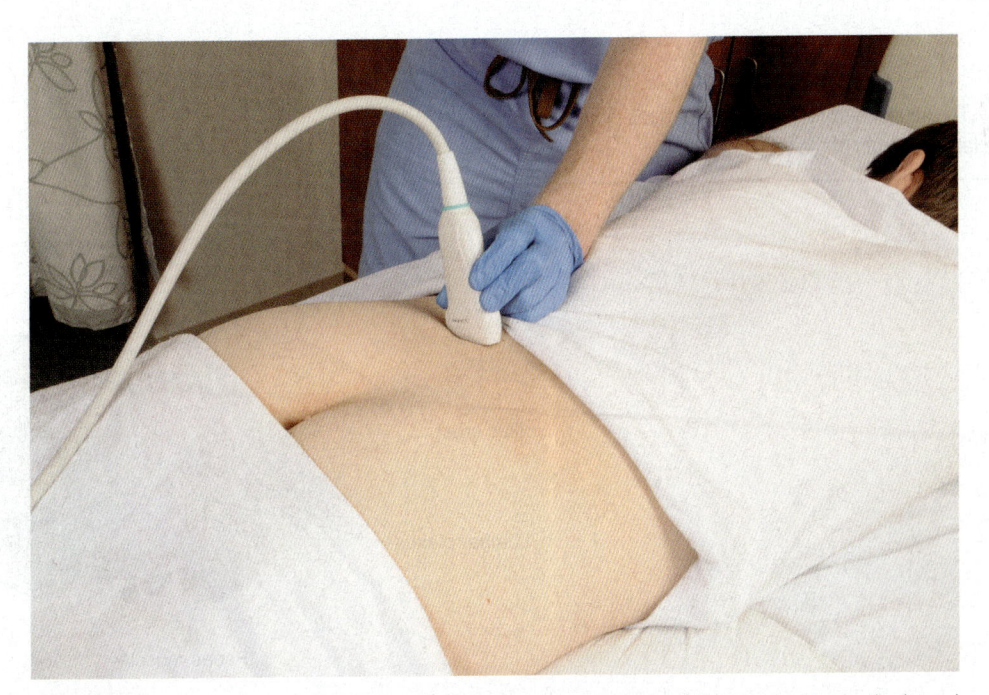

**FIGURE 119.11.** To obtain an ultrasound image of the lateral aspect of the vertebral body, the lateral aspect of the ultrasound transducer is rocked laterally to "see" around the posterior elements of the vertebra.

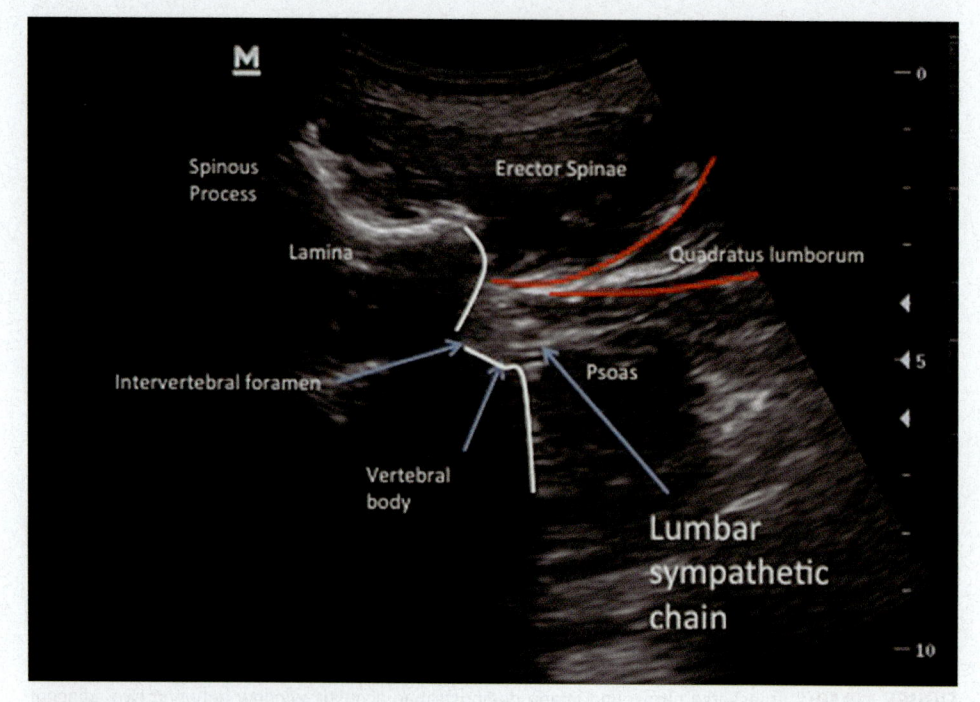

**FIGURE 119.12.** Transverse ultrasound view with transducer rocked laterally to visualize the lateral margin of the vertebral body and the lumbar plexus lying adjacent to it embedded in the psoas muscle.

**FIGURE 119.13.** The lumbar plexus lies within the psoas muscle just lateral to the lateral margin of the vertebral body.

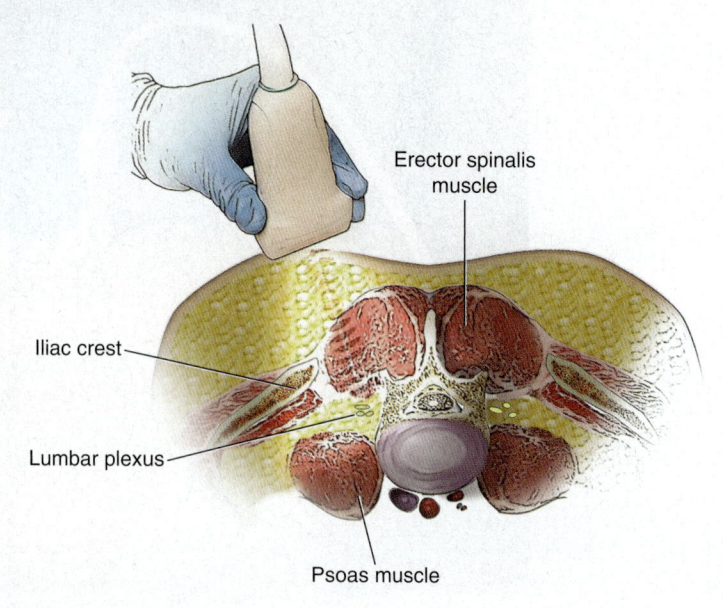

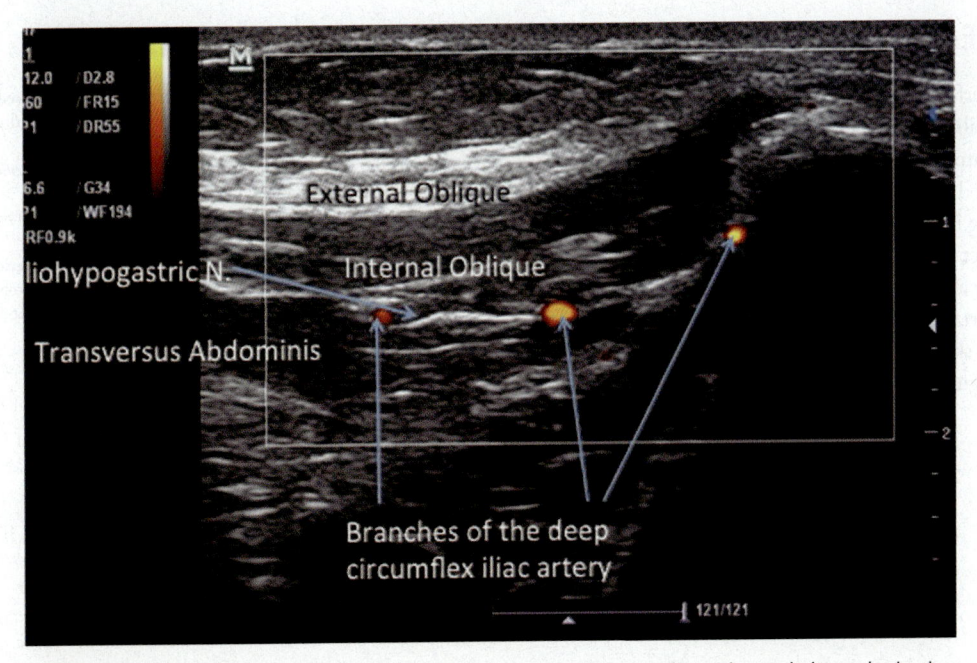

**FIGURE 119.14.** Transverse color Doppler image demonstrating vasculature in proximity to the lumbar plexus.

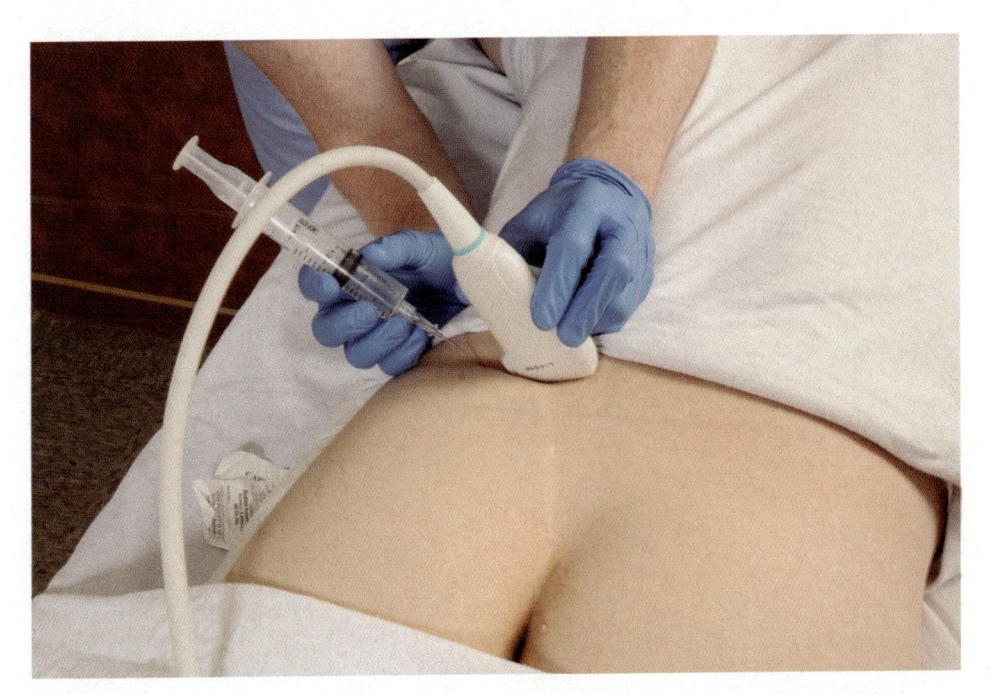

**FIGURE 119.15.** Proper in-plane needle position for performing selective lumbar nerve root block.

## CLINICAL PEARLS

The key to performing successful ultrasound-guided nerve blocks is the ability to properly identify the clinically relevant sonographic anatomy. This should not be a problem if the above technique is used. Any significant pain or sudden increase in resistance during injection when performing ultrasound-guided suggests incorrect needle placement, and one should stop injecting immediately and reassess the position of the needle. Because pain is an important indication of improper needle placement, the practitioner should avoid the use of excessive sedation during ultrasound-guided superior hypogastric plexus block.

## SUGGESTED READINGS

Waldman SD. Superior hypogastric plexus block: single needle paraspinous technique. In: *Atlas of Interventional Pain Management*. 3rd ed. Philadelphia, PA: Saunders Elsevier; 2009:467–471.

Waldman SD. Superior hypogastric plexus block. In: *Pain Review*. Philadelphia, PA: Saunders Elsevier; 2009:538–540.

Waldman SD. The superior hypogastric plexus and nerves. In: *Pain Review*. Philadelphia, PA: Saunders Elsevier; 2009:130–131.

Waldman SD, Wilson WL, Kreps RD. Clinical report: superior hypogastric plexus block utilizing a single needle and computerized tomographic guidance: description of a modified technique. *Reg Anesth* 1991;16:286–287.

# CHAPTER 120

# Ultrasound-Guided Ganglion of Walther (Impar) Block

## CLINICAL PERSPECTIVES

Ultrasound-guided ganglion impar (Walther) block is utilized in a variety of clinical scenarios as a diagnostic, prognostic, and therapeutic maneuver. As a diagnostic tool, ultrasound-guided ganglion impar (Walther) block allows accurate placement of the needle tip within proximity of the ganglion impar when performing differential neural blockade on an anatomic basis in the evaluation of pelvic, bladder, perineal, genital, rectal, and anal pain. As a prognostic tool, ultrasound-guided ganglion impar block can be utilized as a prognostic indicator of the degree of motor and sensory impairment that the patient may experience if the ganglion impar is going to be destroyed in an effort to palliate intractable pain. In the acute pain setting, ultrasound-guided ganglion impar (Walther) block with local anesthetics and/or steroids may be used to palliate acute pain emergencies while waiting for pharmacologic, surgical, and/or antiblastic methods to become effective. This technique has great clinical utility in both children and adults when managing acute postoperative and posttrauma pain. Sympathetically mediated pain syndromes including the pain of acute herpes zoster of the lower sacral and coccygeal dermatomes can also be effectively managed with epidurally administered local anesthetics, steroids, and/or opioids. Additionally, this technique is of value in patients suffering from pain secondary to endometriosis, reflex sympathetic dystrophy, causalgia, proctitis fugax, and radiation enteritis.

Pain of malignant origin involving the pelvis, perineum, rectum, anus, genitals, and lower extremities is also amenable to treatment with local anesthetics and steroids administered by this technique.

## CLINICALLY RELEVANT ANATOMY

The five sacral vertebrae are fused together to form the triangular-shaped sacrum (Fig. 120.1). The dorsally convex sacrum inserts in a wedge-like manner between the two iliac bones with superior articulations with the fifth lumbar vertebra and caudad articulations with the coccyx. On the anterior concave surface, there are four pairs of unsealed anterior sacral foramina that allow passage of the anterior rami of the upper four sacral nerves. The posterior sacral foramina are smaller than their anterior counterparts. Leakage of drugs injected into the sacral canal is effectively prevented by the sacrospinal and multifidus muscles. The vestigial bony remnants that are the result of the incomplete fusion of the inferior articular processes of the lower half of the S4 and all of the S5 vertebrae project downward on each side of the sacral hiatus (see Fig. 120.1). These bony projections are called the sacral cornua and represent important clinical landmarks when performing ultrasound-guided ganglion impar (Walther) nerve block. The U-shaped sacral hiatus is covered posteriorly by the sacrococcygeal ligament, which is also an important clinical landmark when performing ultrasound ganglion impar (Walther) nerve block (Fig. 120.2). Penetration of the sacrococcygeal joint provides direct access to precoccygeal space. The ganglion of impar (Walther) lies in front of the sacrococcygeal joint and is amenable to blockade at this level (Fig. 120.3). The ganglion receives fibers from the lumbar and sacral portions of the sympathetic and parasympathetic nervous system and provides sympathetic innervation to portions of the pelvic viscera and genitalia. Although there are gender- and race-determined differences in the shape of the sacrum, they are of little importance relative to the ultimate ability to successfully perform ganglion impar (Walther) nerve block on a given patient. The triangular coccyx is made up of three to five rudimental vertebrae. Its superior surface articulates with the inferior articular surface of the sacrum.

## ULTRASOUND-GUIDED TECHNIQUE

Ultrasound-guided ganglion impar (Walther) block can be carried out by placing the patient in the prone position with the patient's abdomen resting on a thin pillow (Fig. 120.4). To relax the gluteal muscles, the patient is asked to turn his or her heels outward (Fig. 120.5). A total of 6 mL of local anesthetic suitable for epidural administration is drawn up in a 20-mL sterile syringe. If the painful condition being treated is thought to have an inflammatory component, 40 to 80 mg of depot steroid is added to the local anesthetic. The skin overlying the sacrum, sacral hiatus, and coccyx is then prepped with antiseptic solution, and the sacral hiatus and cornua are palpated using a rocking motion (Fig. 120.6). A high-frequency linear ultrasound transducer is then placed over the lower sacrum in the transverse plane and slowly moved caudally until the sacral cornua

**Sacrum and Coccyx**
(Dorsal Surface)

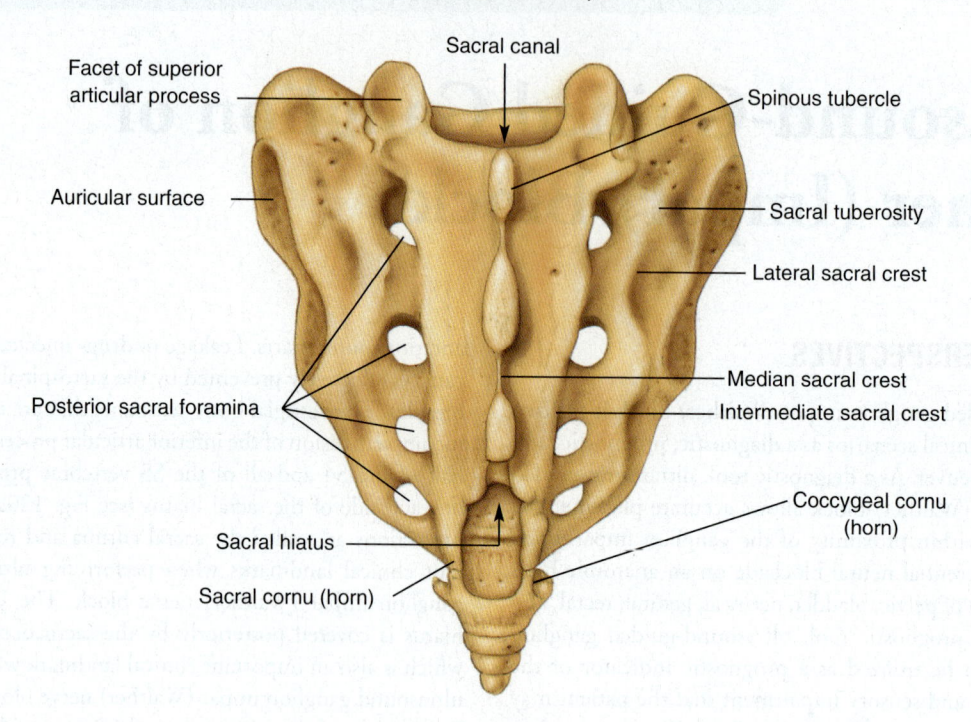

**FIGURE 120.1.** The anatomy of the sacrum. Note the relationship of the sacral cornua and sacral hiatus. (From Anatomical Chart Co., 2013.)

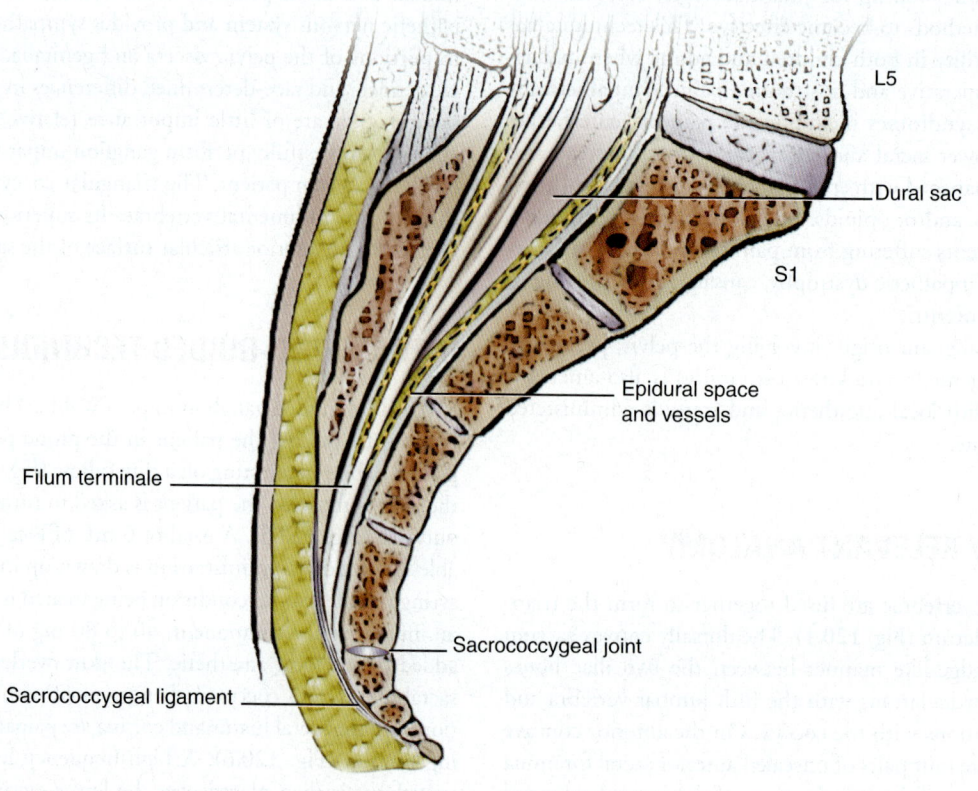

**FIGURE 120.2.** The sacrococcygeal ligament and caudal canal.

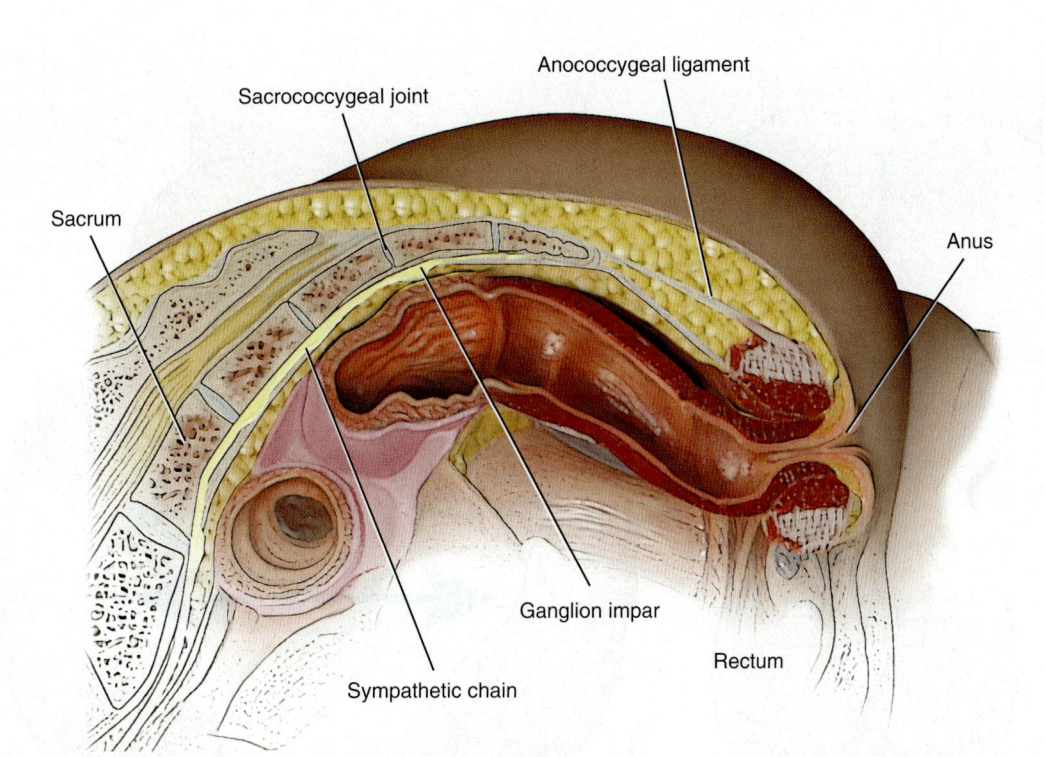

**FIGURE 120.3.** The anatomy of the ganglion impar (Walther).

are visualized (Figs. 120.7 and 120.8). The classic ultrasound appearance of the sacral cornua and their acoustic shadow are reminiscent of two nuns walking down the street (Fig. 120.9). Lying between the two nuns is the sacral hiatus, which provides access to the epidural space (see Fig. 108). Between the necks of the two is the sacrococcygeal ligament, which appears as a hyperechoic band-like structure (Fig. 120.10). Lying just beneath the sacrococcygeal ligament is the hypoechoic caudal canal (see Fig. 120.10). The floor of the caudal canal will appear as a bright hyperechoic line (see Fig. 120.10).

After sacral cornua, sacral hiatus, and the sacrococcygeal ligament are identified, the ultrasound transducer is turned to the longitudinal position and moved slowly caudad until the sacrococcygeal joint and first coccygeal vertebra are visualized (Figs. 120.11 and 120.12). After the sacrococcygeal is identified, a 22- or 25-gauge, 2-inch needle is inserted through

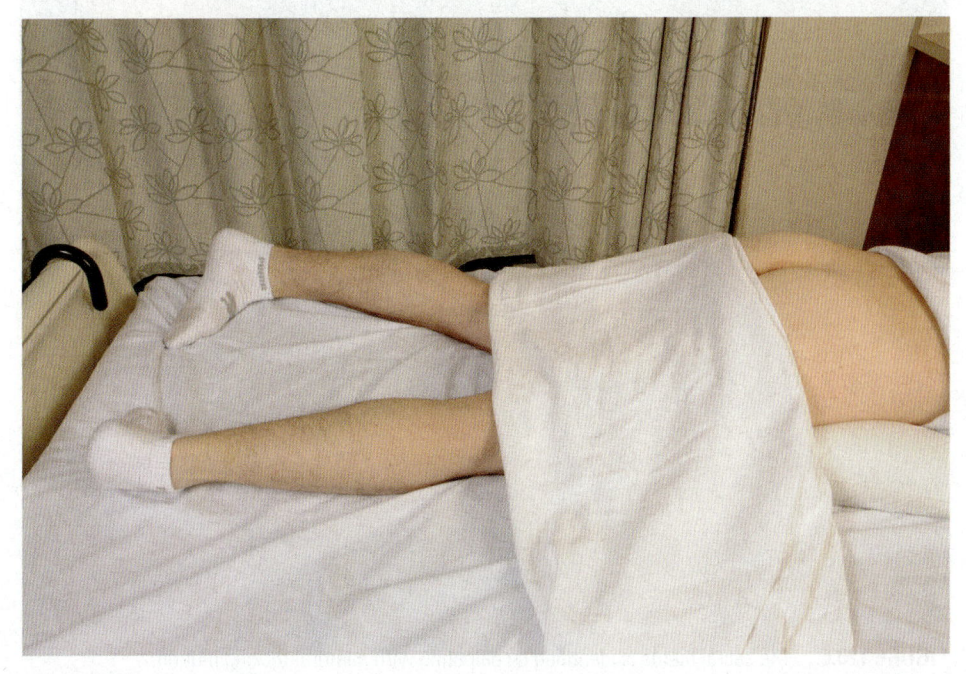

**FIGURE 120.4.** Proper prone patient position for ultrasound-guided ganglion impar (Walther) block.

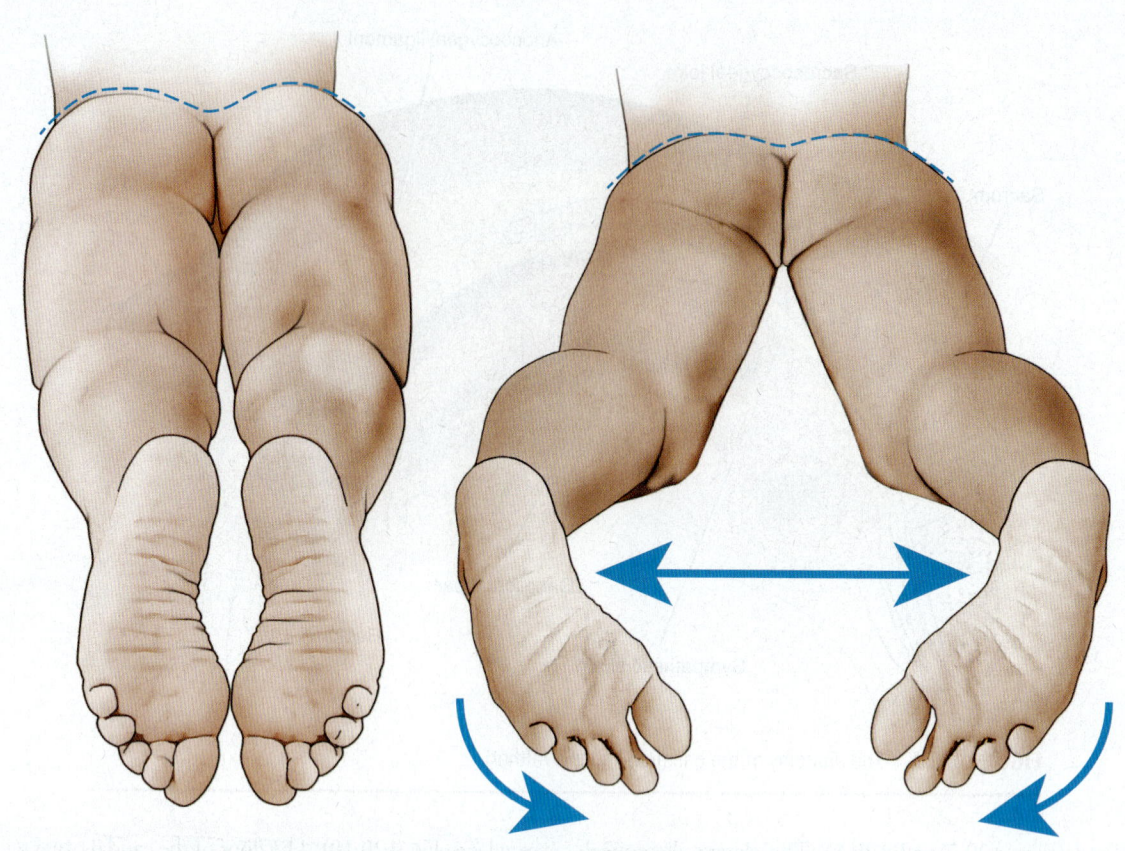

**FIGURE 120.5.** The patient is asked to turn his or her heels outward to relax the gluteal muscles.

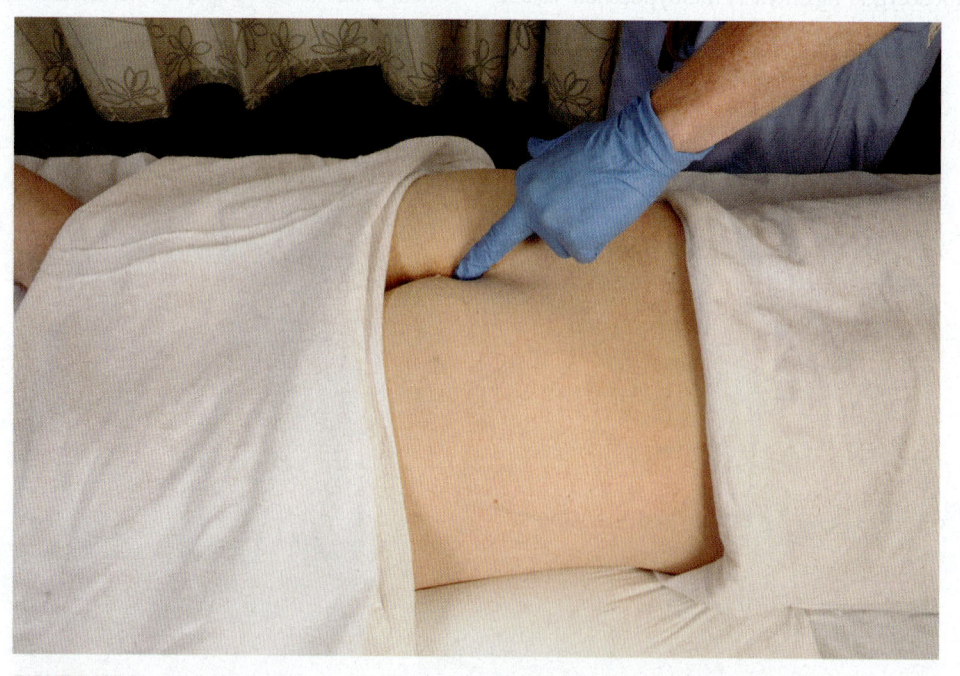

**FIGURE 120.6.** The sacral hiatus is identified by palpating with a lateral rocking motion.

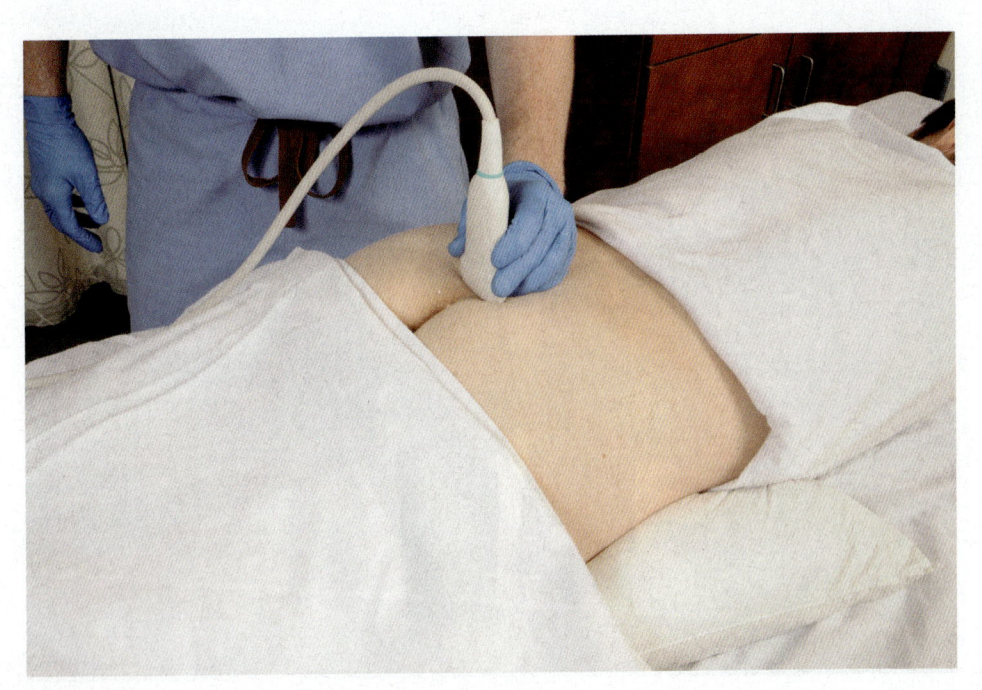

**FIGURE 120.7.** Placement of the ultrasound transducer in the transverse plane across the sacrum to obtain a paramedian sagittal transverse process view.

the skin ~1 cm below the inferior border of the transducer utilizing an in-plane approach and advanced with a 45-degree angle to the skin into the cartilaginous joint. A saline loss of resistance technique is then utilized to allow controlled advancement of the needle through the joint and into the precoccygeal space in proximity to the ganglion impar (Walther) (Fig. 120.13). As the sacrococcygeal joint is penetrated, a "pop" will be felt. The needle tip should only be advanced just beyond the anterior wall of the sacrococcygeal joint to avoid entering the rectum and contaminating the needle. After gentle aspiration is negative for cerebrospinal fluid and blood, 6 mL of solution is injected. The needle is removed and pressure is placed on the injection site to avoid hematoma formation.

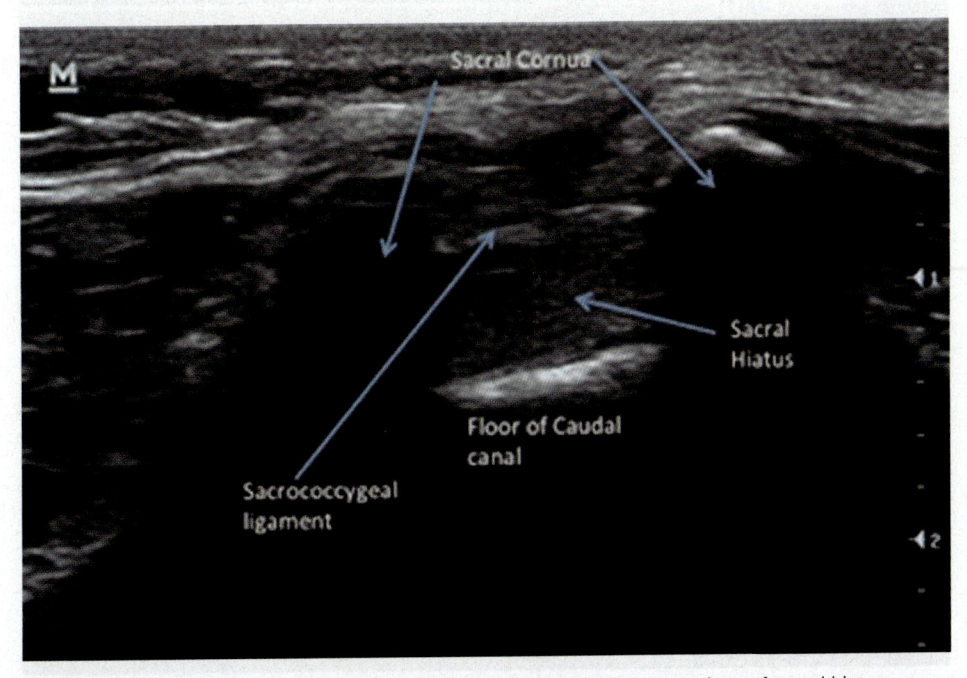

**FIGURE 120.8.** Transverse ultrasound image demonstrating the sacrum and top of sacral hiatus.

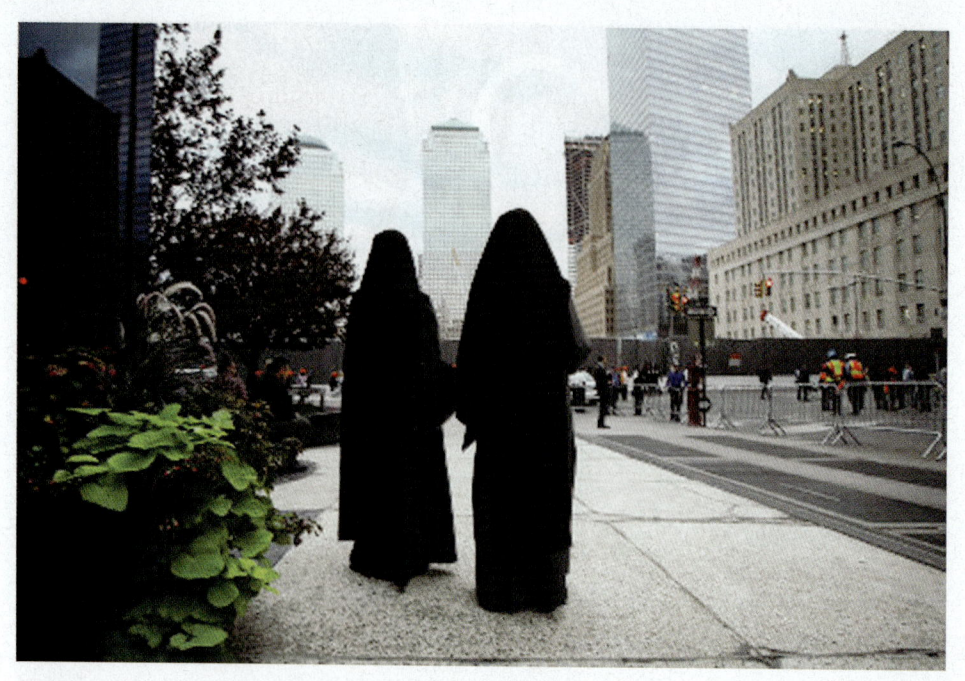

**FIGURE 120.9.** The sacral cornua and their acoustic shadow are reminiscent of two nuns walking down the street.

## COMPLICATIONS

Because of the proximity of the ganglion of impar (Walther) to the rectum makes rectal perforation and subsequent tracking of contaminants back through the needle track during needle removal a distinct possibility, care must be taken that the needle tip is not placed too deeply. Infection and fistula formation, especially in those patients who are immunocompromised or have received radiation therapy to the perineum, can represent a devastating and potentially life-threatening complication to this block if such needle contamination occurs. Although uncommon, infection in the lumbar epidural space remains an ever-present possibility, especially in the immunocompromised AIDS or cancer patient, and should be considered in any patient with fever and the onset

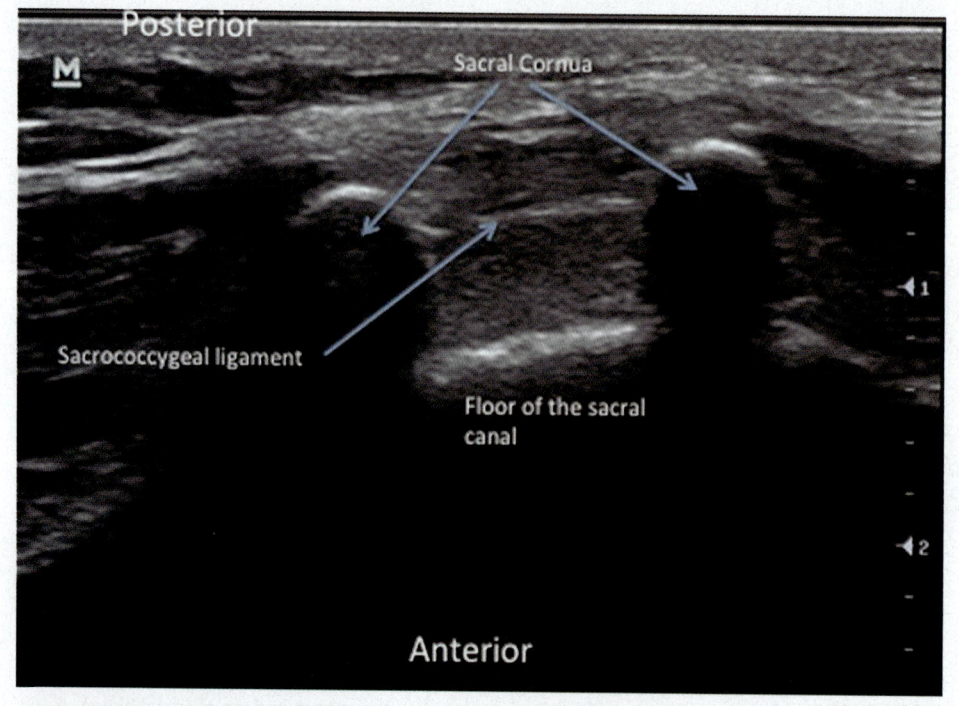

**FIGURE 120.10.** Transverse ultrasound view of the sacral hiatus, sacrococcygeal ligament, and caudal canal.

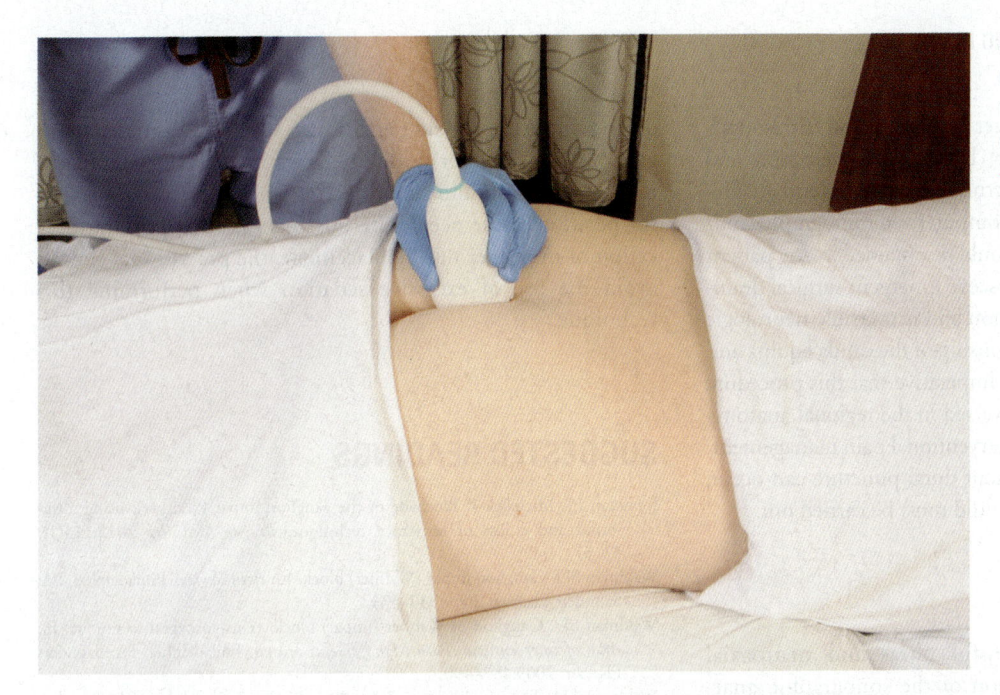

**FIGURE 120.11.** Proper longitudinal ultrasound transducer placement to visualize the sacrococcygeal ligament and caudal canal.

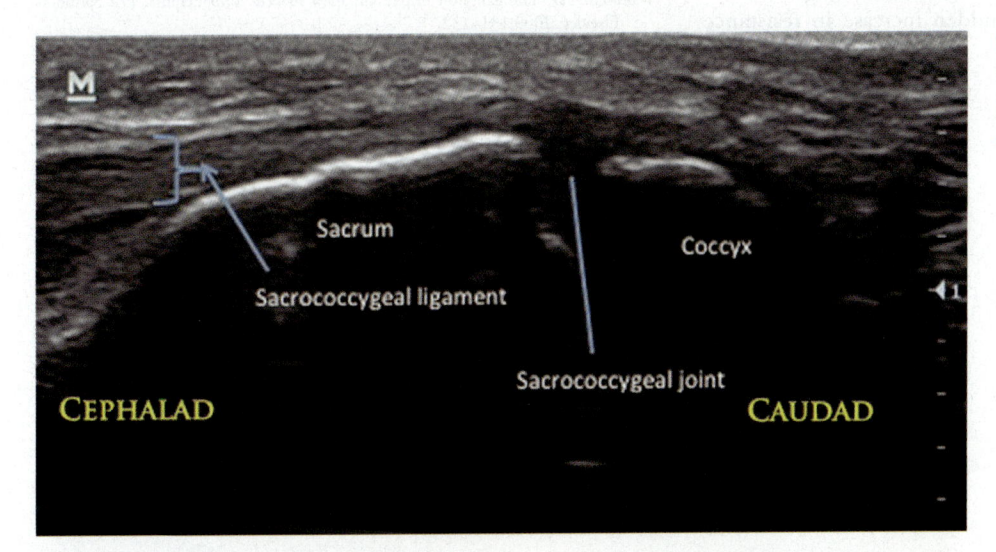

**FIGURE 120.12.** Longitudinal ultrasound image of the sacrococcygeal joint.

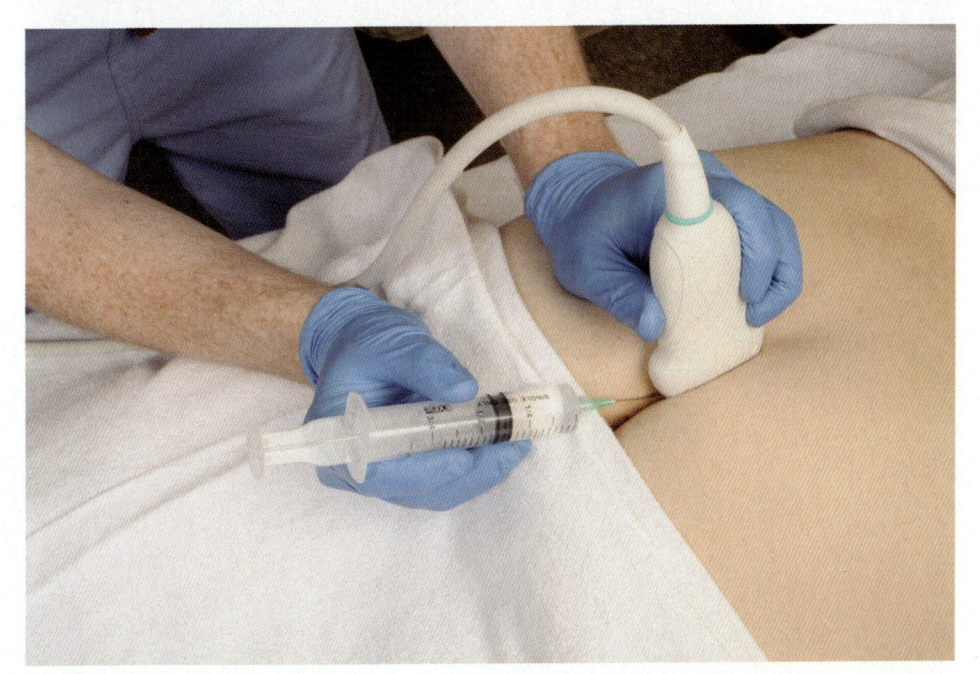

**FIGURE 120.13.** Proper in-plane needle position for performing ultrasound-guided ganglion impar (Walther) block.

of neurologic symptomatology after undergoing an ultrasound-guided ganglion impar (Walther) block. Early detection and treatment of epidural infection is crucial to avoid potentially life-threatening sequelae, and urgent computerized tomography and/or magnetic resonance imaging should be obtained in any patient suspected of having an epidural abscess. Emergent surgical drainage to avoid spinal cord compression and irreversible neurologic deficit is often required. The relationship of the cauda equina and exiting sacral nerve roots makes it imperative that this procedure be carried out only by those well versed in the regional anatomy and experienced in performing interventional pain management. Although exceeding rare, inadvertent dural puncture can occur, and careful observation for spinal fluid must be carried out.

## CLINICAL PEARLS

The key to performing successful ultrasound neuroaxial blocks is the proper identification of the sonographic anatomy. Any significant pain or sudden increase in resistance during injection when performing ultrasound-guided ganglion impar (Walther) block suggests incorrect needle placement, and one should stop injecting immediately and reassess the position of the needle. Because pain is an important indication of improper needle placement, the practitioner should avoid the use of excessive sedation when performing this technique.

## SUGGESTED READINGS

Johnston PJ, Michalek P. Blockade of the ganglion impar (Walther), using ultrasound and a loss of resistance technique. *Prague Med Rep* 2012;113(1): 53–57.

Waldman SD. Ganglion impar (Walther) block. In: *Pain Review*. Philadelphia, PA: Saunders Elsevier; 2009:530–533.

Waldman SD. Ganglion of Walther (impar) block: trans-coccygeal technique. In: *Atlas of Interventional Pain Management*. 3rd ed. Philadelphia, PA: Saunders Elsevier; 2009:487–490.

Waldman SD. The ganglion impar. In: *Pain Review*. Philadelphia, PA: Saunders Elsevier; 2009:131–132.

# CHAPTER 121

# Ultrasound-Guided Injection Technique for Coccydynia

## CLINICAL PERSPECTIVES

Ultrasound-guided injection technique for coccydynia is utilized in the evaluation and treatment of coccydynia. Coccydynia is a common pain syndrome that is characterized by pain localized to the tailbone that radiates into the lower sacrum and perineum. Affecting females more frequently than males, coccydynia most often occurs after direct trauma to the coccyx from a kick or a fall directly onto the coccyx. Coccydynia also can occur in the parturient after a difficult vaginal delivery. The pain of coccydynia is thought to be the result of strain of the sacrococcygeal ligament or occasionally from occult fracture of the coccyx. Less commonly, arthritis of the sacrococcygeal joint can result in coccydynia.

On physical examination, the patient suffering from coccydynia will exhibit point tenderness over the coccyx with the pain being increased with flexion and extension of the coccyx. Any movement of the coccyx also may cause sharp paresthesias into the rectum, which can be quite distressing to the patient. On rectal examination, the levator ani, piriformis, and coccygeus muscles may feel indurated, and palpation of these muscles may induce severe spasm. Sitting may exacerbate the pain of coccydynia, and the patient may attempt to sit on one buttock to avoid pressure on the coccyx.

Plain radiographs are indicated in all patients who present with pain thought to be emanating from the coccyx to rule out fracture, occult bony pathology, and tumor (Fig. 121.1). Based on the patient's clinical presentation, additional testing may be indicated, including complete blood cell count, prostate-specific antigen, sedimentation rate, and antinuclear antibody. Magnetic resonance imaging (MRI) of the pelvis is indicated if occult mass or tumor is suspected (Fig. 121.2). Radionuclide bone scanning may be useful to rule out stress fractures not seen on plain radiographs. The injection technique presented later serves as both a diagnostic and a therapeutic maneuver.

## CLINICALLY RELEVANT ANATOMY

The five sacral vertebrae are fused together to form the triangular-shaped sacrum (Fig. 121.3). The dorsally convex sacrum inserts in a wedge-like manner between the two iliac bones with superior articulations with the fifth lumbar vertebra and caudad articulations with the coccyx. On the anterior concave surface, there are four pairs of unsealed anterior sacral foramina that allow passage of the anterior rami of the upper four sacral nerves. The posterior sacral foramina are smaller than their anterior counterparts. Leakage of drugs injected into the sacral canal is effectively prevented by the sacrospinal and multifidus muscles. The vestigial bony remnants that are the result of the incomplete fusion of the inferior articular processes of the lower half of the S4 and all of the S5 vertebrae project downward on each side of the sacral hiatus (see Fig. 121.3). These bony projections are called the sacral cornua and represent important clinical landmarks when performing ultrasound-guided injection for coccydynia. The U-shaped sacral hiatus is covered posteriorly by the sacrococcygeal ligament, which is also an important clinical landmark when performing ultrasound-guided injection for coccydynia (Fig. 121.4). Penetration of the sacrococcygeal ligament provides direct access to the epidural space of the sacral canal. The triangular coccyx is made up of three to five rudimental vertebrae. Its superior surface articulates with the inferior articular surface of the sacrum.

## ULTRASOUND-GUIDED TECHNIQUE

Ultrasound injection technique for coccydynia can be carried out by placing the patient in the prone position with the patient's abdomen resting on a thin pillow (Fig. 121.5). To relax the gluteal muscles, the patient is asked to turn his or her heels outward (Fig. 121.6). A total of 5 mL of local anesthetic suitable for epidural administration is drawn up in a 12-mL sterile syringe. If the painful condition being treated is thought to have an inflammatory component, 40 to 80 mg of depot steroid is added to the local anesthetic. The skin overlying the sacrum and sacral hiatus are then prepped with antiseptic solution, and the sacral hiatus and cornua are palpated using a rocking motion (Fig. 121.7). A high-frequency linear ultrasound transducer is then placed over the lower sacrum in the transverse plane and slowly moved caudally until the sacral cornua are visualized (Figs. 121.8 and 121.9). The classic ultrasound appearance of the sacral cornua and their acoustic shadow are reminiscent of two nuns walking down the street (Fig. 121.10). Lying between the two nuns is the sacral hiatus, which provides access to the epidural space (see Fig. 121.9). Between the

**FIGURE 121.1.** Ultrasound injection technique for coccydynia is useful in the management of the pain of acute fractures of the coccyx. Plain lateral radiograph of a displaced coccygeal fracture. (From Greenberg MI. *Greenberg's Text-Atlas of Emergency Medicine.* 1st ed. Philadelphia, PA: Lippincott Williams & Wilkins; 2004.)

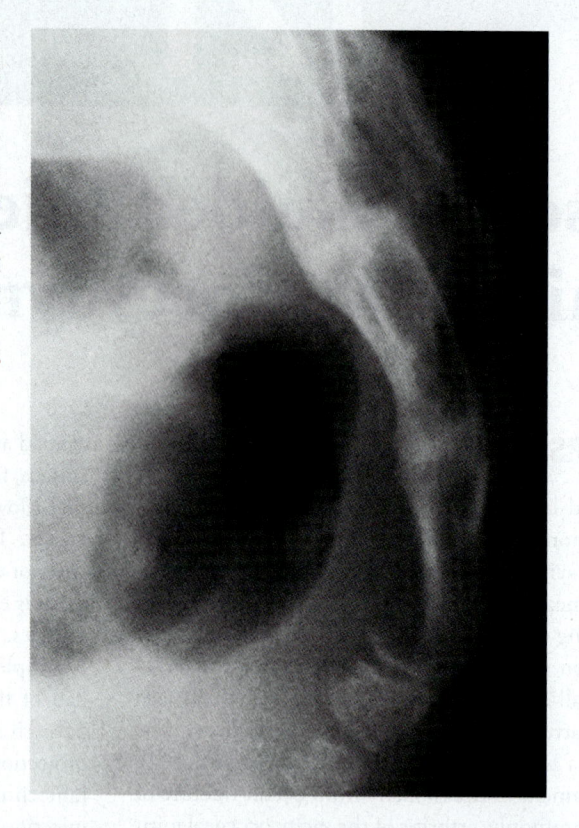

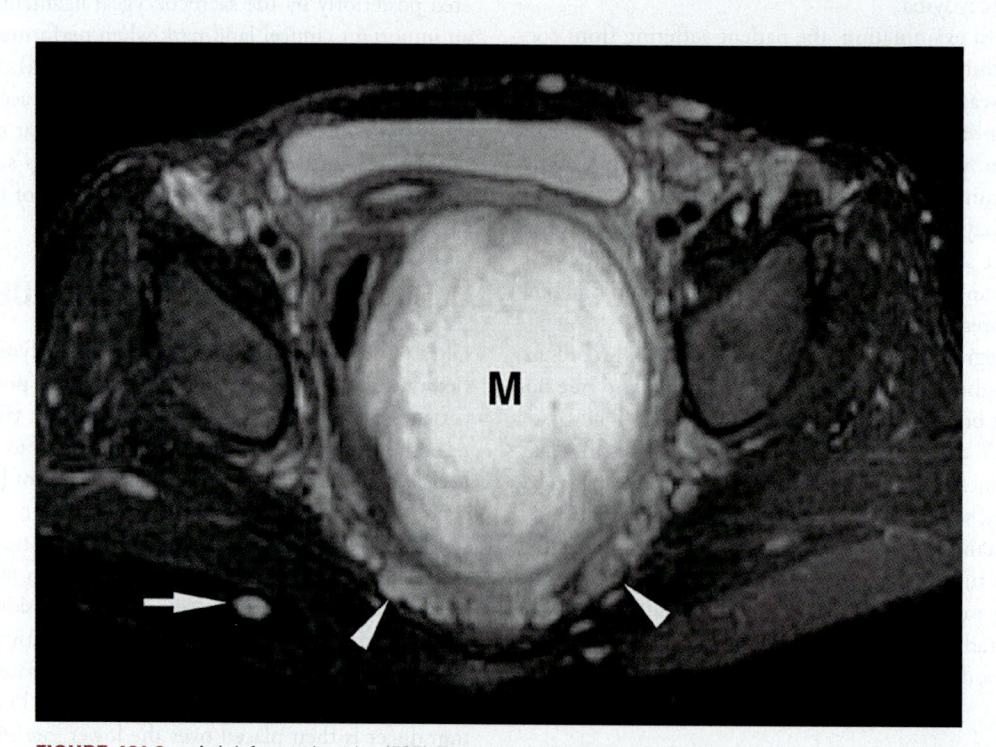

**FIGURE 121.2.** Axial fast spin-echo (FSE) T2-weighted fat-saturated MRI scan in a 16-year-old girl demonstrates multiple neurofibromas along the sacrum (*arrowheads*). The presence of a larger, asymmetric mass (M) with heterogeneous signal intensity is consistent with sarcomatous degeneration. Also note a small neurofibroma (*arrow*) in the subcutaneous tissues. (From Siegel MJ, Coley BD. Adrenal glands, pancreas, and other retroperitoneal structures. In: *The Core Curriculum: Pediatric Imaging.* 1st ed. Philadelphia, PA: Lippincott Williams & Wilkins; 2005.)

**FIGURE 121.3.** The anatomy of the sacrum. Note the relationship of the sacral cornua and sacral hiatus. (From Anatomical Chart Co., 2013.)

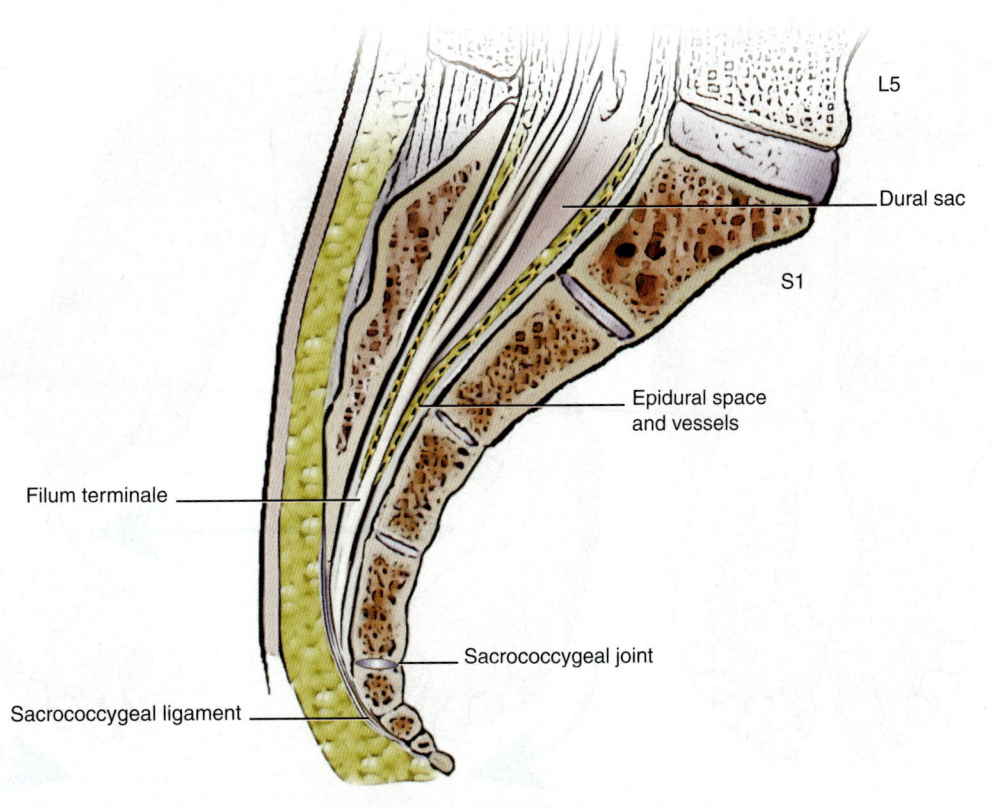

**FIGURE 121.4.** The sacrococcygeal ligament and caudal canal.

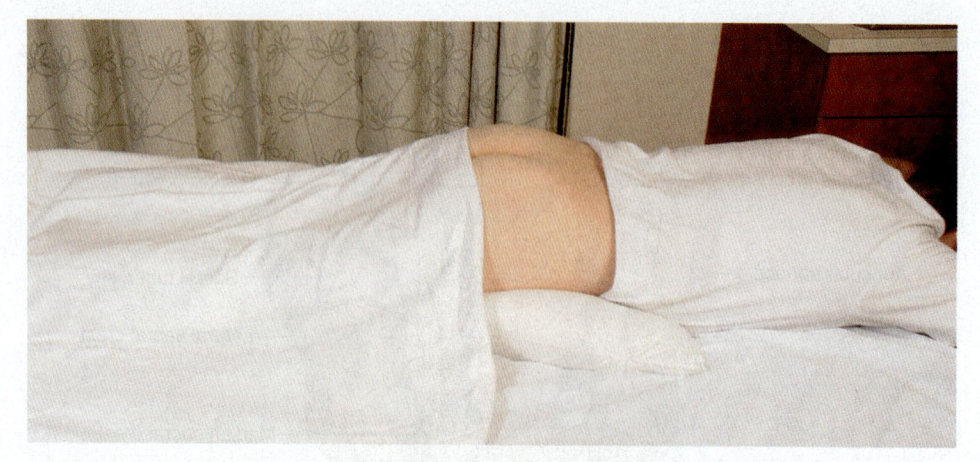

**FIGURE 121.5.** Proper prone patient position for ultrasound injection technique for coccydynia.

necks of the two is the sacrococcygeal ligament, which appears as a hyperechoic band-like structure (Fig. 121.11). Lying just beneath the sacrococcygeal ligament is the hypoechoic caudal canal (see Fig. 121.11). The floor of the caudal canal will appear as a bright hyperechoic line (see Fig. 121.11).

After sacral cornua, sacral hiatus, and the sacrococcygeal ligament are identified, the ultrasound transducer is turned to the longitudinal position and moved slowly cephalad until the inferior portion of the ultrasound transducer lies toward the top of the sacral hiatus (Figs. 121.12 and 121.13). After the sacral hiatus, sacrococcygeal ligament, and caudal canal are reidentified, a 22- or 25-gauge, 2-inch needle is inserted through the skin ~1 cm below the inferior border of the transducer utilizing an in-plane approach and advanced

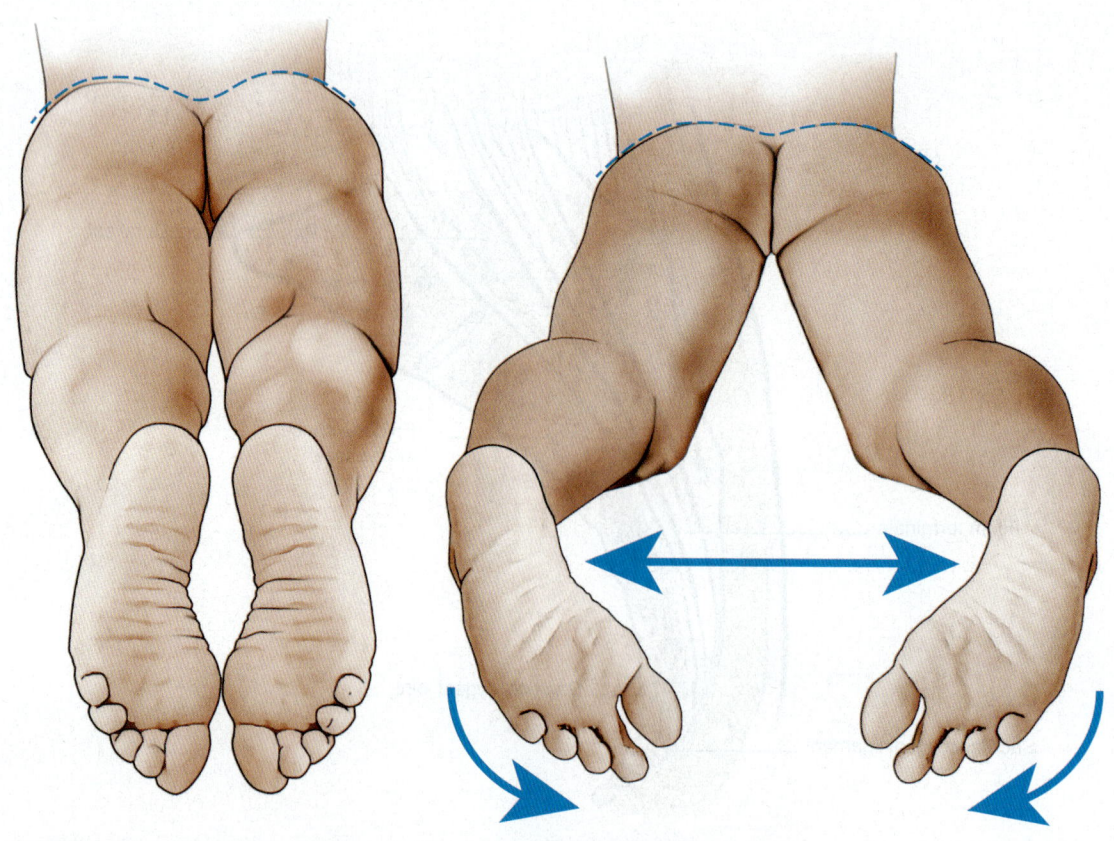

**FIGURE 121.6.** The patient is asked to turn his or her heels outward to relax the gluteal muscles.

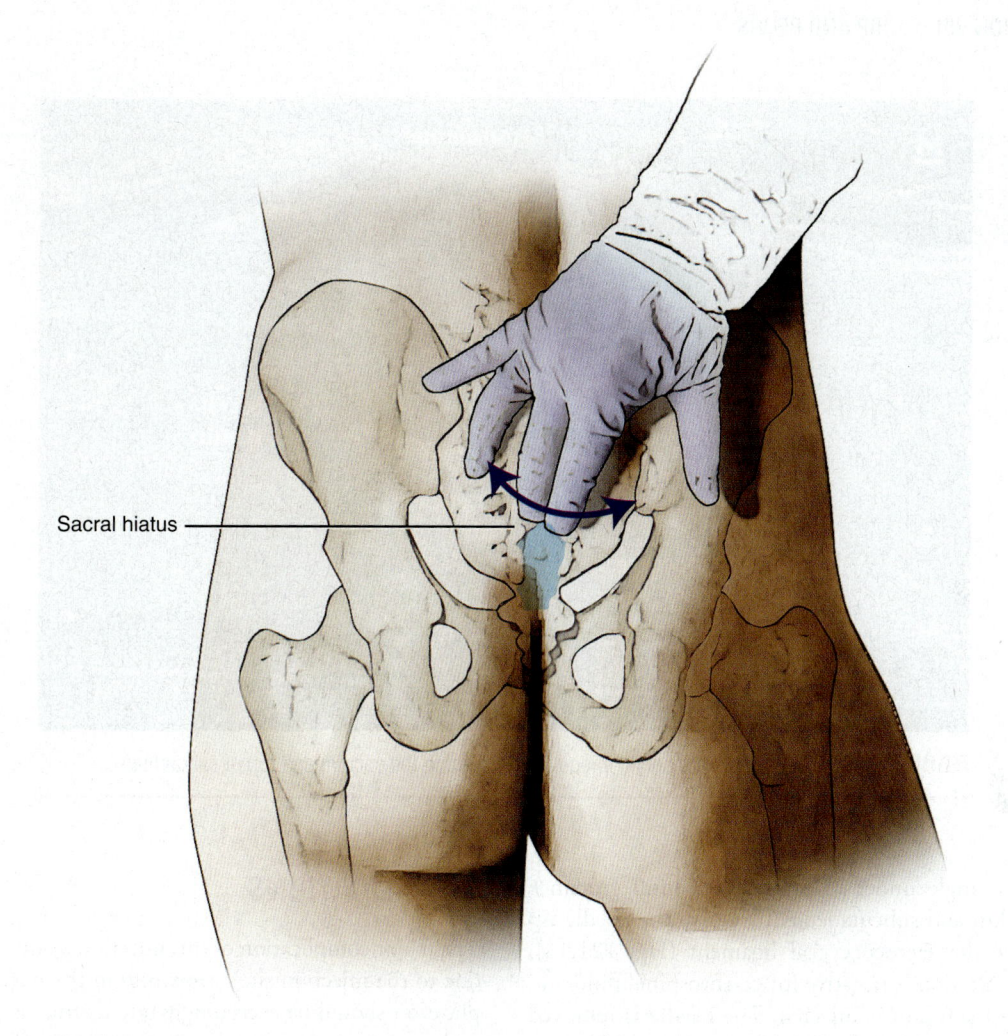

**FIGURE 121.7.** The sacral hiatus is identified by palpating with a lateral rocking motion.

Sacral hiatus

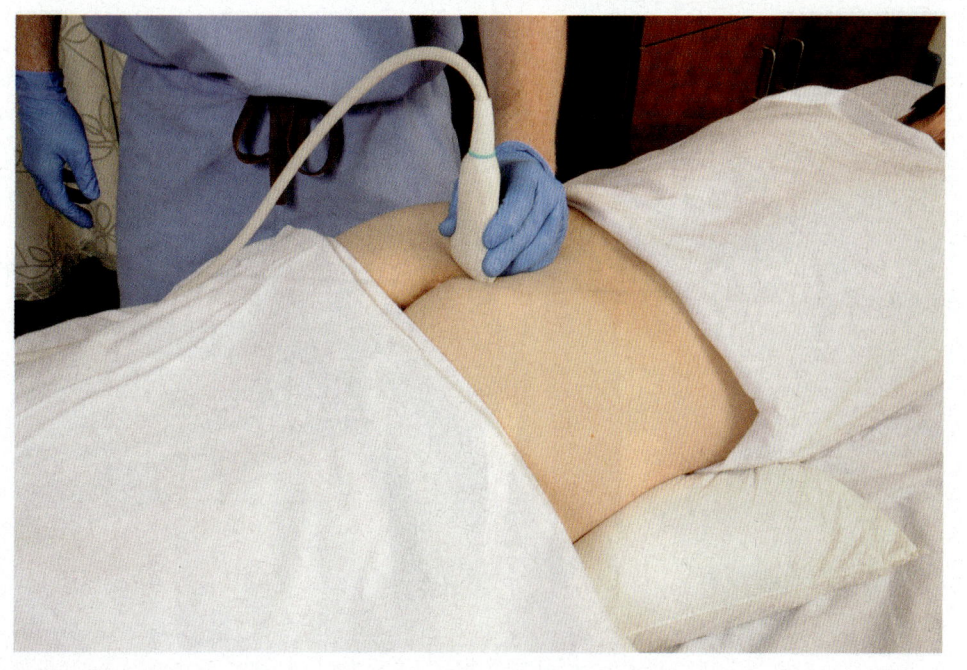

**FIGURE 121.8.** Placement of the ultrasound transducer in the transverse plane across the sacrum to obtain a paramedian sagittal transverse process view.

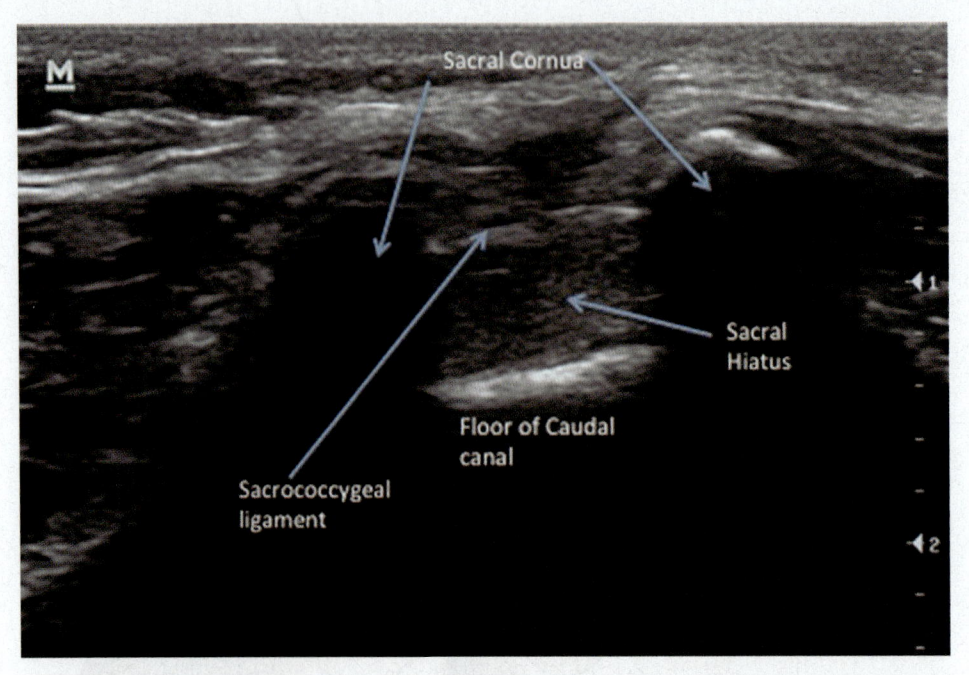

**FIGURE 121.9.** Transverse ultrasound image demonstrating the sacrum and top of sacral hiatus.

at a 45-degree angle under real-time ultrasound guidance through the skin and subcutaneous tissues so the needle tip lies just above the sacrococcygeal ligament (Fig. 121.14). After gentle aspiration is negative for cerebrospinal fluid and blood, 5 mL of solution is injected. The needle is removed and pressure is placed on the injection site to avoid hematoma formation.

## COMPLICATIONS

The major complication of this injection technique is infection due to the injection site's proximity to the rectum. This complication should be exceedingly rare if strict aseptic technique and careful attention to identification of the clinically relevant anatomy is followed. Approximately 25% of patients complain

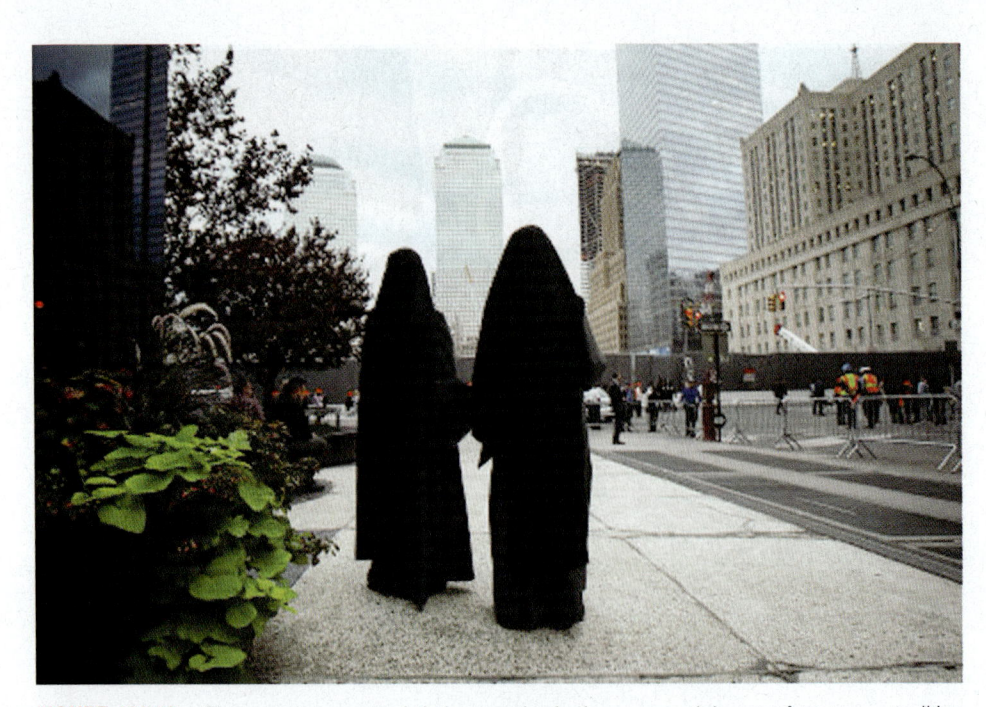

**FIGURE 121.10.** The sacral cornua and their acoustic shadow are reminiscent of two nuns walking down the street.

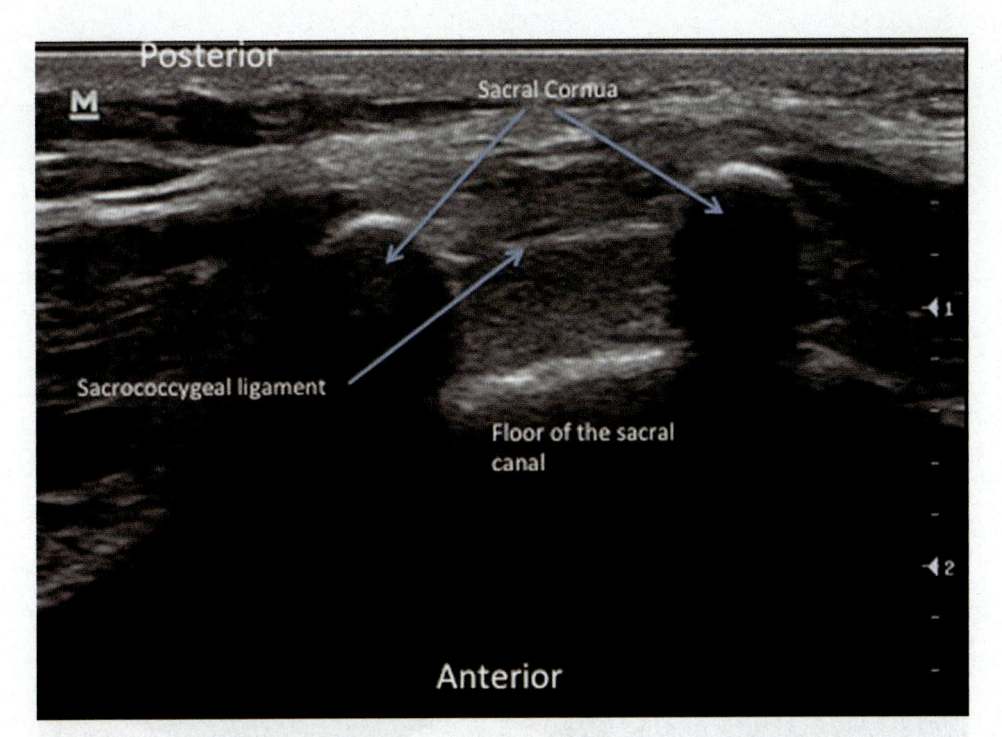

**FIGURE 121.11.** Transverse ultrasound view of sacral hiatus, sacrococcygeal ligament, and caudal canal.

of a transient increase in pain after this injection technique, and the patient should be warned of this. Care must be taken to avoid placing the needle too deeply, or inadvertent caudal epidural placement of the local anesthetic and corticosteroid, with its attendant sensory and motor blockade, could result.

## CLINICAL PEARLS

Ultrasound-guided injection technique for coccydynia is extremely effective in the treatment of coccydynia. In some patients, ganglion of impar block is required to provide long-lasting relief.

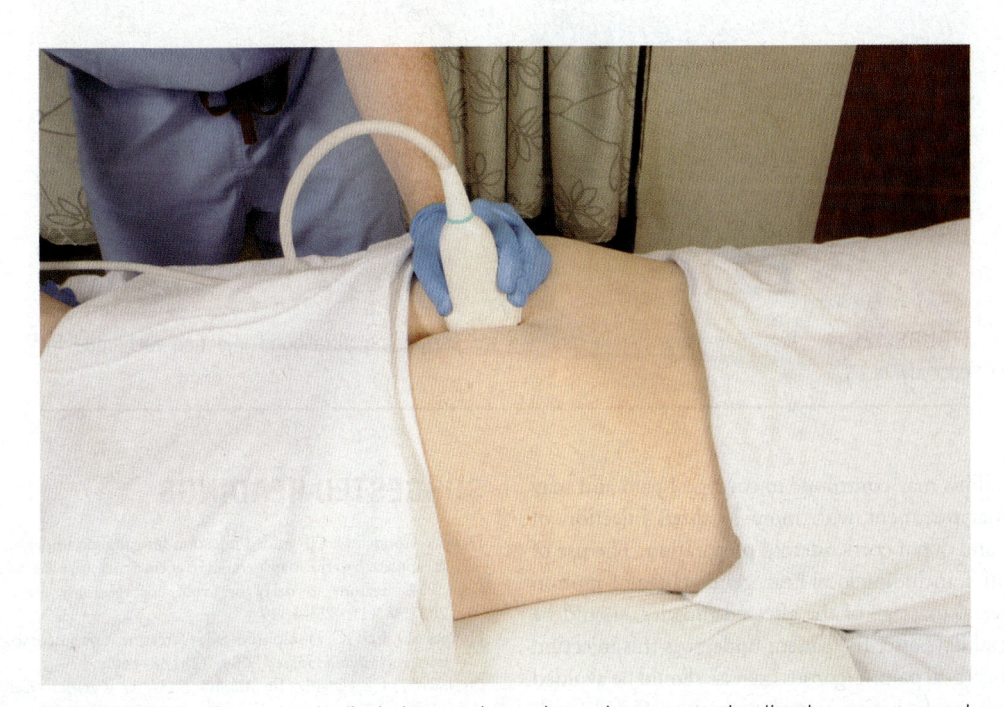

**FIGURE 121.12.** Proper longitudinal ultrasound transducer placement to visualize the sacrococcygeal ligament and caudal canal.

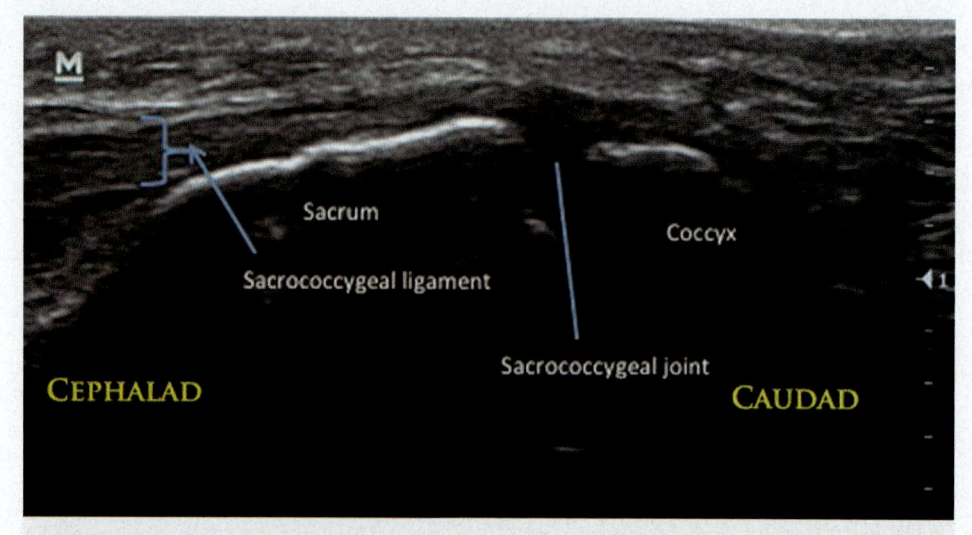

**FIGURE 121.13.** Longitudinal ultrasound image of the sacral hiatus, sacrococcygeal ligament, and caudal canal.

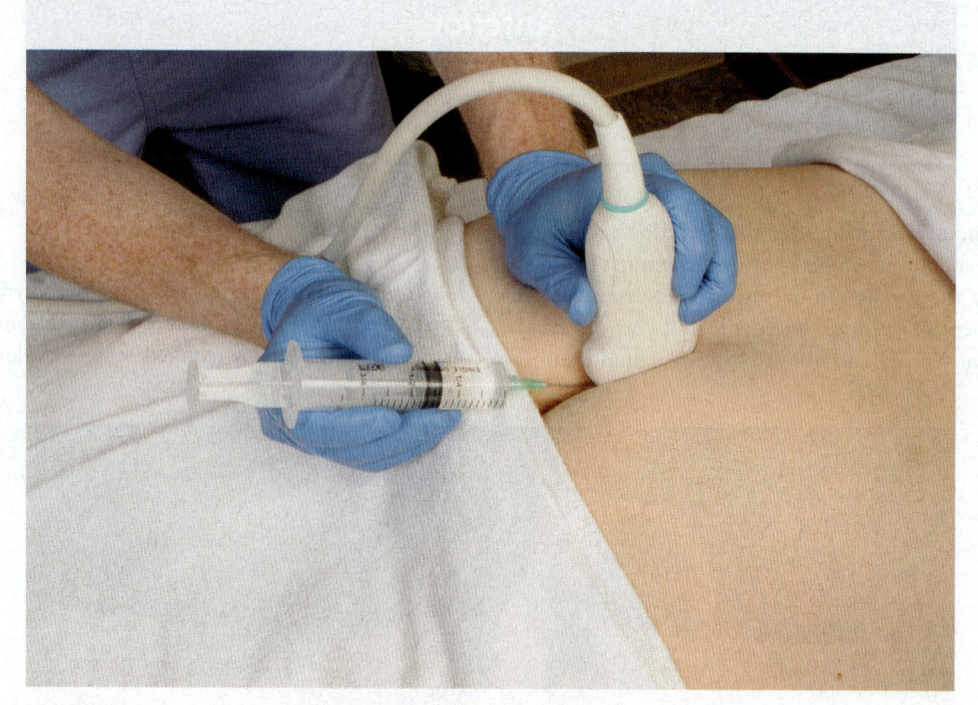

**FIGURE 121.14.** Proper in-plane needle position for performing ultrasound injection technique for coccydynia.

Coexistent sacroiliitis may contribute to coccygeal pain and may require additional treatment with more localized injection of local anesthetic and depot corticosteroid preparation. The use of physical modalities, including local heat, gentle range-of-motion exercises, and rectal massage of the affected muscles, should be introduced several days after the patient undergoes this injection technique for coccygeal pain. Vigorous exercise should be avoided because it exacerbates the patient's symptomatology. Simple analgesics and nonsteroidal anti-inflammatory agents may be used concurrently with this injection technique.

## SUGGESTED READINGS

Datir A, Connell D. CT-guided injection for ganglion impar blockade: a radiological approach to the management of coccydynia. *Clin Radiol* 2010;65(1):21–25.
Foye PM. Reasons to delay or avoid coccygectomy for coccyx pain. *Injury* 2007;38(11):1328–1329.
Hodges SD, Eck JC, Humphreys SC. A treatment of outcomes analysis of patients with coccydynia. *Spine J* 2004;4(2):138–140.
Oyelowo T. Coccydynia. In: *Mosby's Guide to Women's Health*. St. Louis, MO: Mosby; 2007:62–64.
Waldman SD. Coccydynia. In: *Pain Review*. Philadelphia, PA: Saunders Elsevier; 2009:252–253.

# CHAPTER 122

# Ultrasound-Guided Pudendal Nerve Block

## CLINICAL PERSPECTIVES

Ultrasound-guided pudendal nerve block is useful in the management of the pelvic pain subserved by the pudendal nerve. This technique serves as an excellent adjunct to lumbar epidural block in obstetrics and for local or general anesthesia or as a stand-alone surgical anesthetic when performing surgery on the labia or scrotum, for example, Bartholin cyst surgery (Fig. 122.1). Ultrasound-guided pudendal nerve block with local anesthetic may be used to palliate acute pain emergencies, including postoperative pain, pain secondary to traumatic injuries of the pudenda, and cancer pain, while waiting for pharmacologic, surgical, and antiblastic methods to become effective.

Ultrasound-guided pudendal nerve block can also be used as a diagnostic tool when performing differential neural blockade on an anatomic basis in the evaluation of pelvic pain as well as in a prognostic manner to determine the degree of neurologic impairment the patient will suffer when destruction of the pudendal nerve is being considered or when there is a possibility that the nerve may be sacrificed during surgeries in the anatomic region of the pudendal nerve at the level of the hip. This technique may also be useful in those patients suffering symptoms from compromise of the pudendal nerve. Ultrasound-guided pudendal nerve block may also be used to palliate the pain and dysesthesias associated with stretch injuries to the pudendal nerve that can occur after "straddle injuries" or forceps delivery. Pudendal nerve block with local anesthetic and steroid is also useful in the palliation of pain of malignant origin arising from tumors invading the labia or scrotum or the pudendal nerve itself. The technique may also be useful in palliation of persistent rectal, vulvar, or vaginal itching that has not responded to topical therapy. Destruction of the pudendal nerve is occasionally indicated for the palliation of persistent pelvic or rectal pain after blunt or open trauma to the pelvis or persistent pain mediated by the pudendal nerve after obstetric deliveries or transvaginal surgery or in the palliation of pain of malignant origin.

Electrodiagnostic testing should be considered in all patients who suffer from pudendal nerve dysfunction to provide both neuroanatomic and neurophysiologic information regarding nerve function. Magnetic resonance imaging and ultrasound imaging of the lumbar plexus and the pelvis anywhere along the course of the pudendal nerve are also useful in determining the cause of pudendal nerve compromise.

## CLINICALLY RELEVANT ANATOMY

The pudendal nerve is comprised of fibers from the S2, S3, and S4 nerves (Fig. 122.2). The nerve passes inferiorly between the piriformis and coccygeal muscles. The pudendal nerve leaves the pelvis accompanying the pudendal artery and vein via the greater sciatic foramen. It then passes around the medial portion of the ischial spine to reenter the pelvis via the lesser sciatic foramen. At this level, the nerve lies between the sacrospinous and sacrotuberous ligaments (Fig. 122.3). The pudendal nerve is amenable to blockade at this point via the transvaginal or ultrasound-guided approach described below. The nerve then divides into three terminal branches: (1) the inferior rectal nerve, which provides innervation to the anal sphincter and perianal region; (2) the perineal nerve, which supplies the posterior two-thirds of the scrotum or labia majora and muscles of the urogenital triangle; and (3) the dorsal nerve of the penis or clitoris, which supplies sensory innervation to the dorsum of the penis or clitoris.

## ULTRASOUND-GUIDED TECHNIQUE

The benefits, risks, and alternative treatments are explained to the patient and informed consent is obtained. The patient is then placed in the prone position (Fig. 122.4). At the midposterior gluteal region, a low-frequency curvilinear ultrasound transducer is placed over the ilium in the posterior midgluteal region, and an ultrasound survey scan is taken (Figs. 122.5 and 122.6). The medial margin of the ilium will appear as a hyperechoic line that is widest at the level of the ischial spine (Fig. 122.7). The ultrasound probe is slowly moved in a caudad direction along the extent of the medial margin of the ilium until the ischial spine comes into view appearing as a straight hyperechoic line (Figs. 122.8 and 122.9). Just above the ischial spine lies the sacrospinous ligament, and sacrotuberous ligaments lies just above the straight hyperechoic line of the ilium (Fig. 122.10). The pudendal nerve lies between these two ligaments at this level. The sacrospinous ligament

**874** SECTION VIII HIP AND PELVIS

**FIGURE 122.1.** Bartholin cyst marsupialization is amenable to ultrasound-guided pudendal nerve block. (Reused from Rubin E, Farber JL. *Pathology.* 3rd ed. Philadelphia, PA: Lippincott Williams & Wilkins; 1999, with permission.)

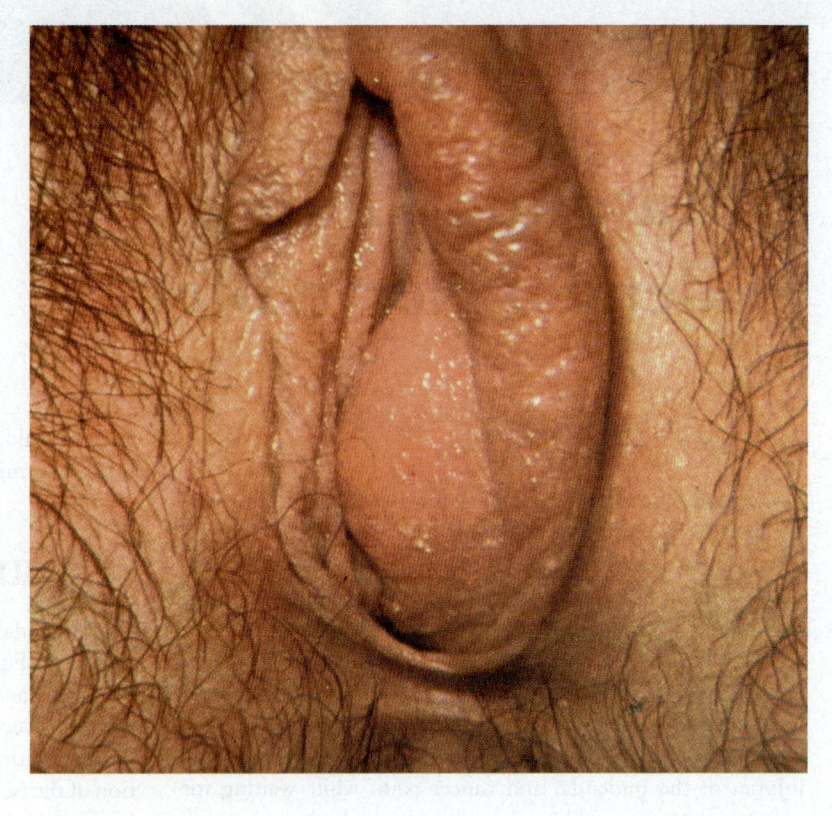

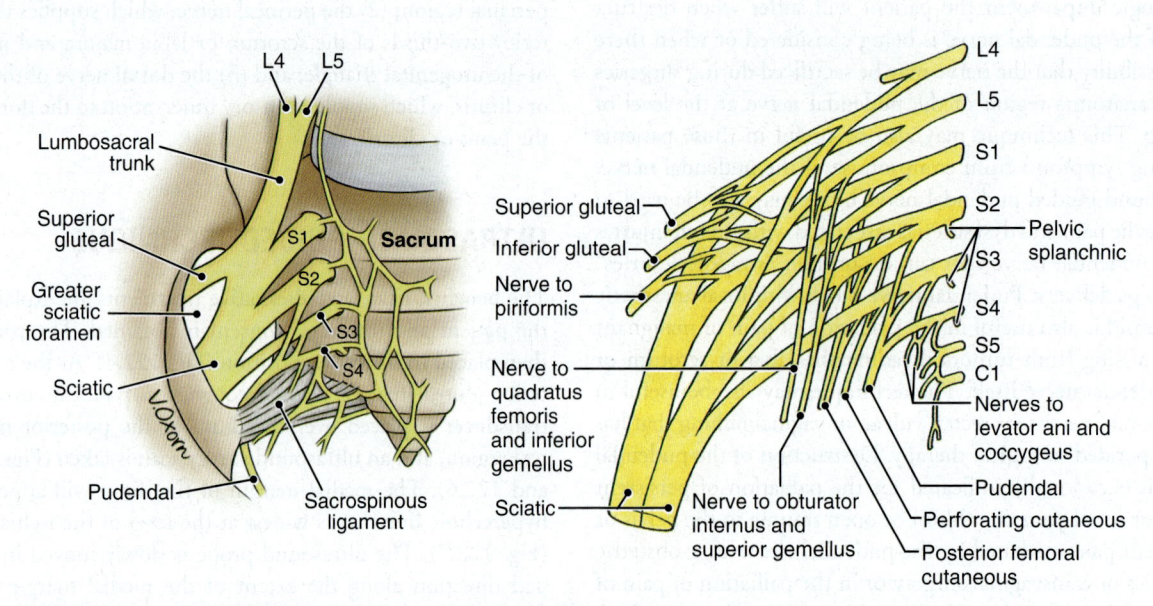

**FIGURE 122.2.** The pudendal nerve is derived from the S2, S3, and S4 nerves. (Reused from Moore KL, Agur AMR. *Essential Clinical Anatomy.* 2nd ed. Baltimore, MD: Lippincott Williams & Wilkins; 2002:220, with permission.)

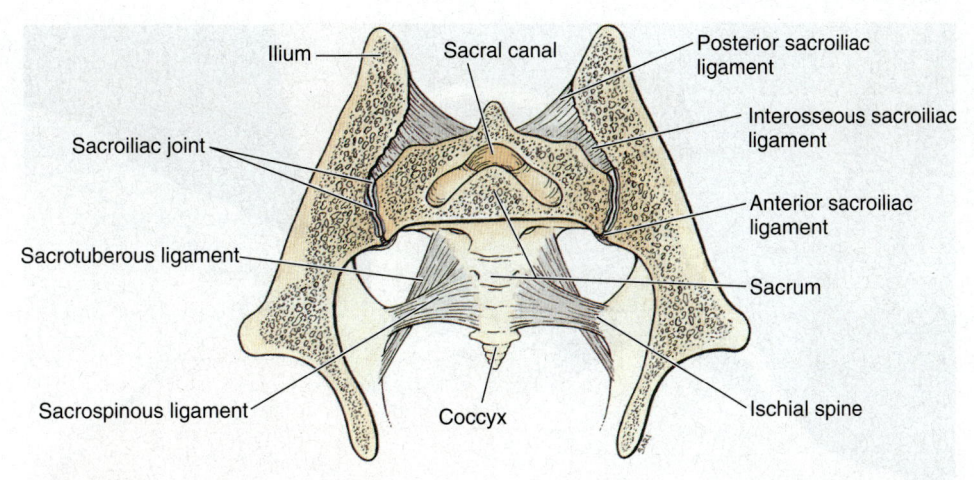

**FIGURE 122.3.** The pudendal nerve lies between the sacrospinous and sacrotuberous ligaments at the level of the ischial spine. (Adapted from Clay JH, Pounds DM. *Basic Clinical Massage Therapy: Integrating Anatomy and Treatment.* 2nd ed. Philadelphia, PA: Lippincott Williams & Wilkins; 2008.)

can be seen as a slightly less hyperechoic line that is confluent with and just above the ischial spine (see Fig. 122.10). The sacrotuberous ligament is seen just above and parallel to the sacrospinous ligament lying deep within the gluteus maximus muscle (see Fig. 122.10). Color Doppler is then utilized to identify the internal pudendal artery, which lies medial to or just above the pudendal nerve (Fig. 122.11). It should be noted that the inferior gluteal artery, which lies lateral to the tip of the ischial spine and in proximity to the sciatic nerve, can be easily mistaken for the internal pudendal artery if the ischial spine is not first identified (Fig. 122.12). The pudendal nerve should be identifiable just medial to or above the inferior pudendal artery (Fig. 122.13). After the internal pudendal artery and adjacent pudendal nerve are identified, the skin overlying the area beneath the ultrasound transducer is prepped with antiseptic solution. A sterile syringe containing 10.0 mL of 0.25% preservative-free bupivacaine is attached to a 3½-inch, 22-gauge needle using strict aseptic technique. If the painful condition being treated is thought to have an inflammatory component, 40 to 80 mg of depot steroid is added to the local anesthetic. The needle is placed through the skin ~1 cm above the medial edge of the transducer and is then advanced using an in-plane approach with the needle trajectory adjusted under real-time ultrasound guidance so that the needle tip rests within proximity, but outside the substance of the pudendal nerve (Fig. 122.14). When the tip of needle is thought to be

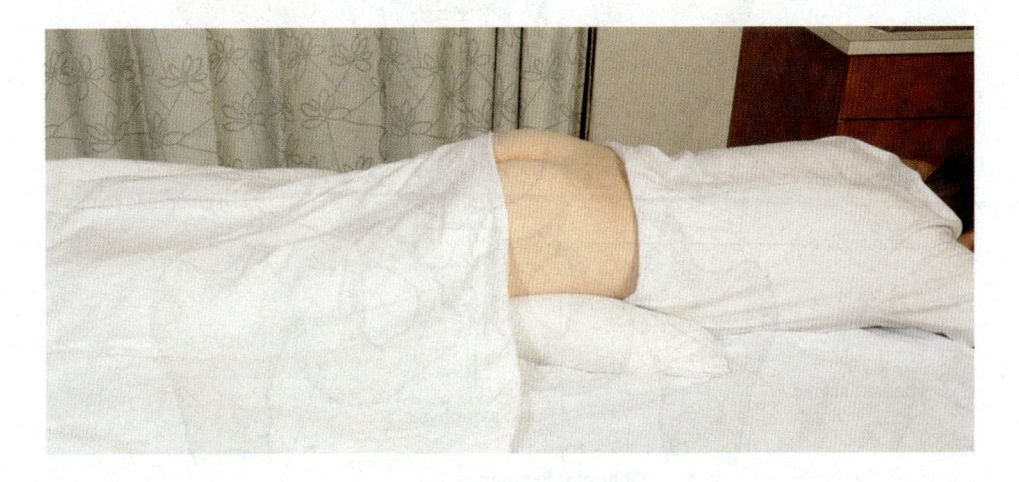

**FIGURE 122.4.** Proper prone patient positioning for ultrasound-guided injection of the pudendal nerve.

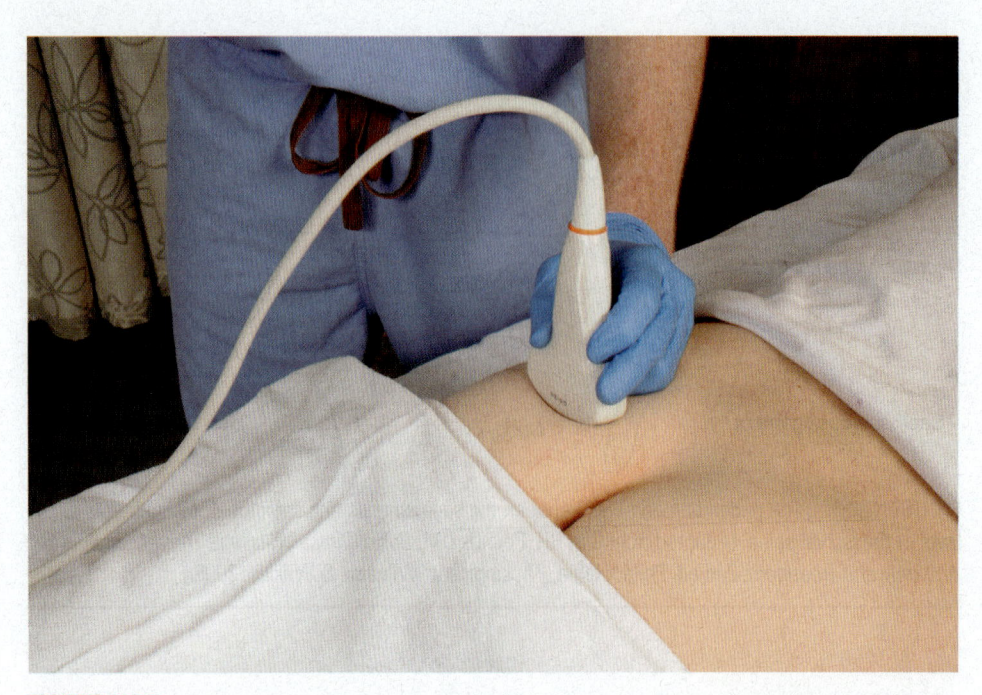

**FIGURE 122.5.** Proper transverse placement of the high-frequency ultrasound transducer over the posterior midgluteal region for ultrasound-guided injection of the pudendal nerve at the hip.

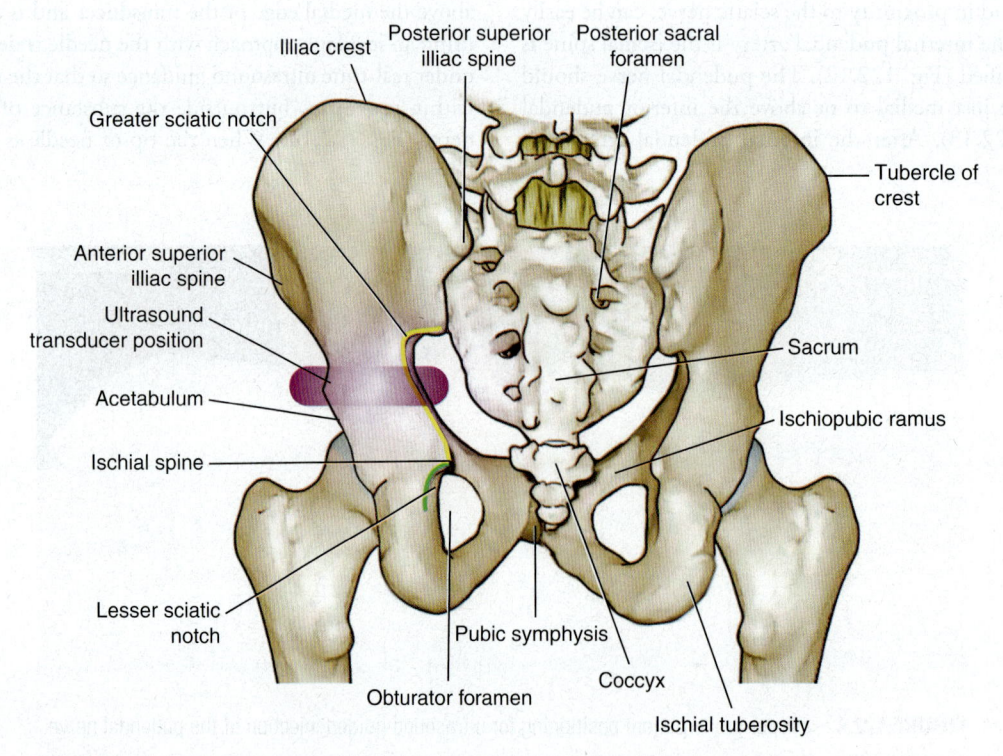

**FIGURE 122.6.** Level of transverse ultrasound transducer placement over ilium.

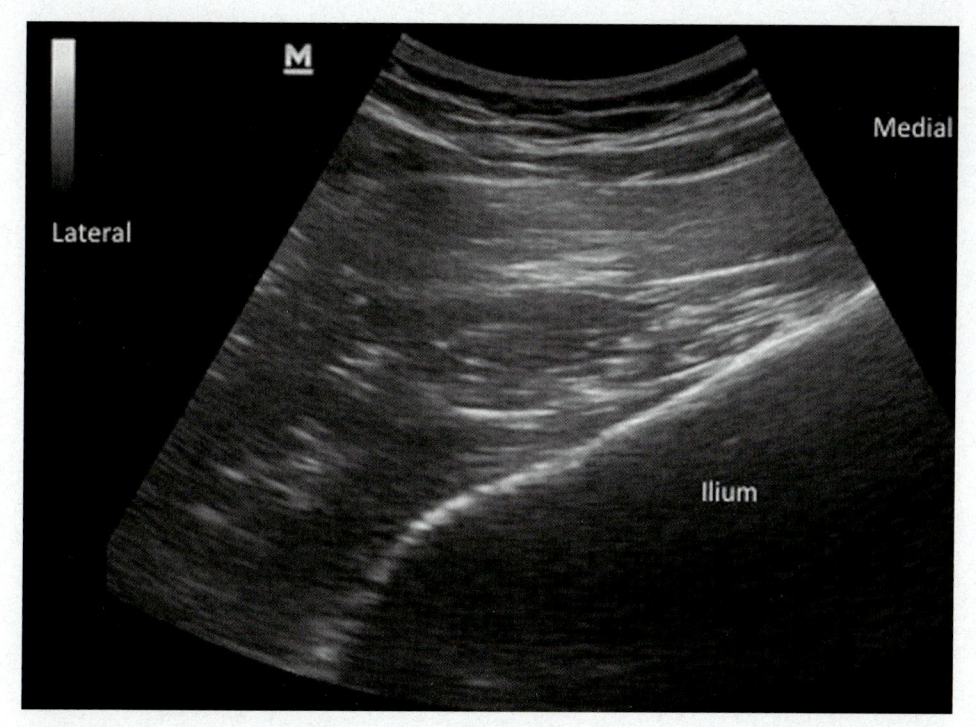

**FIGURE 122.7.** Transverse ultrasound image of the ilium.

in satisfactory position, after careful aspiration, a small amount of local anesthetic and steroid is injected under real-time ultrasound guidance to confirm that the needle tip is lying between the sacrospinous and sacrotuberous ligaments and not within the substance of the nerve. After proper needle tip placement is confirmed, the remainder of the contents of the syringe are slowly injected. There should be minimal resistance to injection, and the clinician should stop injecting immediately if the patient experiences any increase in pain during the injection procedure.

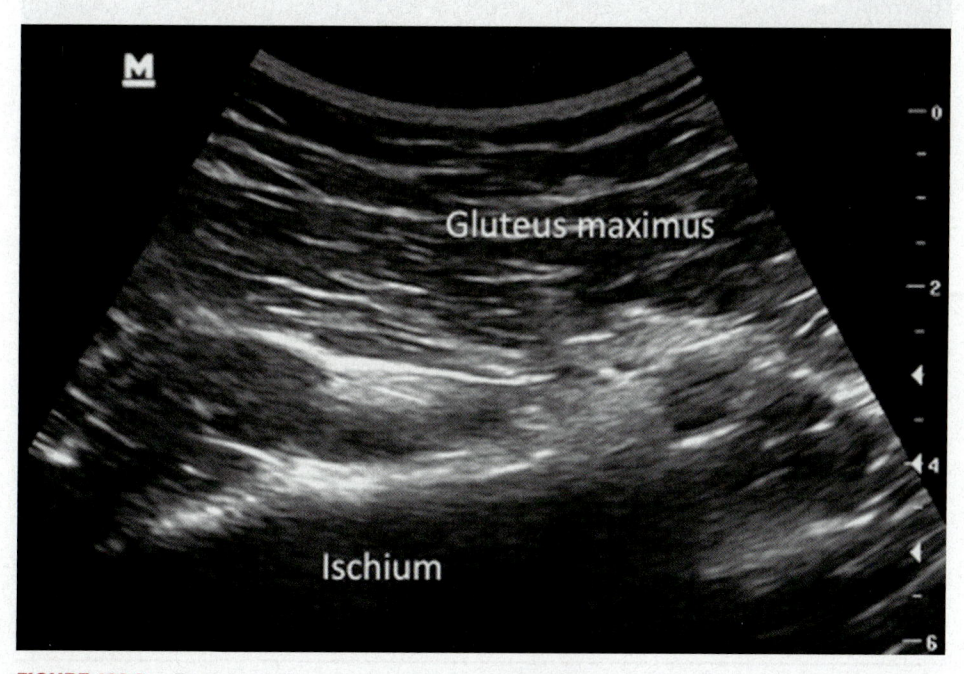

**FIGURE 122.8.** Transverse ultrasound view of the ischial spine.

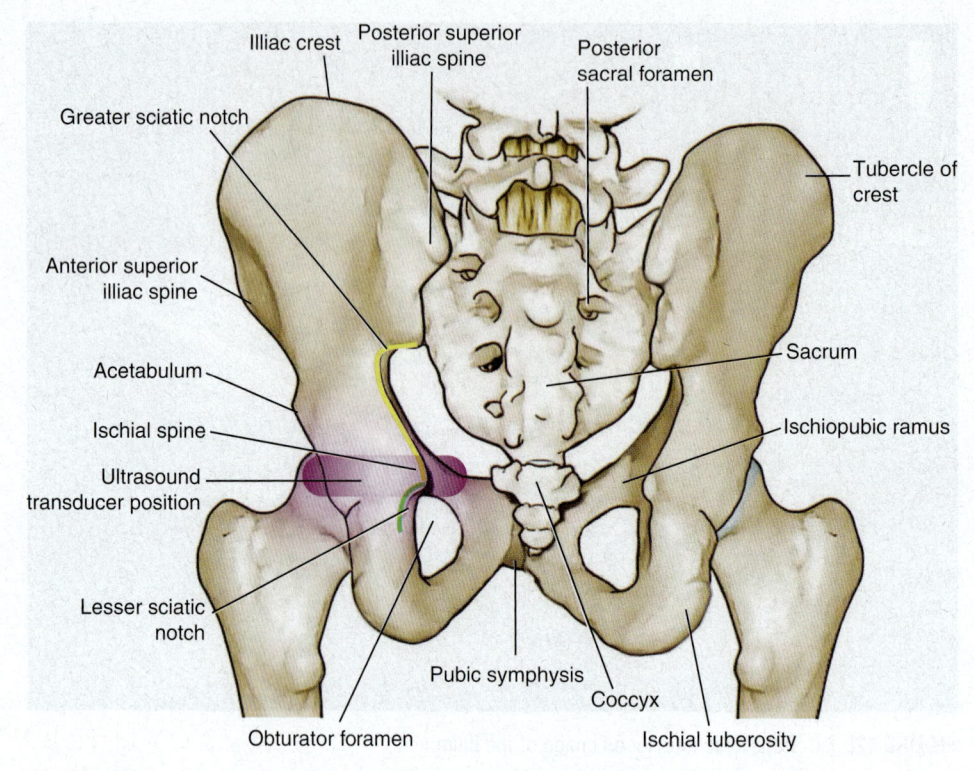

**FIGURE 122.9.** Level of transverse ultrasound transducer placement over ischial spine.

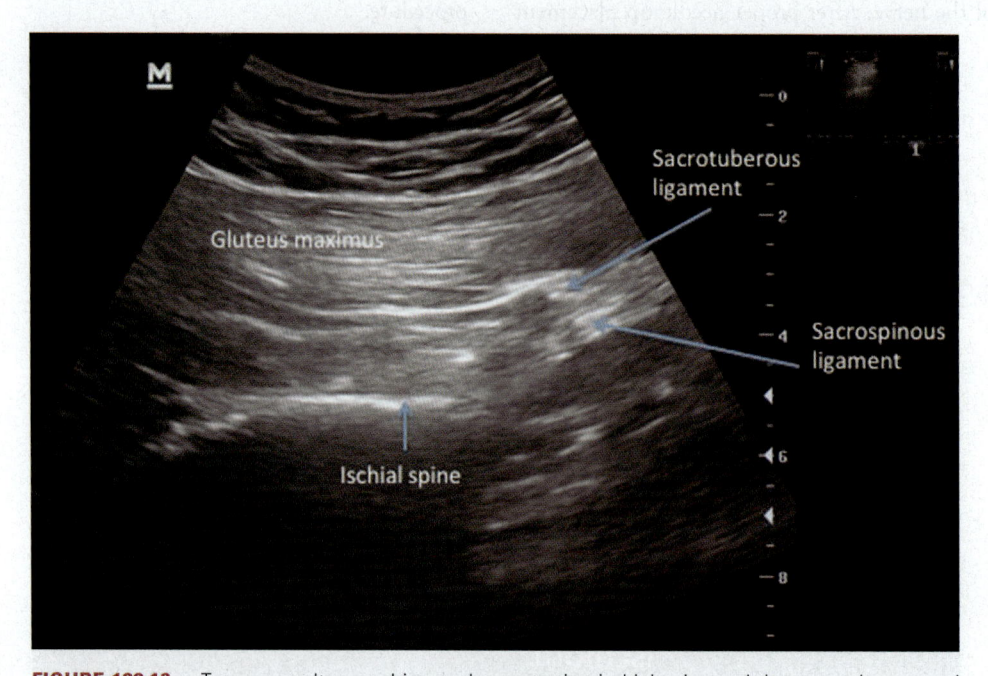

**FIGURE 122.10.** Transverse ultrasound image demonstrating ischial spine and the sacrotuberous and sacrospinous ligaments.

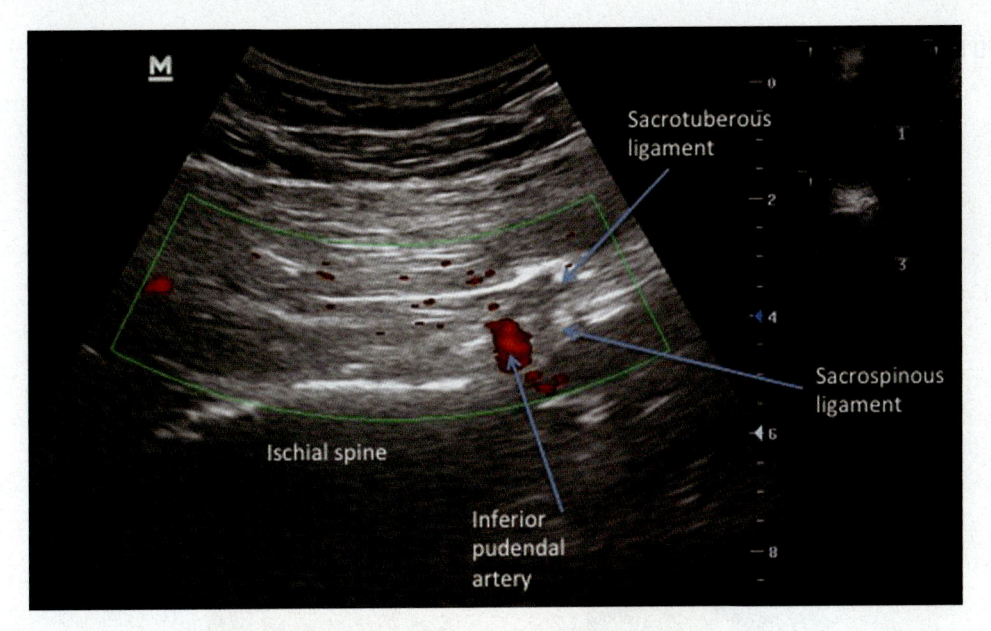

**FIGURE 122.11.** Transverse color Doppler view of the internal pudendal artery and its relationship to the sacrotuberous and sacrospinous ligaments.

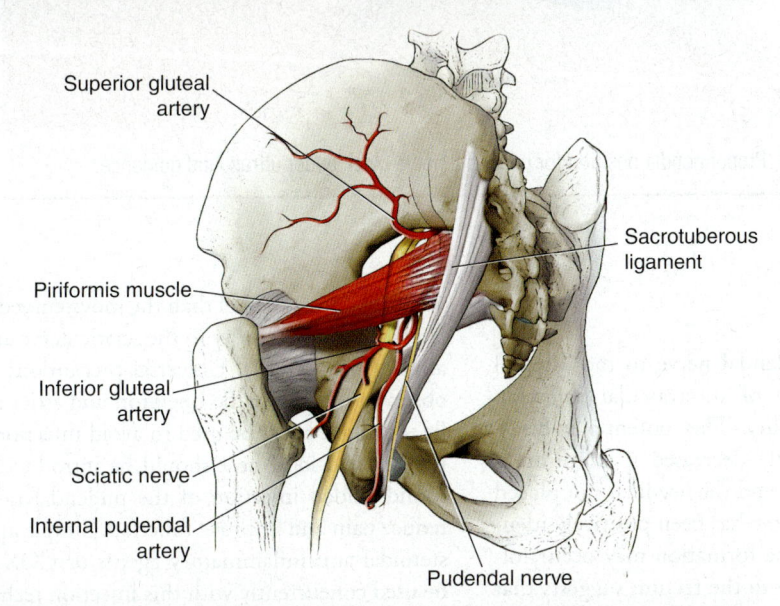

**FIGURE 122.12.** The inferior gluteal artery lies lateral to the ischial spine and can easily be confused with the internal pudendal artery on color Doppler if the ischial spine is not first identified.

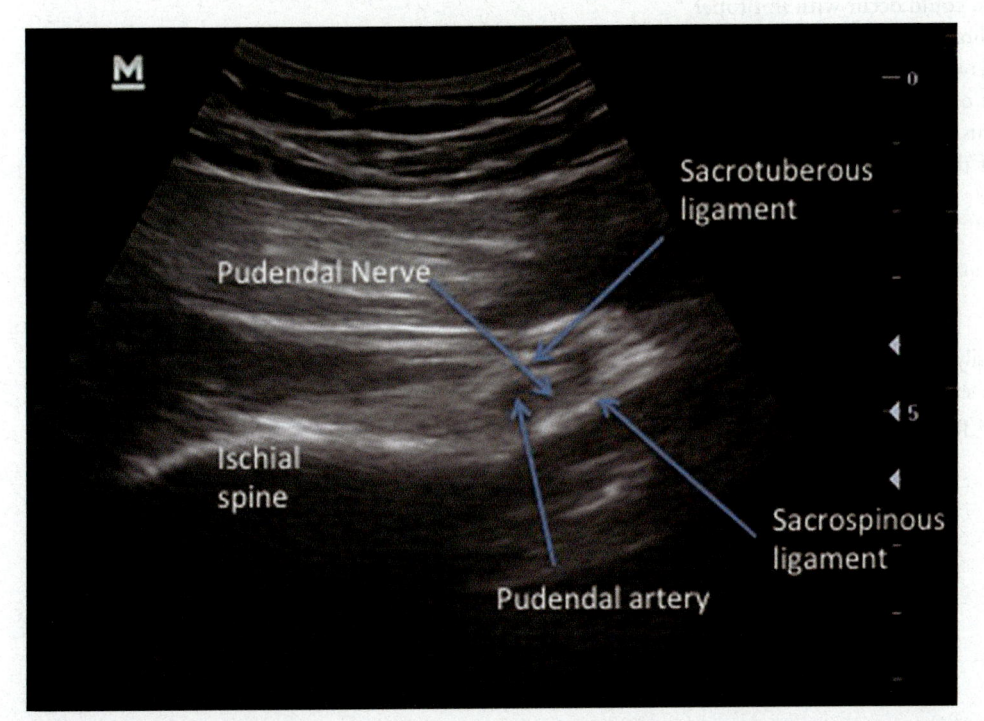

**FIGURE 122.13.** Transverse ultrasound view of the pudendal nerve. Note the relative positions of the internal pudendal artery, the ischial spine, and the sacrotuberous and sacrospinous ligaments.

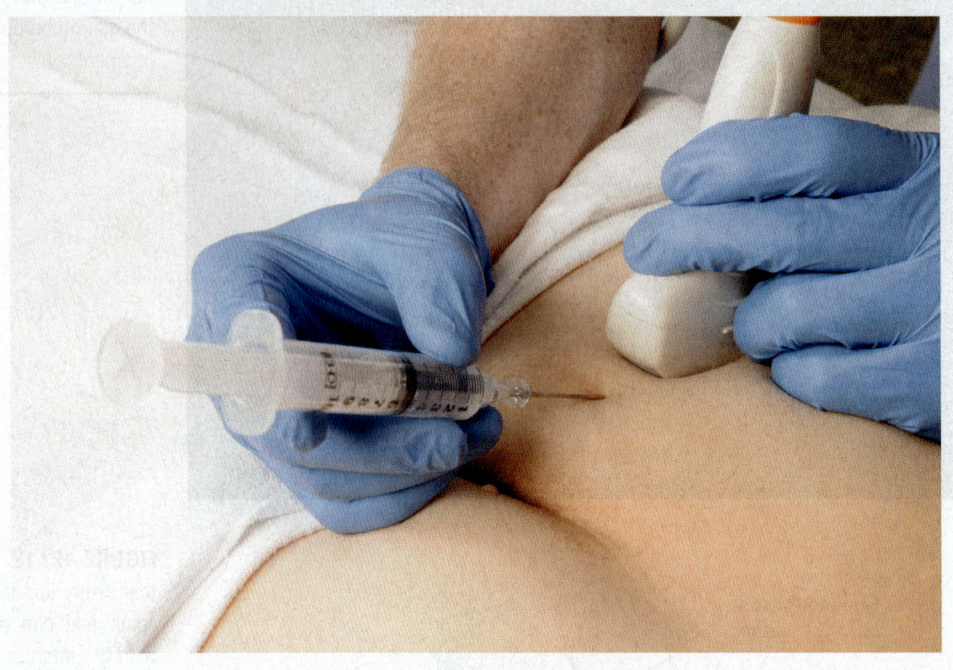

**FIGURE 122.14.** Proper needle position for pudendal nerve block under ultrasound guidance.

## COMPLICATIONS

Given the proximity of the pudendal nerve to the internal pudendal artery, the possibility of intravascular injection remains an ever-present possibility. This potentially disastrous complication can be greatly decreased if attention is paid to the sonographic anatomy and the needle is not placed until the pudendal artery and nerve has been positively identified. Ecchymosis and hematoma formation may occur following this procedure. Proximity to the rectum suggests that infection and/or fistula formation could occur with improper needle placement, especially in those patients who are immunocompromised or have received radiation therapy to the perineum. A transient exacerbation of the patient's pain occurs ~25% of the time following this injection technique, and the patient should be warned of this possibility prior to the procedure.

## CLINICAL PEARLS

The inferior gluteal artery can easily be mistaken for the internal pudendal artery on Doppler examination. It is therefore important to first identify the flat portion of the ischial spine, which lies more medial than the move curved portion, which is lateral and in proximity to the sciatic nerve and inferior gluteal artery (Fig. 122.12). Universal precautions should always be observed to protect the operator, and strict adherence to sterile technique must be used to avoid infection. Gentle physical therapy and local heat should be introduced following ultrasound-guided injection of the pudendal nerve at the hip to reduce pain and improve function. Simple analgesics and nonsteroidal anti-inflammatory agents or COX-2 inhibitors may be used concurrently with this injection technique.

## SUGGESTED READINGS

Beco J, Mouchel J, Mouchel T, et al. Concerns about the use of colour Doppler in the diagnosis of pudendal nerve entrapment. *Pain* 2009;145(1–2):261.
Peng PWH, Tumber PS. Ultrasound-guided interventional procedures for patients with chronic pelvic pain—a description of techniques and review of literature. *Pain Physician* 2008;11:215–224.
Rofaeel A, Peng P, Louis I, et al. Feasibility of real-time ultrasound for pudendal nerve block in patients with chronic perineal pain. *Reg Anesth Pain Med* 2008;33(2):139–145.
Waldman SD. Injection technique for pudendal nerve-transperineal approach. In: *Atlas of Interventional Pain Management Techniques*. 3rd ed. Philadelphia, PA: Saunders Elsevier; 2009:494–496.
Waldman SD. Pudendal nerve block. In: *Pain Review*. Philadelphia, PA: Saunders Elsevier; 2009:543–544.

# CHAPTER 123

# Ultrasound-Guided Sacroiliac Joint Injection

## CLINICAL PERSPECTIVES

The sacroiliac joint is a bicondylar synovial joint that is formed by the articulation between the sacrum and ilium (Fig. 123.1). The articular surface of the sacrum is covered with hyaline cartilage, with the articular surface of the ilium covered with fibrocartilage. The articular surfaces are characterized by irregular elevations and depressions that allow the joints to interlock at numerous points along their articular surface contributing to joint strength. The joint's articular cartilage is susceptible to damage from overuse or misuse, which left untreated, will result in arthritis with its associated pain and functional disability. Osteoarthritis of the joint is the most common form of arthritis that results in sacroiliac joint pain and functional disability, with rheumatoid arthritis, spondyloarthropathies, and post-traumatic arthritis also causing arthritis of the sacroiliac joint. Less common causes of arthritis-induced sacroiliac joint pain include the collagen vascular diseases, infection, villonodular synovitis, and Lyme disease. Acute infectious arthritis of the sacroiliac joint is best treated with early diagnosis, with culture and sensitivity of the synovial fluid, and with prompt initiation of antibiotic therapy. The collagen vascular diseases generally manifest as a polyarthropathy rather than a monoarthropathy limited to the sacroiliac joint, although sacroiliac pain secondary to the collagen vascular diseases responds exceedingly well to ultrasound-guided intra-articular injection of the sacroiliac joint. Occasionally, the clinician encounters patients with iatrogenically induced sacroiliac joint dysfunction due to over-aggressive bone graft harvesting for spinal fusions.

Patients with sacroiliac joint pain secondary to strain or arthritis-related pain complain of pain that is localized to the sacroiliac and proximal lower extremity. The pain of sacroiliac joint strain or arthritis radiates into the posterior buttocks and the back of the legs (Fig. 123.2). The pain does not radiate below the knees. Activity makes the pain worse, with rest and heat providing some relief. The pain is constant and characterized as aching. Sleep disturbance is common with awakening when the patient rolls over onto the affected sacroiliac joint. Spasm of the lumbar paraspinal musculature often is present, as is limitation of range of motion of the lumbar spine in the erect position that improves in the sitting position due to relaxation of the hamstring muscles. Patients with pain emanating from the sacroiliac joint exhibit a positive Yeoman test. The Yeoman test is performed by flexing the knee to 90 degrees and then hyperextending the hip, putting stress on the sacroiliac joint (Fig. 123.3). A positive test is indicated by the production of pain around the sacroiliac joint.

Plain radiographs are indicated in all patients who present with sacroiliac pain as not only intrinsic sacroiliac disease, as well as other regional pathology may be perceived as sacroiliac pain by the patient (Fig. 123.4). Based on the patient's clinical presentation, additional testing may be indicated, including complete blood cell count, sedimentation rate, and antinuclear antibody testing. Magnetic resonance imaging or ultrasound of the sacroiliac is indicated if the diagnosis is in question or infection of the joint is a possibility.

## CLINICALLY RELEVANT ANATOMY

The sacroiliac joint is a bicondylar synovial joint that is formed by the articulation between the sacrum and ilium (see Fig. 123.1). The articular surface of the sacrum is covered with hyaline cartilage, with the articular surface of the ilium covered with fibrocartilage. These articular surfaces have corresponding elevations and depressions, which give the joints their irregular appearance on radiographs. The strength of the sacroiliac joint comes primarily from the posterior and interosseous ligaments, rather than from the bony articulations. The sacroiliac joints bear the weight of the trunk and are thus subject to the development of strain and arthritis. As the joint ages, the intra-articular space narrows, making intra-articular injection more challenging. The ligaments and the sacroiliac joint itself receive their innervation from L3 to S3 nerve roots, with L4 and L5 providing the greatest contribution to the innervation of the joint. This diverse innervation may explain the ill-defined nature of sacroiliac pain. The sacroiliac joint has a very limited range of motion, and that motion is induced by changes in the forces placed on the joint by shifts in posture and joint loading.

## ULTRASOUND-GUIDED TECHNIQUE

The benefits, risks, and alternative treatments are explained to the patient and informed consent is obtained. The patient is then placed in the prone position with a thin pillow under the hips (Fig. 123.5). The skin overlying the sacroiliac joint is

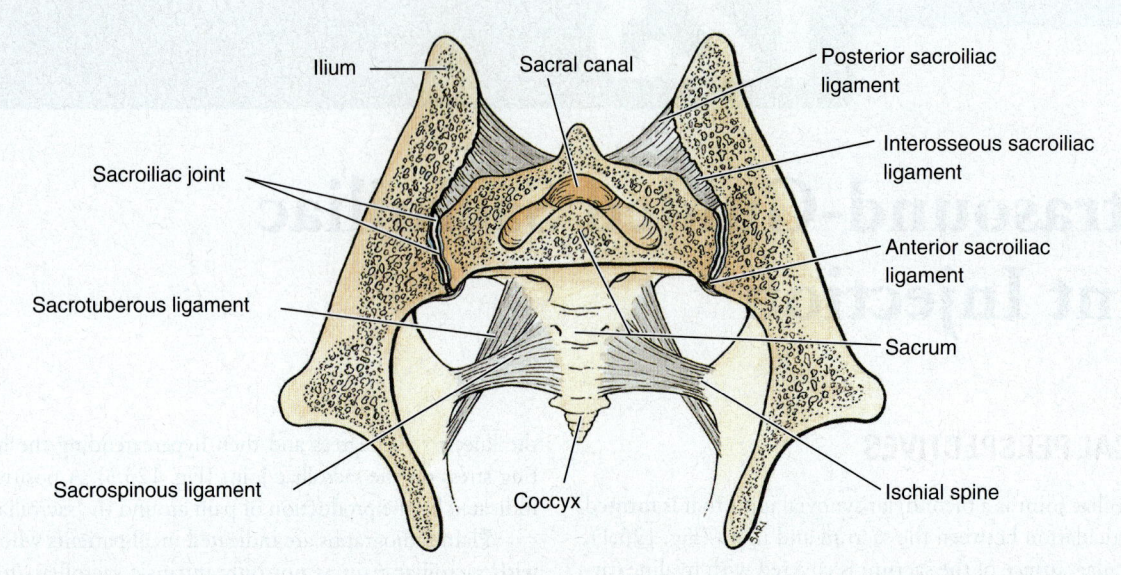

**FIGURE 123.1.** The anatomy of the sacroiliac joint. (Reused from Moore KL, Agur A. *Essential Clinical Anatomy*. 2nd ed. Philadelphia, PA: Lippincott Williams & Wilkins; 2002, with permission.)

then prepped with antiseptic solution. A sterile syringe containing 2.0 mL of 0.25% preservative-free bupivacaine and 40 mg of methylprednisolone is attached to a 3½-inch, 22-gauge needle using strict aseptic technique. A curvilinear low-frequency ultrasound transducer is placed in the transverse plane over the dorsal medial crest of the sacrum, and an ultrasound survey scan is taken (Fig. 123.6). The dorsal medial crest of the sacrum will appear as a hyperechoic structure that looks like batman's head with the resultant acoustic shadow looking like his spread out cape (Fig. 123.7). When the dorsal median

**FIGURE 123.2.** The pattern of pain referred from the sacroiliac joint.

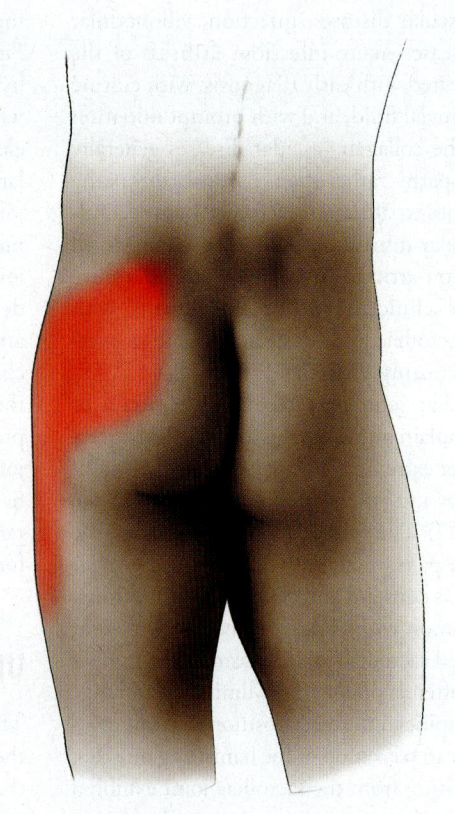

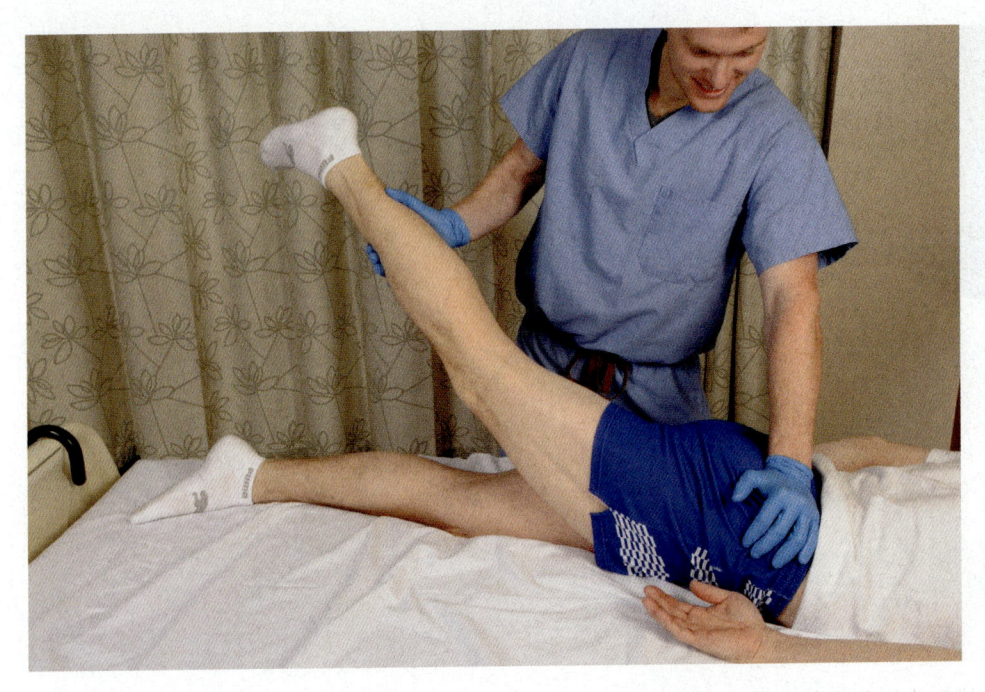

**FIGURE 123.3.** Yeoman test is useful in the diagnosis of sacroiliac pain. It is performed by flexing the knee to 90 degrees and then hyperextending the hip, putting stress on the sacroiliac joint.

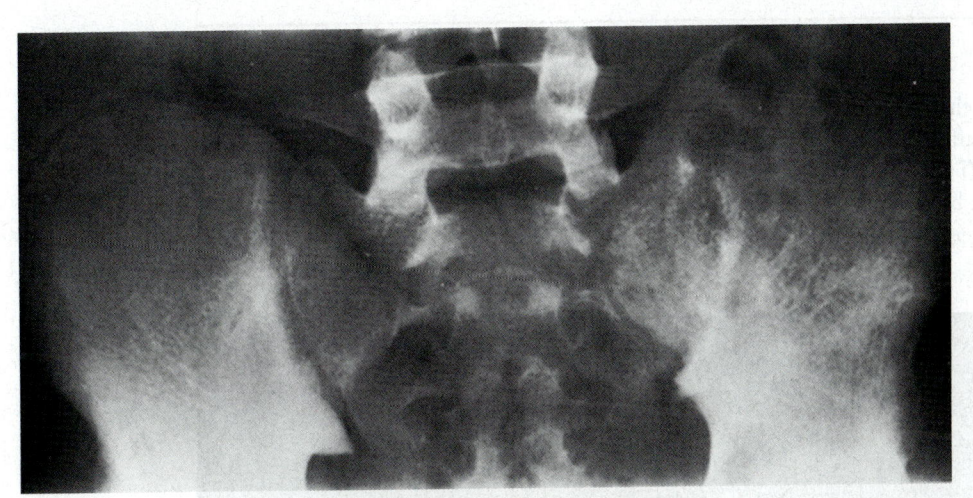

**FIGURE 123.4.** Bilateral, though asymmetric, sclerosis and narrowing of the sacroiliac joints with reactive sclerosis secondary to Reiter syndrome. (From Eisenberg RL. Sacroiliac joint abnormality. In: *Clinical Imaging: An Atlas of Differential Diagnosis*. 4th ed. Philadelphia, PA: Lippincott Williams & Wilkins; 2009.)

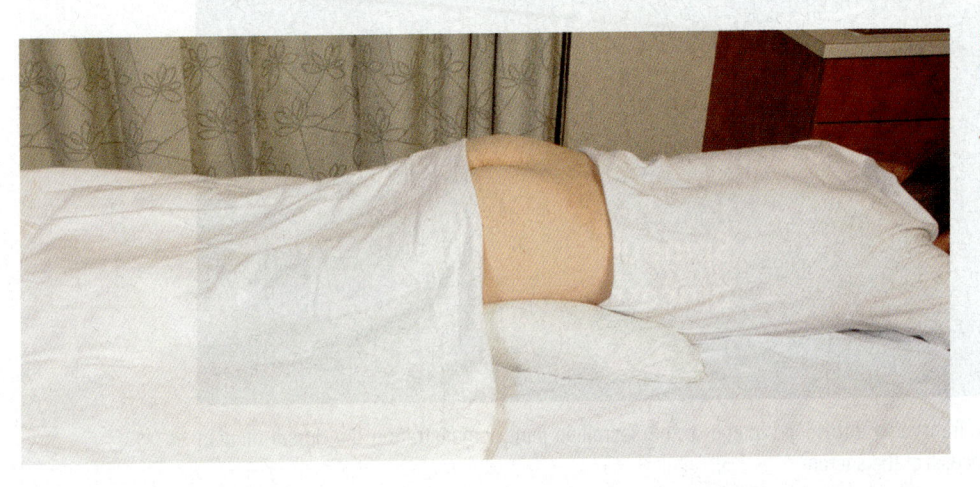

**FIGURE 123.5.** Proper patient position for ultrasound-guided intra-articular sacroiliac injection.

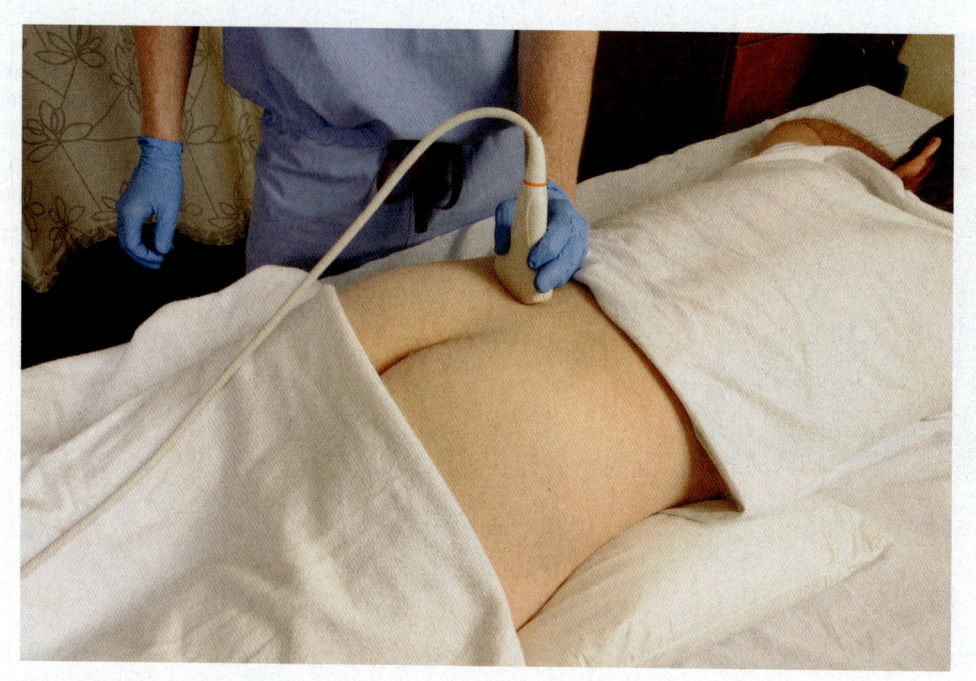

**FIGURE 123.6.** Correct transverse position for ultrasound transducer for ultrasound-guided intra-articular injection of the sacroiliac joint.

crest of the sacrum is identified, the ultrasound transducer is slowly moved laterally toward the affected joint until the medial margin of the ilium is visualized (Figs. 123.8 and 123.9). The sacroiliac joint will be seen to lie between this medial border of the sacrum and the lateral border of the ilium (Fig. 123.10).

After the joint space is identified, the needle is placed through the skin ~1 cm below the middle of the ultrasound transducer and angled ~25 degrees and is then advanced toward the joint using an out-of-plane approach with the needle trajectory adjusted under real-time ultrasound guidance to enter the

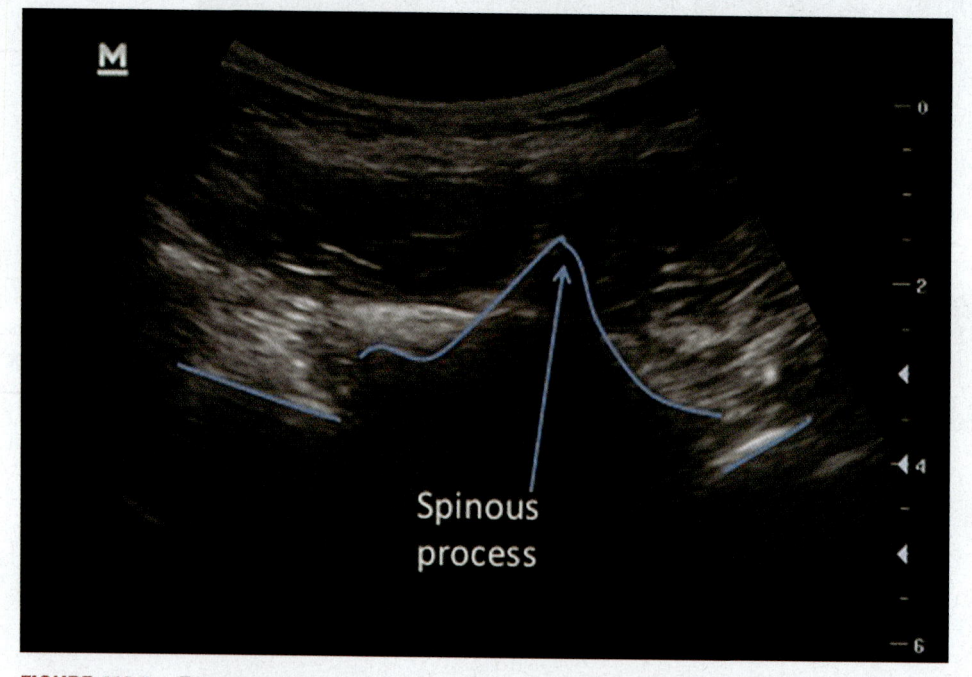

**FIGURE 123.7.** Transverse ultrasound image of the sacroiliac joint demonstrating the dorsal median crest (spinous process) of the sacrum.

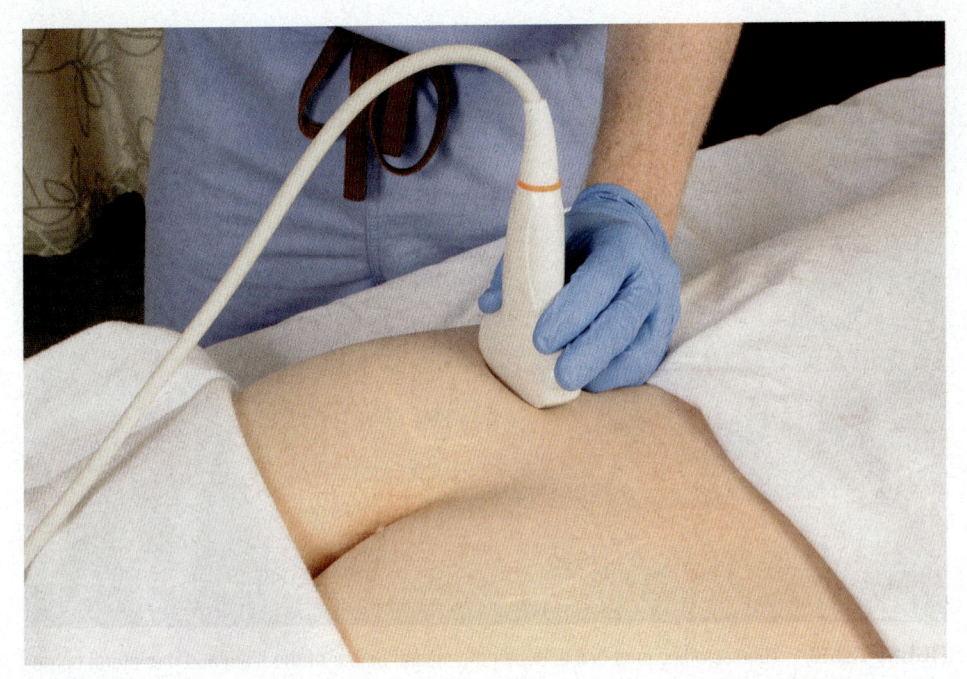

**FIGURE 123.8.** The transversely placed ultrasound transducer is then slowly moved laterally to identify the medial margin of the ilium.

sacroiliac joint (Fig. 123.11). When the tip of needle is thought to be within the joint space, a small amount of local anesthetic and steroid is injected under real-time ultrasound guidance to confirm intra-articular placement. After intra-articular needle tip placement is confirmed, the remainder of the contents of the syringe is slowly injected. There should be minimal resistance to injection. The needle may have to be repositioned to ensure that the entire intra-articular space is treated. The needle is then removed, and a sterile pressure dressing and ice pack are placed at the injection site.

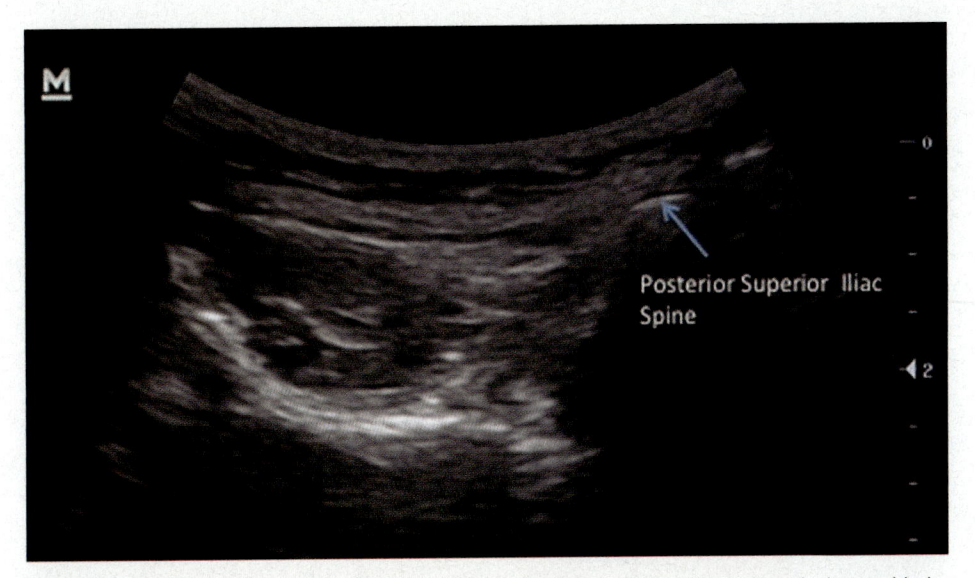

**FIGURE 123.9.** Transverse ultrasound image of the medial border of the ilium as it articulates with the sacrum.

**FIGURE 123.10.** The sacroiliac joint lies between the medial border of the ilium and the lateral border of the sacrum.

## COMPLICATIONS

The major complication of ultrasound-guided injection of the sacroiliac joint is infection. Ecchymosis and hematoma formation may also occur. A transient exacerbation of the patient's pain occurs ~25% of the time following this injection technique, and the patient should be warned of this possibility prior to the procedure.

## CLINICAL PEARLS

Ultrasound-guided injection of the sacroiliac joint is extremely effective in the treatment of sacroiliac joint pain. Coexistent bursitis and tendonitis also may contribute to sacroiliac pain and may require additional treatment with more localized injection of local anesthetic and depot corticosteroid preparation. This technique is safe if careful

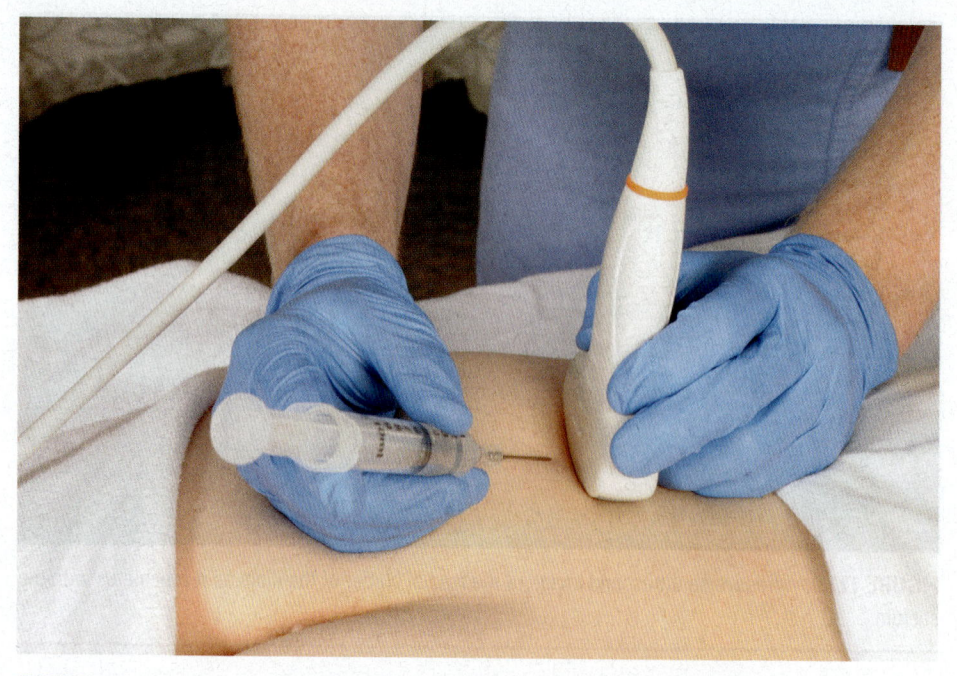

**FIGURE 123.11.** Correct in-plane needle placement for ultrasound-guided sacroiliac joint injection.

attention is paid to the clinically relevant anatomy in the areas to be injected. Care must be taken to use sterile technique to avoid infection; universal precautions should be used to avoid risk to the operator. The incidence of ecchymosis and hematoma formation can be decreased if pressure is placed on the injection site immediately after injection. The use of physical modalities, including local heat and gentle range-of-motion exercises, should be introduced several days after the patient undergoes this injection technique for sacroiliac pain. Vigorous exercise should be avoided because it exacerbates the patient's symptomatology. Simple analgesics and nonsteroidal anti-inflammatory agents may be used concurrently with this injection technique.

## SUGGESTED READINGS

Block BM, Hobelmann JG, Murphy KJ, et al. An imaging review of sacroiliac injection under computer tomography guidance. *Reg Anesth Pain Med* 2005;30(3):295–298.

Vydyanathan A, Samer N. Ultrasound-guided caudal and sacroiliac joint injections. *Tech Reg Anesth Pain Manag* 2009;13(3):157–160.

Waldman SD, Campbell RSD. Sacroiliac joint disorders. In: *Imaging of Pain*. Philadelphia, PA: Saunders Elsevier; 2011:197–199.

Waldman SD, Campbell RSD. Special imaging considerations of the sacroiliac joint and bony pelvis. In: *Imaging of Pain*. Philadelphia, PA: Saunders Elsevier; 2011:193–196.

Waldman SD. Intra-articular injection of the sacroiliac joint. In: *Pain Review*. Philadelphia, PA: Saunders Elsevier; 2009:544–545.

Waldman SD. Intra-articular injection of the sacroiliac joint. In: *Atlas of Pain Management Injection Techniques*. 3rd ed. Philadelphia, PA: Saunders Elsevier; 2012:343–345.

# CHAPTER 124

# Ultrasound-Guided Injection Technique for External Snapping Hip Syndrome

## CLINICAL PERSPECTIVES

Snapping hip is an uncommon cause of lateral hip pain, not a single syndrome, but a group of disorders that have in common abnormal passage of musculotendinous units or fascial bands over the greater trochanter. In an effort to better understand the pathophysiology responsible for snapping hip syndrome in a specific patient, it is helpful to classify the pathology as to the anatomic structures or region responsible for the symptomatology (Table 124.1). To this end, snapping hip syndrome can be classified as external, internal, or intra-articular. The pathophysiology associated with external slipping hip syndrome is related to abnormal passage of the posterior border of the iliotibial band or the anterior border of the gluteus maximus muscle over the greater trochanter (Fig. 124.1). The pathophysiology of internal snapping hip syndrome is thought to be related to the abnormal passage of the iliopsoas tendon over the iliopectineal eminence (Fig. 124.2). Loose bodies, synovial abnormalities, and tears of the labrum have been implicated as the cause of intra-articular snapping hip syndrome.

The constellation of symptoms associated with external snapping hip syndrome includes a snapping, clicking, or grating sensation in the lateral hip associated with sudden, sharp pain in the area of the greater trochanter. The symptomatology of snapping hip syndrome occurs most commonly when the patient rises from a sitting to a standing position or when walking briskly. Often, trochanteric bursitis coexists with snapping hip syndrome, further increasing the patient's pain and disability.

Patients suffering from external snapping hip syndrome can usually recreate the snapping and pain by moving from a sitting to a standing position and by adducting the hip. These patients will also usually exhibit a positive snap test. The snap test is performed by having the patient move rapidly from a squatting to a standing position while the clinician palpates the area over the grater trochanter (Fig. 124.3). Point tenderness over the trochanteric bursa indicative of trochanteric bursitis also is often present.

Plain radiographs are indicated in all patients who present with pain thought to be emanating from the hip to rule out occult bony pathology and tumor. Based on the patient's clinical presentation, additional testing may be indicated, including complete blood cell count, prostate-specific antigen, sedimentation rate, and antinuclear antibody testing. Magnetic resonance and/or ultrasound imaging of the affected hip is indicated to help confirm the diagnosis and identify coexistent trochanteric bursitis, as well as to rule other hip pathology (Fig. 124.4).

## CLINICALLY RELEVANT ANATOMY

The trochanteric bursa lies between the greater trochanter and the tendon of the gluteus medius and the iliotibial tract (Fig. 124.5). The gluteus medius muscle has its origin from the outer surface of the ilium, and its fibers pass downward and laterally to attach on the lateral surface of the greater trochanter. The gluteus medius locks the pelvis in place when walking and

**TABLE 124.1  Causes of Snapping Hip Syndrome**

External causes
- Abnormal passage of iliotibial band over the greater trochanter
- Abnormal passage of the tensor fascia lata over the greater trochanter
- Abnormal passage of the gluteus medius tendon over the grater trochanter
- Trochanteric bursitis

Internal causes
- Abnormal passage of the iliopsoas tendon over the anterior inferior iliac spine
- Abnormal passage of the iliopsoas tendon over the lesser trochanter
- Abnormal passage of the iliopsoas tendon over the over the iliopectineal ridge

Intra-articular causes
- Torn acetabular labrum
- Repeated subluxation of the hip
- Torn ligamentum teres
- Synovial chondromatosis
- Joint mice
- Abnormalities of the articular cartilage

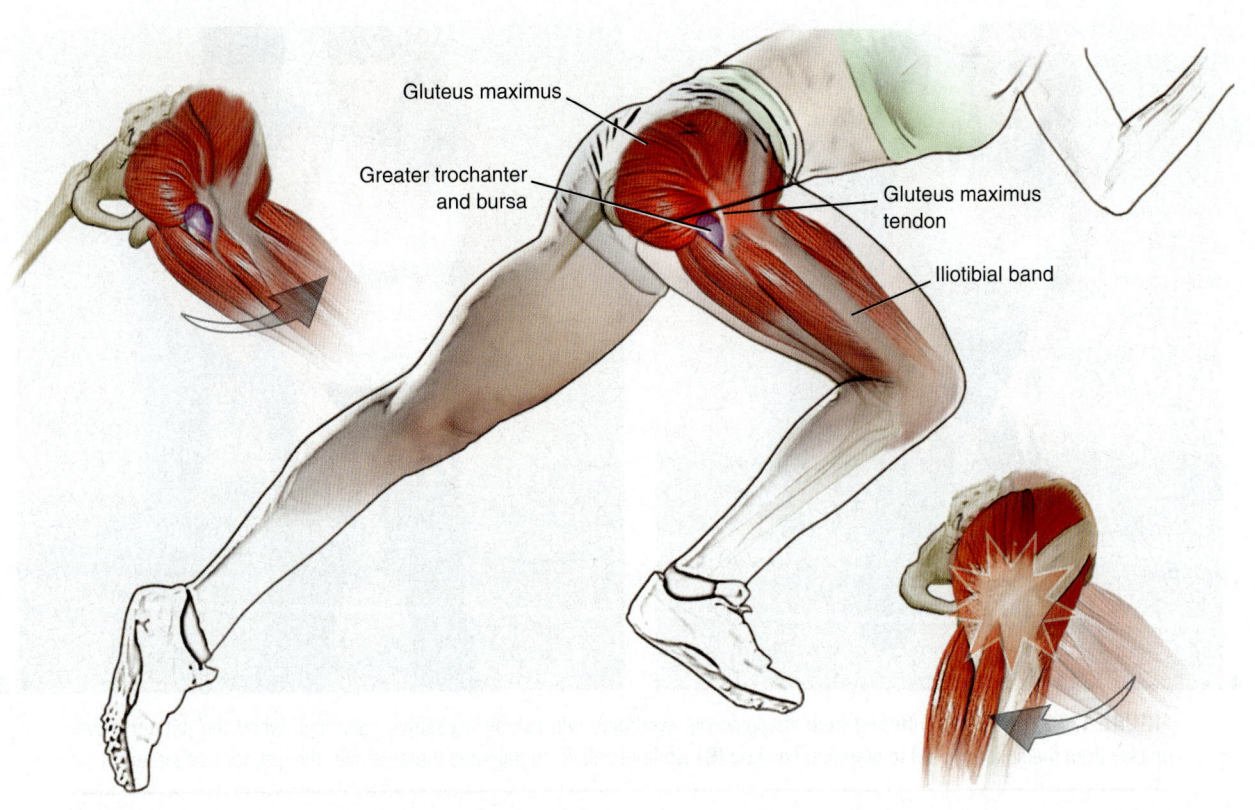

**FIGURE 124.1.** External snapping hip syndrome is caused by abnormal slipping of the iliotibial band or the gluteus maximus iliotibial unit over the trochanteric bursa.

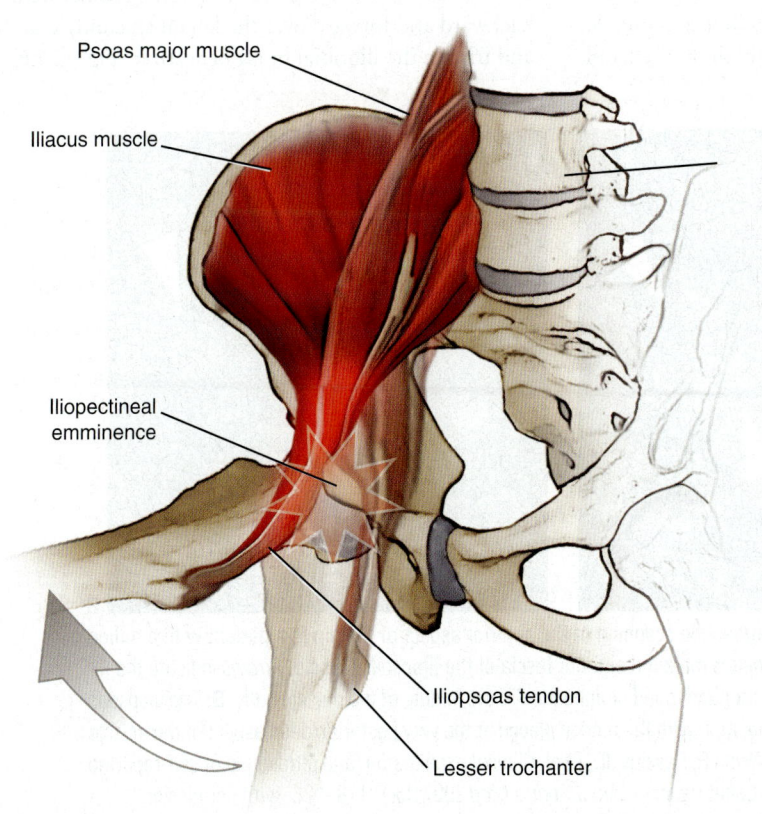

**FIGURE 124.2.** Internal snapping hip syndrome is caused by abnormal slipping of the iliopsoas tendon over the pectineal eminence.

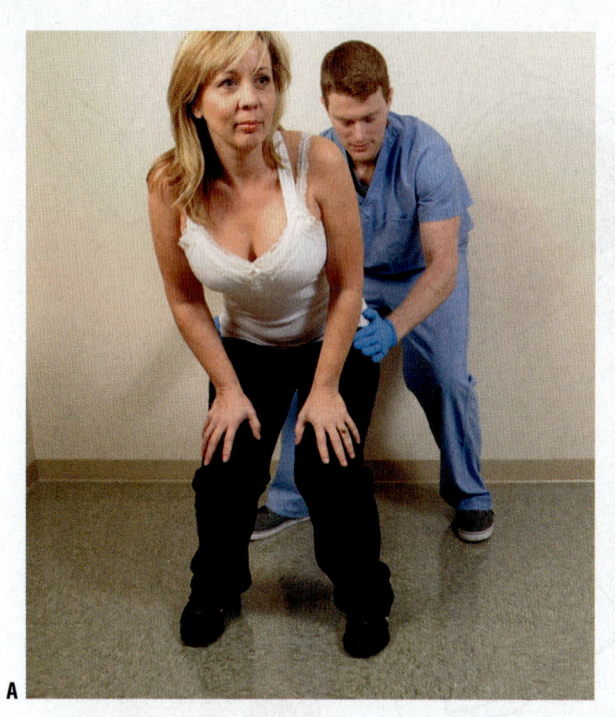

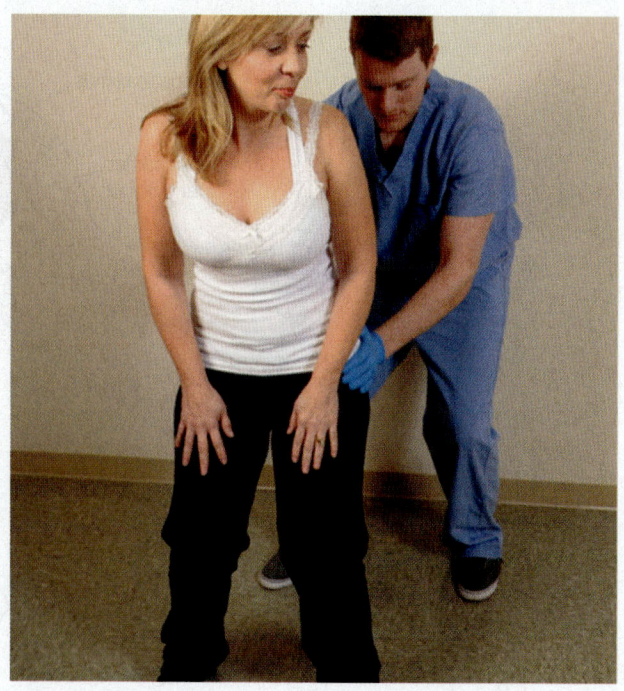

**FIGURE 124.3.** Patients suffering from snapping hip syndrome will exhibit a positive snap sign when the patient moves quickly from the squatting **(A)** to standing position **(B)** while the clinician palpates the area over the greater trochanteric.

running. The gluteus medius muscle is innervated by the superior gluteal nerve. The iliopectineal eminence is the point at which the ilium and the pubis bone merge (see Fig. 124.2). The psoas and iliacus muscles join at the lateral side of the psoas, and the combined fibers are referred to as the iliopsoas muscle. Like the psoas muscle, the iliacus flexes the thigh on the trunk or, if the thigh is fixed, flexes the trunk on the thigh, as when moving from a supine to sitting position. The iliotibial band is an extension of the fascia lata, which inserts at the lateral condyle of the tibia (see Fig. 125.5). The iliotibial band can rub backward and forward over the lateral epicondyle of the femur and irritate the iliotibial bursa beneath it (Fig. 124.6).

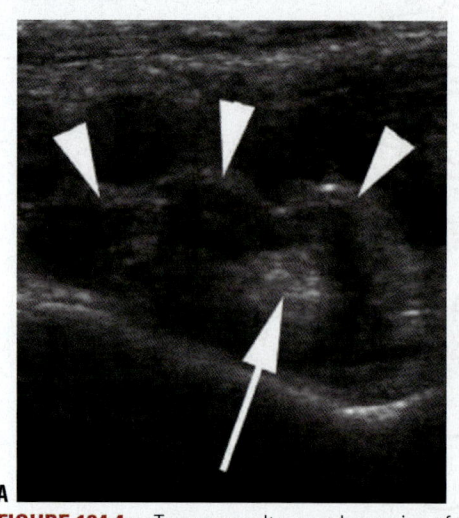

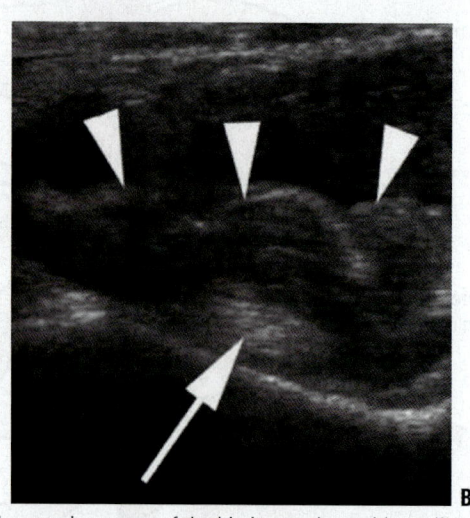

**FIGURE 124.4.** Transverse ultrasound scanning of the anterior aspect of the hip in a patient with a rolling iliopsoas snapping hip. *Arrow heads* mark the anterior fascia of the iliopsoas muscle, *arrows* indicate the iliopsoas tendon. **A:** The iliopsoas tendon rolled or imbedded in the middle of the muscle belly. **B:** The iliopsoas has snapped back to a normal position with the tendon placed at the very posterior/deep aspect of the muscle belly. (Reused from Winston P, Awan R, Cassidy JD, et al. Clinical examination and ultrasound of self-reported snapping hip syndrome in elite ballet dancers. *Am J Sports Med* 2007;35(1):118–126, with permission.)

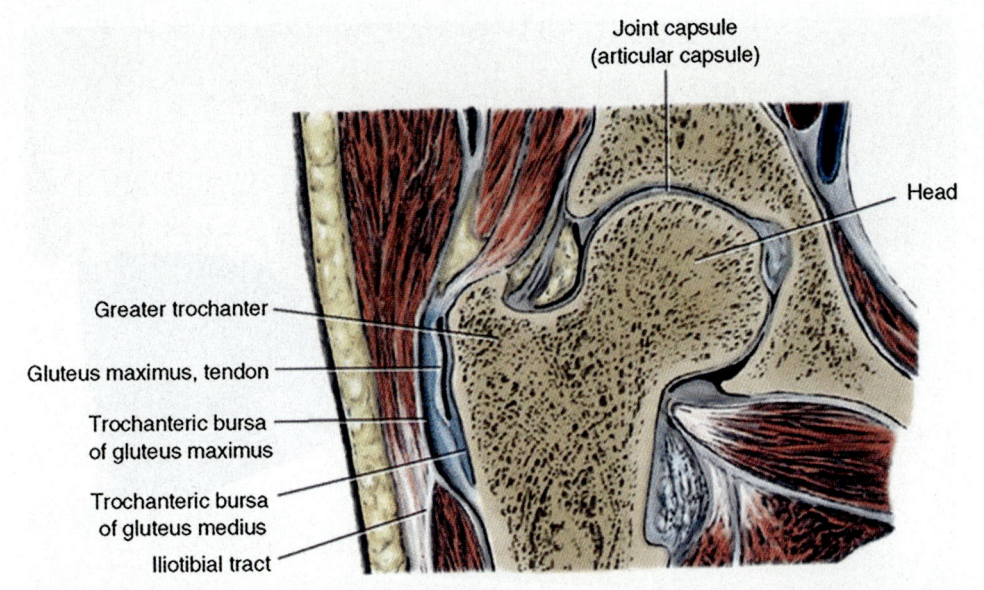

**FIGURE 124.5.** The trochanteric bursa serves to cushion and facilitate sliding of the musculotendinous unit of the gluteus maximus muscle and iliotibial band over the greater trochanter of the femur. (From: McNabb JW. *A Practical Guide to Joint and Soft Tissue Injection and Aspiration Snapping Hip*. 1st ed. Philadelphia, PA: Lippincott Williams & Wilkins; 2005.)

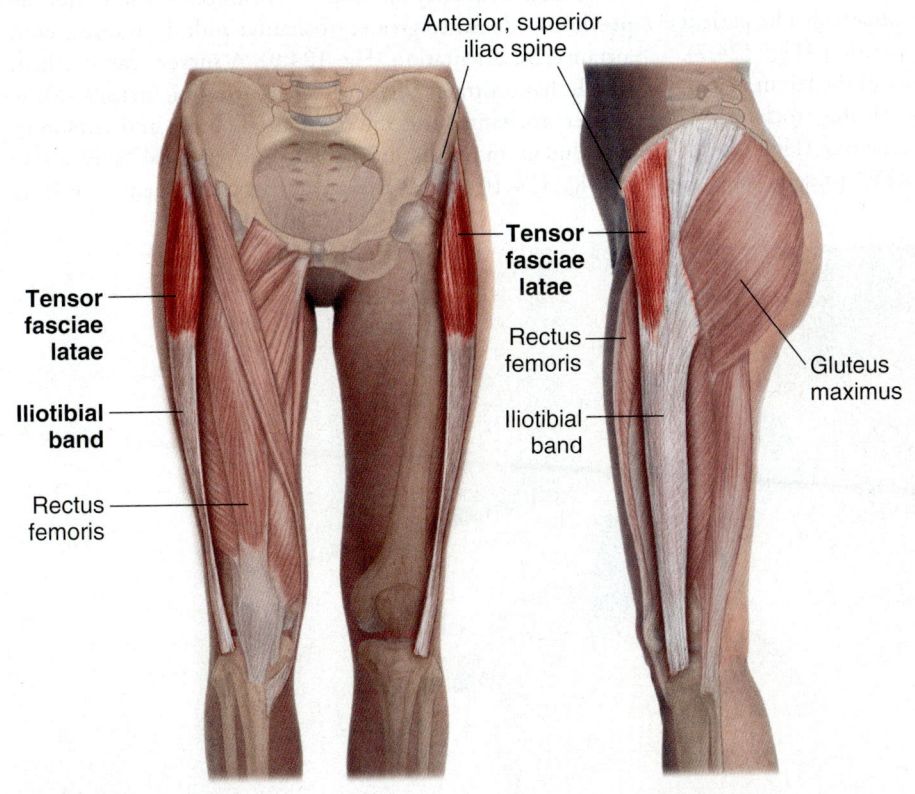

**FIGURE 124.6.** The iliotibial band. (Adapted from Clay JH, Pounds DM. *Basic Clinical Massage Therapy: Integrating Anatomy and Treatment*. 2nd ed. Philadelphia, PA: Lippincott Williams & Wilkins; 2008.)

**TENSOR FASCIAE LATAE**

| | |
|---|---|
| Origin | Outer surface of anterior superior iliac spine, outer lip of anterior iliac crest. |
| Insertion | Lateral condyle of tibia via the iliotibial band. |
| Action | Flex hip, medially rotate hip, abduct hip, anterior pelvic tilt. |
| Nerve | Superior gluteal. |

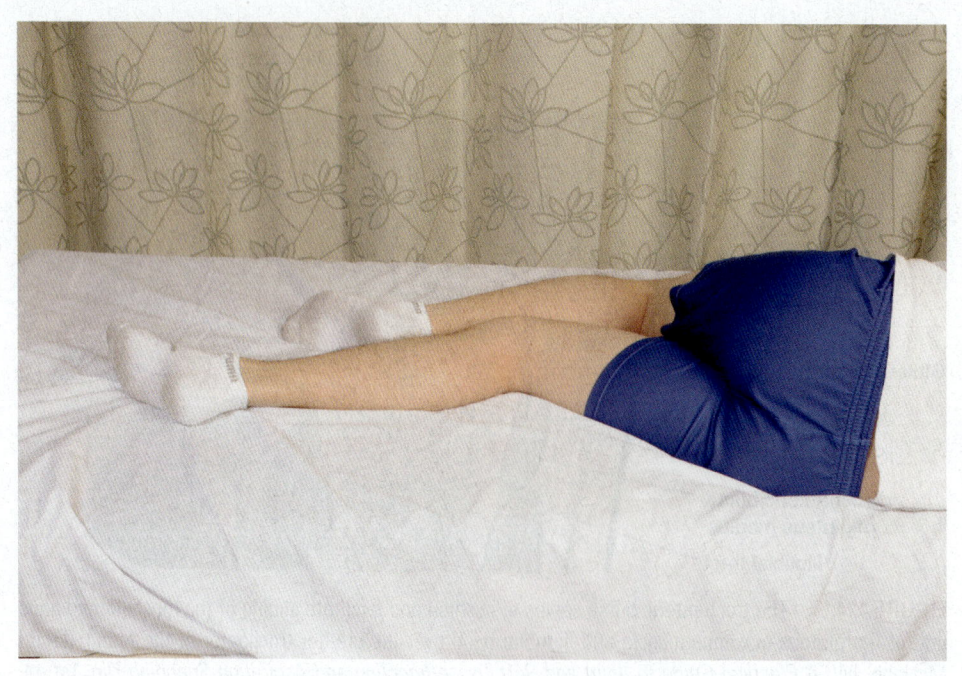

**FIGURE 124.7.** Proper patient position for ultrasound-guided injection of the external snapping hip.

## ULTRASOUND-GUIDED TECHNIQUE

The benefits, risks, and alternative treatments are explained to the patient and informed consent is obtained. The patient is then placed in the modified Sims position (Fig. 124.7). The skin overlying the greater trochanter of the femur is then prepped with antiseptic solution. The greater trochanter is then identified by using a grasping maneuver (Fig. 124.8). A sterile syringe containing 4.0 mL of 0.25% preservative-free bupivacaine and 40 mg of methylprednisolone is attached to a 1½-inch, 22-gauge needle using strict aseptic technique. A linear high-frequency ultrasound transducer is placed over the previously identified greater trochanter with the transducer in a transverse orientation (Fig. 124.9). A survey scan is taken, which demonstrates the irregular hyperechoic margin of the greater trochanter and the trochanteric bursa and tendon of the gluteus maximus muscle and the iliotibial band above it (Fig. 124.10). After the greater trochanter and overlying

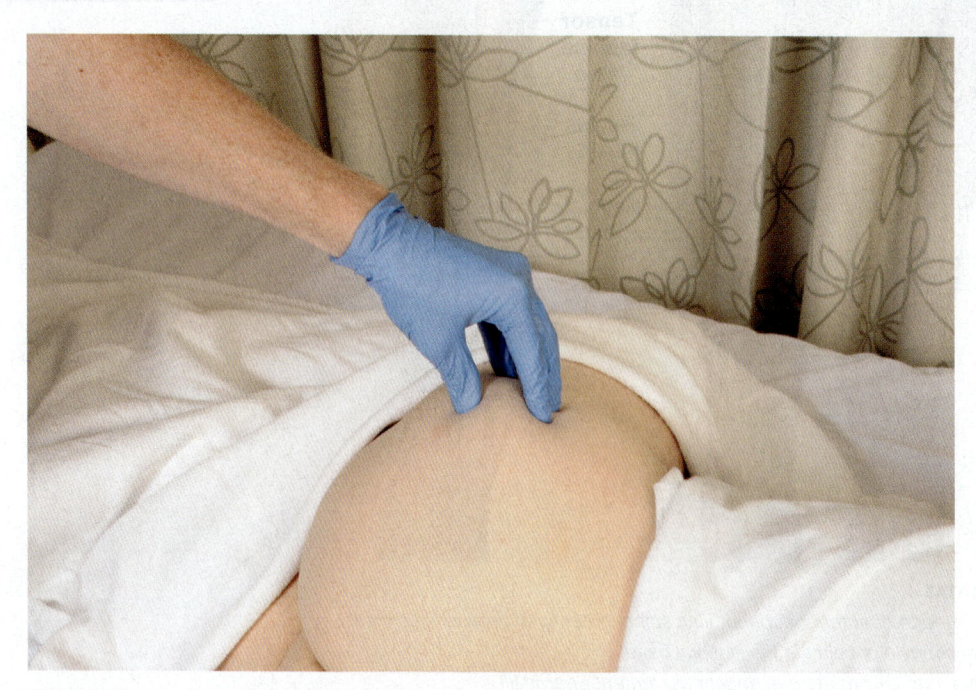

**FIGURE 124.8.** The greater trochanter of the femur is identified by using a grasping maneuver.

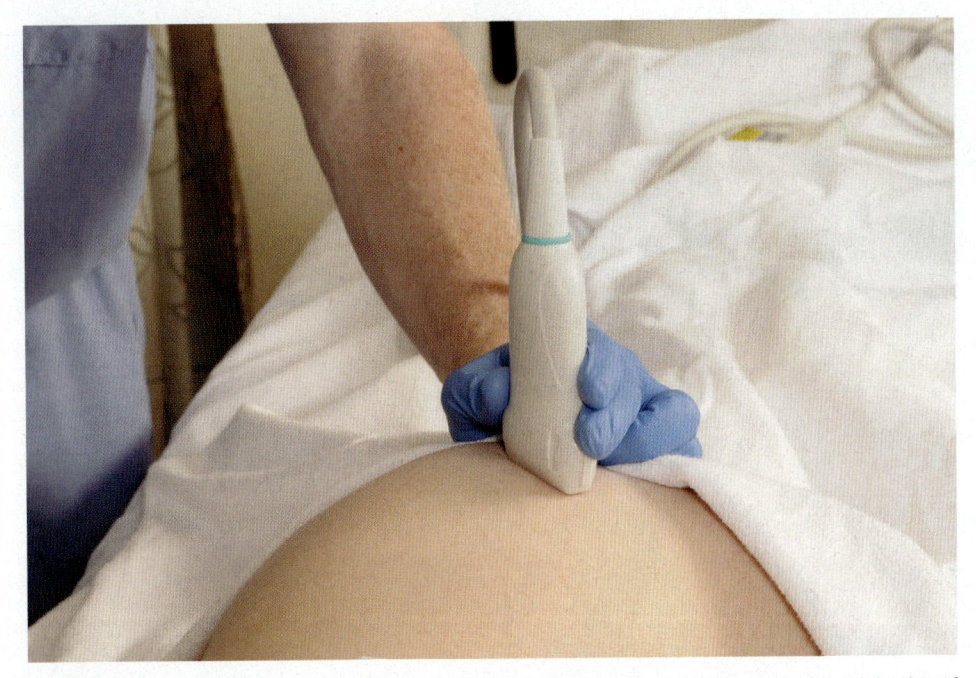

**FIGURE 124.9.** Correct transverse position for ultrasound transducer for ultrasound-guided injection of external snapping hip.

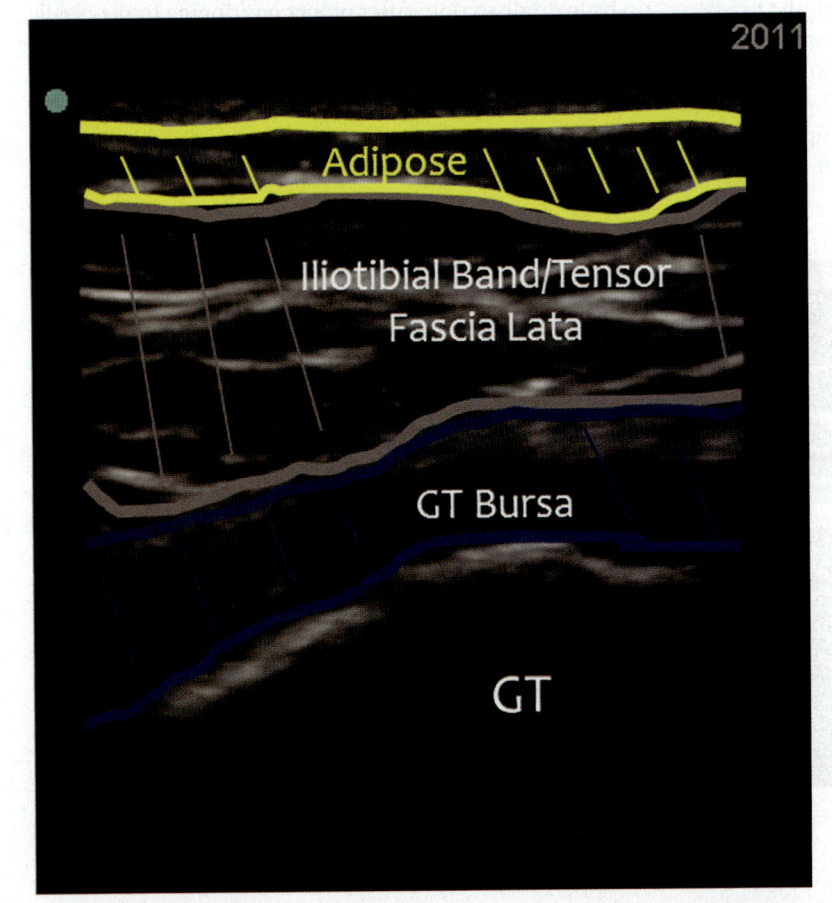

**FIGURE 124.10.** Ultrasound image of the hip joint demonstrating the greater trochanter and overlying trochanteric bursa and iliotibial band.

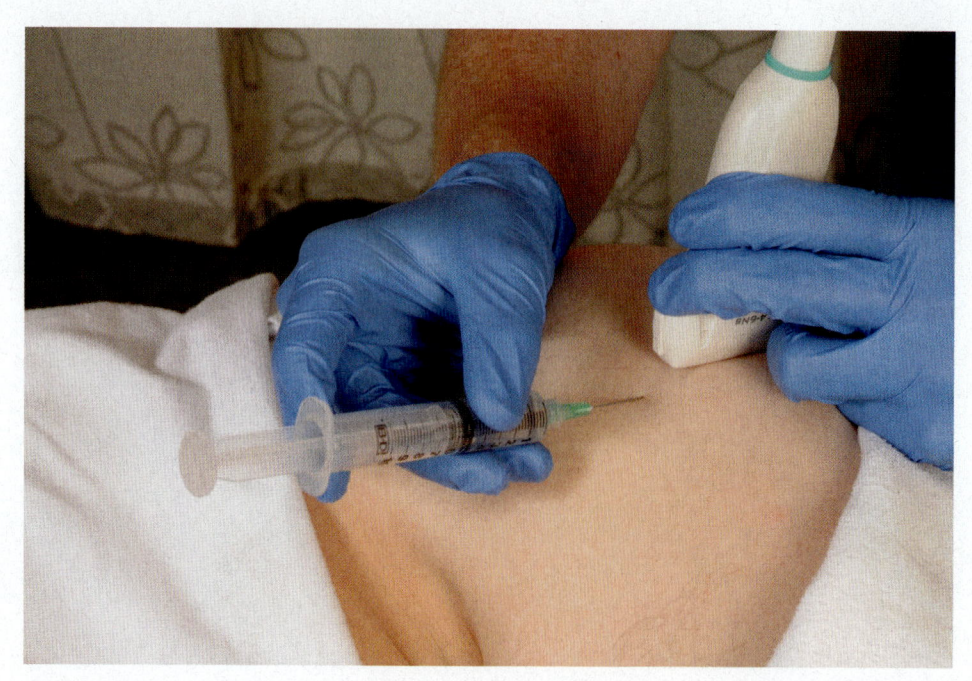

**FIGURE 124.11.** Correct in-plane needle placement for ultrasound-guided injection of external snapping hip.

structures over it are identified, the needle is placed through the skin ~1 cm from the anterior end of the transducer and is then advanced using an in-plane approach with the needle trajectory adjusted under real-time ultrasound guidance to pass through the substance of the gluteus maximus tendon to place the needle tip between the tendon and greater trochanter (Figs. 124.11 and 124.12). When the tip of needle is thought to be in satisfactory position, a small amount of local anesthetic and steroid is injected under real-time ultrasound guidance to confirm proper placement of the needle tip by hydrodissection. After proper positioning of the needle tip placement is confirmed, the remainder of the contents of the syringe are slowly injected. There should be minimal resistance to injection. If significant trochanteric bursitis is identified, the needle may have to be repositioned to ensure that the entire bursa is treated. The needle is then removed,

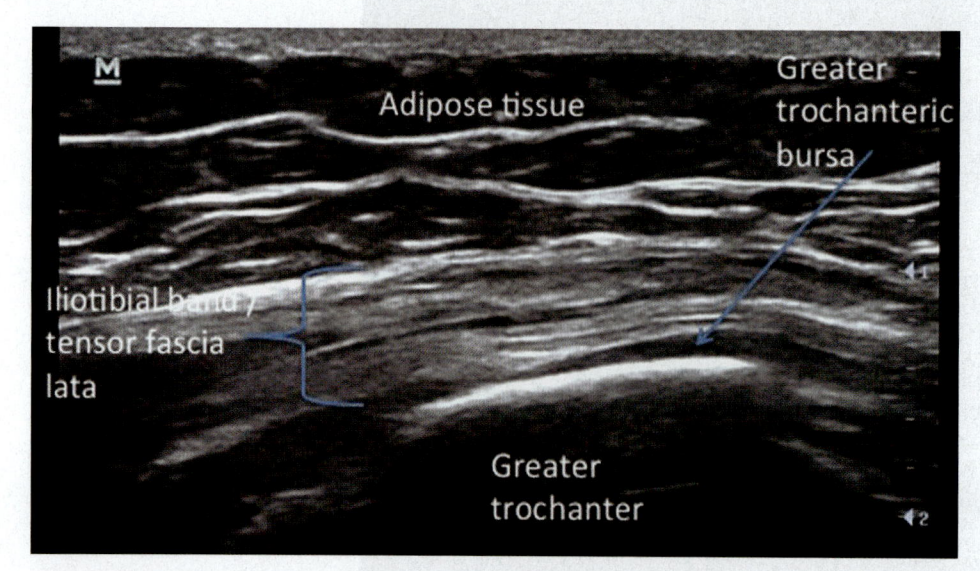

**FIGURE 124.12.** Trajectory of in-plane needle placement for ultrasound-guided injection of the external snapping hip.

and a sterile pressure dressing and ice pack are placed at the injection site.

## COMPLICATIONS

The major complication of ultrasound-guided injection of external snapping hip is infection. Ecchymosis and hematoma formation may also occur. A transient exacerbation of the patient's pain occurs ~25% of the time following this injection technique, and the patient should be warned of this possibility prior to the procedure.

## CLINICAL PEARLS

Bursitis, labral tears, tendinopathy, osteoarthritis, synovitis, nerve entrapment, avascular necrosis of the femoral head, and impingement syndromes may coexist with other hip joint disease and may contribute to the patient's pain symptomatology. Universal precautions should always be observed to protect the operator, and strict adherence to sterile technique must be used to avoid infection. Gentle physical therapy and local heat should be introduced following ultrasound-guided injection of the elbow joint to reduce pain and improve function. Simple analgesics and nonsteroidal anti-inflammatory agents or COX-2 inhibitors may be used concurrently with this injection technique.

## SUGGESTED READINGS

Campbell RSD. Anatomy, special imaging considerations of pelvis, hip, and lower extremity pain syndromes. In: *Imaging of Pain*. Philadelphia, PA: Saunders Elsevier; 2011:335–336.

Ellis R, Hing W, Reid D. Iliotibial band friction syndrome—A systematic review. *Man Ther* 2007;12(3):200–208.

Segal NA, Felson DT, Torner JC, et al. Multicenter Osteoarthritis (MOST) Study Group. Greater trochanteric pain syndrome: epidemiology and associated factors. *Arch Phys Med Rehabil* 2007;88(8):988–992.

Waldman SD. Injection technique for snapping hip. In: *Pain Review*. Philadelphia, PA: Saunders Elsevier; 2009:554–555.

Waldman SD. Snapping hip syndrome. In: *Atlas of Uncommon Pain Syndromes* 2nd ed. Philadelphia, PA: Saunders Elsevier; 2009:257–258.

Waldman SD. The trochanteric bursa. In: *Pain Review*. Philadelphia, PA: Saunders Elsevier; 2009:140–141.

Waldman SD. Injection for snapping hip syndrome. In: *Atlas of Pain Management Injection Techniques* 3rd ed. Philadelphia, PA: Saunders Elsevier; 2012:307–310.

# SECTION IX

# Knee and Lower Extremity

# CHAPTER 125

# Ultrasound-Guided Injection Technique for Intra-articular Injection of the Knee Joint

## CLINICAL PERSPECTIVES

The largest joint in the body, the knee joint, is a trochoginglymus–type joint, which provides flexion and extension as well as a limited range of medial and lateral rotation. The joint has two articulations: (1) between the femur and tibia and (2) between the patella and femur (Fig. 125.1). The joint's articular cartilage is susceptible to damage, which, if left untreated, will result in arthritis with its associated pain and functional disability. Osteoarthritis of the joint is the most common form of arthritis that results in knee joint pain and functional disability, with rheumatoid arthritis and posttraumatic arthritis also causing arthritis of the knee joint. Less common causes of arthritis-induced knee joint pain include the collagen vascular diseases, infection, villonodular synovitis, and Lyme disease. Acute infectious arthritis of the knee joint is best treated with early diagnosis, with culture and sensitivity of the synovial fluid, and with prompt initiation of antibiotic therapy. The collagen vascular diseases generally manifest as a polyarthropathy rather than a monoarthropathy limited to the knee joint, although knee pain secondary to the collagen vascular diseases responds exceedingly well to ultrasound-guided intra-articular injection of the knee joint.

Patients with knee joint pain secondary to arthritis, tears of the menisci, and collagen vascular disease–related joint pain complain of pain that is localized to the knee and surrounding area. Activity makes the pain worse, with rest and heat providing some relief. The pain is constant and characterized as aching. Sleep disturbance is common with awakening when the patient rolls over onto the affected knee. Some patients complain of a grating, catching, or popping sensation with range of motion of the joint, and crepitus may be appreciated on physical examination.

Functional disability often accompanies the pain associated with many pathologic conditions of the knee joint. Patients will often notice increasing difficulty in performing their activities of daily living, and tasks that require walking, climbing stairs, and walking on uneven surfaces are particularly problematic. If the pathologic process responsible for the patient's pain symptomatology is not adequately treated, the patient's functional disability may worsen and muscle wasting, especially of the quadriceps and ultimately a frozen knee, may occur.

Plain radiographs are indicated in all patients who present with knee pain as not only intrinsic knee disease but also other regional pathology may be perceived as knee pain by the patient (Fig. 125.2). Based on the patient's clinical presentation, additional testing may be indicated, including complete blood cell count, sedimentation rate, and antinuclear antibody testing. Magnetic resonance imaging or ultrasound of the knee is indicated if avascular necrosis or meniscal tear is suspected (Fig. 125.3).

## CLINICALLY RELEVANT ANATOMY

The knee joint is comprised of the articulation between the rounded condyles of the distal femur and the condyles of the proximal tibia below and the patella anteriorly (see Fig. 125.1). The articular surface of the knee joint is covered with hyaline cartilage, which is susceptible to arthritis from a variety of causes (Fig. 125.4). Because the vascular supply to the articular cartilage is tenuous, the knee joint is susceptible to avascular necrosis. Posterior and lateral joint support is provided by a dense joint capsule with the suprapatellar and prepatellar bursae taking its place anteriorly. Additional posterior stability is provided by the oblique popliteal ligament as well as the posterior cruciate ligament with the anterior cruciate ligament providing anterior stability. Medial and lateral support is provided by the medial and lateral collateral ligaments (see Fig. 125.4). The knee joint is provided with two unique cartilaginous articular discs, the medial meniscus and lateral meniscus, which partly divide the joint space and serve as both shock absorbers to prevent the condyles of the femur and tibia from abrading each other (see Fig. 125.4).

## ULTRASOUND-GUIDED TECHNIQUE

The benefits, risks, and alternative treatments are explained to the patient and informed consent is obtained. The patient is then placed in the supine position with the lower extremity

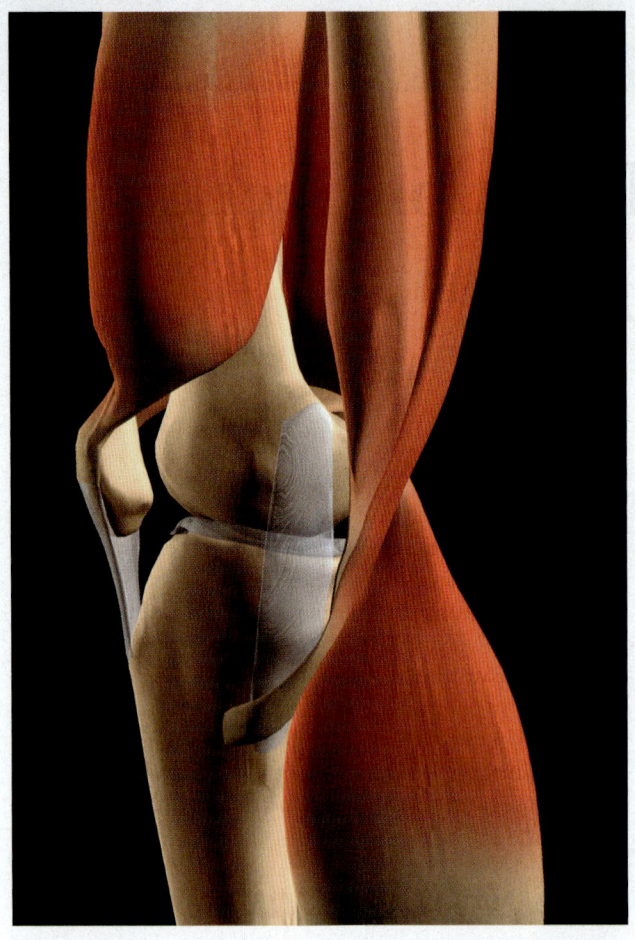

**FIGURE 125.1.** The articulations of the knee. (LifeART, 2013.)

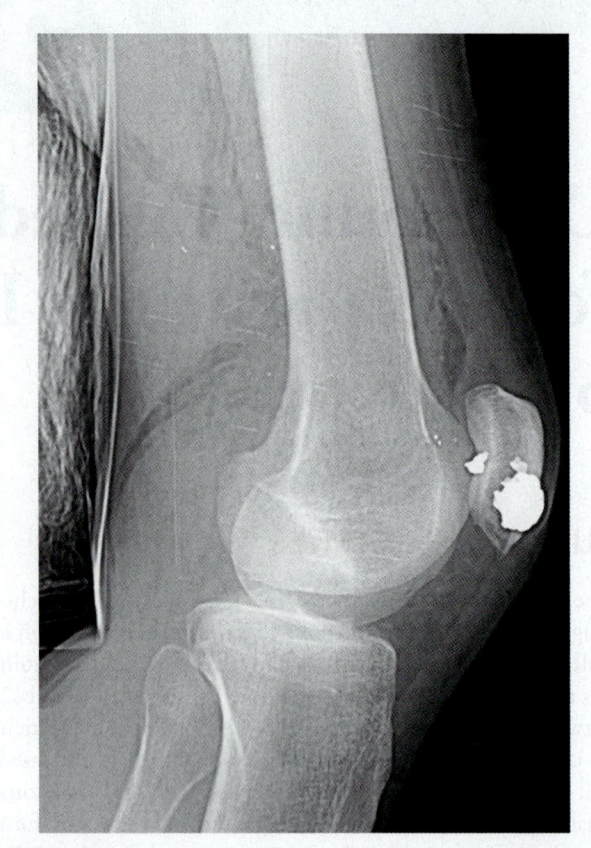

**FIGURE 125.2.** Lateral radiograph demonstrating retained bullet fragment causing knee pain. (Reused from Bucholz RW, Heckman JD. *Rockwood & Green's Fractures in Adults*. 5th ed. Philadelphia, PA: Lippincott Williams & Wilkins; 2001, with permission.)

externally rotated (Fig. 125.5). The skin overlying the medial knee joint is then prepped with antiseptic solution. A sterile syringe containing 2.0 mL of 0.25% preservative-free bupivacaine and 40 mg of methylprednisolone is attached to a 1½-inch, 22-gauge needle using strict aseptic technique. A high-frequency linear ultrasound transducer is placed over the medial knee joint in the longitudinal plane (Fig. 125.6). A survey scan is taken, which demonstrates the thick hyperechoic filaments of the medial collateral ligament and the bony contours of the medial margins of the femur and tibia (Fig. 125.7). The medial meniscus is visualized as a triangular-shaped hyperechoic structure resting between the bony medial margins of the femur and tibia (Fig. 125.8). This triangular space between the bony medial margins of the femur and tibia allows easy access to the joint space under ultrasound guidance (Fig. 125.9). After the medial joint space is identified, the needle is placed through the skin ~1 cm above the middle of the longitudinally placed transducer and is then advanced using an out-of-plane approach with the needle trajectory adjusted under real-time ultrasound guidance to enter the center of the knee joint via the triangular space between the medial borders of the femur and tibia (Fig. 125.10). When the tip of needle is thought to be within the joint space, a small amount of local anesthetic and steroid is injected under real-time ultrasound guidance. There should be minimal resistance to injection. After intra-articular needle tip placement is confirmed, the remainder of the contents of the syringe are slowly injected. If synechiae, loculations, or calcifications are present, the needle may have to be repositioned to ensure that the entire intra-articular space is treated. The needle is then removed, and a sterile pressure dressing and ice pack are placed at the injection site.

## COMPLICATIONS

The major complication of ultrasound-guided injection of the knee joint is infection. Ecchymosis and hematoma formation may also occur. A transient exacerbation of the patient's pain occurs ~25% of the time following this injection technique, and the patient should be warned of this possibility prior to the procedure.

CHAPTER 125  US-GUIDED INTRA-ARTICULAR INJECTION TECHNIQUE OF THE KNEE JOINT   899

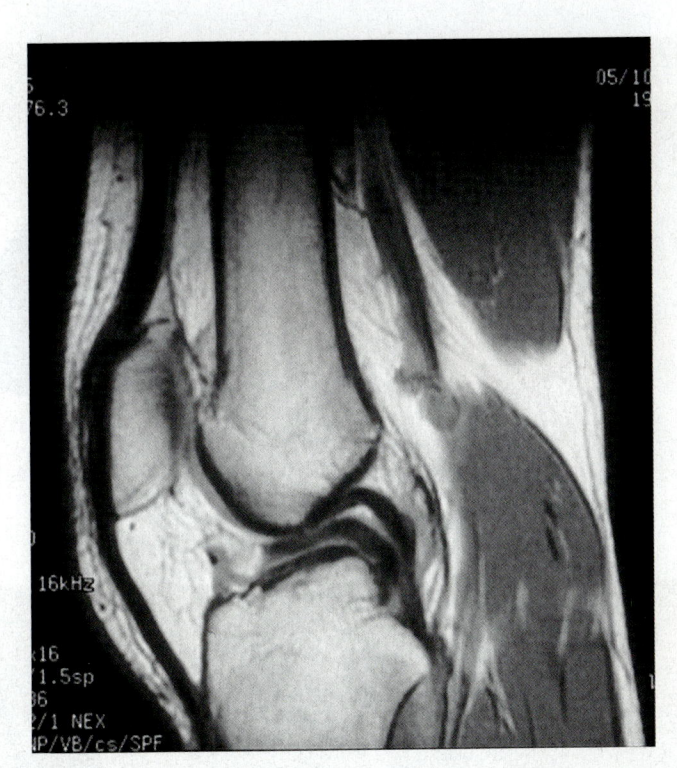

**FIGURE 125.3.** T2-weighted MRI image of the knee demonstrating a locked bucket-handle medial meniscus tear. (Reused from Bucholz RW, Heckman JD. *Rockwood & Green's Fractures in Adults*. 5th ed. Philadelphia, PA: Lippincott Williams & Wilkins; 2001, with permission.)

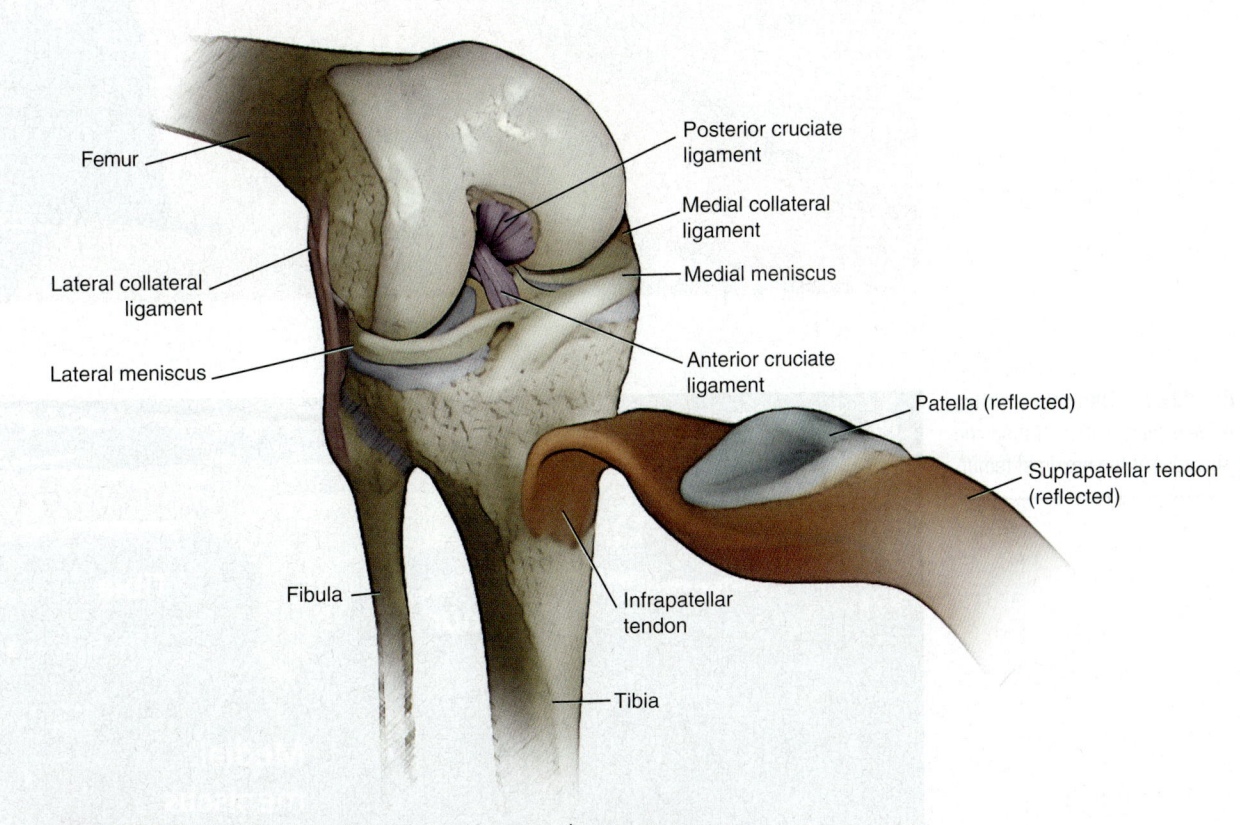

**FIGURE 125.4.** Anterior view of the knee and its supporting structures.

**FIGURE 125.5.** Proper patient position for ultrasound-guided intra-articular knee injection. Note that the affected extremity is externally rotated.

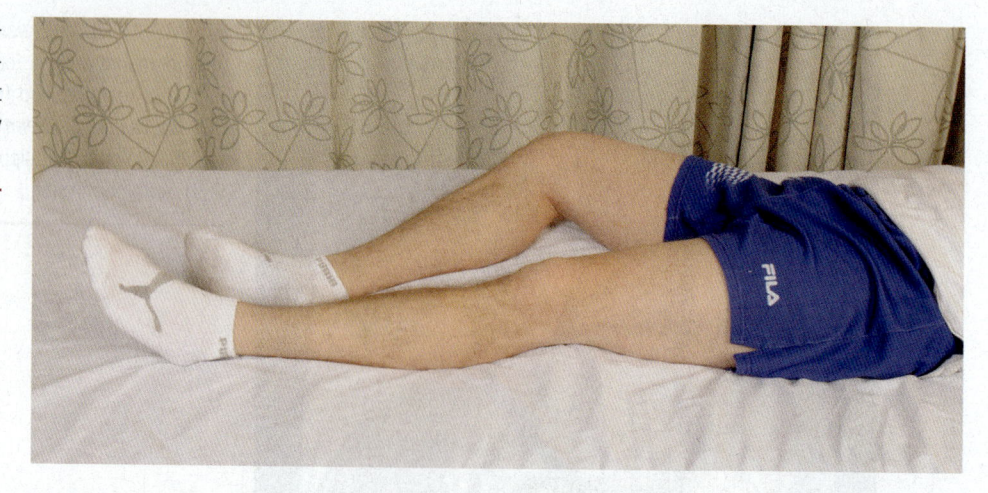

**FIGURE 125.6.** Correct longitudinal position for ultrasound transducer for ultrasound-guided intra-articular injection of the knee joint.

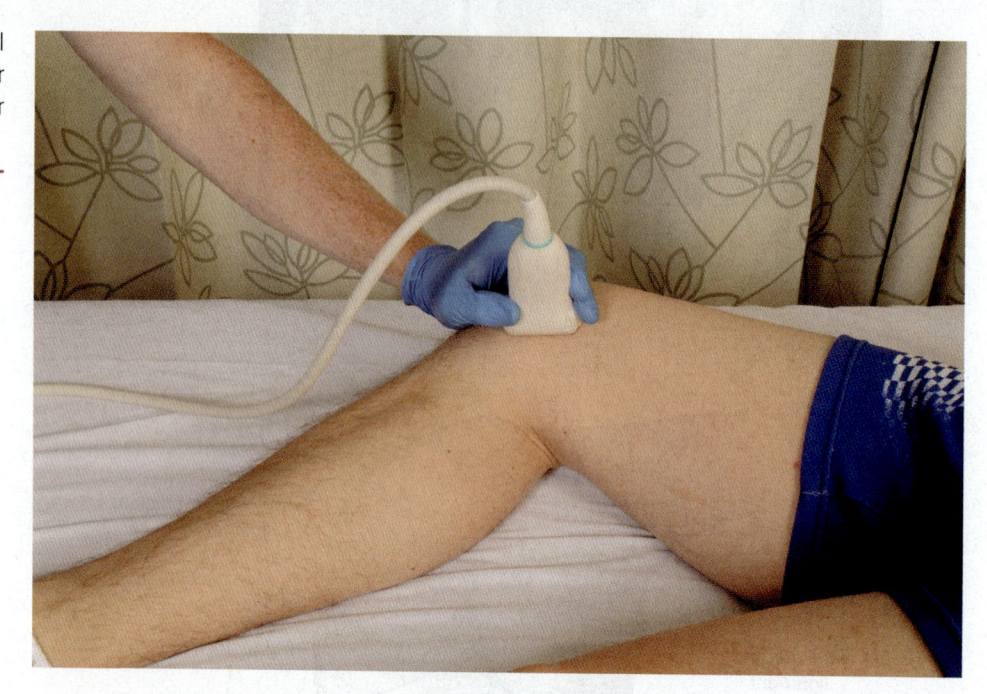

**FIGURE 125.7.** Ultrasound image of the knee joint demonstrating the medial border of the proximal femur.

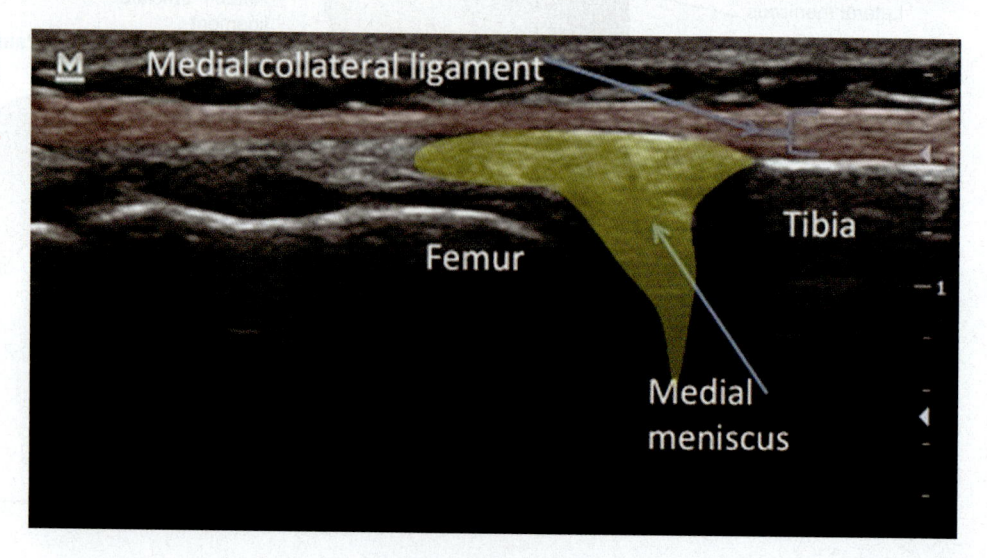

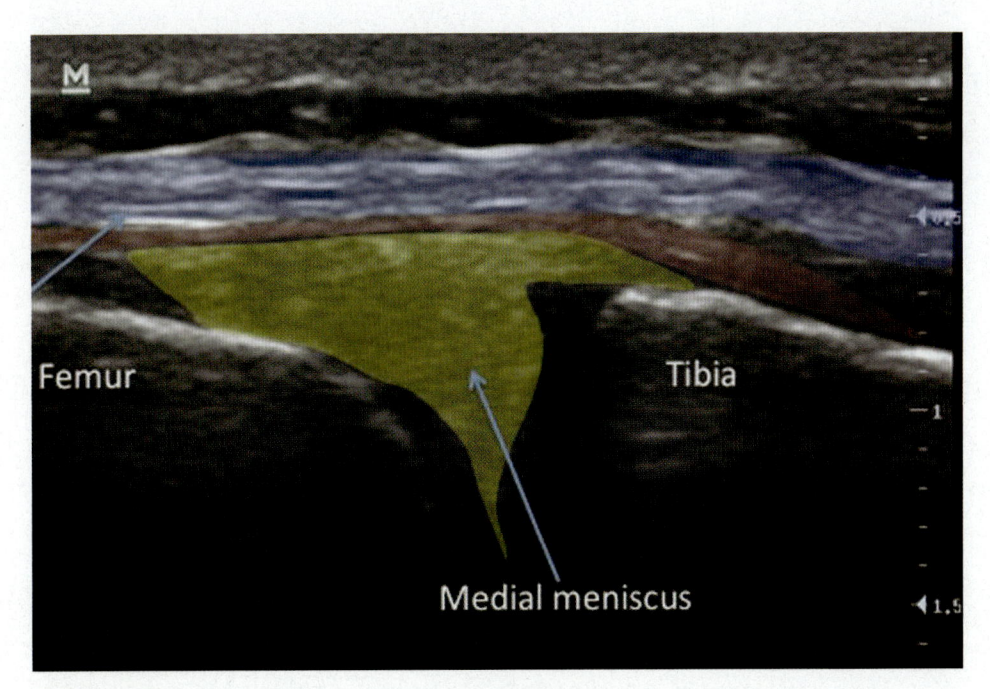

**FIGURE 125.8.** Longitudinal ultrasound image demonstrating the triangular-shaped medial meniscus nestled between the medial borders of the femur and tibia.

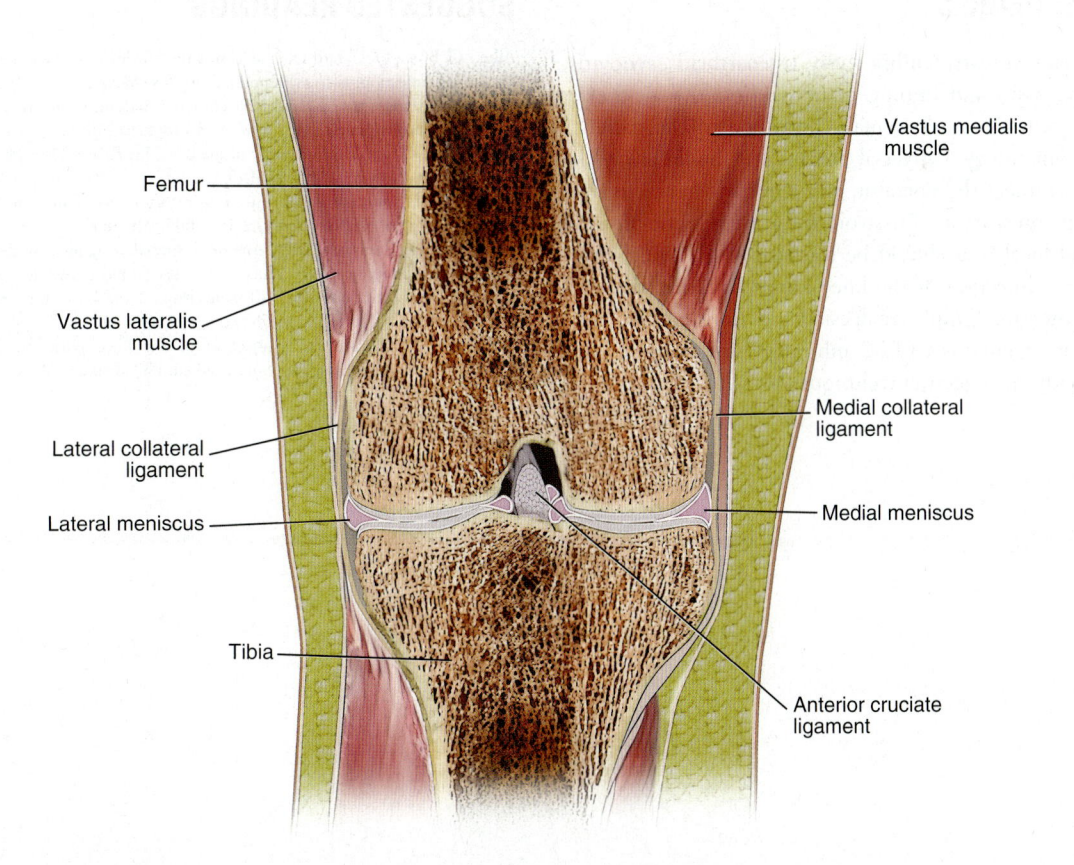

**FIGURE 125.9.** Cross-sectional view of the medial knee joint demonstrating the relationship of the triangular-shaped medial meniscus to the medial margins of the femur and tibia.

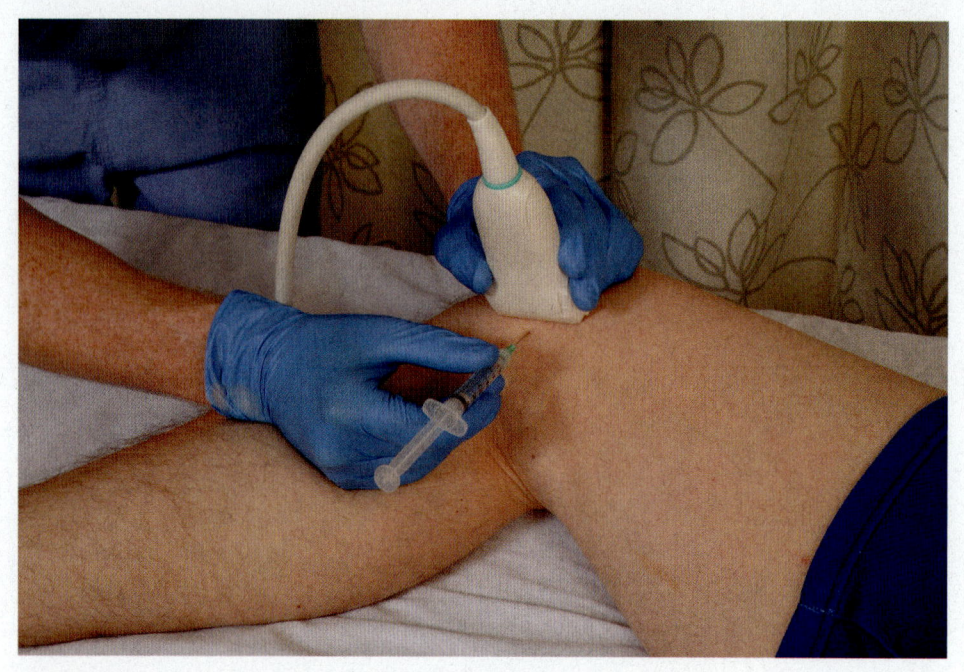

**FIGURE 125.10.** Correct in-plane needle placement for ultrasound-guided knee joint injection.

## CLINICAL PEARLS

Bursitis, meniscal tears, tendinopathy, osteoarthritis, synovitis, avascular necrosis, and impingement syndromes may coexist with knee joint disease and may contribute to the patient's pain symptomatology. Universal precautions should always be observed to protect the operator, and strict adherence to sterile technique must be used to avoid infection. Gentle physical therapy and local heat should be introduced following ultrasound-guided injection of the knee joint to reduce pain and improve function. Simple analgesics and nonsteroidal anti-inflammatory agents or COX-2 inhibitors may be used concurrently with this injection technique.

## SUGGESTED READINGS

Albert C, Brocq O, Gerard D, et al. Septic knee arthritis after intra-articular hyaluronate injection: two case reports. *Joint Bone Spine* 2006;73(2):205–207.

Schumacher HR, Chen LX. Injectable corticosteroids in treatment of arthritis of the knee. Review Article. *Am J Med* 2005;118(11):1208–1214.

Waldman SD. Functional anatomy of the knee. In: *Pain Review*. Philadelphia, PA: Saunders Elsevier; 2009:144–149.

Waldman SD. Intra-articular injection of the knee joint. In: *Pain Review*. Philadelphia, PA: Saunders Elsevier; 2009:583–584.

Waldman SD, Campbell RSD. Anatomy, special imaging considerations of the knee. In: *Imaging of Pain*. Philadelphia, PA: Saunders Elsevier; 2011:367–368.

Waldman SD, Campbell RSD. Osteonecrosis of the knee. In: *Imaging of Pain*. Philadelphia, PA: Saunders Elsevier; 2011:393–396.

Waldman SD. Intra-articular injection of the knee joint. In: *Atlas of Pain Management Injection Techniques*. 3rd ed. Philadelphia, PA: Saunders Elsevier; 2012:346–348.

# CHAPTER 126

# Ultrasound-Guided Injection Technique for Intra-articular Injection of the Superior Tibiofibular Joint

## CLINICAL PERSPECTIVES

The superior tibiofibular joint is an arthrodial-type joint, which allows a very limited range of motion. The joint is comprised of the articulations between lateral condyle of the tibia and the head of the fibula (Fig. 126.1). The joint's articular cartilage is susceptible to damage, which, if left untreated, will result in arthritis with its associated pain and functional disability. Osteoarthritis of the joint is the most common form of arthritis that results in superior tibiofibular joint pain and functional disability, with rheumatoid arthritis and posttraumatic arthritis also causing arthritis of the superior tibiofibular joint. The tibiofibular joint frequently is damaged from falls with the foot fully medially rotated and the superior tibiofibular joint flexed. Less common causes of arthritis-induced superior tibiofibular joint pain include the collagen vascular diseases, infection, villonodular synovitis, and Lyme disease. Acute infectious arthritis of the superior tibiofibular joint is best treated with early diagnosis, with culture and sensitivity of the synovial fluid, and with prompt initiation of antibiotic therapy. The collagen vascular diseases generally manifest as a polyarthropathy rather than a monoarthropathy limited to the superior tibiofibular joint, although superior tibiofibular pain secondary to the collagen vascular diseases responds exceedingly well to ultrasound-guided intra-articular injection of the superior tibiofibular joint. The superior tibiofibular joint is a common site of ganglion cysts.

Patients with superior tibiofibular joint pain secondary to arthritis and collagen vascular disease–related joint pain complain of pain that is localized to the superior tibiofibular joint and lateral knee. Activity, especially involving flexion and medial rotation of the superior tibiofibular joint, makes the pain worse, with rest and heat providing some relief. The pain is constant and characterized as aching. Sleep disturbance is common with awakening when the patient rolls over onto the affected superior tibiofibular. Some patients complain of a grating, catching, or popping sensation with range of motion of the joint, and crepitus may be appreciated on physical examination.

Functional disability often accompanies the pain associated with many pathologic conditions of the superior tibiofibular joint. Patients will often notice increasing difficulty in performing their activities of daily living, and tasks that require walking, climbing stairs, and walking on uneven surfaces are particularly problematic. If the pathologic process responsible for the patient's pain symptomatology is not adequately treated, the patient's functional disability may worsen and muscle wasting may occur.

Plain radiographs are indicated in all patients who present with superior tibiofibular pain as not only intrinsic superior tibiofibular disease but also other regional pathology may be perceived as superior tibiofibular pain by the patient. Based on the patient's clinical presentation, additional testing may be indicated, including complete blood cell count, sedimentation rate, and antinuclear antibody testing. Magnetic resonance imaging, computed tomography (CT), or ultrasound of the superior tibiofibular joint is indicated if avascular necrosis or meniscal tear is suspected or if the diagnosis is unclear (Fig. 126.2).

## CLINICALLY RELEVANT ANATOMY

The lateral epicondyle of the tibia and the head of the fibula articulate at the superior tibiofibular joint (see Fig. 126.1). The flattened articular surfaces are covered with hyaline cartilage, which is susceptible to arthritis. The joint is completely surrounded by a capsule that provides support to the joint. Anterior and posterior ligaments strengthen the joint as does the interosseous membrane, which connects the shafts of the tibia and fibula together (Fig. 126.3). The joint capsule is lined with a synovial membrane that attaches to the articular cartilage and may give rise to bursae. The tibiofibular joint is innervated by the common peroneal nerves. The blood supply to the tibiofibular joint is provided by the inferior lateral genicular and anterior fibula recurrent arteries. In addition to arthritis, the tibiofibular joint is susceptible to the development of tendonitis, bursitis, and disruption of the ligaments, cartilage, and tendons.

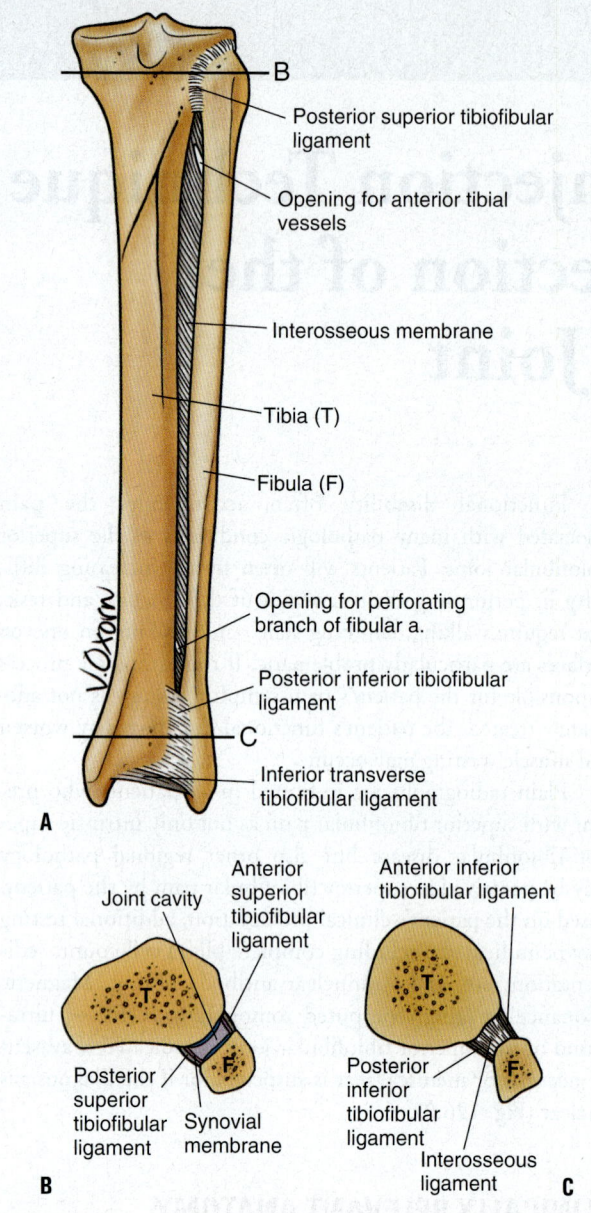

**FIGURE 126.1.** The articulations of the superior tibiofibular joint. (Reused from Moore KL, Agur A. *Essential Clinical Anatomy*. 2nd ed. Philadelphia, PA: Lippincott Williams & Wilkins; 2002, with permission.)

## ULTRASOUND-GUIDED TECHNIQUE

The benefits, risks, and alternative treatments are explained to the patient and informed consent is obtained. The patient is then placed in the curled up on the side position with the superior tibiofibular joint pointed at the ceiling and the knee flexed 30 degrees to relax open the superior tibiofibular joint by relaxing the fibular collateral ligament and the biceps femoris tendon (Fig. 126.4). The skin overlying the superior tibiofibular joint is then prepped with antiseptic solution. A sterile syringe containing 2.0 mL of 0.25% preservative-free bupivacaine and 40 mg of methylprednisolone is attached to a 1½-inch, 22-gauge needle using strict aseptic technique. A high-frequency linear ultrasound transducer is placed over the oblique longitudinal plane with the inferior border of the ultrasound transducer over the fibular head and the superior portion of the ultrasound transducer pointed toward the inferior margin of the patella (Figs. 126.5 and 126.6). A survey scan is taken, which demonstrates the thick anterosuperior tibiofibular ligament that serves as the sonographic landmark for the superior tibiofibular joint (Fig. 126.7). Rotation of the ultrasound transducer in the clockwise and counterclockwise position will aid in optimizing joint visualization (see Fig. 126.6). After the joint space is identified, the needle is placed through the skin ~1 cm above the middle of the obliquely placed transducer and is then advanced using an out-of-plane approach with the needle trajectory adjusted under real-time ultrasound guidance to enter the center of the superior tibiofibular joint via the between the borders of the fibula and tibia (Figs. 126.7 and 126.8). When the tip of needle is thought to be within the joint space, a small amount of local anesthetic and steroid is injected under real-time ultrasound guidance to confirm that the needle tip is within the joint space. There should be minimal resistance to injection. After intra-articular needle tip placement is confirmed, the remainder of the contents of the syringe are slowly injected. Bulging of the anterior superior tibiofibular ligament may be appreciated. If synechiae, loculations, or calcifications are present, the needle may have to be repositioned to ensure that the entire intra-articular space is treated. The needle is then removed, and a sterile pressure dressing and ice pack are placed at the injection site.

## COMPLICATIONS

The major complication of ultrasound-guided injection of the superior tibiofibular joint is infection. Ecchymosis and hematoma formation may also occur. A transient exacerbation of the patient's pain occurs ~25% of the time following this injection technique, and the patient should be warned of this possibility prior to the procedure.

## CLINICAL PEARLS

Bursitis, lateral meniscal tears, tendinopathy, osteoarthritis, synovitis, avascular necrosis, and impingement syndromes may coexist with superior tibiofibular joint disease and may contribute to the patient's pain symptomatology. Universal precautions should always be observed to protect the operator, and strict adherence to sterile technique must be used to avoid infection. Gentle physical therapy and local heat should be introduced following ultrasound-guided injection of the superior tibiofibular joint to reduce pain and improve function. Simple analgesics and nonsteroidal anti-inflammatory agents or COX-2 inhibitors may be used concurrently with this injection technique.

CHAPTER 126    INTRA-ARTICULAR INJECTION TECHNIQUE FOR THE SUPERIOR TIBIOFIBULAR JOINT

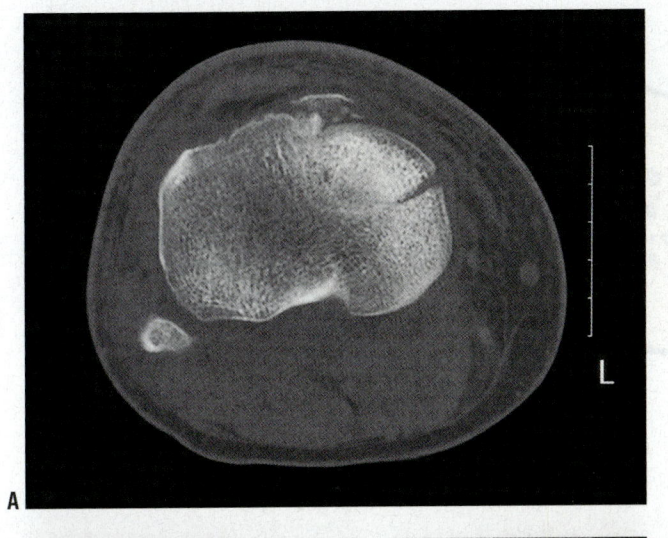

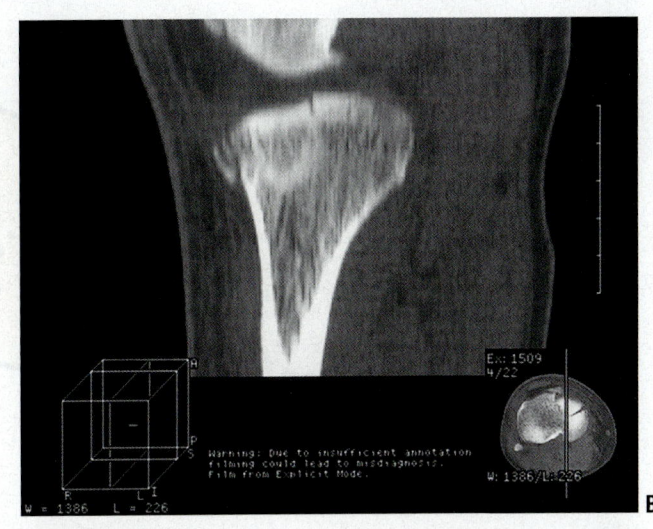

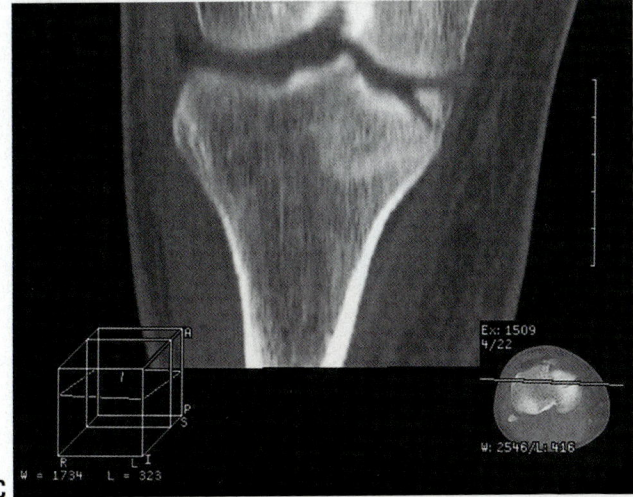

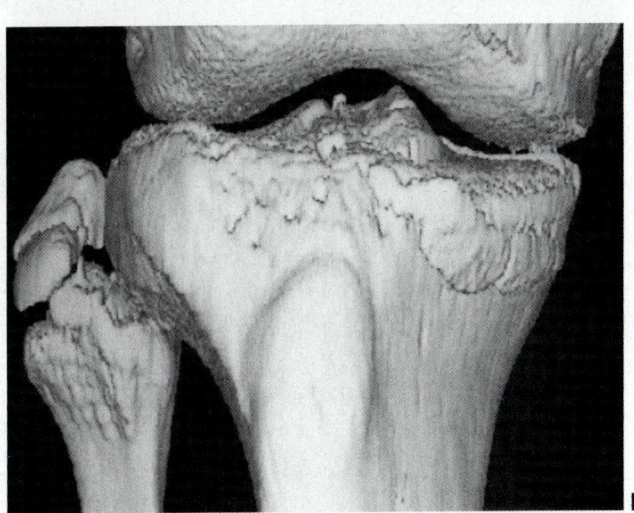

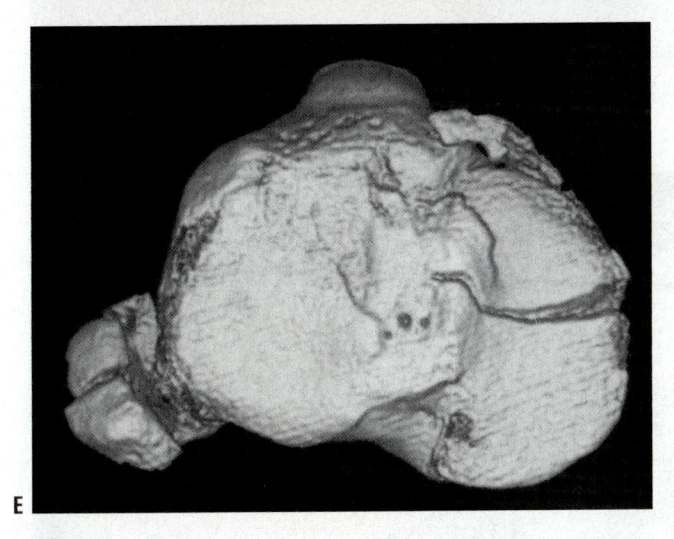

**FIGURE 126.2.** CT of fracture of the tibial plateau. A 23-year-old man was injured in a motorcycle accident. The conventional radiographs of the right knee showed fracture of the tibial plateau. **A:** Axial CT section through the proximal tibia shows a comminuted fracture of the medial tibial plateau. **B:** Sagittal reformatted image shows that the anterior part of the plateau is mainly affected. **C:** Coronal reformatted image demonstrates comminution and depression. **D:** Anterior view of the 3D reconstructed image in addition to depression of the medial anterior tibial plateau shows associated fracture of the proximal fibula. **E:** Bird's-eye view of the 3D reconstructed image shows the spatial orientation of the fracture lines. (Reused from Greenspan A. *Orthopedic Imaging: A Practical Approach.* 5th ed. Philadelphia, PA: Lippincott Williams & Wilkins; 2011, with permission.)

**FIGURE 126.3.** Cross section of the superior tibiofibular joint.

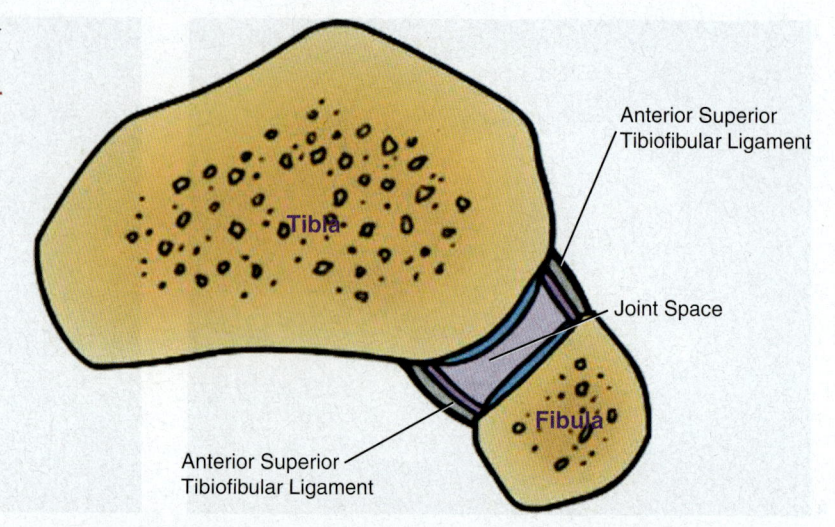

**FIGURE 126.4.** Proper patient position for ultrasound-guided intra-articular superior tibiofibular injection.

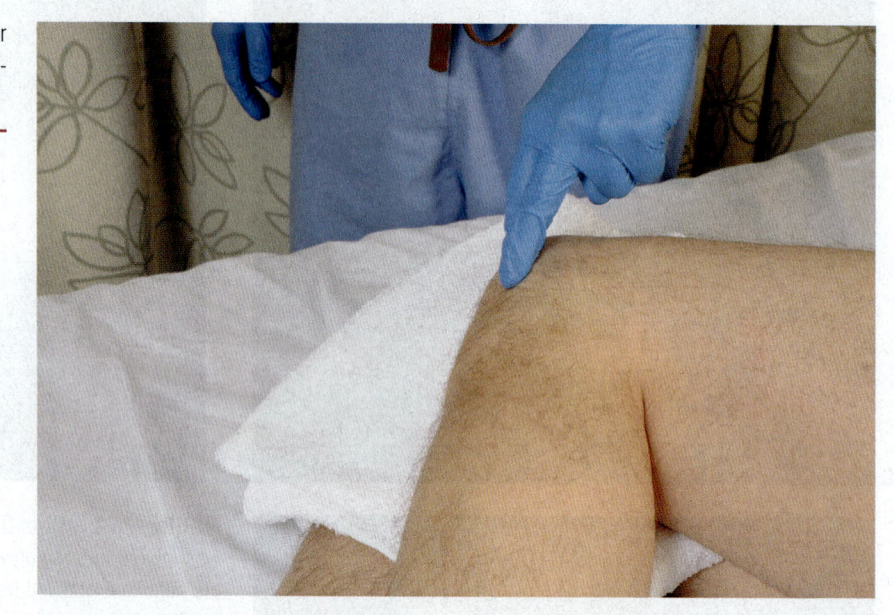

**FIGURE 126.5.** Correct oblique longitudinal position for ultrasound transducer for ultrasound-guided intra-articular injection of the superior tibiofibular joint.

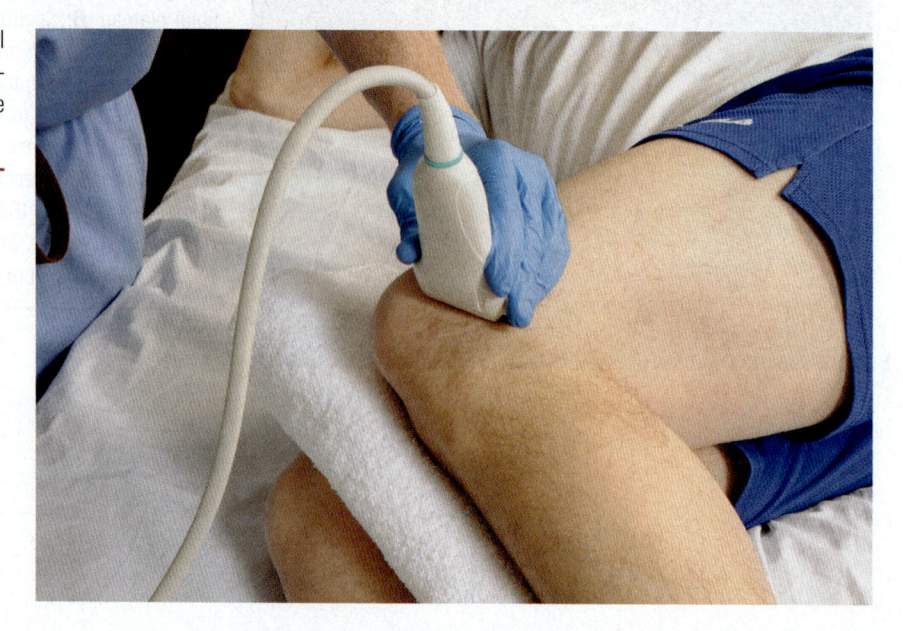

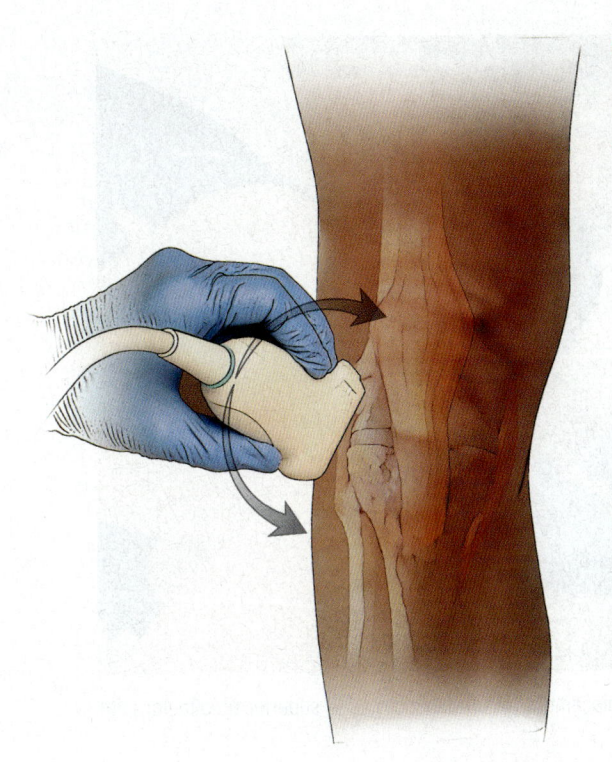

**FIGURE 126.6.** Rotating the obliquely placed ultrasound transducer in a clockwise or counterclockwise will optimize visualization of the superior tibiofibular joint.

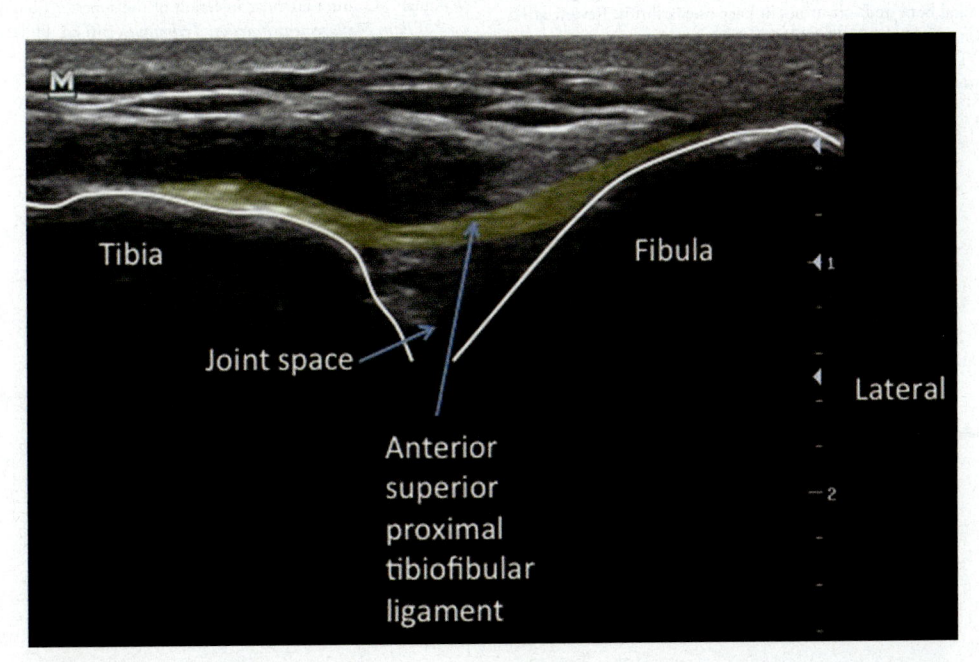

**FIGURE 126.7.** Ultrasound image of the superior tibiofibular joint demonstrating the anterior superior proximal tibiofibular ligament.

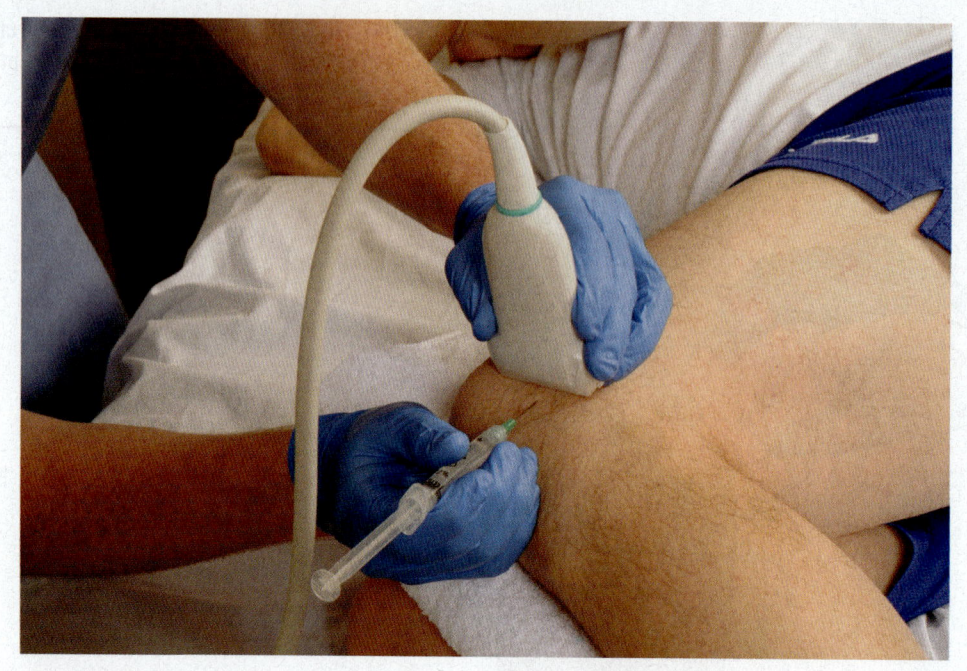

**FIGURE 126.8.** Correct out-of-plane needle placement for ultrasound-guided superior tibiofibular joint injection.

## SUGGESTED READINGS

Bellemans J. Biomechanics of anterior knee pain. *Knee* 2003;10(2):123–126.

Crema MD, Roemer FW, Marra MD, et al. Magnetic resonance imaging assessment of subchondral bone and soft tissues in knee osteoarthritis. Review article. *Rheum Dis Clin North Am* 2009;35(3):557–577.

Kesson M, Atkins E. The superior tibiofibular. In: *Orthopaedic Medicine*. 2nd ed. Oxford, UK: Butterworth-Heinemann; 2005:403–452.

Rethnam U, Sinha A. Instability of the proximal tibiofibular joint, an unusual cause for superior tibiofibular pain. *Inj Extra* 2006;37(5):190–192.

Waldman SD. Functional anatomy of the superior tibiofibular. In: *Pain Review*. Philadelphia, PA: Saunders Elsevier; 2009:144–149.

Waldman SD. Intra-articular injection of the superior tibiofibular Joint. In: *Atlas of Pain Management Injection Techniques*. 3rd ed. Philadelphia, PA: Saunders Elsevier; 2012:349–351.

# CHAPTER 127

# Ultrasound-Guided Injection Technique for Semimembranosus Insertion Syndrome

## CLINICAL PERSPECTIVES

As the most medial of the three muscles that make up the hamstring, the semimembranosus muscle is subjected to an amazing degree of stresses, especially at its distal insertion on the posterior medial condyle of the tibia (Fig. 127.1). When this musculotendinous insertion becomes inflamed, it presents clinically as a constellation of symptoms consisting of localized tenderness over the posterior aspect of the medial knee joint with severe pain being elicited on palpation of the attachment of the semimembranosus muscle at the posterior medial condyle of the tibia. This clinical presentation is known as semimembranosus insertion syndrome. Semimembranosus insertion syndrome most commonly occurs after starting an overaggressive exercise program or following direct blunt trauma to the posterior knee from kicks or tackles during football or rugby.

The semimembranosus bursa that lies between the medial head of the gastrocnemius muscle, the medial femoral epicondyle, and the semimembranosus tendon can become concurrently inflamed further exacerbating the patient's pain and functional disability.

Patients suffering from semimembranosus insertion syndrome will present with point tenderness over the attachment of the semimembranosus muscle at the posterior medial condyle of the tibia. The tenderness may extend to the posteromedial knee. If the symptoms progress, the patient will exhibit a positive twist test for semimembranosus insertion syndrome (Fig. 127.2). The twist test is performed by placing the knee in 20 degrees of flexion and passively rotating the flexed knee. The test is positive if the pain is reproduced. Activity makes the pain worse, with rest and heat providing some relief. The pain is constant and characterized as aching. Sleep disturbance is common with awakening when the patient rolls over onto the affected knee. Some patients complain of a grating, catching, or popping sensation with range of motion of the joint, and crepitus may be appreciated on physical examination. Bursitis, meniscal tears, tendinopathy, osteoarthritis, synovitis, avascular, and impingement syndromes may coexist with semimembranosus insertion syndrome and may contribute to the patient's pain symptomatology and confuse the clinical diagnosis (see Fig. 127.1).

Plain radiographs are indicated in all patients who present with semimembranosus insertion pain as not only semimembranosus insertion pathology, as well as other regional pathology including tibial plateau abnormalities may be perceived as semimembranosus insertion pain by the patient. Based on the patient's clinical presentation, additional testing may be indicated, including complete blood cell count, sedimentation rate, and antinuclear antibody testing. MRI or ultrasound of the semimembranosus tendinous insertion is indicated if the diagnosis is in question or if avascular necrosis, bursitis, or meniscal tear is suspected (Fig. 127.3).

## CLINICALLY RELEVANT ANATOMY

The semimembranosus muscle is the most medial of the three muscles that make up the hamstrings. It finds its origin from the ischial tuberosity and inserts into a groove on the medial surface of the medial condyle of the tibia (Figs. 127.4 and 127.5). The semimembranosus muscle flexes and medially rotates the leg at the knee as well as extending the thigh at the hip joint. A fibrous extension of the muscle called the oblique popliteal ligament extends upward and laterally to provide support to the posterior knee joint. This ligament, as well as the tendinous insertion of the semimembranosus muscle, is prone to the development of inflammation from overuse, misuse, or trauma. The semimembranosus muscle is innervated by the tibial portion of the sciatic nerve. The common peroneal nerve is in proximity to the insertion of the semimembranosus muscle, with the tibial nerve lying more medial. The popliteal artery and vein also lie in the middle of the joint. The semimembranosus bursa, which lies between the medial head of the gastrocnemius muscle, the medial femoral epicondyle, and the semimembranosus tendon, also serves as a source of medioposterior knee pain.

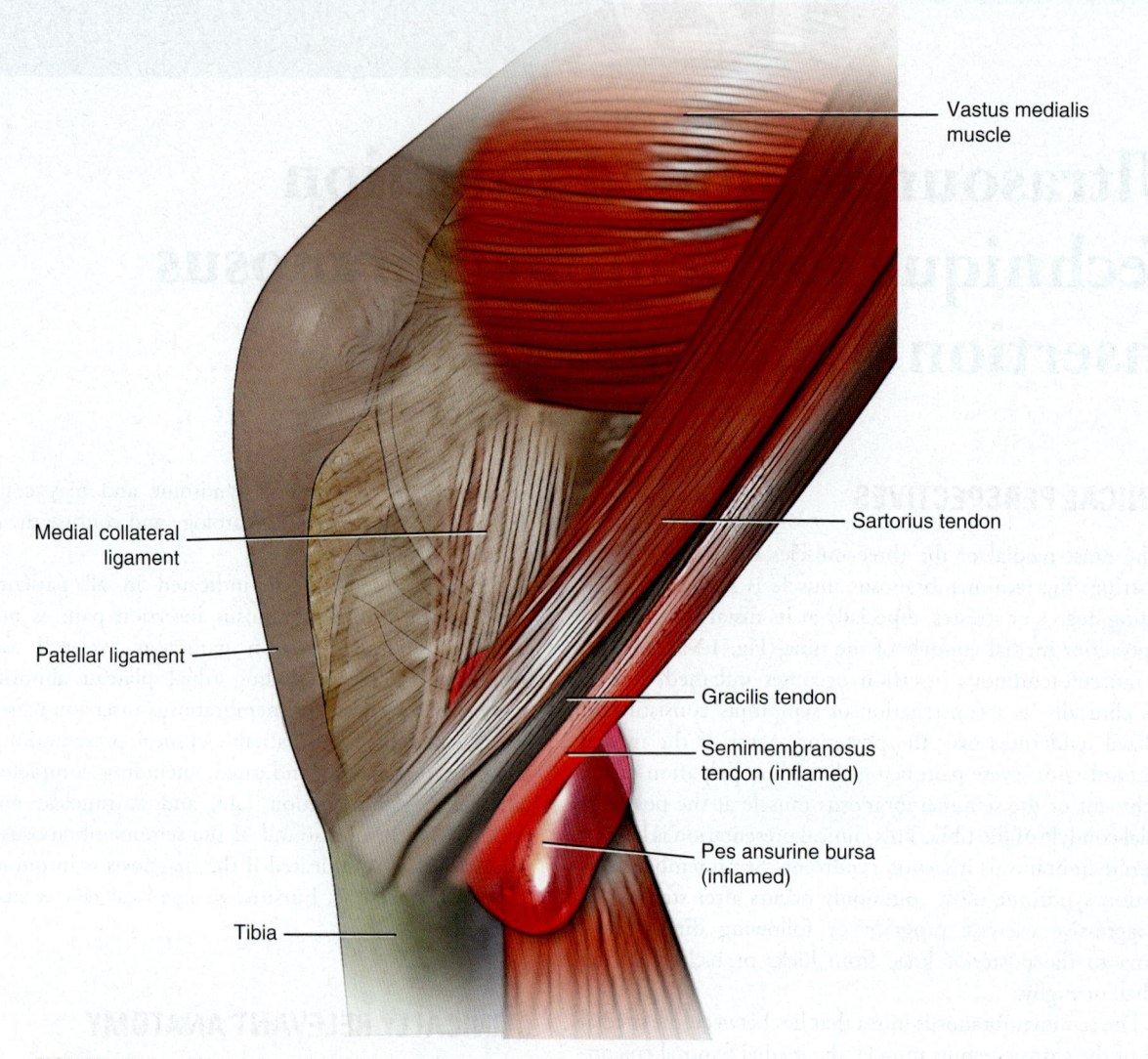

**FIGURE 127.1.** The semimembranosus insertion.

## ULTRASOUND-GUIDED TECHNIQUE

The benefits, risks, and alternative treatments are explained to the patient and informed consent is obtained. The patient is then placed in the supine position with the lower extremity externally rotated (Fig. 127.6). The skin overlying the medioposterior knee is then prepped with antiseptic solution. A sterile syringe containing 4.0 mL of 0.25% preservative-free bupivacaine and 40 mg of methylprednisolone is attached to a 1½-inch, 22-gauge needle using strict aseptic technique. A high-frequency linear ultrasound transducer is placed over the medial semimembranosus insertion joint in the oblique longitudinal plane with the superior portion of the ultrasound transducer turned about 20 degrees toward the patella (Fig. 127.7). A survey scan is taken, which demonstrates the characteristic appearance of the medial joint space with the hyperechoic medial margins of the femur and the tibia with the thick hyperechoic filaments of the medial collateral ligament overlying the triangular-shaped medial meniscus (Fig. 127.8). The medial meniscus is visualized as a triangular-shaped hyperechoic structure resting between the bony medial margins of the femur and tibia (Fig. 127.9). Just inferior to the joint space is the hypoechoic rounded tendon of the semimembranosus muscle at its tibial insertion. The tendon can be seen to lie within the medial contour of the tibia (Fig. 127.10). After the semimembranosus tendon is identified, the needle is placed through the skin ~1 cm above the middle of the longitudinally placed transducer and is then advanced using an out-of-plane approach with the needle trajectory adjusted under real-time ultrasound guidance until the needle tip lies in proximity to the tendon as it lies within

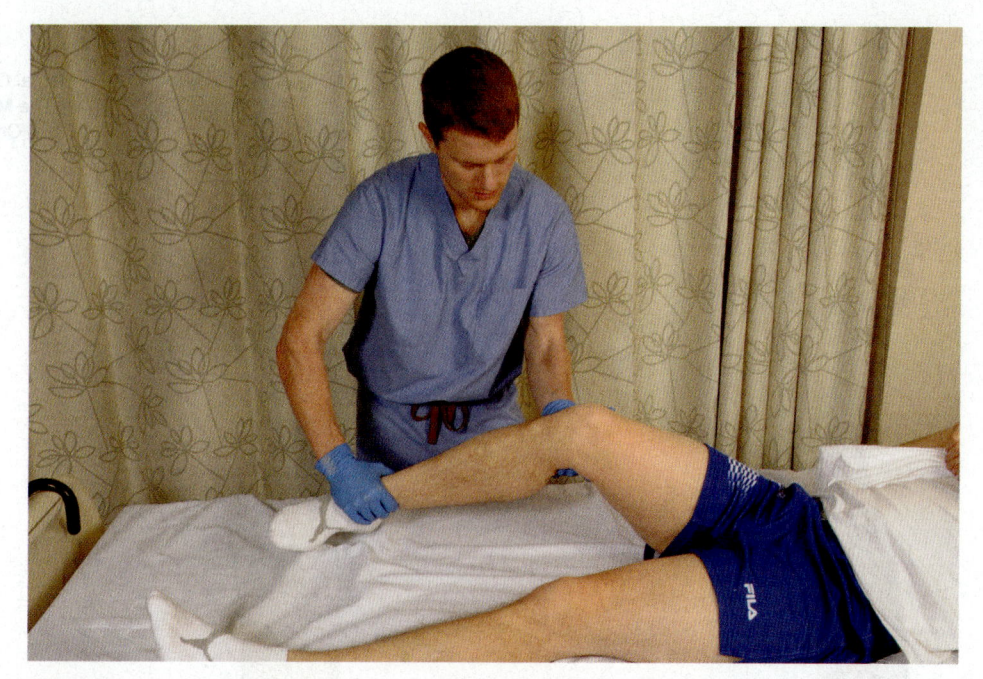

**FIGURE 127.2.** Patients suffering from semimembranosus insertion syndrome will exhibit a positive twist test. The twist test is performed by placing the knee in 20 degrees of flexion and passively rotating the flexed knee. The test is positive if the pain is reproduced.

the contour of the medial tibia (Fig. 127.10). When the tip of needle is thought to be within proximity to the semimembranosus insertion, a small amount of local anesthetic and steroid is injected under real-time ultrasound guidance to confirm that the needle tip is outside the substance of the tendon. There should be minimal resistance to injection. After proper needle tip placement is confirmed, the remainder of the contents of the syringe are slowly injected. If synechiae, loculations, or calcifications are present, the needle may have to be repositioned to ensure that the entire intra-articular space is treated. The needle is then removed, and a sterile pressure dressing and ice pack are placed at the injection site.

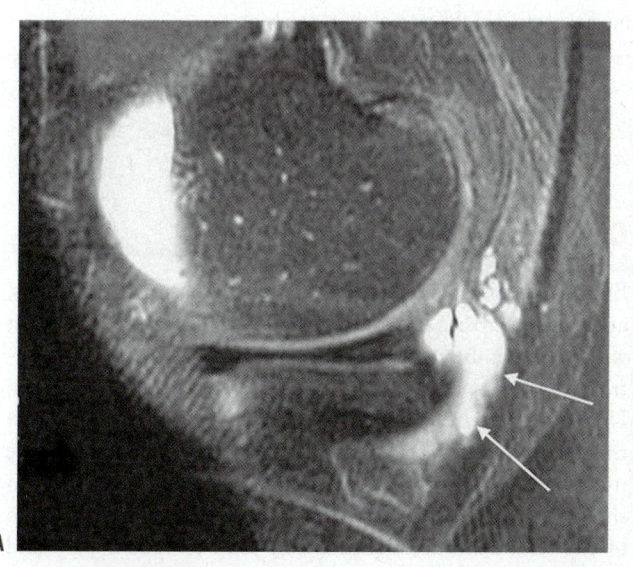

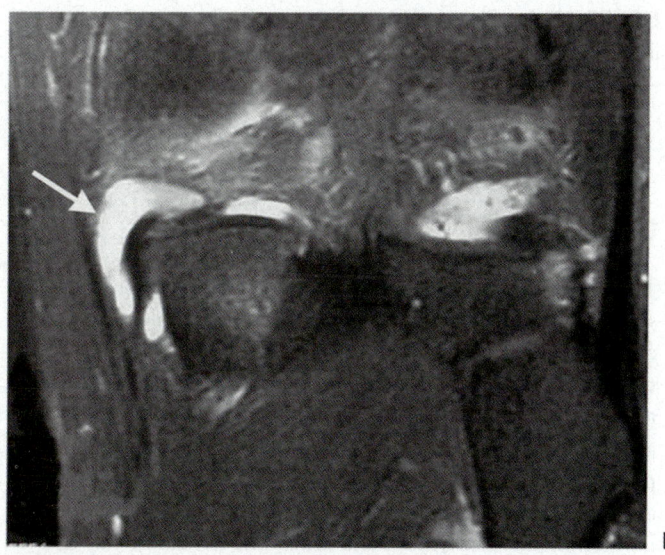

**FIGURE 127.3.** Semimembranosus bursitis frequently coexists with semimembranosus insertion syndrome. **A:** Arrows indicate fluid surrounding the tendon consistent with tendinitis and coexistent bursitis. **B:** Arrow indicates typical "U"-shaped fluid collection associated with semimembranosus bursitis. (Reused from Brant WE, Helms CA. *Fundamentals of Diagnostic Radiology*. 3rd ed. Philadelphia, PA: Lippincott Williams & Wilkins; 2007.)

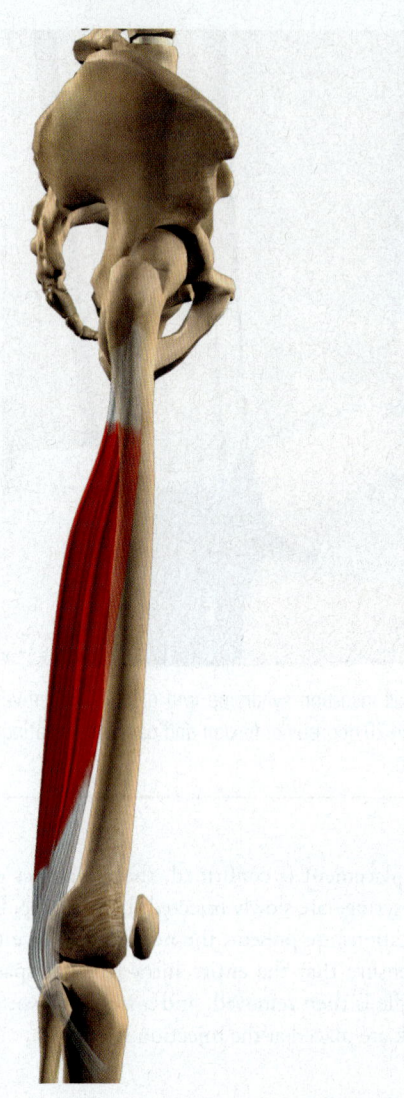

**FIGURE 127.4.** The insertions of the semimembranosus muscle. (LifeART, 2013.)

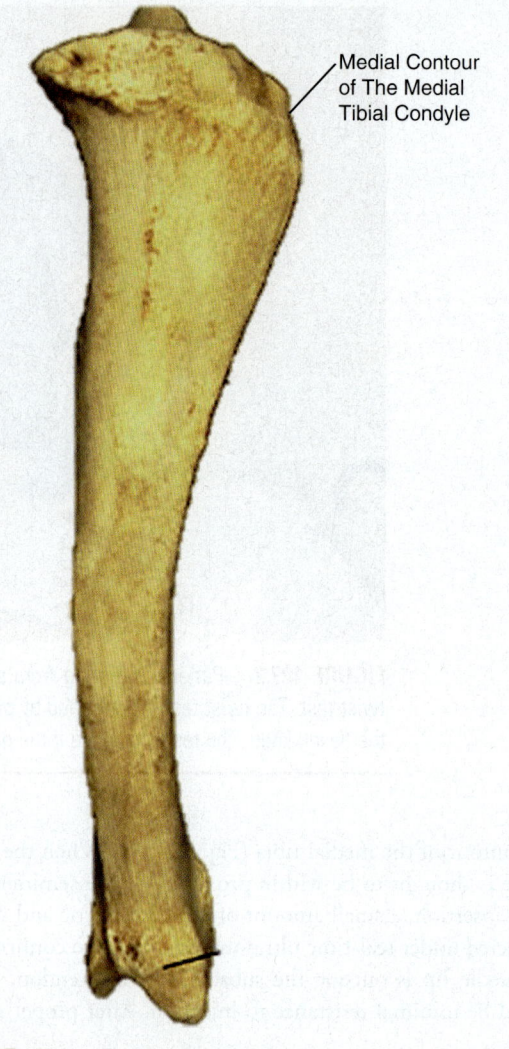

**FIGURE 127.5.** The distal semimembranosus tendon lies within the medial contour of the medial tibial condyle.

## COMPLICATIONS

The major complication of ultrasound-guided injection of the semimembranosus insertion is infection. Highly inflamed tendons are subject to rupture if directly injected, so care must be taken to insure that the needle tip is outside the substance of the tendon. The proximity to the common peroneal and tibial nerve as well as the popliteal artery and vein makes it imperative that this procedure be carried out only by those well versed in the regional anatomy and experienced in performing ultrasound-guided injection techniques. Ecchymosis and hematoma formation may also occur. A transient exacerbation of the patient's pain occurs ~25% of the time following this injection technique, and the patient should be warned of this possibility prior to the procedure.

## CLINICAL PEARLS

Bursitis, meniscal tears, tendinopathy, osteoarthritis, synovitis, avascular necrosis, and impingement syndromes may coexist with semimembranosus insertion joint disease and may contribute to the patient's pain symptomatology (Fig. 127.11). Universal precautions should always be observed to protect the operator, and strict adherence to sterile technique must be used to avoid infection. Gentle physical therapy and local heat should be introduced following ultrasound-guided injection of the semimembranosus insertion joint to reduce pain and improve function. Simple analgesics and nonsteroidal anti-inflammatory agents or COX-2 inhibitors may be used concurrently with this injection technique.

# CHAPTER 127 US-GUIDED INJECTION TECHNIQUE FOR SEMIMEMBRANOSUS INSERTION SYNDROME

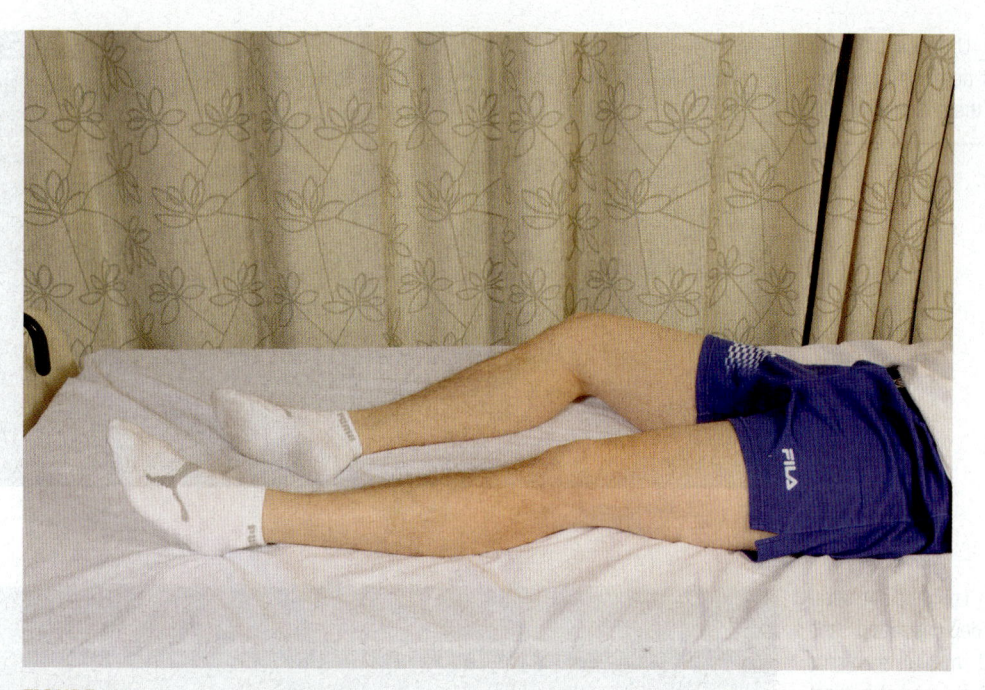

**FIGURE 127.6.** Proper patient position for ultrasound-guided intra-articular semimembranosus insertion injection. Note that the affected extremity is externally rotated.

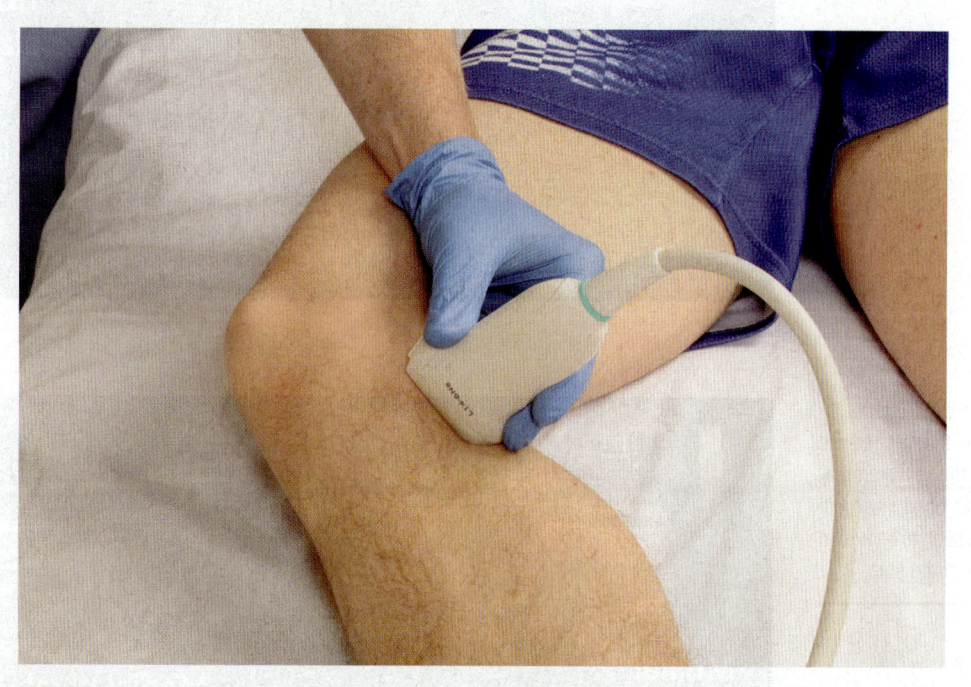

**FIGURE 127.7.** Correct longitudinal position for ultrasound transducer for ultrasound-guided intra-articular injection of the semimembranosus insertion joint.

**FIGURE 127.8.** Ultrasound image of the knee joint demonstrating the medial border of the proximal femur.

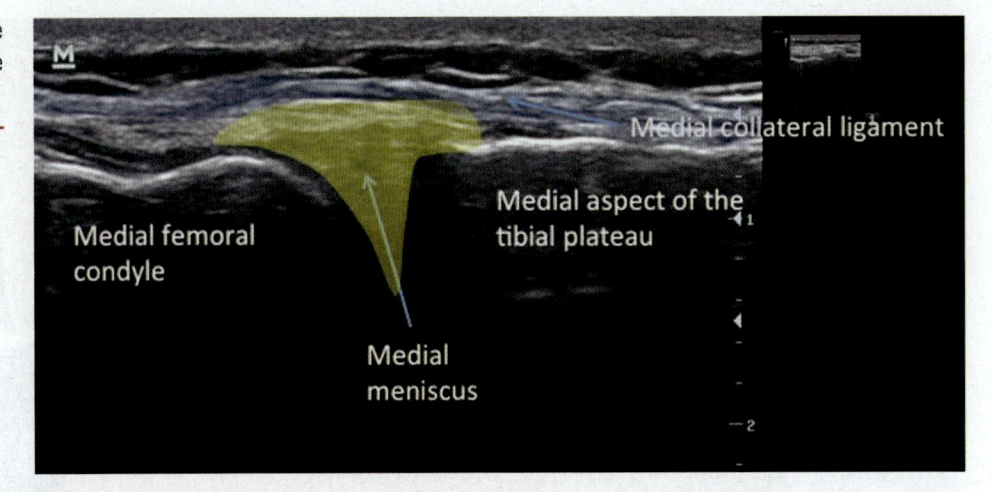

**FIGURE 127.9.** Longitudinal ultrasound image demonstrating the triangular-shaped medial meniscus nestled between the medial borders of the femur and tibia.

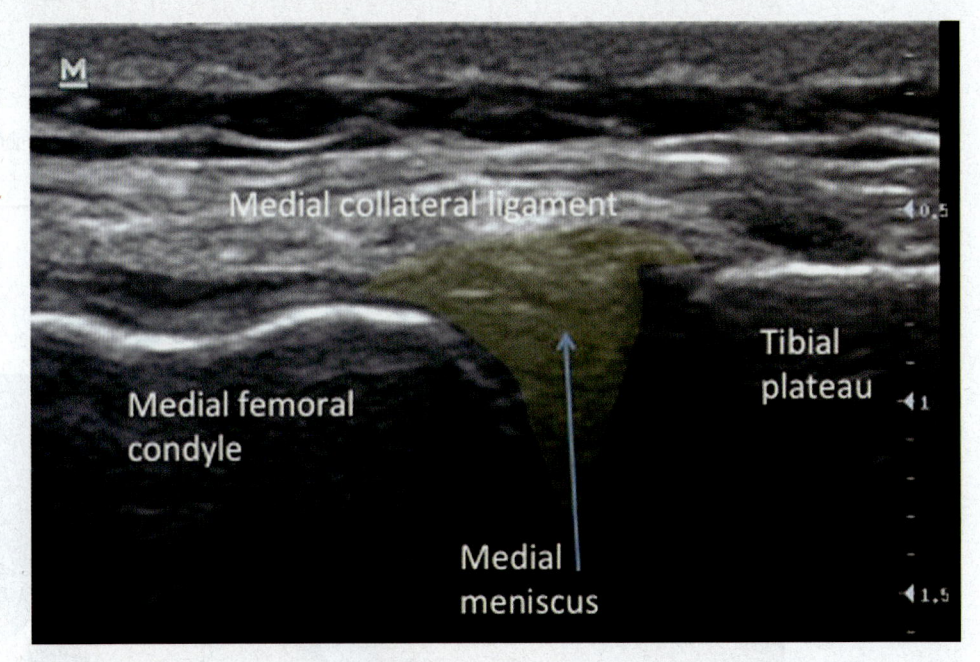

**FIGURE 127.10.** Just inferior to the joint space is the hypoechoic rounded tendon of the semimembranosus muscle at its tibial insertion. The tendon can be seen to lie within the medial contour of the tibia.

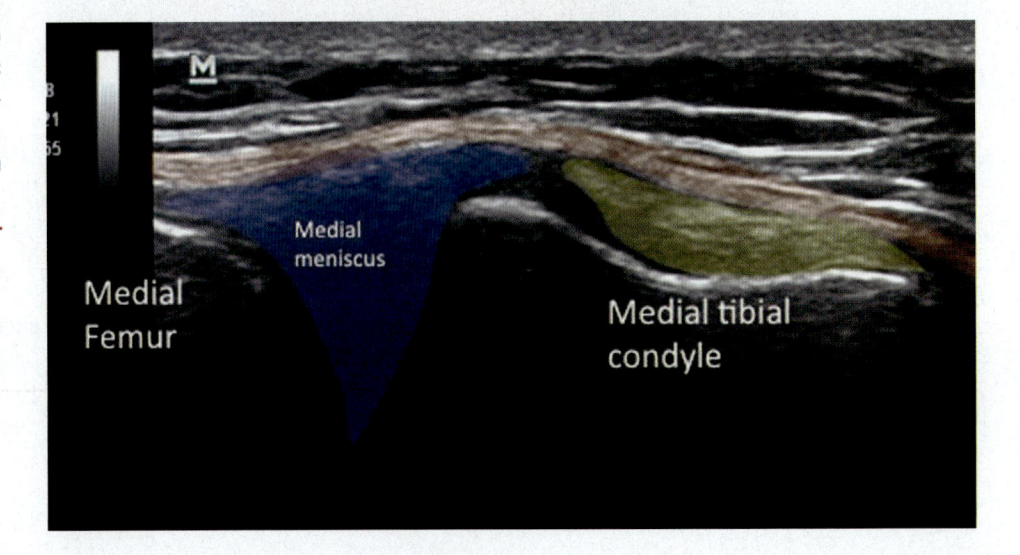

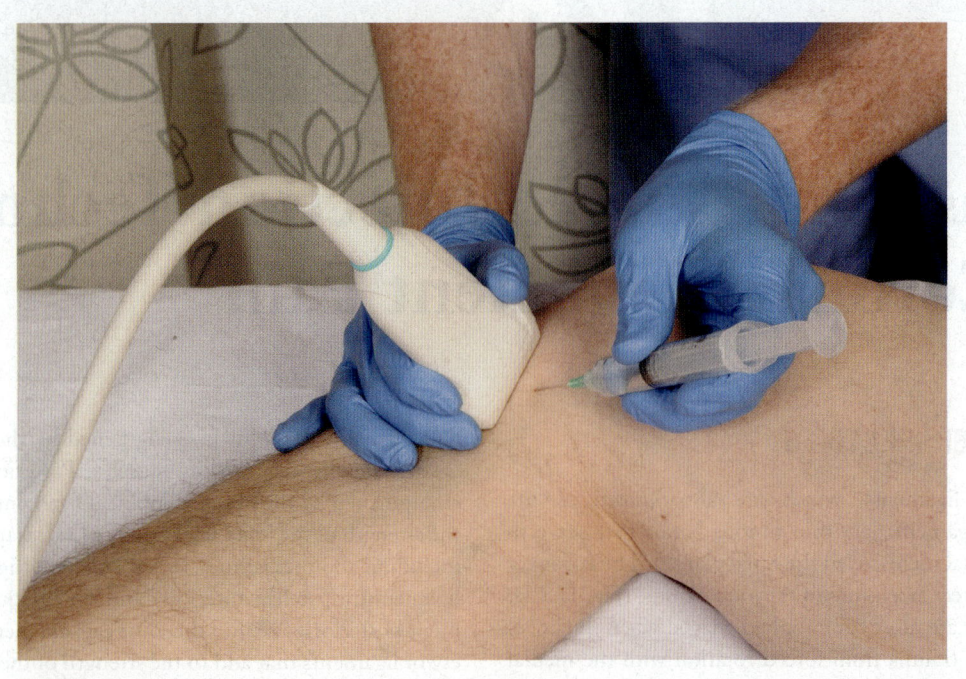

**FIGURE 127.11.** Proper out-of-plane needle placement for ultrasound-guided injection of the semimembranosus insertion.

## SUGGESTED READINGS

Albert C, Brocq O, Gerard D, et al. Septic semimembranosus insertion arthritis after intra-articular hyaluronate injection: two case reports. *Joint Bone Spine* 2006;73(2):205–207.

Schumacher HR, Chen LX. Injectable corticosteroids in treatment of arthritis of the semimembranosus insertion. Review article. *Am J Med* 2005;118(11):1208–1214.

Waldman SD. Functional anatomy of the semimembranosus insertion. In: *Pain Review*. Philadelphia, PA: Saunders Elsevier; 2009:144–149.

Waldman SD. Intra-articular injection of the semimembranosus insertion Joint. In: *Pain Review*. Philadelphia, PA: Saunders Elsevier; 2009:583–584.

Waldman SD, Campbell RSD. Anatomy, Special Imaging Considerations of the Semimembranosus insertion. In: *Imaging of Pain*. Philadelphia, PA: Saunders Elsevier; 2011:367–368.

Waldman SD, Campbell RSD. Osteonecrosis of the Semimembranosus insertion. In: *Imaging of Pain*. Philadelphia, PA: Saunders Elsevier; 2011:393–396.

Waldman SD. Intra-articular injection of the semimembranosus insertion joint. In: *Atlas of Pain Management Injection Techniques*. 3rd ed. Philadelphia, PA: Saunders Elsevier; 2012:346–348.

# CHAPTER 128

# Ultrasound-Guided Injection Technique for Coronary Ligament Pain

## CLINICAL PERSPECTIVES

The coronary ligaments, which are also known as the meniscotibial ligaments, are thin fibrous bands that serve to anchor the medial meniscus to the tibial plateau. The coronary ligaments are direct extensions of the joint capsule (Fig. 128.1). These ligaments are most commonly damaged when the knees are subjected to trauma from forced rotation with the medial coronary ligaments damaged much more frequently than their lateral counterparts. Patients with medial coronary ligament damage present with pain over the medial joint and increased pain on passive external rotation of the knee. Flexion and external rotation of the knee when carrying out the activities of daily living will cause an exacerbation of the patient's pain. Rest and heat may provide some relief. The pain associated with damage to the medial coronary ligaments is characterized as constant and is characterized as aching and may interfere with sleep. Coexistent bursitis, tendonitis, arthritis, or internal derangement of the knee, in particular the medial meniscus, may confuse the clinical picture after trauma to the knee joint.

Plain radiographs are indicated in all patients who present with coronary ligament syndrome pain. Based on the patient's clinical presentation, additional testing may be indicated, including complete blood cell count, sedimentation rate, and antinuclear antibody testing. MRI of the knee is indicated if internal derangement or occult mass or tumor is suspected as well as to confirm the diagnosis of coronary ligament damage or meniscal tears (Fig. 128.2). Bone scan may be useful to identify occult stress fractures involving the medial joint, especially if trauma has occurred.

## CLINICALLY RELEVANT ANATOMY

The rounded condyles of the femur articulate with the condyles of the tibia below and the patella anteriorly. The articular surface is covered with hyaline cartilage, which is susceptible to arthritis. The joint is surrounded laterally and posteriorly by a capsule, which provides support for the joint. As extensions of the joint capsule, the coronary ligaments are thin bands of fibrous tissue that anchor the medial meniscus to the tibial plateau (see Fig. 128.1). The capsule is absent anteriorly and in its place is the suprapatellar and infrapatellar bursa. Laterally and medially, the joint is strengthened by the tendons of the vastus lateralis and medius muscles. Posteriorly, the joint is strengthened by the oblique popliteal ligament. Also adding to the strength of the joint are a variety of extracapsular ligaments, including the medial and lateral collateral ligaments and the ligamentum patellae anteriorly and the oblique popliteal ligament posteriorly. Within the joint capsule there are also a variety of ligaments that add to the strength of the joint, including the anterior and posterior cruciate ligaments (Fig. 128.3). The joint capsule is lined with a synovial membrane that attaches to the articular cartilage and gives rise to a number of bursae, including the suprapatellar and infrapatellar bursae. The knee joint is innervated by the femoral, obturator, common peroneal, and tibial nerves. In addition to arthritis, the knee joint is susceptible to the development of tendonitis, bursitis, and disruption of the ligaments, cartilage, and tendons.

## ULTRASOUND-GUIDED TECHNIQUE

The benefits, risks, and alternative treatments are explained to the patient and informed consent is obtained. The patient is then placed in the supine position with the lower extremity externally rotated (Fig. 128.4). The skin overlying the medioposterior knee is then prepped with antiseptic solution. A sterile syringe containing 4.0 mL of 0.25% preservative-free bupivacaine and 40 mg of methylprednisolone is attached to a 1½-inch, 22-gauge needle using strict aseptic technique. A high-frequency linear ultrasound transducer is placed over the medial coronary ligament joint in the oblique longitudinal plane with the superior portion of the ultrasound transducer turned about 20 degrees toward the patella (Fig. 128.5). A survey scan is taken, which demonstrates the characteristic appearance of the medial joint space with the hyperechoic medial margins of the femur and the tibia with the thick hyperechoic filaments of the medial collateral ligament overlying the triangular-shaped medial meniscus (Fig. 128.6). The medial meniscus is visualized as a triangular-shaped hyperechoic structure resting between the bony medial margins of the femur and tibia (Fig. 128.7). At the superior margin of the hyperechoic medial margin of the tibia lies the medial portion of the coronary ligaments (Fig. 128.8). After the medial margin of the tibia is identified, the needle is placed through

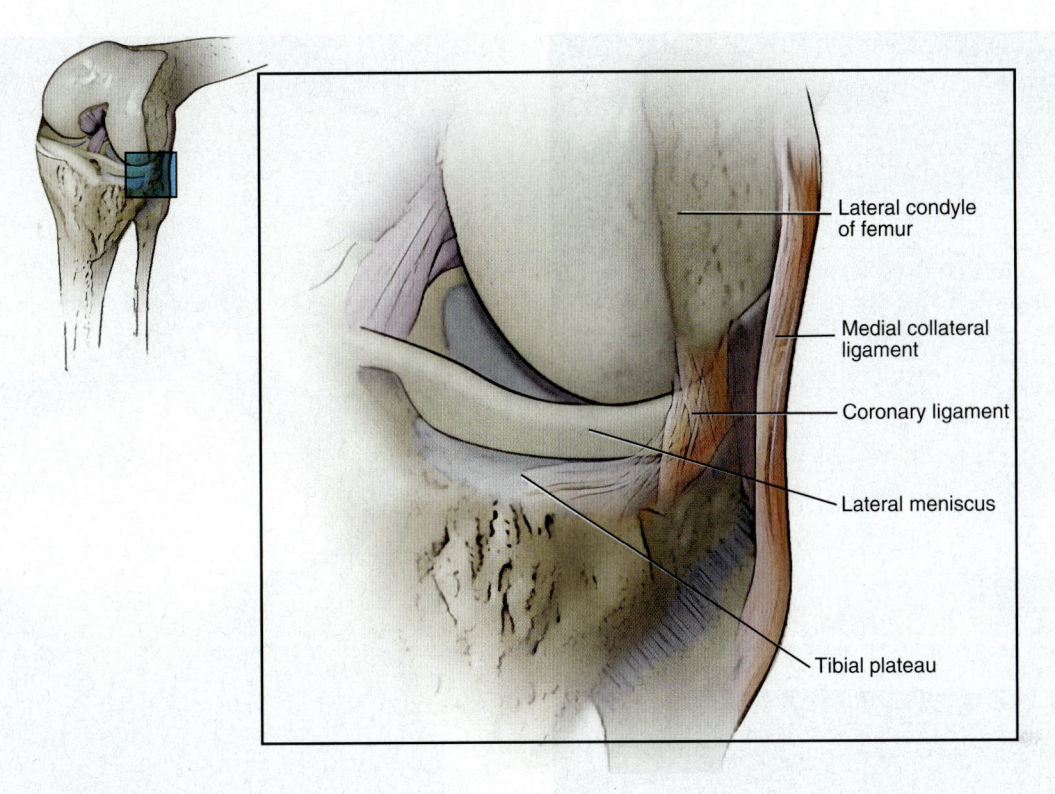

**FIGURE 128.1.** The medial coronary ligaments.

the skin ~1 cm above the middle of the longitudinally placed transducer and is then advanced using an out-of-plane approach with the needle trajectory adjusted under real-time ultrasound guidance until the needle tip lies in proximity to the junction of the medial meniscus as it abuts against the superior tibial margin (Fig. 128.9). When the tip of needle is thought to be within satisfactory position, a small amount of local anesthetic and steroid is injected under real-time ultrasound guidance to confirm that the needle tip is next to the medial coronary ligament. There should be minimal resistance to injection. After intra-articular needle tip placement is confirmed, the remainder of the contents of the syringe is slowly injected. If synechiae, loculations, or calcifications are present, the needle may have to be repositioned to ensure that the entire intra-articular space is treated. The needle is then removed, and a sterile pressure dressing and ice pack are placed at the injection site.

## COMPLICATIONS

The major complication of ultrasound-guided injection of the coronary ligament is infection. Highly inflamed tendons are subject to rupture if directly injected, so care must be taken to insure that the needle tip is outside the coronary ligament itself. The proximity to the common peroneal and tibial nerve as well as the popliteal artery and vein makes it imperative that this procedure be carried out only by those well versed in the regional anatomy and experienced in performing ultrasound-guided injection techniques. Ecchymosis and hematoma formation may also occur. A transient exacerbation of the patient's pain occurs ~25% of the time following this injection technique, and the patient should be warned of this possibility prior to the procedure.

## CLINICAL PEARLS

Bursitis, meniscal tears, tendinopathy, osteoarthritis, synovitis, avascular necrosis, and impingement syndromes may coexist with coronary ligament joint disease and may contribute to the patient's pain symptomatology. Universal precautions should always be observed to protect the operator, and strict adherence to sterile technique must be used to avoid infection. Gentle physical therapy and local heat should be introduced following ultrasound-guided injection of the coronary ligament joint to reduce pain and improve function. Simple analgesics and nonsteroidal anti-inflammatory agents or COX-2 inhibitors may be used concurrently with this injection technique.

**918** SECTION IX  KNEE AND LOWER EXTREMITY

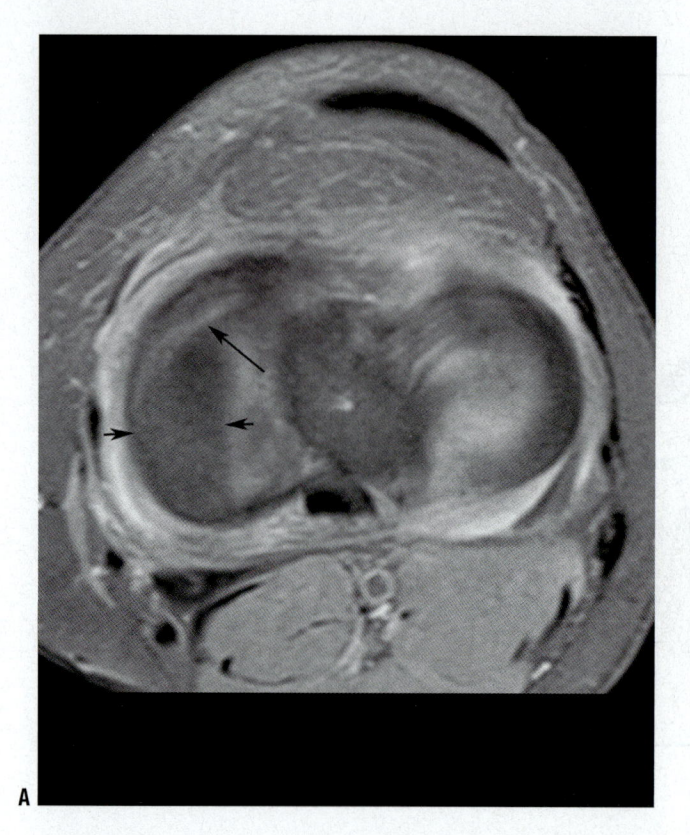

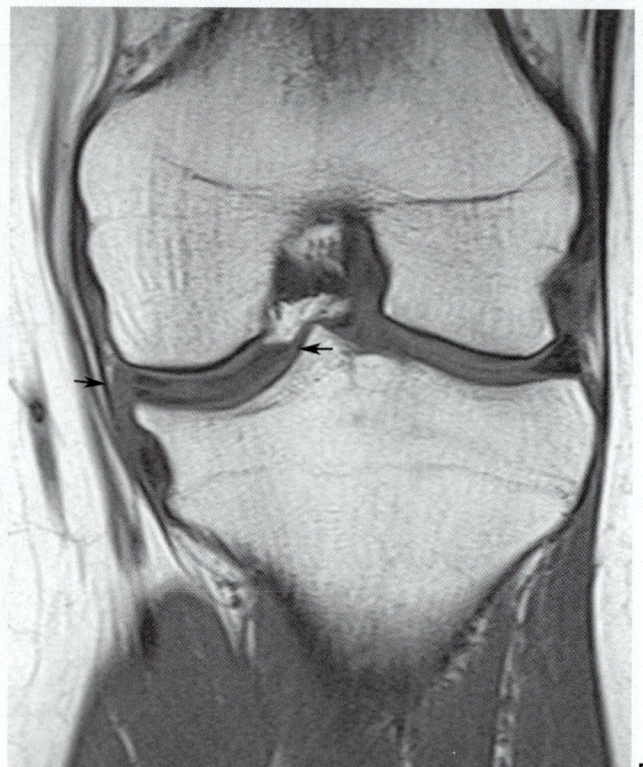

**FIGURE 128.2.** Discoid medial meniscus. **A:** Axial fat-suppressed proton density image demonstrating the size of the discoid meniscus (*short arrows*) with a tear (*long arrow*) anteriorly. Coronal T1-weighted **(B)** and DESS **(C)** images demonstrating the extension of the meniscus into the joint (*short arrows*). (Reused from Berquist TH. *MRI of the Musculoskeletal System.* 6th ed. Philadelphia, PA: Lippincott Williams & Wilkins; 2013.)

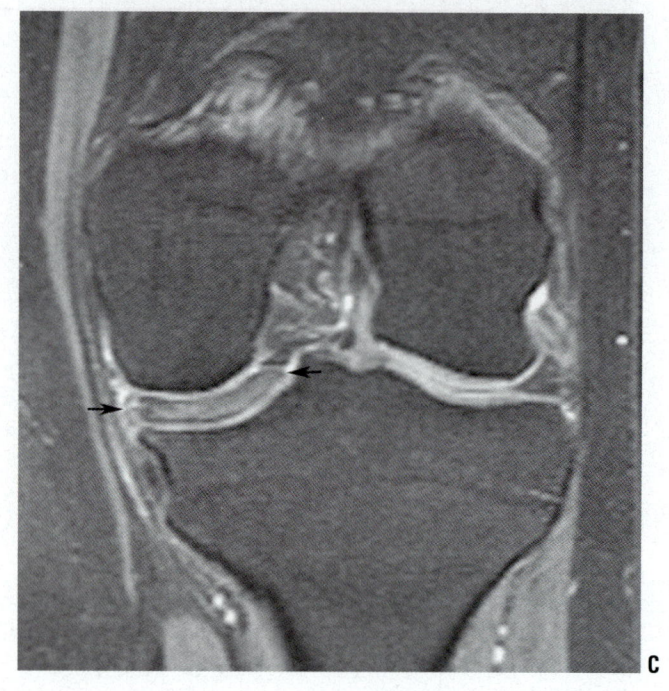

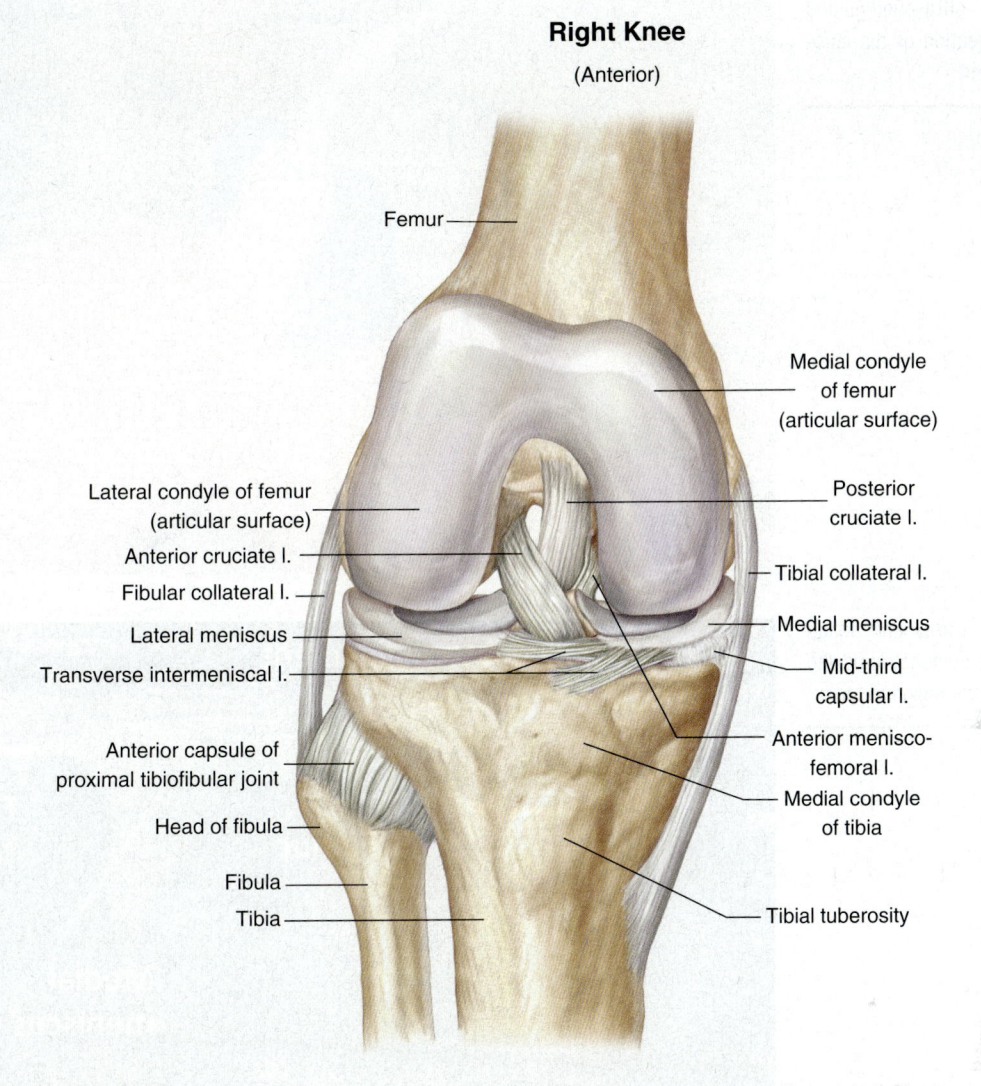

**FIGURE 128.3.** Anterior view of the knee demonstrating supporting ligaments. (Anatomical Chart Company, 2013.)

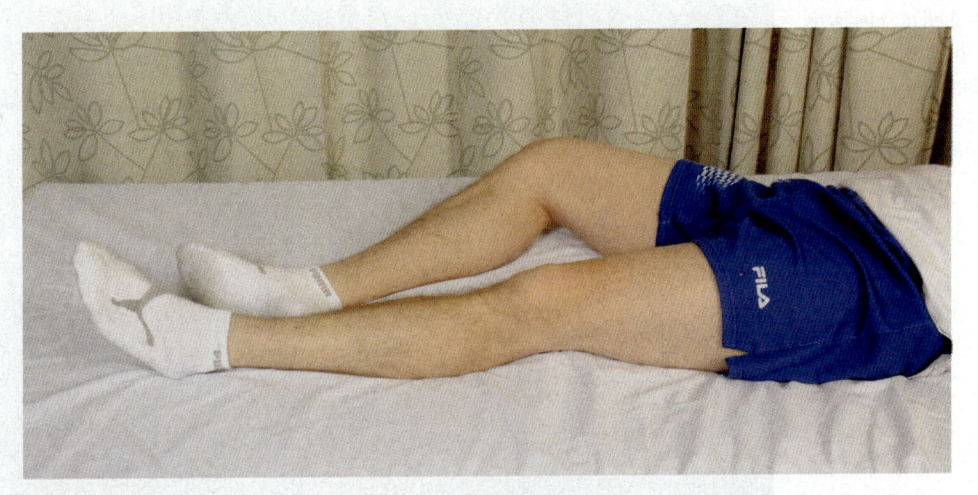

**FIGURE 128.4.** Proper patient position for ultrasound-guided intra-articular coronary ligament injection. Note that the affected extremity is externally rotated.

**FIGURE 128.5.** Correct longitudinal position for ultrasound transducer for ultrasound-guided intra-articular injection of the coronary ligament joint.

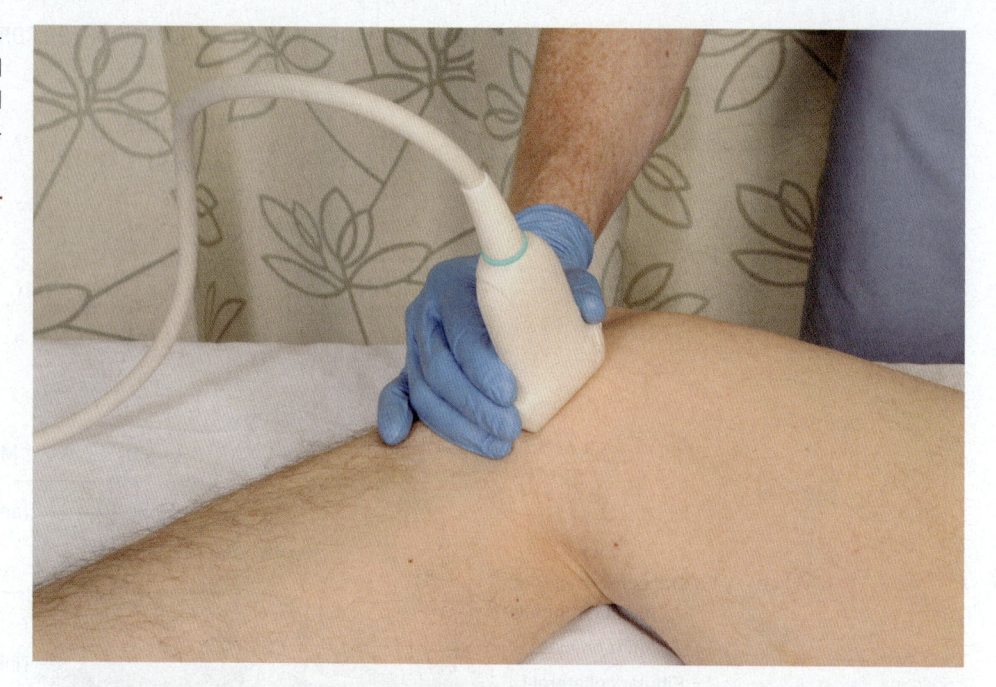

**FIGURE 128.6.** Ultrasound image of the knee joint demonstrating the medial border of the proximal femur.

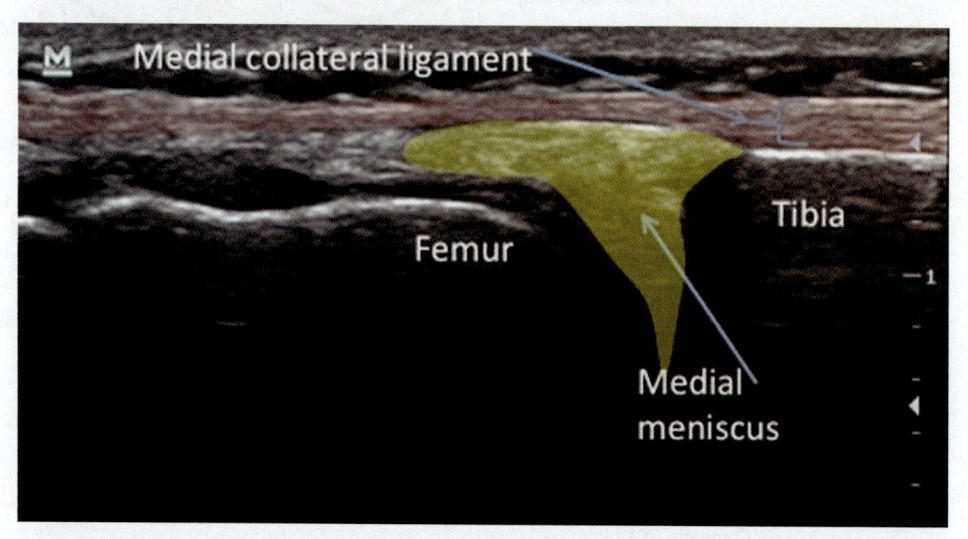

**FIGURE. 128.7.** Longitudinal ultrasound image demonstrating the triangular-shaped medial meniscus nestled between the medial borders of the femur and tibia.

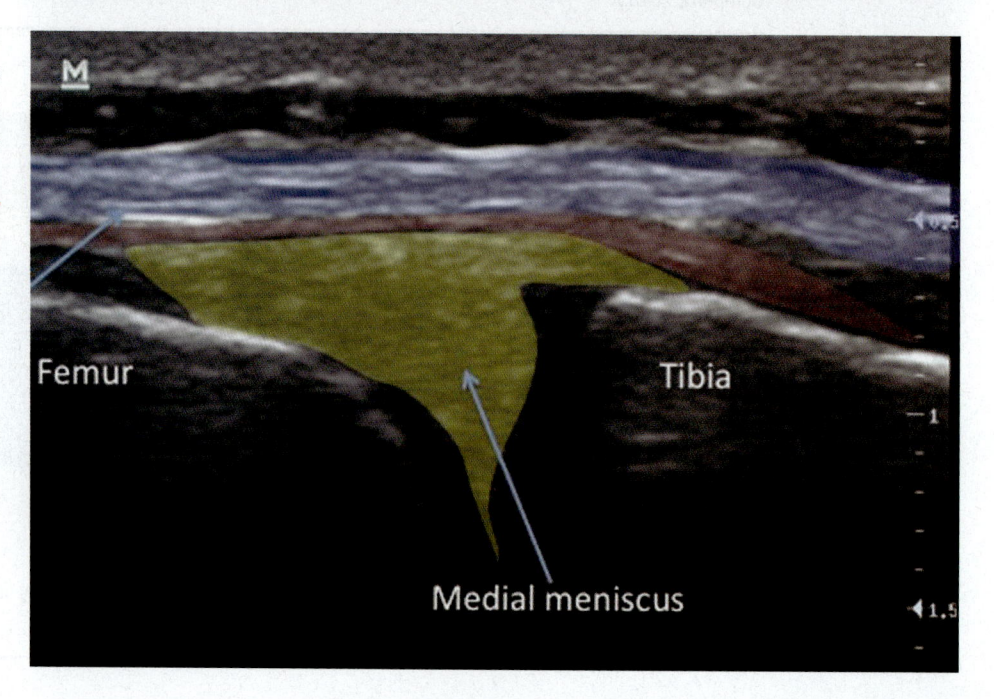

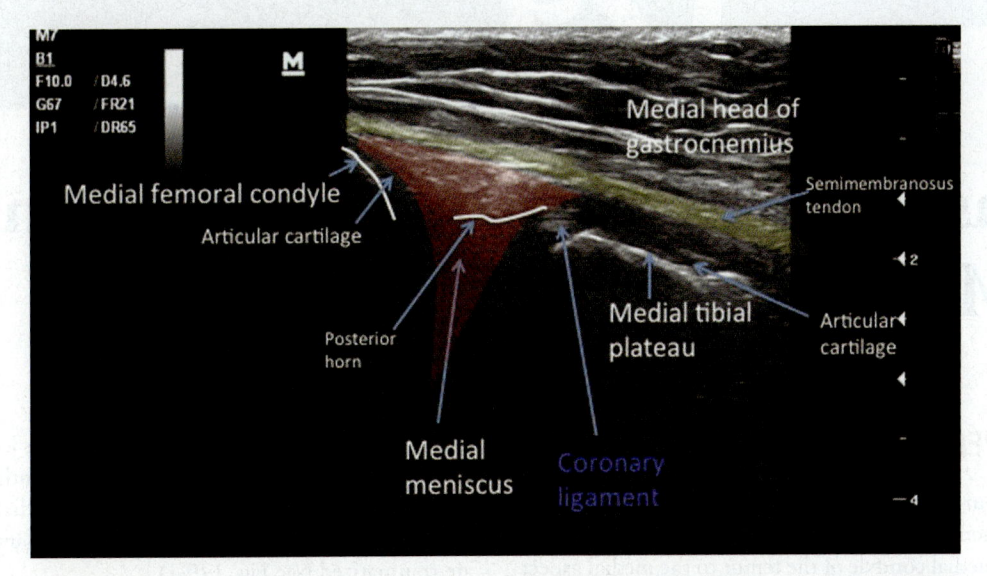

**FIGURE 128.8.** Just inferior to the joint space is the hypoechoic rounded tendon of the semimembranosus muscle at its tibial insertion. The tendon can be seen to lie within the medial contour of the tibia.

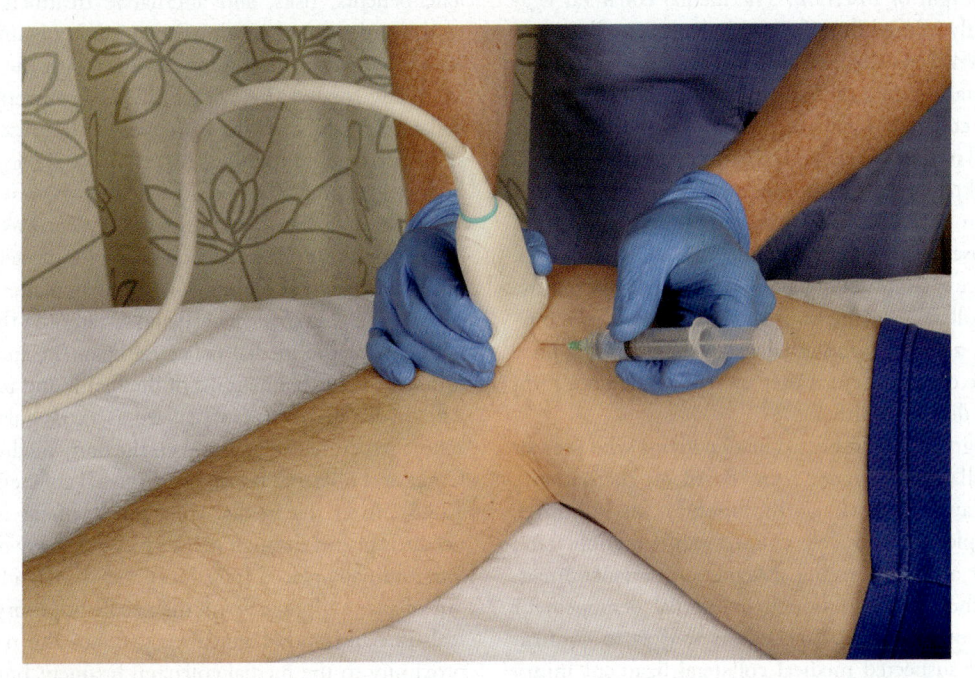

**FIGURE 128.9.** Proper needle placement for ultrasound-guided injection of the semimembranosus insertion.

## SUGGESTED READINGS

Aichroth P. Degenerative meniscal tears. *Knee* 1994;1(3):181–182.

Colletti JE, Kilgore KP, Derrick J. Traumatic knee pain. *Ann Emerg Med* 2009;53(3):403, 409.

Drosos GI, Pozo JL. The causes and mechanisms of meniscal injuries in the sporting and non-sporting environment in an unselected population. [Original Research Article] *Knee* 2004;11(2):143–149.

Loudon JK. Meniscal injuries. In: *Orthopaedic Physical Therapy Secrets*. 2nd ed. Philadelphia, PA: Hanley & Belfus; 2006:564–569.

Waldman SD, Campbell RSD. Osteonecrosis of the knee. In: *Imaging of Pain*. Philadelphia, PA: Saunders Elsevier; 2011:393–396.

Waldman SD. Intra-articular injection of the coronary ligament joint. In: *Atlas of Pain Management Injection Techniques*. 3rd ed. Philadelphia, PA: Saunders Elsevier; 2012:356–357.

# Ultrasound-Guided Injection Technique for Medial Collateral Ligament

## CLINICAL PERSPECTIVES

One of the four major ligaments of the knee, the medial collateral ligament, is a broad, flat, band-like ligament that runs from the medial condyle of the femur to the medial aspect of the shaft of the tibia, where it attaches just above the groove of the semimembranosus muscle attachment (Fig. 129.1). The ligament also attaches to the edge of the medial semilunar cartilage. The ligament is susceptible to strain at the joint line or avulsion at its origin or insertion. The medial collateral ligament is frequently injured from falls with the leg in valgus and externally rotated, typically during snow skiing accidents or as the result of tackles in American football (Fig. 129.2). The pain of medial collateral ligament damage is localized to the medial knee and is made worse with passive valgus and external rotation of the knee. Activity, especially involving flexion and external rotation of the knee, will exacerbate the pain. Local heat and decreased activity may provide a modicum of relief. Sleep disturbance is common in patients suffering from trauma to the medial collateral ligament of the knee. Coexistent bursitis, tendonitis, arthritis, or internal derangement of the knee may confuse the clinical picture after trauma to the knee joint making clinical diagnosis difficult.

Plain radiographs are indicated in all patients who present with medial collateral ligament pain. Based on the patient's clinical presentation, additional testing may be indicated, including complete blood cell count, sedimentation rate, and antinuclear antibody testing. Magnetic resonance imaging (MRI) of the knee is indicated if internal derangement or occult mass or tumor is suspected as well as to confirm the diagnosis of suspected medical collateral ligament injury (Fig. 129.3). Bone scan may be useful to identify occult stress fractures involving the joint, especially if trauma has occurred.

## CLINICALLY RELEVANT ANATOMY

The medial collateral ligament, which is also known as the tibial collateral ligament, is a broad, flat, band-like ligament that runs from the medial condyle of the femur to the medial aspect of the shaft of the tibia, where it attaches just above the groove of the semimembranosus muscle attachment (see Fig. 129.1). It also attaches to the edge of the medial meniscus (Fig. 129.4).

The medial collateral ligament is crossed at its lower part by the tendons of the sartorius, gracilis, and semitendinosus muscles. A bursa is between these tendons and the medial collateral ligament and is subject to inflammation if the ligament or tendons are traumatized (see Fig. 129.1).

## ULTRASOUND-GUIDED TECHNIQUE

The benefits, risks, and alternative treatments are explained to the patient, and informed consent is obtained. The patient is then placed in the supine position with the lower extremity externally rotated (Fig. 129.5). The skin overlying the medial collateral ligament is then prepped with antiseptic solution. A sterile syringe containing 2.0 mL of 0.25% preservative-free bupivacaine and 40 mg of methylprednisolone is attached to a 1½-inch, 22-gauge needle using strict aseptic technique. A high-frequency linear ultrasound transducer is placed over the medial collateral ligament in the longitudinal plane (Fig. 129.6). A survey scan is taken, which demonstrates the thick hyperechoic filaments of the medial collateral ligament and the bony contours of the medial margins of the femur and tibia (Fig. 129.7). The medial meniscus is visualized as a triangular-shaped hyperechoic structure resting between the bony medial margins of the femur and tibia and beneath the medial collateral ligament (Fig. 129.8). After the medial collateral ligament is identified, the needle is placed through the skin ~1 cm above the middle of the longitudinally placed transducer and is then advanced using an out-of-plane approach with the needle trajectory adjusted under real-time ultrasound guidance to place the needle tip within proximity to the medial collateral ligament but not within the substance of the ligament (Fig. 129.9). When the tip of needle is thought to be in satisfactory position, a small amount of local anesthetic and steroid is injected under real-time ultrasound guidance to confirm that the needle tip is not within the substance of the medial collateral ligament. There should be minimal resistance to injection. After intra-articular needle tip placement is confirmed, the remainder of the contents of the syringe is slowly injected. If synechiae, loculations, or calcifications are present, the needle may have to be repositioned to ensure that the entire intra-articular space is treated. The needle is then removed, and a sterile pressure dressing and ice pack are placed at the injection site.

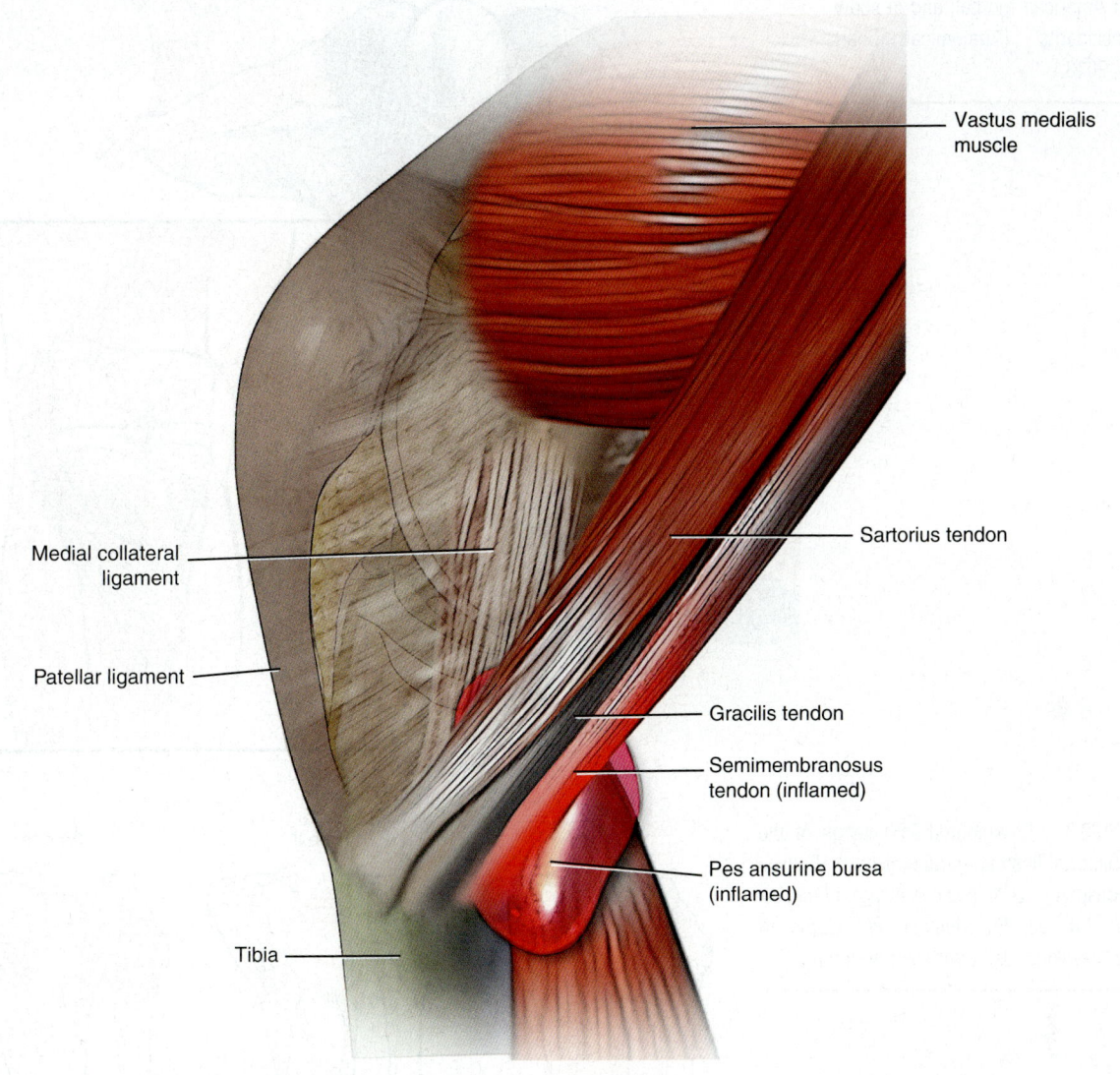

**FIGURE 129.1.** The anatomy of the medial collateral ligament and its relationship with the other musculotendinous units of the medial knee.

## COMPLICATIONS

The major complication of ultrasound-guided injection of the medial collateral ligament is infection. Highly inflamed tendons and ligaments are subject to rupture if directly injected so care must be taken to insure that that the needle tip is outside the substance of the tendon. Ecchymosis and hematoma formation may also occur given proximity to the tibial artery and vein. A transient exacerbation of the patient's pain occurs ~25% of the time following this injection technique, and the patient should be warned of this possibility prior to the procedure.

## CLINICAL PEARLS

Bursitis, meniscal tears, tendinopathy, osteoarthritis, synovitis, avascular necrosis, and impingement syndromes may coexist with medial collateral ligament disease and may contribute to the patient's pain symptomatology. Universal precautions should always be observed to protect the operator, and strict adherence to sterile technique must be used to avoid infection. Gentle physical therapy and local heat should be introduced following ultrasound-guided injection of the medial collateral ligament to reduce pain and improve function. Simple analgesics and nonsteroidal anti-inflammatory agents or COX-2 inhibitors may be used concurrently with this injection technique.

**FIGURE 129.2.** The medial collateral ligament is frequently injured by low tackles in American football and in snow skiing accidents. (Anatomical Chart Company, 2013.)

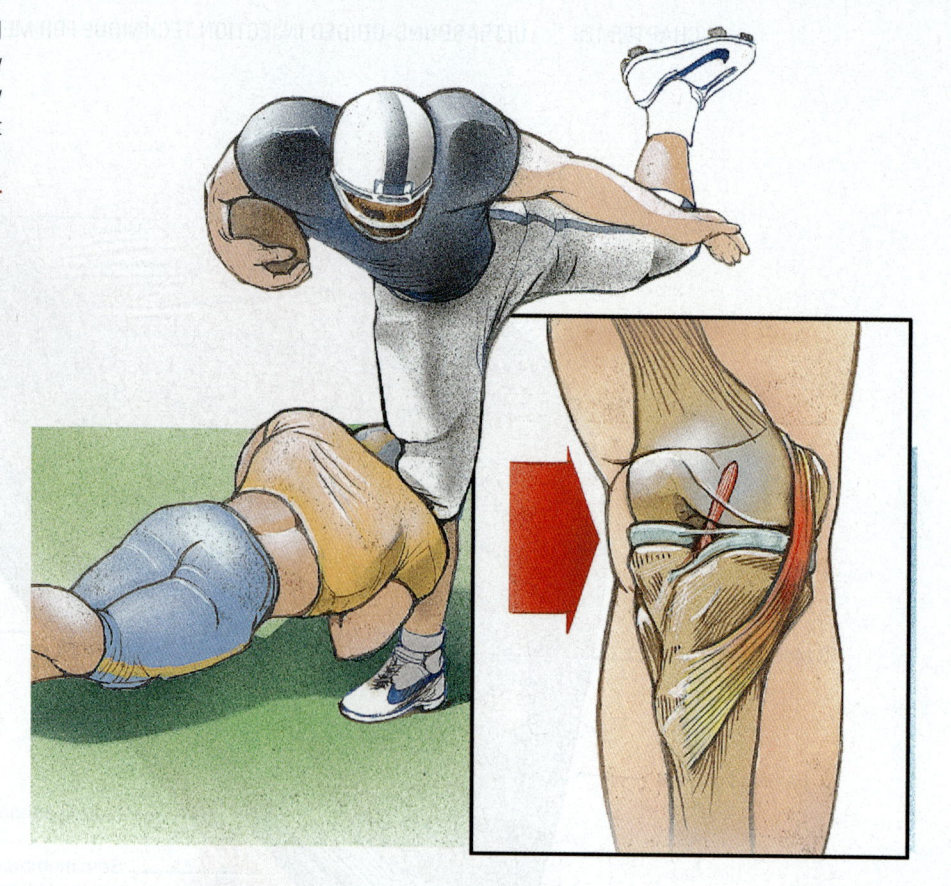

**FIGURE 129.3.** T2-weighted MRI image of the medial collateral ligament strain (*arrows*). (Reused from Greenspan A. *Orthopedic Imaging: A Practical Approach*. 5th ed. Philadelphia, PA: Lippincott Williams & Wilkins; 2011, with permission.)

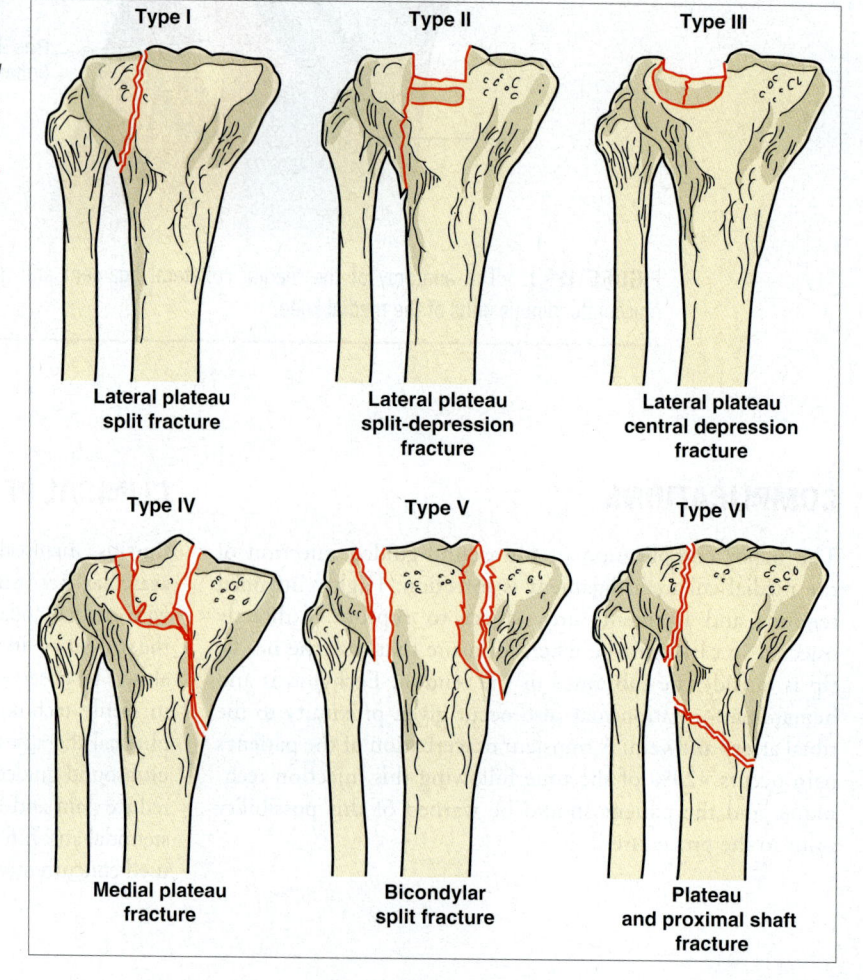

Type I — Lateral plateau split fracture
Type II — Lateral plateau split-depression fracture
Type III — Lateral plateau central depression fracture
Type IV — Medial plateau fracture
Type V — Bicondylar split fracture
Type VI — Plateau and proximal shaft fracture

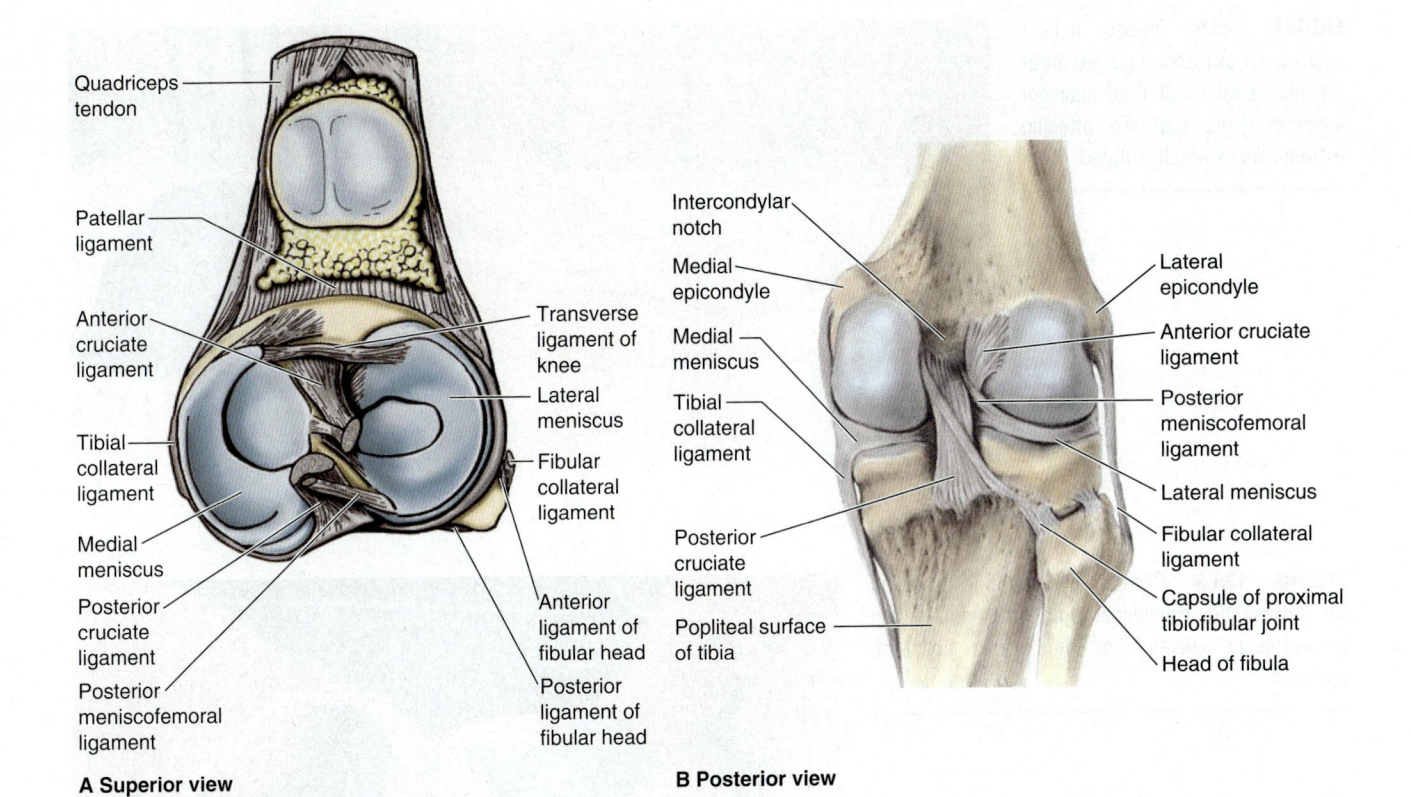

CHAPTER 129  ULTRASOUND-GUIDED INJECTION TECHNIQUE FOR MEDIAL COLLATERAL LIGAMENT

**A** Superior view

**B** Posterior view

**C** Coronal MRI of right knee

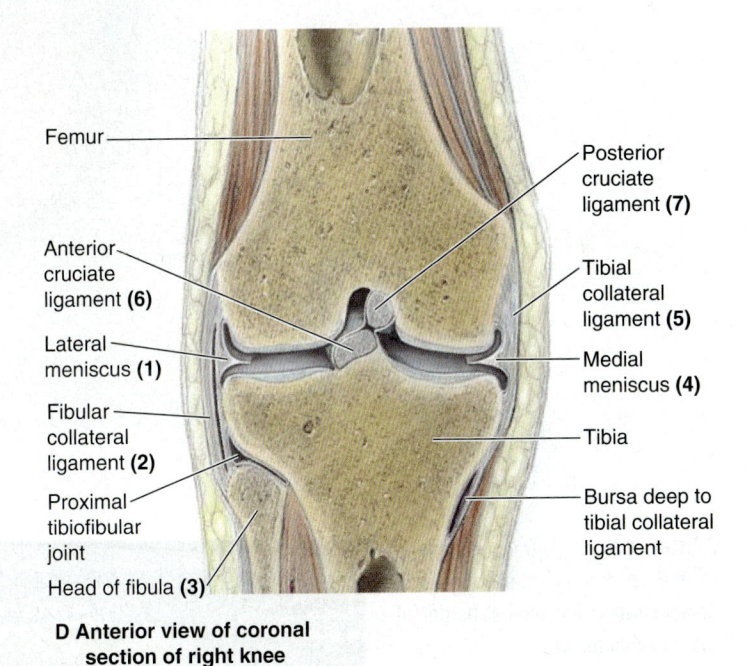

**D** Anterior view of coronal section of right knee

**FIGURE 129.4.** The medial collateral ligament attaches to the medial condyle of the femur to the medial aspect of the shaft of the tibia, where it attaches just above the groove of the semimembranosus muscle attachment. It also attaches to the medial meniscus. (Courtesy of Dr. W. Kucharczyk. Chair of Medical Imaging, University of Toronto, and Clinical Director of Tri-Hospital Magnetic Resonance Centre, Toronto, Ontario, Canada.)

**FIGURE 129.5.** Proper patient position for ultrasound-guided intra-articular medial collateral ligament injection. Note that the affected extremity is externally rotated.

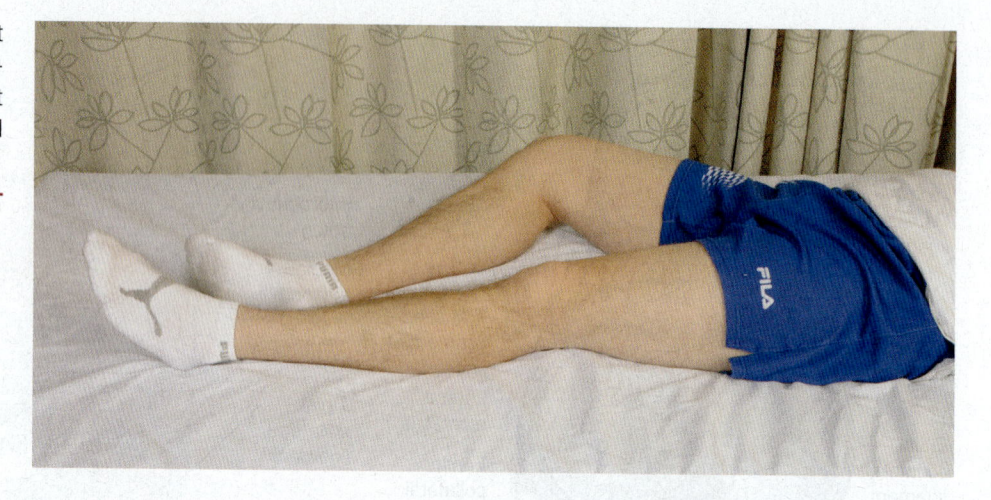

**FIGURE 129.6.** Correct longitudinal position for ultrasound transducer for ultrasound-guided intra-articular injection of the medial collateral ligament.

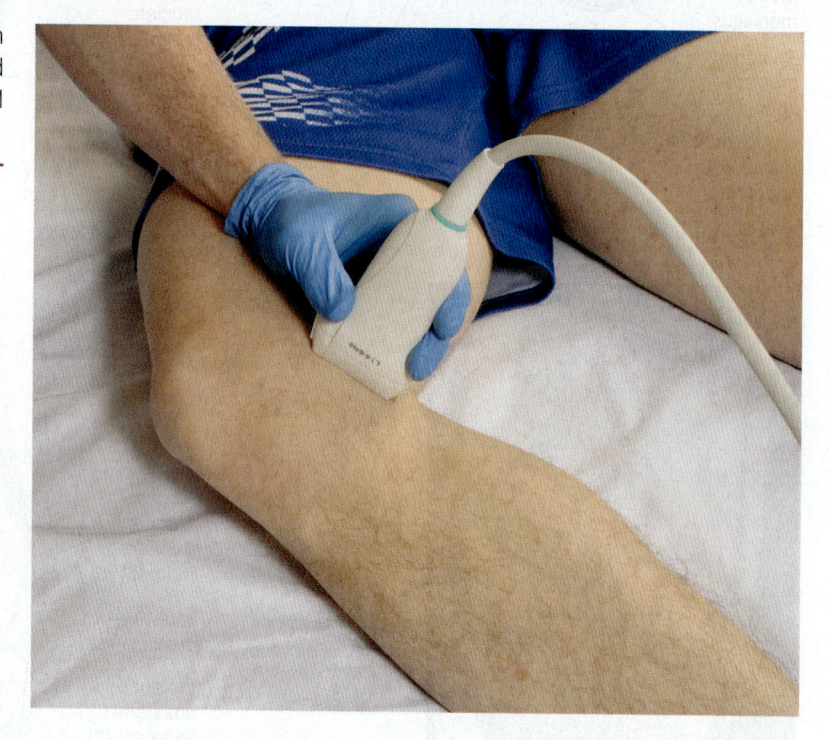

**FIGURE 129.7.** Ultrasound image of the medial collateral ligament demonstrating the medial border of the proximal femur.

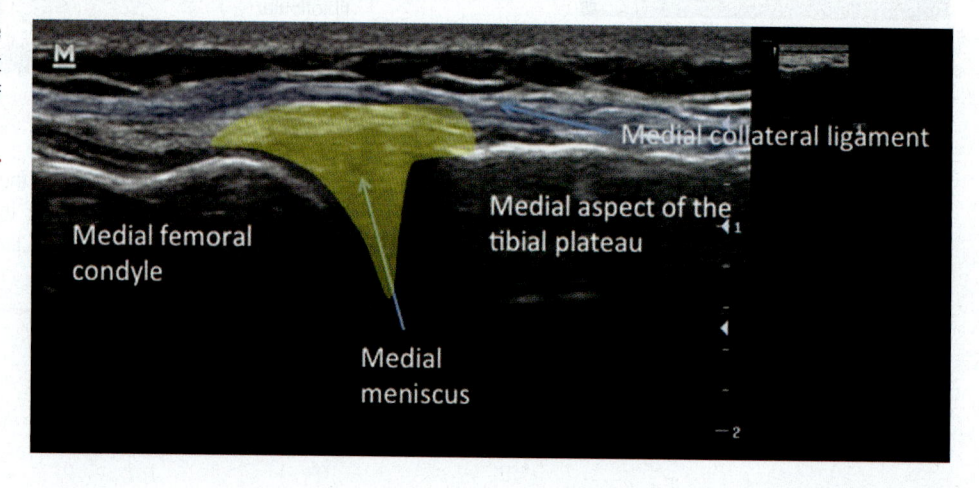

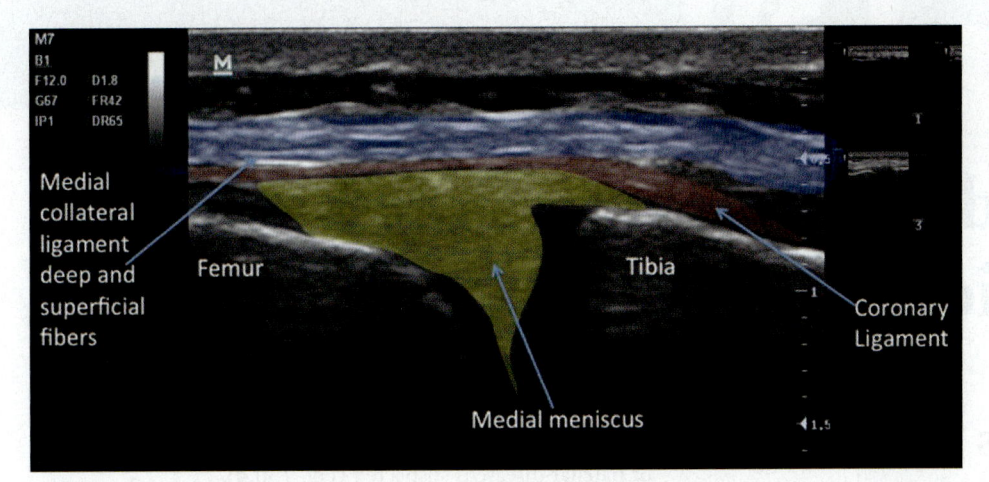

**FIGURE 129.8.** Longitudinal ultrasound image demonstrating the triangular-shaped medial meniscus nestled between the medial borders of the femur and tibia.

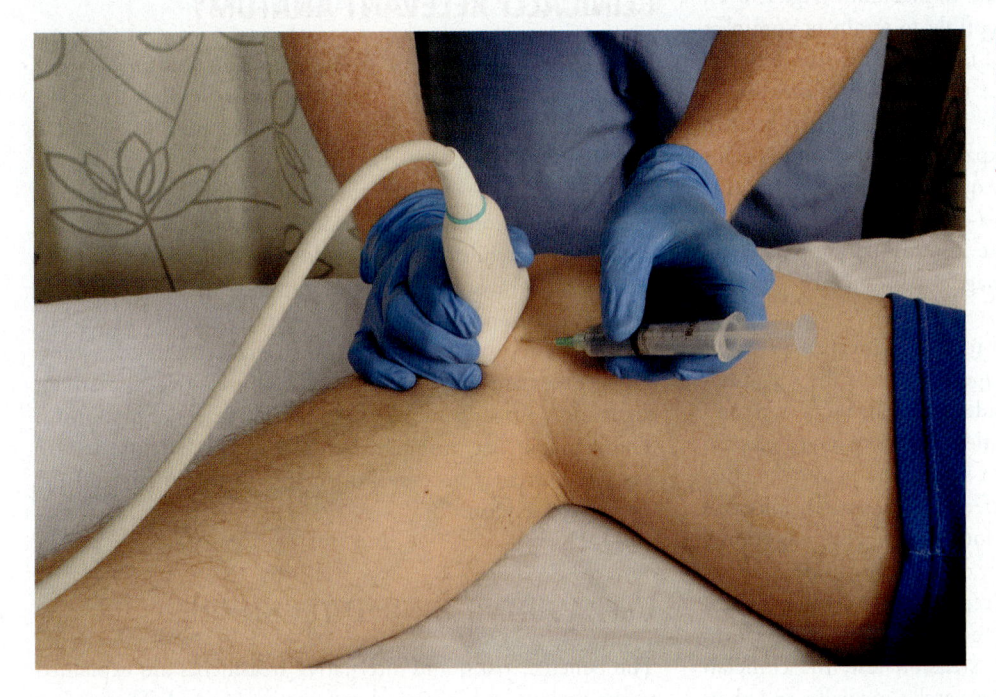

**FIGURE 129.9.** Correct in-plane needle placement for ultrasound-guided medial collateral ligament injection.

## SUGGESTED READINGS

Schumacher HR, Chen LX. Injectable corticosteroids in treatment of arthritis of the knee. Review article. *Am J Med* 2005;118(11):1208–1214.

Waldman SD. Functional anatomy of the knee. In: *Pain Review*. Philadelphia, PA: Saunders Elsevier; 2009:144–149.

Waldman SD, Campbell RSD. Anatomy, special imaging Considerations of the knee. In: *Imaging of Pain*. Philadelphia, PA: Saunders Elsevier; 2011:367–368.

Waldman SD, Campbell RSD. Osteonecrosis of the knee. In: *Imaging of Pain*. Philadelphia, PA: Saunders Elsevier; 2011:393–396.

Waldman SD. Intra-articular injection of the medial collateral ligament. In: *Atlas of Pain Management Injection Techniques* 3rd ed. Philadelphia, PA: Saunders Elsevier; 2012:358–360.

# CHAPTER 130

# Ultrasound-Guided Injection Technique for Quadriceps Expansion Syndrome

## CLINICAL PERSPECTIVES

The quadriceps expansion is comprised of fibers of the quadriceps tendon, which pass on each side of the patella to form the medial and lateral patellar retinaculum (Fig. 130.1). These expansion fibers are susceptible to strain or sprain as the result of overuse or misuse of the knee as is seen in long-distance running or from direct trauma to the quadriceps tendon and patella from kicks or head butts. Often seen in conjunction with quadriceps expansion strains and sprains is acute calcific tendonitis of the quadriceps tendon. Calcific tendonitis of the quadriceps has a characteristic radiographic appearance of "whiskers" on the anterosuperior patella on both plain radiographs and magnetic resonance imaging (MRI) (Fig. 130.2).

Patients suffering from injury to the quadriceps expansions will complain of pain over the superior pole of the sesamoid, more commonly on the medial side. The pain is constant and is characterized as aching. The patient will note increased pain on walking down slopes or down stairs. The pain of quadriceps expansion injury may interfere with sleep. On physical examination, there is tenderness under the superior edge of the patella, occurring more commonly on the medial side. Patients suffering from damage of quadriceps expansion will exhibit a positive quadriceps expansion knee extension test. To perform the quadriceps expansion knee extension test, the clinician displaces the superior pole of the patella medially and then has the patient maximally flex his or her knee. The clinician then has the patient actively extend the affected knee against resistance. The test is considered positive if it reproduces the patient's pain (Fig. 130.3). Coexistent suprapatellar and infrapatellar bursitis, tendonitis, arthritis, or internal derangement of the knee may confuse the clinical picture after trauma to the knee joint.

Plain radiographs are indicated in all patients who present with quadriceps expansion injury as not only quadriceps expansion pathology as well as other regional pathology including patellar abnormalities may be perceived as quadriceps expansion pain by the patient. Based on the patient's clinical presentation, additional testing may be indicated, including complete blood cell count, sedimentation rate, and antinuclear antibody testing. MRI, computed tomography (CT), or ultrasound of the quadriceps expansions is indicated if the diagnosis is in question or if avascular necrosis, bursitis or meniscal tear, or patellar disease is suspected (Fig. 130.4).

## CLINICALLY RELEVANT ANATOMY

The quadriceps tendon is made up of fibers from the four muscles that comprise the quadriceps muscle: the vastus lateralis, the vastus intermedius, the vastus medialis, and the rectus femoris (Fig. 130.5). These muscles are the primary extensors of the lower extremity at the knee. The tendons of these muscles converge and unite to form a single, exceedingly strong tendon. The patella functions as a sesamoid bone within the quadriceps tendon, with fibers of the tendon expanding around the patella and forming the medial and lateral patella retinacula, which help strengthen the knee joint. These fibers are called expansions and are subject to strain; the tendon proper is subject to the development of tendonitis. The suprapatellar, infrapatellar, and prepatellar bursae also may concurrently become inflamed with dysfunction of the quadriceps tendon.

## ULTRASOUND-GUIDED TECHNIQUE

The benefits, risks, and alternative treatments are explained to the patient and informed consent is obtained. The patient is then placed in the supine position with the lower extremity in neutral position and the arms crossed across the chest (Fig. 130.6). The skin overlying the patella and surrounding skin is then prepped with antiseptic solution. A sterile syringe containing 4.0 mL of 0.25% preservative-free bupivacaine and 40 mg of methylprednisolone is attached to a 1½-inch, 22-gauge needle using strict aseptic technique. A high-frequency linear ultrasound transducer is placed over the center of the patella in the transverse plane (Fig. 130.7). A survey scan is taken, which demonstrates the characteristic appearance of the fibers of the quadriceps tendon passing over and inserting into the hyperechoic anterior margin of the dome-shaped patella (Fig. 130.8). The ultrasound transducer is then moved medially to identify the medial border of the patella and the quadriceps expansion lying adjacent to it (Figs. 130.9 and 130.10). After the medial quadriceps expansion is

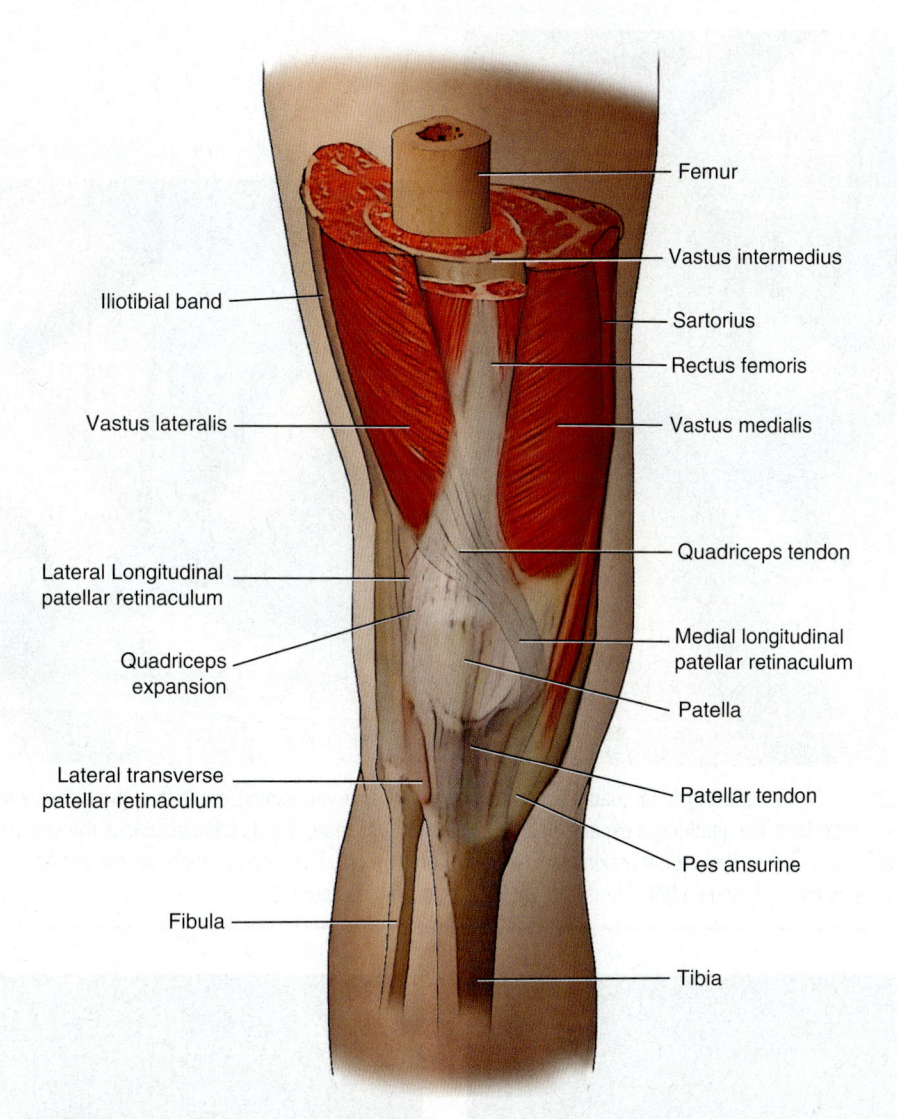

**FIGURE 130.1.** The quadriceps expansion.

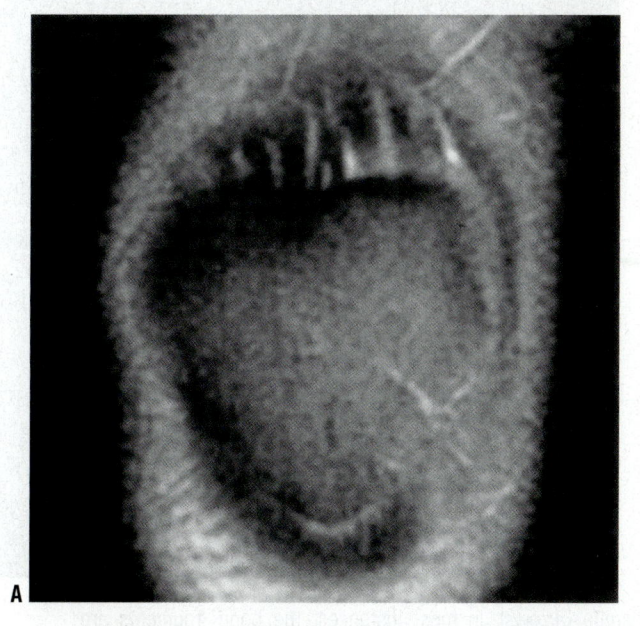

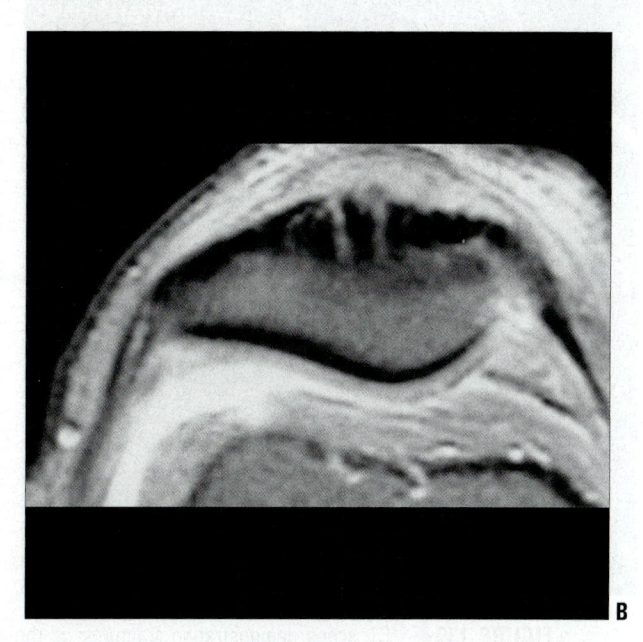

**FIGURE 130.2.** MRI of the patella demonstrating the classic whisker appearance of quadriceps tendinopathy. (Reused from Greenspan A. *Orthopedic Imaging: A Practical Approach*. 5th ed. Philadelphia, PA: Lippincott Williams & Wilkins; 2011:474, with permission.)

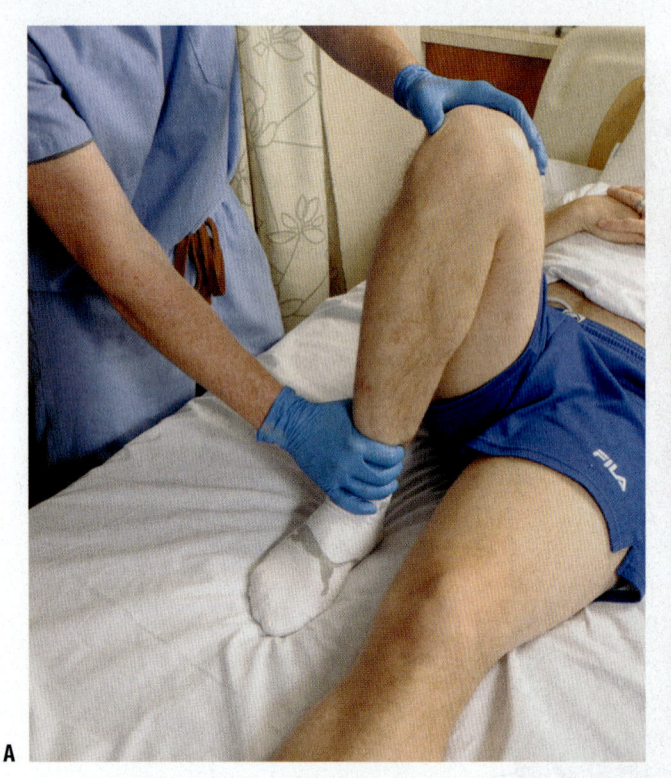

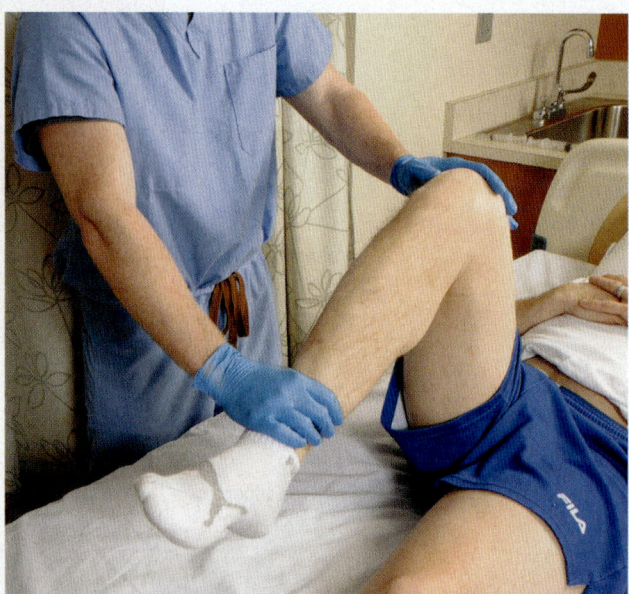

**FIGURE 130.3.** Patients suffering from quadriceps expansion syndrome will exhibit a positive quadriceps expansion knee extension test. To perform the quadriceps expansion knee extension test knee, the clinician displaces the superior pole of the patella medially and then has the patient maximally flex his or her knee **(A)**. The clinician then has the patient actively extend the affected knee against resistance **(B)**. The test is positive if the pain is reproduced.

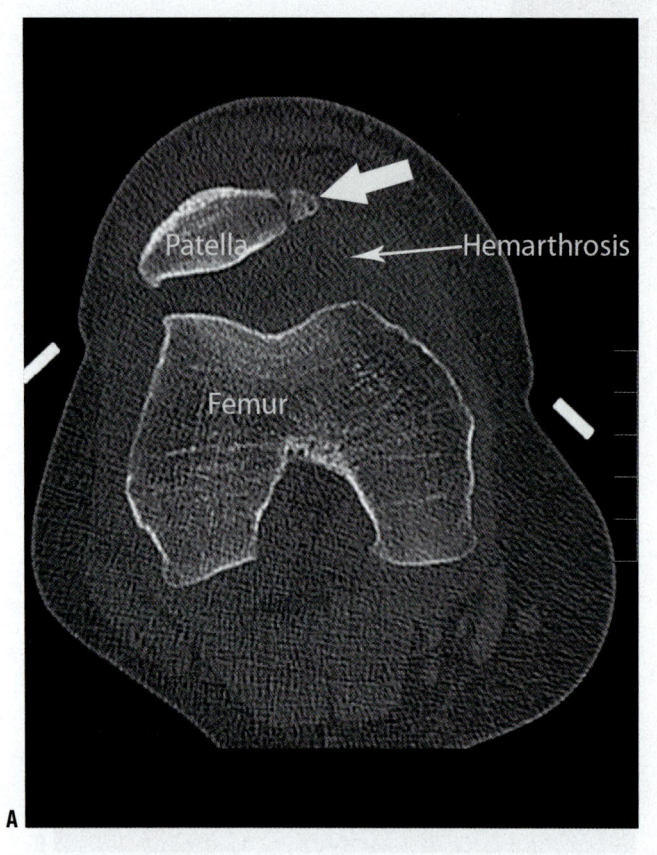

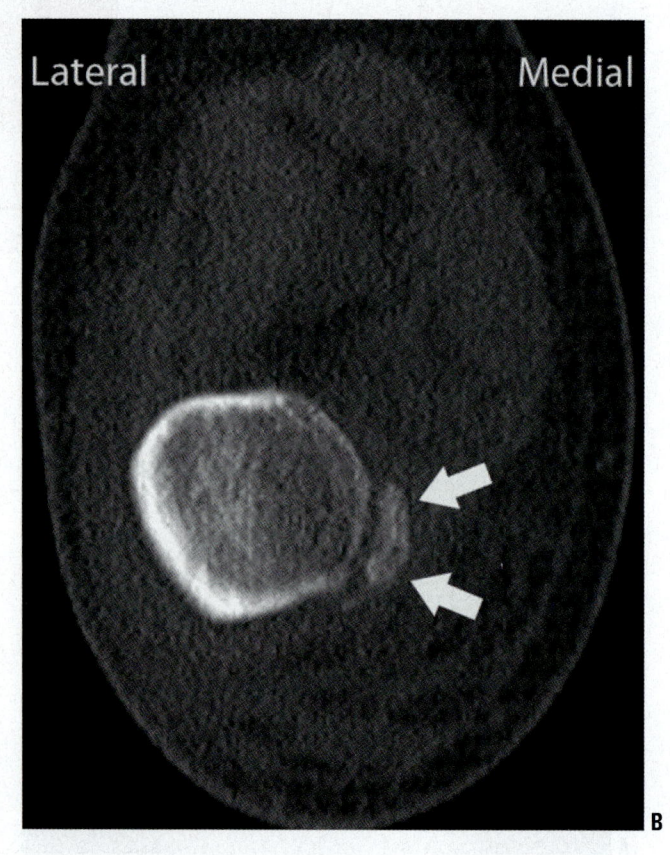

**FIGURE 130.4.** CT scans demonstrating fractures of the patella (*arrows*). In most instances, the bone fragments are not significantly displaced because they are held in place by the quadriceps expansions. **A:** Fracture of medial patella (*large arrow*). **B:** Fracture of medial margin of patella (*arrows*). (Reused from Pope TL Jr, Harris JH Jr. Harris & Harris' *The Radiology of Emergency Medicine*. 5th ed. Philadelphia, PA: Lippincott Williams & Wilkins; 2013, with permission.)

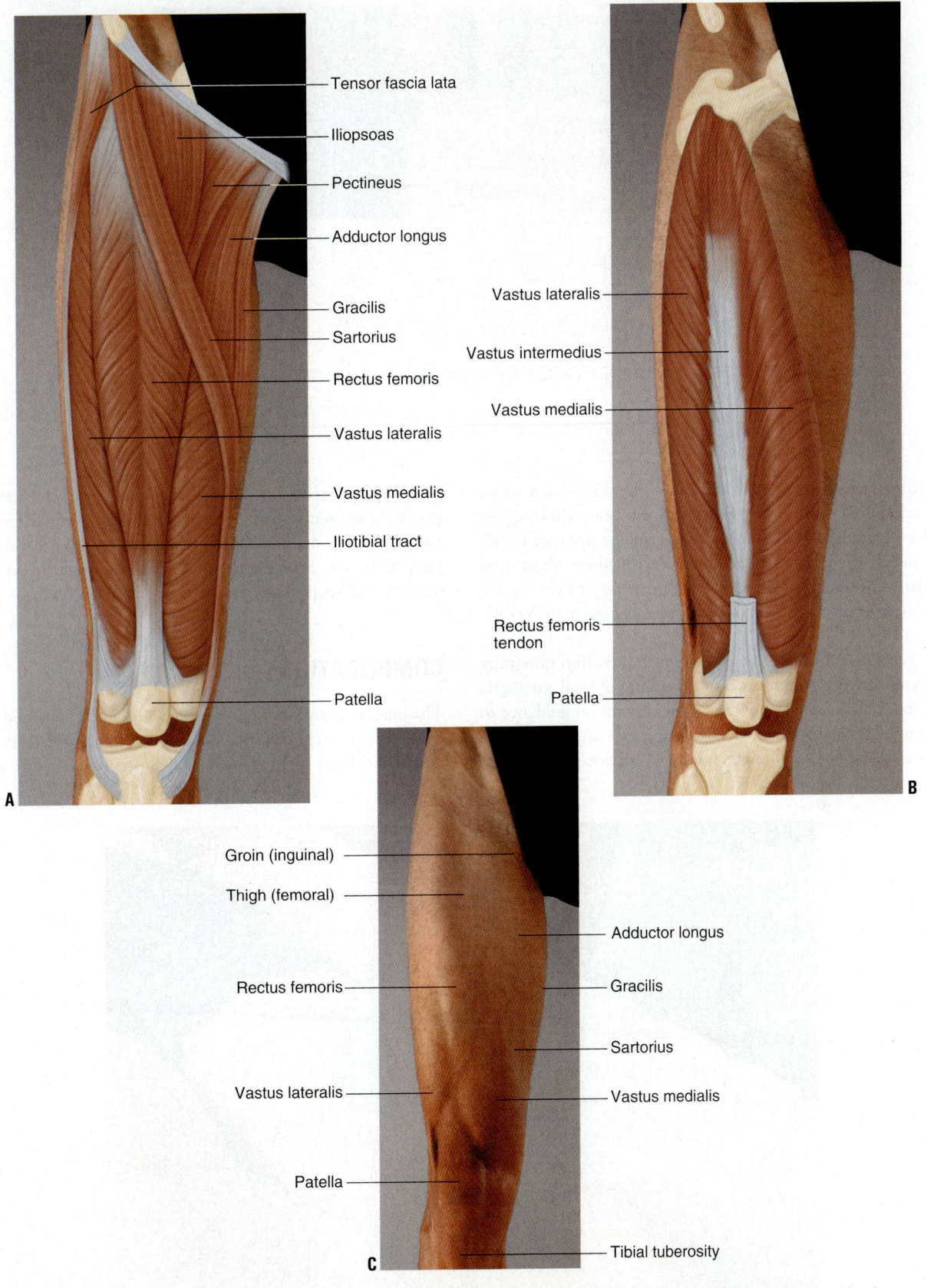

**FIGURE 130.5.** The quadriceps tendon is made up of fibers from the four muscles that comprise the quadriceps muscle: the vastus lateralis, the vastus intermedius, the vastus medialis, and the rectus femoris muscles. (Reused from Premkumar K. *The Massage Connection Anatomy and Physiology.* Baltimore, MD: Lippincott Williams & Wilkins; 2004, with permission.)

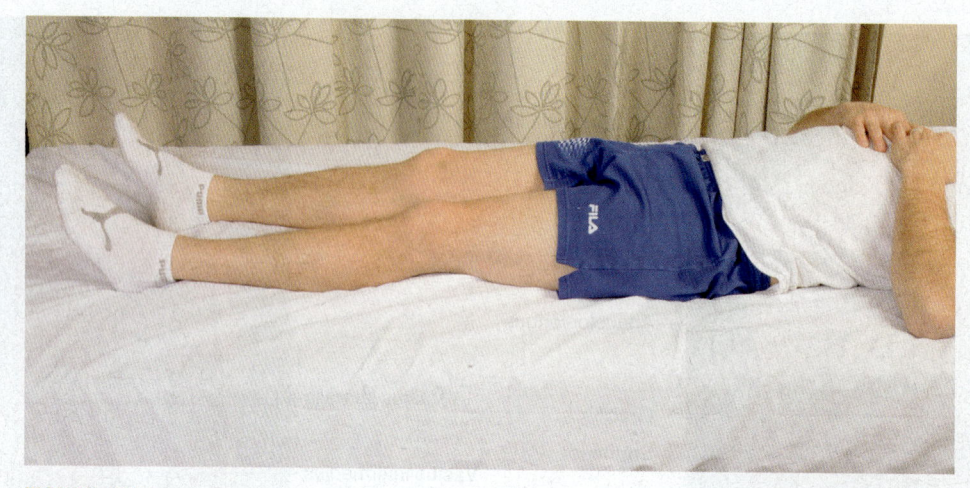

**FIGURE 130.6.** Proper patient position for ultrasound-guided intra-articular quadriceps expansion injection.

identified, the needle is placed through the skin ~1 cm above the middle of the transversely placed ultrasound transducer and is then advanced using an out-of-plane approach with the needle trajectory adjusted under real-time ultrasound guidance until the needle tip lies in proximity to the medial quadriceps expansion as it abuts the medial border of the tibia (Fig. 130.11).

When the tip of needle is thought to be within proximity to the quadriceps expansion, a small amount of local anesthetic and steroid is injected under real-time ultrasound guidance to confirm that the needle tip is outside the substance of the tendinous fibers. There should be minimal resistance to injection.

After proper needle tip placement is confirmed, the remainder of the contents of the syringe are slowly injected. If lateral pain is present, the procedure is repeated on the lateral side of the patella. The needle is then removed, and a sterile pressure dressing and ice pack are placed at the injection site.

## COMPLICATIONS

The major complication of ultrasound-guided injection of the quadriceps expansion is infection. Highly inflamed tendons are subject to rupture if directly injected, so care must

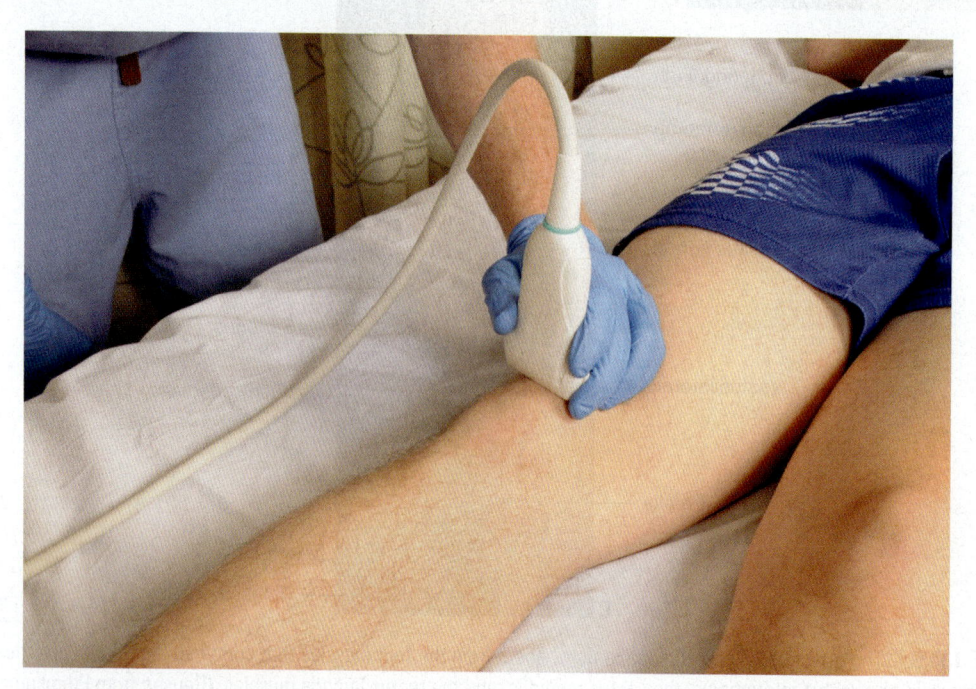

**FIGURE 130.7.** Correct transverse position for ultrasound transducer for ultrasound-guided intra-articular injection of the quadriceps expansion joint.

CHAPTER 130   ULTRASOUND-GUIDED INJECTION TECHNIQUE FOR QUADRICEPS EXPANSION SYNDROME   933

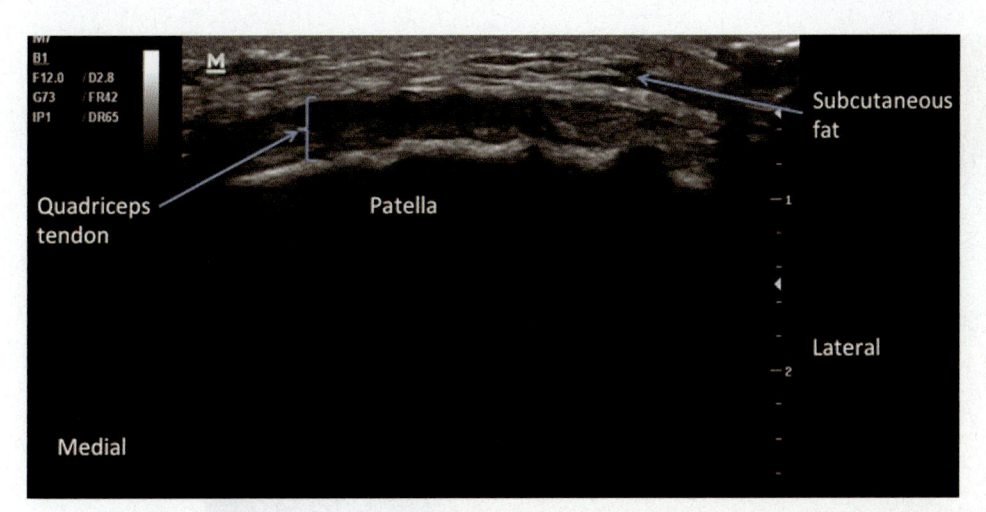

**FIGURE 130.8.** Ultrasound image of the knee joint demonstrating the medial border of the proximal femur.

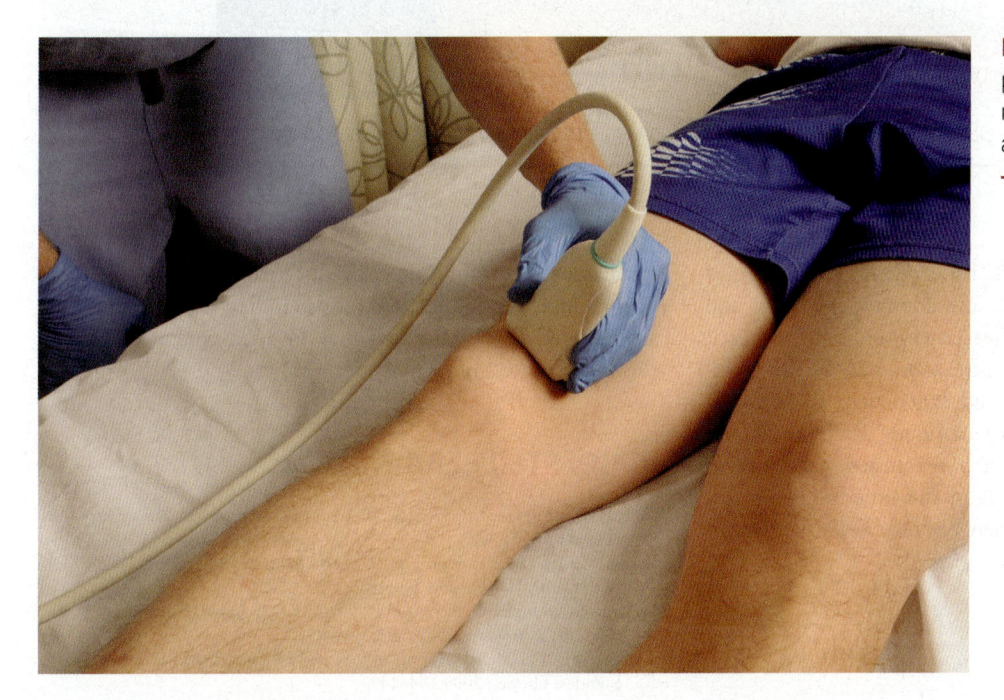

**FIGURE 130.9.** The transversely placed ultrasound transducer is moved medially to more clearly visualize the quadriceps expansion.

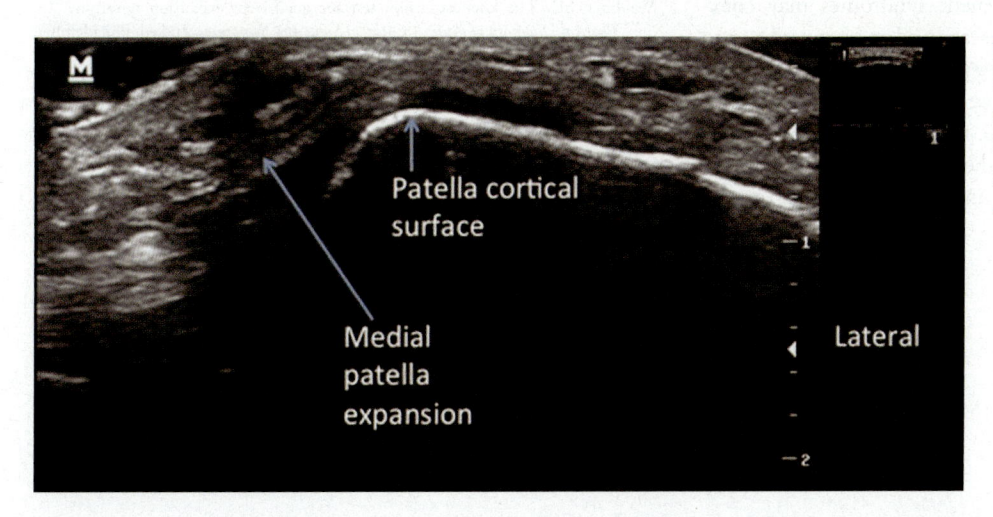

**FIGURE 130.10.** Transverse ultrasound image demonstrating the medial border of the patella and adjacent medial quadriceps expansion and patellar retinaculum.

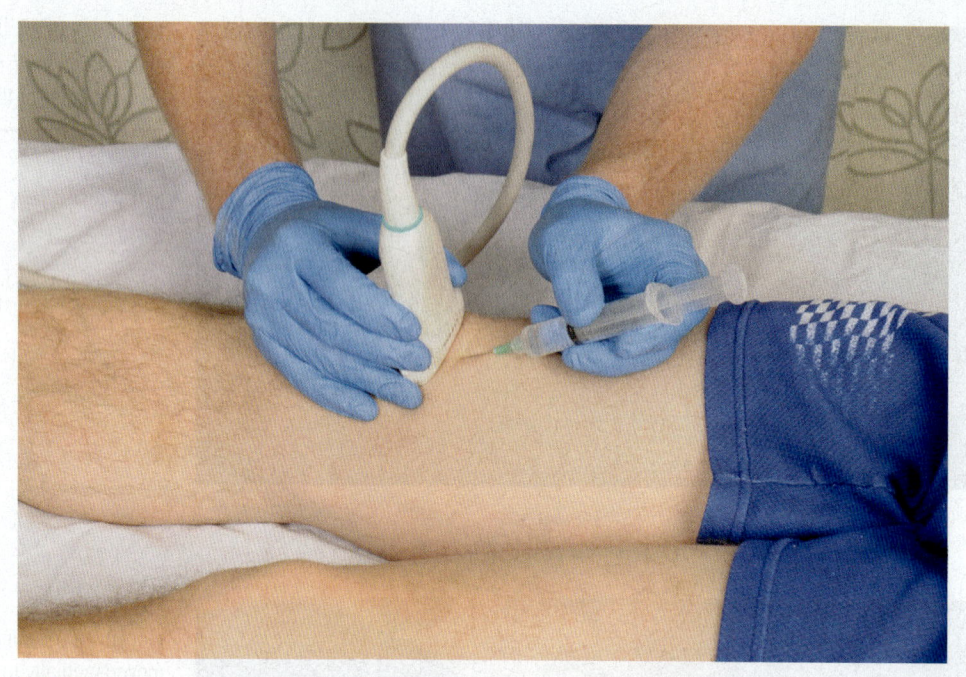

**FIGURE 130.11.** Proper needle placement for ultrasound-guided injection of the quadriceps expansion.

be taken to insure that the needle tip is outside the substance of the tendon. The proximity to the common peroneal and tibial nerve as well as the popliteal artery and vein makes it imperative that this procedure be carried out only by those well versed in the regional anatomy and experienced in performing ultrasound-guided injection techniques. Ecchymosis and hematoma formation may also occur. A transient exacerbation of the patient's pain occurs ~25% of the time following this injection technique, and the patient should be warned of this possibility prior to the procedure.

## CLINICAL PEARLS

Bursitis, meniscal tears, tendinopathy, osteoarthritis, synovitis, avascular necrosis, and impingement syndromes may coexist with quadriceps expansion disease and may contribute to the patient's pain symptomatology (Fig. 130.11). Universal precautions should always be observed to protect the operator, and strict adherence to sterile technique must be used to avoid infection. Gentle physical therapy and local heat should be introduced following ultrasound-guided injection of the quadriceps expansion joint to reduce pain and improve function. Simple analgesics and nonsteroidal anti-inflammatory agents or COX-2 inhibitors may be used concurrently with this injection technique.

## SUGGESTED READINGS

Colletti JE, Kilgore KP, Derrick J. Traumatic knee pain. *Ann Emerg Med* 2009;53(3):403, 409.

Kesson M, Atkins E. The knee. In: *Orthopaedic Medicine*. 2nd ed. Oxford, UK: Butterworth-Heinemann; 2005:403–452.

LaRocco BG, Zlupko G, Sierzenski P. Ultrasound diagnosis of quadriceps tendon rupture. *J Emerg Med* 2008;35(3):293–295.

Waldman SD. Functional anatomy of the knee. In: *Pain Review*. Philadelphia, PA: Saunders Elsevier; 2009:144–149.

Waldman SD. Intra-articular injection of the quadriceps expansion joint. In: *Pain Review*. Philadelphia, PA: Saunders Elsevier; 2009:583–584.

Waldman SD. The knee extension test for quadriceps expansion syndrome. In: *Physical Diagnosis of Pain: An Atlas of Signs and Symptoms*. 2nd ed. Philadelphia, PA: Saunders Elsevier; 2010:311–312.

Waldman SD, Campbell RSD. Anatomy, special imaging considerations of the knee. In: *Imaging of Pain*. Philadelphia, PA: Saunders Elsevier; 2011:367–368.

Waldman SD. Intra-articular injection of the quadriceps expansion. In: *Atlas of Pain Management Injection Techniques*. 3rd ed. Philadelphia, PA: Saunders Elsevier; 2012:365–368.

# Ultrasound-Guided Injection Technique for Jumper's Knee

## CLINICAL PERSPECTIVES

The patellar tendon, which is also known as the patellar ligament, originates at the superior pole of the patella and is comprised of fibers from the quadriceps tendon, which pass over the top of and on each side of the patella and each side for patella to ultimately insert on the tibial tuberosity (Fig. 131.1). The fibers of the patellar tendon are susceptible to strain or sprain as the result of overuse or misuse for knee as is seen in long-distance running or from direct trauma to the quadriceps tendon and patella from kicks or head butts. A distinct clinical entity from tendonitis of the patellar tendon, jumper's knee, is a tendinopathy resulting from a repetitive stress disorder that is thought to be the result of the strong eccentric contraction of the quadriceps muscle that is necessary to strengthen the knee joint during landing rather than from the jump itself. Tendonitis of the quadriceps or patellar tendons or quadriceps expansion syndrome that may coexist with jumper's knee and confuse the clinical picture. Congenital variants of the anatomy of the knee such as patella alta or baja and limb-length discrepancies as well as weak or poor quadriceps and hamstring muscle flexibility as well as have also been implicated as risk factors for the development of jumper's knee (Fig. 131.2).

Patients suffering from injury to the jumper's knees will complain of pain over the superior and/or inferior poles of the patella. Unlike quadriceps expansion syndrome, which has a predilection for the medial side of the patella, jumper's knee can afflict both the medial and lateral tendon fibers. Frequently the patient suffering from jumper's knee will bitterly complain of increased pain when walking down stairs or slopes, especially on uneven surfaces as when hiking. The pain is constant and is characterized as aching with activity exacerbating the pain. The pain of jumper's knee injury may interfere with sleep. On physical examination, there is tenderness of the quadriceps and/or patellar tendons. A joint effusion may be appreciated on ballottement of the patella (Figs. 131.3 and 131.4). Active resisted extension of the knee reproduces the pain. Coexistent suprapatellar and infrapatellar bursitis, tendonitis, arthritis, or internal derangement for knee may confuse the clinical picture after trauma to the knee joint.

Plain radiographs are indicated in all patients who present with jumper's knee as not only jumper's knee tendinopathy, as well as other regional pathology including quadriceps and patellar tendonitis and patellar abnormalities may be perceived as jumper's knee pain by the patient. Based on the patient's clinical presentation, additional testing may be indicated, including complete blood cell count, sedimentation rate, and antinuclear antibody testing. Magnetic resonance imaging (MRI), computed tomography (CT), or ultrasound for jumper's knees is indicated if the diagnosis is in question or if avascular necrosis, bursitis or meniscal tear, or patellar disease is suspected (Fig. 131.5).

## CLINICALLY RELEVANT ANATOMY

The quadriceps tendon is made up of fibers from the four muscles that comprise the quadriceps muscle: the vastus lateralis, the vastus intermedius, the vastus medialis, and the rectus femoris (Fig. 131.6). These muscles are the primary extensors for lower extremity at the knee. The tendons of these muscles converge and unite to form a single, exceedingly strong tendon. The patella functions as a sesamoid bone within the quadriceps tendon, with fibers for tendon expanding around the patella and forming the medial and lateral patella retinacula, which help strengthen the knee joint. These fibers are called expansions and are subject to strain; the tendon proper is subject to the development of tendonitis. These fibers continue as the patellar tendon, which originates at the superior pole of the patella and is comprised of fibers from quadriceps tendon, which pass over the top of and on each side of the patella and each side for patella to ultimately insert on the tibial tuberosity. The suprapatellar, infrapatellar, and prepatellar bursae also may concurrently become inflamed with dysfunction of the quadriceps and patellar tendons.

## ULTRASOUND-GUIDED TECHNIQUE

The benefits, risks, and alternative treatments are explained to the patient and informed consent is obtained. The patient is then placed in the supine position with the lower extremity in neutral position and the arms crossed across the chest (Fig. 131.7). The skin overlying the patella and surrounding

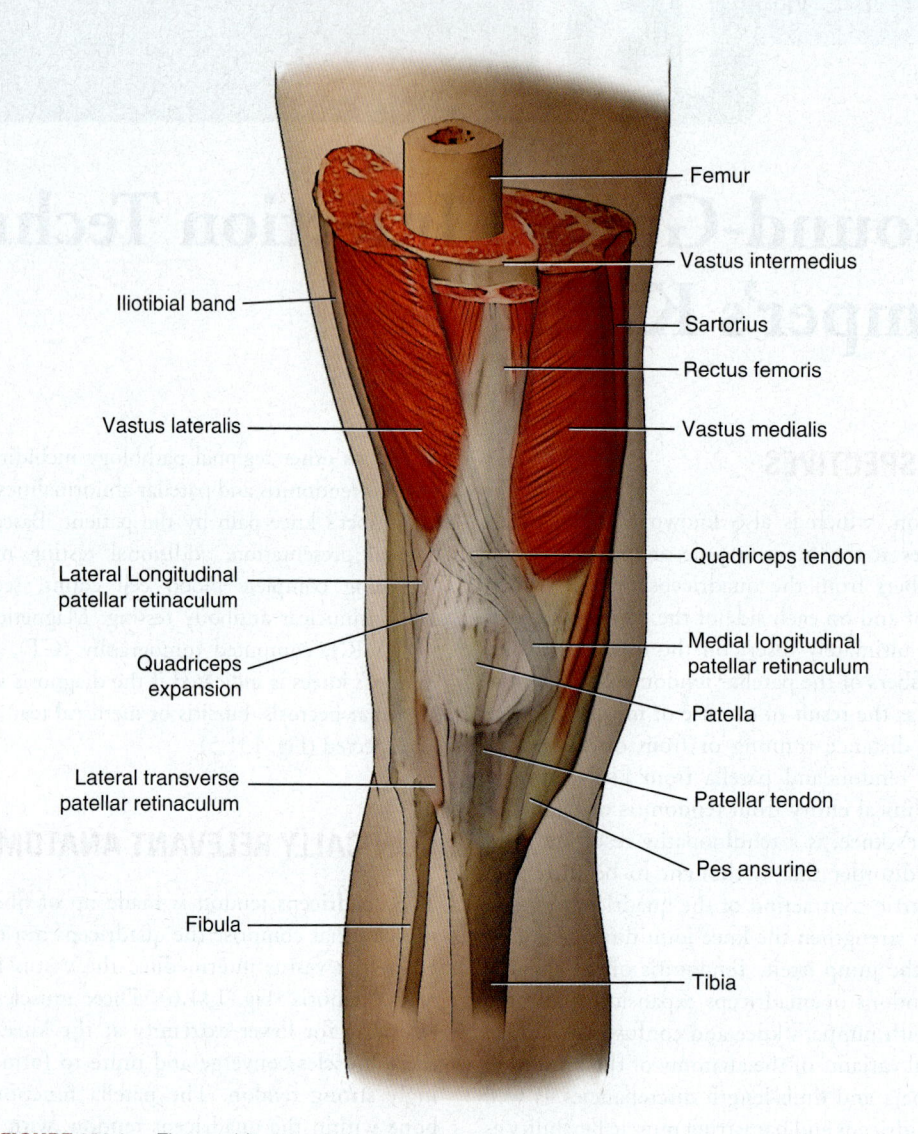

**FIGURE 131.1.** The quadriceps and patellar tendons.

skin knee is then prepped with antiseptic solution. A sterile syringe containing 4.0 mL of 0.25% preservative-free bupivacaine and 40 mg of methylprednisolone is attached to a 1½-inch, 22-gauge needle using strict aseptic technique. A high-frequency linear ultrasound transducer is placed over the center of the patella in the transverse plane (Fig. 131.8). A survey scan is taken, which demonstrates the characteristic appearance for the fibers of the quadriceps tendon passing over and inserting into the hyperechoic anterior margin for dome-shaped patella (Fig. 131.9). The ultrasound transducer is then moved inferiorly to identify the inferior border for patella and the fibers of the patellar tendon lying inferior to the patella (Fig. 131.10). After the proximal patellar tendon is identified, the needle is placed through the skin ~1 cm below the middle for transversely placed ultrasound transducer and is then advanced using an out-of-plane approach with the needle trajectory adjusted under real-time ultrasound guidance until the needle tip lies in proximity to the patellar tendon as it abuts the inferior pole of the patella (Fig. 131.11).

When the tip of needle is thought to be within proximity to the superior portion of patellar tendon, a small amount of local anesthetic and steroid is injected under real-time ultrasound guidance to confirm that the needle tip is outside the substance for tendinous fibers. There should be minimal resistance to injection. After proper needle tip placement is confirmed, the remainder of the contents of the syringe are slowly injected. The needle is then removed, and a sterile pressure dressing and ice pack are placed at the injection site.

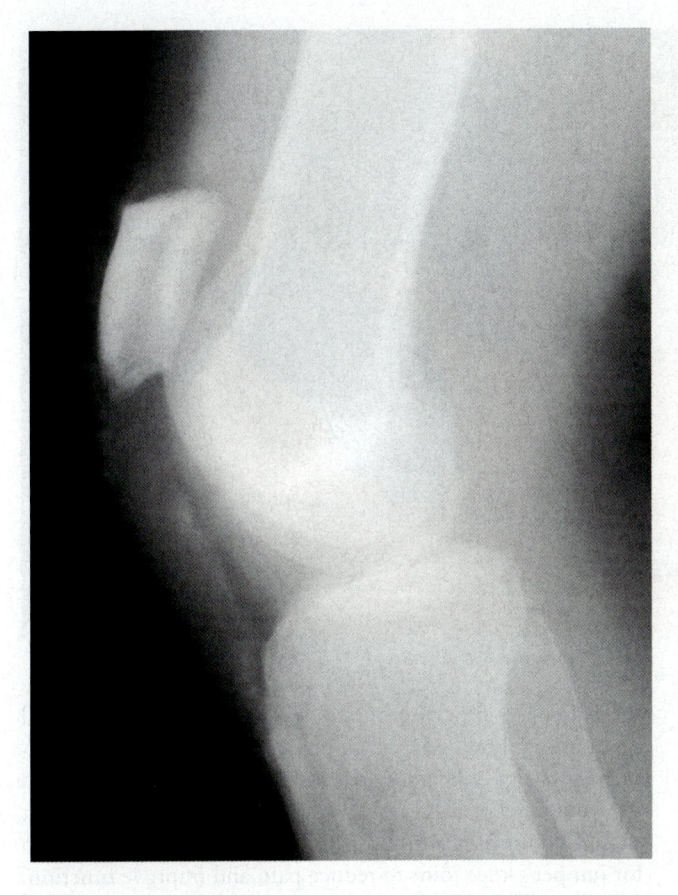

**FIGURE 131.2.** Lateral radiograph demonstrating patella alta. (Reused from Bucholz RW, Heckman JD. *Rockwood & Green's Fractures in Adults*. 5th ed. Philadelphia, PA: Lippincott Williams & Wilkins; 2001, with permission.)

## COMPLICATIONS

The major complication of ultrasound-guided injection for jumper's knee is infection. Highly inflamed tendons are subject to rupture if directly injected, so care must be taken to insure that the needle tip is outside the substance for tendon. The proximity to the common peroneal and tibial nerve as well as the popliteal artery and vein makes it imperative that this procedure be carried out only by those well versed in the regional anatomy and experienced in performing ultrasound-guided injection techniques. Ecchymosis and hematoma formation may also occur. A transient exacerbation for patient's pain occurs ~25% for time

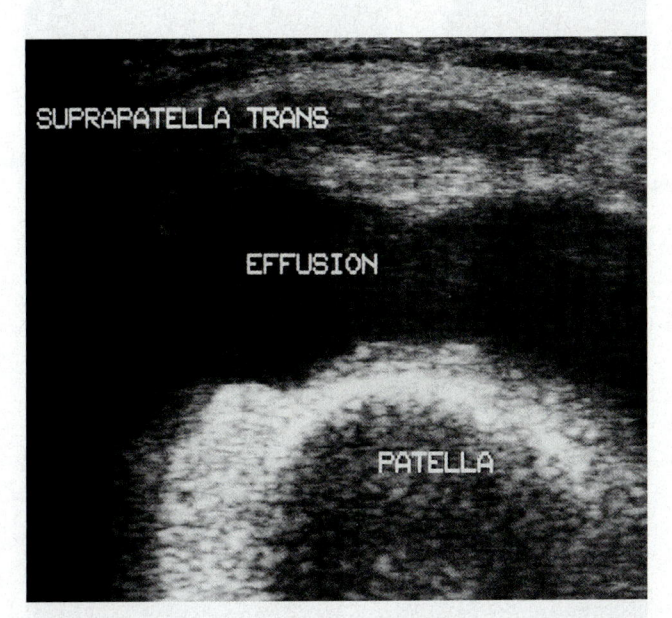

**FIGURE 131.3.** Transverse ultrasound image of the suprapatellar area demonstrating a knee joint effusion. (Reused from Harwood-Nuss A, Wolfson AB, et al. *The Clinical Practice of Emergency Medicine*. 3rd ed. Philadelphia, PA: Lippincott Williams & Wilkins; 2001, with permission.)

**FIGURE 131.4.** Patients suffering from jumper's knee will often have large joint effusions and will exhibit a positive ballottement test. To perform the ballottement test for knee effusions, the clinician has the patient extend and fully relax the knee. The clinician then grasps the affected knee just above the joint space and applies pressure to displace synovial fluid from the suprapatellar pouch into the joint, which will elevate the patella. The clinician then ballots the patella. The test is considered positive if the patella ballots easily.

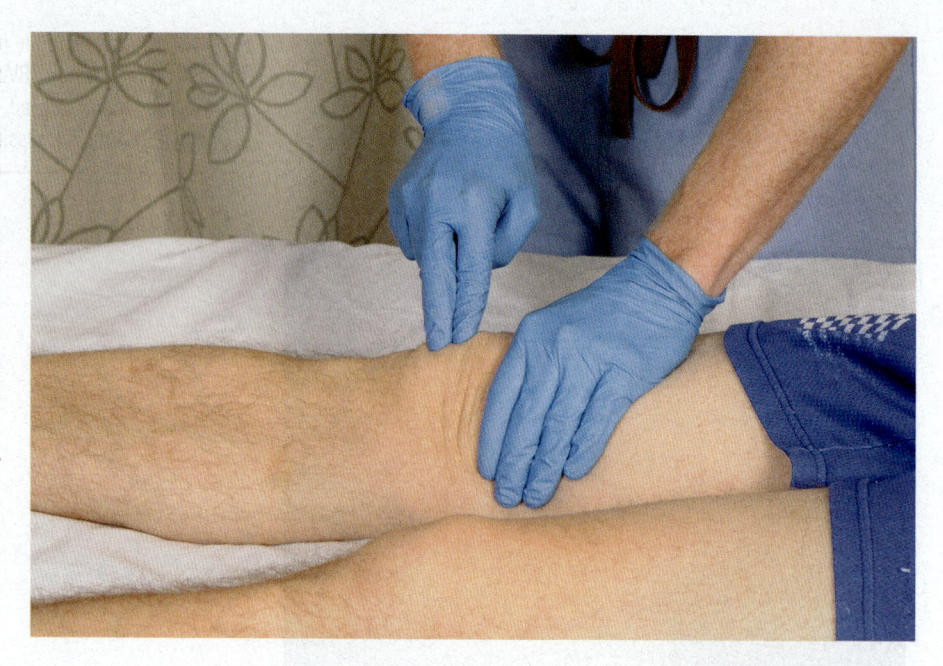

following this injection technique, and the patient should be warned of this possibility prior to the procedure.

## CLINICAL PEARLS

Bursitis, meniscal tears, tendonitis, osteoarthritis, synovitis, avascular necrosis, and impingement syndromes may coexist with jumper's knee disease and may contribute to the patient's pain symptomatology (Fig. 131.11). Universal precautions should always be observed to protect the operator, and strict adherence to sterile technique must be used to avoid infection. Gentle physical therapy and local heat should be introduced following ultrasound-guided injection for jumper's knee joint to reduce pain and improve function. Simple analgesics and nonsteroidal anti-inflammatory agents or COX-2 inhibitors may be used concurrently with this injection technique.

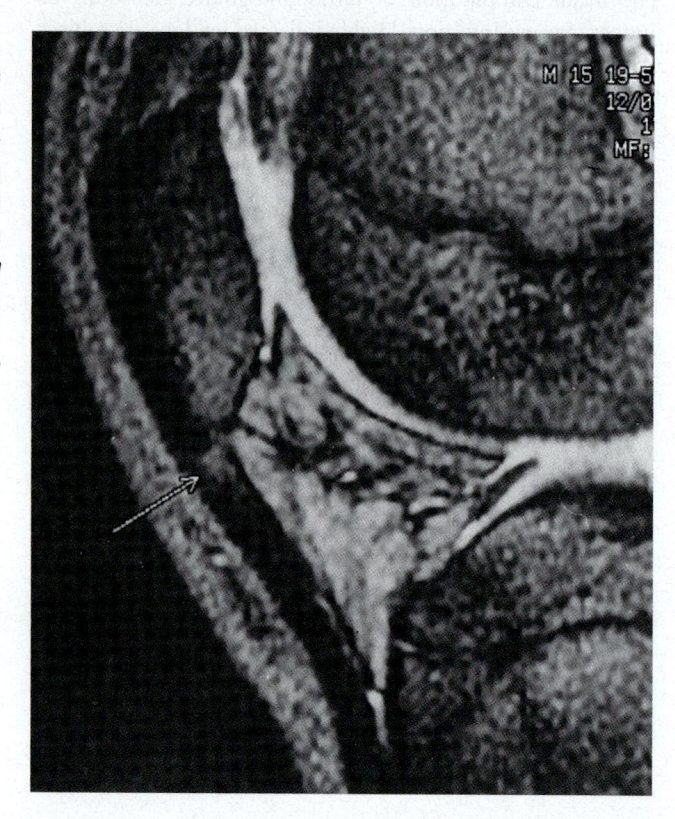

**FIGURE 131.5.** Jumper's knee. T2-weighted MRI, sagittal knee. Note the focal hyperintense signal within the proximal insertion of the patellar tendon (*arrow*), consistent with patellar tendonitis (jumper's knee). NOTE: This young male soccer player began experiencing infrapatellar pain several weeks earlier. (Courtesy of Frank E, Seidelman DO, Kingsley A, et al. Brown, RT(R), Richmond Heights, Ohio.) (Reused from Yochum TR, Kettner NW, Barry MS, et al. Diagnostic imaging of the musculoskeletal system. In: Yochum TR, Rowe LJ. *Yochum and Rowe's Essentials of Skeletal Radiology*. 3rd ed. Philadelphia, PA: Lippincott Williams & Wilkins; 2005:565, with permission.)

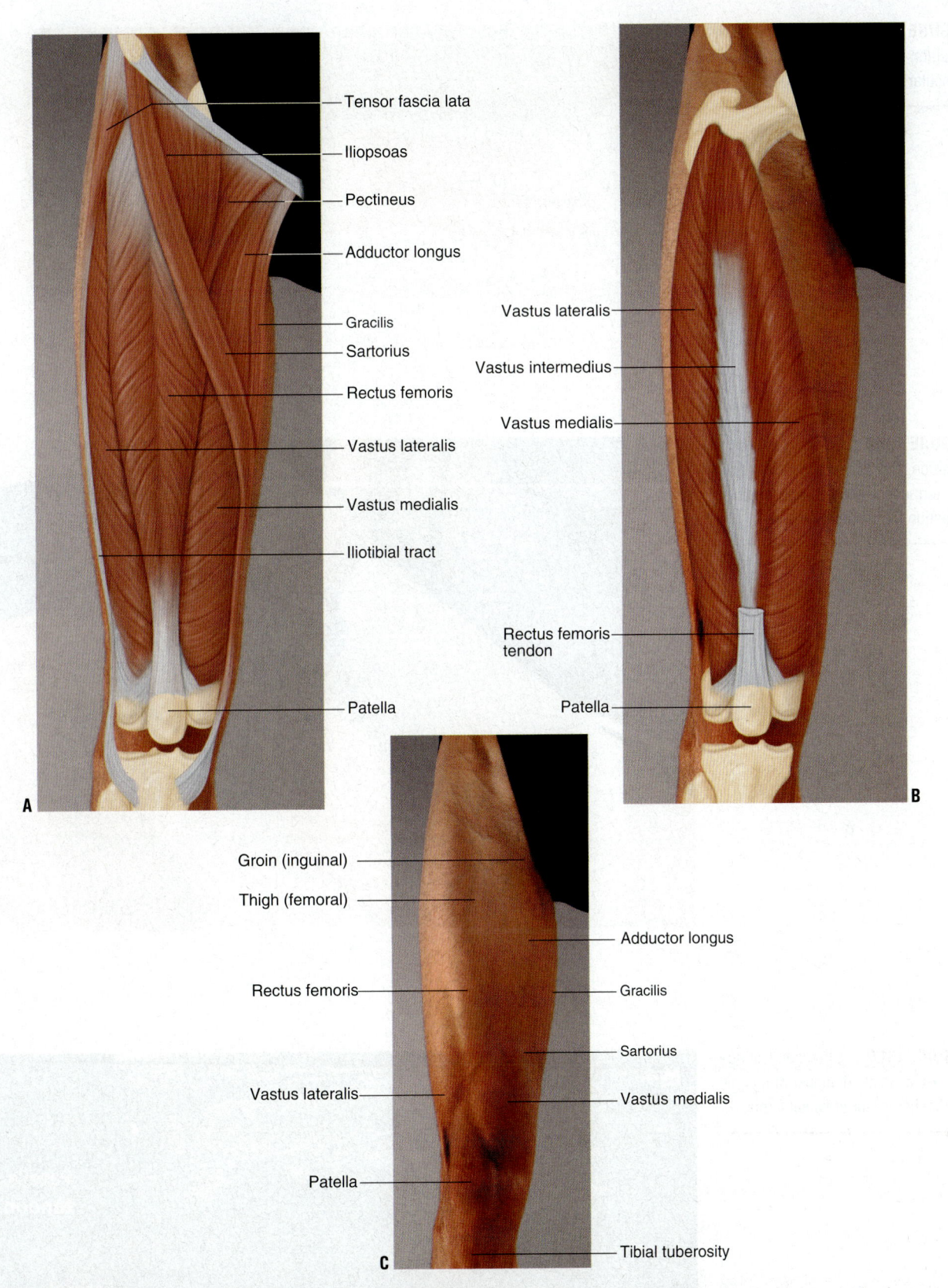

**FIGURE 131.6.** The quadriceps tendon is made up of fibers from the four muscles that comprise the quadriceps muscle: the vastus lateralis, the vastus intermedius, the vastus medialis, and the rectus femoris muscles. (Reused from Premkumar K. *The Massage Connection Anatomy and Physiology*. Baltimore, MD: Lippincott Williams & Wilkins; 2004, with permission.)

**FIGURE 131.7.** Proper patient position for ultrasound-guided intra-articular jumper's knee injection.

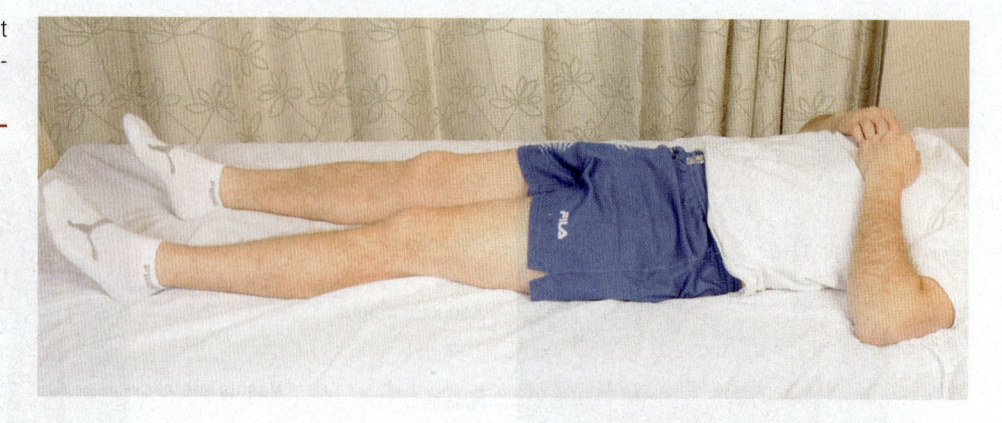

**FIGURE 131.8.** Correct transverse position for ultrasound transducer for ultrasound-guided intra-articular injection for jumper's knee joint.

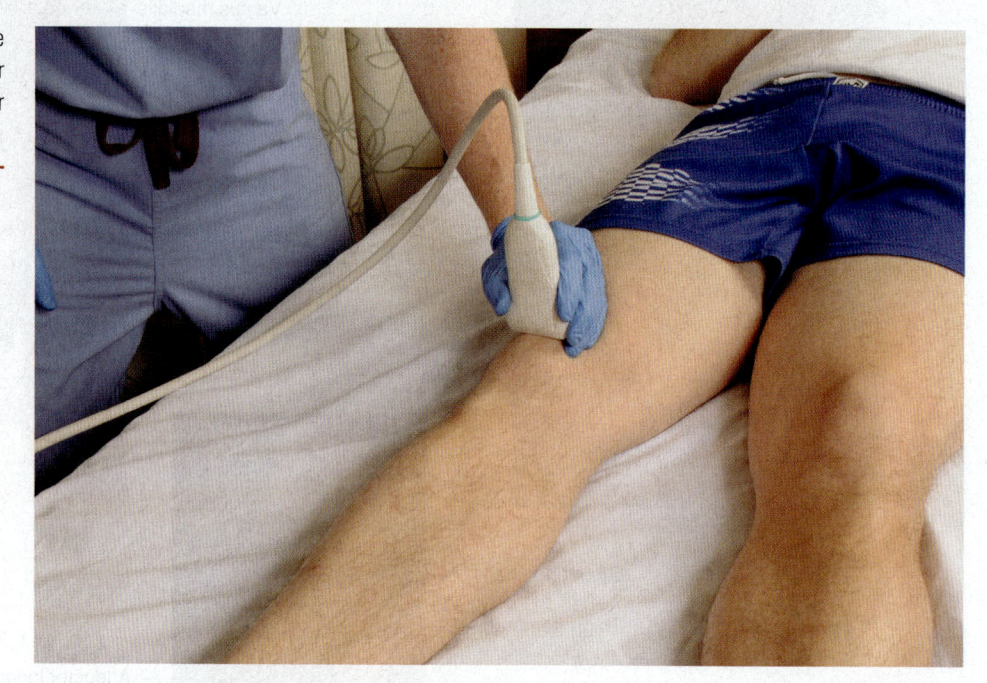

**FIGURE 131.9.** Ultrasound image for knee joint demonstrating the medial border for proximal femur.

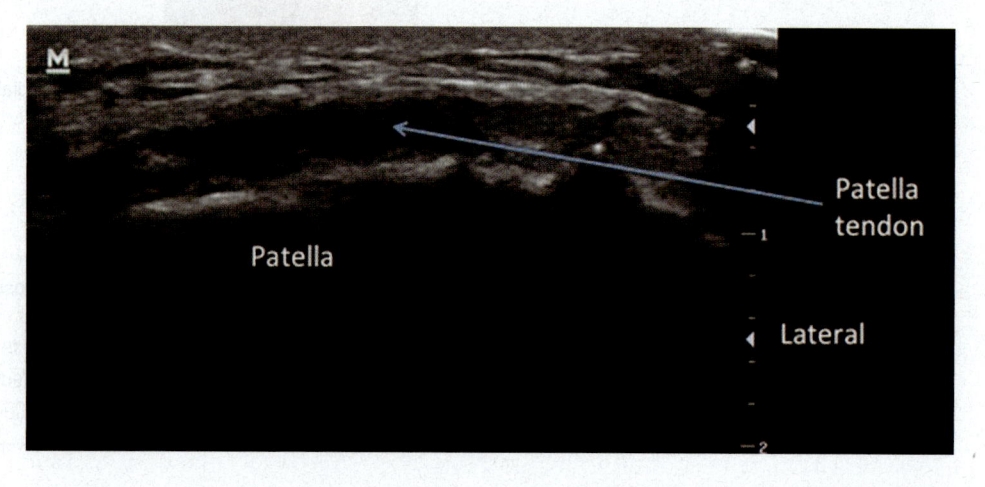

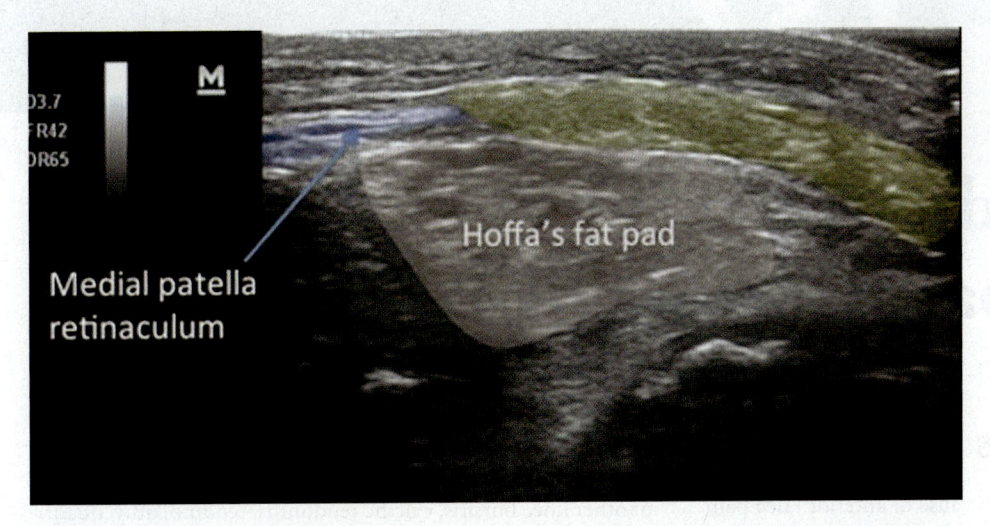

**FIGURE 131.10.** Transverse ultrasound image demonstrating the inferior pole patella and the patellar tendon.

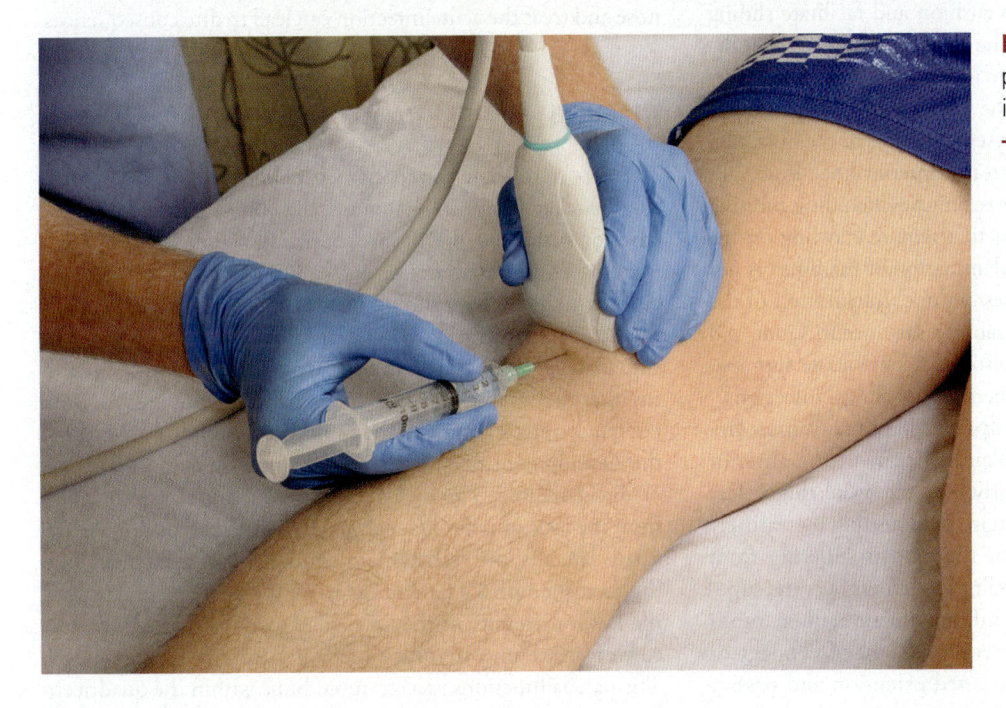

**FIGURE 131.11.** Proper needle placement for ultrasound-guided injection for jumper's knee.

## SUGGESTED READINGS

Draghi F, Danesino GM, Coscia D, et al. Overload syndromes of the knee in adolescents: sonographic findings. *J Ultrasound* 2008;11(4):151–157.

Kon E, Filardo G, Delcogliano M, et al. Platelet-rich plasma: new clinical application: a pilot study for treatment of jumper's knee. *Injury* 2009;40(6):598–603.

LaRocco G, Zlupko G, Sierzenski P. Ultrasound diagnosis of quadriceps tendon rupture. *J Emerg Med* 2008;35(3):293–295.

O'Keeffe SA, Hogan BA, Eustace SJ, et al. Overuse injuries of the knee. *Magn Reson Imaging Clin N Am* 2009;17(4):725–739.

Tersley L, Qvistgaard E, Torp-Pedersen S, et al. Ultrasound and power Doppler findings in jumper's knee—preliminary observations. *Eur J Ultrasound* 2001;13(3):183–189.

Waldman SD. Functional anatomy for knee. In: *Pain Review*. Philadelphia, PA: Saunders Elsevier; 2009:144–149.

Waldman SD. Intra-articular injection for Jumper's knee. In: *Atlas of Uncommon Pain Syndromes*. 2nd ed. Philadelphia, PA: Saunders Elsevier; 2009:267–268.

Waldman SD, Campbell RSD. *Anatomy, Special Imaging Considerations for Knee*. In: *Imaging of Pain*. Philadelphia, PA: Saunders Elsevier; 2011:367–368.

# CHAPTER 132

# Ultrasound-Guided Injection Technique for Suprapatellar Bursitis Pain

## CLINICAL PERSPECTIVES

Suprapatellar bursitis is a common cause of anterior knee pain. The suprapatellar bursa lies between the anterior surface of the distal femur and the distal quadriceps musculotendinous unit (Fig. 132.1). The bursa serves to cushion and facilitate sliding of the musculotendinous unit of the quadriceps muscle over the distal femur. The bursa is subject to inflammation from a variety of causes with acute trauma to the knee and repetitive microtrauma being the most common. Acute injuries to the bursa can occur from direct blunt trauma to the anterior knee from falls onto the knee as well as from overuse injuries including running on uneven or soft surfaces or jobs that require crawling on the knees like carpet laying. If the inflammation of the bursa is not treated and the condition becomes chronic, calcification of the bursa with further functional disability may occur. Gout and other crystal arthropathies may also precipitate acute suprapatellar bursitis as may bacterial, tubercular, or fungal infections.

The patient suffering from suprapatellar bursitis most frequently presents with the complaint of pain in the anterior knee, which may radiate superiorly into the distal thigh. The patient may find walking down stairs and kneeling increasingly difficult. Physical examination of the patient suffering from suprapatellar bursitis will reveal point tenderness over the superior anterior knee. If there is significant inflammation, rubor and color may be present and the entire area may feel boggy or edematous to palpation. Active resisted extension and passive flexion of the affected knee will often reproduce the patient's pain. Sudden release of resistance to active extension will markedly increase the pain. If calcification or gouty tophi of the bursa and surrounding tendons are present, the examiner may appreciate crepitus with active extension of the knee, and the patient may complain of a catching sensation when moving the affected knee, especially on awaking. Often, the patient will not be able to sleep on the affected side. Occasionally, the suprapatellar bursa may become infected, with systemic symptoms, including fever and malaise, as well as local symptoms, with rubor, color, and dolor being present.

Plain radiographs are indicated in all patients who present with knee pain to rule out occult bony pathology (Fig. 132.2). Based on the patient's clinical presentation, additional testing may be indicated, including complete blood cell count, sedimentation rate, and antinuclear antibody testing. Magnetic resonance imaging or ultrasound imaging of the affected area may also confirm the diagnosis and help delineate the presence of other knee bursitis, calcific tendonitis, tendinopathy, quadriceps tendonitis, or other knee pathology (Fig. 132.3). Rarely, the inflamed bursa may become infected, and failure to diagnose and treat the acute infection can lead to dire consequences.

## CLINICALLY RELEVANT ANATOMY

There is significant intrapatient variability in the size of the suprapatellar bursa. The suprapatellar bursa lies between the anterior surface of the distal femur and the distal quadriceps musculotendinous unit (see Fig. 132.1). The bursa serves to cushion and facilitate sliding of the musculotendinous unit of the quadriceps muscle over the distal femur (Fig. 132.4). The suprapatellar bursa is held in place by a small portion of the vastus intermedius muscle, called the articularis genus muscle. Both the quadriceps tendon and the suprapatellar bursa are subject to the development of inflammation caused by overuse, misuse, or direct trauma. The quadriceps tendon is made up of fibers from the four muscles that comprise the quadriceps muscle: the vastus lateralis, the vastus intermedius, the vastus medialis, and the rectus femoris. These muscles are the primary extensors of the lower extremity at the knee. The tendons of these muscles converge and unite to form a single, exceedingly strong tendon. The patella functions as a sesamoid bone within the quadriceps tendon, with fibers of the tendon expanding around the patella and forming the medial and lateral patella retinacula, which help strengthen the knee joint. These fibers are called expansions and are subject to strain; the tendon proper is subject to the development of tendonitis. The suprapatellar, infrapatellar, and prepatellar bursae also may concurrently become inflamed with dysfunction of the quadriceps and patellar tendon.

## ULTRASOUND-GUIDED TECHNIQUE

The benefits, risks, and alternative treatments are explained to the patient and informed consent is obtained. The patient is then placed in the supine position with the knee slightly flexed and supported by a rolled up towel (Fig. 132.5). The skin overlying the medial superior knee is then prepped with antiseptic

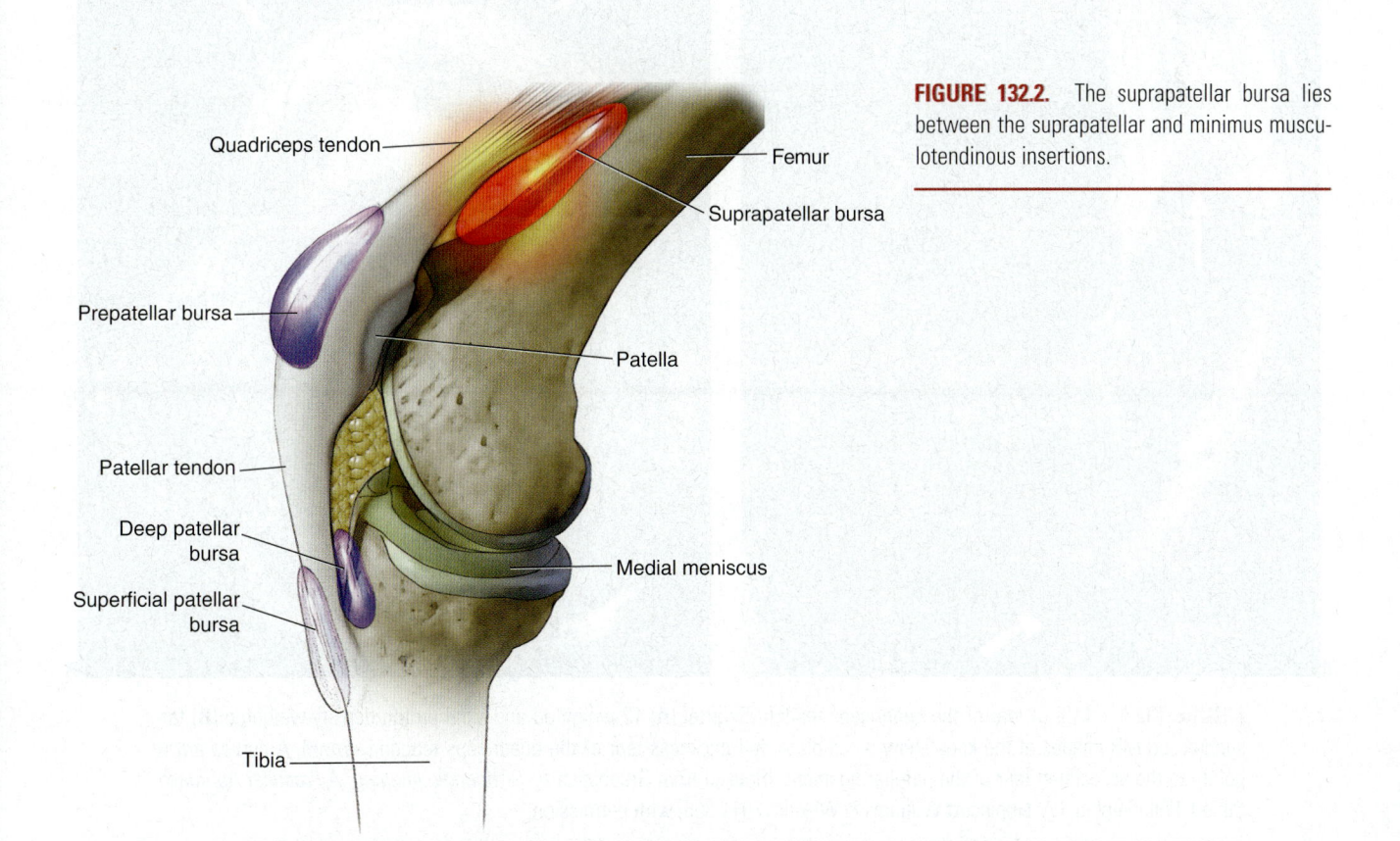

# CHAPTER 132 ULTRASOUND-GUIDED INJECTION TECHNIQUE FOR SUPRAPATELLAR BURSITIS PAIN

**FIGURE 132.1.** The bursa of the knee.

**FIGURE 132.2.** The suprapatellar bursa lies between the suprapatellar and minimus musculotendinous insertions.

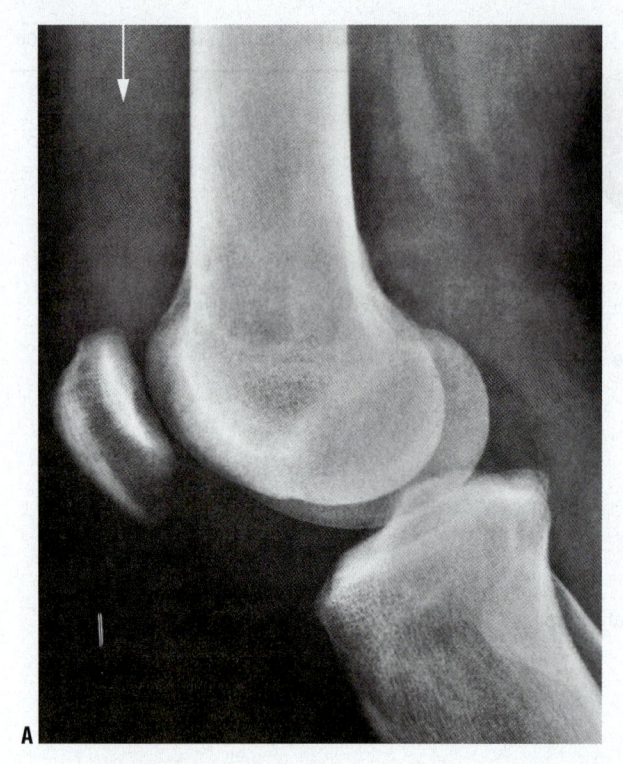

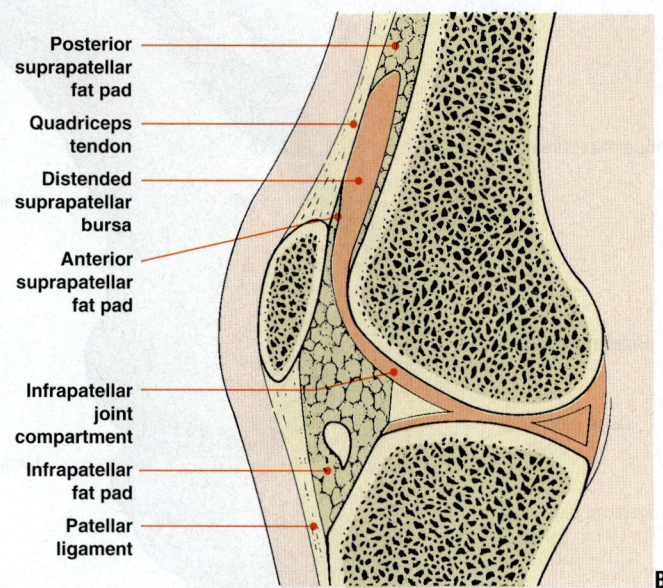

**FIGURE 132.3.** **A,B:** Knee joint effusion. In knee joint effusion, the suprapatellar bursa distends with fluid, thus obliterating the fat space posterior to the quadriceps tendon (*arrow*). (Reused from Greenspan A. *Orthopedic Imaging: A Practical Approach*. 5th ed. Philadelphia, PA: Lippincott Williams & Wilkins; 2011: 293, with permission.)

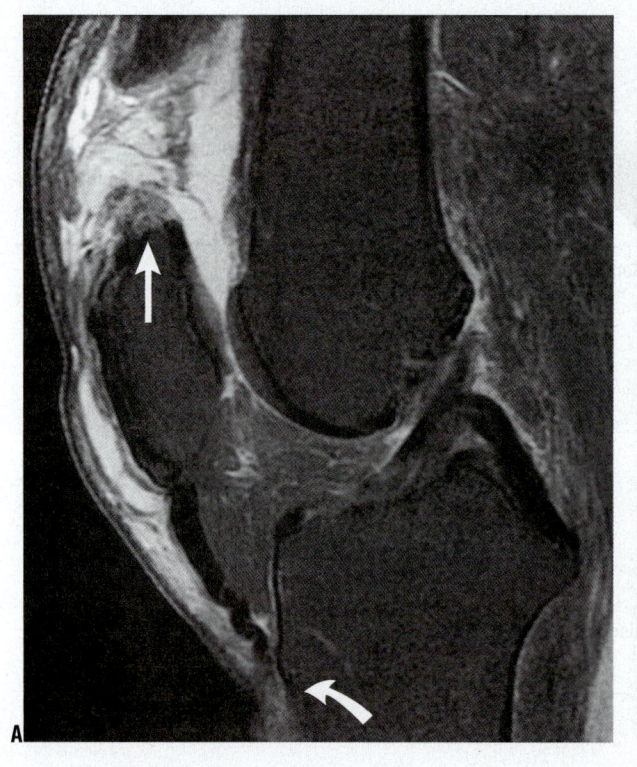

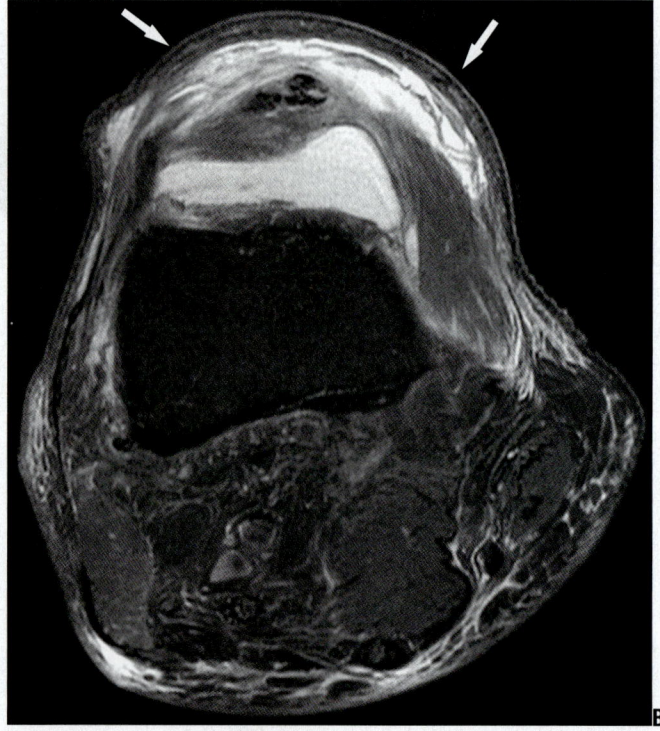

**FIGURE 132.4.** MRI of tear of the quadriceps tendon. Sagittal (**A**) T2-weighted and axial proton density-weighted (**B**) fat-suppressed MR images of the knee show a complete, full-thickness tear of the quadriceps tendon (*arrows*). A *curved arrow* points to the associated tear of the patellar ligament. (Reused from Greenspan A. *Orthopedic Imaging: A Practical Approach*. 5th ed. Philadelphia, PA: Lippincott Williams & Wilkins; 2011:305, with permission.)

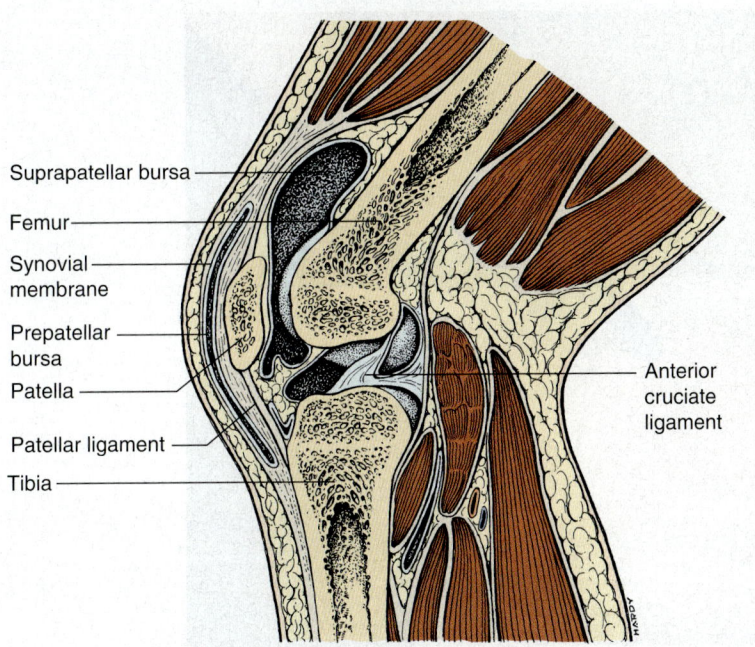

**FIGURE 132.5.** The relationship of the suprapatellar bursa to the femur and quadriceps tendon.

solution. The superior pole of the patella is identified by palpation (Fig. 132.6). A sterile syringe containing 4.0 mL of 0.25% preservative-free bupivacaine and 40 mg of methylprednisolone is attached to a 1½-inch, 22-gauge needle using strict aseptic technique. A linear high-frequency ultrasound transducer is placed over the previously identified superior pole of the patella in a longitudinal orientation (Fig. 132.7). A survey scan is taken, which demonstrates the hyperechoic margin of the superior pole of the patella, the quadriceps tendon, and the suprapatellar bursa beneath it (Fig. 132.8). After the quadriceps tendon and suprapatellar bursa are identified, a 3½-inch needle is placed through the skin ~1 cm from the center of medial aspect of the transducer and is then advanced using an out-of-plane approach with the needle trajectory adjusted under real-time ultrasound guidance to place the needle tip into just beneath the quadriceps tendon within the suprapatellar bursa (Fig. 132.9). When the tip of needle is thought to be in satisfactory position within the suprapatellar bursa, a small amount of local anesthetic and steroid is injected under real-time ultrasound guidance to confirm proper placement of the needle tip by hydrodissection (Fig. 132.10). After proper positioning of the needle tip placement is confirmed, the remainder of the contents of the syringe are slowly injected. There should be minimal resistance to injection. If synechiae, loculations, or calcifications are present, the needle may have to be repositioned to ensure that the entire bursa is treated. The needle is then removed, and a sterile pressure dressing and ice pack are placed at the injection site.

## COMPLICATIONS

The major complication of ultrasound-guided injection of the suprapatellar bursa is infection. Ecchymosis and hematoma formation may also occur. A transient exacerbation of the patient's pain occurs ~25% of the time following this injection technique, and the patient should be warned of this possibility prior to the procedure.

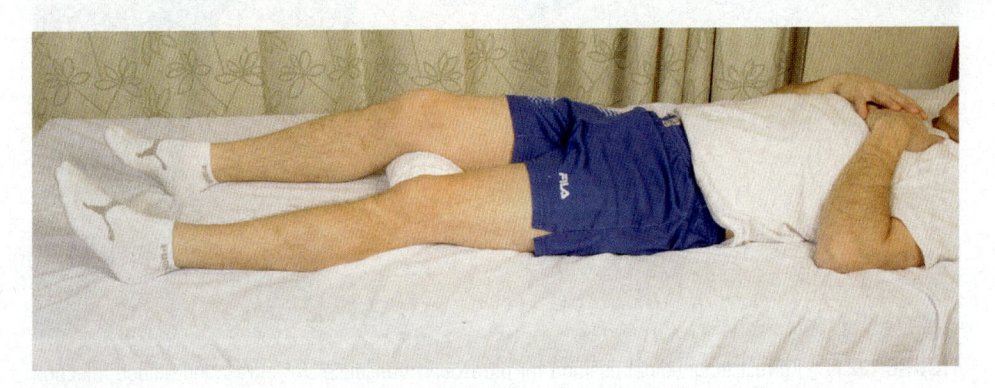

**FIGURE 132.6.** Proper patient position for ultrasound-guided injection of the suprapatellar bursa.

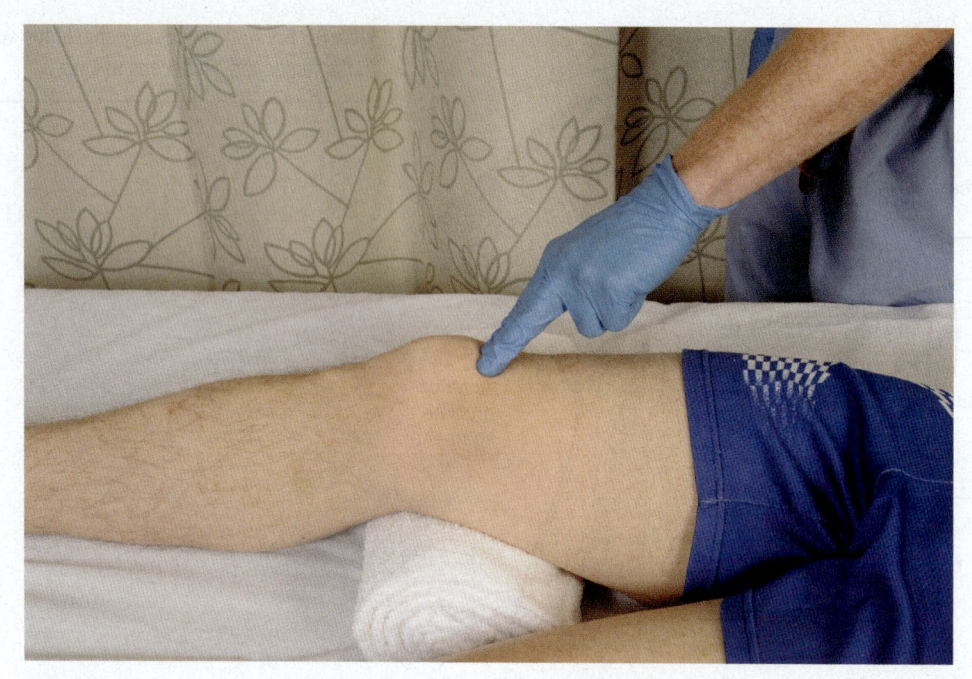

**FIGURE 132.7.** The superior pole of the patella is identified by palpation.

## CLINICAL PEARLS

Bursitis, labral tears, tendinopathy, osteoarthritis, synovitis, nerve entrapment, avascular necrosis of the knee, and impingement syndromes may coexist with other knee joint disease and may contribute to the patient's pain symptomatology. Universal precautions should always be observed to protect the operator, and strict adherence to sterile technique must be used to avoid infection. Gentle physical therapy and local heat should be introduced following ultrasound-guided injection of the elbow joint to reduce pain and improve function. Simple analgesics and nonsteroidal anti-inflammatory agents or COX-2 inhibitors may be used concurrently with this injection technique.

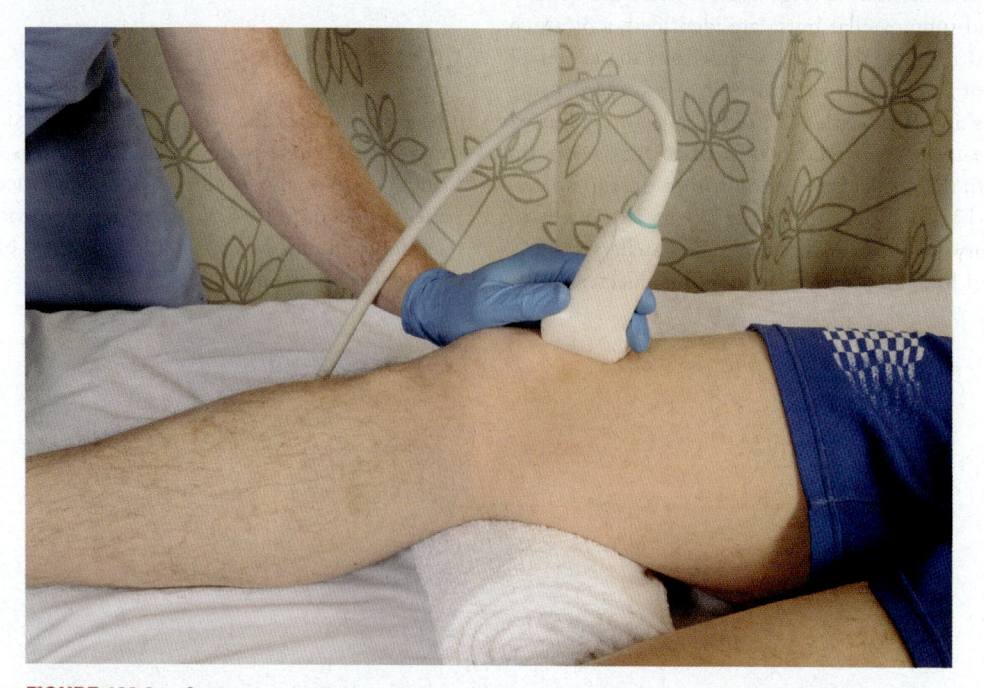

**FIGURE 132.8.** Correct longitudinal position for ultrasound transducer for ultrasound-guided injection of the suprapatellar bursa.

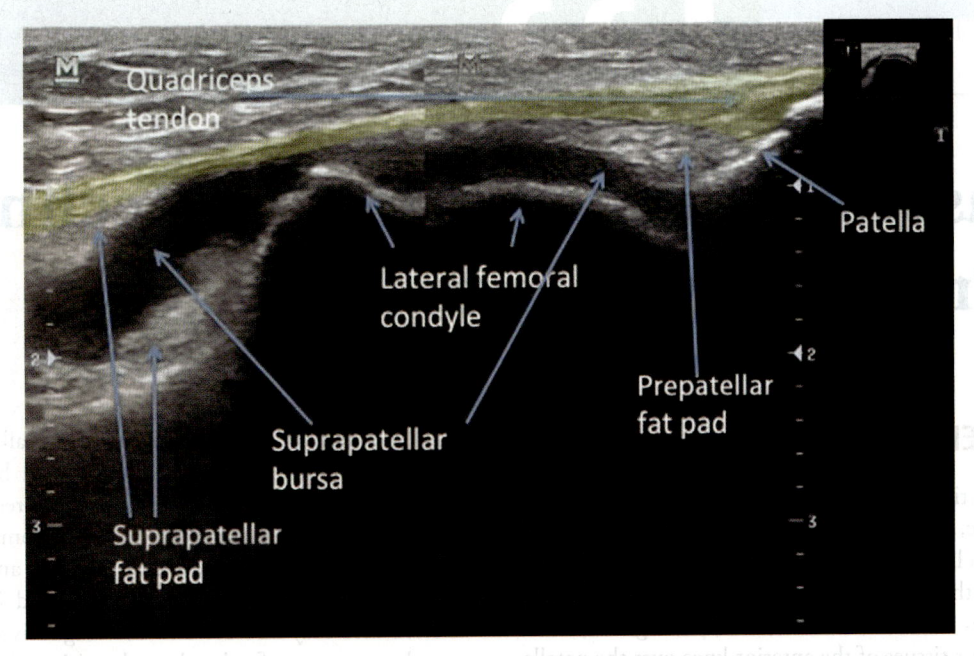

**FIGURE 132.9.** Ultrasound image of the knee joint demonstrating the suprapatellar bursa lying beneath the quadriceps tendon.

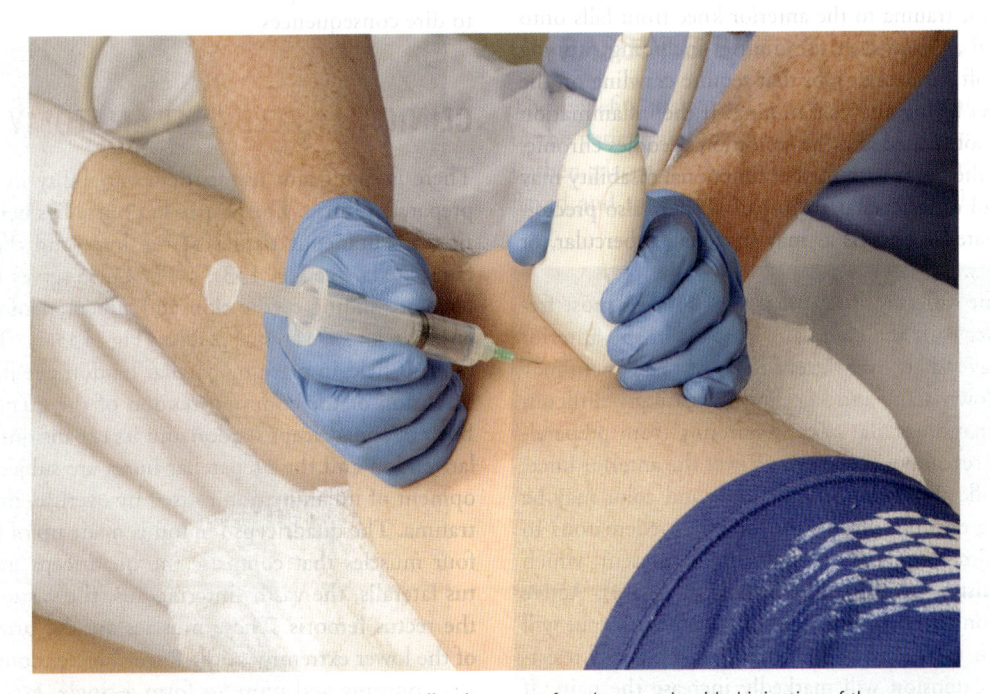

**FIGURE 132.10.** Correct out-of-plane needle placement for ultrasound-guided injection of the suprapatellar bursa.

## SUGGESTED READINGS

Marra MD, Crema MD, Chung M, et al. MRI features of cystic lesions around the knee. *Knee* 2008;15(6):423–438.

Waldman SD. Bursitis syndromes of the knee. In: *Pain Review*. Philadelphia, PA: Saunders Elsevier; 2009:318–322.

Waldman SD. Injection technique for suprapatellar bursitis. In: *Pain Review*. Philadelphia, PA: Saunders Elsevier; 2009:584–585.

Waldman SD. Suprapatellar bursitis. In: *Atlas of Common Pain Syndromes*. 3rd ed. Philadelphia, PA: Saunders Elsevier; 2012:325–328.

Waldman SD. Suprapatellar bursa injection. In: *Atlas of Pain Management Injection Techniques*. 3rd ed. Philadelphia, PA: Saunders Elsevier; 2012:369–371.

Yamamoto T, Akisue T, Marui T, et al. Isolated suprapatellar bursitis: computed tomographic and arthroscopic findings. *Arthroscopy* 2003;19(2):10.

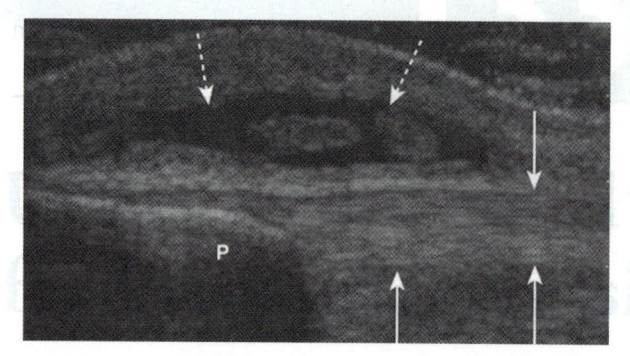

**FIGURE 133.4.** Longitudinal ultrasound image demonstrating prepatellar bursitis. (*Broken arrows*, fluid within bursal sac; *solid arrows*, patellar bursa; P, patella.)

skin overlying the anterior knee is then prepped with antiseptic solution. The patella is identified by palpation (Fig. 133.7). A sterile syringe containing 4.0 mL of 0.25% preservative-free bupivacaine and 40 mg of methylprednisolone is attached to a 1½-inch, 22-gauge needle using strict aseptic technique. A linear high-frequency ultrasound transducer is placed over the previously identified patella in a longitudinal orientation (Fig. 133.8). A survey scan is taken, which demonstrates the hyperechoic margin of the skin and subcutaneous tissues, the prepatellar bursa, and the patella beneath it (Fig. 133.9). After the skin and subcutaneous tissues and the prepatellar bursa are identified, a 3½-inch needle is placed through the skin ~1 cm from the center of medial aspect of the transducer and is then advanced using an out-of-plane approach with the needle trajectory adjusted under real-time ultrasound guidance to place the needle tip into just beneath the skin and subcutaneous tissues within the prepatellar bursa (Fig. 133.10). When the tip of needle is thought to be in satisfactory position within the prepatellar bursa, a small amount of local anesthetic and steroid is injected under real-time ultrasound guidance to confirm proper placement of the needle tip by hydrodissection. After proper positioning of the needle tip placement is confirmed, the remainder of the contents of the syringe are slowly injected. There should be minimal resistance to injection. If synechiae, loculations, or calcifications are present, the needle may have to be repositioned to ensure that the entire bursa is treated. The needle is then removed, and a sterile pressure dressing and ice pack are placed at the injection site.

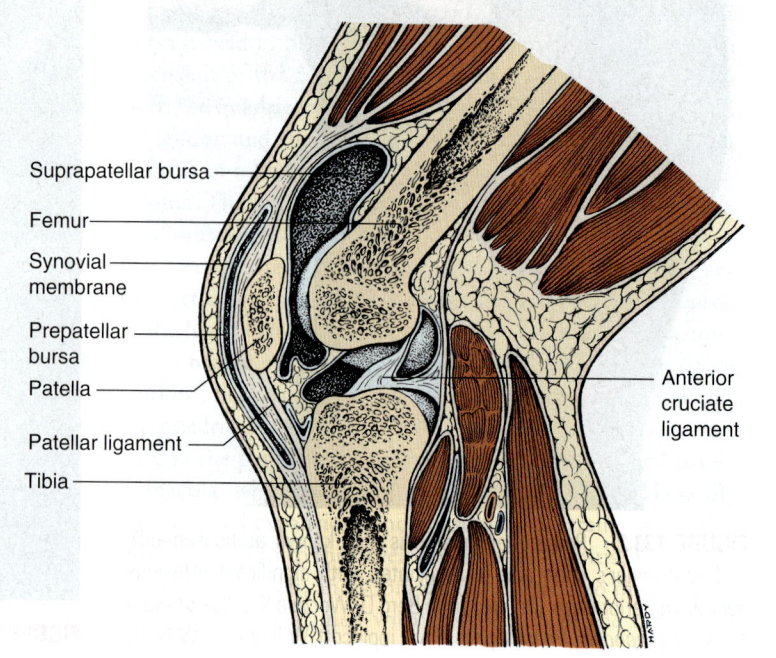

## COMPLICATIONS

The major complication of ultrasound-guided injection of the prepatellar bursa is infection. Ecchymosis and hematoma formation may also occur. A transient exacerbation of the patient's pain occurs ~25% of the time following this injection technique, and the patient should be warned of this possibility prior to the procedure.

## CLINICAL PEARLS

Bursitis, labral tears, tendinopathy, osteoarthritis, synovitis, nerve entrapment, avascular necrosis of the knee, and impingement syndromes may coexist with other knee joint disease

**FIGURE 133.5.** The relationship of the prepatellar bursa to the skin and subcutaneous tissues and patella.

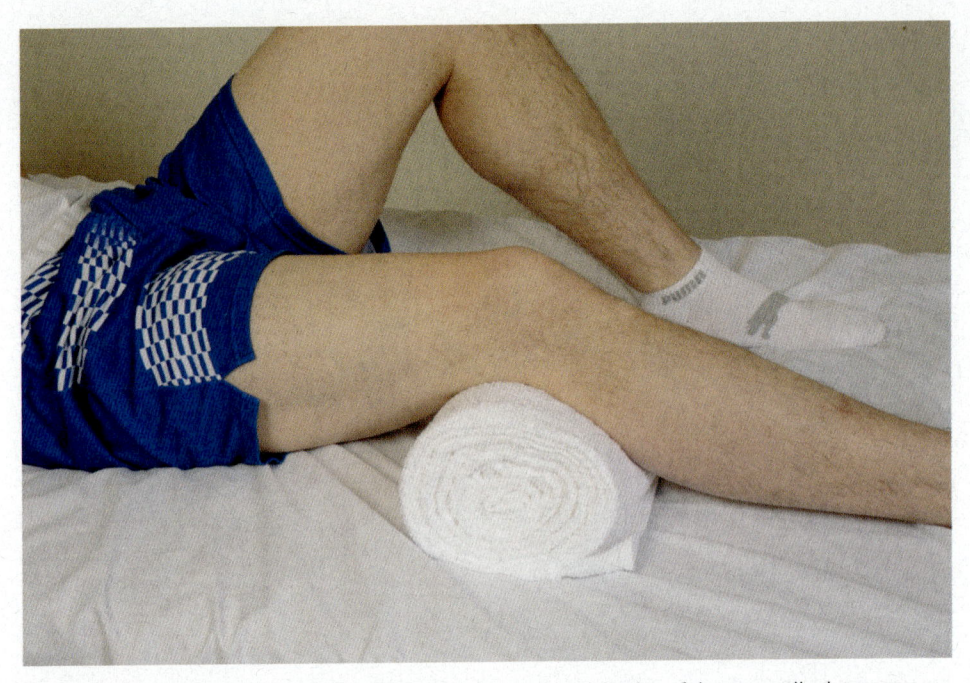

CHAPTER 133 ULTRASOUND-GUIDED INJECTION TECHNIQUE FOR PREPATELLAR BURSITIS PAIN

**FIGURE 133.6.** Proper patient position for ultrasound-guided injection of the prepatellar bursa.

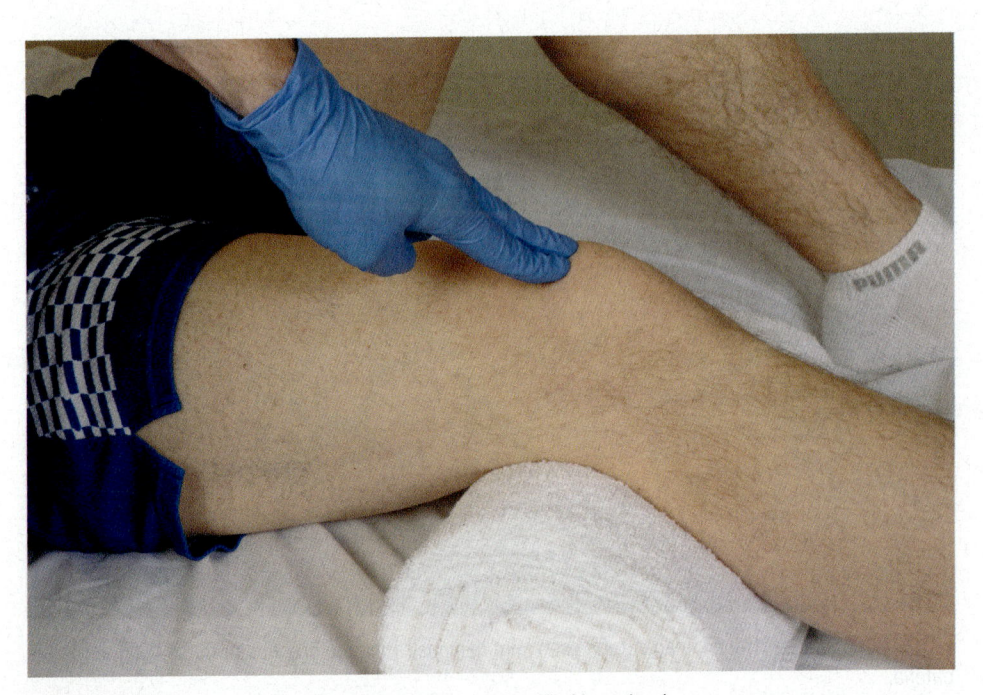

**FIGURE 133.7.** The superior pole of the patella is identified by palpation.

**FIGURE 133.8.** Correct longitudinal position for ultrasound transducer for ultrasound-guided injection of the prepatellar bursa.

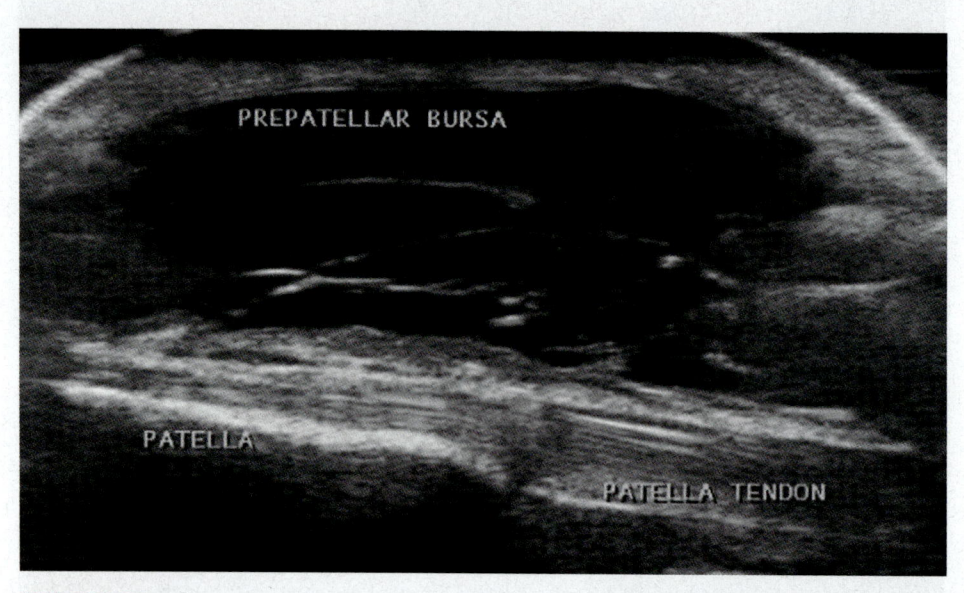

**FIGURE 133.9.** Ultrasound image of the knee joint demonstrating the prepatellar bursa lying above the patella.

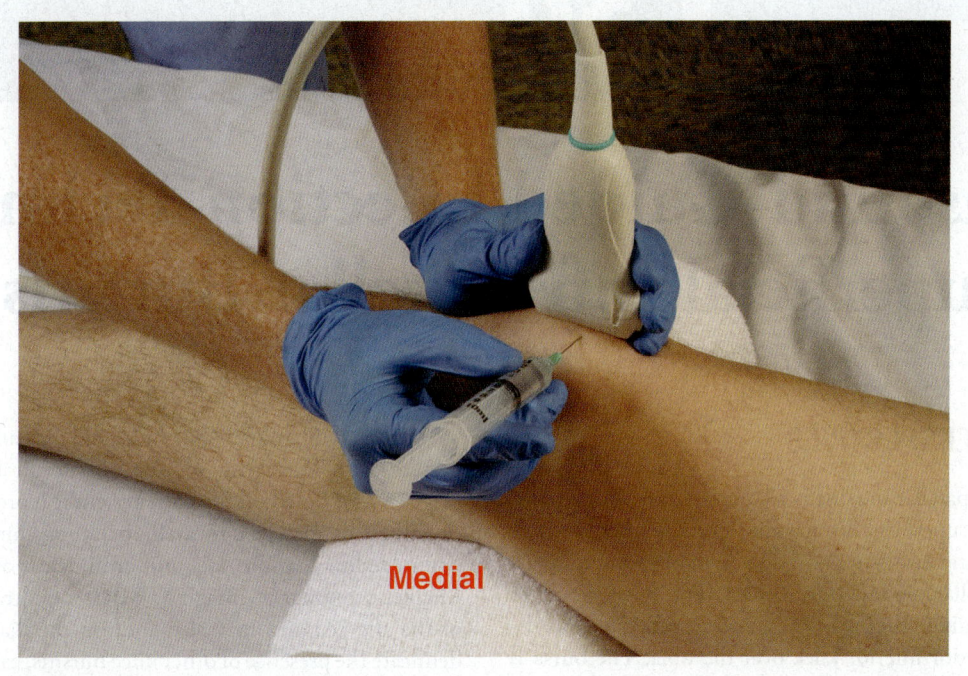

**FIGURE 133.10.** Correct out-of-plane needle placement for ultrasound-guided injection of the prepatellar bursa.

and may contribute to the patient's pain symptomatology. Universal precautions should always be observed to protect the operator, and strict adherence to sterile technique must be used to avoid infection. Gentle physical therapy and local heat should be introduced following ultrasound-guided injection of the elbow joint to reduce pain and improve function. Simple analgesics and nonsteroidal anti-inflammatory agents or COX-2 inhibitors may be used concurrently with this injection technique.

## SUGGESTED READINGS

Marra MD, Crema MD, Chung M, et al. MRI features of cystic lesions around the knee. *Knee* 2008;15(6):423–438.
Waldman SD. Bursitis syndromes of the knee. In: *Pain Review*. Philadelphia, PA: Saunders Elsevier; 2009:318–322.
Wasserman AR, Melville LD, Birkhahn RH. Septic bursitis: a case report and primer for the emergency clinician. *J Emerg Med* 2009;37(3):269–272.
Waldman SD. Prepatellar bursitis. In: *Atlas of Common Pain Syndromes*. 3rd ed. Philadelphia, PA: Saunders Elsevier; 2012:328–330.
Waldman SD. Prepatellar bursa injection. In: *Atlas of Pain Management Injection Techniques*. 3rd ed. Philadelphia, PA: Saunders Elsevier; 2012:372–373.

# Ultrasound-Guided Injection Technique for Superficial Infrapatellar Bursitis Pain

## CLINICAL PERSPECTIVES

Superficial infrapatellar bursitis is a common cause of anterior knee pain. The superficial infrapatellar bursa lies between the anterior subcutaneous tissues of the knee and the anterior surface of the patellar tendon (Fig. 134.1). The bursa serves to cushion and facilitate sliding of the skin and subcutaneous tissues of the anterior inferior knee over the tibia. The bursa is subject to inflammation from a variety of causes with acute trauma to the knee and repetitive microtrauma being the most common. Acute injuries to the bursa can occur from direct blunt trauma to the anterior knee from falls onto the knee as well as from overuse injuries including running on uneven or soft surfaces or jobs that require crawling on the knees like carpet laying and scrubbing floors. If the inflammation of the bursa is not treated and the condition becomes chronic, calcification of the bursa with further functional disability may occur. Gout and other crystal arthropathies may also precipitate acute superficial infrapatellar bursitis as may bacterial, tubercular, or fungal infections.

The patient suffering from superficial infrapatellar bursitis most frequently presents with the complaint of pain in the anterior knee, which may radiate inferiorly over the lower knee. The patient may find walking down stairs and kneeling increasingly difficult. Physical examination of the patient suffering from superficial infrapatellar bursitis will reveal point tenderness over the anterior knee. If there is significant inflammation, rubor and color may be present and the entire area may feel boggy or edematous to palpation. At times massive effusion may be present, which can be quite distressing to the patient (Fig. 134.2). Active resisted extension and passive flexion of the affected knee will often reproduce the patient's pain. Sudden release of resistance to active extension will markedly increase the pain. If calcification or gouty tophi of the bursa and surrounding tendons are present, the examiner may appreciate crepitus with active extension of the knee, and the patient may complain of a catching sensation when moving the affected knee, especially on awaking. Often, the patient will not be able to sleep on the affected side. Occasionally, the superficial infrapatellar bursa may become infected, with systemic symptoms, including fever and malaise, as well as local symptoms, with rubor, color, and dolor being present.

Plain radiographs are indicated in all patients who present with knee pain to rule out occult bony pathology (Fig. 134.3). Based on the patient's clinical presentation, additional testing may be indicated, including complete blood cell count, sedimentation rate, and antinuclear antibody testing. Magnetic resonance imaging (MRI) or ultrasound imaging of the affected area may also confirm the diagnosis and help delineate the presence of other knee bursitis, calcific tendonitis, tendinopathy, patellar tendonitis, or other knee pathology (Fig. 134.4). Rarely, the inflamed bursa may become infected, and failure to diagnose and treat the acute infection can lead to dire consequences.

## CLINICALLY RELEVANT ANATOMY

There is significant intrapatient variability in the size of the superficial infrapatellar bursa. The superficial infrapatellar bursa lies between the anterior subcutaneous tissues of the knee and the anterior surface of the patellar tendon (see Fig. 134.1). The bursa serves to cushion and facilitate sliding of the skin and subcutaneous tissues of the anterior inferior portion of the knee over the tibia. The superficial infrapatellar bursa is held in place by patellar tendon, which is an extension of the common tendon of the quadriceps tendon. Both the quadriceps tendon and its expansions and the patellar tendon and the superficial infrapatellar bursa are subject to the development of inflammation caused by overuse, misuse, or direct trauma. The quadriceps tendon is made up of fibers from the four muscles that comprise the quadriceps muscle: the vastus lateralis, the vastus intermedius, the vastus medialis, and the rectus femoris. These muscles are the primary extensors of the lower extremity at the knee. The tendons of these muscles converge and unite to form a single, exceedingly strong tendon. The patella functions as a sesamoid bone within the quadriceps tendon, with fibers of the tendon expanding around the patella and forming the medial and lateral patella retinacula, which help strengthen the knee joint. These fibers are called expansions and are subject to strain; the tendon proper is subject to the development of tendonitis. The superficial infrapatellar, deep infrapatellar, and prepatellar bursae also may concurrently become inflamed with dysfunction of the quadriceps and patellar tendon.

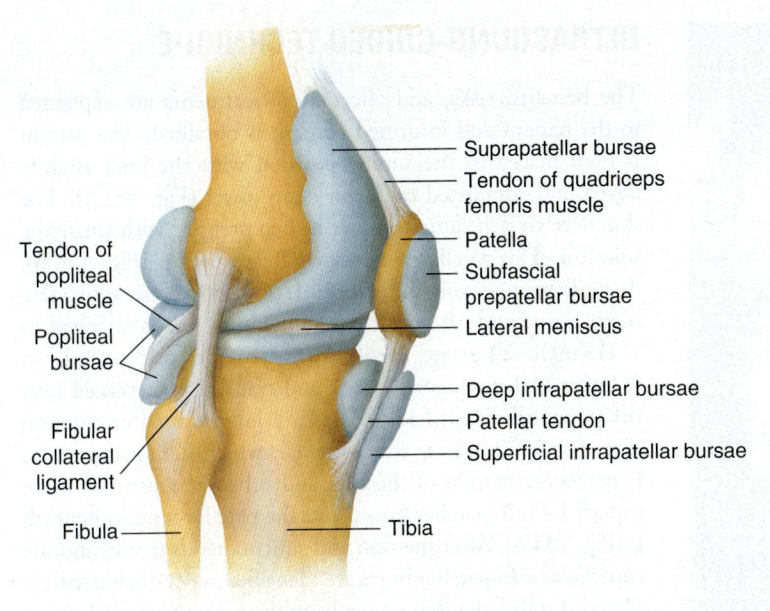

CHAPTER 134  ULTRASOUND-GUIDED INJECTION TECHNIQUE FOR SUPERFICIAL INFRAPATELLAR BURSITIS PAIN    955

**FIGURE 134.1.** The bursa of the knee. (Anatomical Chart Company, 2013.)

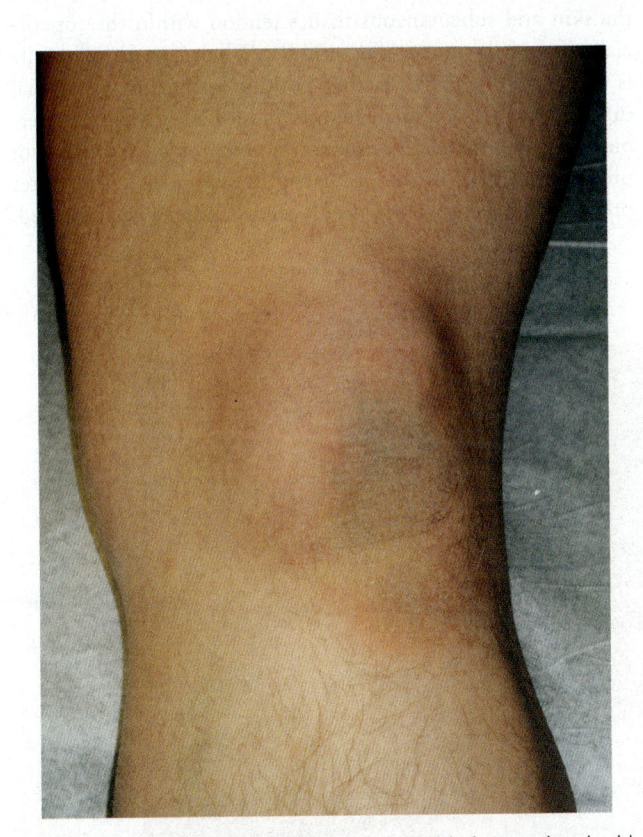

**FIGURE 134.2.** Superficial infrapatellar bursitis is associated with significant effusions over the inferior anterior knee. Note the callus over the superficial infrapatellar bursa. (Reused from Berg D, Worzala K. *Atlas of Adult Physical Diagnosis*. Philadelphia, PA: Lippincott Williams & Wilkins; 2006, with permission.)

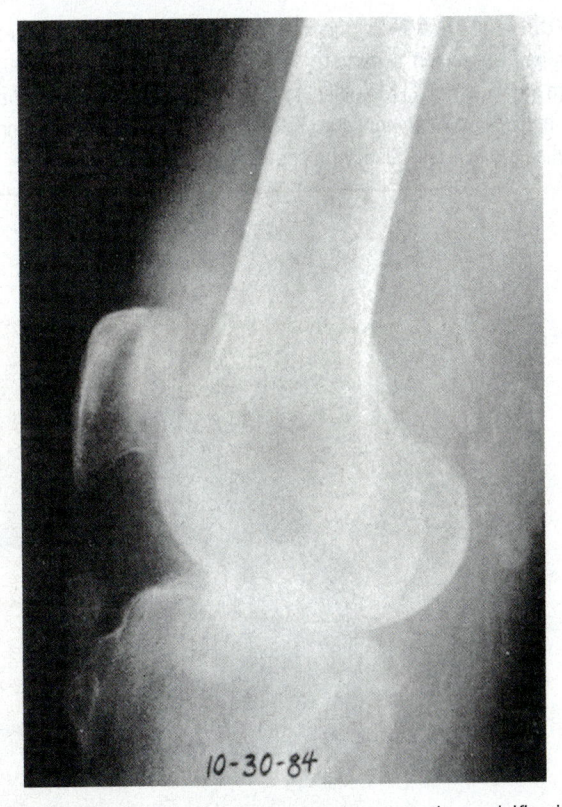

**FIGURE 134.3.** Lateral radiography demonstrating calcifications of the infrapatellar and popliteal spaces in a patient with end-stage renal disease. (Reused from Schumacher HR, Reginato AJ, Pullman S. Synovial fluid oxalate deposition complicating rheumatoid arthritis with amyloidosis and renal failure: demonstration of intracellular oxalate crystals. *J Rheumatol* 1987;4:361–366, with permission.)

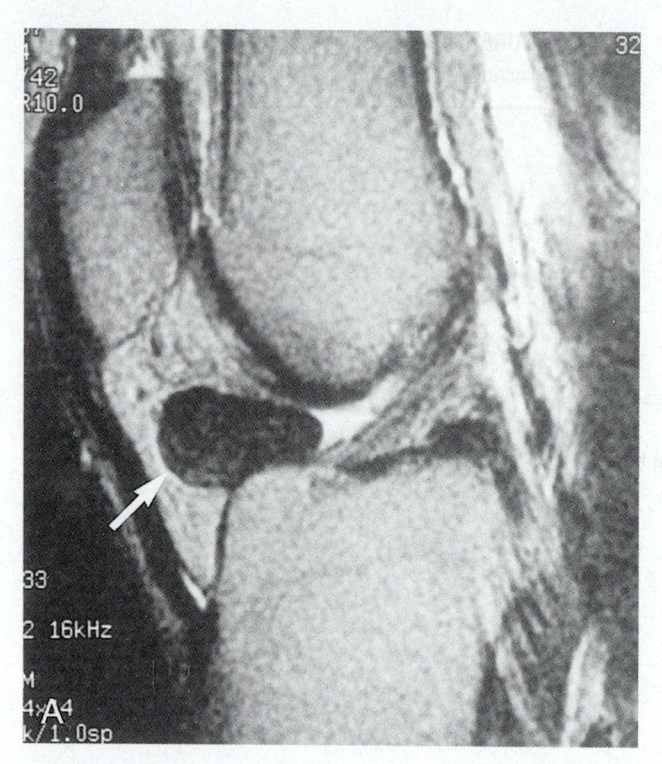

**FIGURE 134.4.** MRI of the knee showing abnormal mass in the infrapatellar region consistent with villonodular synovitis. (Reused from Koopman WJ, Moreland LW. *Arthritis and Allied Conditions: A Textbook of Rheumatology.* 15th ed. Philadelphia, PA: Lippincott Williams & Wilkins; 2005, with permission.)

## ULTRASOUND-GUIDED TECHNIQUE

The benefits, risks, and alternative treatments are explained to the patient and informed consent is obtained. The patient is then placed in the supine position with the knee slightly flexed and supported by a rolled up towel (Fig. 134.5). The skin overlying the anterior knee is then prepped with antiseptic solution. The patella is identified by palpation (Fig. 134.6). A sterile syringe containing 4.0 mL of 0.25% preservative-free bupivacaine and 40 mg of methylprednisolone is attached to a 1½-inch, 22-gauge needle using strict aseptic technique. A linear high-frequency ultrasound transducer is placed over the previously identified patella in a longitudinal orientation (Fig. 134.7). A survey scan is taken, which demonstrates the hyperechoic margin of the skin and subcutaneous tissues, the superficial infrapatellar bursa, and the patellar tendon beneath it (Fig. 134.8). After the skin and subcutaneous tissues and the superficial infrapatellar bursa are identified, a 3½-inch needle is placed through the skin ~1 cm from the center of medial aspect of the transducer and is then advanced using an out-of-plane approach with the needle trajectory adjusted under real-time ultrasound guidance to place the needle tip into just beneath the skin and subcutaneous tissues tendon within the superficial infrapatellar bursa (Fig. 134.9). When the tip of needle is thought to be in satisfactory position within the superficial infrapatellar bursa, a small amount of local anesthetic and steroid is injected under real-time ultrasound guidance to confirm proper placement of the needle tip by hydrodissection. After proper positioning of the needle tip placement is confirmed,

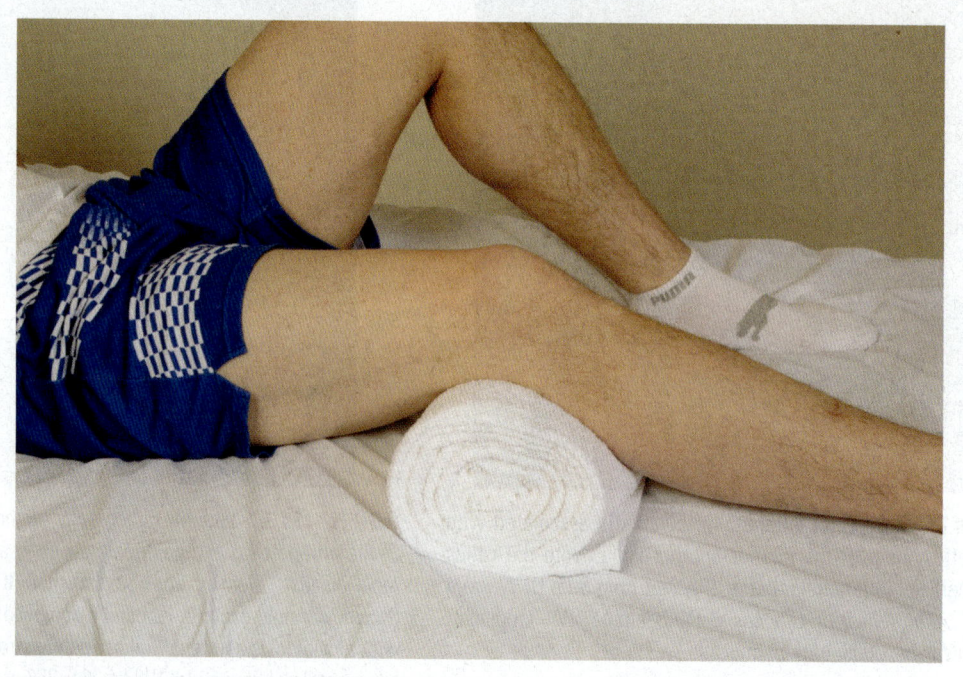

**FIGURE 134.5.** Proper patient position for ultrasound-guided injection of the superficial infrapatellar bursa.

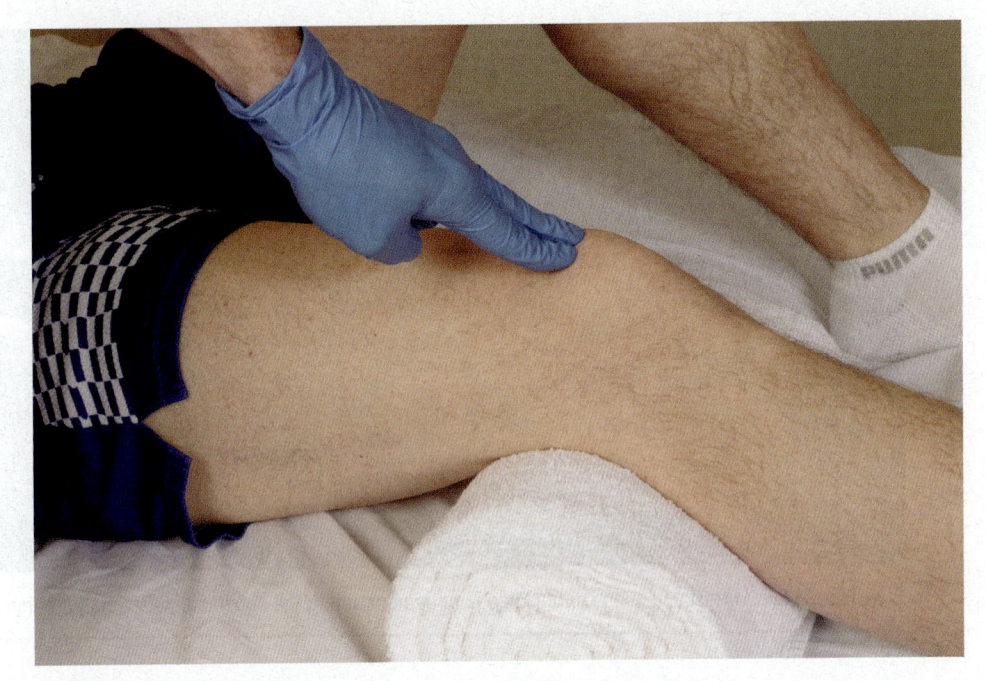

**FIGURE 134.6.** The superior pole of the patella is identified by palpation.

the remainder of the contents of the syringe are slowly injected. There should be minimal resistance to injection. If synechiae, loculations, or calcifications are present, the needle may have to be repositioned to ensure that the entire bursa is treated. The needle is then removed, and a sterile pressure dressing and ice pack are placed at the injection site.

## COMPLICATIONS

The major complication of ultrasound-guided injection of the superficial infrapatellar bursa is infection. Ecchymosis and hematoma formation may also occur. A transient exacerbation of the patient's pain occurs ~25% of the time following this

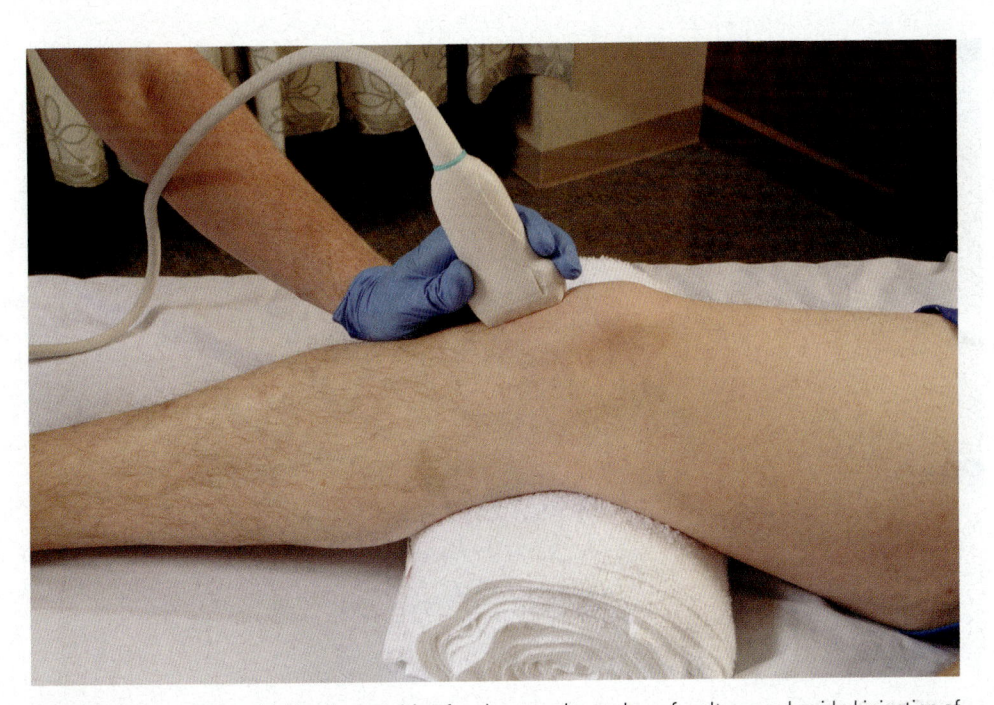

**FIGURE 134.7.** Correct longitudinal position for ultrasound transducer for ultrasound-guided injection of the superficial infrapatellar bursa.

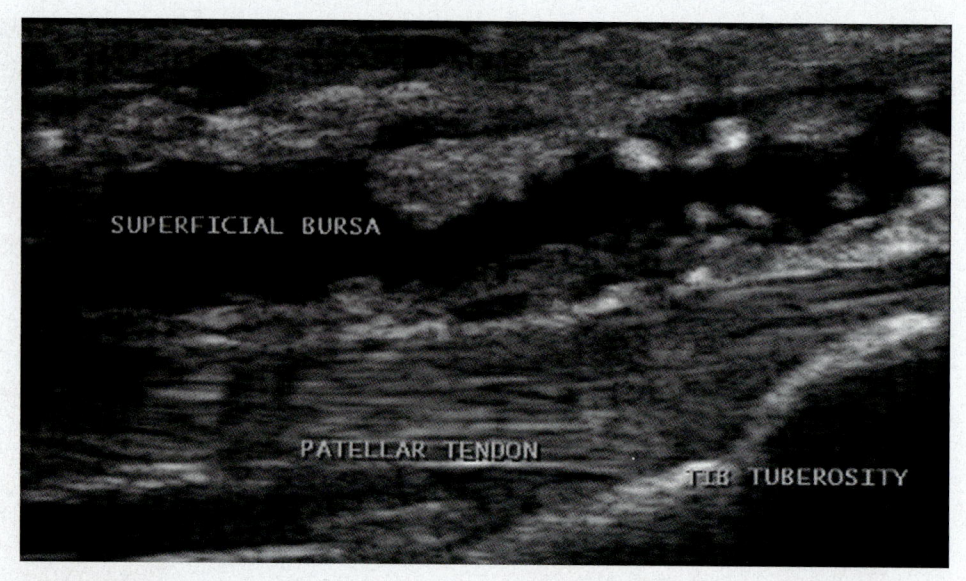

**FIGURE 134.8.** Ultrasound image of the knee joint demonstrating the superficial infrapatellar bursa.

injection technique, and the patient should be warned of this possibility prior to the procedure.

## CLINICAL PEARLS

Bursitis, labral tears, tendinopathy, osteoarthritis, synovitis, nerve entrapment, avascular necrosis of the knee, and impingement syndromes may coexist with other knee joint disease and may contribute to the patient's pain symptomatology. Universal precautions should always be observed to protect the operator, and strict adherence to sterile technique must be used to avoid infection. Gentle physical therapy and local heat should be introduced following ultrasound-guided injection of the elbow joint to reduce pain and improve function. Simple analgesics and nonsteroidal anti-inflammatory agents or COX-2 inhibitors may be used concurrently with this injection technique.

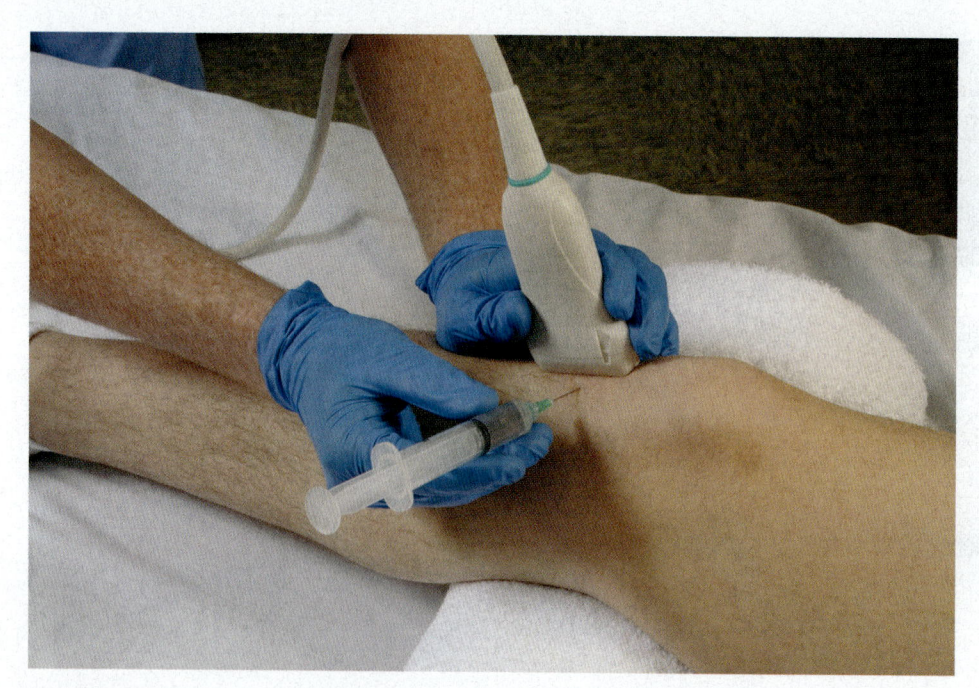

**FIGURE 134.9.** Correct out-of-plane needle placement for ultrasound-guided injection of the superficial infrapatellar bursa.

## SUGGESTED READINGS

Marra MD, Crema MD, Chung M, et al. MRI features of cystic lesions around the knee. *Knee* 2008;15(6):423–438.

Waldman SD. Bursitis syndromes of the knee. In: *Pain Review*. Philadelphia, PA: Saunders Elsevier; 2009:318–322.

Waldman SD. Injection technique for superficial infrapatellar bursitis. In: *Pain Review*. Philadelphia, PA: Saunders Elsevier; 2009:587–588.

Wasserman AR, Melville LD, Birkhahn RH. Septic bursitis: a case report and primer for the emergency clinician. *J Emerg Med* 2009;37(3):269–272.

Waldman SD. Superficial infrapatellar bursitis. In: *Atlas of Common Pain Syndromes*. 3rd ed. Philadelphia, PA: Saunders Elsevier; 2012:331–333.

Waldman SD. Superficial infrapatellar bursa injection. In: *Atlas of Pain Management Injection Techniques*. 3rd ed. Philadelphia, PA: Saunders Elsevier; 2012:375–377.

# Ultrasound-Guided Injection Technique for Deep Infrapatellar Bursitis Pain

## CLINICAL PERSPECTIVES

Deep infrapatellar bursitis, which is also known as clergyman's knee, is a common cause of anterior knee pain. The deep infrapatellar bursa lies between the patellar tendon and the tibia (Fig. 135.1). The bursa serves to cushion and facilitate sliding of the patellar tendon over the tibia. The bursa is subject to inflammation from a variety of causes with acute trauma to the knee and repetitive microtrauma being the most common. Acute injuries to the bursa can occur from direct blunt trauma to the anterior knee from falls onto the knee as well as from overuse injuries including running on uneven or soft surfaces or jobs that require crawling on the knees like carpet laying and scrubbing floors. If the inflammation of the bursa is not treated and the condition becomes chronic, calcification of the bursa with further functional disability may occur. Gout and other crystal arthropathies may also precipitate acute deep infrapatellar bursitis as may bacterial, tubercular, or fungal infections.

The patient suffering from deep infrapatellar bursitis most frequently presents with the complaint of pain in the anterior knee, which may radiate inferiorly over the lower knee. The patient may find walking down stairs and kneeling increasingly difficult. Physical examination of the patient suffering from deep infrapatellar bursitis will reveal point tenderness over the anterior knee. If there is significant inflammation, rubor and color may be present and the entire area may feel boggy or edematous to palpation. At times massive effusion may be present, which can be quite distressing to the patient (Fig. 135.2). Active resisted extension and passive flexion of the affected knee will often reproduce the patient's pain. Sudden release of resistance to active extension will markedly increase the pain. If calcification or gouty tophi of the bursa and surrounding tendons are present, the examiner may appreciate crepitus with active extension of the knee, and the patient may complain of a catching sensation when moving the affected knee, especially on awaking. Often, the patient will not be able to sleep on the affected side. Occasionally, the deep infrapatellar bursa may become infected, with systemic symptoms, including fever and malaise, as well as local symptoms, with rubor, color, and dolor being present.

Plain radiographs are indicated in all patients who present with knee pain to rule out occult bony pathology (Fig. 135.3). Based on the patient's clinical presentation, additional testing may be indicated, including complete blood cell count, sedimentation rate, and antinuclear antibody testing. Magnetic resonance imaging or ultrasound imaging of the affected area may also confirm the diagnosis and help delineate the presence of other knee bursitis, calcific tendonitis, tendinopathy, patellar tendonitis, or other knee pathology (Fig. 135.4). Rarely, the inflamed bursa may become infected, and failure to diagnose and treat the acute infection can lead to dire consequences.

## CLINICALLY RELEVANT ANATOMY

There is significant intrapatient variability in the size of the deep infrapatellar bursa. The deep infrapatellar bursa lies between the anterior subcutaneous tissues of the knee and the anterior surface of the patellar tendon (see Fig. 135.1). The bursa serves to cushion and facilitate sliding of the skin and subcutaneous tissues of the anterior inferior portion of the knee over the tibia. The deep infrapatellar bursa is held in place by patellar tendon, which is an extension of the common tendon of the quadriceps tendon. Both the quadriceps tendon and its expansions and the patellar tendon and the deep infrapatellar bursa are subject to the development of inflammation caused by overuse, misuse, or direct trauma. The quadriceps tendon is made up of fibers from the four muscles that comprise the quadriceps muscle: the vastus lateralis, the vastus intermedius, the vastus medialis, and the rectus femoris. These muscles are the primary extensors of the lower extremity at the knee. The tendons of these muscles converge and unite to form a single, exceedingly strong tendon. The patella functions as a sesamoid bone within the quadriceps tendon, with fibers of the tendon expanding around the patella and forming the medial and lateral patella retinacula, which help strengthen the knee joint. These fibers are called expansions and are subject to strain; the tendon proper is subject to the development of tendonitis. The deep infrapatellar, deep infrapatellar, and prepatellar bursae also may concurrently become inflamed with dysfunction of the quadriceps tendon.

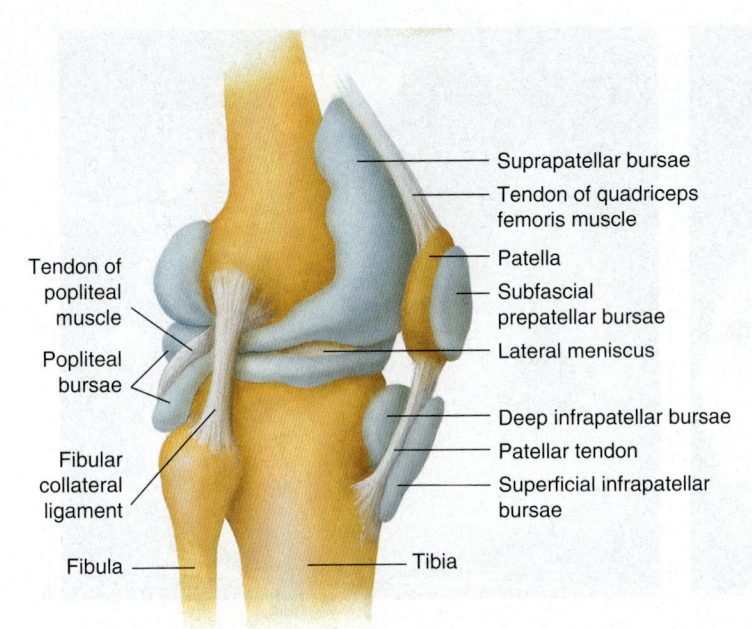

CHAPTER 135    ULTRASOUND-GUIDED INJECTION TECHNIQUE FOR DEEP INFRAPATELLAR BURSITIS PAIN    961

**FIGURE 135.1.** The bursa of the knee. (Anatomical Chart Company, 2013.)

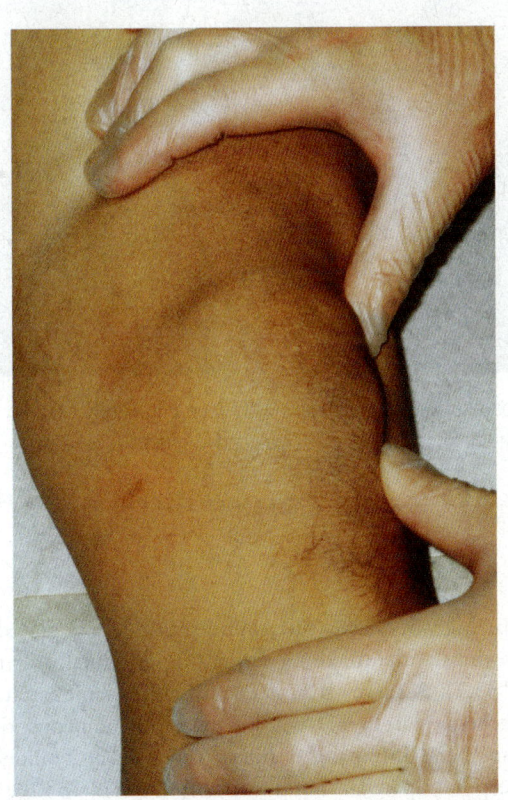

**FIGURE 135.2.** Effusion associated with deep infrapatellar bursitis can be appreciated by displacing the patella. (Reused from Berg D, Worzala K. *Atlas of Adult Physical Diagnosis*. Philadelphia, PA: Lippincott Williams & Wilkins; 2006, with permission.)

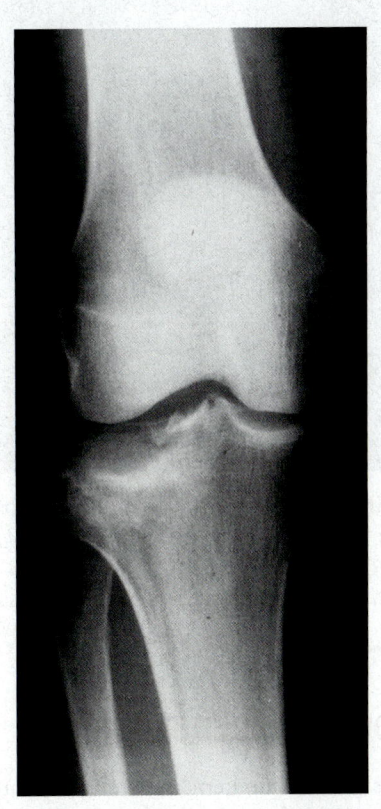

**FIGURE 135.3.** Radiograph demonstrating high-energy *tibial plateau* fractures includes primary fracture lines that involve both tibial condyles, severe impaction and comminution of one or both articular surfaces, and fracture extension into the shaft. (Reused from Bucholz RW, Heckman JD. *Rockwood & Green's Fractures in Adults*. 5th ed. Philadelphia, PA: Lippincott Williams & Wilkins; 2001, with permission.)

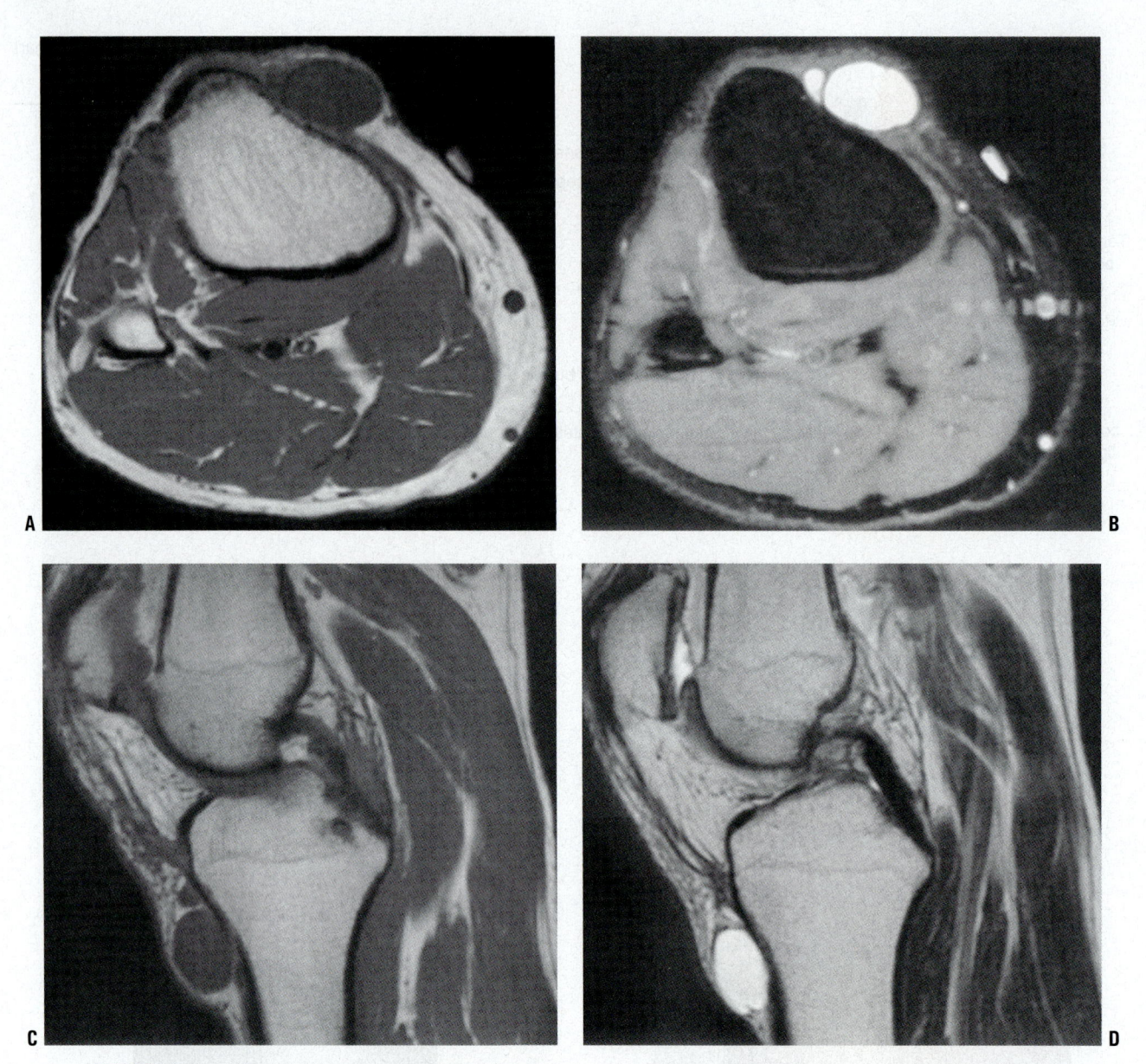

**FIGURE 135.4.** MRI of the knee showing abnormal mass in the infrapatellar region consistent with deep infrapatellar bursitis. (Reused from Berquist TH. *MRI of the Musculoskeletal System*. 6th ed. Philadelphia, PA: Lippincott Williams & Wilkins; 2013, with permission.)

## ULTRASOUND-GUIDED TECHNIQUE

The benefits, risks, and alternative treatments are explained to the patient and informed consent is obtained. The patient is then placed in the supine position with the knee slightly flexed and supported by a rolled up towel (Fig. 135.5). The skin overlying the anterior knee is then prepped with antiseptic solution. The patella is identified by palpation (Fig. 135.6). A sterile syringe containing 4.0 mL of 0.25% preservative-free bupivacaine and 40 mg of methylprednisolone is attached to a 1½-inch, 22-gauge needle using strict aseptic technique.

A linear high-frequency ultrasound transducer is placed over the previously identified patella in a longitudinal orientation (Fig. 135.7). A survey scan is taken, which demonstrates the hyperechoic margin of the skin and subcutaneous tissues, the superficial infrapatellar bursa, the patellar tendon, and the deep infrapatellar bursa beneath it (Fig. 135.8). After the skin and subcutaneous tissues, the patellar tendon, and the deep infrapatellar bursa are identified, a 3½-inch needle is placed through the skin ~1 cm from the center of medial aspect of the transducer and is then advanced using an out-of-plane approach with the needle trajectory adjusted under

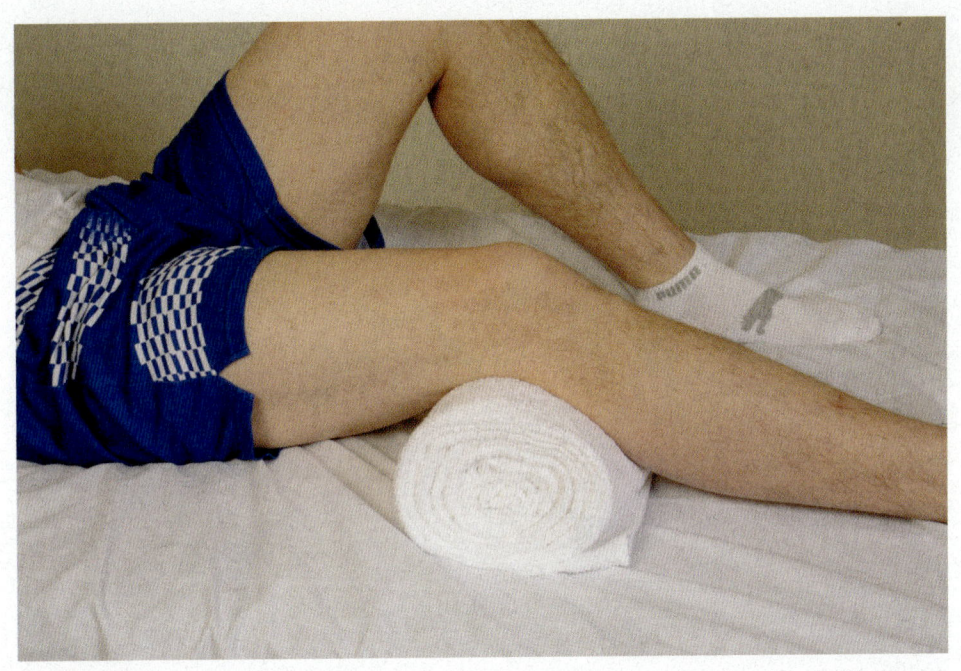

**FIGURE 135.5.** Proper patient position for ultrasound-guided injection of the deep infrapatellar bursa.

real-time ultrasound guidance to place the needle tip into just beneath the patellar tendon within the deep infrapatellar bursa (Fig. 135.9). When the tip of needle is thought to be in satisfactory position within the deep infrapatellar bursa, a small amount of local anesthetic and steroid is injected under real-time ultrasound guidance to confirm proper placement of the needle tip by hydrodissection. After proper positioning of the needle tip placement is confirmed, the remainder of the contents of the syringe are slowly injected. There should be minimal resistance to injection. If synechiae, loculations, or

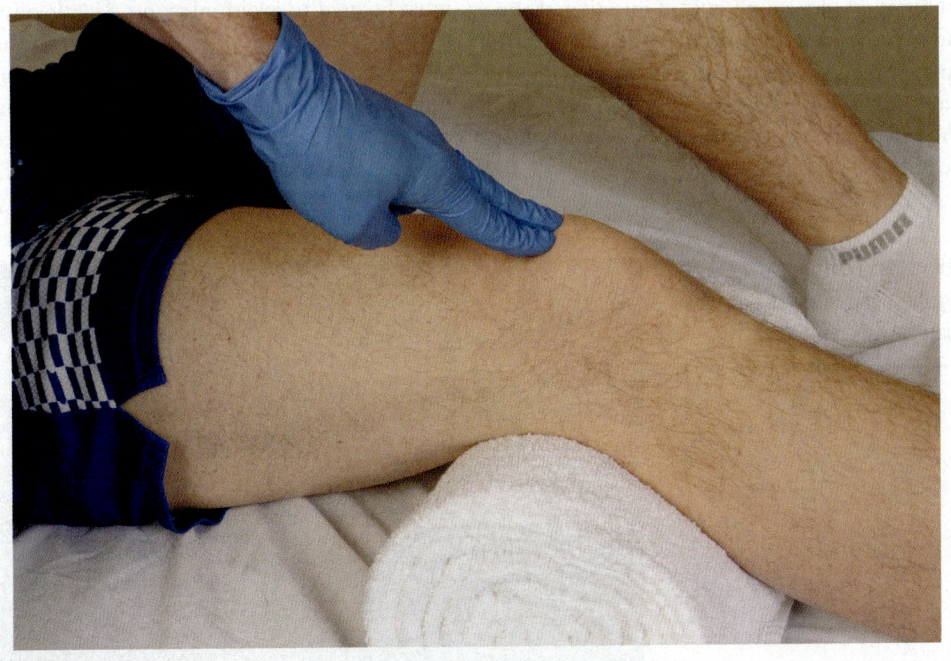

**FIGURE 135.6.** The superior pole of the patella is identified by palpation.

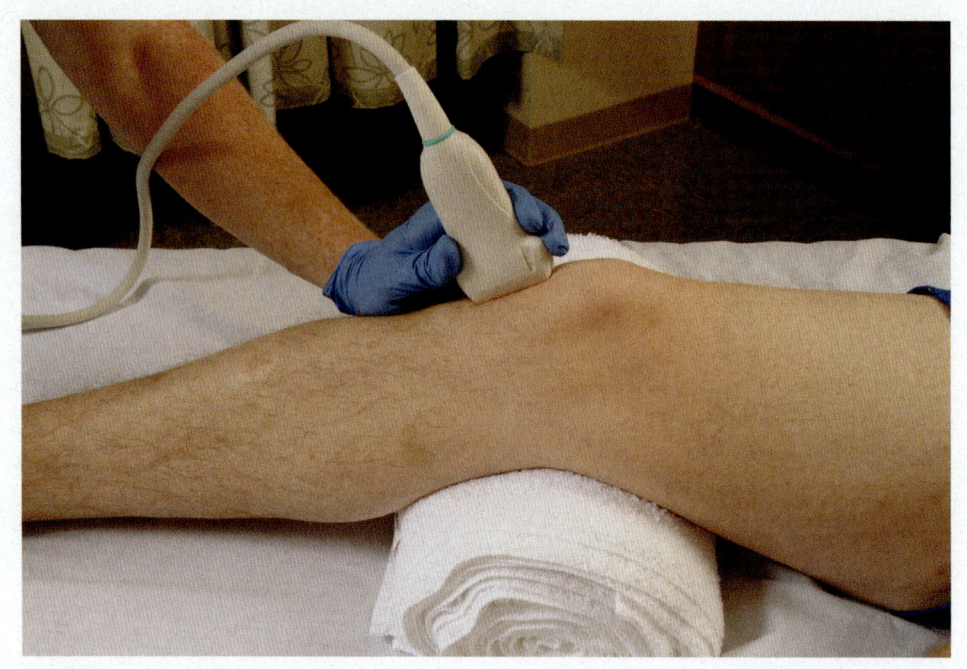

**FIGURE 135.7.** Correct longitudinal position for ultrasound transducer for ultrasound-guided injection of the deep infrapatellar bursa.

calcifications are present, the needle may have to be repositioned to ensure that the entire bursa is treated. The needle is then removed, and a sterile pressure dressing and ice pack are placed at the injection site.

## COMPLICATIONS

The major complication of ultrasound-guided injection of the deep infrapatellar bursa is infection. Ecchymosis and hematoma formation may also occur. A transient exacerbation of the patient's pain occurs ~25% of the time following this injection technique, and the patient should be warned of this possibility prior to the procedure.

## CLINICAL PEARLS

Bursitis, labral tears, tendinopathy, osteoarthritis, synovitis, nerve entrapment, avascular necrosis of the knee, and impingement syndromes may coexist with other knee joint disease and may contribute to the patient's pain symptomatology. Universal precautions should always be observed to protect the operator, and strict adherence to sterile technique must be used to avoid infection. Gentle physical therapy and local heat should be introduced following ultrasound-guided injection of the elbow joint to reduce pain and improve function. Simple analgesics and nonsteroidal anti-inflammatory agents or COX-2 inhibitors may be used concurrently with this injection technique.

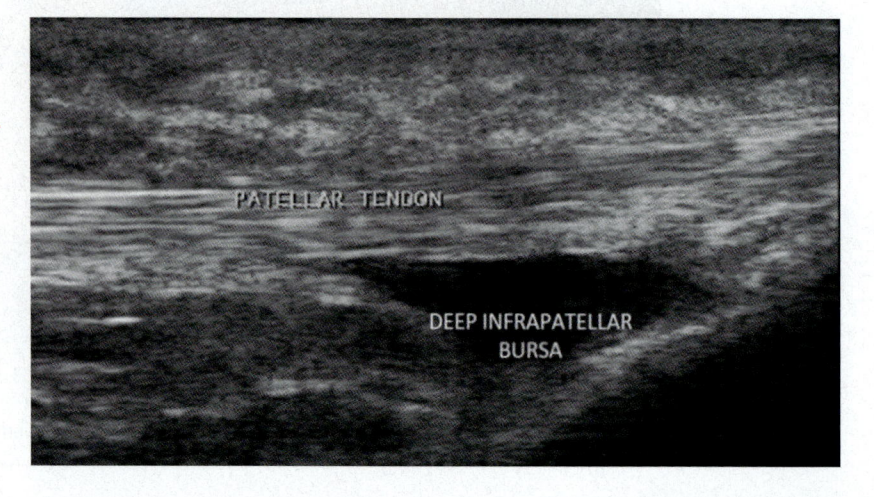

**FIGURE 135.8.** Ultrasound image of the knee joint demonstrating the deep infrapatellar bursa lying beneath the patellar tendon.

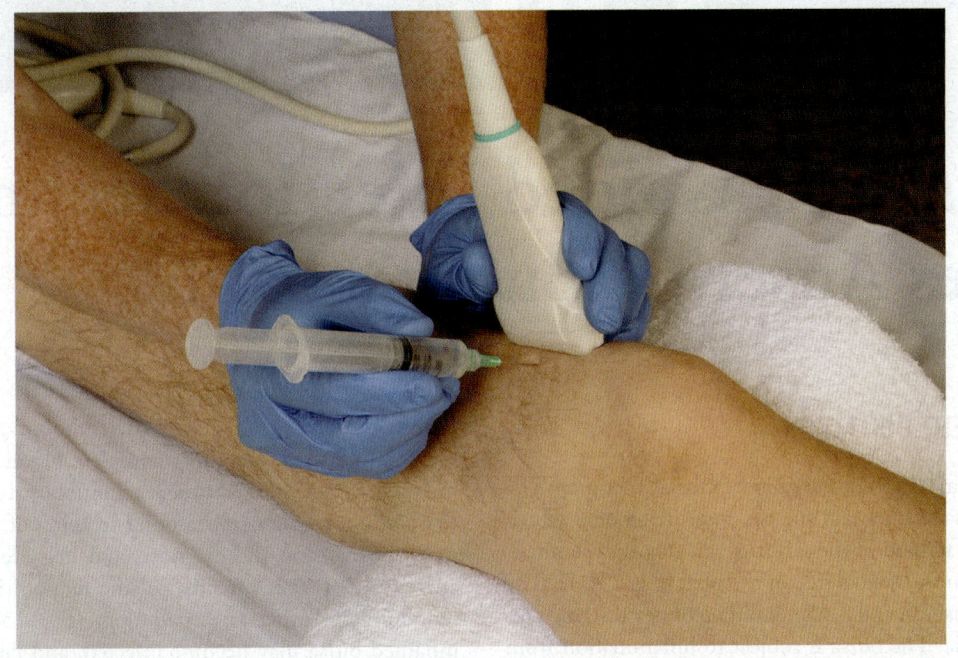

**FIGURE 135.9.** Correct out-of-plane needle placement for ultrasound-guided injection of the deep infrapatellar bursa.

## SUGGESTED READINGS

Marra MD, Crema MD, Chung M, et al. MRI features of cystic lesions around the knee. *Knee* 2008;15(6):423–438.

Waldman SD. Bursitis syndromes of the knee. In: *Pain Review*. Philadelphia, PA: Saunders Elsevier; 2009:318–322.

Wasserman AR, Melville LD, Birkhahn RH. Septic bursitis: a case report and primer for the emergency clinician. *J Emerg Med* 2009;37(3):269–272.

Waldman SD. Deep infrapatellar bursitis. In: *Atlas of Common Pain Syndromes*. 3rd ed. Philadelphia, PA: Saunders Elsevier; 2012:334–336.

Waldman SD. Deep infrapatellar bursa injection. In: *Atlas of Pain Management Injection Techniques*. 3rd ed. Philadelphia, PA: Saunders Elsevier; 2012: 378–380.

# CHAPTER 136

# Ultrasound-Guided Injection Technique for Pes Anserine Bursitis Pain

## CLINICAL PERSPECTIVES

Pes anserine bursitis is a common cause of medial knee pain. The pes anserine bursa lies beneath the pes anserine tendon, which is the insertional tendon of the sartorius, gracilis, and semitendinosus muscle to the medial side of the tibia (Fig. 136.1). The bursa serves to cushion and facilitate sliding of pes anserine tendon over the tibia. The bursa is subject to inflammation from a variety of causes with acute trauma to the knee and repetitive microtrauma being the most common. Acute injuries to the bursa can occur from direct blunt trauma to the medial knee as well as from overuse injuries including running on hills or sudden increases in the distance that one runs. If the inflammation of the bursa is not treated and the condition becomes chronic, calcification of the bursa with further functional disability may occur. Gout and other crystal arthropathies may also precipitate acute pes anserine bursitis as may bacterial, tubercular, or fungal infections.

The patient suffering from pes anserine bursitis most frequently presents with the complaint of pain in the medial knee, which may radiate inferiorly over the medial tibia. The patient may find any activity that involves flexion or external rotation of the knee such as getting in and out of cars increasingly difficult. Physical examination of the patient suffering from pes anserine bursitis will reveal point tenderness over the medial knee just below the medial knee joint. If there is significant inflammation, rubor and color may be present and the entire area may feel boggy or edematous to palpation. At times, significant effusion may be present, which can be quite distressing to the patient (Fig. 136.2). Active resisted flexion and passive external rotation of the affected knee will often reproduce the patient's pain. Sudden release of resistance to active flexion will markedly increase the pain. If calcification or gouty tophi of the bursa and surrounding tendons are present, the examiner may appreciate crepitus with active extension of the knee, and the patient may complain of a catching sensation when moving the affected knee, especially on awaking. Often, the patient will not be able to sleep on the affected side. Occasionally, the pes anserine bursa may become infected, with systemic symptoms, including fever and malaise, as well as local symptoms, with rubor, color, and dolor being present.

Plain radiographs are indicated in all patients who present with knee pain to rule out occult bony pathology (Fig. 136.3). Based on the patient's clinical presentation, additional testing may be indicated, including complete blood cell count, sedimentation rate, and antinuclear antibody testing. Magnetic resonance imaging or ultrasound imaging of the affected area may also confirm the diagnosis and help delineate the presence of other knee bursitis, calcific tendonitis, tendinopathy, tendonitis, or other knee pathology (Fig. 136.4). Rarely, the inflamed bursa may become infected, and failure to diagnose and treat the acute infection can lead to dire consequences.

## CLINICALLY RELEVANT ANATOMY

There is significant intrapatient variability in the size of the pes anserine bursa. The pes anserine bursa lies between the combined tendinous insertion of the sartorius, gracilis, and semitendinosus muscles and the medial tibia (see Fig. 136.1). The bursa is subject to the development of inflammation after overuse, misuse, or direct trauma. The medial collateral ligament often also is involved if the medial knee has been subjected to trauma. The medial collateral ligament is a broad, flat, band-like ligament that runs from the medial condyle of the femur to the medial aspect of the shaft of the tibia, where it attaches just above the groove of the semimembranosus muscle. It also attaches to the edge of the medial semilunar cartilage. The medial collateral ligament is crossed at its lower part by the tendons of the sartorius, gracilis, and semitendinosus muscles.

## ULTRASOUND-GUIDED TECHNIQUE

The benefits, risks, and alternative treatments are explained to the patient and informed consent is obtained. The patient is then placed in the supine position with the knee slightly flexed and supported by a rolled up towel (Fig. 136.5). The skin overlying the medial knee and medial proximal tibia is then prepped with antiseptic solution. A sterile syringe containing 4.0 mL of 0.25% preservative-free bupivacaine and 40 mg of methylprednisolone is attached to a 1½-inch, 22-gauge needle using strict aseptic technique. A high-frequency linear ultrasound transducer is placed over the medial knee joint space in the oblique longitudinal plane with the superior portion of the ultrasound transducer turned about 20 degrees

# CHAPTER 136  ULTRASOUND-GUIDED INJECTION TECHNIQUE FOR PES ANSERINE BURSITIS PAIN

**FIGURE 136.1.** The pes anserine bursa lies between the combined tendinous insertions of the sartorius, gracilis, and semitendinosus muscles and medial tibia.

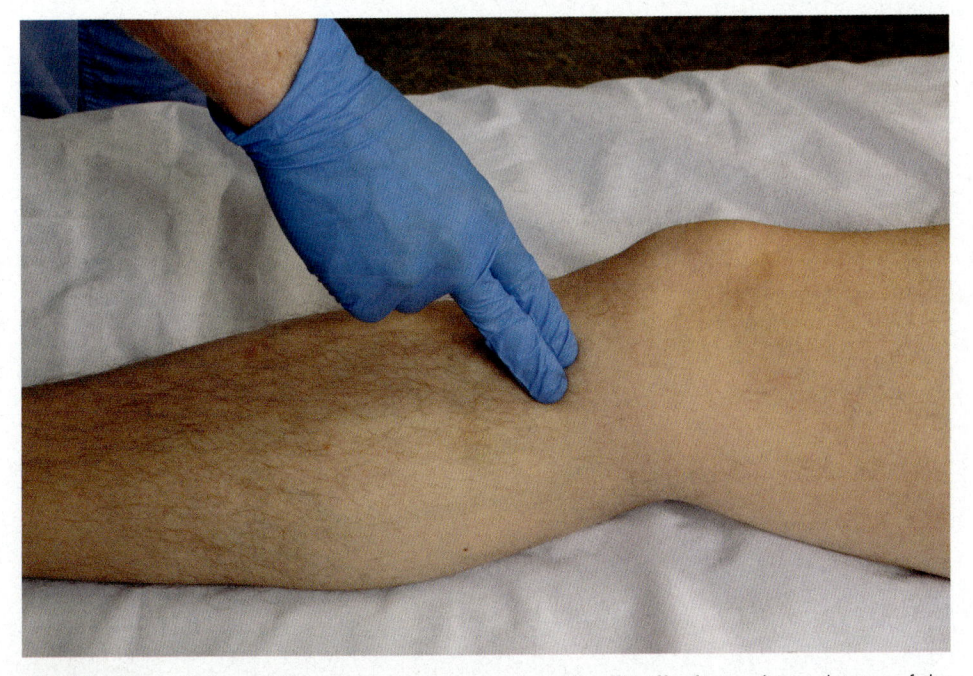

**FIGURE 136.2.** Patients suffering from pes anserine bursitis will suffer from point tenderness of the insertion of the pes anserine tendon.

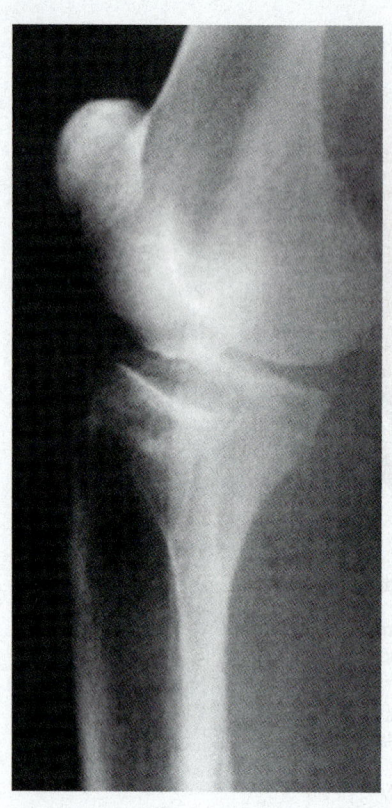

**FIGURE 136.3.** Radiograph demonstrating a depressed *tibial plateau* fracture after an automobile–pedestrian bumper injury. (Reused from Bucholz RW, Heckman JD. *Rockwood & Green's Fractures in Adults.* 5th ed. Philadelphia, PA: Lippincott Williams & Wilkins; 2001, with permission.)

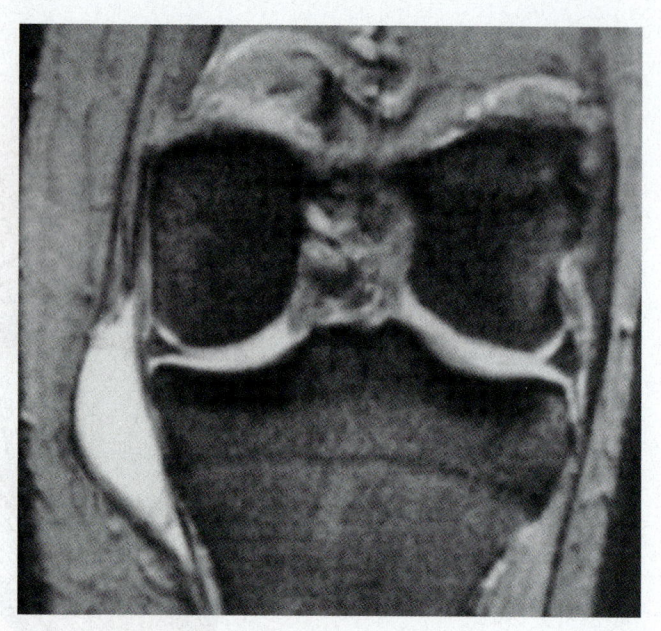

**FIGURE 136.4.** MRI of the knee showing abnormal mass of the proximal medial tibia consistent with pes anserine bursitis. (Reused from Helms CA. *Fundamentals of Diagnostic Radiology.* 3rd ed. Philadelphia, PA: Lippincott Williams & Wilkins; 2007.)

toward the patella (Fig. 136.6). A survey scan is taken, which demonstrates the characteristic appearance of the medial joint space with the hyperechoic medial margins of the femur and the tibia with the thick hyperechoic filaments of the medial collateral ligament overlying the triangular-shaped medial meniscus

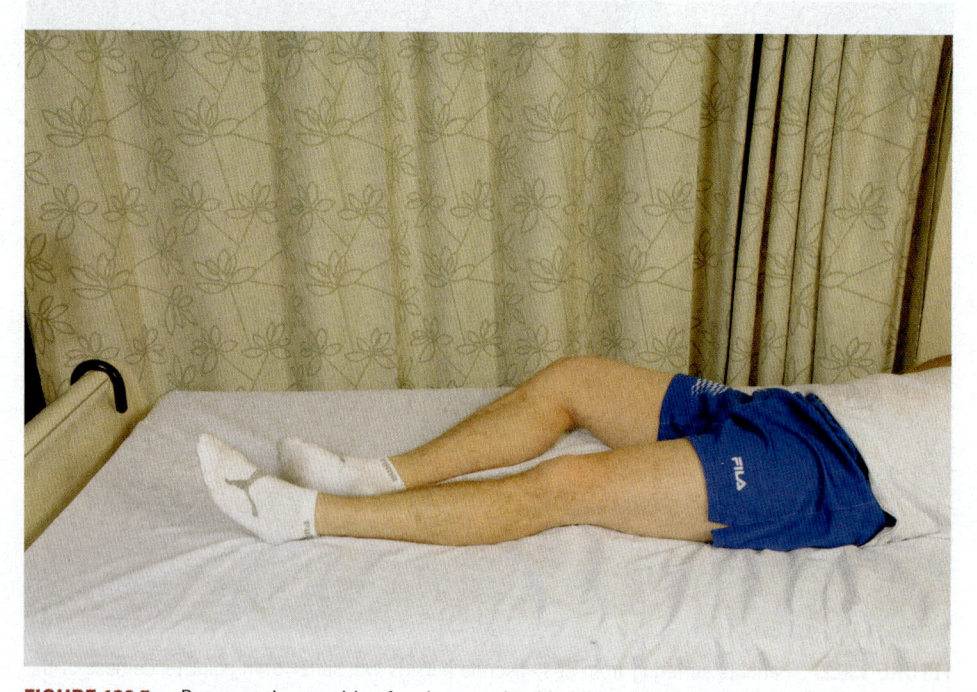

**FIGURE 136.5.** Proper patient position for ultrasound-guided injection of the pes anserine bursa.

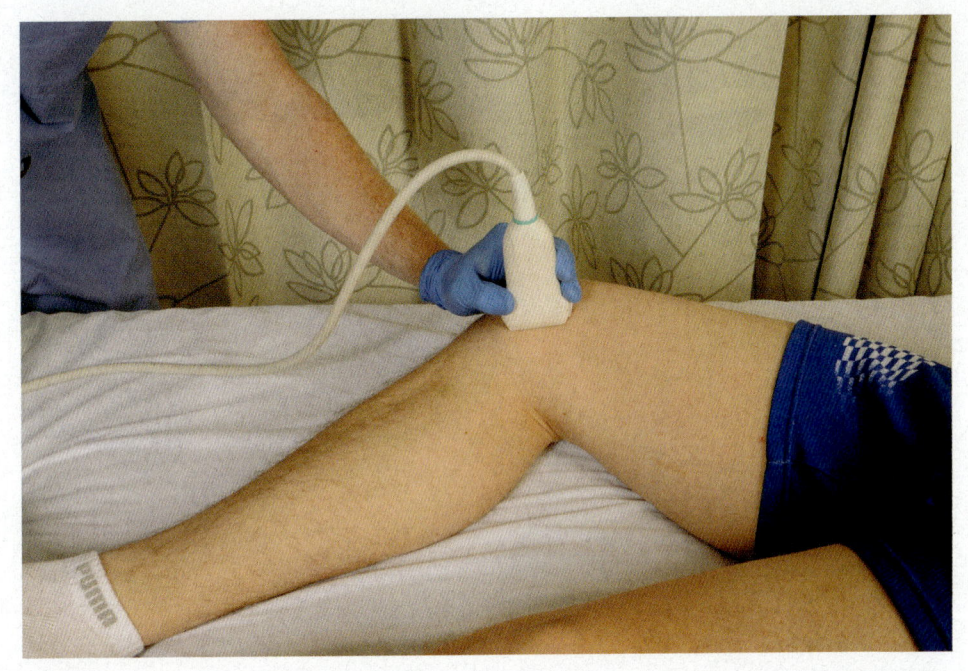

**FIGURE 136.6.** Correct longitudinal position for ultrasound transducer for evaluation of the medial knee joint space.

(Fig. 136.7). The medial meniscus is visualized as a triangular-shaped hyperechoic structure resting between the bony medial margins of the femur and tibia (see Fig. 136.7). After the structures of the medial joint space and proximal tibia are identified, the ultrasound transducer is slowly moved inferiorly while slowly rotating the superior border of the transducer clockwise when imaging the right medial knee and counterclockwise when imaging the medial left knee until the pes anserine tendon is visualized as it is passing over the medial collateral ligament (Figs. 136.8 to 136.10). The pes anserine bursa lies just beneath the pes anserine tendon at this level. When the pes anserine tendon and pes anserine bursa are identified, the needle is placed through the skin ~1 cm above the middle of the superior aspect of the longitudinally placed transducer

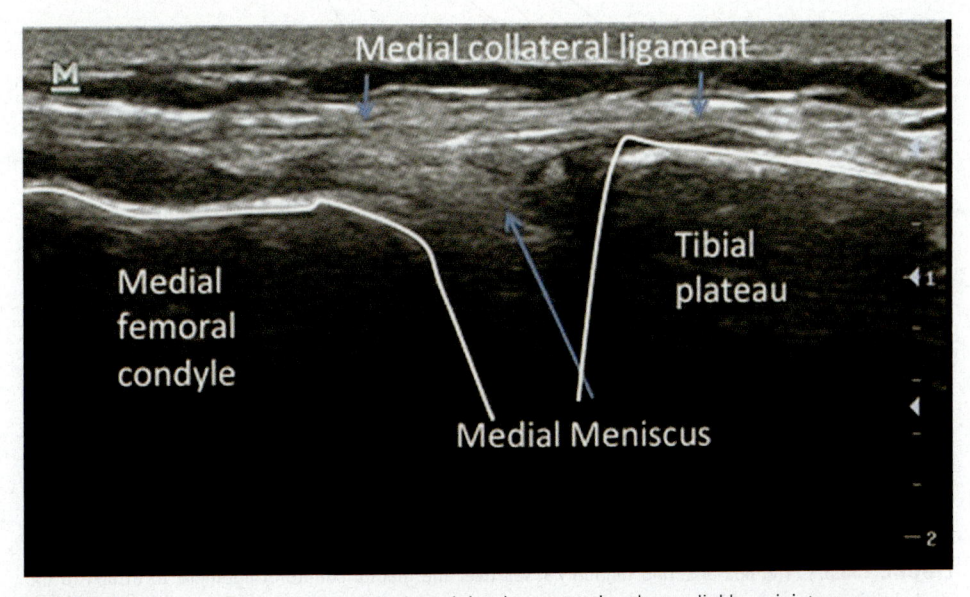

**FIGURE 136.7.** Ultrasound image of the knee joint demonstrating the medial knee joint space.

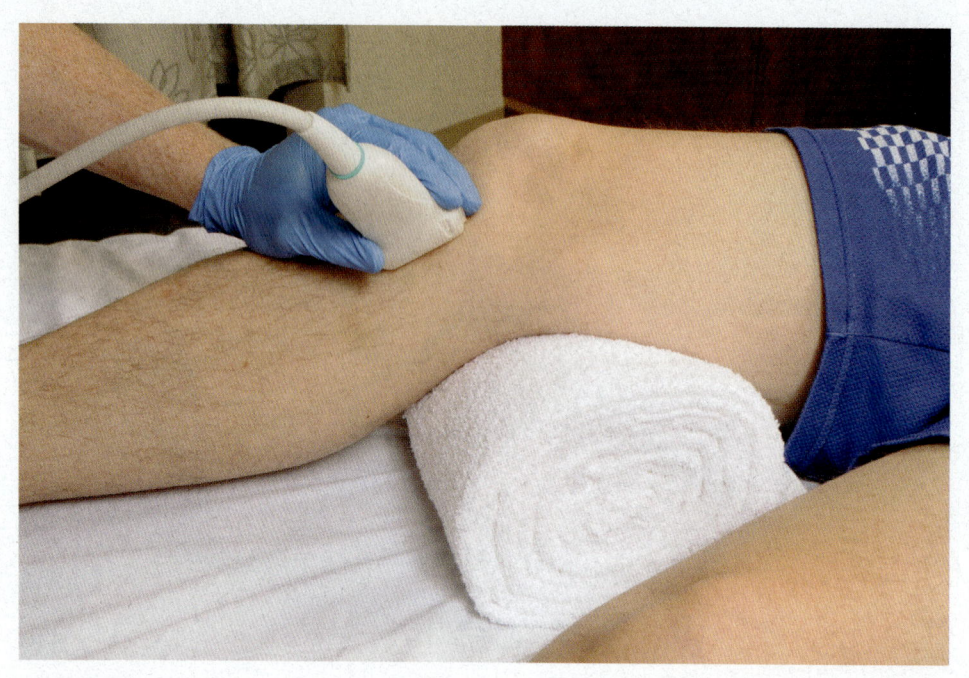

**FIGURE 136.8.** Correct oblique position for ultrasound transducer for ultrasound-guided injection of the pes anserine bursa.

and is then advanced using an out-of-plane approach with the needle trajectory adjusted under real-time ultrasound guidance until the needle tip passes through the pes anserine tendon and lies in between the tendon and the tibia (Fig. 136.11). When the tip of needle is thought to be in satisfactory position, a small amount of local anesthetic and steroid is injected under real-time ultrasound guidance to confirm that the needle tip is outside the substance of the tendon and correctly placed between the tendon and the tibia within the pes anserine bursa. There should be minimal resistance to injection. After needle

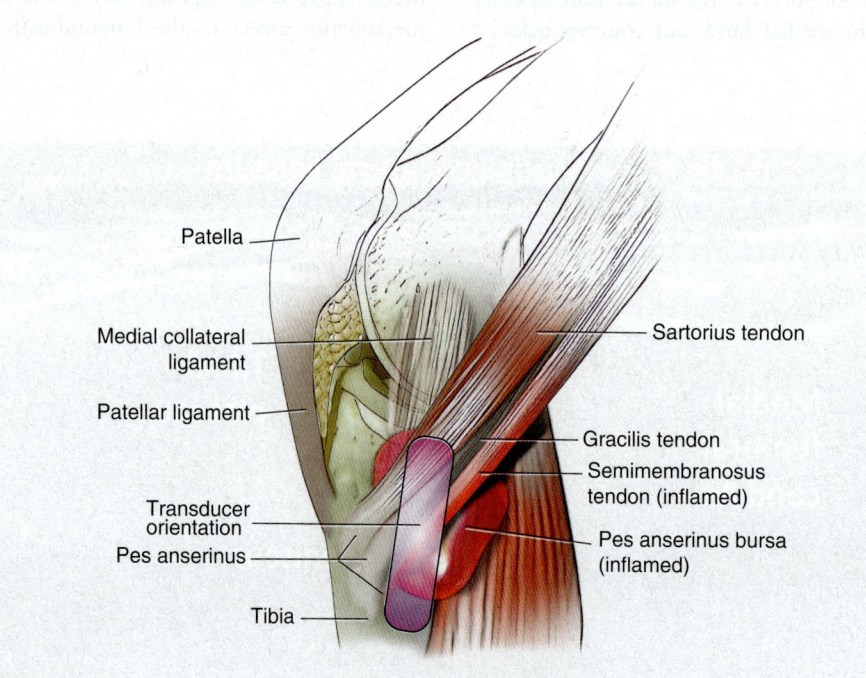

**FIGURE 136.9.** The pes anserine tendon passes over the medial collateral ligament to attach to the medial tibia.

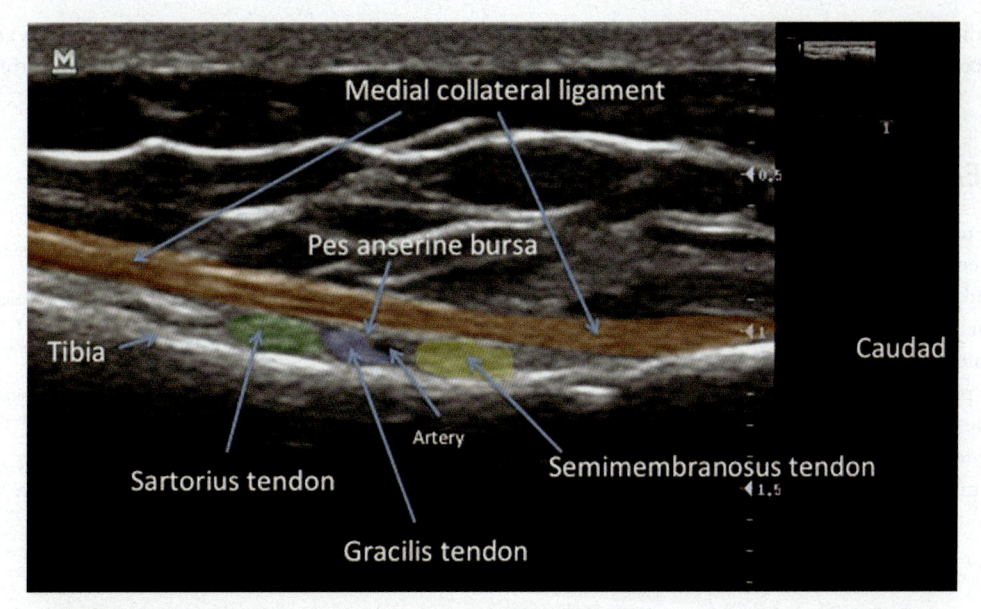

**FIGURE 136.10.** Ultrasound image of the knee joint demonstrating the pes anserine bursa lying beneath the pes anserine tendon.

tip placement is confirmed, the remainder of the contents of the syringe are slowly injected. If synechiae, loculations, or calcifications are present, the needle may have to be repositioned to ensure that the entire intra-articular space is treated. The needle is then removed, and a sterile pressure dressing and ice pack are placed at the injection site.

## COMPLICATIONS

The major complication of ultrasound-guided injection of the pes anserine bursa is infection. Ecchymosis and hematoma formation may also occur. A transient exacerbation of the patient's pain occurs ~25% of the time following this injection

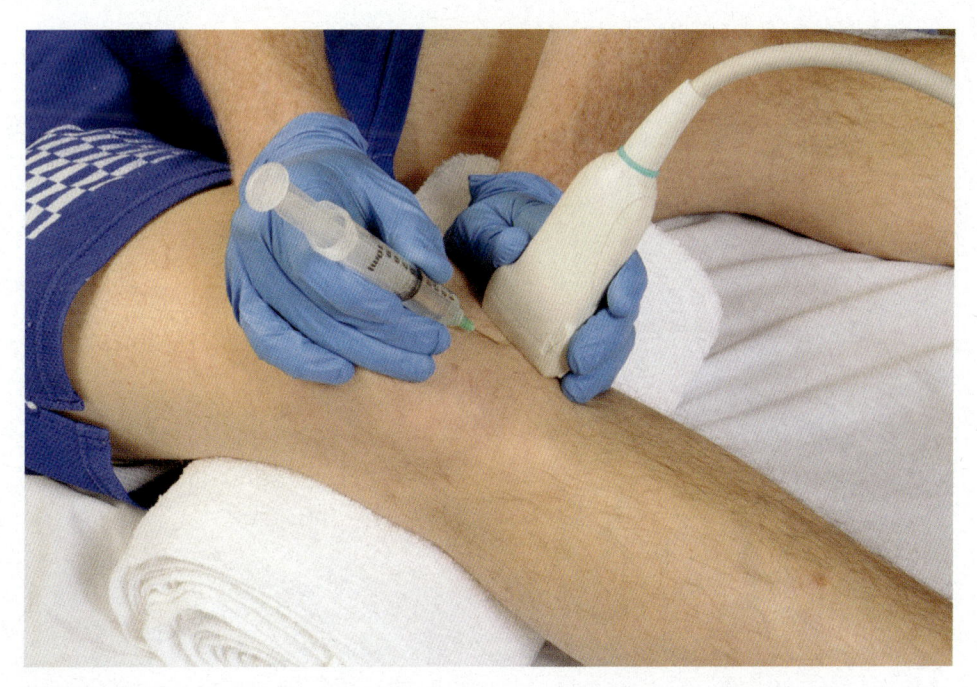

**FIGURE 136.11.** Correct out-of-plane needle placement for ultrasound-guided injection of the pes anserine bursa.

technique, and the patient should be warned of this possibility prior to the procedure.

## CLINICAL PEARLS

Bursitis, labral tears, tendinopathy, osteoarthritis, synovitis, internal derangement, nerve entrapment, avascular necrosis of the knee, and impingement syndromes may coexist with other knee joint disease and may contribute to the patient's pain symptomatology. Universal precautions should always be observed to protect the operator, and strict adherence to sterile technique must be used to avoid infection. Gentle physical therapy and local heat should be introduced following ultrasound-guided injection of the elbow joint to reduce pain and improve function. Simple analgesics and nonsteroidal anti-inflammatory agents or COX-2 inhibitors may be used concurrently with this injection technique.

## SUGGESTED READINGS

Marra MD, Crema MD, Chung M, et al. MRI features of cystic lesions around the knee. *Knee* 2008;15(6):423–438.

Waldman SD. Bursitis syndromes of the knee. In: *Pain Review*. Philadelphia, PA: Saunders Elsevier; 2009:318–322.

Waldman SD. Pes anserine bursitis. In: *Atlas of Uncommon Pain Syndromes*. 2nd ed. Philadelphia, PA: Saunders Elsevier; 2009:290–292.

Wasserman AR, Melville LD, Birkhahn RH. Septic bursitis: a case report and primer for the emergency clinician. [Original Research Article]. The *J Emerg Med* 2009;37(3):269–272.

Waldman SD. Pes anserine bursa injection. In: *Atlas of Pain Management Injection Techniques*. 3rd ed. Philadelphia, PA: Saunders Elsevier; 2012:381–383.

# CHAPTER 137

# Ultrasound-Guided Saphenous Nerve Block at the Knee

## CLINICAL PERSPECTIVES

Ultrasound-guided saphenous nerve block is utilized as a diagnostic and therapeutic maneuver in the evaluation and treatment of distal lower extremity pain thought to be mediated via the saphenous nerve. The most common pain syndrome mediated via the saphenous nerve is a postoperative neuropathy secondary to surgical injuries to the saphenous nerve during vein harvesting procedures for coronary artery bypass surgery or during lower extremity vein stripping procedures. Less commonly, saphenous neuralgia can occur as an isolated mononeuropathy without apparent cause. The symptoms associated with saphenous neuralgia depend on the point at which the nerve is damaged (Fig. 137.1).

Ultrasound-guided saphenous nerve block can also be utilized to provide surgical anesthesia when combined with ultrasound-guided sciatic nerve block for distal lower extremity surgery including distal amputations, debridements, skin grafting procedures, and fracture reductions and fixations. Ultrasound-guided saphenous nerve block with local anesthetics can be employed as a diagnostic maneuver when performing differential neural blockade on an anatomic basis to determine if the patient's distal lower extremity pain is subserved by the saphenous nerve. If destruction of the saphenous nerve is being contemplated, ultrasound-guided saphenous nerve block with local anesthetic can provide prognostic information as to the extent of motor and sensory deficit the patient will experience following nerve destruction.

Ultrasound-guided saphenous nerve block with local anesthetic may also be used to provide postoperative pain relief following distal lower extremity surgeries and is useful in the treatment of persistent postoperative neuropathic pain following vein harvesting and stripping procedures. Electromyography can distinguish saphenous nerve dysfunction from lumbar plexopathy, lumbar radiculopathy, and diabetic polyneuropathy. Plain radiographs of the knee and distal lower extremity are indicated in all patients who present with saphenous neuralgia to rule out occult bony pathology. Based on the patient's clinical presentation, additional testing may be warranted, including a complete blood count, uric acid level, erythrocyte sedimentation rate, and antinuclear antibody testing. Magnetic resonance imaging of the point of suspected nerve compromise is indicated if to clarify the diagnosis or if tumor, infection, or hematoma is suspected (Fig. 137.2). Ultrasound and computerized tomographic scanning are also indicated if mass or tumor is suspected or if the cause of saphenous nerve compromise is in question. The injection technique described later serves as both a diagnostic and a therapeutic maneuver.

## CLINICALLY RELEVANT ANATOMY

The saphenous nerve is the largest sensory branch of the femoral nerve. The saphenous nerve provides sensory innervation to the medial malleolus, the medial calf, and a portion of the medial arch of the foot. The saphenous nerve is derived primarily from the fibers of the L3 and L4 nerve roots. The nerve travels along with the femoral artery through Hunter canal and moves superficially as it approaches the knee (Fig. 137.3). It passes over the medial condyle of the femur, splitting into terminal sensory branches. The saphenous nerve is subject to trauma or compression anywhere along its course. The nerve is frequently traumatized during vein harvest for coronary artery bypass grafting procedures. The saphenous nerve is also subject to compression as it passes over the medial condyle of the femur.

## ULTRASOUND-GUIDED TECHNIQUE

Ultrasound-guided block of the saphenous nerve at the knee can be carried out by placing the patient in the supine position with the arms resting comfortably across the chest and the affected lower extremity externally rotated (Fig. 137.4). A total of 8 mL of local anesthetic is drawn up in a 12-mL sterile syringe. If the painful condition being treated is thought to have an inflammatory component, 40 to 80 mg of depot steroid is added to the local anesthetic. A point ~5 cm above the patella on the anteromedial femur is then identified by palpation (Fig. 137.5). A linear high-frequency ultrasound transducer is placed in a transverse plane over the previously identified point on the anteromedial femur, and an ultrasound survey scan is obtained (Figs. 137.6 and 137.7). The hyperechoic anterior medial border of the femur will be visualized as well as the vastus medialis muscle just anteromedial to it. The ultrasound transducer is then slowly moved in a more medial direction until the sartorius muscle, which lies posteromedial

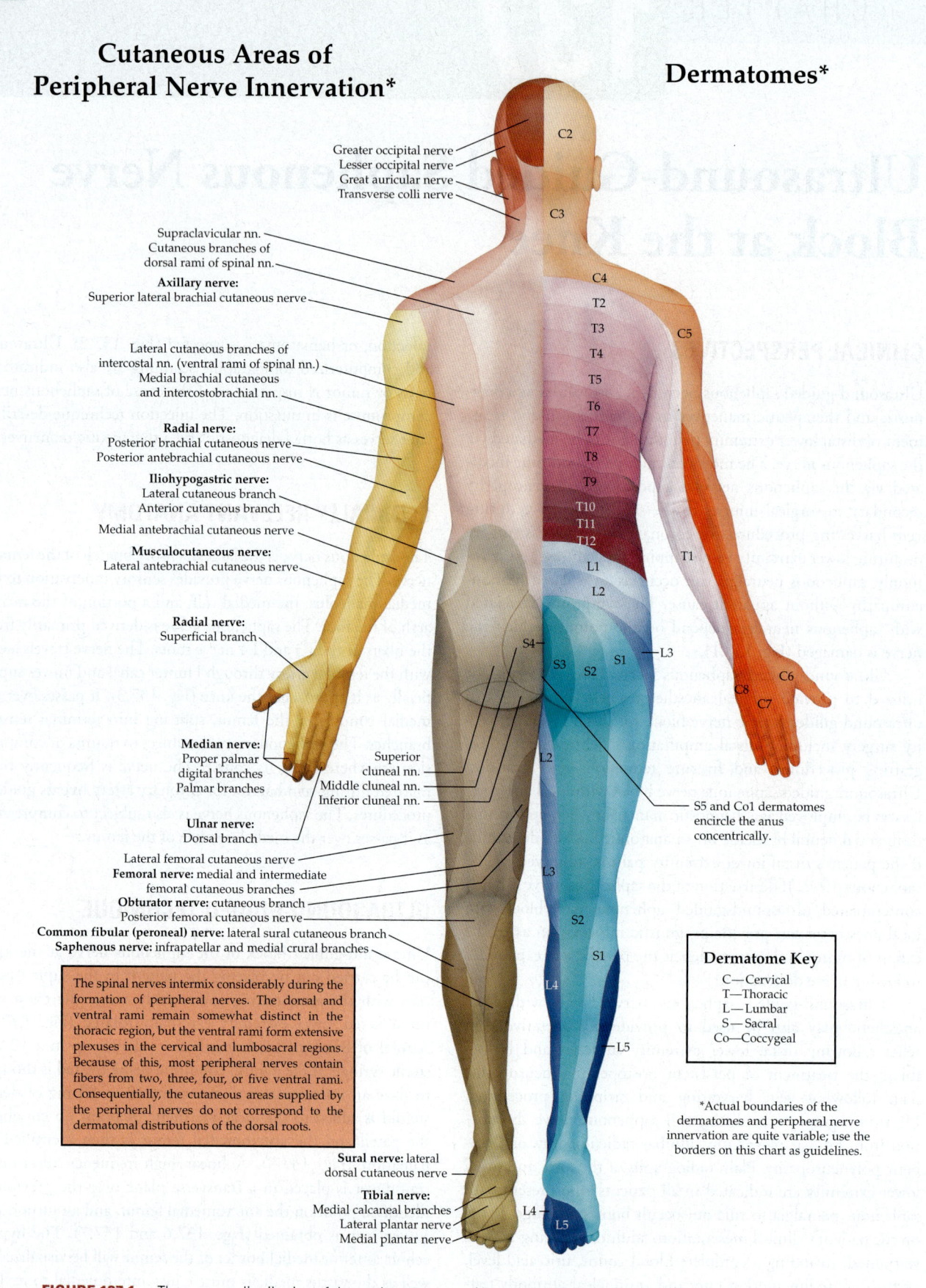

## Cutaneous Areas of Peripheral Nerve Innervation*

## Dermatomes*

- Greater occipital nerve
- Lesser occipital nerve
- Great auricular nerve
- Transverse colli nerve
- Supraclavicular nn.
- Cutaneous branches of dorsal rami of spinal nn.
- **Axillary nerve:** Superior lateral brachial cutaneous nerve
- Lateral cutaneous branches of intercostal nn. (ventral rami of spinal nn.)
- Medial brachial cutaneous and intercostobrachial nn.
- **Radial nerve:** Posterior brachial cutaneous nerve; Posterior antebrachial cutaneous nerve
- **Iliohypogastric nerve:** Lateral cutaneous branch; Anterior cutaneous branch
- Medial antebrachial cutaneous nerve
- **Musculocutaneous nerve:** Lateral antebrachial cutaneous nerve
- **Radial nerve:** Superficial branch
- **Median nerve:** Proper palmar digital branches; Palmar branches
- Superior cluneal nn.
- Middle cluneal nn.
- Inferior cluneal nn.
- **Ulnar nerve:** Dorsal branch
- Lateral femoral cutaneous nerve
- **Femoral nerve:** medial and intermediate femoral cutaneous branches
- **Obturator nerve:** cutaneous branch
- Posterior femoral cutaneous nerve
- **Common fibular (peroneal) nerve:** lateral sural cutaneous branch
- **Saphenous nerve:** infrapatellar and medial crural branches
- **Sural nerve:** lateral dorsal cutaneous nerve
- **Tibial nerve:** Medial calcaneal branches; Lateral plantar nerve; Medial plantar nerve
- S5 and Co1 dermatomes encircle the anus concentrically.

The spinal nerves intermix considerably during the formation of peripheral nerves. The dorsal and ventral rami remain somewhat distinct in the thoracic region, but the ventral rami form extensive plexuses in the cervical and lumbosacral regions. Because of this, most peripheral nerves contain fibers from two, three, four, or five ventral rami. Consequentially, the cutaneous areas supplied by the peripheral nerves do not correspond to the dermatomal distributions of the dorsal roots.

**Dermatome Key**
C—Cervical
T—Thoracic
L—Lumbar
S—Sacral
Co—Coccygeal

*Actual boundaries of the dermatomes and peripheral nerve innervation are quite variable; use the borders on this chart as guidelines.

**FIGURE 137.1.** The sensory distribution of the saphenous nerve. (Anatomical Chart Company, 2013.)

CHAPTER 137 ULTRASOUND-GUIDED SAPHENOUS NERVE BLOCK AT THE KNEE 975

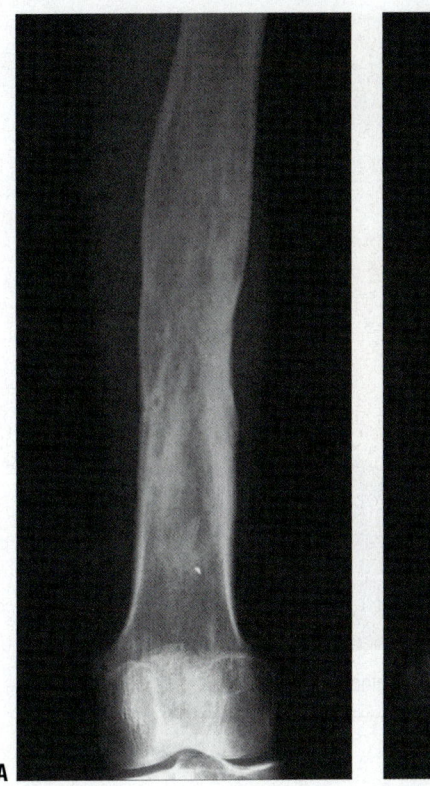

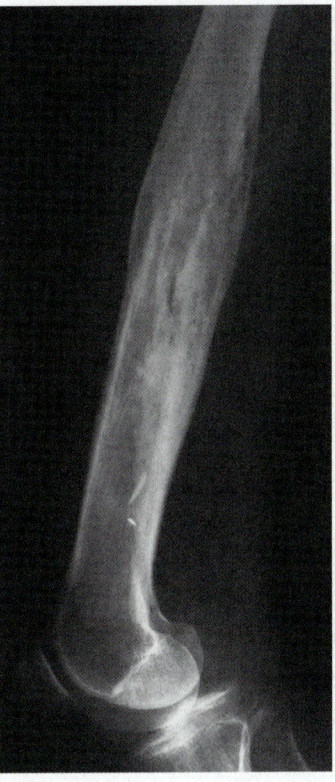

**FIGURE 137.2.** Anteroposterior and lateral radiographs of a patient with osteomyelitis of the femur. **A:** PA view. **B:** Lateral view. (Reused with permission from Berquist TH. *MRI of the Musculoskeletal System*. 6th ed. Philadelphia, PA: Lippincott Williams & Wilkins; 2013; with permission.)

to vastus medialis muscle, is visualized (Fig. 137.8). The saphenous nerve lies just in the fascial plane just below the sartorius muscle (Fig. 137.9). When the fascial plane below the sartorius muscle is identified on ultrasound imaging, the skin is prepped with anesthetic solution, and a 3½-inch, 22-gauge needle is advanced from the lateral border of the ultrasound transducer and advanced utilizing an in-plane approach with the trajectory being adjusted under real-time ultrasound guidance until the needle tip is resting within the facial plane beneath the sartorius muscle in proximity to the saphenous nerve (Fig. 137.10). When the tip of needle is thought to be in satisfactory position, a small amount of local anesthetic and steroid is injected under real-time ultrasound guidance to confirm that the needle tip is correctly beneath the sartorius muscle in proximity to the saphenous nerve. There should be minimal resistance to injection. After needle tip placement is confirmed, the remainder of the contents of the syringe are slowly injected. The needle is then removed, and a sterile pressure dressing and ice pack are placed at the injection site.

## COMPLICATIONS

A failure to accurately assess the correct position of the needle tip when performing ultrasound-guided saphenous nerve block can lead to a failure to block the saphenous nerve. The use of ultrasound guidance when performing saphenous nerve block should markedly decrease this problem. Postblock ecchymosis and hematoma may occur, and the patient should be warned

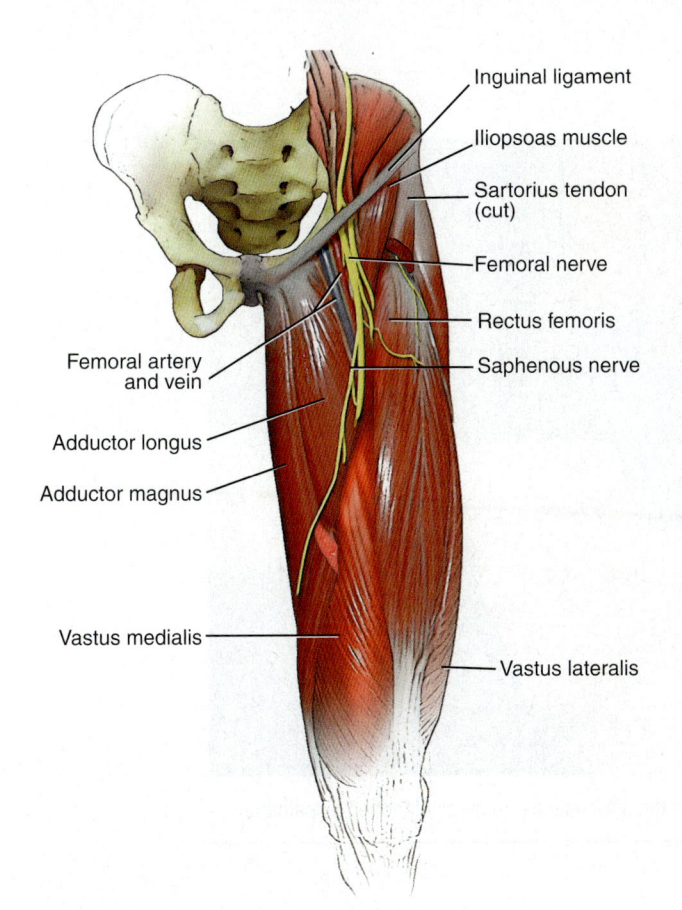

**FIGURE 137.3.** The anatomy of the saphenous nerve.

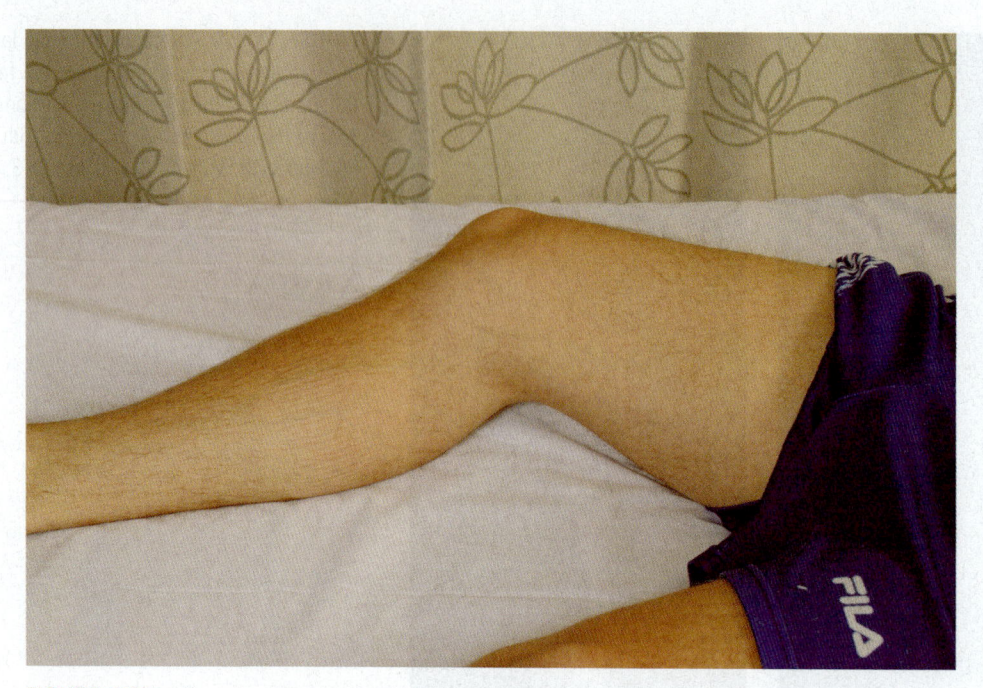

**FIGURE 137.4.** Proper patient position for ultrasound-guided saphenous nerve block.

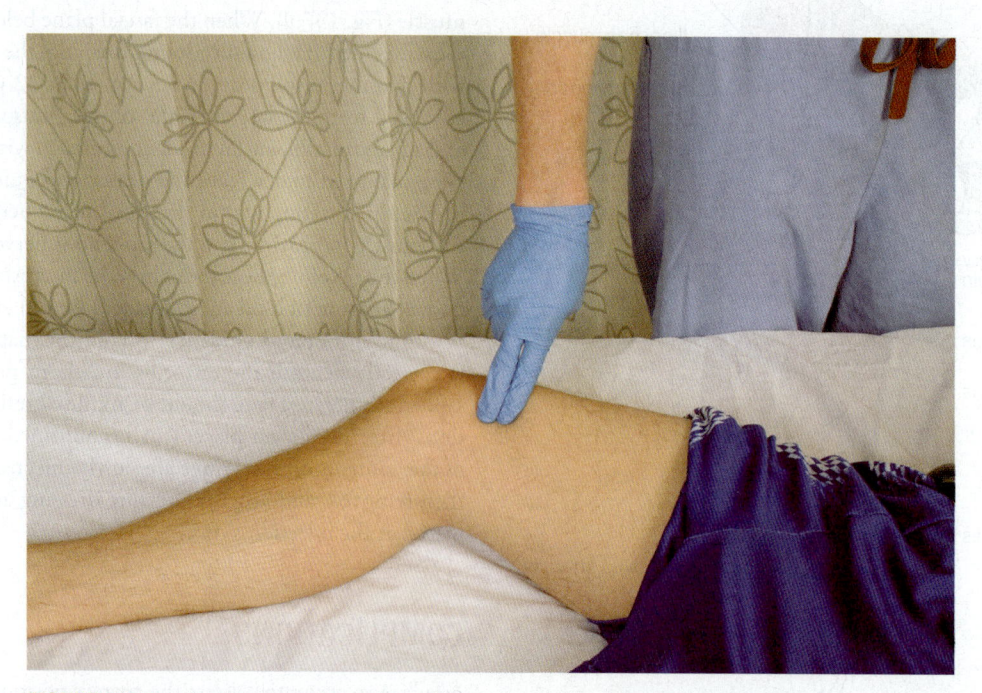

**FIGURE 137.5.** A point ~5 cm above the patella on the anteromedial femur is identified by palpation.

CHAPTER 137    ULTRASOUND-GUIDED SAPHENOUS NERVE BLOCK AT THE KNEE    977

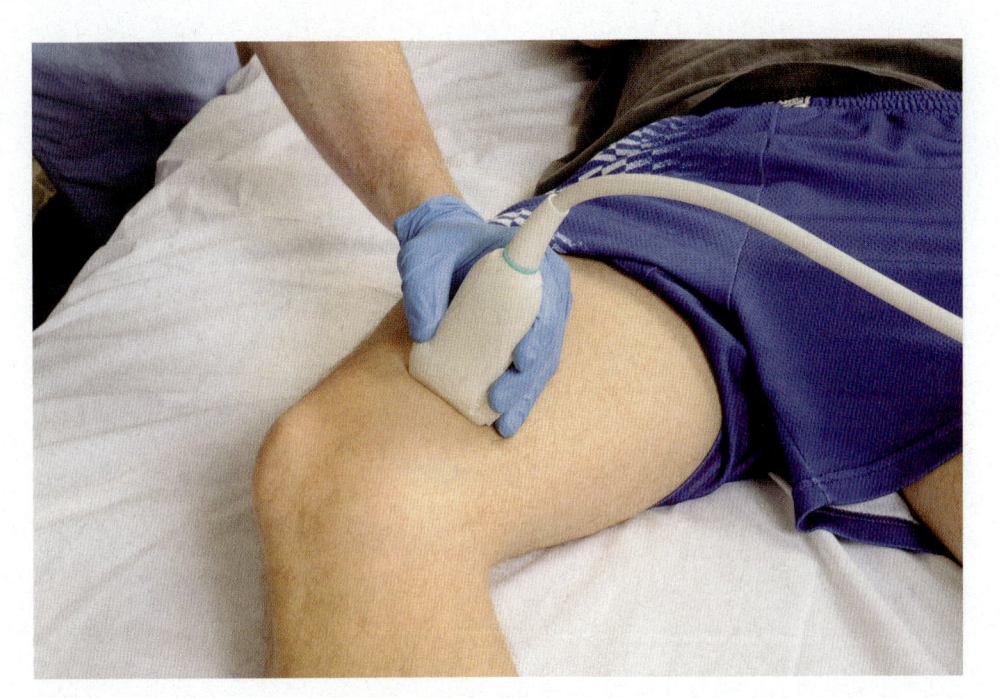

**FIGURE 137.6.** Proper transverse position of the ultrasound transducer for ultrasound-guided saphenous nerve block at the knee.

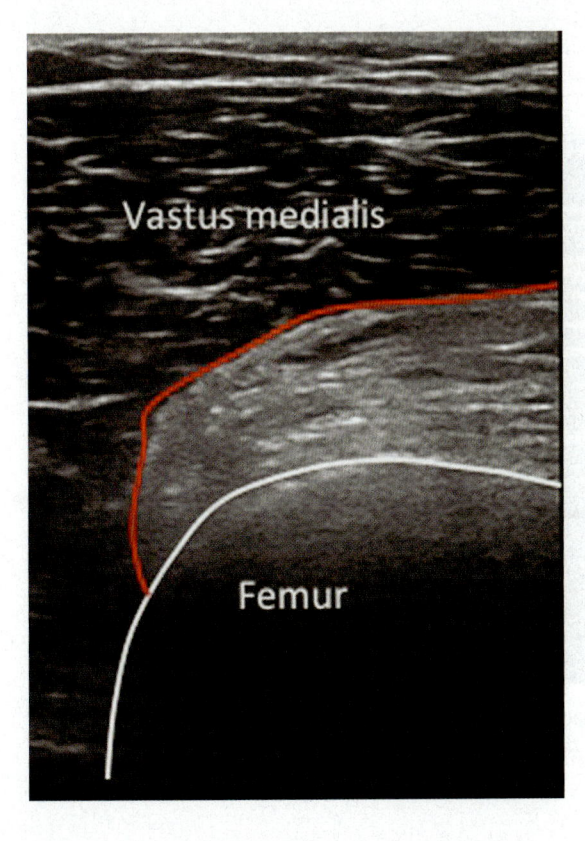

**FIGURE 137.7.** Transverse ultrasound image demonstrating the vastus medialis lying above the anteromedial femur.

**FIGURE 137.8.** The transversely placed ultrasound transducer is moved medially to identify the sartorius muscle and the saphenous nerve beneath it.

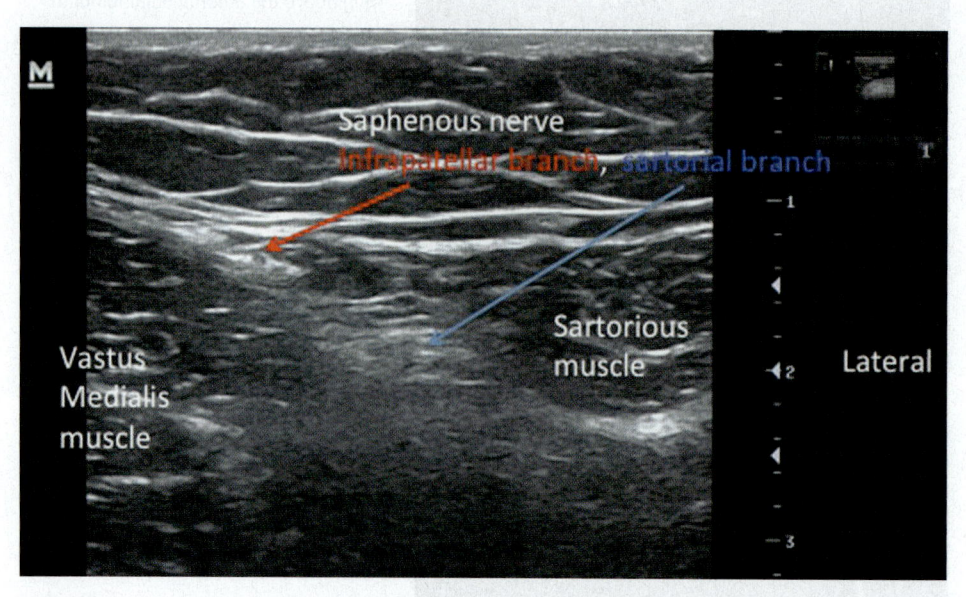

**FIGURE 137.9.** Transverse ultrasound image demonstrating the sartorius muscle.

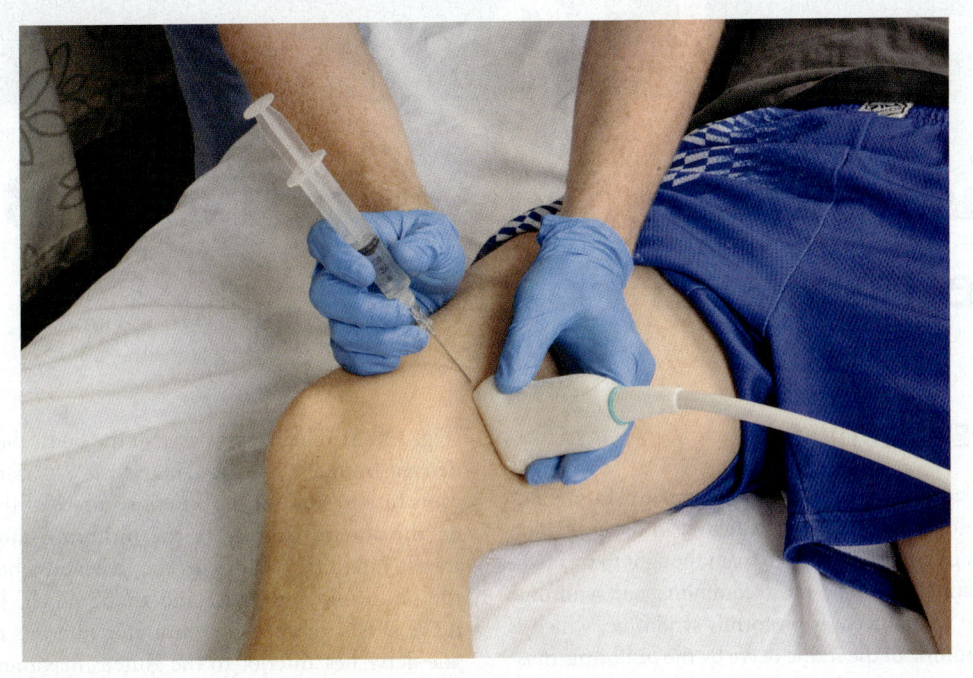

**FIGURE 137.10.** Proper in-plane needle position for performing saphenous nerve block.

of such. These complications can be decreased by the use of a pressure dressing and cold packs applied to the injection site following the procedure.

## CLINICAL PEARLS

The key to performing successful ultrasound saphenous nerve block is the proper identification of the sonographic anatomy and in particular the ability to properly identify the sartorius muscle. This should not be a problem if the above technique is used. Any significant pain or sudden increase in resistance during injection when performing ultrasound-guided suggests incorrect needle placement, and one should stop injecting immediately and reassess the position of the needle.

## SUGGESTED READINGS

Damarey B, Demondion X, Wavreille G, et al. Imaging of the nerves of the knee region. *Eur J Radiol* 2013;82(1):27–37.

Krombach J, Gray AT. Sonography for saphenous nerve block near the adductor canal. *Reg Anesth Pain Med* 2007;32(4):369–370.

Sakura S, Hara K. Using ultrasound guidance in peripheral nerve blocks. *Trends Anaesth Crit Care* 2012;2(6):274–280.

Waldman SD. Saphenous nerve block. In: *Atlas of Interventional Pain Management*. 3rd ed. Philadelphia, PA: Saunders Elsevier; 2009:551–554.

# CHAPTER 138

# Ultrasound-Guided Sciatic Nerve Block at the Popliteal Fossa

## CLINICAL PERSPECTIVES

Ultrasound-guided sciatic nerve block at the popliteal fossa is utilized as a diagnostic and therapeutic maneuver in the evaluation and treatment of distal lower extremity pain thought to be mediated via the sciatic nerve. The most common pain syndrome mediated via the sciatic nerve is piriformis syndrome, which is caused by compromise of the sciatic nerve by the piriformis muscle. The symptoms associated with sciatic neuralgia depend on the point at which the nerve is compromised (Fig. 138.1).

Ultrasound-guided sciatic nerve block at the popliteal fossa can be used for surgical anesthesia for distal lower extremity surgery when combined with lateral femoral cutaneous, femoral, saphenous, and obturator nerve block or lumbar plexus block. Ultrasound-guided sciatic nerve block at the hip with local anesthetic may be used to palliate acute pain emergencies, including postoperative pain, pain secondary to traumatic injuries of the lower extremity, and cancer pain, while waiting for pharmacologic, surgical, and antiblastic methods to become effective.

Ultrasound-guided sciatic nerve block at the popliteal fossa can also be used as a diagnostic tool when performing differential neural blockade on an anatomic basis in the evaluation of lower extremity pain as well as in a prognostic manner to determine the degree of neurologic impairment the patient will suffer when destruction of the sciatic nerve is being considered or when there is a possibility that the nerve may be sacrificed during surgeries in the anatomic region of the sciatic nerve at the level of the popliteal fossa.

Electrodiagnostic testing should be considered in all patients who suffer from sciatic nerve dysfunction to provide both neuroanatomic and neurophysiologic information regarding nerve function. Magnetic resonance imaging and ultrasound imaging of the popliteal fossa as well as anywhere along the course of the sciatic nerve are also useful in determining the cause of sciatic nerve compromise (Fig. 138.2).

## CLINICALLY RELEVANT ANATOMY

The sciatic nerve provides innervation to the distal lower extremity and foot with the exception of the medial aspect of the calf and foot, which are subserved by the saphenous nerve (Fig. 138.3). The largest nerve in the body, the sciatic nerve, is derived from the L4, the L5, and the S1–S3 nerve roots. The roots fuse in front of the anterior surface of the lateral sacrum on the anterior surface of the piriformis muscle. The nerve travels inferiorly and leaves the pelvis just below or through the piriformis muscle via the sciatic notch. Just beneath the nerve at this point is the obturator internus muscle. The sciatic nerve lies anterior to the gluteus maximus muscle; at this muscle's lower border, the sciatic nerve lies halfway between the greater trochanter and the ischial tuberosity. The sciatic nerve courses downward past the lesser trochanter to lie posterior and medial to the femur. In the midthigh, the nerve gives off branches to the hamstring muscles and the adductor magnus muscle. In most patients, the nerve divides to form the tibial and common peroneal nerves in the upper portion of the popliteal fossa, although in some patients these nerves can remain separate through their entire course (see Fig. 138.3). The tibial nerve continues downward to provide innervation to the distal lower extremity, whereas the common peroneal nerve travels laterally to innervate a portion of the knee joint and, via its lateral cutaneous branch, provide sensory innervation to the back and lateral side of the upper calf.

## ULTRASOUND-GUIDED TECHNIQUE

Ultrasound-guided block of the sciatic nerve at the knee can be carried out by placing the patient in the prone position with the arms resting comfortably along the patient's side (Fig. 138.4). A total of 8 mL of local anesthetic is drawn up in a 12-mL sterile syringe. If the painful condition being treated is thought to have an inflammatory component, 40 to 80 mg of depot steroid is added to the local anesthetic. A linear high-frequency ultrasound transducer is placed in a transverse plane ~8 cm above the popliteal crease, and an ultrasound survey scan is obtained (Fig. 138.5). The pulsating popliteal artery should be visualized toward the bottom of the image, with the popliteal vein lying just lateral to the artery (Fig. 138.6). Just superficial and slightly lateral to the popliteal vein is the sciatic nerve, which will appear as a bright hyperechoic structure (see Fig. 138.6). Compression of the popliteal vein with pressure on the ultrasound transducer can aid in identification of the sciatic nerve, which lies just superficial to the vein (Fig. 138.7). Color Doppler can be utilized to

CHAPTER 138   ULTRASOUND-GUIDED SCIATIC NERVE BLOCK AT THE POPLITEAL FOSSA   981

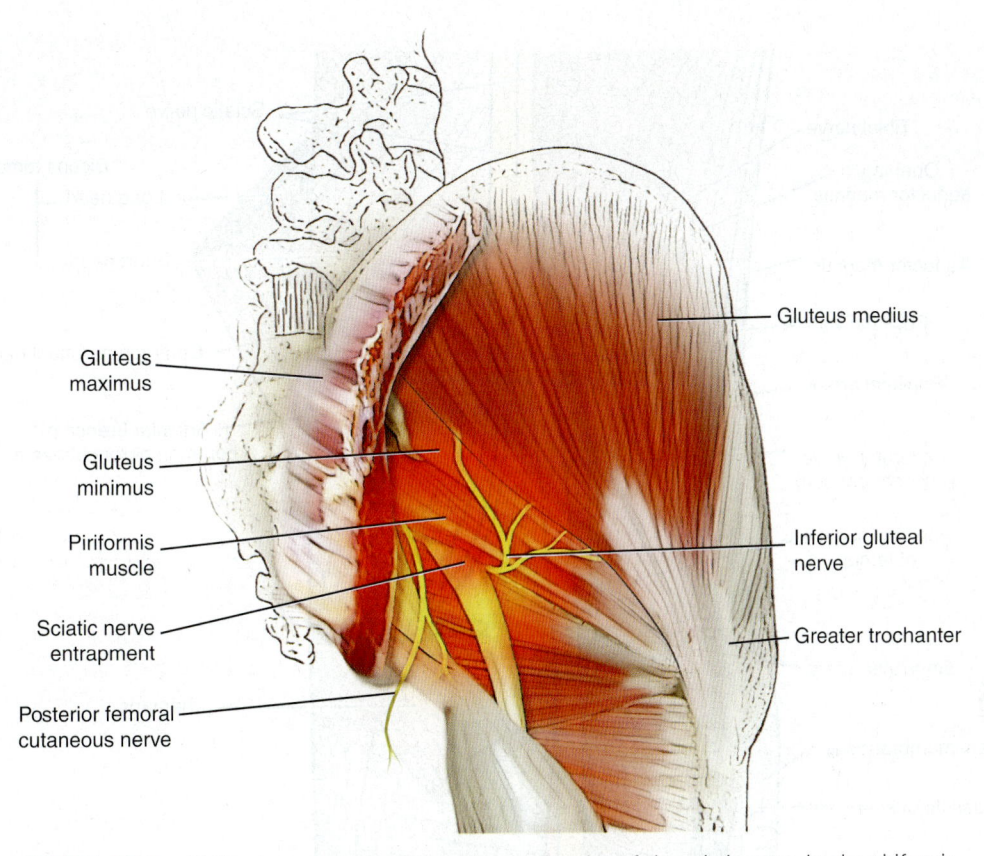

**FIGURE 138.1.** Piriformis syndrome is caused by compression of the sciatic nerve by the piriformis muscle.

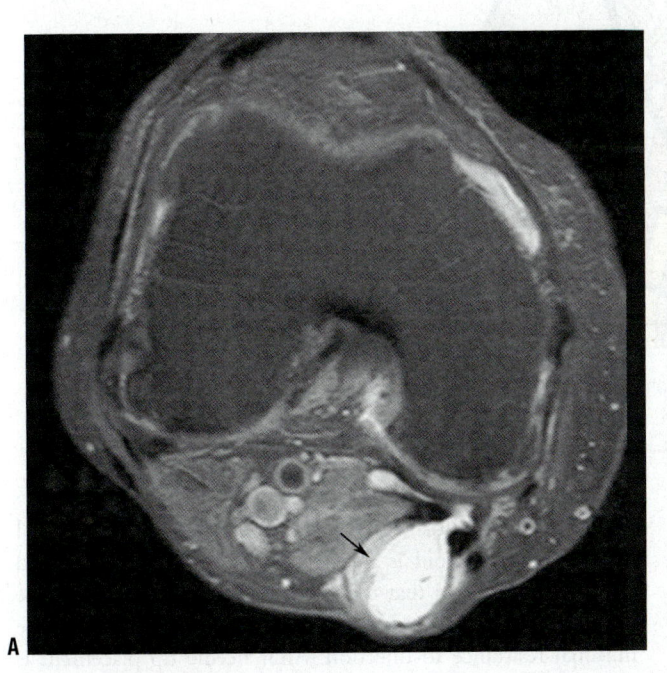

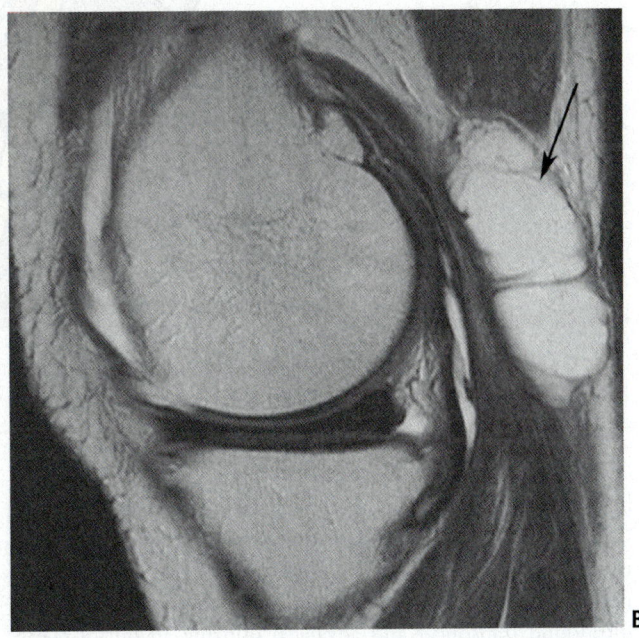

**FIGURE 138.2.** Axial and sagittal MRI images demonstrating popliteal cyst (*arrows*). (Reused from Berquist TH. *MRI of the Musculoskeletal System*. 6th ed. Philadelphia, PA: Lippincott Williams & Wilkins; 2013, with permission.)

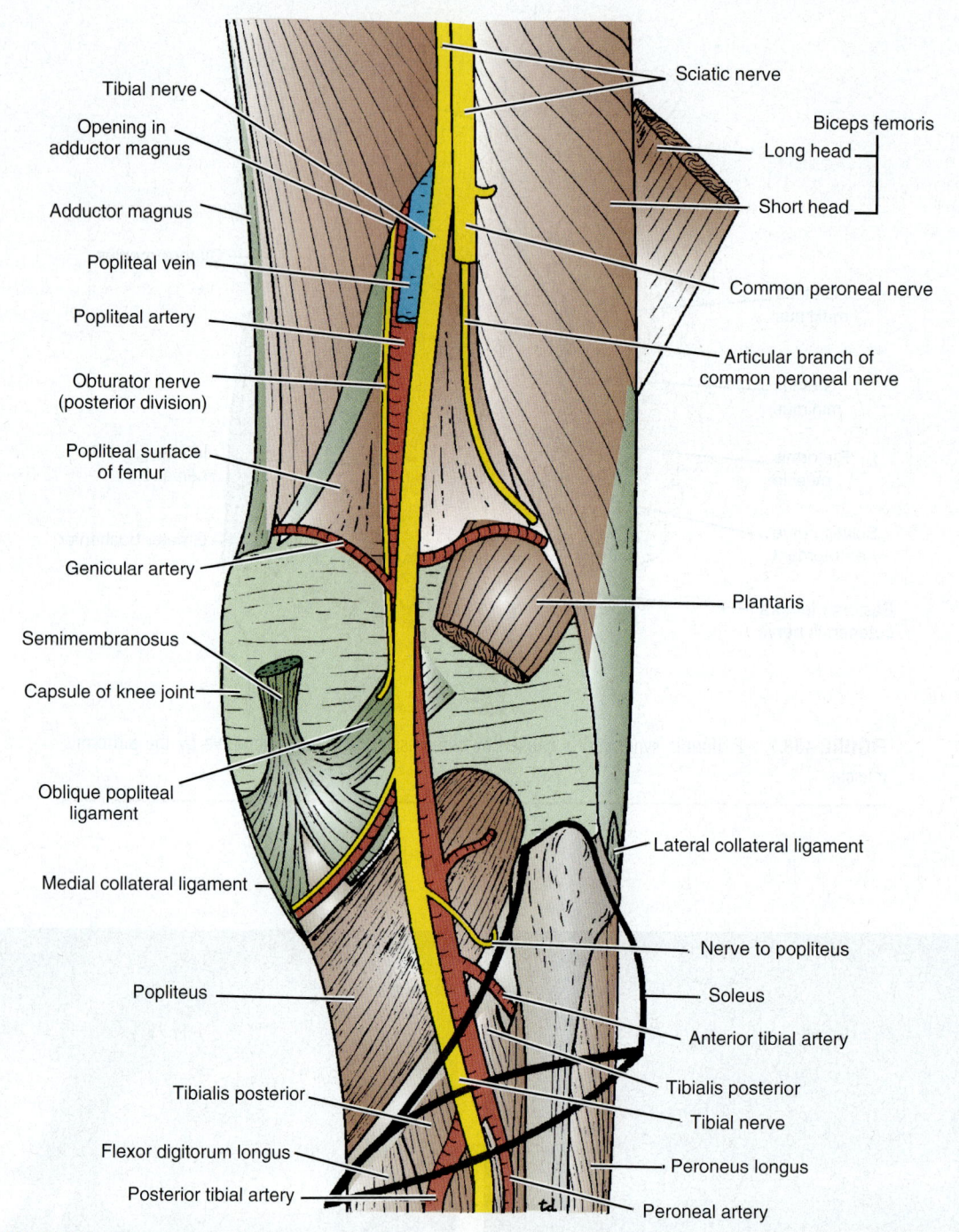

**FIGURE 138.3.** The anatomy of the sciatic nerve. (Reused from Snell RS. *Clinical Anatomy by Regions*. 8th ed. Philadelphia, PA: Lippincott Williams & Wilkins; 2008, with permission.)

help identify the popliteal artery and vein (Fig. 138.8). When the sciatic nerve is identified on ultrasound imaging, the skin is prepped with anesthetic solution, and a 3½-inch, 22-gauge needle is advanced from the middle of the inferior border of the ultrasound transducer and advanced utilizing an out-of-plane approach with the trajectory being adjusted under real-time ultrasound guidance until the needle tip is resting in proximity to the sciatic nerve (Fig. 138.9). When the tip of needle is thought to be in satisfactory position, a small amount of local anesthetic and steroid is injected under real-time ultrasound guidance to confirm that the needle tip is in proximity to the sciatic nerve, but not within the nerve itself. There should be minimal resistance to injection. After needle tip placement is confirmed, the remainder of the contents of the syringe are slowly injected. The needle is then removed, and a sterile pressure dressing and ice pack are placed at the injection site.

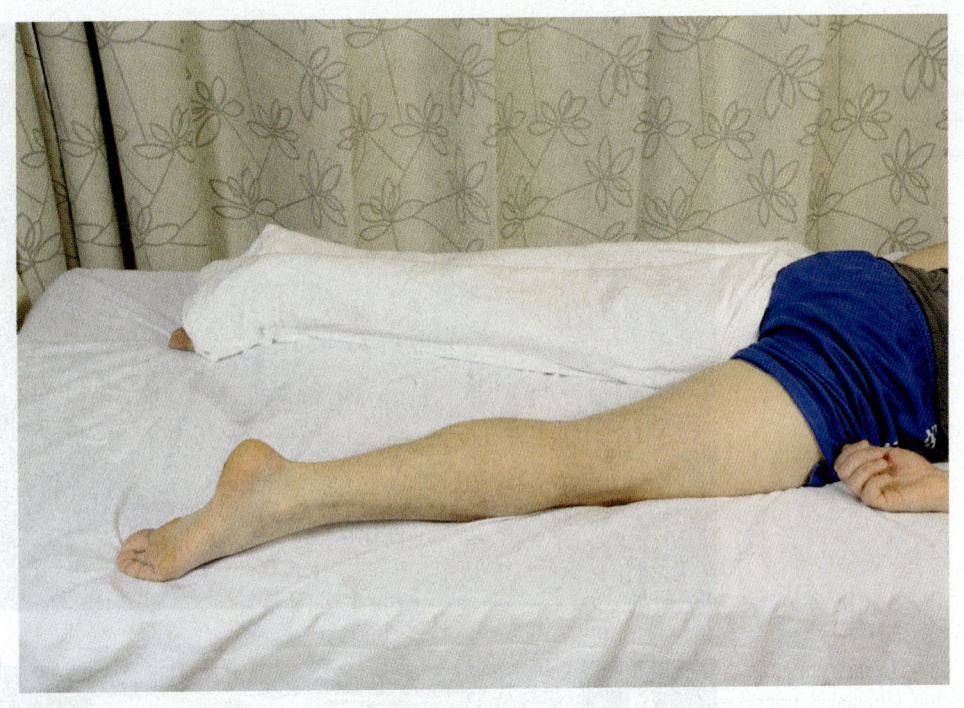

**FIGURE 138.4.** Proper patient position for ultrasound-guided sciatic nerve block.

## COMPLICATIONS

A failure to accurately assess the correct position of the needle tip when performing ultrasound-guided sciatic nerve block at the popliteal fossa can lead to a failure to block the sciatic nerve or needle-induced trauma to the sciatic nerve, popliteal artery, and/or vein. The use of ultrasound guidance when performing sciatic nerve block at the popliteal fossa should markedly decrease these problems. Postblock ecchymosis and hematoma may occur, and the patient should be warned of such. These complications can be decreased by the use of a pressure dressing and cold packs applied to the injection site following the procedure.

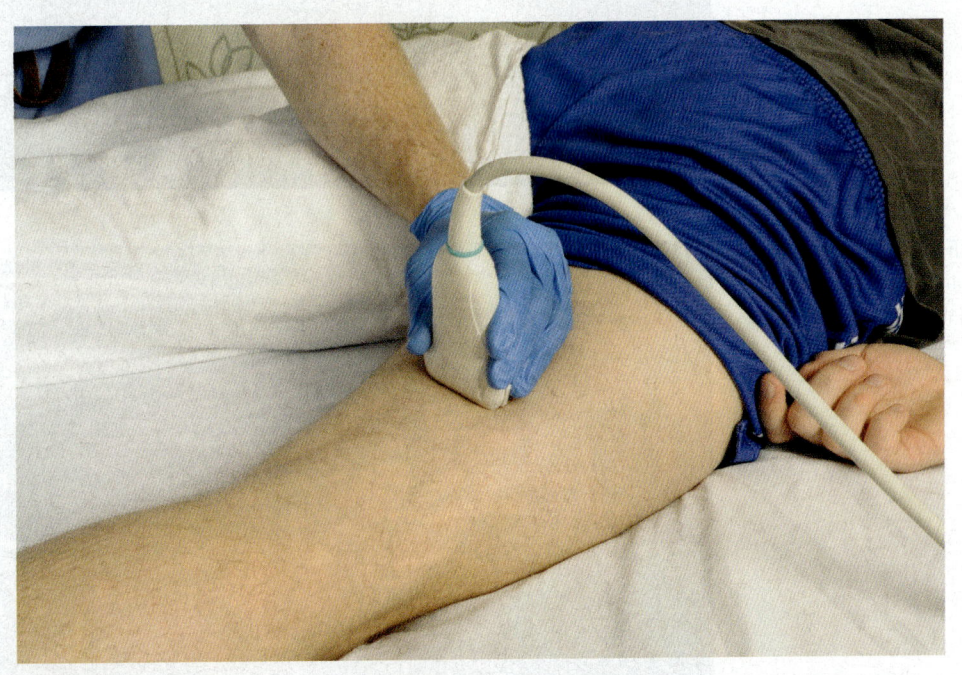

**FIGURE 138.5.** Proper transverse position of the ultrasound transducer ~8 cm above the popliteal crease for ultrasound-guided sciatic nerve block at the popliteal fossa.

**FIGURE 138.6.** Transverse ultrasound image demonstrating the popliteal artery and vein and the sciatic nerve just superficial and lateral to the popliteal vein.

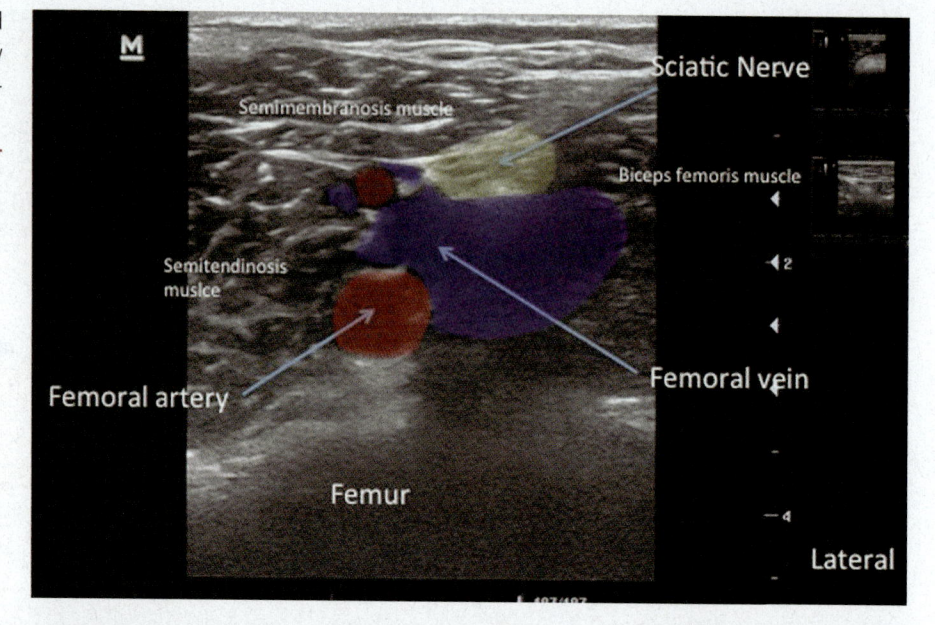

**FIGURE 138.7.** Compression of the popliteal vein with the ultrasound transducer can aid in identification of the sciatic nerve, which is just lateral and superficial to the vein.

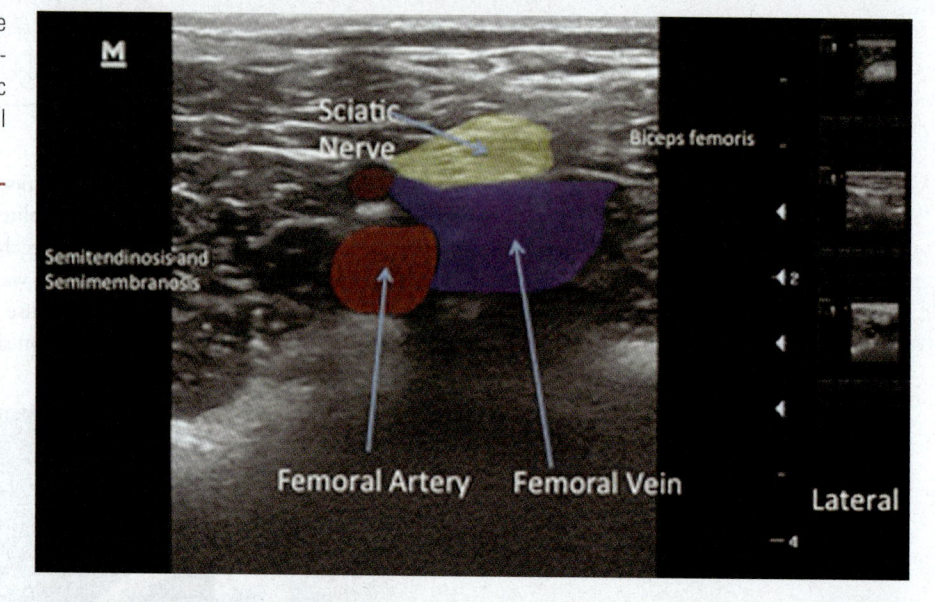

**FIGURE 138.8.** Transverse color Doppler image demonstrating the popliteal vein and artery and the relationship of the vein to the sciatic nerve.

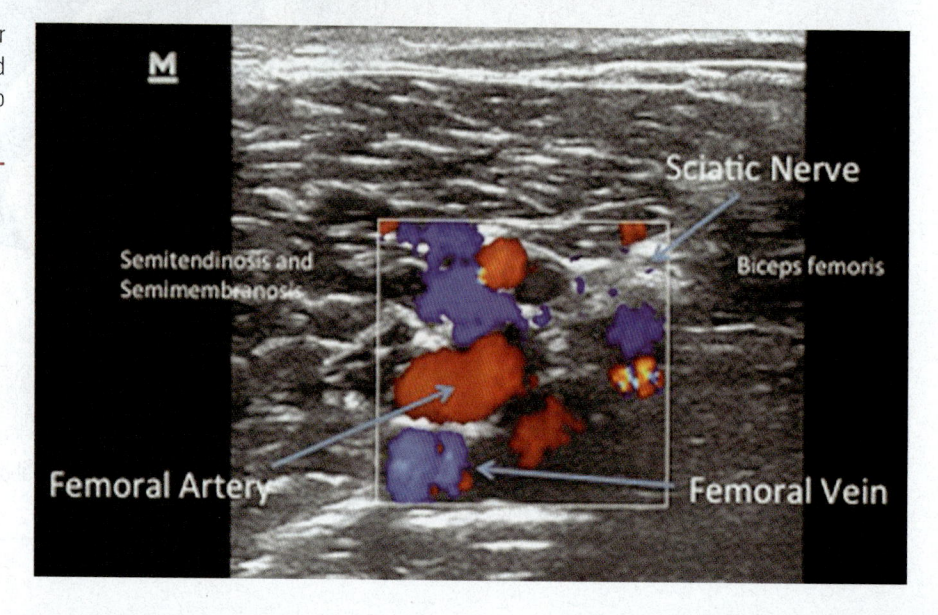

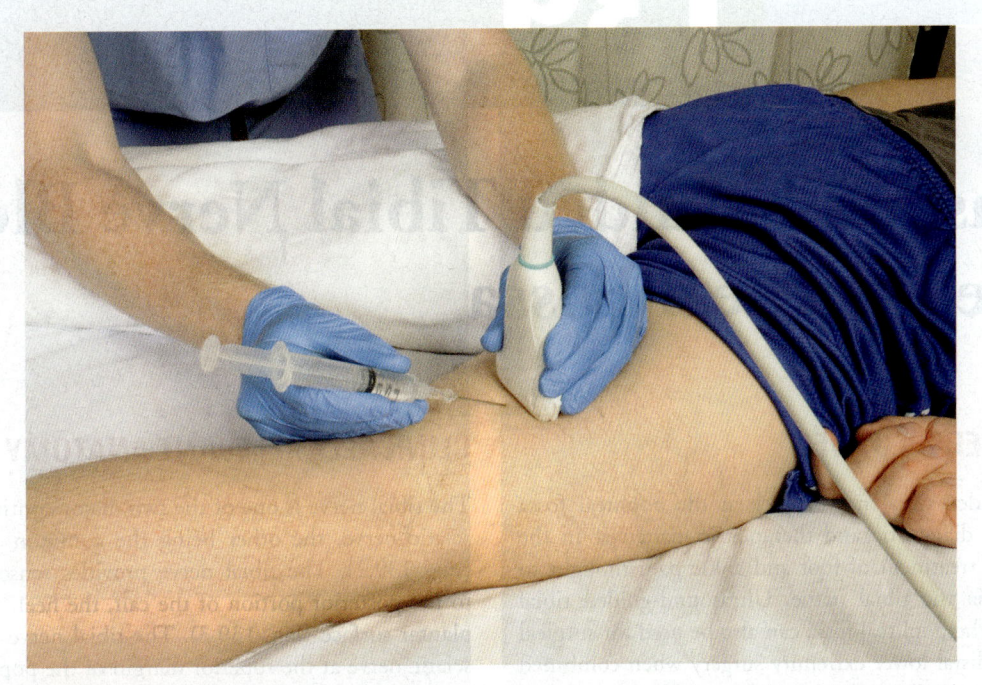

**FIGURE 138.9.** Proper out-of-plane needle position for performing sciatic nerve block at the popliteal fossa.

## CLINICAL PEARLS

The key to performing successful ultrasound sciatic nerve block at the popliteal fossa is the proper identification of the sonographic anatomy and in particular the ability to properly identify the sciatic nerve. This should not be a problem if the above technique is used. Any significant pain or sudden increase in resistance during injection when performing ultrasound-guided suggests incorrect needle placement, and one should stop injecting immediately and reassess the position of the needle.

## SUGGESTED READINGS

Herring AA, Stone MB, Fischer J, et al. Ultrasound-guided distal popliteal sciatic nerve block for ED anesthesia. *Am J Emerg Med* 2011;29(6):697.e3–e5.

Ricci S. Ultrasound observation of the sciatic nerve and its branches at the popliteal fossa: always visible, never seen. *Eur J Vasc Endovasc Surg* 2005;30(6):659–663.

Sinha A, Chan VWS. Ultrasound imaging for popliteal sciatic nerve block. *Reg Anesth Pain Med* 2004;29(2):130–134.

Waldman SD. Piriformis syndrome. In: *Pain Review*. Philadelphia, PA: Saunders Elsevier; 2009:310.

Waldman SD. Sciatic nerve block-posterior approach. In: *Atlas of Interventional Pain Management*. 3rd ed. Philadelphia, PA: Saunders Elsevier; 2009:534–538.

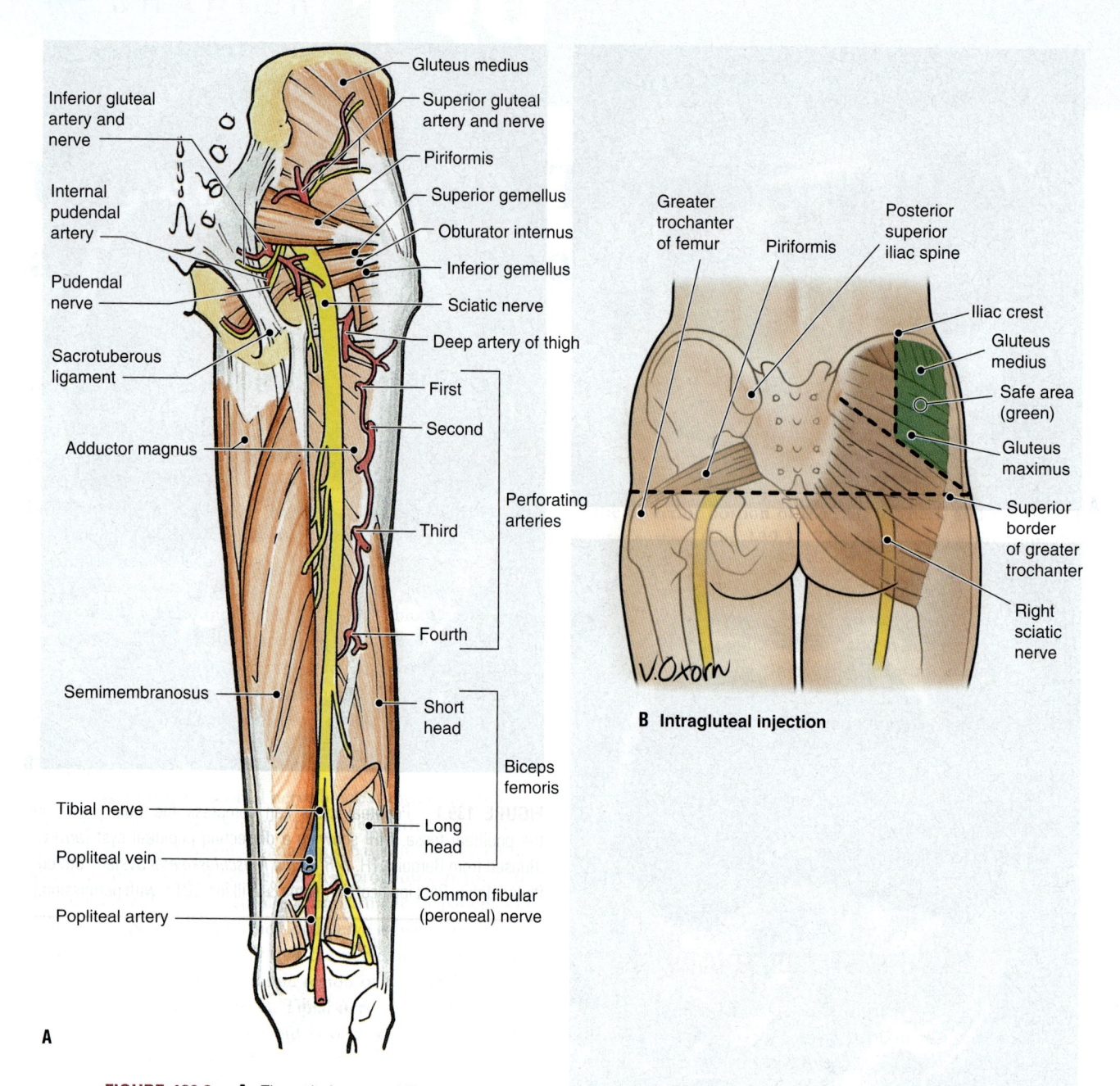

**FIGURE 139.2. A:** The sciatic nerve bifurcates into the tibial and common peroneal nerves within the popliteal fossa. **B:** The safe zone for intragluteal injection. (Reused from Moore KL, Agur AMR. *Essential Clinical Anatomy*. 2nd ed. Baltimore, MD: Lippincott Williams & Wilkins; 2002, with permission.)

solution, and a 3½-inch, 22-gauge needle is advanced from the middle of the inferior border of the ultrasound transducer and advanced utilizing an out-of-plane approach with the trajectory being adjusted under real-time ultrasound guidance until the needle tip is resting in proximity to the tibial nerve (Fig. 139.12). When the tip of needle is thought to be in satisfactory position, a small amount of local anesthetic and steroid is injected under real-time ultrasound guidance to confirm that the needle tip is in proximity to the tibial nerve, but not within the nerve itself. There should be minimal resistance to injection. After needle tip placement is confirmed, the remainder of the contents of the syringe are slowly injected. The needle is then removed, and a sterile pressure dressing and ice pack are placed at the injection site.

CHAPTER 139 ULTRASOUND-GUIDED TIBIAL NERVE BLOCK AT THE POPLITEAL FOSSA 989

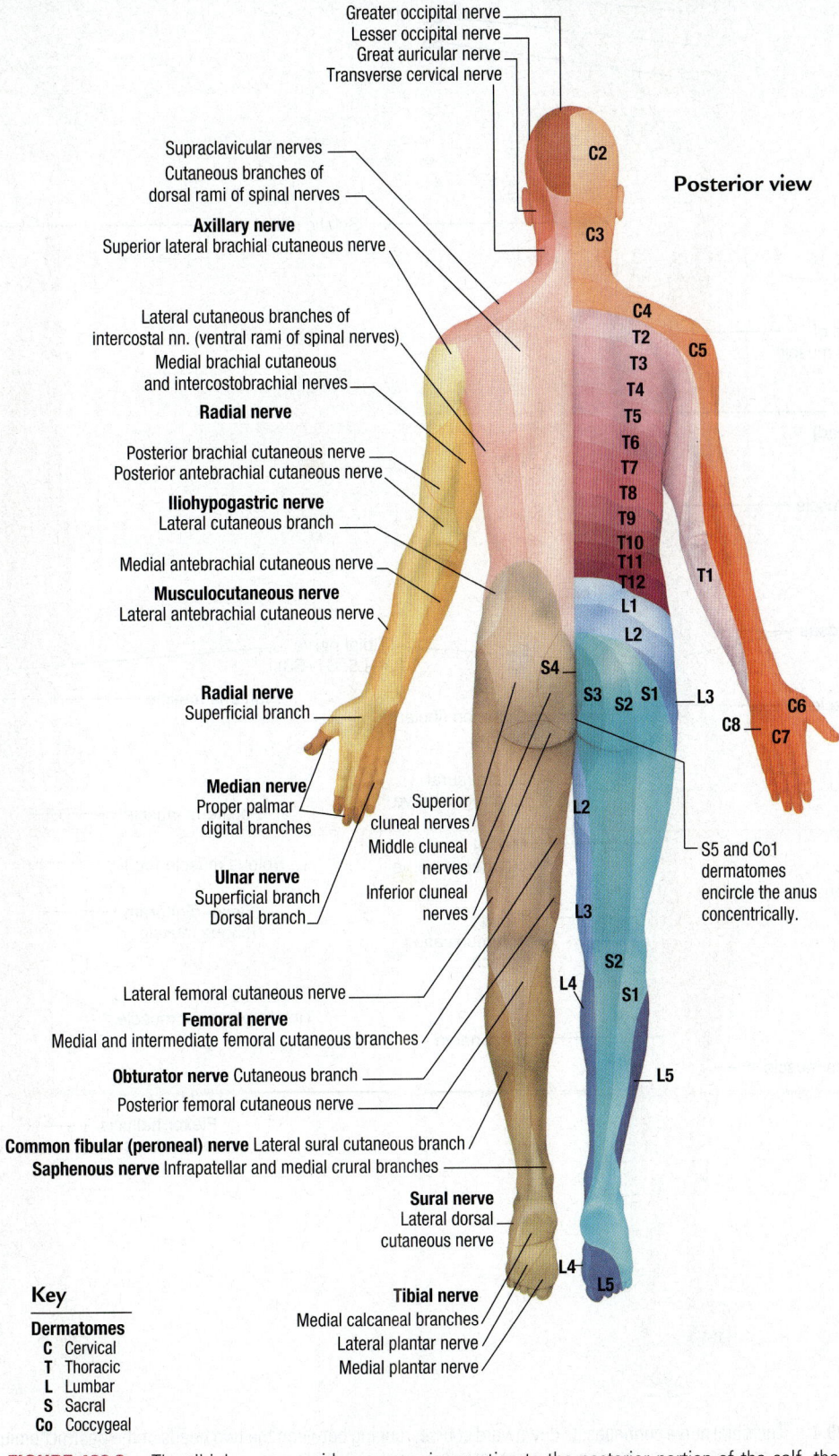

**FIGURE 139.3.** The tibial nerve provides sensory innervation to the posterior portion of the calf, the heel, and the medial plantar surface. (Anatomical Chart Company, 2013.)

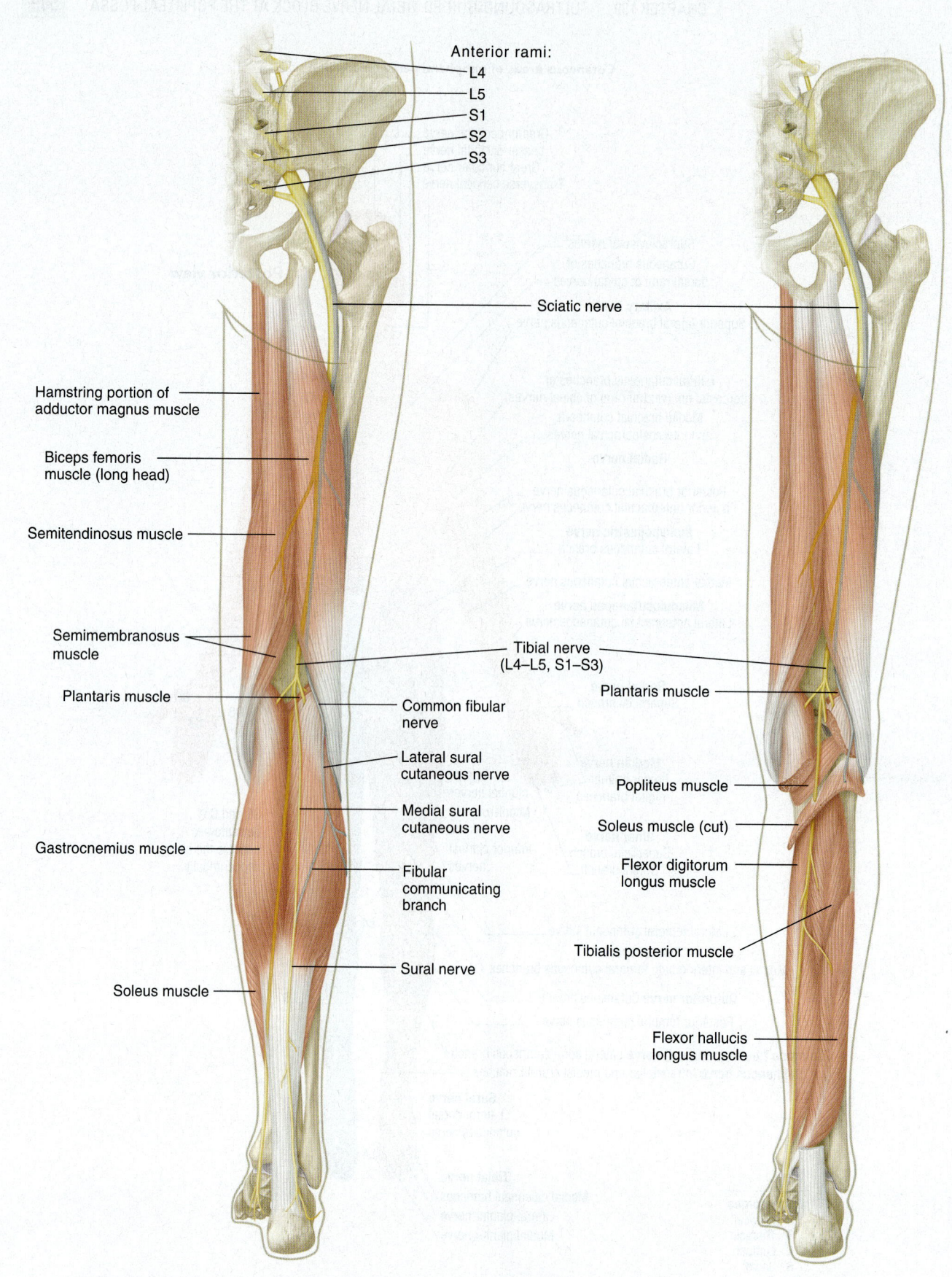

**FIGURE 139.4.** The tibial nerve continues its downward course, running between the two heads of the gastrocnemius muscle, passing deep to the soleus muscle. (Reused from Tank PW, Gest TR. *Atlas of Anatomy*. Baltimore, MD: Lippincott Williams & Wilkins; 2008, with permission.)

CHAPTER 139   ULTRASOUND-GUIDED TIBIAL NERVE BLOCK AT THE POPLITEAL FOSSA

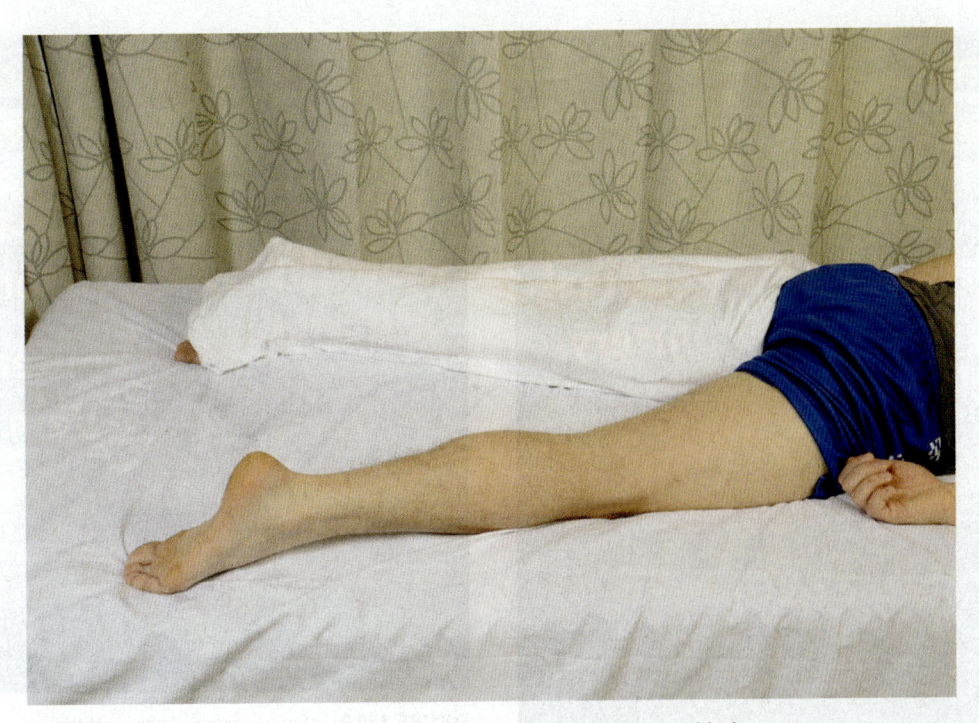

**FIGURE 139.5.** Proper patient position for ultrasound-guided tibial nerve block.

## COMPLICATIONS

A failure to accurately assess the correct position of the needle tip when performing ultrasound-guided tibial nerve block at the popliteal fossa can lead to a failure to block the tibial nerve or needle-induced trauma to the tibial nerve, popliteal artery, and/or vein. The use of ultrasound guidance when performing tibial nerve block at the popliteal fossa should markedly decrease these problems. Postblock ecchymosis and hematoma may occur, and the patient should be warned of such. These complications can be decreased by the use of a pressure dressing and cold packs applied to the injection site following the procedure.

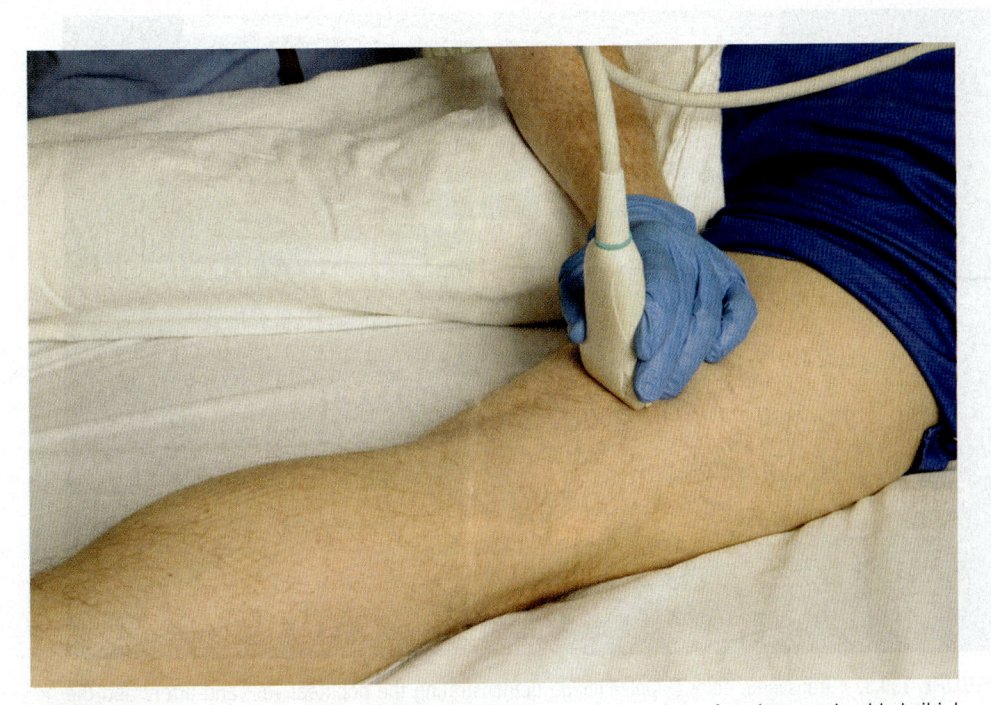

**FIGURE 139.6.** Proper transverse position of the ultrasound transducer for ultrasound-guided tibial nerve block at the popliteal fossa.

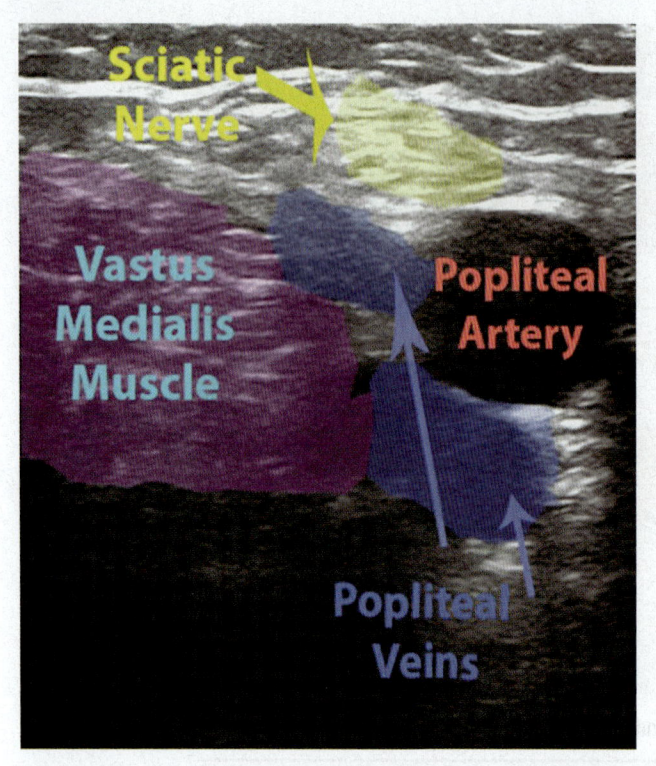

**FIGURE 139.7.** Transverse ultrasound image demonstrating the popliteal artery and vein and the sciatic nerve just above and lateral to the vein. Note the location of the vastus medialis which lies above the anteromedial femur.

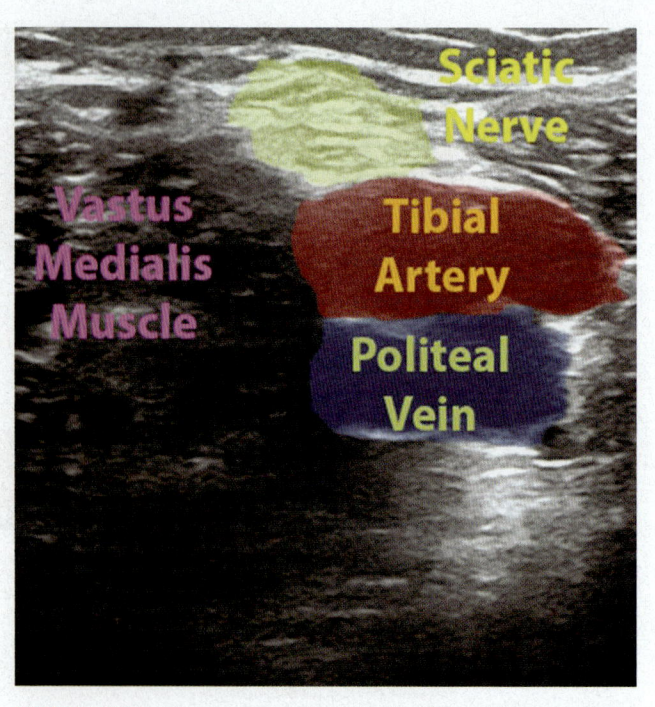

**FIGURE 139.8.** Compression of the popliteal vein with pressure on the ultrasound transducer can aid in identification of the sciatic nerve, which lies just superficial to the vein.

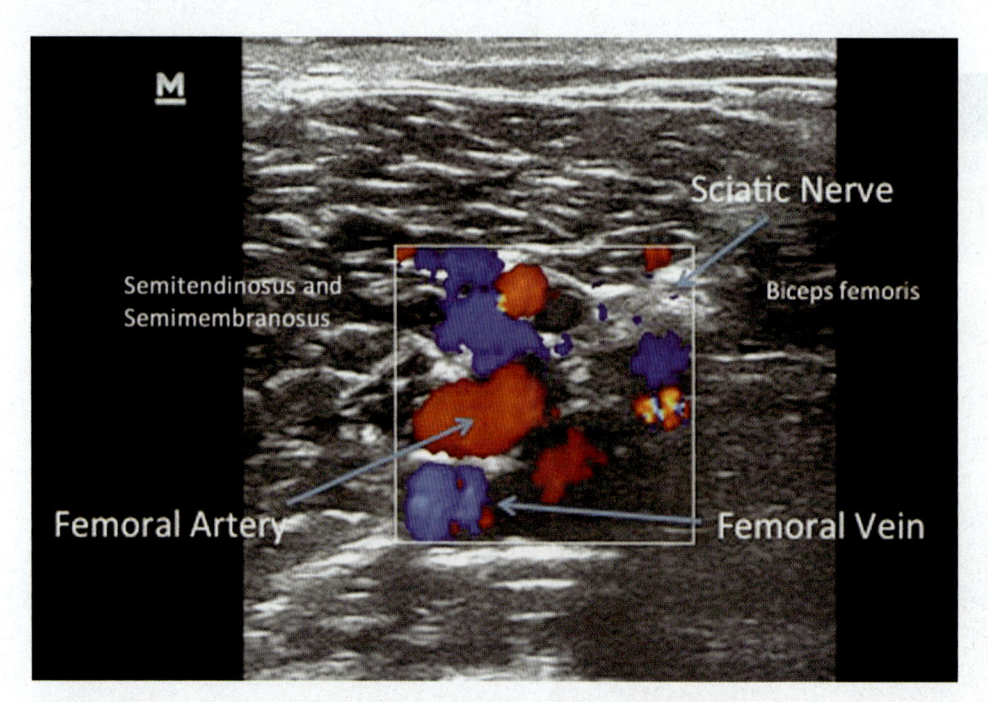

**FIGURE 139.9.** Transverse color Doppler image demonstrating the popliteal vein and artery and the relationship of the vein to the sciatic nerve.

CHAPTER 139  ULTRASOUND-GUIDED TIBIAL NERVE BLOCK AT THE POPLITEAL FOSSA    993

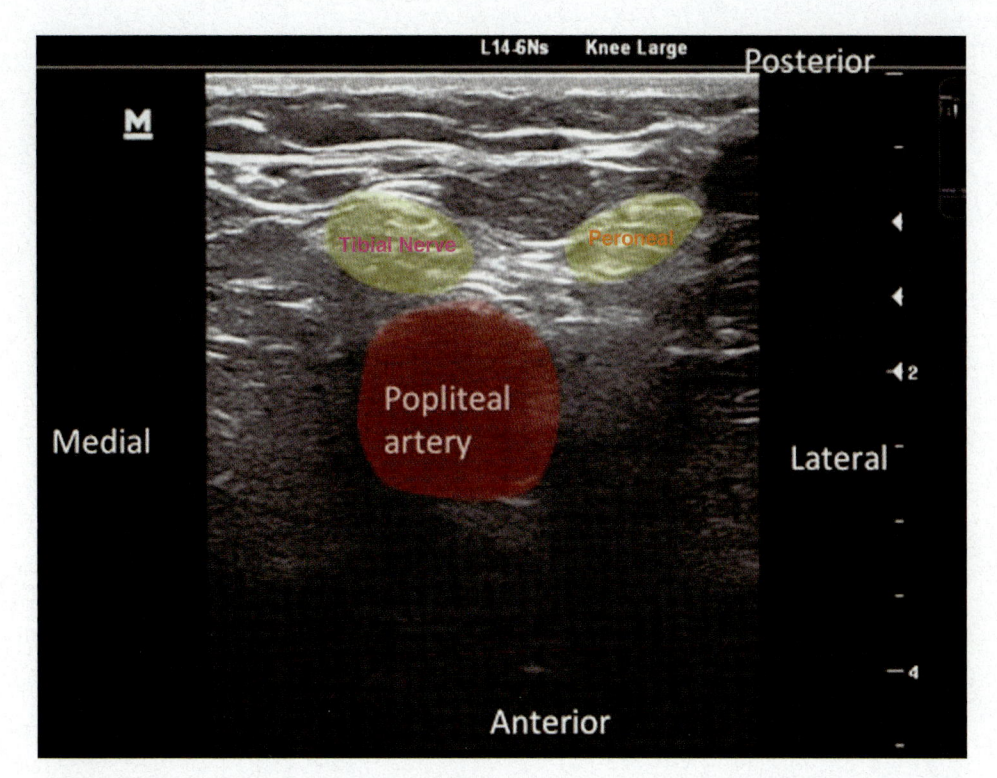

**FIGURE 139.10.** The sciatic nerve bifurcates to form the tibial and common peroneal nerves. Transverse ultrasound image at the bifurcation of the sciatic nerve.

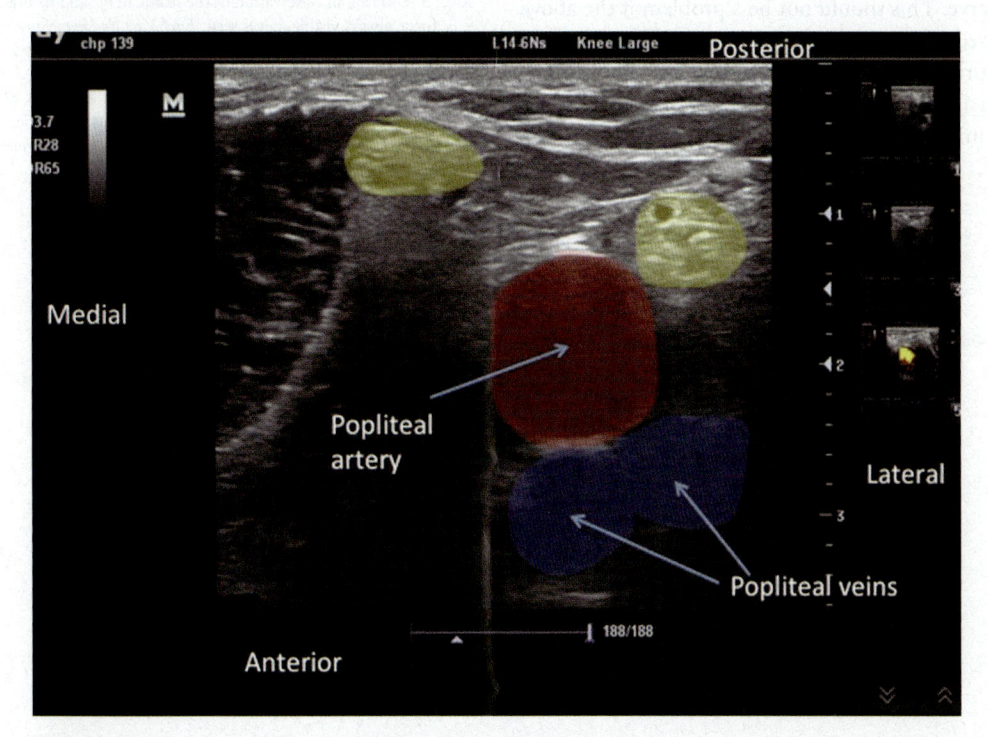

**FIGURE 139.11.** Transverse ultrasound image of the tibial nerve just below the bifurcation of the sciatic nerve. Note the relationship of the artery to the tibial nerve.

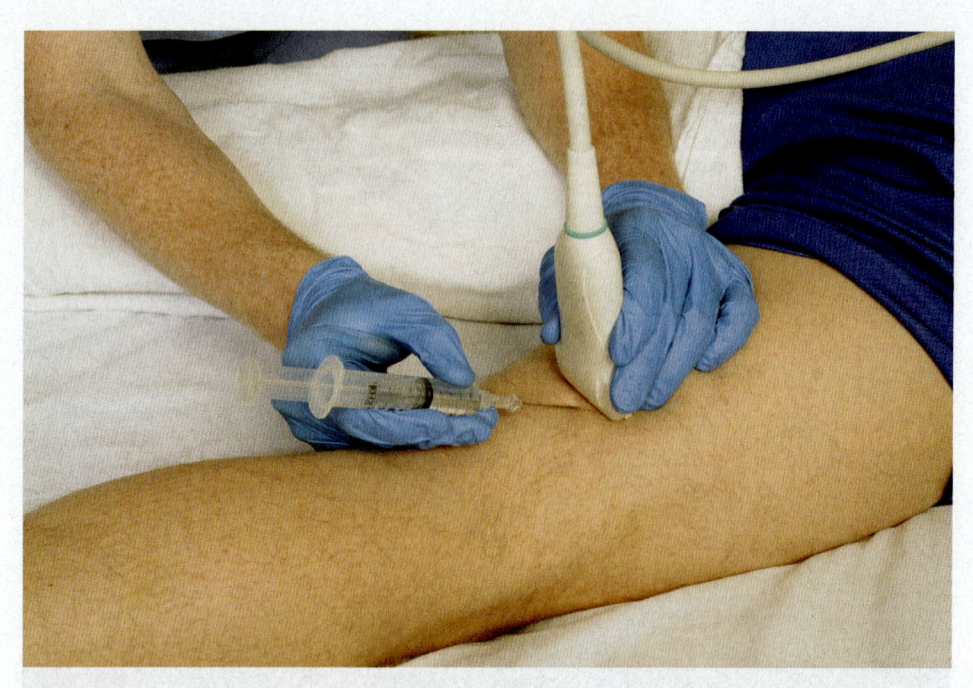

**FIGURE 139.12.** Proper out-of-plane needle position for performing tibial nerve block at the popliteal fossa.

## CLINICAL PEARLS

The key to performing successful ultrasound tibial nerve block at the popliteal fossa is the proper identification of the sonographic anatomy and in particular the ability to properly identify the tibial nerve. This should not be a problem if the above technique is used. Any significant pain or sudden increase in resistance during injection when performing ultrasound-guided suggests incorrect needle placement, and one should stop injecting immediately and reassess the position of the needle.

## SUGGESTED READINGS

Rangel Vde O, Cavalho Rde A, Mandim BL, et al. Tibial and common fibular nerve block in the popliteal fossa with single puncture using percutaneous nerve stimulator: anatomical considerations and ultrasound description. *Rev Bras Anestesiol* 2011;61(5):533–543.

Ricci S. Ultrasound observation of the sciatic nerve and its branches at the popliteal fossa: always visible, never seen. *EurJ Vasc Endovasc Surg* 2005;30(6):659–663.

Sinha A, Chan VWS. Ultrasound imaging for popliteal sciatic nerve block. *Reg Anesth Pain Med* 2004;29(2):130–134.

Waldman SD. Tibial nerve block at the knee. In: *Atlas of Interventional Pain Management*. 3rd ed. Philadelphia, PA: Saunders Elsevier; 2009:542–546.

Waldman SD. Tibial nerve block at the knee. In: *Pain Review*. Philadelphia, PA: Saunders Elsevier; 2009:569–570.

# CHAPTER 140

# Ultrasound-Guided Common Peroneal Nerve Block at the Popliteal Fossa

## CLINICAL PERSPECTIVES

Ultrasound-guided common peroneal nerve block at the popliteal fossa is utilized as a diagnostic and therapeutic maneuver in the evaluation and treatment of distal lower extremity pain thought to be mediated via the common peroneal nerve. Ultrasound-guided common peroneal nerve block at the popliteal fossa can also be used for surgical anesthesia for distal lower extremity surgery when combined with saphenous and tibial nerve block or lumbar plexus block. Ultrasound-guided common peroneal nerve block at the popliteal fossa with local anesthetic may be used to palliate acute pain emergencies, including postoperative pain, pain secondary to traumatic injuries of the distal lower extremity, and cancer pain, while waiting for pharmacologic, surgical, and antiblastic methods to become effective.

Ultrasound-guided common peroneal nerve block at the popliteal fossa can also be used as a diagnostic tool when performing differential neural blockade on an anatomic basis in the evaluation of distal lower extremity pain as well as in a prognostic manner to determine the degree of neurologic impairment the patient will suffer when destruction of the common peroneal nerve is being considered or when there is a possibility that the nerve may be sacrificed during surgeries in the anatomic region of the common peroneal nerve at the level of the popliteal fossa. Common peroneal nerve block at the knee with local anesthetic and steroid is occasionally used in the treatment of persistent ankle and foot pain when the pain is thought to be secondary to inflammation or when entrapment of the common peroneal nerve at the popliteal fossa is suspected. The common peroneal nerve is commonly entrapped or compressed as it crosses the head of the fibula and is known as cross leg or yoga palsy. Symptoms of entrapment of the common peroneal nerve at this anatomic location are numbness and foot drop. Common peroneal nerve block at the knee with local anesthetic and steroid is also indicated in the palliation of pain and motor dysfunction associated with diabetic neuropathy. Destruction of the common peroneal nerve is occasionally used in the palliation of persistent lower extremity pain secondary to invasive tumor that is mediated by the common peroneal nerve and has not responded to more conservative measures.

Electrodiagnostic testing should be considered in all patients who suffer from common peroneal nerve dysfunction to provide both neuroanatomic and neurophysiologic information regarding nerve function. Magnetic resonance imaging and ultrasound imaging of the popliteal fossa as well as anywhere along the course of the common peroneal nerve are also useful in determining the cause of common peroneal nerve compromise (Fig. 140.1).

## CLINICALLY RELEVANT ANATOMY

The common peroneal nerve, which is also known as the common fibular nerve, is one of the two major continuations of the sciatic nerve, the other being the tibial nerve (Fig. 140.2). The common peroneal nerve provides sensory innervation to the inferior portion of the knee joint and the posterior and lateral skin of the upper calf (Fig. 140.3). The common peroneal nerve is derived from the posterior branches of the L4, the L5, and the S1 and S2 nerve roots. The nerve splits from the sciatic nerve at the superior margin of the popliteal fossa and descends laterally behind the head of the fibula (Fig. 140.4). The common peroneal nerve is subject to compression at this point by such circumstances as improperly applied casts and tourniquets. The nerve is also subject to compression as it continues its lateral course, winding around the fibula through the fibular tunnel, which is made up of the posterior border of the tendinous insertion of the peroneus longus muscle and the fibula itself. Just distal to the fibular tunnel, the nerve divides into its two terminal branches, the superficial and the deep peroneal nerves. Each of these branches is subject to trauma and may be blocked individually as a diagnostic and therapeutic maneuver.

## ULTRASOUND-GUIDED TECHNIQUE

Ultrasound-guided block of the common peroneal nerve at the knee can be carried out by placing the patient in the prone position with the arms resting comfortably along the patient's side (Fig. 140.5). A total of 8 mL of local anesthetic is drawn up in a 12-mL sterile syringe. If the painful condition being treated is thought to have an inflammatory component, 40 to 80 mg of depot steroid is added

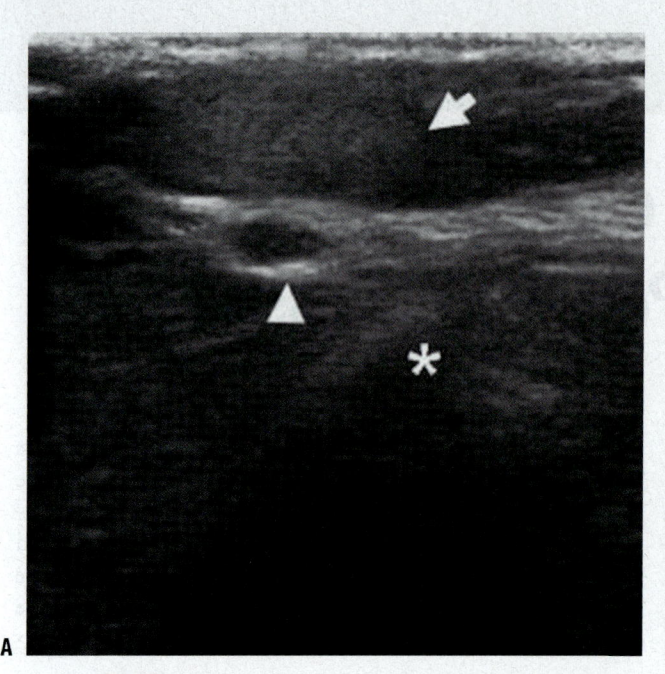

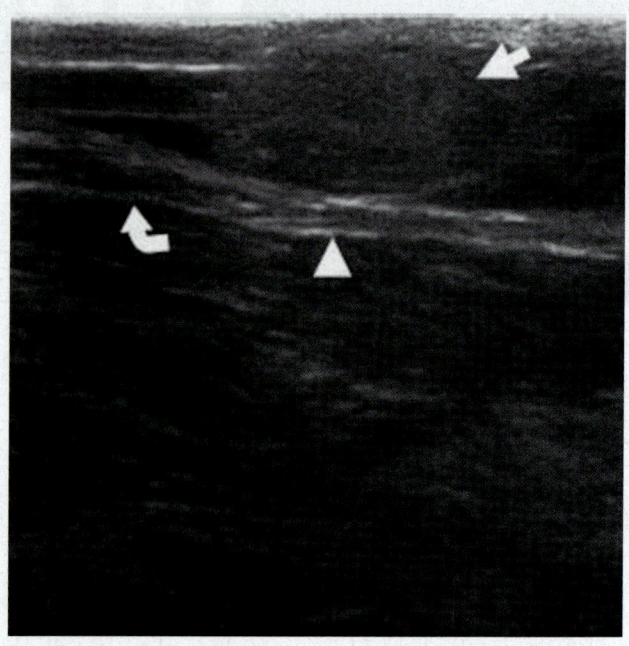

**FIGURE 140.1.** Lipoma can compress the common peroneal nerve against the fibular head. Transverse **(A)** and longitudinal **(B)** sonograms show the relationship between the lipoma (*arrow*) and the common peroneal nerve (*arrowhead*). The subcutaneous lipoma is located lateral to the fibular head (*asterisk*). The nerve proximal to the compression site shows slight swelling with fusiform enlargement of the fascicles (*curved arrow*) on the longitudinal scan. The compressed nerve appears hypoechoic. (Reused from Hsu YC, Shih YY, Gao HW, et al. Subcutaneous lipoma compressing the common peroneal nerve and causing palsy: sonographic diagnosis. *J Clin Ultrasound* 2010;38(2):97–99, with permission.)

to the local anesthetic. A linear high-frequency ultrasound transducer is placed in a transverse plane ~8 cm above the popliteal crease and an ultrasound survey scan is obtained (Fig. 140.6). The pulsating popliteal artery should be visualized toward the bottom of the image, with the popliteal vein lying just lateral to the artery (Fig. 140.7). Just superficial and slightly lateral to the popliteal vein is the sciatic nerve, which will appear as a bright hyperechoic structure (see Fig. 140.7). Compression of the popliteal vein with pressure on the ultrasound transducer can aid in identification of the common peroneal nerve, which lies just superficial to the vein (Fig. 140.8). Color Doppler can be utilized to help identify the popliteal artery and vein (Fig. 140.9). When the sciatic nerve is identified on ultrasound imaging, the ultrasound transducer is slowly moved inferiorly along the course of the sciatic nerve until the bifurcation of the nerve into the tibial and common peroneal nerves occurs (Fig. 140.10). The common peroneal nerve is followed in its downward course until it completely separates from the tibial nerve (Fig. 140.11). When the common peroneal nerve is satisfactorily identified, the skin is prepped with anesthetic solution, and a 3½-inch 22-gauge needle is advanced from the middle of the inferior border of the ultrasound transducer and advanced utilizing an out-of-plane approach with the trajectory being adjusted under real-time ultrasound guidance until the needle tip is resting in proximity to the common peroneal nerve (Fig. 140.12). When the tip of needle is thought to be in satisfactory position, a small amount of local anesthetic and steroid is injected under real-time ultrasound guidance to confirm that the needle tip is in proximity to the common peroneal nerve, but not within the nerve itself. There should be minimal resistance to injection. After needle tip placement is confirmed, the remainder of the contents of the syringe are slowly injected. The needle is then removed, and a sterile pressure dressing and ice pack are placed at the injection site.

CHAPTER 140 ULTRASOUND-GUIDED COMMON PERONEAL NERVE BLOCK AT THE POPLITEAL FOSSA 997

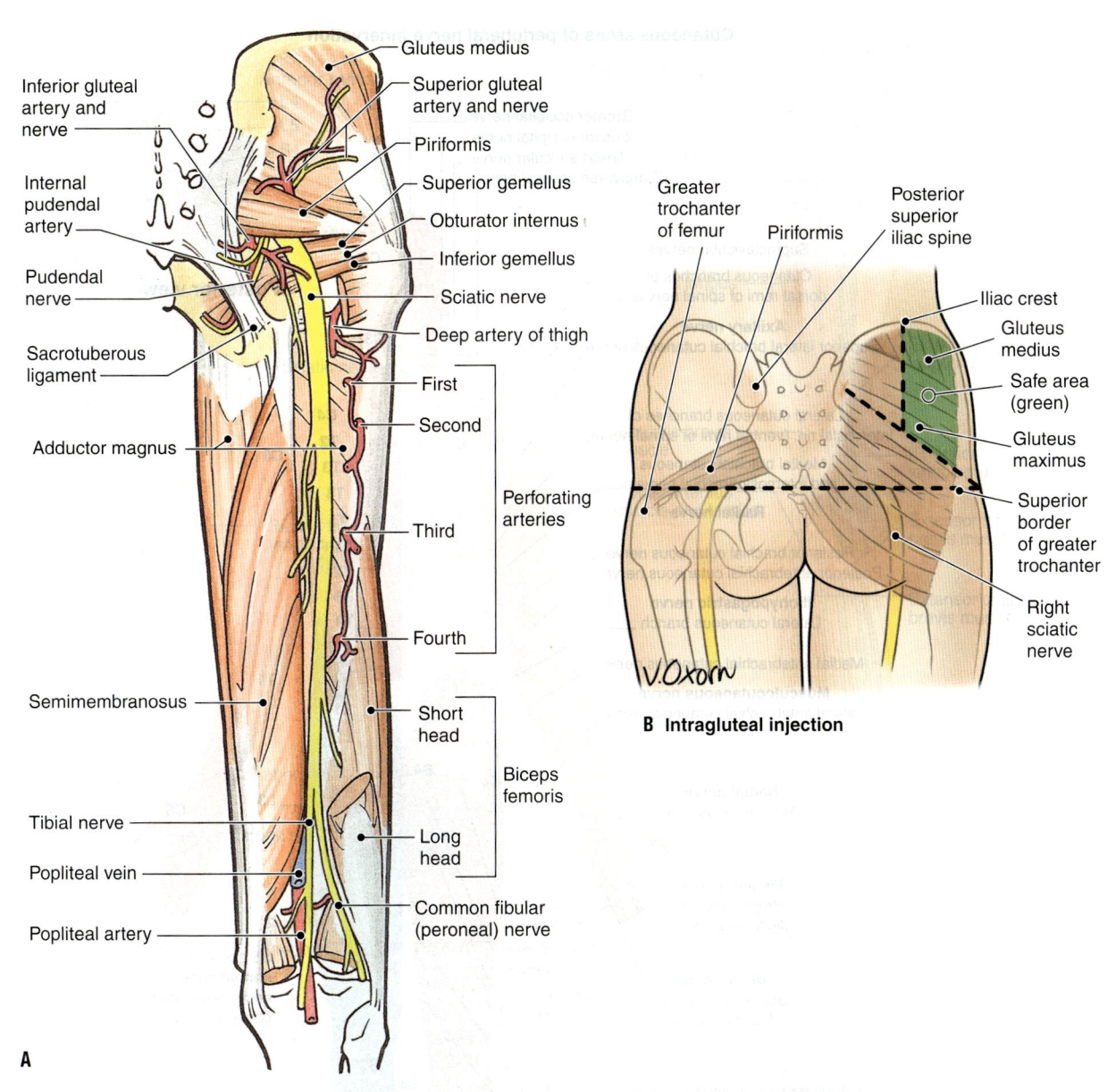

**FIGURE 140.2. A:** The sciatic nerve bifurcates into the tibial and common peroneal (common fibular) nerves within the popliteal fossa. **B:** The safe zone for intragluteal injection. (Reused from Moore KL, Agur AMR. *Essential Clinical Anatomy*. 2nd ed. Baltimore, MD: Lippincott Williams & Wilkins; 2002, with permission.)

## COMPLICATIONS

A failure to accurately assess the correct position of the needle tip when performing ultrasound-guided common peroneal nerve block at the popliteal fossa can lead to a failure to block the common peroneal nerve or needle-induced trauma to the common peroneal nerve, popliteal artery, and/or vein. The use of ultrasound guidance when performing common peroneal nerve block at the popliteal fossa should markedly decrease these problems. Postblock ecchymosis and hematoma may occur, and the patient should be warned of such. These complications can be decreased by the use of a pressure dressing and cold packs applied to the injection site following the procedure.

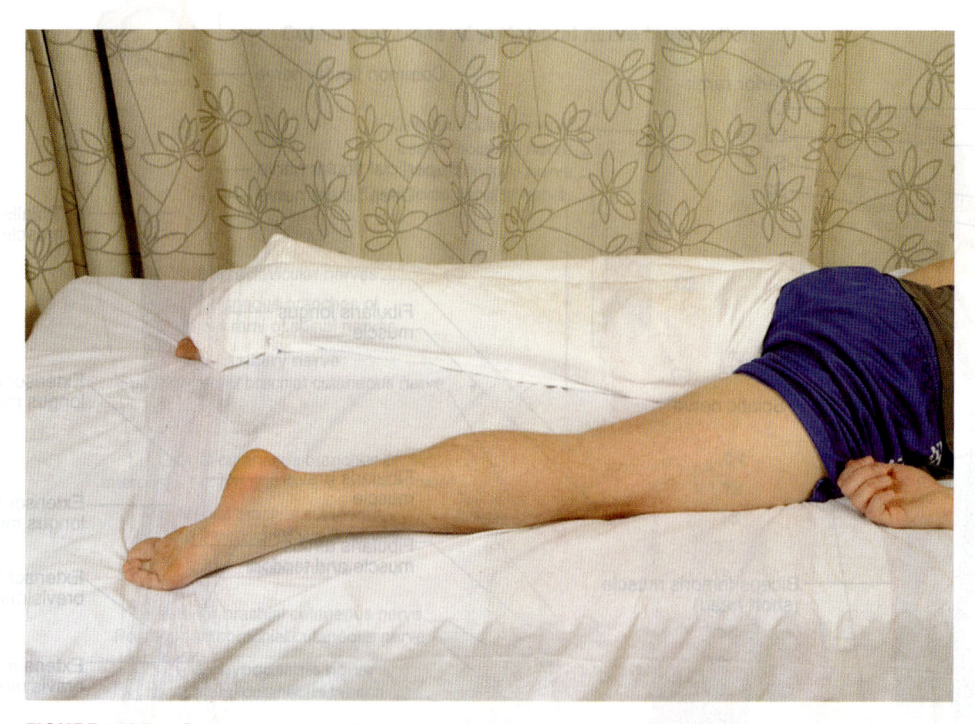

**FIGURE 140.5.** Proper patient position for ultrasound-guided common peroneal nerve block.

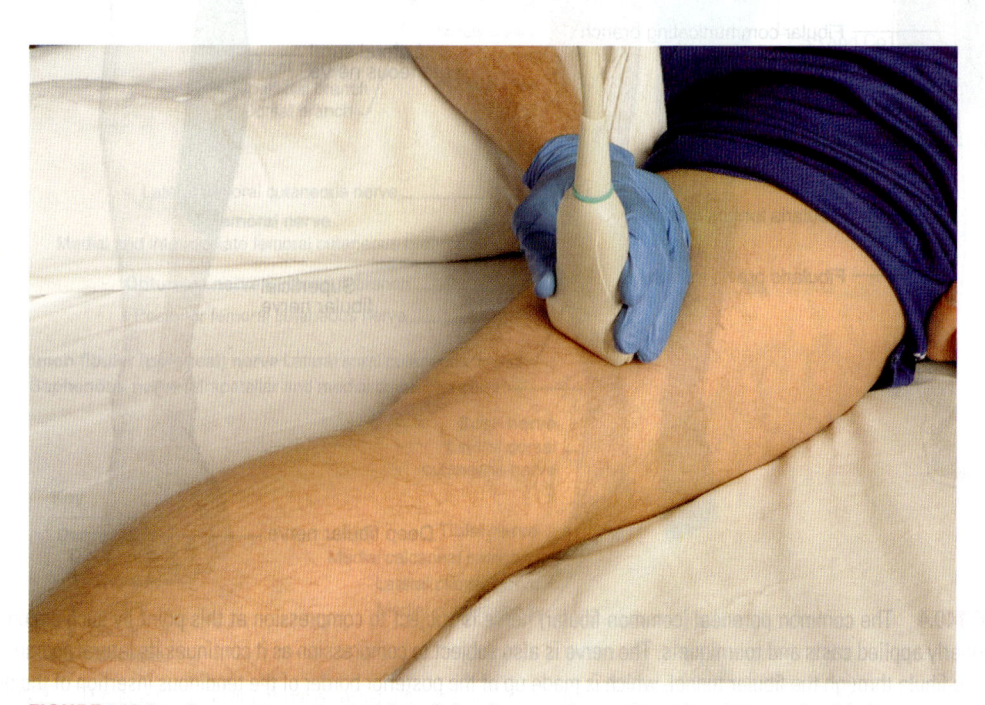

**FIGURE 140.6.** Proper transverse position of the ultrasound transducer for ultrasound-guided common peroneal nerve block at the popliteal fossa.

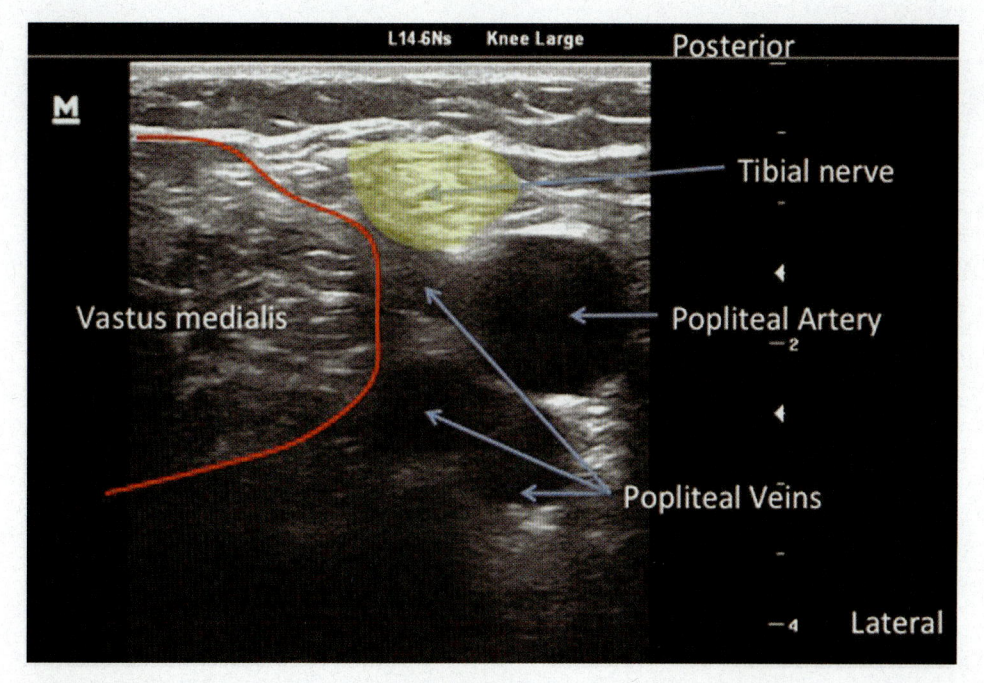

**FIGURE 140.7.** Transverse ultrasound image demonstrating the popliteal artery and vein and the common peroneal nerve just above and lateral to the vein.

## CLINICAL PEARLS

The key to performing successful ultrasound common peroneal nerve block at the popliteal fossa is the proper identification of the sonographic anatomy and in particular the ability to properly identify the common peroneal nerve. This should not be a problem if the above technique is used. Any significant pain or sudden increase in resistance during injection when performing ultrasound-guided suggests incorrect needle placement, and one should stop injecting immediately and reassess the position of the needle.

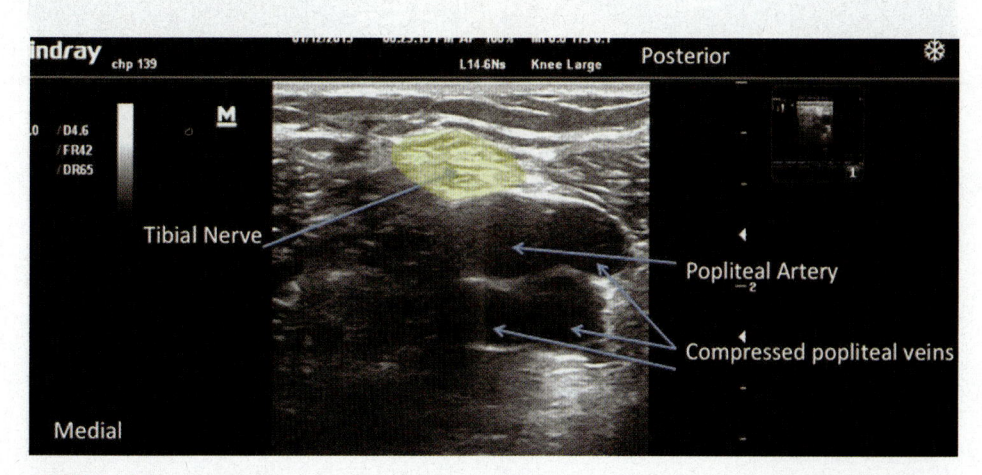

**FIGURE 140.8.** Compression of the popliteal vein can aid in identification of the sciatic nerve, which is just lateral and superficial to the vein.

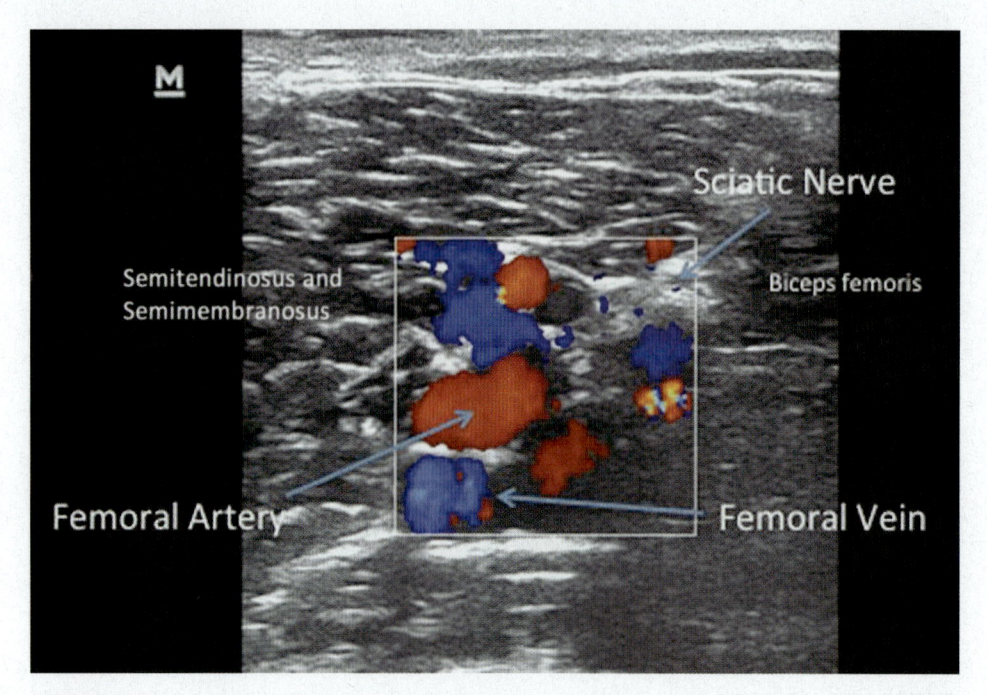

**FIGURE 140.9.** Transverse color Doppler image demonstrating the popliteal vein and artery and the relationship of the vein to the common peroneal nerve.

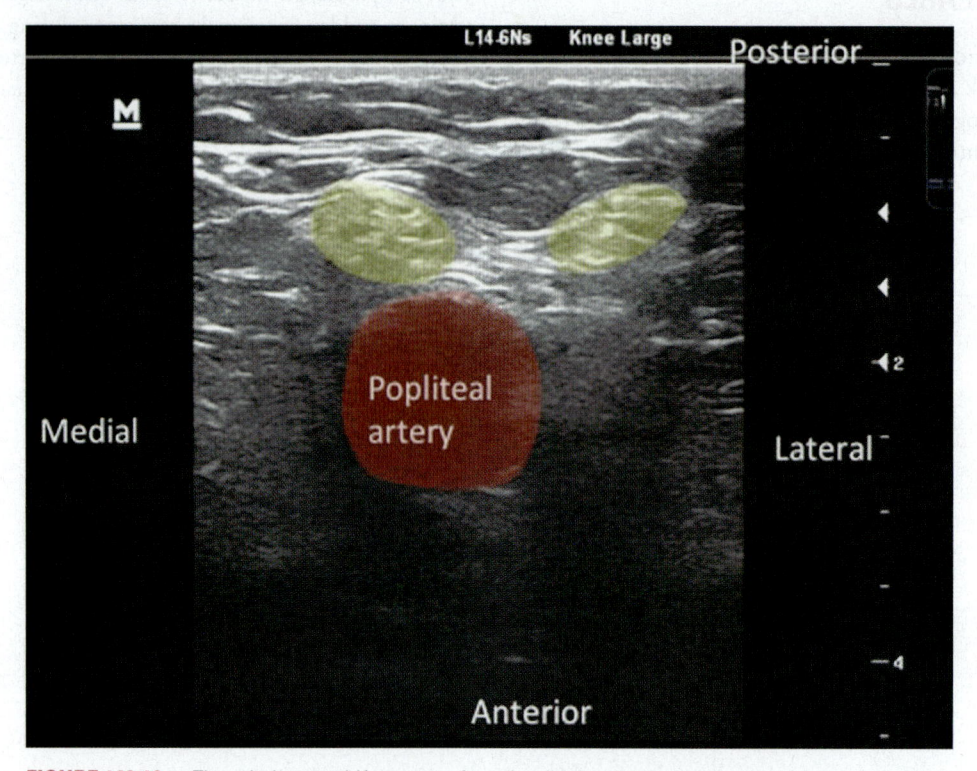

**FIGURE 140.10.** The sciatic nerve bifurcates to form the tibial and common peroneal nerves. Transverse ultrasound image at the bifurcation of the sciatic nerve.

# CHAPTER 140  ULTRASOUND-GUIDED COMMON PERONEAL NERVE BLOCK AT THE POPLITEAL FOSSA

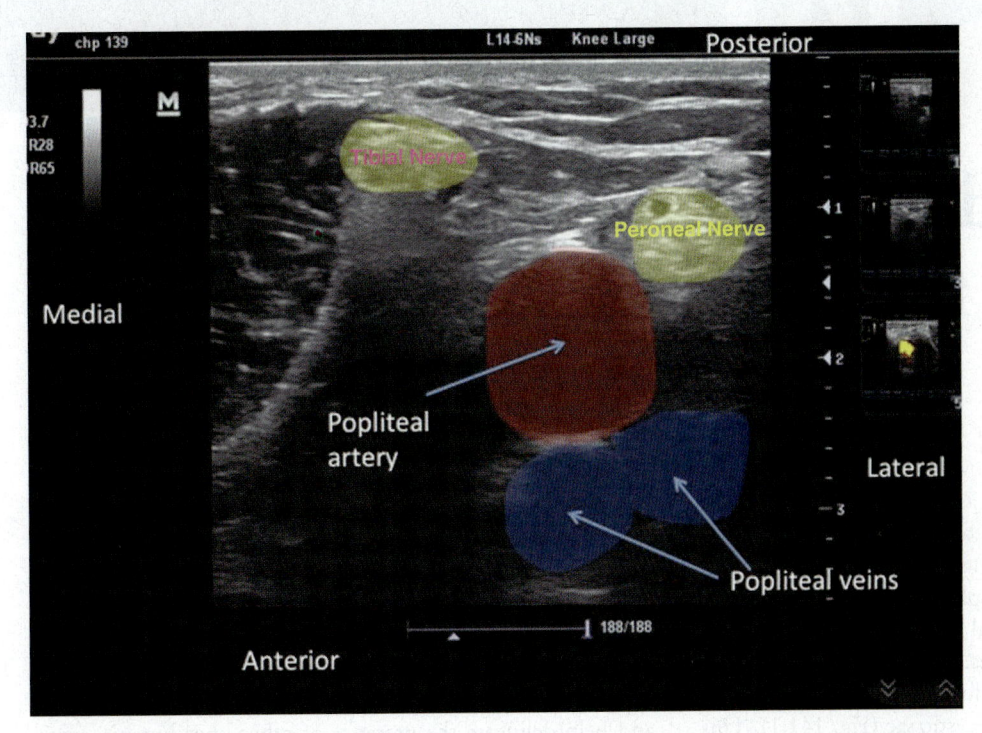

**FIGURE 140.11.** Transverse ultrasound image of the common peroneal nerve just below the bifurcation of the sciatic nerve. Note the relationship of the artery to the common peroneal nerve.

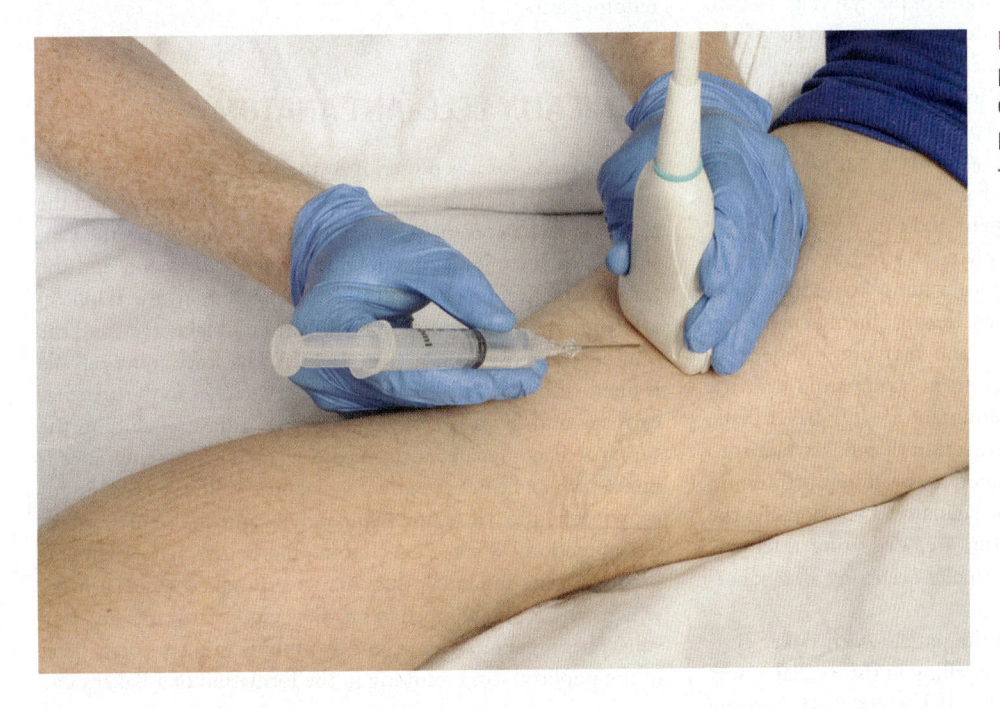

**FIGURE 140.12.** Proper out-of-plane needle position for performing common peroneal nerve block at the popliteal fossa.

## SUGGESTED READINGS

Rangel Vde O, Cavalho Rde A, Mandim BL, et al. Common peroneal and common fibular nerve block in the popliteal fossa with single puncture using percutaneous nerve stimulator: anatomical considerations and ultrasound description. *Rev Bras Anestesiol* 2011;61(5):533–543.

Ricci S. Ultrasound observation of the sciatic nerve and its branches at the popliteal fossa: always visible, never seen. *Eur J Vasc Endovasc Surg* 2005;30(6):659–663.

Sinha A, Chan VWS. Ultrasound imaging for popliteal sciatic nerve block. *Reg Anesth Pain Med* 2004;29(2):130–134.

Waldman SD. Common peroneal nerve block at the knee. In: *Atlas of Interventional Pain Management*. 3rd ed. Philadelphia, PA: Saunders Elsevier; 2009:542–546.

Waldman SD. Common peroneal nerve block at the knee. In: *Pain Review*. Philadelphia, PA: Saunders Elsevier; 2009:569–570.

# CHAPTER 141

# Ultrasound-Guided Injection Technique for Baker Cyst

## CLINICAL PERSPECTIVES

Baker cyst, which is also known as popliteal cyst, is a common cause of posterior knee pain and swelling. Baker cyst of the knee is the result of an abnormal accumulation of synovial fluid in the medial aspect of the popliteal fossa most commonly between the tendons of the medial head of the gastrocnemius and the semimembranosus muscles.

Overproduction of synovial fluid from an inflamed knee joint results in the formation of a cystic sac (Fig. 141.1). This sac often communicates with the knee joint, with a one-way valve effect causing a gradual expansion of the cyst (Fig. 141.2). Often a tear of the medial meniscus or a tendonitis of the medial hamstring tendon is the inciting factor responsible for the development of a Baker cyst. Patients who suffer from rheumatoid arthritis are especially susceptible to the development of Baker cysts, although any form of arthritis or pathology of the synovium can cause a Baker cyst (Fig. 141.3).

Patients suffering from the pain and functional disability associated with Baker cysts complain of a feeling of fullness behind the knee. Often, they notice a lump behind the knee that becomes more apparent when flexing the affected knee. The cyst may continue to enlarge and may dissect inferiorly into the calf. Patients who suffer from rheumatoid arthritis are particularly prone to the development of large Baker cysts. Often the pain associated with dissection of a Baker cyst into the calf may be initially misdiagnosed as thrombophlebitis and inappropriately treated with anticoagulants. Occasionally, the Baker cyst may spontaneously rupture, dissecting inferiorly along the gastrocnemius muscle, usually occurring after squatting (Fig. 141.4).

On physical examination of the patient with Baker cyst, the clinician may identify a cystic swelling in the medial aspect of the popliteal fossa (Fig. 141.5). Baker cysts can become quite large, especially in patients who suffer from rheumatoid arthritis. Activity, including squatting, flexing the affected knee, or walking, makes the pain of Baker cyst worse. Rest and heat may provide a modicum of relief. The pain of Baker cyst is constant and is characterized as aching. Sleep disturbance is common. Baker cyst may spontaneously rupture, and resulting rubor and color in the calf that may mimic thrombophlebitis are frequently present. In contradistinction to thrombophlebitis, Homans sign is negative and no cords are palpable. Occasionally, tendonitis of the medial hamstring tendon may be confused with Baker cyst.

Plain radiographs are indicated in all patients who present with knee pain to aid in the diagnosis and to rule out occult bony pathology (Fig. 141.6). Based on the patient's clinical presentation, additional testing may be indicated, including complete blood cell count, sedimentation rate, and antinuclear antibody testing. Magnetic resonance imaging or ultrasound imaging of the affected area may also confirm the diagnosis and help delineate the presence of other knee bursitis, internal derangement, calcific tendonitis, synovial disease, and tendinopathy.

## CLINICALLY RELEVANT ANATOMY

The popliteal fossa is posterior to the knee joint. The boundaries of the popliteal fossa are the skin, superficial fascia, and the popliteal fascia and the popliteal surface of the femur, the capsule of the knee joint, the oblique popliteal ligament, and the fascia of the popliteus muscle. The fossa contains the popliteal artery and vein, the common peroneal and tibial nerves, and the semimembranosus bursa (Fig. 141.7). The knee joint capsule is lined with a synovial membrane that attaches to the articular cartilage and gives rise to a number of bursae, including the suprapatellar, prepatellar, infrapatellar, and semimembranosus bursae, which lie between the medial head of the gastrocnemius muscle, the medial femoral epicondyle, and the semimembranosus tendon. When these bursae and/or the synovial membrane become inflamed, they may overproduce synovial fluid, which can become trapped in sac-like cysts because of a one-way valve phenomenon. This occurs commonly in the medial aspect of the popliteal fossa resulting in the formation of a Baker cyst.

## ULTRASOUND-GUIDED TECHNIQUE

Ultrasound-guided block of the Baker cyst at the knee can be carried out by placing the patient in the prone position with the arms resting comfortably along the patient's side (Fig. 141.8). A total of 6 mL of local anesthetic is drawn up in a 12-mL sterile syringe. If the painful condition being treated is thought to have an inflammatory component, 40 to 80 mg of depot steroid is

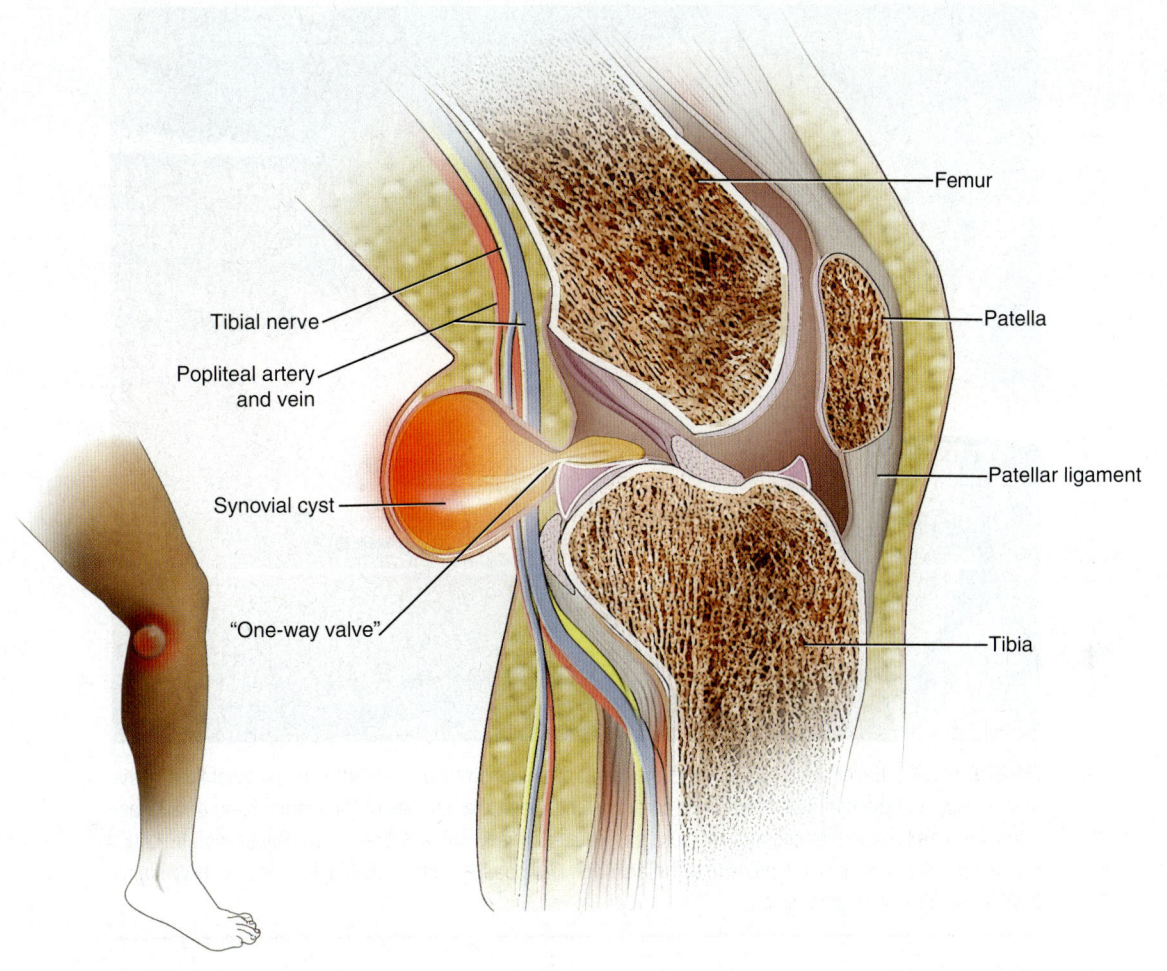

**FIGURE 141.1.** Baker cysts are the result of abnormal production of the synovial fluid. Baker cysts often communicate with the joint space.

added to the local anesthetic. A linear high-frequency ultrasound transducer is placed in a transverse plane at the medial aspect of the popliteal crease, and an ultrasound survey scan is obtained (Fig. 141.9). A characteristic cystic hypoechoic fluid collection will be easily visualized between the gastrocnemius and semimembranosus muscles (Figs. 141.10 and 141.11). When the Baker cyst is satisfactorily identified, the skin is prepped with anesthetic solution, and a 3½-inch, 22-gauge needle is advanced from the middle of the inferior border of the ultrasound transducer and advanced utilizing an out-of-plane approach with the trajectory being adjusted under real-time ultrasound guidance until the needle tip is resting within the Baker cyst (Fig. 141.12). When the tip of needle is thought to be in satisfactory position, a small amount of local anesthetic and steroid is injected under real-time ultrasound guidance to confirm that the needle tip is within the Baker cyst. There should be slight resistance to injection. After needle tip placement is confirmed, aspiration of the fluid within the cyst is carried out, and then the remainder of the contents of the syringe are slowly injected. The needle is then removed, and a sterile pressure dressing and ice pack are placed at the injection site.

## COMPLICATIONS

The proximity to the common peroneal and tibial nerves, as well as the popliteal artery and vein, makes it imperative that this procedure be carried out only by those well versed in the regional anatomy and experienced in performing ultrasound-guided injection techniques. Postblock ecchymosis and hematoma may occur, and the patient should be warned of such. These complications can be decreased by the use of a pressure dressing and cold packs applied to the injection site following the procedure.

## CLINICAL PEARLS

The clinician must rule out the presence of thrombophlebitis in patients thought to be suffering from Baker cyst. Coexistent semimembranosus bursitis, medial hamstring tendonitis, or internal derangement of the knee may contribute to knee pain associated with and may require additional treatment with more localized injection of local anesthetic and depot corticosteroid

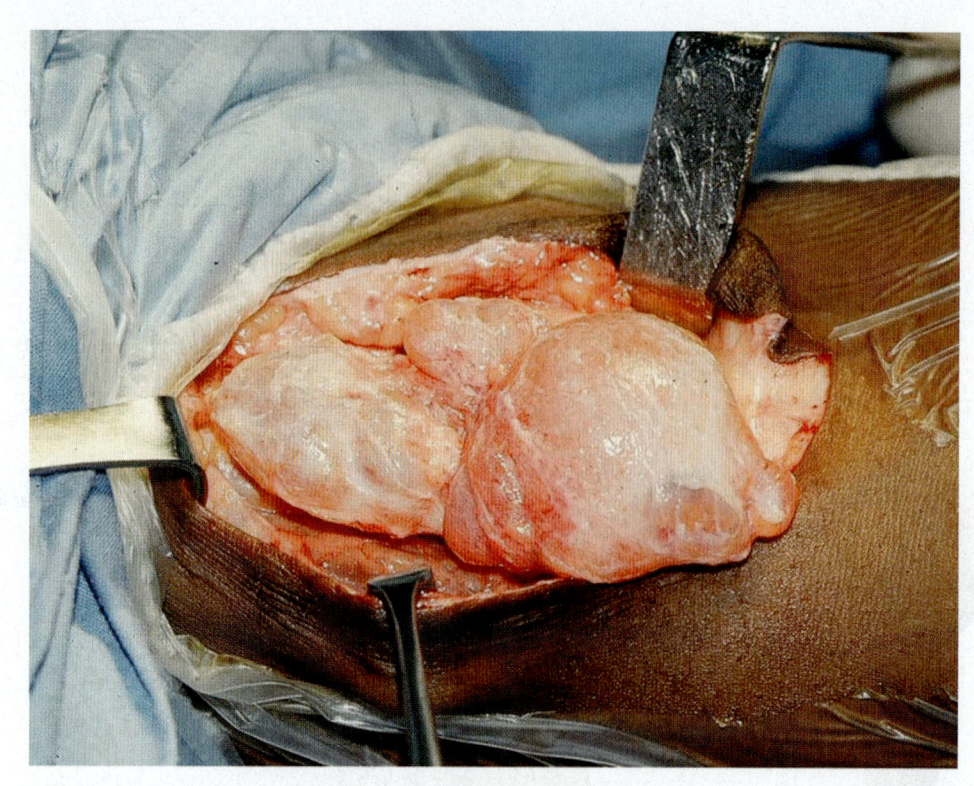

**FIGURE 141.2.** Baker cyst of the knee is the result of an abnormal accumulation of synovial fluid in the medial aspect of the popliteal fossa most commonly between the tendons of the medial head of the gastrocnemius and the semimembranosus muscles. (Reused from Kusuma S, Lonner JH. Baker cyst. In: Lotke PA, Abboud JA, Ende J, eds. *Lippincott's Primary Care: Orthopaedics*. Philadelphia, PA: Lippincott Williams & Wilkins; 2008, with permission.)

**FIGURE 141.3.** Sagittal T2-weighted spin-echo magnetic resonance image of the knee of a patient with a hemorrhagic Baker cyst (*arrows*) containing irregular areas of signal void producing an appearance similar to that of pigmented villonodular synovitis. (Reused from Koopman WJ, Moreland LW. *Arthritis and Allied Conditions: A Textbook of Rheumatology*. 15th ed. Philadelphia, PA: Lippincott Williams & Wilkins; 2005, with permission.)

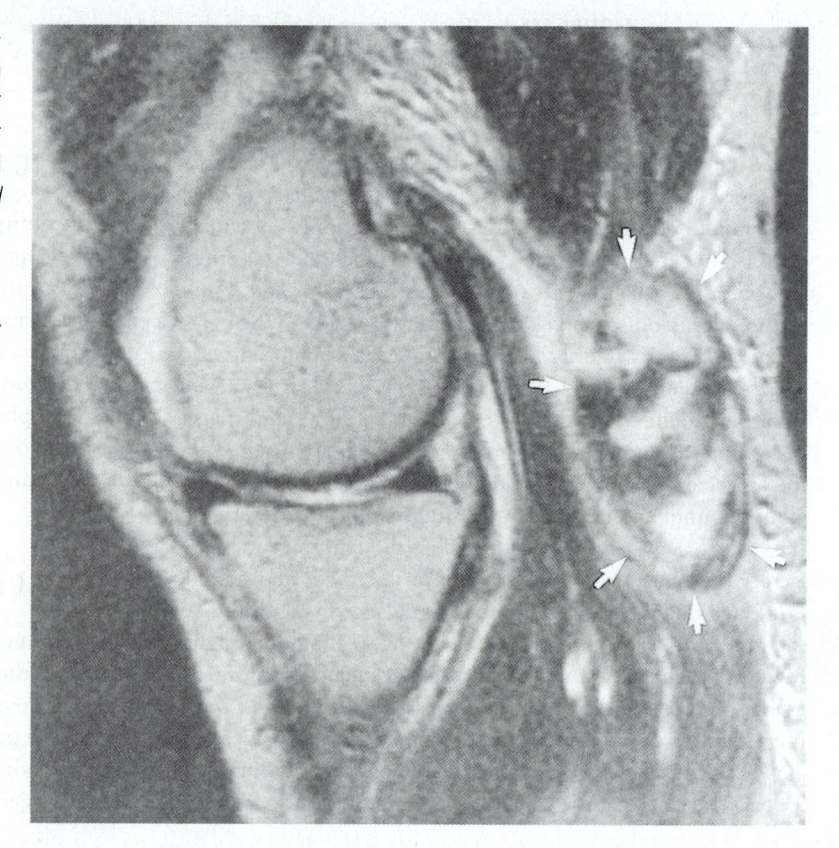

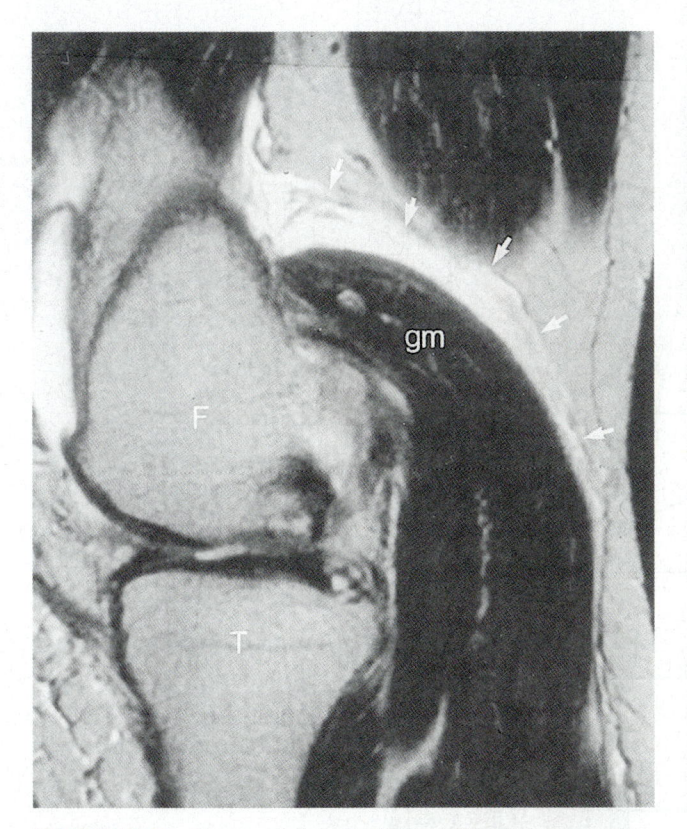

**FIGURE 141.4.** Ruptured Baker cyst. Sagittal T2-weighted spin-echo magnetic resonance image shows free fluid (*arrows*) from a ruptured Baker cyst tracking along fascial planes deep to the gastrocnemius muscle (gm). (F, femur; T, tibia.) (Reused from Koopman WJ, Moreland LW. *Arthritis and Allied Conditions: A Textbook of Rheumatology.* 15th ed. Philadelphia, PA: Lippincott Williams & Wilkins; 2005, with permission.)

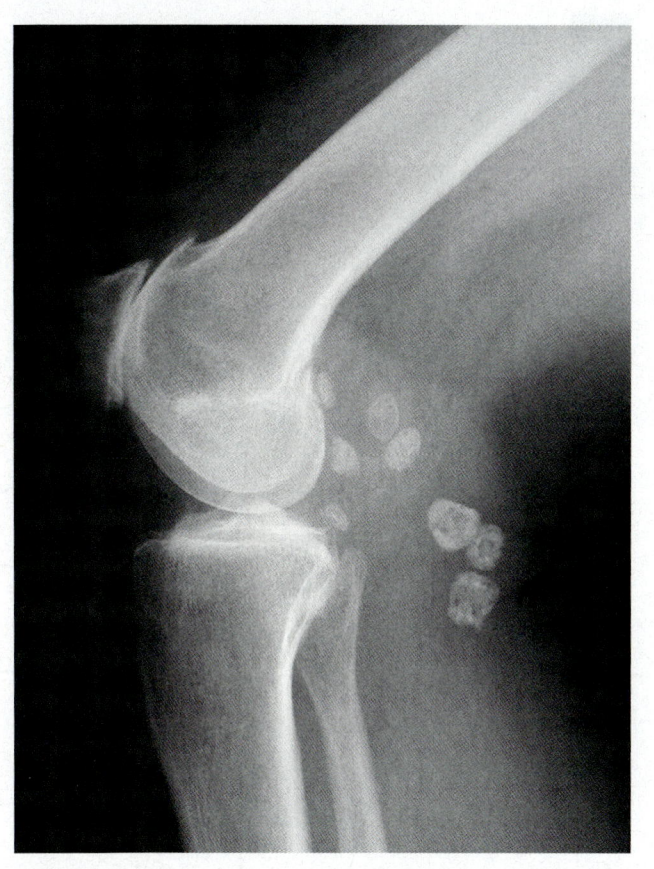

**FIGURE 141.6.** Lateral radiograph demonstrating multiple loose bodies in the popliteal fossa consistent with synovial osteochondromatosis within a Baker cyst. (Reused from Daffner H. *Clinical Radiology: The Essentials.* 3rd ed. Philadelphia, PA: Lippincott Williams & Wilkins; 2007, with permission.)

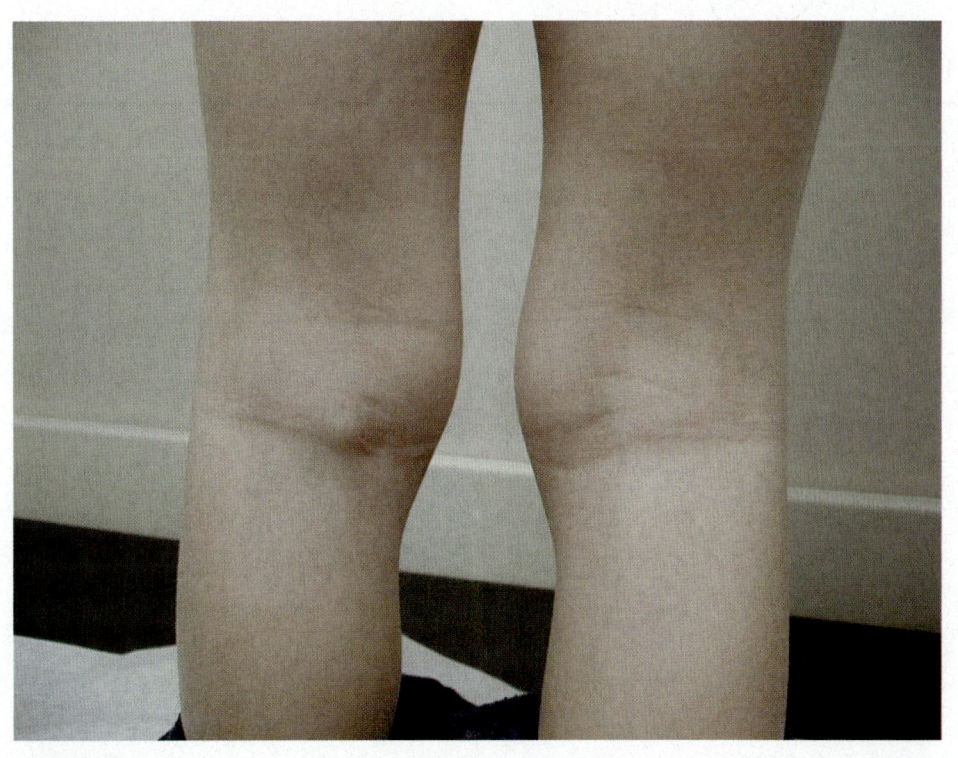

**FIGURE 141.5.** Classic appearance of a Baker cyst. (Courtesy of Mary L. Brandt, MD.)

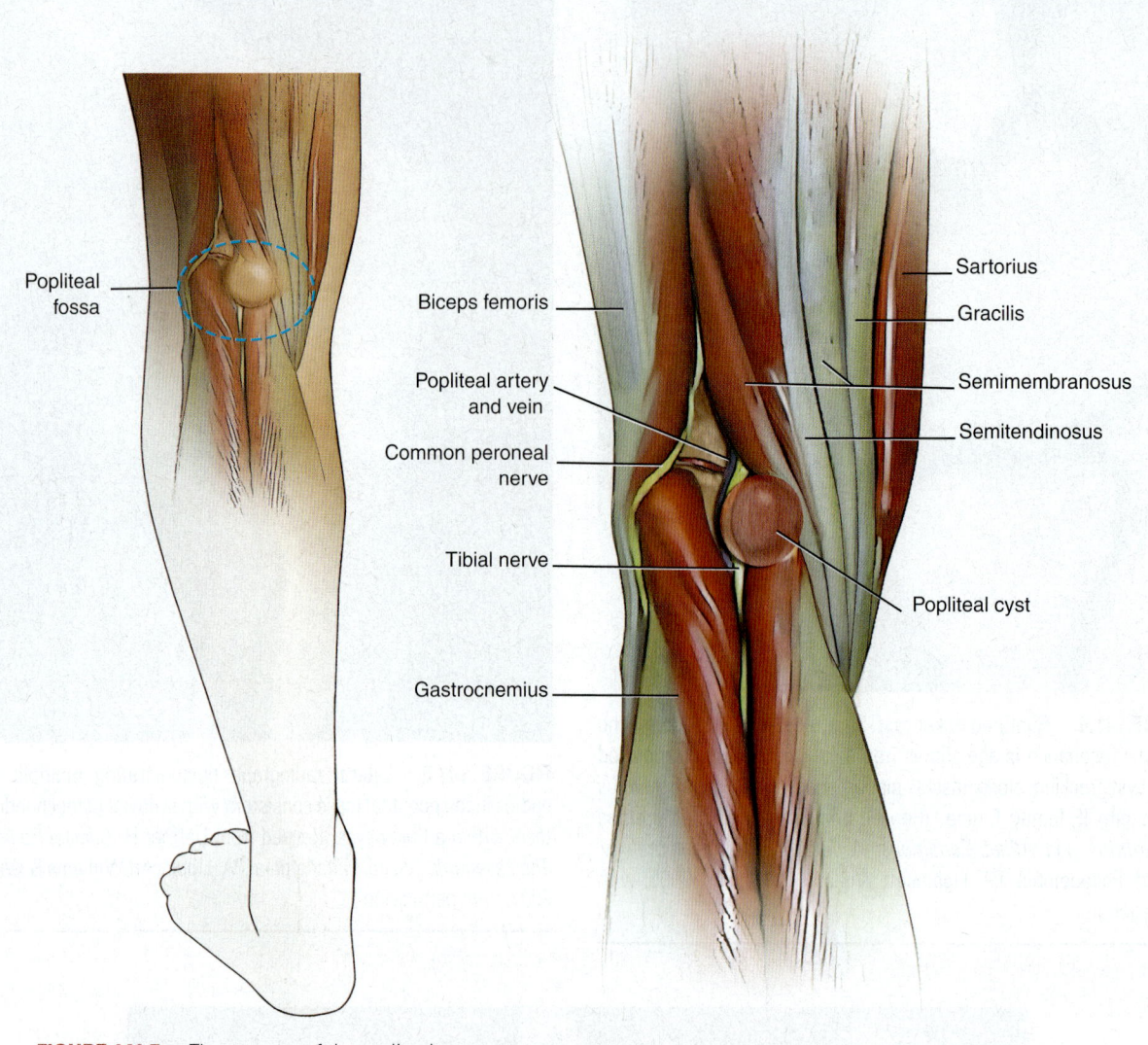

**FIGURE 141.7.** The anatomy of the popliteal space.

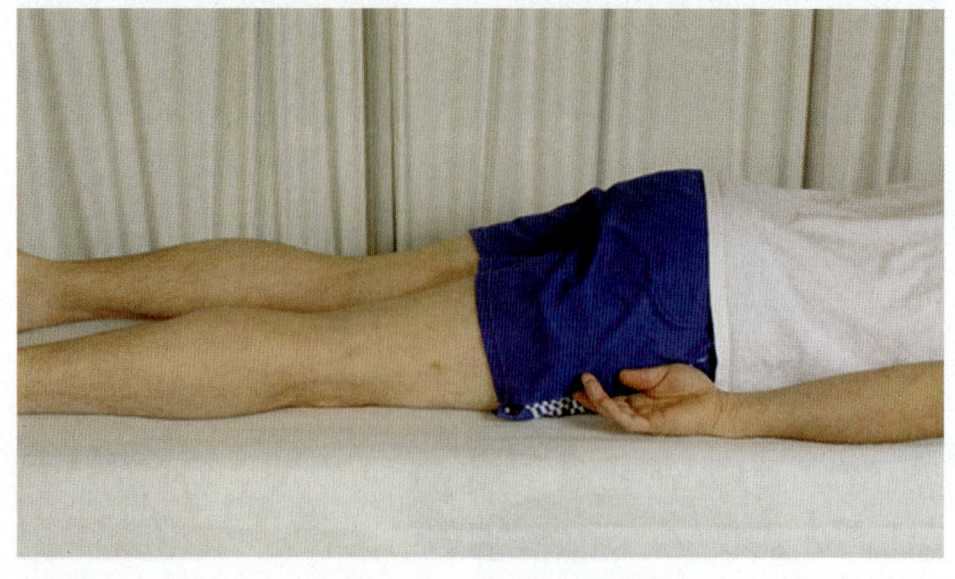

**FIGURE 141.8.** Proper patient position for ultrasound-guided injection technique for Baker cyst block.

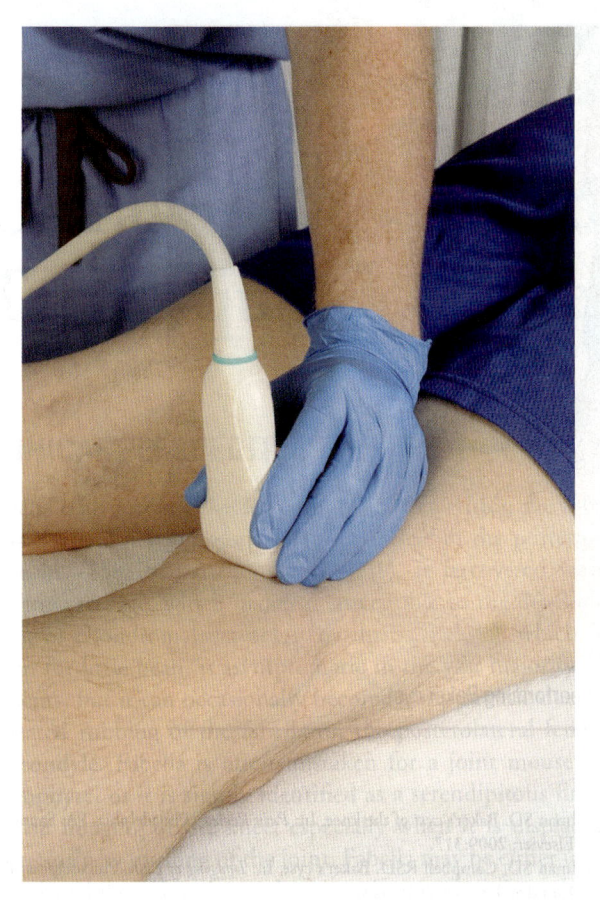

**FIGURE 141.9.** Proper transverse position of the ultrasound transducer for ultrasound-guided injection technique for Baker cyst block at the popliteal fossa.

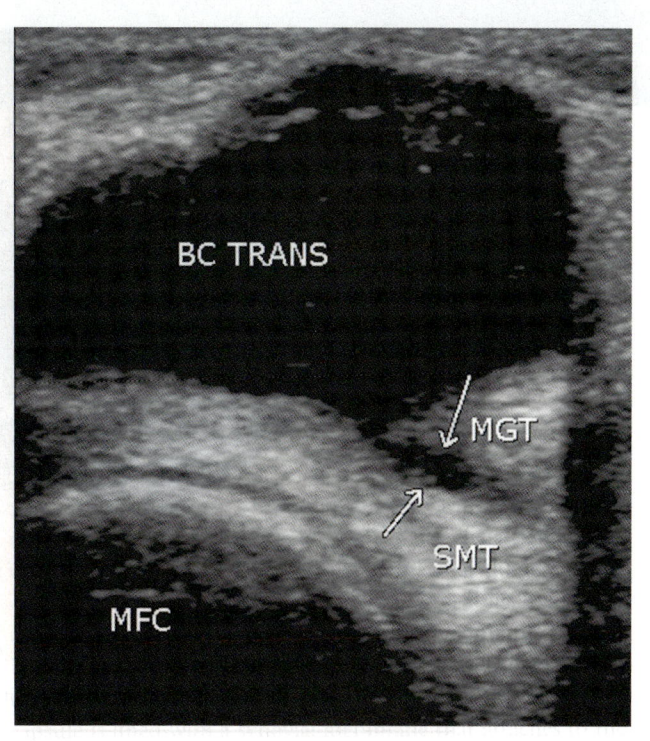

**FIGURE 141.10.** Transverse ultrasound image demonstrating a hypoechoic Baker cyst lying above the denser band of the semimembranosus tendon (*SMT*). The *arrows* point to the neck of the cyst, which leads to the joint. (BC TRANS, Baker cyst transverse view; MFC, medial femoral condyle; MGT, medial head of the gastrocnemius muscle.) (Courtesy of Mihra Taljanovic, MD, University of Arizona, Tucson.) (Reused from Daffner H. *Clinical Radiology: The Essentials*. 3rd ed. Philadelphia, PA: Lippincott Williams & Wilkins; 2007, with permission.)

preparation. This technique is safe if careful attention is paid to the clinically relevant anatomy in the areas to be injected. Care must be taken to use sterile technique to avoid infection; universal precautions should be used to avoid risk to the operator. The incidence of ecchymosis and hematoma formation, as well as reaccumulation of fluid within the Baker cyst, can be decreased if pressure is placed on the injection site immediately after injection. The use of physical modalities, including local heat and gentle range-of-motion exercises, should be introduced several days after the patient undergoes this injection technique for knee pain. Vigorous exercise should be avoided because it exacerbates the patient's symptomatology. Simple analgesics and nonsteroidal anti-inflammatory agents may be used concurrently with this injection technique.

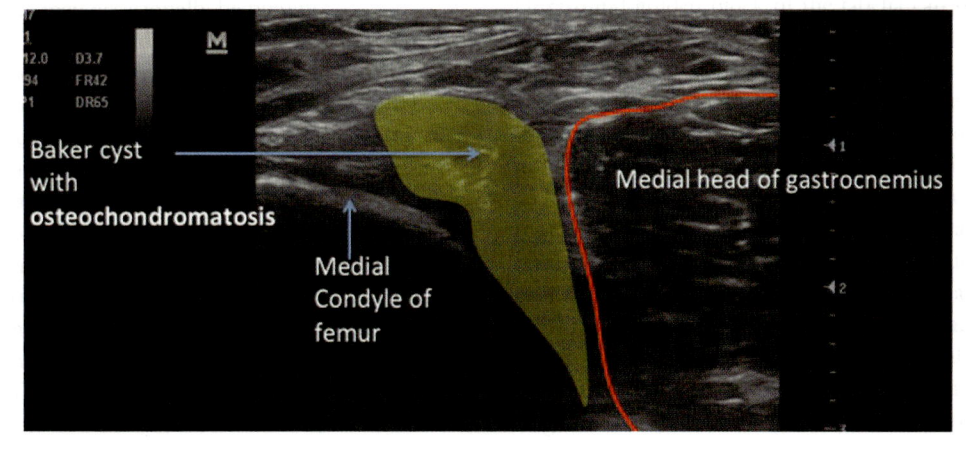

**FIGURE 141.11.** Ultrasound view of a Baker cyst with associated osteochondromatosis.

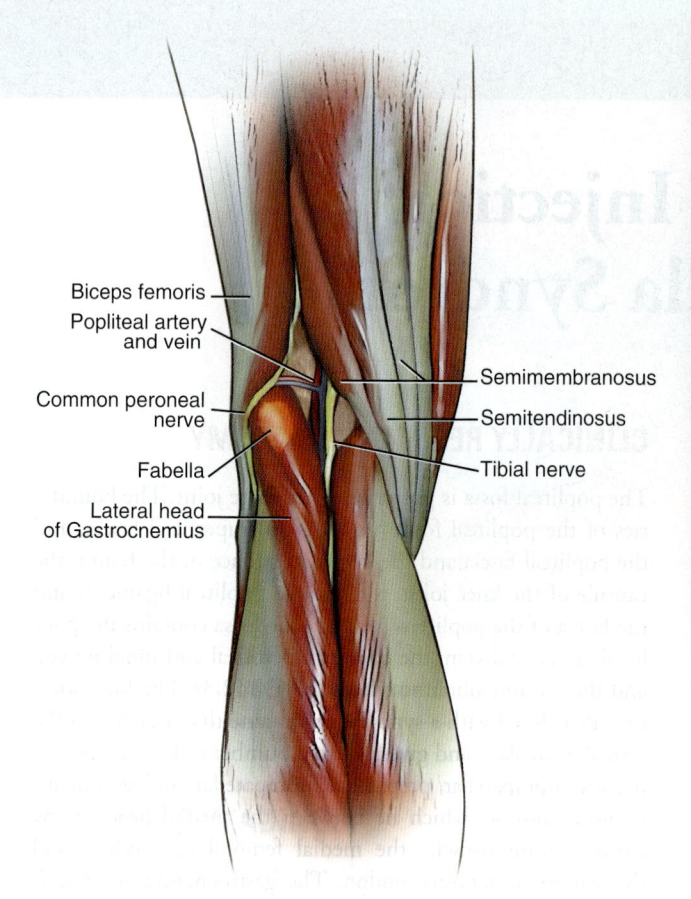

**FIGURE 142.1.** Fabella is an accessory sesamoid bone located within the substance lateral head of gastrocnemius muscle in the posterior knee in ~25% of patients.

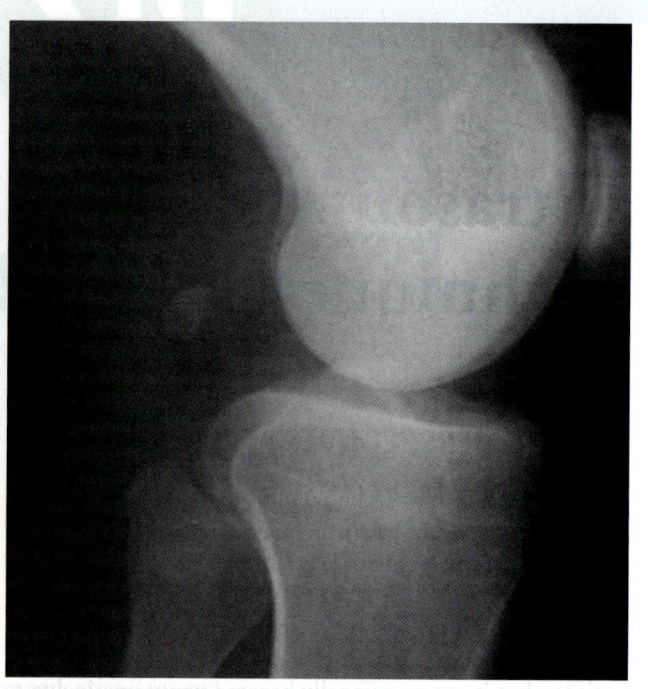

**FIGURE 142.2.** Lateral radiograph of the knee demonstrating flabella.

the gastrocnemius muscle is identified with the ovid, smooth-appearing hyperechoic fabella lying beneath it (Fig. 142.9). When the fabella is satisfactorily identified, the skin is prepped with anesthetic solution, and a 3½-inch, 22-gauge needle is advanced from the inferior border of the ultrasound transducer and advanced utilizing an in-plane approach with the trajectory being adjusted under real-time ultrasound guidance until the needle tip is resting beneath the fabella and above the lateral femoral condyle (Fig. 142.10). When the tip of needle is thought to be in satisfactory position, a small amount of local anesthetic and steroid is injected under real-time ultrasound guidance to confirm that the needle tip is beneath the fabella. There should be minimal resistance to injection. After needle tip placement is confirmed, aspiration of the fluid within the cyst is carried out, and then the remainder of the contents of the syringe are slowly injected. The needle is then removed, and a sterile pressure dressing and ice pack are placed at the injection site.

## COMPLICATIONS

The proximity to the common peroneal and tibial nerves, as well as the popliteal artery and vein, makes it imperative that this procedure be carried out only by those well versed in the regional anatomy and experienced in performing ultrasound-guided injection techniques. Postblock ecchymosis and hematoma may occur, and the patient should be warned of such. These complications can be decreased by the use of a pressure dressing and cold packs applied to the injection site following the procedure.

## CLINICAL PEARLS

The clinician must rule out the presence of joint mice in patients thought to be suffering from fabella. In general, a fabella will have an ovid smooth appearance, while a loose body will appear more jagged. Coexistent bursitis, tendonitis, or internal

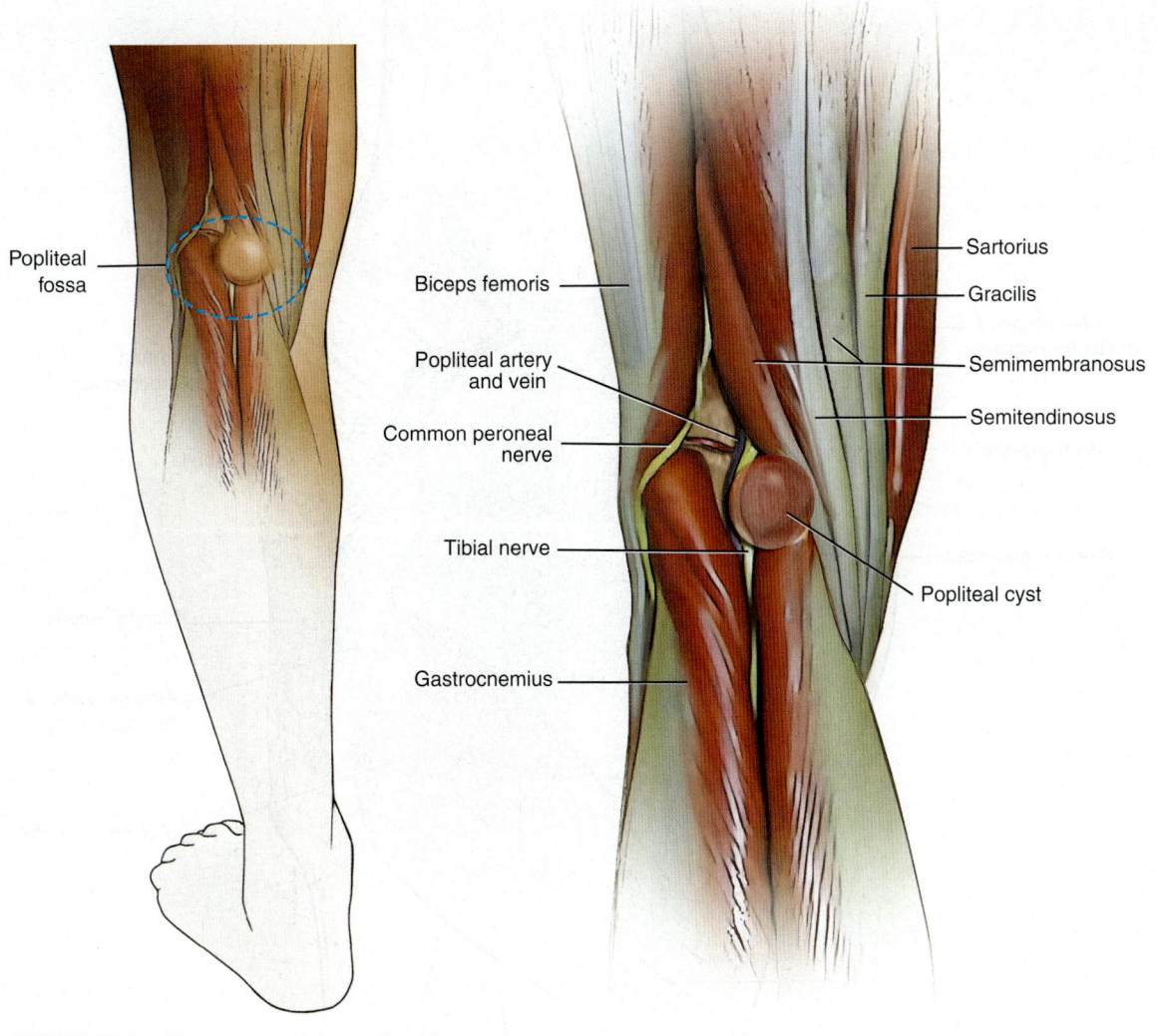

**FIGURE 142.3.** The anatomy of the popliteal fossa.

derangement of the knee may contribute to knee pain associated with and may require additional treatment with more localized injection of local anesthetic and depot corticosteroid preparation. This technique is safe if careful attention is paid to the clinically relevant anatomy in the areas to be injected. Care must be taken to use sterile technique to avoid infection; universal precautions should be used to avoid risk to the operator. The incidence of ecchymosis and hematoma formation can be decreased if pressure is placed on the injection site immediately after injection. The use of physical modalities, including local heat and gentle range-of-motion exercises, should be introduced several days after the patient undergoes this injection technique for knee pain. Vigorous exercise should be avoided because it exacerbates the patient's symptomatology. Simple analgesics and nonsteroidal anti-inflammatory agents may be used concurrently with this injection technique.

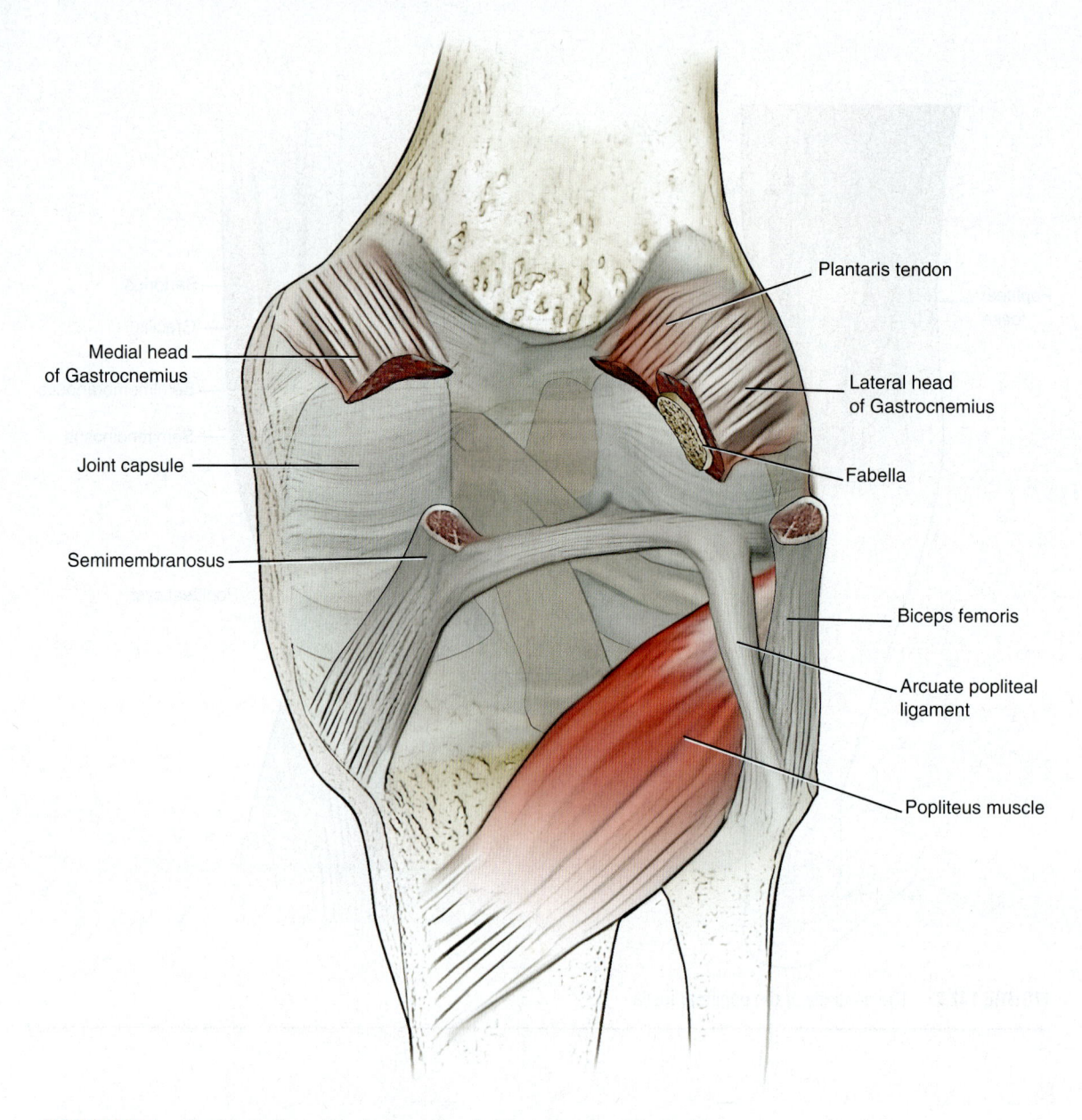

**FIGURE 142.4.** The fabella lies within the lateral head of the gastrocnemius muscle.

**FIGURE 142.5.** Proper patient position for ultrasound-guided injection technique for fabella block.

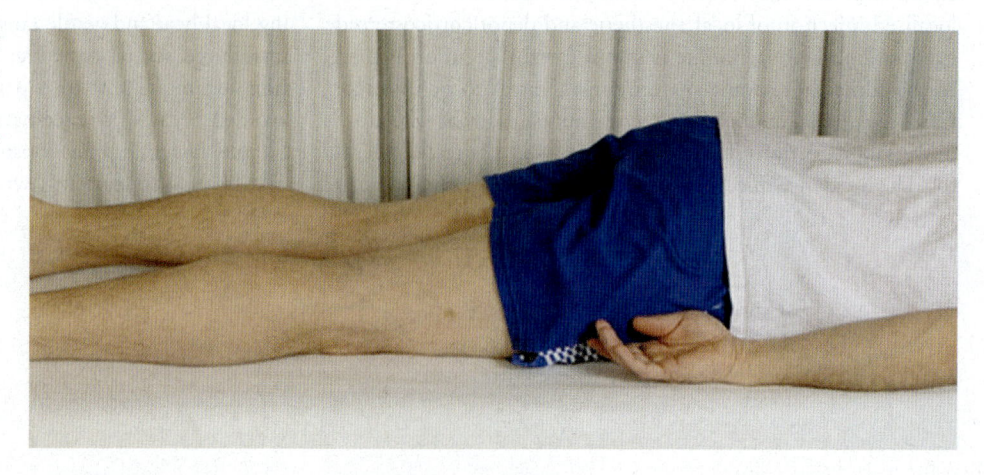

CHAPTER 142 ULTRASOUND-GUIDED INJECTION TECHNIQUE FOR FABELLA SYNDROME 1015

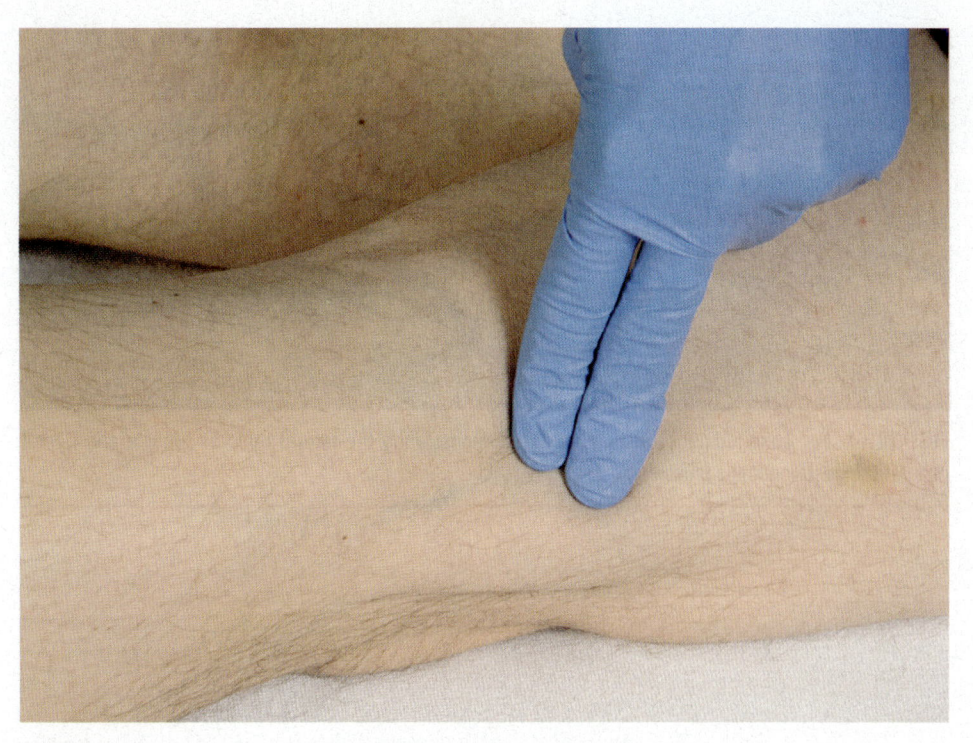

**FIGURE 142.6.** Palpation of the lateral joint space of the knee.

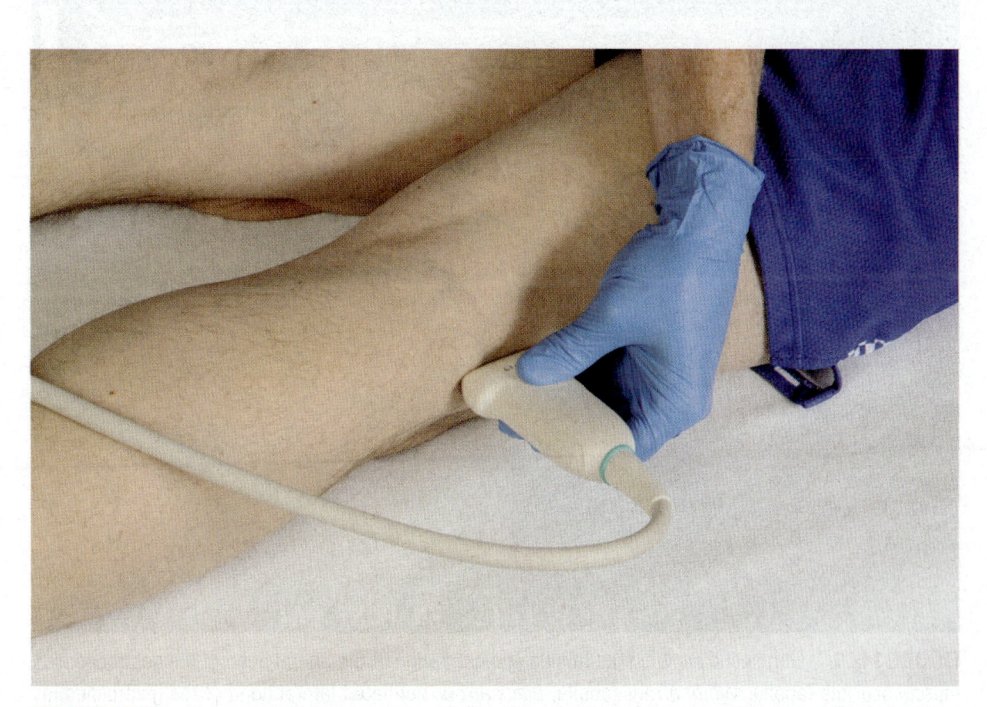

**FIGURE 142.7.** Proper longitudinal position of the ultrasound transducer over the lateral posterior knee at the level of the joint space for ultrasound-guided injection technique for fabella.

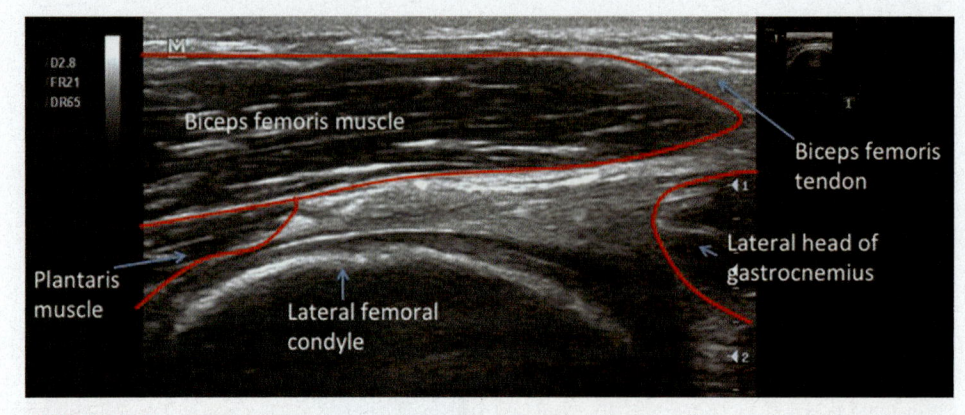

**FIGURE 142.8.** Longitudinal ultrasound image demonstrating the lateral femoral condyle and lateral head of the gastrocnemius muscle.

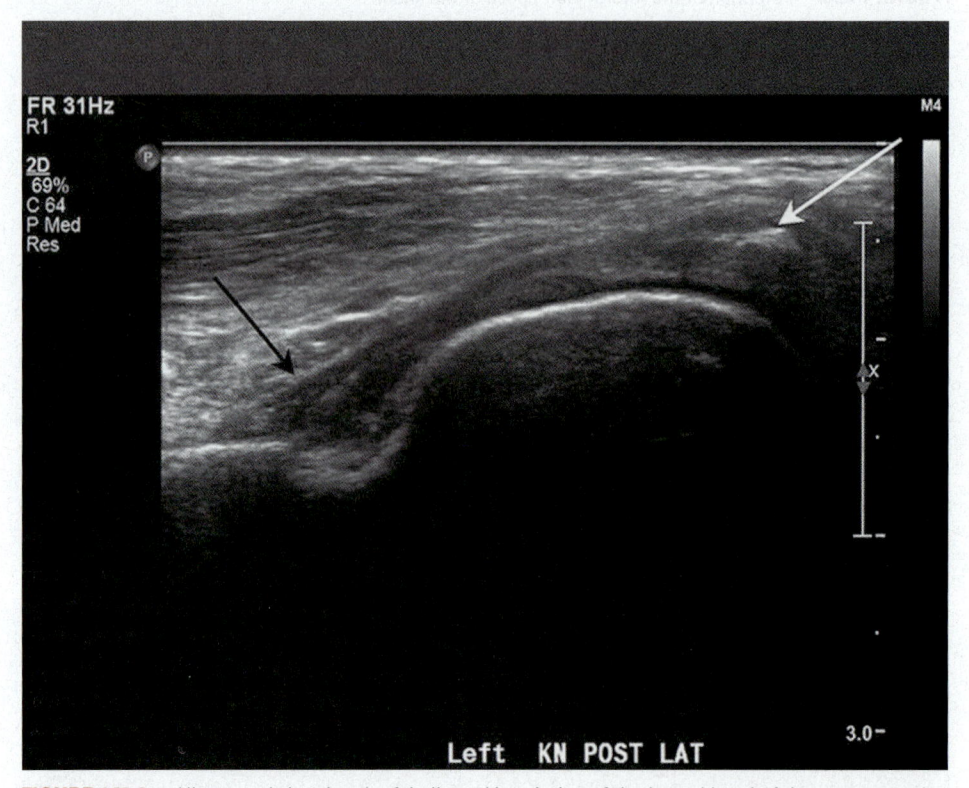

**FIGURE 142.9.** Ultrasound showing the fabella and herniation of the lateral head of the gastrocnemius muscle over the fabella. *White arrow:* fabella, *black arrow:* herniated lateral head of the gastrocnemius muscle. (Reused from Hong JH. Herniation of the lateral head of the gastrocnemius muscle: is it the source of the posterolateral knee pain? *Anesth Analg* 2007;104(5):1310–1311, with permission.)

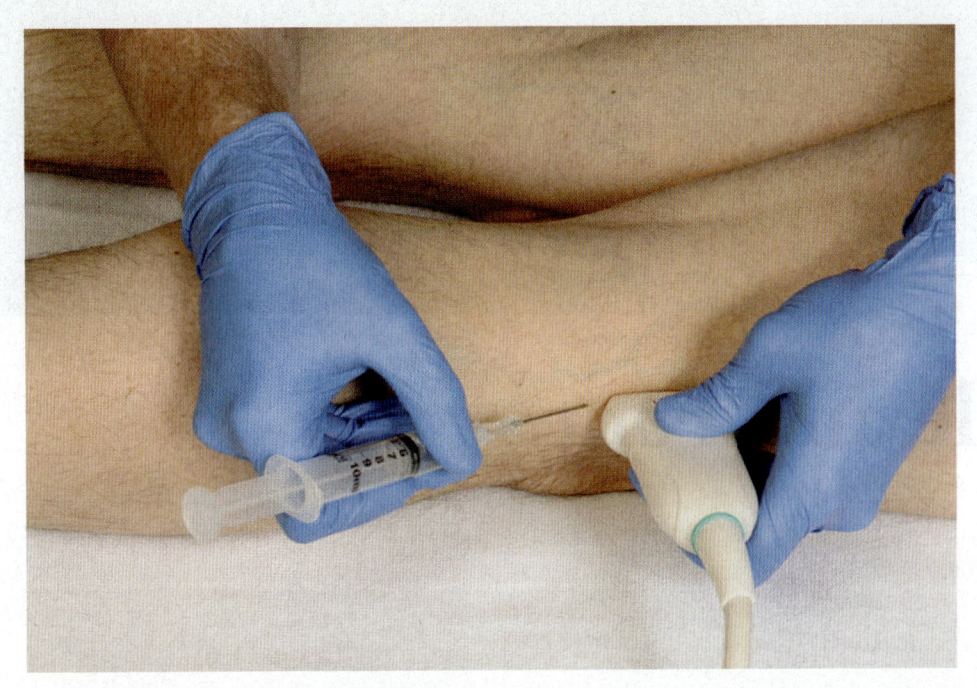

**FIGURE 142.10.** Proper in-plane needle position for performing ultrasound-guided injection of a fabella.

## SUGGESTED READINGS

Clark AM, Matthews JG. Osteoarthritis of the fabella: a fourth knee compartment? *J R Coll Surg Edinb* 1991;36:58.

Franceschi F, Longo UG, Ruzzini L, et al. Dislocation of an enlarged fabella as uncommon cause of knee pain: a case report. *Knee* 2007;14(4):330–332.

Kuur E. Painful fabella: a case report with review of the literature. *Acta Orthop Scand* 1986;57:453–454.

Robertson A, Jones SCE, Paes R, et al. The fabella: a forgotten source of knee pain? *Knee* 2004;11(3):243–245.

Weiner DS, McNab I. The "Fabella syndrome": an update. *J Paediatric Orthop* 1982;2(4):405–408.

# SECTION X

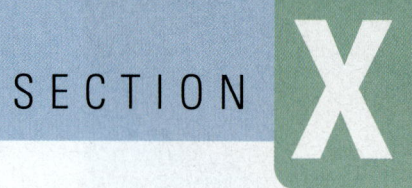

# Ankle and Foot

# CHAPTER 143

# Ultrasound-Guided Intra-articular Injection of the Ankle Joint

## CLINICAL PERSPECTIVES

The ankle joint, which is also known as the tibiotalar or talocrural joint, is a synovial hinge-type joint, which allows dorsiflexion and plantar flexion. The joint is comprised of three bones: (1) the tibia, (2) the fibula, and (3) the talus (Fig. 143.1). The joint's articular cartilage is susceptible to damage, which left untreated, will result in arthritis with its associated pain and functional disability. Osteoarthritis of the joint is the most common form of arthritis that results in ankle joint pain and functional disability, with rheumatoid arthritis and posttraumatic arthritis also causing arthritis of the ankle joint. The joint is the most commonly injured joint in the human body, with sports injuries from basketball, football, tennis, and cross-country running being frequent causes of pain and functional disability. Less common causes of arthritis-induced ankle joint pain include the collagen vascular diseases, infection, villonodular synovitis, and Lyme disease. Acute infectious arthritis of the ankle joint is best treated with early diagnosis, with culture and sensitivity of the synovial fluid, and with prompt initiation of antibiotic therapy. The collagen vascular diseases generally manifest as a polyarthropathy rather than a monoarthropathy limited to the ankle joint, although ankle pain secondary to the collagen vascular diseases responds exceedingly well to ultrasound-guided intra-articular injection of the ankle joint.

Patients with ankle joint pain secondary to arthritis and collagen vascular disease–related joint pain complain of pain that is localized to the ankle joint and distal lower extremity. Activity, especially involving dorsiflexion of the ankle joint, makes the pain worse, with rest and heat providing some relief. The pain is constant and characterized as aching. Sleep disturbance is common with awakening when the patient rolls over onto the affected ankle. Some patients complain of a grating, catching, or popping sensation with range of motion of the joint, and crepitus may be appreciated on physical examination.

Functional disability often accompanies the pain associated with many pathologic conditions of the ankle joint. Patients will often notice increasing difficulty in performing their activities of daily living, and tasks that require walking, climbing stairs, and walking on uneven surfaces are particularly problematic. If the pathologic process responsible for the patient's pain symptomatology is not adequately treated, the patient's functional disability may worsen and muscle wasting may occur.

Plain radiographs are indicated in all patients who present with ankle pain as not only intrinsic ankle disease but also other regional pathology may be perceived as ankle pain by the patient (Fig. 143.2). Based on the patient's clinical presentation, additional testing may be indicated, including complete blood cell count, sedimentation rate, and antinuclear antibody testing. Magnetic resonance imaging, computed tomography, or ultrasound of the ankle joint is indicated if avascular necrosis or meniscal tear is suspected or if the diagnosis is unclear.

## CLINICALLY RELEVANT ANATOMY

The tibia and fibula articulate with the talus at the ankle joint (see Fig. 143.1). The articular surface is dome shaped and referred to as the mortise. The articular surfaces are covered with hyaline cartilage, which are susceptible to arthritis. The joint is completely surrounded by a dense capsule that provides support to the joint. The majority of strength to the ankle joint is provided by the major ligaments, which include the deltoid, anterior talofibular, calcaneofibular, and posterior talofibular ligaments (Fig. 143.3). The joint capsule is lined with a synovial membrane that attaches to the articular cartilage and may give rise to bursae. The tibiofibular joint is innervated by the deep peroneal and tibial nerves. In addition to arthritis, the ankle joint is susceptible to the development of tendonitis and bursitis and disruption of the ligaments, cartilage, and tendons.

## ULTRASOUND-GUIDED TECHNIQUE

The benefits, risks, and alternative treatments are explained to the patient, and informed consent is obtained. The patient is then placed in the supine position with the affected lower extremity flexed at the knee so that the foot rests comfortably on the examination table (Fig. 143.4).

The skin overlying the ankle joint is then prepped with antiseptic solution. A sterile syringe containing 2.0 mL of

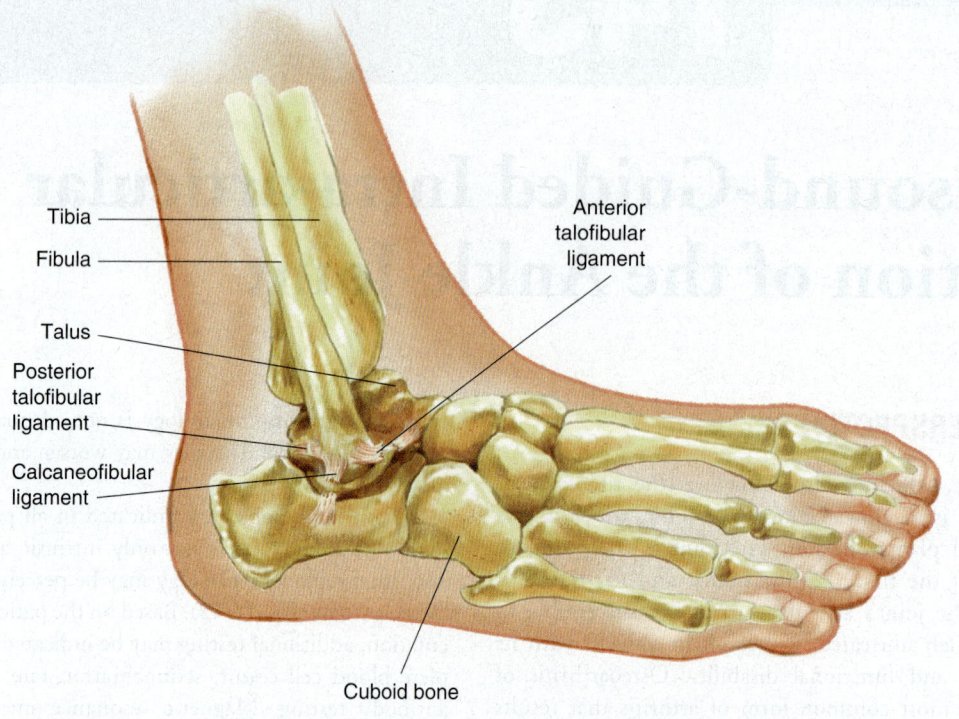

**FIGURE 143.1.** The articulations of the ankle joint. (Anatomical Chart Company, 2013.)

**FIGURE 143.2.** Lateral radiograph demonstrating joint mice, which are causing ankle pain. (Reused from Koval KJ, Zuckerman JD. *Atlas of Orthopaedic Surgery: A Multimedia Reference.* Philadelphia, PA: Lippincott Williams & Wilkins; 2004, with permission.)

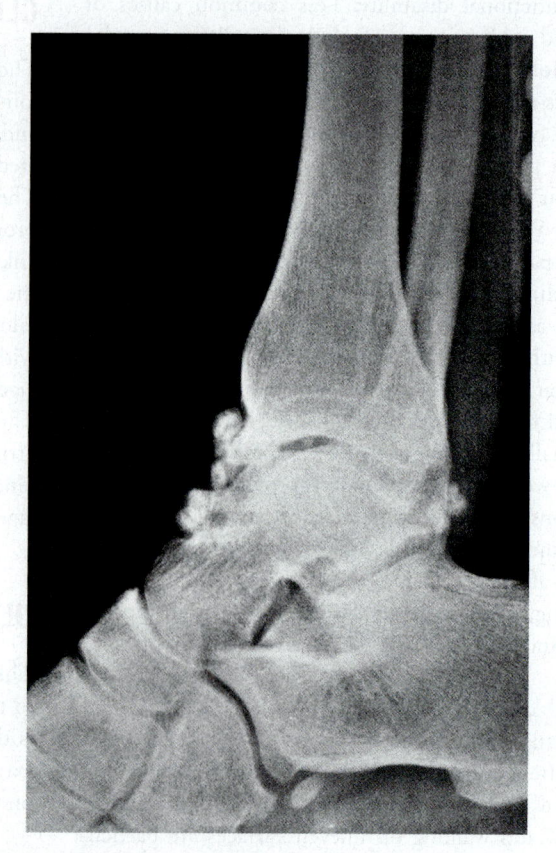

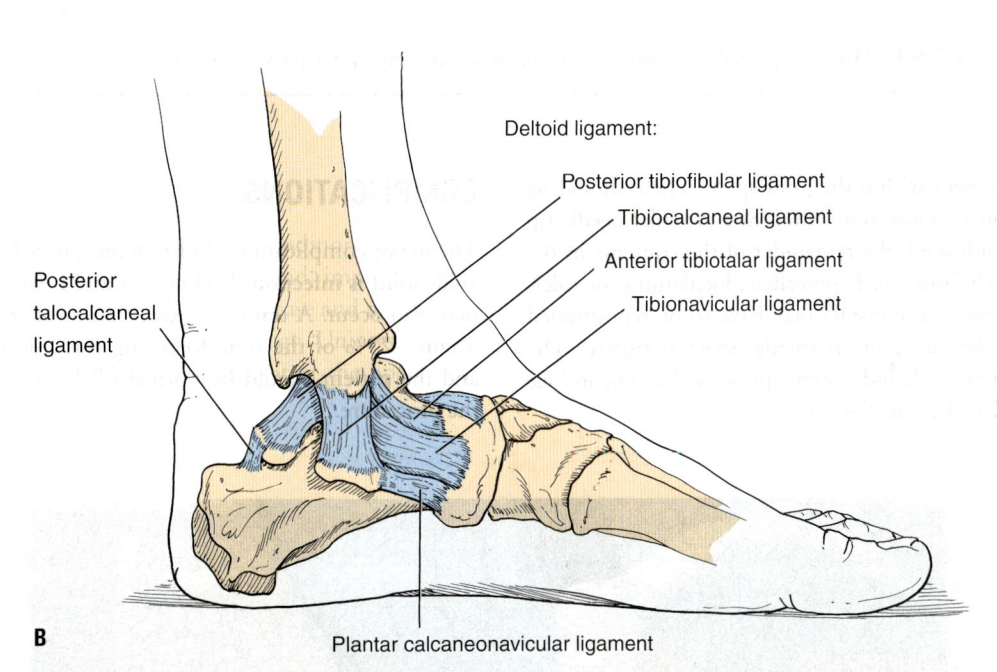

**FIGURE 143.3.** The major ligament of the ankle joint. **A:** Lateral. **B:** Medial. (Reused from Cipriano J. *Photographic Manual of Regional Orthopaedic and Neurological Tests.* 2nd ed. Baltimore, MD: Lippincott Williams & Wilkins; 1991, with permission.)

0.25% preservative-free bupivacaine and 40 mg of methylprednisolone is attached to a 1½-inch, 22-gauge needle using strict aseptic technique. A high-frequency linear ultrasound transducer is placed over the ankle joint in the longitudinal plane over the anterior aspect of the ankle joint (Fig. 143.5). An ultrasound survey scan is obtained, which demonstrates the "V"-shaped anterior tibiotalar joint (Fig. 143.6). After the joint space is identified, color Doppler imaging is utilized to identify major vessels including the dorsalis pedis artery, which frequently runs over the superior aspect of the joint (Fig. 143.7). After the joint space and major vessels are identified, the ultrasound transducer is moved slightly laterally or medially to avoid the identified vessels, and the needle is placed through the skin ~1 cm below the middle of the longitudinally placed transducer. The needle is then advanced using an inplane approach with the needle trajectory adjusted under real-time ultrasound guidance to enter the center of the ankle joint (Fig. 143.8). When the tip of needle is thought to be within the joint space, a small amount of local anesthetic and steroid is injected under real-time ultrasound guidance to confirm

**FIGURE 146.1.** Sagittal, fast, multiplanar inversion recovery (FMPIR) image of the heel depicts water with high signal intensity and fat with low signal intensity and thus shows edema in the local soft tissues and bone marrow (*curved arrow*) with extremely high sensitivity. Fluid can also be seen tracking along the plantar aponeurosis (*long straight arrow*) (*plantar fasciitis*). The arching high-signal-intensity structures (*short straight arrows*) are blood vessels.

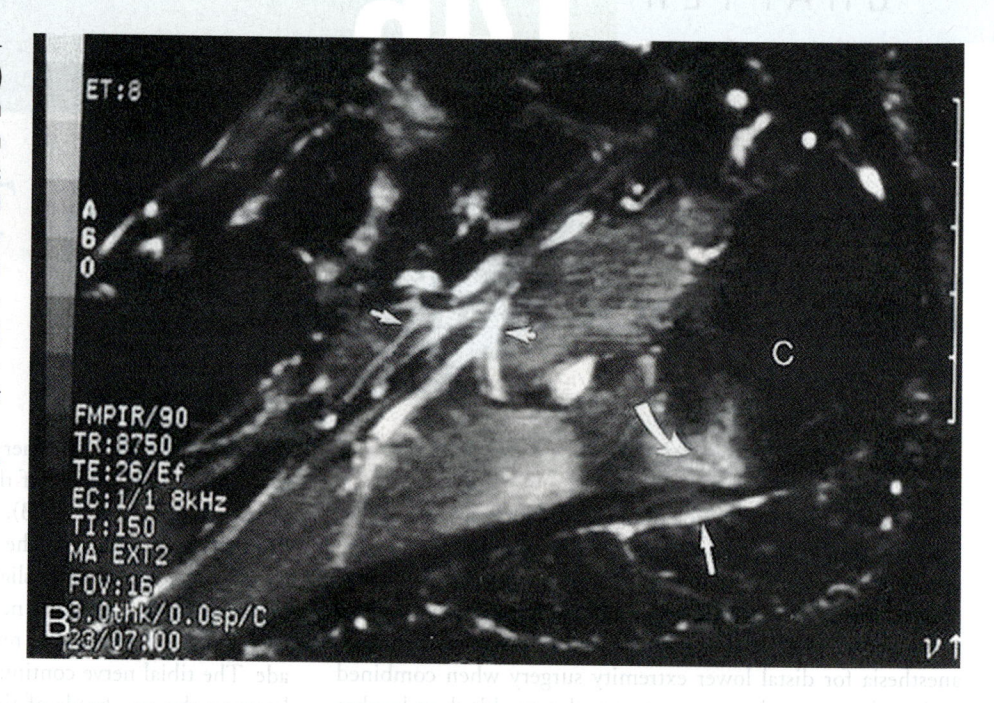

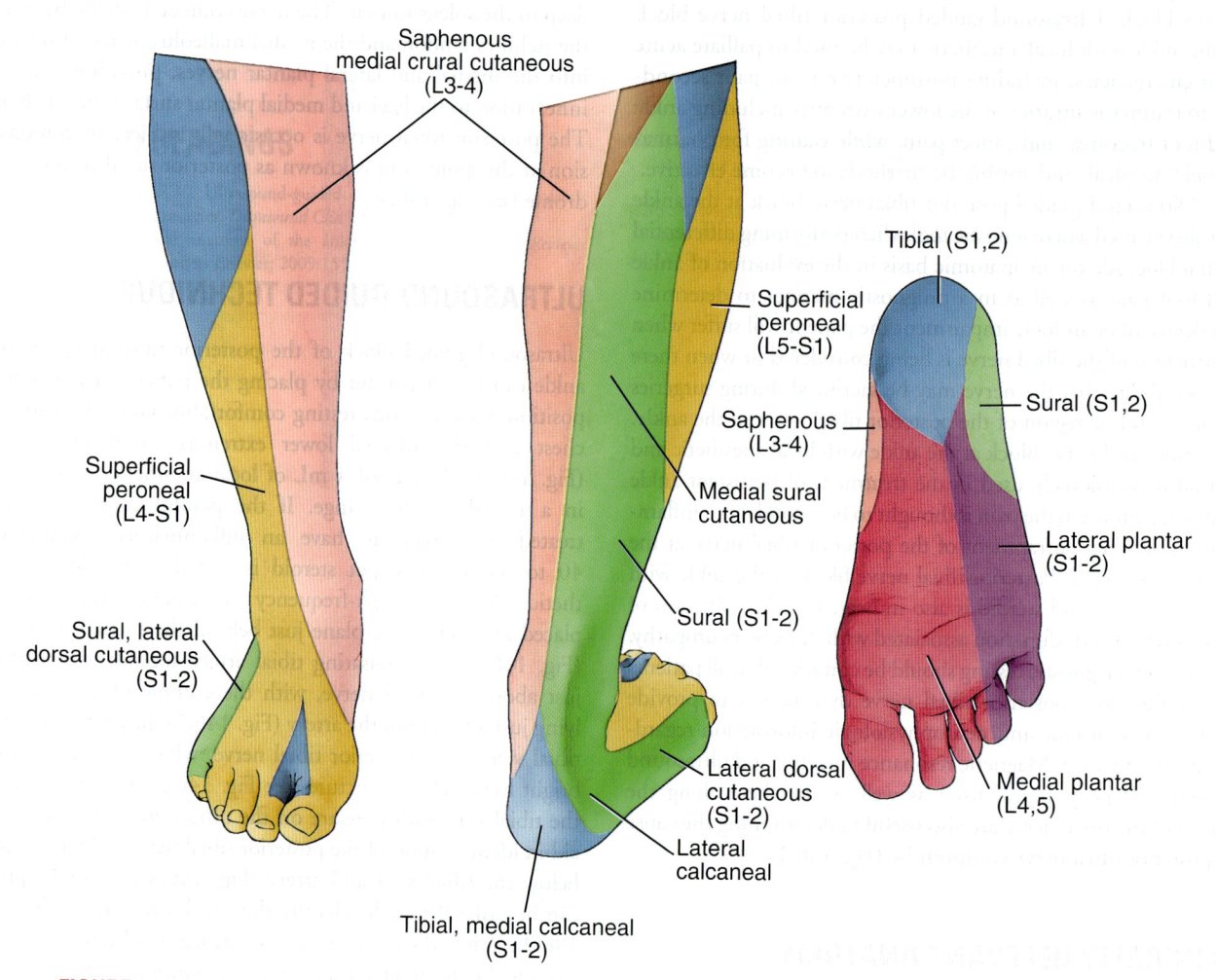

**FIGURE 146.2.** The posterior tibial nerve provides sensory innervation to the posterior portion of the calf, the heel, and the medial plantar surface.

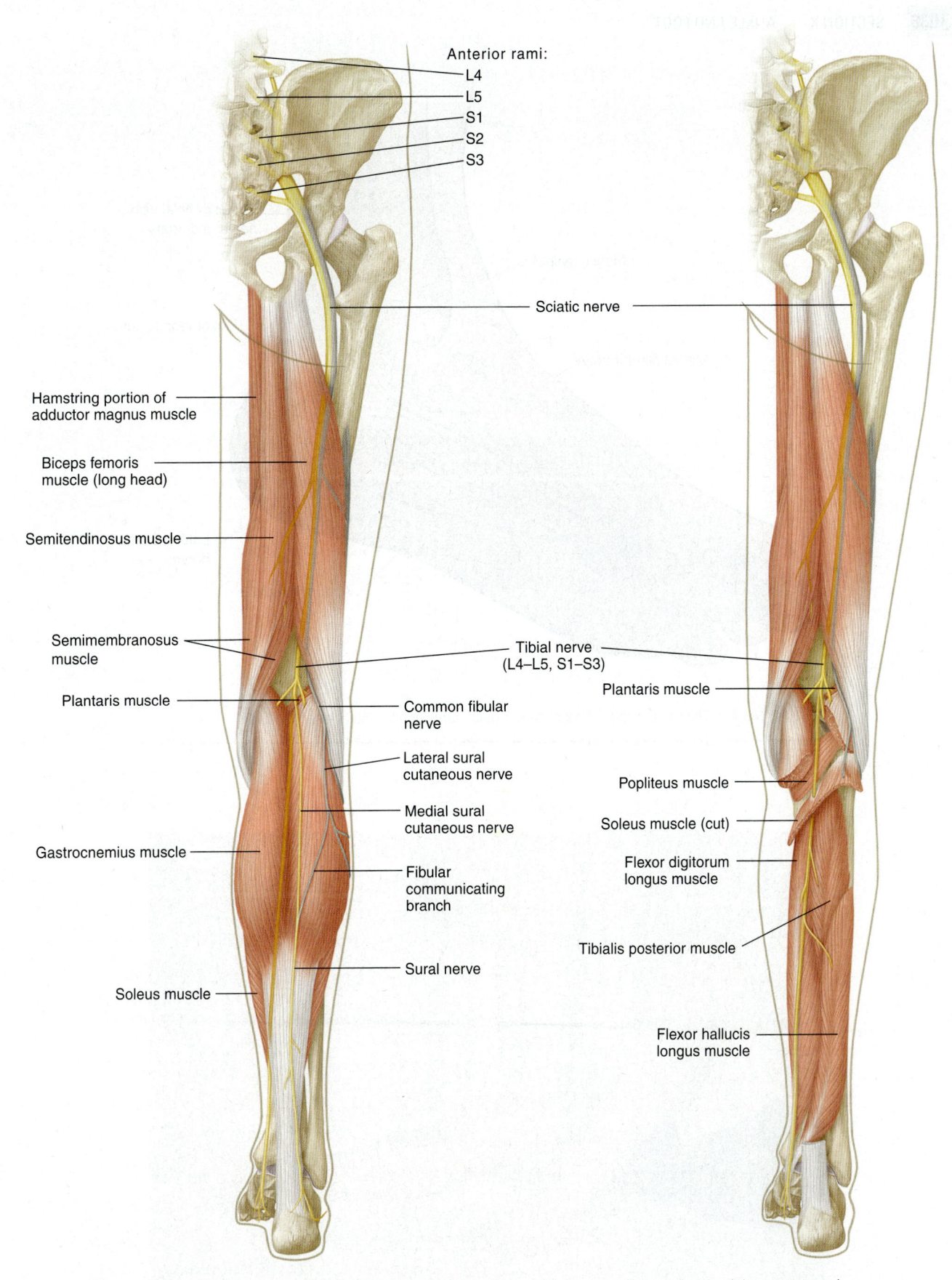

**FIGURE 146.3.** The tibial nerve continues its downward course, running between the two heads of the gastrocnemius muscle, passing deep to the soleus muscle. (Reused from Tank PW, Gest TR. *Atlas of Anatomy.* Baltimore, MD: Lippincott Williams & Wilkins; 2008, with permission.)

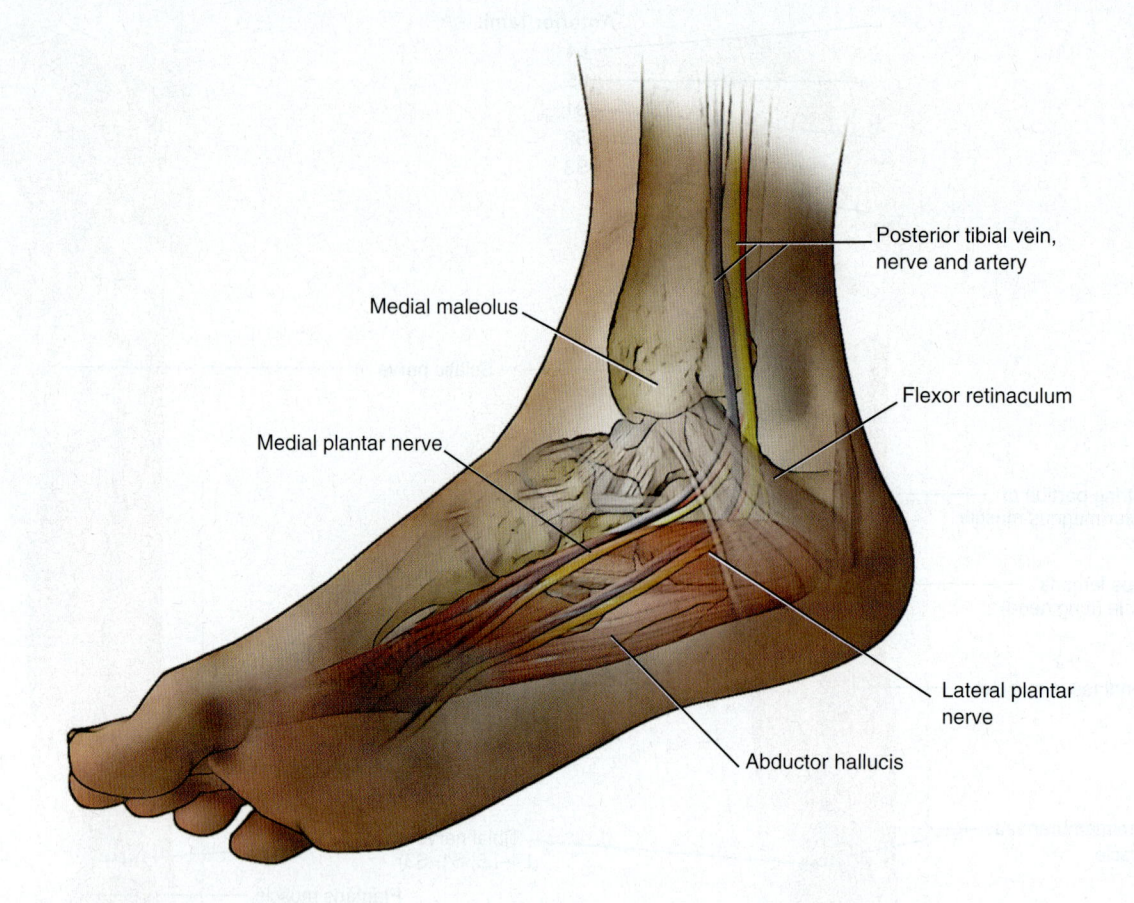

**FIGURE 146.4.** The relationship of the posterior tibial nerve and the tibial artery and vein.

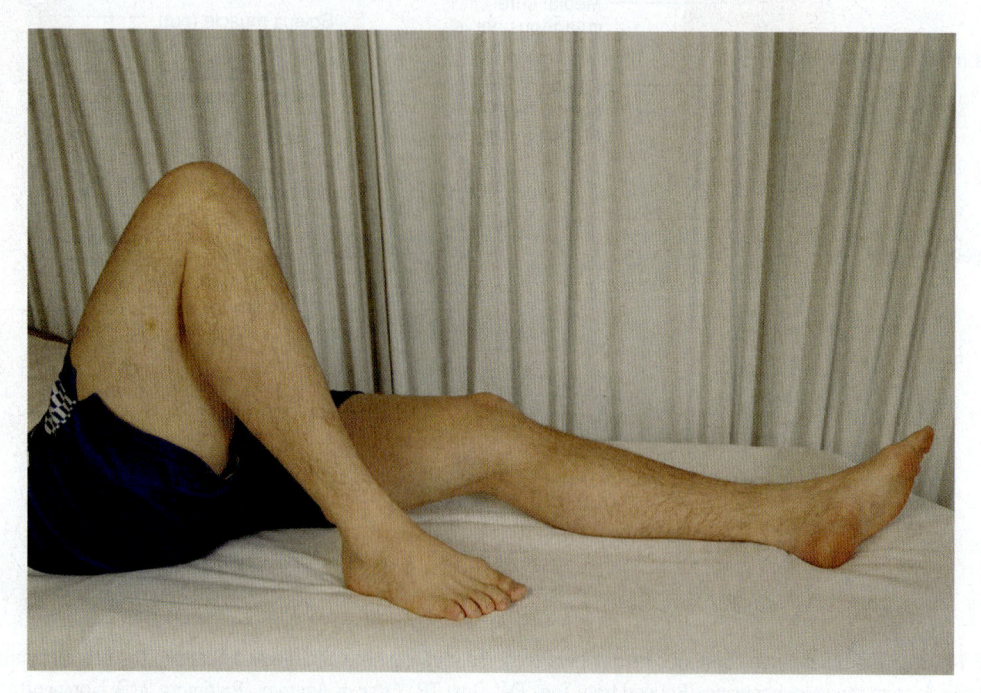

**FIGURE 146.5.** Proper patient position for ultrasound-guided posterior tibial nerve block.

CHAPTER 146    ULTRASOUND-GUIDED POSTERIOR TIBIAL NERVE BLOCK AT THE ANKLE    1039

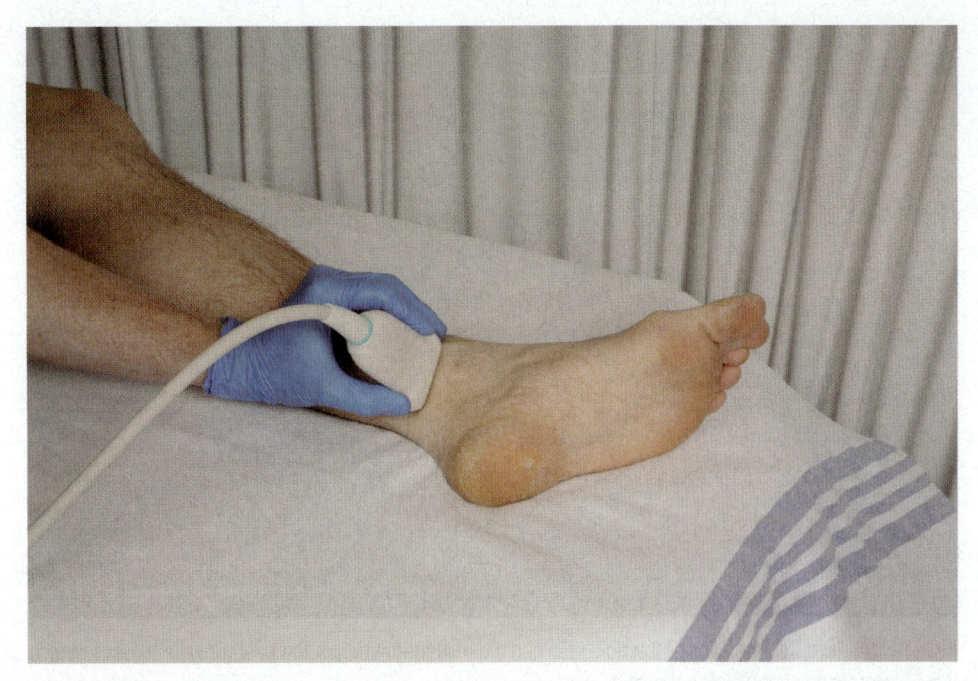

**FIGURE 146.6.** Proper transverse position of the ultrasound transducer for ultrasound-guided posterior tibial nerve block at the ankle.

advanced utilizing an out-of-plane approach with the trajectory being adjusted under real-time ultrasound guidance until the needle tip is resting in proximity to the posterior tibial nerve (Fig. 146.10). When the tip of needle is thought to be in satisfactory position, after careful aspiration, a small amount of local anesthetic and steroid is injected under real-time ultrasound guidance to confirm that the needle tip is in proximity to the posterior tibial nerve, but not within the nerve itself. There should be minimal resistance to injection. After needle tip placement is confirmed, the remainder of the contents of the syringe are slowly injected. The needle is then removed, and a sterile pressure dressing and ice pack are placed at the injection site.

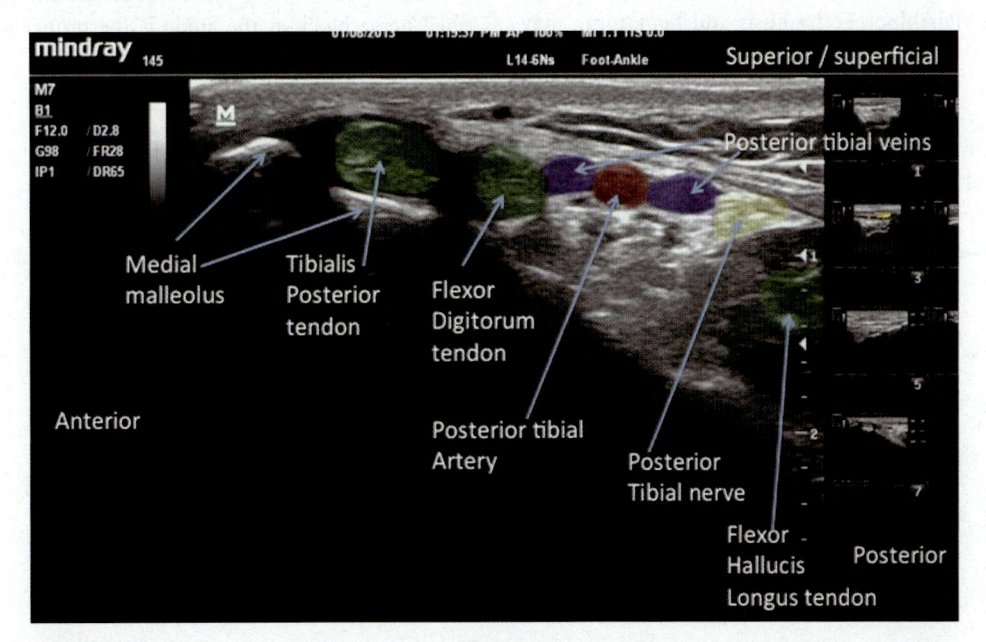

**FIGURE 146.7.** Transverse ultrasound image demonstrating the tibial artery and vein and the posterior tibial nerve just above and lateral to the vein. Vastus medialis lying above the anteromedial femur.

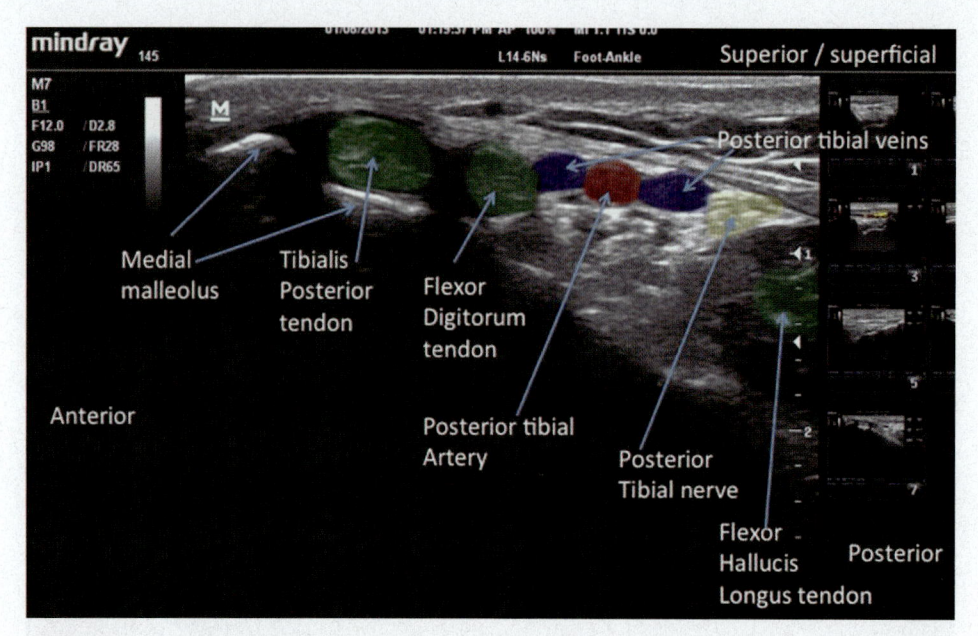

**FIGURE 146.8.** Compression of the tibia vein can aid in identification of the posterior tibial nerve, which is just lateral and superficial to the vein.

## COMPLICATIONS

A failure to accurately assess the correct position of the needle tip when performing ultrasound-guided posterior tibial nerve block at the ankle can lead to a failure to block the posterior tibial nerve or cause needle-induced trauma to the posterior tibial nerve and/or tibial artery and vein. The use of ultrasound guidance when performing posterior tibial nerve block at the ankle should markedly decrease these problems. Postblock ecchymosis and hematoma may occur, and the patient should be warned of such. These complications can be decreased by the use of a pressure dressing and cold packs applied to the injection site following the procedure.

## CLINICAL PEARLS

The key to performing successful ultrasound-guided posterior tibial nerve block at the ankle is the proper identification of

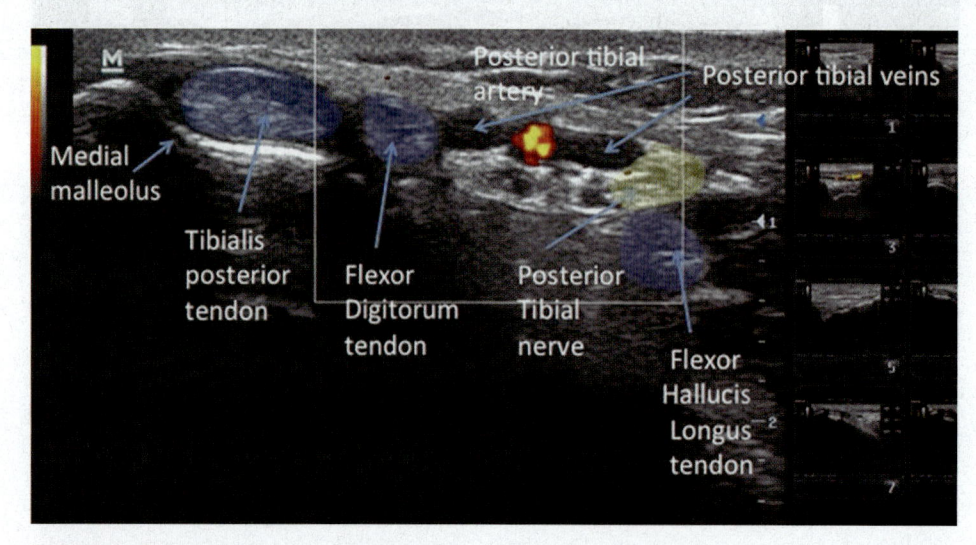

**FIGURE 146.9.** Transverse color Doppler image demonstrating the popliteal vein and artery and the relationship of the vein to the posterior tibial nerve.

CHAPTER 146   ULTRASOUND-GUIDED POSTERIOR TIBIAL NERVE BLOCK AT THE ANKLE   1041

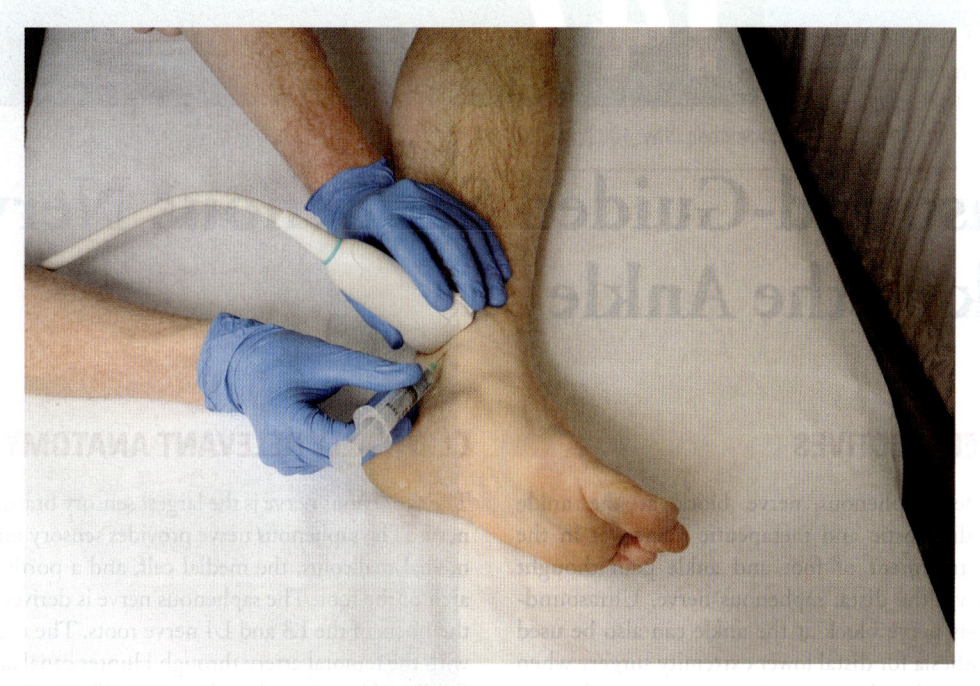

**FIGURE 146.10.** Proper out-of-plane needle position for performing posterior tibial nerve block at the ankle.

the sonographic anatomy and in particular the ability to properly identify the posterior tibial nerve. This should not be a problem if the above technique is used. Any significant pain or sudden increase in resistance during injection when performing this ultrasound-guided technique suggests incorrect needle placement, and one should stop injecting immediately and reassess the position of the needle.

## SUGGESTED READINGS

Cho KH, Wansaicheong GKL. Ultrasound of the foot and ankle. [Review Article.] *Ultrasound Clin* 2012;7(4):487–503.
Lopez-Ben R. Imaging of nerve entrapment in the foot and ankle. [Review Article.] *Foot Ankle Clin* 2011;16(2):213–224.
Milnes HL, Pavier JC. Schwannoma of the tibial nerve sheath as a cause of tarsal tunnel syndrome—a case study. *Foot(Edinb)* 2012;22(3):243–246.
Waldman SD. Posterior tibial nerve block at the ankle. In: *Atlas of Interventional Pain Management*. 3rd ed. Philadelphia, PA: Saunders Elsevier; 2009:547–550.

**FIGURE 147.6.** Proper transverse position of the ultrasound transducer for ultrasound-guided saphenous nerve block at the ankle.

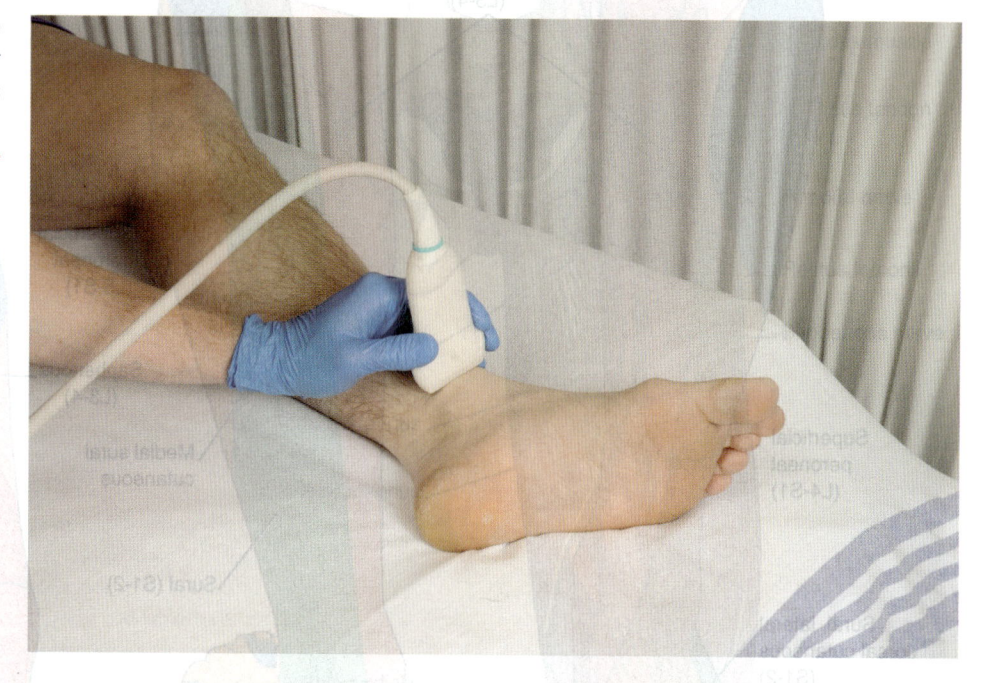

**FIGURE 147.7.** Transverse ultrasound image demonstrating the saphenous vein and the saphenous nerve just above and lateral to the vein.

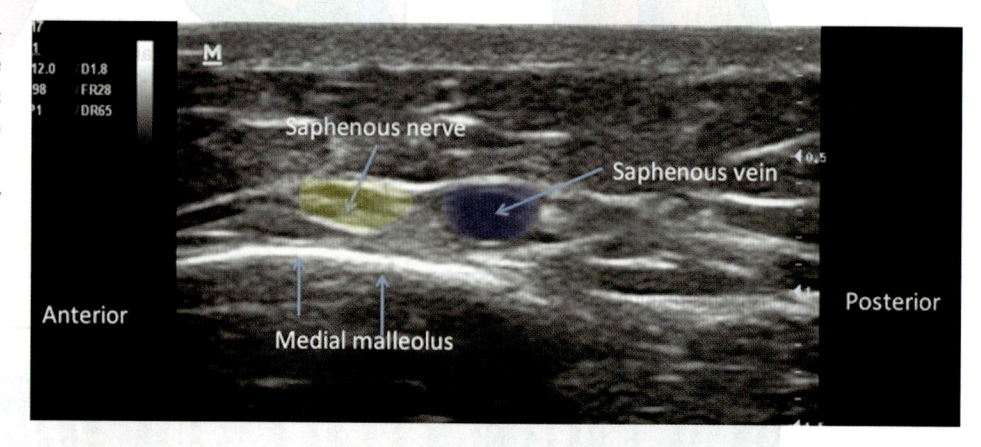

**FIGURE 147.8.** Transverse color Doppler image demonstrating the popliteal vein and artery and the relationship of the vein to the saphenous nerve.

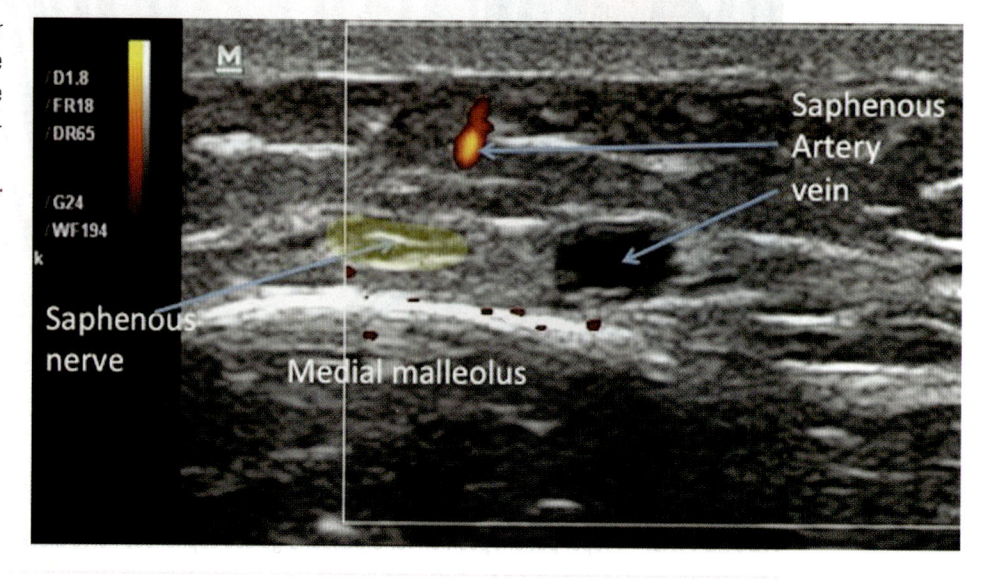

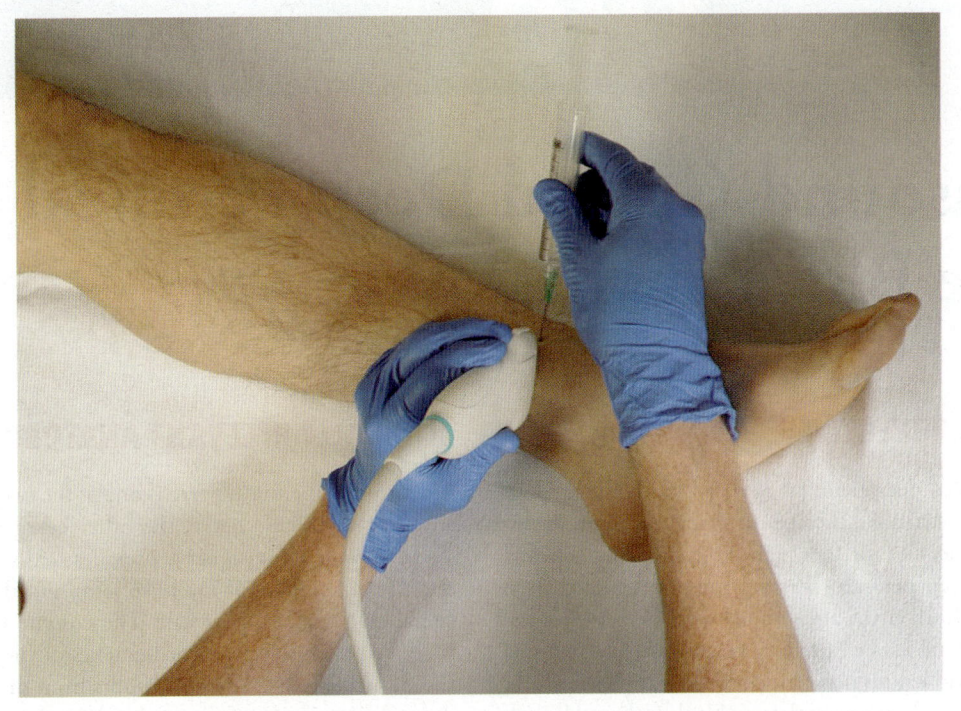

**FIGURE 147.9.** Proper in-plane needle position for performing saphenous nerve block at the ankle.

## SUGGESTED READINGS

Cho KH, Wansaicheong KL. Ultrasound of the foot and ankle. [Review Article.] *Ultrasound Clin* 2012;7(4):487–503.

Lopez-Ben R. Imaging of nerve entrapment in the foot and ankle. [Review Article.] *Foot Ankle Clin* 2011;16(2):213–224.

Sanders B, Rolf R, McClelland W, et al. Prevalence of saphenous nerve injury after autogenous hamstring harvest: an anatomic and clinical study of sartorial branch injury. *Arthroscopy* 2007;23(9):956–963.

Waldman SD. Saphenous nerve block at the ankle. In: *Atlas of Interventional Pain Management*. 3rd ed. Philadelphia, PA: Saunders Elsevier; 2009:555–558.

# CHAPTER 148

# Ultrasound-Guided Deep Peroneal Nerve Block at the Ankle

## CLINICAL PERSPECTIVES

Ultrasound-guided deep peroneal nerve block at the ankle is utilized as a diagnostic and therapeutic maneuver in the evaluation and treatment of forefoot pain thought to be mediated via the distal deep peroneal nerve. Ultrasound-guided deep peroneal nerve block at the ankle can also be used for surgical anesthesia for distal lower extremity surgery when combined with tibial and saphenous nerve block or lumbar plexus block. Ultrasound-guided deep peroneal nerve block at the ankle with local anesthetic may be used to palliate acute pain emergencies, including postoperative pain, pain secondary to traumatic injuries of the lower extremity including forefoot fractures, and cancer pain, while waiting for pharmacologic, surgical, and antiblastic methods to become effective.

Ultrasound-guided deep peroneal nerve block at the ankle can also be used as a diagnostic tool when performing differential neural blockade on an anatomic basis in the evaluation of ankle and foot pain as well as in a prognostic manner to determine the degree of neurologic impairment the patient will suffer when destruction of the deep peroneal nerve is being considered or when there is a possibility that the nerve may be sacrificed during surgeries in the anatomic region of the deep peroneal nerve at the ankle. Deep peroneal nerve block at the ankle with local anesthetic and steroid is occasionally used in the treatment of persistent ankle and foot pain when the pain is thought to be secondary to inflammation or when entrapment of the deep peroneal nerve at the ankle is suspected. Deep peroneal nerve block at the ankle with local anesthetic and steroid is also indicated in the palliation of pain and motor dysfunction associated with diabetic neuropathy.

Electrodiagnostic testing should be considered in all patients who suffer from deep peroneal nerve dysfunction to provide both neuroanatomic and neurophysiologic information regarding nerve function. Magnetic resonance imaging and ultrasound imaging anywhere along the course of the deep peroneal nerve are also useful in determining the cause of deep peroneal nerve compromise. Plain radiographs and/or computerized tomography of the ankle should be obtained in all patients who have trauma to the ankle to rule out fractures of the medial ankle, which can damage the deep peroneal nerve (Fig. 148.1).

## CLINICALLY RELEVANT ANATOMY

The common peroneal nerve is one of the two major continuations of the sciatic nerve, the other being the tibial nerve. The common peroneal nerve provides sensory innervation to the inferior portion of the knee joint and the posterior and lateral skin of the upper calf. The common peroneal nerve is derived from the posterior branches of the L4, L5, and S1 and S2 nerve roots. The nerve splits from the sciatic nerve at the superior margin of the popliteal fossa and descends laterally behind the head of the fibula (Fig. 148.2). The common peroneal nerve is subject to compression at this point by such circumstances as improperly applied casts and tourniquets. The nerve is also subject to compression as it continues its lateral course, winding around the fibula through the fibular tunnel, which is made up of the posterior border of the tendinous insertion of the peroneus longus muscle and the fibula itself. Just distal to the fibular tunnel, the nerve divides into its two terminal branches, the superficial and the deep peroneal nerves. Each of these branches are subject to trauma and may be blocked individually as a diagnostic and therapeutic maneuver.

The deep branch continues down the leg in conjunction with the tibial artery and vein to provide sensory innervation to the web space of the first and second toes and adjacent dorsum of the foot (Figs. 148.3 and 148.4). Although this distribution of sensory fibers is small, this area is often the site of Morton neuroma surgery and thus is important to the regional anesthesiologist. The deep peroneal nerve provides motor innervation to all of the toe extensors and the anterior tibialis muscles. The deep peroneal nerve passes beneath the dense superficial fascia of the ankle, where it is subject to an entrapment syndrome known as the anterior tarsal tunnel syndrome.

## ULTRASOUND-GUIDED TECHNIQUE

Ultrasound-guided block of the deep peroneal nerve at the ankle can be carried out by placing the patient in the supine position with the arms resting comfortably along the patient's chest and the affected lower extremity in neutral position (Fig. 148.5). A total of 4 mL of local anesthetic is drawn up in a 12-mL sterile syringe. If the painful condition being treated is thought to have

CHAPTER 148   ULTRASOUND-GUIDED DEEP PERONEAL NERVE BLOCK AT THE ANKLE   1049

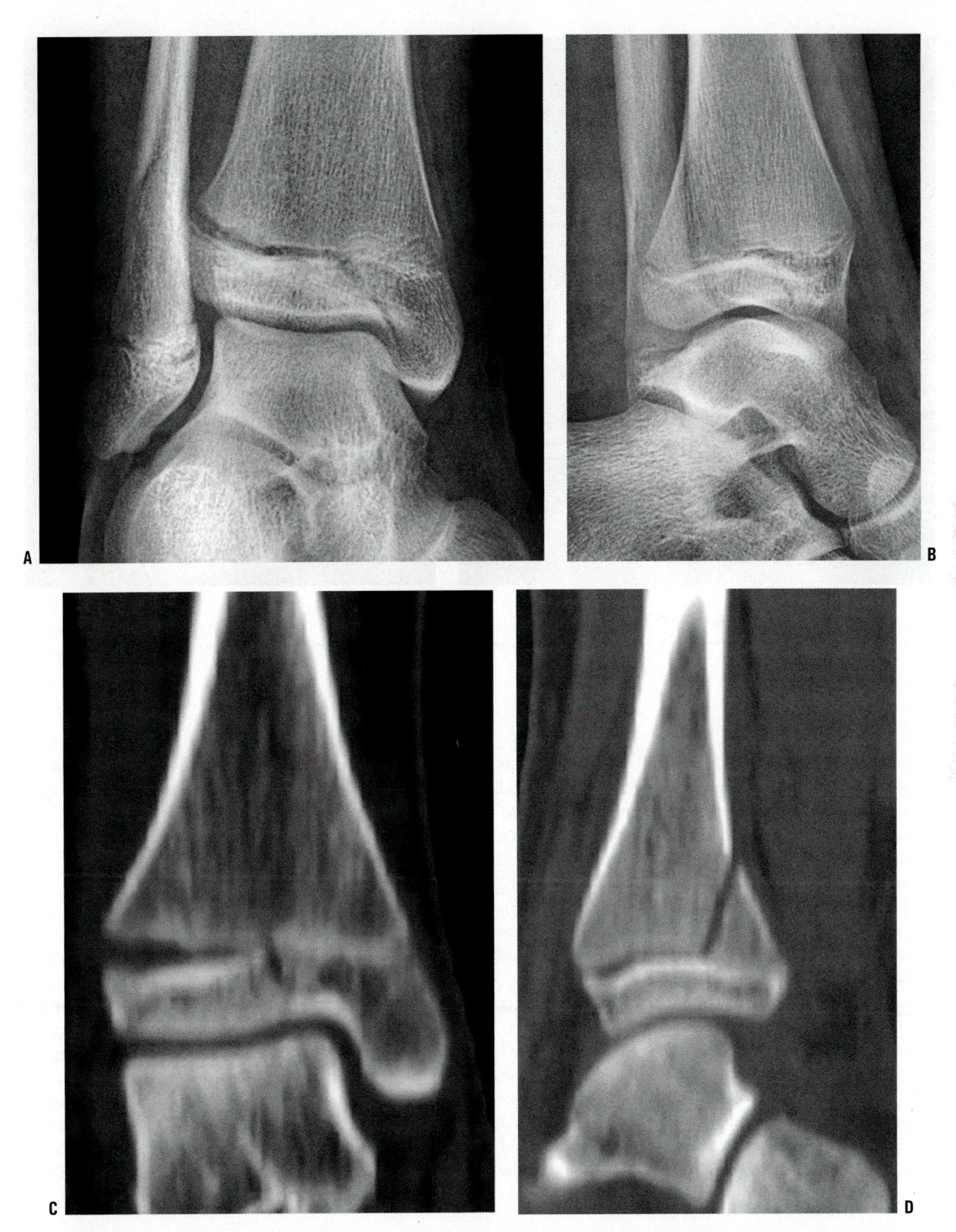

**FIGURE 148.1.** Computed tomography (CT) and 3D CT of triplanar fracture. Anteroposterior **(A)** and lateral **(B)** radiographs of the right ankle show all three components of the triplanar fracture that are more vividly demonstrated on **(C)** coronal and **(D)** sagittal reformatted CT images, and on **(E)** and **(F)** 3D CT reconstruction. (Reused from Greenspan A. *Orthopedic Imaging: A Practical Approach.* 5th ed. Philadelphia, PA: Lippincott Williams & Wilkins; 2011, with permission.)

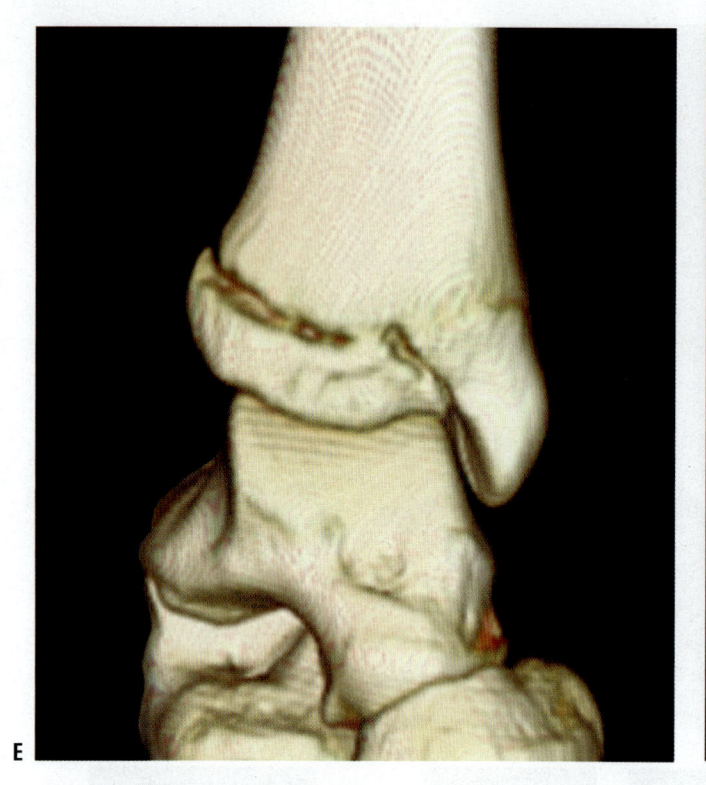

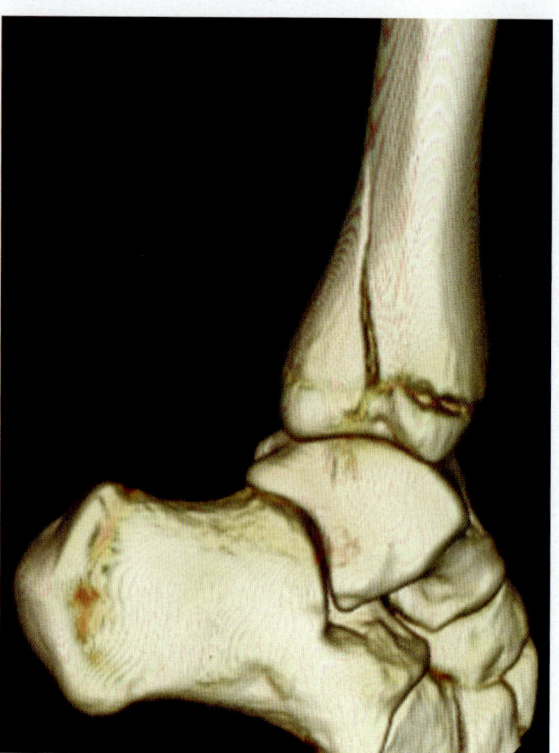

**FIGURE 148.1.** (Continued)

an inflammatory component, 40 to 80 mg of depot steroid is added to the local anesthetic. A linear high-frequency ultrasound transducer is placed in a transverse plane just above the anterior crease of the ankle, and an ultrasound survey scan is taken (Fig. 148.6). The deep peroneal nerve is seen lying just lateral to the anterior tibial artery (Fig. 148.7). Color Doppler can be utilized to help identify the anterior tibial artery (Fig. 148.8). When the anterior tibial artery and adjacent deep peroneal nerve are identified on ultrasound imaging, the skin is prepped with anesthetic solution, and a 1½-inch, 22-gauge needle is advanced from the lateral border of the ultrasound transducer and advanced utilizing an in-plane approach with the trajectory being adjusted under real-time ultrasound guidance until the needle tip is resting in proximity to the deep peroneal nerve (Fig. 148.9). When the tip of needle is thought to be in satisfactory position, after careful aspiration, a small amount of local anesthetic and steroid is injected under real-time ultrasound guidance to confirm that the needle tip is in proximity to the deep peroneal nerve, but not within the nerve itself. There should be minimal resistance to injection. After needle tip placement is confirmed, the remainder of the contents of the syringe are slowly injected. The needle is then removed, and a sterile pressure dressing and ice pack are placed at the injection site.

## COMPLICATIONS

A failure to accurately assess the correct position of the needle tip when performing ultrasound-guided deep peroneal nerve block at the ankle can lead to a failure to block the deep peroneal nerve or cause needle-induced trauma to the deep peroneal nerve and/or dorsalis pedis artery. The use of ultrasound guidance when performing deep peroneal nerve block at the ankle should markedly decrease these problems. Postblock ecchymosis and hematoma may occur, and the patient should be warned of such. These complications can be decreased by the use of a pressure dressing and cold packs applied to the injection site following the procedure.

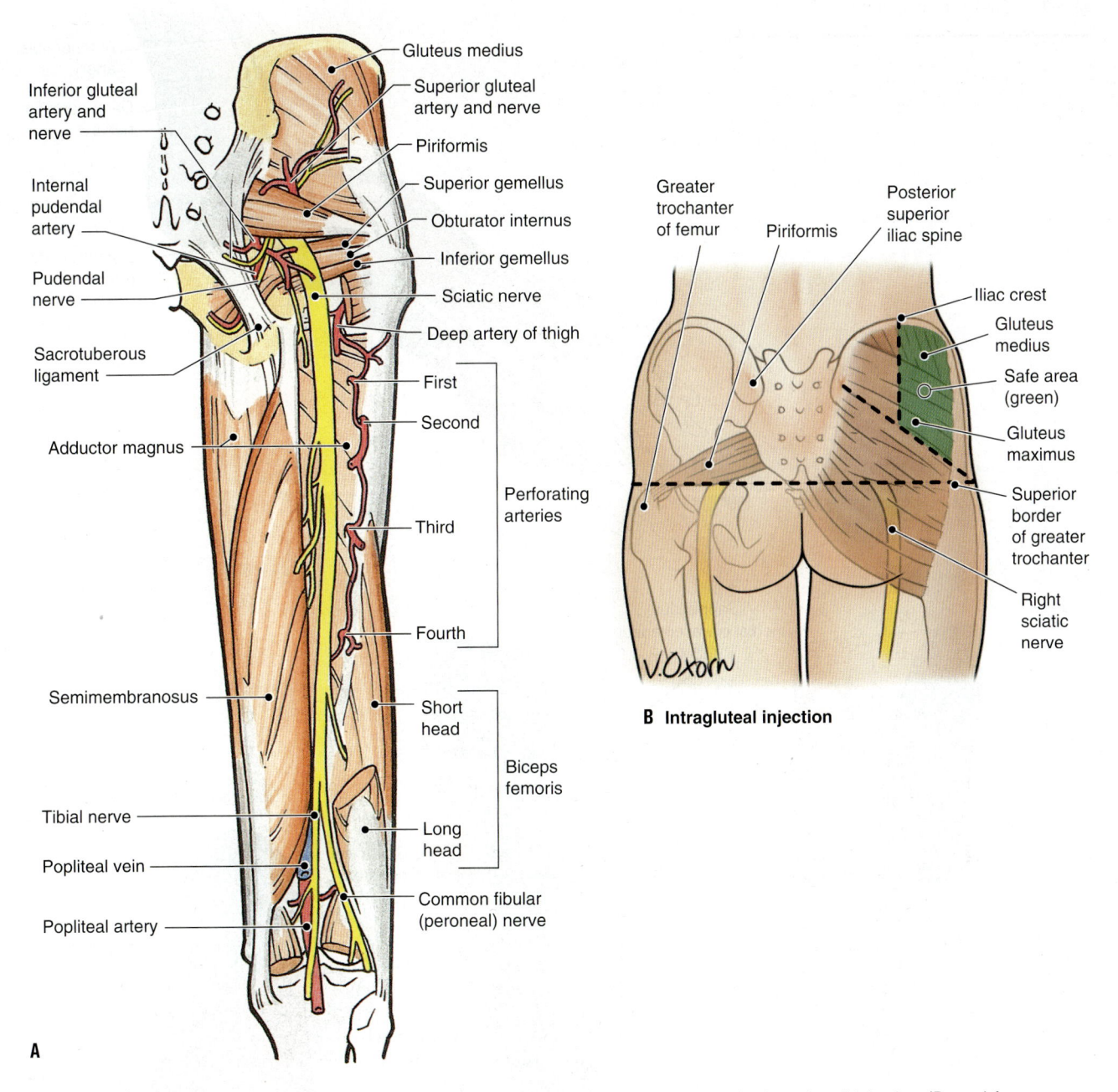

**FIGURE 148.2.** **A:** The anatomy of the common peroneal nerve. **B:** The safe zone for intragluteal injection. (Reused from Moore KL, Agur AMR. *Essential Clinical Anatomy.* 2nd ed. Baltimore, MD: Lippincott Williams & Wilkins; 2002, with permission.)

**FIGURE 148.3.** The anatomy of the distal deep peroneal nerve. Note the relationship of the nerve to the deep peroneal vein.

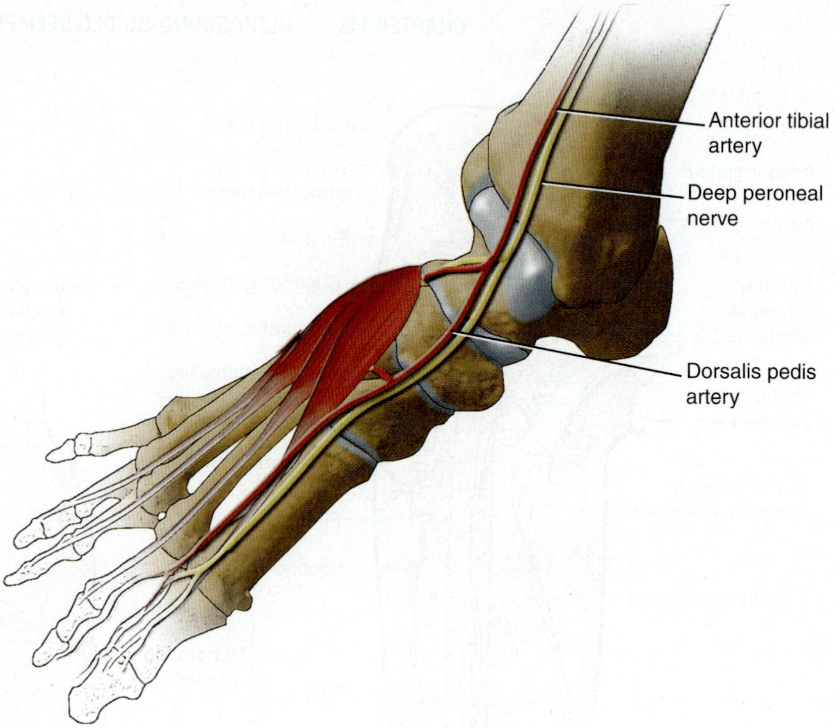

- Anterior tibial artery
- Deep peroneal nerve
- Dorsalis pedis artery

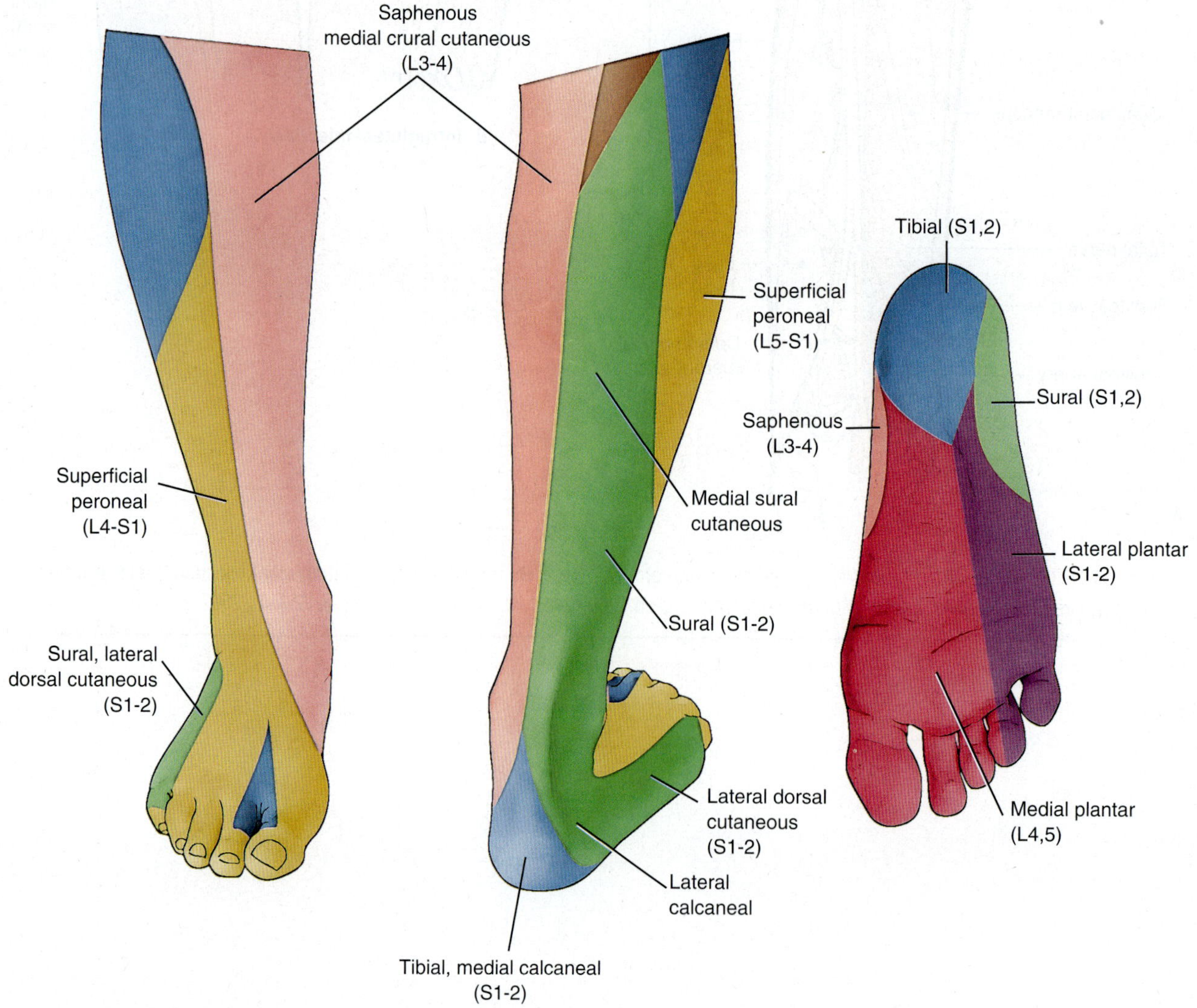

- Saphenous medial crural cutaneous (L3-4)
- Superficial peroneal (L5-S1)
- Saphenous (L3-4)
- Medial sural cutaneous
- Sural (S1-2)
- Superficial peroneal (L4-S1)
- Sural, lateral dorsal cutaneous (S1-2)
- Lateral dorsal cutaneous (S1-2)
- Lateral calcaneal
- Tibial, medial calcaneal (S1-2)
- Tibial (S1,2)
- Sural (S1,2)
- Lateral plantar (S1-2)
- Medial plantar (L4,5)

**FIGURE 148.4.** Sensory distribution of the distal deep peroneal nerve.

CHAPTER 148 ULTRASOUND-GUIDED DEEP PERONEAL NERVE BLOCK AT THE ANKLE 1053

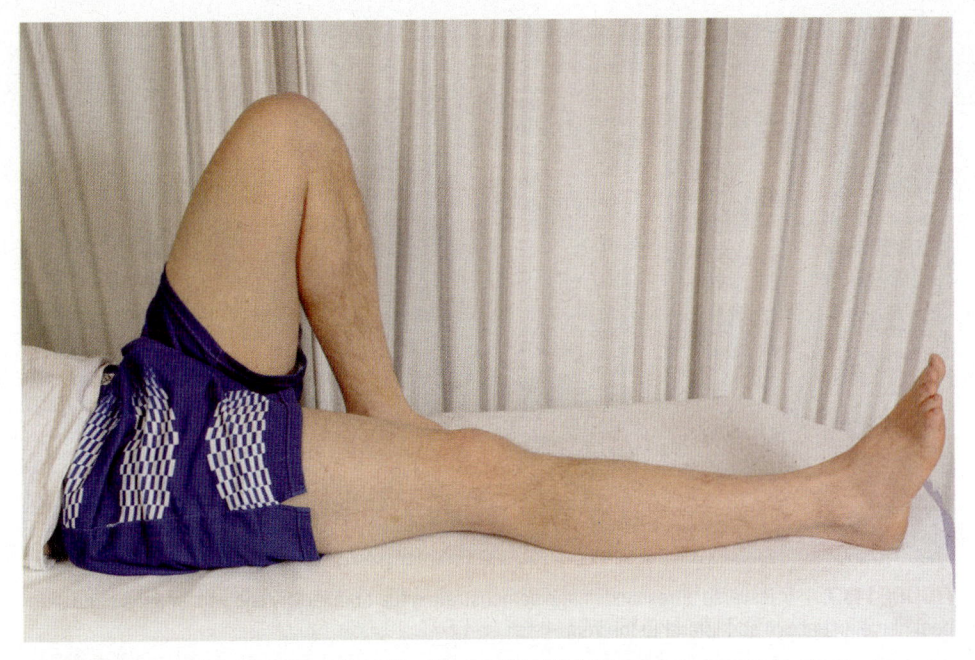

**FIGURE 148.5.** Proper patient position for ultrasound-guided deep peroneal nerve block.

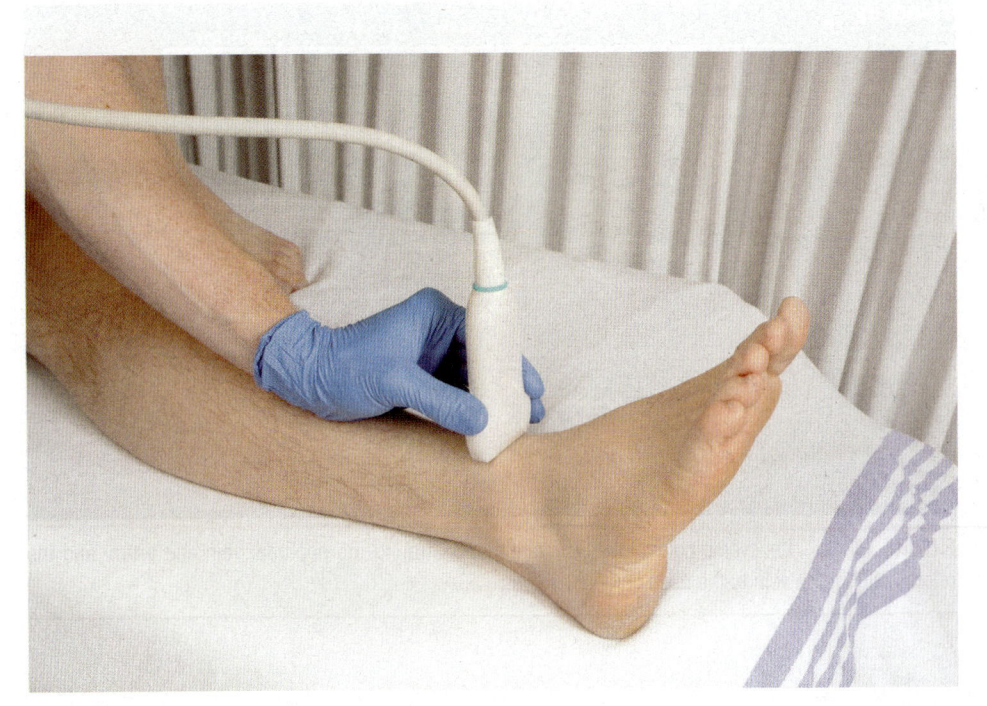

**FIGURE 148.6.** Proper transverse position of the ultrasound transducer for ultrasound-guided deep peroneal nerve block at the ankle.

1054 SECTION X ANKLE AND FOOT

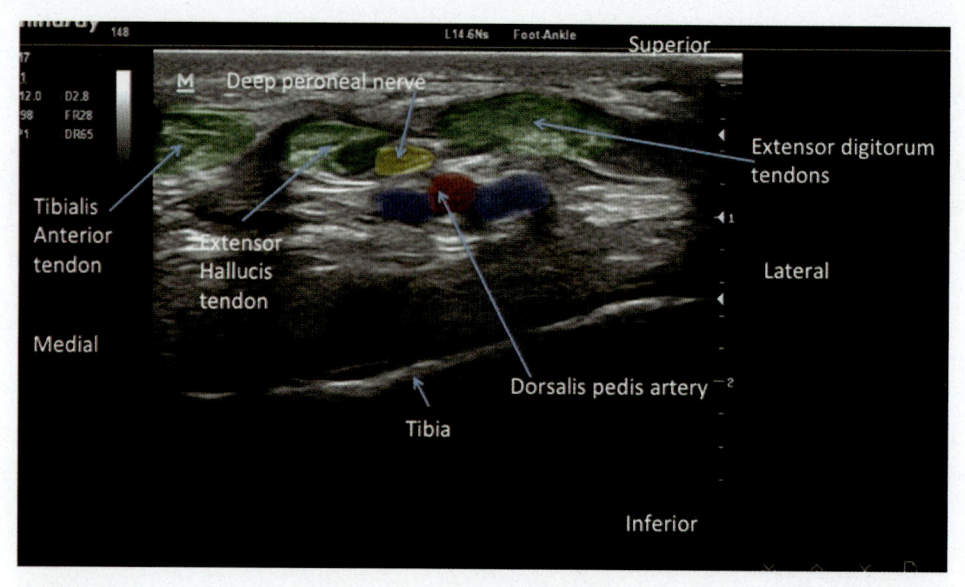

**FIGURE 148.7.** Transverse ultrasound image demonstrating the tibial artery and vein and the deep peroneal nerve just above and lateral to the vein.

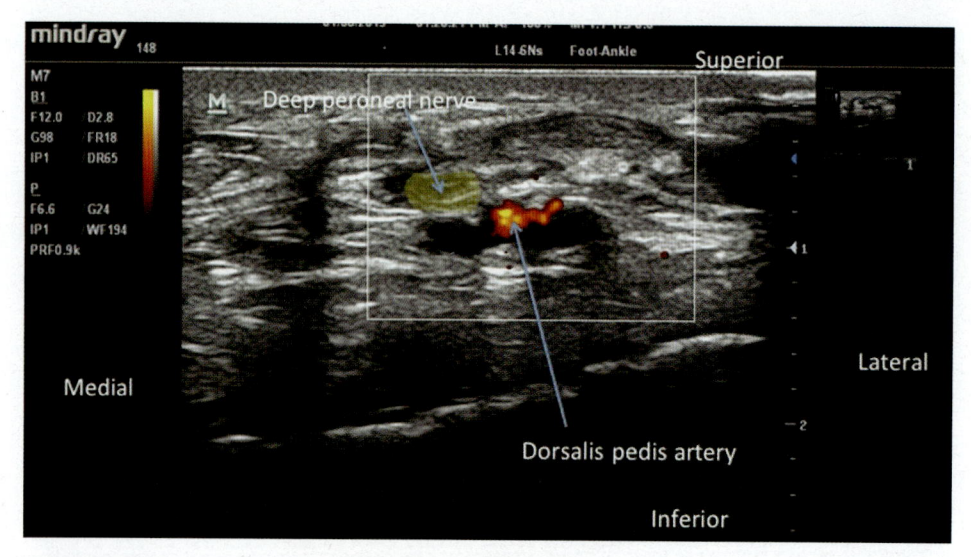

**FIGURE 148.8.** Transverse color Doppler image demonstrating the popliteal vein and artery and the relationship of the vein to the deep peroneal nerve.

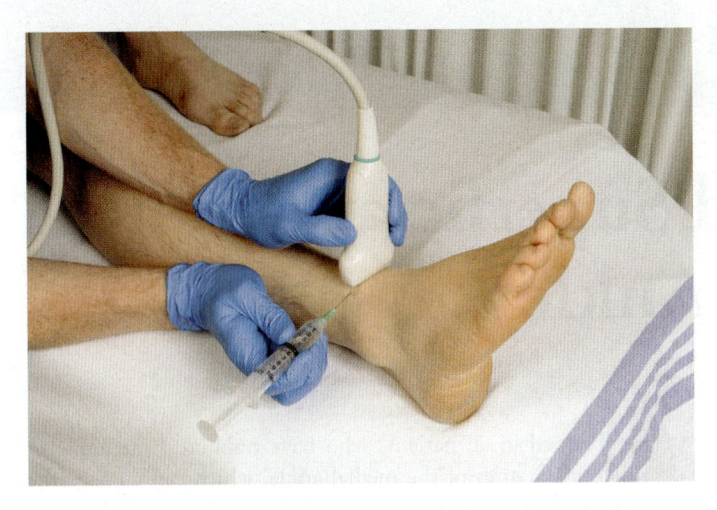

**FIGURE 148.9.** Proper in-plane needle position for performing deep peroneal nerve block at the ankle.

## CLINICAL PEARLS

The key to performing successful ultrasound-guided deep peroneal nerve block at the ankle is the proper identification of the sonographic anatomy and in particular the ability to properly identify the deep peroneal nerve. This should not be a problem if the above technique is used. Any significant pain or sudden increase in resistance during injection when performing ultrasound-guided technique suggests incorrect needle placement, and one should stop injecting immediately and reassess the position of the needle.

## SUGGESTED READINGS

Cho KH, Wansaicheong GKL. Ultrasound of the foot and ankle. Review article. *Ultrasound Clin* 2012;7(4):487–503.

Lopez-Ben R. Imaging of nerve entrapment in the foot and ankle. [Review Article.] *Foot Ankle Clin* 2011;16(2):213–224.

Waldman SD. Deep peroneal nerve block at the ankle. In: *Atlas of Interventional Pain Management*. 3rd ed. Philadelphia, PA: Saunders Elsevier; 2009:563–566.

Waldman SD. Deep peroneal nerve block at the ankle. In: *Pain Review*. Philadelphia, PA: Saunders Elsevier; 2009:576–577.

# CHAPTER 149

# Ultrasound-Guided Superficial Peroneal Nerve Block at the Ankle

## CLINICAL PERSPECTIVES

Ultrasound-guided superficial peroneal nerve block at the ankle is utilized as a diagnostic and therapeutic maneuver in the evaluation and treatment of distal lower extremity pain thought to be mediated via the distal superficial peroneal nerve. Ultrasound-guided superficial peroneal nerve block at the ankle can also be used for surgical anesthesia for distal lower extremity surgery when combined with deep peroneal, tibial, and saphenous nerve block or lumbar plexus block. Ultrasound-guided superficial peroneal nerve block at the ankle with local anesthetic may be used to palliate acute pain emergencies, including postoperative pain, pain secondary to traumatic injuries of the lower extremity including foot and ankle fractures, and cancer pain, while waiting for pharmacologic, surgical, and antiblastic methods to become effective.

Ultrasound-guided superficial peroneal nerve block at the ankle can also be used as a diagnostic tool when performing differential neural blockade on an anatomic basis in the evaluation of ankle and foot pain as well as in a prognostic manner to determine the degree of neurologic impairment the patient will suffer when destruction of the superficial peroneal nerve is being considered or when there is a possibility that the nerve may be sacrificed during surgeries in the anatomic region of the superficial peroneal nerve at the ankle. Superficial peroneal nerve block at the ankle with local anesthetic and steroid is occasionally used in the treatment of persistent ankle and foot pain when the pain is thought to be secondary to inflammation or when entrapment of the superficial peroneal nerve at the ankle is suspected. Superficial peroneal nerve block at the ankle with local anesthetic and steroid is also indicated in the palliation of pain and motor dysfunction associated with diabetic neuropathy.

Electrodiagnostic testing should be considered in all patients who suffer from superficial peroneal nerve dysfunction to provide both neuroanatomic and neurophysiologic information regarding nerve function. Magnetic resonance imaging and ultrasound imaging anywhere along the course of the superficial peroneal nerve are also useful in determining the cause of superficial peroneal nerve compromise. Plain radiographs and/or computerized tomography of the ankle should be obtained in all patients who have trauma to the ankle to rule out fractures of the medial ankle, which can damage the superficial peroneal nerve (Fig. 149.1).

## CLINICALLY RELEVANT ANATOMY

The common peroneal nerve is one of the two major continuations of the sciatic nerve, the other being the tibial nerve. The common peroneal nerve provides sensory innervation to the inferior portion of the knee joint and the posterior and lateral skin of the upper calf. The common peroneal nerve is derived from the posterior branches of the L4, L5, and S1 and S2 nerve roots. The nerve splits from the sciatic nerve at the superior margin of the popliteal fossa and descends laterally behind the head of the fibula (Fig. 149.2). The common peroneal nerve is subject to compression at this point by such circumstances as improperly applied casts and tourniquets. The nerve is also subject to compression as it continues its lateral course, winding around the fibula through the fibular tunnel, which is made up of the posterior border of the tendinous insertion of the peroneus longus muscle and the fibula itself. Just distal to the fibular tunnel, the nerve divides into its two terminal branches, the superficial and the superficial peroneal nerves. Each of these branches are subject to trauma and may be blocked individually as a diagnostic and therapeutic maneuver.

The deep branch continues down the leg in conjunction with the tibial artery and vein to provide sensory innervation to the web space of the first and second toes and adjacent dorsum of the foot (Fig. 149.3). Although this distribution of sensory fibers is small, this area is often the site of Morton neuroma surgery and thus is important to the regional anesthesiologist. The superficial peroneal nerve provides motor innervation to all of the toe extensors and the anterior tibialis muscles. The superficial peroneal nerve passes beneath the dense superficial fascia of the ankle, where it is subject to an entrapment syndrome known as the anterior tarsal tunnel syndrome. The superficial peroneal nerve also provides sensory innervation to the toes except for the area between the first and second toe, which is supplied by the deep peroneal nerve (Fig. 149.4).

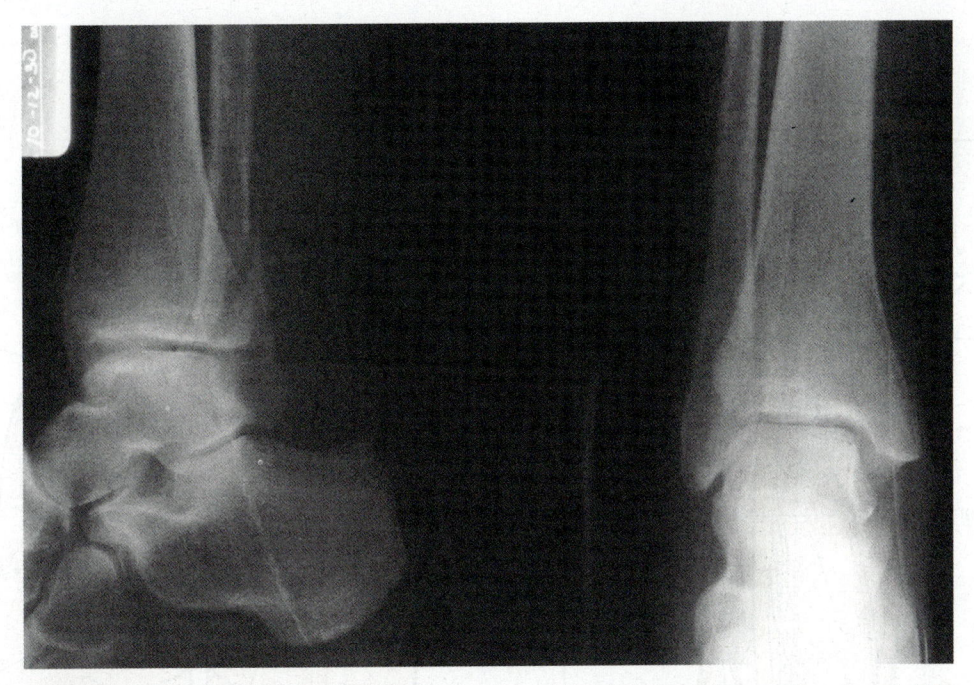

**FIGURE 149.1.** Radiographs demonstrating a fracture of the distal fibula. (Reused from Bucholz RW, Heckman JD. *Rockwood & Green's Fractures in Adults.* 5th ed. Philadelphia, PA: Lippincott Williams & Wilkins; 2001, with permission.)

## ULTRASOUND-GUIDED TECHNIQUE

Ultrasound-guided block of the superficial peroneal nerve at the ankle can be carried out by placing the patient in the lateral curled-up position with the affected leg positioned up on a folded blanket (Fig. 149.5). A total of 4 mL of local anesthetic is drawn up in a 12-mL sterile syringe. If the painful condition being treated is thought to have an inflammatory component, 40 to 80 mg of depot steroid is added to the local anesthetic. A linear high-frequency ultrasound transducer is placed in a transverse plane ~8 cm above the lateral malleolus of the ankle, and an ultrasound survey scan is taken (Fig. 149.6). The superficial peroneal nerve is seen lying just above the fibula and peroneal muscles (Fig. 149.7). Color Doppler imaging can help identify the anterior tibial artery with the superficial peroneal nerve lying just above it (Fig. 149.8). When the superficial peroneal nerve is identified on ultrasound imaging, the skin is prepped with anesthetic solution, and a 1½-inch, 22-gauge needle is advanced from the inferior border of the ultrasound transducer and advanced utilizing an in-plane approach with the trajectory being adjusted under real-time ultrasound guidance until the needle tip is resting in proximity to the superficial peroneal nerve (Fig. 149.9). When the tip of needle is thought to be in satisfactory position, after careful aspiration, a small amount of local anesthetic and steroid is injected under real-time ultrasound guidance to confirm that the needle tip is in proximity to the superficial peroneal nerve, but not within the nerve itself. There should be minimal resistance to injection. After needle tip placement is confirmed, the remainder of the contents of the syringe are slowly injected. The needle is then removed, and a sterile pressure dressing and ice pack are placed at the injection site.

## COMPLICATIONS

A failure to accurately assess the correct position of the needle tip when performing ultrasound-guided superficial peroneal nerve block at the ankle can lead to a failure to block the superficial peroneal nerve or cause needle-induced trauma to the superficial peroneal nerve. The use of ultrasound guidance when performing superficial peroneal nerve block at the ankle should markedly decrease these problems. Postblock ecchymosis and hematoma may occur, and the patient should be warned of such. These complications can be decreased by the use of a pressure dressing and cold packs applied to the injection site following the procedure.

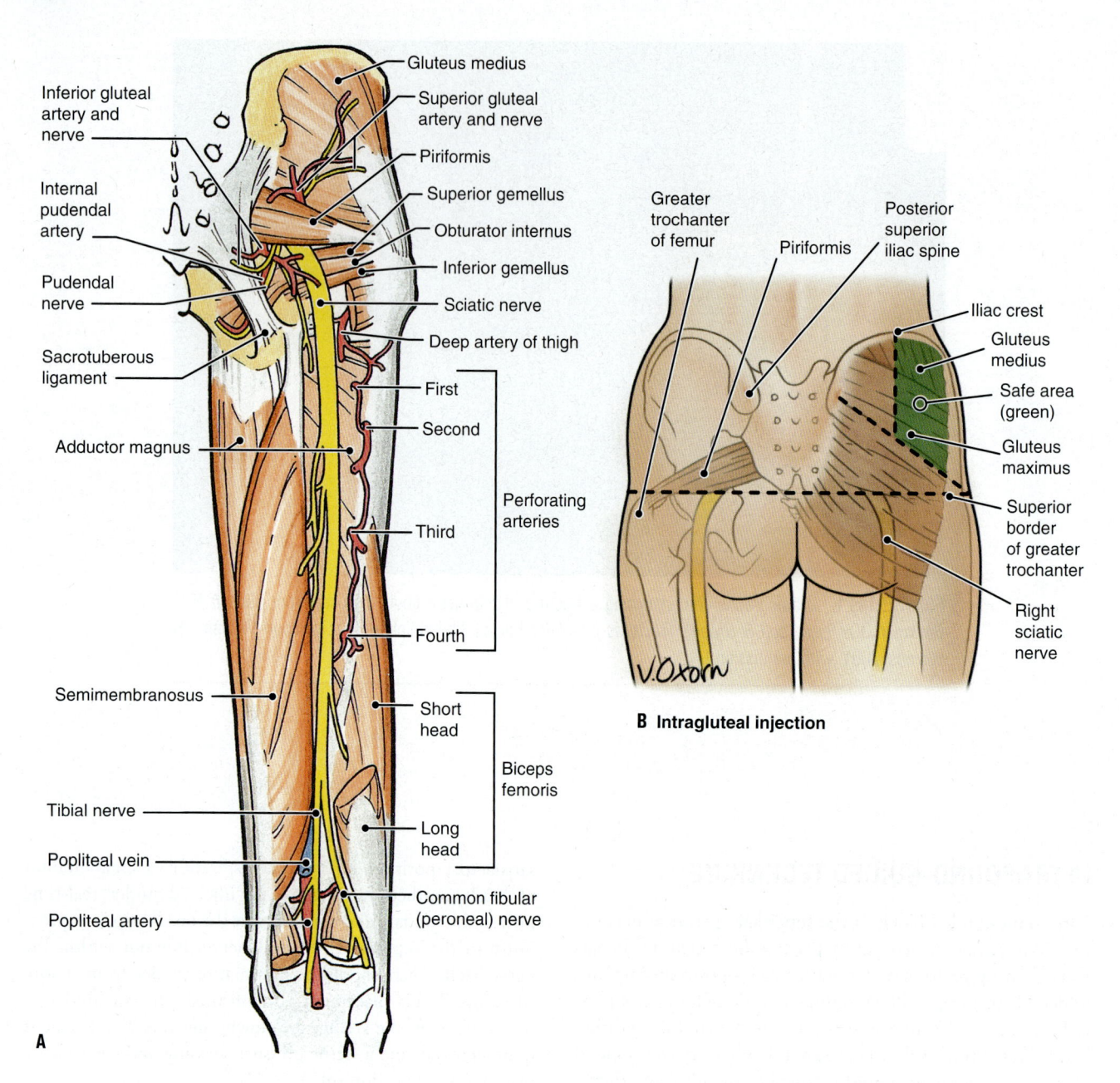

**FIGURE 149.2.** **A:** The anatomy of the common peroneal nerve. **B:** The safe zone for intragluteal injection. (Reused from Moore KL, Agur AMR. *Essential Clinical Anatomy*. 2nd ed. Baltimore, MD: Lippincott Williams & Wilkins; 2002, with permission.)

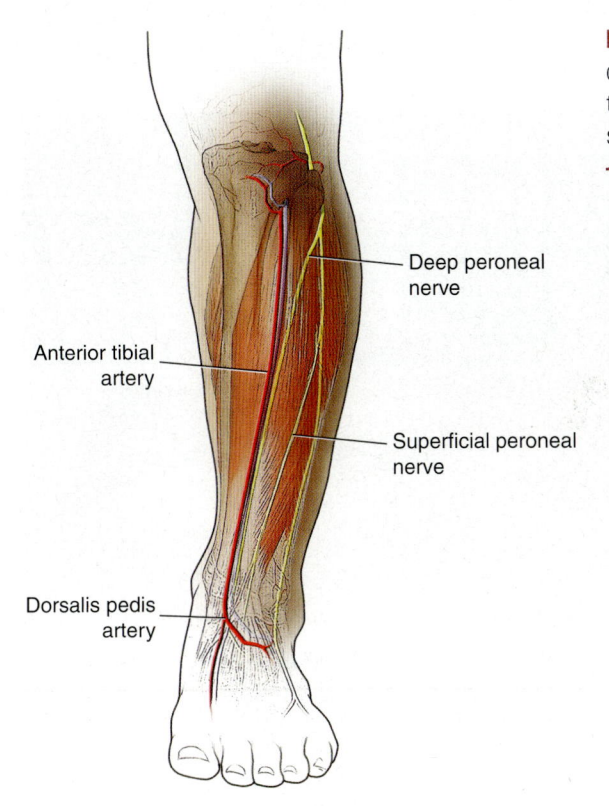

**FIGURE 149.3.** The anatomy of the distal superficial peroneal nerve. Note the relationship of the nerve to the superficial peroneal vein.

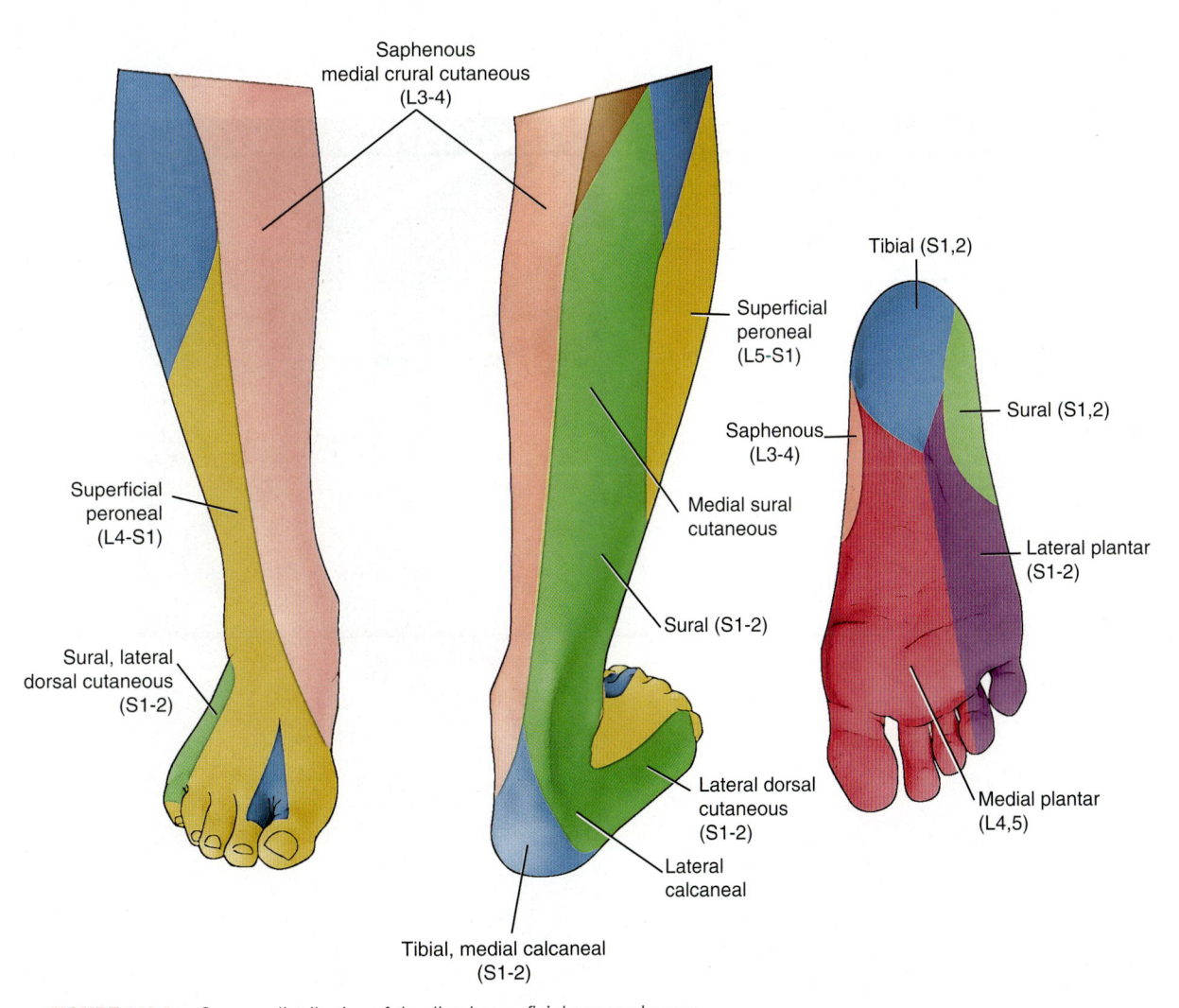

**FIGURE 149.4.** Sensory distribution of the distal superficial peroneal nerve.

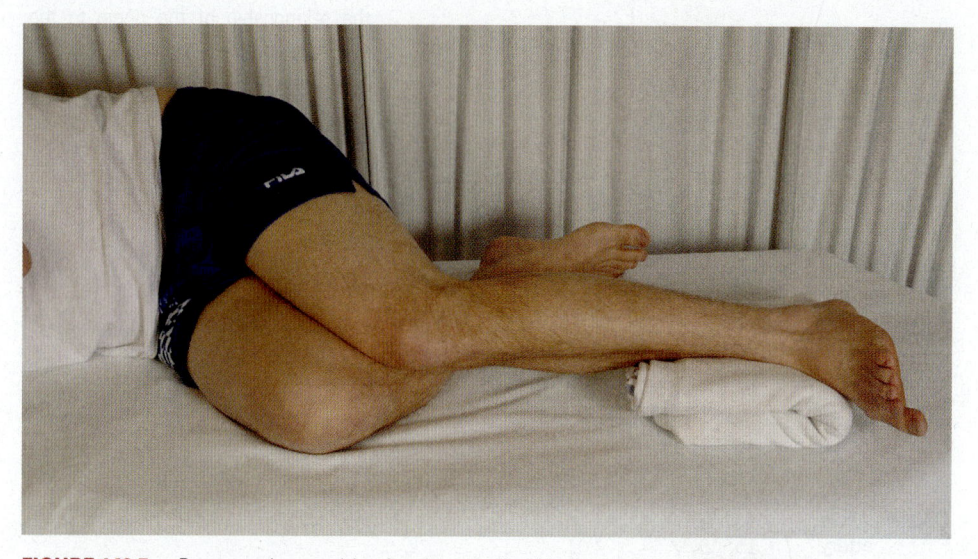

**FIGURE 149.5.** Proper patient position for ultrasound-guided superficial peroneal nerve block.

**FIGURE 149.6.** Proper transverse position of the ultrasound transducer for ultrasound-guided superficial peroneal nerve block at the ankle.

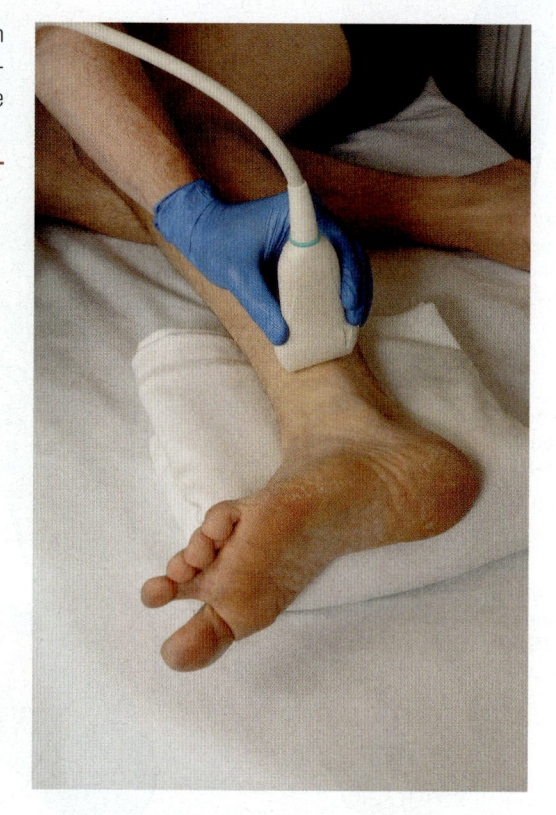

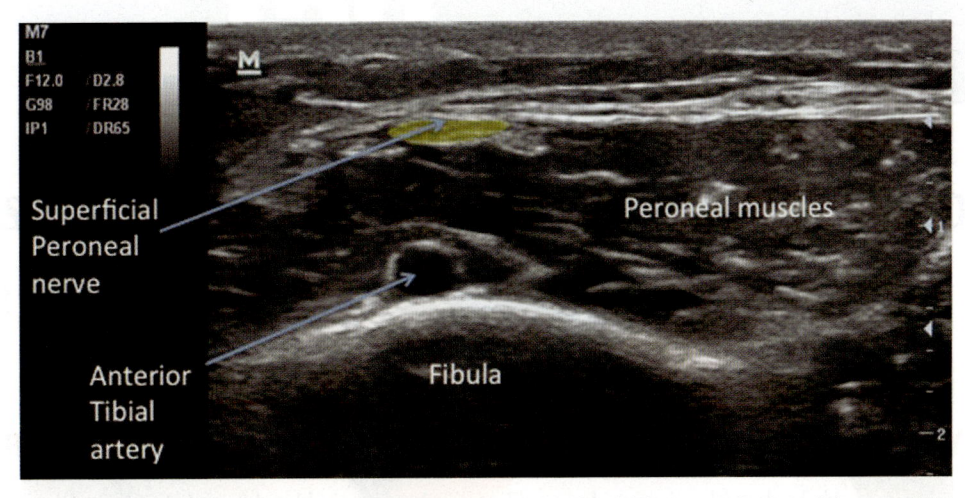

**FIGURE 149.7.** Transverse ultrasound image demonstrating the tibial artery and vein and the superficial peroneal nerve just above and lateral to the vein.

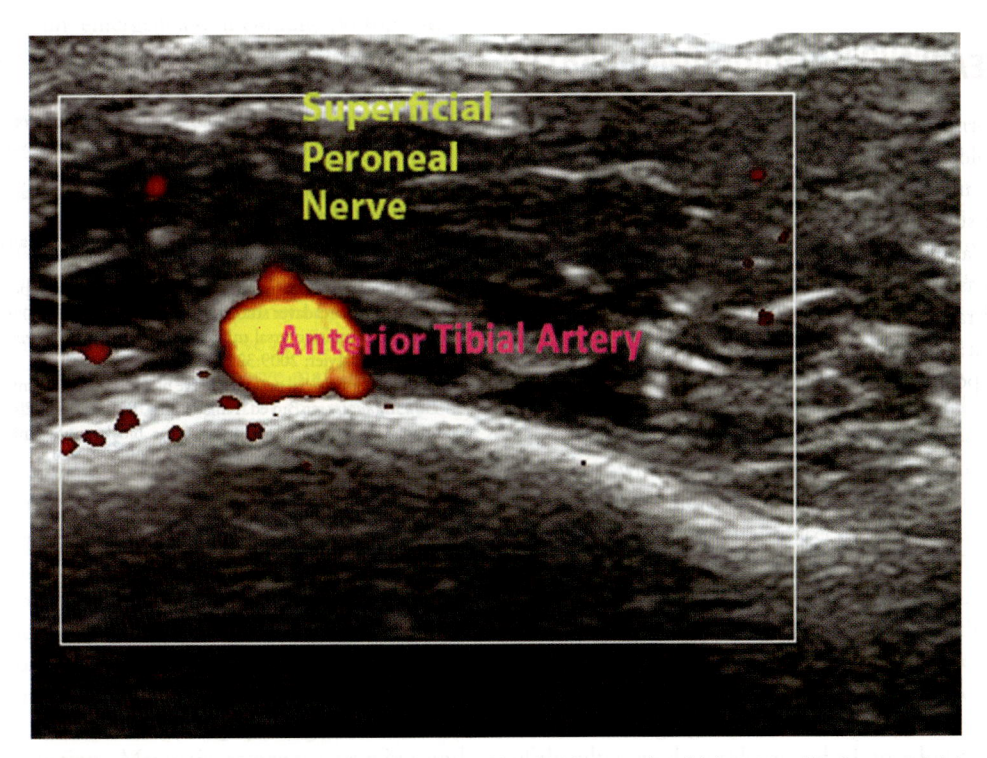

**FIGURE 149.8.** Color Doppler imaging can help identify the anterior tibial artery with the superficial peroneal nerve lying just above it.

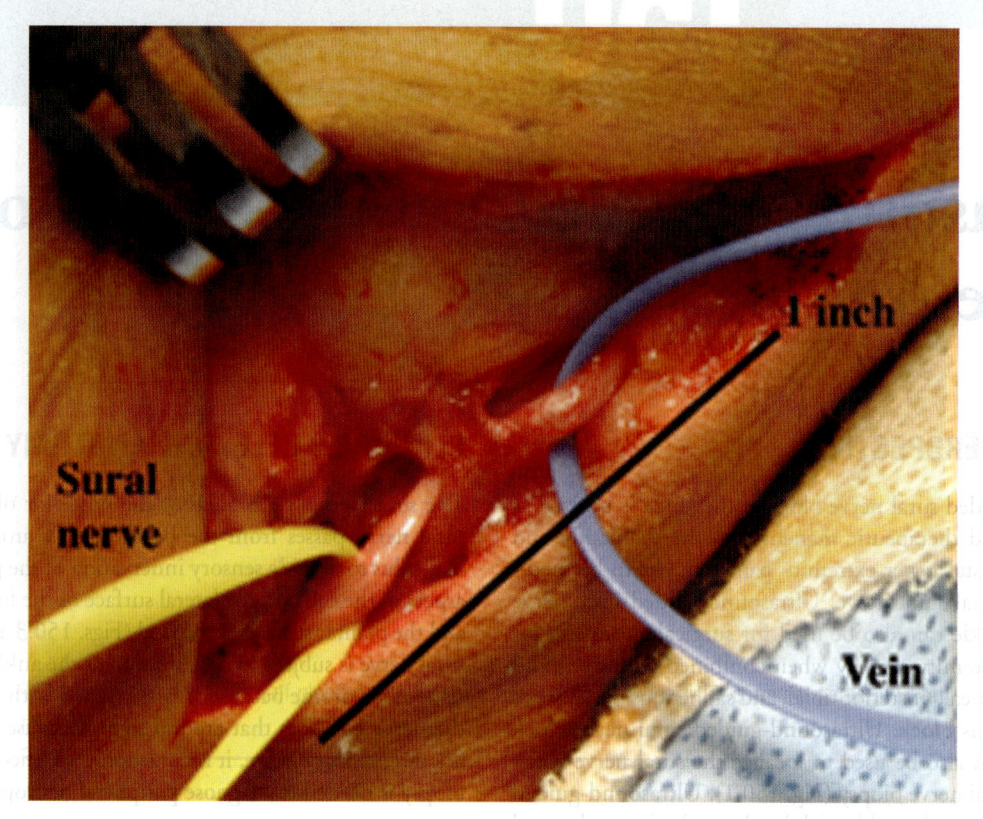

**FIGURE 150.1.** This technique can also be used to localize the sural nerve when performing sural nerve biopsy. Note the anatomic relationship of the sural nerve and the small saphenous vein.

**FIGURE 150.2.** Radiographs demonstrating a fracture of the distal fibula and dislocation of the talus causing damage to the sural nerve. (Reused from Bucholz RW, Heckman JD. *Rockwood & Green's Fractures in Adults*. 5th ed. Philadelphia, PA: Lippincott Williams & Wilkins; 2001, with permission.)

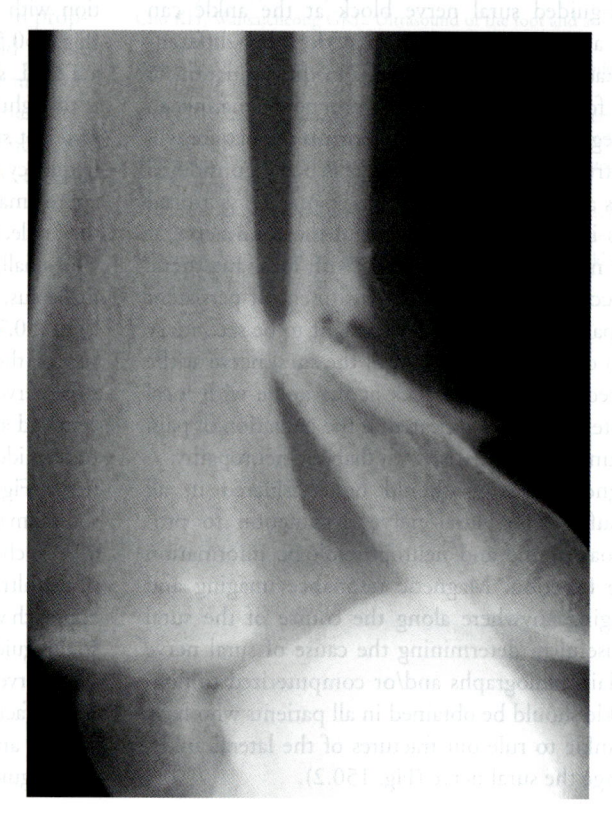

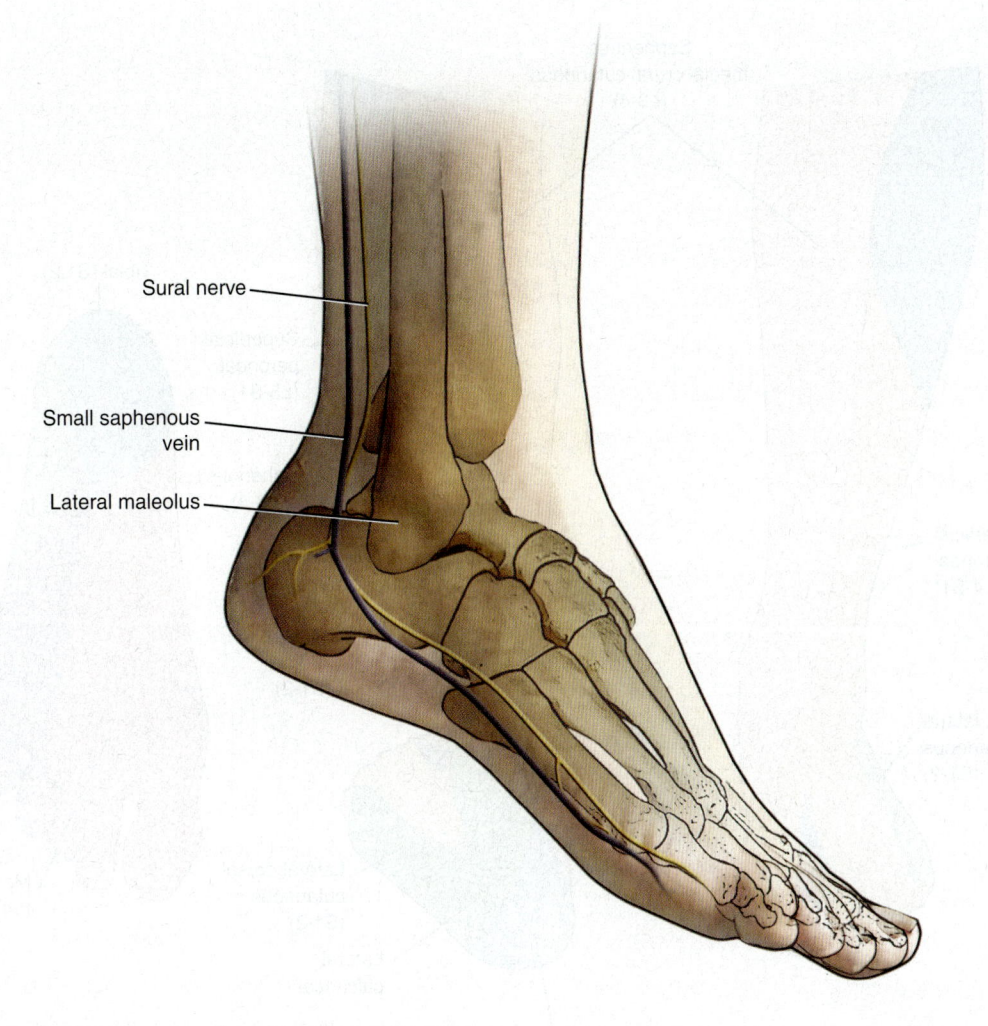

**FIGURE 150.3.** The anatomy of the sural nerve.

Labels: Sural nerve; Small saphenous vein; Lateral maleolus

to the sural nerve, but not within the nerve itself. There should be minimal resistance to injection. After needle tip placement is confirmed, the remainder of the contents of the syringe are slowly injected. The needle is then removed, and a sterile pressure dressing and ice pack are placed at the injection site.

## COMPLICATIONS

A failure to accurately assess the correct position of the needle tip when performing ultrasound-guided sural nerve block at the ankle can lead to a failure to block the sural nerve or cause needle-induced trauma to the sural nerve and adjacent sural vein. The use of ultrasound guidance when performing sural nerve block at the ankle should markedly decrease these problems. Postblock ecchymosis and hematoma may occur, and the patient should be warned of such. These complications can be decreased by the use of a pressure dressing and cold packs applied to the injection site following the procedure.

## CLINICAL PEARLS

The key to performing successful ultrasound-guided sural nerve block at the ankle is the proper identification of the sonographic anatomy and in particular the ability to properly identify the sural nerve. This should not be a problem if the above technique is used. Any significant pain or sudden increase in resistance during injection when performing ultrasound-guided technique suggests incorrect needle placement, and one should stop injecting immediately and reassess the position of the needle.

**1066** SECTION X ANKLE AND FOOT

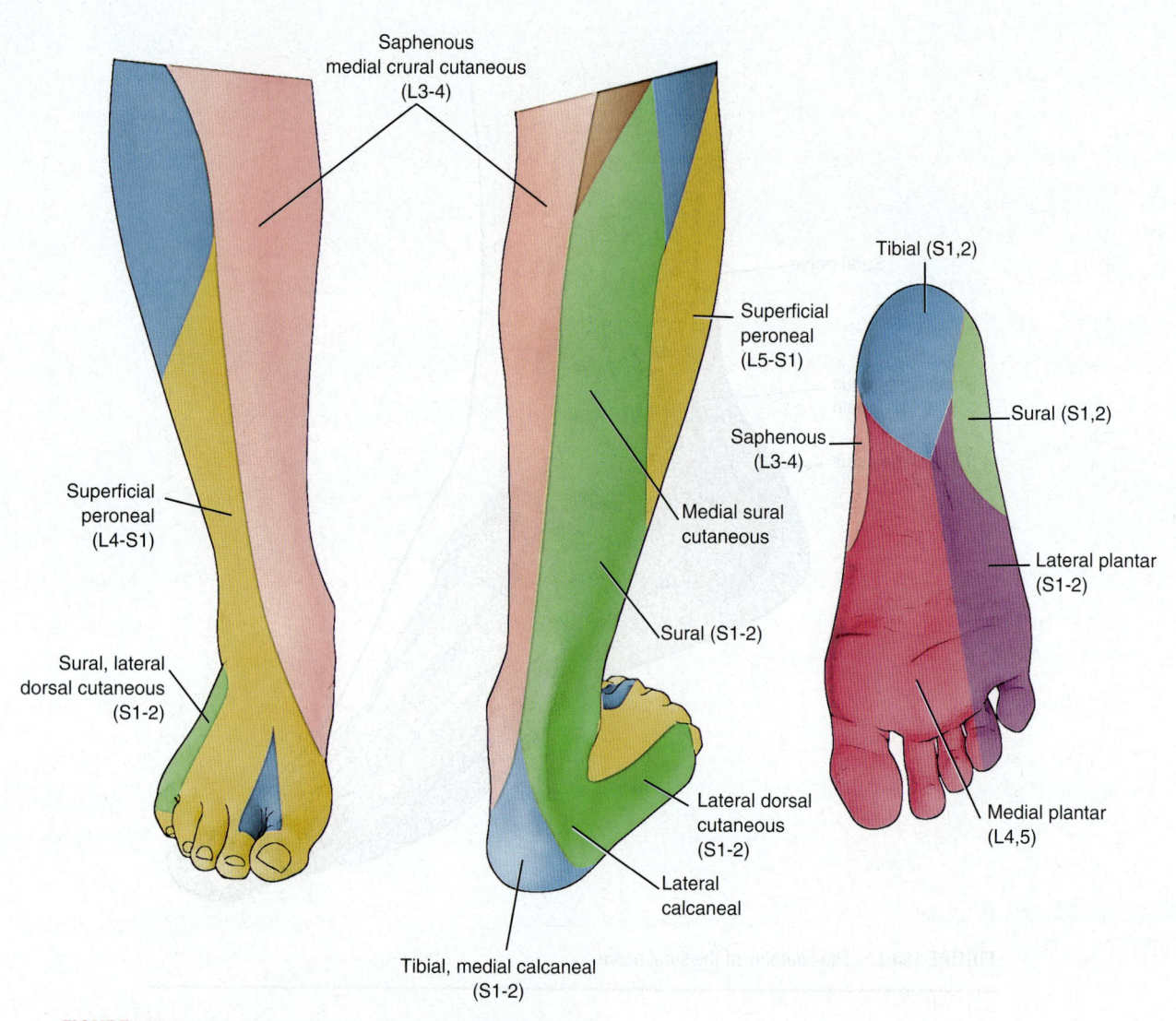

**FIGURE 150.4.** Sensory distribution of the distal sural nerve.

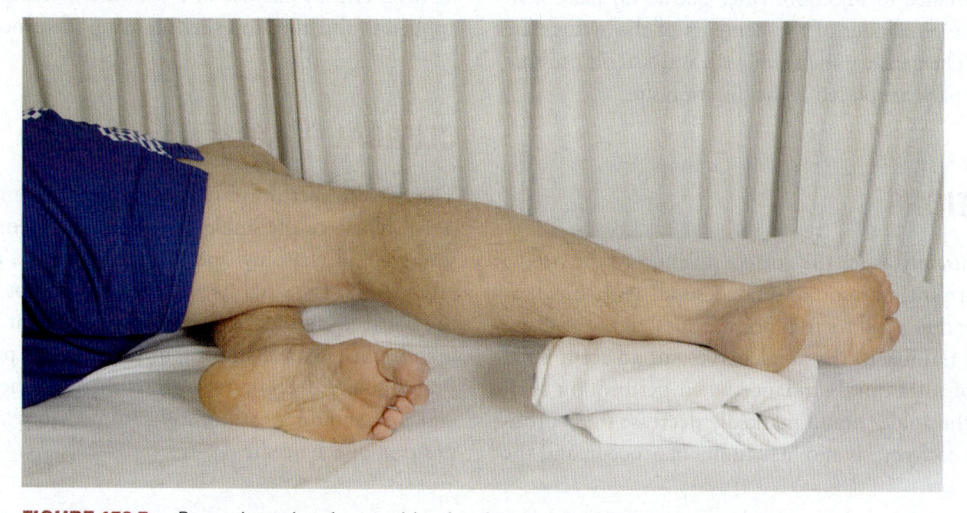

**FIGURE 150.5.** Proper lateral patient position for ultrasound-guided sural nerve block.

CHAPTER 150    ULTRASOUND-GUIDED SURAL NERVE BLOCK AT THE ANKLE    1067

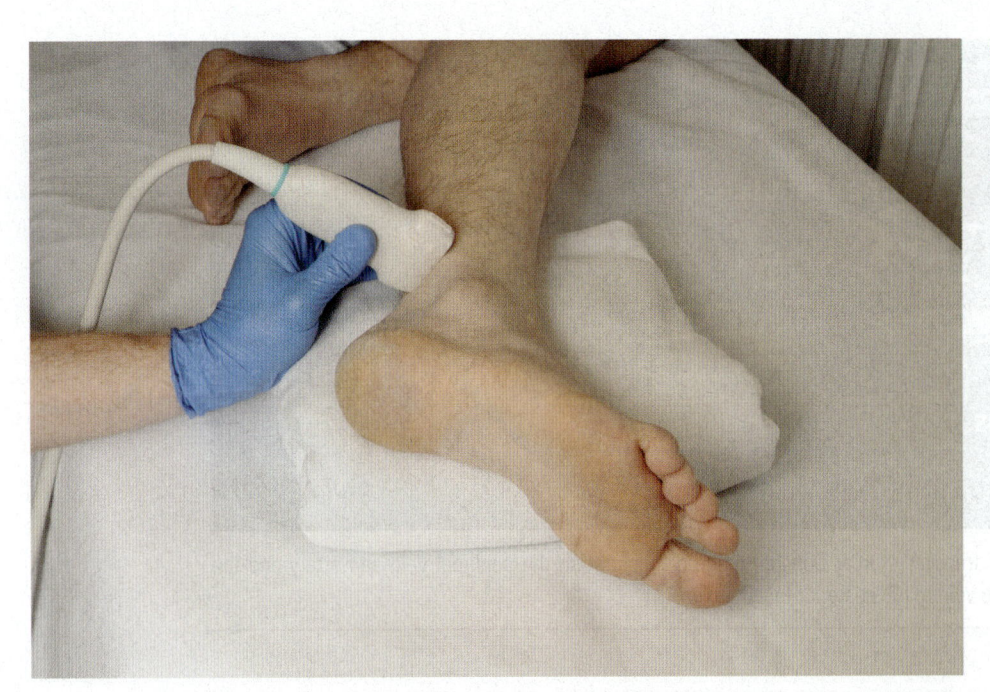

**FIGURE 150.6.** Proper transverse position of the ultrasound transducer for ultrasound-guided sural nerve block at the ankle.

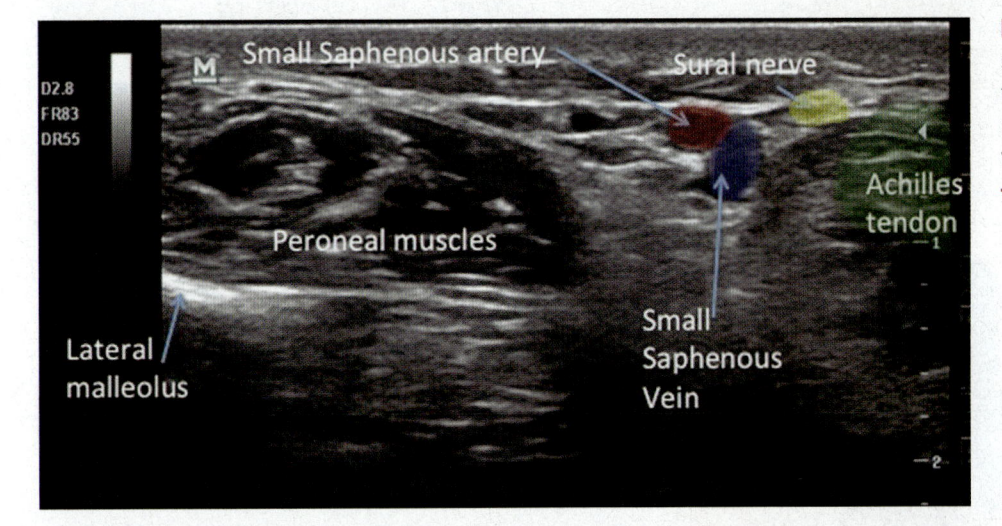

**FIGURE 150.7.** Transverse ultrasound image demonstrating the tibial artery and vein and the sural nerve just above and lateral to the vein.

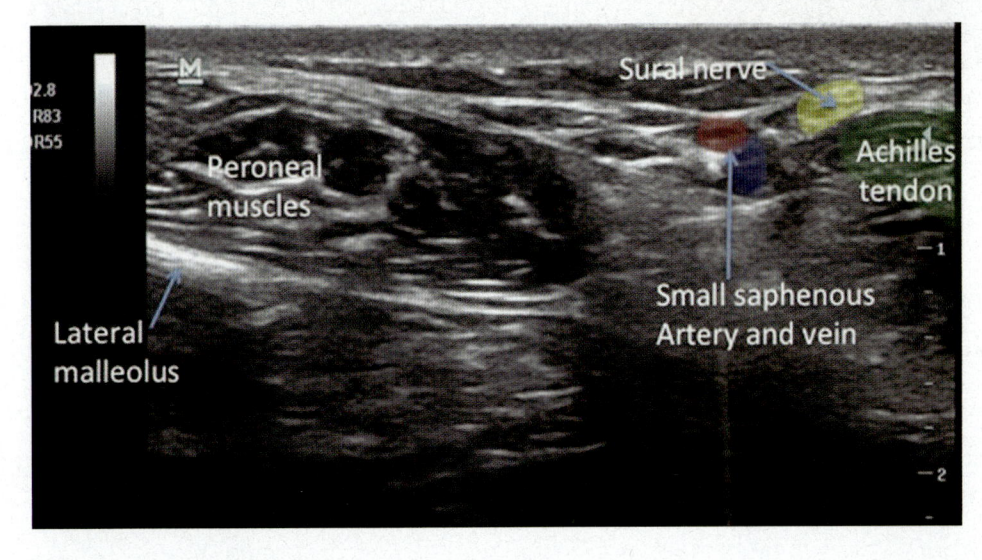

**FIGURE 150.8.** Compression of the small saphenous vein can aid in identification of the sural nerve, which is just posterior to the vein.

**FIGURE 150.9.** Transverse color Doppler image demonstrating the popliteal vein and artery and the relationship of the vein to the posterior tibial nerve.

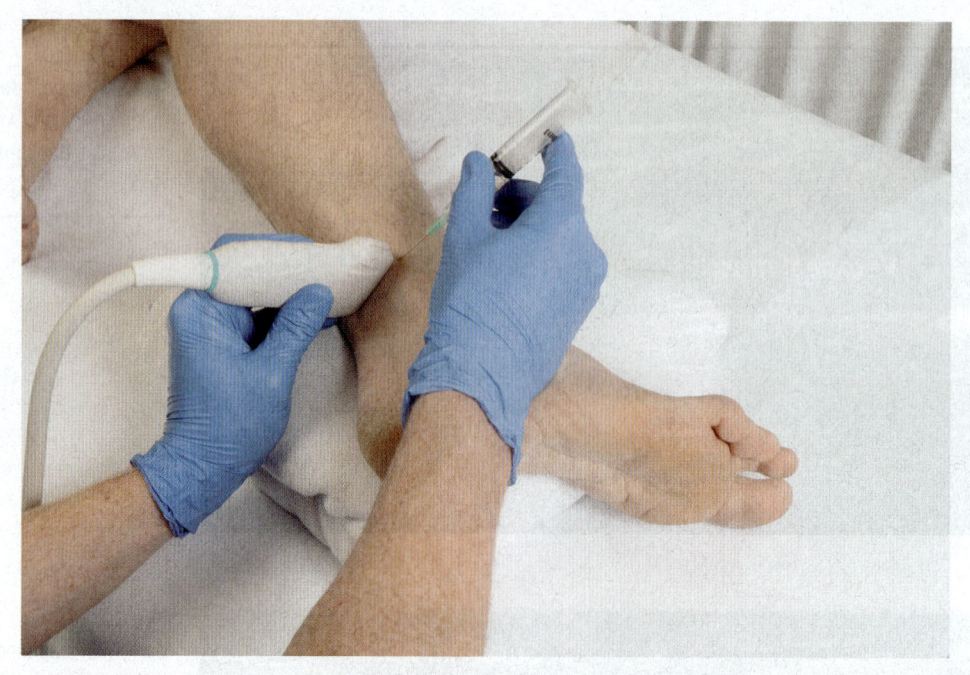

**FIGURE 150.10.** Proper in-plane needle position for performing sural nerve block at the ankle.

## SUGGESTED READINGS

Cho KH, Wansaicheong GKL. Ultrasound of the foot and ankle. [Review Article.] *Ultrasound Clin* 2012;7(4):487–503.

Lopez-Ben R. Imaging of nerve entrapment in the foot and ankle. [Review Article.] *Foot Ankle Clin* 2011;16(2):213–224.

Ricci S, Moro L, Incalzi A. Ultrasound imaging of the sural nerve: ultrasound anatomy and rationale for investigation. *Eur J Vasc Endovasc Surg* 2010;39(5):636–641.

Waldman SD. Sural nerve block at the ankle. In: *Atlas of Interventional Pain Management*. 3rd ed. Philadelphia, PA: Saunders Elsevier; 2009:570–574.

Waldman SD. Sural nerve block at the ankle. In: *Pain Review*. Philadelphia, PA: Saunders Elsevier; 2009:579–580.

# CHAPTER 151

# Ultrasound-Guided Injection Technique for Deltoid Ligament Strain

## CLINICAL PERSPECTIVES

One of the four major ligaments of the ankle joint, the deltoid ligament, is a strong, triangular-shaped, bilaminar ligament that runs from the medial malleolus, with the deep layer of the ligament attaching below to the medial body of the talus and the superficial layer of the ligament attaching to the medial talus, the sustentaculum tali of the calcaneus, and the navicular tuberosity (Fig. 151.1). Also known as the medial ligament of talocrural joint, the deltoid ligament is susceptible to strain at the joint line or avulsion at its origin or insertion. The deltoid ligament is frequently injured from eversion injuries to the ankle that occur when tripping when high heels, landing hard on uneven surfaces, and during dancing, soccer, and American football (Fig. 151.2). The pain of deltoid ligament damage is localized to the medial ankle and is made worse with plantar flexion and eversion of the ankle joint. Significant swelling and ecchymosis are often evident after acute injury (Fig. 151.3). Activity, especially involving weight bearing, plantar flexion, and eversion of the ankle, will exacerbate the pain. Local heat and decreased activity as well as elevation of the affected ankle may provide a modicum of relief. Sleep disturbance is common in patients suffering from trauma to the deltoid ligament of the ankle. Coexistent fracture, bursitis, tendonitis, arthritis, or internal derangement of the ankle may confuse the clinical picture after trauma to the knee joint making clinical diagnosis difficult.

Plain radiographs are indicated in all patients who present with deltoid ligament pain, especially after ankle trauma (Fig. 151.4). Based on the patient's clinical presentation, additional testing may be indicated, including complete blood cell count, sedimentation rate, and antinuclear antibody testing. Magnetic resonance imaging and/or ultrasound imaging of the ankle is indicated if internal derangement or occult mass or tumor is suspected as well as to confirm the diagnosis of suspected deltoid ligament injury (Fig. 151.5). Bone scan may be useful to identify occult stress fractures involving the joint, especially if trauma has occurred.

## CLINICALLY RELEVANT ANATOMY

The ankle is a hinge-type articulation between the distal tibia, the two malleoli, and the talus. The articular surface is covered with hyaline cartilage, which is susceptible to arthritis. The joint is surrounded by a dense capsule that helps strengthen the ankle. The joint capsule is lined with a synovial membrane that attaches to the articular cartilage. The ankle joint is innervated by the deep peroneal and tibial nerves.

The major ligaments of the ankle joint include the deltoid, anterior talofibular, calcaneofibular, and posterior talofibular ligaments, which provide the majority of strength to the ankle joint (see Fig. 151.1). The deltoid ligament is exceptionally strong and is not as subject to strain as the anterior talofibular ligament. The triangular-shaped deltoid ligament is made up of a number of smaller separate ligaments including the anterior tibiotalar ligament, tibiocalcaneal ligament, posterior tibiotalar ligament, and tibionavicular ligament. These ligaments are arranged in two layers. Both layers attach above to the medial malleolus. A deep layer attaches below to the medial body of the talus, with the superficial fibers attaching to the medial talus, the sustentaculum tali of the calcaneus, and the navicular tuberosity.

## ULTRASOUND-GUIDED TECHNIQUE

The benefits, risks, and alternative treatments are explained to the patient, and informed consent is obtained. The patient is then placed in the supine position with the lower extremity externally rotated (Fig. 151.6). The skin overlying the medial deltoid ligament is then prepped with antiseptic solution. A sterile syringe containing 2.0 mL of 0.25% preservative-free bupivacaine and 40 mg of methylprednisolone is attached to a 1½-inch, 22-gauge needle using strict aseptic technique. A high-frequency linear ultrasound transducer is placed in the longitudinal position with the superior aspect of the transducer placed just over the center of the medial malleolus and rotated toward the Achilles tendon (Fig. 151.7). A survey scan is taken, which demonstrates the triangular-shaped deltoid ligament nestled between the medial malleolus and talus (Fig. 151.8). After the deltoid ligament is identified, the needle is placed through the skin ~1 cm above the middle of the superior aspect of the slightly rotated longitudinally placed transducer and is then advanced using an out-of-plane approach with the needle trajectory adjusted under real-time ultrasound guidance to place the needle tip within proximity to the deltoid ligament but not within the substance of the ligament (Fig. 151.9).

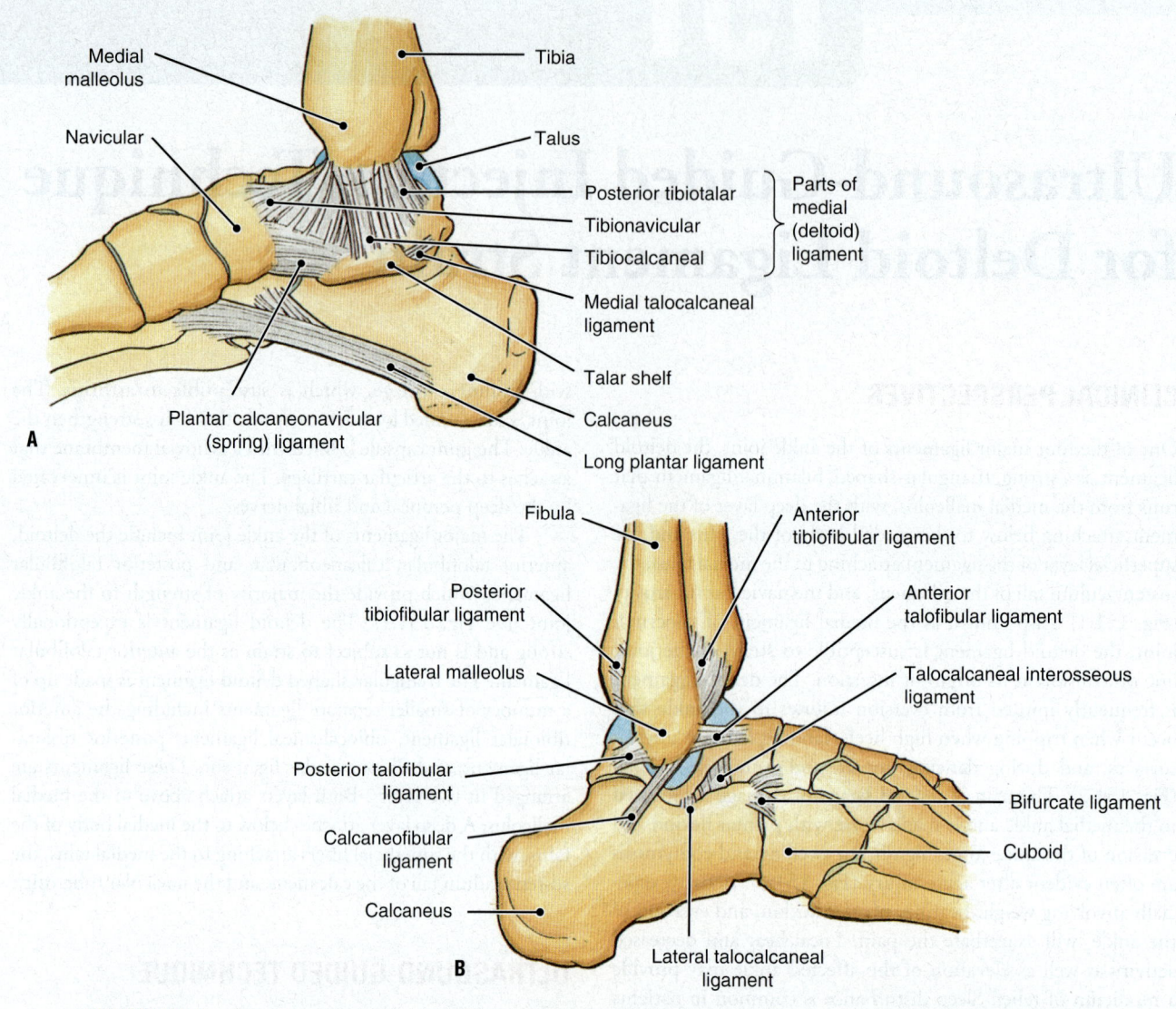

**FIGURE 151.1.** The anatomy of the deltoid ligament and its relationship with the other ligaments of the medial ankle. **A:** Medial view. **B:** Lateral view. (Reused from Moore KL, Agur AMR. *Essential Clinical Anatomy.* 2nd ed. Baltimore, MD: Lippincott Williams & Wilkins; 2002, with permission.)

When the tip of needle is thought to be in satisfactory position, a small amount of local anesthetic and steroid is injected under real-time ultrasound guidance to confirm that the needle tip is not within the substance of the deltoid ligament. There should be minimal resistance to injection. After intra-articular needle tip placement is confirmed, the remainder of the contents of the syringe are slowly injected. If synechiae, loculations, or calcifications are present, the needle may have to be repositioned to ensure that the entire intra-articular space is treated. The needle is then removed, and a sterile pressure dressing and ice pack are placed at the injection site.

## COMPLICATIONS

The major complication of ultrasound-guided injection of the deltoid ligament is infection. Highly inflamed tendons and ligaments are subject to rupture if directly injected so care must be taken to insure that the needle tip is outside the substance of the tendon. Ecchymosis and hematoma formation may also occur. A transient exacerbation of the patient's pain occurs ~25% of the time following this injection technique, and the patient should be warned of this possibility prior to the procedure.

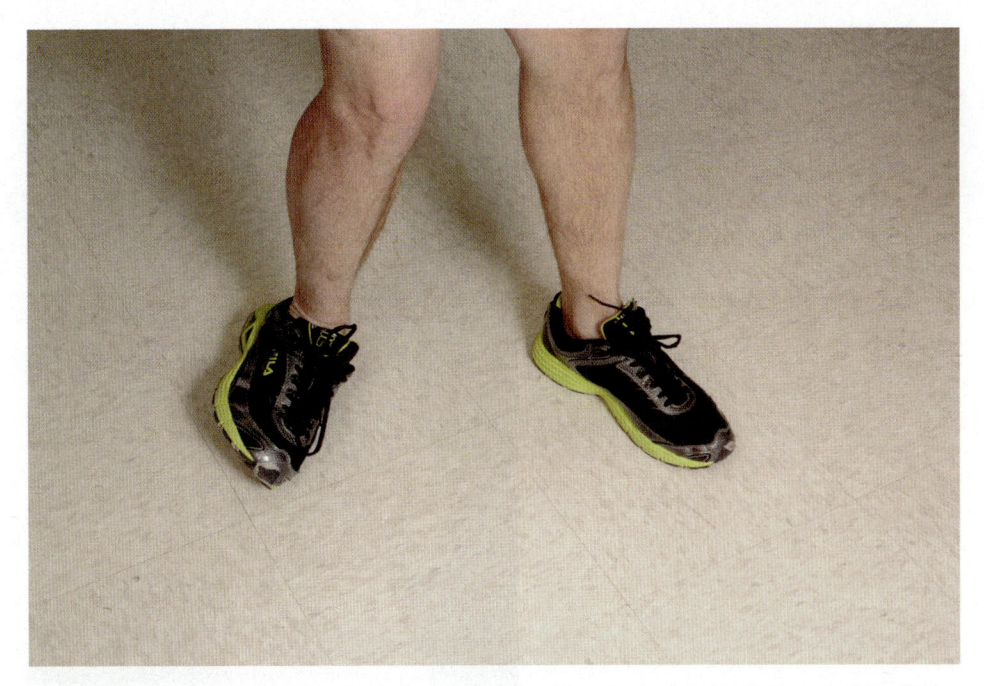

**FIGURE 151.2.** The deltoid ligament is frequently injured by eversion injuries that occur when tripping when high heels, landing hard on uneven surfaces, and during dancing, soccer, and American football.

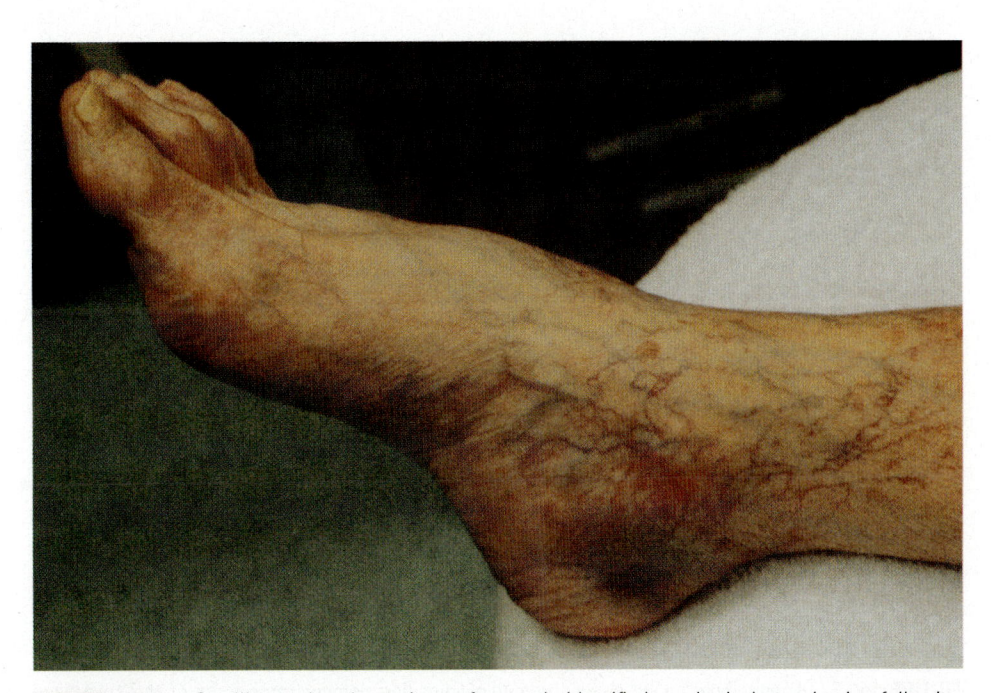

**FIGURE 151.3.** Swelling and ecchymosis are frequently identified on physical examination following deltoid ligament injury. (Reused from Berg D, Worzala K. *Atlas of Adult Physical Diagnosis*. Philadelphia, PA: Lippincott Williams & Wilkins; 2006, with permission.)

**FIGURE 151.4.** Radiograph demonstrating a fracture dislocation of the ankle with complete disruption of the deltoid ligament. (Reused from Mulholland MW, Maier RV, Lillemoe KD, et al. *Greenfield's Surgery: Scientific Principles and Practice.* 4th ed. Philadelphia, PA: Lippincott Williams & Wilkins; 2006, with permission.)

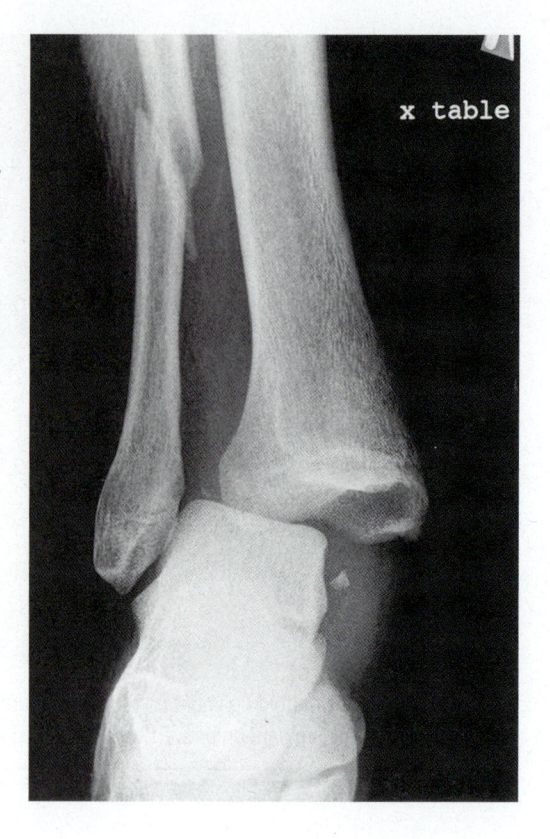

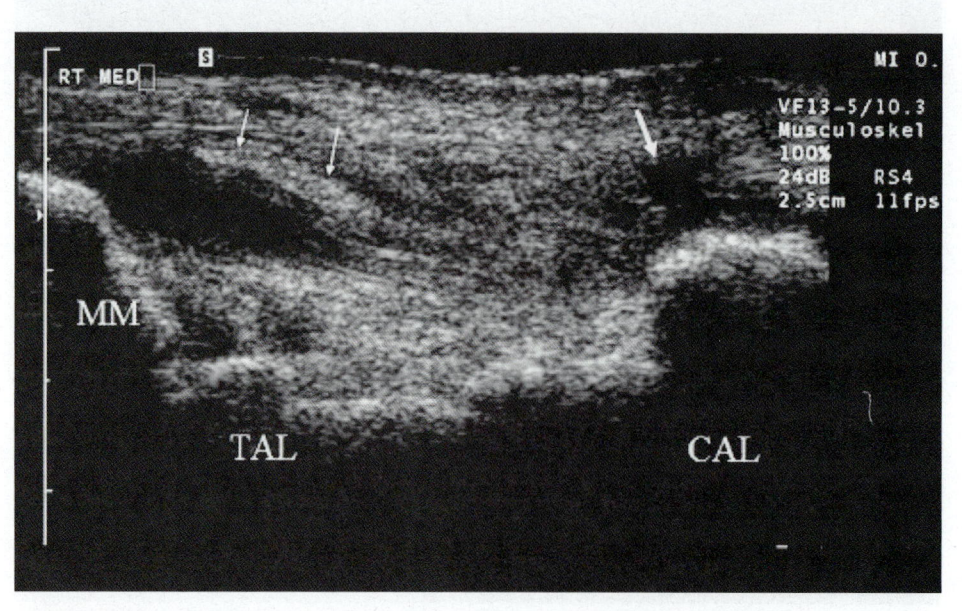

**FIGURE 151.5.** Longitudinal image along the medial joint line demonstrates tears of the superficial (talocalcaneal) and tibionavicular fibers of the deltoid ligament (*arrows*). The medial malleolus (MM), talus (TAL), and calcaneus (CAL) are also indicated. (Reused from Adler RS, Sofka CM, Positano RG. *Atlas of Foot and Ankle Sonography.* Philadelphia, PA: Lippincott Williams & Wilkins; 2004:71, with permission.)

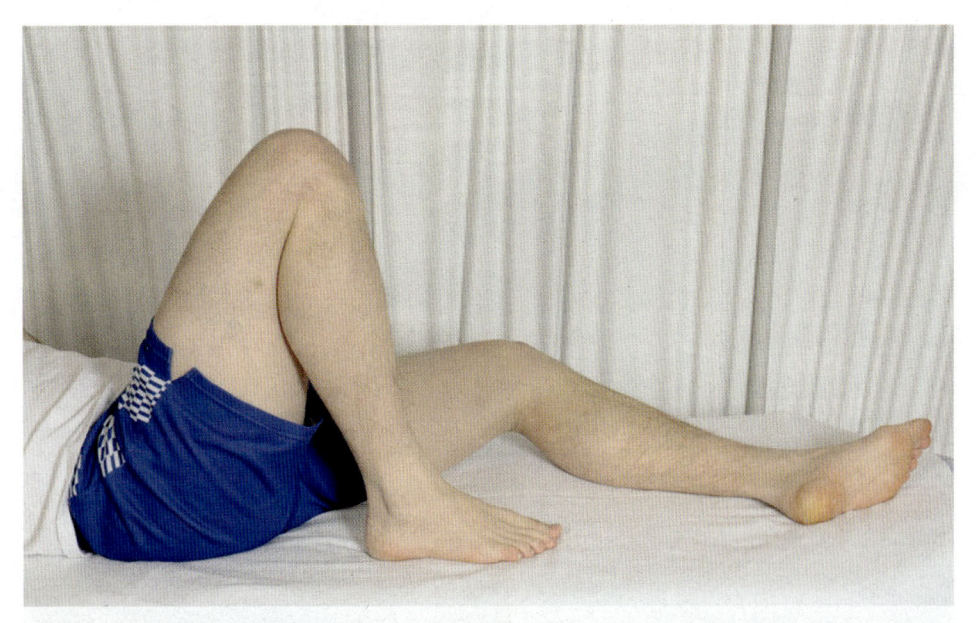

CHAPTER 151 ULTRASOUND-GUIDED INJECTION TECHNIQUE FOR DELTOID LIGAMENT STRAIN 1073

**FIGURE 151.6.** Proper patient position for ultrasound-guided intra-articular deltoid ligament injection. Note that the affected extremity is externally rotated.

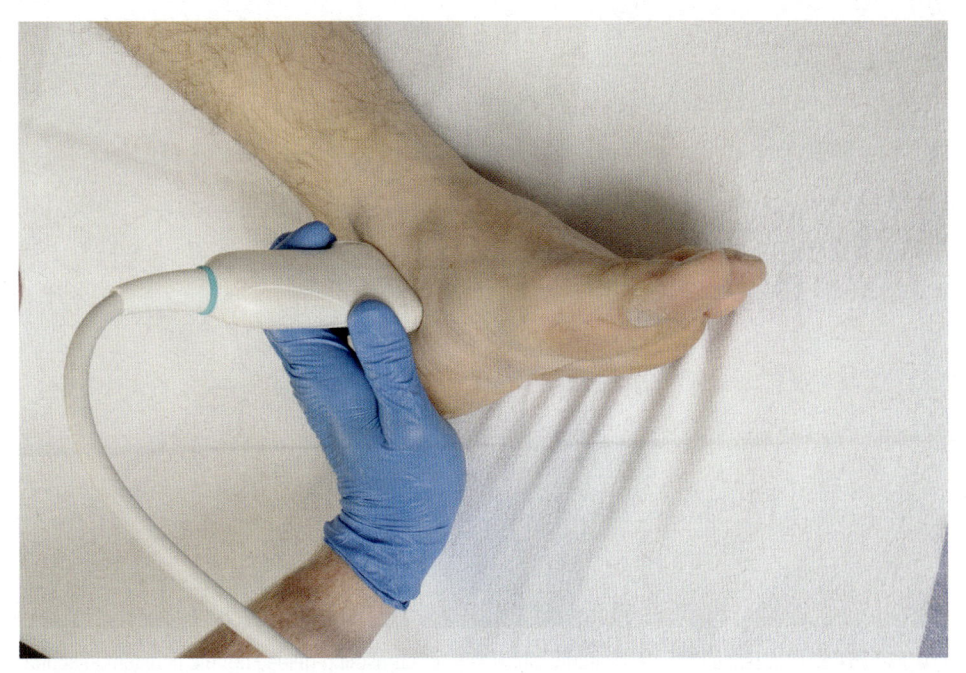

**FIGURE 151.7.** Correct longitudinal position for the ultrasound transducer for ultrasound-guided intra-articular injection of the deltoid ligament. Note that the superior aspect of the ultrasound transducer is slightly rotated toward the Achilles tendon.

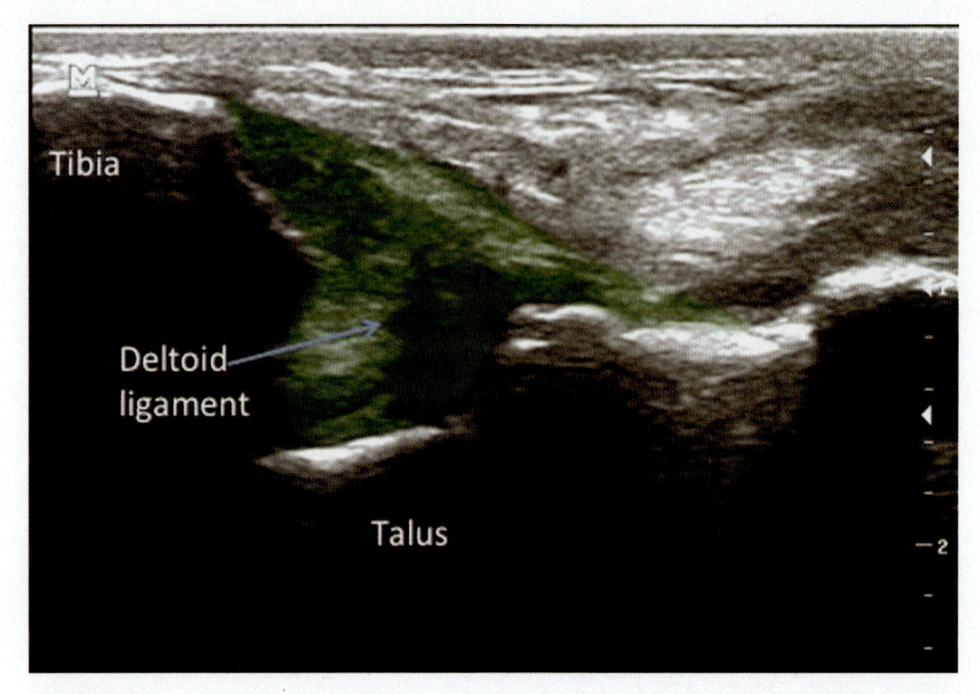

**FIGURE 151.8.** Longitudinal ultrasound image demonstrating the triangular-shaped deltoid ligament.

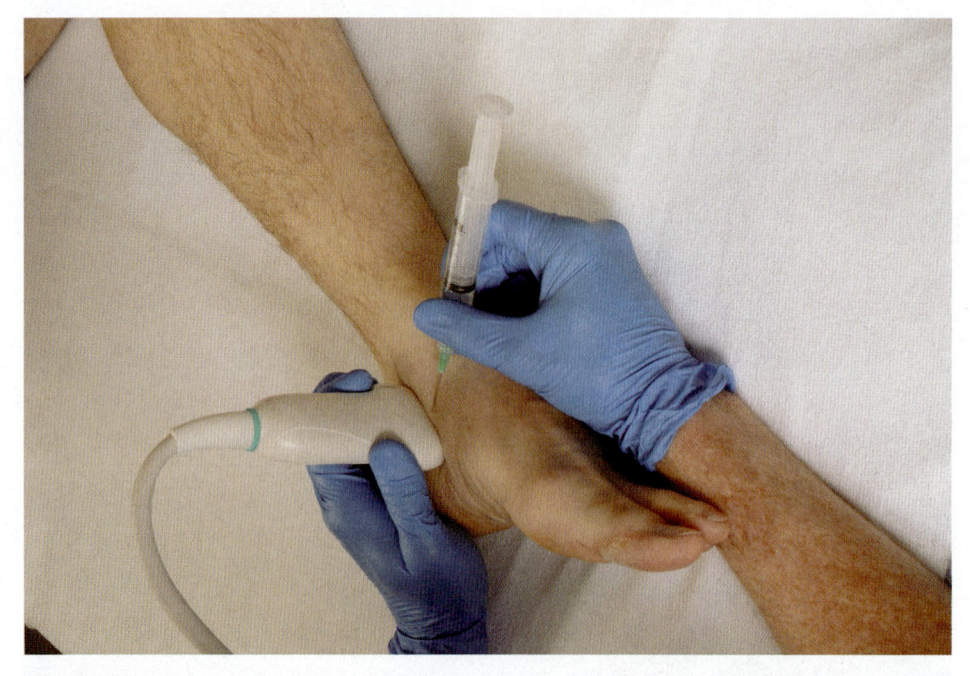

**FIGURE 151.9.** Correct out-of-plane needle placement for ultrasound-guided deltoid ligament injection.

## CLINICAL PEARLS

Bursitis, fractures, tendinopathy, osteoarthritis, synovitis, avascular necrosis, and impingement syndromes may coexist with deltoid ligament pathology and may contribute to the patient's pain symptomatology. Universal precautions should always be observed to protect the operator, and strict adherence to sterile technique must be used to avoid infection. Gentle physical therapy and local heat should be introduced following ultrasound-guided injection of the deltoid ligament to reduce pain and improve function. Simple analgesics and nonsteroidal anti-inflammatory agents or COX-2 inhibitors may be used concurrently with this injection technique.

## SUGGESTED READINGS

Beals TC, Crim J, Nickisch F. Deltoid ligament injuries in athletes: techniques of repair and reconstruction. *Oper Tech Sports Med* 2010;18(1):11–17.

Hintermann B, Knupp M, Pagenstert GI. Deltoid ligament injuries: diagnosis and management. *Foot Ankle Clin* 2006;11(3):625–637.

Waldman SD. Functional anatomy of the ankle and foot. In: *Pain Review*. Philadelphia, PA: Saunders Elsevier; 2009:155–156.

Waldman SD. The deltoid ligament. In: *Pain Review*. Philadelphia, PA: Saunders Elsevier; 2009:157.

Waldman SD, Campbell RSD. Deltoid ligament tear. In: *Imaging of Pain*. Philadelphia, PA: Saunders Elsevier; 2010:439–441.

Waldman SD. Intra-articular injection of the deltoid ligament. In: *Atlas of Pain Management Injection Techniques*. 3rd ed. Philadelphia, PA: Saunders Elsevier; 2012:419–421.

# CHAPTER 152

# Ultrasound-Guided Injection Technique for Anterior Talofibular Ligament Strain

## CLINICAL PERSPECTIVES

One of the four major ligaments of the ankle joint, the anterior talofibular ligament, runs from anterior border of the lateral malleolus to the lateral surface of the talus (Fig. 152.1). Also known as the medial ligament of talocrural joint, the anterior talofibular ligament is susceptible to strain at the joint line or avulsion at its origin or insertion. The anterior talofibular ligament is frequently injured from inversion injuries to the ankle that occur when tripping when high heels, landing hard or running on hard uneven surfaces, and during dancing, soccer, and basketball (Fig. 152.2). The pain of anterior talofibular ligament damage is localized to the lateral ankle and is made worse with inversion of the ankle joint. Point tenderness just below the lateral malleolus is often present on physical examination. Significant swelling and ecchymosis are often evident after acute injury. Activity, especially involving weight bearing, plantar flexion, and inversion of the ankle, will exacerbate the pain. Local heat and decreased activity as well as elevation of the affected ankle may provide a modicum of relief. Sleep disturbance is common in patients suffering from trauma to the anterior talofibular ligament of the ankle. Coexistent fracture, bursitis, tendonitis, arthritis, or internal derangement of the ankle may confuse the clinical picture after trauma to the knee joint making clinical diagnosis difficult.

Plain radiographs and/or arthrography is indicated in all patients who present with anterior talofibular ligament pain, especially after ankle trauma (Fig. 152.3). Based on the patient's clinical presentation, additional testing may be indicated, including complete blood cell count, sedimentation rate, and antinuclear antibody testing. Magnetic resonance imaging (MRI) and/or ultrasound imaging of the ankle is indicated if internal derangement or occult mass or tumor is suspected as well as to confirm the diagnosis of suspected anterior talofibular ligament injury (Figs. 152.4 and 152.5). Bone scan may be useful to identify occult stress fractures involving the joint, especially if trauma has occurred.

## CLINICALLY RELEVANT ANATOMY

The ankle is a hinge-type articulation between the distal tibia, the two malleoli, and the talus. The articular surface is covered with hyaline cartilage, which is susceptible to arthritis. The joint is surrounded by a dense capsule that helps strengthen the ankle. The joint capsule is lined with a synovial membrane that attaches to the articular cartilage. The ankle joint is innervated by the deep peroneal and tibial nerves.

The major ligaments of the ankle joint include the talofibular, anterior talofibular, calcaneofibular, and posterior talofibular ligaments, which provide the majority of strength to the ankle joint. The talofibular ligament is not as strong as the deltoid ligament and is susceptible to strain. The talofibular ligament runs from the anterior border of the lateral malleolus to the lateral surface of the talus (see Fig. 152.1).

## ULTRASOUND-GUIDED TECHNIQUE

The benefits, risks, and alternative treatments are explained to the patient, and informed consent is obtained. The patient is then placed in the supine position with the lateral curled-up position with the affected ankle up (Fig. 152.6). The skin overlying the medial anterior talofibular ligament is then prepped

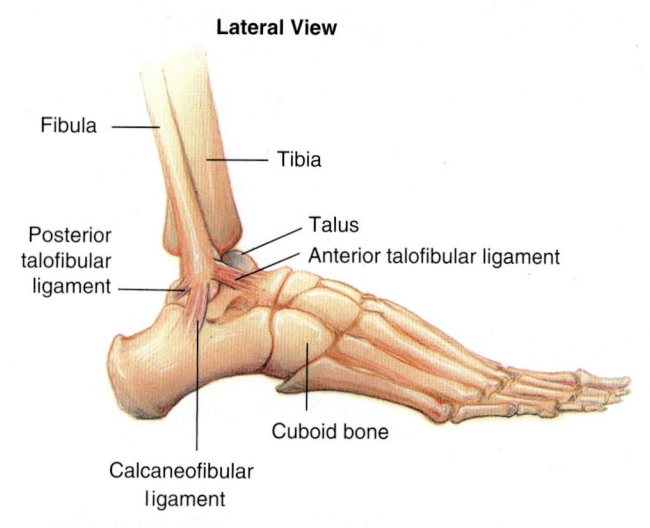

**FIGURE 152.1.** The anatomy of the anterior talofibular ligament and its relationship with the other ligaments of the lateral ankle. (Anatomical Chart Company, 2013.)

# CHAPTER 152   ULTRASOUND-GUIDED INJECTION TECHNIQUE FOR ANTERIOR TALOFIBULAR LIGAMENT STRAIN

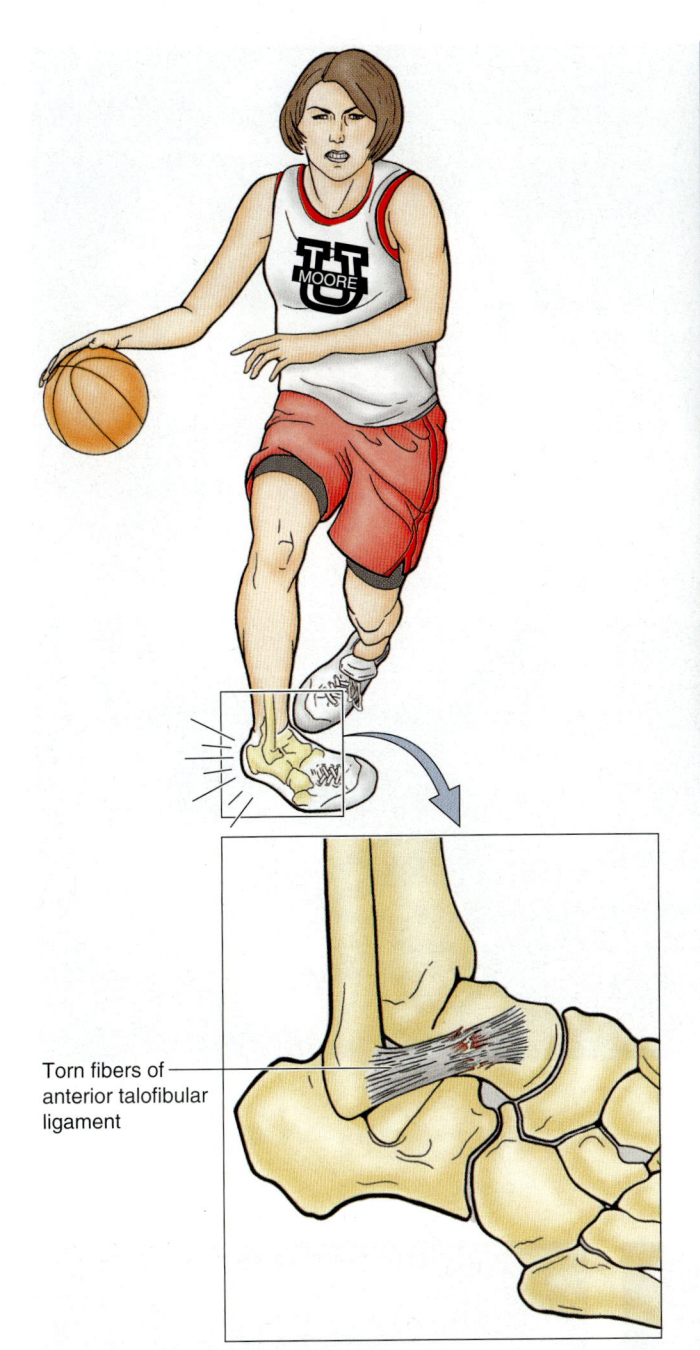

**FIGURE 152.2.** The anterior talofibular ligament is frequently injured by inversion injuries that occur when tripping when high heels, landing hard on uneven surfaces, and during dancing, soccer, and basketball. (Reused from Moore KL, Dalley AF. *Clinical Oriented Anatomy.* 4th ed. Baltimore, MD: Lippincott Williams & Wilkins; 1999, with permission.)

Torn fibers of anterior talofibular ligament

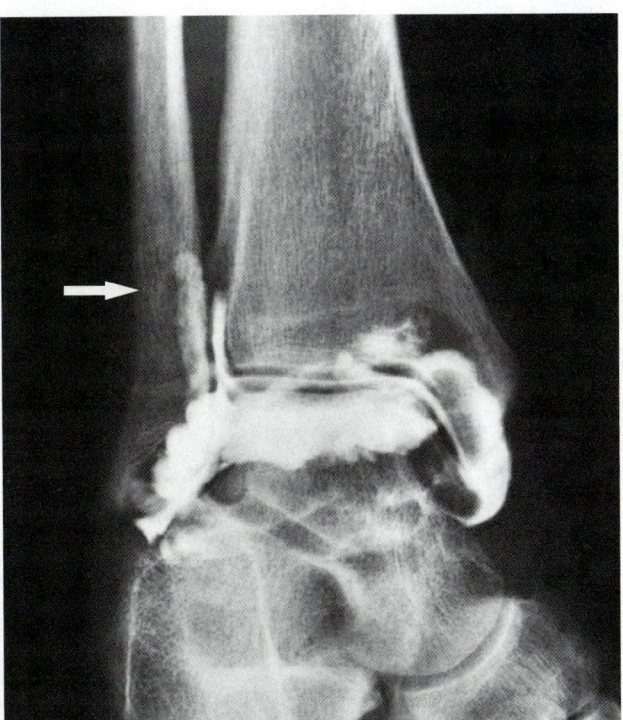

**FIGURE 152.3.** Tear of the distal anterior tibiofibular ligament. A 29-year-old man injured his ankle during a basketball game. Conventional radiograph and stress examination revealed no abnormalities. On arthrography, however, leak of contrast into the region of the tibiofibular syndesmosis (*arrow*) indicates a tear of the distal anterior tibiofibular ligament. (Reused from Greenspan A. *Orthopedic Imaging: A Practical Approach.* 5th ed. Philadelphia, PA: Lippincott Williams & Wilkins; 2011, with permission.)

with antiseptic solution. A sterile syringe containing 2.0 mL of 0.25% preservative-free bupivacaine and 40 mg of methylprednisolone is attached to a 1½-inch, 22-gauge needle using strict aseptic technique. A high-frequency linear ultrasound transducer is then placed in the transverse position with the posterior aspect of the transducer placed just over the bottom of the lateral malleolus (Fig. 152.7). A survey scan is taken, which demonstrates the hyperechoic anterior talofibular ligament running from the talus to the lateral malleolus of the fibula (Fig. 152.8). After the anterior talofibular ligament is identified, the needle is placed through the skin ~1 cm above the middle of the superior aspect of the transversely placed transducer and is then advanced using an out-of-plane approach with the needle trajectory adjusted under real-time ultrasound guidance to place the needle tip within proximity to the anterior talofibular ligament but not within the substance of the ligament (Fig. 152.9). When the tip of needle is thought to be in satisfactory position, a small amount of local anesthetic and steroid is injected under real-time ultrasound guidance to confirm that the needle tip is not within the substance of the anterior talofibular ligament. There should be minimal resistance to injection. After intra-articular needle tip placement is confirmed, the remainder of the contents of the syringe are slowly injected. If synechiae, loculations, or calcifications are present, the needle may have to be repositioned to ensure that the entire intra-articular space is treated. The needle is then removed, and a sterile pressure dressing and ice pack are placed at the injection site.

**FIGURE 152.4.** MRI of the tear of the anterior talofibular ligament. An axial T2-weighted MRI shows disruption of the anterior talofibular ligament resulting in its replacement by high-signal-intensity fluid (*straight arrow*). Note that the intact posterior talofibular ligament shows normal low-signal intensity (*curved arrow*). (Reused from Greenspan A. *Orthopedic Imaging: A Practical Approach.* 5th ed. Philadelphia, PA: Lippincott Williams & Wilkins; 2011, with permission.)

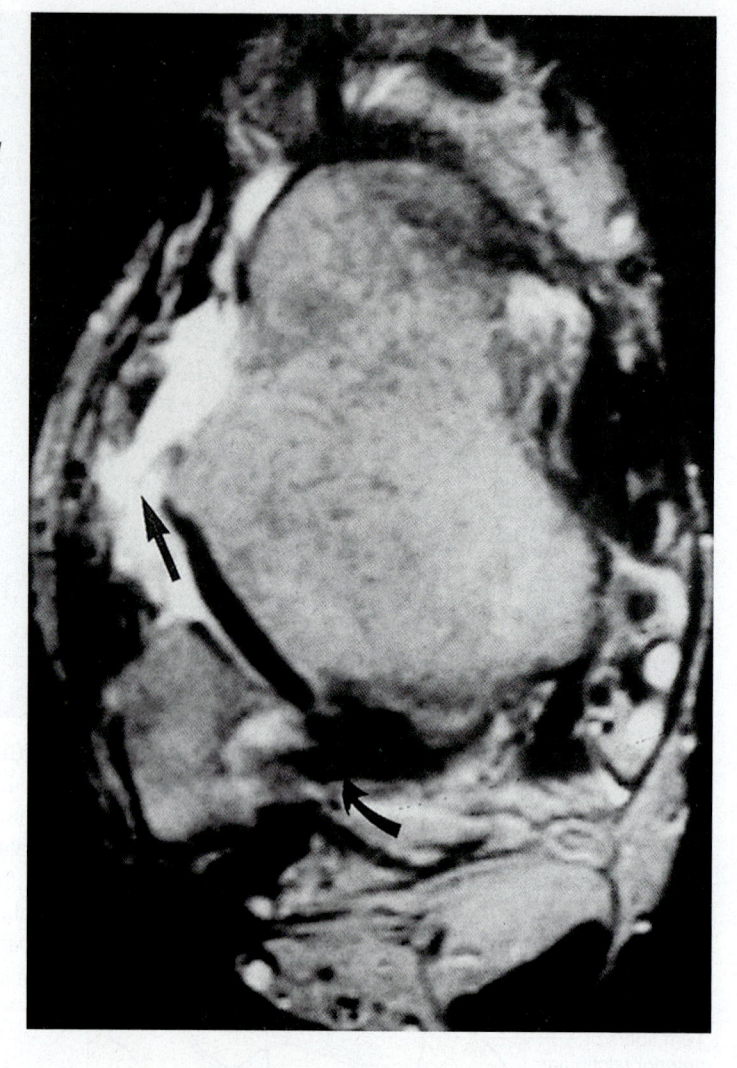

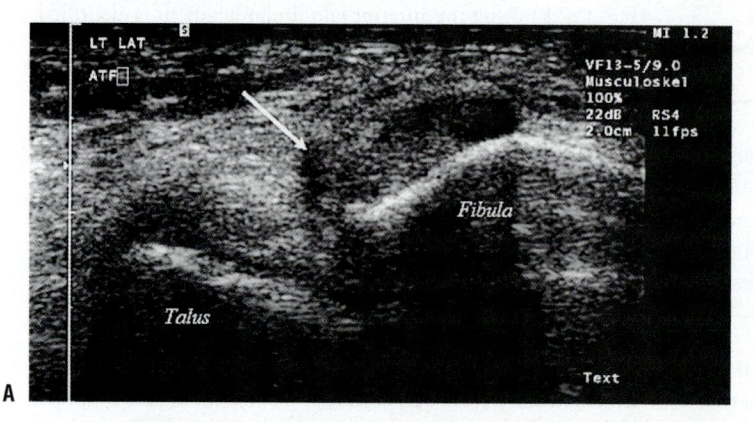

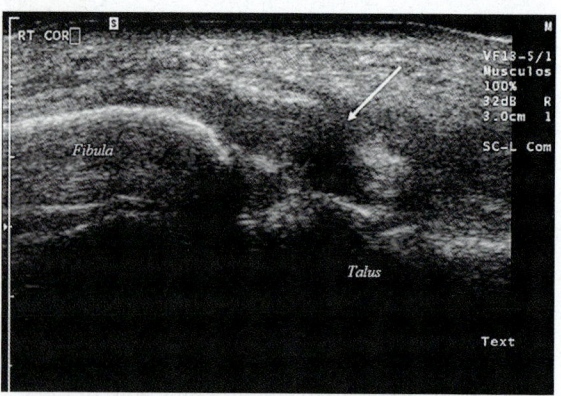

**FIGURE 152.5.** **A:** Ultrasound image along the lateral aspect of the ankle demonstrates a focal tear of anterior talofibular ligament (*arrow*). Note the discontinuity of the ligament apparent as a discrete hypoechoic defect (*arrow*). **B:** Full-thickness tear (*arrow*) of the ATF in another patient. (Reused from Adler RS, Sofka CM, Positano RG. *Atlas of Foot and Ankle Sonography.* Philadelphia, PA: Lippincott Williams & Wilkins; 2004: 69, with permission.)

CHAPTER 152    ULTRASOUND-GUIDED INJECTION TECHNIQUE FOR ANTERIOR TALOFIBULAR LIGAMENT STRAIN    **1079**

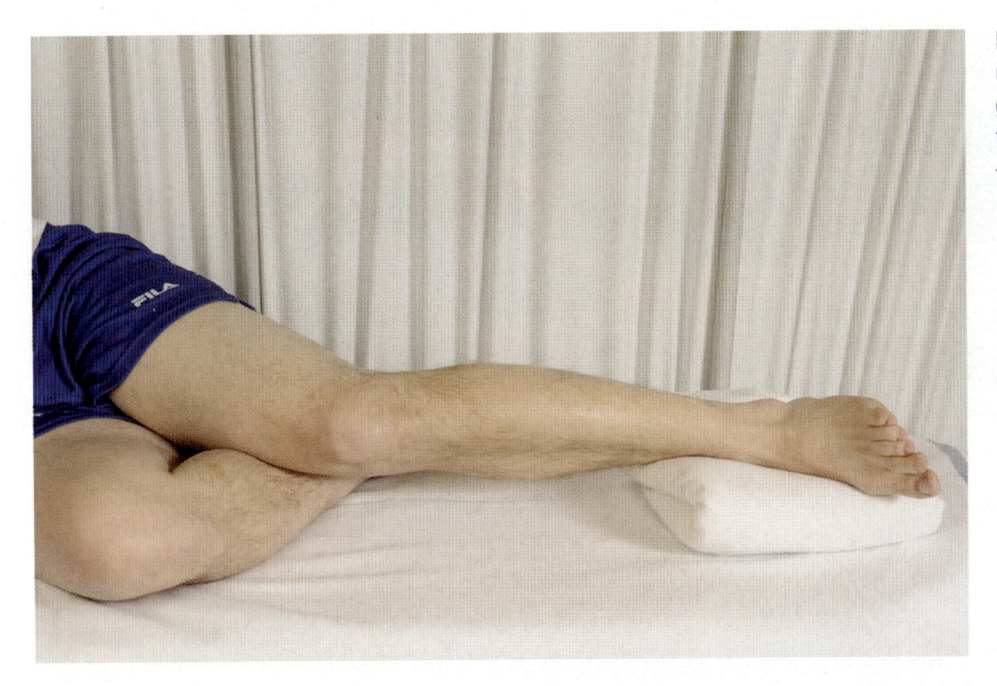

**FIGURE 152.6.** Proper lateral curled-up patient position for ultrasound-guided intra-articular anterior talofibular ligament injection.

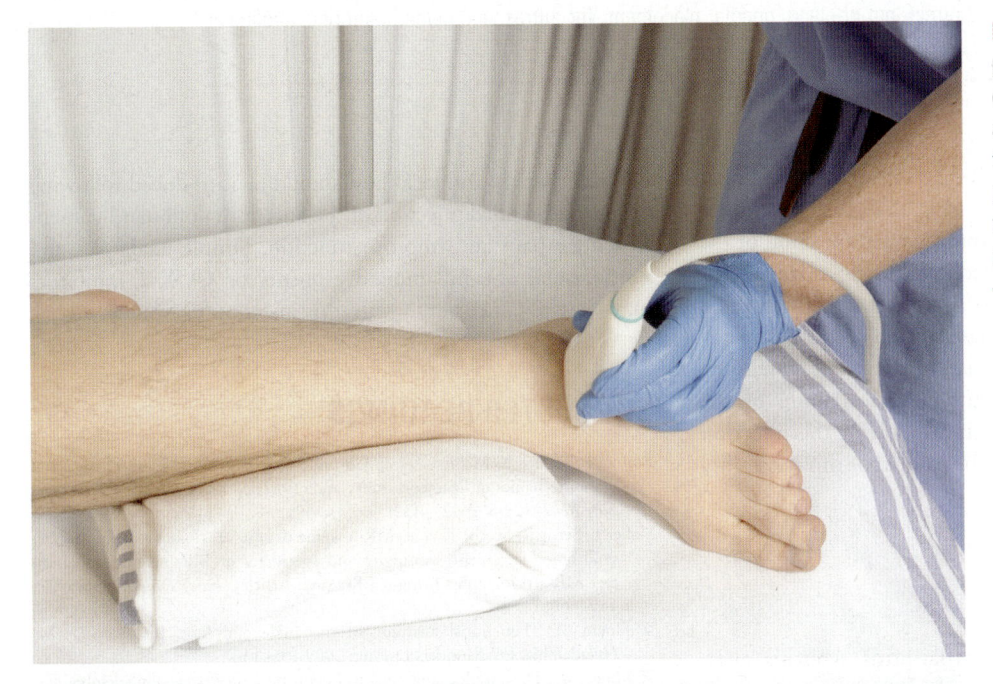

**FIGURE 152.7.** Correct transverse position for the ultrasound transducer for ultrasound-guided intra-articular injection of the anterior talofibular ligament. Note that the posterior aspect of the ultrasound transducer is lying over the bottom of the lateral malleolus.

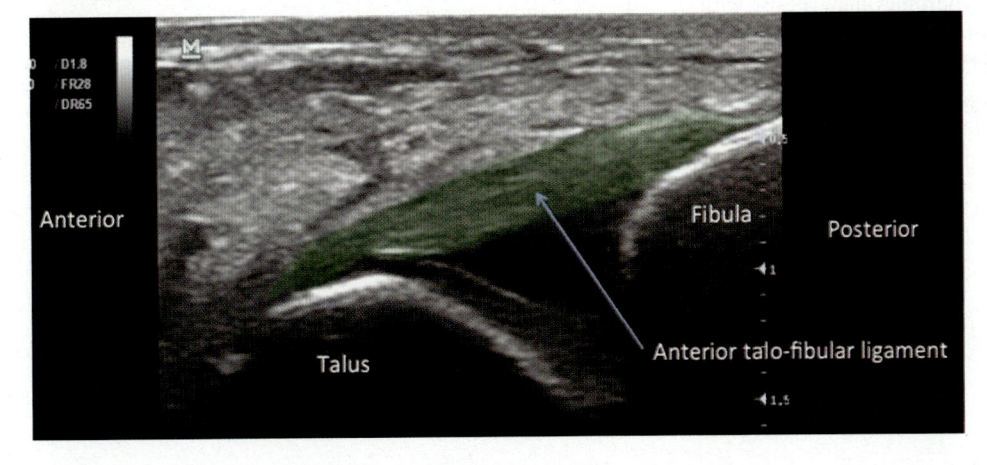

**FIGURE 152.8.** Transverse ultrasound image demonstrating the anterior talofibular ligament.

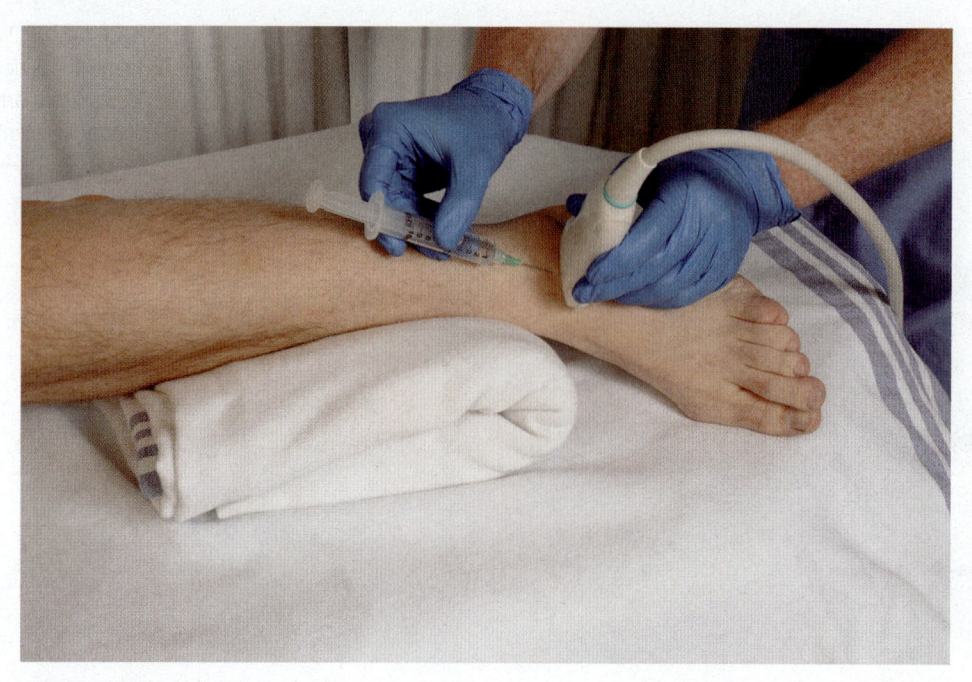

**FIGURE 152.9.** Correct out-of-plane needle placement for ultrasound-guided anterior talofibular ligament injection.

## COMPLICATIONS

The major complication of ultrasound-guided injection of the anterior talofibular ligament is infection. Highly inflamed tendons and ligaments are subject to rupture if directly injected so care must be taken to insure that that the needle tip is outside the substance of the tendon. Ecchymosis and hematoma formation may also occur. A transient exacerbation of the patient's pain occurs ~25% of the time following this injection technique, and the patient should be warned of this possibility prior to the procedure.

## CLINICAL PEARLS

Bursitis, fractures, tendinopathy, osteoarthritis, synovitis, avascular necrosis, and impingement syndromes may coexist with anterior talofibular ligament pathology and may contribute to the patient's pain symptomatology. Universal precautions should always be observed to protect the operator, and strict adherence to sterile technique must be used to avoid infection. Gentle physical therapy and local heat should be introduced following ultrasound-guided injection of the anterior talofibular ligament to reduce pain and improve function. Simple analgesics and nonsteroidal anti-inflammatory agents or COX-2 inhibitors may be used concurrently with this injection technique.

## SUGGESTED READINGS

Bonnel F, Toullec E, Mabit C, et al. Chronic ankle instability: biomechanics and pathomechanics of ligaments injury and associated lesions. *Orthop Traumatol Surg Res* 2012;96(4):424–432.

Haller J, Bernt R, Seeger T, et al. MR-imagine of anterior tibiotalar impingement syndrome: agreement, sensitivity and specificity of MR-imaging and indirect MR-arthrography. [Original Research Article]. *Eur J Radiol* 2006;58(3):450–460.

Waldman SD. Functional anatomy of the ankle and foot. In: *Pain Review*. Philadelphia, PA: Saunders Elsevier; 2009:155–156.

Waldman SD. The anterior talofibular ligament. In: *Pain Review*. Philadelphia, PA: Saunders Elsevier; 2009:158.

Waldman SD, Campbell RSD. Anterior talofibular ligament tear. In: *Imaging of Pain*. Philadelphia, PA: Saunders Elsevier; 2010:437–438.

Waldman SD. Intra-articular injection of the anterior talofibular ligament. In: *Atlas of Pain Management Injection Techniques.* 3rd ed. Philadelphia, PA: Saunders Elsevier; 2012:427–430.

# CHAPTER 153

# Ultrasound-Guided Injection Technique for Anterior Tarsal Tunnel Syndrome

## CLINICAL PERSPECTIVES

An uncommon cause of dorsal foot pain, anterior tarsal tunnel syndrome, is caused by entrapment and compression of the deep peroneal nerve as it passes beneath the superficial fascia of the ankle (Fig. 153.1). Patients suffering from anterior tarsal tunnel syndrome complain of pain, dysesthesias, and numbness of the dorsum of the foot that radiate into the first dorsal web space. The pain associated with anterior tarsal tunnel syndrome may also radiate into the anterior ankle. There is no motor involvement unless the distal lateral division of the deep peroneal nerve is involved. Patients suffering from anterior tarsal tunnel syndrome often report nocturnal foot pain analogous to the nocturnal pain seen in carpal tunnel syndrome sufferers. The patient may report that holding the foot in the everted position may decrease the pain and paresthesias of anterior tarsal tunnel syndrome.

Severe, acute plantar flexion of the foot has been implicated in the evolution of anterior tarsal tunnel syndrome, as has the wearing of overly tight shoes or squatting and bending forward, as when planting flowers. Tumor, osteophyte, ganglion, and synovitis that impinge on the deep peroneal nerve as can cause anterior tarsal tunnel syndrome (Fig. 153.2). Anterior tarsal tunnel syndrome is much less common than posterior tarsal tunnel syndrome.

Patients suffering from anterior tarsal tunnel syndrome will exhibit tenderness on palpation of the deep peroneal nerve at the dorsum of the foot. A positive Tinel sign just medial to the dorsalis pedis pulse over the deep peroneal nerve as it passes beneath the fascia usually is present (Fig. 153.3). The pain of anterior tarsal tunnel syndrome may be elicited by active plantar flexion of the affected foot. Weakness of the extensor digitorum brevis may be identified if the lateral branch of the deep peroneal nerve is affected.

Anterior tarsal tunnel syndrome is frequently misdiagnosed as lumbar radiculopathy or diabetic neuropathy or is attributed to primary ankle pathology leading to both diagnostic and therapeutic misadventures. Plain radiographs of the ankle will help identify primary ankle pathology, and electromyography will help distinguish the compromise of deep peroneal nerve associated with anterior tarsal tunnel syndrome from radiculopathy. Most patients who suffer from lumbar radiculopathy have back pain associated with reflex, motor, and sensory changes that are associated with back pain, whereas patients with anterior tarsal tunnel syndrome have no back pain and no reflex changes. Furthermore, the motor and sensory changes of anterior tarsal tunnel syndrome are limited to the distribution of the deep peroneal nerve. Lumbar radiculopathy and deep peroneal nerve entrapment may coexist as the so-called "double crush" syndrome, and this can further confuse the clinical picture. Based on the patient's clinical presentation, additional testing may be indicated, including complete blood cell count, uric acid, sedimentation rate, and antinuclear antibody testing. Magnetic resonance imaging or computed tomography scanning of the lumbar spine is indicated if a herniated disk, spinal stenosis, or a space-occupying lesion is suspected. MRI and/or ultrasound imaging of the anterior ankle and foot is indicated to confirm the diagnosis of anterior tarsal tunnel syndrome by identifying the pathology responsible for nerve entrapment, for example, tumor, mass, and osteophyte, as well as to identify occult pathology (Fig. 153.4).

## CLINICALLY RELEVANT ANATOMY

The common peroneal nerve is one of the two major continuations of the sciatic nerve, the other being the tibial nerve. The common peroneal nerve provides sensory innervation to the inferior portion of the knee joint and the posterior and lateral skin of the upper calf. The common peroneal nerve is derived from the posterior branches of the L4, L5, and S1 and S2 nerve roots. The nerve splits from the sciatic nerve at the superior margin of the popliteal fossa and descends laterally behind the head of the fibula (Fig. 153.5). The common peroneal nerve is subject to compression at this point by such circumstances as improperly applied casts and tourniquets. The nerve is also subject to compression as it continues its lateral course, winding around the fibula through the fibular tunnel, which is made up of the posterior border of the tendinous insertion of the peroneus longus muscle and the fibula itself. Just distal to the fibular tunnel, the nerve divides into its two terminal branches: the superficial and the deep peroneal nerves. Each of these branches is subject to trauma and may be blocked individually as a diagnostic and therapeutic maneuver.

**FIGURE 153.1.** The deep peroneal nerve can be entrapped at several points beneath the superficial fascia of the dorsum of the foot.

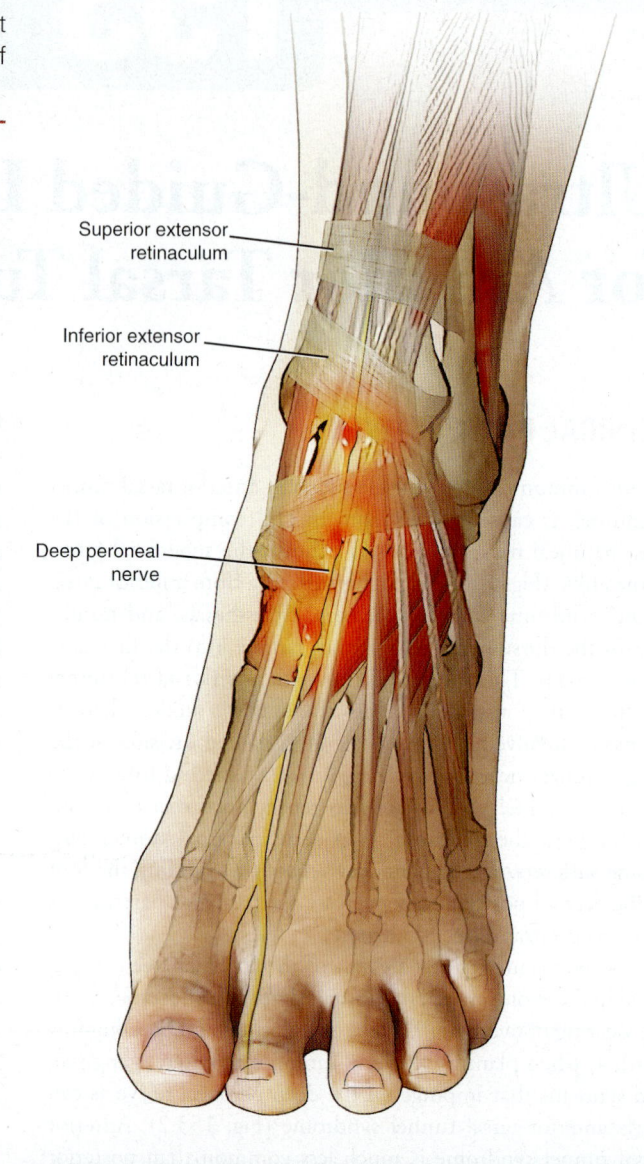

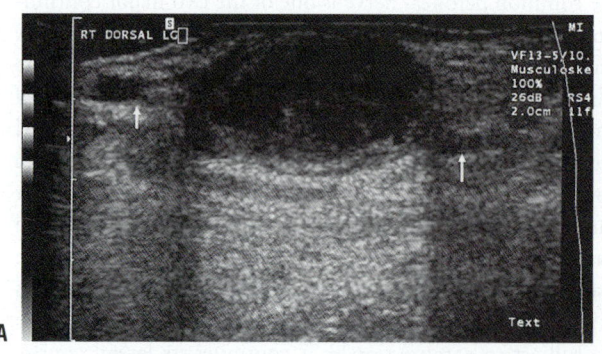

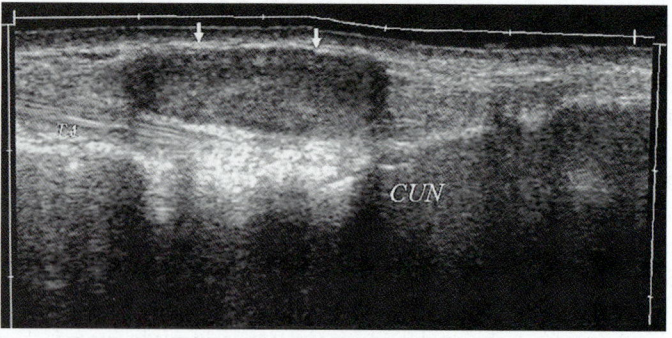

**FIGURE 153.2. A:** The relationship of masses to regional neurovascular structures can be defined with sonography. This longitudinal image demonstrates a well-defined hypoechoic mass within the substance of the deep peroneal nerve (the more normal proximal and distal aspects of the nerve can be seen (*arrows*)) consistent with a neurofibroma. The presence of a nerve having entry and exit points relative to such a mass is pathognomonic for a neural tumor. **B:** The presence of a nerve in relation to a neural tumor is not always evident. Longitudinal extended field of view image of the dorsum of the midfoot demonstrates a well-defined hypoechoic mass consistent with a neurofibroma (*arrows*). Note the proximity of the mass to the medial cuneiform (CUN) and the tibialis anterior tendon (TA). (Reused from Adler R, Sofka CM, Positano RG. *Atlas of Foot and Ankle Sonography.* Philadelphia, PA: Lippincott Williams & Wilkins; 2004:100, with permission.)

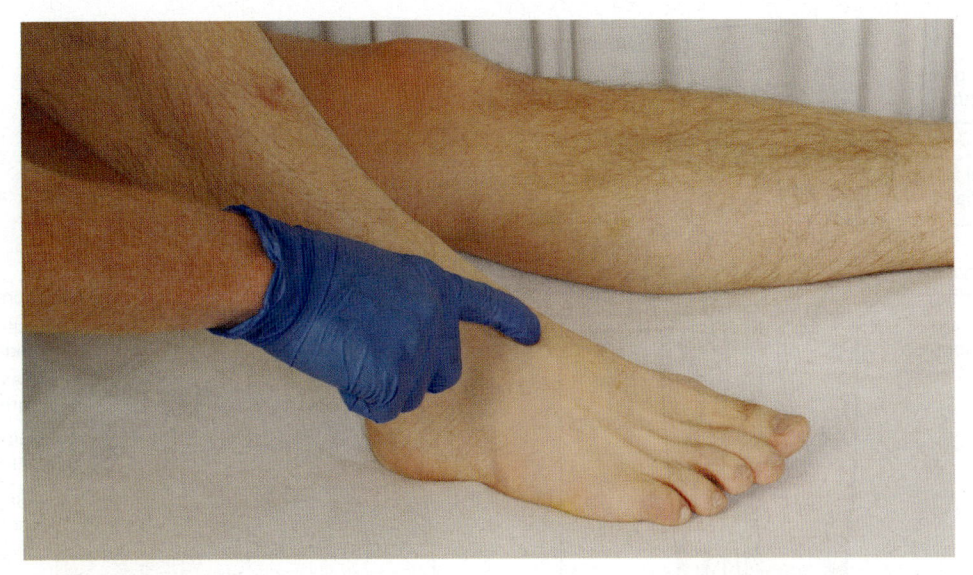

**FIGURE 153.3.** A positive Tinel sign just medial to the dorsalis pedis pulse over the deep peroneal nerve as it passes beneath the fascia is usually present in patient's suffering from anterior tarsal tunnel syndrome.

The deep branch continues down the leg in conjunction with the tibial artery and vein to provide sensory innervation to the web space of the first and second toes and adjacent dorsum of the foot (Figs. 153.6 and 153.7). Although this distribution of sensory fibers is small, this area is often the site of Morton neuroma surgery and thus is important to the regional anesthesiologist. The deep peroneal nerve provides motor innervation to all of the toe extensors and the anterior tibialis muscles. The deep peroneal nerve passes beneath the dense superficial fascia of the ankle, where it is subject to an entrapment syndrome known as the anterior tarsal tunnel syndrome.

## ULTRASOUND-GUIDED TECHNIQUE

Ultrasound-guided injection technique for anterior tarsal tunnel syndrome involves blocking the deep peroneal nerve at the ankle at the site of nerve entrapment. The technique can be carried out by placing the patient in the supine position with the arms resting comfortably along the patient's chest and the affected lower extremity in neutral position (Fig. 153.8). A total of 4 mL of local anesthetic is drawn up in a 12-mL sterile syringe. If the painful condition being treated is thought to have an inflammatory component, 40 to 80 mg of depot steroid is added to the local anesthetic. A linear high-frequency ultrasound transducer is placed in a transverse plane just above the anterior crease of the ankle, and an ultrasound survey scan is taken (Fig. 153.9). The deep peroneal nerve is seen lying just lateral to the anterior tibial artery (Fig. 153.10). Color Doppler can be utilized to help identify the anterior tibial artery (Fig. 153.11). When the anterior tibial artery and adjacent deep peroneal nerve are identified on ultrasound imaging, the skin is prepped with anesthetic solution, and a 1½-inch,

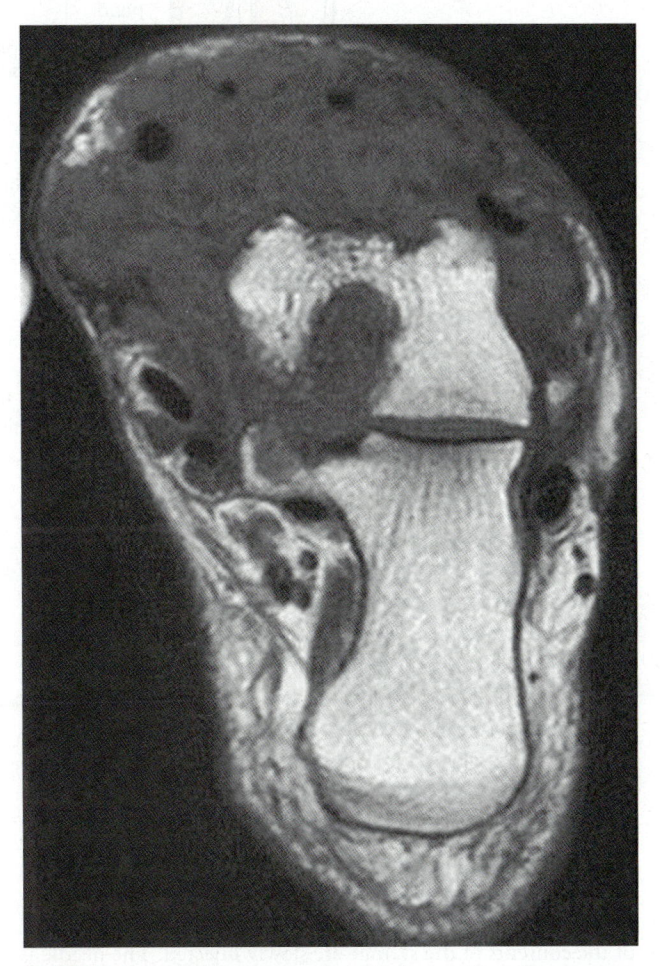

**FIGURE 153.4.** MRI of the anterior ankle in a patient with symptoms of anterior tarsal tunnel syndrome demonstrating a mass, which is consistent with villonodular synovitis.

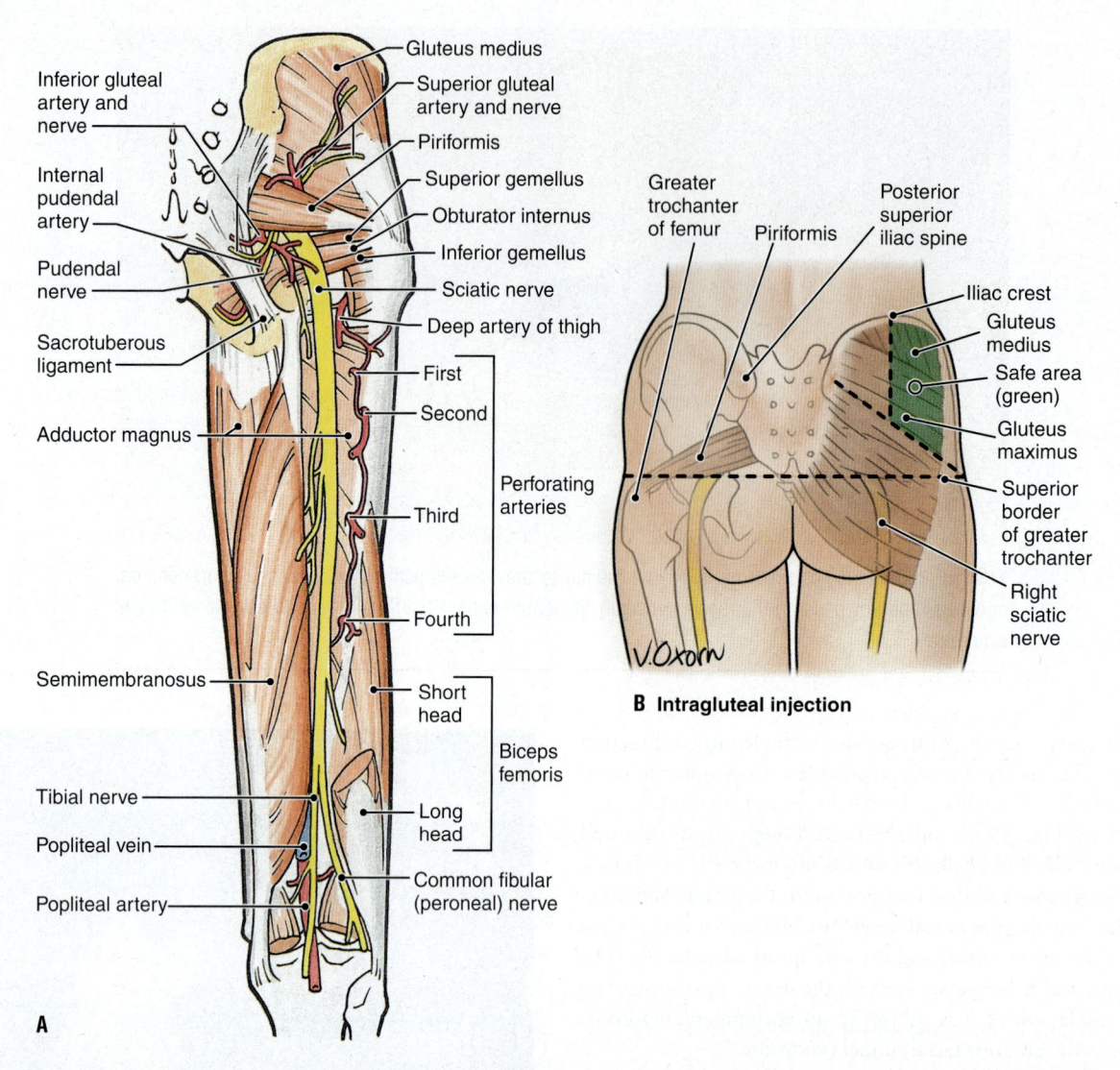

**FIGURE 153.5. A:** The anatomy of the common peroneal nerve. **B:** The safe zone for intragluteal injection. (Reused from Moore KL, Agur AMR. *Essential Clinical Anatomy.* 2nd ed. Baltimore, MD: Lippincott Williams & Wilkins; 2002, with permission.)

22-gauge needle is advanced from the lateral border of the ultrasound transducer and advanced utilizing an in-plane approach with the trajectory being adjusted under real-time ultrasound guidance until the needle tip is resting in proximity to the deep peroneal nerve (Fig. 153.12). When the tip of needle is thought to be in satisfactory position, after careful aspiration, a small amount of local anesthetic and steroid is injected under real-time ultrasound guidance to confirm that the needle tip is in proximity to the deep peroneal nerve, but not within the nerve itself. There should be minimal resistance to injection. After needle tip placement is confirmed, the remainder of the contents of the syringe are slowly injected. The needle is then removed, and a sterile pressure dressing and ice pack are placed at the injection site.

## COMPLICATIONS

A failure to accurately assess the correct position of the needle tip when performing ultrasound-guided injection technique for anterior tarsal tunnel syndrome can lead to a failure to block the deep peroneal nerve or cause needle-induced trauma to the deep peroneal nerve and/or anterior artery. The use of ultrasound guidance when performing injection technique for anterior tarsal tunnel syndrome should markedly decrease these problems. Postblock ecchymosis and hematoma may occur, and the patient should be warned of such. These complications can be decreased by the use of a pressure dressing and cold packs applied to the injection site following the procedure.

**FIGURE 153.6.** The anatomy of the distal deep peroneal nerve. Note the relations hip of the ankle of the nerve to the deep peroneal vein.

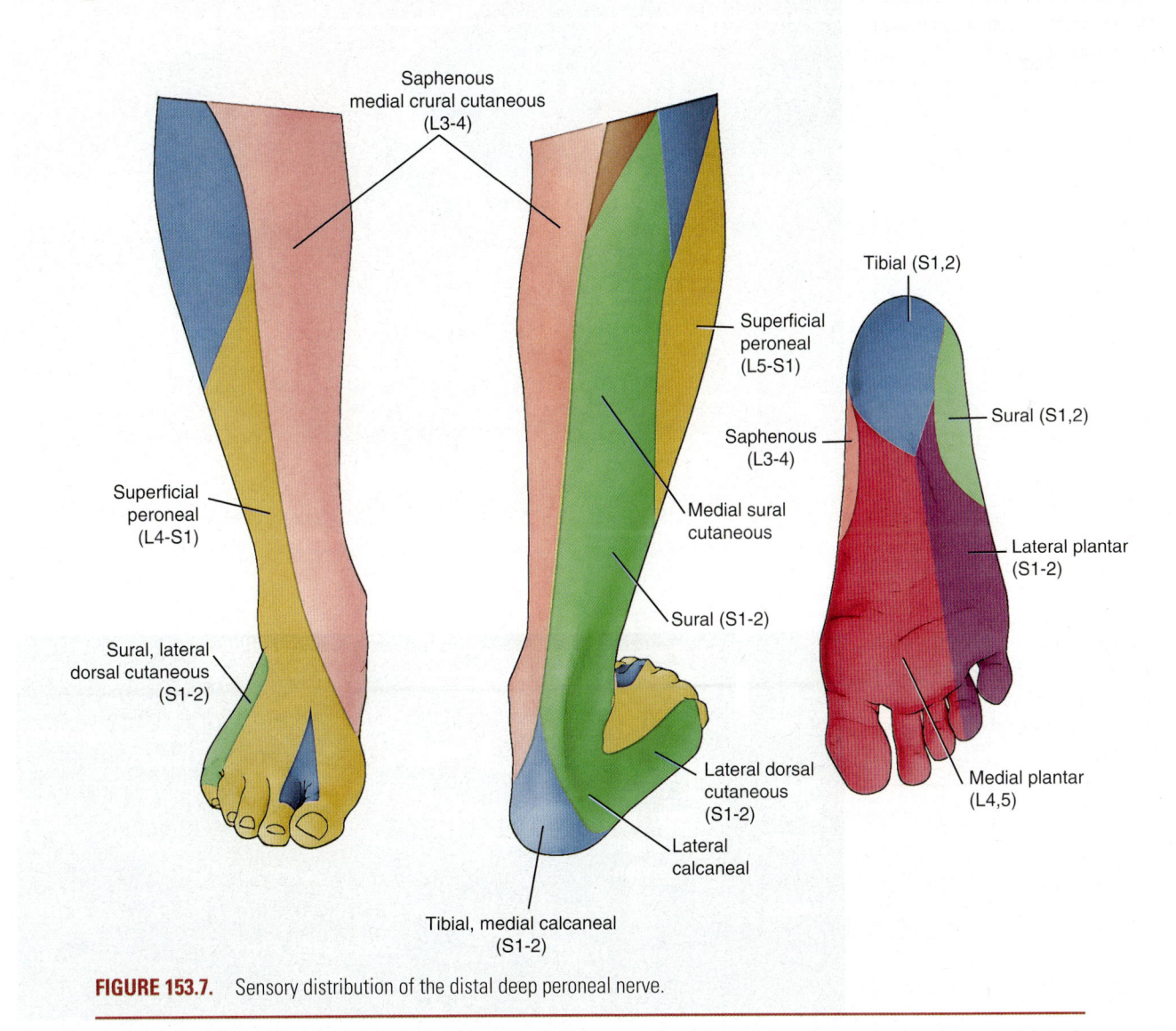

- Anterior tibial artery
- Deep peroneal nerve
- Dorsalis pedis artery

- Saphenous medial crural cutaneous (L3-4)
- Superficial peroneal (L5-S1)
- Saphenous (L3-4)
- Medial sural cutaneous
- Sural (S1-2)
- Lateral dorsal cutaneous (S1-2)
- Lateral calcaneal
- Tibial, medial calcaneal (S1-2)
- Superficial peroneal (L4-S1)
- Sural, lateral dorsal cutaneous (S1-2)
- Tibial (S1,2)
- Sural (S1,2)
- Lateral plantar (S1-2)
- Medial plantar (L4,5)

**FIGURE 153.7.** Sensory distribution of the distal deep peroneal nerve.

1086   SECTION X   ANKLE AND FOOT

**FIGURE 153.8.** Proper patient position for ultrasound-guided deep peroneal nerve block.

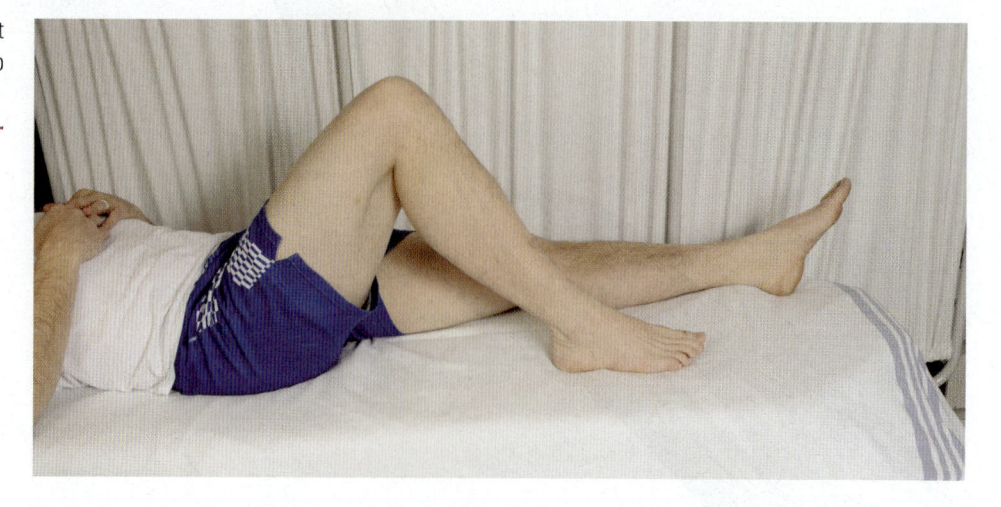

**FIGURE 153.9.** Proper transverse position of the ultrasound transducer for ultrasound-guided deep peroneal nerve block at the ankle.

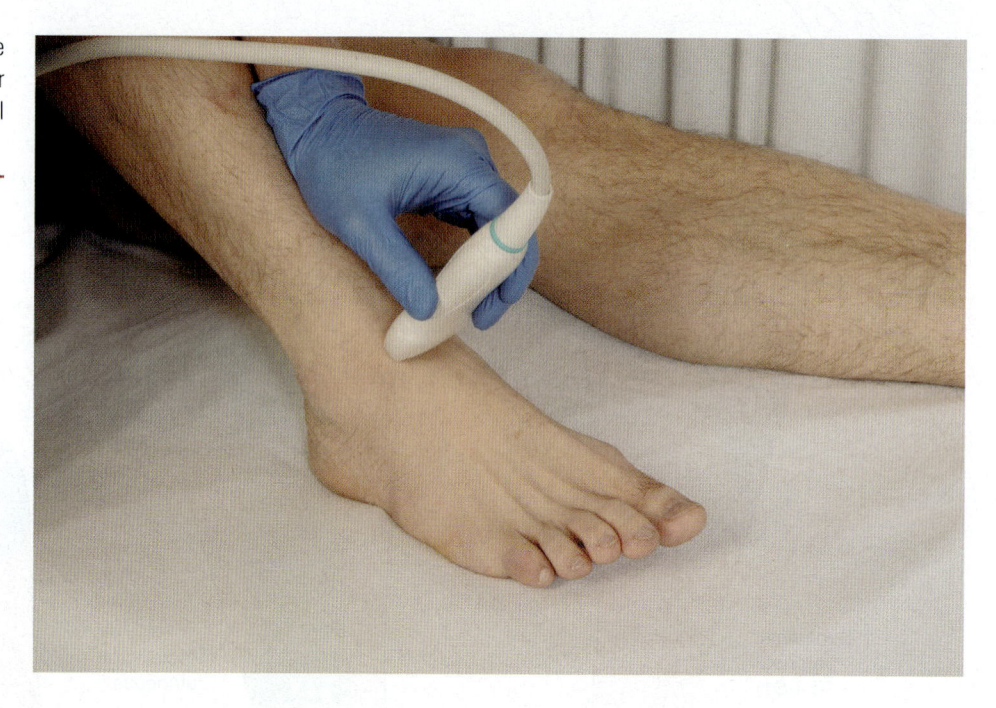

**FIGURE 153.10.** Transverse ultrasound image demonstrating the tibial artery and vein and the deep peroneal nerve just above and lateral to the vein.

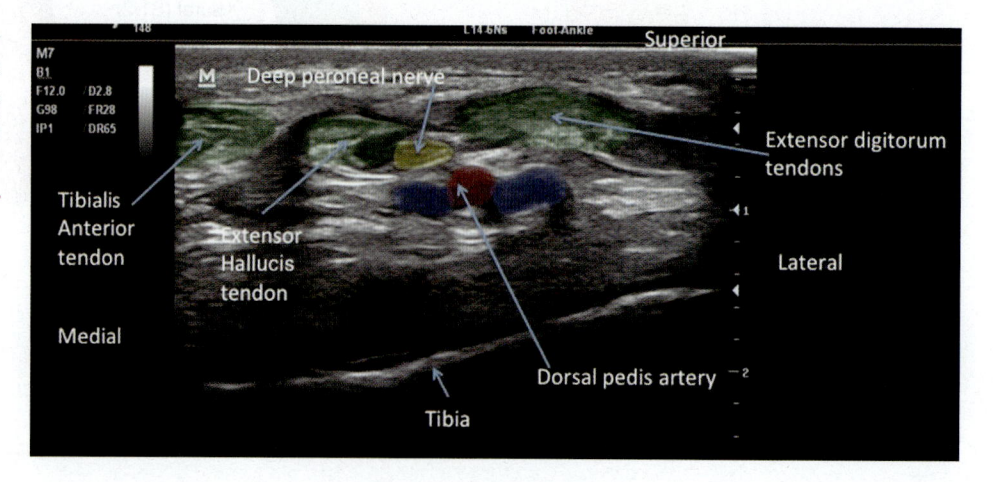

CHAPTER 153  ULTRASOUND-GUIDED INJECTION TECHNIQUE FOR ANTERIOR TARSAL TUNNEL SYNDROME  1087

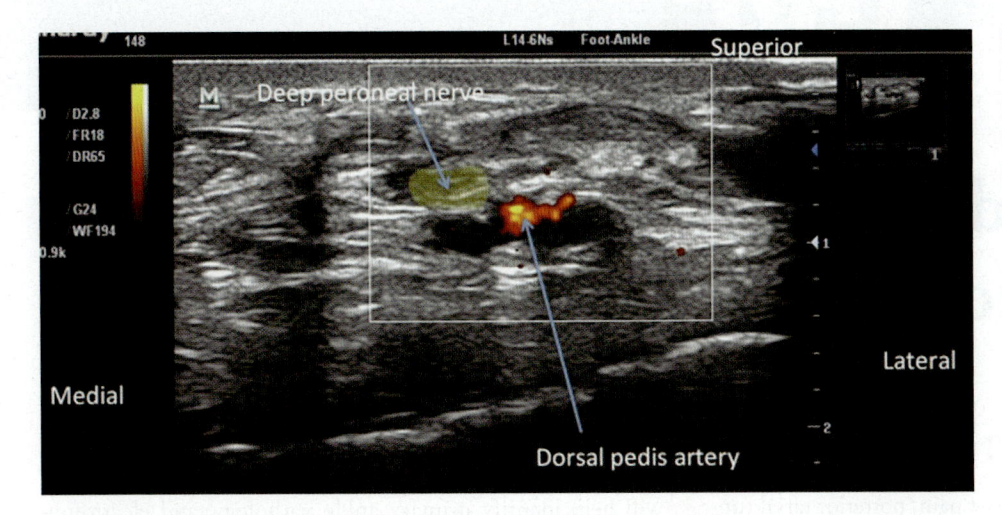

**FIGURE 153.11.** Transverse color Doppler image demonstrating the popliteal vein and artery and the relationship of the vein to the deep peroneal nerve.

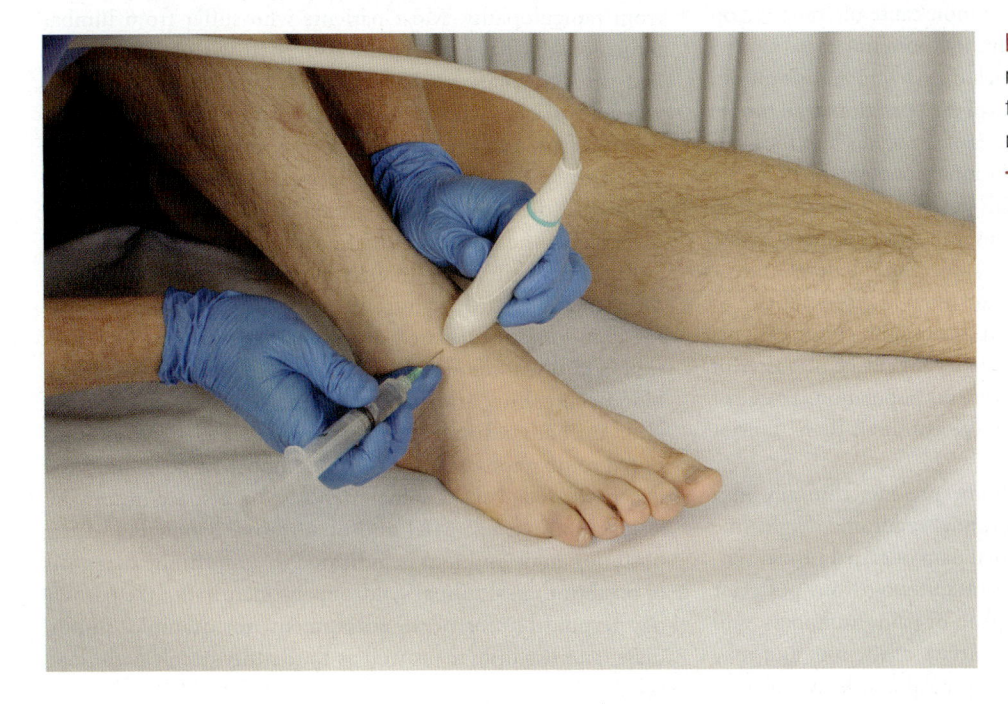

**FIGURE 153.12.** Proper in-plane needle position for performing injection technique for anterior tarsal tunnel syndrome.

## CLINICAL PEARLS

The key to performing successful ultrasound injection technique for anterior tarsal tunnel syndrome is the proper identification of the sonographic anatomy and in particular the ability to properly identify the deep peroneal nerve at the site of nerve entrapment. This should not be a problem if the above technique is used. Any significant pain or sudden increase in resistance during injection when performing ultrasound-guided suggests incorrect needle placement, and one should stop injecting immediately and reassess the position of the needle.

## SUGGESTED READINGS

DiDomenico LA, Masternick EB. Anterior tarsal tunnel syndrome. *Clin Podiatr Med Surg* 2006;23(3):611–620.
Lopez-Ben R. Imaging of nerve entrapment in the foot and ankle. [Review Article.] *Foot Ankle Clin* 2011;16(2):213–224.
Waldman SD. Anterior tarsal tunnel syndrome. In: *Pain Review*. Philadelphia, PA: Saunders Elsevier; 2009:322–323.
Waldman SD. Functional anatomy of the ankle and foot. In: *Pain Review*. Philadelphia, PA: Saunders Elsevier; 2009:155–156.
Waldman SD, Campbell RSD. Anterior tarsal tunnel syndrome. In: *Imaging of Pain*. Philadelphia, PA: Saunders Elsevier; 2010:421–423.
Waldman SD. Anterior tarsal tunnel syndrome. In: *Atlas of Common Pain Syndromes*. 3rd ed. Philadelphia, PA: Saunders Elsevier; 2012:356–358.
Waldman SD. Injection technique for anterior tarsal tunnel syndrome. In: *Atlas of Pain Management Injection Techniques*. 3rd ed. Philadelphia, PA: Saunders Elsevier; 2012:431–434.

# CHAPTER 154

# Ultrasound-Guided Injection Technique for Posterior Tarsal Tunnel Syndrome

## CLINICAL PERSPECTIVES

An uncommon cause of plantar foot pain, posterior tarsal tunnel syndrome, is caused by entrapment and compression of the posterior tibial nerve as it passes through the posterior tarsal tunnel (Fig. 154.1). The most common cause of compression of the posterior tibial nerve within the posterior tarsal tunnel location is trauma to the ankle, including fracture, dislocation, and crush injuries. The boundaries of the posterior tarsal tunnel are the flexor retinaculum, the bones of the ankle, and the lacunar ligament. The posterior tarsal tunnel contains the posterior tibial nerve, vein and artery, tibialis posterior, flexor digitorum longus, and flexor hallucis longus musculotendinous units. These musculotendinous units are subject to the development of tenosynovitis, while the posterior tibial artery is subject to the development of aneurysms and thrombophlebitis. Patients with rheumatoid arthritis have a higher incidence of posterior tarsal tunnel syndrome than the general population. Posterior tarsal tunnel syndrome is much more common than anterior tarsal tunnel syndrome.

Posterior tarsal tunnel syndrome presents clinically in a manner very analogous to carpal tunnel syndrome. Nighttime foot pain analogous to the nocturnal pain of carpal tunnel syndrome often is present. The patient suffering from posterior tarsal tunnel will frequently complain of pain, numbness, and dysesthesias involving the plantar surface of the foot and may radiate into the medial ankle. The medial and lateral plantar divisions of the posterior tibial nerve provide motor innervation to the intrinsic muscles of the foot. The patient may note weakness of the toe flexors and instability of the foot caused by weakness of the lumbrical muscles.

Physical findings include tenderness over the posterior tibial nerve at the medial malleolus. A positive Tinel sign just below and behind the medial malleolus over the posterior tibial nerve usually is present (Fig. 154.2). Active inversion of the ankle often reproduces the symptoms of the posterior tarsal tunnel syndrome. Weakness of the flexor digitorum brevis and the lumbrical muscles may be present if the medial and lateral branches of the posterior tibial nerve are compromised.

Posterior tarsal tunnel syndrome is frequently misdiagnosed as lumbar radiculopathy or diabetic neuropathy or is attributed to primary ankle pathology leading to both diagnostic and therapeutic misadventures. Plain radiographs of the ankle will help identify primary ankle pathology, and electromyography will help distinguish the compromise of posterior tibial nerve associated with posterior tarsal tunnel syndrome from radiculopathy. Most patients who suffer from lumbar radiculopathy have back pain associated with reflex, motor, and sensory changes that are associated with back pain, whereas patients with posterior tarsal tunnel syndrome have no back pain and no reflex changes. Furthermore, the motor and sensory changes of posterior tarsal tunnel syndrome are limited to the distribution of the medial and lateral plantar divisions of the posterior tibial nerve. Lumbar radiculopathy and posterior tibial nerve entrapment may coexist as the so-called "double crush" syndrome, and this can further confuse the clinical picture. Based on the patient's clinical presentation, additional testing may be indicated, including complete blood cell count, uric acid, sedimentation rate, and antinuclear antibody testing. Magnetic resonance imaging or computed tomography scanning of the lumbar spine is indicated if a herniated disk, a spinal stenosis, or a space-occupying lesion is suspected. MRI and/or ultrasound imaging of the posterior ankle and foot is indicated to confirm the diagnosis of posterior tarsal tunnel syndrome by identifying the pathology responsible for nerve entrapment, for example, tumor, mass, and osteophyte, as well as to identify occult pathology (Fig. 154.3).

## CLINICALLY RELEVANT ANATOMY

The tibial nerve is one of the two major continuations of the sciatic nerve, the other being the common peroneal nerve (Fig. 154.4). The tibial nerve provides sensory innervation to the posterior portion of the calf, the heel, and the medial plantar surface. The tibial nerve splits from the sciatic nerve at the superior margin of the popliteal fossa and descends in a slightly medial course through the popliteal fossa. The tibial nerve at the ankle lies just beneath the fascia and is readily accessible for neural blockade. The tibial nerve continues its downward course, running between the two heads of the gastrocnemius muscle and passing deep to the soleus muscle. The

# CHAPTER 154 ULTRASOUND-GUIDED INJECTION TECHNIQUE FOR POSTERIOR TARSAL TUNNEL SYNDROME

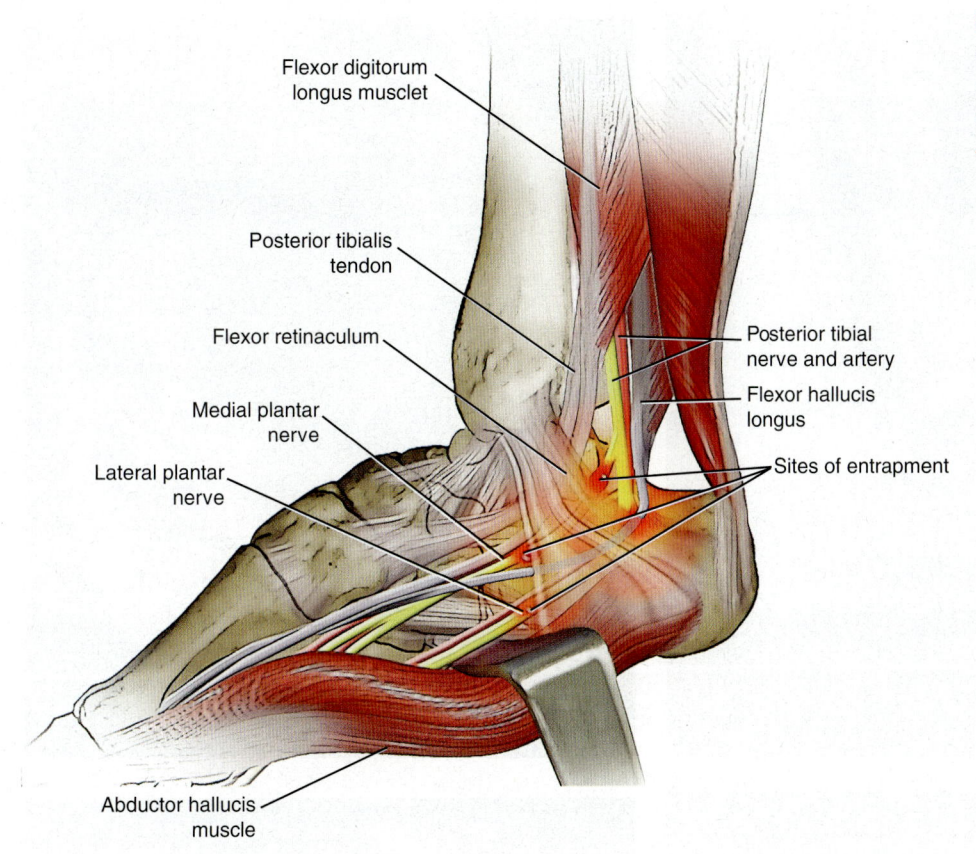

**FIGURE 154.1.** The posterior tibial nerve can be entrapped at several points beneath the superficial fascia of the dorsum of the foot.

nerve courses medially between the Achilles tendon and the medial malleolus, where it divides into the medial and lateral plantar nerves, providing sensory innervation to the heel and medial plantar surface (Fig. 154.5). The tibial nerve is subject to compression at this point as the nerve passes through the posterior tarsal tunnel (see Fig. 154.1). The posterior tarsal tunnel is made up of the flexor retinaculum, the bones of the ankle, and the lacunar ligament. In addition to the posterior tibial nerve, the tunnel contains the posterior tibial artery and vein as well as a number of flexor musculotendinous units.

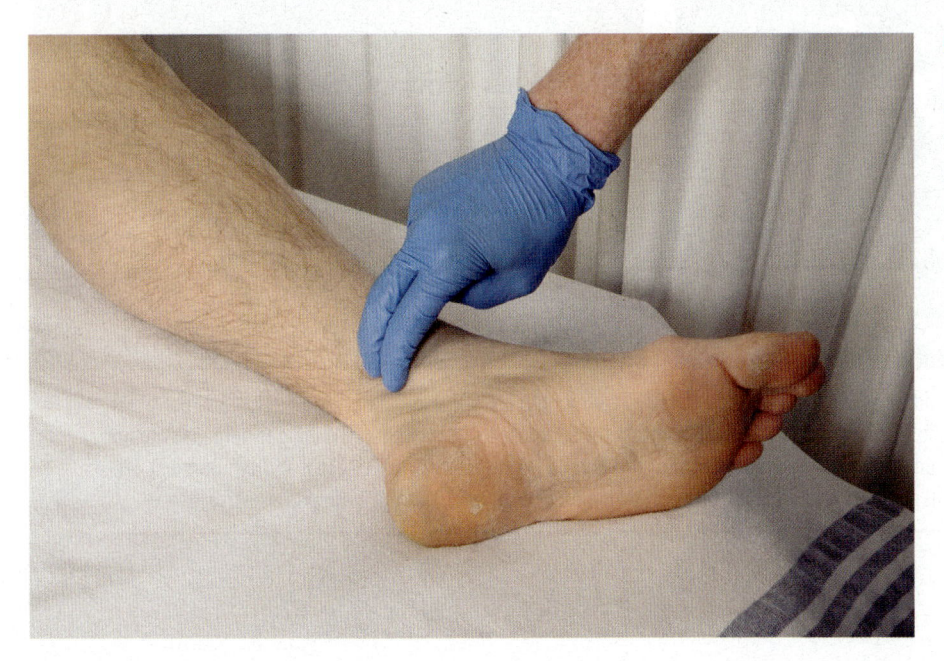

**FIGURE 154.2.** A positive Tinel sign just posterior to the medial malleolus over the posterior tibial nerve as it passes beneath the fascia is usually present in patient's suffering from posterior tarsal tunnel syndrome.

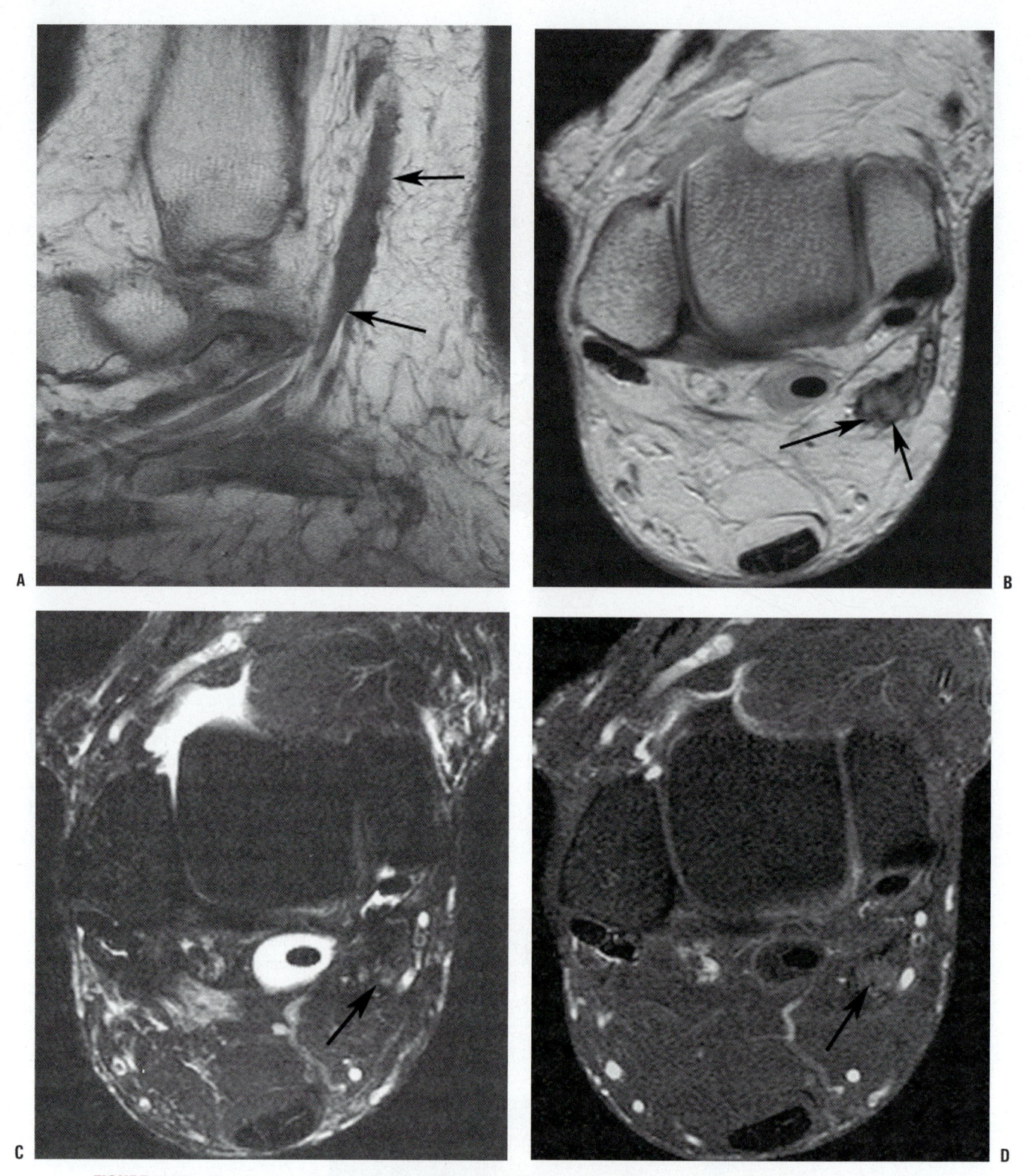

**FIGURE 154.3.** Tarsal tunnel syndrome. Sagittal **(A)** and axial **(B)** T1-weighted images demonstrating a neuroma of the tibial nerve (*arrows*). Axial fast spin-echo T2-weighted **(C)** and postcontrast fat-suppressed T1-weighted **(D)** images demonstrate no increase in signal intensity and minimal contrast enhancement of the fibrous neural lesion (*arrow*). (Reused from Berquist TH. *Imaging of the Foot and Ankle*. 3rd ed. Philadelphia, PA: Lippincott Williams & Wilkins; 2011:182, with permission.)

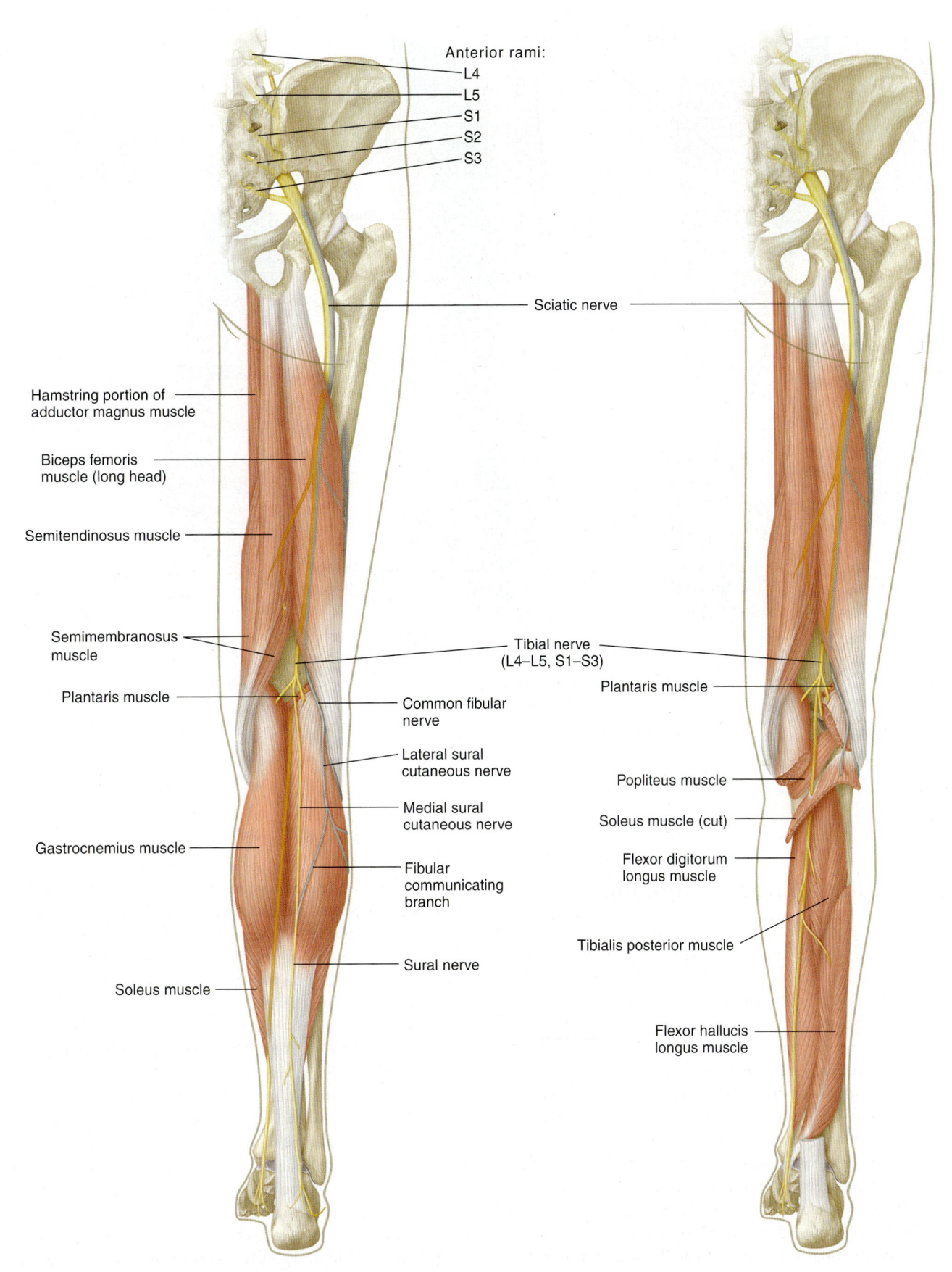

**FIGURE 154.4.** The anatomy of the tibial nerve. (Reused from Tank PW, Gest TR. *Atlas of Anatomy*. Philadelphia, PA: Lippincott Williams & Wilkins; 2008, with permission.)

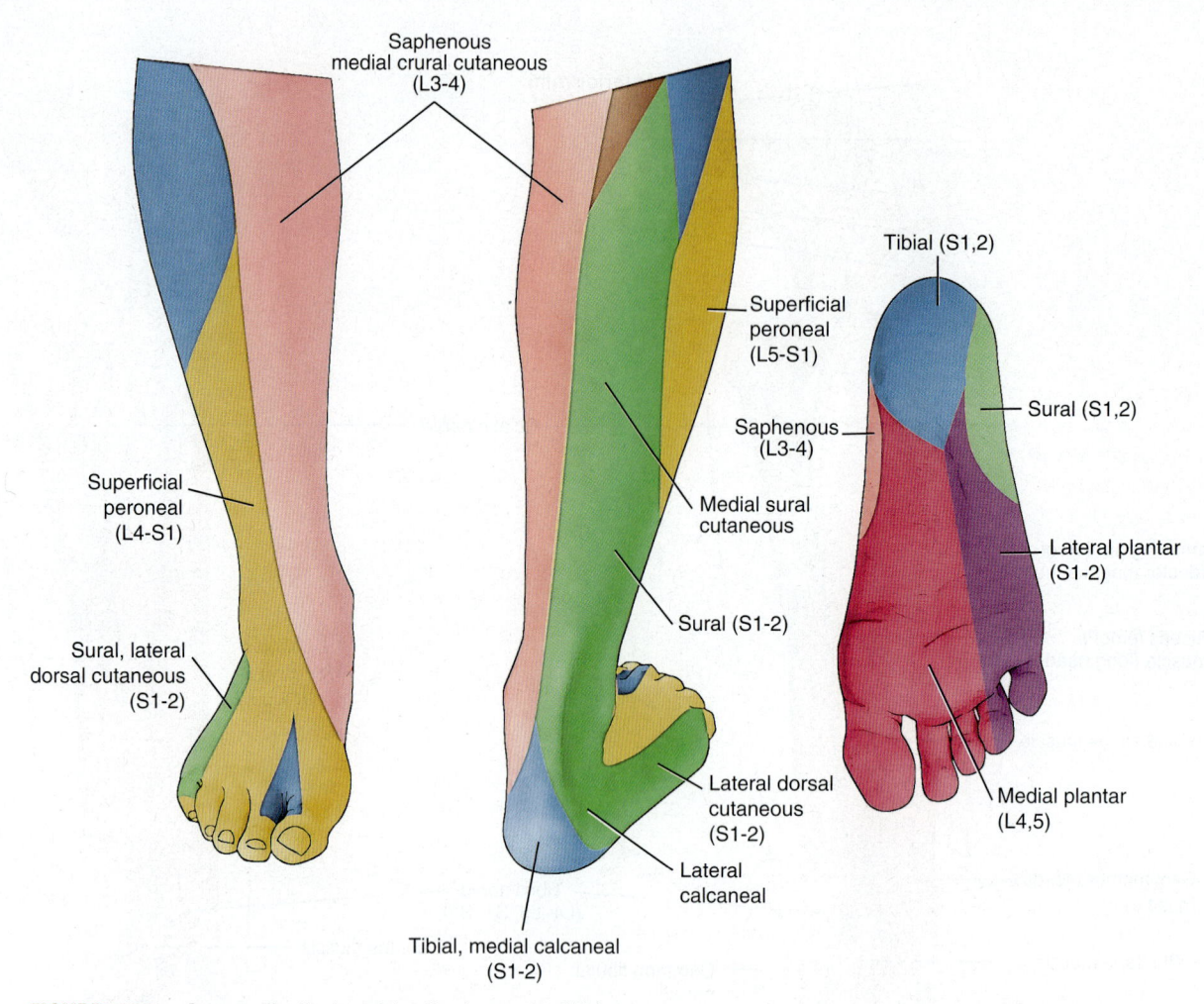

**FIGURE 154.5.** Sensory distribution of the distal posterior tibial nerve.

## ULTRASOUND-GUIDED TECHNIQUE

Ultrasound-guided injection technique for posterior tarsal tunnel syndrome involves blocking the posterior tibial nerve at the ankle as it passes through the posterior tarsal tunnel. The technique can be carried out by placing the patient in the supine position with the arms resting comfortably along the patient's chest and the affected lower extremity externally rotated (Fig. 154.6). A total of 4 mL of local anesthetic is drawn up in a 12-mL sterile syringe. If the painful condition being treated is thought to have an inflammatory component, 40 to 80 mg of depot steroid is added to the local anesthetic. The pulsation of the posterior tibial artery is then identified by palpation (Fig. 154.7). A linear high-frequency ultrasound transducer is placed in a longitudinal plane over the previously identified pulsation of the posterior tibial artery, and then the superior aspect of the transducer is rotated toward the front of the ankle with the superior aspect of the ultrasound transducer lying on the posteroinferior border of the medial malleolus and the inferior aspect of the ultrasound transducer pointed at the calcaneus (Fig. 154.8). This will put the ultrasound transducer perpendicular to the posterior tibial nerve, artery, and vein as they pass through the posterior tarsal tunnel. An ultrasound survey scan is taken. The posterior tibial artery and vein can be seen lying between the skin, subcutaneous tissues, and flexor retinaculum and medial tubercle of the talus (Fig. 154.9). The posterior tibial nerve will be seen to lie just beneath the posterior tibial artery and vein. Color Doppler can be utilized to help identify the posterior tibial artery and vein (Fig. 154.10). When the posterior tibial artery and vein and the posterior tibial nerve lying beneath them are identified on ultrasound imaging, the skin is prepped with anesthetic solution and a 1½-inch, 22-gauge needle is advanced

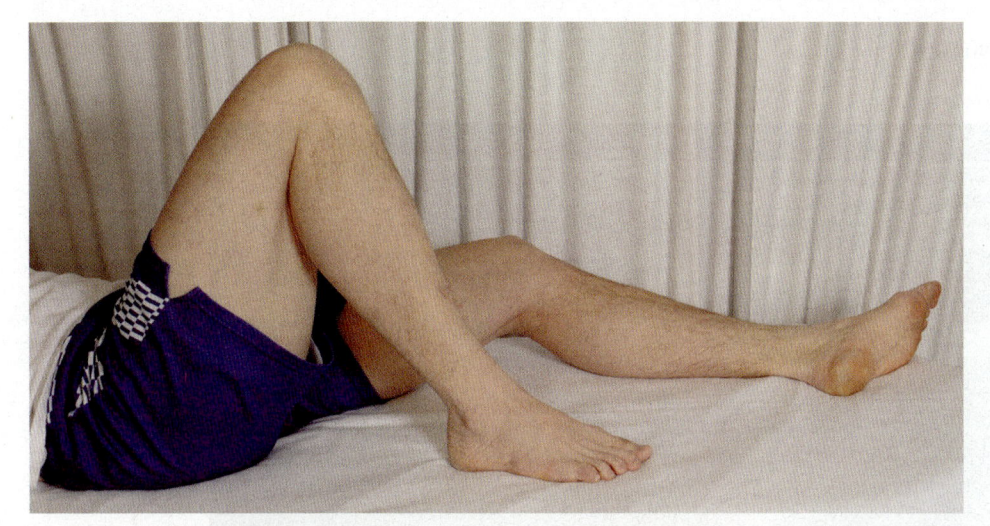

**FIGURE 154.6.** Proper patient position for ultrasound-guided posterior tibial nerve block.

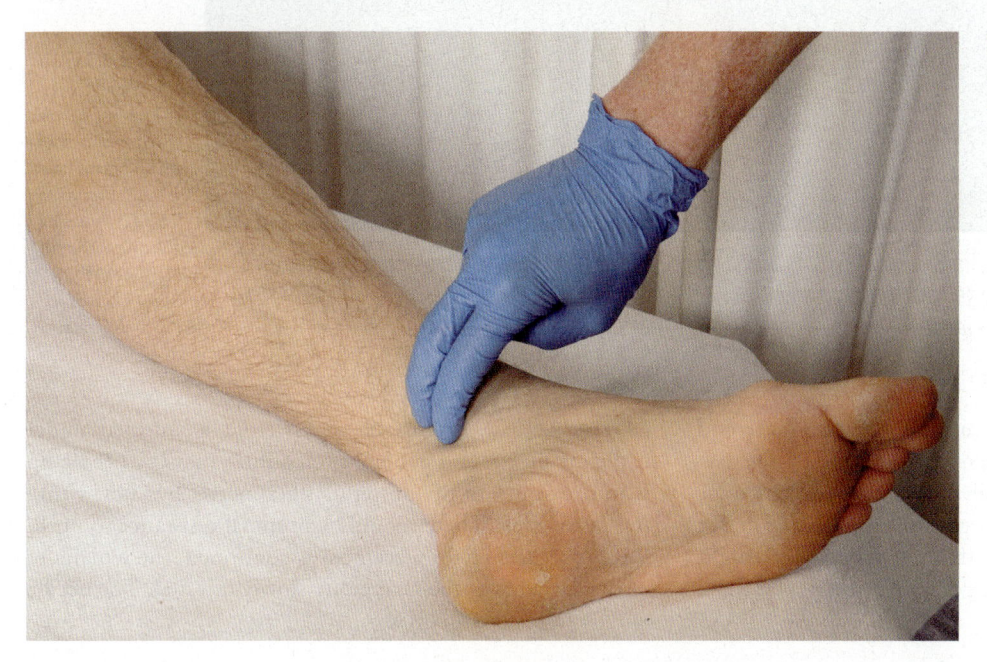

**FIGURE 154.7.** Palpation of the posterior tibial artery.

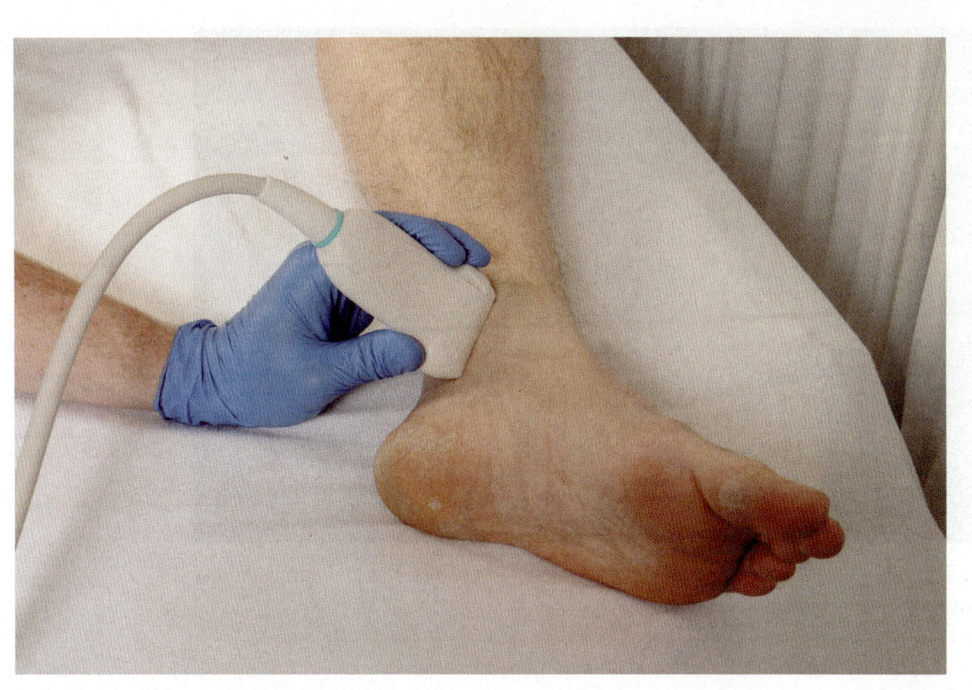

**FIGURE 154.8.** Proper longitudinal position of the ultrasound transducer with the superior aspect of the transducer rotated toward the anterior ankle for ultrasound-guided posterior tibial nerve block at the ankle.

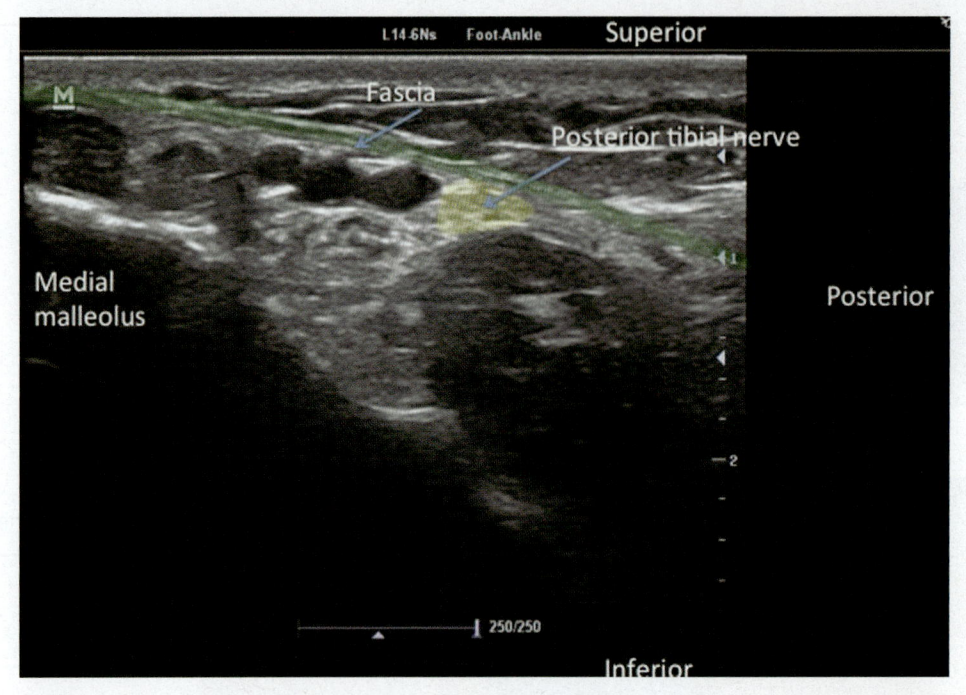

**FIGURE 154.9.** Transverse ultrasound image demonstrating the posterior tibial artery and vein and the posterior tibial nerve adjacent to the vein.

from the inferior border of the ultrasound transducer and advanced utilizing an out-of-plane approach with the trajectory being adjusted under real-time ultrasound guidance until the needle tip is resting in proximity to the posterior tibial nerve (Fig. 154.11). When the tip of needle is thought to be in satisfactory position, after careful aspiration, a small amount of local anesthetic and steroid is injected under real-time ultrasound guidance to confirm that the needle tip is in proximity to the posterior tibial nerve, but not within the nerve itself. There should be minimal resistance to injection. After needle tip placement is confirmed, the remainder of the contents of the syringe are slowly injected. The needle

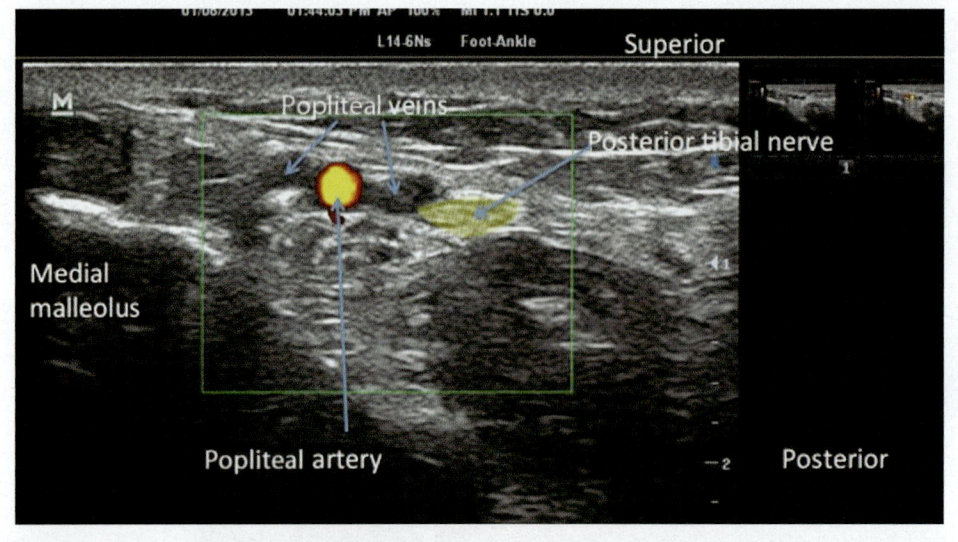

**FIGURE 154.10.** Transverse color Doppler image demonstrating the popliteal vein and artery and the relationship of the vein to the posterior tibial nerve.

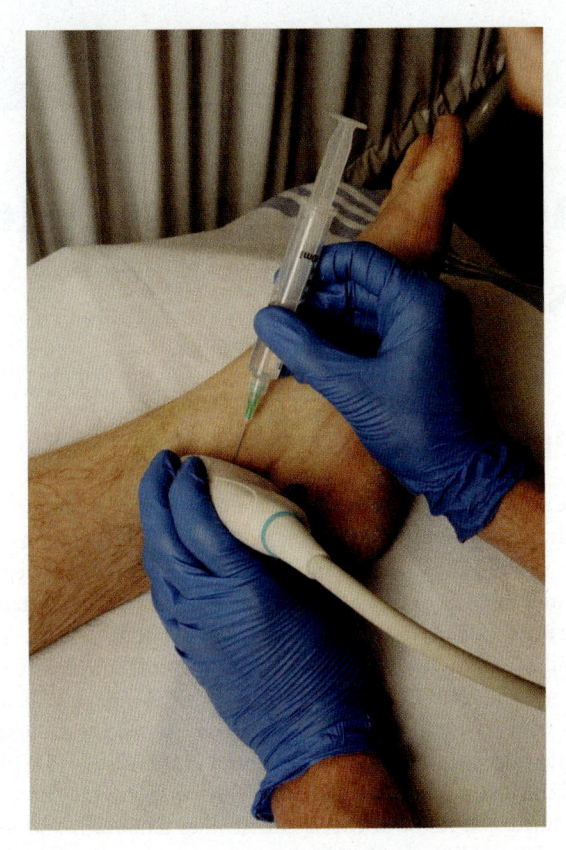

**FIGURE 154.11.** Proper out-of-plane needle position for performing injection technique for posterior tarsal tunnel syndrome.

is then removed, and a sterile pressure dressing and ice pack are placed at the injection site.

## COMPLICATIONS

A failure to accurately assess the correct position of the needle tip when performing ultrasound-guided injection technique for posterior tarsal tunnel syndrome can lead to a failure to block the posterior tibial nerve or cause needle-induced trauma to the posterior tibial nerve and/or posterior artery and vein. The use of ultrasound guidance when performing injection technique for posterior tarsal tunnel syndrome should markedly decrease these problems. Postblock ecchymosis and hematoma may occur, and the patient should be warned of such. These complications can be decreased by the use of a pressure dressing and cold packs applied to the injection site following the procedure.

## CLINICAL PEARLS

The key to performing successful ultrasound injection technique for posterior tarsal tunnel syndrome is the proper identification of the sonographic anatomy and in particular the ability to properly identify the posterior tibial nerve at the site of nerve entrapment. This should not be a problem if the above technique is used. Any significant pain or sudden increase in resistance during injection when performing ultrasound-guided suggests incorrect needle placement, and one should stop injecting immediately and reassess the position of the needle.

## SUGGESTED READINGS

Cancilleri F, Ippolito M, Amato C, et al. Tarsal tunnel syndrome: four uncommon cases. *Foot Ankle Surg* 2007;13(4):214–217.
Fujita I, Matsumoto K, Minami T, et al. Tarsal tunnel syndrome caused by epineural ganglion of the posterior tibial nerve: report of 2 cases and review of the literature. *J Foot Ankle Surg* 2004;43(3):185–190.
Mezrow CK, Sanger JR, Matloub HS. Acute tarsal tunnel syndrome following partial avulsion of the flexor hallucis longus muscle: a case report. *J Foot Ankle Surg* 2002;41(4):243–246.
Waldman SD. Functional anatomy of the ankle and foot. In: *Pain Review*. Philadelphia, PA: Saunders Elsevier; 2009:155–156.
Waldman SD. Injection technique for posterior tarsal tunnel syndrome. In: *Atlas of Pain Management Injection Techniques*. 3rd ed. Philadelphia, PA: Saunders Elsevier; 2012:435–436.
Waldman SD. Posterior tarsal tunnel syndrome. In: *Pain Review*. Philadelphia, PA: Saunders Elsevier; 2009:323–324.
Waldman SD, Campbell RSD. Posterior tarsal tunnel syndrome. In: *Imaging of Pain*. Philadelphia, PA: Saunders Elsevier; 2010:425–426.
Waldman SD. Posterior tarsal tunnel syndrome. In: *Atlas of Common Pain Syndromes*. 3rd ed. Philadelphia, PA: Saunders Elsevier; 2012:359–361.

# CHAPTER 155

# Ultrasound-Guided Injection Technique for Achilles Tendonitis

## CLINICAL PERSPECTIVES

Achilles tendonitis is a clinical syndrome characterized by sharp, constant, and severe posterior ankle pain on plantar flexion of the ankle. Patients suffering from Achilles tendonitis will often splint the inflamed Achilles tendon by adopting a flat-footed gait to avoid plantar flexing the affected tendon. This dysfunctional gait may cause a secondary bursitis and tendonitis around the foot and ankle, which may serve to confuse the clinical picture and further increase the patient's pain and disability. Pain on palpation of the insertion of the Achilles tendon on the calcaneus or at a point ~5 cm above the calcaneus at the narrowest part of the Achilles tendon is a consistent finding in patients with Achilles tendonitis as is exacerbation of pain with active resisted plantar flexion. Patients suffering from Achilles tendonitis will also exhibit a positive creaking tendon test. This test is performed by having the patient sit on the edge of the examination table. The examiner then palpates the Achilles tendon while passively plantar flexing and dorsiflexing the ankle (Fig. 155.1). The test is positive if the examiner appreciates a creaking sensation. Untreated, Achilles tendonitis will result in increasing pain and functional disability calcium deposition around the tendon occurring, making subsequent treatment more difficult. Continued trauma to the inflamed tendon ultimately may result in tendon rupture (Fig. 155.2).

The onset of Achilles tendonitis usually is acute, occurring after overuse or misuse of the ankle joint. Inciting factors may include activities such as running and sudden stopping and starting, as when playing tennis. Improper stretching of the gastrocnemius and Achilles tendon before exercise as well as the use of quinolone antibiotics has also been implicated in the development of Achilles tendonitis, as well as acute tendon rupture.

Plain radiographs are indicated in all patients who present with posterior ankle pain (Fig. 155.3). Based on the patient's clinical presentation, additional testing may be indicated, including complete blood cell count, sedimentation rate, and antinuclear antibody testing. Magnetic resonance imaging and/or ultrasound imaging of the ankle is indicated if Achilles tendonitis, rupture, or joint instability is suggested (Figs. 155.4 and 155.5). Radionuclide bone scanning is useful to identify stress fractures of the tibia not seen on plain radiographs. The injection technique described later serves as both a diagnostic and a therapeutic maneuver.

## CLINICALLY RELEVANT ANATOMY

The Achilles tendon is the thickest and strongest tendon in the body, yet is also very susceptible to rupture. The common tendon of the gastrocnemius muscle, the Achilles tendon, begins at midcalf and continues downward to attach to the posterior calcaneus, where it may become inflamed (Fig. 155.6). The Achilles tendon narrows during this downward course, becoming most narrow at ~5 cm above its calcaneal insertion. It is at this narrowest point that tendonitis also may occur. A bursa is located between the Achilles tendon and the base of the tibia and the upper posterior calcaneus. This bursa also may become inflamed as a result of coexistent Achilles tendonitis and may confuse the clinical picture.

## ULTRASOUND-GUIDED TECHNIQUE

The benefits, risks, and alternative treatments are explained to the patient, and informed consent is obtained. The patient is then placed in the prone position with the patient's ankle hanging off the edge of the table (Fig. 155.7). With the patient in the above position, a high-frequency linear ultrasound transducer is placed in a longitudinal plane with the inferior portion of the ultrasound transducer over the insertion of the Achilles tendon on the calcaneus, and an ultrasound survey scan is taken (Fig. 155.8). The linear Achilles tendon is identified at its insertion on the calcaneus (Fig. 155.9). When the insertion of the Achilles tendon is identified, the skin overlying the area beneath the ultrasound transducer is prepped with antiseptic solution. A sterile syringe containing 3.0 mL of 0.25% preservative-free bupivacaine and 40 mg of methylprednisolone is attached to a 1½-inch, 22-gauge needle using strict aseptic technique. The needle is placed through the skin ~1 cm above the superior border of the ultrasound transducer and is then advanced using an in-plane approach with the needle trajectory adjusted under real-time ultrasound guidance so that the needle tip rests against the site of tendinous insertion (Fig. 155.10). When the tip of needle is thought to be in satisfactory position, a small amount of solution is injected to insure that the needle tip is not in the substance of the tendon. After confirmation that the needle tip is outside the tendon, after careful aspiration, the contents of the syringe are slowly injected.

CHAPTER 155 ULTRASOUND-GUIDED INJECTION TECHNIQUE FOR ACHILLES TENDONITIS 1097

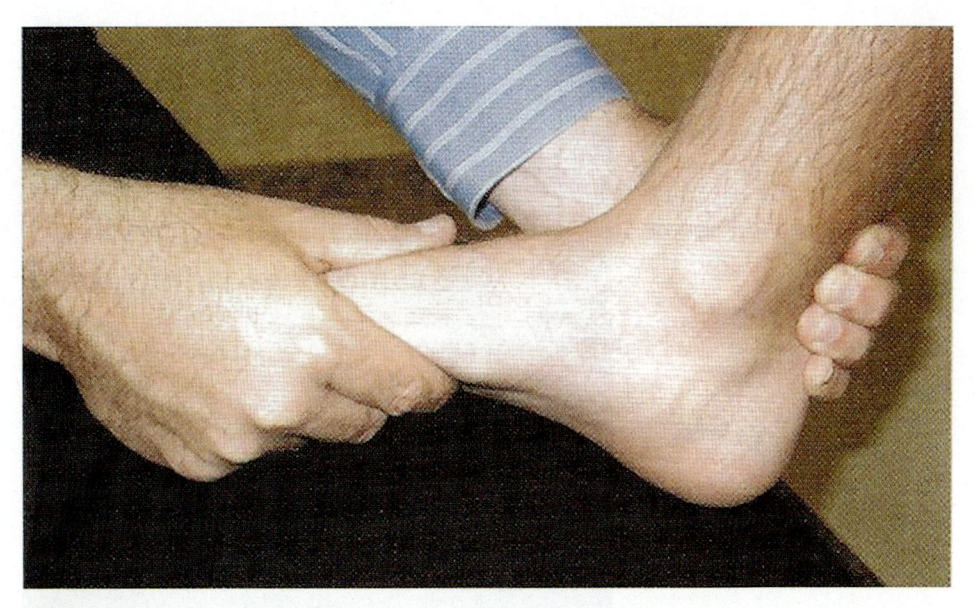

**FIGURE 155.1.** The creaking tendon test is performed by having the patient sit on the edge of the examination table. The examiner then palpates the Achilles tendon while passively plantar flexing and dorsiflexing the ankle. The test is positive if the examiner appreciates a creaking sensation.

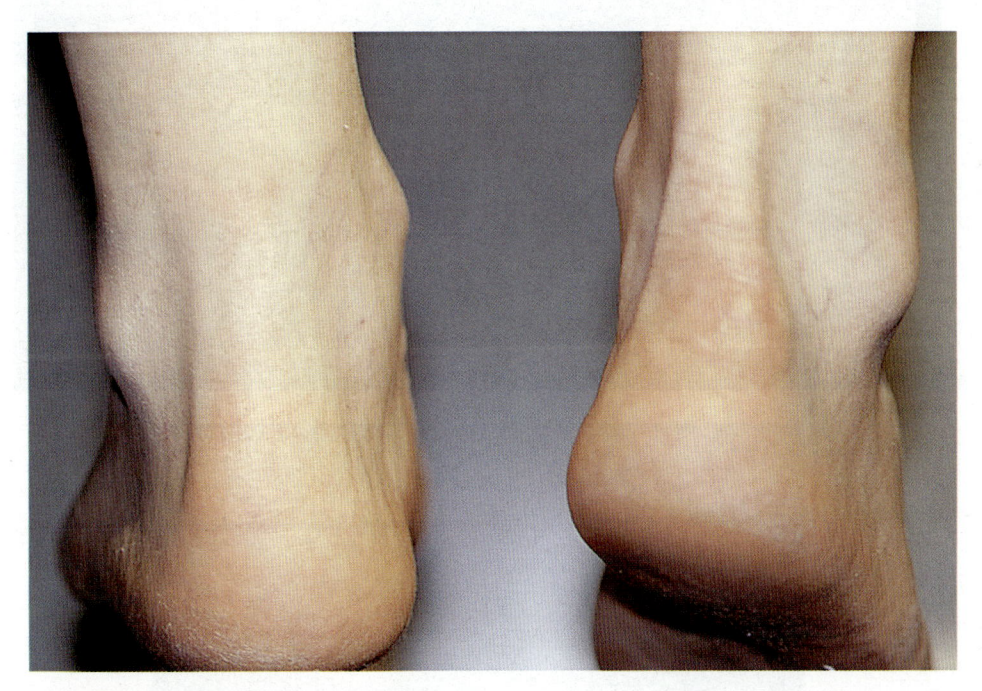

**FIGURE 155.2.** The patient's ruptured left Achilles tendon appears thickened and less distinct than the normal right side, and the patient is unable to plantar flex the left foot. (Reused from Fleisher GR, Ludwig S, et al. *Atlas of Pediatric Emergency Medicine*. Philadelphia, PA: Lippincott Williams & Wilkins; 2004, with permission.)

**FIGURE 155.3.** Lateral view of the ankle demonstrates areas of ossification in the Achilles tendon resulting from recurring injuries. (Reused from Berquist TH. *Imaging of the Foot and Ankle.* 3rd ed. Philadelphia, PA: Lippincott Williams & Wilkins; 2011:145, with permission.)

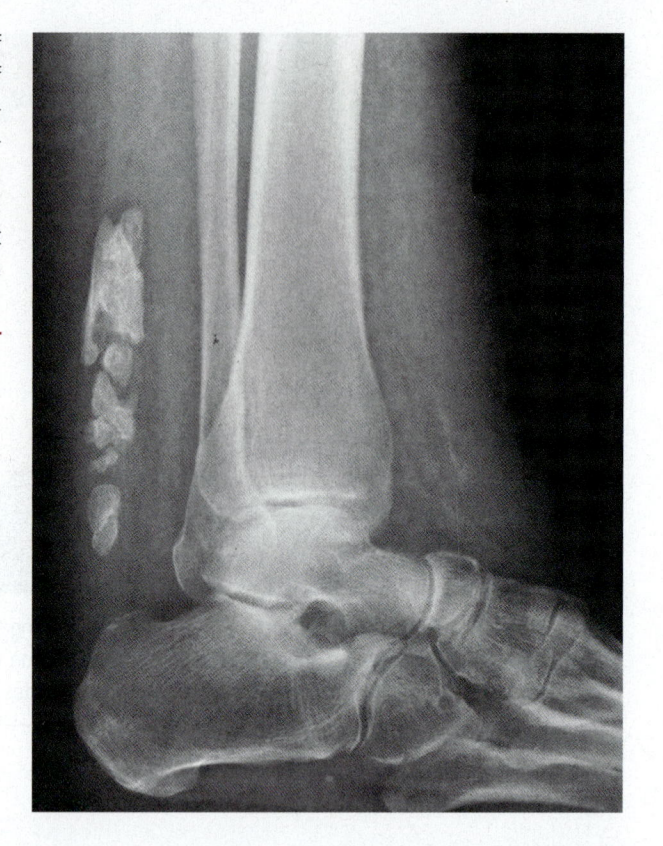

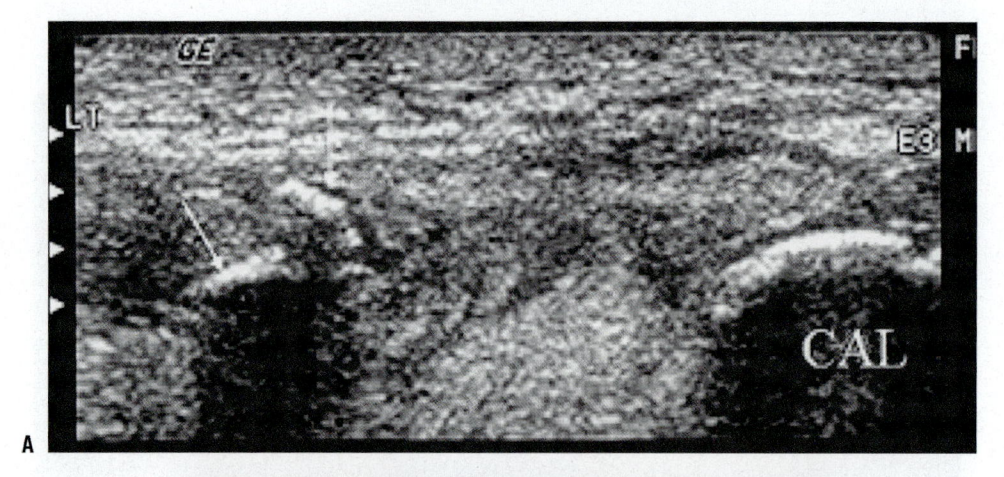

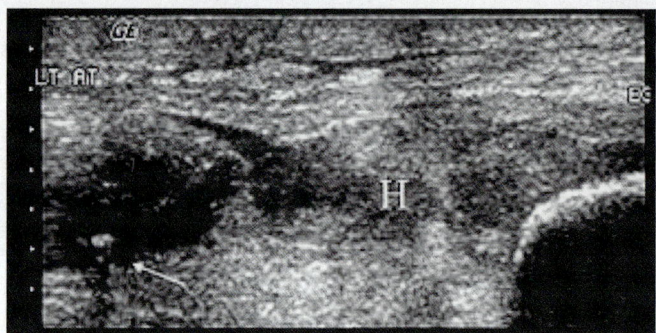

**FIGURE 155.4.** Longitudinal images **(A,B)** demonstrate a complete tear of the Achilles tendon at the calcaneus (CAL). Small avulsion fracture fragments can be seen with the retracted tendon (*arrows*). A complex hematoma (H) replaces the tendon distally. (Reused from Adler RS, Sofka CM, Positano RG. *Atlas of Foot and Ankle Sonography.* Philadelphia, PA: Lippincott Williams & Wilkins; 2004:79, with permission.)

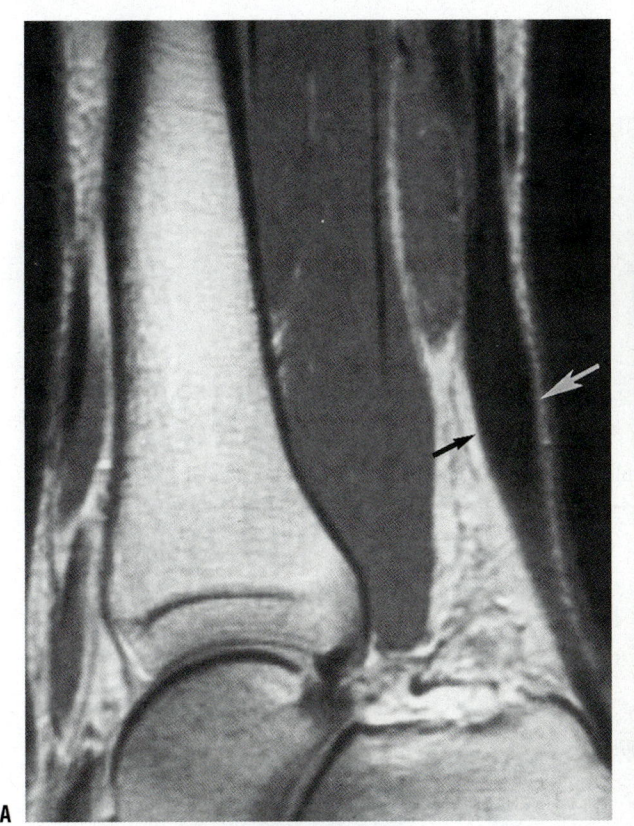

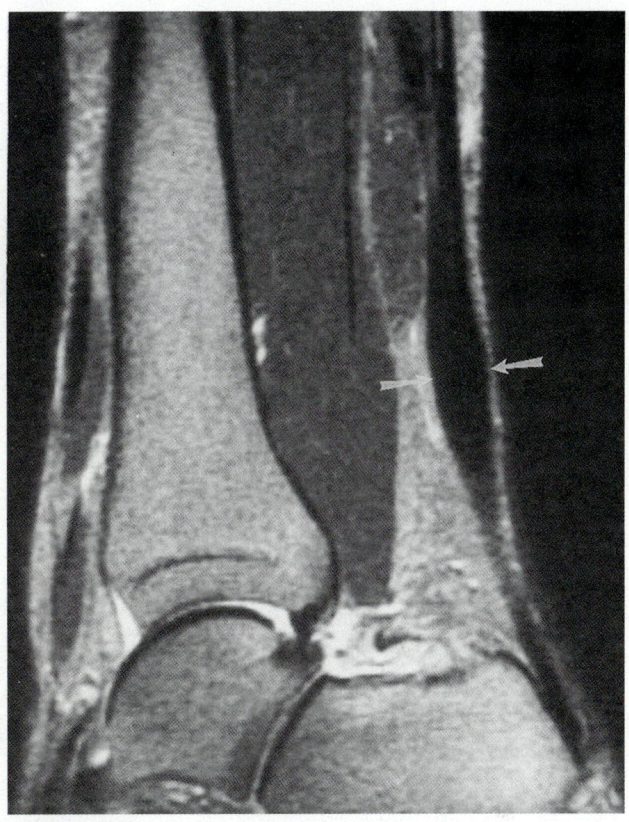

**FIGURE 155.5.** Sagittal proton density **(A)** and T2-weighted **(B)** images of an old low-grade tear that has filled in with scar tissue. There is tendon thickening (*arrows*) but no increased signal intensity. This has the same appearance as hypoxic tendinosis. (Reused from Berquist TH. *Imaging of the Foot and Ankle*. 3rd ed. Philadelphia, PA: Lippincott Williams & Wilkins; 2011, with permission.)

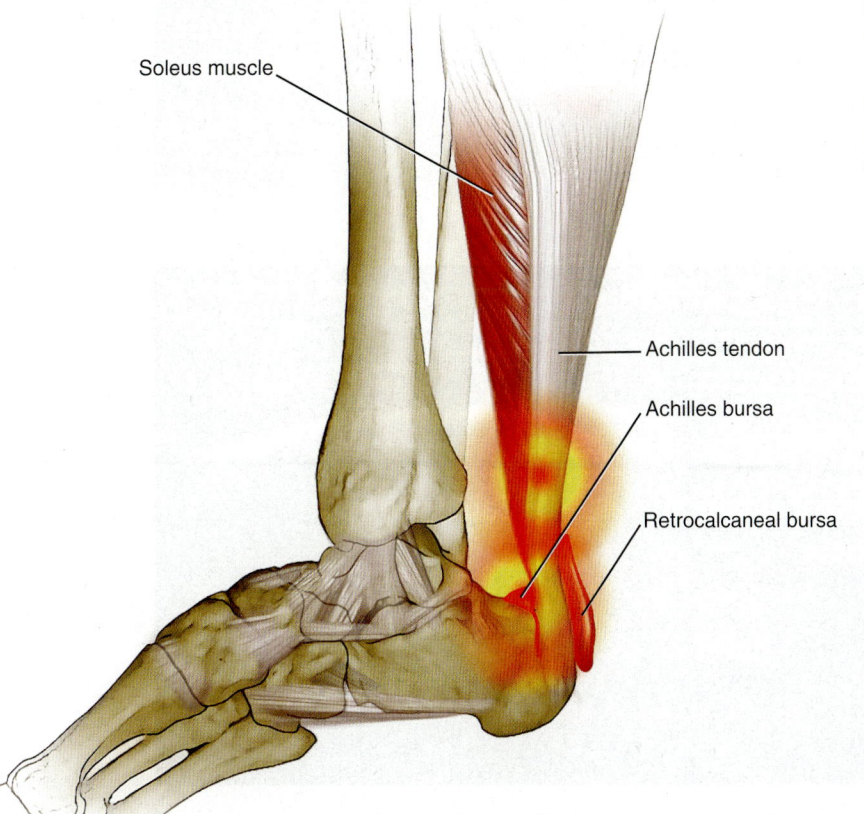

**FIGURE 155.6.** The Achilles tendon is susceptible to the development of tendonitis at its insertion on the calcaneus as well at its narrowest point ~5 cm above the calcaneal insertion.

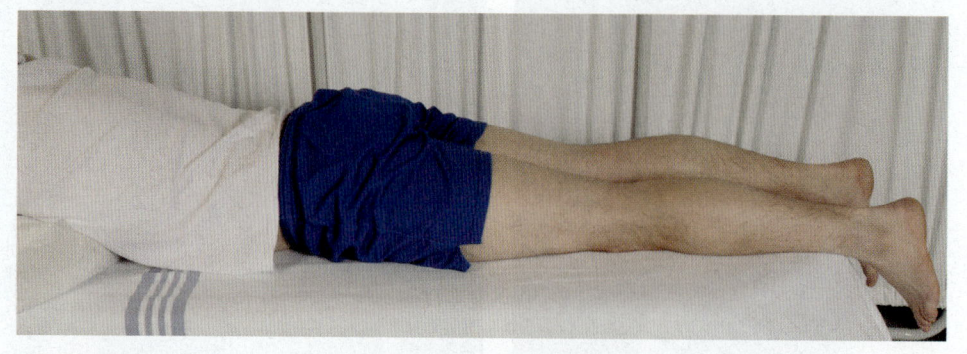

**FIGURE 155.7.** Proper prone patient positioning for ultrasound-guided injection for Achilles tendonitis.

**FIGURE 155.8.** Proper longitudinal ultrasound transducer placement for ultrasound-guided injection for Achilles tendonitis.

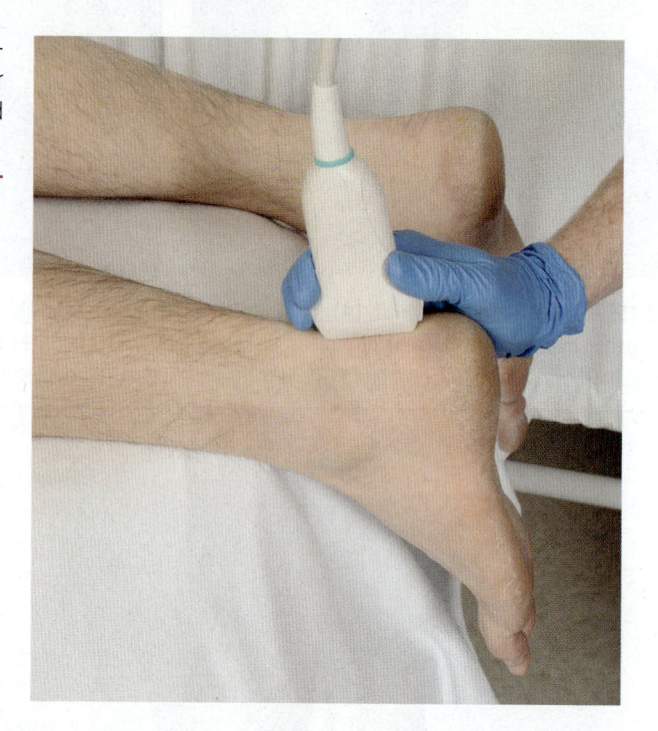

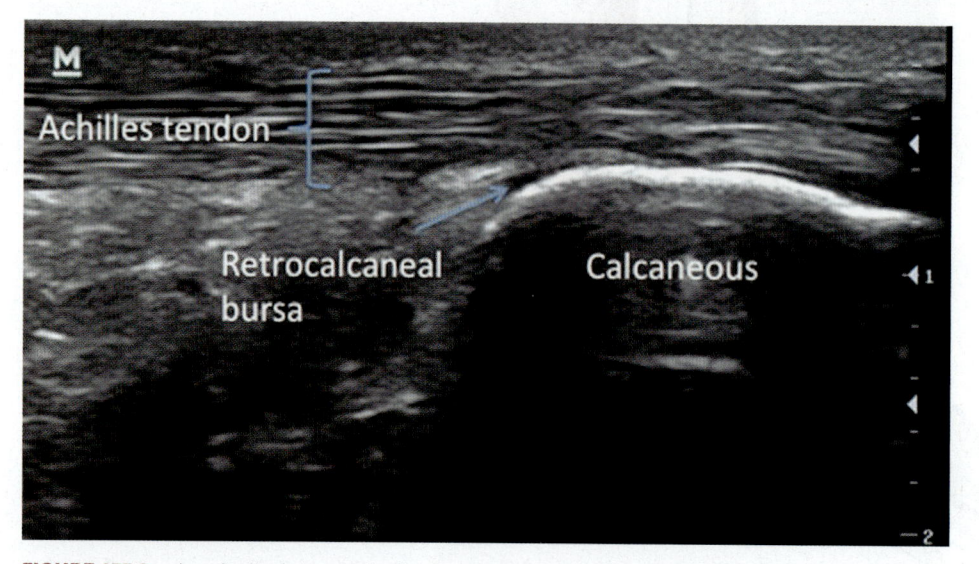

**FIGURE 155.9.** Longitudinal view of the Achilles tendon and its calcaneal insertion.

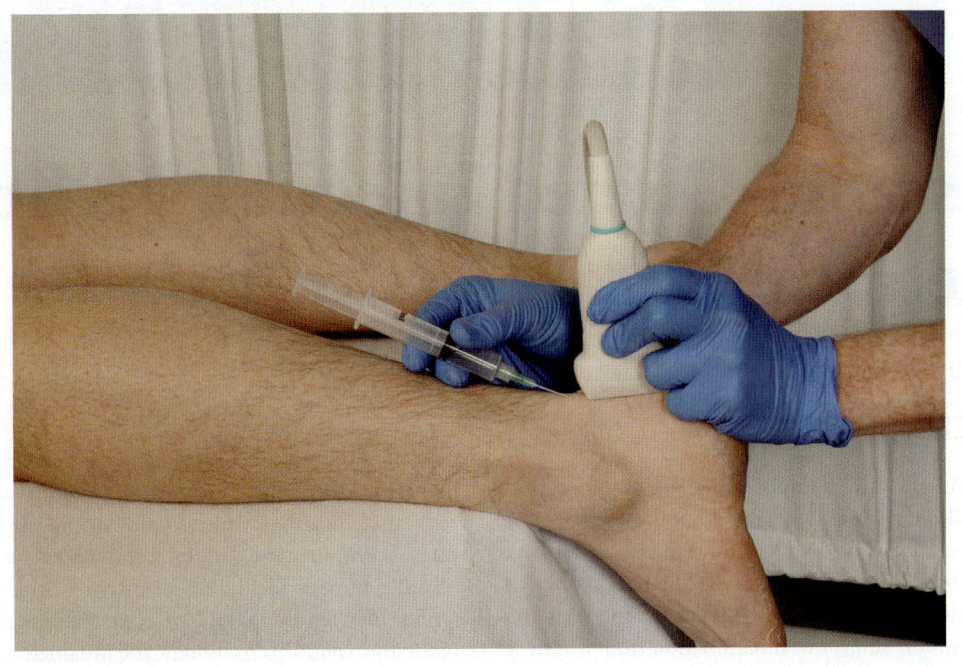

**FIGURE 155.10.** Proper needle placement for an ultrasound-guided in-plane injection for Achilles tendonitis.

There should be minimal resistance to injection. The patient may note an exacerbation of his or her pain during the injection.

## COMPLICATIONS

The major complication of this ultrasound-guided injection technique is infection. Ecchymosis and hematoma formation following this procedure may also occur. The possibility of trauma to the already compromised tendons from the injection itself remains an ever-present possibility, although the risk of this is decreased if the clinician uses gentle technique and stops injecting immediately if significant resistance to injection is encountered. Approximately 25% of patients complain of a transient increase in pain after this injection technique; the patient should be warned of this.

## CLINICAL PEARLS

Bursitis and tendonitis of the ankle and foot may coexist with Achilles tendonitis and may contribute to the patient's pain symptomatology. Universal precautions should always be observed to protect the operator, and strict adherence to sterile technique must be used to avoid infection. Gentle physical therapy and local heat should be introduced following ultrasound-guided injection of Achilles tendonitis to reduce pain and improve function. Simple analgesics and nonsteroidal anti-inflammatory agents or COX-2 inhibitors may be used concurrently with this injection technique.

## SUGGESTED READINGS

Damuth E, Heidelbaugh J, Malani PN, et al. An elderly patient with fluoroquinolone-associated Achilles tendinitis. *Am J Geriatr Pharmacother* 2008; 6(5):264–268.
Lesic A, Bumbasirevic M. Disorders of the Achilles tendon. Original research article. *Curr Orthop* 2004;18(1):63–75.
Waldman SD. Achilles tendinitis. In: *Pain Review*. Philadelphia, PA: Saunders Elsevier; 2009:325.
Waldman SD, Campbell RSD. Achilles tendinitis. In: *Imaging of Pain*. Philadelphia, PA: Saunders Elsevier; 2010:427–428.
Waldman SD, Campbell RSD. Achilles tendon rupture. In: *Imaging of Pain*. Philadelphia, PA: Saunders Elsevier; 2011:431–432.
Waldman SD, Campbell RSD. Achilles tendinitis. In: *Atlas of Common Pain Syndromes*. 3rd ed. Philadelphia, PA: Saunders Elsevier; 2012:362–364.
Waldman SD. Injection technique for Achilles tendinitis. In: *Atlas of Pain Management Injection Techniques*. 3rd ed. Philadelphia, PA: Saunders Elsevier; 2013:439–441.
Waldman SD. The creaking tendon test for Achilles tendinitis. In: *Physical Diagnosis of Pain*. 2nd ed. Philadelphia, PA: Saunders Elsevier; 2010:268–269.

# Ultrasound-Guided Injection Technique for Retrocalcaneal Bursitis Pain

## CLINICAL PERSPECTIVES

Retrocalcaneal bursitis is a common cause of posterior heel pain. The retrocalcaneal bursa, which is also known as the subtendinous calcaneal bursa, lies between the Achilles tendon and its insertion on the calcaneus (Fig. 156.1). The bursa serves to cushion and facilitate sliding of the Achilles tendon over the calcaneus. The bursa is subject to inflammation from a variety of causes with acute trauma to the ankle and repetitive microtrauma being the most common. Acute injuries to the bursa can occur from direct blunt trauma to the posterior ankle kicks while playing sports as well as from overuse injuries including running on uneven or soft surfaces or jobs that require repeated plantar flexion of the ankle. If the inflammation of the bursa is not treated and the condition becomes chronic, calcification of the bursa with further functional disability may occur. Gout and other crystal arthropathies may also precipitate acute retrocalcaneal bursitis as may bacterial, tubercular, or fungal infections.

The patient suffering from retrocalcaneal bursitis most frequently presents with the complaint of pain in the posterior heel, which may radiate into the posterior ankle. The patient may find walking downstairs, standing on tiptoes, and kneeling increasingly difficult. Physical examination of the patient suffering from retrocalcaneal bursitis will reveal point tenderness over the posterior ankle. If there is significant inflammation, rubor and color may be present and the entire area may feel boggy or edematous to palpation. At times massive effusion may be present, which can be quite distressing to the patient. Active plantar flexion of the affected ankle will often reproduce the patient's pain. Sudden release of resistance to active plantar will markedly increase the pain. If calcification or gouty tophi of the bursa and surrounding tendons are present, the examiner may appreciate crepitus with active extension of the ankle, and the patient may complain of a catching sensation when moving the affected ankle, especially on awaking. Often, the patient will not be able to sleep on the affected side. Occasionally, the retrocalcaneal bursa may become infected, with systemic symptoms, including fever and malaise, as well as local symptoms, with rubor, color, and dolor being present.

Plain radiographs are indicated in all patients who present with ankle pain to rule out occult ankle pathology (Fig. 156.2). Based on the patient's clinical presentation, additional testing may be indicated, including complete blood cell count, sedimentation rate, and antinuclear antibody testing. Magnetic resonance imaging or ultrasound imaging of the affected area may also confirm the diagnosis and help delineate the presence of other bursitis including coexistent Achilles bursitis, calcific tendonitis, tendinopathy, triceps tendonitis, or other ankle pathology (Fig. 156.3). Rarely, the inflamed bursa may become infected, and failure to diagnosis and treat the acute infection can lead to dire consequences.

## CLINICALLY RELEVANT ANATOMY

The retrocalcaneal bursa lies between the Achilles tendon and the base of the tibia and the posterior calcaneus (see Fig. 156.1). The bursa is subject to the development of inflammation after overuse, misuse, or direct trauma as is the Achilles bursa, which lies posterior to the Achilles tendon at its insertion on the calcaneus. The Achilles tendon is the thickest and strongest tendon in the body, yet is also very susceptible to rupture. The common tendon of the gastrocnemius muscle, the Achilles tendon, begins at midcalf and continues downward to attach to the posterior calcaneus, where it may become inflamed (see Fig. 156.1). The Achilles tendon narrows during this downward course, becoming most narrow ~5 cm above its calcaneal insertion. It is at this narrowest point that tendonitis also may occur. Tendonitis, especially at the calcaneal insertion, may mimic retrocalcaneal bursitis and may make diagnosis difficult.

## ULTRASOUND-GUIDED TECHNIQUE

The benefits, risks, and alternative treatments are explained to the patient, and informed consent is obtained. The patient is then placed in the prone position with the patient's ankle hanging off the edge of the table (Fig. 156.4). With the patient in the above position, a high-frequency linear ultrasound transducer is placed in a longitudinal plane with the inferior portion of the ultrasound transducer over the insertion of the Achilles tendon on the calcaneus, and an ultrasound survey scan is taken (Fig. 156.5). The linear Achilles tendon is identified

CHAPTER 156 ULTRASOUND-GUIDED INJECTION TECHNIQUE FOR RETROCALCANEAL BURSITIS PAIN 1103

**FIGURE 156.1.** The bursa of the knee.

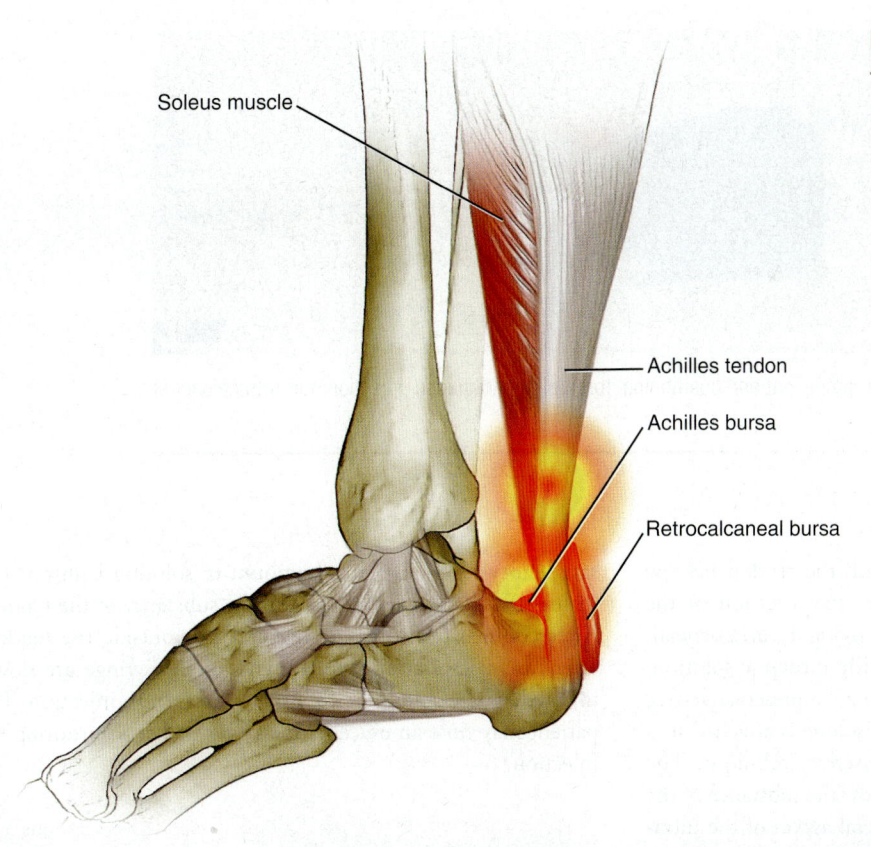

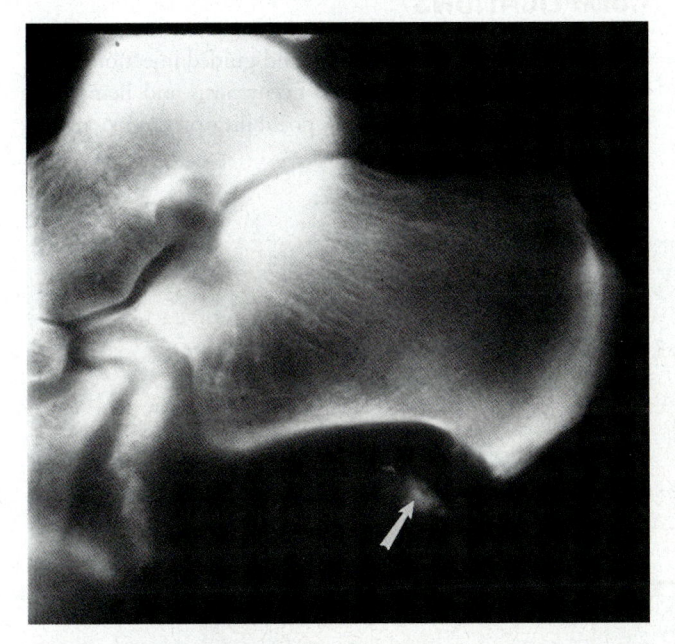

**FIGURE 156.2.** Lateral radiograph demonstrating an avulsed osteophyte in a patient with persistent heel pain. (Reused from Berquist TH. *Imaging of the Foot and Ankle*. 3rd ed. Philadelphia, PA: Lippincott Williams & Wilkins; 2011, with permission.)

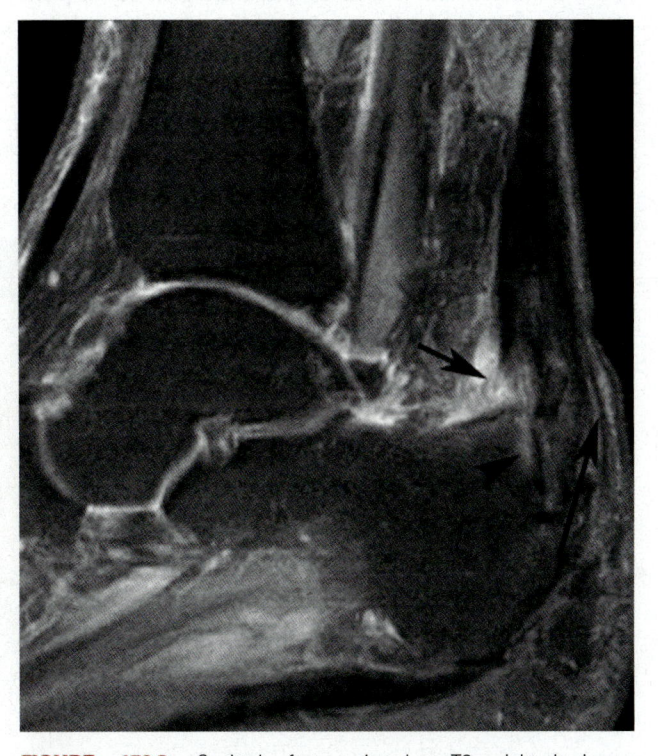

**FIGURE 156.3.** Sagittal fast spin-echo T2-weighted image demonstrates retro-Achilles bursitis (*short arrow*), prominence of the posterior tuberosity with marrow edema (*arrowhead*), thickening and inflammation of the Achilles tendon, and fluid in the superficial bursa (*long arrow*). (Reused from Berquist TH. *Imaging of the Foot and Ankle*. 3rd ed. Philadelphia, PA: Lippincott Williams & Wilkins; 2011, with permission.)

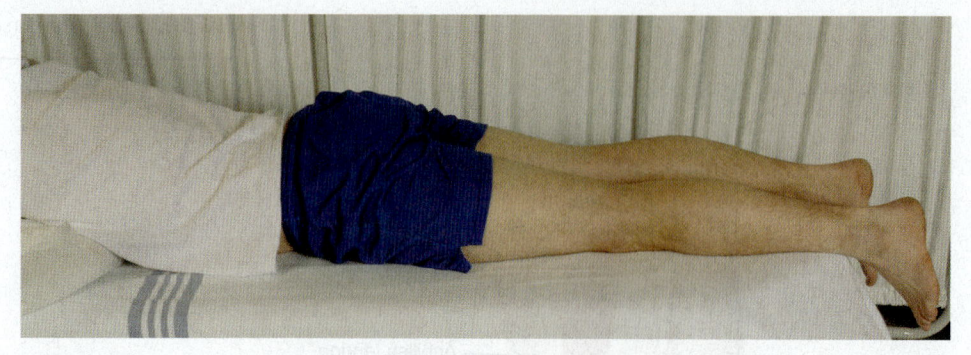

**FIGURE 156.4.** Proper prone patient positioning for ultrasound-guided injection for retrocalcaneal bursitis.

as its insertion on the calcaneus. Beneath the tendon lies the retrocalcaneal bursa (Fig. 156.6). When the insertion of the Achilles tendon is identified, the skin overlying the area beneath the ultrasound transducer is prepped with antiseptic solution. A sterile syringe containing 3.0 mL of 0.25% preservative-free bupivacaine and 40 mg of methylprednisolone is attached to a 1½-inch, 22-gauge needle using strict aseptic technique. The needle is placed through the skin just below the substance of the Achilles tendon at the middle of the lateral aspect of the ultrasound transducer and is then advanced using an out-of-plane approach with the needle trajectory adjusted under real-time ultrasound guidance so that the needle tip rests beneath the substance of the Achilles tendon within the retrocalcaneal bursa (Fig. 156.7). When the tip of needle is thought to be in satisfactory position, a small amount of solution is injected to insure that the needle tip is not in the substance of the tendon. After confirmation that the needle tip is outside the tendon, after careful aspiration, the contents of the syringe are slowly injected. There should be minimal resistance to injection. The patient may note an exacerbation of his or her pain during the injection.

## COMPLICATIONS

The major complication of ultrasound-guided injection of the retrocalcaneal bursa is infection. Ecchymosis and hematoma formation may also occur. The possibility of trauma to the

**FIGURE 156.5.** Proper longitudinal ultrasound transducer placement for ultrasound-guided injection for retrocalcaneal bursitis.

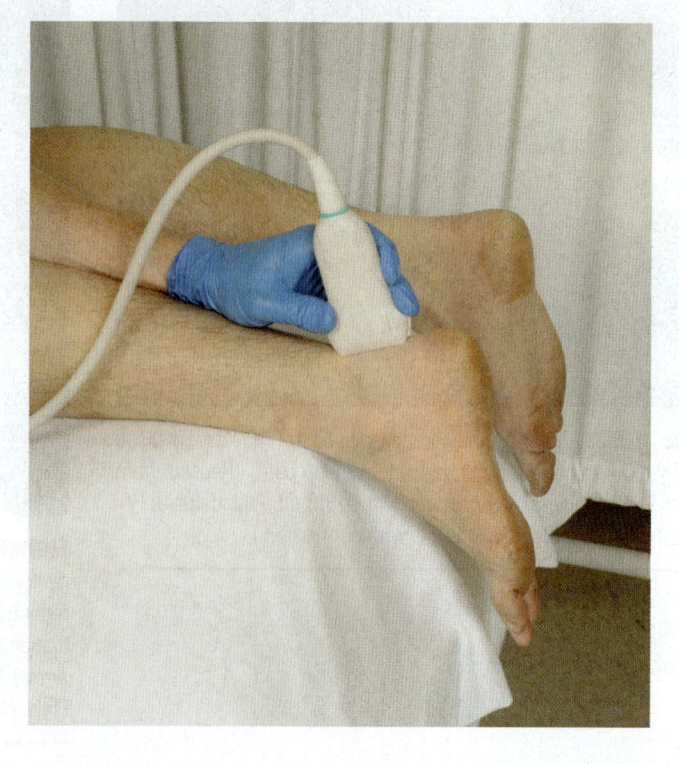

# CHAPTER 156 ULTRASOUND-GUIDED INJECTION TECHNIQUE FOR RETROCALCANEAL BURSITIS PAIN

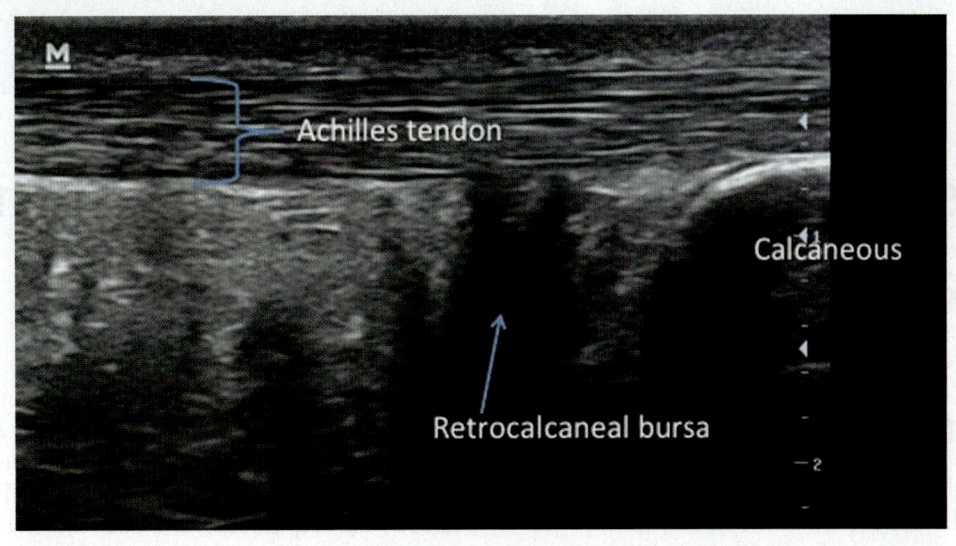

**FIGURE 156.6.** Longitudinal view of the Achilles tendon, its calcaneal insertion, and an enlarged retrocalcaneal bursa.

already compromised tendons from the injection itself remains an ever-present possibility, although the risk of this is decreased if the clinician uses gentle technique and stops injecting immediately if significant resistance to injection is encountered. A transient exacerbation of the patient's pain occurs ~25% of the time following this injection technique, and the patient should be warned of this possibility prior to the procedure.

## CLINICAL PEARLS

Bursitis, labral tears, tendinopathy, osteoarthritis, synovitis, nerve entrapment, avascular necrosis of the knee, and impingement syndromes may coexist with other knee joint disease and may contribute to the patient's pain symptomatology. Universal precautions should always be observed to protect the operator, and strict adherence to sterile technique must be used to avoid infection. Gentle physical therapy and local heat should be introduced following ultrasound-guided injection of the elbow joint to reduce pain and improve function. Simple analgesics and nonsteroidal anti-inflammatory agents or COX-2 inhibitors may be used concurrently with this injection technique.

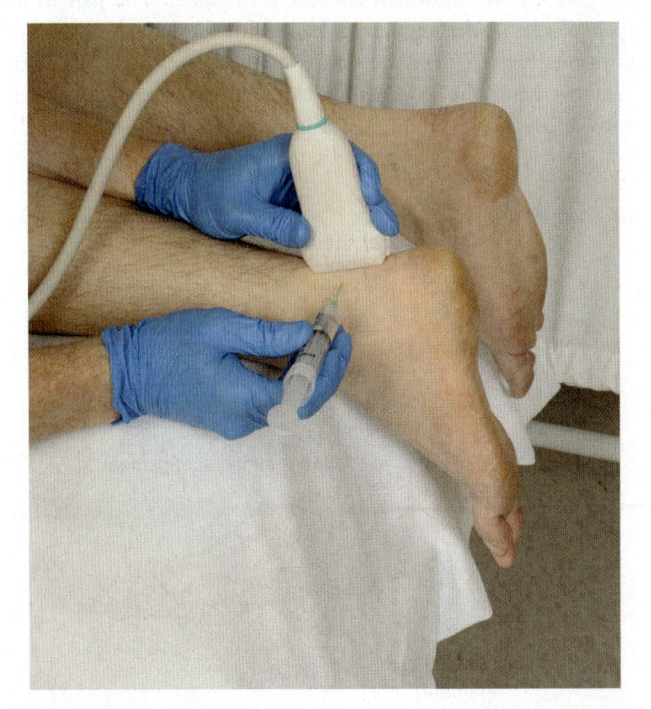

**FIGURE 156.7.** Proper needle placement for an ultrasound-guided out-of-plane injection for Achilles tendonitis.

## SUGGESTED READINGS

Aronow MS. Posterior heel pain (retrocalcaneal bursitis, insertional and noninsertional Achilles tendinopathy). *Clin Podiatr Med Surg* 2005;22(1):19–43.

Hochman MG, Ramappa AJ, Newman JS, et al. Imaging of tendons and bursae. In: *Imaging of Arthritis and Metabolic Bone Disease*. 1st ed. Philadelphia, PA: Saunders Elsevier; 2009:196–238.

Lesic A, Bumbasirevic M. Disorders of the Achilles tendon. *Curr Orthop* 2004; 18(1):63–75.

Van der Wall H, Lee A, Magee M, et al. Radionuclide bone scintigraphy in sports injuries. *Semin Nucl Med* 2010;40(1):16–30.

Vyce SD, Addis-Thomas E, Mathews EE, et al. Painful prominences of the heel. [Review Article.] *Clin Podiatr Med Surg* 2010;27(3):443–462.

Waldman SD. Achilles bursitis. In: *Atlas of Uncommon Pain Syndromes*. 2nd ed. Philadelphia, PA: Saunders Elsevier; 2009:304–306.

Waldman SD. Achilles bursa injection. In: *Atlas of Pain Management Injection Techniques*. 3rd ed. Philadelphia, PA: Saunders Elsevier; 2012:443–445.

# CHAPTER 157

# Ultrasound-Guided Injection Technique for Calcaneofibular Ligament

## CLINICAL PERSPECTIVES

The calcaneofibular ligament runs from the anterior border of the lateral malleolus to the lateral surface of the calcaneus (Fig. 157.1). Also known as the fibulocalcaneal ligament, the calcaneofibular ligament is susceptible to strain at the joint line or avulsion at its origin or insertion. The calcaneofibular ligament is frequently injured from inversion injuries to the ankle that occur when tripping when high heels, stepping off a high curb, landing hard or running on hard uneven surfaces, and during dancing, soccer, and basketball. The pain of calcaneofibular ligament damage is localized anterior and inferior to the lateral malleolus and is made worse with inversion of the ankle joint. Point tenderness just below and behind the lateral malleolus is often present on physical examination. Significant swelling and ecchymosis is often evident after acute injury. Activity, especially involving weight bearing, plantar flexion, and inversion of the ankle, will exacerbate the pain. Local heat and decreased activity as well as elevation of the affected ankle may provide a modicum of relief. Sleep disturbance is common in patients suffering from trauma to the calcaneofibular ligament of the ankle. Coexistent fracture, bursitis, tendonitis, arthritis, or internal derangement of the ankle may confuse the clinical picture after trauma to the knee joint making clinical diagnosis difficult.

Plain radiographs and/or arthrography is indicated in all patients who present with calcaneofibular ligament pain, especially after ankle trauma (Fig. 157.2). Based on the patient's clinical presentation, additional testing may be indicated, including complete blood cell count, sedimentation rate, and antinuclear antibody testing. Magnetic resonance imaging and/or ultrasound imaging of the ankle is indicated if internal derangement or occult mass or tumor is suspected as well as to confirm the diagnosis of suspected calcaneofibular ligament injury (Fig. 157.3). Bone scan may be useful to identify occult stress fractures involving the joint, especially if trauma has occurred.

## CLINICALLY RELEVANT ANATOMY

The ankle is a hinge-type articulation between the distal tibia, the two malleoli, and the talus. The articular surface is covered with hyaline cartilage, which is susceptible to arthritis. The joint is surrounded by a dense capsule that helps strengthen the ankle. The joint capsule is lined with a synovial membrane that attaches to the articular cartilage. The ankle joint is innervated by the deep peroneal and tibial nerves.

The major ligaments of the ankle joint include the talofibular, anterior talofibular, calcaneofibular, and posterior talofibular ligaments, which provide the majority of strength to the ankle joint. The calcaneofibular ligament is not as strong as the deltoid ligament and is susceptible to strain. The calcaneofibular ligament runs from the anterior border of the lateral malleolus to the lateral surface of the calcaneus (see Fig. 157.1).

## ULTRASOUND-GUIDED TECHNIQUE

The benefits, risks, and alternative treatments are explained to the patient, and informed consent is obtained. The patient is then placed in the supine position with the lateral curled-up position (Fig. 157.4). The skin over the lateral malleolus and heel overlying the calcaneofibular ligament is then prepped with antiseptic solution. A sterile syringe containing 2.0 mL

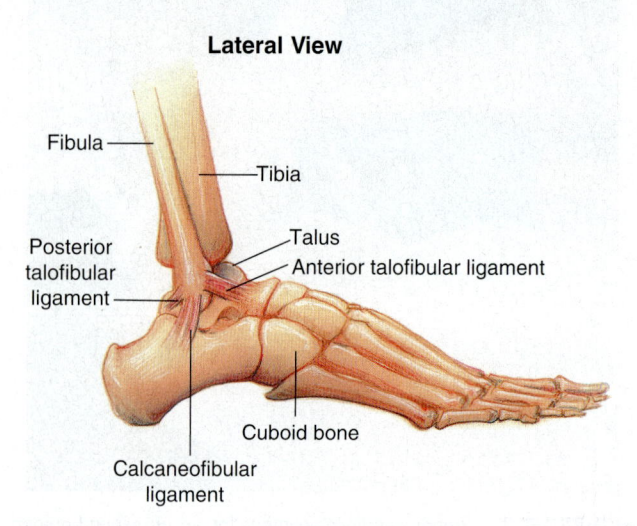

**FIGURE 157.1.** The anatomy of the calcaneofibular ligament and its relationship with the other ligaments of the lateral ankle. (Anatomical Chart Company, 2013.)

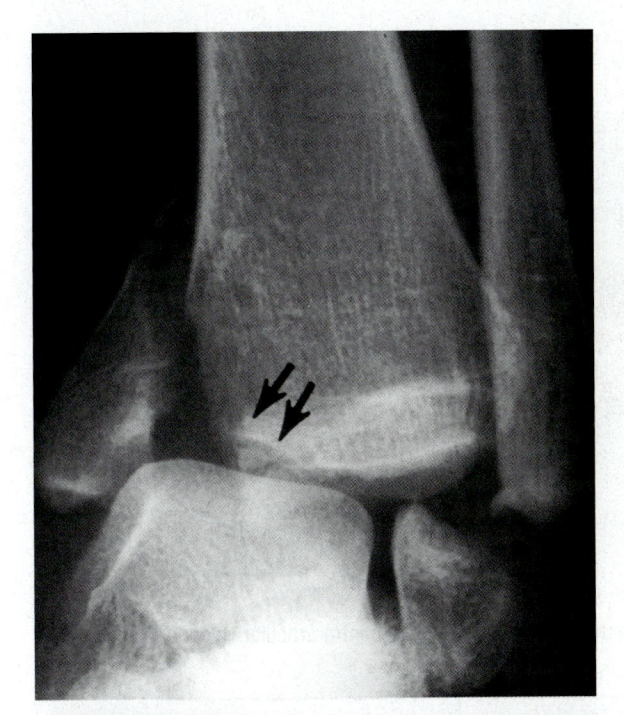

**FIGURE 157.2.** A 45-year-old woman sustained an inversion injury of her ankle. An anteroposterior radiograph illustrates a classic supination–adduction injury pattern. The medial malleolus fracture is vertical, and the fibula fracture is very distal and transverse. There is an impacted fragment in the medial aspect of the remaining tibial plafond (*arrows*). (Reused from Bucholz RW, Heckman JD. *Rockwood & Green's Fractures in Adults*. 5th ed. Philadelphia, PA: Lippincott Williams & Wilkins; 2001, with permission.)

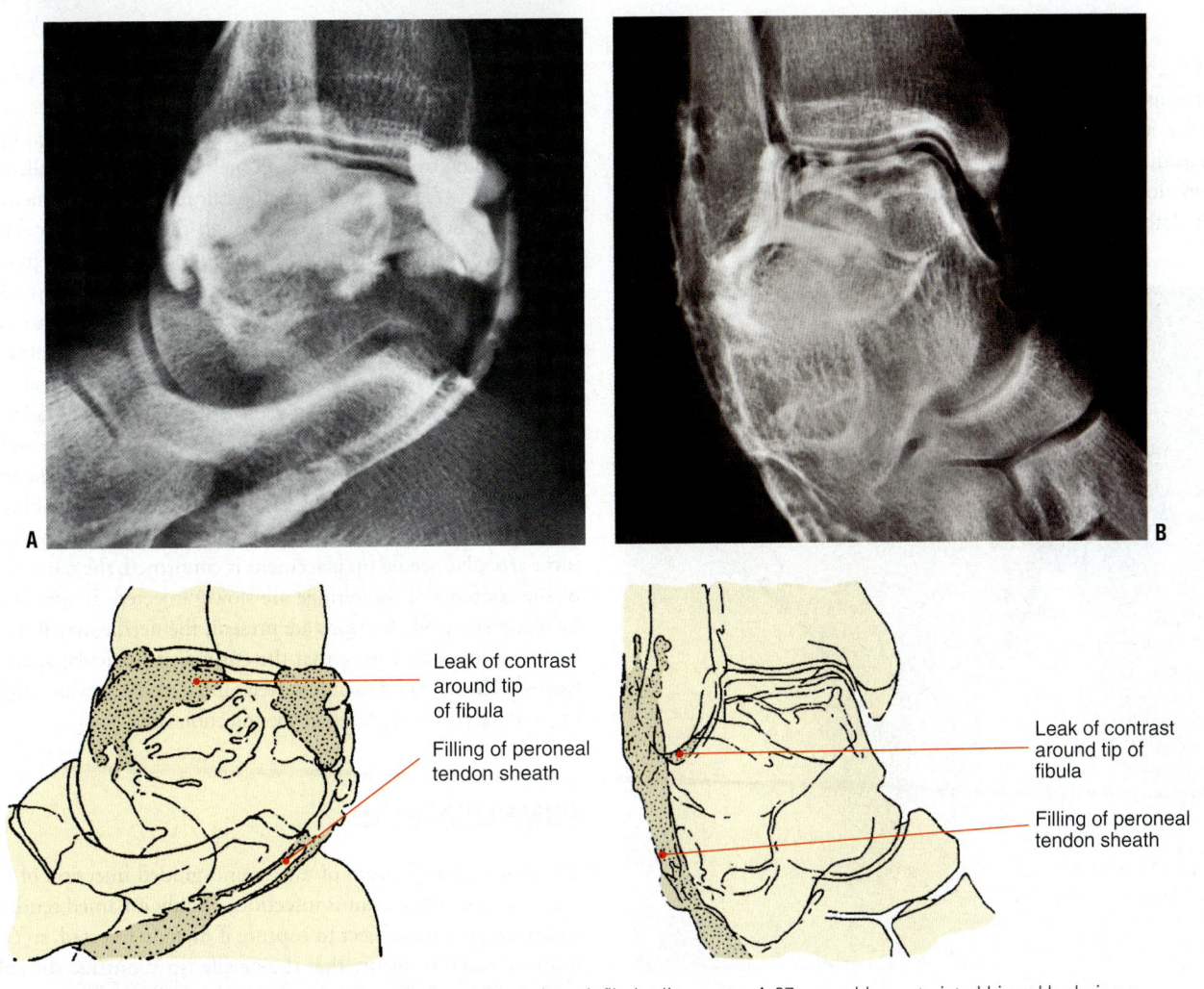

**FIGURE 157-3.** Tear of the calcaneofibular and anterior talofibular ligaments. A 27-year-old man twisted his ankle during a sports activity. Conventional graphs were normal, and stress views were equivocal. Contrast arthrograms in the lateral **(A)** and oblique **(B)** projections of the ankle show opacification of the peroneal tendon sheath, characteristic of tear of the calcaneofibular ligament. Leak of contrast agent along the fibular malleolus, seen on both views, indicates an associated tear of the anterior talofibular ligament. (Reused from Greenspan A. *Orthopedic Imaging: A Practical Approach*. 5th ed. Philadelphia, PA: Lippincott Williams & Wilkins; 2011:345, with permission.)

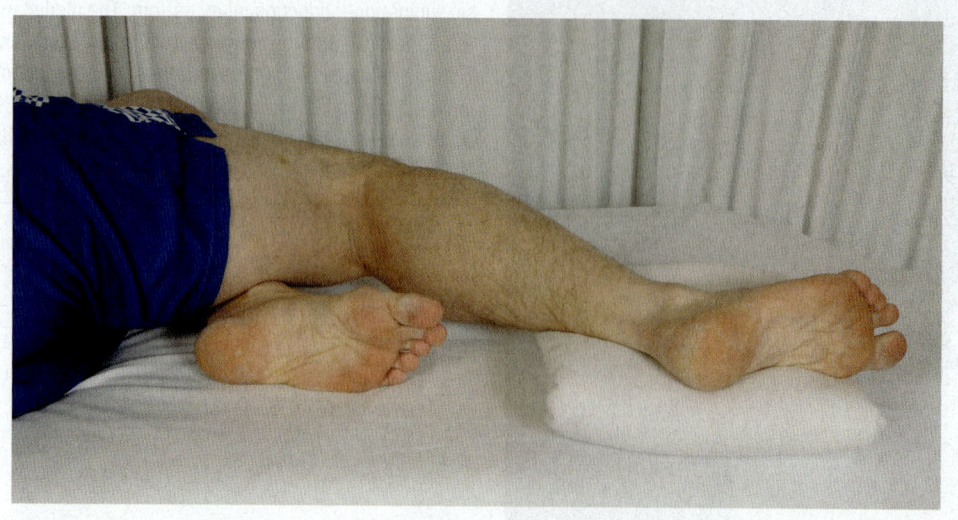

**FIGURE 157.4.** Proper lateral curled-up patient position for ultrasound-guided intra-articular calcaneofibular ligament injection.

of 0.25% preservative-free bupivacaine and 40 mg of methylprednisolone is attached to a 1½-inch, 22-gauge needle using strict aseptic technique. A high-frequency linear ultrasound transducer is then placed in the longitudinal position with the superior aspect of the transducer placed just over the bottom of the lateral malleolus with the superior aspect of the transducer rotated toward the anterior ankle with the inferior aspect of the transducer pointed at the calcaneus (Fig. 157.5). A survey scan is taken, which demonstrates the hyperechoic calcaneofibular ligament running from the lateral calcaneus to the lateral malleolus of the fibula (Fig. 157.6). After the calcaneofibular ligament is identified, the needle is placed through the skin ~1 cm above the middle of the anterior aspect of the longitudinally placed transducer and is then advanced using an out-of-plane approach with the needle trajectory adjusted under real-time ultrasound guidance to place the needle tip within proximity to the calcaneofibular ligament but not within the substance of the ligament (Fig. 157.7). When the tip of needle is thought to be in satisfactory position, a small amount of local anesthetic and steroid is injected under real-time ultrasound guidance to confirm that the needle tip is not within the substance of the calcaneofibular ligament. There should be minimal resistance to injection. After intra-articular needle tip placement is confirmed, the remainder of the contents of the syringe are slowly injected. If synechiae, loculations, or calcifications are present, the needle may have to be repositioned to ensure that the entire intra-articular space is treated. The needle is then removed, and a sterile pressure dressing and ice pack are placed at the injection site.

## COMPLICATIONS

The major complication of ultrasound-guided injection of the calcaneofibular ligament is infection. Highly inflamed tendons and ligaments are subject to rupture if directly injected, so care must be taken to insure that the needle tip is outside the substance of the tendon. Ecchymosis and hematoma formation may also occur. A transient exacerbation of the patient's pain occurs ~25% of the time following this injection technique, and the patient should be warned of this possibility prior to the procedure.

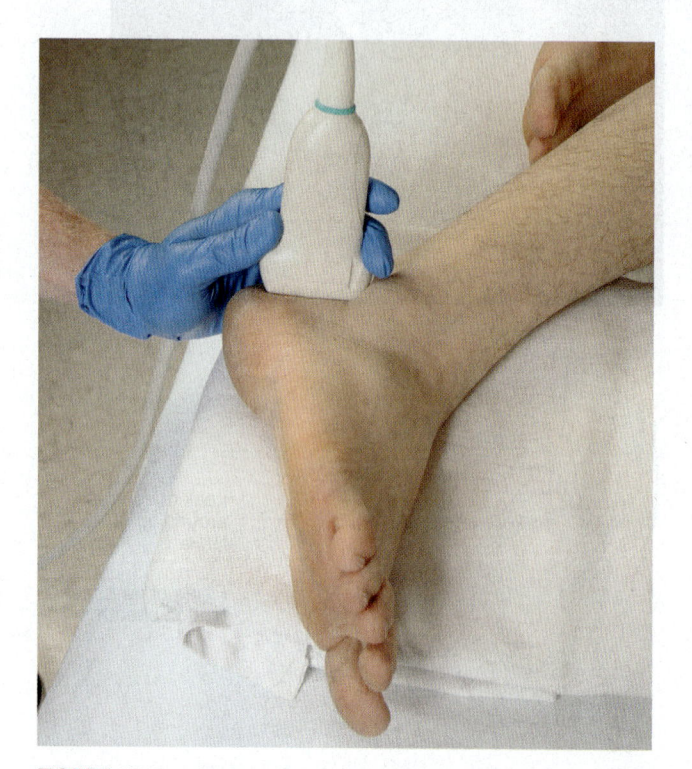

**FIGURE 157.5.** Correct transverse position for the ultrasound transducer for ultrasound-guided intra-articular injection of the calcaneofibular ligament. Note that the posterior aspect of the ultrasound transducer is lying over the bottom of the lateral malleolus.

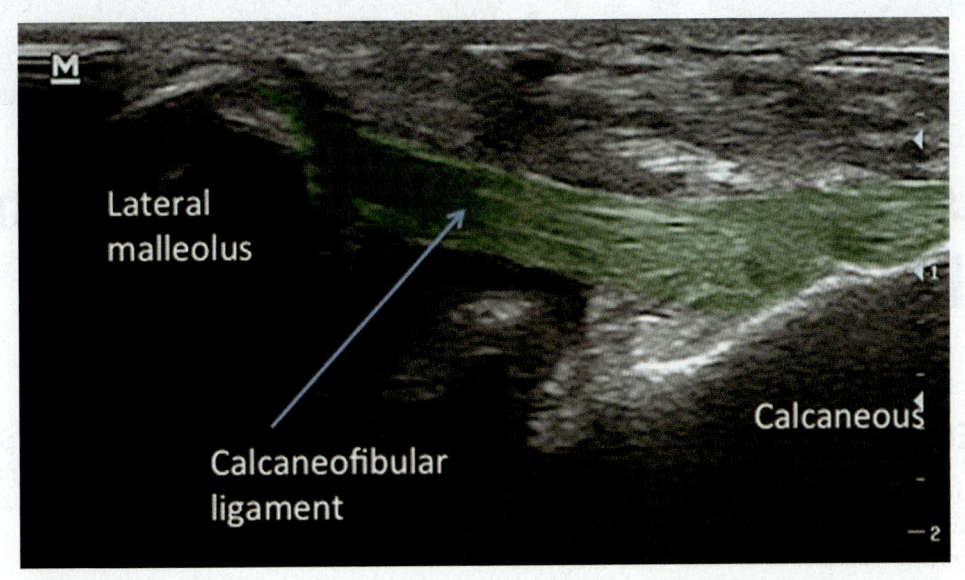

**FIGURE 157.6.** Longitudinal ultrasound image demonstrating the calcaneofibular ligament.

## CLINICAL PEARLS

Bursitis, fractures, tendinopathy, osteoarthritis, synovitis, avascular necrosis, and impingement syndromes may coexist with calcaneofibular ligament pathology and may contribute to the patient's pain symptomatology. Universal precautions should always be observed to protect the operator, and strict adherence to sterile technique must be used to avoid infection. Gentle physical therapy and local heat should be introduced following ultrasound-guided injection of the calcaneofibular ligament to reduce pain and improve function. Simple analgesics and nonsteroidal anti-inflammatory agents or COX-2 inhibitors may be used concurrently with this injection technique.

## SUGGESTED READINGS

Bonnel F, Toullec E, Mabit C, et al. Chronic ankle instability: biomechanics and pathomechanics of ligaments injury and associated lesions. *Orthop Traumatol Surg Res* 2010; 96(4):424–432.

Haller J, Bernt R, Seeger T, et al. MR-imaging of anterior tibiotalar impingement syndrome: agreement, sensitivity and specificity of MR-imaging and indirect MR-arthrography. [Original Research Article.] *Eur J Radiol* 2006;58(3): 450–460.

Waldman SD, Campbell RSD. Calcaneofibular ligament tear. In: *Imaging of Pain*. Philadelphia, PA: Saunders Elsevier; 2010:437–438.

Waldman SD. Functional anatomy of the ankle and foot. In: *Pain Review*. Philadelphia, PA: Saunders Elsevier; 2009:155–156.

Waldman SD. Injection of the calcaneofibular ligament. In: *Atlas of Pain Management Injection Techniques*. 3rd ed. Philadelphia, PA: Saunders Elsevier; 2012:427–430.

Waldman SD. The calcaneofibular ligament. In: *Pain Review*. Philadelphia, PA: Saunders Elsevier; 2009:158.

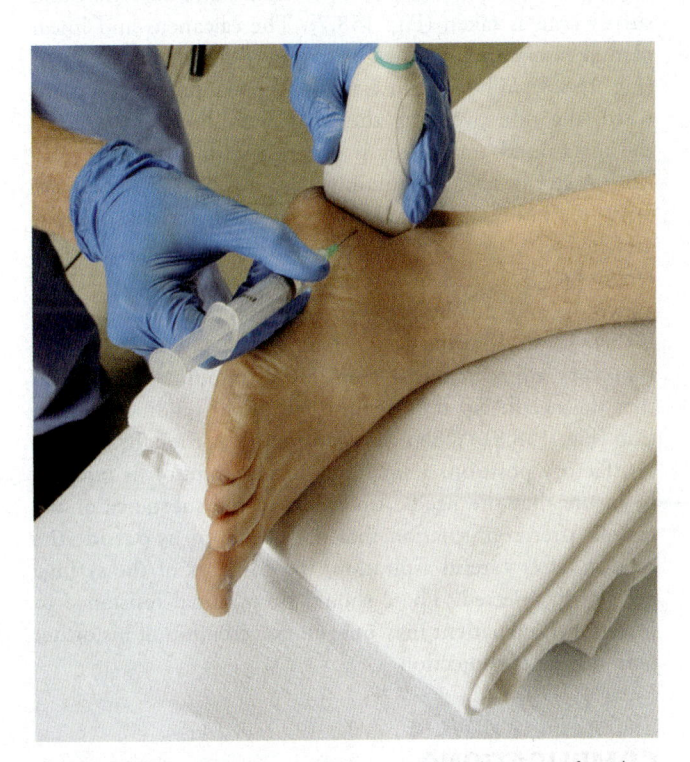

**FIGURE 157.7.** Correct out-of-plane needle placement for ultrasound-guided calcaneofibular ligament injection.

# Ultrasound-Guided Injection Technique for Plantar Fasciitis

## CLINICAL PERSPECTIVES

Plantar fasciitis is a clinical syndrome characterized by pain and tenderness over the plantar surface of the calcaneus made immediately worse by dorsiflexion of the toes. Occurring twice as often in women, plantar fasciitis is thought to be caused by an inflammation of the plantar fascia. Inflammation of the plantar fascia can occur alone or be part of a systemic inflammatory condition, such as rheumatoid arthritis, Reiter syndrome, or gout. Obesity also seems to predispose to the development of plantar fasciitis, as does going barefoot or wearing house slippers for prolonged periods. High-impact aerobic exercise also has been implicated.

Pain on palpation of the insertion of the plantar fascia on the plantar medial calcaneal tuberosity is a consistent finding in patients with plantar fasciitis as is exacerbation of pain with active resisted dorsiflexion of the toes (Fig. 158.1). Patients suffering from plantar fasciitis will also exhibit pain on deep palpation of the plantar fascia, especially when the toes are dorsiflexed pulling the plantar fascia taunt. The pain of plantar fasciitis is most severe on taking the first few steps after having not borne weight and is made worse by prolonged standing or walking.

Plain radiographs are indicated in all patients who present with heel and foot pain (Fig. 158.2). Based on the patient's clinical presentation, additional testing may be indicated, including complete blood cell count, sedimentation rate, and antinuclear antibody testing. Magnetic resonance imaging and/or ultrasound imaging of the ankle is indicated if plantar fasciitis, rupture, or joint instability is suggested (Figs. 158.3 and 158.4). Radionuclide bone scanning is useful to identify stress fractures of the calcaneus and foot not seen on plain radiographs and may aid in the diagnosis as there may be increased uptake of radionuclide at the insertion of the plantar fascia at the calcaneus. The injection technique described later serves as both a diagnostic and a therapeutic maneuver.

## CLINICALLY RELEVANT ANATOMY

The plantar fascia is made up of thick, longitudinally oriented connective tissue that is tightly attached to the plantar skin. It attaches to the medial calcaneal tuberosity and then runs forward, dividing into five bands, one going to each toe (Fig. 158.5). The plantar fascia provides dynamic support in the arch of the foot, tightening as the foot bears weight.

## ULTRASOUND-GUIDED TECHNIQUE

The benefits, risks, and alternative treatments are explained to the patient, and informed consent is obtained. The patient is then placed in the prone position with the patient's ankle hanging off the edge of the table (Fig. 158.6). With the patient in the above position, a high-frequency linear ultrasound transducer is placed in a longitudinal plane with the inferior portion of the ultrasound transducer over plantar surface of the foot with the superior end of the transducer on the anterior portion of the calcaneus, and an ultrasound survey scan is taken (Fig. 158.7). The calcaneus and linear plantar fascia are identified at its insertion on the calcaneus (Fig. 158.8). When the insertion of the plantar fascia is identified, the skin overlying the area of the heel and beneath the ultrasound transducer is prepped with antiseptic solution. A sterile syringe containing 3.0 mL of 0.25% preservative-free bupivacaine and 40 mg of methylprednisolone is attached to a 1½-inch, 22-gauge needle using strict aseptic technique. The needle is placed through the skin ~1 cm above the superior border of the ultrasound transducer and is then advanced using an in-plane approach with the needle trajectory adjusted under real-time ultrasound guidance so that the needle tip rests against the site of tendinous insertion (Fig. 158.9). When the tip of needle is thought to be in satisfactory position, a small amount of solution is injected to insure that the needle tip is not in the substance of the fascia. After confirmation that the needle tip is outside the tendon, after careful aspiration, the contents of the syringe are slowly injected. There should be minimal resistance to injection. The patient may note an exacerbation of his or her pain during the injection.

## COMPLICATIONS

The major complication of this ultrasound-guided injection technique is infection. Ecchymosis and hematoma formation

CHAPTER 158 ULTRASOUND-GUIDED INJECTION TECHNIQUE FOR PLANTAR FASCIITIS 1111

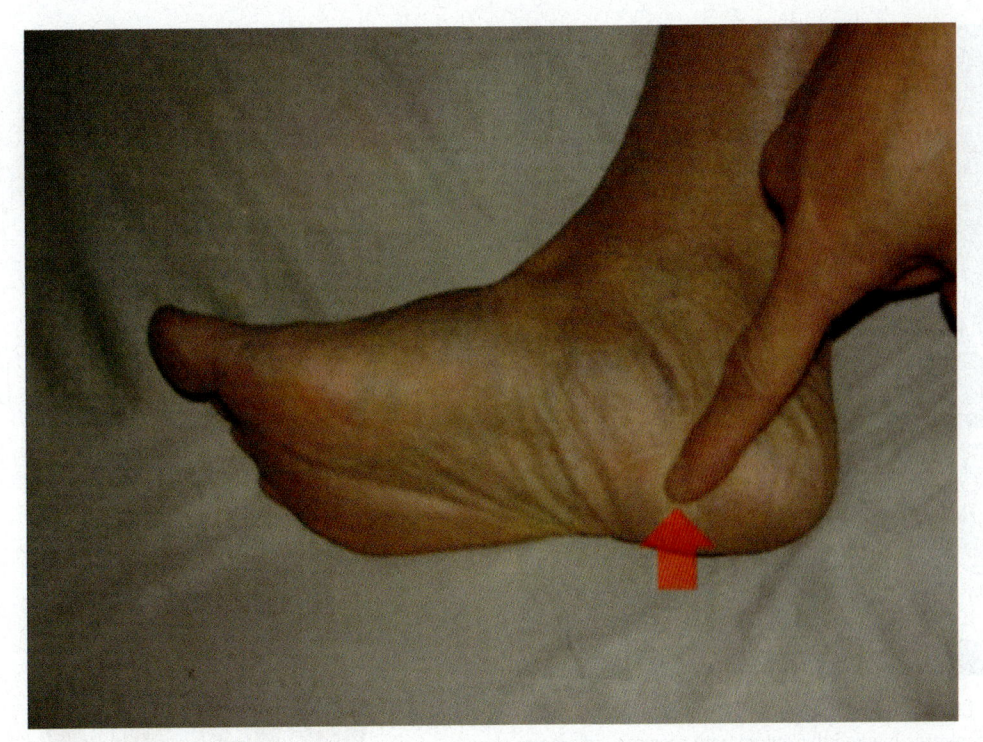

**FIGURE 158.1.** Pain on palpation of the insertion of the plantar fascia on the plantar medial calcaneal tuberosity is a consistent finding in patients with plantar fasciitis as is exacerbation of pain with active resisted dorsiflexion of the toes.

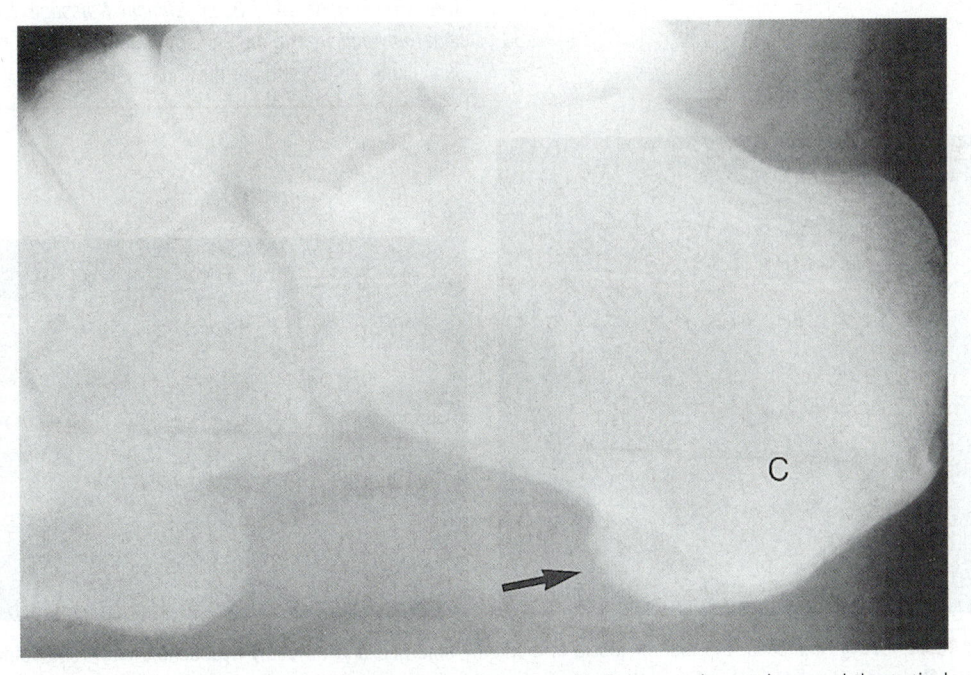

**FIGURE 158.2.** Lateral radiograph of the heel of a man with Reiter syndrome shows subtle cortical irregularity at the calcaneal insertion of the plantar aponeurosis (*arrow*). (Reused from Koopman WJ, Moreland LW. *Arthritis and Allied Conditions: A Textbook of Rheumatology.* 15th ed. Philadelphia, PA: Lippincott Williams & Wilkins; 2005, with permission.)

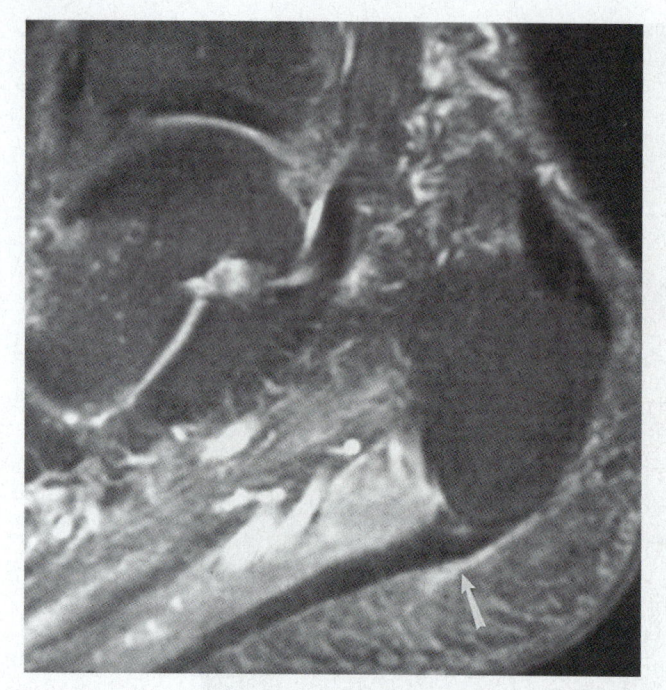

**FIGURE 158.3.** Chronic fasciitis. Sagittal fat-suppressed fast spin-echo image demonstrates marked thickening with proximal inflammation (*arrow*). (Reused from Berquist TH. *Imaging of the Foot and Ankle*. 3rd ed. Philadelphia, PA: Lippincott Williams & Wilkins; 2011:176, with permission.)

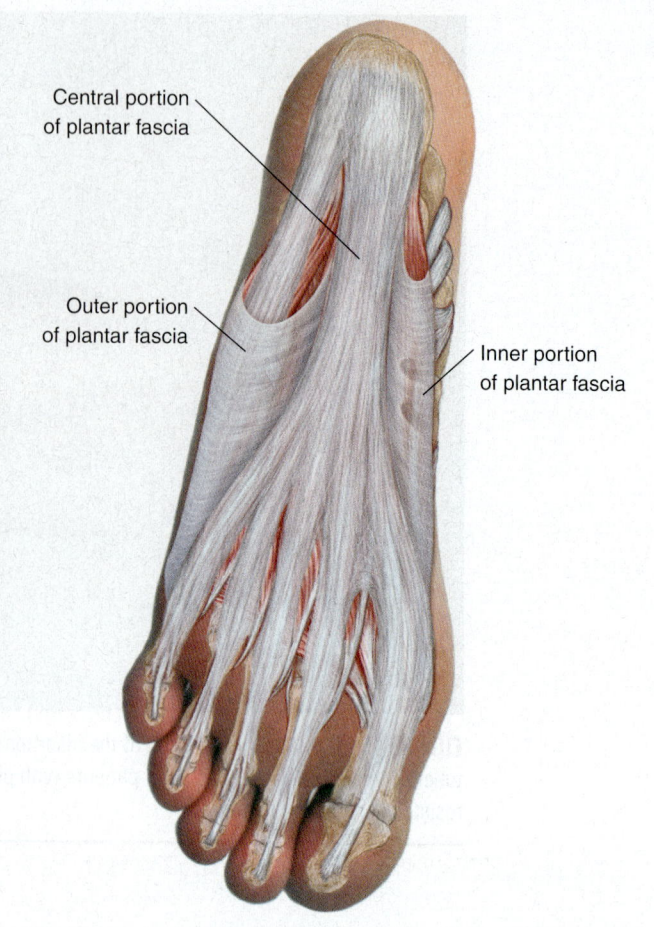

**FIGURE 158.5.** The anatomy of the plantar fascia. (Reused from Clay JH, Pounds DM. *Basic Clinical Massage Therapy: Integrating Anatomy and Treatment*. 2nd ed. Philadelphia, PA: Lippincott Williams & Wilkins; 2008, with permission.)

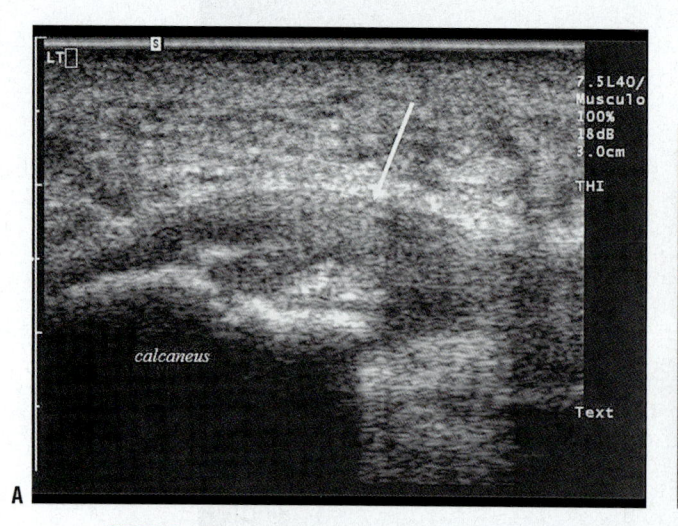

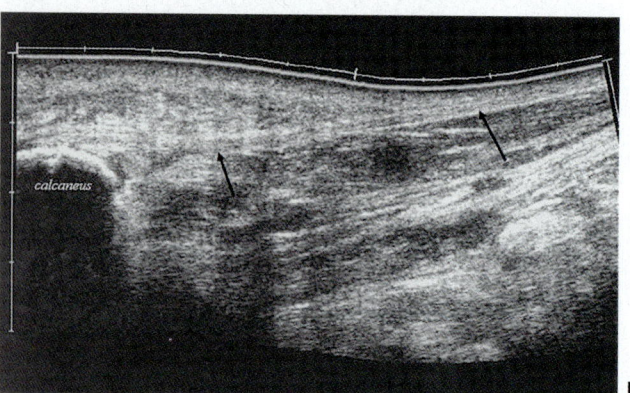

**FIGURE 158.4. A:** In this case, the plantar fascia is markedly enlarged and diffusely hypoechoic with remodeling of the calcaneus. **B:** Longitudinal extended field of view image of the plantar demonstrates moderate plantar fasciitis, with diffused thickening and decreased echogenicity of the proximal plantar fascia. These cases illustrate that most cases of isolated plantar fasciitis are confined to the proximal 2 to 3 cm of the plantar fascia. The distal plantar fascia (*arrows*) retains normal thickness and morphology. (Reused from Adler RS, Sofka CM, Positano RG. *Atlas of Foot and Ankle Sonography*. Philadelphia, PA: Lippincott Williams & Wilkins; 2004:89, with permission.)

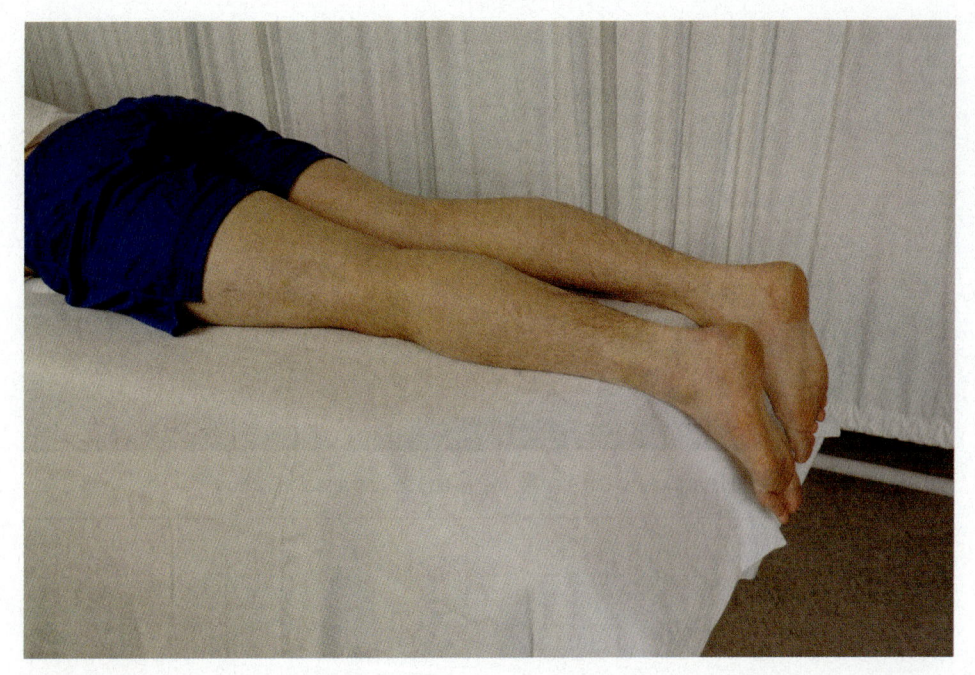

**FIGURE 158.6.** Proper prone patient positioning for ultrasound-guided injection for plantar fasciitis.

following this procedure may also occur. The possibility of trauma to the already compromised fascia from the injection itself remains an ever-present possibility, although the risk of this is decreased if the clinician uses gentle technique and stops injecting immediately if significant resistance to injection is encountered. Approximately 25% of patients complain of a transient increase in pain after this injection technique; the patient should be warned of this.

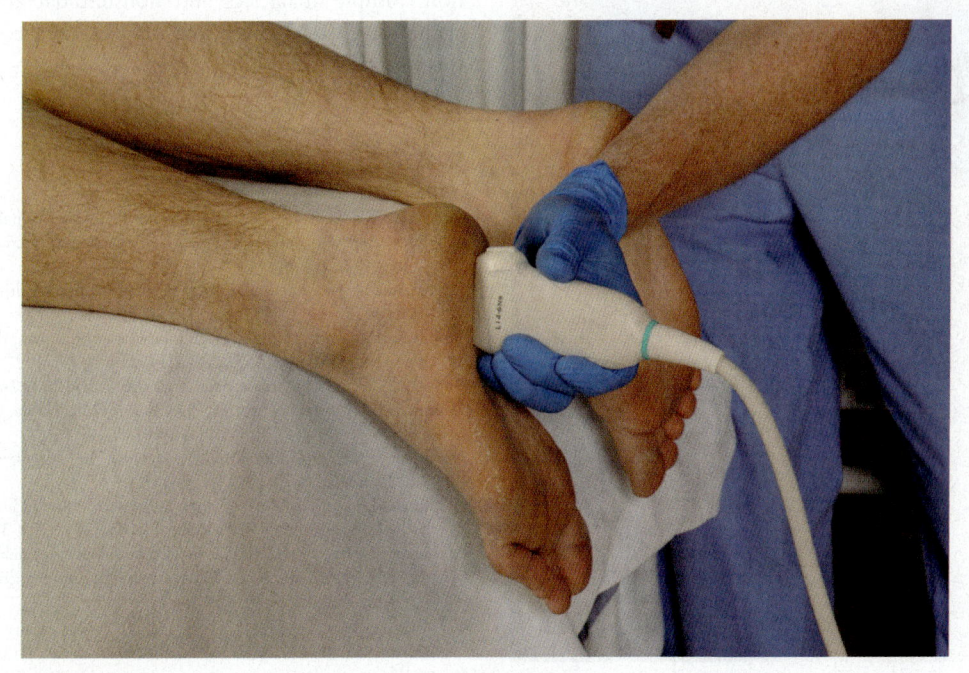

**FIGURE 158.7.** Proper longitudinal ultrasound transducer placement for ultrasound-guided injection for plantar fasciitis.

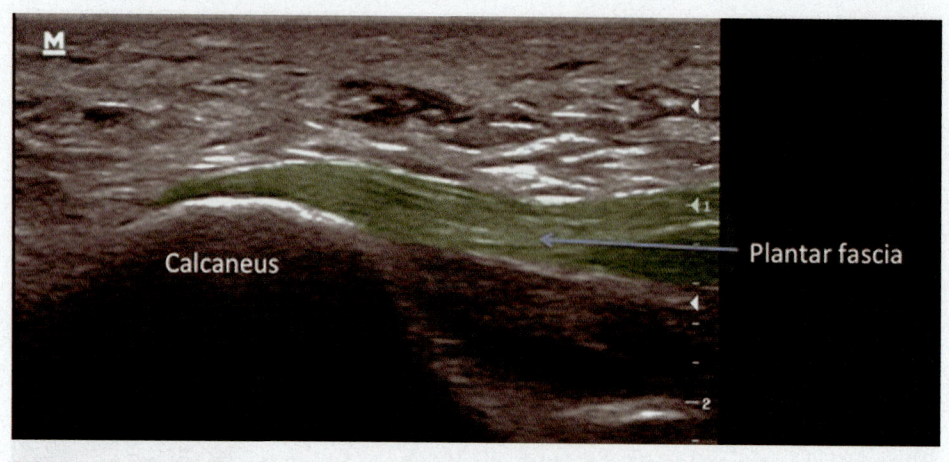

**FIGURE 158.8.** Longitudinal view of the plantar fascia and its calcaneal insertion.

## CLINICAL PEARLS

Bursitis and tendonitis of the ankle and foot may coexist with plantar fasciitis and may contribute to the patient's pain symptomatology. Universal precautions should always be observed to protect the operator, and strict adherence to sterile technique must be used to avoid infection. Gentle physical therapy and local heat should be introduced following ultrasound-guided injection of plantar fasciitis to reduce pain and improve function. Simple analgesics and nonsteroidal anti-inflammatory agents or COX-2 inhibitors may be used concurrently with this injection technique.

## SUGGESTED READINGS

Buccilli Jr TA, Hall HR, Solmen JD. Sterile abscess formation following a corticosteroid injection for the treatment of plantar fasciitis. *J Foot Ankle Surg* 2005;44(6):466–468.
Puttaswamaiah R, Chandran P. Degenerative plantar fasciitis: a review of current concepts. *Foot* 2007;17(1):3–9.
Rajput B, Abboud RJ. Common ignorance, major problem: the role of footwear in plantar fasciitis. *Foot* 2004;14(4):214–218.
Toomey EP. Plantar heel pain. *Foot Ankle Clin N Am* 2009;14(2):229–245.
Waldman SD. Plantar fasciitis. In: *Pain Review*. Philadelphia, PA: Saunders Elsevier; 2009:327.
Waldman SD, Campbell RSD. Plantar fasciitis. In: *Imaging of Pain*. Philadelphia, PA: Saunders Elsevier; 2011:457–459.
Waldman SD, Campbell RSD. Plantar fasciitis. In: *Atlas of Common Pain Syndromes*. 3rd ed. Philadelphia, PA: Saunders Elsevier; 2012:377–379.
Waldman SD. Injection technique for plantar fasciitis. In: *Atlas of Pain Management Injection Techniques*. 3rd ed. Philadelphia, PA: Saunders Elsevier; 2012:453–455.

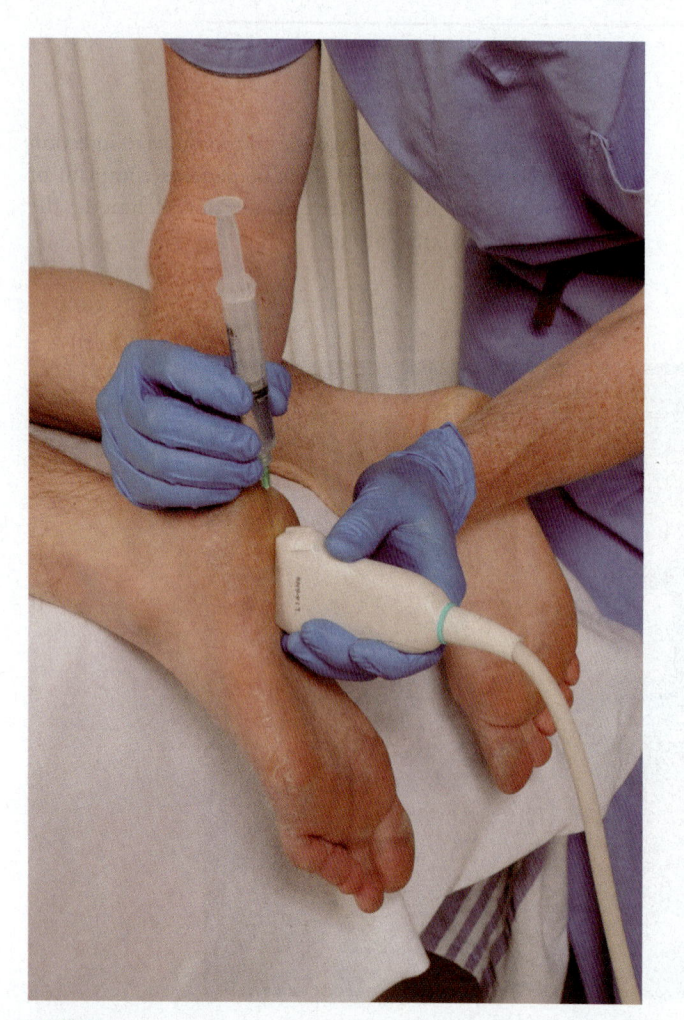

**FIGURE 158.9.** Proper needle placement for an ultrasound-guided out-of-plane injection for plantar fasciitis.

CHAPTER 159

# Ultrasound-Guided Injection Technique for Calcaneal Spurs

## CLINICAL PERSPECTIVES

Calcaneal spurs are a common cause of heel pain. Calcaneal spurs may be asymptomatic or symptomatic. When symptomatic, calcaneal spurs are usually seen in conjunction with plantar fasciitis. The clinical syndrome associated with symptomatic calcaneal spurs is characterized by pain and tenderness over the plantar surface of the calcaneus made immediately worse by dorsiflexion of the toes. Calcaneal spurs are thought to be caused by an inflammation of the insertional fibers of plantar fascia onto the medial tuberosity of the calcaneus (Fig. 159.1). Inflammation of these insertional fibers of the plantar fascia can occur alone or can be part of a systemic inflammatory condition, such as rheumatoid arthritis, plantar fasciitis, Reiter syndrome, or gout (Fig. 159.2). In some patients, suffering from symptomatic heel spurs, there does not appear to be an inflammatory basis for the patient's pain symptomatology, and the etiology of the pain appears to be entirely mechanical as is seen with patients with gait abnormalities that include an excessive heel strike. High-impact aerobic exercise also has been implicated.

Pain on palpation of the insertion of the plantar fascia on the plantar medial calcaneal tuberosity is a consistent finding in patients with calcaneal spurs as is exacerbation of pain with active resisted dorsiflexion of the toes (Fig. 159.3). Patients suffering from calcaneal spurs will also exhibit pain on deep palpation of the plantar fascia, especially when the toes are dorsiflexed pulling the plantar fascia taunt. The pain of calcaneal spurs is most severe on taking the first few steps after having not borne weight and is made worse by prolonged standing or walking. The pain of symptomatic heel spurs is made worse by standing for long periods or by weight bearing and is often relieved by padding of the affected heel.

Plain radiographs are indicated in all patients who present with heel and foot pain (Fig. 159.4). Based on the patient's clinical presentation, additional testing may be indicated, including complete blood cell count, sedimentation rate, and antinuclear antibody testing. Magnetic resonance imaging and/or ultrasound imaging of the ankle is indicated if calcaneal spurs, rupture of the plantar fascia, or joint instability is suggested (Figs. 159.5 and 159.6). Radionuclide bone scanning is useful to identify stress fractures of the calcaneus and foot not seen on plain radiographs and may aid in the diagnosis as there may be increased uptake of radionucleotide at the insertion of the plantar fascia at the calcaneus. The injection technique described later serves as both a diagnostic and a therapeutic maneuver.

## CLINICALLY RELEVANT ANATOMY

The calcaneus is the largest of the tarsal bones. The main function of the calcaneus is to transfer the weight of the body to the ground, as well as to serve as a lever for the muscles of the calf. The plantar surface of the calcaneus is elevated posteriorly to form the calcaneal tuberosity. The calcaneal tuberosity is depressed centrally, with a lateral and medial process. It is at the medial process that symptomatic calcaneal spurs most commonly occur. The plantar fascia is made up of thick, longitudinally oriented connective tissue that is tightly attached to the plantar skin. It attaches to the medial calcaneal tuberosity and then runs forward, dividing into five bands, one going to each toe (see Fig. 159.2). The plantar fascia provides dynamic support in the arch of the foot, tightening as the foot bears weight.

## ULTRASOUND-GUIDED TECHNIQUE

The benefits, risks, and alternative treatments are explained to the patient, and informed consent is obtained. The patient is then placed in the prone position with the patient's ankle hanging off the edge of the table (Fig. 159.7). With the patient in the above position, a high-frequency linear ultrasound transducer is placed in a longitudinal plane with the inferior portion of the ultrasound transducer over plantar surface of the foot with the superior end of the transducer on the anterior portion of the calcaneus, and an ultrasound survey scan is taken (Fig. 159.8). The calcaneus, calcaneal spur, and linear plantar fascia are identified at its insertion on the calcaneus (Fig. 159.9). When the insertion of the plantar fascia is identified, the skin overlying the area of the heel and beneath the ultrasound transducer is prepped with antiseptic solution. A sterile syringe containing 3.0 mL of 0.25% preservative-free bupivacaine and 40 mg of

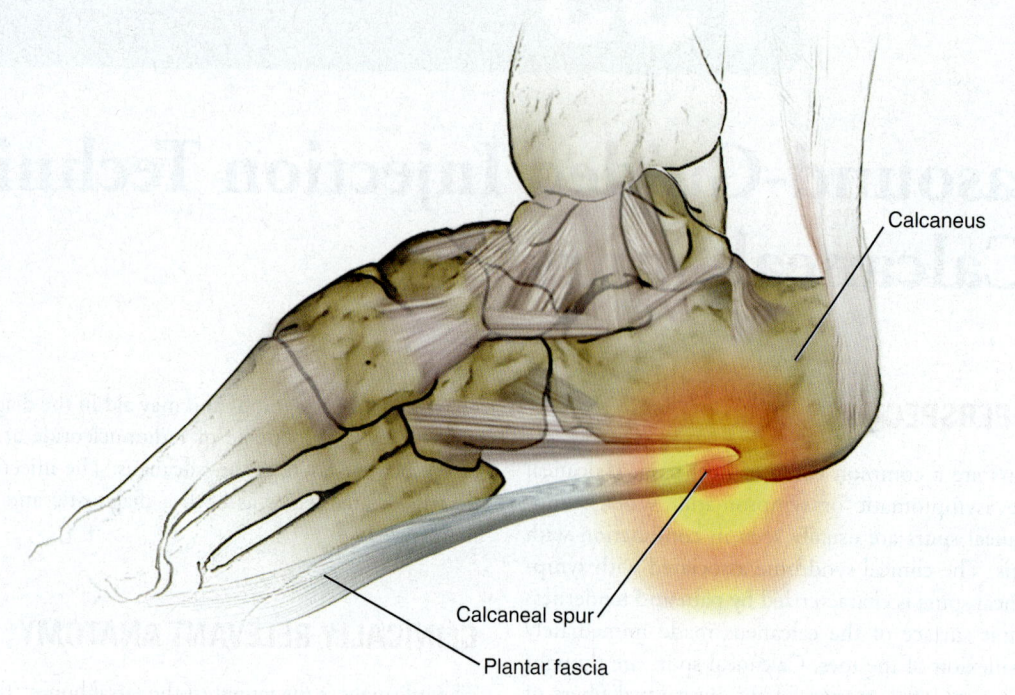

**FIGURE 159.1.** Calcaneal spurs are thought to be caused by an inflammation of the insertional fibers of plantar fascia onto the medial tuberosity of the calcaneus, although in some patients the etiology is purely mechanical.

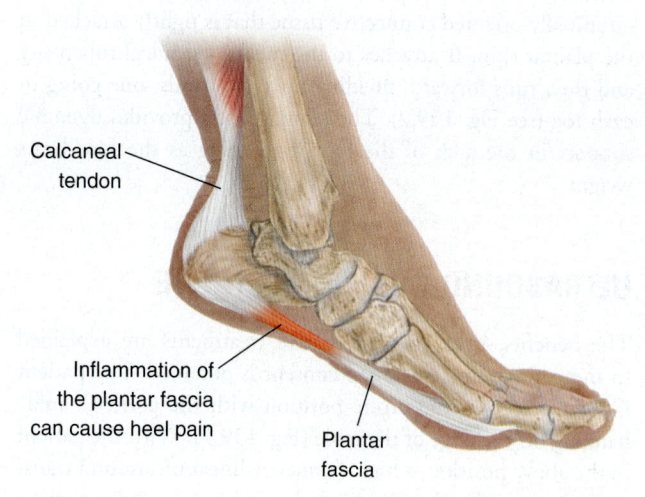

**FIGURE 159.2.** Inflammation of these insertional fibers of the plantar fascia can occur alone or can be part of a systemic inflammatory condition, such as rheumatoid arthritis, plantar fasciitis, Reiter syndrome, or gout, although in some patients the etiology is purely mechanical. (Reused from Bucci C. *Condition-Specific Massage Therapy.* Baltimore, MD: Lippincott Williams & Wilkins; 2012, with permission.)

methylprednisolone is attached to a 1½-inch, 22-gauge needle using strict aseptic technique. The needle is placed through the skin ~1 cm above the superior border of the ultrasound transducer and is then advanced using an in-plane approach with the needle trajectory adjusted under real-time ultrasound guidance so that the needle tip rests against the site of tendinous insertion (Fig. 159.10). When the tip of needle is thought to be in satisfactory position, a small amount of solution is injected to insure that the needle tip is not in the substance of the fascia. After confirmation that the needle tip is outside the tendon, after careful aspiration, the contents of the syringe are slowly injected. There should be minimal resistance to injection. The patient may note an exacerbation of his or her pain during the injection.

## COMPLICATIONS

The major complication of this ultrasound-guided injection technique is infection. Ecchymosis and hematoma formation following this procedure may also occur. The possibility of trauma to the already compromised fascia from the injection

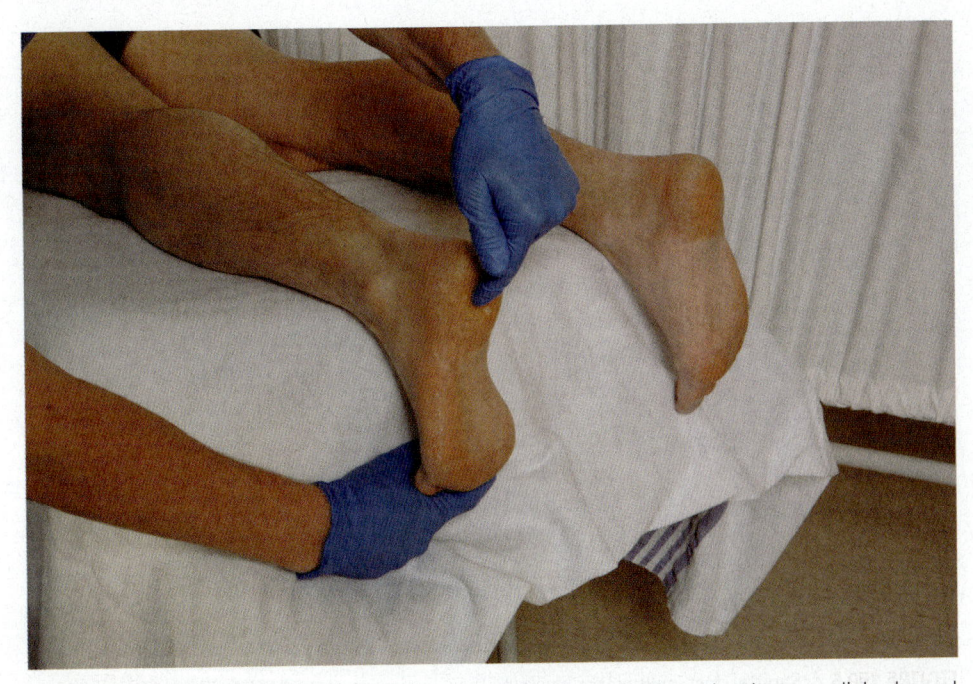

CHAPTER 159 ULTRASOUND-GUIDED INJECTION TECHNIQUE FOR CALCANEAL SPURS 1117

**FIGURE 159.3.** Pain on palpation of the insertion of the plantar fascia on the plantar medial calcaneal tuberosity is a consistent finding in patients with calcaneal spurs as is exacerbation of pain with active resisted dorsiflexion of the toes, especially if the plantar fascia is also inflamed.

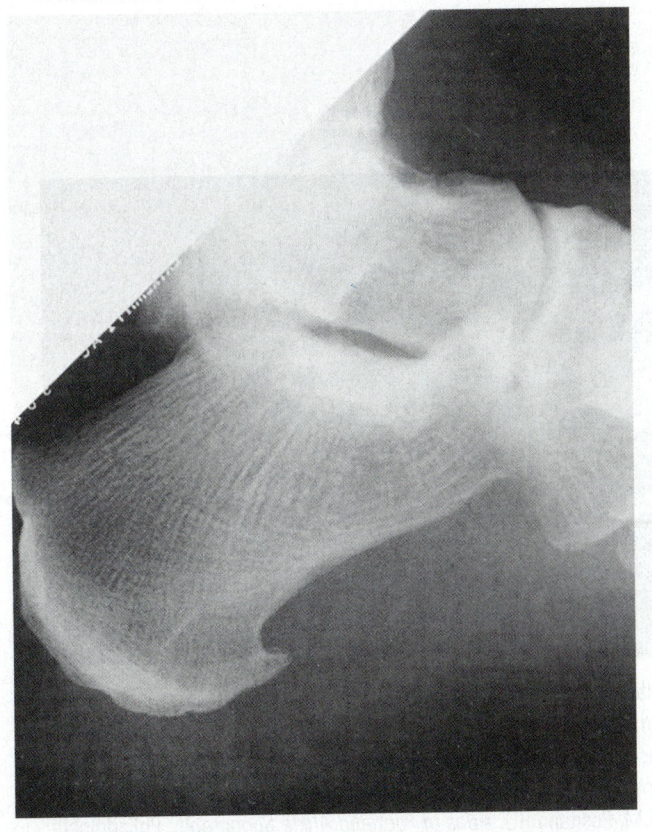

**FIGURE 159.4.** Lateral radiograph demonstrating a calcaneal spur. (Reused from Koopman WJ, Moreland LW. *Arthritis and Allied Conditions: A Textbook of Rheumatology.* 15th ed. Philadelphia, PA: Lippincott Williams & Wilkins; 2005, with permission.)

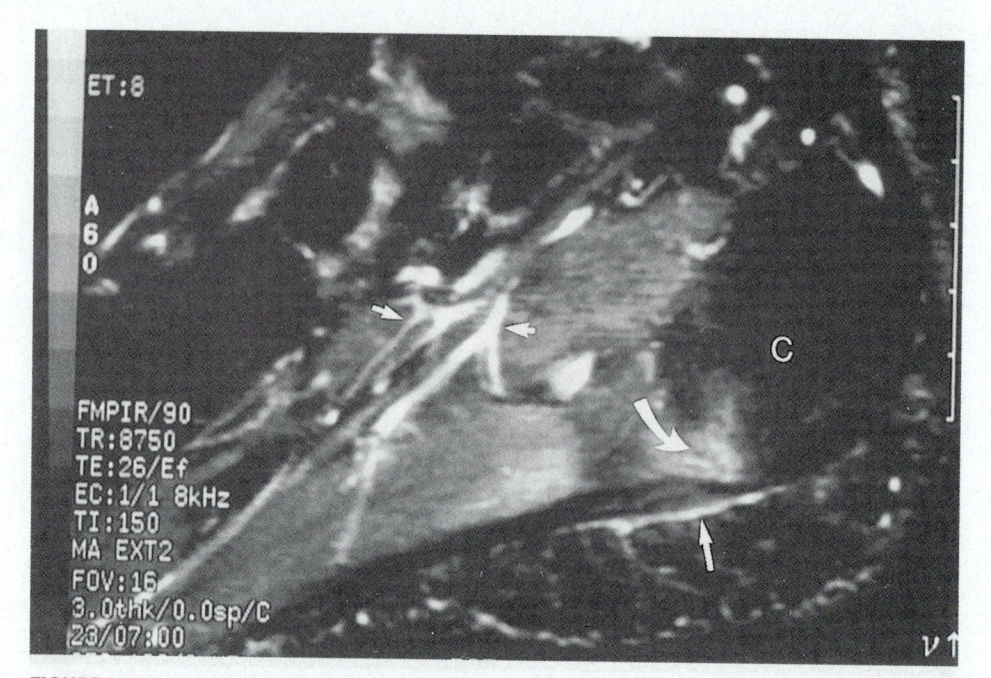

**FIGURE 159.5.** Sagittal, fast, multiplanar inversion recovery image of the heel depicts water with high-signal intensity and fat with low-signal intensity and thus shows edema in the local soft tissues and bone marrow (*curved arrow*) with extremely high sensitivity. Fluid can also be seen tracking along the plantar aponeurosis (*long straight arrow*) (plantar fasciitis). The anching high-signal-intensity structures (*short straight arrows*) are blood vessels. (Reused from Koopman WJ, Moreland LW. *Arthritis and Allied Conditions: A Textbook of Rheumatology.* 15th ed. Philadelphia, PA: Lippincott Williams & Wilkins; 2005, with permission.)

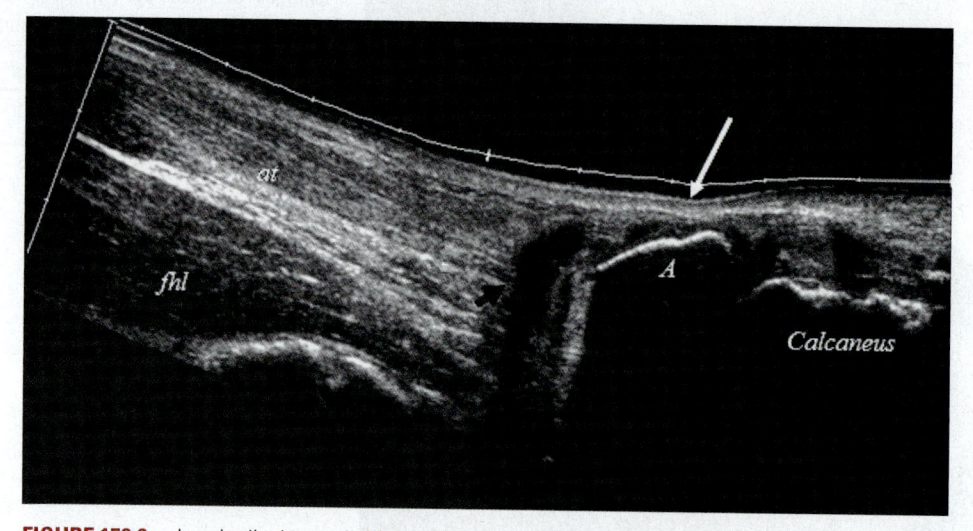

**FIGURE 159.6.** Longitudinal extended field of view image in an adolescent with ankle pain and swelling following a "hard landing" during gymnastics. There is a moderately displaced fracture of the calcaneal apophysis (A, *arrow*). Moreover, a tear at the Achilles tendon (*at*) insertion can be seen (*short black arrow*) and distal to the apophyseal fragment. The flexor hallucis long (*fhl*) and calcaneus are labeled for reference. (Reused from Adler RS, Sofka CM, Positano RG. *Atlas of Foot and Ankle Sonography.* Philadelphia, PA: Lippincott Williams & Wilkins; 2004:82, with permission.)

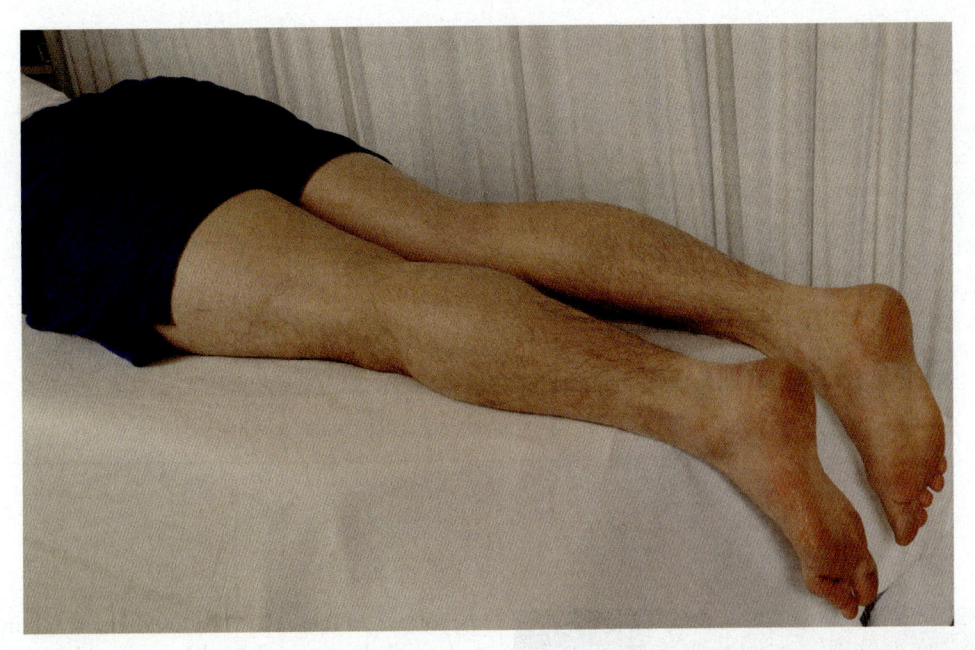

**FIGURE 159.7.** Proper prone patient positioning for ultrasound-guided injection for calcaneal spurs.

itself remains an ever-present possibility, although the risk of this is decreased if the clinician uses gentle technique and stops injecting immediately if significant resistance to injection is encountered. Approximately 25% of patients complain of a transient increase in pain after this injection technique; the patient should be warned of this.

## CLINICAL PEARLS

Bursitis and tendonitis of the ankle and foot may coexist with calcaneal spurs and may contribute to the patient's pain symptomatology. Universal precautions should always be observed to protect the operator, and strict adherence to

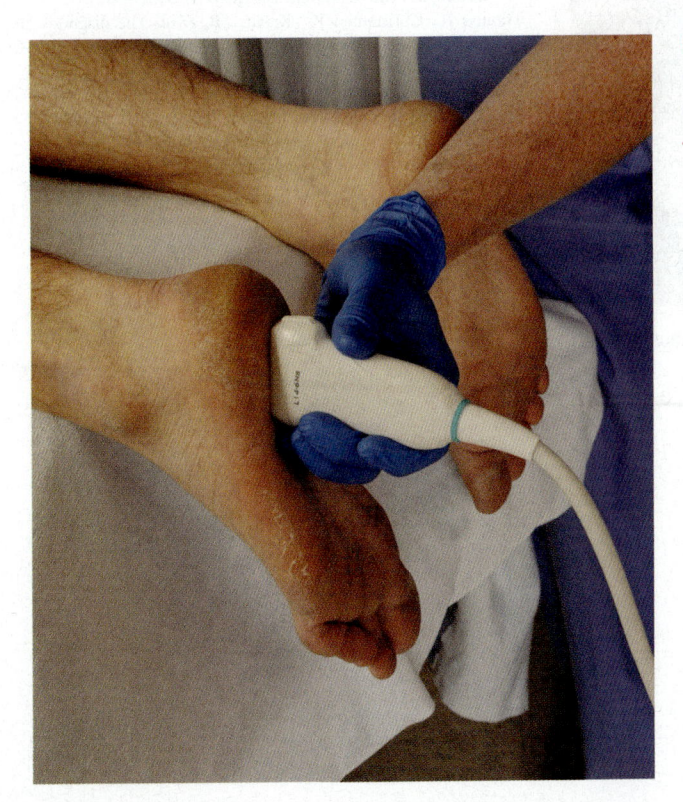

**FIGURE 159.8.** Proper longitudinal ultrasound transducer placement for ultrasound-guided injection for calcaneal spurs.

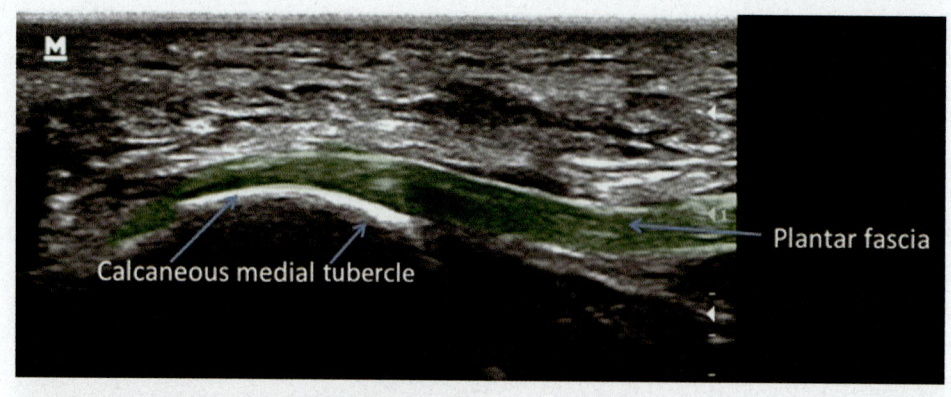

**FIGURE 159.9.** Longitudinal view of the plantar fascia and its calcaneal insertion.

sterile technique must be used to avoid infection. Gentle physical therapy and local heat should be introduced following ultrasound-guided injection of calcaneal spurs to reduce pain and improve function. Simple analgesics and nonsteroidal anti-inflammatory agents or COX-2 inhibitors may be used concurrently with this injection technique.

## SUGGESTED READINGS

Irving DB, Cook JL, Menz HB. Factors associated with chronic plantar heel pain: a systematic review. [Review Article.] *J Sci Med Sport* 2006;9(1–2):11–22.
Onwuanyi ON. Calcaneal spurs and plantar heel pad pain. *Foot* 2000;10(4):182–185.
Smith S, Tinley P, Gilheany M, et al. The inferior calcaneal spur—anatomical and histological considerations. *Foot* 2007;17(1):25–31.
Thomas JL, Christensen JC, Kravitz SR, et al. The diagnosis and treatment of heel pain: a clinical practice guideline–revision 2010. *J Foot Ankle Surg* 2010; 49(3):S1–S19.
Waldman SD, Campbell RSD. Calcaneal spurs. In: *Atlas of Common Pain Syndromes.* 3rd ed. Philadelphia, PA: Saunders Elsevier; 2012:380–382.
Waldman SD. Injection technique for calcaneal spurs. In: *Atlas of Pain Management Injection Techniques.* 3rd ed. Philadelphia, PA: Saunders Elsevier; 2013:456–457.

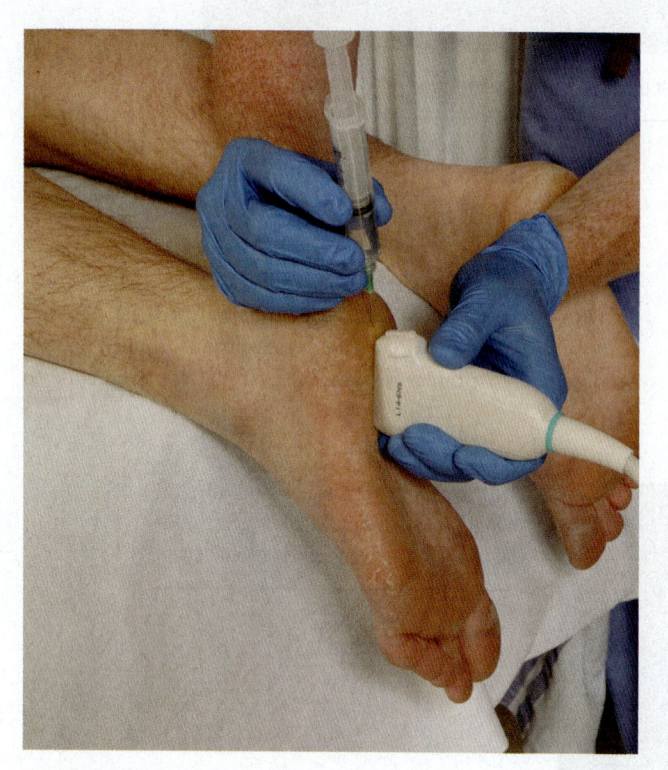

**FIGURE 159.10.** Proper needle placement for an ultrasound-guided out-of-plane injection for calcaneal spurs.

# CHAPTER 160

# Ultrasound-Guided Injection Technique for Posterior Tibialis Tendonitis

## CLINICAL PERSPECTIVES

Posterior tibialis tendonitis is a clinical syndrome characterized by sharp, constant, and severe inner ankle pain. This painful condition is often seen as a result of acute eversion injuries to the ankle although it is also seen with overuse or misuse of the ankle in foot, as seen in long-distance running with improper shoes. Recently, there have been a number of reports of posterior tibialis tendonitis in Irish dancers as a result of the "leap-over move" that is a common part of their dance routine (Fig. 160.1). Patients suffering from posterior tibialis tendonitis will often splint the inflamed posterior tibialis tendon by adopting an antalgic gait to avoid using the affected tendon. This dysfunctional gait may cause a secondary bursitis and tendonitis around the foot and ankle, which may serve to confuse the clinical picture and further increase the patient's pain and disability. Pain on palpation of the posterior tibialis tendon as it passes behind the medial malleolus is a consistent finding in patients with posterior tibialis tendonitis as is exacerbation of pain with active resisted inversion and passive eversion of the ankle (Fig. 160.2). The inner aspect of the ankle may feel hot and appear swollen, which may be misdiagnosed as superficial thrombophlebitis or cellulitis. Patients suffering from posterior tibialis tendonitis will also often complain that it feels like their shoes are rubbing the inside of their ankles raw, although on examination the skin appears normal. A creaking or grating sensation may be palpated when passively inverting and everting the ankle. Untreated, posterior tibialis tendonitis will result in increasing pain and functional disability calcium deposition around the tendon occurring, making subsequent treatment more difficult. Continued trauma to the inflamed tendon ultimately may result in tendon rupture (Fig. 160.3). Rupture of the posterior tibialis tendon will result if disruption of the normal architecture of the foot resulting in the loss of the arch of the foot and development of the pes planus deformity (Fig. 160.4).

Plain radiographs are indicated in all patients who present with medial ankle pain. Based on the patient's clinical presentation, additional testing may be indicated, including complete blood cell count, sedimentation rate, and antinuclear antibody testing. Magnetic resonance imaging and/or ultrasound imaging of the ankle is indicated if posterior tibialis tendonitis, rupture, or joint instability is suggested (Figs. 160.5 and 160.6). Radionuclide bone scanning is useful to identify stress fractures of the tibia not seen on plain radiographs. The injection technique described later serves as both a diagnostic and a therapeutic maneuver.

## CLINICALLY RELEVANT ANATOMY

The posterior tibialis muscle plantar flexes the foot at the ankle and inverts the foot at the subtalar and transverse tarsal joints. The muscle finds its origin from the posterior tibia and fibula. The tendon of the muscle passes behind the medial malleolus, running beneath the flexor retinaculum, and into the sole of the foot where it inserts on the navicular bone (Fig. 160.7). The posterior tibialis tendon is susceptible to the development of tendonitis as it curves around the medial malleolus.

## ULTRASOUND-GUIDED TECHNIQUE

Ultrasound-guided injection technique for posterior tibialis tendonitis involves blocking the inflamed tendon as it passes behind the medial malleolus. The technique can be carried out by placing the patient in the supine position with the arms resting comfortably along the patient's chest and the affected lower extremity externally rotated (Fig. 160.8). A total of 4 mL of local anesthetic and 80 mg of depot steroid is drawn up in a 12-mL sterile syringe. The medial malleolus is then identified by palpation (Fig. 160.9). A linear high-frequency ultrasound transducer is placed in a longitudinal plane, with the middle of the ultrasound transducer lying over the posterior border of the medial malleolus (Fig. 160.10). This will put the ultrasound transducer parallel to the posterior tibialis tendon as it passes behind the medial malleolus. An ultrasound survey scan is taken. The posterior tibialis tendon can be seen lying just behind the medial malleolus as a fibular linear structure (Figs. 160.11 and 160.12). When the posterior tibialis tendon is identified on ultrasound imaging, the skin is prepped with anesthetic solution and a 1½-inch, 22-gauge needle is advanced from the superior border of the

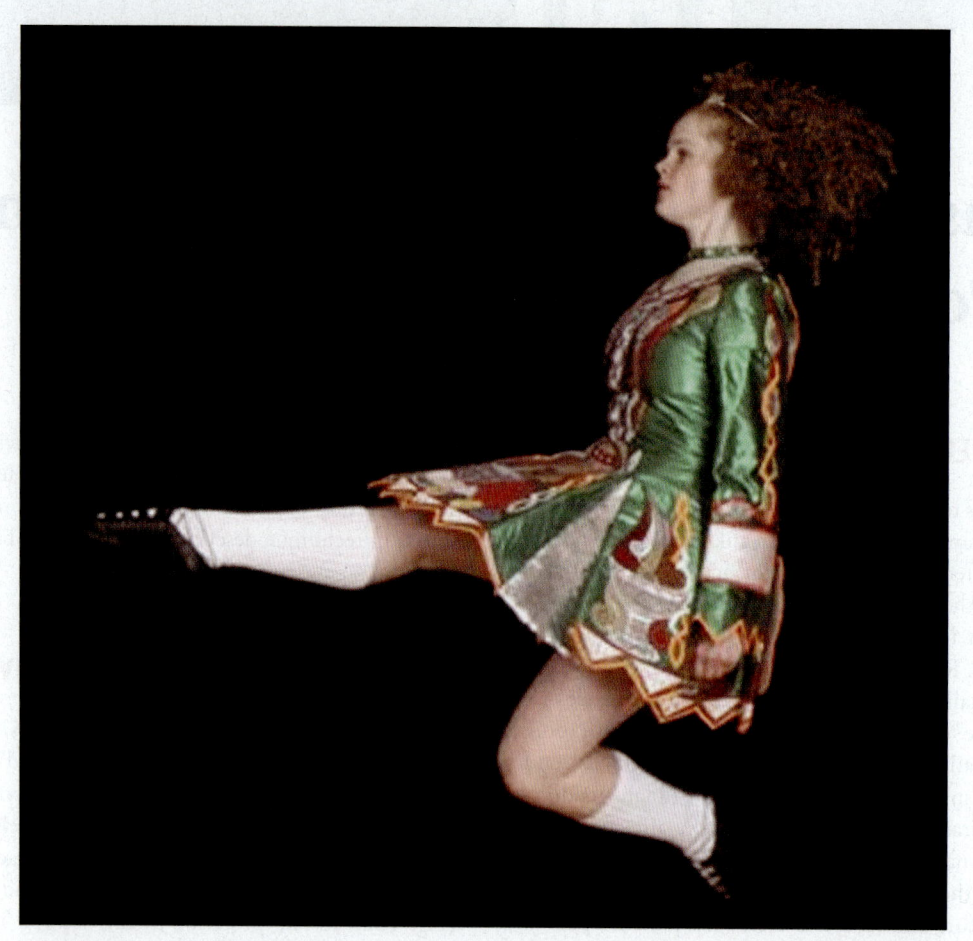

**FIGURE 160.1.** The leap-over move, which is popular in Irish dancing, has been implicated in the development of posterior tibialis tendonitis.

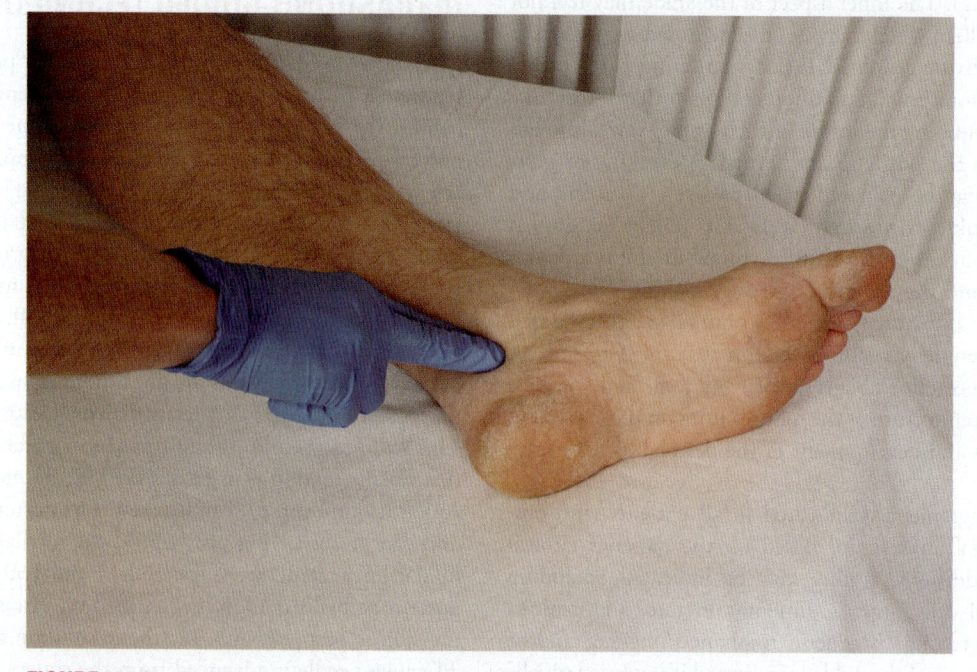

**FIGURE 160.2.** Pain on palpation of the posterior tibialis tendon as it passes behind the medial malleolus is a consistent finding in patients with posterior tibialis tendonitis.

# CHAPTER 160  ULTRASOUND-GUIDED INJECTION TECHNIQUE FOR POSTERIOR TIBIALIS TENDONITIS

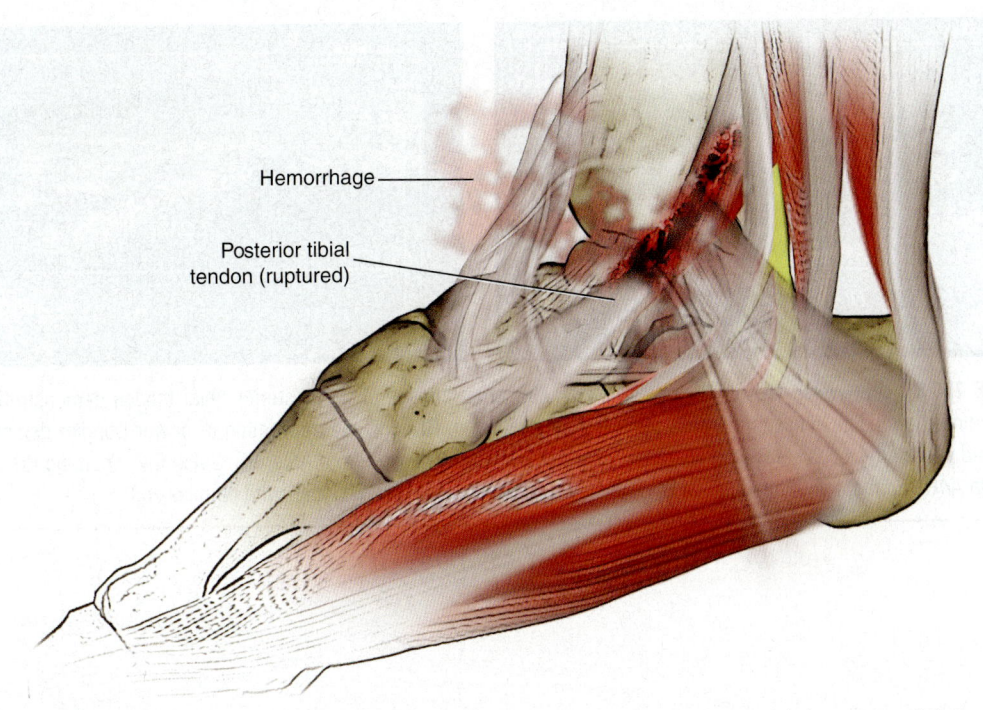

**FIGURE 160.3.** Failure to aggressively treat posterior tibialis tendonitis may result in rupture of the tendon.

ultrasound transducer and advanced utilizing an in-plane approach with the trajectory being adjusted under real-time ultrasound guidance until the needle tip is resting in proximity to the posterior tibialis tendon, but not within the tendon itself (Fig. 160.13). When the tip of needle is thought to be in satisfactory position, after careful aspiration, a small amount of local anesthetic and steroid is injected under real-time ultrasound guidance to confirm that the needle tip is in proximity to the posterior tibialis tendon, but not within the tendon itself. There should be minimal resistance to injection. After needle tip placement is confirmed, the remainder of the contents of the syringe are slowly injected. The needle is then removed, and a sterile pressure dressing and ice pack are placed at the injection site.

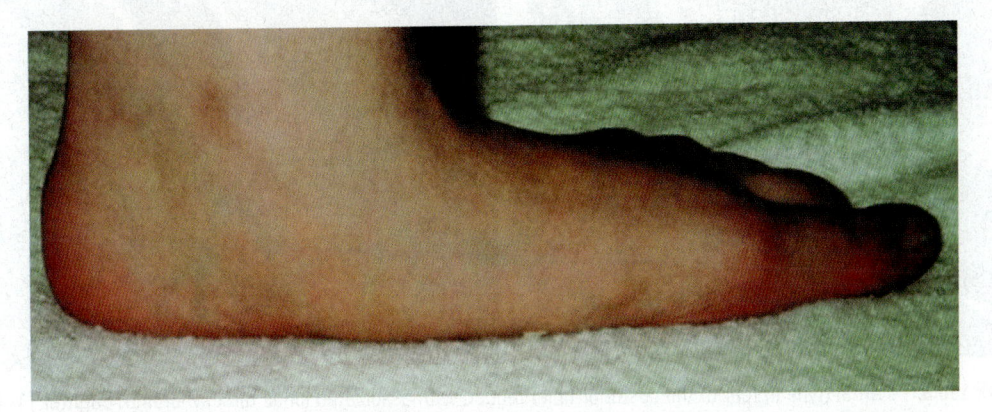

**FIGURE 160.4.** Rupture of the posterior tibialis tendon will result if disruption of the normal architecture of the foot resulting in the loss of the arch of the foot and development of the pes planus deformity.

**1124** SECTION X ANKLE AND FOOT

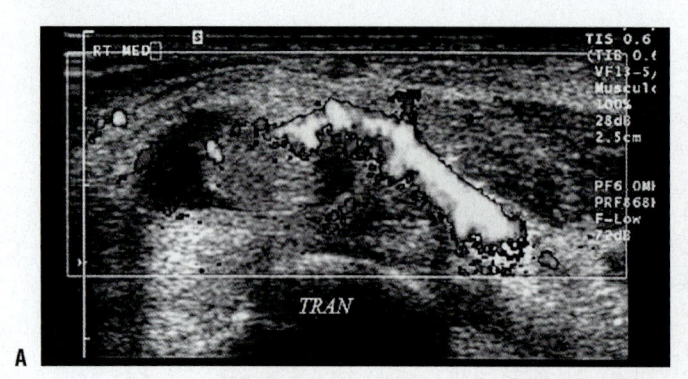

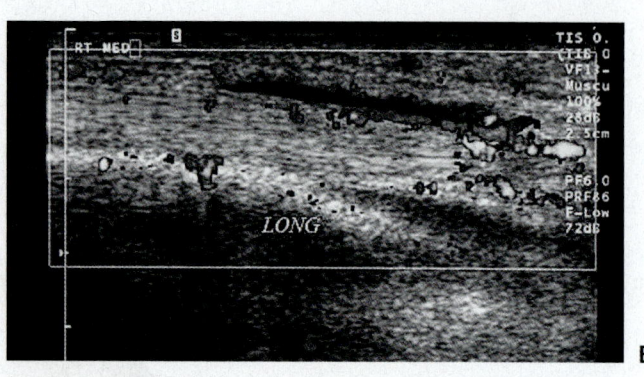

**FIGURE 160.5.** Transverse **(A)** and longitudinal **(B)** ultrasound images of the posterior tibial tendon demonstrating fluid surrounding the tendon, consistent with a tendon sheath effusion. Of note, the application of power Doppler demonstrates increased vascularity, consistent with posterior tibial tenosynovitis. (Reused from Adler RS, Sofka CM, Positano RG. *Atlas of Foot and Ankle Sonography.* Philadelphia, PA: Lippincott Williams & Wilkins; 2004:59, with permission.)

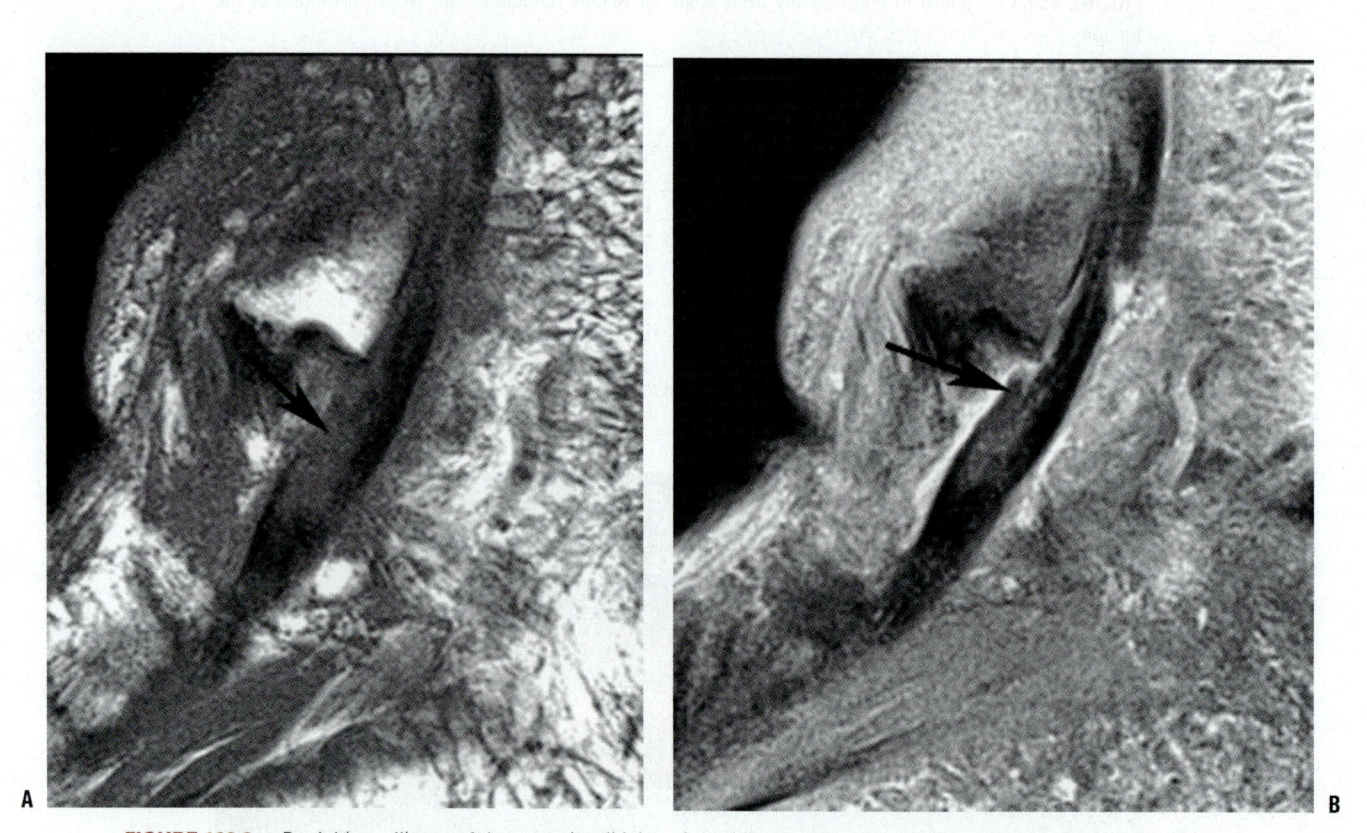

**FIGURE 160.6.** Partial (type II) tear of the posterior tibial tendon with associated sinus tarsi syndrome. Sagittal T1- **(A)** and T2- **(B)** weighted and axial T2-weighted **(C)** images through the posterior tibial tendon demonstrate a tear at the malleolar tip (*arrow*) with thickening of the tendon and fluid in the tendon sheath.

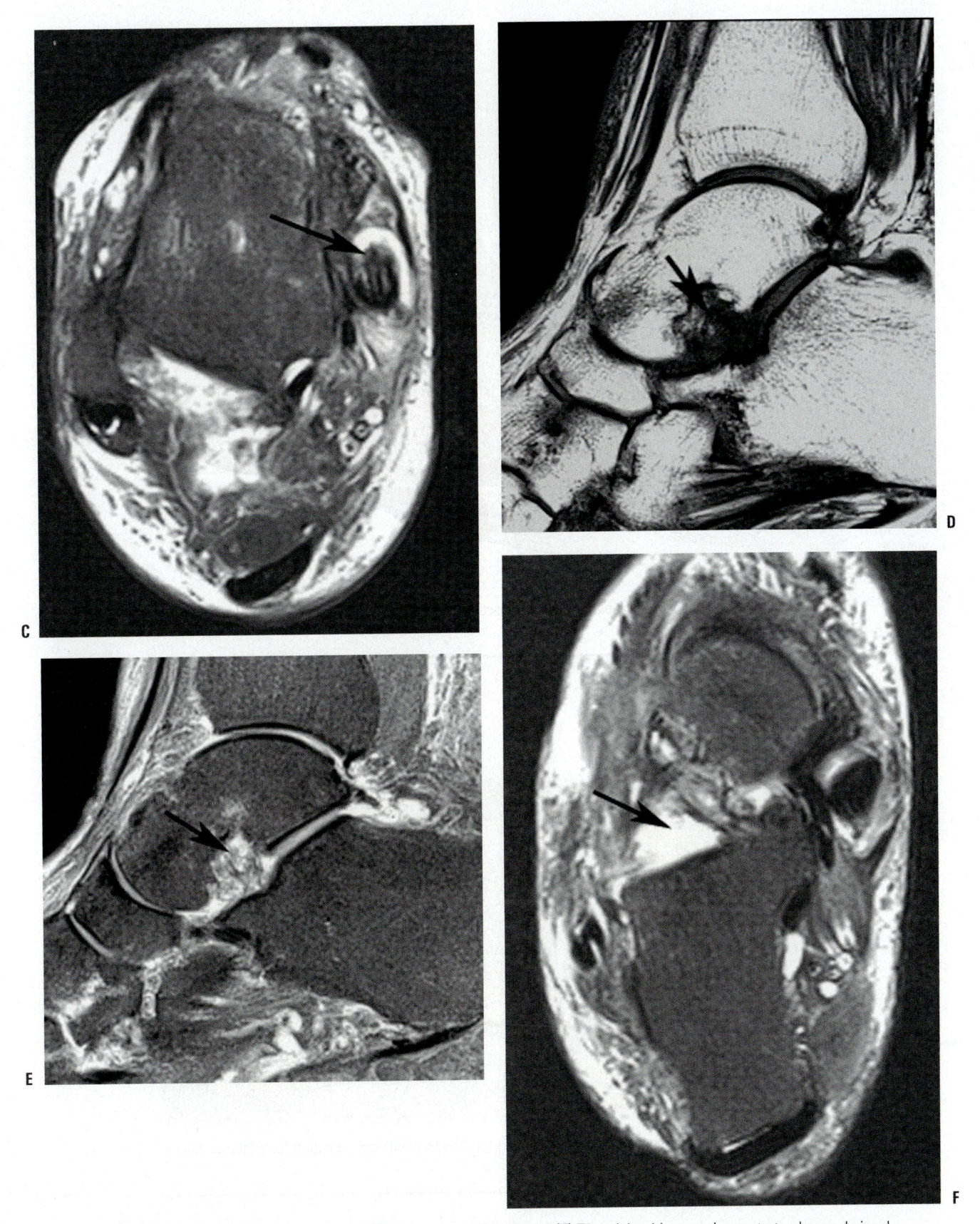

**FIGURE 160.6.** *(Continued)* Sagittal T1- **(D)** and sagittal **(E)** and axial **(F)** T2-weighted images demonstrate abnormal signal intensity in the tarsal canal and sinus (*arrow*) due to associated sinus tarsi syndrome. (Reused from Berquist TH. *Imaging of the Foot and Ankle.* 3rd ed. Philadelphia, PA: Lippincott Williams & Wilkins; 2011:157–158, with permission.)

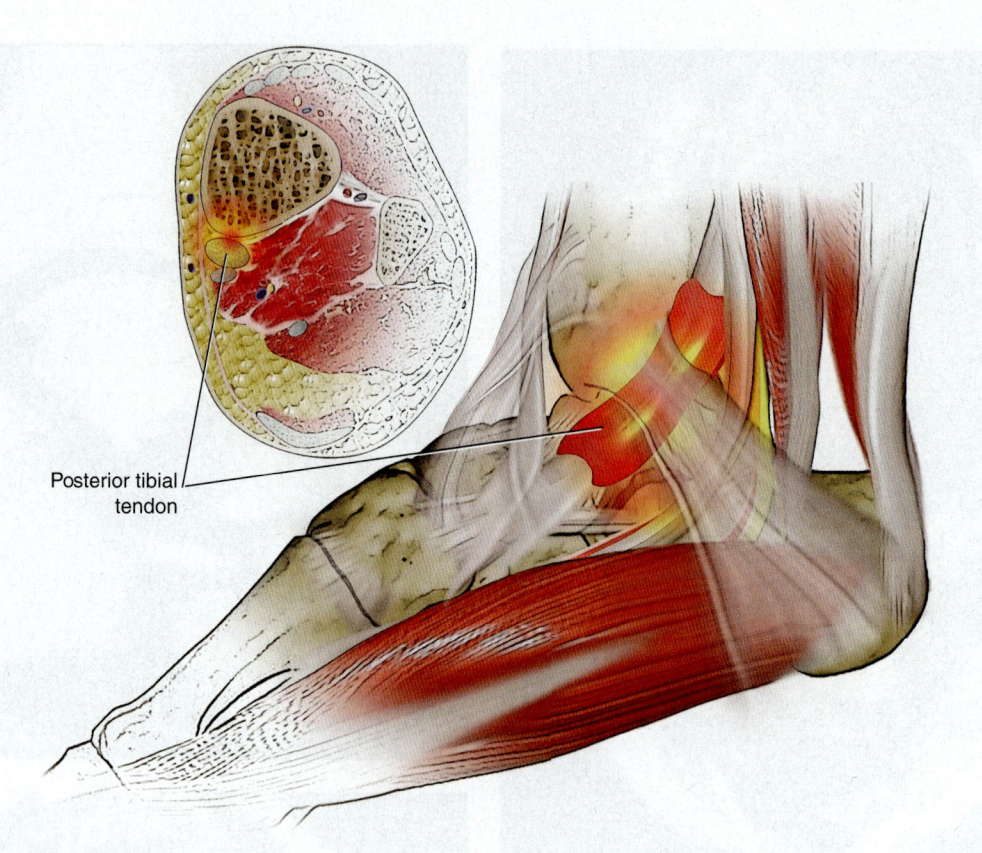

**FIGURE 160.7.** The posterior tibialis tendon is susceptible to the development of tendonitis as it passes behind the medial malleolus.

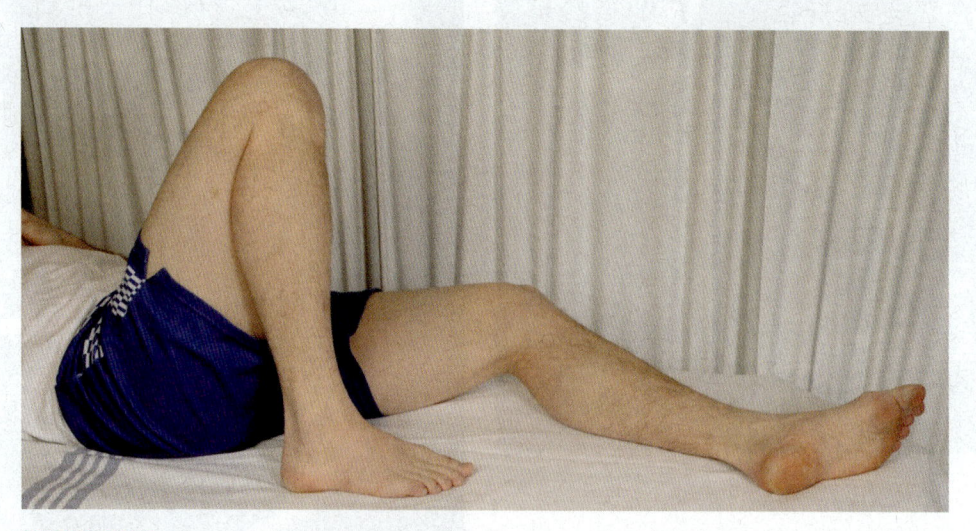

**FIGURE 160.8.** Proper supine patient positioning for ultrasound-guided injection for posterior tibialis tendonitis.

CHAPTER 160   ULTRASOUND-GUIDED INJECTION TECHNIQUE FOR POSTERIOR TIBIALIS TENDONITIS

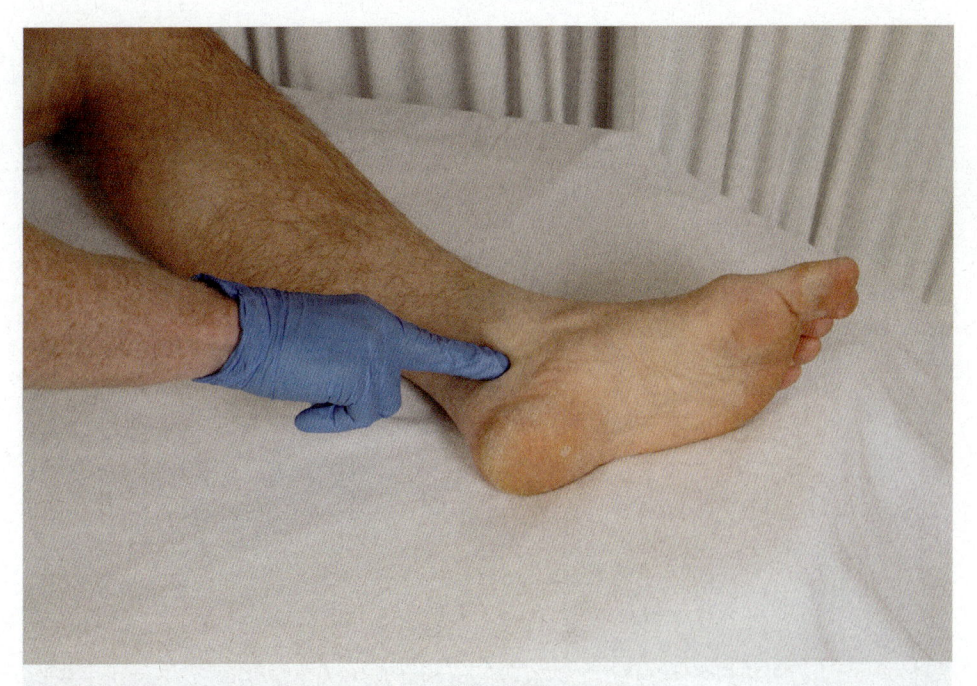

**FIGURE 160.9.** Palpation of the posterior medial malleolus.

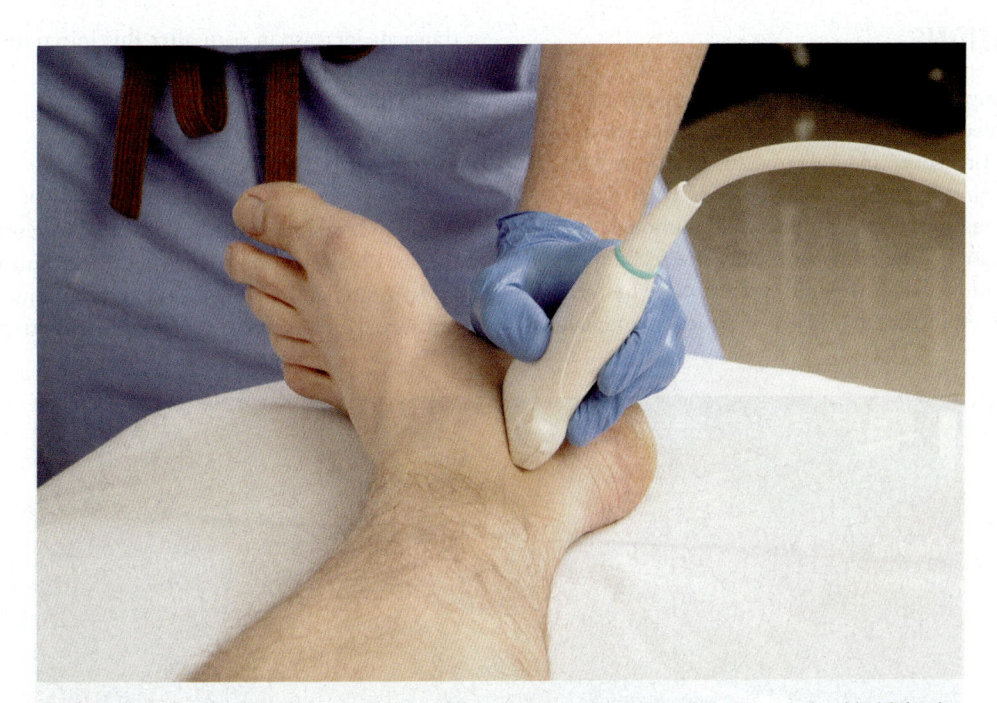

**FIGURE 160.10.** Proper longitudinal ultrasound transducer placement for ultrasound-guided injection for posterior tibialis tendonitis.

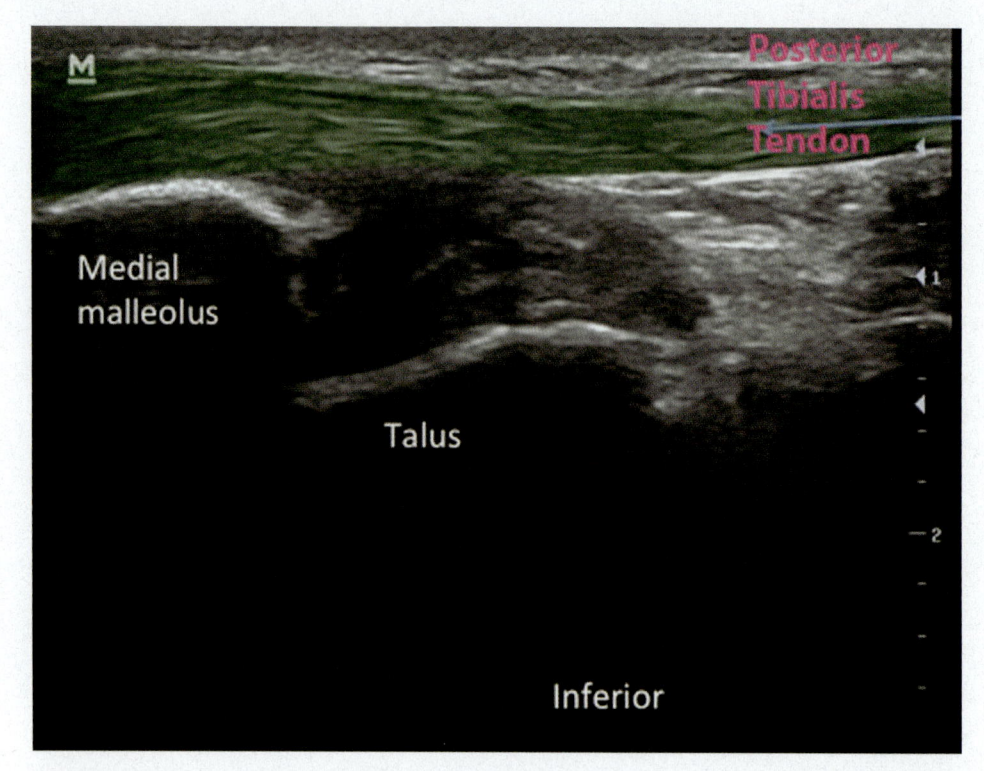

**FIGURE 160.11.** Longitudinal view of the posterior tibialis tendon as it passes behind the medial malleolus.

## COMPLICATIONS

The major complication of this ultrasound-guided injection technique is infection. Ecchymosis and hematoma formation following this procedure may also occur. The possibility of trauma to the already compromised tendons from the injection itself remains an ever-present possibility, although the risk of this is decreased if the clinician uses gentle technique and stops injecting immediately if significant resistance to injection is encountered. Approximately 25% of patients complain of a transient increase in pain after this injection technique; the patient should be warned of this.

## CLINICAL PEARLS

Bursitis and tendonitis of the ankle and foot may coexist with posterior tibialis tendonitis and may contribute to the patient's pain symptomatology. Universal precautions should always be observed to protect the operator, and strict adherence to

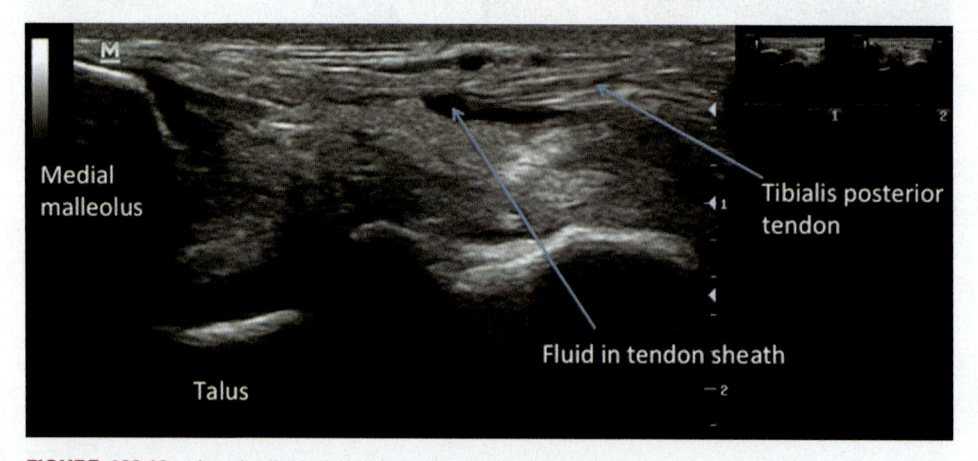

**FIGURE 160.12.** Longitudinal view of the posterior tibialis tendon as it passes behind the medial malleolus demonstrating fluid within the tendon sheath.

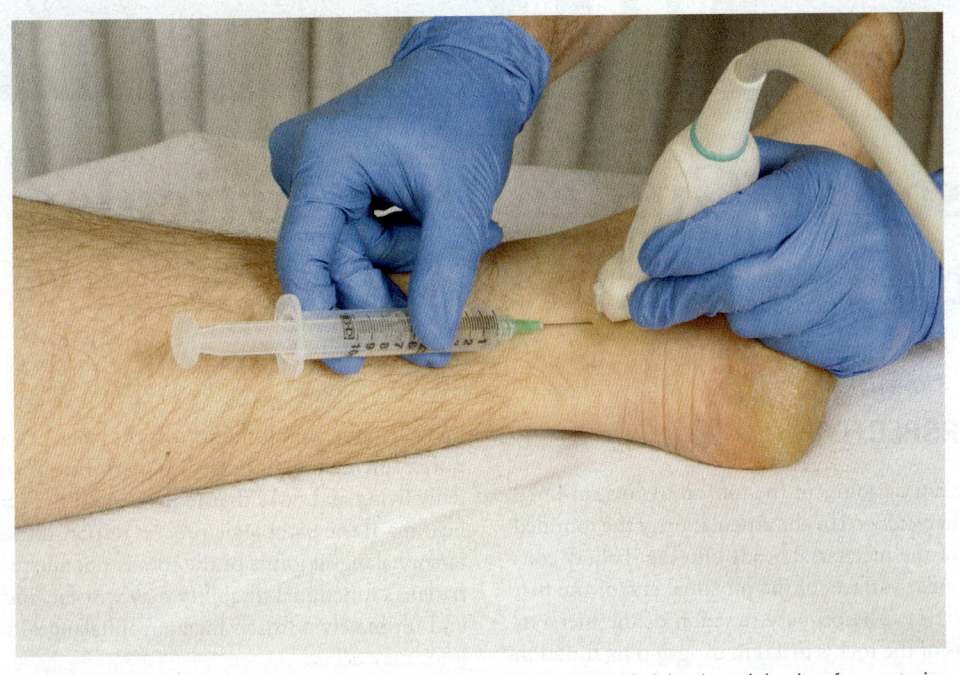

**FIGURE 160.13.** Proper needle placement for an ultrasound-guided in-plane injection for posterior tibialis tendonitis.

sterile technique must be used to avoid infection. Gentle physical therapy and local heat should be introduced following ultrasound-guided injection of posterior tibialis tendonitis to reduce pain and improve function. Simple analgesics and non-steroidal anti-inflammatory agents or COX-2 inhibitors may be used concurrently with this injection technique.

## SUGGESTED READINGS

Bowring B, Chockalingam N. Conservative treatment of tibialis posterior tendon dysfunction—a review. *Foot* 2010;20(1):18–26.

Edwards MR, Jack C, Singh SK. Tibialis posterior dysfunction. *Curr Orthop* 2008;22(3):185–192.

Shibuya N, Ramanujam CL, Garcia GM. Association of tibialis posterior tendon pathology with other radiographic findings in the foot: a case-control study. [Original Research Article]. *J Foot Ankle Surg* 2008;47(6):546–553.

Waldman SD. Posterior tibialis tendonitis. In: *Pain Review*. Philadelphia, PA: Saunders Elsevier; 2009:325.

Waldman SD, Campbell RSD. Posterior tibialis tendonitis. In: *Atlas of Uncommon Pain Syndromes*. 2nd ed. Philadelphia, PA: Saunders Elsevier; 2009:300–304.

Waldman SD, Campbell RSD. Posterior tibialis tendon rupture. In: *Imaging of Pain*. Philadelphia, PA: Saunders Elsevier; 2011:435–436.

Waldman SD. Injection technique for posterior tibialis tendonitis. In: *Atlas of Pain Management Injection Techniques*. 3rd ed. Philadelphia, PA: Saunders Elsevier; 2012:662–663.

# CHAPTER 161

# Ultrasound-Guided Intra-articular Injection of the Toe Joints

## CLINICAL PERSPECTIVES

The metatarsophalangeal joints of the toes are synovium-lined condyloid joints characterized by the articulation of the rounded articular surfaces of the metatarsal heads into the shallow concavities of the articular surfaces of the proximal end of the first phalanges (Fig. 161.1). The primary function of the metatarsophalangeal joints of the toes is to aid in the gripping function of the foot. The articular cartilage of the metatarsophalangeal joints of the toes is susceptible to damage, which, left untreated, will result in arthritis with its associated pain and functional disability. Osteoarthritis is seen in the metatarsophalangeal joints of the toes, which results in pain and functional disability, with rheumatoid arthritis, posttraumatic arthritis, and crystal arthropathy also causing arthritis of the metatarsophalangeal joints of the toes. Gout selectively afflicts the metatarsophalangeal joint of the first toe and is called podagra (Fig. 161.2). Less common causes of arthritis-induced pain of the metatarsophalangeal joints of the toes include the other collagen vascular diseases, infection, villonodular synovitis, and Lyme disease. Acute infectious arthritis of the metatarsophalangeal joints of the toes joint is best treated with early diagnosis, with culture and sensitivity of the synovial fluid, and with prompt initiation of antibiotic therapy. The collagen vascular diseases generally manifest as a polyarthropathy rather than a monoarthropathy limited to the metatarsophalangeal joints of the toes, although pain of the metatarsophalangeal joints of the toes secondary to the collagen vascular diseases responds exceedingly well to ultrasound-guided intra-articular injection.

Patients with pain of the metatarsophalangeal joints of the toes secondary to arthritis, gout, synovitis, and collagen vascular disease–related joint pain complain of pain that is localized to the head of the metatarsals. Activity, including walking and weight bearing, makes the pain worse, with rest and heat providing some relief. The pain is constant and characterized as aching in nature. Sleep disturbance is common with awakening when patients roll over onto the affected foot. Some patients complain of a grating, catching, or popping sensation with range of motion of the joints, and crepitus may be appreciated on physical examination.

Functional disability often accompanies the pain associated with the many pathologic conditions of the metatarsophalangeal joints of the toes. Patients will often notice increasing difficulty in performing their activities of daily living and tasks that require standing, walking, or weight bearing. If the pathologic process responsible for pain of metatarsophalangeal joints of the toes is not adequately treated, the patient's functional disability may worsen, and muscle wasting and ultimately a frozen metatarsophalangeal joints of the toes joint may occur.

Plain radiographs are indicated in all patients who present with pain of the metatarsophalangeal joints of the toes (Fig. 161.3). Based on the patient's clinical presentation, additional testing may be indicated, including complete blood cell count, sedimentation rate, and antinuclear antibody testing. Magnetic resonance imaging or ultrasound of the metatarsophalangeal joints of the toes joint is indicated if fracture, effusion, tendinopathy, crystal arthropathy, joint mice, synovitis, foreign body, bursitis, or ligamentous injury is suspected (Fig. 161.4).

## CLINICALLY RELEVANT ANATOMY

The metatarsophalangeal joints of the toes are condyloid joints characterized by the articulation of the rounded articular surfaces of the metatarsal heads into the shallow concavities of the articular surfaces of the proximal end of the first phalanges (see Fig. 161.1). Each joint is lined with synovium, and the ample synovial space allows for intra-articular placement of needles for injection and aspiration. The metatarsophalangeal joints have a dense joint capsule and strong plantar and collateral ligaments, although fracture and subluxation may still occur. The metatarsophalangeal joints of the toes are also susceptible to overuse and misuse injuries with resultant inflammation and arthritis.

## ULTRASOUND-GUIDED TECHNIQUE

The benefits, risks, and alternative treatments are explained to the patient, and informed consent is obtained. The patient is then placed in the supine position with the knee flexed so that the plantar surface of the affected foot rests comfortably

CHAPTER 161 ULTRASOUND-GUIDED INTRA-ARTICULAR INJECTION OF THE TOE JOINTS 1131

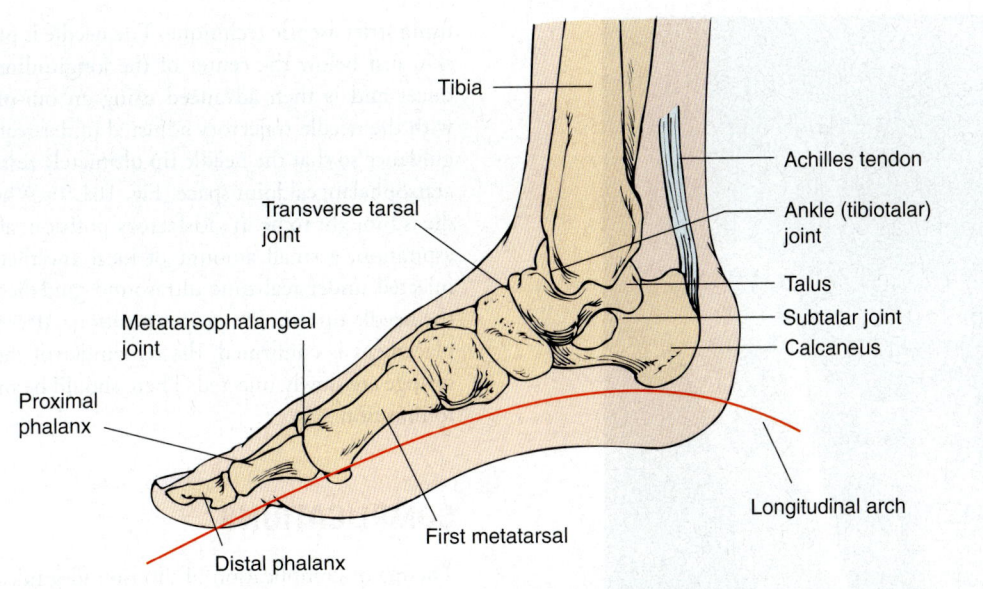

**FIGURE 161.1.** Anatomy of the metatarsophalangeal joints. (Reused from Weber J, Kelley J. *Health Assessment in Nursing*. 2nd ed. Philadelphia, PA: Lippincott Williams & Wilkins; 2003, with permission.)

on the examination table (Fig. 161.5). With the patient in the above position, the dorsal surface of the metatarsophalangeal joint of the affected toe is identified by palpation (Fig. 161.6). A high-frequency small linear ultrasound transducer is placed in a longitudinal position over the metatarsophalangeal joint of the affected toe, and an ultrasound survey scan is taken (Figs. 161.7 and 161.8). The hypoechoic joint space is identified between the head of the metatarsal and the base of the proximal phalanges. When the joint space is identified, the skin overlying the area beneath the ultrasound transducer as well as the skin covering the lateral portion of the joint is then prepped with antiseptic solution. A sterile syringe containing 1.0 mL of 0.25% preservative-free bupivacaine and 40 mg of methylprednisolone is attached to a 1½-inch, 25-gauge needle

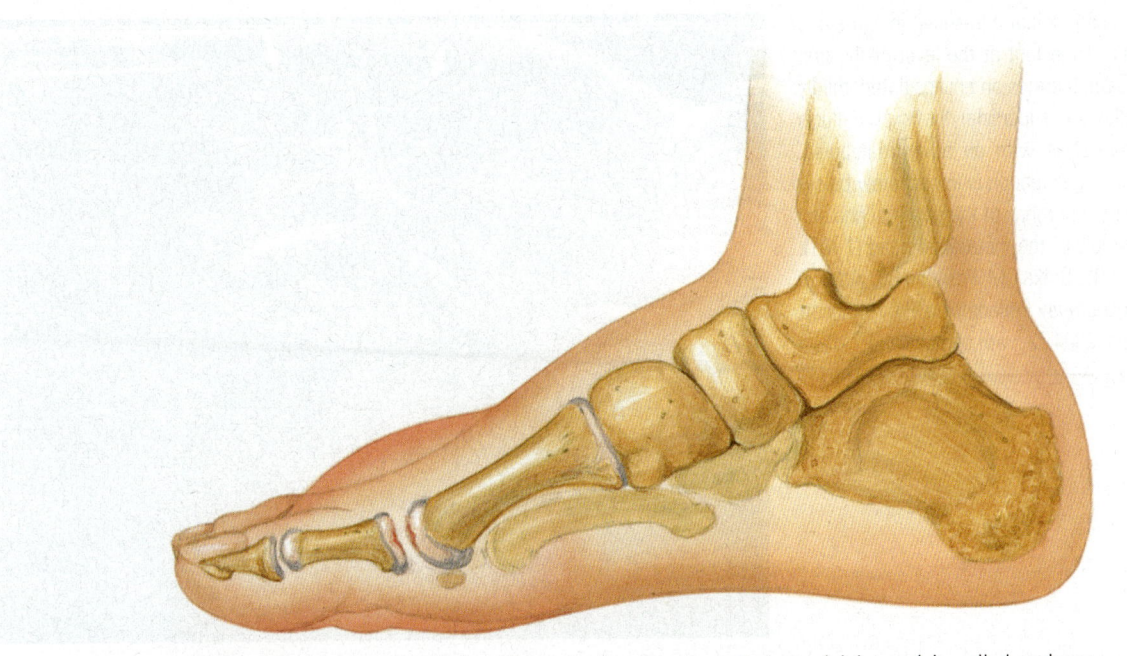

**FIGURE 161.2.** Gout frequently afflicts the first metatarsophalangeal joint and is called podagra. (Anatomical Chart Company, 2013.)

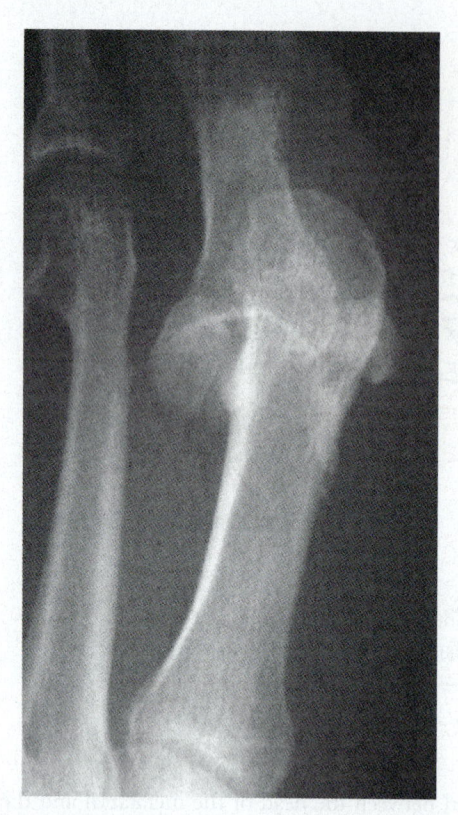

**FIGURE 161.3.** Plain radiograph of metatarsophalangeal joint showing a complete dislocation. (Reused from Bucholz RW, Heckman JD. *Rockwood & Green's Fractures in Adults.* 5th ed. Philadelphia, PA: Lippincott Williams & Wilkins; 2001, with permission.)

using strict aseptic technique. The needle is placed through the skin just below the center of the longitudinally placed transducer and is then advanced using an out-of-plane approach with the needle trajectory adjusted under real-time ultrasound guidance so that the needle tip ultimately rests within the metatarsophalangeal joint space (Fig. 161.9). When the tip of needle is thought to be in satisfactory position, after careful gentle aspiration, a small amount of local anesthetic and steroid is injected under real-time ultrasound guidance to confirm that the needle tip is in the proper position. After proper needle tip placement is confirmed, the remainder of the contents of the syringe are slowly injected. There should be minimal resistance to injection.

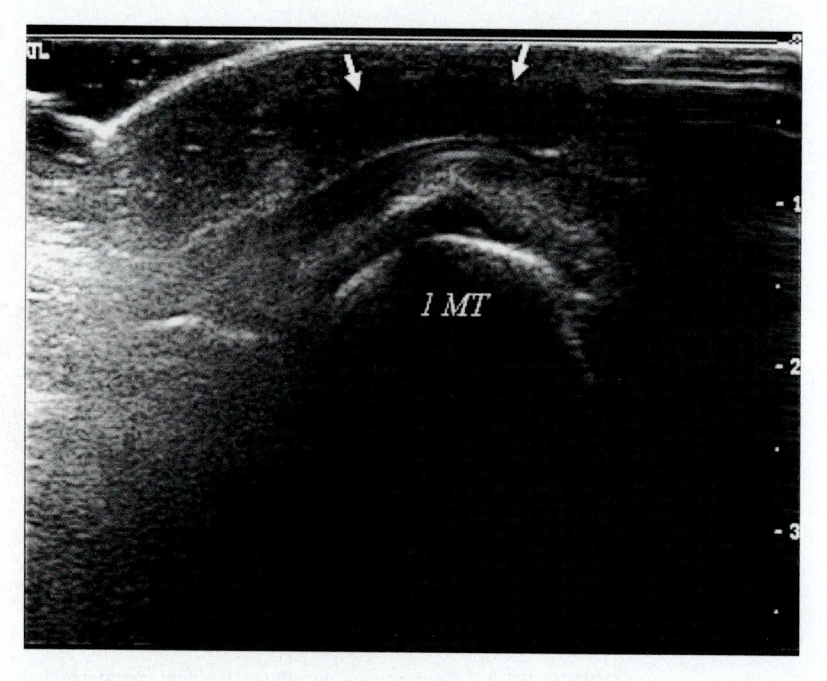

## COMPLICATIONS

The major complication of ultrasound-guided injection of the metatarsophalangeal joints of the toes is infection. Ecchymosis and hematoma formation may also occur. A transient exacerbation of the patient's pain occurs ~25% of the time following this injection technique, and the patient should be warned of this possibility prior to the procedure.

## CLINICAL PEARLS

Toe pathology including tendinopathy, occult fractures, osteoarthritis, rheumatoid arthritis, crystal arthropathies,

**FIGURE 161.4.** Longitudinal ultrasound image along the plantar aspect of the foot at the level of the first metatarsal head demonstrates an encapsulated, mildly heterogenous collection superficial to flexor hallucis longus tendon consistent with an adventitial bursa. The flexor hallucis longus tendon is immediately below the collection, and the portions of the proximal phalanx are present to the left of the metatarsal head (1 MT). (Reused from Adler RS, Sofka CM, Positano RG. *Atlas of Foot and Ankle Sonography.* Philadelphia, PA: Lippincott Williams & Wilkins; 2004:22, with permission.)

CHAPTER 161 ULTRASOUND-GUIDED INTRA-ARTICULAR INJECTION OF THE TOE JOINTS 1133

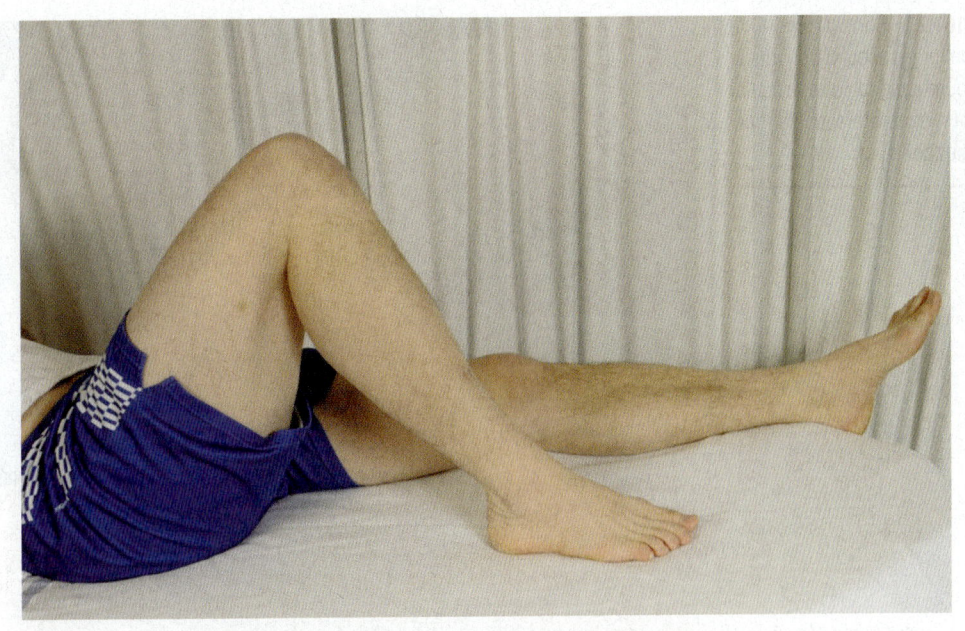

**FIGURE 161.5.** Proper patient position for ultrasound-guided injection of the metatarsophalangeal joint.

avascular necrosis bursitis, synovitis, and impingement syndromes may coexist with disease of the metatarsophalangeal joints of the toes and may contribute to the patient's pain symptomatology. Universal precautions should always be observed to protect the operator, and strict adherence to sterile technique must be used to avoid infection. Gentle physical therapy and local heat should be introduced following ultrasound-guided injection of the metatarsophalangeal joints of the toes to reduce pain and improve function. Simple analgesics and nonsteroidal anti-inflammatory agents or COX-2 inhibitors may be used concurrently with this injection technique.

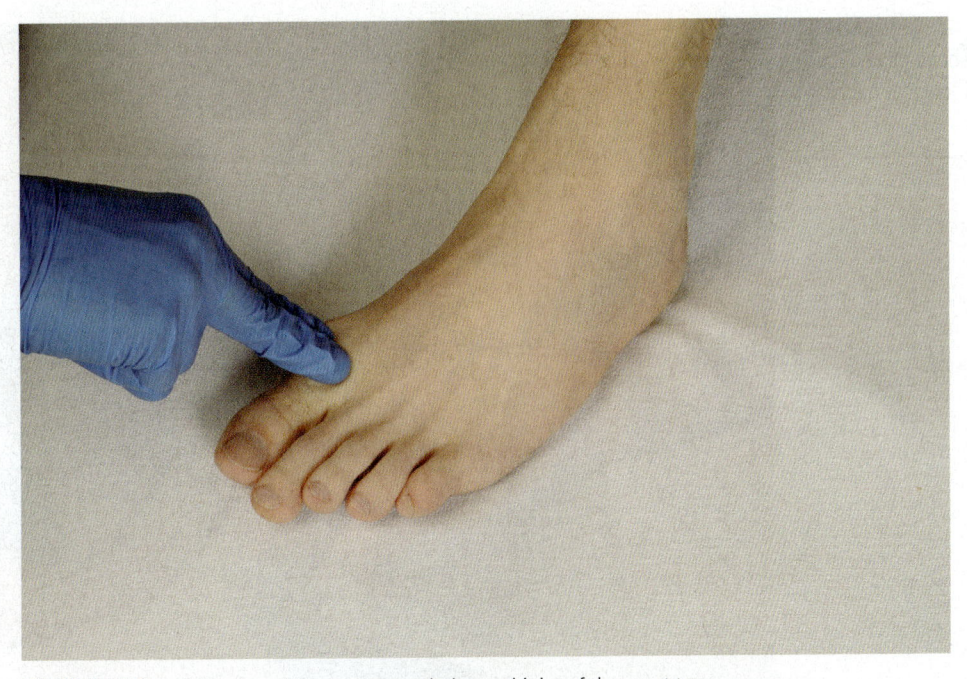

**FIGURE 161.6.** Palpation of the metatarsophalangeal joint of the great toe.

**FIGURE 161.7.** Correct longitudinal position for ultrasound transducer for ultrasound-guided intra-articular injection of the metatarsophalangeal joints of the toes joint.

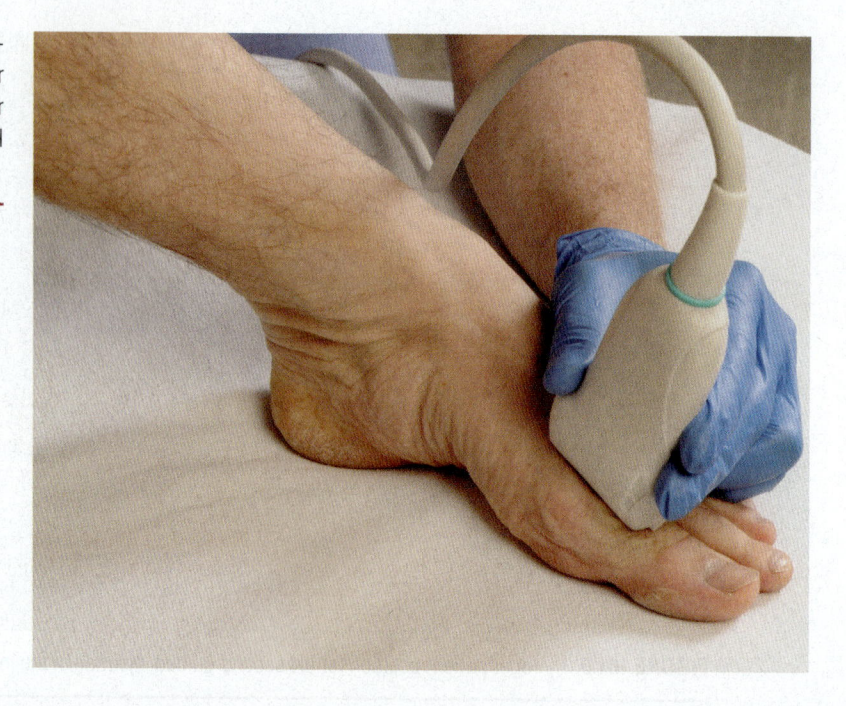

**FIGURE 161.8.** Longitudinal ultrasound view of the metatarsophalangeal joint space.

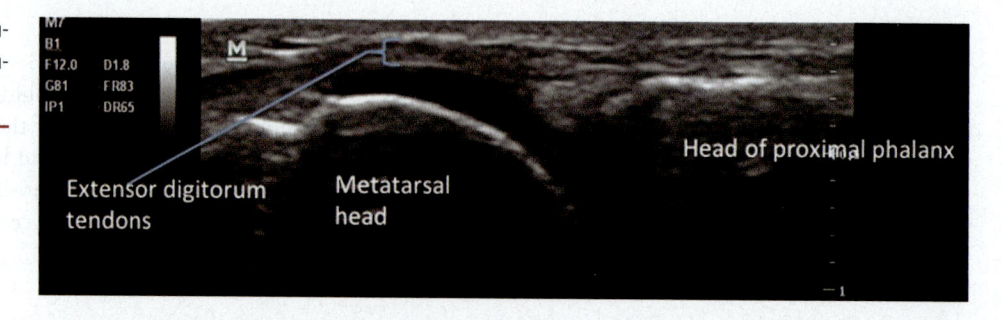

**FIGURE 161.9.** Proper needle position for ultrasound-guided out-of-plane injection of the metatarsophalangeal joint.

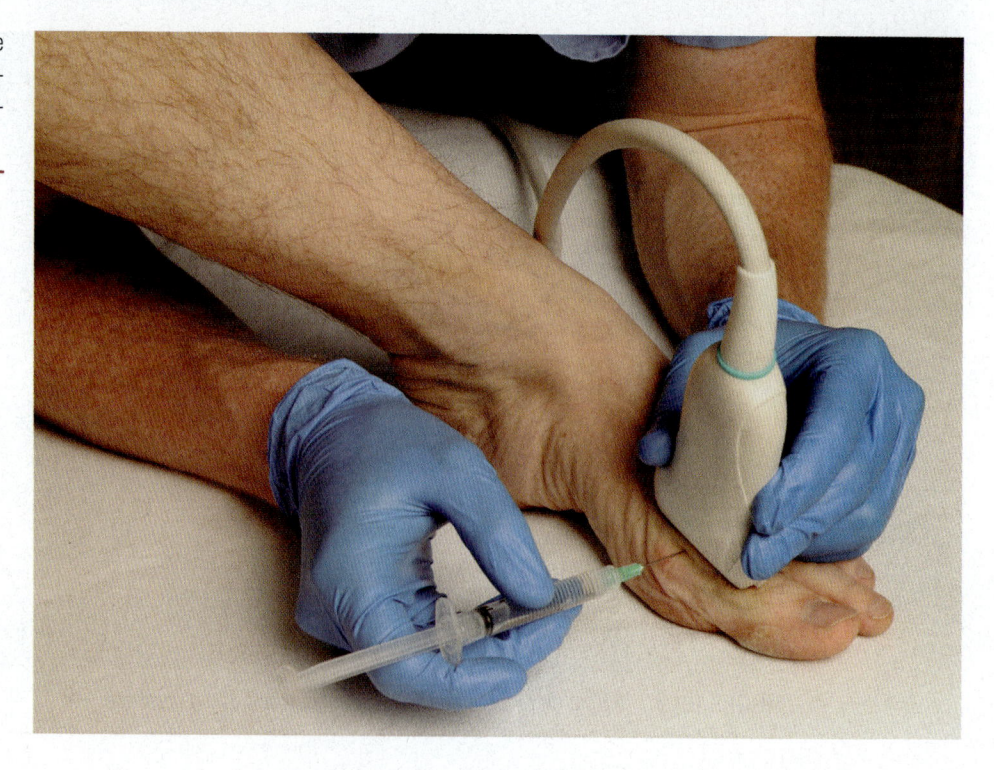

## SUGGESTED READINGS

De Zordo T, Mur E, Bellmann-Weiler R, et al. US guided injections in arthritis. *Eur J Radiol* 2009;71(2):197–203.

Grassi W, Salaffi F, Filipucci E. Ultrasound in rheumatology. *Best Pract Res Clin Rheumatol* 2005;19(3):467–485.

Waldman SD. Intra-articular injection of the toe joints. In: *Pain Review*. Philadelphia, PA: Saunders Elsevier; 2009:591–592.

Waldman SD. Technique for intra-articular injection of the toe joints. In: *Atlas of Pain Management Injection Techniques*. 3rd ed. Philadelphia, PA: Saunders Elsevier; 2012:419–421.

# CHAPTER 162

# Ultrasound-Guided Metatarsal and Digital Nerve Block of the Foot

## CLINICAL PERSPECTIVES

Ultrasound-guided metatarsal and digital nerve block is useful in the management of the pain subserved by the metatarsal and digital nerves. This technique serves as an excellent adjunct to lumbar plexus block and for general anesthesia when performing surgery on the toes and is seeing increased utilization to provide anesthesia for reduction of fractures and dislocations of the metatarsals and phalanges as well as to provide surgical anesthesia for tendon repairs and plastic surgery repairs of complex toe injuries. Ultrasound-guided metatarsal and digital nerve block can also be used to provide postoperative pain relief following total joint arthroplasties of the joints of the toes.

Ultrasound-guided metatarsal and digital nerve block can also be used as a diagnostic tool when performing differential neural blockade on an anatomic basis in the evaluation of foot and toe pain as well as in a prognostic manner to determine the degree of neurologic impairment the patient will suffer when destruction of a metatarsal or digital nerve is being considered or when there is a possibility that the nerve may be sacrificed during surgeries in this anatomic region. This technique may also be useful in those patients suffering symptoms from compression of the metatarsal and digital nerves from tumor, aneurysms of the digital arteries, sesamoid bones, or osteophytes (Fig. 162.1).

Patients suffering from dysfunction of the metatarsal or digital nerve may suffer from pain with pressure on the nerve making it difficult to wear shoes. Dysesthesias are common as is sleep disturbance. On physical examination, pain can be elicited by compression over the affected nerve. Continued compression of the affected nerve may cause numbness distal to the point of compression. Coexistent arthritis, sesamoiditis, gout, other crystal arthropathies, and synovitis of the metatarsal and interphalangeal joints may predispose the patient to the development of entrapment of the metatarsal and digital nerves.

Plain radiographs of the feet are indicated in all patients suspected of suffering from metatarsal and digital nerve dysfunction to rule out occult bony pathology (Fig. 162.2). Based on the patient's clinical presentation, additional testing may be indicated, including complete blood cell count, uric acid, sedimentation rate, and antinuclear antibody testing. Magnetic resonance imaging and ultrasound imaging of the foot are indicated to assess the status of the affected nerves as well as to identify other occult pathology including arthritis, sesamoiditis, and synovitis (Fig. 162.3).

## CLINICALLY RELEVANT ANATOMY

In a manner analogous to that of the digital nerves of the hand, the digital nerves of the foot travel through the intermetatarsal space to innervate each toe. The plantar digital nerves, which are derived from the posterior tibial nerve, provide sensory innervation to the major portion of the plantar surface (Figs. 162.4 and 162.5). These nerves are subject to entrapment and resultant development of perineural fibrosis and degeneration resulting in the clinical syndrome known as Morton neuroma (Fig. 162.6). The dorsal aspect of the foot is innervated by terminal branches of the deep and superficial peroneal nerves. The overlap of the innervation of these nerves may be considerable.

## ULTRASOUND-GUIDED TECHNIQUE

The benefits, risks, and alternative treatments are explained to the patient, and informed consent is obtained. The patient is then placed in the supine position with the knee flexed so that the plantar surface of the affected foot rests comfortably on the examination table (Fig. 162.7). With the patient in the above position, the affected metatarsal or toe is identified, and a high-frequency linear ultrasound transducer is placed in a transverse position over the more distal portion of the metatarsal or the proximal portion of the toe to be blocked, and an ultrasound survey scan is taken (Figs. 162.8 and 162.9). The flexor tendon is identified and the metatarsal or digital nerve will be seen flanking the tendon laterally. A longitudinal view can help confirm the location of the nerve as can the use of color Doppler to identify the metatarsal or digital artery, which both lie just dorsal to their corresponding nerves (Figs. 162.10 and 162.11). After the correct metatarsal or digital nerve is identified, the skin overlying the area beneath the ultrasound transducer as well as the skin on the lateral aspects of the affected toes is then prepped with antiseptic solution. A sterile syringe containing 1.0 mL of 0.25% preservative-free bupivacaine and 40 mg of methylprednisolone is attached to a 1½-inch, 25-gauge needle using strict aseptic technique. The

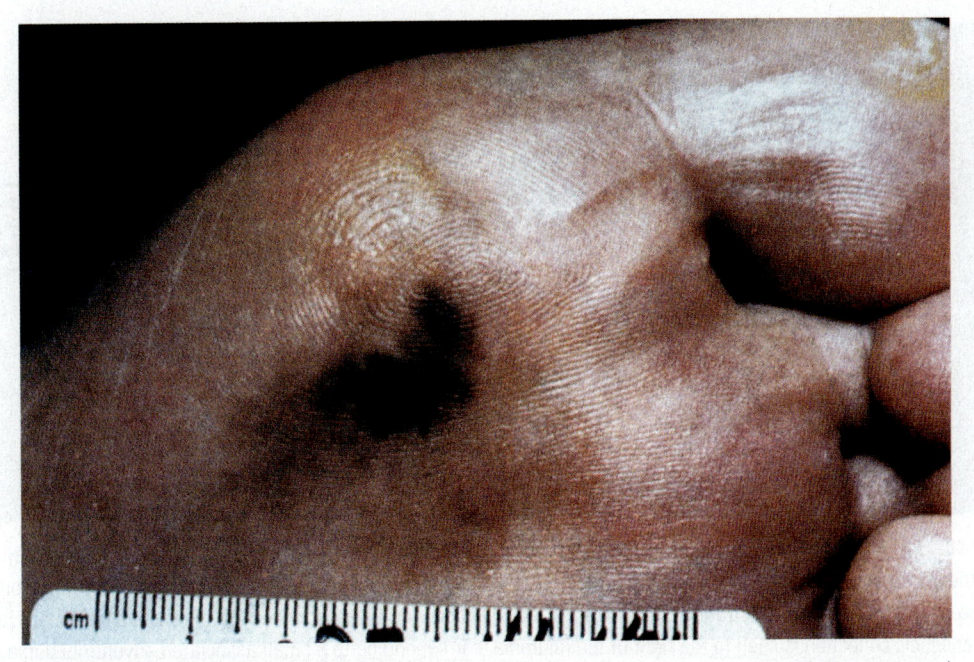

**FIGURE 162.1.** Melanoma of the plantar aspect of the foot causing compression of the metatarsal nerve. (Reused from Rubin E, Farber JL. *Pathology*. 3rd ed. Philadelphia, PA: Lippincott Williams & Wilkins; 1999, with permission.)

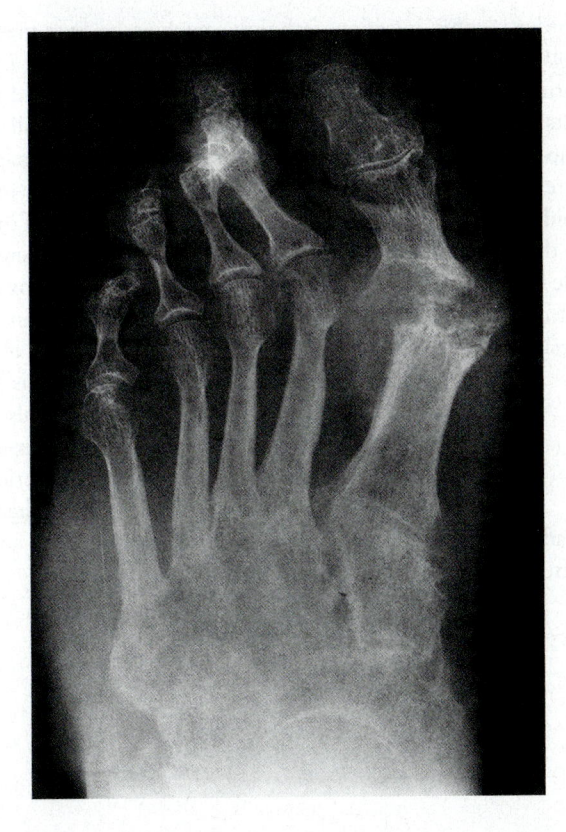

**FIGURE 162.2.** Plain radiograph demonstrating tophaceous gout and a concurrent joint space infection in a diabetic patient. (Reused from Daffner RH. *Clinical Radiology: The Essentials*. 3rd ed. Philadelphia, PA: Lippincott Williams & Wilkins; 2007, with permission.)

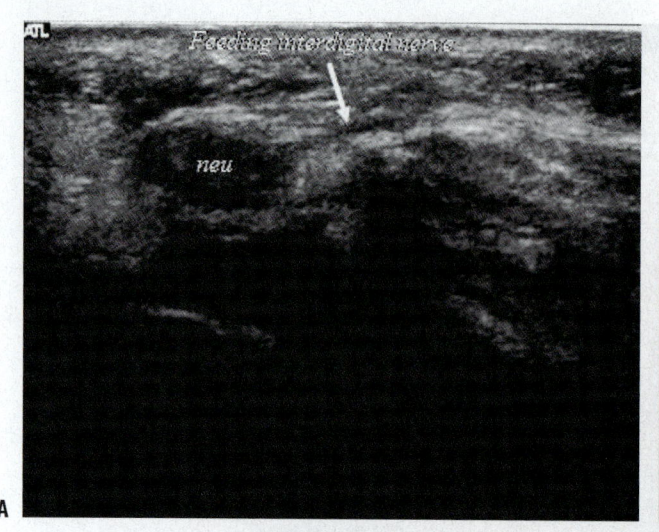

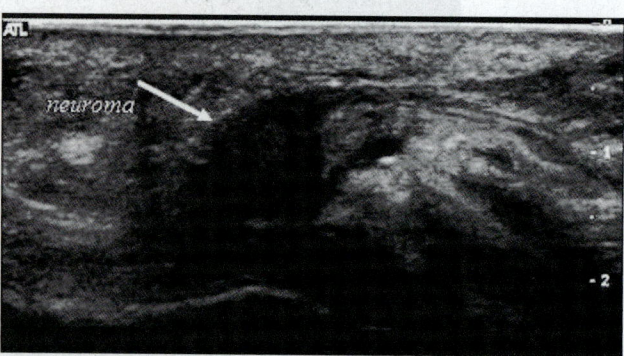

**FIGURE 162.3.** **A:** Longitudinal image of the second web space demonstrating a neuroma (neu). Note the comet tail appearance of the proximal border of the neuroma, consistent with feeding interdigital nerve (*arrow*). **B:** Longitudinal ultrasound image in a different patient again demonstrating a tubular enlarged interdigital nerve associated with the second web space neuroma. A small anechoic collection is seen to the right of the neuroma, corresponding to a small associated adventitial bursa (*arrow*). (Reused from Adler RS, Sofka CM, Positano RG. *Atlas of Foot and Ankle Sonography.* Philadelphia, PA: Lippincott Williams & Wilkins; 2004:18, with permission.)

needle is placed through the skin just below the inferior border of the transducer and is then advanced using an out-of-plane approach with the needle trajectory adjusted under real-time ultrasound guidance so that the needle tip ultimately rests in proximity to the digital nerve (Fig. 162.12). When the tip of needle is thought to be in satisfactory position, after careful aspiration, a small amount of local anesthetic and steroid is injected under real-time ultrasound guidance to confirm that the needle tip is in the proper position. After proper needle tip placement is confirmed, the remainder of the contents of the syringe are slowly injected. There should be minimal resistance to injection.

## COMPLICATIONS

The possibility of trauma to the flexor tendons, the metatarsal or digital nerves, and their corresponding arteries from this injection technique remains an ever-present possibility, although the risk of this is decreased if care is taken to place the needle outside the tendon and nerve and the injection is performed under real-time ultrasound visualization. Tendons that are highly inflamed or previously damaged are subject to rupture if substances are injected directly into the tendon. This complication can be greatly decreased if the clinician uses gentle technique and stops injecting immediately if significant resistance to injection is encountered. Approximately 25% of patients complain of a transient increase in pain after this injection technique; the patient should be warned of this. Infection, although uncommon, can occur. Ecchymosis and hematoma formation following this procedure may also occur. These complications can be decreased if manual pressure is applied to the area of the block immediately after injection. Application of cold packs for 20-minute periods after the block will also decrease the amount of postprocedure pain and bleeding the patient may experience.

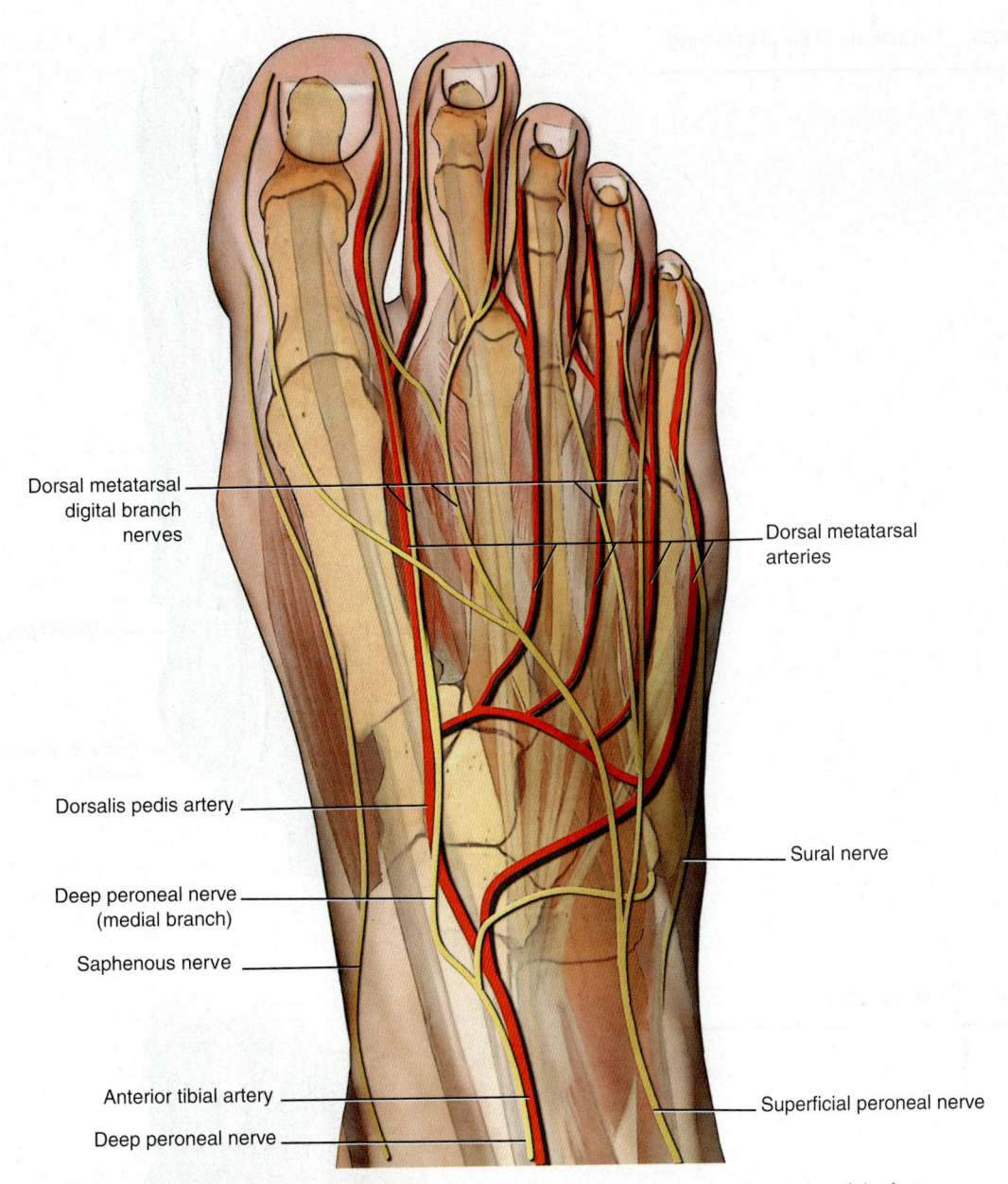

**FIGURE 162.4.** The anatomic relationship of the metatarsal and digital nerves to the arteries of the foot.

## CLINICAL PEARLS

Ultrasound-guided injection of the metatarsal and digital nerves is a straightforward and relatively safe technique if attention is paid to the clinically relevant anatomy. The use of physical modalities, including local heat and gentle range-of-motion exercises, should be introduced several days after the patient undergoes this injection technique. Vigorous exercise should be avoided because it may exacerbate the patient's symptomatology. Simple analgesics and nonsteroidal anti-inflammatory agents may be used concurrently with this injection technique. Careful neurologic examination to identify preexisting nerve compromise that may later be attributed to the procedure should be performed on all patients before beginning ultrasound-guided injection for metatarsal and digital nerves.

**FIGURE 162.5.** The anatomy of the plantar nerves.

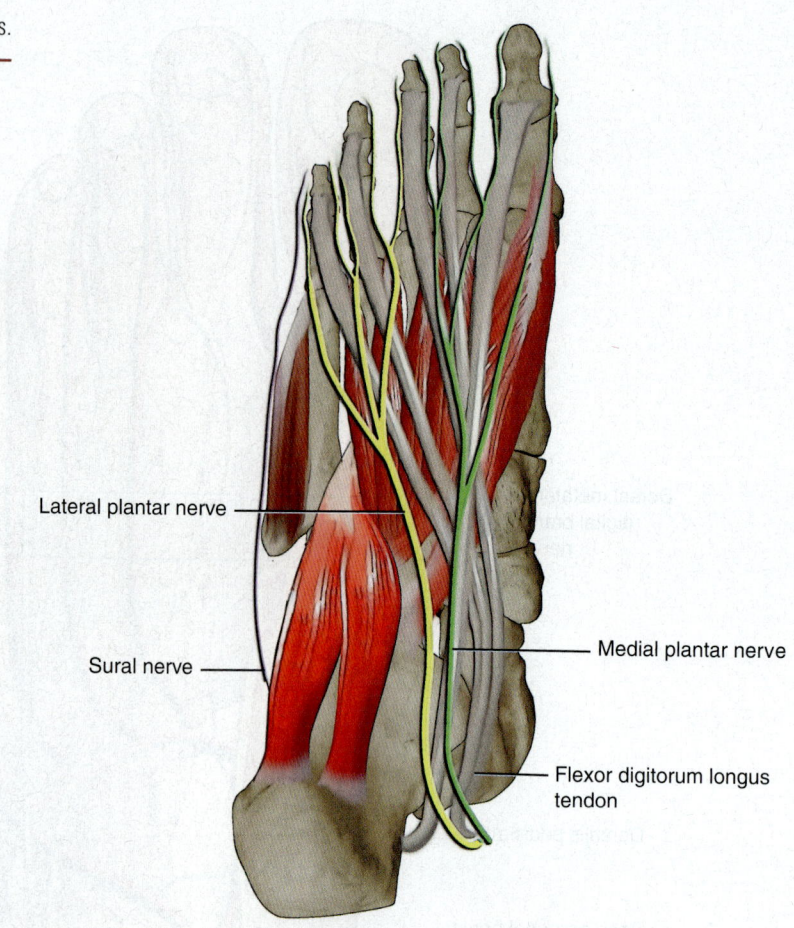

**FIGURE 162.6.** Morton neuroma.

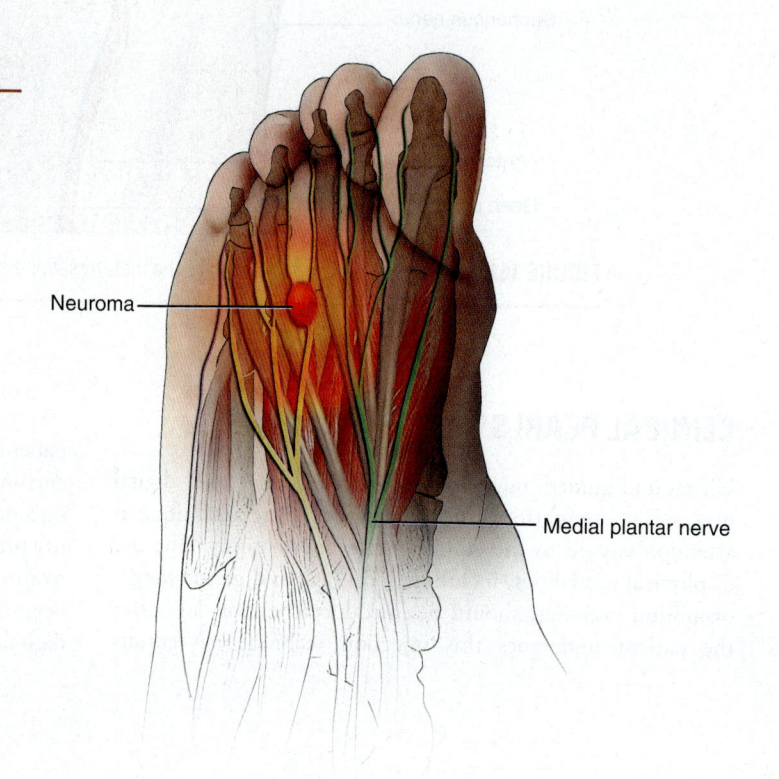

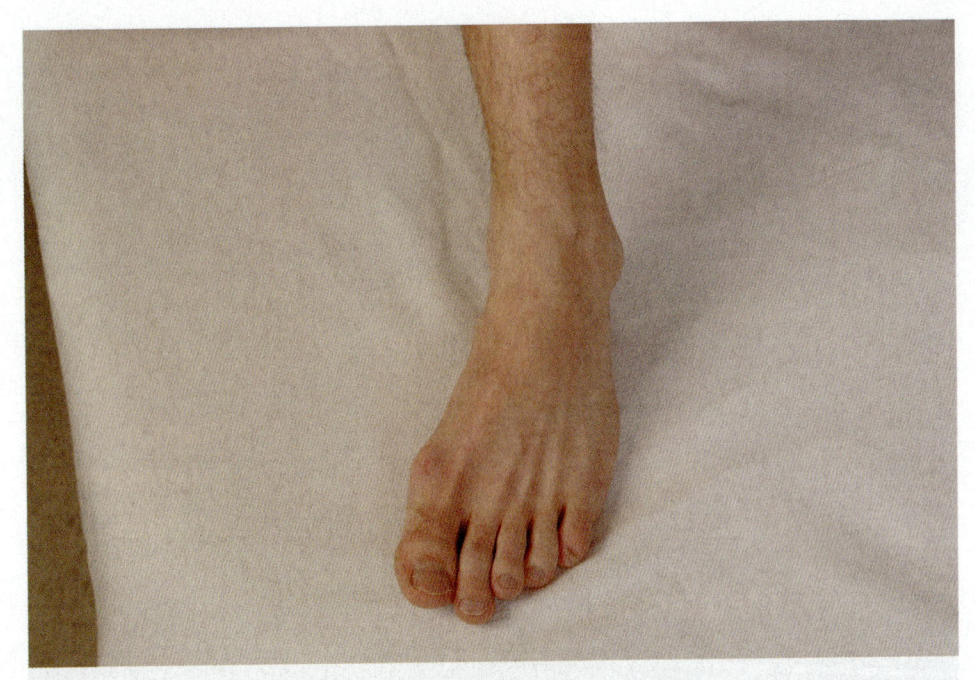

**FIGURE 162.7.** Proper patient position for ultrasound-guided injection for metatarsal and digital nerves.

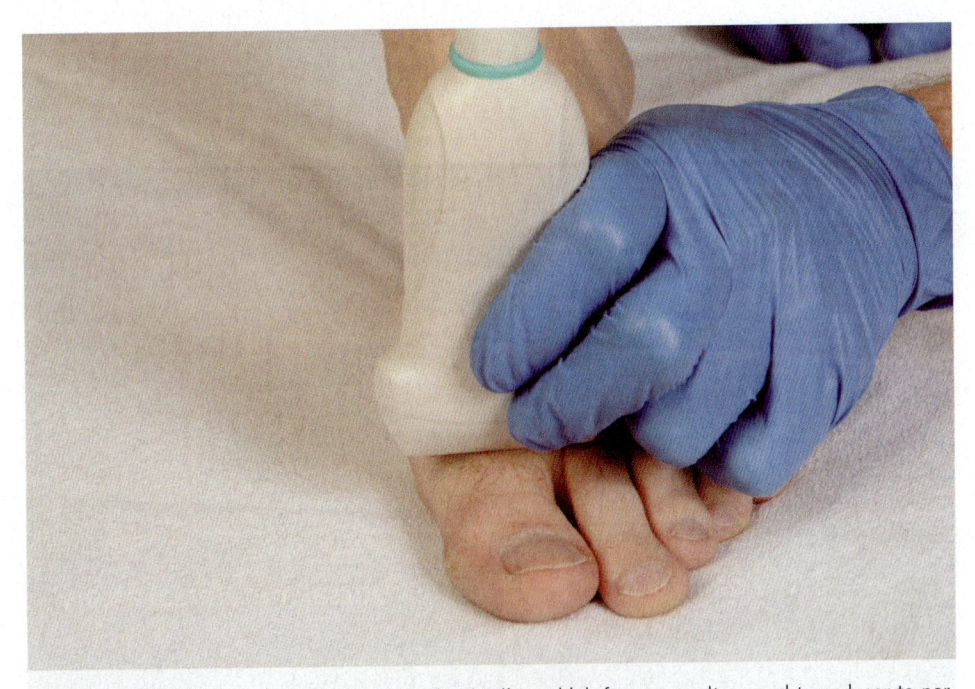

**FIGURE 162.8.** Proper transverse position for the linear high-frequency ultrasound transducer to perform ultrasound-guided metatarsal and digital nerves injection.

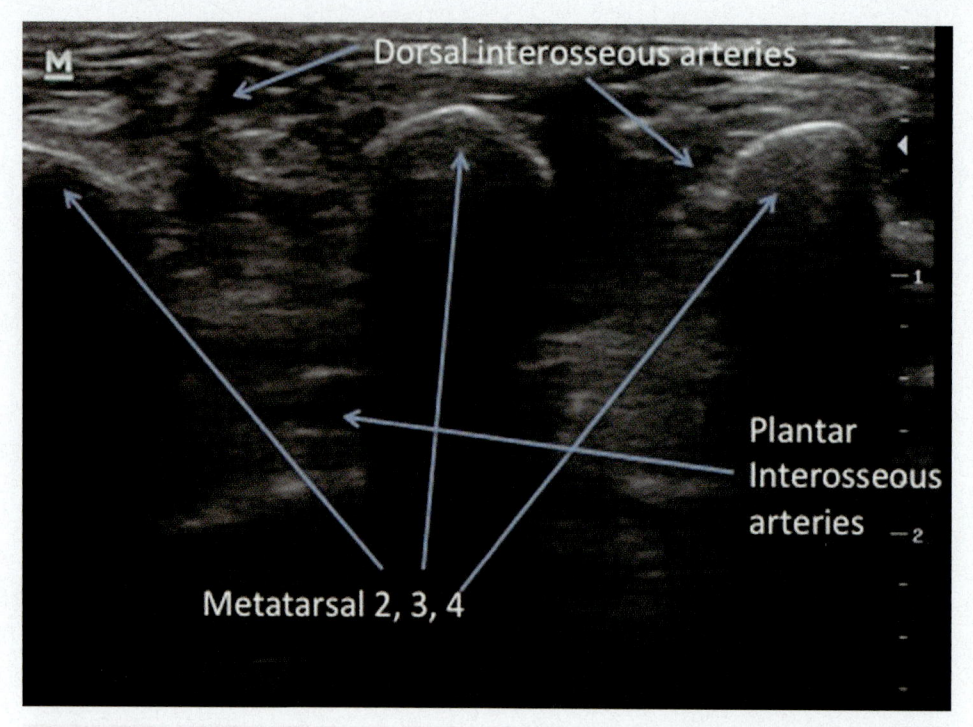

**FIGURE 162.9.** Transverse ultrasound image demonstrating the relationship of the flexor tendons and the dorsal and plantar artery and nerve at the level of the distal metatarsal.

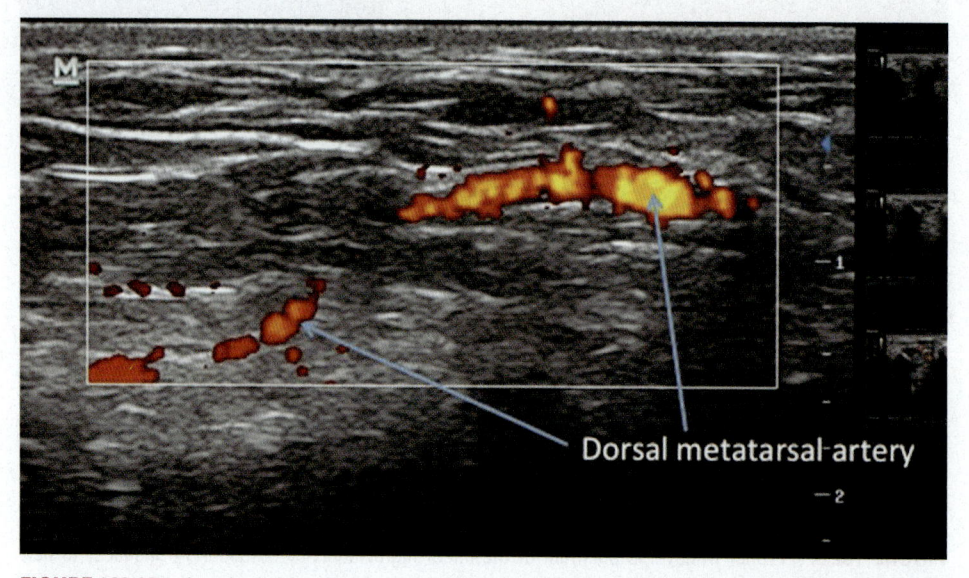

**FIGURE 162.10.** Longitudinal color Doppler view of the metatarsal nerve and artery of the great toe.

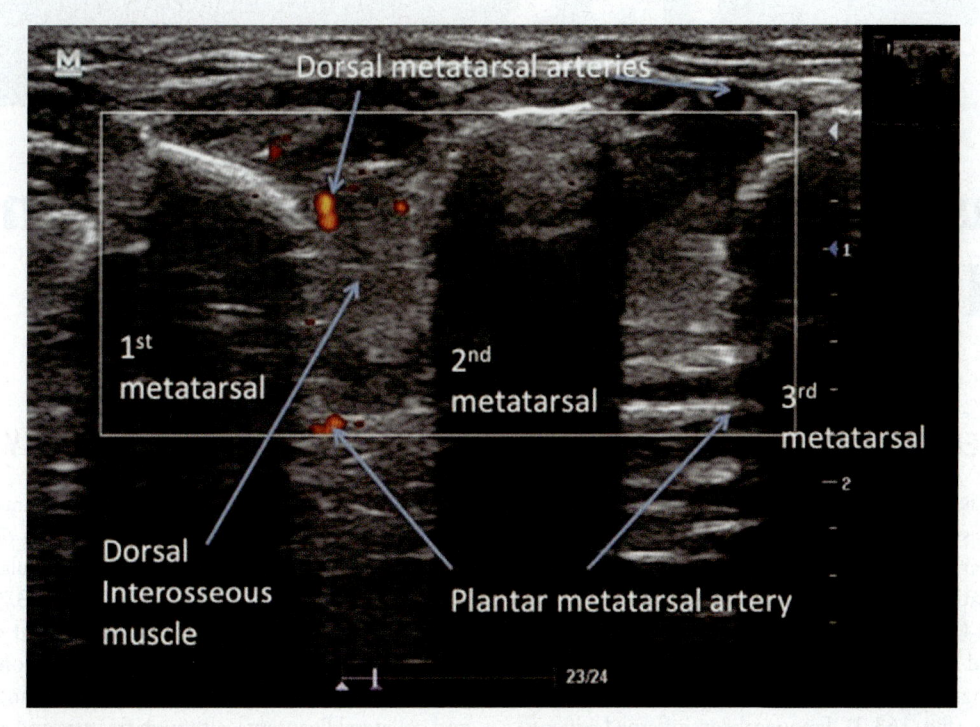

**FIGURE 162.11.** Transverse color Doppler view of the digital artery.

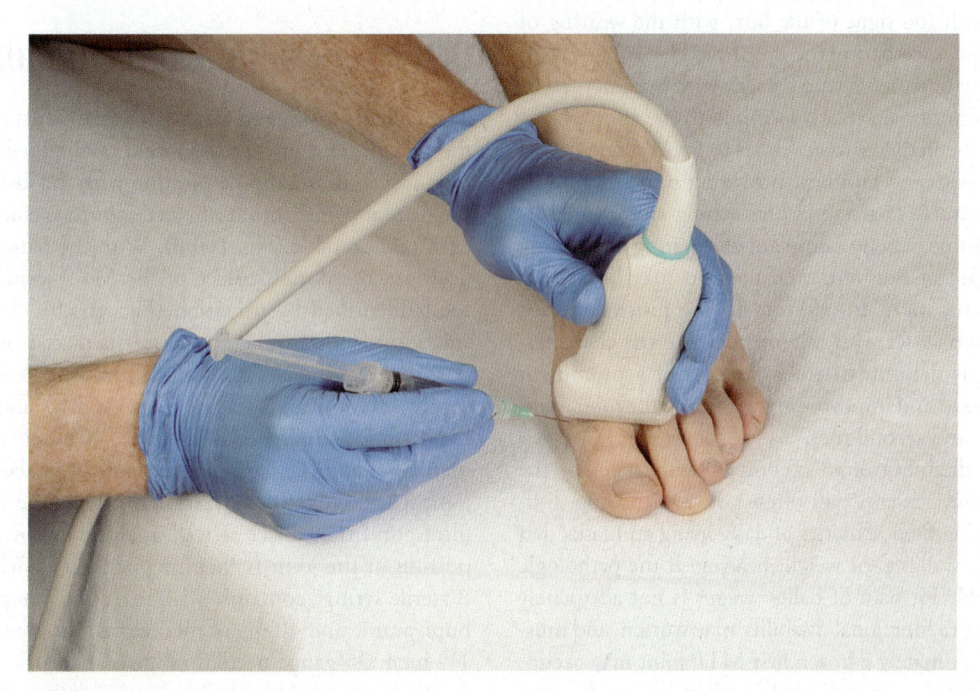

**FIGURE 162.12.** Proper needle placement for ultrasound-guided injection of the digital nerve.

## SUGGESTED READINGS

Bibbo C, Jaffe L, Goldkind A. Complications of digital and lesser metatarsal surgery. *Clin Podiatr Med Surg* 2010;27(4):485–507.

Gregg JM, Schneider T, Marks P. MR imaging and ultrasound of metatarsalgia—the lesser metatarsals. *Radiol Clin North Am* 2008;46(6):1061–1078.

Lopez-Ben R. Imaging of nerve entrapment in the foot and ankle. *Foot Ankle Clin* 2011;16(2):213–224.

Waldman SD. Metatarsal and digital nerves. In: *Atlas of Interventional Pain Management*. 3rd ed. Philadelphia, PA: Saunders Elsevier; 2009:575–580.

# CHAPTER 163

# Ultrasound-Guided Injection Technique for Hallux Valgus Deformity

## CLINICAL PERSPECTIVES

Bunion, which is also known as the hallux valgus, refers to a constellation of symptoms including soft tissue swelling over the first metatarsophalangeal (MTP) joint associated with abnormal angulation of the joint that results in a prominent first metatarsal head (Fig. 163.1). Ultimately, the first MTP joint may sublux, and the overlapping of the first and second toes worsens resulting in a painful condition known as the hallux valgus deformity (Fig. 163.2). Frequently an inflamed adventitious bursa may coexist with the bunion, further exacerbating the pain and cosmetic deformity (Fig. 163.3). Occurring more commonly in women, bunion is most commonly the result of wearing shoes with too tight of toe box, with the wearing of high-heeled shoes exacerbating the problem (Fig. 163.4).

The majority of patients who present with bunion present with the complaint of pain that is localized to the affected first MTP joint and the inability to get shoes to fit. Walking makes the pain worse, with rest and heat providing some relief. The pain is constant and is characterized as aching and may interfere with sleep. Some patients complain of a grating or popping sensation with use of the joint, and crepitus may be present on physical examination. In addition to the just-mentioned pain, patients who suffer with bunions develop the characteristic hallux valgus deformity, which consists of a prominent first metatarsal head and improper angulation of the joint, with overlapping first and second toes.

Functional disability often accompanies the pain of the hallux valgus joint. Patients will often notice increasing difficulty in performing their activities of daily living and tasks that require standing, walking, or weight bearing. If the pathologic process responsible for pain of hallux valgus is not adequately treated, the patient's functional disability may worsen, and muscle wasting and ultimately a frozen first MTP joint may occur.

Plain radiographs are indicated in all patients who present with pain of the hallux valgus (Fig. 163.5). Based on the patient's clinical presentation, additional testing may be indicated, including complete blood cell count, sedimentation rate, and antinuclear antibody testing. Magnetic resonance imaging or ultrasound of the hallux valgus joint is indicated if fracture, effusion, tendinopathy, crystal arthropathy, joint mice, synovitis, foreign body, bursitis, or ligamentous injury is suspected (Fig. 163.6).

## CLINICALLY RELEVANT ANATOMY

The MTP joints are condyloid joints characterized by the articulation of the rounded articular surfaces of the metatarsal heads into the shallow concavities of the articular surfaces of the proximal end of the first phalanges (Fig. 163.7). Each joint is lined with synovium, and the ample synovial space allows for intra-articular placement of needles for injection and aspiration. The MTP joints have a dense joint capsule and strong plantar and collateral ligaments, although fracture and subluxation may still occur. The MTP joints are also susceptible to overuse and misuse injuries with resultant inflammation and arthritis.

## ULTRASOUND-GUIDED TECHNIQUE

The benefits, risks, and alternative treatments are explained to the patient, and informed consent is obtained. The patient is then placed in the supine position with the knee flexed so that the plantar surface of the affected foot rests comfortably on the examination table (Fig. 163.8). With the patient in the above position, the dorsal surface of the MTP joint of the affected toe is identified by palpation (Fig. 163.9). A high-frequency small linear ultrasound transducer is placed in a longitudinal position over the MTP joint of the affected toe, and an ultrasound survey scan is taken (Figs. 163.10 and 163.11). The hypoechoic joint space is identified between the head of the metatarsal and the base of the proximal phalanges. When the joint space is identified, the skin overlying the area beneath the ultrasound transducer as well as the skin covering the lateral portion of the joint is then prepped with antiseptic solution. A sterile syringe containing 1.0 mL of 0.25% preservative-free bupivacaine and 40 mg of methylprednisolone is attached to a 1½-inch, 25-gauge needle using strict aseptic technique. The needle is placed through the skin just below the center of the longitudinally placed transducer and is then advanced using an out-of-plane approach with the needle trajectory adjusted under real-time ultrasound guidance so that the needle tip ultimately rests within the MTP joint space (Fig. 163.12). When the tip of needle is thought to be in satisfactory position, after careful gentle aspiration, a small amount of local anesthetic and steroid is injected under real-time ultrasound guidance to confirm that the needle tip is in the proper position (Fig. 163.13).

CHAPTER 163    ULTRASOUND-GUIDED INJECTION TECHNIQUE FOR HALLUX VALGUS DEFORMITY

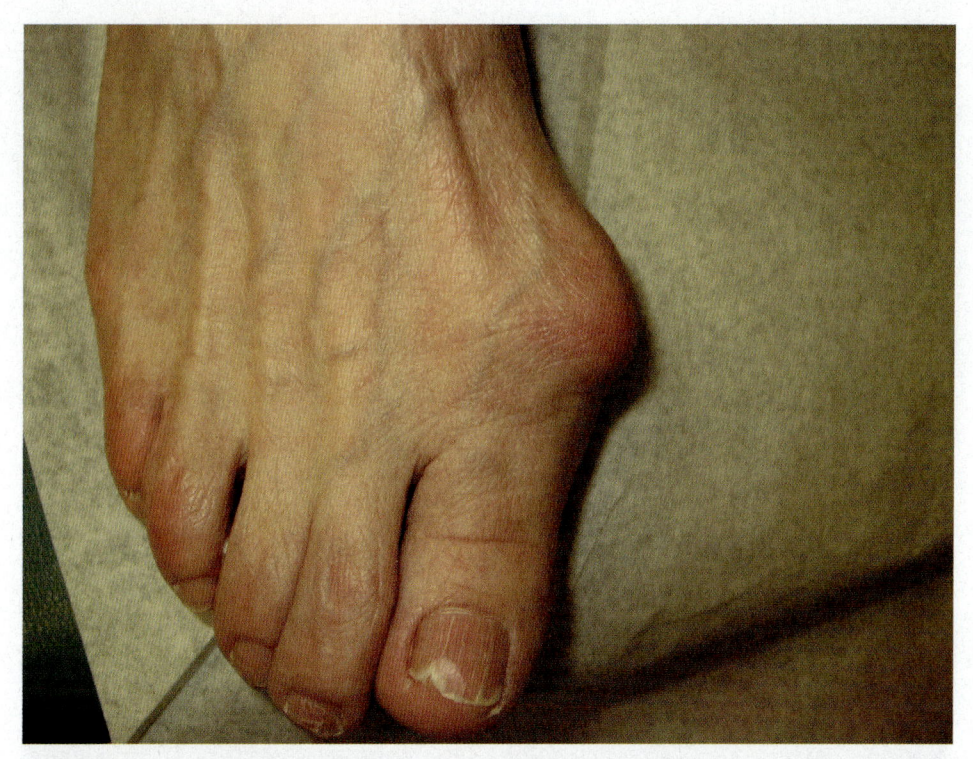

**FIGURE 163.1.** The classic appearance of bunion. (Image provided by Stedman's Medical Dictionary, 2013.)

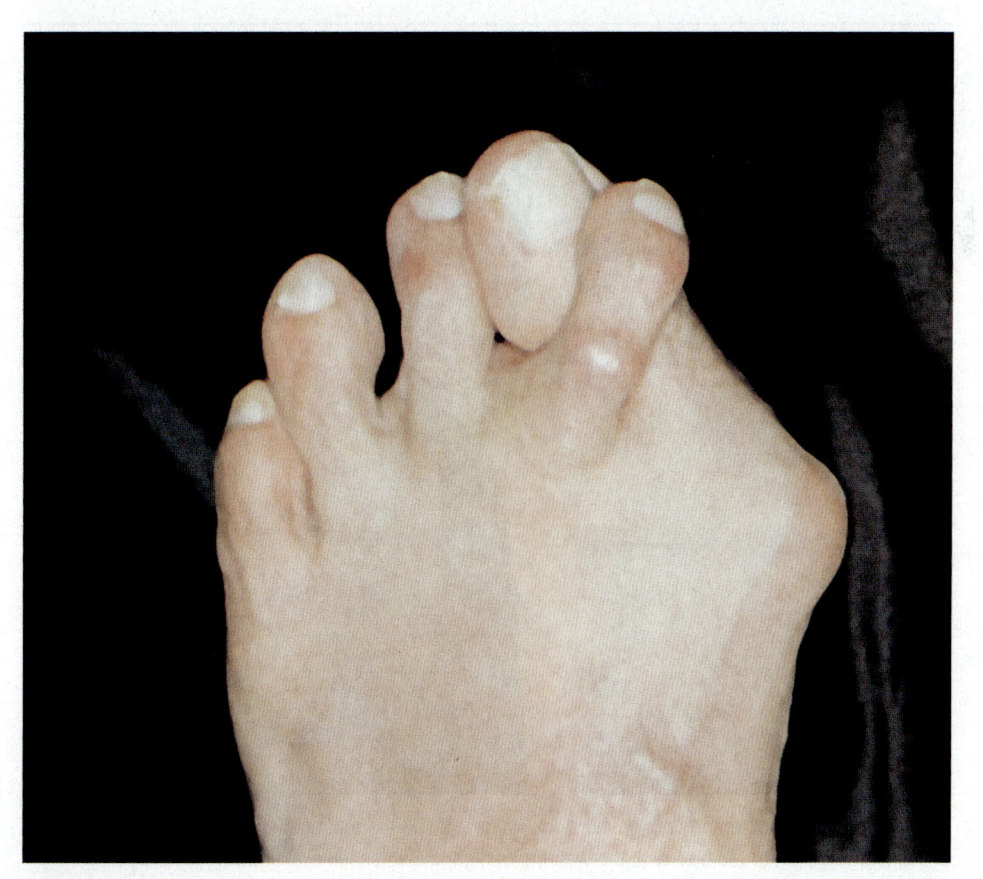

**FIGURE 163.2.** The hallux valgus deformity. (Reused from Weber J, Kelley J. *Health Assessment in Nursing*. 2nd ed. Philadelphia, PA: Lippincott Williams & Wilkins; 2003, with permission.)

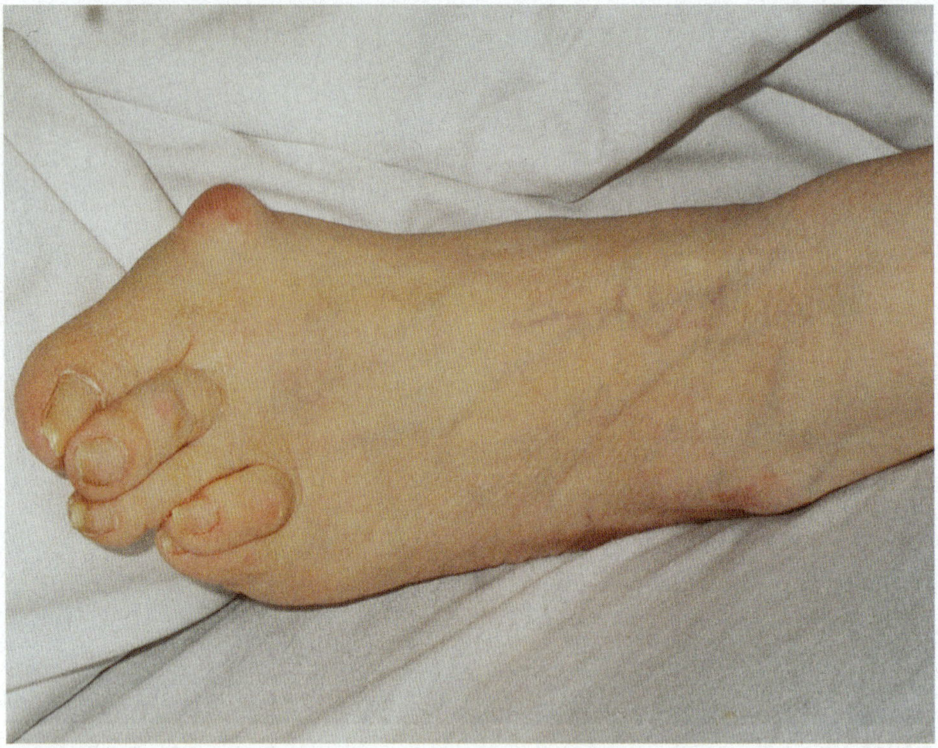

**FIGURE 163.3.** An inflamed adventitial bursa frequently accompanies the pain and functional disability associated with bunion. (Reused from Berg D, Worzala K. *Atlas of Adult Physical Diagnosis.* Philadelphia, PA: Lippincott Williams & Wilkins; 2006, with permission.)

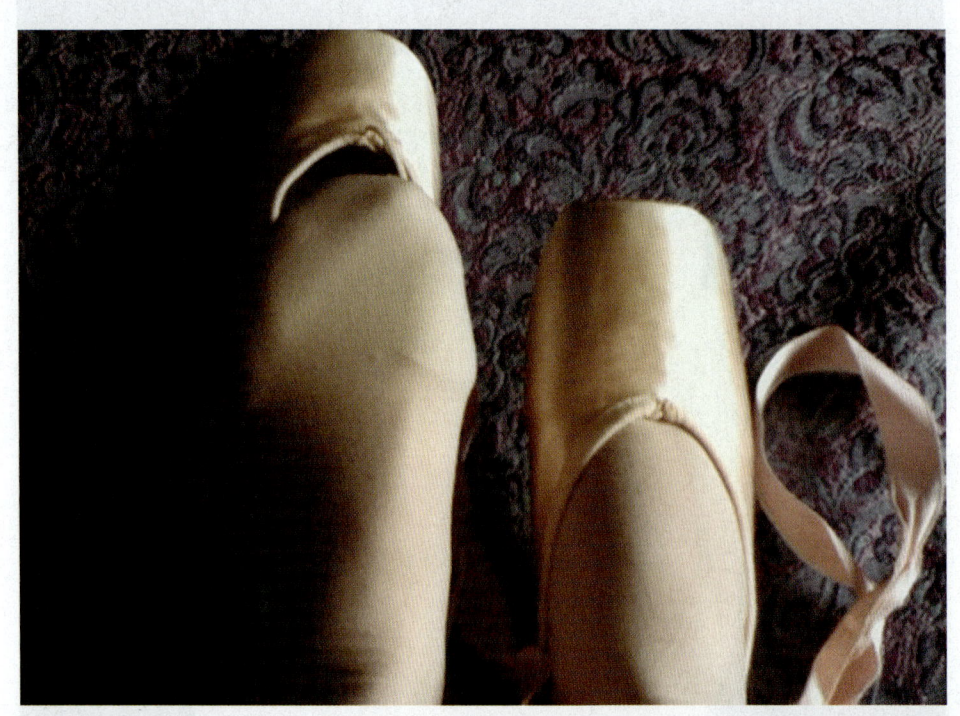

**FIGURE 163.4.** Occurring more commonly in women, bunion is most commonly the result of wearing shoes with too tight of toe box, with the wearing of high-heeled shoes exacerbating the problem.

# CHAPTER 163 ULTRASOUND-GUIDED INJECTION TECHNIQUE FOR HALLUX VALGUS DEFORMITY

After proper needle tip placement is confirmed, the remainder of the contents of the syringe are slowly injected. There should be minimal resistance to injection.

## COMPLICATIONS

The major complication of ultrasound-guided injection of the hallux valgus is infection. Ecchymosis and hematoma formation may also occur. A transient exacerbation of the patient's pain occurs ~25% of the time following this injection technique, and the patient should be warned of this possibility prior to the procedure.

## CLINICAL PEARLS

Toe pathology including tendinopathy, occult fractures, osteoarthritis, rheumatoid arthritis, crystal arthropathies, avascular necrosis bursitis, synovitis, and impingement syndromes may coexist with disease of the hallux valgus and may contribute to the patient's pain symptomatology. Universal precautions should always be observed to protect the operator, and strict adherence to sterile technique must be used to avoid infection. Gentle physical therapy and local heat should be introduced following ultrasound-guided injection of the hallux valgus to reduce pain and improve function. Simple analgesics and nonsteroidal anti-inflammatory agents or COX-2 inhibitors may be used concurrently with this injection technique.

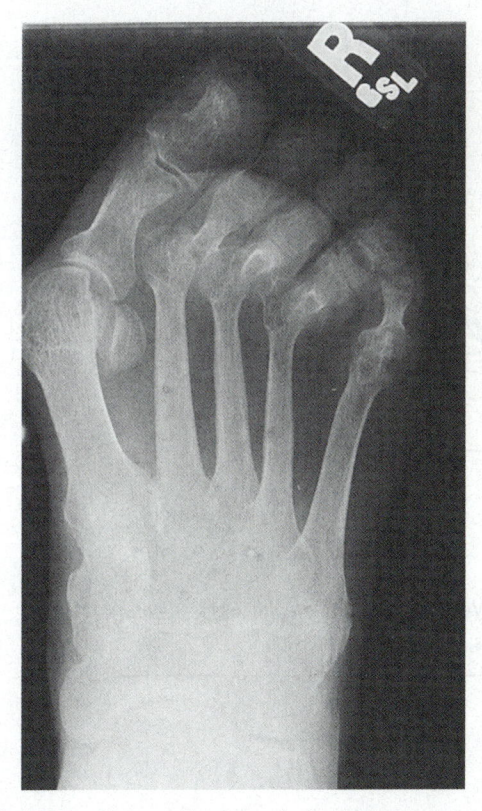

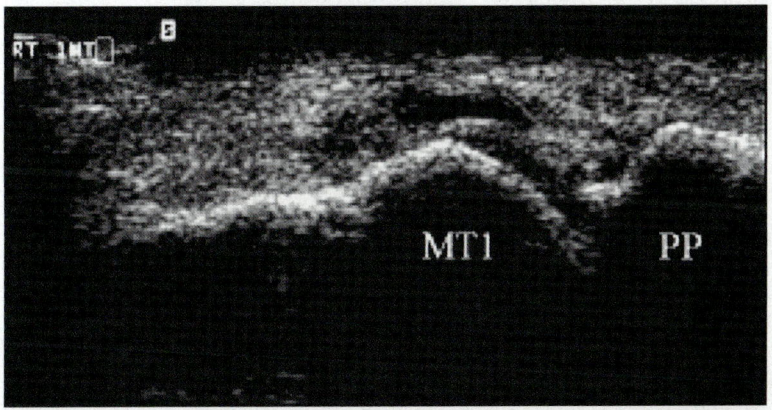

**FIGURE 163.5.** Plain radiograph of the hallux valgus deformity. (Reused from Koopman WJ, Moreland LW. *Arthritis and Allied Conditions: A Textbook of Rheumatology.* 15th ed. Philadelphia, PA: Lippincott Williams & Wilkins; 2005, with permission.)

**FIGURE 163.6.** **A:** Longitudinal image of the first MTP joint in a patient with hallux valgus deformity demonstrating a small effusion. The first metatarsal (MT1) and proximal phalanx (PP) are labeled. **B:** Long axis view of the first MTP joint in the same patient, scanned along the medial joint line, demonstrates cystic change in the first metatarsal head (*arrow*). (Reused from Adler RS, Sofka CM, Positano RG. *Atlas of Foot and Ankle Sonography.* Philadelphia, PA: Lippincott Williams & Wilkins; 2004:29, with permission.)

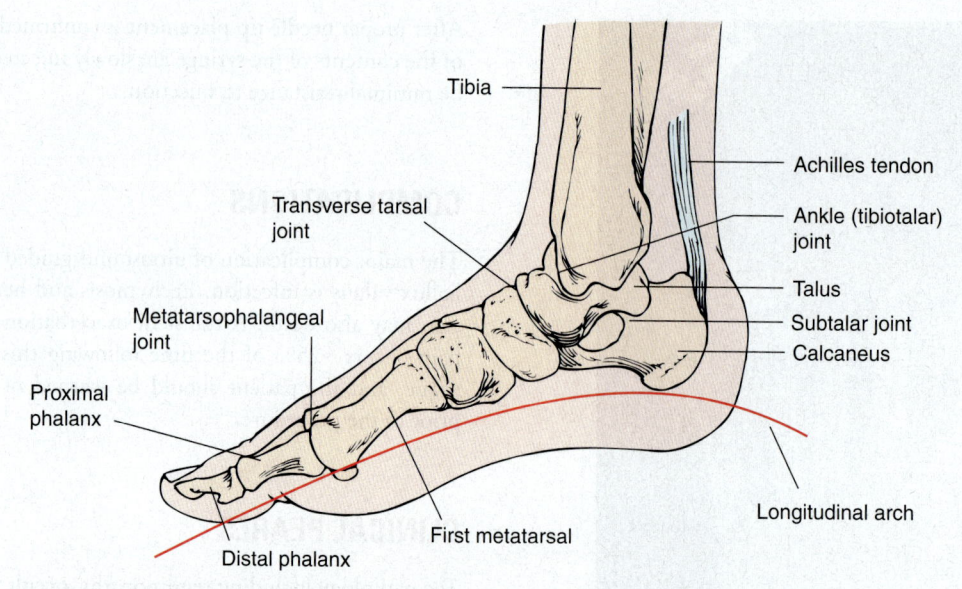

**FIGURE 163.7.** Anatomy of the MTP joints. (Reused from Weber J, Kelley J. *Health Assessment in Nursing.* 2nd ed. Philadelphia, PA: Lippincott Williams & Wilkins; 2003, with permission.)

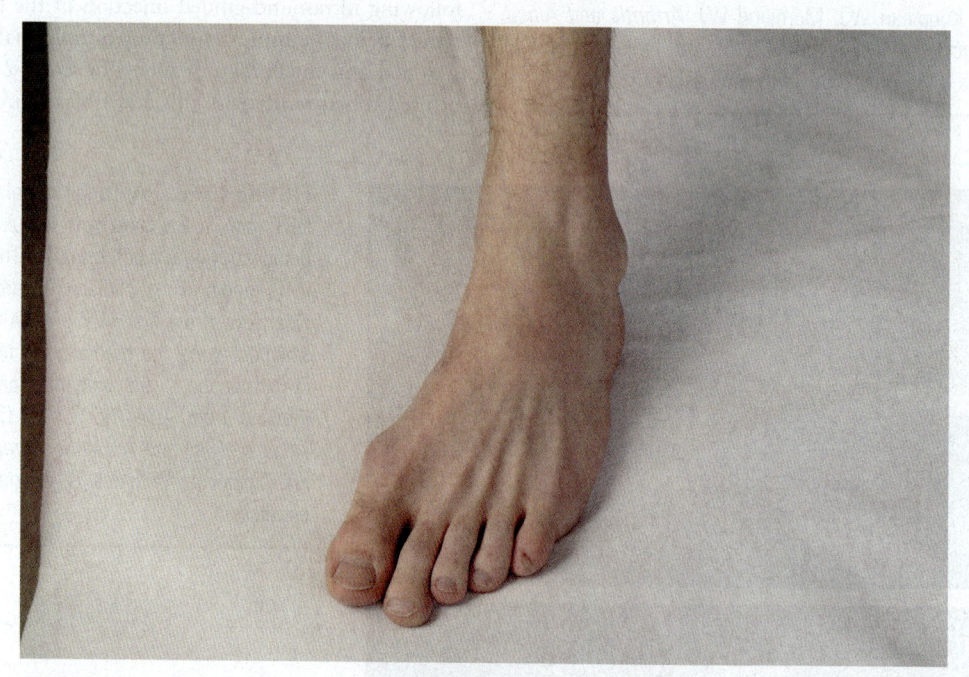

**FIGURE 163.8.** Proper patient position for ultrasound-guided injection of hallux valgus.

CHAPTER 163  ULTRASOUND-GUIDED INJECTION TECHNIQUE FOR HALLUX VALGUS DEFORMITY   1149

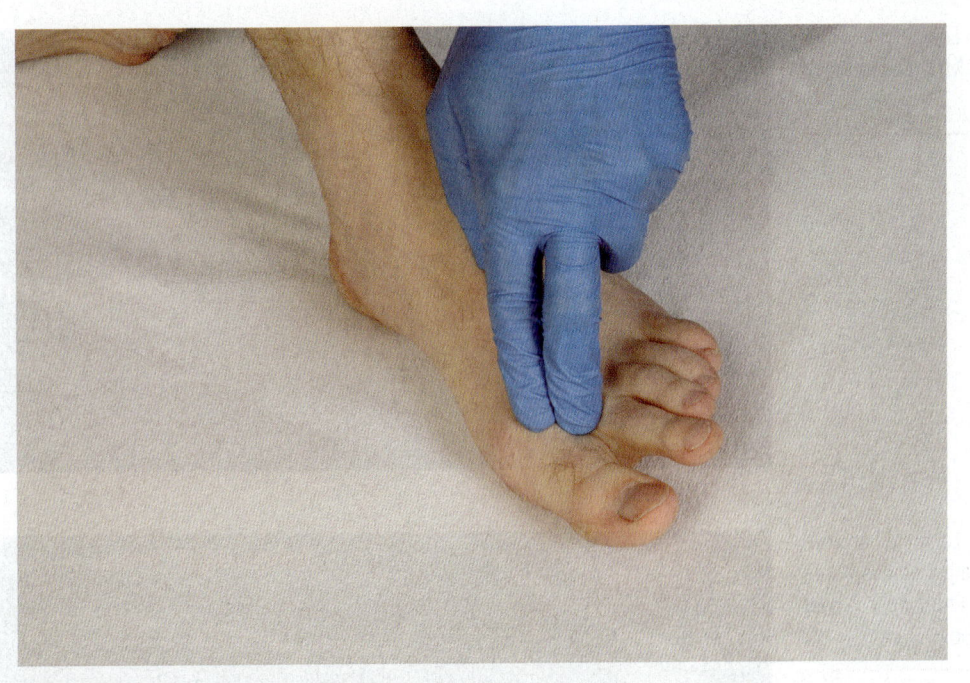

**FIGURE 163.9.** Palpation of the MTP joint.

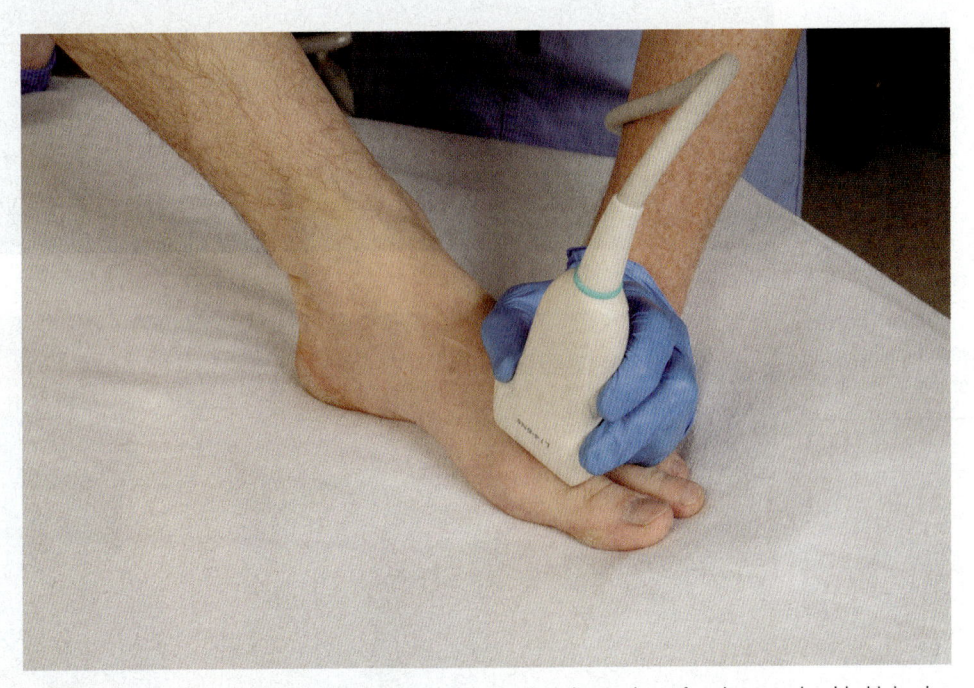

**FIGURE 163.10.** Correct longitudinal position for ultrasound transducer for ultrasound-guided injection technique for hallux valgus joint.

**FIGURE 163.11.** Longitudinal ultrasound view of the MTP joint space of the great toe.

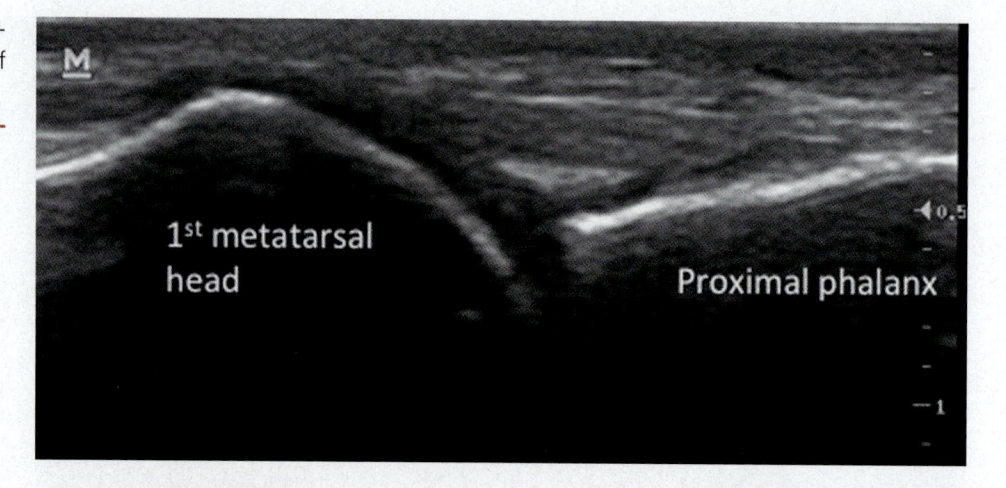

**FIGURE 163.12.** Longitudinal ultrasound view of hallux valgus. Note the significant adventitial tissue over the lateral great toe.

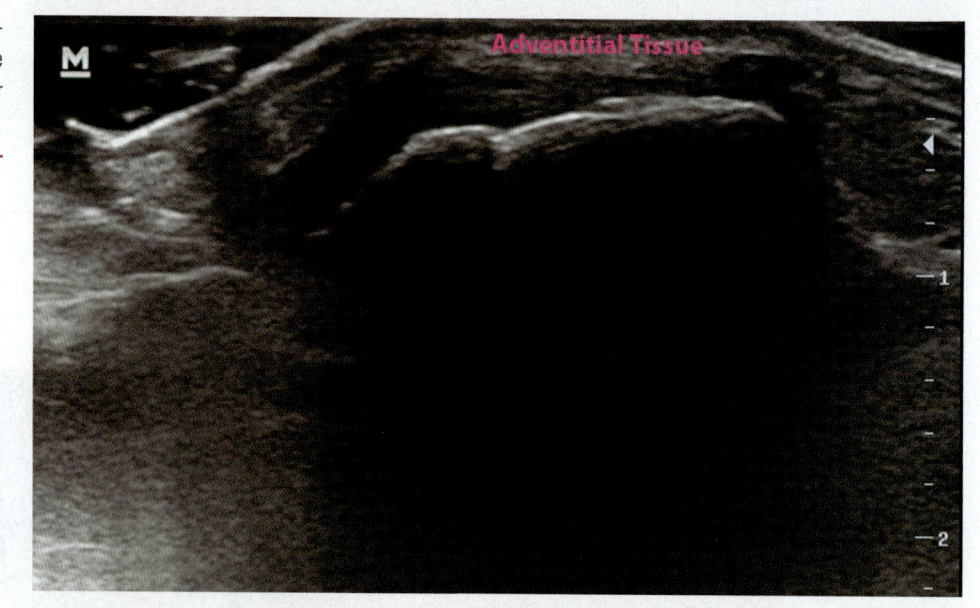

**FIGURE 163.13.** Proper needle position for ultrasound-guided out-of-plane injection of the MTP joint.

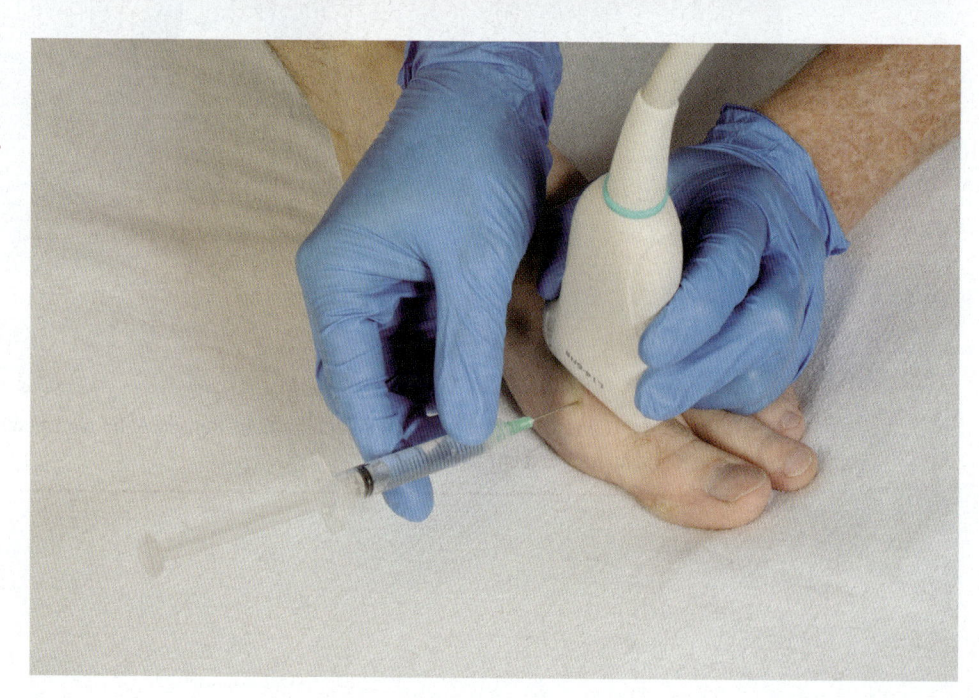

## SUGGESTED READINGS

Albert A, Leemrijse T. The dorsal bunion: an overview. *Foot Ankle Surg* 2005; 11(2):65–68.

Kennedy JG, Collumbier JA. Bunions in Dancers. *Clin Sports Med* 2008; 27(2):321–328.

Mann R. Bunion deformity in elite athletes. In: *Baxter's the Foot and Ankle in Sport*. 2nd ed. Philadelphia, PA: Mosby; 2008:435–443.

Mann RA, Horton GA. Management of the foot and ankle in rheumatoid. [Original Research Article]. *Rheum Dis Clin North Am* 1996;22(3):457–476.

Motta-Valencia K. Dance-Related Injury. *Phys Med Rehabil Clin N Am* 2006; 17(3):697–723.

Waldman SD. Intra-articular injection of the toe joints. In: *Pain Review*. Philadelphia, PA: Saunders Elsevier; 2009:591–592.

Waldman SD. Technique for injection technique of the toe joints. In: *Atlas of Pain Management Injection Techniques*. 3rd ed. Philadelphia, PA: Saunders Elsevier; 2012:419–421.

# CHAPTER 164

# Ultrasound-Guided Injection Technique for Bunionette Pain Syndrome

## CLINICAL PERSPECTIVES

Bunionette, which is also known as the tailor's bunion, refers to a constellation of symptoms including soft tissue swelling over the fifth metatarsophalangeal joint associated with abnormal angulation of the joint that results in a prominent fifth metatarsal head (Fig. 164.1). Ultimately, the fifth metatarsophalangeal joint may sublux, and a corn overlying the metatarsal head will develop. An inflamed adventitious bursa may also coexist with the bunionette, further exacerbating the pain and cosmetic deformity (Fig. 164.2). Occurring more commonly in women, bunionette is most commonly the result of wearing shoes with too tight of toe box, with the wearing of high-heeled shoes exacerbating the problem.

The majority of patients who present with bunionette present with the complaint of pain that is localized to the affected fifth metatarsophalangeal joint and the inability to get shoes to fit. Walking makes the pain worse, with rest and heat providing some relief. The pain is constant and is characterized as aching and may interfere with sleep. Some patients complain of a grating or popping sensation with use of the joint, and crepitus may be present on physical examination. In addition to the just-mentioned pain, patients who suffer with bunionette develop the characteristic bunionette deformity, which consists of a prominent fifth metatarsal head and improper angulation of the fifth metatarsal.

Functional disability often accompanies the pain of the bunionette joint. Patients will often notice increasing difficulty in performing their activities of daily living and tasks that require standing, walking, or weight bearing. If the pathologic process responsible for pain of bunionette is not adequately treated, the patient's functional disability may worsen and muscle wasting and ultimately a frozen fifth metatarsophalangeal joint may occur.

Plain radiographs are indicated in all patients who present with pain of the bunionette (Fig. 164.3). Based on the patient's clinical presentation, additional testing may be indicated, including complete blood cell count, sedimentation rate, and antinuclear antibody testing. Magnetic resonance imaging or ultrasound of the bunionette joint is indicated if fracture, effusion, tendinopathy, crystal arthropathy, joint mice, synovitis, foreign body, bursitis, or ligamentous injury is suspected.

## CLINICALLY RELEVANT ANATOMY

The metatarsophalangeal joints are condyloid joints characterized by the articulation of the rounded articular surfaces of the metatarsal heads into the shallow concavities of the articular surfaces of the proximal end of the phalanges (Fig. 164.4). Each joint is lined with synovium, and the ample synovial space allows for intra-articular placement of needles for injection and aspiration. The metatarsophalangeal joints have a dense joint capsule and strong plantar and collateral ligaments, although fracture and subluxation may still occur. The metatarsophalangeal joints are also susceptible to overuse and misuse injuries with resultant inflammation and arthritis.

## ULTRASOUND-GUIDED TECHNIQUE

The benefits, risks, and alternative treatments are explained to the patient, and informed consent is obtained. The patient is then placed in the supine position with the knee flexed so that the plantar surface of the affected foot rests comfortably on the examination table (Fig. 164.5). With the patient in the above position, the dorsal surface of the metatarsophalangeal joint of the affected toe is identified by palpation (Fig. 164.6). A high-frequency small linear ultrasound transducer is placed in a longitudinal position over the metatarsophalangeal joint of the affected toe, and an ultrasound survey scan is taken (Figs. 164.7 and 164.8). The hypoechoic joint space is identified between the head of the metatarsal and the base of the proximal phalanges. When the joint space is identified, the skin overlying the area beneath the ultrasound transducer as well as the skin covering the lateral portion of the joint is then prepped with antiseptic solution. A sterile syringe containing 1.0 mL of 0.25% preservative-free bupivacaine and 40 mg of methylprednisolone is attached to a 1½-inch, 25-gauge needle using strict aseptic technique. The needle is placed through the skin just below the center of the longitudinally placed transducer and is then advanced using an out-of-plane approach with the needle trajectory adjusted under real-time ultrasound guidance so that the needle tip ultimately rests within the metatarsophalangeal joint space (Fig. 164.9). When the tip of needle is thought to be in satisfactory position, after careful gentle aspiration, a small amount of local anesthetic and steroid is

CHAPTER 164    ULTRASOUND-GUIDED INJECTION TECHNIQUE FOR BUNIONETTE PAIN SYNDROME

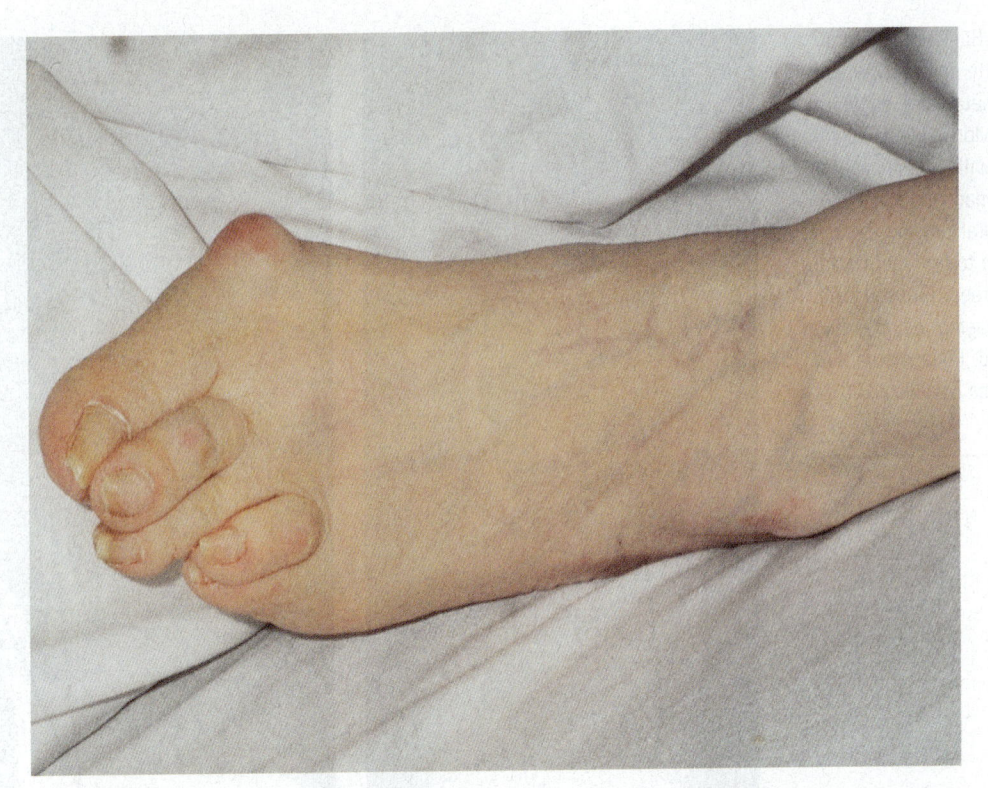

**FIGURE 164.1.** Bunionette affects the fifth metatarsophalangeal joint. This patient also suffers from hallux valgus with a significantly inflamed adventitial bursa of the first metatarsophalangeal joint. (Reused from Berg D, Worzala K. *Atlas of Adult Physical Diagnosis.* Philadelphia, PA: Lippincott Williams & Wilkins; 2006, with permission.)

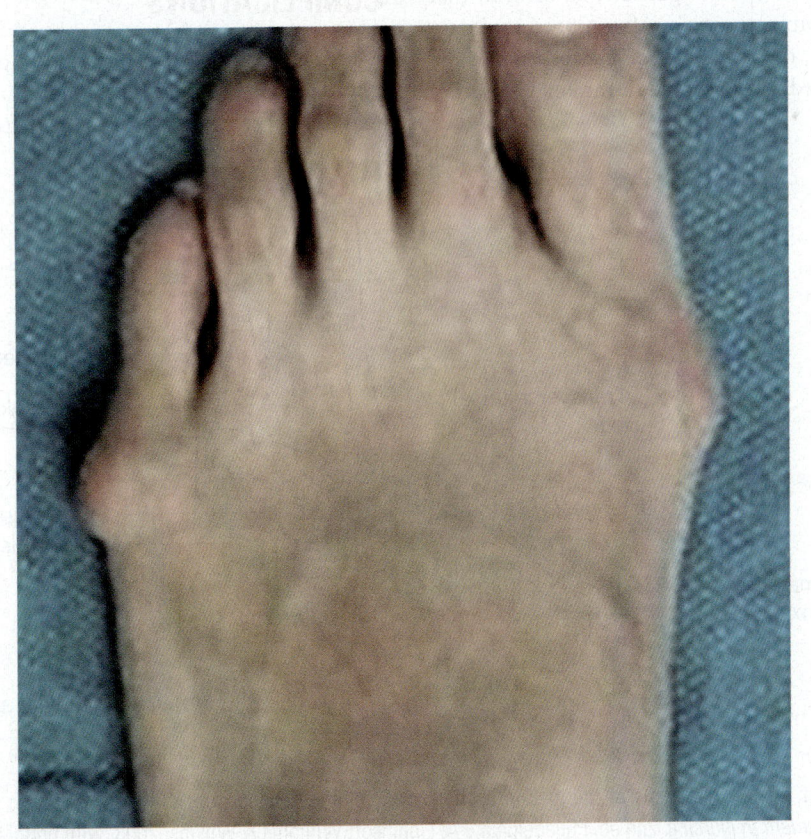

**FIGURE 164.2.** Significant corn development can accompany the bunionette deformity.

**FIGURE 164.3.** Bunionette deformities. **A:** Bunionette deformity with a fourth to fifth metatarsal angle of 15 degrees. **B:** More severe bunionette deformity with prominence of the metatarsal head and bone erosion (*arrow*), lateral bowing (*broken line*), and a fourth to fifth metatarsal angle of 18 degrees. (Reused from Berquist TH. *Imaging of the Foot and Ankle*. 3rd ed. Philadelphia, PA: Lippincott Williams & Wilkins; 2011, with permission.)

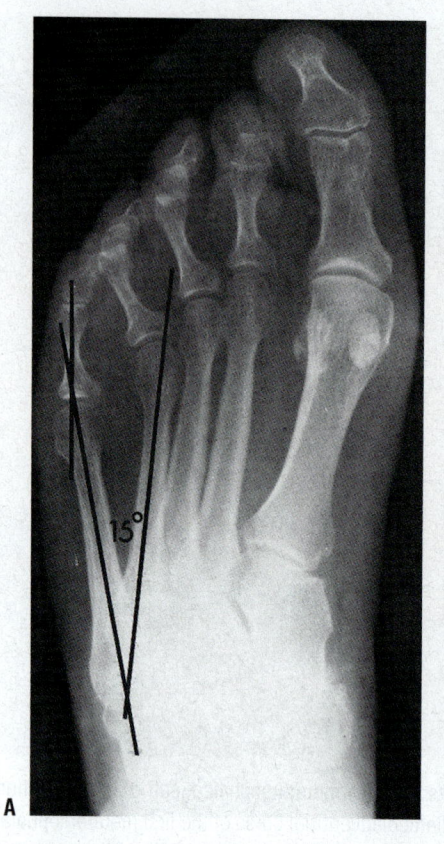

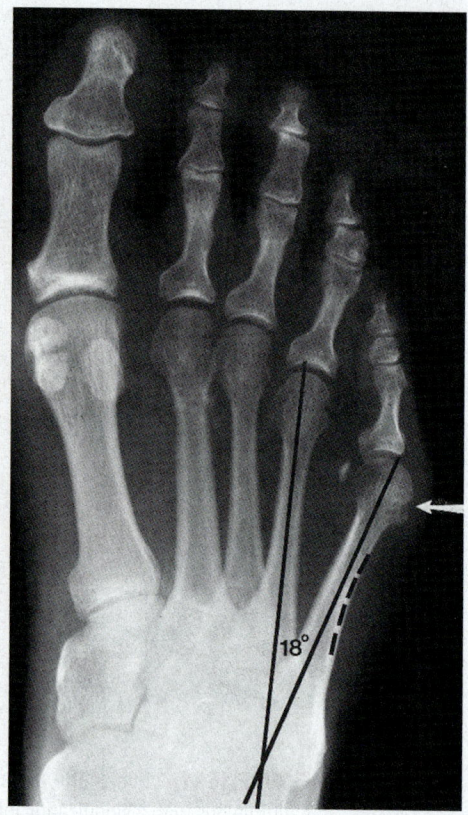

injected under real-time ultrasound guidance to confirm that the needle tip is in the proper position. After proper needle tip placement is confirmed, the remainder of the contents of the syringe are slowly injected. There should be minimal resistance to injection.

## COMPLICATIONS

The major complication of ultrasound-guided injection of the bunionette is infection. Ecchymosis and hematoma formation may also occur. A transient exacerbation of the patient's pain

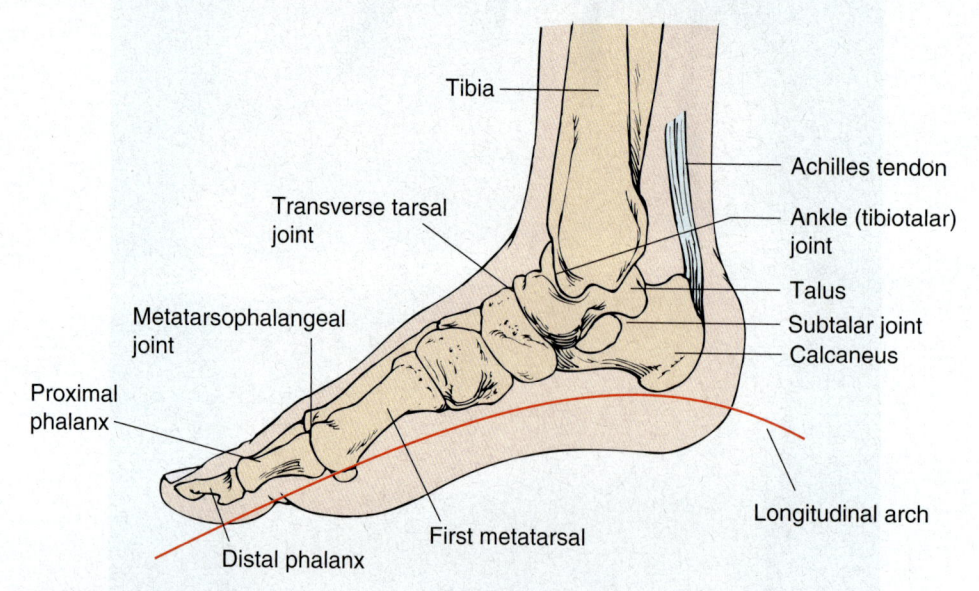

**FIGURE 164.4.** Anatomy of the metatarsophalangeal joints. (Reused from Weber J, Kelley J. *Health Assessment in Nursing*. 2nd ed. Philadelphia, PA: Lippincott Williams & Wilkins; 2003, with permission.)

CHAPTER 164 ULTRASOUND-GUIDED INJECTION TECHNIQUE FOR BUNIONETTE PAIN SYNDROME

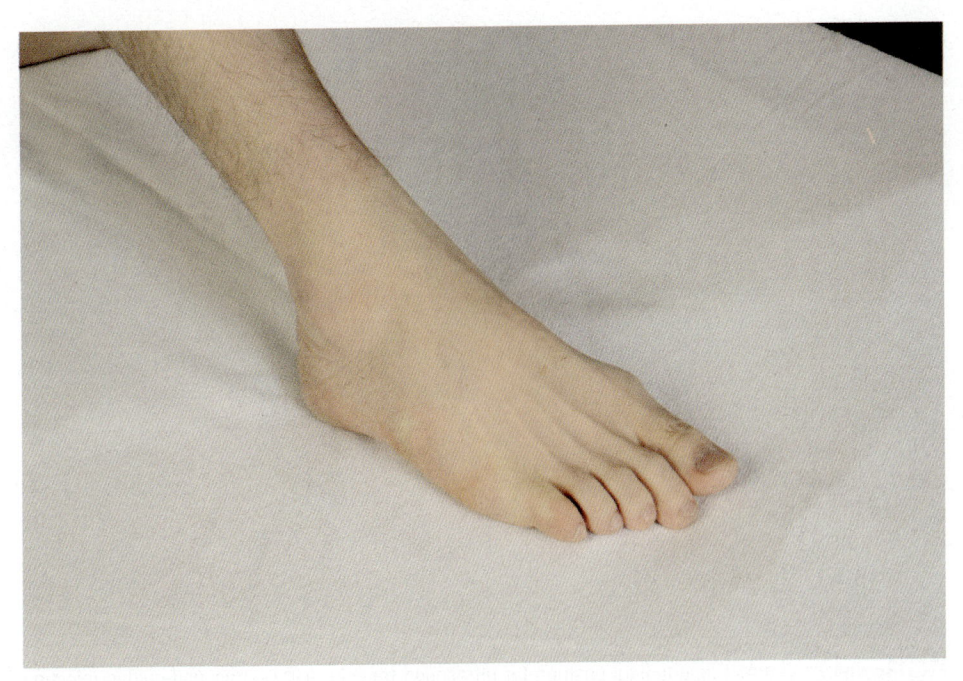

**FIGURE 164.5.** Proper patient position for ultrasound-guided injection of the metatarsophalangeal joint.

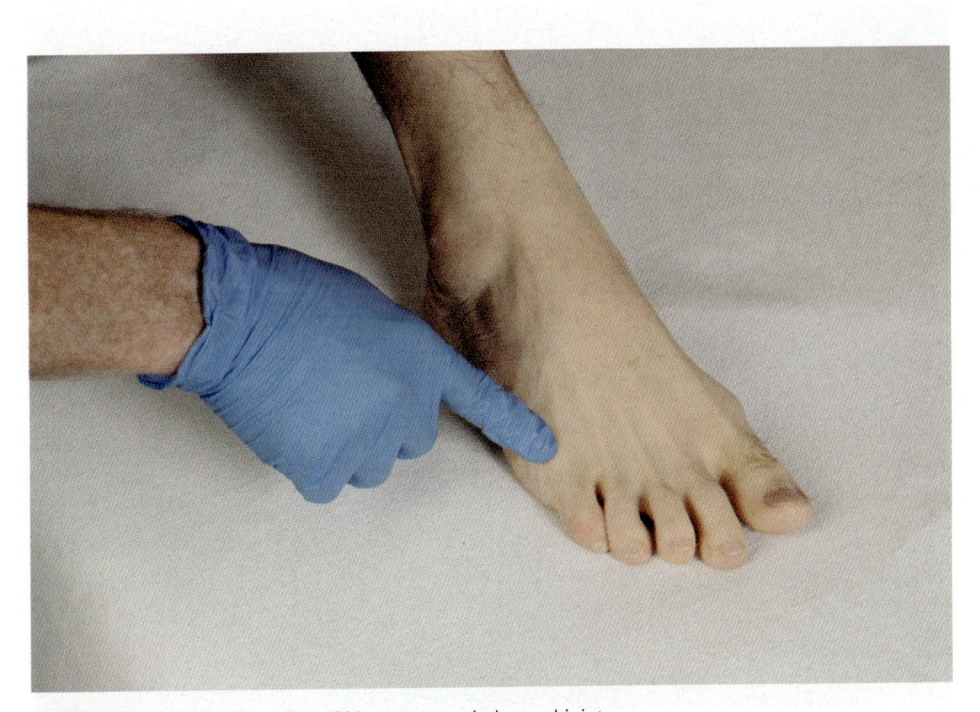

**FIGURE 164.6.** Palpation of the fifth metatarsophalangeal joint.

1156  SECTION X  ANKLE AND FOOT

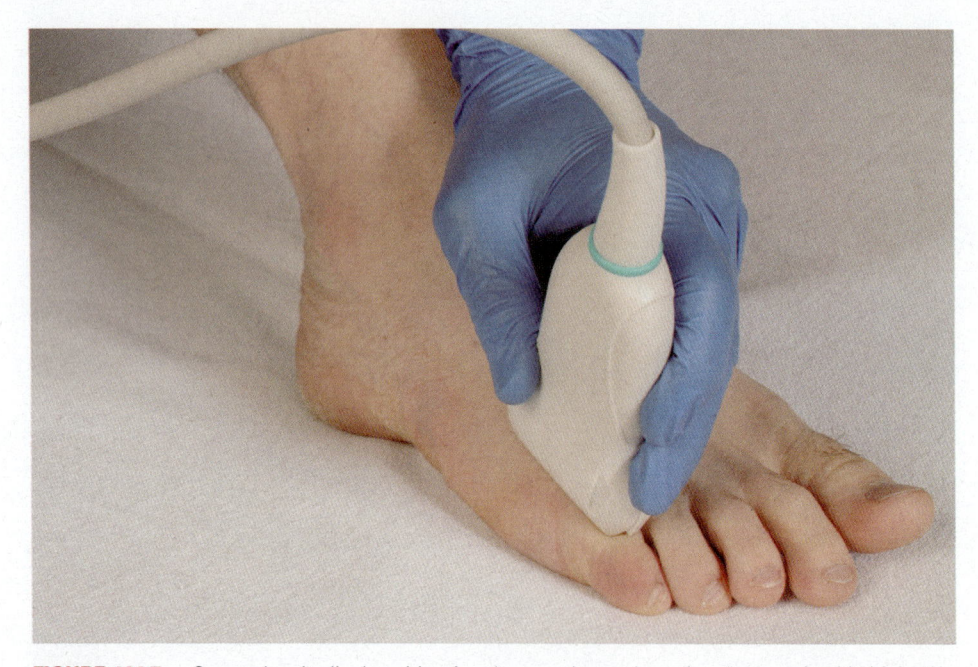

**FIGURE 164.7.** Correct longitudinal position for ultrasound transducer for ultrasound-guided injection technique for bunionette joint.

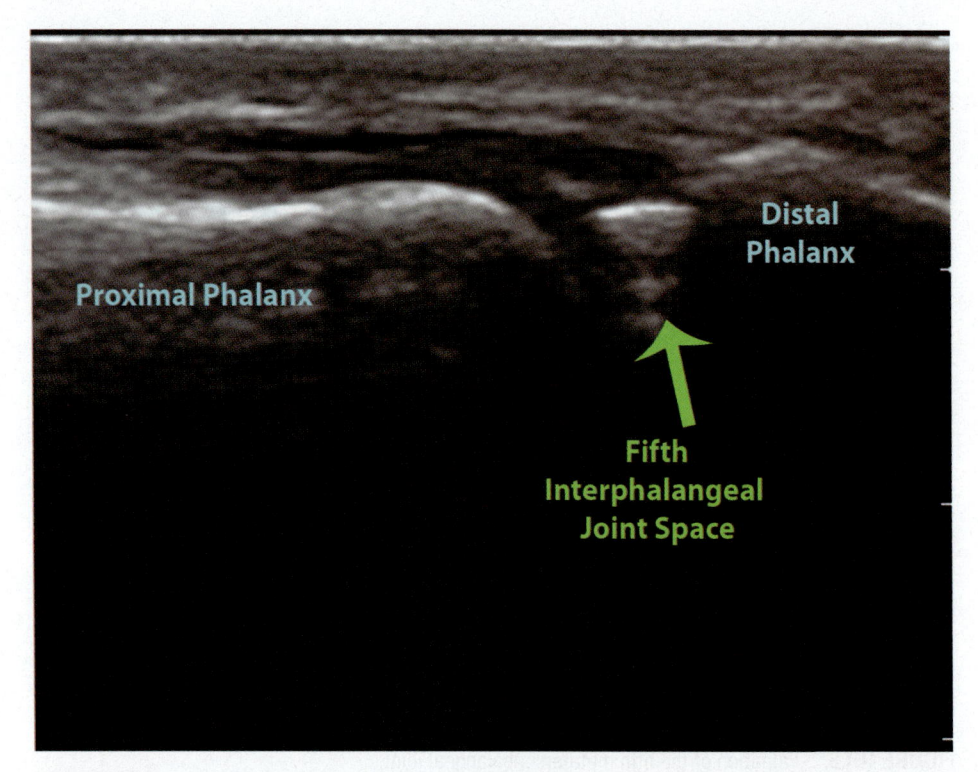

**FIGURE 164.8.** Longitudinal ultrasound view of the metatarsophalangeal joint space of the great toe.

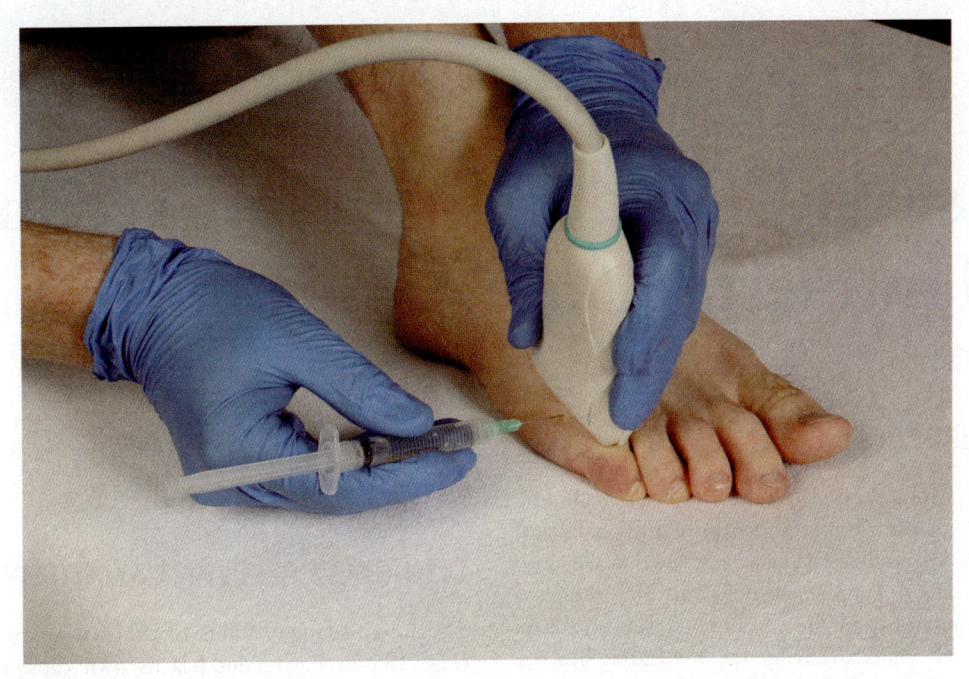

**FIGURE 164.9.** Proper needle position for ultrasound-guided out-of-plane injection of the metatarsophalangeal joint.

occurs ~25% of the time following this injection technique, and the patient should be warned of this possibility prior to the procedure.

## CLINICAL PEARLS

Toe pathology including tendinopathy, occult fractures, osteoarthritis, rheumatoid arthritis, crystal arthropathies, avascular necrosis bursitis, synovitis, and impingement syndromes may coexist with disease of the bunionette and may contribute to the patient's pain symptomatology. Universal precautions should always be observed to protect the operator, and strict adherence to sterile technique must be used to avoid infection. Gentle physical therapy and local heat should be introduced following ultrasound-guided injection of the bunionette to reduce pain and improve function. Simple analgesics and nonsteroidal anti-inflammatory agents or COX-2 inhibitors may be used concurrently with this injection technique.

## SUGGESTED READINGS

Ajis A, Koti M, Maffulli N. Tailor's bunion: a review. *J Foot Ankle Surg* 2005; 44(3):236–245.

Mann RA, Horton GA. Management of the foot and ankle in rheumatoid arthritis. [Original Research Article.] *Rheum Dis Clin North Am* 1996; 22(3): 457–476.

Motta-Valencia K. Dance-related Injury. *Phys Med Rehabil Clin N Am* 2006; 17(3):697–723.

Thomas JL, Blitch IV EL, Chaney DM, et al. Diagnosis and treatment of forefoot disorders. *J Foot Ankle Surg* 2009;48(2):239–250.

Thomas JL, Blitch IV EL, Chaney DM, et al. Diagnosis and treatment of forefoot disorders. *J Foot Ankle Surg* 2009;48(2):264–272.

Waldman SD. Intra-articular injection of the toe joints. In: *Pain Review*. Philadelphia, PA: Saunders Elsevier; 2009:591–592.

Waldman SD. Technique for injection technique for bunionette. In: *Atlas of Pain Management Injection Techniques*. 3rd ed. Philadelphia, PA: Saunders Elsevier; 2012:446–448.

# CHAPTER 165

# Ultrasound-Guided Injection Technique for Hammertoe Pain Syndrome

## CLINICAL PERSPECTIVES

Hammertoe refers to a constellation of symptoms including a painful flexion deformity of the proximal interphalangeal joint with the middle and distal phalanges flexed down onto the proximal phalanges. Hammertoe deformity almost always involves the second toe, and the condition is almost always bilateral. A plantar callus overlying the metatarsal head is usually present as is an inflamed adventitious bursa, further exacerbating the pain and cosmetic deformity (Figs. 165.1 and 165.2). Occurring more commonly in women, like hallux valgus, hammertoe is most commonly the result of wearing shoes with too tight of toe box, with the wearing of high-heeled shoes exacerbating the problem (Fig. 165.3).

The majority of patients who present with hammertoe present with the complaint of pain that is localized to the affected proximal interphalangeal joint and the inability to get shoes to fit. Walking makes the pain worse, with rest and heat providing some relief. The pain is constant and is characterized as aching and may interfere with sleep. Some patients complain of a grating or popping sensation with use of the joint, and crepitus may be present on physical examination. In addition to the just-mentioned pain, patients who suffer with hammertoes develop the characteristic hammertoe deformity, which consists of a painful flexion deformity of the proximal interphalangeal joint with the middle and distal phalanges flexed down onto the proximal phalanges.

Functional disability often accompanies the pain of the hammertoe joint. Patients will often notice increasing difficulty in performing their activities of daily living and tasks that require standing, walking, or weight bearing. If the pathologic process responsible for pain of hammertoe is not adequately treated, the patient's functional disability may worsen and muscle wasting and ultimately a frozen interphalangeal joint may occur.

Plain radiographs are indicated in all patients who present with pain of the hammertoe (Fig. 165.4). Based on the patient's clinical presentation, additional testing may be indicated, including complete blood cell count, sedimentation rate, and antinuclear antibody testing. Magnetic resonance imaging or ultrasound of the hammertoe joint is indicated if fracture, effusion, tendinopathy, crystal arthropathy, joint mice, synovitis, foreign body, bursitis, or ligamentous injury is suspected.

## CLINICALLY RELEVANT ANATOMY

The interphalangeal joints of the foot are ginglymoid joints (Fig. 165.5). Each joint has its own capsule. The articular surface of these joints is covered with hyaline cartilage that is susceptible to arthritis. The toe joint capsules are lined with a synovial membrane that attaches to the articular cartilage. The deep transverse ligaments connect the joints of the five toes and provide the majority of strength to the toe joints. The muscles of the toe joint and their attaching tendons are susceptible to trauma and to wear and tear from overuse and misuse. These joints are also susceptible to overuse and misuse injuries with resultant inflammation and arthritis.

## ULTRASOUND-GUIDED TECHNIQUE

The benefits, risks, and alternative treatments are explained to the patient, and informed consent is obtained. The patient is then placed in the supine position with the knee flexed so that the plantar surface of the affected foot rests comfortably on the examination table (Fig. 165.6). With the patient in the above position, the dorsal surface of the metatarsophalangeal joint of the affected toe is identified by palpation (Fig. 165.7). A high-frequency small linear ultrasound transducer is placed in a longitudinal position over the proximal interphalangeal joint of the affected toe, and an ultrasound survey scan is taken (Figs. 165.8 and 165.9). The hypoechoic joint space is identified between the phalanges. When the joint space is identified, the skin overlying the area beneath the ultrasound transducer as well as the skin covering the lateral portion of the joint is then prepped with antiseptic solution. A sterile syringe containing 1.0 mL of 0.25% preservative-free bupivacaine and 40 mg of methylprednisolone is attached to a 1½-inch, 25-gauge needle using strict aseptic technique. The needle is placed through the skin just below the center of the longitudinally placed transducer and is then advanced using an out-of-plane approach with the needle trajectory adjusted under real-time ultrasound guidance

CHAPTER 165   ULTRASOUND-GUIDED INJECTION TECHNIQUE FOR HAMMERTOE PAIN SYNDROME   1159

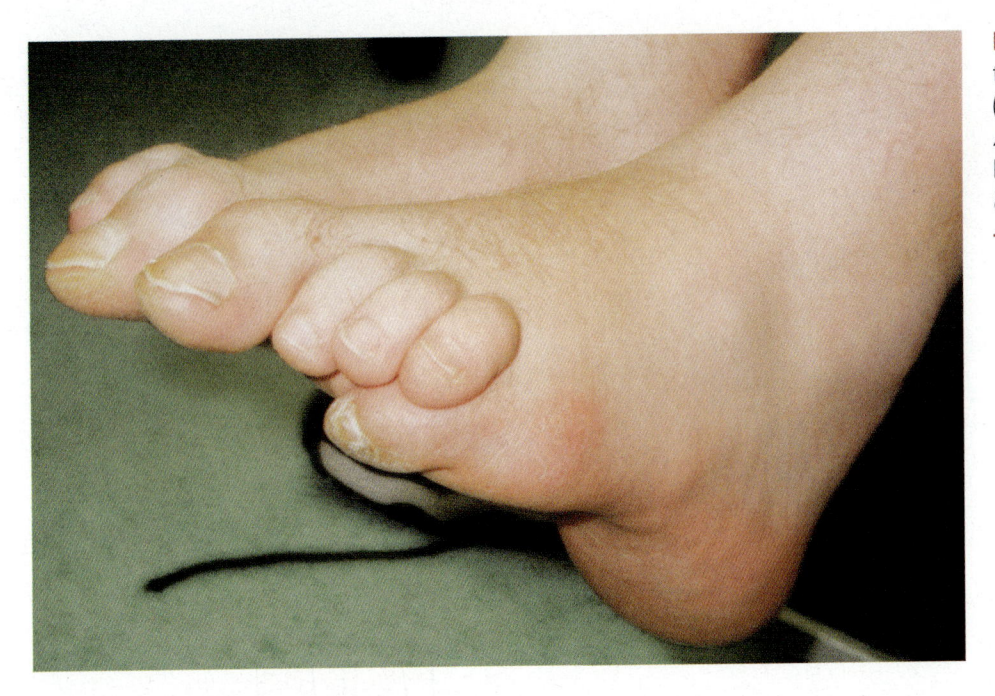

**FIGURE 165.1.** Hammertoe affects the proximal interphalangeal joints. (Reused from Berg D, Worzala K. *Atlas of Adult Physical Diagnosis*. Philadelphia, PA: Lippincott Williams & Wilkins; 2006, with permission.)

so that the needle tip ultimately rests within the proximal interphalangeal joint space (Fig. 165.10). When the tip of needle is thought to be in satisfactory position, after careful gentle aspiration, a small amount of local anesthetic and steroid is injected under real-time ultrasound guidance to confirm that the needle tip is in the proper position. After proper needle tip placement is confirmed, the remainder of the contents of the syringe are slowly injected. There should be minimal resistance to injection.

## COMPLICATIONS

The major complication of ultrasound-guided injection of the hammertoe is infection. Ecchymosis and hematoma formation may also occur. A transient exacerbation of the patient's pain

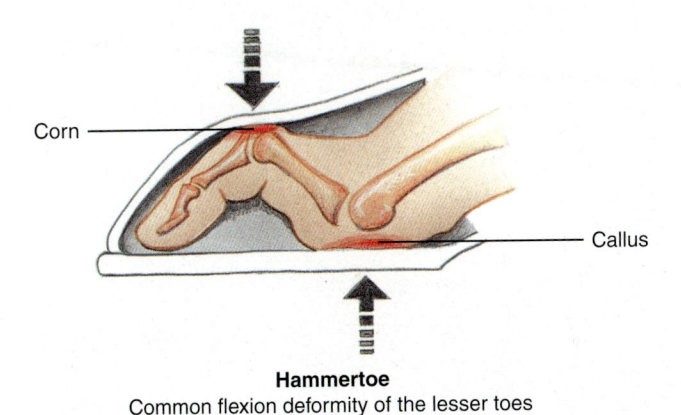

**FIGURE 165.2.** Significant callus development can accompany the hammertoe deformity. (Anatomical Chart Company, 2013.)

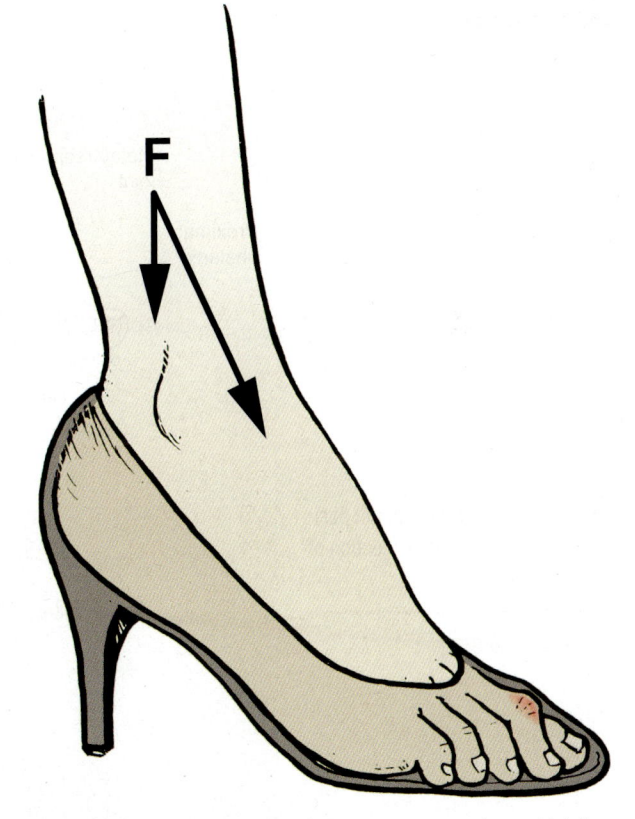

**FIGURE 165.3.** Poor-fitting shoe with a narrow toe box, which forces proximal phalanx into extension and proximal interphalangeal joint into flexion, and an excessively high heel, which allows the toes to slide forward into the narrow toe box. (Reused from Koval KJ, Zuckerman JD. *Atlas of Orthopaedic Surgery: A Multimedia Reference*. Philadelphia, PA: Lippincott Williams & Wilkins; 2004, with permission.)

**FIGURE 165.4.** Lateral radiograph demonstrating the flexion deformity associated with hammertoe. (Reused from Koval KJ, Zuckerman JD. *Atlas of Orthopaedic Surgery: A Multimedia Reference*. Philadelphia, PA: Lippincott Williams & Wilkins; 2004, with permission.)

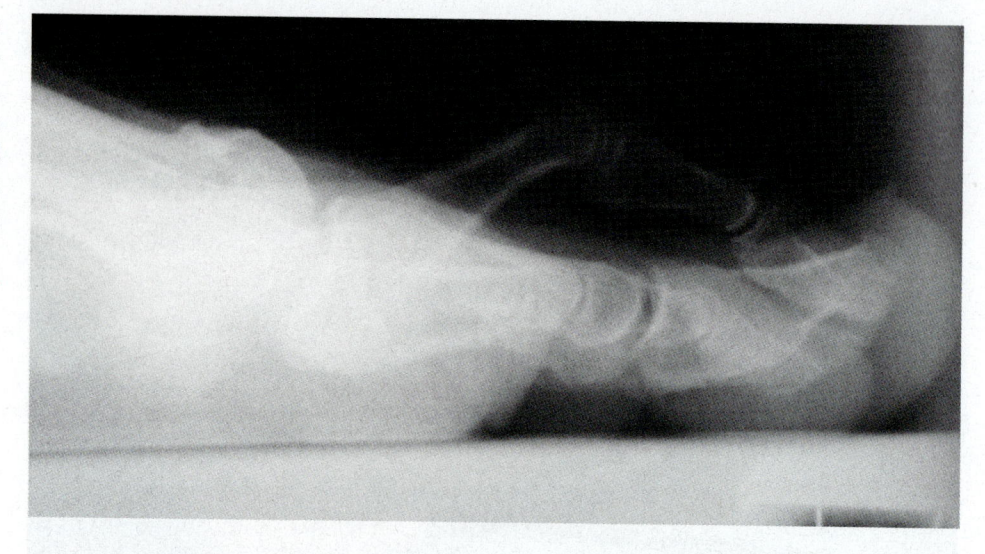

**FIGURE 165.5.** Anatomy of the metatarsophalangeal joints. (Weber J, Kelley J. *Health Assessment in Nursing*. 2nd ed. Philadelphia, PA: Lippincott Williams & Wilkins; 2003, with permission).

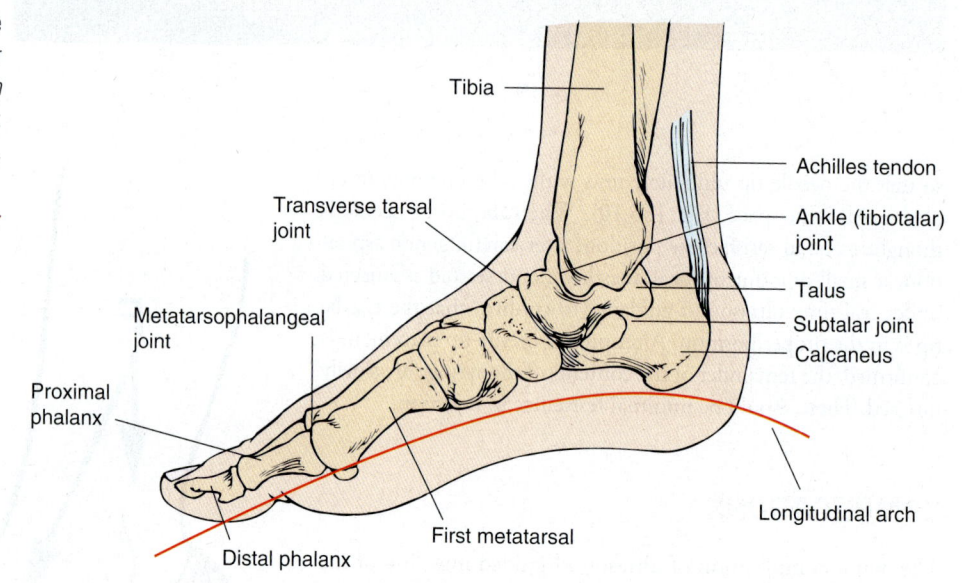

**FIGURE 165.6.** Proper patient position for ultrasound-guided injection of hammertoe.

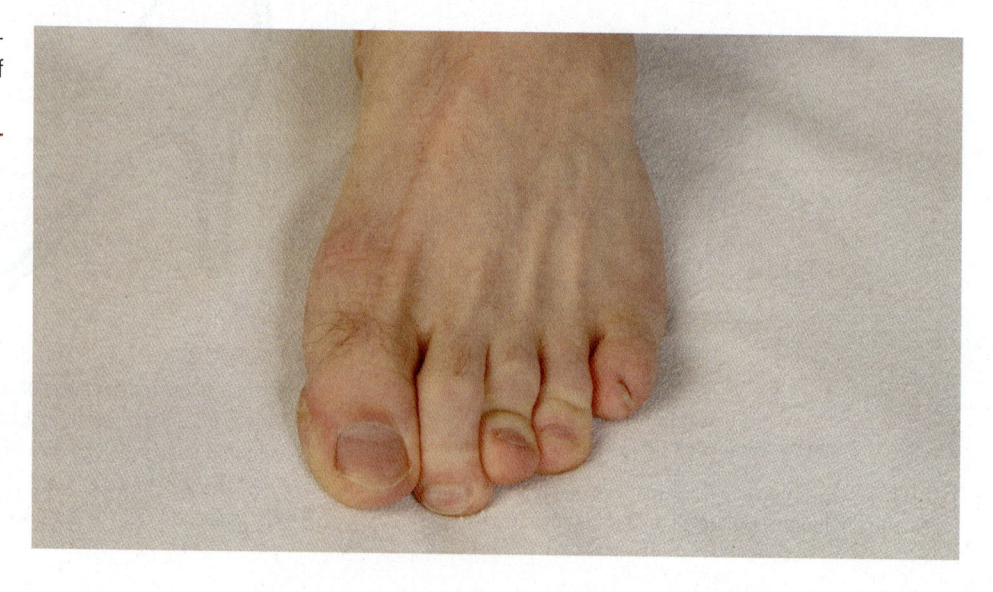

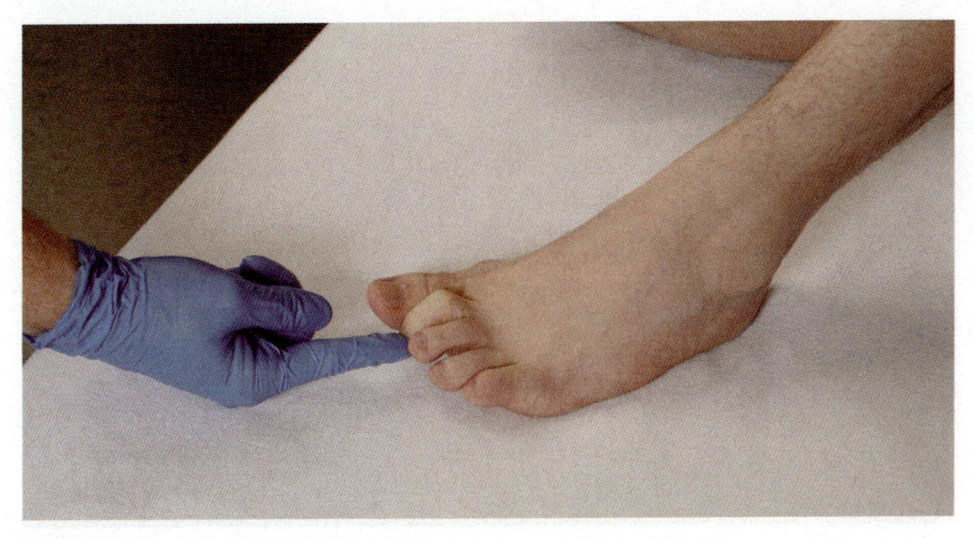

**FIGURE 165.7.** Palpation of the hammertoe.

occurs ~25% of the time following this injection technique, and the patient should be warned of this possibility prior to the procedure.

## CLINICAL PEARLS

Toe pathology including tendinopathy, occult fractures, osteoarthritis, rheumatoid arthritis, crystal arthropathies, avascular necrosis bursitis, synovitis, and impingement syndromes may coexist with disease of the hammertoe and may contribute to the patient's pain symptomatology. Universal precautions should always be observed to protect the operator, and strict adherence to sterile technique must be used to avoid infection. Gentle physical therapy and local heat should be introduced following ultrasound-guided injection of the hammertoe to reduce pain and improve function. Simple analgesics and nonsteroidal anti-inflammatory agents or COX-2 inhibitors may be used concurrently with this injection technique.

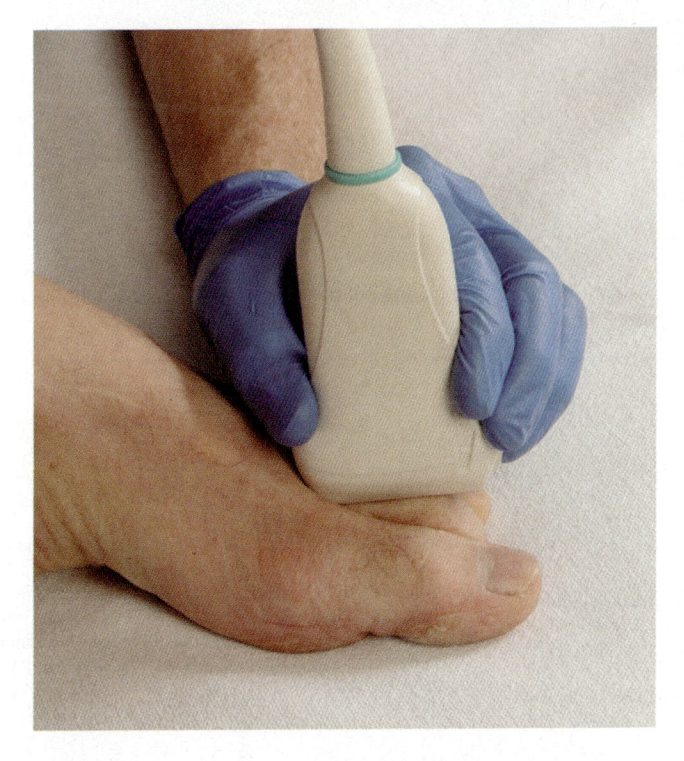

**FIGURE 165.8.** Correct longitudinal position for ultrasound transducer for ultrasound-guided injection technique for hammertoe joint.

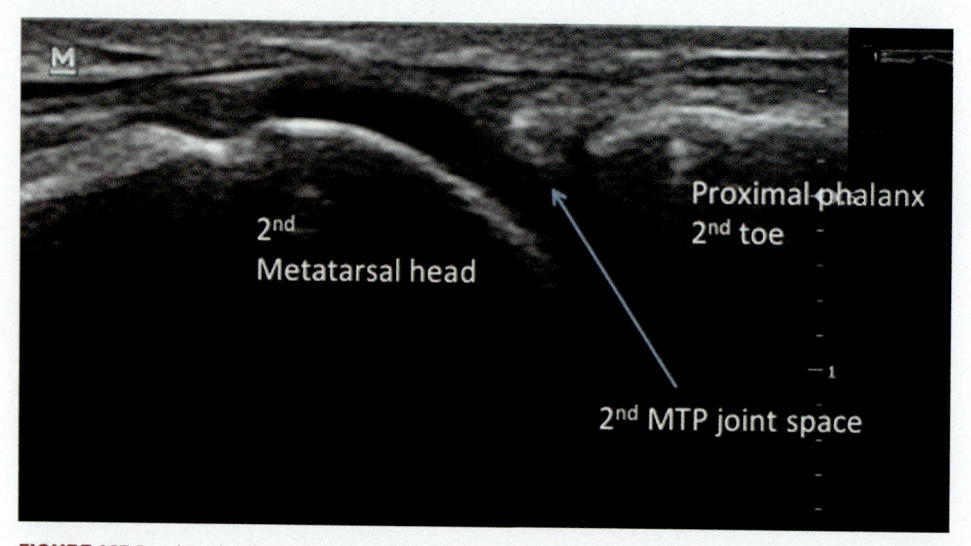

**FIGURE 165.9.** Longitudinal ultrasound view of the metatarsophalangeal joint space of the great toe.

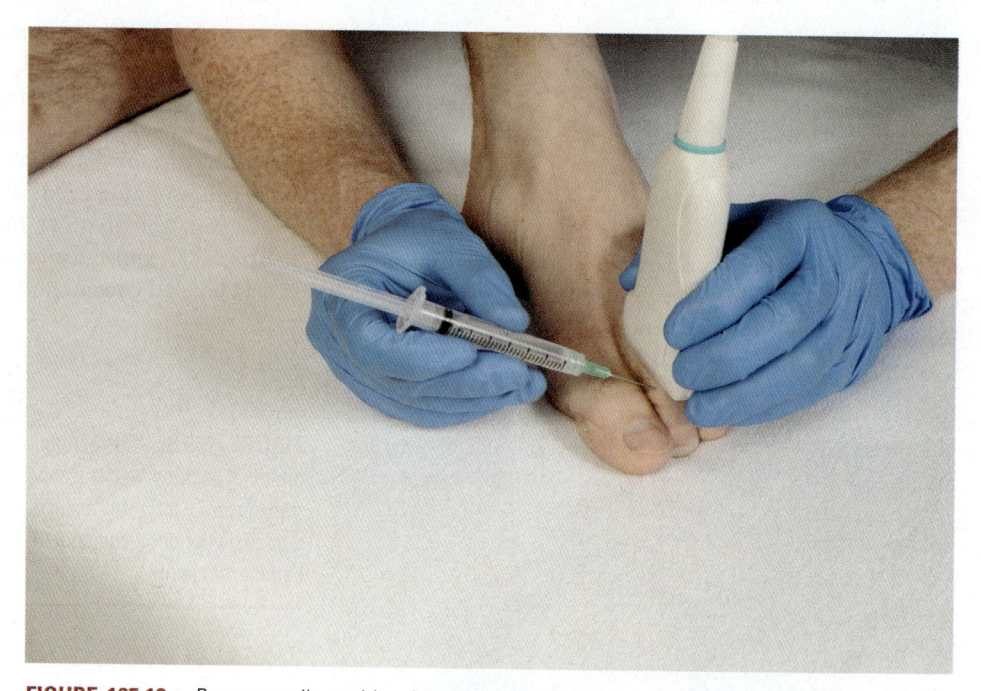

**FIGURE 165.10.** Proper needle position for ultrasound-guided out-of-plane injection of the metatarsophalangeal joint.

## SUGGESTED READINGS

Mann Ra, Horton GA. Management of the foot and ankle in rheumatoid arthritis. [Original Research Article.] *Rheum Dis Clin North Am* 1996;22(3):457–476.

Motta-Valencia K. Dance-related injury. *Phys Med Rehabil Clin N Am* 2006;17(3): 697–723.

Thomas JL, Blitch IV EL, Chaney DM, et al. Diagnosis and treatment of forefoot disorders. *J Foot Ankle Surg* 2009;48(2):239–250.

Thomas JL, Blitch IV EL, Chaney DM, et al. Diagnosis and treatment of forefoot disorders. *J Foot Ankle Surg* 2009;48(2):264–272.

Waldman SD. Intra-articular injection of the toe joints. In: *Pain Review*. Philadelphia, PA: Saunders Elsevier; 2009:591–592.

Waldman SD. Technique for Injection technique for hammertoe. In: *Atlas of Pain Management Injection*. 3rd ed. Philadelphia, PA: Saunders Elsevier; 2012:471–472.

CHAPTER 166

# Ultrasound-Guided Injection Technique for Morton Neuroma Syndrome

## CLINICAL PERSPECTIVES

Morton neuroma, which was first described by Thomas Morton in 1876, refers to a constellation of symptoms including tenderness and burning pain in the plantar surface of the forefoot, with associated painful dysesthesias into the affected two toes. This pain syndrome is thought to be caused by perineural fibrosis of the interdigital nerves (Fig. 166.1). There is often coexistent intermetatarsal bursitis as the pathogenesis of both pathologic conditions is similar. Although the nerves between the third and fourth toes most often are affected, the second and third toes and, rarely, the fourth and fifth toes can be affected.

The majority of patients who present with Morton neuroma present with the complaint of pain in the plantar surface with associated dysesthesias radiating into the adjacent toes. Patients commonly complain that it feels like they are walking with a stone caught in their shoe. Walking, standing, or wearing tight shoes makes the pain worse, with rest and heat providing some relief. The pain is constant and is characterized as aching and may interfere with sleep.

On physical examination, the pain associated with Morton neuroma can be reproduced by performing the Mulder maneuver. This is accomplished by firmly squeezing the two metatarsal heads together with one hand while placing firm pressure on the interdigital space with the other hand (Fig. 166.2). A palpable click may also be appreciated as the neuroma is forced from between the metatarsals. The patient with Morton neuroma often exhibits an antalgic gait in an effort to reduce weight bearing during walking.

Plain radiographs are indicated in all patients who present with Morton neuroma. Based on the patient's clinical presentation, additional testing may be indicated, including complete blood cell count, sedimentation rate, and antinuclear antibody testing. Magnetic resonance imaging (MRI) or ultrasound of the Morton neuroma is indicated to help confirm the diagnosis and if fracture, effusion, tendinopathy, crystal arthropathy, joint mice, synovitis, foreign body, bursitis, or ligamentous injury is suspected (Figs. 166.3 and 166.4).

## CLINICALLY RELEVANT ANATOMY

In a manner analogous to that of the digital nerves of the hand, the digital nerves of the foot travel through the intrametatarsal space to innervate each toe. The plantar digital nerves, which are derived from the posterior tibial nerve, provide sensory innervation to the major portion of the plantar surface (Fig. 166.5). These nerves are subject to entrapment and resultant development of perineural fibrosis and degeneration

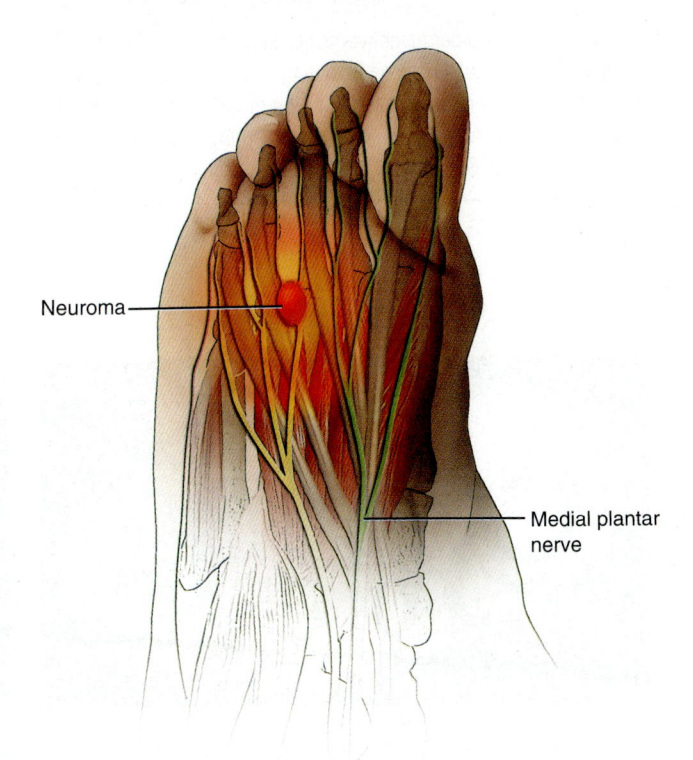

**FIGURE 166.1.** Patients suffering from Morton neuroma present with the complaint of pain in the plantar surface with associated dysesthesias radiating into the adjacent toes.

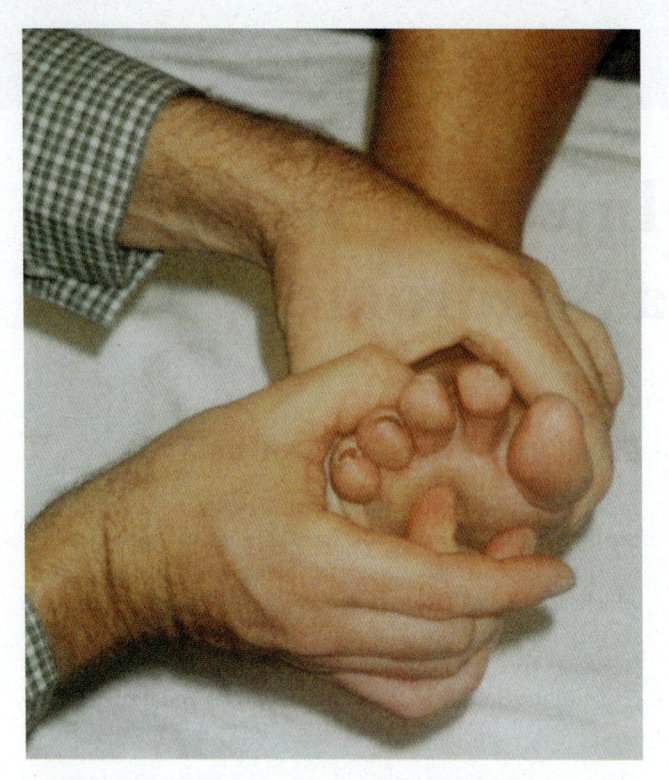

**FIGURE 166.2.** Mulder maneuver is accomplished by firmly squeezing the two metatarsal heads together with one hand while placing firm pressure on the interdigital space with the other hand. (Reused from Berg D, Worzala K. *Atlas of Adult Physical Diagnosis*. Philadelphia, PA: Lippincott Williams & Wilkins; 2006, with permission.)

resulting in the clinical syndrome known as Morton neuroma (see Fig. 166.1). The dorsal aspect of the foot is innervated by terminal branches of the deep and superficial peroneal nerves. The overlap of the innervation of these nerves may be considerable.

## ULTRASOUND-GUIDED TECHNIQUE

The benefits, risks, and alternative treatments are explained to the patient, and informed consent is obtained. The patient is then placed in the prone position with the affected foot hanging comfortably over the edge of the examination table (Fig. 166.6). With the patient in the above position, a high-frequency small linear ultrasound transducer is placed in a transverse position over the metatarsophalangeal heads, and an ultrasound survey scan is taken (Fig. 166.7). The intermetatarsal space is identified between the heads of the metatarsals, and the homogeneous-appearing intermetatarsal soft tissue is searched for the appearance of a rounded hyperechoic Morton neuroma (see Fig. 166.4). Dynamic scanning while performing the Mulder maneuver may help identify the neuroma as it is forced from between the metatarsal heads (Fig. 166.8). When the intermetatarsal space containing the Morton neuroma is identified, the skin on the plantar surface of the foot overlying the area containing the Morton neuroma is then prepped with antiseptic solution. A sterile syringe containing 3.0 mL of 0.25% preservative-free bupivacaine and 40 mg of methylprednisolone is attached to a 1½-inch, 25-gauge needle using strict aseptic technique. The needle is placed through the skin just

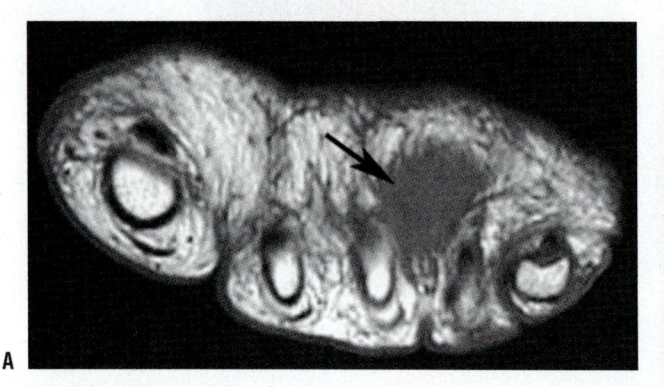

**FIGURE 166.3.** Axial T1-weighted **(A)**, T2-weighted **(B)**, and postcontrast-enhanced fat-suppressed T1-weighted **(C)** images demonstrate a Morton neuroma between the third and fourth metatarsals that extends dorsally (*arrow*). Note the mixed signal intensity on the T2-weighted image (B) and intense enhancement (C). (Berquist TH, Kransdorf MJ. Bone and soft tissue tumors and tumor-like conditions. In: Berquist TH, ed. *Imaging of the foot and ankle*. 3rd ed. Philadelphia, PA: Lippincott Williams & Wilkins; 2011:426, with permission.)

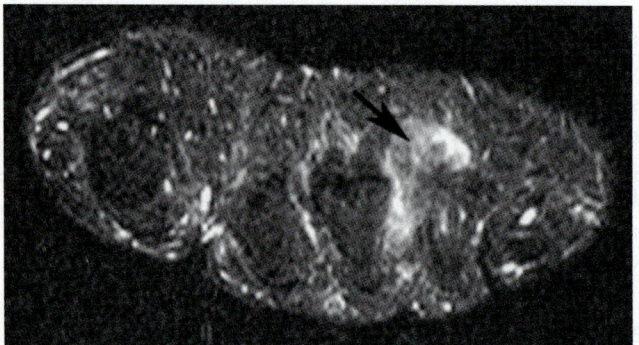

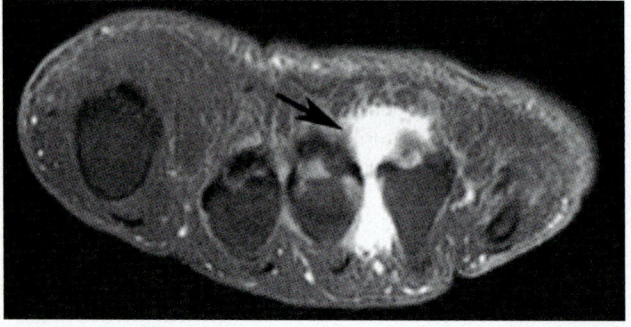

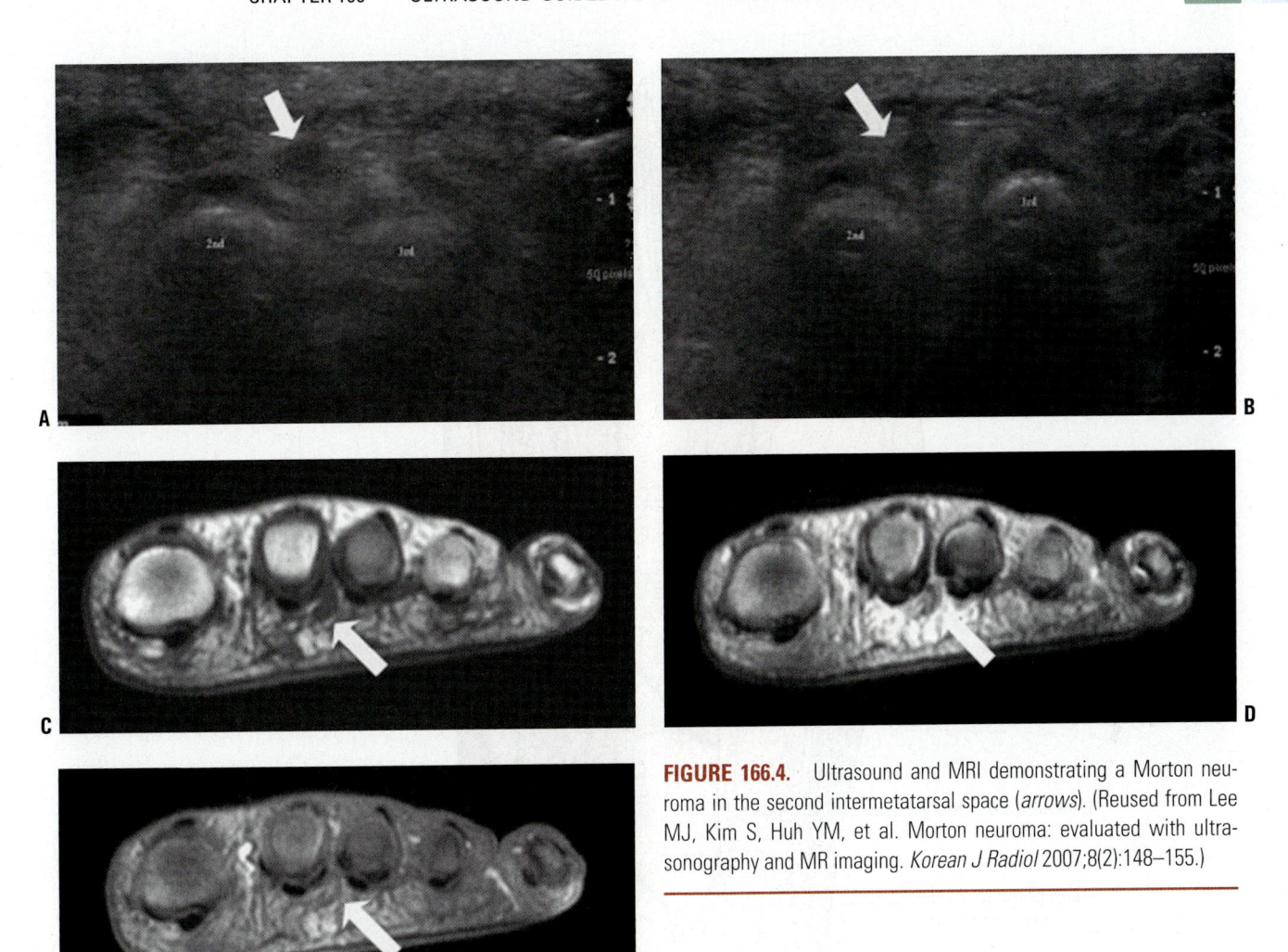

**FIGURE 166.4.** Ultrasound and MRI demonstrating a Morton neuroma in the second intermetatarsal space (*arrows*). (Reused from Lee MJ, Kim S, Huh YM, et al. Morton neuroma: evaluated with ultrasonography and MR imaging. *Korean J Radiol* 2007;8(2):148–155.)

above the center of the transversely placed transducer and is then advanced using an out-of-plane approach with the needle trajectory adjusted under real-time ultrasound guidance so that the needle tip ultimately rests within the intermetatarsal space in proximity to the Morton neuroma (Fig. 166.9). When the tip of the needle is thought to be in satisfactory position, after careful gentle aspiration, a small amount of local anesthetic and steroid is injected under real-time ultrasound guidance to confirm that the needle tip is in the proper position in proximity to the neuroma. After proper needle tip placement is confirmed, the remainder of the contents of the syringe are slowly injected. There should be minimal resistance to injection.

## COMPLICATIONS

The major complication of ultrasound-guided injection of the Morton neuroma is infection. Ecchymosis and hematoma formation may also occur. A transient exacerbation of the patient's pain occurs ~25% of the time following this injection technique, and the patient should be warned of this possibility prior to the procedure.

## CLINICAL PEARLS

Toe pathology including tendinopathy, occult fractures, osteoarthritis, rheumatoid arthritis, crystal arthropathies, avascular necrosis bursitis, synovitis, and impingement syndromes may coexist with disease of the Morton neuroma and may contribute to the patient's pain symptomatology. Universal precautions should always be observed to protect the operator, and strict adherence to sterile technique must be used to avoid infection. Gentle physical therapy and local heat should be introduced following ultrasound-guided injection of the Morton neuroma to reduce pain and improve function. Simple analgesics and nonsteroidal anti-inflammatory agents or COX-2 inhibitors may be used concurrently with this injection technique.

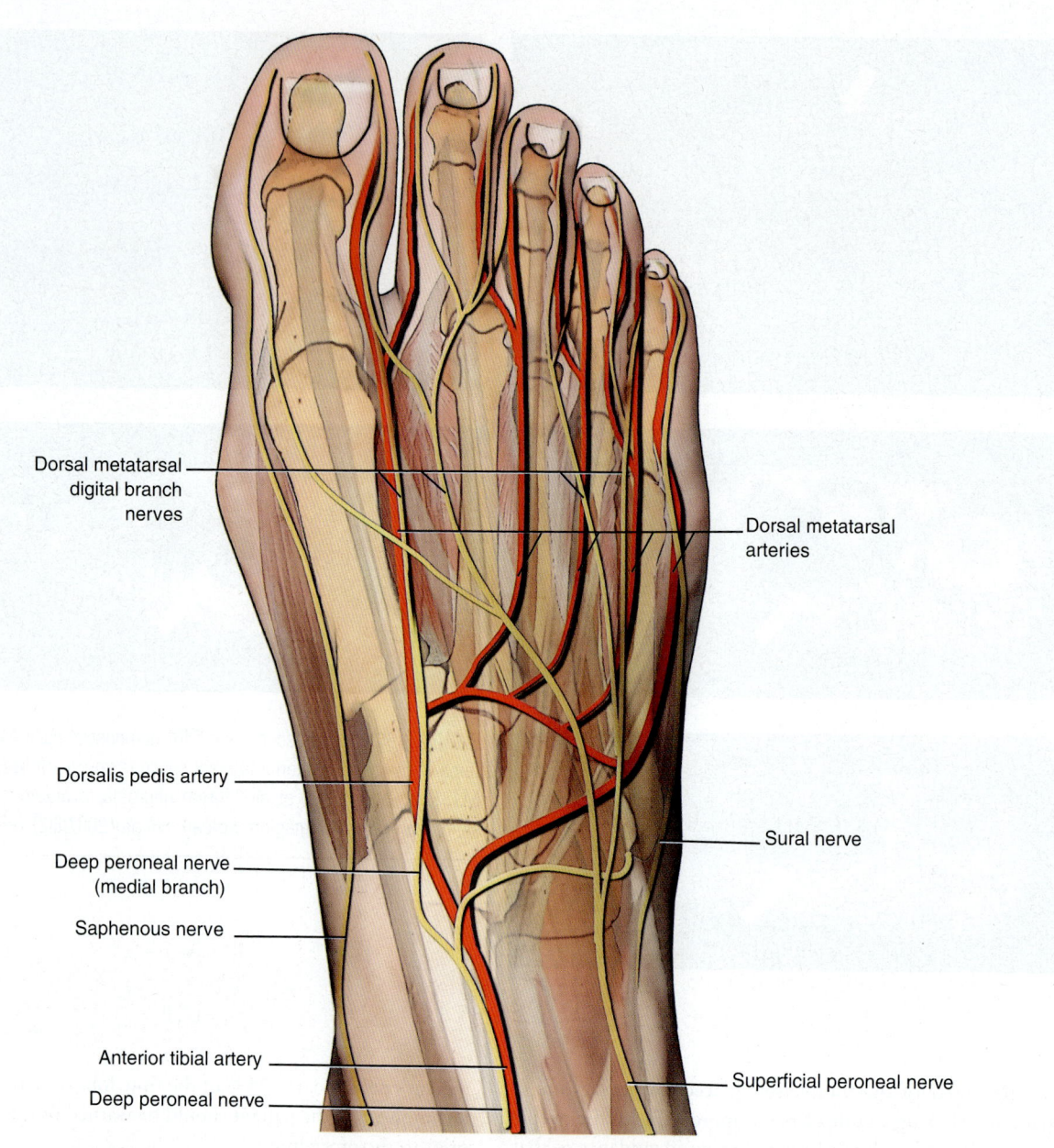

**FIGURE 166.5.** Anatomy of the metatarsophalangeal and digital nerves.

CHAPTER 166 ULTRASOUND-GUIDED INJECTION TECHNIQUE FOR MORTON NEUROMA SYNDROME 1167

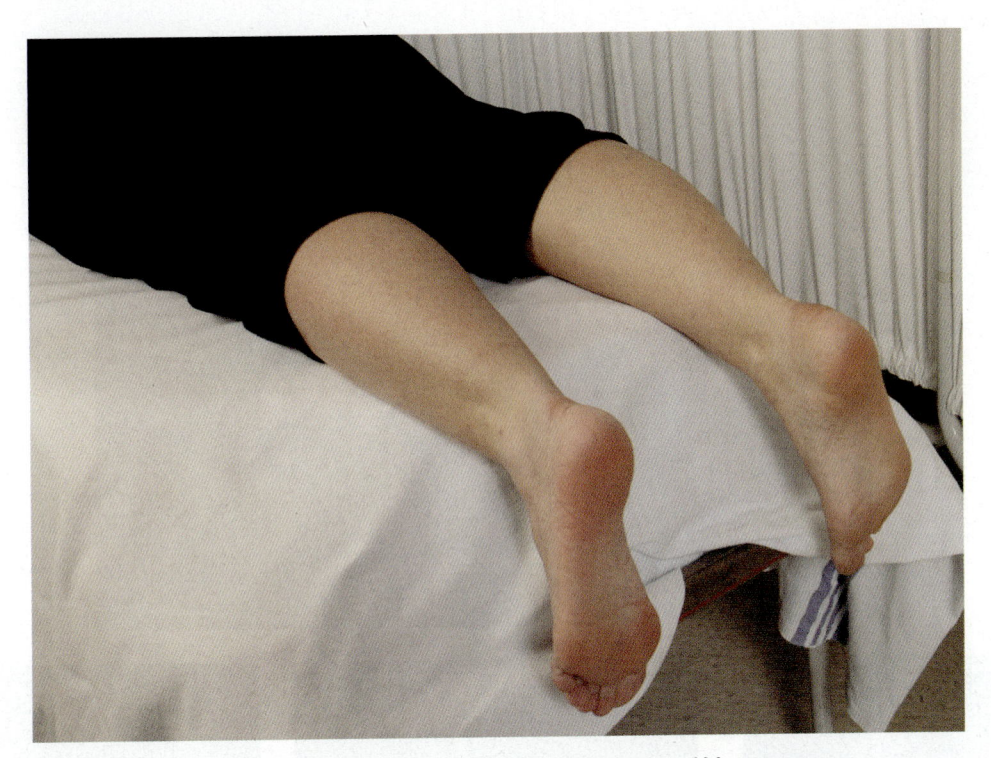

**FIGURE 166.6.** Proper patient position for ultrasound-guided injection of Morton neuroma.

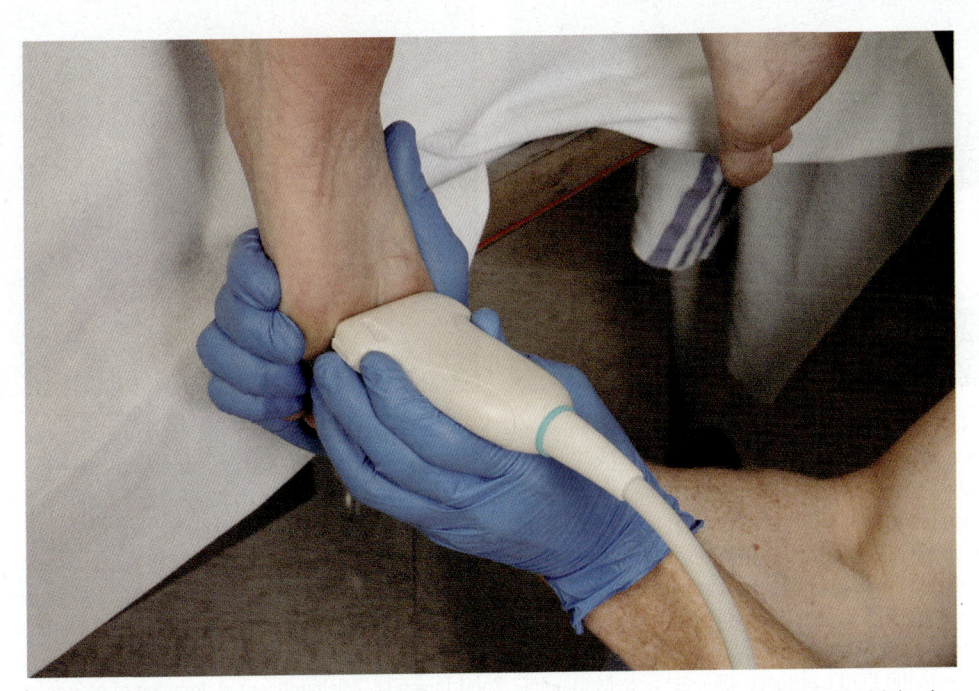

**FIGURE 166.7.** Correct transverse position for ultrasound transducer for ultrasound-guided injection technique for Morton neuroma while performing Mulder maneuver.

**1168** SECTION X ANKLE AND FOOT

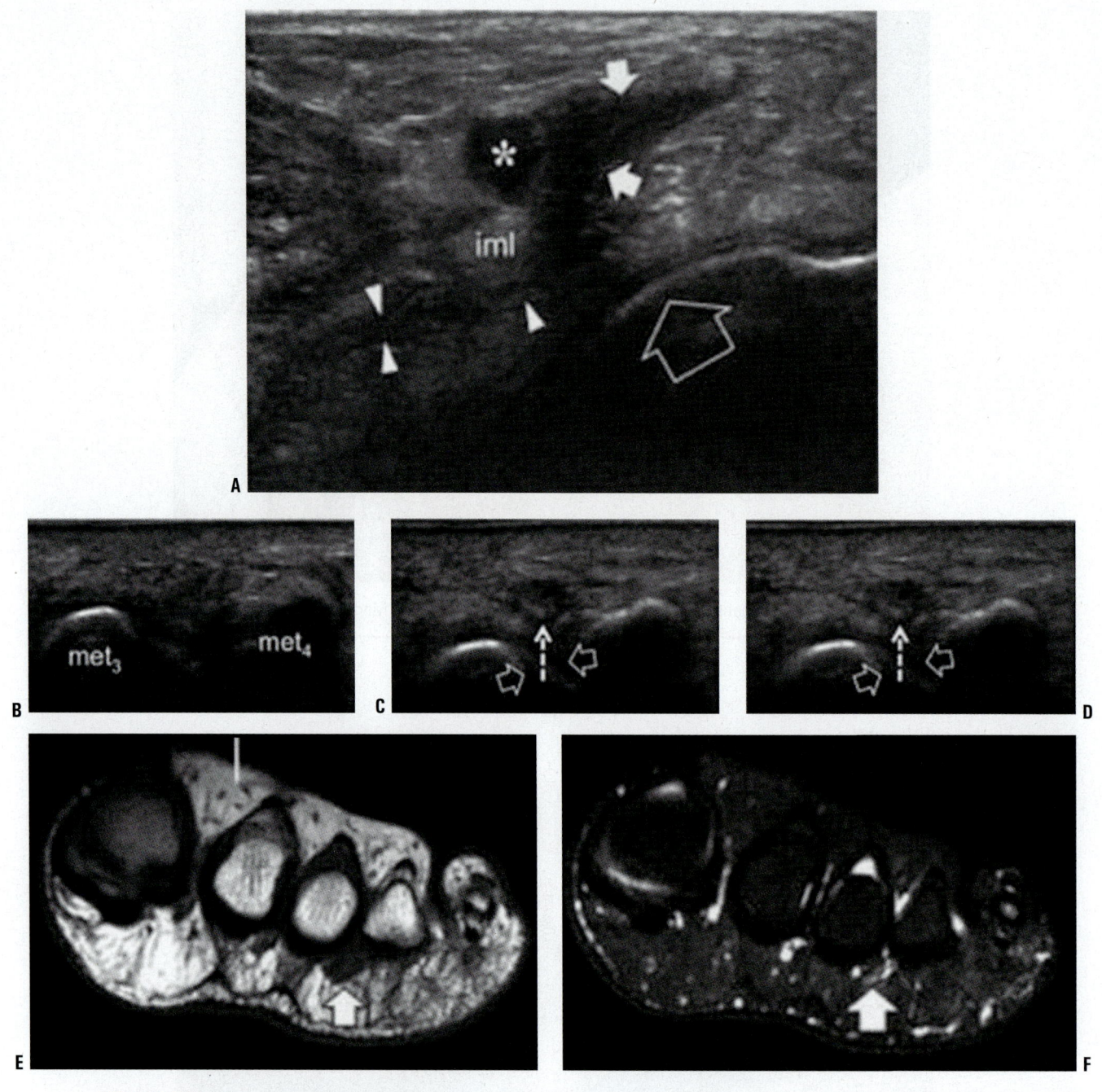

**FIGURE 166.8.** Morton neuroma. **A:** Longitudinal ultrasound image of the third webspace obtained with a dorsal approach while pressing with the thumb (*large void arrow*) from the plantar aspect of the foot shows the interdigital nerve (*arrowheads*) as it passes underneath the intermetatarsal ligament (iml) before deflecting dorsally and continuing in a fusiform hypoechoic Morton neuroma (*white arrows*). A fluid-filled intermetatarsal bursa (*asterisk*) can be appreciated dorsal to the neuroma. **B,C:** Sonographic Mulder's test. Transverse ultrasound images of the third webspace obtained **(B)** in a resting state and **(C)** while squeezing the third ($met_3$) and fourth ($met_4$) metatarsals together. With this maneuver, the metatarsal gets closer (*arrows*) and a mushroom-like hypoechoic neuroma is seen popping up (*dashed arrow*) from the intermetatarsal space. **D:** Short-axis T1-weighted and **(E,F)** fat-suppressed T2-weighted MRI of the forefoot demonstrate a hypointense neuroma (*arrow*) of the interdigital nerve to the third webspace. (Reused from Martinoli C, Court-Payen M, Michaud J, et al. Imaging of neuropathies about the ankle and foot. *Semin Musculoskelet Radiol* 2010;14(3):344–356, with permission.)

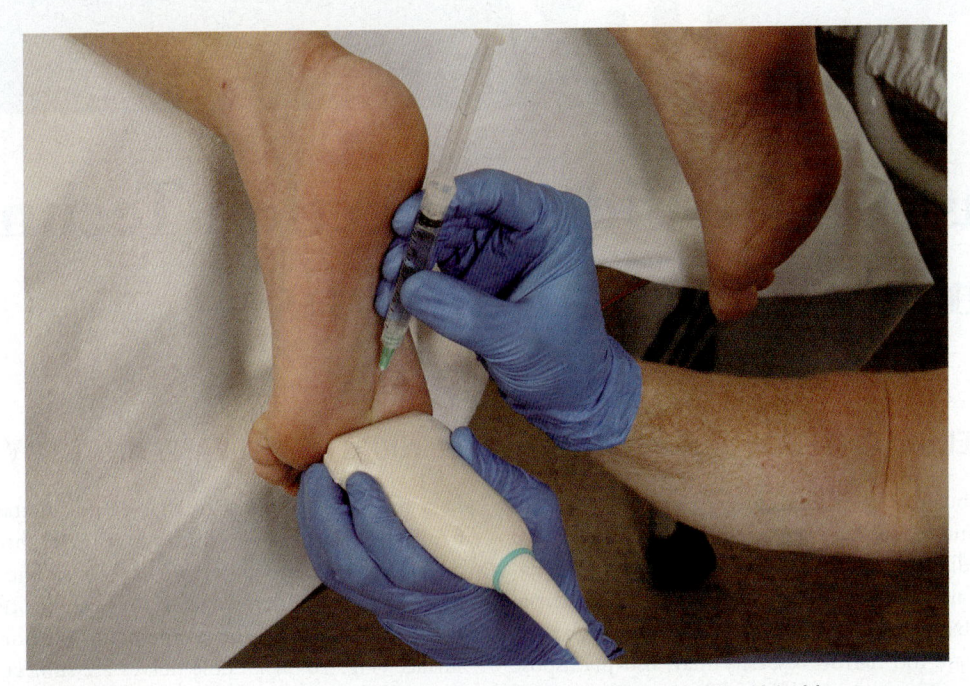

**FIGURE 166.9.** Proper needle position for ultrasound-guided out-of-plane injection of the Morton neuroma.

## SUGGESTED READINGS

Adams II WR. Morton's neuroma. *Clin Podiatr Med Surg* 2010;27(4):535–545.
Betts RP, Bygrave CJ, Jones S, et al. Ultrasonic diagnosis of Morton's neuroma: a guide to problems, pointers, pitfalls and prognosis. [Original Research Article.] *Foot* 2003;13(2):92–99.
George VA, Khan AM, Hutchinson CE, et al. Morton's neuroma: the role of MR scanning in diagnostic assistance. [Original Research Article.] *Foot* 2005;15(1):14–16.
Kay D, Bennett GL. Morton's neuroma. *Foot Ankle Clin* 2003;8(1):49–59.
Waldman SD. Technique for injection technique for Morton's neuroma. In: *Atlas of Pain Management Injection Techniques*. 3rd ed. Philadelphia, PA: Saunders Elsevier; 2012:473–474.

# CHAPTER 167

# Ultrasound-Guided Injection Technique for Intermetatarsal Bursitis

## CLINICAL PERSPECTIVES

Intermetatarsal bursitis refers to a constellation of symptoms including pain and tenderness over the affected intermetatarsal spaces, which radiate distally into the toes especially if the adjacent interdigital nerve is inflamed. The pain of intermetatarsal bursitis is exacerbated by weight bearing and wearing high heels or shoes which are too narrow. Obesity may also predispose to this condition. The patient suffering from intermetatarsal bursitis is often unable to stand on tiptoes or walk up stairs. Walking and standing for long periods make the pain worse. The pain of intermetatarsal bursitis is constant and is characterized as sharp and may interfere with sleep. Coexistent neuritis, neuropathy, Morton neuroma formation, stress fractures, metatarsalgia, and synovitis may confuse the clinical picture. As the bursitis worsens, the affected intermetatarsal bursae tend to expand surrounding the adjacent interdigital nerves making the patients clinical presentation indistinguishable from the pain of Morton neuroma. If the inflammation of the intermetatarsal bursae becomes chronic, calcification of the bursae and fibrosis of the surrounding interdigital space may occur.

On physical examination, pain can be reproduced by squeezing the affected web space between the index finger and thumb. If the interdigital nerve is involved or if a Morton neuroma has developed, a positive Mulder sign can be elicited by firmly squeezing the two metatarsal heads together with one hand while placing firm pressure on the interdigital space with the other hand (Fig. 167.1). The patient with intermetatarsal bursitis often exhibits an antalgic gait in an effort to reduce weight bearing during walking.

Plain radiographs are indicated in all patients who present with intermetatarsal bursa. Based on the patient's clinical presentation, additional testing may be indicated, including complete blood cell count, sedimentation rate, and antinuclear antibody testing. Magnetic resonance imaging or ultrasound of the intermetatarsal bursa is indicated to help confirm the diagnosis and if fracture, effusion, tendinopathy, crystal arthropathy, joint mice, synovitis, foreign body, bursitis, or ligamentous injury is suspected (Figs. 167.2 and 167.3).

## CLINICALLY RELEVANT ANATOMY

In a manner analogous to that of the digital nerves of the hand, the digital nerves of the foot travel through the intermetatarsal space to innervate each toe. The plantar digital nerves, which are derived from the posterior tibial nerve, provide sensory innervation to the major portion of the plantar surface (Fig. 167.4). These nerves are subject to entrapment and resultant development of perineural fibrosis and degeneration resulting in the clinical syndrome known as Morton neuroma (Fig. 167.5). The dorsal aspect of the foot is innervated by terminal branches of the deep and superficial peroneal nerves. The overlap of the innervation of these nerves may be considerable. The intermetatarsal bursa lies between the metatarsal phalangeal joints in a position that is just dorsal to the interdigital nerves (Fig. 167.6). The bursae extend ~1 cm beyond the distal border of the ligament in the web spaces between the second and third and third and fourth digits.

## ULTRASOUND-GUIDED TECHNIQUE

The benefits, risks, and alternative treatments are explained to the patient, and informed consent is obtained. The patient is then placed in the prone position with the affected foot hanging comfortably over the edge of the examination table (Fig. 167.7). With the patient in the above position, a high-frequency small linear ultrasound transducer is placed in a transverse position over the metatarsophalangeal heads, and an ultrasound survey scan is taken (Fig. 167.8). The intermetatarsal space is identified between the heads of the metatarsals, and the homogeneous-appearing intermetatarsal soft tissue is searched for the appearance of a rounded hypoechoic intermetatarsal bursa (see Fig. 167.3). Dynamic scanning while performing the Mulder maneuver may help identify the inflamed and enlarged bursa as it is forced from between the metatarsal heads (Fig. 167.9). When the intermetatarsal space containing the symptomatic intermetatarsal bursa is identified, the skin on the plantar surface of the foot overlying the area containing the intermetatarsal bursa is then prepped with antiseptic solution. A sterile syringe containing 3.0 mL of 0.25% preservative-free bupivacaine and 40 mg of methylprednisolone is attached to a 1½-inch, 25-gauge needle using strict aseptic technique. The needle is placed through the skin just above the center of the transversely placed transducer and is then advanced using an out-of-plane approach with the needle trajectory adjusted under real-time ultrasound guidance so that the needle tip ultimately rests within the intermetatarsal bursa (Fig. 167.10). When the tip of needle is thought to be in satisfactory position, after careful gentle aspiration, a small amount of local anesthetic and steroid is injected under real-time ultrasound guidance to confirm that the needle tip is in the proper position within the bursa. After proper needle tip placement is confirmed, the remainder of the contents of the syringe are slowly injected. There should be minimal resistance to injection.

## COMPLICATIONS

The major complication of ultrasound-guided injection of intermetatarsal bursitis is infection. Ecchymosis and hematoma formation may also occur. A transient exacerbation of the patient's pain occurs ~25% of the time following this injection technique, and the patient should be warned of this possibility prior to the procedure.

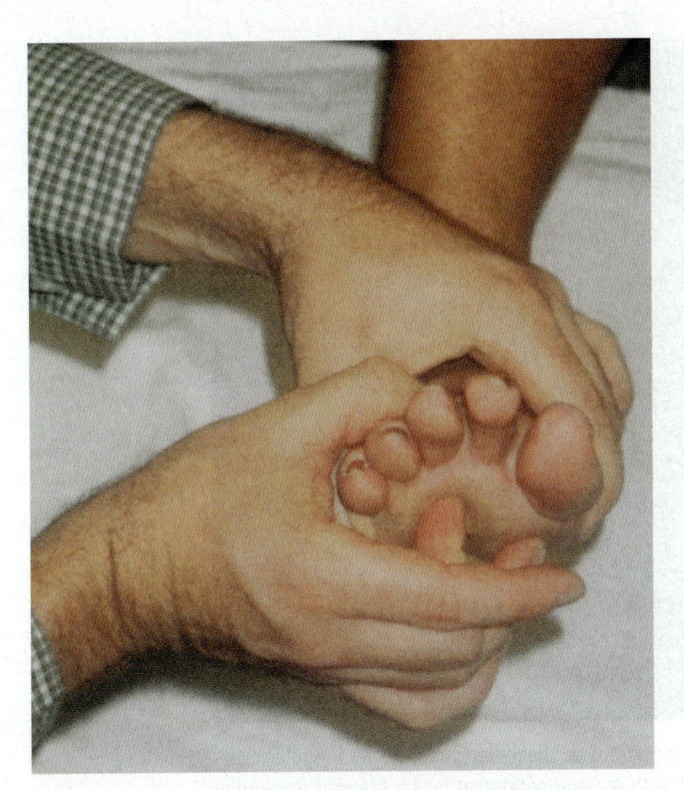

**FIGURE 167.1.** Mulder maneuver is accomplished by firmly squeezing the two metatarsal heads together with one hand while placing firm pressure on the interdigital space with the other hand. (Reused from Berg D, Worzala K. *Atlas of Adult Physical Diagnosis*. Philadelphia, PA: Lippincott Williams & Wilkins; 2006, with permission.)

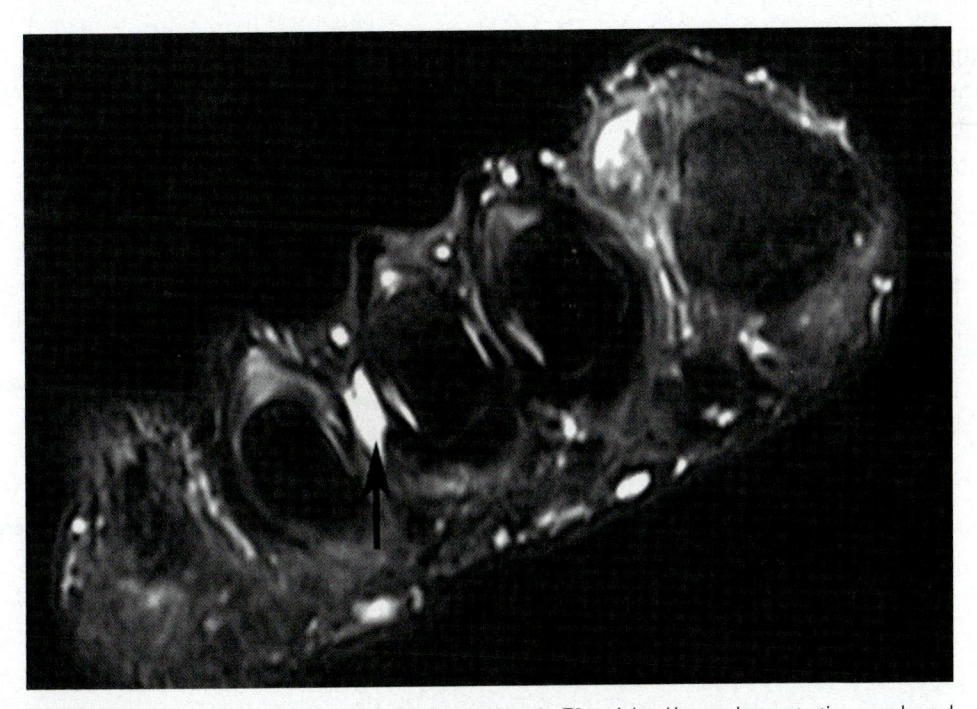

**FIGURE 167.2.** Intermetatarsal bursa. Coronal fast spin-echo T2-weighted image demonstrating an enlarged intermetatarsal (*arrow*) bursa between the third and fourth metatarsals. (Reused from Berquist TH. *Imaging of the Foot and Ankle*. 3rd ed. Philadelphia, PA: Lippincott Williams & Wilkins; 2011:196, with permission.)

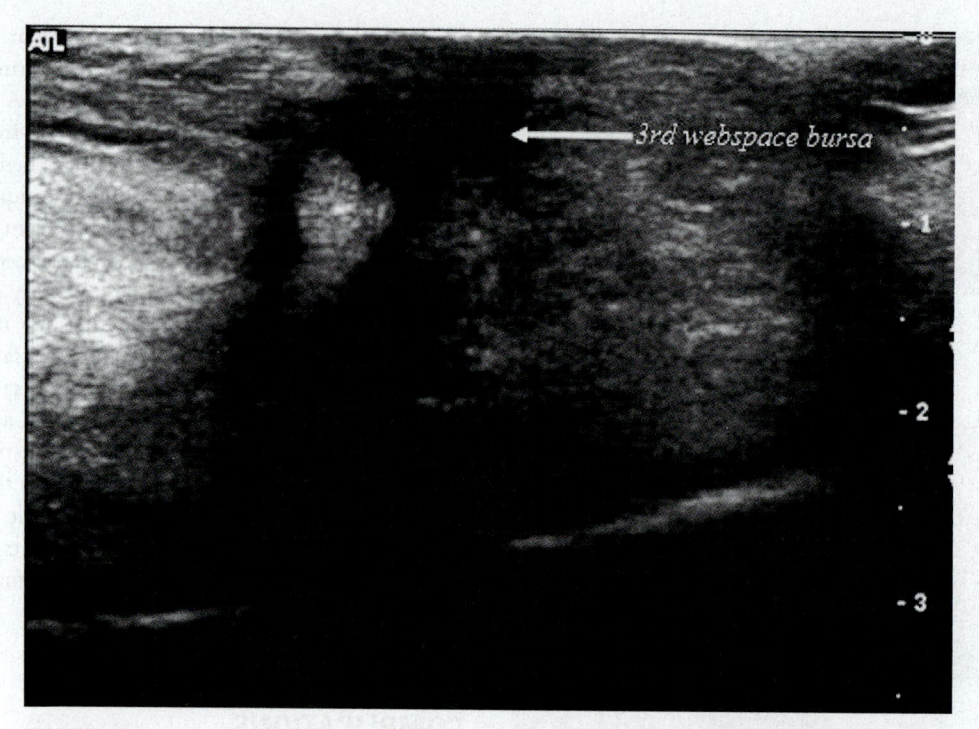

**FIGURE 167.3.** Longitudinal ultrasound image of the third web space demonstrates an irregular hypoechoic collection that was compressible, consistent with an intermetatarsal bursa. (Reused from Adler RS, Sofka CM, Positano RG. *Atlas of Foot and Ankle Sonography*. Philadelphia, PA: Lippincott Williams & Wilkins; 2004:19, with permission.)

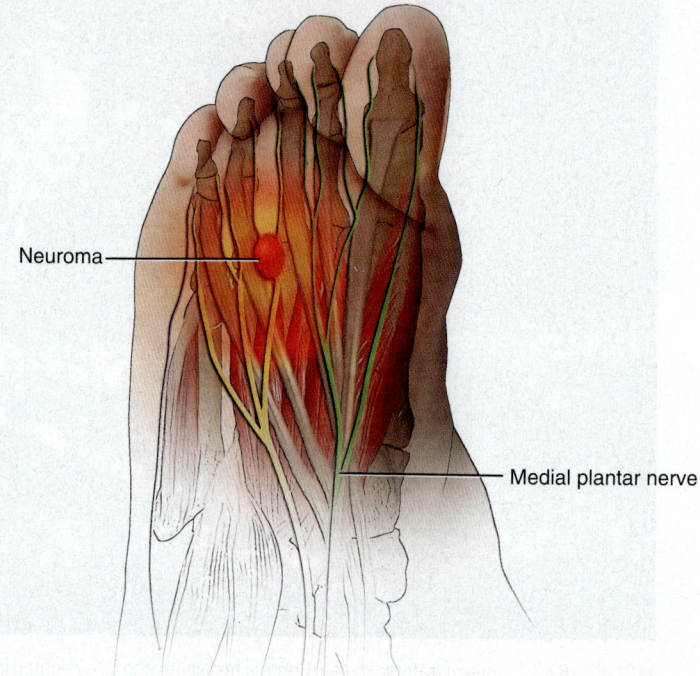

**FIGURE 167.4.** The anatomy of the metatarsal and digital nerves.

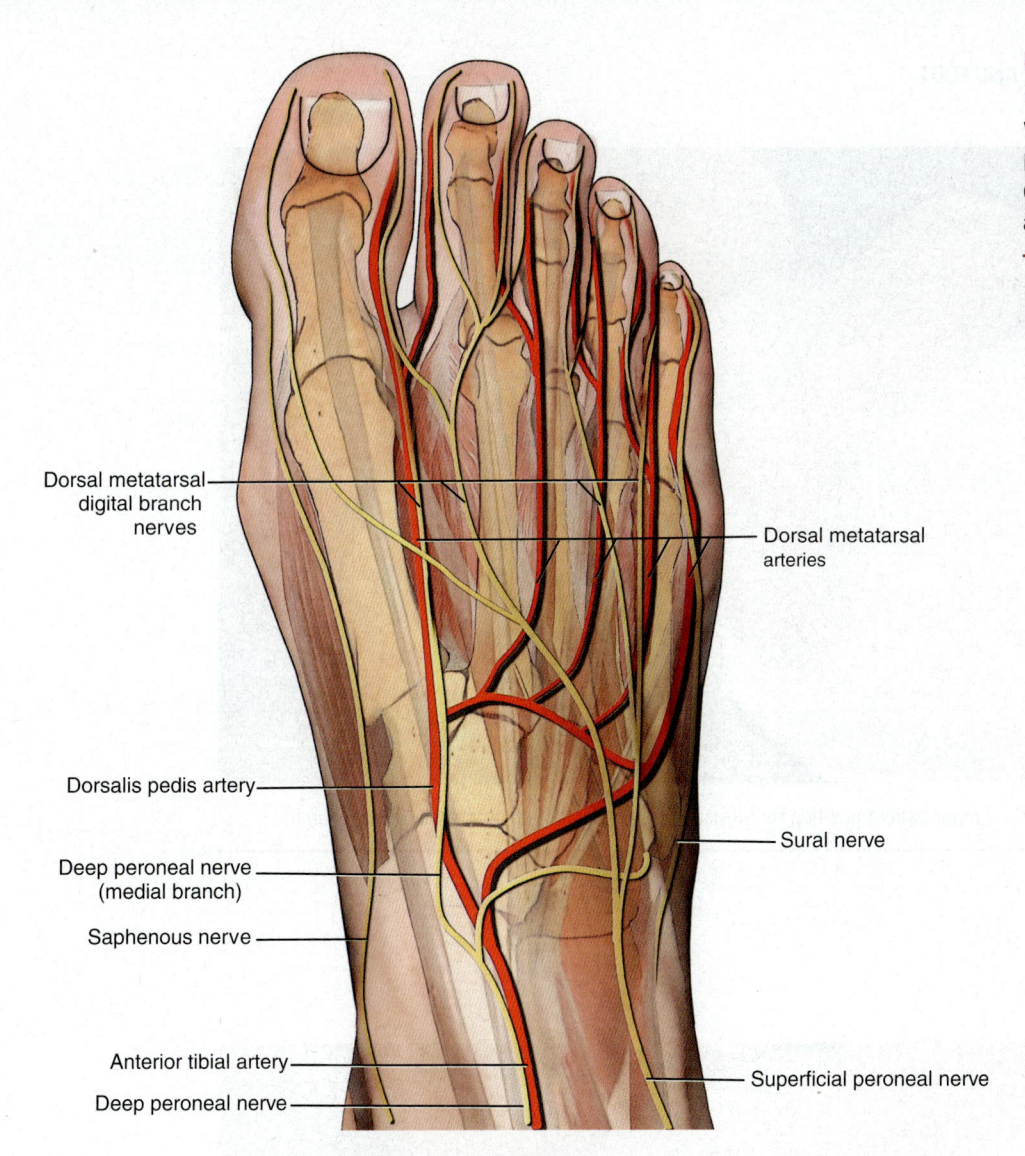

**FIGURE 167.5.** Patients suffering from Morton neuroma present with the complaint of pain in the plantar surface with associated dysesthesias radiating into the adjacent toes.

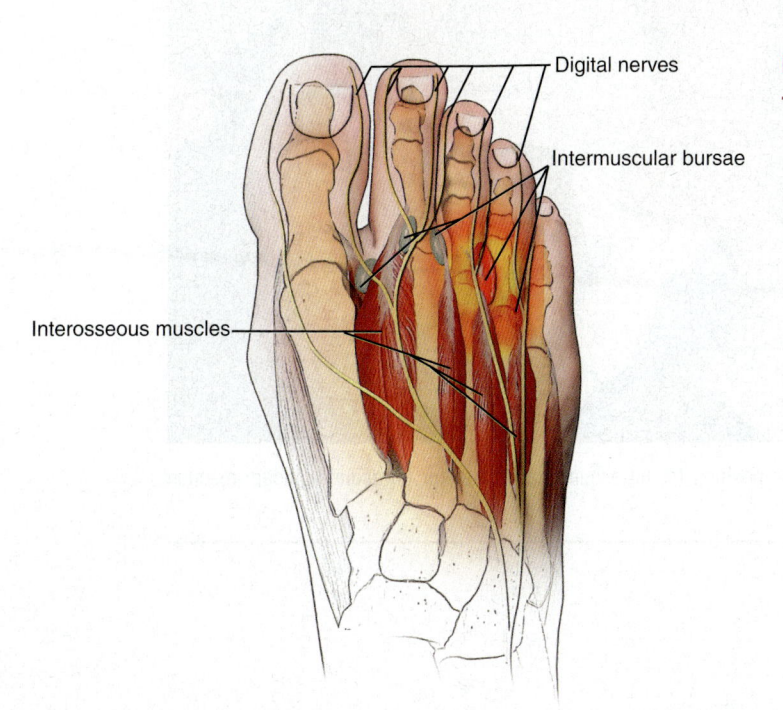

**FIGURE 167.6.** Anatomy of the intermetatarsal bursa.

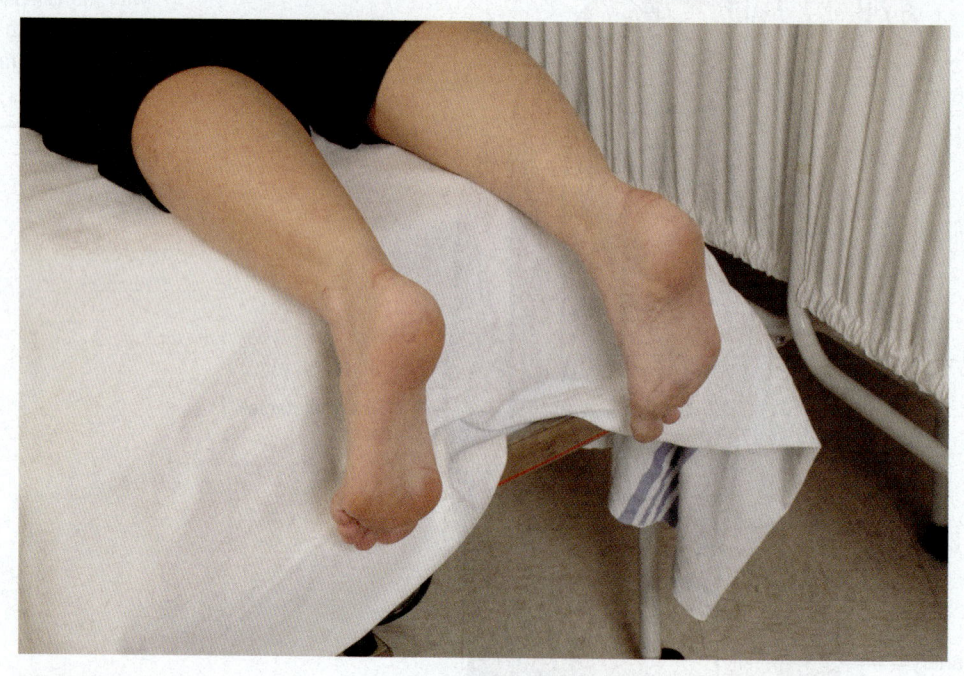

**FIGURE 167.7.** Proper patient position for ultrasound-guided injection of intermetatarsal bursa.

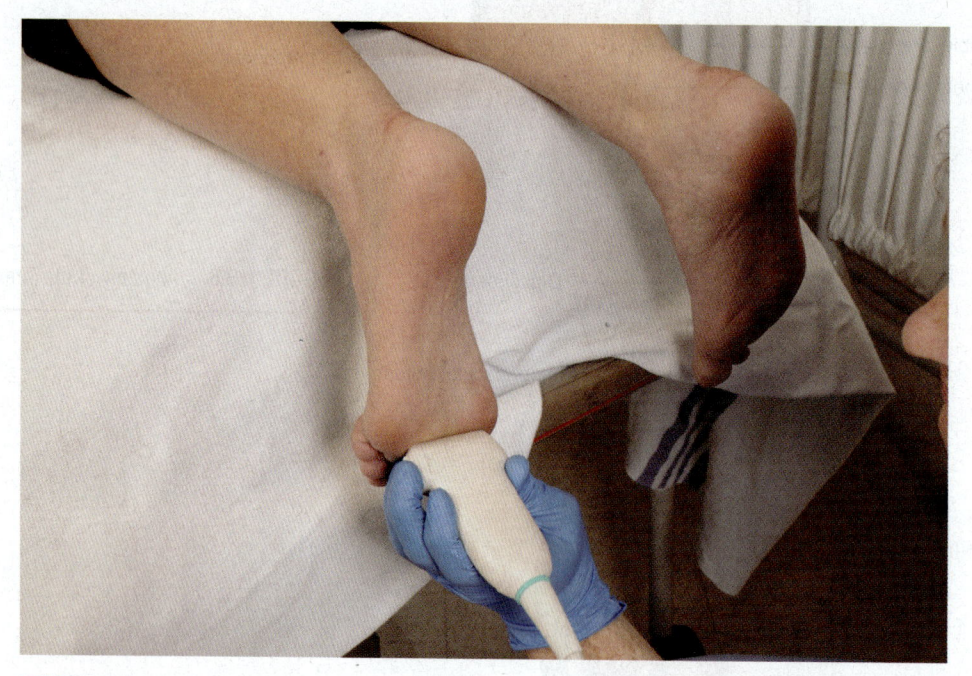

**FIGURE 167.8.** Correct transverse position for ultrasound transducer for ultrasound-guided injection technique for intermetatarsal bursa.

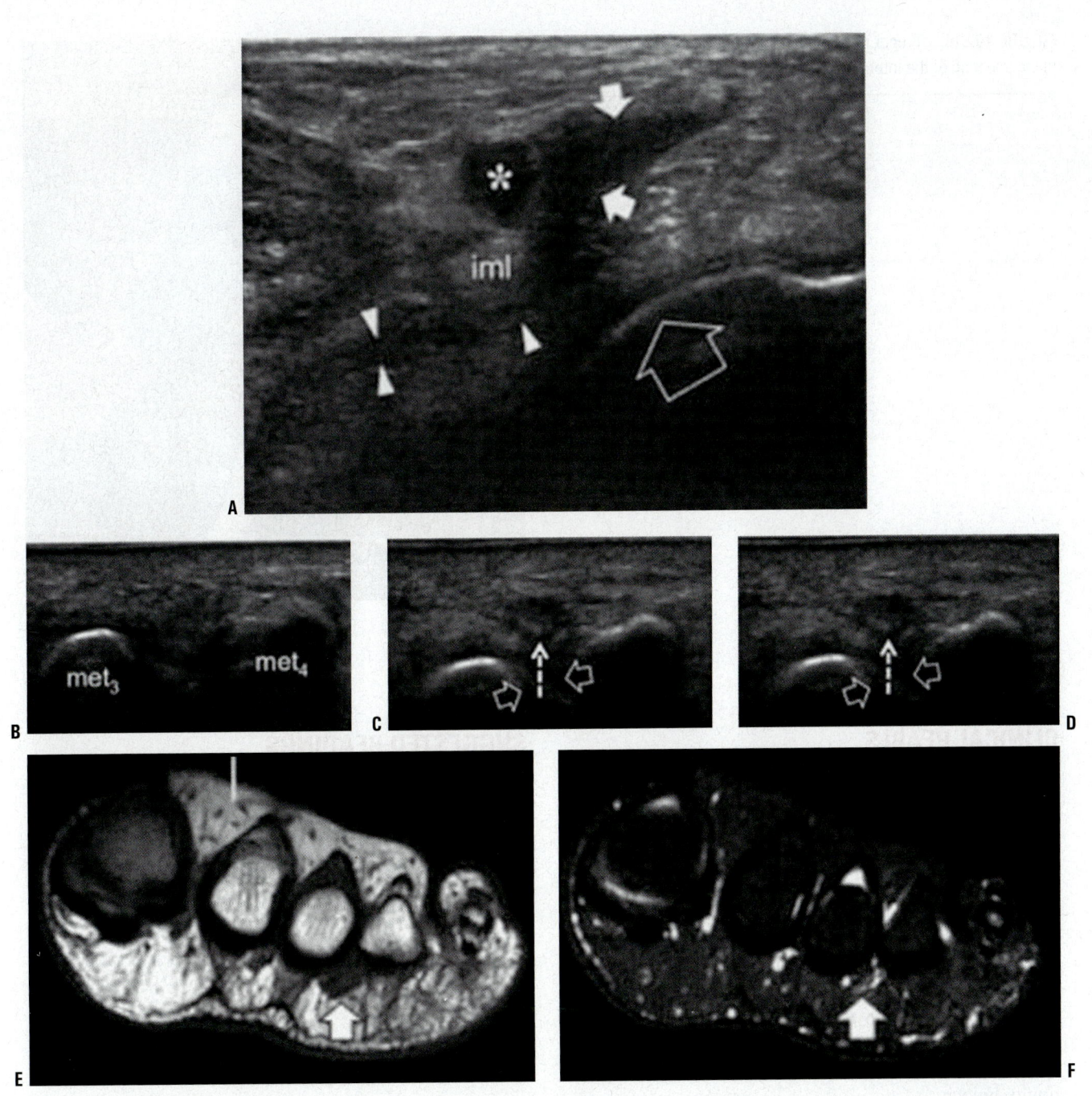

**FIGURE 167.9.** Morton neuroma. **A:** Longitudinal ultrasound (US) image of the third webspace obtained with a dorsal approach while pressing with the thumb (*large void arrow*) from the plantar aspect of the foot shows the interdigital nerve (*arrowheads*) as it passes underneath the intermetatarsal ligament (iml) before deflecting dorsally and continuing in a fusiform hypoechoic Morton neuroma (*white arrows*). A fluid-filled intermetatarsal bursa (*asterisk*) can be appreciated dorsal to the neuroma. **B,C:** Sonographic Mulder's test. Transverse ultrasound images of the third webspace obtained **(B)** in a resting state and **(C)** while squeezing the third ($met_3$) and fourth ($met_4$) metatarsals together. With this maneuver, the metatarsal gets closer (*arrows*) and a mushroom-like hypoechoic neuroma is seen popping up (*dashed arrow*) from the intermetatarsal space. **D:** Short-axis T1-weighted and **(E,F)** fat-suppressed T2-weighted MRI of the forefoot demonstrate a hypointense neuroma (*arrow*) of the interdigital nerve to the third webspace. (Reused from Martinoli C, Court-Payen M, Michaud J, et al. Imaging of neuropathies about the ankle and foot. *Semin Musculoskelet Radiol* 2010;14(3):344–356, with permission.)

**FIGURE 167.10.** Proper needle position for ultrasound-guided out-of-plane injection of the intermetatarsal bursa.

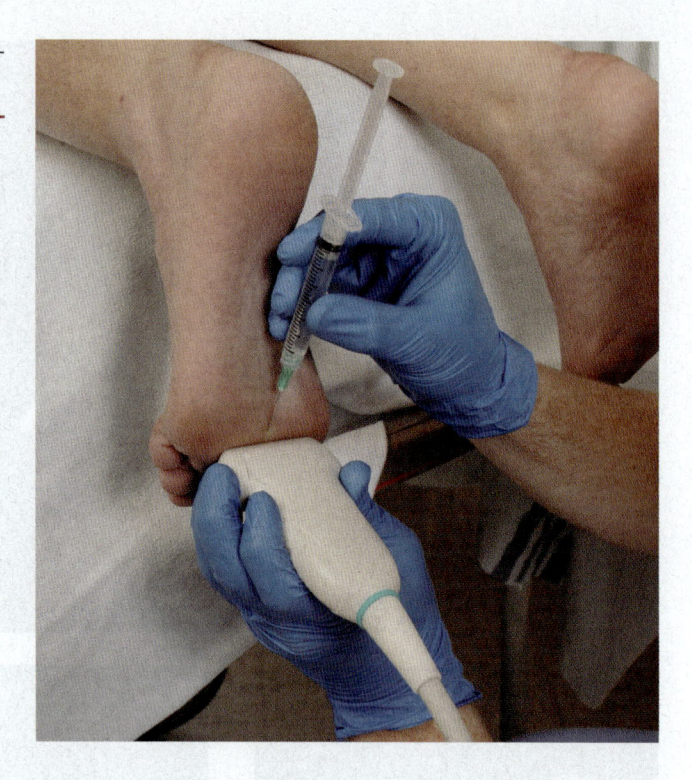

## CLINICAL PEARLS

Toe pathology including tendinopathy, occult fractures, osteoarthritis, rheumatoid arthritis, crystal arthropathies, avascular necrosis bursitis, synovitis, and impingement syndromes may coexist with disease of intermetatarsal bursitis and may contribute to the patient's pain symptomatology. Universal precautions should always be observed to protect the operator, and strict adherence to sterile technique must be used to avoid infection. Gentle physical therapy and local heat should be introduced following ultrasound-guided injection of the intermetatarsal bursa to reduce pain and improve function. Simple analgesics and nonsteroidal anti-inflammatory agents or COX-2 inhibitors may be used concurrently with this injection technique.

## SUGGESTED READINGS

Franson J, Baravarian B. Intermetatarsal compression neuritis. *Clin Podiatr Med Surg* 2006;23(3):569–578.

Lento PH, Strakowski JA. The use of ultrasound in guiding musculoskeletal interventional procedures. *Phys Med Rehabil Clin N Am* 2010;21(3):559–583.

Menz HB. *Disorders of the Forefoot. Foot Problems in Older People*. Philadelphia, PA: Churchill Livingstone; 2008:179–189.

Waldman SD. Technique for injection technique for intra metatarsal bursa. In: *Atlas of Pain Management Injection Techniques*. 3rd ed. Philadelphia, PA: Saunders Elsevier; 2012:476–479.

Wessely MA. MR imaging of the ankle and foot—A review of the normal imaging appearance with an illustration of common disorders. *Clin Chiroprac* 2007; 10(2):101–111.

# CHAPTER 168

# Ultrasound-Guided Injection Technique for Sesamoiditis Pain

## CLINICAL PERSPECTIVES

Sesamoiditis is one of the most common pain syndromes that affects the forefoot. Caused by inflammation of the sesamoid bones, sesamoiditis is characterized by tenderness and pain over the metatarsal heads. The first sesamoid bone of the first metatarsal head is most commonly affected, although the sesamoid bones of the second and fifth metatarsal heads also are subject to the development of sesamoiditis (Fig. 168.1). The patient suffering from sesamoiditis frequently complains that it feels like he or she is walking with a stone in his or her shoe. The pain of sesamoiditis worsens with prolonged standing or walking for long distances and is exacerbated by improperly fitting or padded shoes. Sesamoiditis is most often associated with pushing-off injuries during football or repetitive microtrauma from running or dancing.

On physical examination, the pain of sesamoiditis can be reproduced by pressure on the affected sesamoid bone. Metatarsalgia is frequently confused with sesamoiditis. In contradistinction to metatarsalgia where the tender area of palpation remains over the metatarsal heads, with sesamoiditis, the tender area moves with the flexor tendon when the patient is asked to actively flexes his or her toe. The patient with sesamoiditis often exhibits an antalgic gait in an effort to reduce weight bearing during walking. With acute trauma to the sesamoid, ecchymosis over the plantar surface of the foot may be present, and on occasion fracture of the sesamoid bone may occur (Fig. 168.2).

Plain radiographs are indicated in all patients who present with sesamoiditis. Based on the patient's clinical presentation, additional testing may be indicated, including complete blood cell count, sedimentation rate, and antinuclear antibody testing. Magnetic resonance imaging or ultrasound of the sesamoid bone is indicated to help confirm the diagnosis and if fracture, effusion, tendinopathy, crystal arthropathy, joint mice, synovitis, foreign body, bursitis, or ligamentous injury is suspected (Figs. 168.3 and 168.4).

## CLINICALLY RELEVANT ANATOMY

The sesamoid bones are small, rounded structures that are embedded in the flexor tendons of the foot and usually are in close proximity to the joints. Sesamoid bones of the first metatarsal occur in almost all patients, with sesamoid bones being present in the flexor tendons of the second and fifth metatarsals in a significant number of patients (see Fig. 168.1). These sesamoid bones serve to decrease friction and pressure of the flexor tendon as it passes in proximity to a joint.

## ULTRASOUND-GUIDED TECHNIQUE

The benefits, risks, and alternative treatments are explained to the patient, and informed consent is obtained. The patient is then placed in the supine position with the patients arms folded comfortably across their chest (Fig. 168.5). With the patient in the above position, a high-frequency small linear ultrasound transducer is placed in a longitudinal plane over the painful metatarsophalangeal (MTP) head, and an ultrasound survey scan is taken (Fig. 168.6).

The hypoechoic joint space is identified between the head of the metatarsal, and the base of the proximal phalanges and the curvilinear sesamoid bone with its acoustic shadow are identified (Figs. 168.7 and 168.8). When the sesamoid bone is identified, the skin overlying the area above and beneath the ultrasound transducer is then prepped with antiseptic solution. A sterile syringe containing 1.0 mL of 0.25% preservative-free bupivacaine and 40 mg of methylprednisolone is attached to a 1½-inch, 25-gauge needle using strict aseptic technique. The needle is placed through the skin just above the center of the longitudinally placed transducer and is then advanced using an out-of-plane approach with the needle trajectory adjusted under real-time ultrasound guidance so that the needle tip ultimately rests within proximity to the sesamoid bone (Fig. 168.9). When the tip of needle is thought to be in satisfactory position, after careful gentle aspiration, a small amount of local anesthetic and steroid is injected under real-time ultrasound guidance to confirm that the needle tip is in the proper position. After proper needle tip placement is confirmed, the remainder of the contents of the syringe are slowly injected. There should be minimal resistance to injection.

## COMPLICATIONS

The major complication of ultrasound-guided injection for sesamoiditis is infection. Ecchymosis and hematoma formation

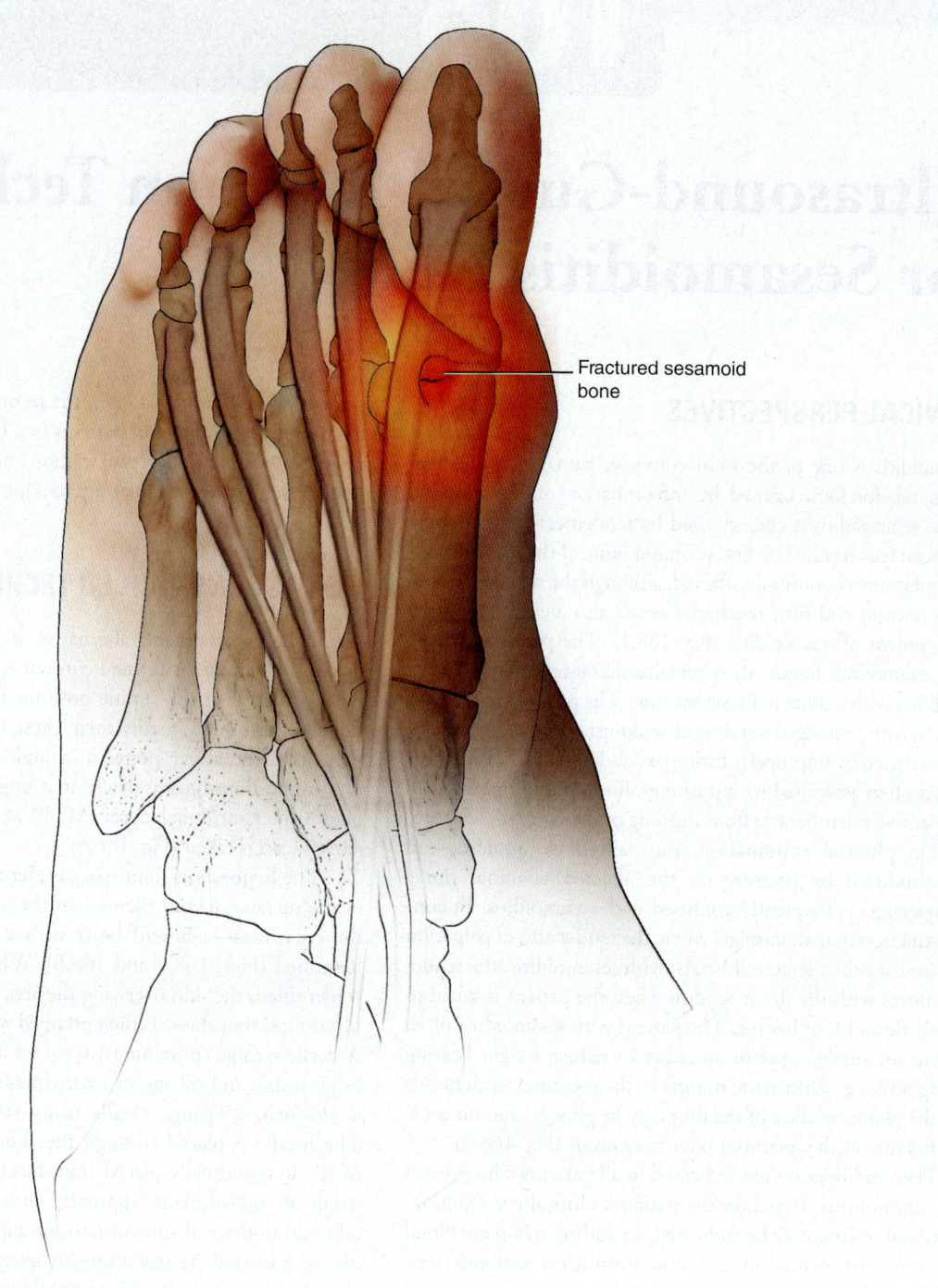

**FIGURE 168.1.** Sesamoiditis most commonly affects the first sesamoid bone of the first metatarsal head, although the sesamoid bones of the second and fifth metatarsal heads also are subject to the development of sesamoiditis.

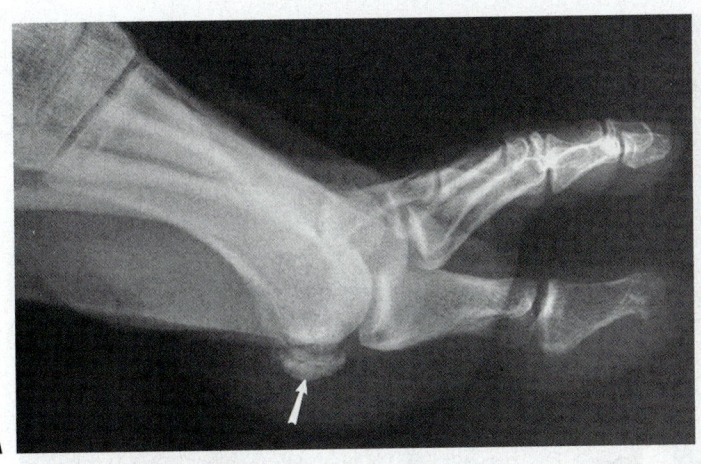

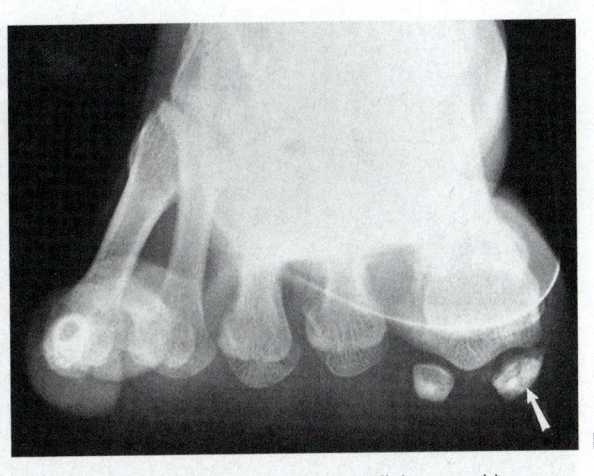

CHAPTER 168  ULTRASOUND-GUIDED INJECTION TECHNIQUE FOR SESAMOIDITIS PAIN  1179

**FIGURE 168.2.** Lateral **(A)** and sesamoid **(B)** views demonstrating sclerosis and fragmentation of the medial sesamoid (*arrow*) due to the fracture with avascular necrosis. (Berquist TH. *Imaging of the Foot and Ankle*. 3rd ed. Philadelphia, PA: Lippincott Williams & Wilkins; 2011:194, with permission.)

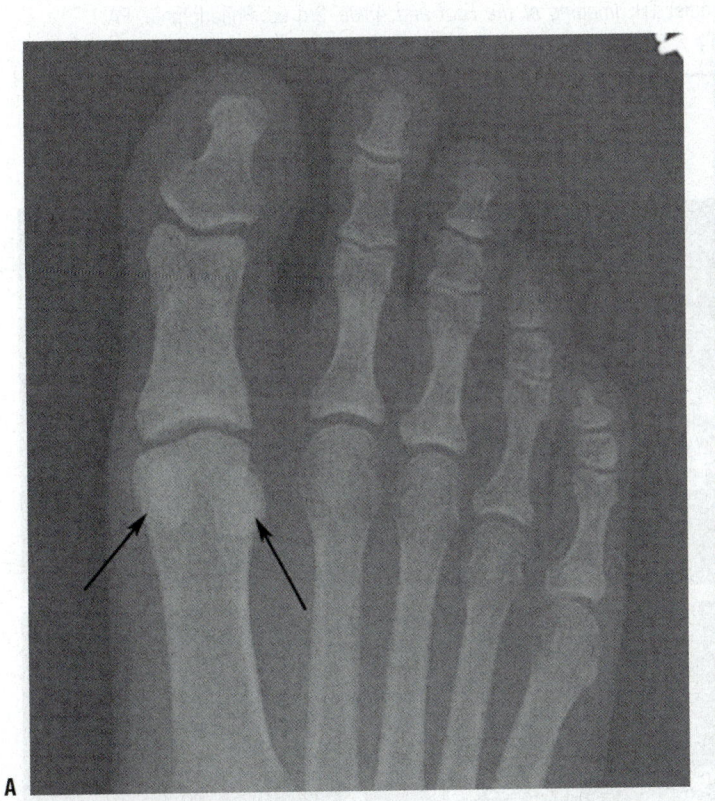

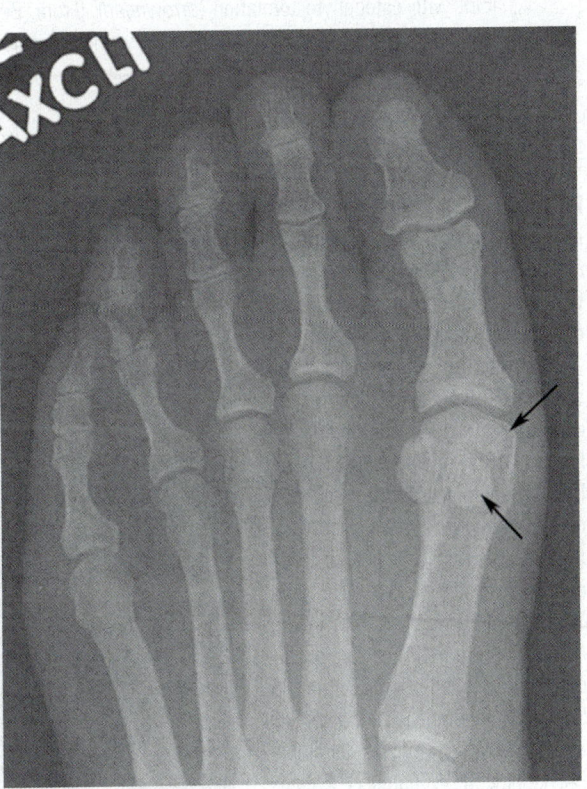

**FIGURE 168.3.** **A:** Radiograph demonstrating medial and lateral sesamoids (*arrows*) formed from single ossification centers. **B:** Radiograph demonstrating a bipartite medial sesamoid (*arrows*) with the lateral sesamoid formed from a single ossification center.

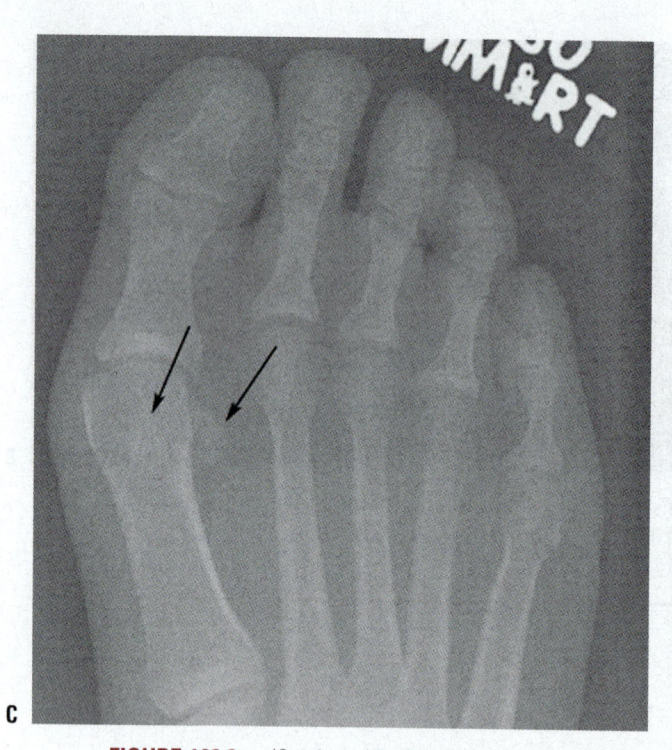

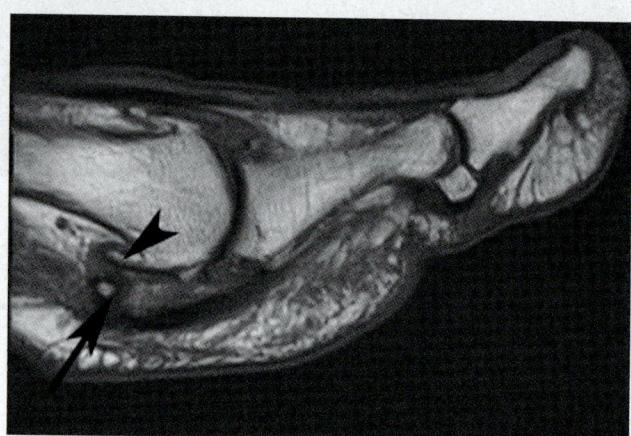

**FIGURE 168.3.** *(Continued)* **C:** Hallux valgus with rotation of the sesamoids laterally out of the normal metatarsal grooves. **D:** T1-weighted MR image demonstrating fragmentation of the sesamoid (*arrow*) and degenerative changes in the first MTP joint with osteophyte formation (*arrowhead*). (From, Berquist TH. *Imaging of the Foot and Ankle*. 3rd ed. Philadelphia, PA: Lippincott Williams & Wilkins; 2011:193, with permission.)

**FIGURE 168.4.** **A:** Longitudinal image over the medial joint line of the first MTP joint depicts cortical irregularity (*long arrow*) of the first metatarsal head (MT). A well-defined heterogenous soft tissue mass (*short arrows*) abuts the cortical surface of the metatarsal head. (P1, 1st phalanges). **B:** Power Doppler imaging of the same area displays abnormal vascularity within the mass as well as adjacent to the cortical surface of the MTP joint. These features reflect the inflammatory nature of this tophaceous deposit. (Reused from Adler RS, Sofka CM, Positano RG. *Atlas of Foot and Ankle Sonography*. Philadelphia, PA: Lippincott Williams & Wilkins; 2004:28, with permission.)

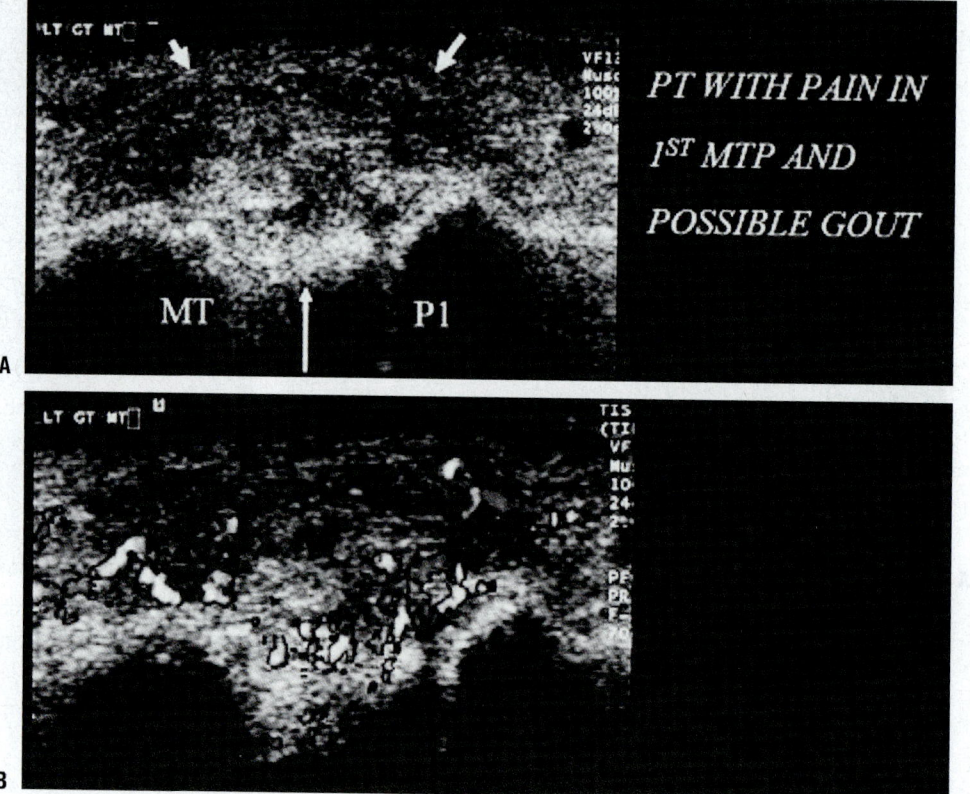

CHAPTER 168  ULTRASOUND-GUIDED INJECTION TECHNIQUE FOR SESAMOIDITIS PAIN  1181

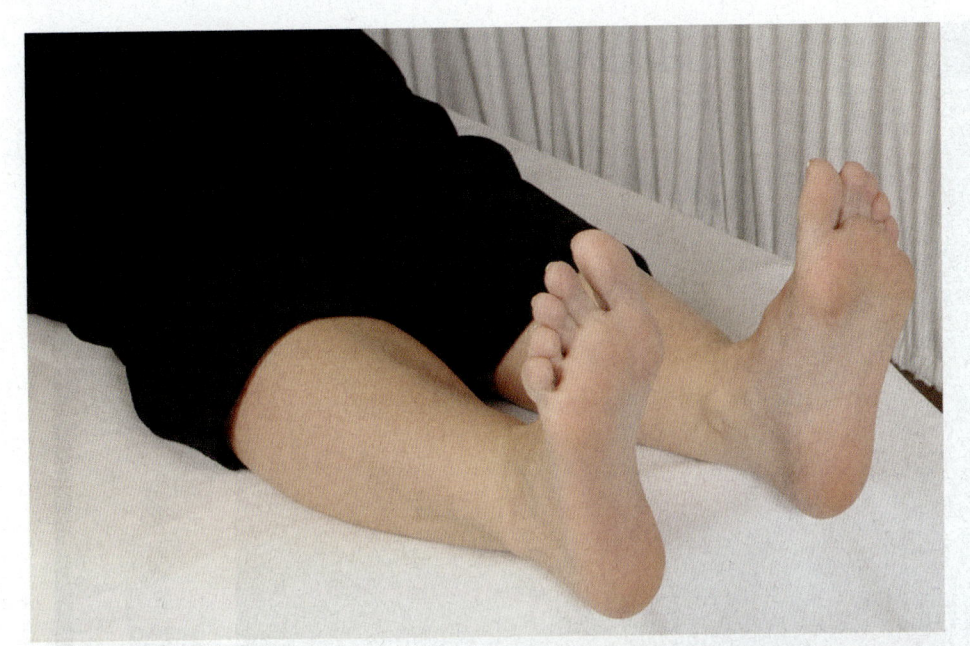

**FIGURE 168.5.** Proper supine position for ultrasound-guided injection for sesamoiditis.

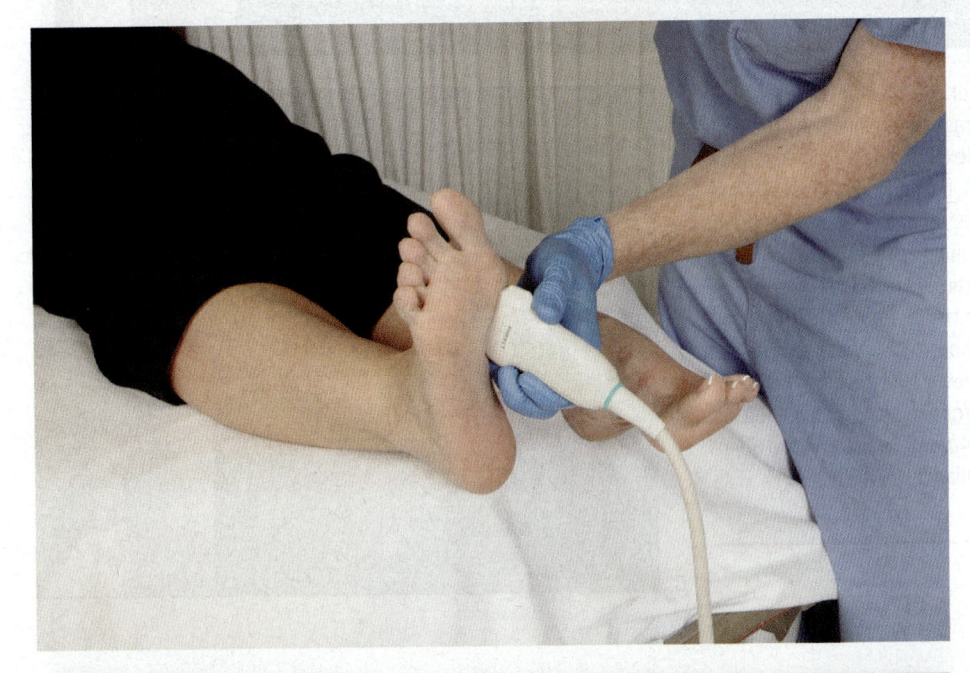

**FIGURE 168.6.** Correct longitudinal position for ultrasound transducer for ultrasound-guided injection technique for sesamoiditis.

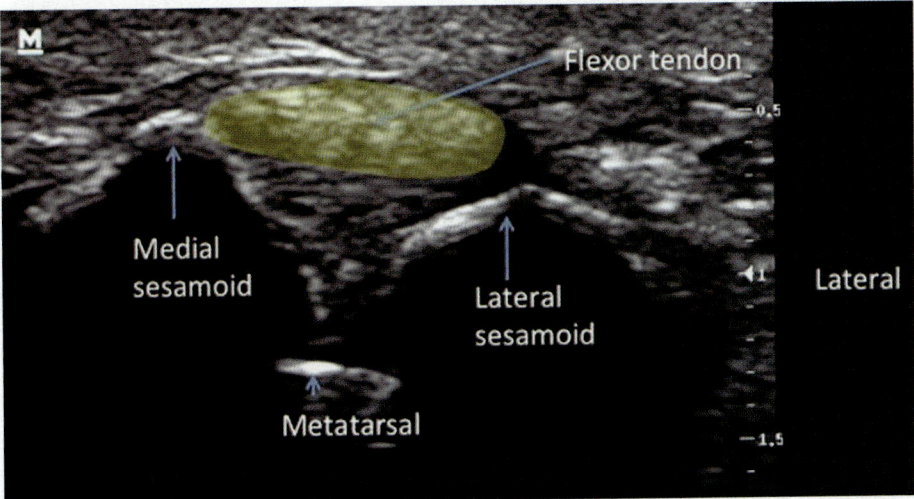

**FIGURE 168.7.** The lateral and medial sesamoids overlying the metatarsals (*blue ovals*).

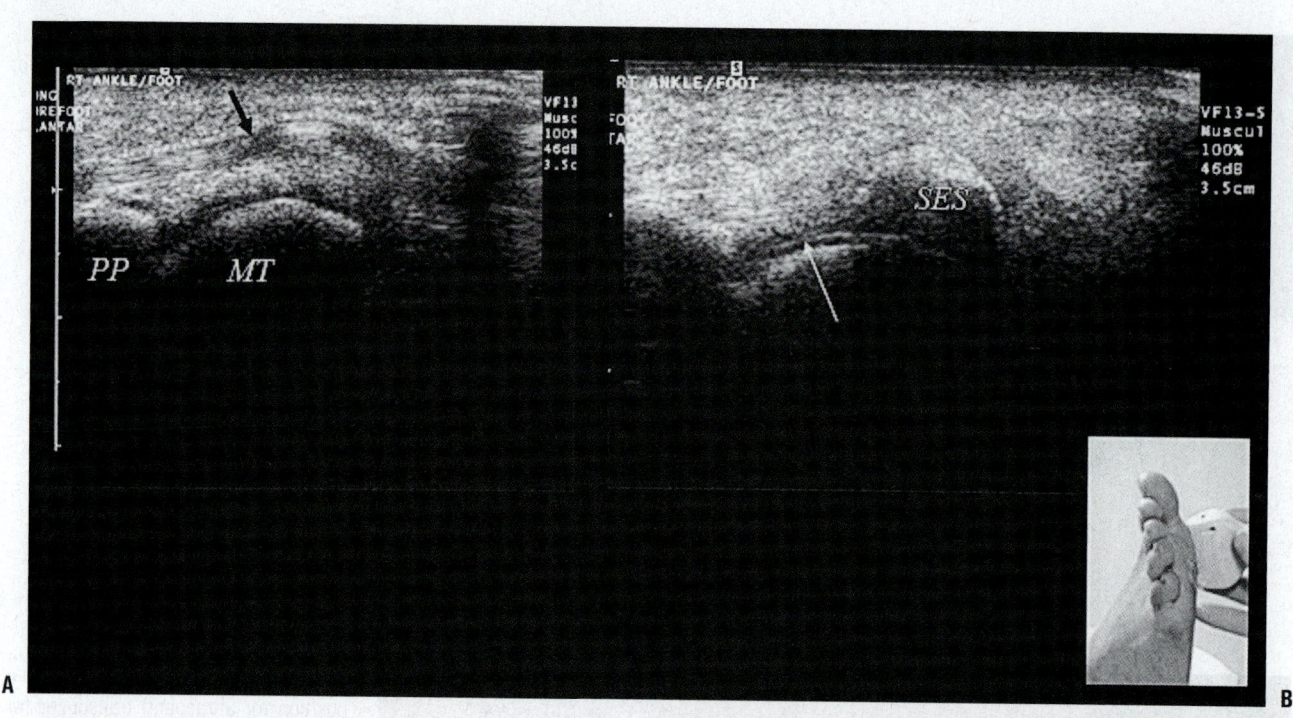

**FIGURE 168.8.** Longitudinal images of the plantar aspect of the first MTP joint at two slightly offset parasagittal planes. **A:** The first image on the left demonstrates the flexor hallucis longus tendon (*black arrow*). The first metatarsal and proximal phalanx (MT and PP, respectively, are indicated). **B:** The second image (transducer slightly more medial) demonstrates the medial sesamoid (SES). The normal uniformly hypoechoic articular cartilage over the first metatarsal head can also be seen (*long thin white arrow*). **C:** Transverse ultrasound image of the sesamoids. Note the normal, curvilinear sesamoids demonstrating posterior acoustic shadowing. The flexor hallucis longus tendon can be seen in cross section (*arrow*). (Reused from Adler RS, Sofka CM, Positano RG. *Atlas of Foot and Ankle Sonography*. Philadelphia, PA: Lippincott Williams & Wilkins; 2004, with permission.)

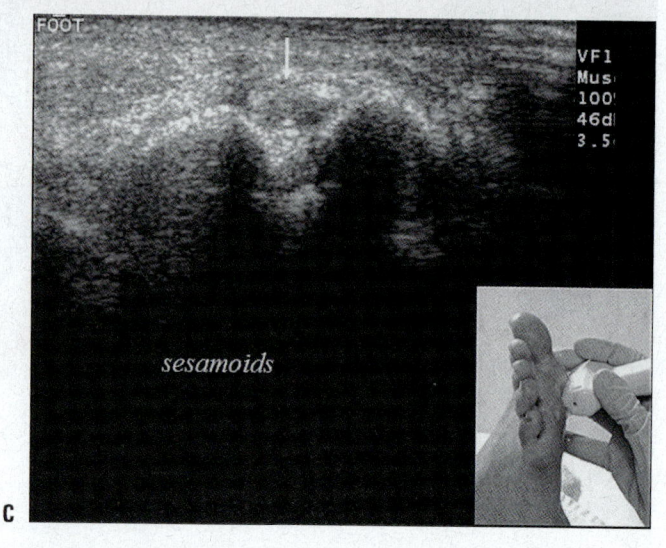

may also occur. A transient exacerbation of the patient's pain occurs ~25% of the time following this injection technique, and the patient should be warned of this possibility prior to the procedure.

## CLINICAL PEARLS

Toe pathology including tendinopathy, occult fractures, osteoarthritis, rheumatoid arthritis, crystal arthropathies, avascular necrosis bursitis, synovitis, and impingement syndromes may coexist with sesamoiditis and may contribute to the patient's pain symptomatology. Universal precautions should always be observed to protect the operator, and strict adherence to sterile technique must be used to avoid infection. Gentle physical therapy and local heat should be introduced following ultrasound-guided injection of the intermetatarsal bursa to reduce pain and improve function. Simple analgesics and nonsteroidal anti-inflammatory agents or COX-2 inhibitors may be used concurrently with this injection technique.

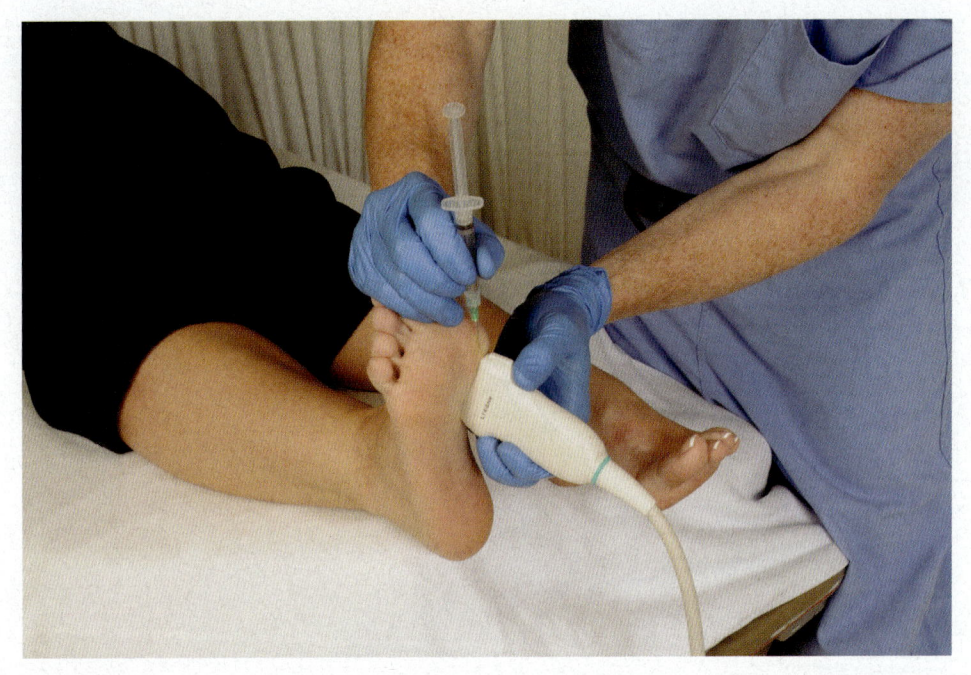

**FIGURE 168.9.** Proper needle position for ultrasound-guided plane injection of the sesamoiditis.

## SUGGESTED READINGS

Anwar R, Anjum SN, Nicholl JE. Sesamoids of the foot. *Curr Orthop* 2005; 19(1):40–48.

Cohen BE. Hallux sesamoid disorders. *Foot Ankle Clin* 2009;14(1):91–104.

Lento PH, Strakowski JA. The use of ultrasound in guiding musculoskeletal interventional procedures. *Phys Med Rehab Clin N Am* 2010;21(3):559–583.

Menz HB. Disorders of the forefoot. In: *Foot Problems in Older People*. Philadelphia, PA: Churchill Livingstone; 2008:179–189.

Sanders TG, Rathur SK. Imaging of painful conditions of the hallucal sesamoid complex and plantar capsular structures of the first metatarsophalangeal joint. *Radiol Clin North Am* 2008;46(6):1079–1092.

Waldman SD. Technique for injection technique for sesamoiditis. In: *Atlas of Pain Management Injection Techniques*. 3rd ed. Philadelphia, PA: Saunders Elsevier; 2012:476–479.

Wessely MA. MR imaging of the ankle and foot—A review of the normal imaging appearance with an illustration of common disorders. *Clin Chiroprac* 2007;10(2):101–111.

# INDEX

Note: Page numbers followed by the letter "f" refer to figures and those followed by the letter "t" refer to tables

## A

Abdominal pain
  anterior cutaneous nerve block, 621
  celiac plexus block (see Celiac plexus block, anterior approach)
  sternoclavicular joint pain
    anatomy, 544, 546
    clinical presentation, 544
    complications, 548–549
    Doppler image, 544, 545f
    informed consent, 544
    needle placement, 547, 548f
    palpation, 544
    patient position, 544, 546f
    position identification, 544, 546f, 547f
    precautions, 549
    radiographs, 544, 545f
    symptoms, 544
    ultrasound transducer position, 547, 547f, 548f
  upper (see Thoracic epidural block)
  xiphisternal joint (see Xiphisternal joint pain)
Abductor pollicis longus tendons
  function, de Quervain's tenosynovitis, 486, 488f
  identification, 486, 488f
  image, 487, 489f, 490f
Achilles tendon
  anatomy of, 1096, 1099f
  deltoid ligament strain
    clinical presentation, 1069, 1070f–1072f
    complications, 1070
    needle placement, 1070, 1074f
    patient position, 1069, 1073f
    physical examination, 1069
    precautions, 1075
    radiographs, 1069, 1072f
    transducer placement, 1069, 1073f
    triangular-shaped, 1069, 1074f
  retrocalcaneal bursa and (see Retrocalcaneal bursitis pain)
Achilles tendonitis
  calcaneal insertion, 1096, 1099f, 1100f
  clinical presentation, 1096, 1097f–1099f
  complications, 1101
  creaking tendon test, 1096, 1097f
  needle placement, 1096, 1101, 1101f
  patient position, 1096, 1100f
  precautions, 1101
  radiographs, 1096, 1198f
  transducer placement, 1096, 1100f
Acrocyanosis, scleroderma patient, 156, 157f
Acromioclavicular joint. See Subacromial impingement syndrome
Acromioclavicular (AC) joint
  anatomy, 221, 223f
  clinical presentation, 221
  complications, 224
  fracture, 221, 222f
  palpation, 221, 224f
  precautions, 225
  radiographs, 221, 222f
  ultrasound anatomy, 221, 224f
  ultrasound-guided technique
    informed consent, 221
    needle placement, 221, 224, 225f
    patient position, 221, 224f
    position identification, 221, 224f, 225f
    transducer placement, 221, 224f
Acromion. See also Subacromial impingement syndrome
  congenital/acquired abnormalities, 227, 230f
  humeral head and impingement, 254, 255f
Acute herpes zoster infection
  auricular nerve block, 33, 33f
  caudal epidural block, 710, 711f
  hypogastric plexus block, 549f
  infraorbital nerve block, 66
  lumbar sympathetic block, 736, 737f
  maxillary nerve block, 46, 47f
  sphenopalatine ganglion block, 14
  stellate ganglion block, 156
  supraorbital nerve block, 60, 61f
  thoracic paravertebral nerve block, 583, 584f
Acute infectious arthritis. See also Arthritis
  ankle joint, 1019
  sacroiliac joint injection, 881
  subtalar joint, 1025
  superior tibiofibular joint, 903
Adductor tendonitis
  anatomy, 782, 784f
  complications, 785
  dysfunctional gait, 782
  musculotendinous units, 782
  precautions, 785
  radiographs, 782, 783f
  tendons of, 782
  ultrasound-guided technique
    appearance, 782, 786f, 787f
    bupivacaine and methylprednisolone, 782
    needle placement, 782 787f
    patient position, 782, 784f
    pubic symphysis insertion view, 782, 786f, 787f
    pubic symphysis location, 782, 785f
    transducer placement, 782, 786f
  Waldman knee squeeze test, 782, 783f
Ankle joint
  anatomy, 1019, 1020f, 1021f
  articulations, 1019, 1020f
  deep peroneal nerve block (see Deep peroneal nerve block, at ankle)
  intra-articular injection of
    clinical presentation, 1019, 1020f
    complications, 1022
    dorsalis pedis artery, 1021, 1023f
    needle placement, 1021, 1024f
    patient position, 1019, 1022f
    precautions, 1023
    radiographs, 1019, 1020f
    transducer placement, 1021, 1022f
    V shape, 1021, 1023f
  ligament, 1019, 1021f
  saphenous nerve block at (see Saphenous nerve block)
  superficial peroneal nerve block at (see Superficial peroneal nerve block, at ankle)
  sural nerve block at (see Sural nerve block, at ankle)
  tibial nerve block (see Tibial nerve block)
Anterior cutaneous nerve block
  abdominal pain, 621
  acute cholecystitis, 621, 622f
  anatomy, 621, 623, 623f
    anterior division, 621
    fibrous ring, 621, 624f
    paravertebral nerve, 621
    posterior division, 621
    subcostal nerve, 621
  complications, 624–625
  mechanism of, 621, 622f
  precautions, 628
  radiographs, 621
  subcapsular hematoma, 627f
  ultrasound-guided technique
    color Doppler image, epigastric artery identification, 623, 626f
    needle placement, 624, 627f
    pain identification point, 623, 625f
    patient position, 623, 624f
    transducer placement, 623, 625f
Anterior interosseous syndrome
  anatomic abnormalities, 401
  antecubital fossa, 404, 405
  axillary artery, 404
  brachial artery, 404
  clinical diagnosis, 404
  complications, 409–410
  double crush syndrome, 403
  forearm, 401
  median nerve, 401
  nerve anatomy, 404, 405f
  nerve compression, 404f
  persistent neurologic deficits, in patients, 410
  Playboy bunny sign, 401, 403f
  sites of compression, 401, 402f
  Spinner sign, 401, 403f
  ulnar artery, 404
  ultrasound-guided technique
    artery vs. nerve, color Doppler image, 406, 409f
    median nerve, transverse image, 407f
    nerve bifurcation, 406, 408f
    patient position, 405, 406f
    proper needle placement, 406, 409f
    ultrasound transducer, 406, 407f
  wrist, 404

Anterior talofibular ligament strain
    clinical presentation, 1076, 1086f–1078f
    complications, 1080
    needle placement, 1077, 1080f
    patient position, 1076, 1079f
    precautions, 1080
    radiographs, 1076, 1077f
    transducer placement, 1077, 1079f
Anterior talofibular ligaments
    anatomy of, 1076, 1076f
    inversion injuries, 1076, 1077f
    tear of, 1106, 1107f
Anterior tarsal tunnel syndrome
    clinical presentation, 1081, 1082f, 1083f
    complications, 1084
    needle placement, 1084, 1087f
    patient position, 1083, 1086f
    precautions, 1087
    radiographs, 1081
    tibial artery and vein, 1083, 1086f
    Tinel sign, 1081, 1083f
    transducer placement, 1084, 1086f
Arnold-Chiari malformation with syrinx, 169f, 170
Arthritis
    acute infectious, 501, 507, 525, 531, 745, 881
        carpometacarpal joints (*see* Carpometacarpal joints, intra-articular injection)
        distal radioulnar joint, 412
        first carpometacarpal joint (*see* First carpometacarpal joint, intra-articular injection)
        hip joint (*see* Hip joint)
        radiocarpal joint, intra-articular injection, 417
    baker cyst, 1004, 1006f
    hip joint, intra-articular injection, 745
    osteoarthritis, 881
    psoriatic, 532f
    rheumatoid, 525, 526f, 775
    thoracic facet block, 589
    treatment, 664, 665f, 673, 674f
Arthrodial-type joint. *See* Superior tibiofibular joint
Arthrosis, 665f, 674f
Articularis genus muscle, 942
Atlantoaxial block
    anatomy, 6
    C2 nerve root, 11f, 12f
    complications, 8
    Jefferson fracture, 6, 7f–8f
    joint instability, diseases associated with, 6, 7t
    pain distribution, 6, 7f
    sleep disturbance, 6
    symptoms, 6
    ultrasound-guided technique
        C1 and C2 vertebral body, 6, 10f
        transducer position, 6, 10f
    *vs.* vertebral artery, 9f
Atlanto-occipital joint injection
    anatomy, joint, 2, 3f
    blockade, 5
    complications, 4–5
    longitudinal ultrasound image, 3f
    pain distribution, 2, 2f
    symptoms, 2
    ultrasound-guided technique
        color Doppler image, 5, 5f
        patient position, 2
        transducer position, 2, 4f
        vertebral artery relationship, 3f
Auricular nerve block. *See* Greater auricular nerve block
Auriculotemporal nerve block
    anatomy, 27, 28f
    causes, 27
    complications, 27
    physical examination, 27
    precautions, 31–32
    symptoms, 27
    ultrasound-guided technique
        informed consent, 27
        needle placement, 27, 31f
        patient position, 27, 30f
        position identification, 27, 29f
        ultrasound transducer position, 27, 31f
Avascular necrosis
    femoral head, 750
    humeral head, 219, 220f
    radiocarpal joint, intra-articular injection, 420, 422f
Axillary brachial plexus block
    anatomy, 209, 210f
    clinical presentation, 209
    complications, 213–214
    Doppler image, 211, 213f
    precautions, 214
    radiographs, 209, 210f–211f
    Raynaud disease symptom management, 209, 210f
    ultrasound-guided technique
        needle placement, 211, 213f
        palpation identification, 209, 211f
        patient position, 209, 211f
        position identification, 209, 212f, 213f
        transducer placement, 209, 212f
Axillary nerve block, quadrilateral space
    anatomy, 297, 299f
    complications, 303
    Doppler image, superior circumflex humeral artery, 298, 302f
    imaging, 297, 300f
    palpation, 297
    precautions, 303
    radiographs, 297
    symptoms, 297
    T1-weighted magnetic resonance image, 298f
    ultrasound-guided technique
        bupivacaine and methylprednisolone administration, 298
        color Doppler image, superior circumflex humeral artery, 298, 302f
        needle placement, 298, 302f, 303
        patient position, 298, 299f
        transducer position, 298, 300f, 301f

## B

Baker cyst
    arthritis, 1004, 1006f
    clinical presentation, 1004, 1005f–1008f
    complications, 1005
    cyst expansion, 1004, 1006f
    cystic sac, 1004, 1005f
    hypoechoic, 1005, 1009f
    needle placement, 1005, 1010f
    with osteochondromatosis, 1005, 1009f
    patient position, 1004, 1008f
    physical examination, 1004, 1007f
    precautions, 1005, 1009
    radiographs, 1004, 1007f
    rupture of, 1004, 1007f
    transducer placement, 1005, 1009f
Ballottement test, 413f, 935, 938f
Bell palsy. *See* Facial nerve block
Bernhardt-Roth syndrome, 758. *See also* Lateral femoral cutaneous nerve block
Bicipital tendonitis
    anatomy, 288, 291f
    clinical presentation, 288
    complications, 296
    Popeye sign, 288, 292f
    precautions, 296
    radiographs, 288, 289f–290f
    rupture, 288, 290f, 292f
    ultrasound-guided technique
        bupivacaine and methylprednisolone, 292
        informed consent, 289
        needle placement, 292, 295f
        palpation identification, 289, 293f
        patient position, 289, 293f
        transducer position, 289, 292, 293f, 294f
        ultrasound image, 292, 294f, 295f
    untreated, 288, 290f
    Yergason sign, 288, 290f
Bouchard nodes, 531, 533f
Brachial plexus block
    axillary
        anatomy, 209, 210f
        clinical presentation, 209
        complications, 213–214
        Doppler image, 211, 213f
        needle placement, 211, 213f
        palpation identification, 209, 211f
        patient position, 209, 211f
        position identification, 209, 212f, 213f
        precautions, 214
        radiographs, 209, 210f–211f
        Raynaud disease symptom management, 209, 210f
        transducer placement, 209, 212f
    infraclavicular
        anatomy, 204, 205f
        clinical presentation, 204
        complications, 205–206
        Doppler image, 204, 208f
        needle placement, 205
        patient position, 204, 207f
        position identification, 204, 207f, 208f
        precautions, 206–207
        radiographs, 204, 205f–206f
        transducer placement, 204, 207f
    interscalene (*see* Interscalene brachial plexus block)
    supraclavicular
        anatomy, 198, 199f
        clinical presentation, 198
        complications, 202–203
        corner pocket, 198, 202
        Doppler image, 198, 202f
        needle placement, 198, 203f

patient position, 198, 201f
position identification, 198, 201f, 202f
precautions, 203
radiographs, 198, 199f–200f
symptoms, 198
transducer placement, 198, 201f
Bunion. *See* Hallux valgus deformity
Bunionette pain syndrome
  clinical presentation, 1152
  complications, 1154, 1157
  functional disability, 1152
  needle placement, 1152, 1157f
  patient position, 1152, 1155f
  precautions, 1157
  radiographs, 1152
  transducer placement, 1152, 1156f
Bursitis. *See also* Intermetatarsal bursitis
  deep infrapatellar pain
    bupivacaine and methylprednisolone, 962
    clinical presentation, 960, 961f
    complications, 964
    needle placement, 963, 965f
    palpation, 963f
    patient position, 962, 963f
    precautions, 964
    radiographs, 960, 961f
    transducer placement, 962, 964f
  iliopectineal pain (*see* Iliopectineal bursitis pain)
  intermetatarsal
    anatomy, 1170, 1172f, 1173f
    chronic, 1170
    complications, 1171
    informed consent, 1170
    Morton neuroma, 1175f
    Mulder maneuver, 1170, 1171f, 1175f
    needle placement, 1171, 1176f
    obesity, 1170
    patient position, 1170, 1174f
    physical examination, 1170, 1171f
    position identification, 1175f
    precautions, 1176
    radiographs, 1170, 1171f
    symptoms, 1170
    ultrasound transducer position, 1174f
  olecranon (*see* Olecranon bursitis)
  subcoracoid pain (*see* Subcoracoid bursitis pain)
  trochanteric pain
    anatomy, 810, 813f
    anteroposterior plain, 810, 812f
    bupivacaine and methylprednisolone, 812
    causes of, 810
    complications, 813
    electromyography, 810
    femur identification, 812, 814f
    gluteus minimus tendon, 810, 813f
    in hip region, 810, 811f
    hydrodissection, 813
    musculotendinous unit, 810, 811f
    needle position, 813, 816f
    patient position, 810, 814f
    physical examination, 810
    precautions, 814
    radiographs, 810, 812f
    resisted abduction test, 810, 812f
    transducer placement, 812, 815f
Buttocks pain. *See* Gluteus medius bursitis pain

## C

Calcaneal spurs
  clinical presentation, 1115, 1116f–1118f
  complications, 1116, 1119
  needle placement, 1116, 1120f
  pain on palpation, 1116, 1117f
  patient position, 1115, 1119f
  plantar fascia and calcaneal insertion, 1120f
  precautions, 1119–1120
  radiographs, 1115, 1117f
  transducer placement, 1116, 1119f
Calcaneofibular ligament
  anatomy of, 1106, 1106f
  tear of, 1106, 1107f
Calcaneofibular ligament strain
  clinical presentation, 1106
  complications, 1108
  needle placement, 1108, 1109f
  patient position, 1106, 1108f
  precautions, 1109
  radiographs, 1106, 1107f
  transducer placement, 1108, 1108f
Calcific tendonitis, 234, 236f
Camper line, 81, 87f
Carpal tunnel syndrome
  anatomy, 446
  complications, 448
  differential diagnosis, 342t
  fluid shifts balance conditions, 448
  inflammatory conditions, 448
  neuropathic/ischemic conditions, 448
  pathologic conditions, 446, 447f
  Phalen test, 446, 449f
  repetitive stress related conditions, 448
  sensory distribution, 446, 449f
  structural/anatomic conditions, 448
  Tinel sign, 446, 448f
  ultrasound-guided technique
    color Doppler image, ulnar artery identification, 447, 452f
    distal crease identification, 446, 450f
    flexor tendons, 446, 450f
    median nerve, transverse image, 451f
    patient position, 450f
    proper needle placement, 447, 453f
    transverse position, 446, 451f
    ulnar artery identification, 447, 452f
    ultrasound transducer, 446, 451f
Carpometacarpal joints, intra-articular injection. *See also* First carpometacarpal joint, intra-articular injection
  acute infectious arthritis, 507
  anatomy, 507, 510
  anterior view of, 508f
  articulations of, 507, 509f
  complications, 512
  first metacarpal joint *vs.* carpometacarpal joints, 507, 510f
  metacarpals location, 507
  osteoarthritis, 507
  precautions, 512
  radiographs, 507, 509f
  ultrasound-guided technique
    hypoechoic cleft, 510, 511f
    needle placement, 512, 512f
    patient position, 510, 510f
    ultrasound transducer, 510, 511f

Caudal epidural block
  acute herpes zoster, 710
  in acute pain setting, 710
  acute vaso-occlusive disease, 711f
  anatomy, 710, 711f
  complications
    epidural veins, 713
    infection, 716–717
    misplacement, 715
    neurologic deficit, 715
  diagnostic tool, 710
  precautions, 717–718
  prognostic tool, 710
  sacral cornua, 710, 711f
  sacrococcygeal ligament, 710, 712f
  treatment of, 710
  ultrasound-guided technique
    appearance, 713, 715f, 716f
    gluteal muscles relax, 710, 713f
    needle position, 713, 717f
    patient position, 710, 712f
    sacral cornua view, 712–713, 715f
    sacral hiatus identification, 712, 714f
    transducer placement, 712, 713, 714f, 716f, 717f
  U-shaped sacral hiatus, 710
Celiac plexus block, anterior approach
  advantages, 629, 630t
  anatomy, 629–630, 632f
  celiac ganglia, 629
  chronic pancreatitis, 629, 630f
  complications, 637
  diagnostic tool, 629
  diaphragm, crura of, 630, 633f
  pancreatic cancer, CT image, 629, 630f
  *vs.* posterior approach, 630t
  postganglionic fibers, 629
  precautions, 637
  single *vs.* two-needle approach, 637
  ultrasound-guided technique
    color Doppler image, 632, 635f, 636f
    needle position, 636, 637f
    palpation identification, 632, 634f
    patient position, 630, 634f
    shofar/ram's horn appearance, 632, 636f
    transducer placement, 632, 634f
    transverse ultrasound image, 632, 635f
Cervical intra-articular facet block
  anatomy, 179, 180f, 181f
  clinical presentation, 179
  complications, 180
  precautions, 180
  radiographs, 179, 180f–181f
  ultrasound-guided technique
    needle placement, 179, 184f
    patient position, 179, 181f
    position identification, 179, 181f, 182f
    transducer placement, 179, 182f
    wavy/sawtooth appearance, 179, 183f
Cervical medial branch block
  anatomy, 171, 172f
  calvarium in Paget disease, 171, 177f
  clinical presentation, 171
  complications, 175
  Paget disease, 177, 177f
  precautions, 177
  ultrasound-guided technique

Cervical medial branch block (*Continued*)
   needle placement, 171
   palpation identification, 171, 173f
   patient position, 171
   transducer placement, 171, 173f, 174f
Cervical plexus block. *See* Deep cervical plexus block
Cervical selective nerve root block
   anatomy, 186, 187f
   clinical presentation, 186
   complications, 187, 190
   Doppler image, 187, 189f
   precautions, 190
   symptoms, 186
   ultrasound-guided technique
      needle placement, 186, 190f
      patient position, 186, 188f
      position identification, 186, 188f, 189f
      transducer placement, 186, 188f
Cheiralgia paresthetica, 424, 425f, 428, 487, 492
Chest wall
   costosternal joint (*see* Costosternal joint, intra-articular injection)
   mediastinum (*see* Manubriosternal joint pain)
   rib tip syndrome (*see* Slipping rib syndrome)
   sternoclavicular joint (*see* Abdominal pain, sternoclavicular joint pain)
   trauma (*see* Costotransverse and costovertebral joint pain)
   xiphisternal joint
      anatomy, 560, 562f
      complications, 564
      cosmetic defect, 560, 561f
      hypoechoic joint, 560, 564f
      mediastinum tumors, 560, 561f
      needle placement, 560, 563, 565f
      palpation identification, 560, 563f
      patient position, 560, 563f
      precautions, 565
      radiographs, 560, 561f
      transducer placement, 560, 564f
Cholecystitis, 921, 922f
Chopart joint, 1030, 1031f
Clergyman's knee. *See* Deep infrapatellar bursitis pain
Coal miner's knee. *See* Prepatellar bursitis pain
Coccydynia
   anatomy, 865, 867f
   anterior concave surface, 865
   complications, 870–871
   physical examination, 865
   precautions, 871–872
   radiographs, 865, 866f
   radionuclide bone, 865
   rectal examination, 865
   sacral cornua, 865, 870f
   sacral hiatus, 865, 868, 869f–872f
   sacrococcygeal ligament, 865, 867f, 868, 871f, 872f
   tailbone, 865
   triangular-shaped sacrum, 865, 867f
   T2-weighted scan, 865, 866f
   ultrasound-guided technique
      gluteal muscles relax, 865, 868f
      hematoma formation, 870
      needle position, 870–871, 872f
      palpation identification, 865, 869f
      patient position, 865, 868f
      ultrasound transducer, 865, 868, 869f, 871f
   U-shaped sacral hiatus, 865
   vigorous exercise, 872
Collagen vascular diseases
   sacroiliac joint injection, 881
   superior tibiofibular joint, 903
   talonavicular joint, 1030
Convention spin echo (CSE) *vs.* fast spin echo (FSE), 234, 237f
Coronary ligament
   anatomy of, 916, 917f, 919f
   medial, 916, 917f (*see also* Medial collateral ligament)
Coronary ligament pain
   clinical presentation, 916, 918f
   complications, 917
   discoid medial meniscus, 918f
   hyperechoic medial margin, 916, 921f
   medial border of proximal femur, 916, 920f
   needle placement, 917, 921f
   patient position, 916, 919f
   precautions, 917
   transducer placement, 916, 920f
   triangular space, 916, 920f
Coronoid approach. *See* Mandibular nerve block, coronoid approach; Maxillary nerve block, coronoid approach; Trigeminal nerve block, coronoid approach
Costosternal joint, intra-articular injection
   anatomy, 550, 551f
   complications, 553
   costochondritis, 551f
   differential diagnosis, 551f
   ligamentous injury, 550
   precautions, 553, 554
   radiographs, 550
   Tietze syndrome, 550
   ultrasound-guided technique
      manubrium identification, 550, 553f
      needle placement, 552, 554f
      palpation identification, 550, 552f
      patient position, 550, 552f
      transducer placement, 550, 553f
Costotransverse and costovertebral joint pain
   anatomy, 566, 567f
   articulations of, 568f
   complications, 567
   computed tomography image, 567f
   precautions, 568
   radiographs, 566
   T12 image, 567f
   thoracic vertebra, 566, 567f, 568f
   ultrasound-guided technique
      needle placement, 567, 571f
      palpation identification, 566, 569f
      patient position, 566, 568f
      transducer placement, 566, 569f
Crass position, 237, 238f, 239, 239f
Creaking tendon test, 1096, 1097f
Cruciate ligaments, 916, 919f
Cubital tunnel syndrome
   anatomy, 351–352, 354f, 355f
   causes, 351, 352f
   complications, 353
   double crush syndrome, 351
   Egawa tests, 351, 354f
   Froment test, 351, 353f
   golfer's elbow, 351
   imaging, 351, 354f
   physical findings, 351, 352f
   precautions, 356
   Tinel test, 351, 352f
   ultrasound-guided technique
      bupivacaine and methylprednisolone, 353
      informed consent, 352
      needle placement, 353, 358f
      patient position, 352, 356f
Cystic sac, 1004, 1005f

## D

de Quervain's tenosynovitis
   abductor pollicis longus function, 486, 488f
   anatomy, 486
   cheiralgia paresthetica, 487, 492
   complications, 487
   coronal fat-suppressed T2-weighted image, 486f
   extensor pollicis brevis tendons function, 486, 488f
   Finkelstein test, 485, 486f
   first dorsal compartment tendons image, 487f, 490f
   inflammation of the tendons, 485, 485f
   intersection syndrome (*see* Intersection syndrome)
   radiographs, 485
   tendon sheath, 485, 485f
   ultrasound-guided technique
      abductor pollicis longus, 486, 487, 488f, 489f, 490f
      color Doppler image, radial artery, 487, 490f
      extensor pollicis brevis tendons, 486, 487, 488f, 489f, 490f, 491f
      needle placement, 487, 491f, 492f
      patient position, 486, 488f
      ultrasound transducer, 487, 489f
Deep cervical plexus block
   anatomy, deep cervical plexus, 137, 138f
   complications, 141
   cross-sectional anatomy, deep cervical plexus, 137, 139f
   Doppler image, 137, 139f
   Horner syndrome, 137
   physical examination, 137
   precautions, 142
   symptoms, 137
   ultrasound-guided technique
      patient position, 137
      position identification, 137, 139f, 140f
      ultrasound transducer position, 137, 139f
Deep infrapatellar bursitis pain
   anatomy of, 960, 961f
   bupivacaine and methylprednisolone, 962
   clinical presentation, 960, 961f
   complications, 964
   needle placement, 963, 965f

palpation, 963f
patient position, 962, 963f
precautions, 964
radiographs, 960, 961f
transducer placement, 962, 964f
Deep peroneal nerve block, at ankle
    anatomy of, 1048, 1052f
    clinical presentation, 1048, 1049f–1050f
    complications, 1050
    electrodiagnostic testing, 1048
    needle placement, 1050, 1055f
    patient position, 1048, 1053f
    precautions, 1055
    radiographs, 1048, 1049f
    sensory distribution, 1048, 1052f
    tibial artery and vein, 1048, 1054f
    transducer placement, 1050, 1053f
Deltoid ligament strain
    anatomy of, 1069, 1070f
    clinical presentation, 1069, 1070f–1072f
    complications, 1070
    eversion injuries, 1069, 1071f
    needle placement, 1070, 1074f
    patient position, 1069, 1073f
    physical examination, 1069
    precautions, 1075
    radiographs, 1069, 1072f
    transducer placement, 1069, 1073f
    triangular-shaped, 1069, 1074f
Dental pain. See Mandibular nerve block, coronoid approach
Digital and metatarsal nerve block, of foot. See Metatarsal and digital nerve block
Digital nerves
    anatomy of, 1163, 1166f
    and metacarpal (see Metacarpal and digital nerve block)
    and metatarsal (see Metatarsal and digital nerve block)
    metatarsophalangeal
        anatomy of, 1130, 1131f, 1144, 1148f, 1163, 1166f
        bunion (see Bunionette pain syndrome)
Discoid medial meniscus, coronary ligament, 918f
Distal deep peroneal nerve, 1085f. See also Anterior tarsal tunnel syndrome
Distal radioulnar joint, intra-articular injection
    anatomy, 412, 414f
    anterior interosseous nerve, 412
    arthritis, acute infectious, 412
    clinical presentation, 412
    collagen vascular diseases, 412
    complications, 416
    COX-2 inhibitors, after injection, 416
    distal forearm, 412
    distal radius, 413f
    effusion, T2-weighted MRI, 413f
    hyaline cartilage, 412
    osteoarthritis joint, 412
    posterior interosseous nerve, 412
    precautions, 416
    radioulnar ballottement test, 413f
    ultrasound-guided technique
        identification, recess, 415, 415f

needle position, 415, 416f
patient position, 412, 414f
transverse view, 415f
ultrasound transducer, 414f, 415
Dorsal foot pain. See Anterior tarsal tunnel syndrome
Double crush syndrome, 403, 1081
    anterior interosseous syndrome, 403
    cubital tunnel syndrome, 351
    pronator syndrome, 393
    radial tunnel syndrome, 372
    sciatic nerve entrapment (see Piriformis syndrome)
    tennis elbow syndrome, 359
Dupuytren contracture
    anatomy, 520
    axial T1-weighted image, 522f
    Clostridium histolyticum, 523
    complications, 522
    flexion contracture character, 521f
    palmar aponeurosis, 520
    radiographs, 520
    sagittal T1-weighted image, 522f
    tender fibrotic nodules, 520
    ultrasound-guided technique
        affected tendons identification, 520, 523f
        needle placement, 521, 524f
        patient position, 520, 522f
        transducer position, 520, 523f
Dysfunctional gait
    Achilles tendonitis
        calcaneal insertion, 1096, 1099f, 1100f
        clinical presentation, 1096, 1097f–1099f
        complications, 1101
        creaking tendon test, 1096, 1097f
        needle placement, 1096, 1101, 1101f
        patient position, 1096, 1100f
        precautions, 1101
        radiographs, 1096, 1198f
        transducer placement, 1096, 1100f
    adductor tendonitis, 782 (see also Adductor tendonitis)
    osteitis pubis
        anatomy, 775, 777f
        anterior pelvis, 775
        bupivacaine and methylprednisolone, 776
        causes, 775, 776t
        complications, 781
        cutting and kicking maneuvers, 781, 781f
        diagnosis, 775
        dysfunctional gait, 775
        interpubic fibroelastic cartilage, 775, 776, 780f
        location, 775
        magnetic resonance imaging, 775
        needle placement, 776, 780f
        noninfectious inflammation of, 775, 776f
        patient position, 775, 778f
        physical examination, 775
        precautions, 781
        pubic symphysis location, 775, 777f, 778f
        radiographic findings of, 775, 776f
        radionuclide bone, 775, 777f
        rheumatoid arthritis, 775
        superior pubic ligament, 775
        ultrasound transducer, 775, 779f

x-rays, 777f
posterior tibialis tendonitis (see Posterior tibialis tendonitis)

E
Eagle syndrome
    anatomy, 90
    bilateral hypertrophied styloid process, CT, 91f–92f
    causes, 90
    complications, 92, 96
    3D CT, 94f
    extralaryngeal spread, 97f
    precautions, 96
    symptoms, 90
    ultrasound-guided technique
        needle placement, 96f
        patient position, 90, 94f
        position identification, 90, 94f, 95f
        ultrasound transducer position, 90, 96f
Elbow
    cubital tunnel syndrome
        anatomy, 351–352, 354f, 355f
        bupivacaine and methylprednisolone, 353
        causes, 351, 352f
        complications, 353
        double crush syndrome, 351
        Egawa test, 351, 354f
        Froment test, 351, 353f
        golfer's elbow, 351
        imaging, 351, 354f
        informed consent, 352
        needle placement, 353, 358f
        patient position, 352, 356f
        physical findings, 351, 352f
        precautions, 356
        Tinel test, 351, 352f
    golfer's elbow (see Golfer's elbow)
    intra-articular technique
        anatomy, 325, 326f, 327f
        bupivacaine and methylprednisolone, 328
        causes, 325
        complications, 330
        functional disability, 325
        informed consent, 327
        needle position, 330, 330f
        osteoarthritis, 325
        patient position, 327, 327f
        precautions, 330
        radiographs, 325, 326f
        tendon identification, 328, 328f
        ultrasound transducer position, 327f, 328, 328f
        V-shaped intra-articular space, 328f, 329, 329f
    joint anatomy, olecranon bursitis, 386, 389f
    median nerve block
        anatomy, 336, 338f, 339f
        bupivacaine and methylprednisolone, 336
        causes, 336
        color Doppler image, antecubital fossa, 341
        complications, 337
        needle placement, 336–337, 342f
        palpation identification, 336, 340f
        patient position, 336, 340f

Elbow (*Continued*)
  precautions, 337, 342
  sensory innervation, median nerve, 339f
  olecranon bursa (*see* Olecranon bursitis)
  pronator syndrome (*see* Pronator syndrome)
  radial nerve block (*see* Radial nerve block)
  radial tunnel syndrome
    anatomy, 372, 374, 374f
    arcade of Frohse, 372, 373f
    causes, 372
    complications, 375, 379
    double crush syndrome, 372
    electromyography, 372
    needle position, 375, 378f
    patient position, 374, 375f
    physical finding, 372, 373f
    precautions, 379
    sagittal T1-weighted magnetic resonance image, 372, 373f
    symptoms, 372, 373f
    ultrasound transducer placement and nerve identification, 374–375, 375f–378f
  tennis elbow (*see* tennis elbow syndrome)
  ulnar nerve block (*see* ulnar nerve block, elbow)
Entrapment syndrome. *See* Anterior cutaneous nerve block
Extensor pollicis brevis tendons
  effusion, 487, 491f
  function, de Quervain's tenosynovitis, 486, 488f
  identification, 486, 488f, 490f
  image, 487, 489f
Extensor tendon compartments, 493, 494t
External snapping hip syndrome
  causes, 888t
  clinical presentation, 888, 889f, 890f
  complications, 895
  greater trochanter identification, 892, 892f, 893f
  needle placement, 894, 894f
  patient position, 892, 892f
  positive snap sign, 888, 890f
  precautions, 895
  radiographs, 888, 891f
  transducer placement, 892, 893f
Extremity pain. *See* Femoral nerve block

**F**
Fabella syndrome
  anatomy of, 1011, 1013f, 1014f
  clinical presentation, 1011, 1012f
  complications, 1012
  femoral condyle and gastrocnemius muscle, 1011, 1016f
  needle placement, 1011, 1017f
  palpation, 1011, 1015f
  patient position, 1011, 1014f
  precautions, 1012–1013
  radiographs, 1011, 1012f
  transducer placement, 1011, 1015f
Facial nerve block
  anatomy, 125, 126f, 127f
  Bell's palsy, 125, 128f
  carotid artery and jugular vein, Doppler image, 125, 131f
  complications, 125, 127
  hemifacial spasm, 125, 126f
  palpation, 125
  precautions, 127, 132
  Ramsay Hunt syndrome, 125, 126f
  symptoms, 125
  ultrasound-guided technique
    needle placement, 125, 131
    patient position, 125, 129f
    position identification, 125, 128f, 129f
    ultrasound transducer position, 125, 129f, 130f
Facial pain. *See* Maxillary nerve block, coronoid approach
Femoral nerve block
  anatomy, 752, 754f
  complications, 753
  destruction of, 752
  diabetic amyotrophy, 752
  electromyography, 752
  motor and sensory distribution of, 752, 753f
  pharmacologic method, 752
  precautions, 756
  radiographs, 752, 753f
  transcervical fracture, 753f
  treatment of, 752
  ultrasound-guided technique
    color Doppler image, femoral artery, 753, 756f
    compressibility, 753, 756f
    iliacus muscle identification, 752–753, 755f
    needle position, 753, 757f
    patient position, 752, 754f
    transducer placement, 752, 755f
  utilization, 752
Fibulocalcaneal ligament. *See* Calcaneofibular ligament
Finkelstein test, 485, 486f
First carpometacarpal joint, intra-articular injection
  acute infectious arthritis, 501
  anatomy, 501, 504
  arthritis development, 504, 504f
  calcium pyrophosphate dihydrate deposition, 503f
  complications, 506
  inflammation and arthritis of, 501, 503f
  needle position, 505, 506f
  osteoarthritis joint, 501
  patient position, 501, 504f
  precautions, 506
  radiographs, 501
  saddle-type joint, 501, 502f
  thumb movements, 501, 502f
  transducer position, 505f
  ulnar collateral ligament, 504f
  Watson stress test, 501, 503f
Flexor carpi radialis tendonitis
  acute tendon rupture, 463
  anatomy, 463, 465f
  complications, 466
  dorsoradial aspect location, 463
  flexor retinaculum, 466f
  precautions, 469
  radiographs, 463
  T2-weighted magnetic resonance image, 463, 464f
  ultrasound-guided technique
    color Doppler image, hyperemia identification, 464
    distal crease identification, 463, 467f
    flexor retinaculum, 464, 469f
    needle placement, 464
    patient position, 463, 467f
    trapezium, insertion, 464, 469f
    ultrasound transducer, 464, 468f
Flexor carpi ulnaris tendonitis
  acute tendon rupture, 471
  anatomy, 471
  complications, 473, 475
  distal tendinous insertion, 471, 473f
  dorso-ulnar aspect location, 471
  precautions, 476
  radiographs, 471
  T2-weighted magnetic resonance image, 472f
  ultrasound-guided technique
    color Doppler image, ulnar artery identification, 472, 476f
    distal crease identification, 471, 474f
    needle placement, 473, 477f
    patient position, 471, 474f
    trapezium, insertion, 472, 476f
    ulnar nerve and artery, relationship, 471, 475f
    ultrasound transducer, 472, 475f
Foot. *See also* Ankle
  Achilles tendonitis
    calcaneal insertion, 1096, 1099f, 1100f
    clinical presentation, 1096, 1097f–1099f
    complications, 1101
    creaking tendon test, 1096, 1097f
    needle placement, 1096, 1101, 1101f
    patient position, 1096, 1100f
    precautions, 1101
    radiographs, 1096, 1198f
    transducer placement, 1096, 1100f
  anterior talofibular ligament strain (*see* Anterior talofibular ligament strain)
  calcaneal spurs (*see* Calcaneal spurs)
  calcaneofibular ligament (*see* Calcaneofibular ligament strain)
  hallux valgus
    clinical presentation, 1144, 1145f–1147f
    complications, 1147
    needle placement, 1144, 1150f
    patient position, 1144, 1148f
    precautions, 1147
    radiographs, 1144, 1147f
    transducer placement, 1144, 1149
  metatarsal and digital nerve block
    clinical presentation, 1136
    color Doppler image, 1136, 1142f
    complications, 1138
    needle placement, 1136, 1143f
    patient position, 1136, 1141f
    precautions, 1139
    radiographs, 1136, 1137f
    transducer placement, 1136, 1141f
  plantar fasciitis (*see* Plantar fasciitis)
  posterior tibialis tendonitis
    clinical presentation, 1121, 1122f–1124f
    complications, 1128
    medial malleolus, 1121, 1127f
    needle placement, 1123, 1129f
    patient position, 1121, 1126f

precautions, 1128–1129
radiographs, 1121
transducer placement, 1121, 1127f
retrocalcaneal bursitis (*see* Retrocalcaneal bursitis)
tarsal tunnel syndrome
anterior (*see* Anterior tarsal tunnel syndrome)
posterior (*see* Posterior tarsal tunnel syndrome)
toe joints
clinical presentation, 1130, 1131f, 1132f
complications, 1132
functional disability, 1130
needle placement, 1132, 1134f
patient position, 1132, 1133
precautions, 1132–1133
radiographs, 1130, 1132f
transducer placement, 1132, 1134f
Forearm
anterior interosseous nerve syndrome (*see* Anterior interosseous syndrome)
cubital tunnel syndrome
anatomy, 351–352, 354f, 355f
bupivacaine and methylprednisolone, 353
causes, 351, 352f
complications, 353
double crush syndrome, 351
Egawa tests, 351, 354f
Froment test, 351, 353f
golfer's elbow, 351
imaging, 351, 354f
informed consent, 352
needle placement, 353, 358f
patient position, 352, 356f
physical findings, 351, 352f
precautions, 356
Tinel test, 351, 352f
distal radioulnar joint (*see* Distal radioulnar joint, intra-articular injection)
pronator syndrome
abnormalities, 393
anatomy, 393–394, 396, 396f
brachial artery identification, 396, 398f
bupivacaine and methylprednisolone, 396
causes, 393
clinical diagnosis, 393
complications, 400
differential diagnosis, 342t
double crush syndrome, 393
honeycombed appearance, 399f
needle placement, 396, 400f
patient position, 396, 398f
physical findings, 393
precautions, 400
sensory innervation, 397f
sites of compression, 393, 394f, 394t
symptoms, 393
tests for, 393, 395f
transverse ultrasound image, 399f
Fracture
acromioclavicular joint (*see* Subacromial impingement syndrome)
avulsion, 747f, 819f
elbow, 331, 332f
Galeazzi, 331, 332f
mandibles, 58f

metacarpal, 438, 439f
phalanges, 438, 439
ribs and flail chest, 598, 599f
Frey syndrome. *See* Auriculotemporal nerve block

## G
Gait. *See* Dysfunctional gait
Ganglia cysts
anatomy, 478
classic dorsal view, 482f
complications, 481
cyst-like cavities, 478
diagnosis, 478
dorsal scapholunate joint, 482f
flexor sheath, 482f
precautions, 481, 484
predilection, 478, 483f
proximal phalanx lesions, 479f
radiographs, 478
simple *vs.* complex multiloculated, 478
solid tumor, 478
synovial sarcoma, 483f
T1-and T2-weighted images, 483f
ultrasound-guided technique
dorsal ganglion identification, 478
multiloculated, 478, 480f
needle tip position, 481
patient position, 478, 484f
posterior acoustic enhancement, 478, 480f, 481f
ultrasound transducer, 478, 479
Ganglion impar (Walther) block. *See* Impar block, ganglion
Gasserian ganglion
mandibular nerve block, 52, 54f
maxillary nerve block, 46, 47f
trigeminal nerve block, 39, 44f
Gastrocnemius muscle, 909, 1011, 1014f, 1016f
Genitofemoral nerve block
anatomy, 655, 657f
complications, 660
destruction of, 655
electromyography, 655
femoral branch, 655
genital branch, 655
orchitis, 656f
precautions, 660
radiographs, 655
sensory distribution of, 655, 656f
surgical anesthesia, 655
traction neuropathy nerve, 655
ultrasound-guided technique
color Doppler image, spermatic cord, 657, 660, 660f, 662f
femoral and external iliac artery image, 657, 659f
inguinal canal and round ligament view, 657, 661f
inguinal canal and spermatic cord view, 657, 661f
needle position, 657, 662f
palpation identification, 655, 658f
patient position, 655, 658f
transducer placement, 657, 659f
Glaucoma, 61, 65f. *See also* Supraorbital nerve block

Glenohumeral joint, intra-articular injection
anatomy, 215, 216f, 217f
clinical presentation, 215
complications, 219
osteoarthritis, 215, 216f
precautions, 219
radiographs, 215, 216f–217f
ultrasound anatomy, 217, 218f
ultrasound-guided technique
informed consent, 215
needle placement, 219, 219f
patient position, 215, 217f
position identification, 215, 217, 217f, 219f
transducer placement, 217, 217f
Glossopharyngeal nerve block
anatomy, 100, 101f
carotid artery and jugular vein, Doppler image, 101f, 102, 104f
complications, 101
left tympanic cavity and mastoid area, lateral view, 102f
multiple sclerosis, 104, 105f
physical examination, 100
precautions, 101, 102, 104
submucosal supraglottic mass and vocal cord dysfunction, 105f
symptoms, 100
ultrasound-guided technique
needle placement, 104f
patient position, 100, 103f
position identification, 100, 103f, 104f
ultrasound transducer position, 100, 104f
Gluteus medius bursitis pain
anatomy, 817, 819f
avulsion fracture, 819f
calcific tendinosis, 819f
causes of, 817
complications, 820
distal insertional tendons, 817, 818f
electromyography, 817
flexed position, 817
injury, 817
musculotendinous units, 817, 818, 823f
physical examination, 817
precautions, 820–821
radiographs, 817
resisted abduction test, 817
signification, 817, 819f
ultrasound-guided technique
bupivacaine and methylprednisolone, 817–818
femur identification, 818, 821f
hydrodissection, 818
needle placement, 818, 823f
patient position, 817, 820f
transducer placement, 818, 821f
ultrasound image, 818, 822f, 823f
Gluteus medius muscle anatomy, 888, 891f
Golfer's elbow
causes, 366, 367f
complications, 371
cubital tunnel syndrome, 351
grip strength, 366
imaging, 366, 368f
physical examination, 366
precautions, 371

Golfer's elbow (*Continued*)
  signs and symptoms, 366
  treatment, 366, 367f
  ultrasound-guided technique
    bupivacaine and methylprednisolone, 367
    location identification, 367, 369f, 370f
    needle placement, 371, 371f
    palpation, medial epicondyle, 367, 369f
    patient position, 367, 369f
Greater auricular nerve block
  anatomy, 33, 34f
  causes, 33
  complications, 33
  physical examination, 33
  precautions, 35
  Ramsay Hunt syndrome, 33, 34f
  sensory distribution, 36f
  sternocleidomastoid muscle, 36f, 37f
  ultrasound-guided technique
    needle placement, 38f
    patient position, 33, 36f
Greater occipital nerve block
  anatomy, 19
  causes, 19
  complications, 20–21
  Doppler image, 19, 23f
  occipital neuralgia, 19, 21
  physical examination, 19
  precautions, 21
  symptoms, 19
  ultrasound-guided technique
    classic technique, 19, 23f, 24f
    obliquus capitis inferior muscle approach, 19–20, 25f
    patient position, 19, 22f
Groin pain
  genitofemoral nerve block (*see* Genitofemoral nerve block)
  iliohypogastric nerve block
    anatomy, 647, 649f
    anesthesia surgical, 647
    complications, 654
    destruction of, 647
    electromyography, 647
    ilioinguinal and iliohypogastric nerve relationship, 647, 650f
    needle placement, 652, 654f
    patient position, 648, 650f
    precautions, 654
    radiographs, 647
    retroperitoneal lymphoma scan, 647, 649f
    sensory distribution of, 647, 648f
    transducer placement, 648, 651f
    visual inspection identification, 648, 651f, 652f
  ilioinguinal nerve block (*see* Ilioinguinal nerve block)
Guyon tunnel syndrome. *See* Ulnar tunnel syndrome

**H**
Hallux valgus deformity
  clinical presentation, 1144, 1145f–1147f
  complications, 1147
  needle placement, 1144, 1150f
  patient position, 1144, 1148f
  precautions, 1147
  radiographs, 1144, 1147f

  transducer placement, 1144, 1149
Hammertoe pain syndrome
  clinical presentation, 1158, 1159f, 1160f
  complications, 1159, 1161
  functional disability, 1158
  needle placement, 1158, 1159, 1162f
  patient position, 1158, 1160f
  precautions, 1161
  radiographs, 1158, 1160
  transducer placement, 1158, 1161f
Hand
  finger (*see* Metacarpal and digital nerve block)
  ganglia cysts
    anatomy, 478
    classic dorsal view, 482f
    complications, 481
    cyst-like cavities, 478
    diagnosis, 478
    dorsal ganglion identification, 478
    dorsal scapholunate joint, 482f
    flexor sheath, 482f
    multiloculated, 478, 480f
    needle tip position, 481
    patient position, 478, 484f
    posterior acoustic enhancement, 478, 480f, 481f
    precautions, 481, 484
    predilection, 478, 483f
    proximal phalanx lesions, 479f
    radiographs, 478
    simple *vs.* complex multiloculated, 478
    solid tumor, 478
    synovial sarcoma, 483f
    T1-and T2-weighted images, 483f
    ultrasound transducer, 478, 479
  pain (*see* Dupuytren contracture; Trigger finger syndrome)
  tendonitis (*see* Flexor carpi ulnaris tendonitis)
Head
  atlantoaxial joint (*see* Atlantoaxial block)
  auriculotemporal nerve (*see* Auriculotemporal nerve block)
  Eagle syndrome
    anatomy, 90
    bilateral hypertrophied styloid process, CT, 91f–92f
    causes, 90
    complications, 92, 96
    3D CT, 94f
    extralaryngeal spread, 97f
    needle placement, 96f
    patient position, 90, 94f
    position identification, 90, 94f, 95f
    precautions, 96
    symptoms, 90
    ultrasound transducer position, 90, 96f
  greater auricular nerve block (*see* Greater auricular nerve block)
  infraorbital nerve block
    anatomy, 66
    brain tumor, MRI, 70, 72f
    complications, 68
    extraoral approach, ultrasound-guided technique, 66–67, 69f–71f
    infraorbital foramen, nerve, 66, 67f, 68f
    intraoral approach, ultrasound-guided technique, 67, 71f, 72f
    palpation, 66

    precautions, 70
    sensory distribution, 66, 67f
    symptoms, 66
  mandibular nerve block
    anatomy, 52, 53f
    complications, 55
    coronoid notch and lateral pterygoid plate, 52
    fracture, radiographs, 58f
    gasserian ganglion and trigeminal nerve, 52
    needle placement, 58f
    palpation, 52
    patient position, 56f
    position identification, 55f
    precautions, 55
    sensory distribution, 54f
    symptoms, 52
    ultrasound transducer position, 56f
  maxillary nerve block
    acute herpes zoster infection, 46, 47f
    anatomy, 46, 47f
    complications, 50
    coronoid notch and pterygoid plate, 46
    gasserian ganglion, 46
    needle placement, 50f
    patient position, 46, 48f
    position identification, 48f
    precautions, 50
    sensory distribution, 46, 47f
    ultrasound transducer position, 48f
  mental nerve block
    anatomy, 74
    anesthesia in cotton ball, 74, 78f
    complications, 80
    3D CT, volume-rendered reconstruction, 75f
    Doppler image, 74, 78f
    extraoral approach, ultrasound-guided technique, 74, 76f–78f
    intraoral approach, ultrasound-guided technique, 74, 78f, 79f
    mental foramen view, 74, 75f
    palpation, mental foramen, 74, 76f
    precautions, 80
    sensory distribution, 74, 76f
    symptoms, 74
  occipital neuralgia (*see* Greater occipital nerve block)
  supraorbital nerve block
    acute herpes zoster, 60, 61f
    anatomy, 60, 61f, 62f
    complications, 60–61
    Doppler image, 64f
    gauze sponge usage, 64f
    needle placement, 64f
    palpation, 62f
    patient position, 62f, 63f
    position identification, 62f
    precautions, 61
    sensory distribution, 62f
    symptoms, 60
    ultrasound transducer position, 63f
  temporomandibular joint (*see* Temporomandibular joint (TMJ) injection)
Headache. *See* Sphenopalatine ganglion block
Heberden nodes, 531, 533f
Heel pain. *See* Calcaneal spurs; Retrocalcaneal bursitis

Hemifacial spasm, 125, 126f. *See also* Facial nerve block
Hiccups, 123t. *See also* Phrenic nerve block
Hip joint pain
   anterior (*see* Iliopsoas bursitis pain)
   bursitis (*see* Iliopectineal bursitis pain)
   extension test, 788, 791f
   intra-articular injection
      acetabular labrum, 745
      acute infectious arthritis, 745
      anatomy, 745, 746f
      arthritis, 745
      articular cartilage, 745, 747f
      avascular necrosis, 745, 747f
      avulsion fracture, 747f
      bupivacaine and methylprednisolone, 746
      collagen vascular diseases, 745
      complications, 749
      femoral neck and head, 746, 749, 750f
      femur medial margin identification, 746, 749f
      ligaments of, 745, 748f
      location, 745
      needle position, 746, 749, 751f
      osteoarthritis, 745, 751f
      pathologic conditions, 745
      patient position, 745–746, 748f
      physical examination, 745
      precautions, 750
      radiographs, 745
      ultrasound transducer, 746, 749f
   lateral (*see* Trochanteric bursitis pain)
   sciatic nerve block (*see* Sciatic nerve block)
   sciatic nerve entrapment (*see* Piriformis syndrome)
Hooking maneuver test, 606, 607f
Horner syndrome. *See* Deep cervical plexus block
Housemaid's knee. *See* Prepatellar bursitis pain
Hyaline cartilage, 916
Hypoechoic baker cyst, 1005, 1009f
Hypogastric plexus block
   anatomy, 848
   complications, 852
   destruction of, 848
   diagnostic tool, 848
   herpes zoster, 848, 849f
   L5-S1 interspace, 848, 849f
   pelvic viscera, 848
   postganglionic fibers, 848
   precautions, 856
   preganglionic fibers, 848
   sacral dermatomes, 848, 849f
   ultrasound-guided technique
      appearance, 848, 851f
      color Doppler image, lumbar plexus, 849, 855
      hematoma formation, 849
      L4-L5 interspace view, 848, 851f
      lumbar plexus, 849, 852f, 854f, 855f
      median sacral crest, 848, 850f
      needle position, 849, 855f
      patient position, 848, 850f
      ultrasound transducer, 848–849, 850f, 851f

## I

Iliohypogastric nerve block
   anatomy, 647, 649f
   anesthesia surgical, 647
   complications, 654
   destruction of, 647
   electromyography, 647
   ilioinguinal and iliohypogastric nerve relationship, 647, 650f
   precautions, 654
   radiographs, 647
   retroperitoneal lymphoma scan, 647, 649f
   sensory distribution of, 647, 648f
   ultrasound-guided technique
      needle placement, 652, 654f
      patient position, 648, 650f
      transducer placement, 648, 651f
      visual inspection identification, 648, 651f, 652f
Ilioinguinal nerve block
   anatomy, 639, 641f
   complications, 640
   destruction of, 639
   electromyography, 639
   novice skier position, 639, 640f
   precautions, 640
   radiographs, 639
   rectus abdominis muscle, 639
   retroperitoneal liposarcoma scan, 639, 641f
   sensory distribution of, 639, 642f
   Tinel sign, 639
   ultrasound-guided technique
      color Doppler image, circumflex iliac artery, 640, 645f
      needle position, 640, 646f
      patient position, 639, 642f
      transducer placement, 640, 643f
      visual inspection identification, 640, 643f, 644f, 645f
Ilioinguinal neuralgia, 655
Iliopectineal bursitis pain
   anatomy, 803
   causes of, 802
   complications, 804
   in hip region, 802, 802f
   iliopectineal eminence point, 802, 803f, 805f
   inflammation of, 802, 803
   musculotendinous unit, 802, 803f
   physical examination, 802
   precautions, 804
   radiographs, 802, 805f
   ultrasound-guided technique
      appearance, 802, 804f
      bupivacaine and methylprednisolone, 803
      needle placement, 803–804, 809f
      patient position, 803, 806f
      pubic symphysis location, 803, 806f
      transducer placement, 803, 807f, 808f
Iliopsoas bursitis pain
   anatomy, 795, 798f
   causes of, 795
   complications, 797
   CT, hip, 801f
   in hip region, 795, 796f
   injury of, 795
   intracapsular osteoid osteoma, 801f
   musculotendinous unit, 795, 796f
   physical examination, 795
   precautions, 801
   radiographs, 795, 798f
   ultrasound-guided technique
      bupivacaine and methylprednisolone, 795
      needle placement, 796–797, 800f
      patient position, 795, 799f
      transducer placement, 796, 799f
Iliotibial band, 889f, 890, 891f
Ilium
   iliohypogastric nerve block, 647
   ilioinguinal nerve block, 639
   iliopectineal eminence, 803, 805f, 890
   piriformis syndrome, 825
   sacroiliac joint injection, 881, 884, 885f, 886f
   transverse ultrasound image, 877f, 885f
   trochanteric bursitis pain, 810
Impar block, ganglion
   acute pain setting, 857
   anatomy, 857, 858f, 859f
   complications, 862, 864
   diagnostic tool, 857
   malignant pain, 857
   precautions, 864
   prognostic tool, 857
   sacral cornua, 857, 858f, 859, 862f
   sacral hiatus, 857, 858f, 860f–862f
   sacrococcygeal ligament, 857, 858f
   triangular coccyx, 857
   triangular-shaped sacrum, 857
   ultrasound-guided technique
      gluteal muscles relax, 857, 860f
      needle position, 861, 863f
      palpation identification, 857, 860f
      patient position, 857, 859f
      sacrococcygeal joint, 859, 861, 863f
      transducer placement, 857, 861f
   U-shaped sacral hiatus, 857
Infraclavicular brachial plexus block
   anatomy, 204, 205f
   clinical presentation, 204
   complications, 205–206
   Doppler image, 204, 208f
   precautions, 206–207
   radiographs, 204, 205f–206f
   ultrasound-guided technique
      needle placement, 205
      patient position, 204, 207f
      position identification, 204, 207f, 208f
      transducer placement, 204, 207f
Infraorbital nerve block
   anatomy, 66
   brain tumor, MRI, 70, 72f
   complications, 68
   infraorbital foramen, nerve, 66, 67f, 68f
   palpation, 66
   precautions, 70
   sensory distribution, 66, 67f
   symptoms, 66
   ultrasound-guided technique
      extraoral approach, 66–67, 69f–71f
      intraoral approach, 67, 71f, 72f
Infraspinatus tendonitis
   anatomy, 241, 243f, 244f
   causes, 241
   clinical presentation, 241
   complications, 243, 246
   precautions, 246
   radiographs, 241, 242f–243f
   ultrasound-guided technique
      informed consent, 241
      needle placement, 241, 246f

Infraspinatus tendonitis (*Continued*)
    patient position, 241, 245f
        position identification, 241, 245f, 246f
        transducer placement, 241, 245f
Intercostal nerve block
    anatomy, 598, 600f
    complications, 599
    diagnostic tool, 598
    intercostal vein and artery, relationship, 598, 601f
    paravertebral nerves, 598
    precautions, 599
    prognostic tool, 598
    ribs and flail chest fracture, 598, 599f
    subcostal nerve, 598
    ultrasound-guided technique
        color Doppler image, intercostal artery, 598, 603f
        flying bat, 599, 603f
        needle placement, 599, 604f
        palpation identification, 598, 601f
        patient position, 598, 601f
        rib identification, 598, 601f, 602f
        sandy beach appearance, 599, 604f
        transducer placement, 598, 601f
Intercostobrachial nerve block
    anatomy, 274, 276f
    clinical presentation, 274
    complications, 274
    Doppler image, 274, 278f
    precautions, 275
    radiographs, 274, 275f–276f
    sensory distribution, 274, 275f
    ultrasound-guided technique
        informed consent, 274
        needle placement, 274, 279f
        palpation, axillary artery, 274, 277f
        patient position, 274, 276f
        position identification, 274, 276f, 277f
        transducer placement, 274, 277f
Intermetatarsal bursitis
    anatomy, 1170, 1172f, 1173f
    chronic, 1170
    complications, 1171
    obesity, 1170
    physical examination, 1170, 1171f
    precautions, 1176
    radiographs, 1170, 1171f
    symptoms, 1170
    ultrasound-guided technique
        informed consent, 1170
        Morton neuroma, 1175f
        Mulder maneuver, 1170, 1171f, 1175f
        needle placement, 1171, 1176f
        patient position, 1170, 1174f
        position identification, 1175f
        ultrasound transducer position, 1174f
Interphalangeal joints
    anatomy of, 531, 532f, 1158, 1160
    intra-articular injection
        acute infectious arthritis, 531
        articular cartilage, 531
        Bouchard nodes, 531, 533f
        bupivacaine and methylprednisolone, 531, 533
        complications, 533, 535
        flexion of, 531, 534f
        Heberden nodes, 531, 533f
        hypoechoic joint space, 531, 535f
        needle position, 533, 535f, 536f
        palpation identification, 531
        patient position, 531, 534f
        precautions, 535
        psoriatic arthritis, 532f
        radiographs, 531, 533f
        ultrasound transducer, 531, 534f
Interscalene brachial plexus block
    anatomy, 192
    clinical presentation, 192
    complications, 196
    Doppler image, 192, 195f
    precautions, 196
    ultrasound-guided technique
        needle placement, 192, 196f
        patient position, 192, 193f
        position identification, 192, 193f, 194f
        transducer placement, 192, 194f
Intersection syndrome
    anatomy, 493
    causes, 493
    clinical presentation, 493
    complications, 496
    creaking tendon sign, 495f
    physical examination, 493
    precautions, 498
    radiographs, 493, 494f–495f
    symptoms, 493
    ultrasound-guided technique
        informed consent, 493
        needle placement, 495, 500f
        patient position, 493, 497f
        position identification, 493, 496f, 497f
        ultrasound transducer position, 493, 496f
Intra-articular injection
    anatomy, 325, 326f, 327f
    of ankle joint (*see* Ankle joint)
    carpometacarpal joints (*see* Carpometacarpal joints, intra-articular injection)
    causes, 325
    complications, 330
    costosternal joint (*see* Costosternal joint, intra-articular injection)
    distal radioulnar joint (*see* Distal radioulnar joint, intra-articular injection)
    first carpometacarpal joint (*see* First carpometacarpal joint, intra-articular injection)
    functional disability, 325
    glenohumeral joint (*see* Glenohumeral joint, intra-articular injection)
    hip (*see* Hip joint)
    interphalangeal joints (*see* Interphalangeal joints, intra-articular injection)
    of knee joint
        clinical perspectives, 897, 898f
        complications, 898
        medial border of proximal femur, 898, 900f
        medial meniscus, 898, 899f, 901f
        needle placement, 898, 902f
        patient position, 897–898, 900f
        precautions, 902
        transducer placement, 898, 900f
        triangular space, 898, 901f
    lumbar facet block, 673
    metacarpophalangeal joints (*see* Metacarpophalangeal joints, intra-articular injection)
    osteoarthritis, 325
    precautions, 330
    radiocarpal joint (*see* Radiocarpal joint, intra-articular injection)
    radiographs, 325, 326f
    of subtalar joint (*see* Subtalar joint)
    of superior tibiofibular joint (*see* Superior tibiofibular joint)
    of talonavicular joint (*see* Talonavicular joint)
    thoracic facet block, 589, 590f
    of toe joints (*see* Toe joint)
    ultrasound-guided technique
        bupivacaine and methylprednisolone, 328
        informed consent, 327
        needle position, 330, 330f
        patient position, 327, 327f
        tendon identification, 328, 328f
        ultrasound transducer position, 327f, 328, 328f
        V-shaped intra-articular space, 328f, 329, 329f
Intractable hiccups, 123t. *See also* Phrenic nerve block
Intraoral approach. *See* Mental nerve block
Inversion injuries, 1076, 1077f
Ischial bursitis pain
    anatomy, 788, 789f
    causes of, 788
    complications, 789
    development of, 788
    hamstring muscles, 788
    hip extension test, 788, 791f
    hydroxyapatite deposition, 788, 789f
    MRI images
        post-gadolinium, 788, 791f
        pre-gadolinium, 788, 791f
    physical examination, 788, 790f
    precautions, 790
    radiographs, 788
    ultrasound-guided technique
        bupivacaine and methylprednisolone, 789
        needle position, 789, 794f
        patient position, 788, 792f
        Sims position, 788, 792f
        ultrasound transducer, 789, 793f
    weaver's bottom, 788, 790f

## J

Jefferson fracture, 6, 7f–8f
Jump sign, 727
Jumper's fracture. *See* Sacral nerve block
Jumper's knee
    clinical presentation, 935, 936f, 937f
    complications, 937–938
    medial border of proximal femur, 936, 940f
    needle placement, 936, 941f
    patient position, 935, 940f
    precautions, 938
    radiographs, 935, 938f
    transducer placement, 936, 940f

## K

Keratitis, 61, 65f. *See also* Supraorbital nerve block

Knee extension test, 928, 930f
Knee joint
 anatomy, 897, 898f, 925f
 articulations, 897, 898f
 bursa of, 943f, 949f
 coronal MRI, 925f
 functional disability, 897
 intra-articular injection for (see Intra-articular injection, of knee joint)
 ligaments, 919f
 medial and lateral support, 897, 899f
 plain radiographs, 897, 898f
 saphenous nerve block at (see Saphenous nerve block)
 T2-weighted MRI image, 897, 899f

## L

Larynx
 nerve block (see Recurrent laryngeal nerve block)
 nerves and vessels, 144f
Lateral epicondylitis. See Tennis elbow syndrome
Lateral femoral cutaneous nerve block
 anatomy, 758, 760f
 anterior branch, 758, 761f
 Bernhardt-Roth syndrome, 758
 complications, 760
 computed tomography scan, 2f
 destruction of, 758
 diagnosis, 764
 electromyography, 758
 lumbar plexus, 758, 760f
 meralgia paresthetica, 758, 759f
 posterior branch, 758, 761f
 procedures, 758
 radiographs, 758, 759f
 sensory examination, 758
 skinny pants syndrome, 758
 symptoms, 758
 ultrasound-guided technique
  color Doppler image, femoral nerve, 759, 764f
  honeycombed appearance, 759, 763f
  needle position, 759, 764f
  palpation identification, 759, 762f
  patient position, 758, 761f
  transducer placement, 759, 762f
  utilization, 758
Lateral infrazygomatic approach. See Sphenopalatine ganglion block
Lesser auricular nerve block
 anatomy, 33, 34f
 causes, 33
 complications, 33
 physical examination, 33
 precautions, 35
 Ramsay Hunt syndrome, 33, 34f
 sensory distribution, 36f
 sternocleidomastoid muscle, 36f, 37f
 ultrasound-guided technique
  needle placement, 38f
  patient position, 33, 36f
Low back pain
 caudal pain (see Caudal epidural block)
 lumbar plexus nerve (see Lumbar plexus nerve block)
 lumbar sympathetic block
  anatomy, 736–737, 737f
  color Doppler image, vasculation, 738, 739, 742f
  complications, 738–739
  computed tomography scan, 738f
  destruction of, 736
  diagnosis and treatment of, 736
  distant ganglia, 737
  indications for, 736t
  needle position, 738, 743f
  palpation identification, 738
  patient position, 738, 738f
  precautions, 743
  psoas muscle, 738, 741f
  stellate ganglion block, 736
  transducer placement, 738, 739f
  transverse process, 738, 739f, 740f
  ureteral calculi, 736, 736f
 myofascial pain (see Myofascial pain syndrome)
Lower extremity
 anatomy of, 925f
 knee joint (see Knee joint)
 tibiofibular joint (see Superior tibiofibular joint)
Lumbar epidural block
 acute pain setting, 682
 anatomy, 682, 684f
 complications, 685–687
 development paraplegia, 686
 diagnostic tool, 682
 herpes zoster, 682
 local anesthetic toxicity, 686
 lumbar spine lateral view, 682, 685f
 malignant pain, 682
 phantom limb pain, 682
 precautions, 687
 prognostic tool, 682
 sagittal T1-and T2-weighted image, 683f
 treatment of, 682
 trident sign, 684, 687f
 ultrasound-guided technique
  articular process view, paramedian sagittal, 684–685, 688f, 689f
  needle position, 685, 692f
  oblique view, paramedian sagittal, 685, 689f–692f
  patient position, 682, 685f
  transverse process view, paramedian sagittal, 684, 686f, 687f
Lumbar facet block
 intra-articular technique
  acute pain setting, 673
  anatomy, 673, 676f
  arthritis treatment, 673, 674f
  complications, 674–675
  diagnostic tool, 673
  facet arthrosis, 673, 674f
  innervation of, 673, 676f
  precautions, 675
  symptoms, 673, 675f
  trident sign, 673, 678f
  ultrasound-guided technique, 673–674, 676f–681f
 medial branch technique
  anatomy, 664, 667f
  arthritis treatment, 664, 665f
  complications, 665–666
  diagnostic tool, 664
  facet arthrosis, 664, 665f
  innervation of, 664, 667f
  precautions, 666
  symptoms, 664, 666f
  trident sign, 664, 669f
  ultrasound-guided technique, 664–665, 667f–672f
Lumbar myofascial pain syndrome. See Myofascial pain syndrome
Lumbar plexus
 anatomy, 758, 760f
 hypogastric plexus block, 849, 852f, 854f, 855f
 lateral femoral cutaneous nerve block, 758, 760f
Lumbar plexus nerve block
 anatomy, 719, 720f
 complications, 726
 destruction of, 719
 femoral cutaneous nerve, 719
 genitofemoral nerve, 719
 invasion tumor, 719
 obturator nerve, 719
 precautions, 726
 ultrasound-guided technique
  anteriorly rocked identification, 719, 723f, 724f
  color Doppler image, 719, 725f, 726
  decubitus patient position, 719, 721f
  needle position, 719, 725f, 726
  palpation identification, 719
  psoas muscle, 719, 724f
  transducer placement, 719, 721f
  transverse process, 719, 722f, 723f
Lumbar selective nerve root block
 anatomy, 693, 694f
 color Doppler image, 694
 complications, 694
 diagnostic neuraxial block, 693
 precautions, 694–695
 symptoms, 693
 ultrasound-guided technique
  needle position, 693, 698f
  patient position, 693, 694f
  spinous processes image, 693, 695f
  transverse view, 693, 696f, 697f
Lumbar subarachnoid block
 in acute pain setting, 699
 anatomy, 699–700, 701f
 complications
  hypotension, 702–703
  infection, 703
  meningitis, 703
  in needle placement, 702
  neurologic, 703
  sepsis and local infection, 702
 diagnostic tool, 699
 precautions, 703
 prognostic tool, 699
 spinal cord, 699, 700f
 subarachnoid space, 699–700, 702f
 trident sign, 700, 704f, 705f
 ultrasound-guided technique
  articular process view, paramedian sagittal, 700, 705f, 706f

Lumbar subarachnoid block (*Continued*)
  needle placement, 701, 702, 708f
  oblique view, paramedian sagittal, 700–702, 706f–708f
  patient position, 700, 703f
  transverse process view, paramedian sagittal, 700, 703f–704f
Lumbar sympathetic block
  anatomy, 736–737, 737f
  complications, 738–739
  computed tomography scan, 738f
  destruction of, 736
  diagnosis and treatment of, 736
  distant ganglia, 737
  indications for, 736t
  precautions, 743
  stellate ganglion block, 736
  ultrasound-guided technique
    color Doppler image, vasculation, 738, 739, 742f
    needle position, 738, 743f
    palpation identification, 738
    patient position, 738, 738f
    psoas muscle, 738, 741f
    transducer placement, 738, 739f
  ureteral calculi, 736, 736f

# M

Mandibular nerve block, coronoid approach
  anatomy, 52, 53f
  complications, 55
  coronoid notch and lateral pterygoid plate, 52
  fracture, radiographs, 58f
  gasserian ganglion and trigeminal nerve, 52
  palpation, 52
  precautions, 55
  sensory distribution, 54f
  symptoms, 52
  ultrasound-guided technique
    needle placement, 58f
    patient position, 56f
    position identification, 55f
    ultrasound transducer position, 56f
Manubriosternal joint pain
  anatomy, 555, 557f
  angle of Louis, 555
  aorta arch, 555
  blunt chest trauma, 556f
  complications, 559
  mediastinum tumors, 555, 556f
  precautions, 559
  radiographs, 555, 556f
  ultrasound-guided technique
    hypoechoic joint, 555, 558f
    needle placement, 555, 559f
    patient position, 555, 557f
    transducer placement, 555, 558f
Maxillary nerve block, coronoid approach
  acute herpes zoster infection, 46, 47f
  anatomy, 46, 47f
  complications, 50
  coronoid notch and pterygoid plate, 46
  gasserian ganglion, 46
  precautions, 50
  sensory distribution, 46, 47f
  ultrasound-guided technique

    needle placement, 50f
    patient position, 46, 48f
    position identification, 48f
    ultrasound transducer position, 48f
Medial brachial cutaneous nerve block
  anatomy, 281
  clinical presentation, 281
  color Doppler image, 281, 285f
  complications, 282
  precautions, 282
  sensory distribution, 281, 282
  ultrasound-guided technique
    informed consent, 281
    needle placement, 281, 287f
    patient position, 281, 283f
    position identification, 281, 283f, 284f
    transducer placement, 281, 284f–286f
Medial branch block
  cervical (*see* Cervical medial branch block)
  lumbar facet block (*see* lumbar facet block)
Medial collateral ligament pain
  anatomy of, 922, 923f
  clinical presentation, 922, 923f, 924f
  complications, 923
  medial border of proximal femur, 922, 926f
  needle placement, 922, 927f
  patient position, 922, 926f
  precautions, 923
  radiographs, 922, 924f
  transducer placement, 922, 926f
  triangular space, 922, 927f
Medial epicondylitis. *See* Golfer's elbow
Medial ligament, of talocrural joint. *See* Anterior talofibular ligaments; Deltoid ligament
Median nerve
  anterior interosseous syndrome (*see* Anterior interosseous syndrome)
  brachial artery, 406, 407f
  carpal tunnel syndrome (*see* Carpal tunnel syndrome)
  honeycombed appearance, 408f
  needle, proper placement, 406, 409f
  nerve bifurcation, 406, 408f
  Phalen test, 446, 449f
  pronator syndrome (*see* Pronator syndrome)
  proximal forearm, 407f
  sensory distribution, 446, 449f
  susceptible to compression, 446, 449f
  Tinel sign, 446, 448f
  ulnar artery, 406, 408f, 447, 452f
  ultrasound transducer, 406
Median nerve block
  anatomy, 430
  axial T2 image, 431f
  bupivacaine and methylprednisolone, 435
  carpal tunnel syndrome, 430, 431f, 432f
  complications, 437
  diagnostic tool, 430
  distal forearm, 430
  elbow
    anatomy, 336, 338f, 339f
    bupivacaine and methylprednisolone, 336
    causes, 336
    color Doppler image, antecubital fossa, 341
    complications, 337
    needle placement, 336–337, 342f

    palpation identification, 336, 340f
    patient position, 336, 340f
    precautions, 337, 342
    sensory innervation, median nerve, 339f
  entrapment neuropathy, 430
  Phalen test, 430, 432f
  physical findings, 430
  precautions, 437
  sensory distribution of, 430, 433f
  sensory innervation of, 430
  Tinel sign, 430, 431f
  ultrasound-guided technique
    color Doppler image, ulnar artery, 435, 436f
    distal crease identification, 434, 434f
    needle placement, 435, 436f, 437f
    patient position, 430, 434f
    transverse position, 434, 435f
    ulnar artery identification, 435, 436f
    ultrasound transducer, 434, 435, 435f
Meniscotibial ligaments. *See* Coronary ligament
Mental nerve block
  anatomy, 74
  anesthesia in cotton ball, 74, 78f
  complications, 80
  3D CT, volume-rendered reconstruction, 75f
  Doppler image, 74, 78f
  mental foramen view, 74, 75f
  palpation, mental foramen, 74, 76f
  precautions, 80
  sensory distribution, 74, 76f
  symptoms, 74
  ultrasound-guided technique
    extraoral approach, 74, 76f–78f
    intraoral approach, 74, 78f, 79f
Metacarpal and digital nerve block
  anatomy, 537, 539f
  bowler's thumb, 537, 538f
  complications, 541, 542
  diagnostic tool, 537
  precautions, 541, 542
  radiographs, 537, 538f
  tophaceous gout, 538f
  ultrasound-guided technique
    color Doppler view, digital artery, 537, 541f
    digital nerve identification, 537, 541f
    flexor tendon identification, 537, 540f
    needle placement, 541, 542f
    patient position, 537, 539f
    transducer placement, 537, 540f
Metacarpophalangeal joints, intra-articular injection
  acute infectious arthritis, 525
  anatomy, 525, 526f
  complications, 529, 530
  osteoarthritis, 525
  precautions, 530
  radiographs, 525, 527f
  rheumatoid arthritis, 525, 526f, 527f
  ultrasound-guided technique
    hypoechoic joint identification, 527, 529f
    needle position, 527, 529f, 530f
    palpation identification, 527, 528f
    patient position, 527, 527f
    transducer position, 527, 528f

Metatarsal and digital nerve block
  clinical presentation, 1136
  color Doppler, 1136, 1142f
  complications, 1138
  intermetatarsal bursitis, 1170, 1172f
  needle placement, 1136, 1143f
  patient position, 1136, 1141f
  precautions, 1139
  radiographs, 1136, 1137f
  transducer placement, 1136, 1141f
Metatarsalgia. See Sesamoiditis pain
Metatarsophalangeal (MTP) joint
  anatomy of, 1130, 1131f, 1144, 1148f, 1163, 1166f
  bunion (see Bunionette pain syndrome)
Migraine headache. See Sphenopalatine ganglion block
Mommy's thumb/wrist. See de Quervain's tenosynovitis
Morton neuroma, 1136, 1140f. See also Metatarsal and digital nerve block
Morton neuroma syndrome
  clinical presentation, 1163, 1164f, 1165f
  complications, 1165
  needle placement, 1164, 1169f
  patient position, 1164, 1167f
  physical examination, 1163, 1164f
  precautions, 1165
  radiographs, 1164f
  symptoms, 1163
  transducer placement, 1164, 1167f
Myofascial pain syndrome
  anatomy, 727, 729f, 730f
  complications, 730
  CT scan, 727, 730f
  jump sign, 727
  location of, 727
  palpation identification, 727, 728f
  physical examination, 727
  precautions, 730
  predisposing factor, 727
  quadratus lumborum muscle, 727, 728f
  stiffness and fatigue, 727
  treatment of, 727
  ultrasound-guided technique
    anteriorly rocked view, 730, 733f
    color Doppler image vasculation, 730, 734f
    needle position, 730, 735f
    palpation identification, 727, 728f
    patient position, 727, 731f
    psoas muscle, 730, 733f
    transducer placement, 729, 730, 731f
    transverse process, 729, 730, 731f, 732f

## N
Neck
  cervical medial branch (see Cervical medial branch block)
  cervical plexus block
    deep (see Deep cervical plexus block)
    superficial (see Superficial cervical plexus block)
  cervical vertebra (see also Cervical selective nerve root block)
    anatomy, 186, 187f
    cross-sectional view, 186, 187f

facial nerve block
  anatomy, 125, 126f, 127f
  Bell palsy, 125, 128f
  carotid artery and jugular vein, Doppler image, 125, 131f
  complications, 125, 127
  hemifacial spasm, 125, 126f
  needle placement, 125, 131
  palpation, 125
  patient position, 125, 129f
  position identification, 125, 128f, 129f
  precautions, 127, 132
  Ramsay Hunt syndrome, 125, 126f
  symptoms, 125
  ultrasound transducer position, 125, 129f, 130f
ganglion block (see Stellate ganglion block)
glossopharyngeal nerve block
  anatomy, 100, 101f
  carotid artery and jugular vein, Doppler image, 101f, 102, 104f
  complications, 101
  left tympanic cavity and mastoid area, lateral view, 102f
  multiple sclerosis, 104, 105f
  needle placement, 104
  patient position, 100, 103f
  physical examination, 100
  position identification, 100, 103f, 104f
  precautions, 101, 102, 104
  submucosal supraglottic mass and vocal cord dysfunction, 105f
  symptoms, 100
  ultrasound transducer position, 100, 104f
hiccups (see Phrenic nerve block)
intra-articular facet block (see Cervical intra-articular facet block)
laryngeal nerve block
  recurrent (see Recurrent laryngeal nerve block)
  superior (see Superior laryngeal nerve block)
  nerve root block (see Cervical selective nerve root block)
  occipital nerve block (see Third occipital nerve block)
  pain (see Stellate ganglion block; Vagus nerve block)
Neer test, 227, 228f

## O
Obesity, 1110, 1170
Oblique popliteal ligament, 909
Obliquus capitis inferior muscle approach. See Greater occipital nerve block
Obturator nerve block
  anatomy, 766, 767f
  anterior branch, 766, 768, 773f
  block adductor spasm, 766
  causes of, 766
  complications, 770
  destruction of, 766
  diagnosis, 766
  electromyography, 766, 774
  motor and sensory distribution of, 768f
  pelvis brim, 766
  posterior branch, 766, 773f

precautions, 770, 774
radiographs, 766, 767f
signification, 766
treatment of, 766
ultrasound-guided technique
  breaching whale view, 768, 771f, 772f
  color Doppler image, femoral artery, 768, 771f
  double-decker sandwich, 768, 772f
  femoral vein compression, 768, 770f
  needle position, 768–769, 773f
  patient position, 766, 769f
  transducer placement, 768, 769f
utilization, 766
Occipital nerve block/ neuralgia. See Greater occipital nerve block
Olecranon bursitis
  anatomy, 386, 387f
  complications, 391
  elbow joint anatomy, 386, 389f
  location, 386
  physical examination, 386
  precautions, 392
  radiographs, 386, 388f
  swelling, 386, 387f
  symptoms, 386
  ultrasound-guided technique
    fluid-filled olecranon bursa, 391f
    high-frequency ultrasound transducer placement, 390, 390f
    needle placement, 390–391, 392f
    patient position, 390, 390f
Osteitis pubis
  anatomy, 775, 777f
  anterior pelvis, 775
  causes, 775, 776t
  complications, 781
  cutting and kicking maneuvers, 781, 781f
  diagnosis, 775
  dysfunctional gait, 775
  interpubic fibroelastic cartilage, 775, 776, 780f
  location, 775
  magnetic resonance imaging, 775
  noninfectious inflammation of, 775, 776f
  physical examination, 775
  precautions, 781
  radiographic findings of, 775, 776f
  radionuclide bone, 775, 777f
  rheumatoid arthritis, 775
  superior pubic ligament, 775
  ultrasound-guided technique
    bupivacaine and methylprednisolone, 776
    interpubic fibroelastic cartilage identification, 776, 780f
    needle placement, 776, 780f
    patient position, 775, 778f
    pubic symphysis, 775, 777f, 778f
    ultrasound transducer, 775, 779f
  x-rays, 777f
Osteoarthritis
  advanced, 751f
  ankle joint, 1019
  carpometacarpal joints, 507
  distal radioulnar joint, intra-articular injection, 412
  glenohumeral joint, 215, 216f

Osteoarthritis (*Continued*)
   hip joint, intra-articular injection, 745
   intra-articular injection, 325
   radiocarpal joint, intra-articular injection, 417
   sacroiliac joint injection, 881
   subtalar joint, 1025
   superior tibiofibular joint, 903
   toe joints, 1130
Osteochondromatosis, 1005, 1009f
Osteonecrosis, 420, 422f
Osteophytes
   acromion, 227, 229f
   coronoid, 325, 326f
   multiple, 589, 590f

## P

Paget disease, 177, 177f
Palmar aponeurosis, 520
Paramedian sagittal approach
   lumbar epidural block
      articular process view, 684–685, 688f, 689f
      oblique view, 685, 689f–692f
      transverse process view, 684, 686f, 687f
   lumbar facet block, intra-articular technique
      articular process view, 673–674, 679f, 680f
      transverse process view, 673, 677f, 678f
   lumbar facet block, medial branch technique
      articular process view, 665, 670f, 671f
      transverse process view, 664, 668f, 669f
   lumbar subarachnoid block
      articular process view, 700, 705f, 706f
      oblique view, 700–702, 706f–708f
      transverse process view, 700, 703f–704f
   thoracic epidural block
      articular process view, 573–574, 578f, 579f
      oblique view, 574, 577, 579f, 580f, 581f
      transverse process view, 573, 575f, 576f
   thoracic facet block, intra-articular technique
      articular process view, 589, 591, 595f, 596f
      transverse process view, 589, 592f–594f
Paravertebral nerves, 598
Patellar tendon. *See also* Jumper's knee
   anatomy of, 935, 936f
   ballottement of, 935, 938f
   MRI of, 929f
Pectoralis major tear syndrome
   anatomy, 316, 318f
   functions, 316
   imaging, 316
   musculotendinous junction injury, 316, 317f
   precautions, 323
   ultrasound-guided technique
      bupivacaine and methylprednisolone, 318
      complications, 318, 323
      informed consent, 316
      needle placement, 318, 323f
      palpation identification, bicipital groove, 316, 319f
      patient position, 316, 319f
Pediatrics, intraoral approach
   infraorbital nerve block, 67, 71f, 72f
   mental nerve block, 74
Pelvis
   anterior (*see* Osteitis pubis)
   coccyx, 865, 866f (*see also* Coccydynia)
   pain (*see* Hip joint pain; Hypogastric plexus block)
   sacrum (*see* Sacral nerve block)
Peroneal nerve. *See also* Anterior tarsal tunnel syndrome
   anatomy of, 995, 997f–999f, 1048, 1051f, 1056, 1058f, 1081, 1084f
   sciatic nerve bifurcation, 995, 997f, 1002f, 1003f
   sensory distribution, 1085f
   sensory innervation, 995, 998f
Peroneal nerve block, at popliteal fossa
   clinical presentation, 995, 996f
   complications, 997
   needle placement, 996, 1003f
   patient position, 995, 1000f
   popliteal artery and vein, 996, 1001f, 1002f
   precautions, 1001
   radiographs, 995, 996f
   transducer placement, 996, 1000f
Pes anserine bursitis pain
   anatomy of, 966, 967f
   bupivacaine and methylprednisolone, 966
   clinical presentation, 966, 967f
   complications, 971–972
   discoid medial meniscus, 969, 969f
   hyperechoic medial margin, 968
   medial, 966, 969, 969f
   medial border of proximal femur
   needle placement, 970–971, 971f
   patient position, 966, 968f
   precautions, 972
   radiographs, 966, 968f
   transducer placement, 969, 969f, 970f
   triangular space, 969, 969f
Phalen test, 430, 432f, 446, 449f
Phrenic nerve block
   anatomy, 118, 119f
   causes, 118
   complications, 123
   internal jugular view, Doppler image, 118, 122f
   neurodestruction, 118
   precautions, 123
   sonogram of, 119f
   sternocleidomastoid muscle identification, 118, 121f
   symptoms, 118
   ultrasound-guided technique
      needle placement, 122f
      patient position, 118, 121f
      position identification, 118, 121f, 122f
      ultrasound transducer position, 118, 122f
Piriformis muscle
   anterior sacrum, 835
   sciatic nerve block (*see* Sciatic nerve block)
Piriformis syndrome
   anatomy, 824–825
   causes, 824, 825f, 826f
   clinical presentation, 824
   color Doppler image, pudendal artery, 829, 833f
   complications, 830, 834
   lumbar disc protrusion, 824, 827f
   precautions, 834
   provocation test, 824, 826f
   radiographs, 824, 825f–826f
   sciatic nerve entrapment, 824, 825f
   symptoms, 824
   ultrasound-guided technique
      informed consent, 825
      needle placement, 829, 834f
      patient position, 825, 830f
      position identification, 824, 827f, 828f
      ultrasound transducer position, 825, 830f
Plantar fasciitis. *See also* Calcaneal spurs
   anatomy of, 1110, 1112f
   chronic fasciitis, 1110, 1112f
   clinical presentation, 1110, 1111f–1112f
   complications, 1110, 1113
   needle placement, 1110, 1114f
   pain on palpation, 1110, 1111f
   patient position, 1110, 1113f
   precautions, 1114
   radiographs, 1110, 1111f
   transducer placement, 1110, 1113f
Plantar foot pain. *See* Posterior tarsal tunnel syndrome
Plantar nerves, 1136, 1140f
Playboy bunny sign, 401, 403f
Pneumoperitoneum. *See* Transversus abdominis plane block
Popeye sign, 288, 292f. *See also* Bicipital tendonitis
Popliteal cyst. *See* Baker cyst
Popliteal fossa
   anatomy of, 1004, 1008f, 1011, 1013f
   peroneal nerve block at (*see* Peroneal nerve block, at popliteal fossa)
   sciatic nerve block at (*see* Sciatic nerve block)
   tibial nerve block at (*see* Tibial nerve block)
Posterior tarsal tunnel syndrome
   clinical presentation, 1088, 1089f, 1090f
   complications, 1095
   needle placement, 1094, 1095f
   patient position, 1092, 1093f
   physical findings, 1088
   precautions, 1095
   radiographs, 1088
   tibial artery and vein, 1092, 1094f
   Tinel sign, 1088, 1089f
   transducer placement, 1092, 1093f
Posterior tibial nerve block. *See* Tibial nerve block
Posterior tibialis tendon
   anatomy of, 1121, 1126f
   tear of, 1124f
Posterior tibialis tendonitis
   clinical presentation, 1121, 1122f–1124f
   complications, 1128
   medial malleolus, 1121, 1127f
   needle placement, 1123, 1129f
   patient position, 1121, 1126f
   precautions, 1128–1129
   radiographs, 1121
   transducer placement, 1121, 1127f
Pregnancy
   genitofemoral neuralgia, 655
   iliohypogastric nerve block, 647
   osteitis pubis, 775, 776t
Prepatellar bursitis pain
   anatomy of, 948, 950f
   bupivacaine and methylprednisolone, 950
   clinical presentation, 948, 949f
   complications, 950
   needle placement, 950, 953f

palpation, 951f
patient position, 949, 951f
physical examination, 948
precautions, 950, 953
radiographs, 948, 949f
transducer placement, 950, 952f
Pronator syndrome. See also Median nerve
    block, elbow
  abnormalities, 393
  anatomy, 393–394, 396, 396f
  causes, 393
  clinical diagnosis, 393
  complications, 400
  differential diagnosis, 342t
  double crush syndrome, 393
  median nerve
    entrapment, 393
    honeycombed appearance, 399f
    sensory innervation, 397f
    transverse ultrasound image, 399f
  physical findings, 393
  precautions, 400
  sites of compression, 393, 394f, 394t
  symptoms, 393
  tests for, 393, 395f
  ultrasound-guided technique
    brachial artery identification, 396, 398f
    bupivacaine and methylprednisolone, 396
    needle placement, 396, 400f
    patient position, 396, 398f
Psoas muscle, 890
Pudendal nerve block
  anatomy, 873
  bartholin cyst surgery, 873, 874f
  complications, 880
  destruction of, 873
  diagnostic tool, 873
  Doppler examination, 880
  dorsal nerve, 873
  electrodiagnostic testing, 873
  inferior rectal nerve, 873
  ischial spine, 873, 875f
  perineal nerve, 873
  precautions, 880
  straddle injury, 873
  ultrasound-guided technique
    bupivacaine, 875
    color Doppler image, pudendal artery, 875, 879f
    ilium image, 873, 876f, 877f
    inferior gluteal artery, 875, 879f, 880
    ischial spine view, 873, 875, 877f
    needle position, 875, 880f
    patient position, 873, 875f
    transducer placement, 873, 875, 876f, 878f

## Q

Quadriceps expansion syndrome
  clinical presentation, 928, 929f
  complications, 932, 934
  knee extension test, 928, 930f
  medial border of proximal femur, 928, 933f
  needle placement, 932, 934f
  patella and, 928, 929f, 930f, 933f
  patient position, 928, 932f
  physical examination, 928

  precautions, 934
  radiographs, 928
  transducer placement, 928, 932f
Quadriceps tendon
  anatomy of, 928, 931f, 935, 939f
  with suprapatellar bursa, 942, 945f
  tear of, 944f
Quadrilateral space syndrome. See Axillary nerve
    block, quadrilateral space

## R

Radial nerve block
  anatomy, 424
  brachial plexus block, 424
  cheiralgia paresthetica, 424, 425f, 428
  complications, 427
  diagnostic tool, 424
  elbow
    anatomy, 331, 332f
    bupivacaine and methylprednisolone, 331
    complications, 335
    Galeazzi fracture, 331, 332f
    informed consent, 331
    needle placement, 331, 335, 335f
    patient position, 331, 333f
    precautions, 335
    radial tunnel syndrome, 331
    transverse position, ultrasound transducer, 331, 333f, 334f
  handcuff/prisoner's palsy, 424, 425f, 428
  humerus
    acute displaced distal radius fracture, 266, 267f
    anatomy, 266
    clinical presentation, 266
    complications, 268
    Doppler image, 266, 272f
    informed consent, 266
    needle placement, 266, 268, 272f
    patient position, 266, 269f
    position identification, 266, 269f, 270f
    precautions, 268
    radiographs, 266, 267f–268f
    transducer placement, 266, 270f
  radial artery, 424, 426f, 427f
  superficial radial nerve, 424, 426f, 427f
  Tinel sign, 424, 425f
  ulnar nerve, 424, 425f
  ultrasound-guided technique
    color Doppler image, radial artery, 427, 428f
    proper needle placement, 427, 428f
    radial artery, palpated, 426f, 427
    transverse position, distal radius, 426f, 427
    ultrasound transducer, 426f, 427
  wristwatch test, 424, 425f
Radial tunnel syndrome
  anatomy, 372, 374, 374f
  arcade of Frohse, 372, 373f
  causes, 372
  double crush syndrome, 372
  electromyography, 372
  physical finding, 372, 373f
  precautions, 379
  sagittal T1-weighted magnetic resonance image, 372, 373f
  symptoms, 372, 373f

  ultrasound-guided technique
    complications, 375, 379
    needle position, 375, 378f
    patient position, 374, 375f
    ultrasound transducer placement and nerve identification, 374–375, 375f–378f
Radiocarpal joint, intra-articular injection
  anatomy, 417f, 418
  anterior interosseous nerve, 418
  arthritis, acute infectious, 417
  avascular necrosis, 420, 422f
  collagen vascular diseases, 417
  complications, 420
  distal forearm, 417
  dorsovolar radiograph of hand, 418f
  osteoarthritis joint, 417
  osteonecrosis, MRI staging, 422f
  posterior interosseous nerve, 418
  ultrasound-guided technique
    distal radius and scaphoid bone identification, 419, 421f
    needle position, 421f
    patient position, 419, 420f
    real-time ultrasound guidance, 419, 420
    ultrasound transducer, 419, 420f
Radionuclide bone scanning, 1115
Radioulnar joint. See Distal radioulnar joint, intra-articular injection
Ramsay Hunt syndrome, 33, 34f, 125, 126f. See also Facial nerve block; Greater auricular nerve block
Raynaud disease, 209, 210f
Recurrent laryngeal nerve block. See also Superior laryngeal nerve block
  anatomy, 150, 151f, 152f
  complications, 150, 155
  Doppler image, 150
  precautions, 155
  symptoms, 150
  ultrasound-guided technique
    needle placement, 150, 155f
    patient position, 150
    position identification, 150, 153f, 154f
    ultrasound transducer position, 150, 155f
Retrocalcaneal bursitis pain
  anatomy of, 1102, 1103f
  clinical presentation, 1102, 1103f
  complications, 1104–1105
  needle placement, 1104, 1105f
  patient position, 1102, 1104f
  physical examination, 1102
  precautions, 1105
  radiographs, 1102, 1103f
  transducer placement, 1104, 1104f
Rheumatoid arthritis, 525, 526f, 527f
  Baker cyst, 1004, 1006f
  glenohumeral joint, 215, 216f
  metacarpophalangeal joints, 525, 526f, 527f
  osteitis pubis, 775
  shoulder, 220f
Rib tip syndrome. See Slipping rib syndrome
Rotator cuff disease
  anatomy, 254
  clinical presentation, 254
  complications, 258, 260
  drop-arm test, 254, 256f
  muscles and tendons of, 254, 256f

Rotator cuff disease (*Continued*)
  precautions, 260
  radiographs, 254, 255f
  supraspinatus tendon, 234
  ultrasound-guided technique
    informed consent, 255
    needle placement, 256, 260f
    patient position, 255, 258f
    position identification, 255, 257f, 258f
    transducer placement, 255, 258f
Rotator cuff tendinopathy, 227, 228f, 229f, 233t

**S**

Sacral nerve block
  anatomy, 841, 843f
  coccyx, 841
  complications
    aspiration test, 846
    devastating, 843
    foraminal branch, 842
    paraplegia development, 843
  destruction of, 841
  diagnostic tool, 841
  dorsally convex sacrum, 841
  electrodiagnostic testing, 841
  precautions, 846
  radiographs, 841, 842f
  sacrococcygeal ligament, 841
  treatment of, 841
  ultrasound-guided technique
    color Doppler image, foraminal artery, 842, 847f
    gluteal muscles, 842, 844f
    hyperechoic curve, 842, 846f
    needle position, 842, 847f
    patient position, 842, 843f
    rocking motion, 842, 844f
    transducer placement, 842, 845f
  U-shaped sacral hiatus, 841
Sacroiliac joint
  anatomy, 881, 882f
  articular cartilage, 881
Sacroiliac joint injection
  articulation, 885f
  bupivacaine and methylprednisolone, 882
  complications, 886
  ilium view, 884, 885f
  needle placement, 884–885, 886f
  patient position, 881, 884f
  pattern of pain, 881, 882f
  precautions, 886–887
  radiographs, 881, 883f
  transducer placement, 882, 884, 884f, 885f
  ultrasound image, 881, 884f, 885f
  vigorous exercise, 887
  Yeoman test, 881, 883f
Saphenous nerve
  anatomy of, 973, 975f
    distal, 1042, 1044f
    proximal, 1042, 1044f
  sensory distribution, 1042, 1045f
Saphenous nerve block
  ankle
    clinical presentation, 1042, 1043f
    complications, 1043
    electrodiagnostic testing, 1042

local anesthetic and steroid, 1042
needle placement, 1043, 1047f
patient position, 1042, 1045f
popliteal vein and artery, 1042, 1046f
precautions, 1043
radiographs, 1042, 1043f
transducer placement, 1042, 1046f
knee
  anteromedial femur, 973, 976f
  clinical presentation, 973, 974f, 975f
  complications, 975, 979
  needle placement, 975, 979f
  patient position, 973, 976f
  precautions, 979
  radiographs, 973, 975f
  sartorius muscle, 975, 978f
  transducer placement, 973, 977f, 978f
  vastus medialis, 973, 977f
Sartorius muscle, 975, 978f
Sciatic nerve
  anatomy of, 980, 982f
  bifurcation, tibial nerve, 987, 993f
Sciatic nerve block
  amputations foot, 835, 836f
  anatomy, 835, 836f
  common peroneal nerves, 835
  complications, 837
  destruction of, 835
  diagnostic tool, 835
  electrodiagnostic testing, 835
  mycetoma of, 835, 836f
  piriformis muscle, 835, 837f
  popliteal fossa
    clinical presentation, 980, 981f
    complications, 983
    electrodiagnostic testing, 980
    medial border of proximal femur
    needle placement, 982, 985f
    patient position, 980, 983f
    popliteal artery and vein, 982, 984f
    precautions, 985
    radiographs, 980, 981f
    transducer placement, 980, 983f
  position of, 836, 839f
  precautions, 840
  radiographs, 838
  sacral plexus, 835
  stretch injury, 835
  surgical anesthesia, 835
  tibial nerves, 835
  ultrasound-guided technique
    bupivacaine, 836
    color Doppler image, gluteal artery, 836, 839f
    needle placement, 836, 840f
    patient position, 836, 837f, 838f
    position of, 836, 839f
    transducer placement, 836, 838f
Sciatic nerve entrapment. *See* Piriformis syndrome
Semimembranosus bursa, 909
Semimembranosus insertion syndrome
  bursitis, 909, 911f
  clinical presentation, 909, 910f, 911f
  complications, 912
  knee joint, medial border, 910, 914f
  needle placement, 910, 915f

patient position, 910, 913f
precautions, 912
radiography, 909
symptoms, 909
transducer placement, 910, 913f
triangular space, 910, 914f
twist test, 909, 911f
Semimembranosus muscle
  anatomy of, 909, 912f
  distal insertion, 909, 910f
  insertions of, 912f
Sesamoiditis pain
  anatomy, 1177, 1178f
  causes, 1177
  complications, 1177, 1182
  Doppler image, 1177, 1180f
  physical examination, 1177
  precautions, 1182
  radiographs, 1177, 1179f–1180f
  sports injury, 1177
  symptoms, 1177
  ultrasound-guided technique
    informed consent, 1177
    needle placement, 1177, 1183f
    patient position, 1177, 1181f
    position identification, 1177, 1180f, 1181f
    ultrasound transducer position, 1177, 1181f
Shoulder
  acromioclavicular joint, 228, 232f (*see also* Acromioclavicular (AC) joint)
  anatomy, 248, 249f, 250f
    brachial plexus (*see* Interscalene brachial plexus block)
    CT images, 241, 243f–244f
    glenohumeral joint, 215, 216f, 217f
    infraclavicular brachial plexus (*see* Infraclavicular brachial plexus)
    normal, 241, 243f–244f
    subacromial space, 227, 228f, 229, 229f, 231f
  arthroplasty, 250, 252f
  bicipital tendonitis (*see* Bicipital tendonitis)
  brachial plexus block
    axillary (*see* Axillary brachial plexus block)
    infraclavicular (*see* Infraclavicular brachial plexus block)
    interscalene (*see* Interscalene brachial plexus block)
    supraclavicular (*see* Supraclavicular brachial plexus block)
  glenohumeral joint (*see* Glenohumeral joint, intra-articular injection)
  infraspinatus tendonitis
    anatomy, 241, 243f, 244f
    causes, 241
    clinical presentation, 241
    complications, 243, 246
    informed consent, 241
    needle placement, 241, 246f
    patient position, 241, 245f
    position identification, 241, 245f, 246f
    precautions, 246
    radiographs, 241, 242f–243f
    transducer placement, 241, 245f
  intercostobrachial cutaneous nerve block
    anatomy, 274, 276f

clinical presentation, 274
complications, 274
Doppler image, 274, 278f
informed consent, 274
needle placement, 274, 279f
palpation, axillary artery, 274, 277f
patient position, 274, 276f
position identification, 274, 276f, 277f
precautions, 275
radiographs, 274, 275f–276f
sensory distribution, 274, 275f
transducer placement, 274, 277f
ligaments, 215, 217f
medial brachial cutaneous nerve block
anatomy, 281
clinical presentation, 281
complications, 282
Doppler image, 281, 285f
informed consent, 281
needle placement, 281, 287f
patient position, 281, 283f
position identification, 281, 283f, 284f
precautions, 282
sensory distribution, 281, 282
transducer placement, 281, 284f–286f
pathology, 265
pathology, subcoracoid bursitis pain (*see* Subcoracoid bursitis pain)
radial nerve anatomy
rheumatoid arthritis, 220f
rotator cuff, supraspinatus tendon, 234
rotator cuff tendinopathy, 227, 228f, 229f, 233t
scapular and acromioclavicular joint pain, 261
subacromial impingement (*see* Subacromial impingement syndrome)
suprascapular nerve (*see* Suprascapular nerve block)
supraspinatus musculotendinous tear, 254, 257f (*see also* Rotator cuff disease)
supraspinatus tendonitis (*see* Supraspinatus tendonitis)
ultrasound images, 217, 218f, 220f
upper arm anatomy, 274, 276f, 281, 283f
Skinny pants syndrome, 758. *See also* Lateral femoral cutaneous nerve block
Sleep disturbance, 2, 6, 215, 227, 234, 241, 254, 288, 325, 417, 903, 1030, 1069, 1106, 1130, 1136
Slipping rib syndrome
abdominal trauma view, 606, 610f
anatomy, 606, 611f
appearance, 609
articular capsule, 606
complications, 608
computed tomography view, 606, 610f
costal cartilages, 606, 607
diagnosis of, 606
floating ribs, 606
hooking maneuver test, 606, 607f
pneumothorax, 609
positive test, 606, 607f
precautions, 609
radiographs, 606
seventh and eighth ribs, transverse sections, 607f, 608f–610f

ultrasound-guided technique
needle position, 608, 614f
palpation identification, 606, 612f
patient position, 606, 612f
transducer placement, 606, 613f
Valsalva maneuver, 606, 609f, 610f
Snapping hip syndrome
external (*see* External snapping hip syndrome)
internal, 888, 889f
Soleus muscle, 1011
Sphenopalatine ganglion block
anatomy, 14, 15f
causes, 14
complications, 18
Doppler image, 14, 16f
headache treatment, 14
indications, 14, 14t
physical examination, 14
precautions, 18
symptoms, 14
ultrasound-guided technique
needle placement, 17f
patient position, 14, 16f
position identification, 14, 16f, 17f
Spinal accessory nerve block
anatomy, 112, 113f
botulinum toxin use, 117
causes, 112
complications, 112, 115–116
intra-axial disease, 112, 116f
precautions, 116–117
styloid process nerve, 115f
symptoms, 112
ultrasound-guided technique
needle placement, 115f
patient position, 112, 114f
position identification, 112, 114f
ultrasound transducer position, 112, 114f
Spinal cord
lateral view, 682, 685f (*see also* Lumbar epidural block)
lumbar subarachnoid block, 699, 700f
Spinner sign, 401, 403f
Spinous process. *See* Thoracic paravertebral nerve block
Sports injury
American football, medial collateral ligament pain, 922, 924f
sesamoiditis pain, 1177
Stellate ganglion block
acrocyanosis, scleroderma patient, 156, 157f
anatomy, 156, 157f, 158f
C6 level, 156, 157f, 158, 159f
C7 vertebral body, 158, 161f
clinical presentation, 156
complications, 161–162
Doppler image, 162f
indications, 156t
lumbar sympathetic block, 736
precautions, 162
symptoms, 156
ultrasound-guided technique
patient position, 156, 159f
position identification, 156, 159f, 160f
transducer placement, 156, 159f
Sternoclavicular (SC) joint pain
anatomy, 544, 546

clinical presentation, 544
complications, 548–549
Doppler image, 544, 545f
palpation, 544
precautions, 549
radiographs, 544, 545f
symptoms, 544
ultrasound-guided technique
informed consent, 544
needle placement, 547, 548f
patient position, 544, 546f
position identification, 544, 546f, 547f
ultrasound transducer position, 547, 547f, 548f
Sternocleidomastoid (SCM) muscle pain, 112, 113f
Stylohyoid syndrome. *See* Eagle syndrome
Subacromial impingement syndrome
anatomy, 227, 228f
causes, 233t
clinical presentation, 227
complications, 230
Neer test, 227, 228f
palpation, 228, 231
precautions, 230, 233
radiographs, 230, 233f
rotator cuff tendinopathy, 227, 228f, 229f, 233t
supraspinatus tendon, 233f
ultrasound-guided technique
informed consent, 227
needle placement, 229, 232f
patient position, 227–228, 231f
position identification, 228, 230f, 231f
transducer placement, 228, 231f
Subcoracoid bursitis pain
anatomy, 310, 311f, 313f
causes, 310
physical examination, 310, 311f
precautions, 311
radiographs, 310, 312f
ultrasound-guided technique
bupivacaine and methylprednisolone, 310
complications, 311
needle position, 311, 315f
patient position, 310, 313f
ultrasound transducer position, 310, 314f
Subcostal nerve, 583, 598, 621
Subdeltoid bursitis pain
anatomy, 304, 305f
causes, 304, 305t
physical examination, 304
precautions, 308–309
radiographs, 304, 305f, 306f
ultrasound-guided technique
bupivacaine and methylprednisolone, 305
complications, 308
informed consent, 304
needle position, 305, 306, 308f
palpation identification, acromion, 305, 307f
patient position, 304, 306f
subdeltoid bursa *vs.* deltoid muscle image, 305, 307f, 308f
ultrasound transducer position, 305, 307f
ultrasound view, needle within subdeltoid bursa, 309f

Subscapularis tendonitis
  anatomy, 248, 249f, 250f
  clinical presentation, 248
  complications, 253
  precautions, 253
  radiographs, 248, 249f–250f
  ultrasound-guided technique
    informed consent, 250
    needle placement, 250, 253f
    patient position, 250, 251f
    position identification, 250, 251f, 252f
    transducer placement, 250, 251f
Subtalar joint
  anatomy of, 1025, 1026f, 1027f
  functional disability, 1025
  intra-articular injection
    clinical presentation, 1025, 1026f
    complications, 1028
    needle placement, 1027, 1029f
    patient position, 1025, 1027f
    precautions, 1029
    radiographs, 1025, 1026f
    transducer placement, 1027, 1028f
    V shape, 1027, 1028f
  inversion and eversion, 1025, 1026f
  ligaments of, 1025, 1027f
Subtendinous calcaneal bursa. *See* Retrocalcaneal bursitis pain
Superficial cervical plexus block
  anatomy, 133, 134f
  complications, 133
  pain palliation, 133, 134f
  precautions, 133, 136
  symptoms, 133
  ultrasound-guided technique
    needle placement, 136f
    patient position, 133, 135f
    position identification, 133, 135f, 136f
    ultrasound transducer position, 133, 136f
Superficial infrapatellar bursitis pain
  anatomy of, 954, 955f
  bupivacaine and methylprednisolone, 956
  clinical presentation, 954, 955f
  complications, 957–958
  needle placement, 956, 958f
  palpation, 957f
  patient position, 956, 956f
  precautions, 958
  radiographs, 954, 955f, 956f
  transducer placement, 956, 957f
Superficial peroneal nerve
  anatomy of, 1056, 1059f
  sensory distribution, 1056, 1059f
Superficial peroneal nerve block, at ankle
  clinical presentation, 1056, 1057f
  complications, 1057
  electrodiagnostic testing, 1056
  needle placement, 1056, 1062f
  patient position, 1057, 1060f
  precautions, 1062
  radiographs, 1056, 1057f
  tibial artery and vein, 1056, 1061f
  transducer placement, 1057, 1060f
Superior laryngeal nerve block
  anatomy, 142, 144f, 145f
  complications, 142
  Doppler image, 142, 149f
  physical examination, 142
  precautions, 144
  radiographs, 142
  symptoms, 142
  ultrasound-guided technique
    needle placement, 142, 148f
    patient position, 142, 146f
    position identification, 142, 146f
    ultrasound transducer position, 142, 146f
Superior tibiofibular joint
  anatomy of, 903, 904f, 906f
  articulations of, 903, 904f
  clinical perspectives, 903
  CT of fracture, 903, 905f
  functional disability, 903
  intra-articular injection for (*see* Intra-articular injection)
  precautions, 904
  ultrasound-guided technique
    complications, 904
    needle placement, 904, 908f
    patient position, 904, 906f
    space identification, 904
    superior tibiofibular ligament, 904, 907f
    transducer placement, 904, 906f
    transducer rotation, 904, 907f
Supraclavicular brachial plexus block
  anatomy, 198, 199f
  clinical presentation, 198
  complications, 202–203
  corner pocket, 198, 202
  Doppler image, 198, 202f
  precautions, 203
  radiographs, 198, 199f–200f
  symptoms, 198
  ultrasound-guided technique
    needle placement, 198, 203f
    patient position, 198, 201f
    position identification, 198, 201f, 202f
    transducer placement, 198, 201f
Supraorbital nerve block
  acute herpes zoster, 60, 61f
  anatomy, 60, 61f, 62f
  complications, 60–61
  Doppler image, 64f
  palpation, 62f
  precautions, 61
  sensory distribution, 62f
  symptoms, 60
  ultrasound-guided technique
    gauze sponge usage, 64f
    needle placement, 64f
    patient position, 62f, 63f
    position identification, 62f
    ultrasound transducer position, 63f
Suprapatellar bursitis pain
  anatomy of, 942, 945f
  bupivacaine and methylprednisolone, 945
  clinical presentation, 942, 943f
  complications, 945
  knee joint effusion, 944f
  needle placement, 945, 947f
  palpation, 946f
  patient position, 942, 945f
  physical examination, 942
  precautions, 946
  radiographs, 942, 943f
  transducer placement, 945, 946f
Suprascapular nerve block
  anatomy, 261
  clinical presentation, 261
  complications, 265
  Doppler image, 261, 264f
  precautions, 265
  radiographs, 261, 262f–263f
  ultrasound-guided technique
    informed consent, 261
    needle placement, 265, 265f
    patient position, 261, 263f
    position identification, 261, 263f
    transducer placement, 261, 263f
Supraspinatus musculotendinous, tear, 254, 257f
Supraspinatus tendonitis
  anatomy, 234, 237f
  clinical presentation, 234
  complications, 240
  convention spin echo (CSE) *vs.* fast spin echo (FSE), 237f
  precautions, 240
  radiographs, 234, 235f–236f
  ultrasound-guided technique
    Crass position, 237, 238f, 239, 239f
    informed consent, 234
    needle placement, 240, 240f
    patient position, 234, 237, 238f
    position identification, 237, 238f, 239f
    transducer placement, 237, 239f
Sural nerve
  anatomy of, 1063, 1065f
  sensory distribution, 1063, 1066
Sural nerve block, at ankle
  clinical presentation, 1063, 1064f
  color Doppler image, 1063, 1068f
  complications, 1065
  needle placement, 1065, 1068f
  patient position, 1063, 1066f
  precautions, 1065
  radiographs, 1063
  tibial artery and vein, 1063, 1067f
  transducer placement, 1067f
Swelling
  acromioclavicular joint pain, 221, 222f
  deltoid ligament strain, 1069, 1071f

# T

Tailbone pain. *See* Coccydynia
Tailor's bunion. *See* Bunionette pain syndrome
Talocrural joint. *See* Anterior talofibular ligaments; Deltoid ligament
Talofibular ligament. *See* Anterior talofibular ligaments
Talonavicular joint
  anatomy of, 1030, 1031f, 1032f
  articulations of, 1030, 1031f
  functional disability, 1030
  intra-articular injection
    clinical presentation, 1030, 1031f
    complications, 1031
    needle placement, 1031, 1034f
    patient position, 1030, 1032f
    precautions, 1032
    radiographs, 1030, 1031f
    transducer placement, 1031, 1033f
    V shape, 1031, 1033f

ligament of, 1030, 1032f
Tarsal tunnel syndrome. *See* Anterior tarsal tunnel syndrome; Posterior tarsal tunnel syndrome
Temporal artery. *See* Auriculotemporal nerve block
Temporomandibular joint (TMJ) injection
  anatomy, 81, 82f
  Camper line, 81, 87f
  causes, 81, 83t
  complications, 83
  dysfunction, 83t
  precautions, 83
  symptoms, 81
  ultrasound-guided technique
    needle placement, 81
    palpation, 81, 87f
    patient position, 81, 88f
    ultrasound transducer position, 81, 88f
Tendonitis
  Achilles
    calcaneal insertion, 1096, 1099f, 1100f
    clinical presentation, 1096, 1097f–1099f
    complications, 1101
    creaking tendon test, 1096, 1097f
    needle placement, 1096, 1101, 1101f
    patient position, 1096, 1100f
    precautions, 1101
    radiographs, 1096, 1198f
    transducer placement, 1096, 1100f
  adductor
    anatomy, 782, 784f
    appearance, 782, 786f, 787f
    bupivacaine and methylprednisolone, 782
    complications, 785
    dysfunctional gait, 782
    musculotendinous units, 782
    needle placement, 782 787f
    patient position, 782, 784f
    precautions, 785
    pubic symphysis insertion view, 782, 786f, 787f
    pubic symphysis location, 782, 785f
    radiographs, 782, 783f
    tendons of, 782
    transducer placement, 782, 786f
    Waldman knee squeeze test, 782, 783f
  bicipital
    anatomy, 288, 291f
    bupivacaine and methylprednisolone, 292
    clinical presentation, 288
    complications, 296
    informed consent, 289
    needle placement, 292, 295f
    palpation identification, 289, 293f
    patient position, 289, 293f
    Popeye sign, 288, 292f
    precautions, 296
    radiographs, 288, 289f–290f
    rupture, 288, 290f, 292f
    transducer position, 289, 292, 293f, 294f
    ultrasound image, 292, 294f, 295f
    untreated, 288, 290f
    Yergason sign, 288, 290f
  calcific, 234, 236f
  flexor carpi radialis
    acute tendon rupture, 463
    anatomy, 463, 465f
    color Doppler image, hyperemia identification, 464
    complications, 466
    distal crease identification, 463, 467f
    dorsoradial aspect location, 463
    flexor retinaculum, 464, 466f, 469f
    needle placement, 464
    patient position, 463, 467f
    precautions, 469
    radiographs, 463
    trapezium, insertion, 464, 469f
    T2-weighted magnetic resonance image, 463, 464f
    ultrasound transducer, 464, 468f
  flexor carpi ulnaris
    acute tendon rupture, 471
    anatomy, 471
    color Doppler image, ulnar artery identification, 472, 476f
    complications, 473, 475
    distal crease identification, 471, 474f
    distal tendinous insertion, 471, 473f
    dorso-ulnar aspect location, 471
    needle placement, 473, 477f
    patient position, 471, 474f
    precautions, 476
    radiographs, 471
    trapezium, insertion, 472, 476f
    T2-weighted magnetic resonance image, 472f
    ulnar nerve and artery, relationship, 471, 475f
    ultrasound transducer, 472, 475f
  infraspinatus
    anatomy, 241, 243f, 244f
    causes, 241
    clinical presentation, 241
    complications, 243, 246
    informed consent, 241
    needle placement, 241, 246f
    patient position, 241, 245f
    position identification, 241, 245f, 246f
    precautions, 246
    radiographs, 241, 242f–243f
    transducer placement, 241, 245f
  musculotendinous unit, 234, 235f, 236f
  posterior tibialis
    clinical presentation, 1121, 1122f–1124f
    complications, 1128
    medial malleolus, 1121, 1127f
    needle placement, 1123, 1129f
    patient position, 1121, 1126f
    precautions, 1128–1129
    radiographs, 1121
    transducer placement, 1121, 1127f
  subscapularis
    anatomy, 248, 249f, 250f
    clinical presentation, 248
    complications, 253
    informed consent, 250
    needle placement, 250, 253f
    patient position, 250, 251f
    position identification, 250, 251f, 252f
    precautions, 253
    radiographs, 248, 249f–250f
    transducer placement, 250, 251f
  supraspinatus
    anatomy, 234, 237f
    clinical presentation, 234
    complications, 240
    convention spin echo (CSE) *vs.* fast spin echo (FSE), 237f
    Crass position, 237, 238f, 239, 239f
    informed consent, 234
    needle placement, 240, 240f
    patient position, 234, 237, 238f
    position identification, 237, 238f, 239f
    precautions, 240
    radiographs, 234, 235f–236f
    transducer placement, 237, 239f
  triceps
    anatomy, 380, 382f, 383f
    bupivacaine and methylprednisolone, 381
    causes, 380
    complications, 381, 383
    in-plane injection, 385f
    needle placement, 381, 384f, 385f
    from overuse/misuse, 380, 381f
    patient position, 380, 384f, 385f
    precautions, 383
    radiographs, 380, 382f
    symptoms, 380
Tennis elbow. *See* Radial tunnel syndrome
Tennis elbow syndrome
  anatomy, 360
  biomechanics, 359
  causes, 359, 360f
  double crush syndrome, 359
  electromyography, 359
  imaging, 359, 362f
  nerve conduction velocity testing, 359
  palpation, 359, 362f
  precautions, 362–363
  signs and symptoms, 359
  tendon rupture, in untreated, 359, 360f
  tests, 359, 361f
  ultrasound-guided technique
    bupivacaine and methylprednisolone administration, 362
    complications, 362
    needle placement, 361, 364f, 365f
    palpation, lateral epicondyle, 361, 363f
    patient position, 361, 363f
Tenosynovitis. *See* Intersection syndrome
Third occipital nerve block
  anatomy, 163
  Arnold-Chiari malformation with syrinx, 169f, 170
  clinical presentation, 163
  complications, 163
  precautions, 170
  sensory distribution, 165, 165f
  symptoms, 163
  ultrasound-guided technique
    C1 and C2 pillar, 163, 167f
    C2–C3 facet, 163, 168f
    mastoid process, image, 163, 166f
    needle placement, 163
    palpation identification, 163, 165f
    patient position, 163, 165f
    transducer placement, 163, 166f, 167f
    vertebral artery *vs.* cervical facet joints, 163, 169f

Thoracic epidural block
 anatomy, 572, 574f
 complications
  distended epidural veins, 578
  paraplegia, 578
  procedure, 577
  surgical drainage, 579
 epidural space, 572
 precautions, 580
 prognostic tool, 572
 sonography, 579
 spinal metastatic disease, 572, 573f
 spinous processes, 572, 575f
 trident sign, 573, 577f
 T1-weighted MRI image, 573f
 ultrasound-guided technique
  articular process view, paramedian sagittal, 573–574, 578f, 579f
  critical anatomic structures identification, 573
  needle position, 577, 582f
  oblique view, paramedian sagittal, 574, 577, 579f, 580f, 581f
  patient position, 572, 575f
  transverse process view, paramedian sagittal, 573, 575f, 576f
Thoracic facet block, intra-articular technique
 anatomy, 589, 590f
 arthritis, 589
 complications, 591–592
 innervation of, 589, 590f
 osteoarthritis, 590f
 pharmacologic methods, 589
 precautions, 592
 radiographs, 590f
 sonography, 592
 trident sign, 589, 594f
 ultrasound-guided technique
  articular process view, paramedian sagittal, 589, 591, 595f, 596f
  needle position, 591, 597f
  patient position, 589, 591f
  transverse process view, paramedian sagittal, 589, 592f–594f
Thoracic paravertebral nerve block
 anatomy, 583
 anterior division, 583, 584f
 complications
  pneumothorax, 586
  procedures, 585
 herpes zoster, 583, 584f
 intervertebral foramen, 583, 584f
 posterior division, 583, 584f
 precautions, 587
 prognostic tool, 583
 spinal metastatic disease, 583
 subcostal nerve, 583
 thoracic dermatomes, 583, 584f
 ultrasound-guided technique
  needle placement, 585, 587f
  palpation identification, 585, 586f
  patient position, 583, 585f
  spinous process, 585, 586f
  transducer placement, 585, 586f
  transverse processes, 585, 587f
Thorax
 intercostal nerve block

  acute pain setting, 598
  anatomy, 598, 600f
  color Doppler image, intercostal artery, 598, 603f
  complications, 599
  diagnostic tool, 598
  flying bat, 599, 603f
  intercostal vein and artery, relationship, 598, 601f
  needle placement, 599, 604f
  palpation identification, 598, 601f
  paravertebral nerves, 598
  patient position, 598, 601f
  precautions, 599
  prognostic tool, 598
  rib identification, 598, 601f, 602f
  ribs and flail chest fracture, 598, 599f
  sandy beach appearance, 599, 604f
  subcostal nerve, 598
  transducer placement, 598, 601f
 intra-articular facet block (see Cervical intra-articular facet block)
 paravertebral nerve block
  anatomy, 583
  anterior division, 583, 584f
  complications, 585–586
  herpes zoster, 583, 584f
  intervertebral foramen, 583, 584f
  needle placement, 585, 587f
  palpation identification, 585, 586f
  patient position, 583, 585f
  posterior division, 583, 584f
  precautions, 587
  prognostic tool, 583
  spinal metastatic disease, 583
  spinous process, 585, 586f
  subcostal nerve, 583
  thoracic dermatomes, 583, 584f
  transducer placement, 585, 586f
  transverse processes, 585, 587f
Tibial collateral ligament. See Medial collateral ligament
Tibial nerve
 anatomy of, 986, 988f–990f, 1035, 1037f, 1088, 1091f
 sciatic nerve bifurcation, 987, 993f
 sensory distribution, 1088, 1092f
 sensory innervation, 986, 989f, 1035, 1036f
Tibial nerve block
 ankle
  clinical presentation, 1035, 1036f
  complications, 1040
  needle placement, 1035, 1039, 1041f
  patient position, 1035, 1038f
  popliteal vein and artery, 1035, 1040f
  precautions, 1040f–1041f
  transducer placement, 1035, 1039, 1039f
 popliteal fossa
  clinical presentation, 986, 987f
  color Doppler image, popliteal vein, 987, 992f
  complications, 991
  needle placement, 988, 994f
  patient position, 986, 991f
  popliteal artery and vein, 986, 992f
  precautions, 994
  radiographs, 986, 987f

  sciatic nerve bifurcation, 987, 993f
  transducer placement, 986, 991f
Tibialis tendon anatomy, 1121, 1126f
Tibiofibular joint, superior. See Superior tibiofibular joint
Tibiotalar/talocrural joint. See Ankle joint
Tietze syndrome, 550
Tinel sign, 430, 431f, 454
 carpal tunnel syndrome, 446, 448f, 448t
 ilioinguinal nerve block, 639
 median nerve block, 430, 431f
 radial nerve block, 424, 425f
 ulnar nerve block, 438, 440f
 ulnar tunnel syndrome, 454
Toe joint
 hammertoe (see Hammertoe pain syndrome)
 intra-articular injection
  clinical presentation, 1130, 1131f, 1132f
  complications, 1132
  functional disability, 1130
  needle placement, 1132, 1134f
  patient position, 1132, 1133
  precautions, 1132–1133
  radiographs, 1130, 1132f
  transducer placement, 1132, 1134f
Transversus abdominis plane block
 anatomy, 615, 616f
 anterior abdominal wall, 615
 complications, 618
 diagnostic tool, 615
 fascial plane, 615, 617f
 intercostal nerves, 615, 617f
 paravertebral nerve, 615
 pneumoperitoneum in, 618, 620f
 posterior division, 615
 precautions, 619
 subcostal nerve, 615
 ultrasound-guided technique
  needle placement, 615, 616, 619f
  palpation identification, 615, 618f
  patient position, 615, 617f
  transducer, midaxillary line, 615, 618f
Trapeziometacarpal joint. See First carpometacarpal joint, intra-articular injection
Trapezius muscle pain, 112, 113f
Triceps tendonitis
 anatomy, 380, 382f, 383f
 causes, 380
 complications, 381, 383
 from overuse/misuse, 380, 381f
 precautions, 383
 radiographs, 380, 382f
 symptoms, 380
 ultrasound-guided technique
  bupivacaine and methylprednisolone, 381
  in-plane injection, 385f
  needle placement, 381, 384f, 385f
  patient position, 380, 384f, 385f
Trident sign
 lumbar epidural block, 684, 687f
 lumbar facet block
  intra-articular technique, 673, 678f
  medial branch technique, 664, 669f
 lumbar subarachnoid block, 700, 704f, 705f
 thoracic epidural block, 573, 577f
 thoracic facet block, intra-articular technique, 589, 594f

Trigeminal nerve block, coronoid approach
　anatomy, 39, 40f
　complications, 43
　gasserian ganglion, 39
　indications, 39t
　needle placement, 43, 43f
　palpation, 41f
　patient position, 42f
　position identification, 42f
　precautions, 43
Trigger finger syndrome
　anatomy, 513
　complications, 518–519
　direct trauma, 513, 514f
　flexor tendons location, 513
　metacarpal/sesamoid bones, 513, 514f
　nodule, 513, 514f
　precautions, 519
　pulley system view, 513, 515f
　radiographs, 513
　tenosynovitis, 513, 514f
　ultrasound-guided technique
　　A1 pulley identification, 513, 517f
　　needle placement, 518, 518f
　　palpation identification, 513, 516f
　　patient position, 513, 516f
　　transducer position, 513, 516f
Trochanteric bursitis pain
　anatomy, 810, 813f, 888, 890, 891f
　anteroposterior plain, 810, 812f
　causes of, 810
　complications, 813
　electromyography, 810
　gluteus minimus tendon, 810, 813f
　in hip region, 810, 811f
　musculotendinous unit, 810, 811f
　physical examination, 810
　precautions, 814
　radiographs, 810, 812f
　resisted abduction test, 810, 812f
　ultrasound-guided technique
　　bupivacaine and methylprednisolone, 812
　　femur identification, 812, 814f
　　hydrodissection, 813
　　needle position, 813, 816f
　　patient position, 810, 814f
　　transducer placement, 812, 815f
Trocho-ginglymus-type joint, 897
Trunk. See Celiac plexus block, anterior approach
Tumors
　brachial plexus block, 209
　ganglia cysts, 478
　infraclavicular approach, 204
　mediastinum, 555, 556f, 560, 561f
　Pancoast superior sulcus, 199f
　TMJ pain, 82, 83t
Twist test, 909, 911f

**U**

Ulnar nerve block
　anatomy, 438, 441f
　complications, 441
　diagnostic tool, 438
　dorsal branch, 438
　elbow
　　anatomy, 344, 345f
　　bupivacaine and methylprednisolone, 344
　　complications, 350
　　needle placement, 344, 350, 350f
　　palpation, 344, 347f
　　patient position, 344, 347f
　　precautions, 350
　　sensory innervation, 344, 3467f
　　symptoms, 344, 345f
　fifth metacarpal fracture, 438, 439f
　palmar branch, 438
　pathologic processes, 438, 439f
　phalanges fracture, 438, 439f
　physical findings, 438
　precautions, 445
　sensory distribution of, 442f
　sensory innervation, 351–352, 355f
　spread sign test, 438, 440f
　Tinel sign, 438, 440f
　treatment of, 445
　ulnar tunnel syndrome, 438, 439f, 440f
　ultrasound-guided technique
　　bupivacaine and methylprednisolone, 441
　　color Doppler image, ulnar artery, 440–441, 444f
　　distal crease identification, 440, 443f
　　needle placement, 440, 445f
　　patient position, 440, 443f
　　ultrasound image, 440, 444f
　　ultrasound transducer, 440, 444f
Ulnar tunnel syndrome, 438, 439f, 440f
　anatomy, 454
　clinical presentation, 454, 455f
　complications, 455, 457
　Guyon canal, 454
　hyperechoic nerve, 455
　nerve bifurcation, 454
　permanent disability and deformity, 454, 456f
　sensory distribution, 454, 458f
　spread sign test, 454
　Tinel sign, 454
　ulnar artery, 454, 455, 457f, 460f, 461f
　ulnar nerve, 454, 455f
　ultrasound-guided technique
　　color Doppler image, ulnar artery identification, 455, 461f
　　distal crease identification, 454, 459f
　　needle placement, 455, 461f
　　patient position, 454, 459f
　　ultrasound transducer, 454, 455, 460f

**V**

Vagus nerve block
　anatomy, 107, 108f
　complications, 107–108
　Doppler image, 107, 110f
　physical examination, 107
　precautions, 110
　symptoms, 107
　ultrasound-guided technique
　　needle placement, 110f
　　patient position, 107, 109f
　　position identification, 107, 109f, 110f
　　ultrasound transducer position, 107, 110f
　vs. vagus neuralgia, 110
Vastus medialis, 973, 977f
Vocal cord dysfunction, 105f. See also Glossopharyngeal nerve block

**W**

Waldman knee squeeze test, 782, 783f
Walther block. See Impar block, ganglion
Watson stress test, 501, 503f
Weaver's bottom, 788, 790f. See also Ischial bursitis pain
Wrist
　anterior interosseous syndrome, 404
　carpal (see Carpal tunnel syndrome)
　carpometacarpal joint (see First carpometacarpal joint, intra-articular injection)
　carpometacarpal joints (see Carpometacarpal joints, intra-articular injection)
　de Quervain's tenosynovitis (see de Quervain's tenosynovitis)
　distal crease identification, 434, 434f
　extensor tendon compartments, 493, 494t
　ganglia cysts (see Ganglia cysts)
　interphalangeal joints (see Interphalangeal joints, intra-articular injection)
　median nerve block (see Median nerve block)
　misuse (see Flexor carpi radialis tendonitis)
　radial nerve block (see Radial nerve block)
　radiocarpal joint
　　anterior interosseous nerve, 418
　　direct trauma, 418
　　posterior interosseous nerve, 418
　　synovial sarcoma, MRI T1-and T2-weighted image, 419f
　radioulnar joint (see Distal radioulnar joint, intra-articular injection)
　ulnar nerve block (see Ulnar nerve block)
　ulnar tunnel syndrome (see Ulnar tunnel syndrome)

**X**

Xiphisternal joint pain
　anatomy, 560, 562f
　complications, 564
　cosmetic defect, 560, 561f
　mediastinum tumors, 560, 561f
　precautions, 565
　radiographs, 560, 561f
　ultrasound-guided technique
　　hypoechoic joint, 560, 564f
　　needle placement, 560, 563, 565f
　　palpation identification, 560, 563f
　　patient position, 560, 563f
　　transducer placement, 560, 564f
Xiphoid process, 632, 634f. See also Celiac plexus block, anterior approach

**Y**

Yeoman test, 881, 883f

**Z**

Zygapophyseal joints. See Cervical intra-articular facet block